Obstetrics

Obstetrics

Edited by

Sir Alec Turnbull CBE MD MB ChB FRCOG
Professor and Head of Nuffield Department of Obstetrics and Gynaecology,
University of Oxford,
John Radcliffe Hospital,
Oxford,
UK

Geoffrey Chamberlain RD MD FRCS FRCOG
Professor and Head of Department of Obstetrics and Gynaecology,
St George's Hospital Medical School,
London,
UK

CHURCHILL LIVINGSTONE
EDINBURGH LONDON MELBOURNE AND NEW YORK 1989

CHURCHILL LIVINGSTONE
Medical Division of Longman Group UK Limited

Distributed in the United States of America by Churchill Livingstone Inc., 1560 Broadway, New York, NY 10036, and by associated companies, branches and representatives throughout the world.

First published 1989

ISBN 0–443–03539–3

British Library Cataloguing in Publication Data
Obstetrics
1. Obstetrics
I. Turnbull, Sir Alec
II. Chamberlain, Geoffrey 1930–
618.2

Library of Congress Cataloging in Publication Data available

Printed in Great Britain at The Bath Press, Avon

Preface

In obstetrics there have been great advances in knowledge over the past 30 years while more has changed in the last decade than in the whole of the history of the subject. Advance has been particularly rapid in the prenatal diagnosis of fetal anomaly, the assessment of intrauterine fetal growth retardation, the detection and effective augmentation of slow labour and the treatment of many neonatal disorders.

Although many books have been written about specialized aspects of obstetrics, there is a dearth of major books covering the whole modern field. *Obstetrics* provides a comprehensive account of current knowledge and practice in the specialty by choosing a full spectrum of experts. Authors have shown how their field has developed over the years, described the present scene and, by providing extensive references to the literature, given readers an opportunity to achieve deeper knowledge. We are proud to have such a distinguished team of authors.

Both the editors are consultants in active clinical practice, looking after patients while teaching undergraduate and postgraduate students. Not only are we kept aware of new developments in the clinical field by our junior staffs but we learn of topics about which there is controversy, argument and confusion. In planning this book, we have ensured that new developments and obstetric controversies are covered. We have also included chapters presenting the views of women themselves on their care in labour and on the role of the modern midwife for we consider these issues of importance to the contemporary obstetrician. We believe that *Obstetrics* will make a major contribution to the training of young specialists.

Advances in clinical practice should depend on new scientific knowledge which itself is based upon appropriate and valid measurements. A strong basic science foundation has been provided in the first quarter of the book. Subsequent chapters deal with normal pregnancy, labour and the puerperium, each section being followed by consideration of abnormal variations of these processes. There are two important groups of chapters on fetal assessment: the first deals with fetal monitoring up to 28 weeks, covering the new areas of prenatal diagnosis, including biophysical and biochemical methods as well as molecular biology and DNA technology; the second group is on fetal diagnosis in late pregnancy and draws attention to the recent trend away from biochemical assessment towards the modern biophysical methods which have revolutionized antenatal care of the fetus at higher risk of various unfavourable outcomes.

Obstetrics includes a large section on the care of the newborn, indicating our opinion that obstetricians need to have a good working knowledge of neonatal disorders and of advances in neonatal care. We also consider it important to include two chapters on assisted fertility, while three chapters on perinatal epidemiology emphasize how correct interpretation of vital statistics can help clinical practice. The book is completed by a major chapter on contraception in relation to the recently pregnant and by another on the vitally important topic of medicolegal problems in obstetrics.

We are grateful to all our authors for the work they have done in preparing the chapters. Our publishers have been particularly helpful and we are especially grateful to Mrs Elif Fincanci-Smith who has survived the brunt of being our real working editor. Mrs Anne Fraser at St George's Hospital has been the stage manager, expertly juggling the various drafts of 80 chapters. We are grateful to Jonathan Frappell and Richard de Chazal, also of St George's Hospital, for proofreading under pressure.

It is our hope that *Obstetrics* will provide a comprehensive account well into the 1990s of the knowledge and practice of the specialty for young obstetricians in training, for practising clinicians and for undergraduates who wish to take a special interest.

Oxford and London 1989

A.T.
G.C.

Contributors

Eva Alberman MD MB BChir FRCP MMRCP
Professor of Clinical Epidemiology, The London Hospital Medical College, London, UK

Lindsay Staubus Alger MD
Associate Professor, Department of Obstetrics and Gynaecology, University of Maryland School of Medicine and Hospital, Baltimore, Maryland, USA

Alan G. Amias FRCS FRCOG
Consultant Obstetrician and Gynaecologist, St George's Hospital, London, UK

Kenneth D. Bagshawe MD MB BS FRCP FRCR FRCOG
Professor of Medical Oncology, Charing Cross and Westminster Medical School, London, UK

David H. Barlow MA BSc MD MRCOG
Clinical Reader, Nuffield Department of Obstetrics and Gynaecology, University of Oxford; Honorary Consultant Obstetrician and Gynaecologist, John Radcliffe Hospital, Oxford, UK

S. Leonard Barron MB FRCS FRCOG
Consultant Obstetrician and Gynaecologist, Princess Mary Maternity Hospital, Newcastle upon Tyne, UK

John M. Beazley MD FRCOG
Professor of Obstetrics and Gynaecology, University of Liverpool, Royal Liverpool Hospital, Liverpool, UK

Felix Beck DSc MD ChB
Foundation Professor and Head, Department of Anatomy, University of Leicester Medical School, Leicester, UK

John Bonnar MA MD FRCOG
Professor and Head, Trinity College Department of Obstetrics and Gynaecology, University of Dublin; Consultant Obstetrician and Gynaecologist, St James's Hospital, Adelaide Hospital and Coombe Lying-in Hospital, Dublin, Eire

Michael Brudenell MB BS FRCS FRCOG
Senior Consultant Obstetrician and Gynaecologist, King's College Hospital, London; Senior Gynaecologist, Queen Victoria Hospital, East Grinstead; Consultant Gynaecologist, King Edward VII Hospital, London, UK

Andrew A. Calder MD FRCP(Glas) FRCOG
Professor of Obstetrics and Gynaecology, University of Edinburgh, Edinburgh, UK

Philippa Cardale SCM ADM
Midwife, St Mary's Hospital, London, UK

Geoffrey Chamberlain RD MD FRCS FRCOG
Professor of Obstetrics and Gynaecology, St George's Hospital Medical School, London, UK

David Charles MD FRCS(C) FRCOG
Emeritus Professor of Obstetrics and Gynaecology, Marshall University School of Medicine, Huntington, West Virginia, USA

James Clinch MA MD FRCOG
Consultant Obstetrician and Gynaecologist, Coombe Lying-in Hospital, Dublin; Clinical Lecturer in Obstetrics and Gynaecology, Trinity College, University of Dublin, Dublin, Eire

Cecil J. T. Craig MD FRCOG
Senior Lecturer in Obstetrics and Gynaecology, University of Cape Town; Senior Specialist in Obstetrics and Gynaecology, Groote Schuur Hospital, Heerengracht, Cape Town, South Africa

Martin d'A. Crawfurd MB BS FRCPath
Consultant Clinical Geneticist, Kennedy-Galton Centre, and Clinical Scientist, Clinical Research Centre, Harrow, UK

Carlyle Crenshaw Jr MD
Professor and Chairman, Department of Obstetrics and Gynaecology, University of Maryland School of Medicine and Hospital, Baltimore, Maryland, USA

Howard S. Cuckle BA MSc DPhil
Cancer Research Campaign Senior Lecturer, Medical College of St Bartholomew's Hospital, London, UK

John M. Davison MD FRCOG
Scientific Staff Consultant Obstetrician and Gynaecologist, MRC Human Reproduction Group, Princess Mary Maternity Hospital, Newcastle upon Tyne, UK

Geoffrey S. Dawes CBE DM FRCOG FRS
Director of the Charing Cross Lumley Research Centre, Oxford, UK

K. John Dennis MB FRCS(Ed) FRCOG
Professor of Human Reproduction and Obstetrics, University of Southampton, Southampton, UK

Noel Dilly GM MB BF BSc PhD DO FCOphth
Professor and Chairman, Department of Anatomy, St George's Hospital Medical School, London, UK

Michael Dooley MMs MRCOG
Senior Registrar in Obstetrics and Gynaecology, St Thomas' Hospital, London, UK

William Dunlop PhD MB ChB FRCOG FRCS(Ed)
Professor and Head, Department of Obstetrics and Gynaecology, Princess Mary Maternity Hospital, Newcastle upon Tyne, UK

Denys V. I. Fairweather MD FRCOG
Professor and Head, Department of Obstetrics and Gynaecology, University College and Middlesex School of Medicine, London, UK

Gillian C. Forrest MB BS MRCPsych MRCGP
Consultant Child Psychiatrist, Park Hospital for Children, Oxford, UK

Harold Fox MD FRCPath FRCOG
Professor of Reproductive Pathology, University of Manchester; Honorary Consultant Pathologist, St Mary's Hospital, Manchester, UK

Donald M. F. Gibb MB ChB MRCP MRCOG
Senior Lecturer and Honorary Consultant, Department of Obstetrics and Gynaecology, King's College Medical School, London, UK

J. Gedis Grudzinskas BSc MB BS MD FRCOG FRACOG
Professor and Honorary Consultant, Joint Academic Unit of Obstetrics and Gynaecology, The London Hospital and St Bartholomew's Hospital Medical Colleges, London, UK

John Guillebaud MA FRCS(Ed) FRCOG
Medical Director, Margaret Pyke Centre for Study and Training in Family Planning; Senior Lecturer, Department of Obstetrics and Gynaecology, University College and Middlesex School of Medicine, London, UK

Marion Hall MD FRCOG
Consultant Obstetrician and Gynaecologist, Aberdeen Maternity Hospital, Aberdeen, UK

Chris Harman MD
Division of Maternal and Fetal Medicine, Department of Obstetrics, Gynaecology and Reproductive Sciences, University of Manitoba, Winnipeg, Manitoba, Canada

Michael Harmer MB BS MRCS LRCP FFA RCS
Consultant Anaesthetist, University Hospital of Wales, Cardiff, UK

David Harvey FRCP
Senior Lecturer in Paediatrics, Royal Postgraduate Medical School's Institute of Obstetrics and Gynaecology, Queen Charlotte's & Chelsea Hospital, London, UK

David L. Healy B Med Sci MB BS PhD FRACOG
Wellcome Trust Senior Research Fellow, Medical Research Centre, Prince Henry's Hospital, Melbourne, Australia

Bryan M. Hibbard MD PhD FRCOG
Professor and Head, Department of Obstetrics and Gynaecology, University of Wales College of Medicine, Cardiff, UK

E. Wren Hoskyns MB BS MRCP
MRC Research Fellow, Department of Child Health, City Hospital, Nottingham, UK

Peter W. Howie MD FRCOG
Professor of Obstetrics and Gynaecology, Ninewells Hospital and Medical School, Dundee, UK

David Hull MSc MB ChB FRCP
Professor of Child Health, University Hospital, Queen's Medical Centre, Nottingham, UK

Rosalinde Hurley DBE LLB MD FRCPath
Professor of Microbiology, Royal Postgraduate Medical School's Institute of Obstetrics and Gynaecology, London, UK

David Isaacs MD MRCP
Wellcome Trust Lecturer and Honorary Consultant Paediatrician, John Radcliffe Hospital, Oxford, UK

Peter M. Johnson MA PhD MRCPath
Professor of Immunology, University of Liverpool, Liverpool, UK

Colin T. Jones MA PhD
Director, Laboratory of Cellular and Developmental Physiology, Institute for Molecular Medicine, University of Oxford, Oxford, UK

Arnold Klopper PhD MD FRCOG
Professor of Reproductive Endocrinology, Department of Obstetrics and Gynaecology, University of Aberdeen, Aberdeen, UK

Ismail Kola PhD
Senior Research Fellow, Centre for Early Human Development, Monash University, Clayton, Victoria, Australia

Bryan Larsen PhD
Professor of Microbiology and Obstetrics and Gynaecology, Marshall University School of Medicine, Huntington, West Virginia, USA

Sylvia D. Lawler MD FRCP FRCPath
Professor Emeritus, Institute of Cancer Research, London, UK

Elizabeth A. Letsky MB BS FRCPath
Consultant Haematologist, Queen Charlotte's Hospital for Women; Honorary Senior Lecturer, Royal Postgraduate Medical School; Honorary Consultant Haematologist, Hospitals for Sick Children, London, UK

Tom Lissauer MA MB MRCP
Consultant Paediatrician, St Mary's Hospital, London, UK

Andres López Bernal DM(Murcia) DPhil(Oxon)
Research Fellow, Nuffield Department of Obstetrics and Gynaecology, University of Oxford, John Radcliffe Hospital, Oxford, UK

Ian MacGillivray MD FRCP(Glas) FRCOG
Emeritus Professor of Obstetrics and Gynaecology, University of Aberdeen, Aberdeen, UK

Iain R. McFadyen MB ChB FRCOG
Honorary Consultant and Senior Lecturer, Department of Obstetrics and Gynaecology, Royal Liverpool Hospital, Liverpool, UK

John Malvern BSc FRCS(Ed) FRCOG
Consultant Obstetrician, Queen Charlotte's Hospital for Women; Honorary Senior Lecturer, Royal Postgraduate Medical School's Institute of Obstetrics and Gynaecology, London, UK

Frank Arthur Manning MD MSc(Oxon) FRCS(C) FACOG FSOGC
Professor and Chairman, Department of Obstetrics, Gynaecology and Reproductive Sciences, University of Manitoba, Winnipeg, Manitoba, Canada

Savas Menticoglou MD
Division of Maternal and Fetal Medicine, Department of Obstetrics, Gynaecology and Reproductive Sciences, University of Manitoba, Winnipeg, Manitoba, Canada

Anthony D. Milner MD FRCP DCH
Professor of Paediatric Respiratory Medicine, University of Nottingham; Consultant Paediatrician, University and City Hospitals, Nottingham, UK

E. Richard Moxon MB FRCP
Professor of Paediatrics, John Radcliffe Hospital, Oxford, UK

Philip Myerscough FRCS(Ed) FRCP(Ed) FRCOG
Deputy Chief of Services (Obstetrics and Gynaecology), Royal Hospital, Sultanate of Oman

Kenneth R. Niswander MD
Professor of Obstetrics and Gynaecology, University of California, Sacramento, California, USA

Ann Oakley MA PhD
Deputy Director, Thomas Covam Research Unit, London, UK

Niall O'Brien FRCPI DCH
Consultant Paediatrician, National Maternity Hospital and The Children's Hospital, Dublin, Eire

Roy N. Palmer LLB MB BS DObstRCOG Barrister
Secretary, The Medical Protection Society, London, UK

Naren Patel FRCOG
Consultant Obstetrician and Honorary Senior Lecturer, Division of Obstetrics and Gynaecology, University of Dundee, Ninewells Hospital and Medical School, Dundee, UK

J. Malcolm Pearce MD FRCS MRCOG
Senior Lecturer and Consultant Obstetrician, Department of Obstetrics and Gynaecology, St George's Hospital, London, UK

Tim J. Peters BSc MSc PhD FSS
Lecturer in Medical Statistics, University of Wales College of Medicine, Cardiff, UK

Shan S. Ratnam MB BS MD FRCS FRCS(Ed) FRCSG FRACS FRCOG FRACOG FWACS FACOG
Professor and Head, Department of Obstetrics and Gynaecology, and Director, School of Postgraduate Medical Studies, National University of Singapore; Consultant, National University Hospital, Singapore

Mary Rauff MB BS MMED(Obst & Gynae) FRCOG
Associate Professor, Department of Obstetrics and Gynaecology, National University of Singapore; Consultant, National University Hospital, Singapore

Christopher W. G. Redman MA MB BChir FRCP
Clinical Reader and Consultant in Obstetric Medicine, Nuffield Department of Obstetrics and Gynaecology, John Radcliffe Hospital, Oxford, UK

Margaret C. P. Rees MB BS BSc DPhil MRCOG
Parke Davis Medical Research Fellow, Nuffield Department of Obstetrics and Gynaecology, John Radcliffe Hospital, Oxford, UK

J. S. Robinson BSc MB BCh BAO FRACOG FRCOG
Professor of Obstetrics and Gynaecology, University of Adelaide, Adelaide, South Australia

Charles H. Rodeck BSc MB BS FRCOG
Professor of Obstetrics and Gynaecology, Royal Postgraduate Medical School's Institute of Obstetrics and Gynaecology, Queen Charlotte's Hospital for Women, London, UK

Peter A. W. Rogers PhD
Senior Research Fellow, Department of Obstetrics and Gynaecology, Monash University, Clayton, Victoria, Australia

Michael Rosen MB ChB FFARCS
Honorary Professor and Consultant Anaesthetist, Department of Anaesthetics, University Hospital of Wales, Cardiff, UK

A. Henry Sathananthan PhD
Senior Lecturer, La Trobe University; Senior Research Associate, Centre for Early Human Development, Monash University, Clayton, Victoria, Australia

Wendy D. Savage BA MB BCh FRCOG
Senior Lecturer in Obstetrics and Gynaecology, Joint Department of General Practice and Primary Care, St Bartholomew's Hospital and London Hospital Medical Colleges, London, UK

Hugh F. Seeley MA MSc MB BS FFARCS
Consultant Anaesthetist and Honorary Senior Lecturer, St George's Hospital and Medical School, London, UK

Albert Singer PhD(Syd) DPhil(Oxon) FRCOG
Consultant Obstetrician and Gynaecologist, Whittington and Royal Northern Hospitals, London, UK

Philip J. Steer BSc MD MRCOG
Professor and Head of Department, Westminster and Charing Cross Hospital Medical School, London, UK

Gordon M. Stirrat MA MD FRCOG
Professor of Obstetrics and Gynaecology, University of Bristol, Bristol Maternity Hospital, Bristol, UK

John Studd MD FRCOG
Consultant Obstetrician and Gynaecologist, King's College Hospital and Dulwich Hospital, London, UK

Michael de Swiet MD FRCP
Consultant Physician, Queen Charlotte's Hospital for Women, London, UK

William Thompson BSc MD FRCOG
Professor of Obstetrics and Gynaecology, Queen's University of Belfast; Consultant Obstetrician, Royal Maternity Hospital, Belfast; Consultant Gynaecologist, Royal Victoria Hospital, Belfast, Northern Ireland

Alan Trounson PhD
Director, Centre for Early Human Development, Monash University, Clayton, Victoria, Australia

Alec Turnbull CBE MD MB ChB FRCOG
Professor of Obstetrics and Gynaecology, Nuffield Department of Obstetrics and Gynaecology, University of Oxford, John Radcliffe Hospital, Oxford, UK

Gillian Turner FRCOG
Consultant and Senior Lecturer in Obstetrics, University of Bristol, Southmead Hospital, Bristol, UK

Nicholas J. Wald DSc(Med) FFCM FRCP
Professor and Head, Department of Environmental and Preventive Medicine, St Bartholomew's Hospital Medical College, London, UK

Andrew R. Wilkinson MB FRCP DCH
Consultant Paediatrician and Lecturer, University of Oxford, John Radcliffe Hospital, Oxford, UK

Carlyle Wood CBE FRCS FRACOG
Professor and Chairman, Department of Obstetrics and Gynaecology, Monash University, Monash Medical Centre, Melbourne, Australia

Contents

SECTION 1

Basic Sciences

1

Geoffrey Chamberlain and Alec Turnbull

The continuum of obstetrics

Obstetrics is the art and science of caring for women and their unborn progeny during pregnancy, labour and continuing into the immediate puerperium. In earlier times there was much craft and not much science. Now there is an increasing amount of well understood science but a lot of the craft is still required; the one has not given way to the other; rather, science has augmented craft.

THE PAST

Early times

Long before physicians took an interest in obstetrical matters, midwives or guid women were supervising labour. With no formal training but a variable heritage of experience, such women have been working since biblical times (Genesis 35.17 and Genesis 38.27) and were well known in the Egyptian and Greek civilizations. Training was usually obtained by learning from another more experienced guid woman—an apprentice system—and there was usually no checking of standards. The first formal training for midwives was laid down by Hippocrates in the fifth century B.C., followed by intermittent efforts in Italy and Greece in the second and third century A.D. In the United Kingdom, William Chamberlin, father of Chamberlin the forceps, started a midwifery school in Southampton; however, a uniform formalization of midwifery training was not undertaken until the Midwives Acts were passed in the early days of this century.

Doctors came into obstetrics comparatively late. At first they were resisted by midwives who saw them as competition, but gradually a team approach evolved so that both professionals worked together. One feature which may have catalysed this was the abundant extramarital activity of the courts of France and England during the later 17th century. In both countries, monarchs and their imitators led a merry life of multiple coitus which, in the days before contraception, led to many pregnancies. In both countries, in consequence, obstetricians were used because of the confidentiality and secrecy required to handle the results of royal dalliance. From such unsalubrious beginnings rose to fame several of the great obstetricians of the 17th and 18th centuries.

The first aid service for delivery

Forceps came into use with Peter Chamberlin, although possibly as a re-invention of a much earlier instrument used for extracting dead babies. A century of manipulative skills then followed with increasingly complex instruments evolved to help deal with problems. A woman did not have access to powerful anaesthesia at this time and so a vaginal delivery had to be successful, even at the expense of the baby's life. Nearly all manipulations were very intrusive, requiring long apprenticeship and practice for training. Hence obstetricians were great mechanists, inventing ingenious instruments to extract babies from awkward corners. Some appliances were modifications of existing tools and the destructive instruments of the previous generation. Most well known obstetricians had their trained mechanic (often the blacksmith) around the corner to make their own variation of the various vaginal instruments. With the aid of personalized tools, these obstetricians would go on using their own eponymous variant. If they were influential and had apprentices, the latter would be taught their skills on their master's instruments, thus perpetuating the innumerable ramifications of the obstetrical armamentorium which flourished into the 19th and early 20th centuries.

Safer Caesarean section came in the mid 1800s (inhalation anaesthesia was first used in 1851); the increase in the use of this route, bypassing the more difficult vaginal procedures, sounded the knell of mechanistic obstetrics. The attitude of 'vaginal delivery or bust' still persisted for a few decades since obstetricians were still concerned about infection. Puerperal sepsis (childbed fever) killed some women after vaginal delivery but peritoneal infection after abdominal operative delivery was a death sentence with no cure until chemotherapy and antibiotics were introduced in the 1930s. Maternal mortality was sharply reduced as a result and only then could obstetricians start to consider a Caesarean section as a comparatively safe substitute for a vaginal delivery.

The beginnings of science

All science depends upon measurement. Among the first steps in obstetrics was the measurement of various aspects of the pelvis by Levret in 1753. Like many enthusiasts, he over-elaborated the complexities of pelvic axes and planes, and Smellie, in the following year, first proposed a measurement which has been continued into current obstetrics, the diagonal conjugate anterioposterior diameter of the pelvis. All sorts of measuring instruments were used and external pelvimetry became fashionable, but was mostly dismissed after the analysis of Michaelis in 1851. In vivo measurements followed the invention of Roentgen when the first X-ray pelvimetries were performed by Albert in 1897.

The more recent surge in biophysical estimations in obstetrics may be considered to have started with fetal heart auscultation in the early 19th century but really came to prominence with the work of the Glaswegian obstetrician, Ian Donald. He, more than any other single person, led biophysics into obstetrics with the use of ultrasound and his work will always be acknowledged. He was a pioneer in all ultrasound measurement of the fetus. Dynamic measurements of blood flow in the placental bed and the fetal blood vessels followed the static ones which provided a system of measuring fetal growth from serial readings.

Biochemistry in medicine owes much to another obstetrician, Robert Barnes of St George's Hospital, London. He was an obstetric physician and then consultant from 1875 to 1907. In this time he set up the first biochemical laboratory in the world for the measurement of levels of body constituents such as sodium, potassium, proteins and urea in human blood. Another great advance came after the Second World War when miniaturization of biochemical processes, automation and the use of radioactive labels allowed steroid biochemistry to forge ahead. Again, measurement led research.

Epidemiology, the measurement of numbers of people, has been a major part of modern obstetrics. The counting of heads started with epidemics of infectious diseases in the Victorian days and went on to quantify birth rates and death rates; from 1830 these measurements were under the control of the Registrar General's Office in England and equivalent bodies in other countries. More recently, the Office of Population Censuses and Surveys has taken over this task for England and Wales. This is an important area: epidemiology in this country has led obstetrics in the rest of the world. Measures of fetal and antenatal outcome can be firmly established, so providing a rapid medical audit of procedures or of doctor groups. Comparisons can be made from one centre to another or even from one country to another, provided the data compare like with like. The ready acceptance of randomized controlled trials by obstetricians has allowed even more sophisticated analyses with more valid results.

Clinical care

Epidemiology however has not always been used in the evaluation of systems of management; antenatal care, for example, evolved piecemeal. Starting in Edinburgh at the turn of the century, current practice owes much to Doreen Campbell in the mid 1920s; it was she who in London laid down the pattern of antenatal visits followed today in most of the western world.

The place of delivery has shifted from the home to the institution. This is partly following the trend of hospitalization of much western medicine, with primary care becoming a service dealing mostly with ambulatory care and a diagnosis only. Further, most obstetricians, concerned with the unexpected serious complications to mother and baby which arise suddenly in labour, wish to have close access to the full facilities which will be required if labour deviates from the normal. Institutional delivery in the United Kingdom has increased from 20% in the 1920s to 99% currently.

CONTEMPORARY OBSTETRICS

The years of the Second World War (1939–1945) provide a convenient division between the end of a long-standing period of conservative maternity care and the beginning of contemporary obstetrics. The older practice was dominated by fear of maternal death: rightly so — the maternal mortality rate in England and Wales remained between 4 and 5 per 1000 births until 1937. The introduction of sulphonamides in 1937 and subsequently newer antibiotics, safe blood transfusion and other advances led to the dramatic reduction in maternal mortality rates (see Chapter 78). As a result, obstetricians returning to practice after the end of the war in 1945 began to realize that the maternal mortality rate had fallen to such an extent that they could now concentrate more on improving perinatal mortality and morbidity.

Perinatal medicine

One of the earliest obstetricians practising in what developed into perinatal medicine was Dugald Baird in Aberdeen; he classified the clinical causes of perinatal death and demonstrated the importance of good maternal health as well as expert perinatal care in achieving a low perinatal mortality rate. By describing the circumstances of perinatal death, he drew attention to those obstetric conditions for which better management was needed to improve fetal outcome. The conditions initially stressed were labour disorders such as prolonged first stage, manipulative vaginal delivery, preterm labour and prolonged pregnancy. Disorders of pregnancy carrying special risks for the fetus included severe pre-eclampsia, antepartum haemorrhage, rhesus disease and maternal medical disorders such as diabetes. He naturally recognized fetal abnormality as a major cause of fetal death, but like others at the same time, regarded this as entirely unavoidable.

ADVANCES IN PERINATAL CARE

Biochemical assessment of fetus and placenta

For many years it was recognized that poor placental function was the probable explanation for complications such as intrauterine fetal death in pregnancy, intrauterine death of the fetus during labour or unexpected birth asphyxia. However it was not possible to make any measurements of placental function or fetal well-being until the mid 1950s, when reliable methods were developed by Arnold Klopper and Jim Brown in Edinburgh for measurement of pregnanediol and oestrogens in urine. At first, urinary pregnanediol was used to assess placental function, but this was soon superseded by urinary oestriol which gave an indication not only of placental function but also of fetal well-being. Scientists made great efforts to provide quicker and simpler methods to measure oestriol in urine and blood, and clinicians hastened to apply these methods even more widely in practice. Other hormones, such as human placental lactogen, were measured in the quest for the best biochemical method for assessing the condition of the fetus and placenta. After about 20 years the popularity of this biochemical approach waned because of the increasing realization that the assessment provided was inconsistent: with urinary oestriol, for example, the daily background coefficient of variation was almost 40%.

Nevertheless, attempts to assess the condition of the fetus by biochemical means did show obstetricians how important it was to have reliable knowledge of the condition of the intrauterine fetus; better biophysical methods became available and finally one of us (GC) formally reported that discontinuing oestriol assay in the third trimester in clinical practice in his unit had no effect on perinatal outcome.

Many biochemical measurements however are of proven value, including serum alpha-fetoprotein assay in maternal blood and amniotic fluid. High levels in early second-trimester pregnancy indicate increased risks of fetal neural tube defect and of later fetal compromise. Recently it has been shown that unduly low levels of serum alpha-fetoprotein, serum oestriol and human chorionic gonadotrophin in early second-trimester pregnancy indicate increased risks of Down's syndrome in the fetus.

Biophysical assessment of fetus and placenta

Biophysical methods of making direct observation of intrauterine conditions have proved more valuable than biochemical methods, which tend to be indirect. Diagnostic ultrasound, pioneered by Ian Donald in Glasgow, has made possible accurate measurements of the parameters of normal and abnormal fetal growth with advancing pregnancy. Pathological growth retardation of the intrauterine fetus is readily detectable by measurements made by serial scans. The first scanners provided only a static picture but now most function in real time and can assess fetal function in dynamic fashion. Frank Manning and Larry Platt in the USA utilized real-time ultrasound to derive a fetal biophysical profile, which gives a dynamic assessment of the fetus.

Another important biophysical measurement, first developed in Germany by Fred Hammacher, is fetal cardiotocography. Fetal heart rate is recorded continuously and the tracing is related to a recording of uterine contractions, originally measured by the changes in intrauterine pressure. Although this method was first developed for use in labour, the application of sophisticated ultrasound techniques has enabled it to be used during pregnancy. It is now a technique of major importance for assessment of the fetus during pregnancy.

Even more recent is the introduction of cordocentesis, by which samples of blood are taken from the umbilical artery or vein through a needle passed, under ultrasound control, through the maternal abdomen into the uterus and then into the cord. This was first developed in France by Daffos in the early 1980s and has since been used extensively in the UK, USA, Europe and Scandinavia in the intrauterine assessment of the potentially jeopardized fetus. Doppler ultrasound techniques now enable the characteristics of blood flow in specific vessels of the fetal and placental circulation to be assessed with considerable accuracy.

While it is now possible to assess the condition of the intrauterine fetus with considerable precision in most cases, it must be remembered that in a minority, possibly 10% of cases, even the most careful and skilful assessment may be misleading, and that repeated assessment is especially important when there is any uncertainty.

Antenatal diagnosis

Interauterine diagnosis of the sex of the fetus was first reported by Fritz Fuchs in Copenhagen in the mid 1950s when he performed amniocentesis, enabling cells of fetal origin in the amniotic fluid to be cultured and the fetal karyotype determined. Progress was initially slow but improvements in amnion cell culture meant that by the mid 1960s the method was reliable enough for clinical application of amniocentesis. National studies on the safety of genetic amniocentesis in the USA, Canada and the UK indicated that the risks were low enough to be clinically acceptable. Since then, amniocentesis has become the standard technique for prenatal diagnosis. Initially used mainly for the diagnosis of chromosomally determined abnormalities such as Down's syndrome, this application has been rather patchy and, disappointingly, the incidence of Down's syndrome at birth has not been reduced over the past 20 years or so.

By contrast, the first demonstration that serum and amniotic fluid alpha-fetoprotein levels were elevated in women carrying a baby with an open neural tube defect (NTD) led to the rapid application of maternal serum alpha-fetoprotein screening. This, coupled with ultrasonic confirmation of the diagnosis, made possible screening programmes which have been associated with a considerable reduction in the incidence of NTD. Although this reduction had started spontaneously, availability of NTD screening procedures has contributed to the reduced incidence of these disorders. Since ultrasound examination can detect NTD by itself, many units have given up the alpha-fetoprotein screening and depend entirely on routine fetal anomaly scanning at about 18 weeks to detect NTD and other fetal abnormalities. However, the association between elevated alpha-fetoprotein at 16 weeks and later pregnancy complications, such as fetal growth retardation and preterm labour, and between very low alpha-fetoprotein at 16 weeks and Down's syndrome represent additional reasons for maintaining alpha-fetoprotein screening at 16–18 weeks' gestation.

DNA technology in prenatal diagnosis

In recent years advances have been made in the application of DNA technology to clinical diagnosis. As a result, disorders associated with gene abnormalities and deletions are now increasingly detectable. Fetal cells can be obtained at amniocentesis while the technique of chorionic villus sampling, performed transcervically or transabdominally, provides small samples of fetal tissue. From these samples results can be obtained rapidly and a reliable diagnosis can be made of fetal disorders such as thalassaemia major, Duchenne's muscular dystrophy, cystic fibrosis or Huntington's chorea.

CONTROL OF EXCESSIVE FERTILITY

Scientific advances are making it increasingly possible for women to bear the number of children they wish, rather than being at the mercy of their own fertility. In the mid 1950s the first combined oral contraceptive preparations became available and were improved rapidly; as major side-effects were found to be dose-related, equally effective lower-dose preparations were introduced. Improved intrauterine devices also became available but medicolegal problems are now causing the manufacturers to reduce production. The technique of laparoscopic sterilization was pioneered in France by Raoul Palmer and popularized in the UK by Patrick Steptoe. This quickly replaced laparotomy for sterilization. Therapeutic abortion for a series of indications was legalized in England, Wales and Scotland in 1967.

The UK birth rate reached its peak in 1964 and then fell steadily to 1977 as a result of many factors, helped by the increased availability of contraception, sterilization and pregnancy termination. From 1978 the rate increased by about 15% up to 1980 and since then has been maintained at around this level with small fluctuations. The increase in births from 1978 occurred first in older women.

PERINATAL MORTALITY AND MORBIDITY

In the UK perinatal mortality has continued to fall steadily. Surveys performed in 1958 and 1970 clarified many aspects of causation and pointed to the directions in which further improvements could be achieved. Improved methods for control of fertility helped women to avoid pregnancy at extremes of age and parity or if there was an unduly high risk of perinatal death. The perinatal mortality rate combines the stillbirth and first week neonatal death rates and is therefore expressed as the rate per 1000 live and stillbirths. In 1987 the rate in England and Wales was 8 per 1000 (see Chapter 77).

NEONATAL INTENSIVE CARE

Among the many specialties on which obstetricians and midwives collaborate in none do they work closer than neonatology. Peter Dunn carried out much of the pioneering work in the UK, and the clinical use of new knowledge of neonatal cardiorespiratory and metabolic functions, combined with impressive technology, has made possible an increasing rate of high quality survival of extremely premature babies. Advances in neonatal surgery have made possible the correction of many congenital fetal disorders previously thought to be lethal.

OBSTETRIC ANAESTHESIA

Anaesthesia and analgesia are essential for good obstetric practice. Although the number of women having general anaesthesia for vaginal operative delivery has been reduced in recent years, there has been an increase in the use of regional methods, especially epidural anaesthesia: currently 17% of women in the UK use this form of analgesia. In the early 1960s the technique of paracervical block was popular but proved dangerous to the fetus and has largely been abandoned in this country. Apart from providing anaesthesia for operative delivery, anaesthetists are often involved with intensive care in obstetrics, for conditions such as severe pre-eclampsia or eclampsia, excessive bleeding with or without coagulation defect and many other conditions requiring intensive care.

CONTROL OF LABOUR

Although the use of a continuous intravenous oxytocin infusion was first reported in 1947 by Geoffrey Theobald in the UK, and in the same year by Louis Helman in the USA, it was not widely used at first because of the relative unreliability of the preparations of oxytocin available. With the synthesis of oxytocin in 1962, various investigators recognized that intravenous administration could be used more efficiently than was previously the case for the induction of labour and to augment uterine contractions in slowly progressing labour of spontaneous onset. One of us (AT) published in 1967 and 1968 studies in Aberdeen which pioneered the use of oxytocin titration for induction and augmentation of labour. The philosophy of active management of labour, in which almost 50% of primigravidae may have their labour augmented by intravenous oxytocin to ensure normal progress, was pioneered at the National Maternity Hospital in Dublin by Kieran O'Driscoll. Oxytocin works best when the membranes are ruptured. Amniotomy and intravenous oxytocin administration remained popular for over 10 years until the mid 1970s, when local administration of prostaglandins proved able to initiate labour without amniotomy and more gradually and physiologically than amniotomy and oxytocin. Prostaglandin E_2 proved to have fewer side-effects than prostaglandin $F_{2\alpha}$. Given intravenously, prostaglandins have no advantages over oxytocin but administered extra-amniotically, intracervically or intravaginally in appropriate doses they are effective and more acceptable to women than the more invasive amniotomy and intravenous oxytocin administration.

WOMEN'S WISHES

Throughout the 1960s, advances in obstetric care involved the introduction of many technological innovations. The continuing fall in perinatal mortality reassured obstetricians that these innovations were beneficial. However, many women were frightened by what they regarded as unnecessary interference in the physiological process of birth and concerned by the potentially serious complications of some of the technology. They felt that women were no longer in control of their own labour. The Caesarean section rate rose steadily and although perinatal mortality fell, the two rates were not necessarily related to each other.

In the UK, obstetricians and women's organizations continued on a collision course until the mid 1970s when there was a major confrontation. Women's organizations vilified obstetric technology on the television, radio and in the newspapers, while obstetricians defended their record of improving results. It became clear that many innovations had not been subjected to trials to assess their efficacy. Subsequently there was a significant reduction in the use of interventions which could not be clearly justified. Obstetricians recognized that they had failed to convince women of the value of many useful advances in technique and so have now involved women increasingly in the decision-making processes of pregnancy management. They need to convince women of the necessity of relevant high technology methods when there is a high risk for the mothers or their infants.

In many units there has been a considerable reduction in the use of interventions previously thought to be essential, including episiotomy, epidural anaesthesia, induction of labour and electronic fetal heart rate monitoring in labour. Women have been encouraged to ensure that their husband or partner is present during labour and at the birth of the baby. Analgesic drug use in labour has been reduced, with many multiparous women requiring no analgesia at all. Ambulation in labour has been encouraged, as has delivery with the mother in any position she cares to adopt. The use of birth chairs has been evaluated and, in general, has not proved to have any genuine advantage over standard methods in the management of the second stage of labour and delivery.

All these changes in practice seem to have lightened the atmosphere in UK maternity hospitals, with many now more orientated towards fulfilling the expectations of pregnant women and their families, even when this involves accepting requests for unusual forms of management. Pregnancy and labour are important days for women and must be seen to be so. It is important that the woman is centre-stage and all the attendants, their equipment and their science are supportive.

BEREAVEMENT COUNSELLING

While most pregnancies end with mother and baby fit and well, the baby may be born dead or may die in the neonatal period. Years ago, it was customary to try to protect such mothers from as much of the experience as possible by not letting her see the dead baby, discharging her from hospital as soon as possible so that she would not be upset by hearing other babies crying and perhaps not bringing her back to the hospital for follow-up since that would remind her of the baby's death. Although this was meant well, it is now recognized that this management caused untold misery to bereaved mothers. Many were uncertain if they had ever had a baby. Grief is normally an intense process but once completed, normal life can start again.

It is now widely recognized that it is important for the

mother to see and hold her dead baby, even if it is abnormal. She should name the baby, ensure that the name is on the birth certificate and have a photograph of the baby. The baby should be buried and its grave marked so that she can return later, if necessary. She should be properly counselled and given an opportunity to talk about her feelings of loss in the weeks or months after the baby's death.

THE FUTURE

Women in the developed world will be having fewer babies; obstetricians will continue to add the fine tuning of safety and comfort to the natural process. With fewer perinatal and maternal deaths, even more individual attention will be paid to those women at higher risk and perhaps fetal and maternal monitoring will be applied more rationally. Individual methods will be more carefully assessed so that we reject the less useful tests but apply more widely those investigations which can be shown to be powerful in their capacity to predict with reasonable precision. If obstetricians concentrate on detecting and protecting this smaller group of higher-risk pregnancies, the majority of healthy women will be cared for by other members of the obstetric team. In the British Commonwealth, these will be the midwives whose natural place in caring for the normal will be better fulfilled.

In providing better support for the woman who is having a baby, a new wave of education and understanding is starting in the developed world. This will spread so that women are more aware and in a better position to discuss with their doctor or midwife what is happening. The Victorian barriers between the professional and the woman will continue to break down and a wider and better understanding will take their place. In non-drug analgesic techniques, we will refine and use what can be more widely applied.

The most important problems facing obstetricians are the prevention of preterm delivery and of intrauterine growth retardation. These two overlapping but separate conditions need much more research into their causes before correct preventive measures can be applied; this will be much more effective than the current emphasis of treating the established conditions.

The precise tests which will be used by obstetricians in the next century have not yet been developed. They will probably involve non-invasive techniques with a biophysical basis. Functions of fetal heart and brain and of uterine muscle will be more precisely measured; so possibly a better understanding of fetal and maternal physiology in pregnancy will follow. The indirect assessment of the body state from blood gas levels and acidaemia will have to continue until better measures are perfected. Probably these too will be derived non-invasively by magnetic resonance imaging rather than blood samples taken from the body.

In the developing world, many of the obstetrical problems are political ones. The provision of health care for such large numbers so widely spread may seem to be the major hurdle, but those who come from countries that went through the Industrial Revolution over a century ago must remember that improvements in health care must take their place among other social priorities in building a country's economy. Politicians perceive different goals from those seen by the medical profession. Maternal and child health preventive measures will in the long run yield greater returns per unit of money spent than will expenditure in the clinical field. Some politicians grasp this principle, forgetting that they must also provide some care for the present generation of women and their babies. They must build for the future but not turn their backs on the present.

Noel Dilly

Female pelvic anatomy

INTRODUCTION

This chapter contains a clinically oriented introduction to functional anatomy and histology of the female genital organs. The tract has been approached from the vulva upwards as it is seen in clinical medicine. Some areas such as lymphatic drainage and nerve supply will be discussed in two contexts, once as a general overview, then in a more specific context of individual regions.

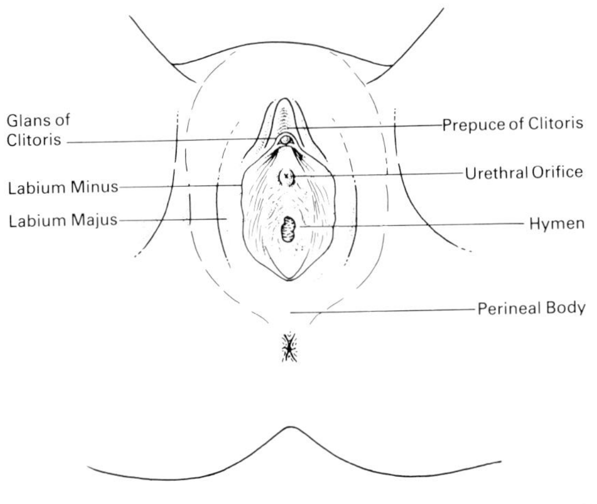

Fig. 2.1 The female external genitalia. This represents the classical portrait of the female external genitalia, but in life the labia majora are normally in contact with each other except during intercourse and labour.

THE VULVA

The vulva consists of the vaginal orifice, the urethral orifice and those structures associated with them which make up the floor of the anterior part of the pelvic outlet. It extends upwards to include the mons pubis (Fig. 2.1). It is supported by the largely transverse fibres of the inferior fascia of the urinogenital diaphragm, a part of the perineal membrane. This fascia has three holes, one just behind the pubic bone, one for the urethra and one for the vagina. It is strengthened posteriorly by the perineal body, an aponeurosis for the fibres of the perineal, levator ani and external and internal anal sphincter muscles.

Above this membrane lies the deep perineal pouch and beneath it the superficial pouch that contains the terminal portions of the vagina and urethra as well as their associated structures, the clitoris, the bulb of the vestibule, the vestibular glands, the superficial perineal muscles and their nerves and vessels.

The perineum

The perineum is the pelvic outlet below the pelvic diaphragm. It is usually divided by a line joining the anterior end of the ischial tuberosities into an anterior urogenital area and a posterior anal triangle. The anal triangle contains the anal canal and the surrounding ischiorectal fossae. It is bound posterolaterally by the sacrotuberous ligaments. The fossa itself is filled with fat. Its lateral wall is the fascia over obturator internus and the edge of the sacrotuberous ligaments; medially the fossae are separated by the perineal body, the anal canal and the anococcygeal body (Fig. 2.2).

The pudendal nerve and vessels leave the pelvis through the greater sciatic foramen then hook around the ischial spine. They enter the perineum through the lesser sciatic

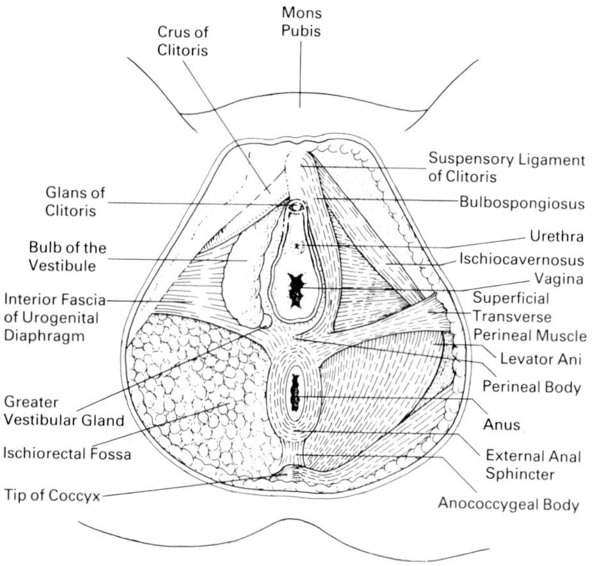

Fig. 2.2 The perineum. A view from below of the pelvic outlet showing its boundaries and triangles.

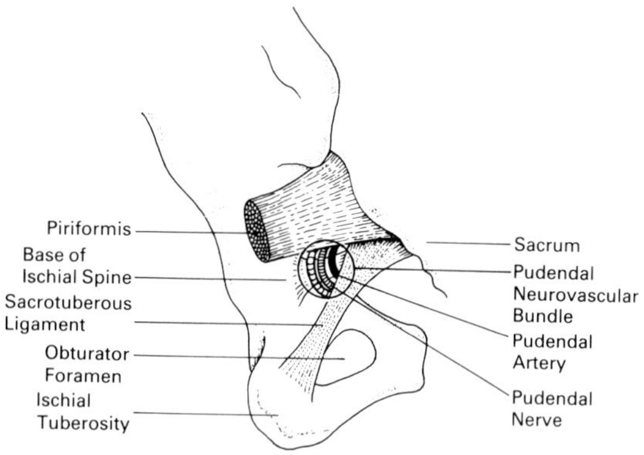

Fig. 2.3 Nerve supply of the perineum. The pudenal nerve usually leaves the pelvis via the greater sciatic foramen and enters the perineum via the lesser sciatic foramen, running forwards along its lateral wall in the pudendal canal.

foramen into the pudendal canal where they run forwards to supply the perineum (Fig. 2.3). The pudendal canal runs on the lateral wall of the fossa from the lesser sciatic foramen to the perineal membrane.

The urogenital triangle

The perineal membrane is a narrow shelf of fibrous tissue attached along the pubic rami. Anteriorly the crurae of the clitoris are attached to it. Each crus is covered by the ischiocavernosus muscle. Medial to each crus is the erectile tissue of the bulb of the vestibule and separating the bulbs on either side are the openings of the urethra and vagina. The bulbs fuse anteriorly in front of the urethral orifice and extend to the glans of the clitoris. The bulbospongiosus

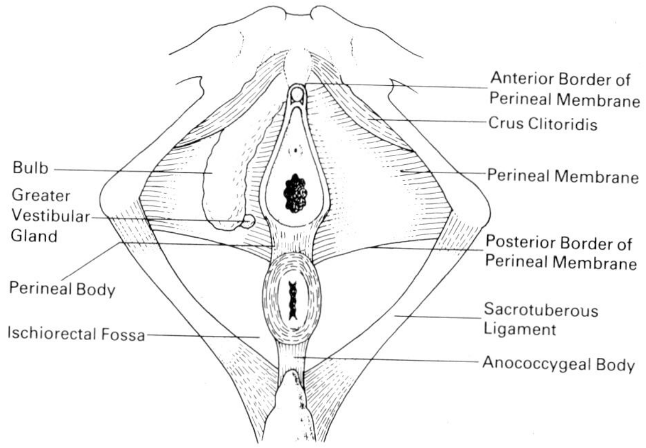

Fig. 2.4 Diagram of the superficial layers of the urogenital triangle. The bulbospongiosus and ischiocavernosus muscles have been removed to reveal the structure of the clitoris and the glands associated with it.

muscle lies superficial to the bulb, extending from the perineal body where it also covers the vestibular glands forwards around the vagina and urethra to the clitoris (Fig. 2.2, 2.4).

The deep perineal pouch is also perforated by the vagina and urethra. The perineal body is the fibrous tissue aponeurosis of the fibres of the bulbospongiosus, the transverse perinei, the sphincter vaginae and the external anal sphincter. It is somewhat mobile but provides support for the levator ani above.

The nerve supply of the urogenital triangle is derived from the ilioinguinal nerve, the perineal branch of the posterior cutaneous nerve of the thigh, and the pudendal nerve. The ilioinguinal nerve supplies the anterior part of the labia majora, the posterior part being supplied by the posterior cutaneous nerve of the thigh laterally. Its remaining area together with the labia minora is supplied medially by branches of the pudendal nerve. The clitoris is supplied by one of the terminal branches of the pudendal nerve, the dorsal nerve of the clitoris. It runs forwards along the ischiopubic ramus above the inferior fascia of the urogenital diaphragm, and reaches the dorsum of the clitoris through the gap between the anterior end of the inferior fascia and the inferior pubic ligament. The major specialized receptors in the clitoris are Pacinian corpuscles.

The mons pubis

The mons pubis is an area over the pubic bone which develops at puberty secondary as a sexual characteristic. The pubic hair is usually distributed upon its surface in a characteristic triangular fashion but a significant proportion of normal woman have male-type distribution with the hair extending up the midline of the lower abdomen. The probable functions of the mons include acting as a buffer between the male and female pubic bones during intercourse and as a source of arousal responses when stimulated. It is also said to provide tissue for the increase in size of the labia minora as they expand during coitus.

The labia majora

The labia are a pair of fatty folds which are continuous anteriorly with the mons. Posteriorly they peter out but a small continuation comes together between the vagina and the anus. Their outer surfaces are covered with pubic hair and their medial surfaces are usually in apposition, closing off a potential aperture called the pudendal cleft. They are sometimes separated by a piece of the labia minora. This surface contains many large sebaceous and sweat glands.

The labia consist of skin-covered loose fibrofatty tissue similar to that of the mons, but containing some muscle, as well as the termination of the round ligament of the uterus.

The labia minora

The labia minora are a pair of erectile fleshy folds usually contained within the folds of the labia majora and separated from them by a deep cleft. They surround the vestibule of the vagina. Posteriorly in the virgin the labia minora join each other with a delicate fold of skin called the fourchette just deep to the labia majora. Anteriorly they divide into a pair of folds that split to enclose the clitoris. The outer surface is hairy and contains many sweat and sebaceous glands but the inner hairless surface is covered by a poorly keratinized stratified squamous epithelium with sweat and sebaceous glands. The labia minora contain extensive vascular spaces surrounded by delicate connective tissue and a little smooth muscle. Their probable functions are to increase the depth of the vaginal canal during intercourse and afterwards probably to help in maintaining the vaginal continence to the ejaculate. They are a potent source of stimuli resulting in sexual arousal.

The vestibule

The vestibule is the space between the labia minora bounded anteriorly by the clitoris and posteriorly by the fold of skin joining the labia minora, the fourchette. Opening into the vestibule are the vagina, the urethra and the ducts of the great and lesser vestibular glands. The bulborectal glands with their alkaline mucus secretion also drain into the vestibule posteriorly. The vaginal orifice may contain a hymen or hymenal remnants. Its lining is similar to the vaginal epithelium and is stratified squamous non-keratinized epithelium. Its glands are one of the two major natural sources of lubrication during coitus.

The clitoris

The clitoris is a small but variable-sized organ made mainly of erectile tissue situated at the anterior end of the vestibule. It is suspended from the lower border of the pubic arch by a small triangular ligament. It is made from two corpora cavernosa, the cavernous blood spaces of which are separated from each other by fibromuscular trabeculae. Each corpus cavernosum arises from a crus near the ischiopubic ramus and this crus is palpable. The free extremity of the clitoris is made up of a rounded mass of erectile tissue — the glans — which, when not aroused, is normally covered by the anterior folds of the labia minora to form a prepuce. This prepuce contains vast numbers of sebaceous and sweat glands. However the glans of the clitoris has neither sweat nor sebaceous glands.

The clitoris is an important source of stimuli and is responsible for sexual arousal and reflex lubrication; it contains a considerable number of mechanoreceptors.

Vestibular bulb

The vestibular bulb consists of two masses of erectile tissue, one on either side of the vaginal orifice. They are covered by the bulbospongiosus muscle and lie deep in the labia majora. They are joined by a commissure in front of the vagina, which is in contact with the lower surface of the urinogenital diaphragm.

Musculature of the vulva

Superficially these muscles are the transverse perinei, the bulbospongiosus and the ischiocavernosus muscles, and deeper, the parts of the urinogenital diaphragm surrounded by the superficial and deep layers of fascia. The deeper muscles are the deep transverse perinei and the sphincter urethrae. The superficial muscles are slender and delicate; the transverse perinei run horizontally from the inferior ramus of the ischium to the perineal body superficial to the posterior part of the inferior fascia of the urinogenital diaphragm. On each side the bulbospongiosus comes from the perineal body and passes forwards encircling the external end of the vagina, superficial to the bulb and the greater vestibular glands. It ends in the dorsal aspect of the connective tissue capsule of the corpus cavernosus of the clitoris.

The deep transverse perinei also meet at the perineal body. The sphincter urethrae fibres not only encircle the anterior and lateral parts of the urethra but also the corresponding parts of the vagina.

Nerve supply

Nerves come from the anterior divisions of the anterior rami of the second, third and fourth sacral spinal nerves. The principal named nerve is the pudendal nerve but the labia and the adjacent skin of the perineum also have a sensory supply from the perineal branch of the posterior cutaneous nerve of the thigh.

The pudendal nerve is a mixed nerve and travels together with the internal pudendal artery in the fascial canal on the

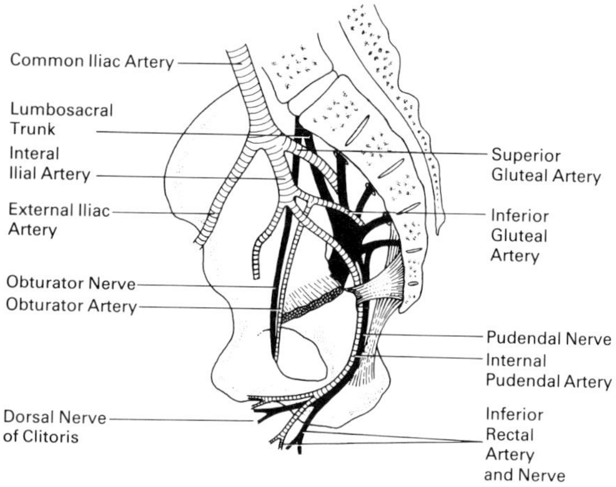

Fig. 2.5 Pelvic nerves and blood supply of the pudenda. The major nerve is the pudendal, but it is supplemented by the posterior cutaneous nerve of the thigh and the ilioinguinal and genitofemoral nerves.

lateral wall of the ischiorectal fossa. In this region it usually branches away from the inferior rectal branch, that is crossing to provide the sensory supply to perianal skin and the lower part of the anal canal, and the vital motor supply to the external anal sphincter.

The pudendal nerve itself divides into two branches in the anterior part of the pudendal canal. The terminal branches are the dorsal nerve of the clitoris and the perineal nerve (Fig. 2.5). The dorsal nerve of the clitoris runs above the inferior fascia of the urinogenital diaphragm alongside the ischiopubic ramus. It then passes out between the anterior border of the urogenital diaphragm and the pubis to reach the clitoris and glans (Fig. 2.5).

The perineal nerve gives motor branches to the striated muscles of the vulva, some of the anterior fibres of the external anal sphincter and the levator ani. Its sensory terminations are a pair of posterior labial nerves.

The vulva contains large numbers of special nerve endings and a corresponding rich supply of sensory nerves. Many of these specialized endings are mechanoreceptors, but they are absent from the region of the vestibule surrounding the vagina where there is a dense arborization of free nerve endings.

Most of the sensory fibres are conveyed by the pudendal nerve, but those in the mons and the anterior parts of the labia major go to the lumbar plexus via the ilioinguinal and genitofemoral nerves. Some fibres from the posterior parts of the labia major are conveyed with the perineal branch of the posterior femoral cutaneous nerve to the sacral plexus.

There is also a dense autonomic nerve supply — the postganglionic sympathetic fibres arising from the hypogastric plexus, and the pelvis plexus; these are distributed to their endings via the pudendal nerve. The parasympathetic fibres come from S2, S3 and S4, as the nervae erigentes to join with the pelvic plexus; they are distributed with either the pelvic blood vessels or the pudendal nerves.

Blood supply

The arteries spring mainly from the internal iliac artery with a significant contribution from the femoral artery. The internal pudendal artery arises from the internal iliac artery and runs in the pudendal canal to the labia majora where it forms a very rich anastomosis with the deep external pudendal branches from the femoral artery. There are also communications between the vessels on either side (Fig. 2.5).

The pudendal artery gives off the inferior rectal artery which supplies the skin and musculature around the anal canal but provides blood for only a small area — the posterior aspect of the lower end of the vagina. Although the pudendal artery is near the ischiopubic ramus, it gives off branches that penetrate the inferior fascia of the urinogenital diaphragm to supply the labia, the erectile tissue of the bulb, the lower end of the vagina and associated muscles. Its final branches are the deep and dorsal arteries of the clitoris. It is the deep branch that is the main supply to the corpus cavernosus. The branches of the femoral artery, the superficial and deep external pudendal vessels, pass medially to reach the anterior portion of the labia majora.

The venous drainage of this area is basically a vast intercommunicating plexus that drains to the internal pudendal veins and hence to the internal iliac veins, with a small part of the anterior region of the labia majora draining to the greater saphenous vein.

Lymphatic drainage

The initial drainage from the vulva, the lower part of the urethra, the vagina and anal canal is mostly to the medial group of superficial inguinal lymph nodes. From here they drain into the deep inguinal lymph nodes in the femoral canal. The glans clitoridis drains directly into these nodes. There is considerable overlap in the drainage, which must be considered bilateral when radical surgery for malignant diseases is considered.

THE VAGINA

The vagina is a distensible fibromuscular tube extending from the vestibule to the cervix of the uterus. It runs backwards and upwards with the anterior and posterior walls in close contact reducing the lumen to a mere slit. The lining epithelium is thrown into transverse folds or rugae. It is probably the slack in these folds that accommodates the considerable distension of the vagina during copulation and, later, parturition so that the vagina does not tear.

The vagina is related anteriorly to the base of the bladder and the urethra. It is separated from the bladder base by loose connective tissue, but the urethra is firmly bound to the adventitia of the anterior surface of the lower two-thirds of the vagina. Where the vagina is related to the bladder

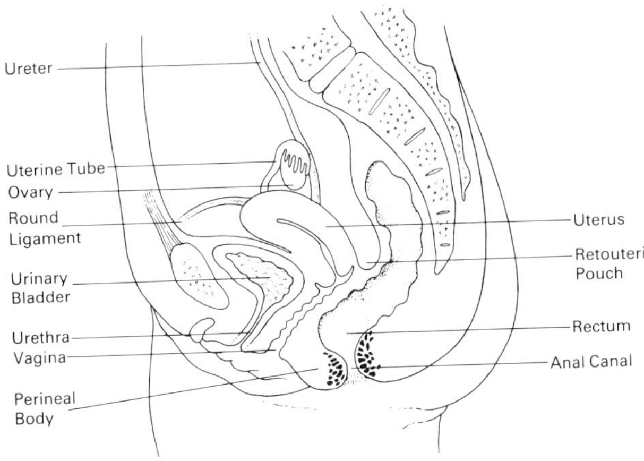

Fig. 2.6 Sagittal section of the female pelvis. The peritoneal covering of the pelvic organs is organized much as if a cover had been draped over them. Note the close relationship between the posterior fornix of the vagina and the rectouterine pouch.

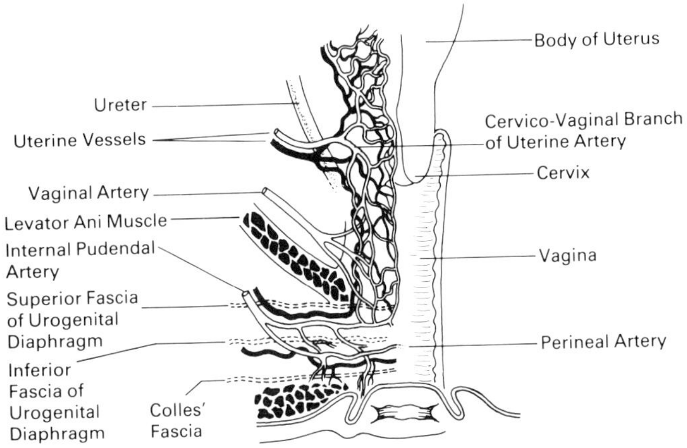

Fig. 2.7 Blood supply to the vagina. The deeper structures are supplied mainly from the uterine vessels, whereas the more superficial structures have a complex supply from the rectal and pudendal arteries.

base it is separated from it in part by the two ureters, as their terminal portions pass in front of the anterior fornix.

Posteriorly the vagina is related to the rectum and the retrouterine pouch of Douglas. The lowermost part of the vagina is separated from the anal canal by the mass of dense connective tissue, the perineal body (Fig. 2.6).

Laterally the upper vagina is related to the pelvic fascia and the lower part is embraced by the anteromedial fibres of pubococcygeus and the urinogenital diaphragm. Near its outermost extremity the bulb of the vestibule, the greater vestibular glands and the bulbospongiosus muscles are its lateral relations.

The epithelium lining the vagina lies upon a dense fibrous lamina propria. The epithelium is stratified, squamous and non-keratinized and does not contain mucus glands. It is unusual in that even the most superficial shrunken cells retain their nuclei. The apparent emptiness of many of the cells in the epithelium results from the fact that they contain glycogen which does not show up on routine histological stains.

The submucosa consists of loosely arranged connective tissue with many elastic fibres and numerous large venous spaces together with occasional lymphoid patches. The muscularis is relatively thin, with both longitudinal and circular smooth muscle and is continuous above with the uterine muscle. The outer layer of the vagina, the adventitia, is a fibrous tissue coat that binds the vagina to the surrounding structures.

Blood supply

The vagina has a rich and variable blood supply. The major vessels are the uterine arteries and the vaginal branches of the internal iliac arteries. From the anastomosis of these vessels, azygos arteries extend on the anterior and posterior surfaces of the vagina. Other contributions, especially to the lower end of the vagina, are from the artery to the bulb, the pudendal arteries, and the middle and inferior rectal vessels. Because the vagina is distensible these vessels have a very tortuous course in its contracted state. The venous drainage, in common with the other pelvic viscera, starts as a series of plexuses associated with the vesicle, rectal and uterine plexuses and drains eventually by vaginal veins to the internal iliac veins (Fig. 2.7).

Lymphatic drainage

Drainage differs for the upper two-thirds compared with the lower third and for the anterior wall as opposed to the posterior wall. From the upper two-thirds the drainage is to the internal and external iliac lymph nodes. The difference between the anterior and posterior walls is that while drainage from the anterior wall is direct to the internal iliac nodes, that from the posterior wall relays first in a node lying in the connective tissue between the vagina and rectum. From the lower third of the vagina, lymph drains to the superficial inguinal nodes on both sides.

Nerve supply

The major nerve supply to the vagina is autonomic from the pelvic plexuses, but the lower end has a sensory supply from the pudendal nerve.

The sympathetic fibres come from the lower lumbar sympathetic ganglia via the hypogastric plexus. The parasympathetic outflow is through the second, third and fourth sacral nerves. The fibres are distributed mainly in company with the arterial supply. The parasympathetic ganglia are found between the bladder and vagina and in association with the lateral walls of the vagina. The majority of nerve endings are undecorated, but Pacinian corpuscles are found within the vaginal adventitia.

THE UTERUS

The uterus is usually described in terms of cervix, body and fundus. In the nulliparous woman it is pear-shaped and measures about $7.5 \times 5 \times 2.5$ cm. There is a cavity which communicates with the peritoneal cavity via the Fallopian tubes and with the cavity of the vagina via the cervical canal. The fundus is that part of the uterus which lies above the openings of the tubes, while the tapering body lies below the fundus. It is somewhat flattened anteroposteriorly and is continuous with the cervix below. The cervix protrudes into the vault of the vagina. The gap between the cervix and the vaginal wall is called the fornix of the vagina; it is deepest posteriorly.

The uterus is described as having four layers—firstly, there is an outer peritoneal or serous coat below which is a subserous connective tissue layer that is densest where the various ligaments attach to the cervix. Third is the myometrium, the muscle layer of the uterus; it is the thickest layer, made up of interlacing bundles of smooth muscle fibres separated by connective tissue sheets containing blood vessels. This layer is about 15 mm thick in the adult nulliparous uterus. The fourth, innermost layer is the endometrium, surrounding the cavity of the uterus; the endometrium undergoes considerable changes during the menstrual cycle.

The cervix has a central canal that extends from the internal os, where it becomes continuous with the cavity of the uterus, to the external os, where it becomes continuous with the cavity of the vagina. It forms a narrow bottleneck between these two organs.

The cervix is divided from the corpus by a fibromuscular junction which acts as a sphincter; its competence is important, especially during the second trimester of pregnancy.

The cervix projects into the vagina, surrounded by a gutter-like fornix. The vaginal cervix has a short anterior lip and a longer posterior lip. It is penetrated by the endocervical canal which joins the uterine cavity to the vagina. The canal is fusiform in shape, flattened from front to back and measures 7 mm across at its widest part and about 3 cm long.

Anteriorly the supravaginal part is separated from the bladder by the connective tissue layer, the parametrium. The uterine arteries run in this tissue while the ureter runs downwards and forwards within the parametrium about 2 mm from the cervix.

Posteriorly the supravaginal cervix is covered with the peritoneum lining the rectouterine pouch of Douglas. The cervix is supported posteriorly by the uterosacral ligaments which extend from this part of the cervix to the second, third and fourth sacral vertebrae. The cardinal ligaments support the cervix laterally and are the major support of the cervix and uterus.

The cervix shares its blood supply with that of the body of the uterus. Coming from the uterine artery, the cervicovaginal branch runs down the lateral margin of the cervix where it anastomoses with branches of the vaginal artery, forming a rich plexus of vessels (Fig. 2.7). The venous drainage is lateral into a plexus on either side of the cervix and from there into veins that follow the arteries.

The nerve supply to the cervix is autonomic, with the densest innervation being at the level of the internal os and most of these fibres supplying the smooth muscle in this region. The fibres appear to follow the arterially derived vessels. In contrast with the body of uterus, many of these nerve fibres are cholinesterase-positive. There are both adrenergic and cholinergic fibres within the cervix: their distribution is very similar, but overall there are fewer cholinergic fibres. Most of these fibres disappear after the menopause. Sensory fibres travel with both divisions of the autonomic nervous system.

The cervix has a rich lymphatic drainage with a three-layered arrangement of beds of vessels: a subepithelial bed, a stromal bed and a serosal bed which gives rise to a series of larger vessels that drain along the base of the broad ligament. The most anterior are closely related to the uterine artery and eventually reach the external iliac nodes. Slightly posteriorly the vessels also follow the uterine artery to its origin where they join the internal iliac nodes. The most posterior group leave the cervix posterolaterally and pass along the uterosacral fold to reach the nodes situated over the sacrum.

The bulk of the cervix consists mainly of fibrous tissue containing varying proportions of smooth muscle—usually about 10%, but it can vary between 2 and 40%.

The vast amount of collagen is probably the reason for the rapid dilatation of the cervix during labour. It may be that during the later stages of pregnancy, the ratio of glycosaminoglycans to collagen exceeds some critical level when there is an influx of water into the tissues. There is also a reduction in the cohesive forces between cervical collagen filaments, so that the adhesion between the fibrils breaks down, producing a soft tissue which is dilated by the mechanical forces of uterine contraction during labour.

Blood supply

This is through the uterine arteries supported superiorly by the terminal branches of the ovarian arteries. The uterine artery arises from the internal iliac artery, passing medially across the pelvic floor and lying in the base of the broad ligament. As the artery reaches the uterus near the supravaginal part of the cervix, it passes above the ureter and turns upwards to pass close to the lateral side of the body of the uterus as far as the entrance of the Fallopian tube into the uterus. Here it anastomoses with the ovarian artery. Throughout its course it gives off many branches that penetrate the wall of the uterus (Fig. 2.8).

The venous drainage of the uterus consists of a plexus of veins that starts in the broad ligament, spreading out across the pelvic floor to communicate with the rectal and vesicle plexuses and draining into the internal iliac veins.

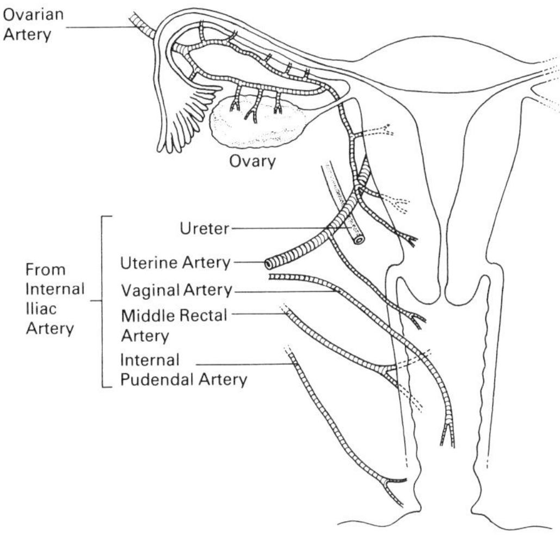

Fig. 2.8 Blood supply of the genitalia. The uterus has an anastomotic supply from both the ovarian and uterine arteries, both vessels running in the broad ligament.

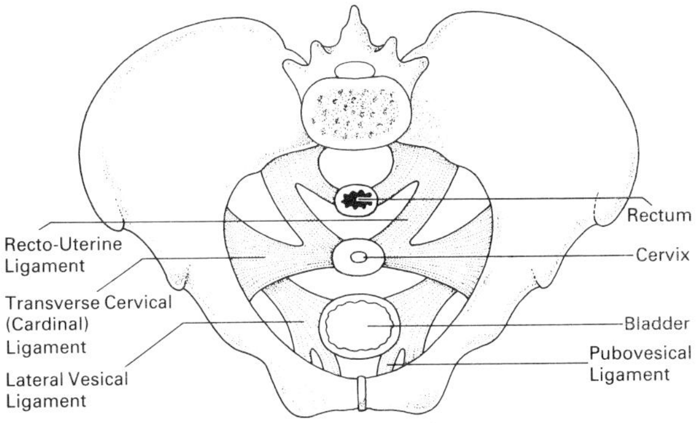

Fig. 2.9 Pelvic ligaments. The transverse or cardinal ligament is probably the major supporting structure of the cervix.

Lymphatic drainage

In general this follows the arteries.

Nerve supply

This system is poorly understood. The main sensory fibres from the cervix run in the nervi erigentes from the sacral segments 2 and 3, while those from the body of the uterus travel with the hypogastric plexus to the lower thoracic segments. Some sensory fibres from the fundus travel in the ovarian and renal plexuses to reach their dorsal nerve roots of T11 and T12.

Peritoneal relations

The uterus is draped in a fold of peritoneum which extends forwards to cover the bladder and backwards to the rectum. It spreads laterally as the broad ligament, and the peritoneum then spreads to cover the pelvic wall. It is as if these organs had been pushed up into the pelvic cavity from below, carrying the peritoneum to various degrees into the cavity of the pelvis.

Anteriorly the peritoneum extends downwards as far as the attachment of the base of the bladder at the level of the internal os, whereas posteriorly the bladder is completely covered by peritoneum.

Fascia and ligaments of the uterus

These ligaments contain a remarkably high proportion of smooth muscle besides the usual collection of collagen. The cardinal and uterosacral ligaments assist the fibrous tissue in fixing the anterior aspect of the uterus to the bladder base and in maintaining the stability of the bladder. This connective tissue extends inferiorly to bind the urethra to the anterior wall of the vagina. It is probable that the broad and round ligaments have little function in uterine stability.

The uterosacral ligaments, arising from the supravaginal part of the cervix, pass backwards, embracing the rectum, to be attached to the front of the lower part of the sacrum. Posteriorly the vagina and anal canals are separated but bound together by the fibromuscular mass of the perineal body. The lateral ligaments, the main ligaments of uterine stability, extend laterally from the cervix to the side wall of the pelvis (Fig. 2.9). The round and broad ligaments are associated with the body of the uterus. The round ligament arises from the junction between the body of the uterus and the uterine tube passes via the broad ligament where it raises a ridge on the anterior surface. It eventually runs along the inguinal canal to the labium majus of the vulva. It is mostly made up of smooth muscle. It probably functions as an anchor for the uterus in the anteverted position during recumbent sleep and against the pressure of a full bladder.

The broad ligament is no ligament: it is little more than a fold of peritoneum extending between the lateral aspect of the body of the uterus and the lateral wall of the pelvis. Superiorly, there is a free border, while inferiorly it merges with the pelvic floor. It contains the ovarian artery and uterine tube, the round and ovarian ligaments superiorly, and the uterine artery medially. There are extensive lymphatics associated with the arteries. The ovary is attached to the posterior surface of the broad ligament by the mesovarium, a fold of peritoneum from the posterior side of the ligament (Fig. 2.10).

MENSTRUATION

In the prepubertal period the epithelium lining the uterine cavity is only a single layer of cuboidal cells and the mucosal glands are simple unbranched tubes. For two or three years before puberty there is considerable growth of the uterus in line with the increased ovarian activity. By menarche the uterus has almost reached its adult size.

The menstrual debris comes from the endometrium above

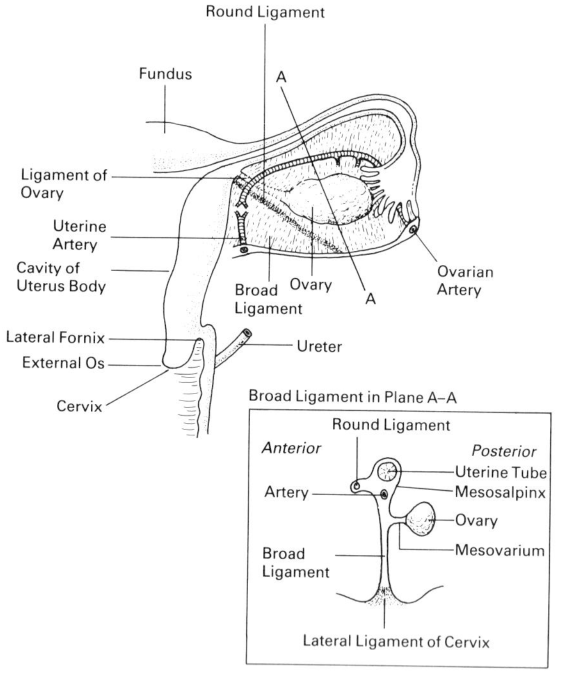

Fig. 2.10 Ovary and broad ligament from the back showing the relations of structures within the broad ligament. There are multiple small branches from the ovarian artery to the Fallopian tube.

the internal os. It is composed of blood and epithelial detritus and averages between 50 and 60 ml in healthy adults. The cyclical changes of the endometrium are directly related to changes occurring in the ovary. It is easiest to consider the menstrual changes from the end of menstruation, that is about day 5 of a 28-day cycle. At this stage the endometrium consists of little else but the stumps of glands in a dense stroma. This part of the lining, the stratum basale, usually has variable amounts of stratum spongiosum on its surface. There is a very rapid spread of epithelial cells from the mouths of the gland remnants so that by the end of the first week of the cycle the surface has a complete epithelial cover (Fig. 2.11).

The second week of the cycle is a time of considerable growth and cell division. The glands increase in size, the blood vessels dilate and the stroma becomes oedematous as a result of the oestrogens secreted by the ovary.

During the third week of the cycle, after ovulation and under the influence of progesterone from the corpus luteum, the endometrium becomes even more oedematous, boggy and pale. The cells in the stroma enlarge and fill with glycogen, the glands become more coiled and swollen and some begin to release their contents into the lumen of the glands.

In the last week of the cycle the endometrium is at its thickest — some 10 times thicker than at the beginning — and is described as having three layers; a narrow stratum compactum below the surface of the epithelium, a thick stratum spongiosum occupying most of the endometrium, and the inactive stratum basale. At the end of this time the strata compactum and spongiosum are shed and the whole cycle begins again.

These cyclical changes, under the control of the ovarian hormones, are brought about by changes in the arterioles supplying the endometrium. There are two types of arterioles — the straight and the spiral. The straight arterioles only supply the basal layer, but the spiral ones supply the whole thickness of the endometrium. It is ischaemia of the spiral arteries which produces the necrosis that results in the menstrual discharge. By the second day of menstruation the endometrium has been lost down to the basal layer.

THE UTERINE TUBES

The uterine (Fallopian) tubes are between 10 and 14 cm long, lying for the middle three-quarters in the upper border of the broad ligament. The lateral extremity is free of the broad ligament and is in close association with the surface of the ovary. The end is opened and expanded with a bunch of finger-like processes, the fimbriae (Fig. 2.12). There can be more than one ostium to a Fallopian tube. It is said that one of the fimbriae — the ovarian fimbria — is longer than the others and is attached by its tip to the ovary.

The uterine tube is usually considered to have four regions — the fimbriated infundibulum outside the broad ligament, a dilated ampulla, followed by a narrow isthmus with a lumen 1–2 mm in diameter within the broad ligament, and finally an intramural part of the tube which lies within the muscular wall of the uterus. Thus the cavity of the uterus is continuous with the peritoneal cavity. However the circular muscle at the uterine end of the Fallopian tube is thickened and is regarded by some as a sphincter controlling the flow of fluids from the uterus into the tube. The tube is capable of producing secretions; the nature of these secretions is poorly known, but the amounts vary during the ovarian cycle, being greatest in the post-ovulation phase.

The tube consists of smooth muscle surrounding a mucous membrane which is ciliated and thrown into many complex longitudinal folds. The isthmus differs in that here the lumen is narrow, the folds disappear and there are only a few cilia.

The tube has a rich blood supply via many small branches from the ovarian artery and its inner end from the uterine artery. The veins of the tube drain to the pampiniform plexus, while the lymphatics follow the course of the ovarian arteries.

THE OVARIES

The ovaries lie free within the cavity of the pelvis; they are without a covering of peritoneum except along the equatorial attachment of the mesovarium. The ovary is attached

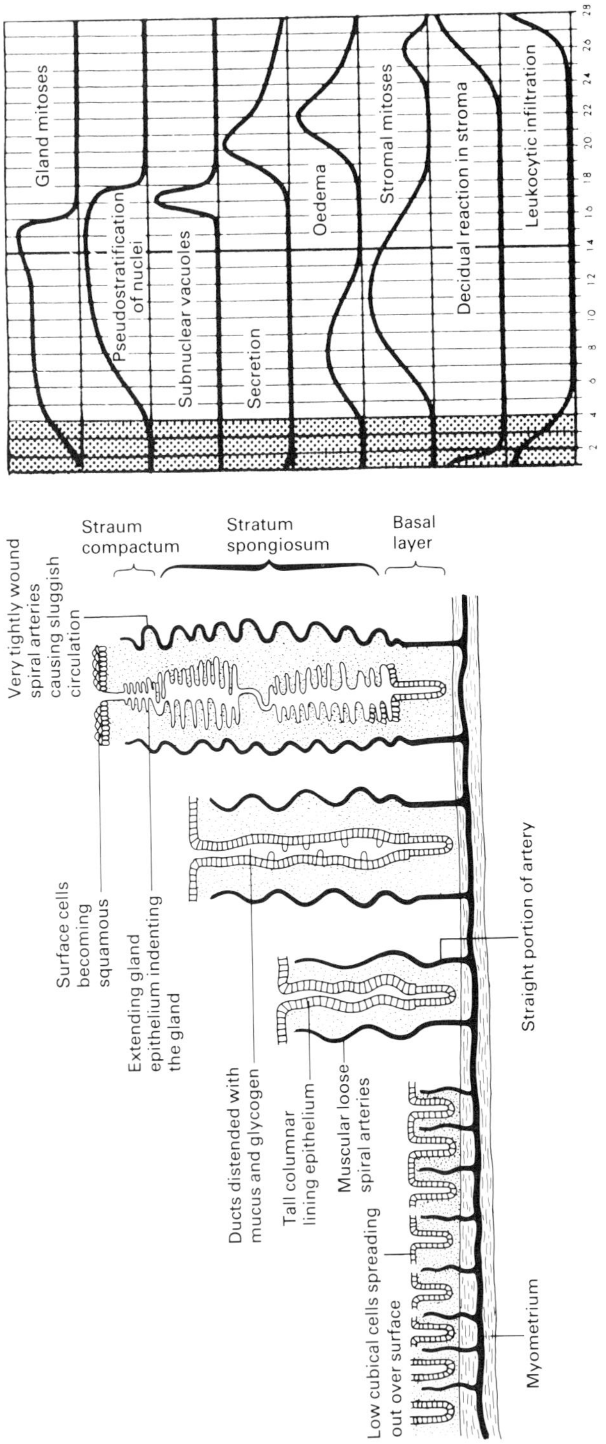

Cyclic changes in endometrium. Approximate relationship of useful microscopic changes

Fig. 2.11 Diagram of the menstrual cycle.

to the uterus at its upper angle by the ligament of the ovary. This mass of fibrous tissue and smooth muscle lies between the two layers of the broad ligament.

The ovary lies obliquely, with its upper pole medial and its lower pole lateral. It touches the side wall of the pelvis between the internal and external iliac vessels and lies upon the obturator nerve. The peritoneum, against which the ovary lies, is supplied by the obturator nerve. The ovary receives its blood from the ovarian arteries — direct branches of the abdominal aorta — while the ovarian veins form a plexus in the mesovarium that eventually drains into a pair of veins which run with the ovarian artery. Those from the left unite to form a single vein that drains into the left renal vein. Those on the right fuse and join the inferior vena cava.

The ovarian lymph drainage follows the course of the ovarian artery.

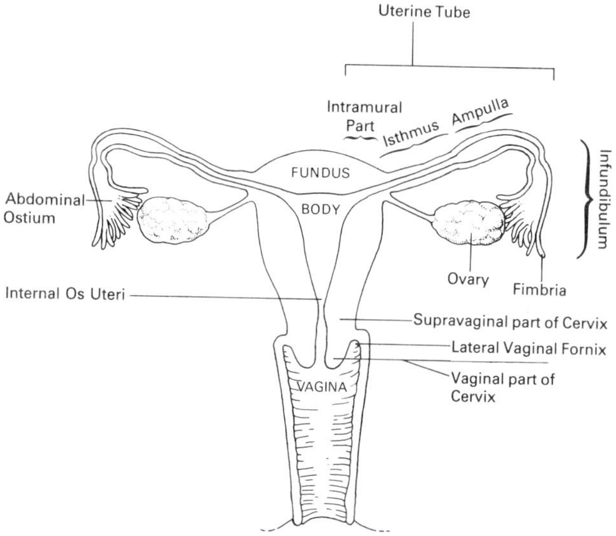

Fig. 2.12 Uterine (Fallopian) tubes. The functional anatomy of the tube is poorly understood. The variations in lumen size probably act as a baffle to stop too large objects passing and the highly convoluted wall with ciliated crests to the folds function to allow sperm to move in one direction and the egg in the opposite way.

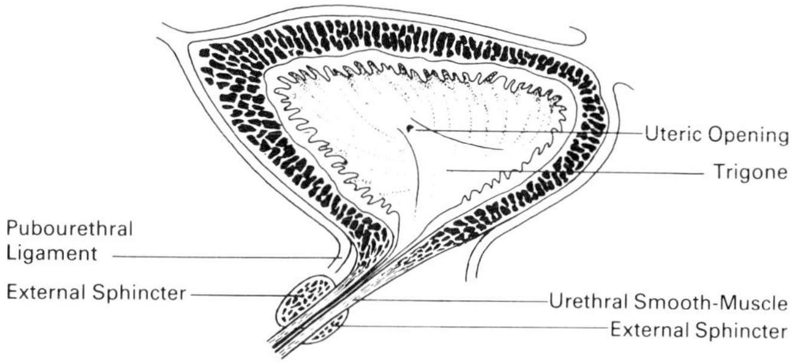

Fig. 2.13 Except where it is fixed at its base, the bladder is a highly distensible structure, and urinary continence probably depends upon the physical relations of the fixed/mobile junction.

Structure

The ovary consists of a cuboidal epithelium surrounding a fibrous stroma. Initially each ovary contains about 3 million potential ova which have migrated along the dorsal mesentery during development.

In the newborn baby the ovaries are very large compared with the uterus. They increase in weight some 20 times before maturity, but the relative growth of the uterus is such that by puberty they are relatively much smaller than the uterus. There is practically no recognizable germinal tissue in the fully involuted ovary after the menopause.

THE BLADDER

The bladder is fixed at the trigone and has a mobile and distensible fundus above it. The trigone is generally immobile; it is attached by ligaments and tough fascia to the cervix and anterior fornix, as well as by the lateral ligaments which pass across the pelvic floor covering the vesicle veins, the inferior vesicle artery and its associated lymphatics, together with the nerves of the bladder.

There are three ligaments extending from the fundus of the bladder to the umbilicus — the median umbilical ligament, the remains of the urachus in the midline, and a pair of lateral umbilical ligaments (the remains of the umbilical arteries of the fetus) extending obliquely upwards to the umbilicus. Each of these ligaments is retroperitoneal and raises a ridge of peritoneum on the internal surface of the anterior abdominal wall. Only the superior surface of the bladder is firmly attached to peritoneum; elsewhere it is surrounded by loose areolar tissue. The potential space between the anterior aspect of the bladder and the pubic symphysis is the cave of Retzius. Posteriorly lies the uterus. Between the uterus and the trigone of the bladder the fascia is strong and it is this fascia that helps the ligaments to anchor the bladder (Fig. 2.13).

The triangular trigone lies between the openings of the ureters into the bladder and the midline internal urethral orifice. The openings of the two ureters are found at either end of a transverse ridge, the interureteric bar. The track of the ureters through the muscle of the bladder wall is oblique, and it is debated whether it is this oblique course or the flap of mucous membrane associated with the opening that has the major role in preventing urinary reflux.

In life, the base of the bladder lies flat; this flat area is greater than the area of the trigone but is of prime importance in maintaining urinary continence. There are said to be three sphincters controlling micturition — an internal, urethral and external urinary sphincter. The internal sphincter is complex. It probably does not exist as such but its effect is produced by a series of muscle actions. It is really the tone of the detrusor loop from the outer longitudinal layer of bladder muscle that forces the urethra backwards and it is the tone of the base plate that forces the trigone forwards into the concavity formed by the circular fibres of the fundus. Thus the trigone comes to lie in front of the urethral orifice, so that as long as the base plate remains flat the bladder neck remains closed.

In order to convert the base plate into a funnel-like tube during voiding, considerable force is required. The human is probably alone amongst animals in being able to hold urine for a considerable time after bladder-filling has reached the point where the bladder would empty reflexly. This can even be achieved during sleep. At birth this bladder control is not possible because the base plate is rounded and does not fit into the concavity formed by the detrusor. In stress incontinence it is probably a sagging of the anterior vaginal wall that causes a descent of the bladder, distorting it in the base and so reducing its ability to resist increases in intra-abdominal pressure.

The bladder wall is made of smooth muscle fibres which run in spirals. The apparently randomly arranged muscle fibres produce a series of trabeculated ridges which at cystoscopy show through the mucous membrane. The muscle as a whole is called the detrusor. The mucous membrane of the bladder is thick and lax and lined with a transitional epithelium which is urine-proof because of the specialized junctions between the inner edges of the adjacent cells. There is said to be a ring of fibres around the internal urethral orifice. The membrane has neither glands nor muscularis mucosa.

The blood supply to the bladder is from the superior and inferior vesicle arteries, assisted by a few branches from the pubic branch of the inferior epigastric artery.

The veins of the bladder become a plexus at the base of the bladder. The vesicle plexus communicates with veins in the broad ligament, and drains to the internal iliac veins.

The lymph drainage follows the course of the arteries. Its nerve supply is autonomic from the pelvic plexus, the parasympathetic segments are S2, S3 and S4 and the fibres reach the plexus via the nervi erigentes. The sympathetic nerves are inhibitory to the detrusor muscle and motor nerves to the internal sphincter.

THE URETHRA

This tube extends from the bladder to the vestibule — a distance in the normal non-pregnant adult female of about 5 cm. It penetrates the urinogenital diaphragm. The vagina is closely related to it posteriorly and the urethra is closely bound to the vagina in its lower two-thirds; the upper part is loose and held only by loose connective tissue. The urethra is a very distensible organ which has muscular, submucous and mucous layers; the smooth muscle is made up of an outer circular and inner longitudinal layer. In its lower part there is a ring of striated muscle fibres, the sphincter urethrae. The submucosa is remarkable in that it contains numerous venous channels surrounded by loose elastic connective tissue. The mucous membrane itself is thrown into a series of longitudinal folds with an especially prominent one posteriorly.

The epithelium is stratified and columnar in the middle third of the urethra, merging with bladder epithelium upwards and with the stratified squamous non-keratinized epithelium of the vestibule inferiorly. There are numerous small and a pair of large periurethral glands that drain via short ducts into its lumen.

The blood supply of the main part of the urethra is from branches of the vaginal vessels and the upper part is supplied by terminations of the vesicle arteries. The venous plexuses have a corresponding drainage, either to the vesicle veins or to the venous plexuses of the vulva.

The urethral sphincter has inner longitudinal and outer circular smooth muscle layers around the urethra and some striated paraurethral muscle. It is normally closed except during micturition when the inner longitudinal muscle contracts, shortening the urethra and therefore increasing the bore of its lumen.

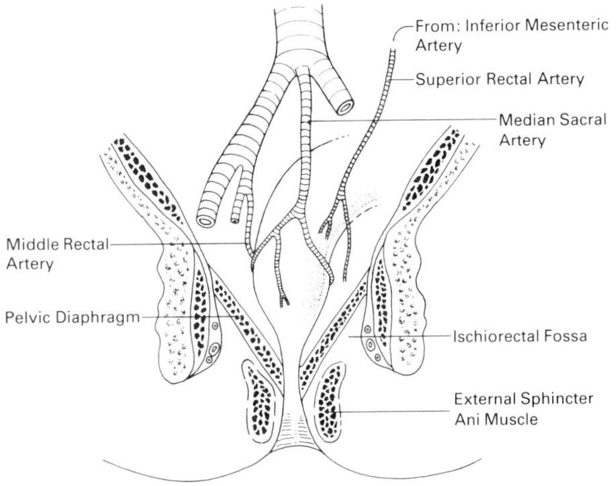

Fig. 2.14 The rectum has a rich anastomotic blood supply, from the median sacral, the internal iliac and the inferior mesenteric arteries and this arrangement is reflected in its venous drainage.

The external urinary sphincter is located between the layers of the urinogenital diaphragm. It is made up of striated muscle innervated by the pudendal nerve. It can stop the voluntary urinary stream.

The lymph drainage is either to inguinal nodes or to the internal and external iliac nodes. The nerve supply is autonomic from the pelvic and hypogastric plexuses.

THE RECTUM

The rectum — despite its name — is anything but straight. It curves to follow the anterior curve of the sacrum and also deviates towards the left in its middle part, whereas the upper and lower thirds lie in the midline. The rectum begins at the level of the third segment of the sacrum and extends as far as the perineal body, where it becomes the anal canal. The rectum has no mesentery but its upper third has pelvic peritoneum on its anterior and lateral surfaces, the middle third only on its anterior surface and the lowest third has no contact with the peritoneum.

Unlike the large intestine, the external layer of longitudinal muscle is complete over the surface of the rectum. Internally the junctions between the curves of the rectum are marked by horizontal folds, the valves of Houston. These folds contain circular muscle of the gut.

Three arteries contribute to the blood supply of the rectum. The principal supply is from the inferior mesenteric artery via the superior rectal branch which supplies the mucous membrane of the organ as far as the rectoanal junction. At the beginning of the rectum the superior rectal arteries divide into a left and right branch. The right branch soon divides into anterior and posterior branches (Fig. 2.14). The venous return mimics the arterial supply but there are considerable anastomoses between the vessels. The

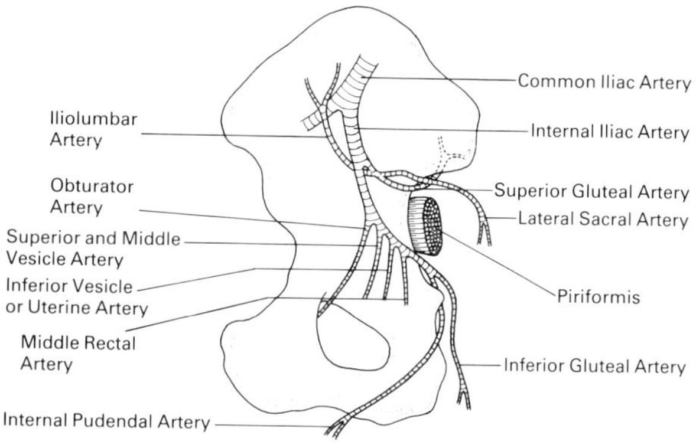

Fig. 2.15 The blood supply to the pelvic viscera is derived in the main from the internal iliac artery.

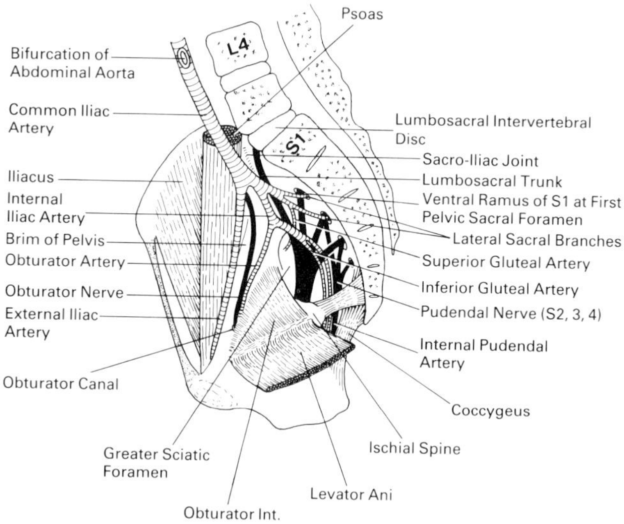

Fig. 2.16 Pelvic musculature. Muscles leave the pelvis either above the superior ramus of the pubis or through the greater or lesser sciatic foramina. Nerves and vessels also leave via the obturator foramen.

submucous plexus of veins communicates with the venous plexus at the base of the broad ligament. This venous plexus is the site both of haemorrhoidal dilation and of porto-systemic anastomosis.

Anorectal lymphatic drainage

The rectosigmoid and upper rectum drain via the mesentery to the inferior mesenteric group of nodes. The middle and lower part of the rectum drains both to the mesenteric group and to the internal iliac nodes. The anal canal below the levator ani muscle drains across the thigh to the inguinal and gluteal nodes.

The rectum has an autonomic nerve supply which is sympathetic directly from the pelvic plexus and parasympathetic via S2 and S3 and the nervi erigentes.

BLOOD VESSELS OF THE PELVIS

The pelvic contents and walls are supplied by branches of the internal iliac artery and are drained to the internal iliac veins. The vessels lie with the parietal pelvic fascia and only those branches that leave the pelvis pierce this membranous structure. The obturator vessels leave the obturator foramen via the obturator canal, which is a hole in this fascia. The internal iliac artery divides into a large anterior branch and a smaller posterior branch, the anterior branch supplying the pelvic viscera (Fig. 2.15).

The venous drainage is via the internal iliac veins to the inferior vena cava, but there are anastomoses through the superior rectal and inferior mesenteric veins to the portal system. There is also a drainage passage of the internal vertebral plexus via the lateral sacral veins to the internal iliac veins, the flow in which can be reversed by raised intra-abdominal pressure. This may be a potential route of spread of pelvic inflammatory and malignant disease.

THE NERVES OF THE PELVIS

Besides nerves of passage such as the obturator nerve, the nerves whose function lie with the pelvis are branches of the sacral plexus and the pelvic autonomic system. The sacral plexus is a broad structure formed by the fusion of nerves from L4 to S4 and lies lateral to the anterior sacral foramina. It lies upon the piriformis muscle and is covered anteriorly by the parietal pelvic fascia (Fig. 2.16).

The parasympathetic nerves travel with some branches of this plexus and arise by several rootlets from the anterior surfaces of S2, S3 and sometimes S4. They are called the nervi erigentes.

The pudendal nerve which is sensory to pudenda arises from S2, S3 and S4; it then passes backwards between the piriformis and coccygeus to round the sacrospinous ligament and enter the ischiorectal fossa. The perineal branch of S4 passes between the coccygeus and iliococcygeus to be distributed to the external anal sphincter and the perianal skin.

The pelvic autonomic plexus lies on the side wall of the pelvis lateral to the rectum. The sympathetic fibres are derived from the hypogastric plexus as well as a contribution from the upper sacral ganglia of the sympathetic trunk. The plexus is ganglionated. About half of the fibres in the hypogastric plexus are preganglionic and synapse in these ganglia; the rest are post-ganglionic and do not synapse. The parasympathetic fibres of the nervi erigentes do not synapse here but in the walls of the viscera.

The autonomic system is organized so that the sympathetic fibres are vasoconstrictor and the parasympathetic fibres are motor to the smooth muscle of the bladder and gut, and secretomotor to the gut glands. The sympathetic fibres are motor to the bladder and anal canal sphincters as well as to the smooth muscle of the seminal vesicles in the male.

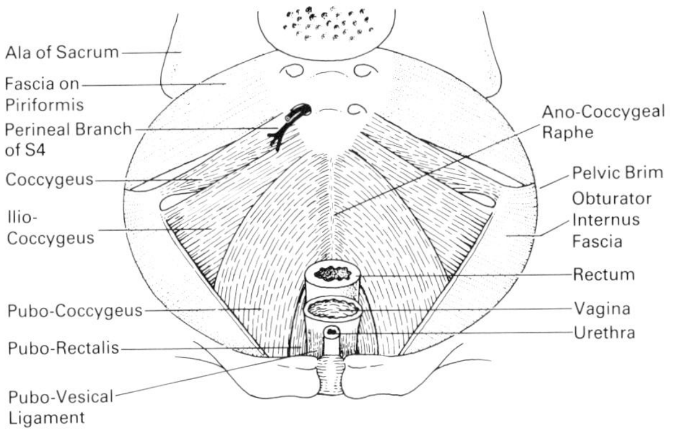

Fig. 2.17 The urogenital diaphragm. The floor of the pelvis slopes steeply forwards and plays an important role in continence and childbirth.

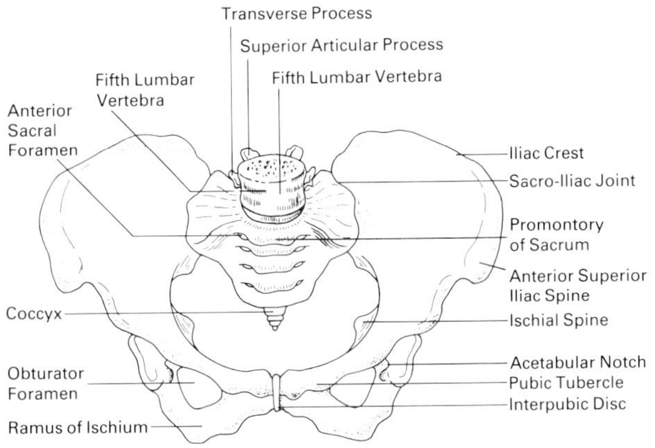

Fig. 2.18 The bony pelvis. The bones both enclose the birth canal and provide support for the body on the legs. There are notable sexual differences between the male and female bony pelvis.

The course of pain and sensory fibres is complex and not fully understood. Most pain fibres travel with the sympathetic system, especially those from the gut and the gonads. However, pain fibres from the bladder and rectum as well as those conveying the sensation of distension probably travel in the nervi erigentes. Pain fibres from the cervix also follow this course, but those from the body of the uterus travel mainly in the hypogastric nerves, especially to thoracic 11 and 12.

THE PELVIC CAVITY

The pelvic cavity is a part of the abdominal cavity surrounded by the bony pelvis. It is bound inferiorly by the urogenital diaphragm separating the pelvis from the perineum. In the female the pelvis contains the organs of reproduction as well as the bladder and the terminal portion of the alimentary canal.

The urogenital diaphragm and perineum are penetrated in the midline by three tubes. From before backwards, they are the urethra, the vagina and the anal canal. The urethra and vagina are surrounded by a series of structures which together constitute the vulva (Fig. 2.17).

The bony pelvis surrounds a cavity shaped like a pudding basin lying on its side, such that the anterior superior iliac spine and the pubic symphysis are in the same vertical plane. The brim of the cavity is made from the promontory and alae of the sacrum, the arcuate line of the ilium, the pectineal line of the pubis; the pubic crest lies at about 30° to this plane. The upper border of the symphysis pubis, the spine of the ischium and the tip of the coccyx define a plane that can just be reached by the tip of a finger placed in the vagina (Fig. 2.18).

The pelvic cavity aspect of the bony pelvis is mostly covered by muscles—superiorly by the psoas and iliacus muscles, below the pelvic brim by the obturator internus muscle and posteriorly by pyriformis and coccygeus muscles arising from the anterior surface of the sacrum (see Fig.

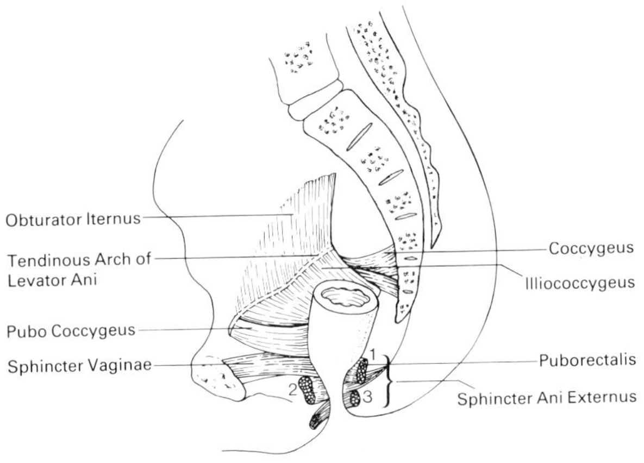

Fig. 2.19 Muscles of the pelvic floor. The slings of muscle that surround and separate the major body effluents have an important role as sphincters.

2.16). The fascia covering these muscles is a tough membrane attached to the periosteum at the edges. The bare bone of the pelvic wall is not covered by fascia.

The pelvic floor is a V-shaped gutter of muscles which is higher posteriorly than anteriorly to produce the base of the V, formed by the midline raphe of these muscles. The raphe and muscles are penetrated by the urethra, vagina and rectum. The direction of the muscle fibres forming the anterior part of this diaphragm of muscles is backwards and medially, such that they form a series of slings encircling the posterior aspects of the penetrating structures and thus have a potential sphincter-like action (Fig. 2.19). There is a hole anteriorly between the muscles arising from the posterior aspect of the pubis. This gap is closed by the pubovesical ligaments, between which passes the deep dorsal vein of the clitoris.

The muscles arise peripherally from a continuous line starting at the spine of ischium, which proceeds as the white line over the fascia covering the medial aspect of

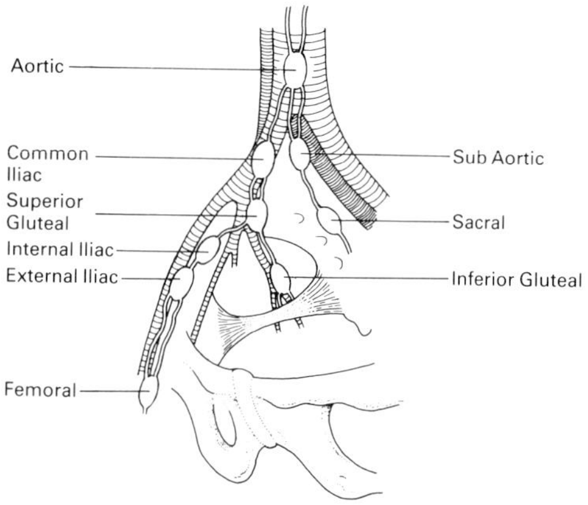

Fig. 2.20 The lymphatic drainage of the pelvis and associated structures.

obturator internus, and from the body of the pubis. The midline raphe extends from the coccyx forwards.

The function of this gutter during labour is to deflect anteriorly the first part of the baby which comes into contact with it and later to rotate the head or buttocks so that the shortest diameter lies transversely at the brim of the bony pelvis. The muscles of the pelvic diaphragm are supplied in the main by the perineal branch of S4, and anteriorly by branches from the inferior rectal and perineal nerves.

The function of these muscles is to respond to changes in intra-abdominal pressure, assisting in maintaining faecal and urinary continence. In micturition and defecation the relevant portion of the muscle is relaxed, but the remainder maintains its tone to prevent prolapse of the pelvic organs. Most of the weight of the gut is borne by the superior aspect of the pubic symphysis.

The fascia of the pelvic floor is little more than loose areolar tissue. Separating the pelvic floor from the pelvic peritoneum are the pelvic viscera. The space around these organs provides room for distension of the bladder and rectum.

THE LYMPHATIC DRAINAGE OF THE PELVIS

The lymphatics in the pelvis originate as tiny lymphocapillaries that form complex nets of interconnecting vessels. They are without valves and their walls consist solely of endothelial plates. These networks join to form lymphatic vessels with smooth muscle in their walls and have valves. Eventually lymph vessels lead to lymph nodes. The lymphatics of the perineum, together with those of the lower limb, go to a collection of lymph nodes below the inguinal ligament. Some of the deeper lymphatics of the buttock follow the superior and inferior gluteal arteries and penetrate into the pelvic cavity (Fig. 2.20). In general these lymphatics are found between the membranous layer of superficial fascia and the deep fascia. The nodes are classified into three major groups—superficial inguinal, deep inguinal and pelvic lymph nodes.

Superficial drainage

The superficial inguinal nodes radiate outwards from the saphenous opening, in the form of the letter T. The stem of the T is made by the group associated with the terminal part of the great saphenous vein, while the arms of the T follow the inguinal ligament. The vulva drains initially to the medial horizontal group. In most cases the vulval lymphatics do not cross the labia crural fold, but reach the nodes by traversing the mons pubis.

From the posterior part of the vulva and the perineum the lymphatics drain into the thigh and the lower lymph nodes, together with those from the lower limb. The deep inguinal nodes lie in relation to the junction between the femoral vein and the great saphenous vein after it has passed through the deep fascia at the saphenous opening. It is no longer believed that all efferents from the inguinal region pass through this group.

Internal iliac system

The pelvic lymph nodes are usually related to the major blood vessels and are named after them. The internal iliac vessels drain the pelvic contents. Unfortunately there are several common variations amongst the veins, and the distribution of the lymphatics may vary with the veins. Usually the internal iliac vein is formed from an anterior, a middle and a posterior branch. Variations include how the vessels join with each other and the territories they drain. There is frequently variation between the two sides of the pelvis. Usually nodes are named external iliac when related to the external iliac artery. All nodes inferior to the external iliac vein and anterior to the internal iliac artery are named inter-iliac. Lymph nodes behind the anterior division of the internal iliac artery are called the internal iliac group. Since there are three main arteries entering the pelvis—one paired, the common iliac arteries, and two single, the median sacral and the superior haemorrhoidal arteries—there are three possible routes for lymphatic drainage.

The external iliac nodes

This system is much confused, as several surgical and anatomical descriptions describe the same structures, giving them differing names. Basically there is a system of chains of nodes and vessels surrounding the external iliac artery and vein with a few related nodes associated with them. Although these lymph chains are interconnected it is usual to describe them as anterior–superior, intermediate and posteromedial (Fig. 2.21).

The associated glands are those within the inguinal canal, those associated with the inferior epigastric artery and those associated with the first part of the obturator artery. They are named after their associated vessels. It is the posteromedial group that is the important lymphatic relay for the genital tract and the cervix.

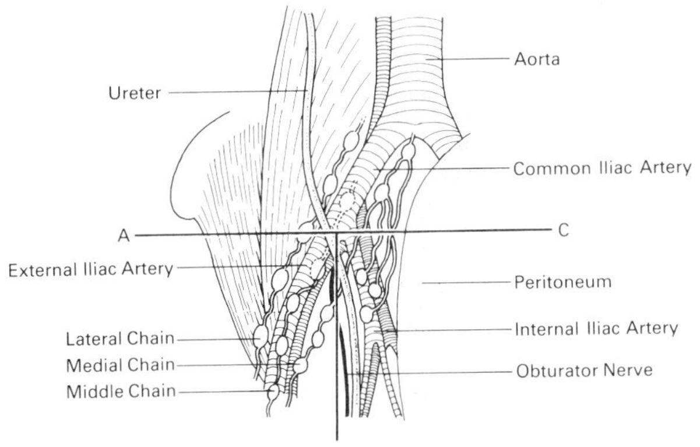

Fig. 2.21 The iliac group of lymph nodes and their related structures. The complex system of interconnections between individual nodes probably precludes any functional significance being correlated with concise anatomical localization.

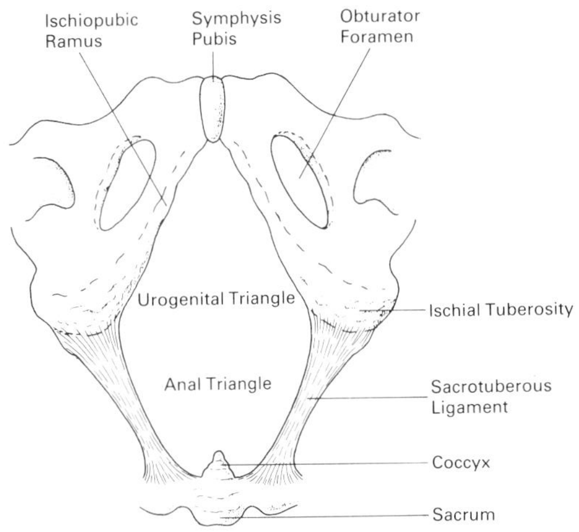

Fig. 2.22 Boundaries of the pelvic outlet. By the time the fetal head reaches this region it has usually been orientated by the pelvic diaphragm such that its long axis is antero-posterior and the face faces posteriorly.

The internal iliac nodes, like the arterial supply, are in two main divisions: those from the pelvic viscera and those from the buttock and leg. Since the viscera within the pelvis are separated from the pelvic wall, the peripheral lymph nodes are associated with the walls of the organs rather than with the pelvic wall. Both the internal and external iliac system of lymphatics drain to the common iliac nodes. They are most easily visualized as a continuation of the three chains of nodes surrounding the external iliac vessels. These chains continue to the bifurcation of the aorta where they anastomose freely with each other and with those from the other side. The symmetry of the two sides is disturbed by the left common iliac vein.

Besides this system there are a few nodes associated with the median sacral artery, and with the superior haemorrhoidal artery. The median sacral vessels join the common iliac lymphatics at the bifurcation of the aorta.

It is important to realize that this classification in terms of adjacent vessels gives very little clue to the drainage of these nodes; structures like the urethra and vagina straddle the territories of several vessels. Even structures such as the bladder and uterus, which are supplied by the visceral division of the internal iliac artery, drain to nodes associated with other vessels. Indeed the ovary can drain almost anywhere — to the renal region via the gonadal vessels; to the iliac nodes via the uterine vessels; to the adjacent pelvic wall, and even to the inguinal nodes via the round ligament.

Nevertheless it is a reasonable generalization that the lymphatic drainage of the pelvic viscera follows the vessels that supply them. The posteromedial group of the external iliac lymph nodes is functionally more related to the visceral branches of the internal iliac artery than to external iliac artery territory.

THE BONY PELVIS

The pelvis is constructed from the two innominate bones and posteriorly, the sacrum, wedged like a keystone between them. Each innominate bone is divided into three parts — an ilium, an ischium and a pubis. The innominate bones come together anteriorly at the symphysis pubis.

The pelvic brim comprises the promontory of the sacrum, the alae of the sacrum, the arcuate line of the ilium, the iliopubic eminence, the pectineal line and the pubic crest, which, together with the upper surface of the symphysis pubis, separates the false pelvis above from the true pelvis below. The outlet of the pelvis is diamond-shaped, bound in front by the lower surface of the symphysis pubis and the ischiopubic ramus, laterally by the ischial tuberosities, posterolaterally by the sacrotuberous ligament and posteriorly by the tip of the coccyx (Fig. 2.22).

The planes of the anterior urogenital triangle and the posterior anal triangle lie at about 150° to each other.

The sacrum is formed by the fusion of the five sacral vertebrae. This classical condition is frequently changed, either by the fusion of the fifth lumbar vertebra to the sacrum, or when the fifth sacral is separated and fused with the coccyx. The sacral hiatus — the inferior opening of the sacral canal — is very variable in size but the two bony prominences on either side of the aperture are usually felt easily — a fact which is of importance when performing caudal anaesthesia. The sacrum joins the innominate bones at the sacroiliac joints.

The major obstetric interest in the bony pelvis is that it is not distensible; only minor degrees of movement are possible at the pubic and sacroiliac joints. Its dimensions are therefore critical during childbirth. Furthermore the diameters of the true pelvis vary in different parts of the pelvis. The pelvic cavity is widest transversely at the inlet and anteroposteriorly at the outlet. Most attempts to classify the shape of the pelvis fail because there appears to be a continuous series of pelves extending from the classical gynaecoid, the anteroposteriorly flattened and platypelloid. Although it is possible to list the salient features of the classical female

Table 2.1 Comparison between the male and female pelvis

	Male	Female
Subpubic angle	45–55°	70–80°
Ratio of width of acetabulum to distance from anterior edge to the symphysis pubis	<1	1
Sciatic notch	75°	50°
Ischial spines point	Inwards	Downwards
Shape of obturator foramen	Triangular	Oval
Sacral index: $\frac{\text{width}}{\text{height}} \times 100$	115	105
Ratio of ala of sacrum to width of body of S1	1	<1
Cavity	Short segment of wide cone	Long segment of narrow cone

pelvis and contrast them with the male pelvis, in a large series the differences are by no means always apparent. The commonly quoted distinctive features of the female pelvis are given in Table 2.1.

The pelvic joints

The sacroiliac joint is a synovial joint between the articular surfaces of the ilium and the sacrum. The facets have interlocking facies and, at least posterosuperiorly, the two bones are united by fibrous tissue typical of a fibrous joint, especially in later life. Indeed, in old age bony fusion may take place. The joint has considerable support from its associated ligaments. The strong posterior superior interosseous ligaments and the posterior sacroiliac ligaments prevent the weight of the body pushing the sacrum downwards and forwards. The sacrotuberous and sacrospinous ligaments also contribute to this stability.

The symphysis pubis is a secondary cartilaginous joint. The adjoining surfaces of the pubic bones are covered with hyaline cartilage, between which there is a disc of fibrocartilage joining the two bones. The joint is further strengthened by ligaments superiorly, and inferiorly by direct fibres, but anteriorly and obliquely by interdigitating fibres that interlace with fibres from the rectus abdominis and external oblique muscles.

There is an increase in movements of these joints, especially during the third trimester of pregnancy. The net result is to increase the sagittal diameter of the outlet and true conjugate. Studies of these movements suggest that as far as pelvic capacity is concerned, squatting during uterine contractions and lying recumbent between them may provide a helpful routine during labour.

CONCLUSIONS

The anatomy of the female urogenital tract is highly dynamic and undergoes vast changes at all stages of the reproductive cycle, from the vast increase in size of the labia minora during copulation to the recovery of the prepregnant uterine size after parturition. The tract is under the control of multiple influences—psychogenic, emotional, sensory, autonomic and hormonal—but seems capable of fulfilling its role in reproduction in the absence of many of them. Its design faults, if they may be considered as such, are the narrowness of the bony pelvic canal and the great vulnerability of the narrow lumen of the Fallopian tubes.

Acknowledgements

I have borrowed heavily from the standard anatomical textbooks and from the advice of my colleagues. The standard diagrams are in such a highly evolved state that it would be a research project in itself to trace them to their origins. I have done little except tinker with their details. To these unknown original artists and ancestors I offer my sincere thanks.

3

Margaret C. P. Rees and David H. Barlow

Ovulation and the endometrial cycle

INTRODUCTION

In mammals two types of cycles have been described. These are the oestrus and menstrual cycles; the latter are confined to humans and subhuman primates. Studies on menstruation were initiated in 1793 when Davidge speculated that ovaries are necessary for the process of menstruation. However, little work was undertaken until the late 19th century when the precise relation of the human menstrual cycle to the oestrous cycle of non-menstruating animals was elucidated. Before then it was thought that the menstrual flow in humans was comparable to the oestrous phase of the animal cycle, since both are conspicuous events in mammalian reproductive cycles. This notion was soon abandoned as a result of work on subhuman primates, notably when Heape (1897) reported that ovulation is not necessarily coincident with menstruation. Furthermore, he emphasized the similarities in the reproductive cycle between monkeys and humans and noted that ovulation does not invariably occur during each menstrual cycle. Consequently our scientific understanding of the physiological mechanisms involved in the ovarian and endometrial cycles is based on animal as well as human data.

Studies on the endometrial cycle have been performed since the 19th century but scientific examination of the ovarian cycle was not commenced until the middle of the 20th century when hormone assays were developed. The rapid acceleration in our knowledge of ovarian function over the past two decades has resulted from the introduction of new techniques, of which the most significant have been radioimmunoassay, laparoscopy, ovarian ultrasound and in vitro fertilization. Ovulation and the endometrial cycle will be discussed as individual topics in two separate sections.

OVULATION

The ovarian follicle

Although some degree of follicular development may be observed in the ovary during childhood (Gougeon & Lefevre 1983), the full span of follicular development is only possible following maturation of the hypothalamic pituitary axis at puberty, at which time the ovary contains approximately 500 000 primordial follicles. These have the basic immature follicular form consisting of the oocyte, arrested in meiotic prophase, surrounded by a single layer of granulosa cells and encircled by a distinct membrane, the basal lamina, which separates the follicle from the adjacent stromal cells. There is communication between the granulosa cells and the oocyte via cytoplasmic processes which form a union with the oocyte plasma membrane, thus providing a route for the passage of nutrients to the oocyte (Brower & Schultz 1982) and possibly facilitating inhibition of oocyte maturation.

Once embarked on the process of maturation a follicle will either mature to ovulation or become atretic. Before the menarche all follicles which start to develop undergo atresia; thus, between birth and the menarche follicular atresia removes up to 90% of the initial complement of primordial follicles (Baker 1963; Fig. 3.1). Even when ovulation is established after the menarche the vast majority of the remaining follicles will eventually become atretic (Tsafriri & Braw 1984).

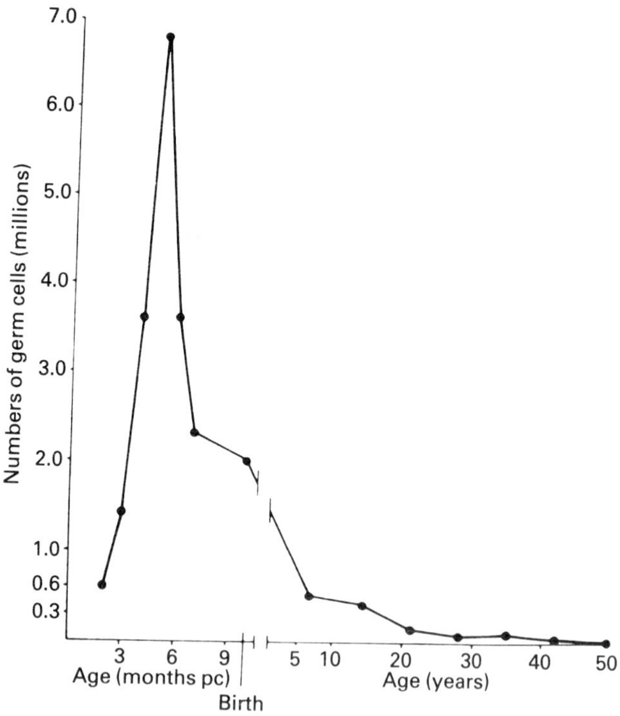

Fig. 3.1 Fluctuations in the total population of germ cells in the human ovary during reproductive life. From Baker (1963).

Follicular structural development

The sequence of follicular development is shown in Figure 3.2. The first phase of follicular development is the transition to a primary follicle. The granulosa layer proliferates to become a multiple cell layer surrounding an enlarged oocyte and mucopolysaccharide is secreted to surround the oocyte and form the zona pellucidum. This has a fenestrated structure which permits continued communication between granulosa cells and the oocyte. Stromal fibroblasts adjacent to the follicle become arranged in concentric layers to form the theca cell layer.

Continued granulosa cell proliferation results in an enlarged follicle in which the granulosa cells are the largest component. Within the granulosa layers follicular fluid collects, then coalesces to form the antrum, the presence of which marks the transition to the Graafian follicle. As the antrum enlarges the granulosa cells adjacent to the basal lamina become separated from those adjacent to the oocyte. These two complements of granulosa cells become the membranum granulosum and the cumulus oophorous respectively. Antrum formation in the granulosa layer is accompanied by the formation of the theca interna in which thecal fibroblasts accumulate cytoplasm and exhibit cellular organelles characteristic of steroid-secreting cells, and theca layer blood vessels and lymphatics proliferate. The less closely associated theca cells retain their fibroblast appearance to become the theca externa.

The maturing follicle is prepared for ovulation by mechanisms which will be discussed below and the oocyte and cumulus oophorus are released. Ovulation is accompanied by morphological changes in the theca and granulosa layers. The cells exhibit cytoplasmic lipid droplets, extensive smooth endoplasmic reticulum and free ribosomes. Angiogenesis leads to penetration of the basal lamina and vascularization of the granulosa, giving an intermingling of theca lutein cells, new blood vessels and granulosa lutein cells. The corpus luteum thus formed will function for 10–12 days supported by the luteotrophic gonadotrophin environment but if pregnancy has not occurred luteolysis is inevitable with degeneration of the structure.

Follicular atresia

Follicles which do not mature to ovulation exhibit major changes in all follicular components as atresia develops. There is degeneration of the oocyte, eventual replacement of granulosa cells by fibroblasts and return of the theca cells to the stromal fibroblast-like pattern. The processes of atresia vary with the different stages of follicular development when atresia commences, and have been described in detail (Ingram 1962, Guraya 1985).

DYNAMICS OF FOLLICULAR DEVELOPMENT

The phases of follicular development may be summarized as the recruitment of early antral follicles, selection of a dominant follicle, followed by preparation for ovulation. The transition from primordial follicle to an early antral follicle which is capable of being recruited into the active growth phase takes about 85 days. This early antral follicle contains approximately 1 000 000 granulosa cells and measures 2–5 mm in diameter (McNatty et al 1983). The production of follicles which may develop further is a continuous process but subsequent recruitment is dependent on exposure to the appropriate gonadotrophin stimulus.

Ultrasonic studies reveal that follicular enlargement proceeds at 1–3 mm (diameter) per day (Bomsel-Helmreich 1985) to attain a mean diameter of approximately 20 ± 3 mm (Hackeloer et al 1979, Marinho et al 1982) at the luteinizing hormone surge. The range of follicle size at this stage is wide, varying from a minimum of 13 mm (Marinho et al 1982) to a maximum of 29 mm (O'Herlihy et al 1980). During the phase of active follicular growth the dominant follicle may be observed to be accompanied by a cohort of other follicles which do not usually ovulate and do not become larger than 16 mm (O'Herlihy et al 1980). Kerin et al (1981) noted at least three developing follicles in 80% of cycles studied and observed that the second-order follicle on the same ovary as the dominant follicle was larger than that on the other ovary, suggesting an influence of the dominant follicle on the response of surrounding follicles.

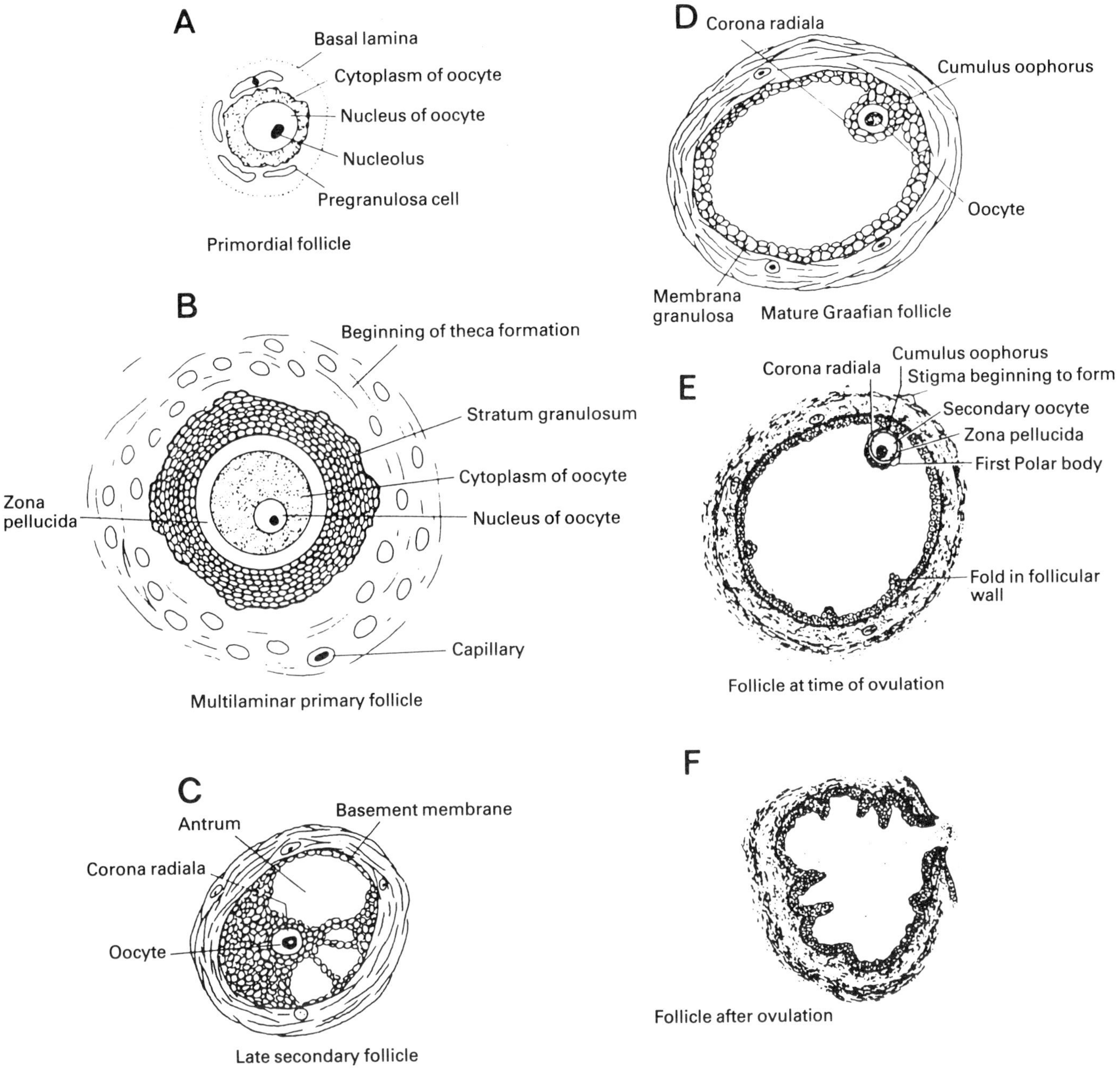

Fig. 3.2 Sequence of follicular development. From Martin (1985).

THE PITUITARY–FOLLICULAR INTERACTION

Gonadotrophin stimulus

An appropriate gonadotrophin stimulus is essential for full follicular development and the pattern of this stimulus is governed to a large extent by ovarian follicular feedback. In order for pituitary gonadotrope cells to produce follicle-stimulating hormone (FSH) and luteinizing hormone (LH) it is essential for these cells to be exposed to pulses of hypothalamic gonadotrophin-releasing hormone (GnRH). The demonstration that in primates it is possible to block the passage of hypothalamic GnRH to the pituitary yet reproduce the events of the cycle, including the LH surge and ovulation, by providing an unvarying GnRH pulsatile stimulus (Knobil et al 1980) emphasizes ovarian feedback as a major determinant of the changes in gonadotrophin secretion and that much of this feedback acts at the level of the pituitary. This work does not negate the evidence that ovarian influences and neurotransmitters, particularly opiates, affect hypothalamic GnRH output, the level of which may be a further modulating influence on the secretion of FSH and LH. Discussion of this extensive field lies outside the scope of this chapter.

Throughout the cycle ovarian follicles are exposed to pulses of FSH and LH and, with the exception of the mid-cycle surge, the FSH levels exceed those of LH. In the follicular phase FSH secretion is influenced by both oestrogen-negative feedback and inhibin. After ovulation the combined negative feedback of oestradiol and progesterone results in a low level of gonadotrophin output in which pulse frequency and amplitude are reduced (Yen et al 1972). The events controlling the mid-cycle surge of gonadotrophins have yet to be fully determined but it is known that as the dominant follicle approaches ovulation the sustained high oestradiol levels produce an accumulation of LH at the gonadotrope cells and increase gonadotrope sensitivity to GnRH (Yen & Lein 1976). As the follicle approaches maturity there is a detectable rise in circulating progesterone and 17α-hydroxyprogesterone, closely associated with the start of the massive release of gonadotrophins (Hoff et al 1983) and which may further sensitize the gonadotrope cells to facilitate the LH surge (Chang & Jaffe 1978).

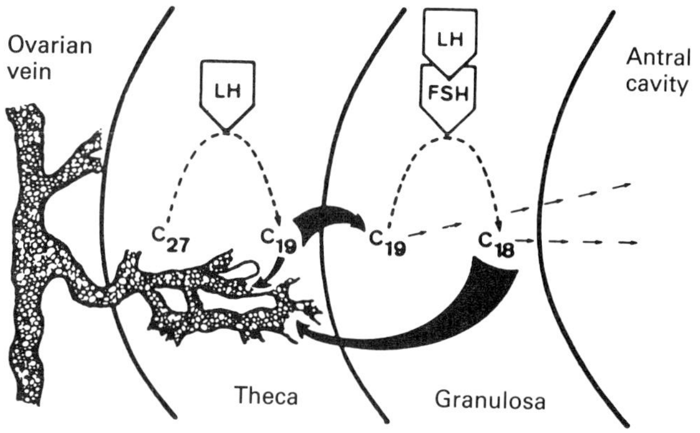

Fig. 3.3 Current concept of gonadotrophin-controlled cellular functions which co-ordinate follicular oestrogen biosynthesis. Androgen (C_{19}) is biosynthesized from cholesterol (C_7) in the vascularized theca. Thecal androgen serves as aromatase substrate in the granulosa to produce oestrogen (C_{18}) which diffuses into blood stream and antral cavity. From Hillier (1985).

Prolactin

The role of prolactin in the physiology of human follicular maturation remains ill defined but it is well established that hyperprolactinaemic states result in failure of follicular development. Prolactin can be identified in follicular fluid throughout the follicular phase but is found in highest concentrations in small follicles (McNatty et al 1975a). One role may be to prevent biosynthesis of progesterone by granulosa cells until a mature follicle has developed, since prolactin inhibits progesterone production by cultured granulosa cells at concentrations found in small follicles but not at concentrations found in large follicles (McNatty & Sawers 1975).

FOLLICULAR ENDOCRINE FUNCTION

Steroidogenesis

Sex steroids are the major product of the developing follicle and the subsequent corpus luteum; the cyclic pattern of sex steroid secretion dominates circulating oestradiol and progesterone profiles. Baird & Fraser (1975) estimated that the dominant follicle is responsible for 90% of oestradiol output thus making possible follicular feedback on the gonadotrophin stimulus via the level of circulating oestradiol.

The mechanism whereby gonadotrophins interact with the follicular cells involves a classic hormone receptor system. Gonadotrophins interact with high-affinity membrane receptors specific for FSH or LH. Formation of the hormone receptor complex causes adenyl cyclase activation. This facilitates production of cyclic adenosine monophosphate (cAMP) which acts in turn as an intermediate messenger within the cell, one of its actions being enhancement of steroidogenesis via activation of calcium-dependent protein kinase.

Follicular steroidogenesis depends on the integrated function of the theca and granulosa cell compartments influenced by gonadotrophins (Fig. 3.3). The theca interna is a major site of biosynthesis of the androgens (C_{19}), androstenedione and testosterone; biosynthesis is regulated by LH acting via the theca cell membrane receptors (Tsang et al 1979). Thecal androgen synthesis involves both de novo biosynthesis from acetate or cholesterol or metabolism of C_{21} steroids (pregnenolone, progesterone) which may originate in the adjacent granulosa layer. Regulation by LH occurs at the rate-limiting 17-hydroxylase and $C_{17,20}$ lyase steps (Bogovich & Richards 1982).

In the granulosa cell layer the pathway for biosynthesis of C_{21} steroids is intact, as is the enzymic capacity (aromatase) to convert C_{19} androgens to oestrogens (C_{18}). However, 17-hydroxylase, $C_{17,20}$ lyase activity is deficient; thus significant amounts of C_{21} steroids cannot be converted to C_{19} androgens. The theca cells are thus the dominant androgen-producing component of the follicle and therefore small follicle antral fluid is predominantly androgenic. Transformation of the follicular fluid into a predominantly oestrogenic environment depends on the level of granulosa cell aromatase activity. The induction of aromatase to produce oestradiol therefore governs both the endocrine activity of the ovary and the paracrine role of oestrogen in promoting follicular maturation and preventing atresia.

Control of aromatase activity

This subject has been the focus of a considerable body of human and animal research, much of which relates to in vitro studies in culture systems. These limitations must be borne in mind when conclusions are drawn concerning human aromatase control and other aspects of ovarian follicular physiology, discussed below.

Gonadotrophins and oestrogen

The principal regulator of granulosa cell aromatase induction is FSH via the membrane receptor mechanism (Tsang et al 1980). As the dominant follicle matures LH receptors develop on granulosa cells influenced by FSH. Once the follicle has been FSH-primed LH will maintain aromatase activity (Wang et al 1981). The appearance of FSH receptors on granulosa cells is stimulated by oestrogen (Richards 1980) and oestrogen may also augment the FSH-mediated induction of granulosa LH receptors (Kessel et al 1985). These actions indicate an oestrogenic paracrine amplification of the responsiveness of the dominant follicle to gonadotrophins. FSH and oestrogen also stimulate granulosa cell proliferation, thus greatly increasing the number of cells producing oestradiol as well as the amount of oestradiol synthesis per cell (Rao et al 1978).

Other factors

The importance of granulosa cell aromatase in follicular function is demonstrated by the influences which apply fine control to its activity. The need for fine control possibly relates to dominant follicle selection mechanisms and to a need for close coupling between thecal androgen production and granulosa androgen aromatization (Hillier 1985). Factors, other than oestrogen, influencing FSH-stimulated aromatase activity include GnRH, follicular regulatory protein and somatomedins.

GnRH. It is likely that a GnRH-like peptide of ovarian origin participates in the paracrine control of the follicle. GnRH receptors occur on granulosa cells (Jones et al 1980) and in rat granulosa cell cultures GnRH treatment inhibits FSH-stimulated aromatase activity (Hseuh & Erickson 1979). Similar experiments reveal that GnRH treatment also suppresses LH receptor generation on granulosa cells.

Follicular regulatory protein (FRP). This protein (molecular weight 16 500) may represent an ovarian paracrine factor. Production appears to increase with follicular maturation in parallel with increasing inhibin activity (Di Zerega et al 1984), and in culture systems FRP inhibits FSH-induced aromatase activity (Di Zerega et al 1983).

Somatomedins. This family of peptides mediates the action of growth hormone on cell growth by acting via specific receptors which also have weak insulin affinity. Davroen & Hsueh (1984) demonstrated that supraphysiological insulin doses augment FSH-stimulated oestrogen production, possibly acting via somatomedin receptors. Subsequently somatomedin C administration has been shown to augment FSH-stimulated oestrogen production in cultured granulosa cells (Davroen et al 1985). Another peptide growth factor which may also potentiate FSH action is platelet-derived growth factor (Mondschien & Schomberg 1981). The complex chemistry of these peptides remains to be clarified. At present it is not clear whether their effects relate to blood-borne factors or ovarian products.

SELECTION OF A DOMINANT FOLLICLE

The interactions between feedback and controlling factors and FSH secretion and stimulation of follicular development have been described. These are the basis for the current understanding of dominant follicle selection, with the additional role of follicular inhibin.

Inhibin has been isolated from follicular extracts in many species and is produced by granulosa cells (Channing et al 1982). It is a peptide (molecular weight >70 000) which will suppress FSH production by rat pituitary cells in culture. Inhibin is produced in greatest amounts by the developing dominant follicle (Channing et al 1982) and human follicular inhibin and oestradiol levels are positively correlated (Marrs et al 1984).

When small antral follicles enter the recruitment phase of development at the end of the preceding luteal phase or early follicular phase, FSH stimulation is essential to promote granulosa cell differentiation and steroidogenesis. Influenced by FSH and follicular oestradiol, the leading follicles will develop the greatest granulosa cell FSH receptor content and those granulosa cells will gain LH receptors. By this stage of development these follicles can continue to mature when the circulating FSH level falls and additionally granulosa cell aromatase can now be stimulated by LH via the adenyl cyclase mechanism. Less mature follicles remain dependent on circulating FSH and cannot respond to LH. As the dominant follicle matures its oestradiol production reduces circulating FSH by negative feedback at the pituitary and higher centres and its output of inhibin reinforces this effect. The less mature follicles are deprived of the FSH stimulus necessary to maintain aromatase-mediated oestradiol production; they become predominantly androgenic as a result of continuing LH stimulation and undergo atresia.

PERIOVULATORY EVENTS

As the dominant follicle approaches ovulation its maturation involves integration of several processes necessary for successful ovulation and luteal function. These are:

1. Ovum maturation.
2. Follicular rupture and ovum expulsion.
3. Granulosa cell luteinization and corpus luteum formation.

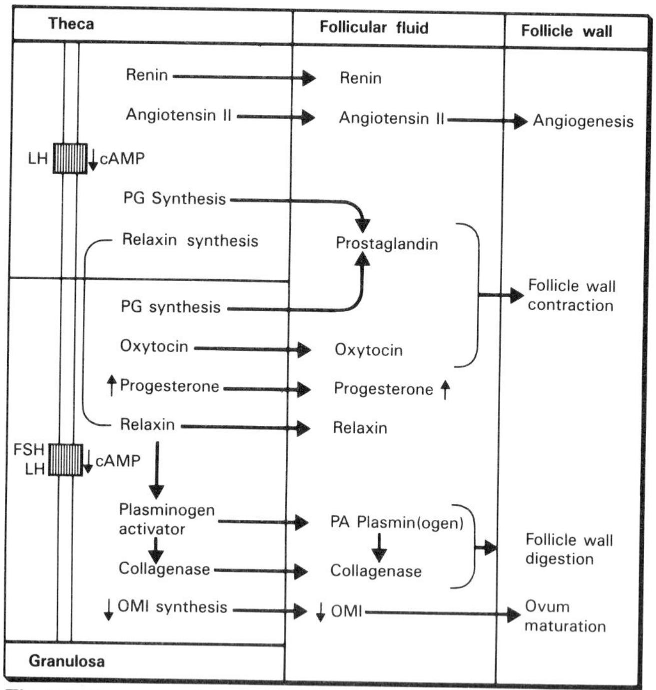

Fig. 3.4 Summary of the periovulatory follicular events resulting in ovum maturation, follicle rupture and angiogenesis.

The interactions involved in these processes are summarized in Figure 3.4.

Ovum maturation

From the time of enclosure of oocytes in primordial follicles during fetal life until the start of the LH surge preceding ovulation, the oocyte remains arrested at the dictyate stage of the first meiotic division. Soon after the start of the LH surge germinal vesicle breakdown occurs and the oocyte completes the first maturation division and ovulation occurs at the metaphase II stage in second meiotic arrest to await sperm penetration.

The prevention of oocyte maturation over the decade before ovulation is mediated by a factor or factors originating in granulosa cells. Removal of the oocyte from a maturing follicle will result in spontaneous resumption of meiosis in culture (Pincus and Enzmann 1935, Schultz 1974) but addition of granulosa cells or follicular fluid to the culture system prevents the resumption of meiosis (Tsafriri & Channing 1975). The granulosa cell-derived factor, oocyte maturation inhibitor (OMI), has been characterized as having a molecular weight below 2000 and exhibits characteristic features of a peptide (Stone et al 1978). However, Downs et al (1985) have suggested that the principal low molecular weight OMI in porcine follicular fluid is hypoxanthine. It is possible that further purification and characterization of OMI will reveal it to be a group of factors.

An intact cumulus appears to be necessary for the action of OMI, suggesting that cumulus cells may mediate OMI activity (Hillensjo et al 1979). It is also apparent that cAMP acts synergistically with OMI in some models to potentiate its effect on the in vitro cumulus oocyte complex (Eppig et al 1983).

LH appears to be the principal trigger to resumption of meiosis (Tsafriri et al 1982) and the presence of LH receptors on cumulus cells but not on the oocyte (Amsterdam & Tsafriri 1979) suggests that the LH effect may be mediated by cumulus cells, perhaps interfering with cumulus–oocyte communication (Gilula et al 1978). Current evidence relating to OMI activity in different animal models has yielded conflicting results; thus, a clear presentation of the mechanisms involving LH, cAMP and cumulus–oocyte communication is not yet possible.

Follicular rupture and ovum expulsion

Espey (1980) has drawn attention to the similarity between the processes of ovulation and the inflammatory response: both involve release of proteolytic enzymes and prostaglandins, hyperaemia, increased capillary permeability and fibroblast proliferation. There is evidence to suggest that prostaglandins E_2 (PGE_2) and $F_{2\alpha}$ ($PGF_{2\alpha}$), relaxin and oxytocin participate in the paracrine control of these events, which remain only partially understood.

Prostaglandins

The structure and biosynthesis of these substances are described below, in the section on the endometrial cycle. The considerable stimulation of PGE_2 and $PGF_{2\alpha}$ biosynthesis in the preovulatory follicle results from gonadotrophin stimulation of the theca and granulosa layers (Plunkett et al 1975) to give cAMP-dependent protein kinase augmentation of cyclo-oxygenase activity.

Studies of the effect of prostaglandin action on the ovary using inhibitors of prostaglandin synthesis or immunological blockage of prostaglandin action suggest that the periovulatory endocrine changes and oocyte maturation do not significantly involve prostaglandin action. The principal effects of the increased prostaglandin activity are on proteolytic enzyme activation (predominantly PGE_2) and smooth muscle contraction (predominantly $PGF_{2\alpha}$). Preovulatory follicles have more recently been shown to contain significant quantities of prostacyclin (Koos & Clark 1982) which may mediate some of the periovulatory vascular changes.

Oxytocin

Although the best evidence for an intraovarian role for a peptide showing oxytocin immunoreactivity relates to luteal cells, oxytocin-like material has also been reported in preovulatory human follicles (Khan-Dawood & Dawood 1983). It is possible that during ovulation this oxytocin-like peptide and $PGF_{2\alpha}$ act synergistically to stimulate follicular wall smooth muscles.

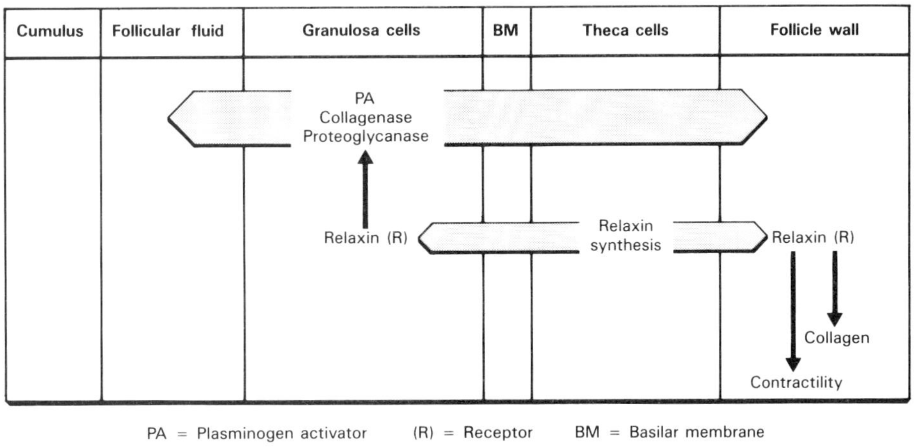

Fig. 3.5 Suggested role for relaxin in ovarian paracrine control. From Bagnell et al (1984).

Relaxin

This two-chain polypeptide, of estimated approximate molecular weight of 6000, exhibits considerable interspecies heterogeneity. It bears some structural resemblance to insulin and the somatomedins and its principal role appears to be in the regulation of collagen physiology, particularly in pregnancy. There is evidence to suggest that relaxin acts as a paracrine regulator of the mechanisms leading to follicle wall rupture at ovulation. Relaxin has been identified in porcine follicular fluid (Bryant-Greenwood et al 1980) and can be identified in the granulosa cell layer (Yki-Jarvinen et al 1984) but the principal source appears to be the theca layer with increased production near to ovulation (Evans et al 1983), at least in the pig. The suggested role for relaxin is stimulation of release of the proteolytic enzymes, plasminogen activator, collagenase and proteoglycanase, by the granulosa cell layer (Too et al 1984; Fig. 3.5). It is not clear whether this paracrine action is restricted to the granulosa cell layer or if relaxin present in follicular fluid is active within that compartment.

Proteolytic enzymes

Formation of the raised hyperaemic stigma preceding follicle rupture is influenced by proteolytic digestion of the follicle wall and the action of histamine and prostaglandins in inducing local hyperaemia. Further subsequent digestion of the wall is determined by proteolytic enzyme activity, both in the follicle wall cells and in the follicular fluid compartment. Follicular fluid contains a variety of proteolytic enzyme activators and inhibitors; these activities are in balance but as ovulation approaches the balance is shifted to activation, principally by stimulation of plasminogen activator (PA) secretion by granulosa cells, mediated by relaxin and prostaglandin at the gonadotrophin surge (Canipari & Strickland 1986). Although it is clear that granulosa cells produce tissue-type PA there is conflicting evidence concerning the origin of urokinase-type PA, which may be a granulosa cell product (Knecht 1986) or of thecal origin (Canipari & Strickland 1985). The PA converts blood-borne plasminogen to plasmin which digests the follicle wall and activates latent collagenase secreted by fibroblasts (Espey 1971) and granulosa cells (Too et al 1984). The activated collagenase achieves a dissociation of the collagen of the follicle wall, thus permitting considerable thinning of the follicular apex leading to ovulation (Espey 1967). The importance of collagenase in follicular rupture is illustrated by ovulation in the rat being blocked by collagenase inhibitors. Serine protease inhibitors, which inhibit PA activity, will inhibit ovulation (Reich et al 1985a,b). Similarly arachidonic acid metabolism inhibitors of the cyclo-oxygenase or lipoxygenase pathways inhibit both collagenases and ovulation (Reich et al 1983, 1985b).

Follicular rupture

The reason for rupture occurring at the apex is probably because this is the site of the greatest mechanical stress, particularly as the dissociation of collagen is accompanied by increased capillary permeability and accumulation of fluid at the apex itself (Cherney et al 1975).

In human ovulation observed ultrasonically the expulsion ranges from a process lasting less than 1 minute to a more protracted expulsion after an initial rapid phase (De Crespigny et al 1981). This expulsion of the oocyte and surrounding cumulus is aided by a slight excess of intrafollicular pressure over intra-abdominal pressure.

Intrafollicular pressure is influenced by the contraction of smooth muscle cells in the follicle wall, and both $PGF_{2\alpha}$ and oxytocin have been shown to increase the pressure (Stahler et al 1977). Although the adrenergic innervation of the ovary is probably the principal mediator of the smooth muscle tone in the follicle wall, the periovulatory increase in $PGF_{2\alpha}$ and oxytocin may be important in determining intrafollicular tone near to ovulation. In some species smooth muscle cells are concentrated in the base of the follicle, thus accentuating the stress at the apex (Martin & Talbot 1981).

Granulosa cell luteinization and corpus luteum formation

Shift in steroidogenesis

As the dominant follicle aproaches the mid-cycle LH surge, granulosa cell oestradiol biosynthesis is maximal and progesterone production is minimal but may be stimulated in vitro by gonadotrophins (Hillier & Wickings 1985). In the 12 hours preceding the onset of the LH surge a rise in circulating progesterone and 17α-hydroxyprogesterone is detectable (Hoff et al 1983), probably reflecting the acquisition of LH receptors by granulosa cells (McNatty et al 1979). The onset of the LH surge is accompanied by a major shift in granulosa cell steroidogenesis from oestradiol to progesterone production, so that circulating progesterone rises rapidly and oestradiol falls (Hoff et al, 1983). The reduction in oestradiol biosynthesis is not primarily due to a fall in granulosa lutein cell aromatase activity (Hillier & Wickings 1985) although a transient reduction in aromatase activity is observed in culture (Wickings et al 1986). It probably reflects lack of availability of androgen substrate during the massive gonadotrophin exposure at the LH surge, perhaps due to desensitization of the theca lutein cells to LH stimulation of androgen synthesis. In contrast, both LH and FSH stimulate side chain cleavage of cholesterol to progesterone in granulosa lutein cells, thus favouring the shift to progesterone synthesis.

The principal factor governing the considerable increase in progesterone biosynthesis in the luteal phase appears to be availability of cholesterol substrate. Endogenous granulosa cell cholesterol is insufficient to support the observed output; thus, the elements which control the access of exogenous cholesterol precursor have a major influence on granulosa lutein cell progesterone output. Before ovulation the basal lamina acts like a molecular sieve, restricting passage of large proteins such as low density lipoprotein (LDL) but not of smaller proteins including high density lipoprotein (HDL) (Shalgi et al 1973). The LDL is a rich source of cholesterol compared with HDL and granulosa lutein cells have been shown to be able to utilize LDL in this way (Tureck & Strauss 1982) since they have specific LDL binding sites (Ohashi et al 1982). The process which makes possible the utilization of blood-borne LDL is the neovascularization of the granulosa cell layer at luteinization (Carr et al 1982).

Angiogenesis

The angiogenic factors which initiate the neovascularization are not yet clarified but angiogenic activity has been demonstrated in human follicular fluid (Frederick et al 1984). Culler et al (1986) have suggested that angiotensin II may be an ovarian angiogenic factor since it is known to have this property in other organs and has been demonstrated in human follicular fluid. Follicular fluid has also been shown to be rich in renin-like activity which would be important in the production of angiotensin II (Fernandez et al 1985).

CONTROL OF LUTEAL STEROIDOGENESIS

Gonadotrophins

Once provided with an adequate supply of cholesterol precursor the granulosa lutein cells will maintain progesterone biosynthesis if the gonadotrophin stimulus is maintained. The main luteotrophic influence is LH, with each LH pulse being followed by increases in circulating progesterone and oestradiol (Backstrom et al 1982). The necessary duration of dependence on LH stimulation during the luteal phase in women is not yet clear since there are conflicting results from clinical studies of ovulation induced in hypophysectomy cases and studies using GnRH analogues. Studies of granulosa lutein cell steroidogenesis in culture indicate that both progesterone production and particularly aromatase activity are considerably enhanced by gonadotrophin exposure (Polan et al 1986, Wickings et al 1986). In the rhesus monkey there is good evidence for corpus luteum dependence on ganadotrophin stimulation throughout the luteal phase (Hutchison & Zeleznik 1984).

Although gonadotrophins are likely to be the major determinants of luteal cell steroid biosynthesis there are other regulating factors which modulate these processes and which may influence luteolysis. These factors include adenosine, oestradiol, prolactin, oxytocin, GnRH and prostaglandins (Fig. 3.6).

Adenosine

The action of LH on the luteal cell is dependent on LH receptor-mediated activation of the adenyl cyclase system to convert adenosine triphosphate (ATP) to cAMP. The addition of adenosine increases the adenyl cyclase substrate pool and thus amplifies LH stimulation of cAMP production and consequent progesterone production by luteal cells in vitro (Hall et al 1981). The luteotrophic influence of adenosine opposes the luteolytic influence of $PGF_{2\alpha}$, at least in the rat.

Oestradiol

Oestradiol is a major product of the luteal cell but in women it may have a role in the control of luteal steroidogenesis as an inhibitory influence. At the ovarian level there is in vitro evidence for oestradiol inhibition of 3β-hydroxysteroid dehydrogenase which converts pregnenolone to progesterone (Williams et al 1979). Oestradiol also stimulates ovarian $PGF_{2\alpha}$ production, at least in primates (Aluetta et al 1978). Oestradiol may also function as a luteolytic influence by negative feedback on pituitary LH secretion.

Prolactin

In the rat corpus luteum prolactin has an important luteotrophic role. It activates cholesterol esterases making choles-

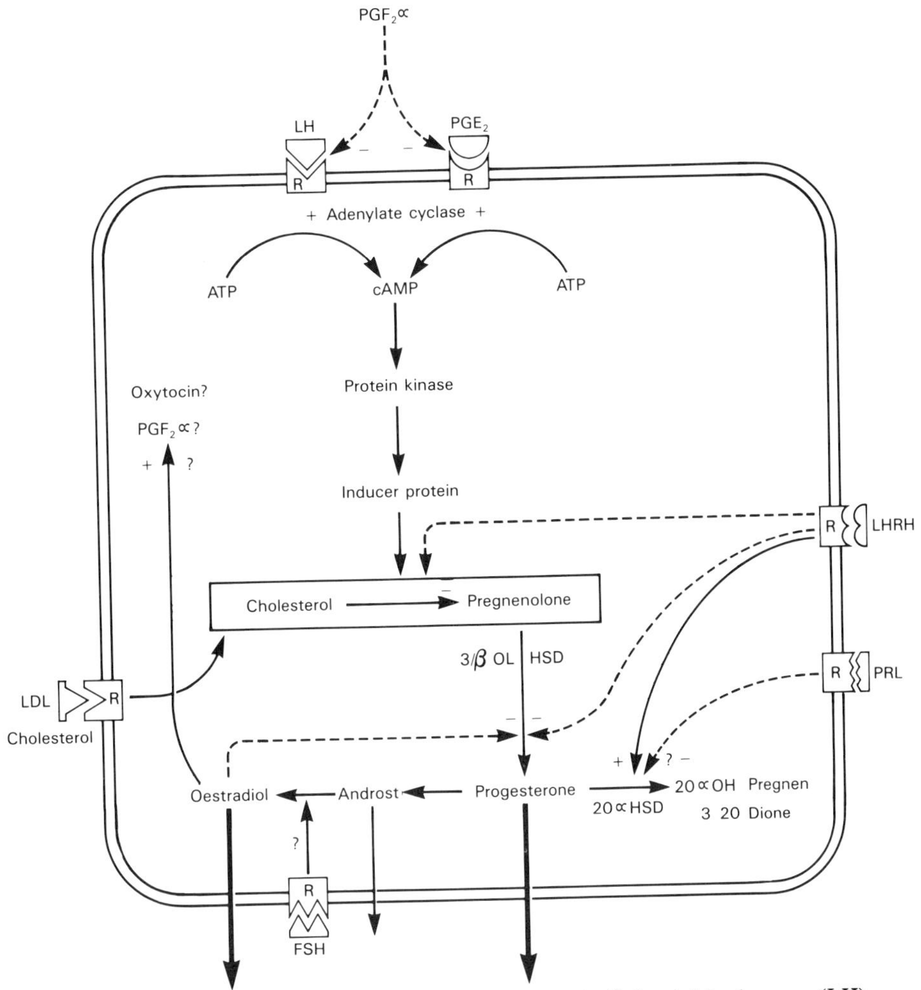

Fig. 3.6 Factors regulating the synthesis of steroids by the luteal cell. Luteinizing hormone (LH) interacts with its receptor (R) to stimulate the production of cyclic adenosine monophosphate (cAMP) and eventually the conversion of cholesterol to pregnenolone within the mitochondrion. Although receptors (R) for luteinizing hormone-releasing hormone (LHRH), follicle-stimulating hormone (FSH) and prolactin (PRL) have been identified in the human luteal cell their physiological role is still unknown. $PGF_{2\alpha}$ = prostaglandin $F_{2\alpha}$; PGE_2 = prostaglandin E_2; ATP = adenosine triphosphate; LDL = low density lipoprotein; HSD = hydroxysteroid dehydrogenase. From Baird (1985).

terol available for progesterone biosynthesis (Hashimoto & Wiest 1969) and inhibits 20α-hydroxysteroid dehydrogenase, thus reducing metabolism of progesterone (Wiest et al 1968). Although prolactin receptors have been demonstrated on human luteal cells (Poindexter et al 1979) a role for prolactin in these cells remains uncertain.

GnRH-like peptide

The effect of GnRH-like peptides on luteal cell steroidogenesis is inhibitory, thus in the rat GnRH is luteolytic. However, clinical studies using GnRH or GnRH analogue agonists in women have produced conflicting results with luteolysis suggested by Casper and Yen (1979) and Lemay et al (1979) but a luteotrophic response reported by Fleming and Coutts (1982b). Laboratory studies on isolated human luteal cells (Casper et al 1984) did not demonstrate a direct effect of GnRH or its agonist in contrast to the stituation in the rat. The inhibitory actions of GnRH-like peptides in the rat include suppression of 3β-hydroxysteroid dehydrogenase which converts pregnenolone to progesterone (Jones & Hsueh 1982) and stimulation of 20α-hydroxysteroid dehydrogenase, which converts progesterone to an inactive metabolite (Jones & Hsueh 1981). It is likely that GnRH-like peptides of ovarian origin will be shown to have a paracrine role in the fine control of luteal steroidogenesis in humans.

Prostaglandins

Despite the considerable evidence that $PGF_{2\alpha}$ is the major luteolysin of many species this has not been proven for humans. Certainly the source of such $PGF_{2\alpha}$ in humans can hardly be uterine, as it is in many species including the ewe, since hysterectomy has little effect on human luteal function (Beiling et al 1970). The probable source of $PGF_{2\alpha}$ in women is the corpus luteum itself (Swanston et al 1977).

It is possible that prostaglandins mediate both luteotrophic (PGE_2) and luteolytic ($PGF_{2\alpha}$) activity. PGE_2 has been shown to stimulate progesterone production by luteal cells, whereas $PGF_{2\alpha}$ suppresses gonadotrophin-stimulated progesterone secretion; however, this effect of $PGF_{2\alpha}$ is blocked by PGE_2 (McNatty et al 1975b). A shift in the relative balance of PGE_2 and $PGF_{2\alpha}$ in favour of $PGF_{2\alpha}$ as the corpus luteum ages have been reported in the rhesus monkey (Balmeceda et al 1979) and may explain the increasing sensitivity of luteal cells to $PGF_{2\alpha}$ as the luteal phase proceeds (Dennefors et al 1982).

Oxytocin

Immunoreactive oxytocin or oxytocin-like material has been isolated from the human corpus luteum (Khan-Dawood & Dawood 1983) and is likely to originate in the corpus luteum (Dawood & Khan-Dawood 1986). The role of oxytocin in human luteal function is not defined but there may be a dose-related effect on progesterone production with low early luteal oxytocin concentrations luteotrophic, but high concentrations luteolytic (Tan et al 1982). In primates in vivo evidence suggests a luteolytic role for oxytocin (Aluetta et al 1984). Ovine data also suggest a luteolytic role for oxytocin, indicating an oestrogen-dependent oxytocin-mediated stimulation of $PGF_{2\alpha}$ output, which in turn increases oxytocin production (Roberts et al 1976). In the ewe the principal source of $PGF_{2\alpha}$ is the endometrium but in primates it is possible that oxytocin stimulates ovarian $PGF_{2\alpha}$ production.

LUTEOLYSIS

During the functional life of the corpus luteum luteal cells are influenced by the luteotrophic and luteolytic stimuli previously described. It is likely that luteolysis is determined by the relative balance of these influences and that this is dependent on the changing sensitivity of the luteal cells as the luteal phase proceeds. Although control of the human corpus luteum is not yet clarified in detail, animal data suggest that the influence of LH, via membrane receptor activation of adenyl cyclase, is critical to luteal cell function and that some of the modulating factors act by interfering with this mechanism. One possibility is that occupation of specific membrane receptors for $PGF_{2\alpha}$ or GnRH-like peptides leads to calcium-mediated uncoupling of the LH receptor mechanism from the adenyl cyclase complex.

PREDICTION OF OVULATION

An ability to predict or detect the occurrence of spontaneous ovulation is of value to women practising natural family planning methods and to those requiring treatment for infertility from ovulatory causes. In infertility management knowing the time of spontaneous ovulation facilitates an assessment of ovulation, the timing of coitus itself as well as post-coital testing and particularly artificial insemination by donor (AID) therapy. Ovulation monitoring is also required in the management of ovulation induction therapy and in in vitro fertilization superovulation practice, but the particular requirements of these techniques will not be considered, since the ovarian processes are not physiological, involving multiple follicular development and altered pituitary ovarian feedback interactions.

Methods of practical value in ovulation prediction include simple biophysical observations such as basal body temperature charting and cervical mucus assessment, both of which can be performed by patients; biochemical assays of oestradiol, progesterone or LH in urine or blood, which demand laboratory facilities; and ovarian ultrasound scanning which employs expensive equipment and trained staff.

Biophysical methods

Basal body temperature (BBT)

Although BBT charts may be useful to assess retrospectively whether a rise in circulating progesterone has occurred by means of the biphasic BBT pattern, they are of limited use in accurate ovulation prediction. Even when ovulation occurs a significant proportion of charts may fail to give a biphasic pattern (Moghissi 1976); where a temperature rise is seen this can be out of step with ovulation by several days (Hilgers & Bailey 1980). The occurrence of a drop in temperature prior to the mid-cycle rise is often regarded as the BBT feature which is most useful as an indicator of impending ovulation, but this is clearly observed in less than 20% of cycles (Marshall 1963).

Cervical mucus assessment

Rising circulating oestrogen in the days preceding ovulation stimulates endocervical epithelial glands to produce watery mucus which is receptive to sperm. The periovulatory rise in progesterone and transient fall in oestrogen cause an abrupt change to a highly viscous mucus which resists sperm penetration. The peak day of watery mucus generally occurs on the day of ovulation (Depares et al 1986) and use of this peak is a better predictor of ovulation than the BBT rise (Hilgers & Bailey 1980). Since these mucus changes can be recognized at the vulva by the woman herself (Hilgers & Prebil 1979) this phenomenon forms the basis of many natural family planning methods, including a major World Health Organization study (Bonnar 1983). Cervical mucus assessment is sufficiently accurate to be employed in ovulation prediction in some AID programmes but remains less accurate than the more expensive biochemical or ultrasonic methods.

Ultrasonic assessment

Ovarian ultrasonic observation of growth of the dominant follicle indicates when the follicular diameter is approaching the ovulatory size, e.g. approximately 20 ± 3 mm (Hackeloer et al 1979, Marinho et al 1982). Unfortunately the range of diameter at ovulation is too large to guarantee that the specific day of ovulation will be pinpointed, but when the diameter exceeds 20 mm, ovulation is very likely to occur in the subsequent 24-hour period.

A further ultrasonic parameter which confirms proximity to ovulation is visualization of the ovarian vessels which distend near to ovulation (Hackeloer & Nitschke-Dabelstein 1980). Although ovarian ultrasound has limitations where accurate pinpointing of time of physiological ovulation is concerned, it remains a fundamental technique in the pre-ovulation monitoring of stimulated cycles since it indicates the extent of multiple follicular growth.

Ultrasound provides an accurate retrospective indication that ovulation has taken place, since formation of the corpus luteum is accompanied by increase in ultrasonic density. This is seen as infilling by echoes of the previously translucent follicle prior to the structure becoming ultrasonically indistinguishable from the rest of the ovary (Hackeloer et al 1979).

Biochemical methods

A range of peripheral hormonal changes have been studied near to ovulation to determine the most useful predictor of the impending event. These include LH, sex steroids and their metabolites in blood, urine and saliva. The most important are oestradiol, progesterone and LH.

Oestradiol

Oestradiol is predominantly a product of the dominant follicle (Baird & Fraser 1975) with circulating oestradiol correlating well with the diameter of that follicle (Hackeloer et al 1979). As a result oestradiol is useful in monitoring the multiple follicles of stimulated cycles but of more limited value in prediction of ovulation in natural cycles. Where plasma oestradiol is measured daily, it may be possible to use the fall in oestradiol production which accompanies the LH surge as a predictor of ovulation. In practical terms progesterone and LH are more useful predictors of physiological ovulation than oestradiol.

Progesterone

A small but significant rise in circulating progesterone precedes the onset of the LH surge by some hours, with plasma progesterone more than doubling between days −3 and −1, but since the rise is within a relatively low range compared with the luteal phase, detection of the rise demands assay sensitivity at low levels. Kerin et al (1981) quote the rise as from 1.4 ± 0.1 ng/ml (day −3) to 3.0 ± 0.3 ng/ml (day −1), whereas mid-luteal phase progesterone will exceed 10 ng/ml. Rapid radioimmunoassays sensitive at low levels of progesterone have been developed (Fleming & Coutts 1982a) and, more recently, commercial radioimmunometric assays have become available with high sensitivity and short assay time. It is therefore possible to use daily plasma progesterone assays near mid-cycle to detect the initial progesterone rise as a reliable predictor that ovulation will occur between 24 and 48 hours later. This is of use in ovulation prediction for AID (Fleming & Coutts 1982a).

Luteinizing hormone

Measurement of LH remains the principal laboratory method for ovulation prediction since the LH surge is closely linked to the time of ovulation; the large change in the hormone level does not demand high assay sensitivity and current assays permit rapid analysis of plasma or urine samples. It is not possible to carry out a quantitative blood or urine LH radioimmunomagnetic assay in less than 1 hour but semi-quantitative or qualitative methods employing haemagglutination inhibition or colorimetric reactions can be performed as side-room tests on urine.

Where the requirement is to pinpoint the day of ovulation then a daily LH assessment will suffice. The daily sample will not indicate closely when the rise commenced in the preceding 24 hours but does indicate that ovulation is likely between 24 and 36 hours after the rise was detected. In in vitro fertilization it is necessary to have a close indication of the time of onset of the LH surge because of the requirement to link the time of oocyte recovery to that event. Three-hourly sampling intervals have been employed by some groups. This pattern of sampling suggests that in a majority of women the onset of the LH surge is between midnight and 8 a.m. (Baird 1983) and that the interval between the onset of the LH surge and ovulation is usually in the range of 24 to 32 hours (Lemay et al 1982).

THE ENDOMETRIAL CYCLE

The endometrial changes which culminate in menstruation, if conception does not occur, are a result of the changes in circulating steroid hormones produced by the ovary during the ovarian cycle (Fig. 3.7). For more than a century it has been known that there is a link between ovarian function and menstruation, since oophorectomy was employed to abolish a variety of menstrual disorders (Battey 1876). Ovarian steroids acting via steroid receptors produce histo-

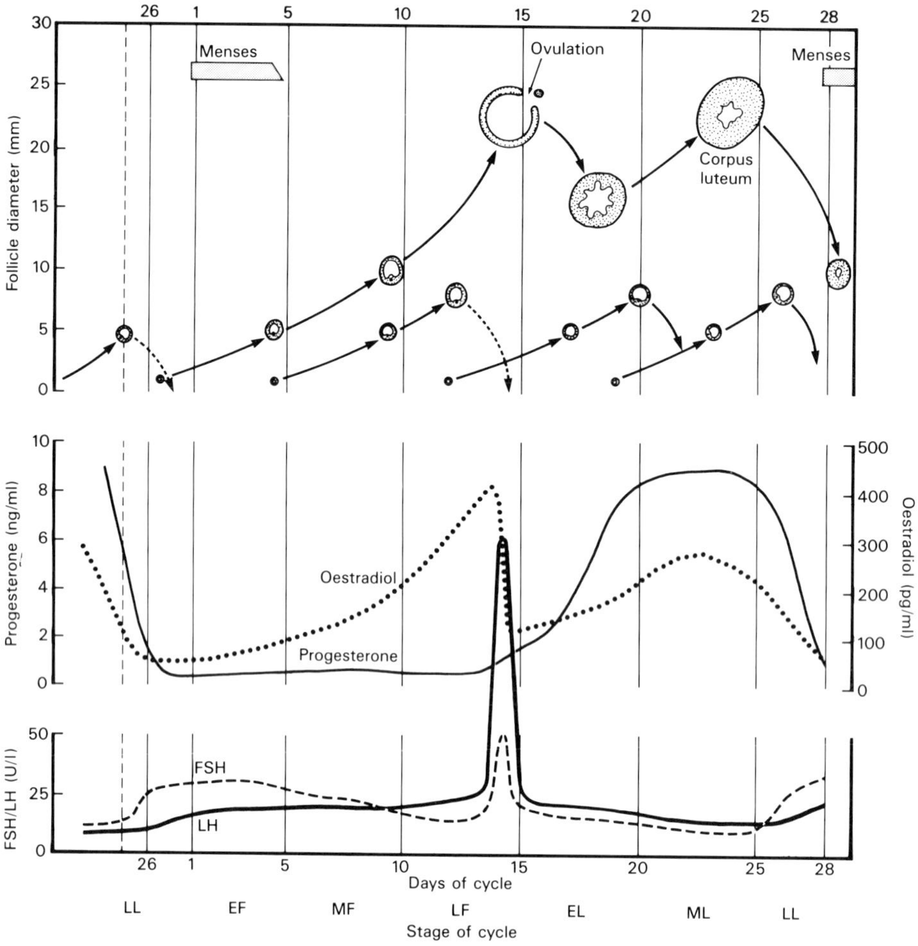

Fig. 3.7 Changes in pituitary and ovarian hormone concentrations and follicular growth throughout the ovarian cycle, resulting in menstruation. From Baird (1983).

logical and biochemical endometrial changes, which will be described below.

ENDOMETRIAL HISTOLOGY

The histology of the endometrium changes throughout the menstrual cycle. Since these have been extensively described (Noyes et al 1950, Demopoulos 1977, Robertson 1981) only a brief description will follow.

Follicular phase

Following endometrial bleeding and shedding during menstruation, rapid resurfacing occurs and a new epithelial surface is produced. In the early follicular phase the glands are small, tubular and short. The lining epithelium is cuboidal to columnar and the nuclei are ovoid and basally or centrally located. Mitoses increase both in the glands and the stroma throughout the follicular phase. In the mid and late follicular phases the glands become elongated and tortuous; the lining cells are columnar and pseudostratification of nuclei is seen.

Luteal phase

The first evidence of ovulation is seen 48 hours later in the endometrium, when small subnuclear vacuoles appear in some of the glands. These vacuoles are clear, rich in glycogen and lipid and located beneath the nucleus, misplacing it to a mid-zonal position. Four days after ovulation the secretory vacuoles have largely migrated to a supranuclear or luminal position. Mitoses are not seen either in glands or stroma in this phase of the cycle. By day 20 the secretions are released into the lumina of the glands and at the same time the glands become so tortuous, due to an increase in length and coiling, that they give the appearance of having serrated margins. Endometrial morphometry shows an increased density of glandular tissue in the luteal phase: consequently, the greater endometrial thickness at that time is due to an increase in the volume occupied by glandular rather than stromal tissue (Fig. 3.8; Rees et al 1984d). Stromal oedema increases simultaneously, reaching a maximum on day 21.

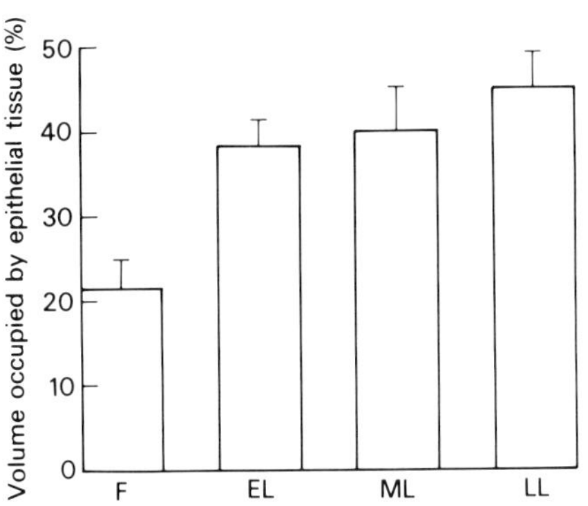

Fig. 3.8 Change in glandular epithelial density throughout the menstrual cycle. Values are means ± SD. F = follicular; EL = early luteal; ML = mid-luteal; LL = late luteal phases of the menstrual cycle. From Rees et al (1984a).

The next change, predecidualization, starts on day 23; it consists of enlargement of cytoplasm of stromal cells around the spiral arterioles. The predecidual changes spread rapidly through the stroma and by the time of menstruation nearly all of the tissue is altered in this way. Simultaneously with predecidualization occurs infiltration with granulocytes and lymphocytes. Finally menstruation ensues.

Menstruation

The extent of endometrial shedding during menstruation has been disputed. It was originally suggested that all of the endometrium except the basal layer was lost (Bohnen 1927). However, more recent studies indicate that the superficial functional layer is only partially shed (McLennan & Rydell 1965).

ENDOMETRIAL VASCULATURE

The vasculature of the endometrium has a characteristic structure which changes throughout the cycle in menstruating species (human and subhuman primates). The endometrial arteries in most species which menstruate are distinctive in that they are profusely coiled into spirals as they run through the tissue (Fig. 3.9). As early as 1774, Hunter demonstrated the presence of tortuous arteries in decidua from the human pregnant uterus. More recently the uterine vasculature has been extensively investigated and the following description is based on these papers (Daron 1936, Bartelmez 1957, Fanger & Barker 1961, Farrer-Brown et al 1970a,b).

The uterus is supplied by the uterine arteries which run a tortuous course in the broad ligament along the lateral side of the uterus and terminate by joining the ovarian arteries. Branches of the main uterine arteries penetrate the lateral margins of the uterine wall, pass through the outer third of the myometrium and then ramify into a ring of vessels to form the arcuate arteries running at the junction of the

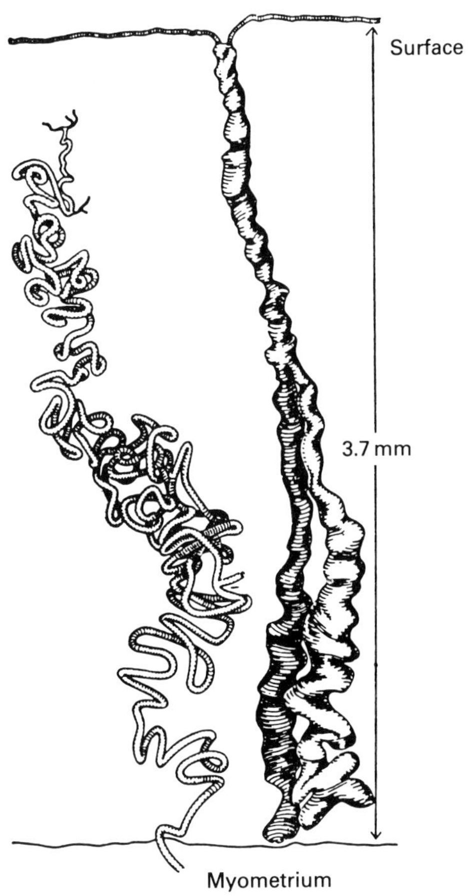

Fig. 3.9 Diagrammatic representation of an endometrial spiral artery. From Daron (1936).

outer and middle thirds of the myometrium. Radial arteries arising from the arcuate arteries pass through the inner myometrium. Just before crossing the myometrial–endometrial junction, the radial artery divides into spiral and basal arterioles. The basal arterioles supply only the basal endometrium, appear to be unaffected by hormonal stimuli and maintain the basal layer throughout the menstrual cycle. In contrast, the spiral arterioles are markedly influenced by the changes of the menstrual cycle: they supply the superficial capillary bed of the endometrium and are end arterioles. Capillaries arise from spiral arterioles at all levels and supply the endometrial glands and stroma in the luteal phase; these capillaries end in the subepithelial capillary plexus. The main veins in the endometrium run parallel to the endometrial glands and in addition there are numerous intercommunicating channels. The veins then enter the myometrium and converge to form larger collecting vessels which in turn drain into arcuate veins, which run with the arcuate arteries and terminate in the uterine veins.

The role of the endometrial vasculature in menstruation was extensively studied by Markee (1940) using rhesus monkeys, in which he transplanted pieces of endometrium into the anterior chamber of the eye where the menstrual process could be observed. He demonstrated that menstruation is preceded by a period of rapid endometrial regression resulting in increased coiling of the spiral arterioles. Before menstruation two different vascular changes may occur:

1. Stasis with or without vasodilatation, which begins 1–5 days before the onset of bleeding;
2. Vasoconstriction of spiral arterioles, which begins 4–24 hours before the onset of bleeding and persists throughout that period, and terminates stasis. This vasoconstriction, which lasts until the end of menstrual bleeding, is interrupted by brief periods of relaxation of the spiral arterioles, usually resulting in haemorrhages. These haemorrhages continue as long as an individual arteriole is relaxed and appear to be terminated through its contraction.

The basal arterioles do not undergo the same vascular changes which occur in the spiral arterioles. It has been estimated that bleeding from arterioles accounts for 50% of the total blood loss during menstruation. Venous bleeding accounts for 25% of blood loss, but it lasts longer than arterial bleeding. The remainder of the bleeding occurs from capillaries or results from diapedesis.

STEROID RECEPTORS AND METABOLISM

The effects of oestradiol and progesterone are mediated by specific high-affinity receptor sites, detected in both cell nuclei and cytoplasm, which exhibit cyclical changes (Bayard et al 1978, Levy et al 1980, Press et al 1984). Recently the complementary DNA sequence of oestrogen receptors has been determined (Green et al 1986). Oestradiol receptor concentrations increase in the follicular phase, reaching a peak before ovulation. Levels decrease in the luteal phase to a nadir in the late luteal phase. Progesterone receptor concentrations are low in the follicular phase, show a preovulatory rise and then decrease after ovulation. A difference has been noted between cytoplasmic and nuclear progesterone receptor concentrations after ovulation — the former decrease immediately, whereas the concentration of the latter is at its highest in the early luteal phase. In the later luteal phase nuclear receptor concentrations decrease to values similar to those found in the follicular phase.

Endometrial receptor concentrations are affected by circulating oestradiol and progesterone levels (Tseng & Gurpide 1975, Kreitman et al 1979, Levy et al 1980, Eckert & Katzenellenbogen 1981). During the follicular phase there is a direct relationship between plasma oestradiol levels and oestradiol and progesterone receptor concentrations. In contrast, during the luteal phase no such correlation is found with either circulating steroid; here progesterone acts both to decrease oestradiol receptor content and influence in situ metabolism of oestradiol. These multiple interactions may explain the absence of a direct relationship between plasma progesterone and progesterone receptor concentrations in endometrium.

The cellular localization of steroid receptors has received attention (Satyaswaroop et al 1982, Press et al 1984). Oestradiol receptors are found both in epithelial and stromal cells, and progesterone receptors principally in glandular epithelium. In addition the intracellular site of oestradiol receptors has been examined: it appears that they are mainly confined to nuclei; this challenges the initial distinction between nuclear and cytoplasmic receptors (King & Greene 1984, Press et al 1984).

Endometrial tissue concentrations of oestradiol and progesterone are dependent not only on circulating plasma levels but also on in situ metabolism. Endometrium can synthesize oestrogen from androstenedione and testosterone and the capacity is higher in the follicular than in the luteal phase (Tseng et al 1982). Oestradiol is converted to:

1. Oestrone by 17β-oestradiol dehydrogenase;
2. Oestrone sulphate by oestrogen sulphotransferase (Tseng & Liu 1981, Clarke et al 1982, Satyaswaroop et al 1982).

The activities of these two enzymes, principally found in glandular epithelium, are coupled, increased in the luteal phase and stimulated by progesterone. Similarly, 20α-hydroxysteroid dehydrogenase, which converts 20α-dehydroprogesterone to progesterone, is also found in higher levels in luteal glandular epithelium and is stimulated by progesterone.

PEPTIDE HORMONES

Relaxin

Immunohistochemical studies have shown that relaxin is present in luteal endometrial glandular epithelium (Yki-Jarvinen et al 1985). It is thought to be involved in the processes of implantation and menstruation (Yki-Jarvinen et al 1985) by causing stromal dissolution (Dallenbach-Hellweg et al 1966).

Prolactin

Prolactin is synthesized by human endometrium during the latter half of the luteal phase, correlating with the appearance of decidualization. It has thus been suggested that prolactin may function in either an immunological role or as a growth-promoting factor for the trophoblast. Prolactin is known to have growth-promoting activity in a variety of lower animals (Riddick et al 1983).

ENDOMETRIAL ENZYMES

Enzymatic changes occur throughout the endometrial cycle (Boutselis 1973). In general two types of enzyme activities

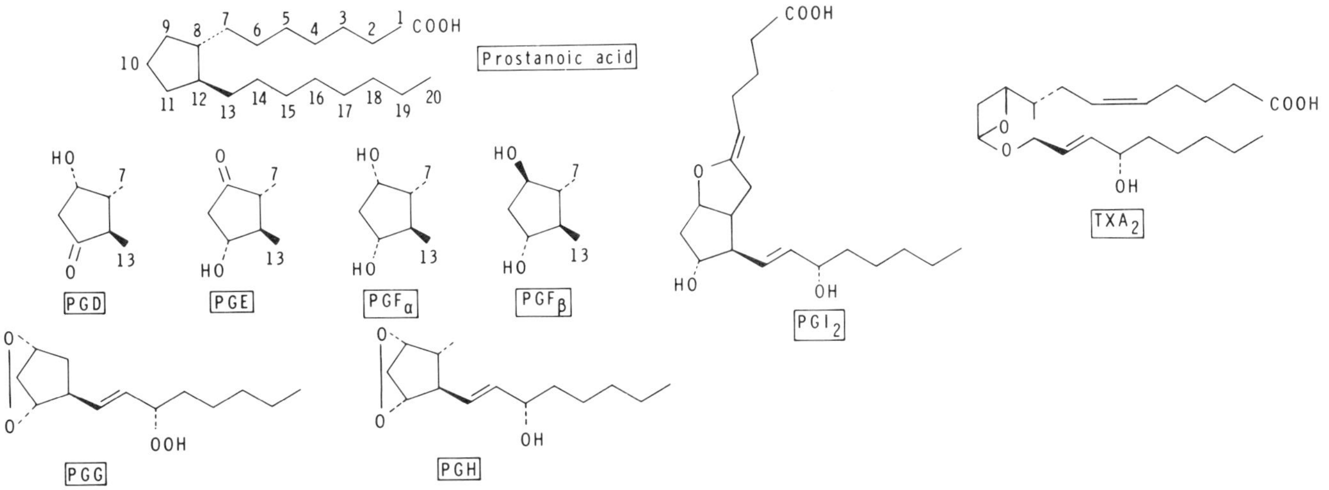

Fig. 3.10 Basic prostaglandin structures.

can be detected: oestrogen-dependent with highest activity at ovulation and progesterone-dependent with highest activity in the luteal phase. The oestrogen-related enzymes are alkaline phosphatase, β-glucuronidase, glucose-6-phosphatase, non-specific esterase, and glucose-6-phosphate dehydrogenase. Progesterone-related enzymes include acid phosphatase, lactic dehydrogenase and diphosphopyridine nucleotide diaphorase.

PROSTAGLANDINS

The role of prostaglandins in endometrium has received considerable attention since 1965 when Pickles et al found high concentrations of PGE_2 and $PGF_{2\alpha}$ in endometrium and menstrual fluid.

Structure

Prostaglandins are C_{20} carboxylic acids consisting of a five-membered carbon ring with two seven- and eight-membered carbon side chains (Bergstrom et al 1963; Fig. 3.10). Different prostaglandins are classified according to the functional groups attached at C_9 and C_{11} in the five-membered ring. Depending on the ring structure, prostaglandins are named prostaglandin A to I. Prostaglandins belong to the 1, 2 or 3 series depending on whether they contain 1, 2 or 3 double bonds in their side chains. Prostaglandins of the 2 series are the most abundant in mammalian tissues. The name thromboxane A_2 (TXA_2) was introduced to describe an unstable vasoconstrictor substance which does not have the basic prostanoic acid structure: it has an oxane–oxetane ring structure and contains two double bonds in its side chain (Hamberg et al 1974).

Biosynthesis

Prostaglandins are not stored in cells but are rapidly synthesized once the substrate essential polyunsaturated fatty acid precursors become available. Prostaglandin biosynthetic pathways have been extensively reviewed (Granstrom 1979, Vane 1982, Green 1986) and this short description is based on these papers (Fig. 3.11). The prostaglandin precursor fatty acids are dihomo-γ-linoleic acid for the 1 series, arachidonic acid for the 2 series, and 5,8,11,14,17-eicosapentaenoic acid for the 3 series. Arachidonic acid is the most common fatty acid present in mammalian tissues. It is not present as a free carboxylic acid in cells but is abundant in ester linkage at the 2 position of phospholipids. Consequently before commencement of prostanglandin biosynthesis arachidonic acid must be liberated from cellular phospholipids by the action of phospholipases, which are activated by changes in their chemical environment (Bonney 1985). Once released from phospholipids, free arachidonic acid is metabolized either by a cyclo-oxygenase-mediated pathway to form prostaglandins, or by a lipoxygenase pathway leading to leukotrienes (Demers et al 1984; Fig. 3.12). Leukotrienes have recently been detected in endometrium (Rees et al 1986).

The first step in the conversion of arachidonic acid to prostaglandins is the formation of PGG_2 and PGH_2 endoperoxide intermediates mediated by the enzyme prostaglandin endoperoxide synthetase, which has both cyclo-oxygenase and peroxidase activity (Fig. 3.11). PGH_2 is then converted to PGE_2, $PGF_{2\alpha}$ and prostaglandin D_2 (PGD_2)— the primary prostaglandins. PGH_2 can also be converted by the enzyme thromboxane synthetase into TXA_2: it is very labile and is rapidly converted into the more stable thromboxane B_2 (TXB_2). Through the agency of prostacyclin synthetase PGH_2 can also be converted into prostacyclin (PGI_2): this is chemically unstable and is rapidly hydrolysed to the more stable 6-keto-prostaglandin $F_{1\alpha}$ (6-keto-$PGF_{1\alpha}$).

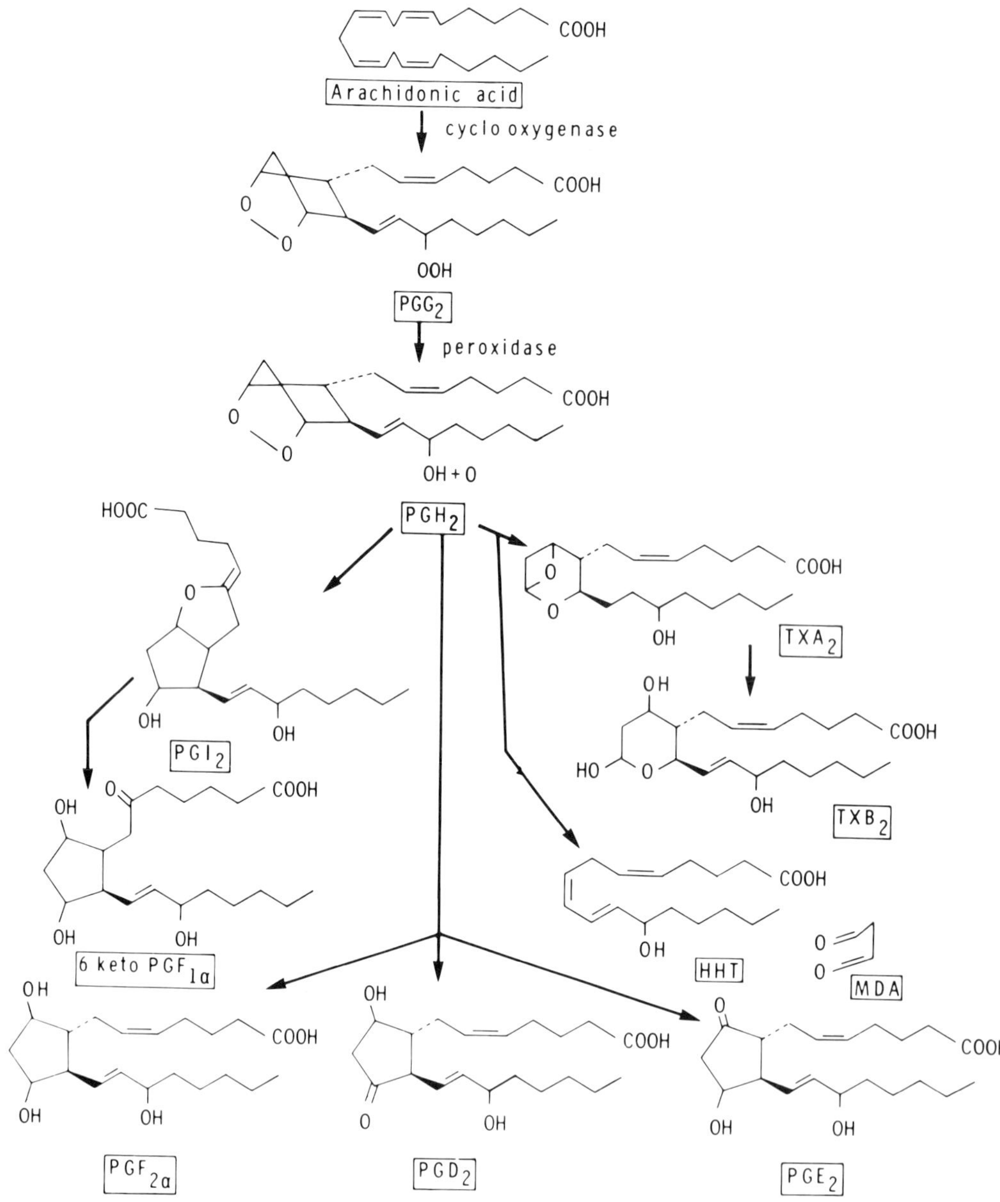

Fig. 3.11 Prostaglandin biosynthetic pathways.

Prostaglandins, endometrium and menstruation

Individual prostaglandins have differing effects on haemostasis and myometrial activity and consequently may be involved in menstruation and the control of menstrual bleeding. With regard to haemostasis, while PGE_2 and PGI_2 cause vasodilatation $PGF_{2\alpha}$ and TXA_2 produce vasoconstriction. In addition TXA_2 and PGI_2 promote and inhibit platelet aggregation respectively (Moncada & Vane 1979).

With regard to myometrial activity the effect of different prostaglandins has been studied both in vitro and in vivo. In vitro, PGE_2 generally inhibits and $PGF_{2\alpha}$ stimulates human myometrial strip contractility (Wiqvist et al 1983). In vivo, $PGF_{2\alpha}$ administration stimulates uterine contractility during all phases of the menstrual cycle, while PGE_2 may produce both inhibition during menstruation and stimulation during the follicular and luteal phases (Bygdeman et al 1979). In vitro, PGI_2 and TXA_2 have inhibitory and stimulatory effects respectively (Wilhelmsson et al 1981). However, in vivo uterine injection of PGI_2 stimulates contractility (Swann & Lundstrom 1983).

The site of prostaglandin production has been localized in human endometrium to glandular epithelium using both immunohistochemical and cell separation techniques (Rees et al 1982, Lumsden et al 1984; Fig. 3.13). Prostaglandin production also varies throughout the menstrual cycle with increased levels in the luteal phase and during menstruation (Maathuis & Kelly 1978, Rees et al 1984a; Fig. 3.14).

Prostaglandins have been implicated in menstruation since Wiqvist et al (1971) found that administration of $PGF_{2\alpha}$ in

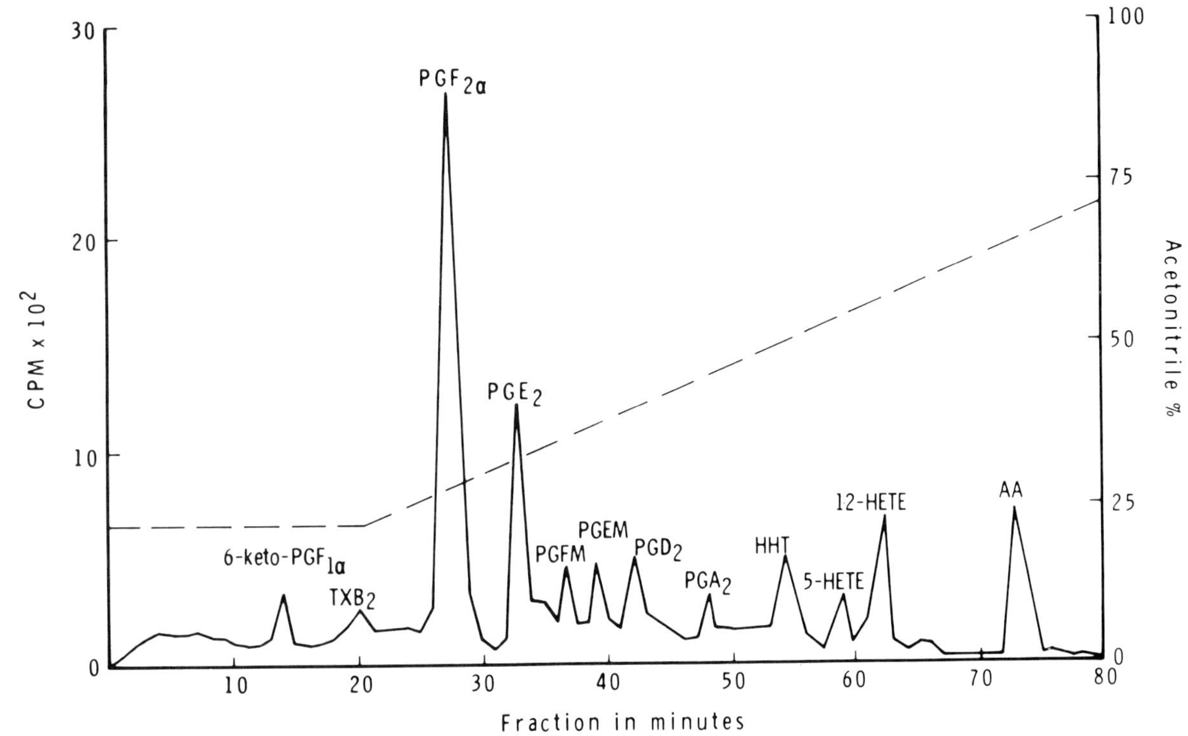

Fig. 3.12 High-pressure liquid chromatography profile of arachidonic acid metabolites from human endometrium incubations. TX = thromboxane; PG = prostaglandins; HETE = lipoxygenase products. Dashed line is indicative of the acetonitrile percentage in the mobile phase of the chromatogram. From Demers et al (1984).

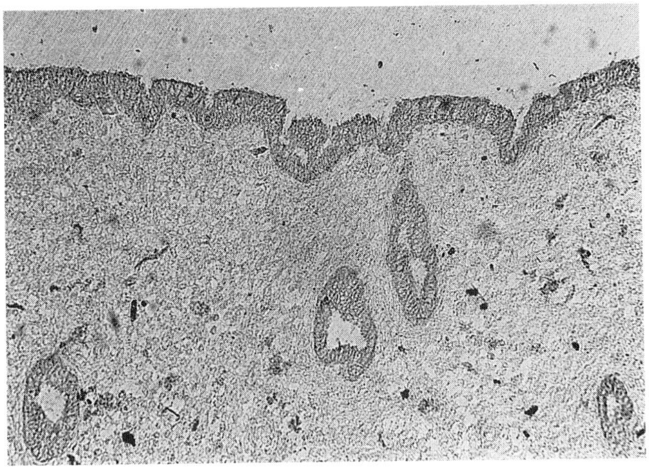

Fig. 3.13 Photomicrograph of a cross-section of human endometrium in the luteal phase treated with anticyclo-oxygenase antiserum. Specific staining is seen in the surface and glandular epithelium. Enlargement ×5. From Rees et al (1982.)

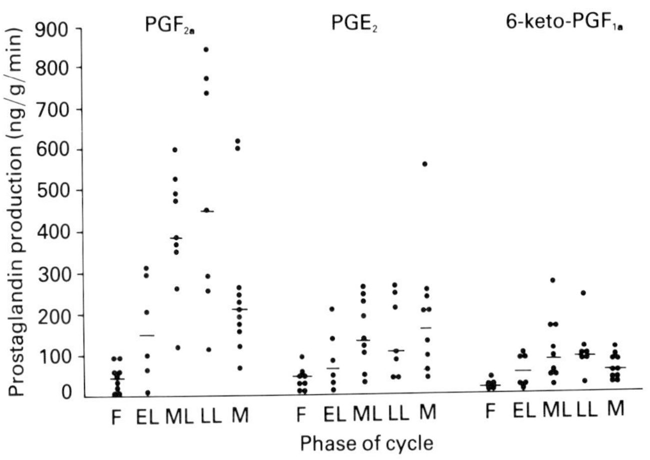

Fig. 3.14 Endometrial prostaglandin release. Bars represent median values. F = follicular; EL = early luteal; ML = mid-luteal; LL = late luteal; M = menstrual phases of the menstrual cycle. From Rees et al (1984a).

the luteal phase induced menstrual bleeding. The overproduction of prostaglandins has been implicated in two menstrual disorders: menorrhagia and dysmenorrhoea (Pickles et al 1965, Smith et al 1981, Rees et al 1984b). Reduction of menstrual blood loss and relief of dysmenorrhoeic symptoms can be achieved by the administration of prostaglandin synthetase inhibitors which inhibit the enzyme prostaglandin endoperoxide synthetase (Anderson et al 1976, 1978).

UTERINE HAEMOSTASIS

It has been apparant for many years that the mechanisms by which uterine haemostasis is achieved differ from those found in other tissue systems. Schickele in 1912 was the first to observe that menstrual fluid could be kept for several weeks without any obvious clotting being detected. In most tissue systems, haemostasis consists of five overlapping phenomena: localized vasoconstriction; platelet adhesion to the lips of a wound; formation of the platelet plug; reinforcement of the platelet plug with fibrin and finally the removal of deposited material via fibrinolytic mechanisms (Vermylen 1978).

In the uterus haemostatic plugs are only present for a limited time: few are seen from 20 hours after the onset of menstruation and they are smaller than in other tissues (Christiaens et al 1980, 1982). This suggests that the contribution of haemostatic mechanisms in menstruating endometrium differs from that usually found in peripheral haemostasis.

The coagulation and fibrinolytic systems have received considerable attention. With regard to fibrinolysis, plasminogen activator has been demonstrated in menstrual fluid and endometrium with increased levels during menstruation (Rybo 1966, Rees et al 1985).

Examination of menstrual fluid indicates that both the coagulation and fibrinolytic enzyme systems are activated during menstruation: thrombin-generating activity is virtually absent and there are high levels of fibrinogen-related antigen, plasmin and plasminogen activator, differing markedly from serum obtained from the clotting of peripheral venous blood (Rees et al 1985). In addition, heparin-like activity has been found in uterine fluid (Foley et al 1978).

Degranulated platelets have been observed in endometrial haemostatic plugs and menstrual fluid (Christiaens et al 1982, Sheppard et al 1983), suggesting that they have been involved in the haemostatic process. In addition menstrual fluid platelets are unable to aggregate and metabolize arachidonic acid via the cyclo-oxygenase pathway (Rees et al 1984c). Thus spent platelets are shed from the endometrium into menstrual fluid.

Excessive menstrual bleeding in the absence of pelvic pathology has been associated with increased levels of fibrinolytic activity in endometrium and menstrual fluid and antifibrinolytic agents have been used successfully to reduce menstrual blood loss (Rybo 1966, Nilsson & Rybo 1967).

MENSTRUATION

Menstruation is the conspicuous visible event of the endometrial cycle. It has been defined as a periodic discharge of sanguinous fluid and a sloughing of the uterine lining in a female; it is an event characteristic of the reproductive cycle in humans and most subhuman primates (Scommegna & Dmowski 1977). Consequently our scientific understanding of the physiological mechanisms involved in the process of menstruation is based on animal as well as on human data.

Hypothetical factors regulating menstruation

Since the original work on menstruation was performed the underlying cause of the process of menstruation has been the subject of numerous hypotheses (Shaw and Roche 1980, Christiaens et al 1982) which are summarized below.

Oestrogen and progesterone withdrawal

This theory was proposed from studies using the castrate monkey model (Allen 1927, Corner 1951). Here a castrate female monkey was administered with sufficient oestrogen to build up the endometrium to a level at which sudden oestrogen deprivation would cause menstruation-like bleeding. To this was added a course of progesterone: the discontinuation of progesterone was always followed after 3–8 days by bleeding, in spite of the continuation of oestrogen in quantities ordinarily sufficient to prevent oestrogen deprivation bleeding. It is hence assumed that the fall in the levels of progesterone and oestrogen prior to menstruation is responsible for the endometrial changes resulting in the onset of menstrual bleeding.

Uterine vasculature

Uterine blood vessels are thought to play an important role in the process of menstruation since most species which menstruate, except for New World monkeys, have spiral arterioles. Their role has already been described (see above).

Inadequate lymphatic drainage

This factor has been proposed as an additional element involved in the aetiology of menstruation. According to this theory, catabolites accumulate due to an inadequate lymphatic system in the superficial endometrium and cause tissue destruction until the endometrium is shed. The theory is based on rhesus monkey experiments in which Wislocki & Dempsey (1939), using an injection technique, showed that lymphatics are confined to the deeper half of the endometrium, whereas the outer half is devoid of lymphatic channels. On the other hand in humans (Rouviere 1932) injection studies suggest that endometrial lymphatic capillaries originate just below the surface epithelium. However, this observation in humans does not appear to have been confirmed histologically (Sheppard & Bonnar 1979). Therefore the role of the lymphatic drainage in the process of menstruation remains difficult to ascertain.

Subcellular mechanisms

More recently three subcellular mechanisms of menstruation have been suggested:

1. Tissue digestion by lysosomal enzymes.
2. The process of apoptosis.
3. Stromal dissolution by the hormone relaxin.

Lyosomal enzymes. Probably the first experimentally supported suggestion that lysosomal enzymes might be involved in the dissolution of endometrium at the time of menstruation came from Cohen et al (1964) and Bitensky & Cohen (1965). These workers proposed that an increase in the activity of the lysosomal enzyme acid phosphatase at the end of the luteal phase results in endometrial breakdown: acid phosphatase is a commonly used marker of lysosomal function, and is an acid hydrolase. This group of enzymes is thought to function as an intracellular digestive system. The lysosomal concept of menstruation was further developed by Henzl et al (1972) using ultrastructural techniques to study acid phosphatase activity. These authors observed that the largest enzymorphological changes occur during the late luteal phase and early menstrual bleeding. These changes are characterized by an increase in acid phosphatase staining within the intercellular spaces of the stromal and epithelial layer; gradual penetration of acid phosphatase into junctional complexes of the surface and glandular epithelium; swelling of arteriolar endothelia; and the finding of acid phosphatase reaction product on the arteriolar basement membranes and between adjacent endothelial cells. Towards menstruation more autophagic bodies with sequestered organelles are seen. Based on these observations Henzl et al (1972) concluded that changes in lysosomal activity may represent important steps in the sequence of events culminating in endometrial regression and bleeding.

Apoptosis. The mechanism of apoptosis, which may be involved in endometrial regression and reorganization during menstruation, was first described by Kerr et al (1972). These authors used the term to describe a process of controlled cell deletion and structural changes which takes place in two discrete stages. The first comprises nuclear and cytoplasmic condensation and breaking up of the cell into a number of membrane-bound fragments. In the second stage these apoptotic bodies are shed from epithelial lined surfaces or taken up by other cells, where they undergo changes resembling in vitro autolysis within phagosomes and are rapidly degraded by lysosomal enzymes from the ingesting cells. Apoptotic bodies in human endometrium were later investigated using electron and light microscopy by Hopwood & Levison (1976). It was found that while these bodies are relatively scarce during the follicular phase they are present with increasing frequency towards and during menstruation, suggesting that the process of apoptosis may play a role in menstration.

Relaxin. The hormone relaxin may affect the process of menstruation (Dallenbach-Hellweg 1975). According to this theory relaxin is liberated at the end of the menstrual cycle. The release of relaxin would initiate premenstrual stromal dissolution and disintegration.

Prostaglandins

The involvement of prostaglandins in menstruation is one of the most recent hypotheses. Their role in haemostatic mechanisms and smooth muscle has already been described.

Blood loss during menstruation

The amount of blood lost during menstruation has received considerable attention since 1814 when John Davidge showed that a woman might lose about 8 ounces of blood in a typical menstrual flow. Population studies in which menstrual blood has been measured (Hallberg et al 1966) show a skewed distribution with 90% of blood losses less than 80 ml (mean 43 ml; median 30 ml). The upper limit of normal blood loss per menstruation is usually considered to be 80 ml, since this is the 90th percentile; above this level of blood loss there is an increased incidence of iron deficiency anaemia.

REFERENCES

Allen E 1927 The menstrual cycle of the monkey *Macacus rhesus*: Observations on normal animals, the effects of removal of the ovaries and the effects of injections of ovarian and placental extracts into the spayed animals. Contributions to Embryology, Carnegie Institute 19: 1–44

Aluetta F J, Agins H, Scommegna A 1978 Prostaglandin F mediation of the inhibitory effect of estrogen on the corpus luteum of the rhesus monkey. Endocrinology 103: 1183–1189

Aluetta F J, Paradis D K, Wesley M, Duby R T 1984 Oxytocin is luteolytic in the rhesus monkey (*Macaca mulatta*). Journal of Reproduction and Fertility 72: 401–406

Amsterdam A, Tsafriri A 1979 In vitro binding of ^{125}I-human chorionic gonadotrophin in the preovulatory follicle: absence of receptor sites on oocytes. Journal of Cell Biology 83: 255A

Anderson A B M, Haynes P J, Guillebaud J, Turnbull A C 1976 Reduction of menstrual blood loss by prostaglandin synthetase inhibition. Lancet i: 774–776

Anderson A B M, Haynes P J, Fraser I S, Turnbull A C 1978 Trial of prostaglandin synthetase inhibitors in primary dysmenorrhoea. Lancet i: 345–347

Bäckström C T, McNeilly A S, Leask R M, Baird D T 1982 Pulsatile secretion of LH, FSH, prolactin, oestradiol and progesterone during the human menstrual cycle. Clinical Endocrinology 17: 29–42

Bagnell C A, Greenwood F C, Bryant-Greenwood G D 1984 A paracrine role for follicular relaxin. In: Sairam M R, Atkinson L (eds) Gonadal proteins and peptides and their biological significance. World Publishing, Singapore, pp 299–308

Baird D T 1983 Prediction of ovulation: biophysical, physiological and biochemical coordinates. In: Jeffcoate S L (ed) Ovulation: methods for its prediction and detection. Wiley, Chichester, pp 1–17

Baird D T 1985 Control of luteolysis. In: Jeffcoate S L (ed) The luteal phase. Wiley, Chichester, pp 25–42

Baird D T, Fraser I S 1975 Concentration of oestrone and oestradiol in follicular fluid and ovarian venous blood of women. Clinical Endocrinology 4: 259–266

Baker T G 1963 A quantitative and cytological study of germ cells in human ovaries. Proceedings of the Royal Society (Biology) 158: 417–433

Baker T G 1971 Radiosensitivity of mammalian oocytes with particular reference to the human female. American Journal of Obstetrics and Gynecology 110: 746–761

Balmeceda J P, Asch R H, Fernandez E O, Eddy C A, Pauerstein C J 1979 Prostaglandin production by the rhesus monkey corpus luteum in vitro. Fertility and Sterility 31: 214–216

Bartelmez G W 1957 The form and functions of the uterine blood vessels in the rhesus monkey. Contributions to Embryology, Carnegie Institute 36: 155–185

Battey R 1876 Extirpation of the functionally active ovaries for the remedy of otherwise incurable diseases. Transactions of the American Gynecological Society 1: 101–120

Bayard F, Danilano S, Robel P, Baulieu E E 1978 Cytoplamic and nuclear estradiol and progesterone receptors in human endometrium. Journal of Clinical Endocrinology and Metabolism 46: 635–648

Beiling C G, Marcus S L, Markam S M 1970 Functional activity of the corpus luteum following hysterectomy. Journal of Clinical Endocrinology and Metabolism 30: 30–39

Bergstrom S, Ryhage R, Samuelsson B, Sjorall J 1963 Prostaglandins and related factors 15: The structures of prostaglandin E_1, $F_{1\alpha}$ and $F_{1\beta}$. Journal of Biological Chemistry 238: 3555–3557

Bitensky L, Cohen S 1965 The variation of endometrial acid phosphatase activity with the menstrual cycle. Journal of Obstetrics and Gynaecology of the British Commonwealth 72: 769–774

Bogovich K, Richards J S 1982 Androgen biosynthesis in developing ovarian follicles: evidence that luteinizing hormone regulates thecal 17α hydroxylase and C_{17-20} lyase activities. Endocrinology 111: 1201–1208

Bohnen P 1927 Wie weit wird das Endometrium bie der Menstruation abgestossen? Archivs der Gynaekologie 129: 459–472

Bomsel-Helmreich O 1985 Ultrasound and the preovulatory human follicle. In: Clarke J R (ed) Oxford reviews of reproductive biology, vol 7. Clarendon Press, Oxford, pp 1–72

Bonnar J 1983 Biological approaches to ovulation detection. In: Jeffcoate S L (ed) Ovulation — methods for its prediction and detection. Wiley, Chichester, pp 41–44

Bonney R C 1985 Measurement of phospholipase A_2 activity in human endometrium during the menstrual cycle. Journal of Endocrinology 107: 183–189

Boutselis J G 1973 Histochemistry of the normal endometrium. In: Norris H J, Hertig A T, Abel M R (eds) The uterus. Williams & Wilkins, Baltimore, pp 175–184

Brower P T, Schultz R M 1982 Intercellular communication between granulosa cells and mouse oocytes: existence and possible nutritional role during oocyte growth. Developmental Biology 90: 144–153

Bryant-Greenwood G D, Jeffrey R, Ralph M M, Seamark R F 1980 Relaxin production by the porcine ovarian follicle in vitro. Biology of Reproduction 23: 792–800

Bygdeman M, Bremme K, Gillespie A, Lundstrom V 1979 Effects of prostaglandins on the uterus. Prostaglandins and uterine contractility. Acta Obstetricia et Gynecologica Scandinavica (suppl) 87: 33–38

Canipari R, Strickland S 1985 Plasminogen activator in the rat ovary. Journal of Biological Chemistry 260: 5121-5125

Canipari R, Strickland S 1986 Studies on the hormonal regulation of plasminogen activator production in the rat ovary. Endocrinology 118: 1652–1659

Carr B R, MacDonald P C, Simpson E R 1982 The role of lipoproteins in the regulation of progesterone secretion by the human corpus luteum. Fertility and Sterility 38: 303–311

Casper R F, Yen S S C 1979 Induction of luteolysis in the human with a long-acting analog of luteinizing hormone-releasing factor. Science 205: 408–410

Casper R F, Erickson G F, Yen S S C 1984 Studies on the effect of gonadotropin-releasing hormone and its agonist on human luteal steroidogenesis in vitro. Fertility and Sterility 42: 39–43

Chang R J, Jaffe R B 1978 Progesterone effects on gonadotrophin release in women pretreated with estradiol. Journal of Clinical Endocrinology and Metabolism 47: 119–125

Channing C P, Anderson L D, Hoover D J et al 1982 The role of non-steroidal regulators in control of oocyte and follicular maturation. Recent Progress in Hormone Research 38: 331–408

Cherney D D, Didio L J A, Motta P 1975 The development of rabbit ovarian follicles following copulation. Fertility and Sterility 26: 257–270

Christiaens G C M L, Sixma J J, Haspels A A 1980 Morphology of haemostasis in menstrual endometrium. British Journal of Obstetrics and Gynaecology 87: 425–432

Christiaens G C M L, Sixma J J, Haspels A A 1982 Haemostasis in menstrual endometrium: a review. Obstetrical and Gynecological Survey 37: 281–303

Clarke C L, Adams J B, Wren B G 1982 Induction of estrogen sulfotransferase in the human endometrium by progesterone in organ culture. Journal of Clinical Endocrinology and Metabolism 55: 70–75

Cohen S, Bitensky L, Chayen L, Cunningham G J, Russell J K 1964 Histochemical studies on the human endometrium. Lancet ii: 56–59

Corner G W 1951 Our knowledge of the menstrual cycle 1910–1950. Lancet i: 919–923

Culler M D, Tarlatzis B C, Lightman A et al 1986 Angiotension II-like immunoreactivity in human ovarian follicular fluid. Journal of Clinical Endocrinology and Metabolism 62: 613–615

Dallenbach-Hellweg G 1975 Histopathology of the endometrium, 2nd edn. Springer-Verlag, New York, pp 72–75

Dallenbach-Hellweg G, Dawson A B, Hisaw F L 1966 The effect of relaxin on the endometrium of monkeys. Histological and histochemical studies. American Journal of Anatomy 119: 61–78

Daron G H 1936 The arterial pattern of the tunica mucosa of the uterus in *Macacus rhesus*. American Journal of Anatomy 58: 349–419

Davidge J B 1793 cited in Corner G W 1951 Our knowledge of the menstrual cycle 1910–1950. Lancet i: 919–923

Davidge J B 1814 cited in Short R V Oestrous and menstrual cycles. In: Austin C R, Short R V (eds) Hormonal control of reproduction, vol 3. Cambridge University Press, Cambridge, pp 115–152

Davroen J B, Hsueh A J W 1984 Insulin enhances FSH-stimulated steroidogenesis by cultured rat granulosa cells. Molecular and Cellular Endocrinology 35: 97–105

Davroen J B, Hsueh A J W, Li C H 1985 Somatomedin-C augments FSH induced differentiation of cultural rat granulosa cells. American Journal of Physiology, Endocrinology and Metabolism 249: E26–E33

Dawood M Y, Khan-Dawood F S 1986 Human ovarian oxytocin: its source and relationship to steroid hormones. American Journal of Obstetrics and Gynecology 154: 756–763

De Crespigny L C, O'Herlihy C, Robinson H P 1981 Ultrasonic observation of the mechanism of human ovulation. American Journal of Obstetrics and Gynecology 139: 636–639

Demers L M, Rees M C P, Turnbull A C 1984 Arachidonic acid metabolism by the non pregnant human uterus. Prostaglandins, Leukotrienes and Medicine 14: 175–180

Demopoulos R I 1977 Normal endometrium. In: Blaustein A Pathology of the female genital tract. Springer Verlag, New York, pp 211–242

Dennefors B L, Sjogren A, Hamberger L 1982 Progesterone and adenosine 3′, 5′-monophosphate formation by isolated human corpus luteum at different ages: influence of human chorionic gonadotrophin and prostaglandins. Journal of Clinical Endocrinology and Metabolism 55: 102–107

Depares J, Ryder R E, Walker S M, Scanlon M F, Normal C M 1986 Ovarian ultrasound highlights precision of symptoms of ovulation as markers of ovulation. British Medical Journal 1: 1562

Di Zerega G S, Marrs R P, Roche P C, Campeau J D, Kling O R 1983 Identification of proteins in pooled human follicular fluid which suppress follicular response to gonadotrophins. Journal of Clinical Endocrinology and Metabolism 56: 35–41

Di Zerega G S, Marrs R P, Lobo R, Ujita E L, Brown J, Campeau J D 1984 Correlation of inhibin and follicle regulatory protein activities with follicular fluid steroid levels in anovulatory patients. Fertility and Sterility 41: 849–855

Downs S M, Coleman D L, Ward-Bailey P W, Eppig J J 1985 Hypoxanthine is the principal inhibitor of murine oocyte maturation in a low molecular weight fraction of porcine follicular fluid. Proceedings of the National Academy of Sciences (USA) 82: 454–458

Eckert R L, Katzenellenbogen B S 1981 Human endometrial cells in primary tissue culture: modulation of the progesterone receptor level by natural and synthetic estrogens in vitro. Journal of Clinical Endocrinology and Metabolism 52: 699–704

Eppig J J, Freter R R, Ward-Bailey R F, Schultz R M 1983 Inhibition of oocyte maturation in the mouse: participation of cAMP, steroid hormones and a putative maturation inhibitory factor. Developmental Biology 100: 39–49

Espey L L 1967 Ultrastructure of the apex of the rabbit graafian follicle during the ovulatory process. Endocrinology 81: 267–276

Espey L L 1971 Decomposition of connective tissue in rabbit ovarian follicles by multivesicular structures of thecal fibroblasts. Endocrinology 88: 437–444

Espey L L 1980 Ovulation as an inflammatory reaction — a hypothesis. Biology of Reproduction 22: 73–106

Evans G, Wathes D C, King G J, Armstrong D R, Porter D G 1983 Changes in relaxin production by the theca during the preovulatory period in the pig. Journal of Reproduction and Fertility 69: 677–683

Fanger H, Barker B E 1961 Capillaries and arterioles in normal endometrium. Obstetrics and Gynecology 17: 543–550

Farrer-Brown G, Beilby J O W, Tarbit M H 1970a The blood supply of the uterus 1. Arterial vascular. Journal of Obstetrics and Gynaecology of the British Commonwealth 77: 687–681

Farrer-Brown G, Beilby J O W, Tarbit M H 1970b The blood supply of the uterus 2. Venous patterns. Journal of Obstetrics and Gynaecology of the British Commonwealth 77: 682–689

Fernandez L A, Tarlatyes B, Rzasa P J et al 1985 Renin-like activity in ovarian follicular fluid. Fertility and Sterility 44: 219–223

Fleming R, Coutts J R T 1982a Prediction of ovulation in women using a rapid progesterone radioimmunoassay. Clinical Endocrinology 16: 171–176

Fleming R, Coutts J R T 1982b LHRH analogues can be luteotrophic. Clinical Endocrinology 17: 593–599

Foley M E, Griffin M D, Zuzel M et al 1978 Heparin like activity in uterine fluid. British Medical Journal 2: 322–323

Frederick J L, Shimanuki T, de Zerega G S 1984 Initiation of angiogenesis by human follicular fluid. Science 224: 389–390

Gilula N B, Epstein M L, Beers W H 1978 Cell-to-cell communication and ovulation: a study of the cumulus-oocyte complex. Journal of Cell Biology 78: 58–75

Gougeon A, Lefevre B 1983 Evolution of the largest healthy and atretic follicles during the menstrual cycle. Journal of Reproduction and Fertility 69: 497–502

Granstrom E 1979 Biosynthesis of prostaglandins and thromboxanes. In: Berti F, Velo G P (eds) The prostaglandin system. Nato Advanced Study Institutes Series. Plenum Press, New York, pp 15–45

Green K 1986 Structure, biosynthesis and metabolism. In: Bygdeman M, Berger G S, Keith L G (eds) Prostaglandins and their inhibitors in clinical obstetrics and gynaecology. MTP Press, Lancaster, pp 13–28

Green S, Walter P, Kumar V et al 1986 Human oestrogen receptor c DNA: sequence, expression and homology to v-εib-A. Nature 320: 134–139

Guraya S S 1985 Follicular atresia 1985. In: Guraya S S (ed) Biology of ovarian follicles in mammals. Springer-Verlag, Berlin, pp 228–275

Hackeloer B J, Fleming R, Robinson H P, Adam A H, Coutts J R T 1979 Correlation of ultrasonic and endocrinologic assessment of human follicular development. American Journal of Obstetrics and Gynecology 135: 122–128

Hackeloer B J, Nitschke-Dabelstein S 1980 Ultrasonographic monitoring of ovarian structural changes. Progress in Medical Ultrasound 1: 141–149

Hall A K, Preston S L, Behrman H R 1981 Purine amplification of luteinising hormone action in ovarian luteal cells. Journal of Biological Chemistry 256: 10390–10398

Hallberg L, Högdahl A, Nilsson L, Rybo G 1966 Menstrual blood loss — a population study. Acta Obstetricia et Gynecologica Scandinavica 45: 320–351

Hamberg M, Svensson J, Samuelsson B 1974 Thromboxanes — a new group of biologically active compounds derived from prostaglandin endoperoxides. Proceedings of the National Academy of Sciences (USA) 72: 2994–2998

Hashimoto I, Wiest W G 1969 Luteotrophic and luteolytic mechanisms in rat corpora lutea. Endocrinology 84: 886–892

Heape W 1897 The menstruation and ovulation of *Macacus rhesus* with observations on the changes undergone by the discharged follicle. Part II. Philosophical Transactions of the Royal Society of London 188B: 135–166

Henzl M R, Smith R E, Boost G, Tyler E T 1972 Lysosomal concept of menstrual bleeding in human. Journal of Clinical Endocrinology and Metabolism 34: 860–875

Hilgers T W, Bailey A J 1980 Natural family planning. II. Basal body temperature and estimated time of ovulation. Obstetrics and Gynecology 55: 333–339

Hilgers T W, Prebil A M 1979 The ovulation method — vulvar observations as an index of fertility/infertility. Obstetrics and Gynecology 53: 12–22

Hillensjo T, Kripner A S, Pomerantz S H, Channing C P 1979 Action of porcine follicular fluid oocyte maturation in vitro: possible role of the cumulus cells. In: Channing C P, Marsh J M, Sadler W A (eds) Ovarian follicular and corpus luteum function. Plenum Press, New York, pp 283–291

Hillier S G 1985 Sex steroid metabolism and follicular development in the ovary. In: Clarke J R (ed) Oxford reviews of reproductive biology, vol 7. Clarendon Press, Oxford, pp 168–222

Hillier S G, Wickings E J 1985 Cellular aspects of corpus luteum function. In: Jeffcoate S L (ed) The luteal phase. Wiley, Chichester, pp 1–23

Hoff J D, Quigley M E, Yen S S C 1983 Hormonal dynamics at midcycle: a reevaluation. Journal of Clinical Endocrinology and Metabolism 57: 792–796

Hopwood D, Levison D A 1976 Atrophy and apoptosis in the cyclical human endometrium. Journal of Pathology 119: 159–166

Hunter W 1774 Anatomia uteri humani gravidi tubulis illustrata. Cited in Daron G H 1936 The arterial pattern of the tunica mucosa of the uterus in *Macacus rhesus*. American Journal of Anatomy 58: 349–419

Hutchison J S, Zeleznik A J 1984 The rhesus monkey corpus luteum is dependent on pituitary gonadotropin secretion throughout the luteal phase of the menstrual cycle. Endocrinology 115: 1780–1786

Hsueh A J W, Erickson G F 1979 Extrapituitary action of gonadotropin-releasing hormone: direct inhibition of ovarian steroidogenesis. Science 204: 854–855

Ingram D L 1962 Atresia. In: Zuckerman S, Mandl A M, Eckstein P (eds) The ovary. Academic Press, London, pp 247–273

Jones P B C, Hsueh A J W 1981 Direct stimulation of ovarian progesterone metabolizing enzyme by gonadotropin-releasing hormone in cultured granulosa cells. Journal of Biological Chemistry 256: 1248–1254

Jones P B C, Hsueh A J W 1982 Regulation of ovarian 3β-hydroxysteroid dehydrogenase by gonadotropin-releasing hormone and follicle stimulating hormone in cultured rat granulosa cells. Endocrinology 110: 1663–1671

Jones P B C, Conn P M, Marian J, Hsueh A J W 1980 Binding of gonadotropin-releasing hormone agonist to rat ovarian granulosa cells. Life Sciences 27: 2125–2132

Kerin J F, Edmonds D K, Warnes G M et al 1981 Morphological and functional relationships of Graafian follicle growth to ovulation in women using ultrasonic, laparoscopic and biochemical measurements. British Journal of Obstetrics and Gynaecology 88: 81–90

Kerr J F R, Wyllie A H, Currie A R 1972 Apoptosis: a basic biological phenomenon with wide ranging implications in tissue kinetics. British Journal of Cancer 26: 239–257

Kessel B, Liu Y X, Jia X-C, Hsueh A J W 1985 Autocrine role of oestrogens in the augmentation of LH receptor formation in cultured rat granulosa cells. Biology of Reproduction 32: 1038–1050

Khan-Dawood F S, Dawood M Y 1983 Human ovaries contain immunoreactive oxytocin. Journal of Clinical Endocrinology and Metabolism 57: 1129–1132

King W J, Greene G L 1984 Monoclonal antibodies localise oestrogen receptor in the nuclei of target cells. Nature 307: 745–750

Knecht M 1986 Production of a cell-associated and secreted plasminogen activator by cultured rat granulosa cells. Endocrinology 118: 348–353

Knobil E, Plant T M, Wildt L, Belchetz P E, Marshall G 1980 Control of the rhesus monkey menstrual cycle: permissive role of hypothalamic gonadotropin-releasing hormone. Science 207: 1371–1373

Koos R O, Clark M R 1982 Production of 6-keto-prostaglandin $F_{1\alpha}$ by rat granulosa cells in vitro. Endocrinology 111: 1513–1518

Kreitman B, Bugdt R, Bayard F 1979 Estrogen and progestin regulation of the progesterone receptor concentration in human endometrium. Journal of Clinical Endocrinology and Metabolism 49: 926–929

Lemay A, Labrie F, Ferland L, Raynaud J P 1979 Possible luteolytic effects of luteinizing hormone-releasing hormone in normal women. Fertility and Sterility 31: 29–34

Levy C, Robel P, Gautray J P et al 1980 Estradiol and progesterone receptors in human endometrium: normal and abnormal menstrual cycles and early pregnancy. American Journal of Obstetrics and Gynecology 136: 646–651

Lumsden M A, Brown A, Baird D T 1984 Prostaglandin production from homogenates of separated glandular epithelium and stroma from human endometrium. Prostaglandins 28: 485–496

Maathuis J B, Kelly R W 1978 Concentration of prostaglandins $F_{2\alpha}$ and E_2 in endometrium throughout the human menstrual cycle, after the administration of clomiphene or an oestrogen–progesterone pill and in early pregnancy. Journal of Endocrinology 77: 361–371

Marinho A O, Sallam H N, Goessens L K V, Collins W P, Rodeck C H H, Campbell S 1982 Real time pelvic ultrasonography during the preovulatory period of patients attending an artificial insemination clinic. Fertility and Sterility 37: 633–638

Markee J E 1940 Menstruation in intraocular endometrial transplants in the rhesus monkey. Contributions to Embryology, Carnegie Institute 28: 219–308

Marrs R P, Lobo R, Campeau J D et al 1984 Correlation of human

follicular fluid inhibin activity and spontaneous and induced follicle maturation. Journal of Clinical Endocrinology and Metabolism 58: 704–709
Marshall J 1963 Thermal changes in the normal menstrual cycle. British Medical Journal 1: 102–104
Martin C 1985 Endocrine physiology. Oxford University Press, New York, pp 626–631
Martin G G, Talbot P 1981 The role of follicular smooth muscle cells in hamster ovulation. Journal of Experimental Zoology 216: 469–482
McLennan C E, Rydell A H 1965 Extent of endometrial shedding during normal menstruation. Obstetrics and Gynecology 26: 605–621
McNatty K P, Sawers R S 1975 Relationship between the endocrine environment within the graafian follicle and the subsequent secretion of progesterone by human granulosa cells in culture. Journal of Endocrinology 66: 391–400
McNatty K P, Hunter W N, McNeilly A S, Sawers R S 1975a Changes in the concentration of pituitary and steroid hormones in the follicular fluid of human graafian follicles throughout the menstrual cycle. Journal of Endocrinology 64: 555–571
McNatty K P, Henderson K M, Sawers R S 1975b Effects of $PGF_{2\alpha}$ and E_2 on the production of progesterone in human granulosa cells in tissue culture. Journal of Endocrinology 67: 231–240
McNatty K P, Makris A, de Grazia C, Osathanondh R, Ryan K J 1979 The production of progesterone, androgens and oestrogens by human granulosa cells, thecal tissue and stromal tissue from human ovaries in vitro. Journal of Clinical Endocrinology and Metabolism 49: 687–699
McNatty K P, Hillier S G, van den Boogaard A M J, Trimbos-Kemper T C M, Reichert L E, van Hall E V 1983 Follicular development during the luteal phase of the human menstrual cycle. Journal of Clinical Endocrinology and Metabolism 56: 1022–1031
Moghissi K S 1976 Accuracy of basal body temperature for ovulation detection. Fertility and Sterility 27: 1415–1421
Moncada S, Vane J R 1979 Pharmacology and endogenous roles of prostaglandin endoperoxides, thromboxane A_2 and prostacyclin. Pharmacology Reviews 30: 293–332
Mondschein J S, Schomberg D W 1981 Growth factors modulate gonadotropin receptor induction in granulosa cell cultures. Science 211: 1179–1180
Nilsson L, Rybo G 1967 Treatment of menorrhagia with an antifibrinolytic agent, tranexamic acid (AMCA). A double blind investigation. Acta Obstetricia et Gynecologica Scandinavica 46: 572–577
Noyes R W, Hertig A I, Rock J 1950 Dating the endometrial biopsy. Fertility and Sterility 1: 3–25
Ohashi M, Carr B R, Simpson E R 1982 Lipoprotein binding sites in human corpus luteum membrane fractions. Endocrinology 110: 1477–1482
O'Herlihy C, de Crespigny L Ch, Lopata A, Johnston I, Hault I, Robinson H 1980 Preovulatory follicular size: a comparison of ultrasonic and laparoscopic measurements. Fertility and Sterility 34: 24–26
Pickles V R, Hall W J, Best F A, Smith G W 1965 Prostaglandins in endometrium and menstrual fluid from normal and dysmenorrhoeic subjects. Journal of Obstetrics and Gynaecology of the British Commonwealth 72: 185–192
Pincus G, Enzmann E V 1935 The comparative behaviour of mammalian eggs in vivo and in vitro. Journal of Experimental Medicine 62: 655–675
Plunkett E R, Moon Y S, Zamecnik J, Armstrong D T 1975 Preliminary evidence of a role for prostaglandin F in human follicular function. American Journal of Obstetrics and Gynecology 123: 391–397
Poindexter A N, Buttram V C, Besch P K, Smith R G 1979 Prolactin receptors in the ovary. Fertility and Sterility 31: 273–277
Polan M L, Seu D, Tarlatzis B 1986 Human chorionic gonadotrophin stimulation of estradiol production and androgen antagonism of gonadotrophin-stimulated responses in cultured human granulosa-lutein cells. Journal of Clinical Endocrinology and Metabolism 62: 628–633
Press M F, Nousek Goebl N, King W J, Herbst A L, Greene G L 1984 Immunohistochemical assessment of estrogen receptor distribution in the human endometrium throughout the menstrual cycle. Laboratory Investigation 51: 495–503
Rao M C, Midgley A R, Richards J S 1978 Hormonal regulation of ovarian cellular proliferation. Cell 14: 71–78
Rees M C P, Parry D M, Anderson A B M, Turnbull A C 1982 Immunohistochemical localisation of cyclooxygenase in the human uterus. Prostaglandins 23: 207–214
Rees M C P, Anderson A B M, Demers L M, Turnbull A C 1984a Endometrial and myometrial prostaglandin release during the menstrual cycle in relation to menstrual blood loss. Journal of Clinical Endocrinology and Metabolism 58: 813–818
Rees M C P, Anderson A B M, Demers L M, Turnbull A C 1984b Prostaglandins in menstrual fluid in menorrhagia and dysmenorrhoea. British Journal of Obstetrics and Gynaecology 91: 673–680
Rees M C P, Demers L M, Anderson A B M, Turnbull A C 1984c A functional study of platelets in menstrual blood. British Journal of Obstetrics and Gynaecology 91: 667–672
Rees M C P, Dunnill M S, Anderson A B M, Turnbull A C 1984d Quantitative endometrial histology during the menstrual cycle in relation to measured menstrual blood loss. British Journal of Obstetrics and Gynaecology 91: 662–666
Rees M C P, Cederholm-Williams S A, Turnbull A C 1985 Coagulation factors and fibrinolytic proteins in menstrual fluid collected from normal and menorrhagic women. British Journal of Obstetrics and Gynaecology 92: 1164–1168
Rees M C P, Di Marzo V, Tippins J R, Morris H R, Turnbull A C 1986 Human endometrium and myometrium release leukotrienes. British Journal of Clinical Pharmacology 21: 585
Reich R, Kohen F, Naor Z, Tsafriri A 1983 Possible involvement of lipoxygenase products of arachidonic acid pathway in ovulation. Prostaglandins 26: 1011–1020
Reich R, Miskin R, Tsafriri A 1985a Follicular plasminogen activator: involvement in ovulation. Endocrinology 116: 516–521
Reich R, Tsafrri A, Mechanic G L 1985b The involvement of collagenolysis in ovulation in the rat. Endocrinology 116: 522–527
Richards J S 1980 Maturation of ovarian follicles: actions and interactions of pituitary and ovarian hormones on follicular cell differentiation. Physiology Reviews 60: 51–89
Riddick D H, Daly D C, Walters C A 1983 The uterus as an endocrine compartment. Clinics in Perinatology 10: 627–639
Roberts J S, McCracken J A, Gavagan J E, Soloff M E 1976 Oxytocin stimulated release of prostaglandin $F_{2\alpha}$ from ovine endometrium in vitro: correlation with estrous cycle and oxytocin-receptor binding. Endocrinology 99: 1107–1114
Robertson W B 1982 The endometrium. Butterworths, London
Rouviere H 1932 Anatomie des lymphatiques de l'homme. Masson, Paris, pp 404–405
Rybo G 1966 Plasminogen activators in the endometrium. Acta Obstetricia et Gynecologica Scandinavica 45: 429–450
Satyaswaroop P G, Wastell D J, Mortel R 1982 Distribution of progesterone receptor, estradiol dehydrogenase and 20α-dihydroprogesterone dehydrogenase activities in human endometrial glands and stroma: progestin induction of steroid dehydrogenase activities in vitro is restricted to the glandular epithelium. Endocrinology 111: 743–749
Schickele G 1912 Biochemische Zeitschrift 38: 169 cited in Bartelmez G W 1937 Menstruation. Physiology Review 17: 28–72
Schultz A W 1974 Role of hormones in oocyte maturation. Biology of Reproduction 10: 150–178
Scomnegna A, Dmowski W P 1977 Menstruation. In: Philipp E E, Barnes J, Newton M (eds) Scientific foundations of obstetrics and gynaecology. Heinemann Medical Books, London, pp 127–136
Shalgi R, Kraicer P, Rimon A, Pinto M, Sofermann N 1973 Proteins of human follicular fluid: the blood–follicle barrier. Fertility and Sterility 24: 429–434
Shaw S T, Roche P C 1980 Menstruation. In: Finn C A (ed) Oxford reviews of reproductive biology. Clarendon Press, Oxford, pp 41–96
Sheppard B L, Bonnar J 1979 Development of vessels of the endometrium during the menstrual cycle in endometrial bleeding and steroidal contraception. In: Diczfalusy E, Fraser I S, Webb F T G (eds) Endometrial bleeding and steroidal contraception. Pitman Press, Bath, pp 65–85
Sheppard B L, Docheray C J, Bonnar J 1983 An ultrastructural study of menstrual blood in normal menstruation and dysfunctional uterine bleeding. British Journal of Obstetrics and Gynaecology 90: 259–265
Smith S K, Abel M H, Kelly R W, Baird D T 1981 Prostaglandin synthesis in the endometrium of women with ovular dysfunctional uterine bleeding. British Journal of Obstetrics and Gynaecology 88: 434–442
Stahler E, Spaetling L, Dauhe E, Buchholz R 1977 Untersuchungen uber das Verhalten des intrafollikulren Druckes in Abhangigkeit vom Druck

im ovariellen Gefassystem und Sewebe. Durchgefuhrt an in vitro perfundierten menschlichen Ovarian. Archiv für Gynäkologie 223: 41–53

Stone S L, Pomerantz S H, Schwartz-Kripner A, Channing C P 1978 Inhibitor of oocyte maturation from porcine follicular fluid: further purification and evidence for reversible action. Biology of Reproduction 19: 585–592

Swann M L, Lundstrom V 1983 The effect of intravenous and intrauterine administration of prostacyclin on non-pregnant uterine contractility in vivo. Acta Obstetricia et Gynecologica Scandinavica (suppl) 113: 47–50

Swanston I A, McNatty K P, Baird D T 1977 Concentration of prostaglandin $F_{2\alpha}$ and steroids in the human corpus luteum. Journal of Endocrinology 73: 115–122

Tan G J S, Tweedale R, Biggs J S G 1982 Oxytocin may play a role in the control of the human corpus luteum. Journal of Endocrinology 95: 65–70

Too C K L, Bryant-Greenwood G D, Greenwood F C 1984 Relaxin increases the release of plasminogen activator collagenase and proteoglycanase from rat granulosa cells in vitro. Endocrinology 115: 1043–1052

Tsafriri A, Braw R H 1984 Experimental approaches to atresia. In: Clarke J R (ed) Oxford reviews of reproductive biology, vol 6. Clarendon Press, Oxford, pp 226–265

Tsafriri A, Channing C P 1975 Inhibitory influence of granulosa cells and follicular fluid upon porcine oocyte meiosis in vitro. Endocrinology 96: 922–927

Tsafriri A, Dekel N, Bar-Ami S 1982 The role of oocyte maturation inhibitor in follicular regulation of oocyte maturation. Journal of Reproduction and Fertility 64: 541–551

Tsang B K, Moon Y S, Simpson C W, Armstrong D T 1979 Androgen biosynthesis in human ovarian follicles: cellular source, gonadotrophic control and adenosine 3′,5′-monophosphate mediation. Journal of Clinical Endocrinology and Metabolism 48: 153–158

Tsang B K, Armstrong D T, Whilfield J F 1980 Steroid biosynthesis by isolated follicular cells in vitro. Journal of Clinical Endocrinology and Metabolism 51: 1407–1411

Tseng L, Gurpide E 1975 Effects of progestins on estradiol receptor levels in human endometrium. Journal of Clinical Endocrinology and Metabolism 41: 402–407

Tseng L, Liu H C 1981 Stimulation of arylsulfotransferase activity by progestins in human endometrium in vitro. Journal of Clinical Endocrinology and Metabolism 53: 418–423

Tseng L, Mazella J, Mann W J, Chumas J 1982 Estrogen synthesis in normal and malignant human endometrium. Journal of Clinical Endocrinology and Metabolism 55: 1029–1030

Tureck R W, Strauss J F 1982 Progesterone synthesis by luteinized human granulosa cells in culture: the role of de novo sterol synthesis and lipoprotein-carried sterol. Journal of Clinical Endocrinology and Metabolism 54: 367–373

Vane J R 1982 Prostacyclin: a hormone with a therapeutic potential. Journal of Endocrinology 95: 3P–43P

Vermylen J 1978 Physiology of haemostasis. In: de Gaetano G, Garattini S (eds) Platelets: a multidisciplinary approach. Raven Press, New York, pp 3–15

Wang C, Hsueh A J W, Erickson G F 1981 LH stimulation of estrogen secretion in cultured granulosa cells. Molecular and Cellular Endocrinology 24: 17–28

Wickings E J, Hillier S G, Reichert L E 1986 Gonadotrophic control of steroidogenesis in human granulosa lutein cells. Journal of Reproduction and Fertility 76: 677–684

Wiest W G, Kidwell W R, Baloch K 1968 Progesterone catabolism in the rat ovary: a regulatory mechanism for progesterone potency during pregnancy. Endocrinology 82: 844–859

Wilhelmsson L, Wikland M, Wiqvist N 1981 PGH_2, TXA_2 and PGT_2 have potent and differentiated actions on human uterine action. Prostaglandins 21: 277–286

Williams M T, Rath M S, Marsh J M, Lemaire W J 1979 Inhibition of human chorionic gonadotrophin induced progesterone synthesis by oestradiol in isolated human luteal cell. Journal of Clinical Endocrinology and Metabolism 48: 437–440

Wiqvist N, Bygdeman M, Kirton K 1971 Non steroidal infertility agents in the female. In: Diczfalusy E, Barell V (eds) Nobel symposium 15. Control of human fertility. Almquist & Wiskell, Stockholm, pp 137–167

Wiqvist N, Lindblom B, Wikland M, Wilhelmsson L 1983 Prostaglandins and uterine contractility. Acta Obstetricia et Gynecologica Scandinavica (suppl) 113: 23–29

Wislocki G B, Dempsey E W 1939 Lymphatics of the reproductive tract of the female monkey (*Macaca mulatta*). Anatomical Record 75: 341–363

Yen S S C, Lein A 1976 The apparent paradox of the negative and positive feedback control system on gonadotrophin secretion. American Journal of Obstetrics and Gynecology 126: 942–954

Yen S S C, Tsai C C, Naftolin F, Vandenberg G, Ajabor L 1972 Pulsatile patterns of gonadotrophin release in subjects with and without ovarian function. Journal of Clinical Endocrinology and Metabolism 34: 671–675

Yki-Jarvine H, Wahlstrom T, Tenhunen A, Koskimies A, Seppala M 1984 The occurrence of relaxin in hyperstimulated human preovulatory follicles collected in an in vitro fertilization programme. Journal of In Vitro Fertilization and Embryo Transfer 1: 180–182

Yki-Jarvinen H, Wahlstrom T, Seppala M 1985 Human endometrium contains relaxin that is progesterone dependent. Acta Obstetricia et Gynecologica Scandinavica 64: 663–665

4

Alan Trounson, Peter A. W. Rogers, Ismail Kola and A. Henry Sathananthan

Fertilization, development and implantation

INTRODUCTION

The events which mark the onset of embryonic development are exceedingly complex and finely balanced between continuation, abnormal change and cessation of development. Given the understanding that a minor modification to one of the composite events could be an effective contraceptive it is slightly easier to comprehend the genesis of infertility. In this chapter we explore the events which determine normal fertilization and embryo development and try to illustrate how these events are controlled by many other interacting factors. We have attempted to simplify the technical language which abounds in this area in order to increase the palatability of this fascinating story which we ourselves are still struggling to comprehend.

THE OVULATED OOCYTES

Oocyte maturation

Fertilization and normal embryonic development can only be achieved if the ovulated oocyte has progressed through complete maturation within the ovarian follicle. It is not known whether immature oocytes may be ovulated in the spontaneous menstrual cycle but in the artificially manipulated and superovulated cycles of treatment for in vitro fertilization (IVF), incomplete oocyte maturation is frequently observed. Immature oocytes may be obtained even after administration of large doses (10 000 iu) of human chorionic gonadotrophin (hCG) (Veek et al 1983) which could be expected to saturate all luteinizing hormone (LH) receptor sites on growing ovarian follicles and thereby initiate the final phase of oocyte maturation. There are maturation inhibitors within follicular fluid which maintain even fully grown oocytes in meiotic arrest; for example, hypoxanthine, a purine found in murine and porcine follicular fluid maintains oocyte–granulose cell coupling (Eppig et al 1985), enabling the oocyte to maintain elevated levels of cyclic adenosine monophosphate (cAMP) essential in at least many rodent species for meiotic arrest (Dekel et al 1981).

The induction of the normal process of oocyte maturation is mediated by the signals from granulosa cells (Moor et al 1981) and involves the action of follicle-stimulating hormone (FSH) as well as specific changes in ovarian steroids. Absence of the granulosa cells, inhibition of their normal function or alteration to the sequence of hormonal changes and cytological events may result in incomplete oocyte maturation, despite the completion of chromosomal changes which are frequently used as indicators of oocyte maturity (Moor et al 1981, Staigmiller & Moor 1984). The sequelae of incomplete or incorrect oocyte maturation are: failure of fertilization and pronuclear formation (Thibault 1977); polyspermic fertilization (Sathananthan & Trounson 1982); oocyte or embryo fragmentation; retardation of embryonic cleavage and inviability of early cleavage stage embryos (Moor & Trounson 1977, Moor et al 1980, Crosby et al 1981).

If, in spontaneous ovulation, oocytes which have not completely matured are produced at times, this will be a source of reproductive failure. In the case of superovulation and IVF, the wastage will be exaggerated by the lack of synchrony in the growth of multiple follicles and the aspiration of oocytes from follicles which would not normally be ovulated. Despite attempts to identify follicular components which completely identify mature oocytes (Carson et al 1982) there is no consensus on any single parameter which can completely identify viable oocytes (Hillier et al 1985). As a result of this difficulty all oocytes obtained for IVF are normally inseminated so that the regularly cleaving embryos can be selected for transfer to the uterus. Since there is no information on the incidence of abnormally matured oocytes and premature or postmature oocytes in natural ovulatory cycles, the contribution of this factor to human reproductive failure cannot be estimated.

Chromosomal abnormalities of human oocytes

The most complete study of chromosomal abnormality in human oocytes has been published by Martin et al (1986). The authors found that in 50 oocytes which were quinicrine-banded to determine structural normality of chromosomes, 16 (32%) had abnormal chromosome numbers or had chromosomal structural abnormalities. The data were obtained from karyotyping spare oocytes from an IVF programme in which the patients were superovulated with fertility drugs. The chromosomal abnormalities observed in this study may include a component due to superovulation. However, it is difficult with hypoploidy to be certain that the absence of chromosomes is not due to technical artefacts, so that conservative estimates of aneuploidy are usually based on a doubling of the incidence of hyperploidy. This would estimate aneuploidy as 4% rather than 28% in the study by Martin et al (1986). The real figure for oocyte chromosomal abnormality must lie somewhere between 8 and 32% when chromosome structural abnormalities are also considered. A recent estimate of 50% chromosomal abnormality in human oocytes (11 of 23 had abnormal chromosome numbers) by Wramsby et al (1987) is almost certainly an overestimate due to technical artefact because in four oocytes only 1–5 chromosomes were located. These authors reported two hyperploid oocytes; this gives a minimum estimate of aneuploidy at about 9%. Rudak et al (1984) reported an incidence of 22% chromosomal abnormality in individual pronuclei of multipronuclear oocytes, and an aneuploidy rate of 17%.

Aneuploidy in human spermatozoa is more consistently estimated at about 9% (Martin 1984) which means that there is probably a higher incidence of chromosomal abnormalities in human oocytes than in sperm. The excessive loss of chromosomes in oogenesis could be due to anomalies in meiosis, such as anaphase lag, and excess hypoploidy has been observed in females of other species. There is a concern about the accumulation of chemicals collectively referred to as biozides in the follicular fluid of women (Trapp et al 1984), which may increase the possibility of chromosomal aberrations. This becomes more concerning if the higher estimates of oocyte abnormality of around 30% are correct because this is substantially higher than for other species. The human female is also unusual in that oocytes formed before birth are not used for reproduction on average for 20 to 25 years which represents a very long period for the accumulated effects of any biozides. It would certainly be of interest to know whether oocyte chromosomal abnormalities vary according to the type of environmental exposure or community in which women are living.

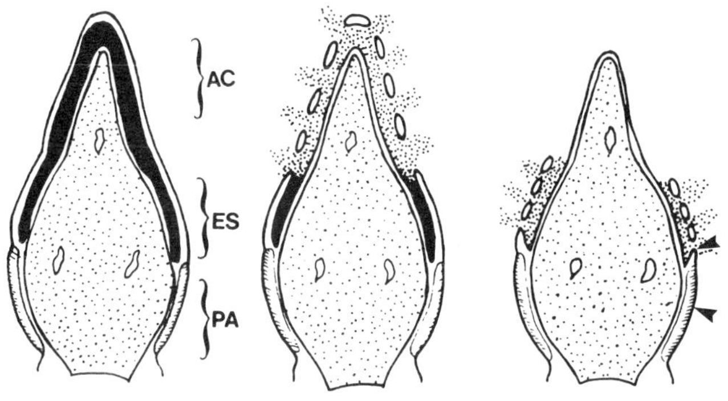

Fig. 4.1 Human sperm acrosome reaction. The illustration of sperm heads shows progressive vesiculation of surface membranes caused by fusion of the plasma and outer acrosomal membranes. The acrosome is the dark structure and consists of a cap (AC) and and equatorial segment (ES). The anterior region of the postacrosomal region (PA) is the fusogenic midsegment of the spermhead (arrowheads). The acrosomal enzymes are shown diffusing out of the acrosome after vesiculation. The nucleus (stippled) occupies most of the head region of the sperm. Reproduced with permission from Sathananthan et al (1986b).

FERTILIZATION

Sperm capacitation

Human sperm, unlike those of many other species, develop the ability to fertilize the oocyte under relatively non-specific conditions. Removal of the seminal plasma component of the ejaculate will result in the progressive capacitation of human sperm and, at any time during incubation after separation of the sperm from seminal plasma, highly motile and acrosome-reacted sperm may be observed to be present. Capacitation includes specific morphological, biochemical and physiological changes in the membranes of the sperm head (Meizel 1978, Yanagimachi 1981).

During capacitation there are marked changes in sperm membrane binding of many substances, including immunoglobulins and lectins (Koehler 1978) and these changes involve glycosylation in order to transform surface glycoproteins into those which enable sperm to bind and fertilize oocytes (Ahuja 1985a). There is also increased sperm motility observed during capacitation and finally the acrosome reaction occurs (Fig. 4.1, 4.2). The acrosome reaction involves the fusion and vesiculation of the plasma membrane with the outer acrosomal membrane (Soupart 1980, Sathananthan 1984). The acrosome consists of a cap and an equatorial segment and the acrosome reaction may occur in two stages, with the cap reacting first followed by the equatorial segment (Fig. 4.1).

Capacitation usually occurs within the female reproductive tract and is difficult to initiate in vitro in many species. Human sperm capacitate spontaneously in vitro in chemically very simple culture media. It is not necessary

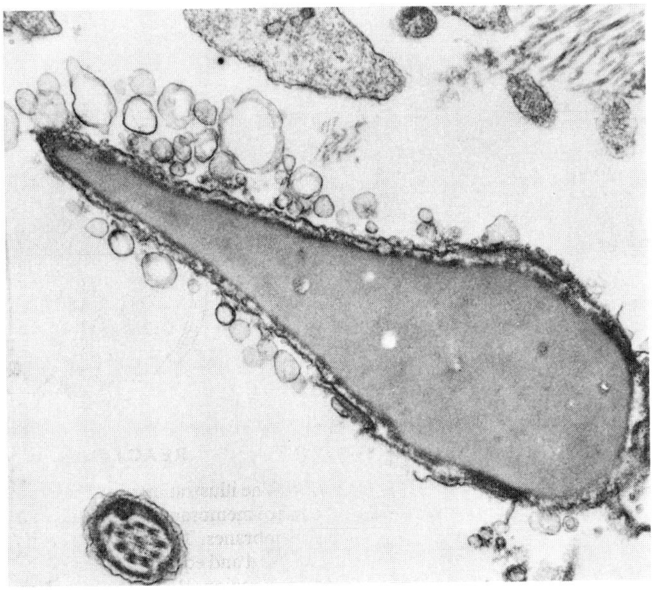

Fig. 4.2 Human sperm head, entering the zona pellucida and undergoing the acrosome reaction by vesiculation of surface membranes. Electron micrograph ×44 100.

for human sperm to be exposed to follicle cells or to follicular fluid for fertilization to occur (Mahadevan & Trounson 1985) nor to supplement culture medium which contains oocytes surrounded by follicle cells with any other protein (Caro & Trounson 1986). A comprehensive review of conditions which enable human sperm to fertilize zona-free hamster oocytes has been published by Yanagimachi (1984). These conditions appear to be the same as those required for human sperm to fertilize human oocytes in vitro.

There are sufficient levels of the enzyme hyaluronidase in seminal plasma or released by the sperm themselves during the acrosome reaction to digest the cumulus oophorus, which is a complex of granulosa and corona radiata cells embedded in a matrix of hyaluronic acid. In fact, the acrosome releases two major enzymes, hyaluronidase and acrosin, a protein-digesting enzyme which is believed to be involved in sperm penetration of the zona pellucida. Both acrosome-reacted and unreacted sperm can be observed in the close vicinity of the zona pellucida but it is only the acrosome-reacted sperm that are capable of penetrating through the glycoprotein matrix of the zona. Prior to zona penetration there is evidently some binding of human sperm that are in close contact with the zona pellucida. The attachment of sperm to the zona is species-specific, involving the binding of specific glycoprotein moieties of the zona and sperm surface membranes (Yanagimachi 1981, Ahuja 1985b).

Sperm transport can also be influenced by a number of conditions within the female reproductive tract. Sperm more readily capacitate under alkaline conditions than in acid conditions which prevail in the vagina. Sperm may be quickly immobilized by immunoglobulins in cervical mucus or by subtle changes in the physical and chemical nature of cervical mucus. It has been reported that a reduction in sialic acid levels in mucus may also be associated with human infertility (Lutjen et al 1985). It is considered that abnormalities of sperm transport are probably responsible for idiopathic (undiagnosed) infertility because both IVF and gamete intrafallopian tube transfer (GIFT), where sperm and oocytes are transferred together into the Fallopian tube (Asch et al 1984), are effective therapies for this type of infertility. Subtle changes in the chemical composition of cervical mucus and in uterine and tubal secretions may reduce the number of capacitated sperm in the tubal ampulla, reducing the chance of fertilization.

The process of fertilization

Fertilization normally occurs in the ampulla of the Fallopian tube. The actual fertilizable lifespan of the human oocyte after ovulation is not known precisely, but apparently mature oocytes obtained for IVF may be inseminated with sperm 19 to 25 hours after aspiration from the follicle. They can be fertilized and develop normally to term when transferred to the uterus (Fishel et al 1984). Fertilization may also occur outside the Fallopian tube, for example in the uterus (Craft et al 1982), and very rarely, intraovarian pregnancies may occur when the oocyte is retained in the ruptured follicle. Sperm can be found in the pouch of Douglas within a few hours of intercourse or artificial insemination (Templeton & Mortimer 1980). There are no accurate data on the fertilizable lifespan of human sperm in vivo, but they may retain their capacity to fertilize zona-denuded hamster oocytes for 6 to 14 days when kept at room temperatures and human oocytes for 5 days (Cohen et al 1985).

There are relatively few sperm at the site of fertilization in most species following natural intercourse, in contrast with the number of sperm (10 000–200 000/ml) used in IVF or transferred with oocytes to the ampulla in the GIFT technique. Reduction of sperm concentration below 10 000/ml in vitro may result in a lowering of fertilization rate (Wolf et al 1984) and the apparent difference in sperm concentrations required for fertilization in vivo and in vitro may be due to selection of sperm by the natural barriers in vivo and more effective capacitation of sperm which migrate to the ampulla in vivo. The presence of the large sticky cumulus at the time of ovulation is important for transport of the oocyte from the surface of the ovary into the ampulla. Cilia on the surface of the fimbria of the Fallopian tube sweep the oocyte cumulus mass into the ciliated ampulla and may assist in moving the oocyte towards the ampulla–isthmus junction. The oocyte is progressively denuded of follicle cells by tubal proteases and never remains stationary because of cilial agitation and ampullary contractions. These movements effectively increase the chance of the few sperm present making contact with the oocyte. Damage to the tubal

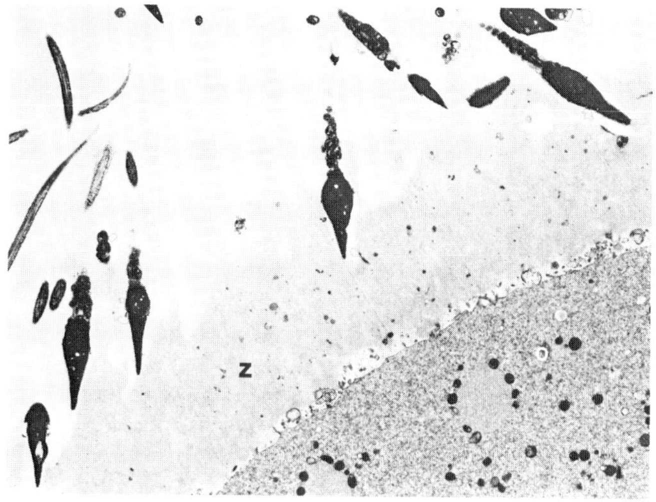

Fig. 4.3 Acrosome-reacted sperm penetrating the outer zona of a polyspermic ovum denuded of its cumulus cells. The sperm are penetrating at all angles and have evidently digested pathways around their heads. These supernumerary sperm have been 'blocked' just outside the inner zona. O = ooplasm; Z = zona pellucida. Electron micrograph ×7000. Reproduced with permission from Sathananthan et al (1986b).

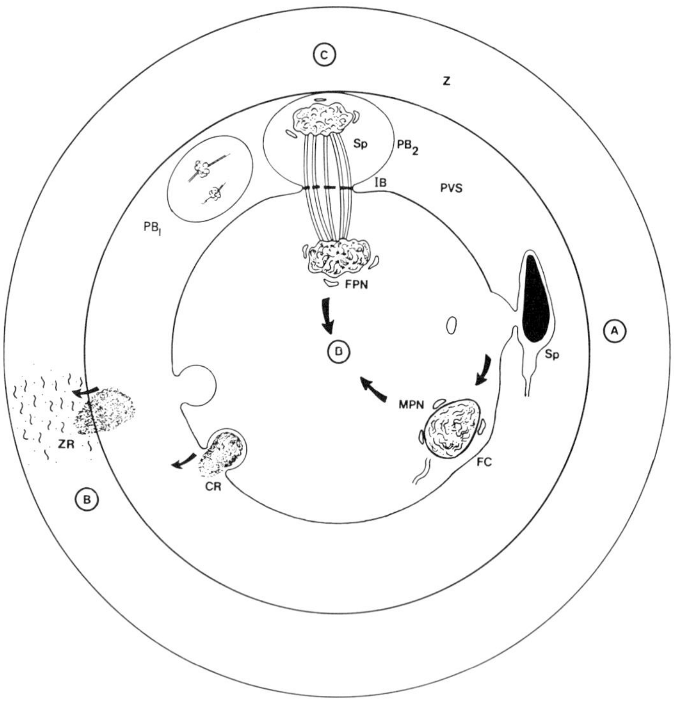

Fig. 4.5 Illustration of the morphological events of fertilization: Ⓐ Sperm–egg fusion and sperm incorporation. Ⓑ Cortical and zona reactions. Ⓒ Completion of meiotic maturation by extrusion of the second polar body. Ⓓ Early formation and association of pronuclei. CR = cortical reaction; FC = fertilization cone; FPN = female pronculeus; IB = interbody; MPN = male pronculeus; PB_1 = first polar body; PB_2 = second polar body; PVS = perivitelline space; Sp = maturation spindle; Z = zona pellucida; ZR = zona reaction. Reproduced with permission Sathananthan et al (1986b).

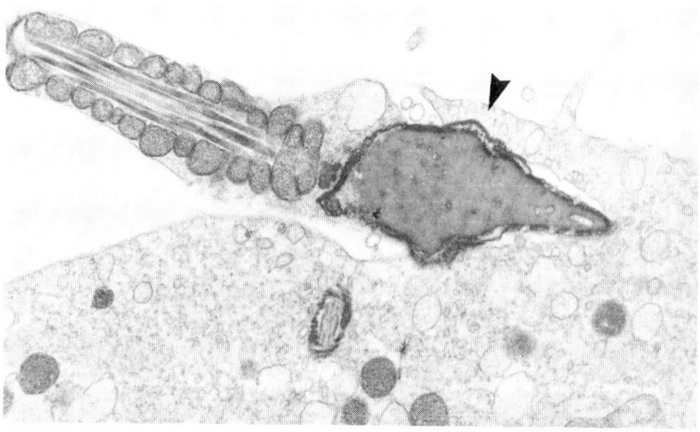

Fig. 4.4 Sperm–egg fusion in the human: the spermhead has been engulfed by a tongue-like process extended from the egg-surface (arrowhead) and the midsegment of the sperm plasma membrane has fused with the oolemma on either side. Electron micrograph ×27 300. Reproduced with permission from Sathananthan et al (1986a).

transport mechanisms may reduce the chance of fertilization and may contribute to the incidence of infertility.

The initial process of fertilization involves passage of the sperm through the cumulus and zona pellucida (Fig. 4.3), entry of the sperm into the perivitelline space, fusion of the mid-segment of the sperm head to oocyte plasma membrane (oolemma; Fig. 4.4), release of cortical granules at the surface of the oolemma (Sathananthan & Trounson 1982), and the gradual incorporation of the whole sperm including the flagellum into the ooplasm. These events have been described at the ultrastructural level in an atlas of human IVF by Sathananthan et al (1986b) and are summarized in Figure 4.5.

During fertilization in vitro, sperm enter the zona pellucida obliquely or tangentially but may be observed entering at all angles in the absence of the cumulus (Fig. 4.3). The acrosomal enzymes help to digest a furrow around the apical and lateral segments of the head in the direction of motion propagated by the vigorously moving flagellum. High sperm concentrations around the oocyte result in many sperm entering the zona and may increase the incidence of polyspermic fertilization (Wolf et al 1984). Incomplete zona formation or incomplete oocyte maturation, where cortical granules have not distributed under the surface of the oolemma, also results in polyspermy (Sathananthan & Trounson 1982). This defect may also include abnormalities of zona glycoproteins which do not enable the normal attachment of sperm as the preliminary step for sperm penetration.

The mature oocyte has many microvilli on the surface of the oolemma which make the initial contact with the sperm head. Sperm incorporation after the initial contact and fusion appears to be an active process because sperm are engulfed by extrusions of the oocyte (Fig. 4.4) and are taken into the ooplasm by the process of phagocytosis (Sathananthan

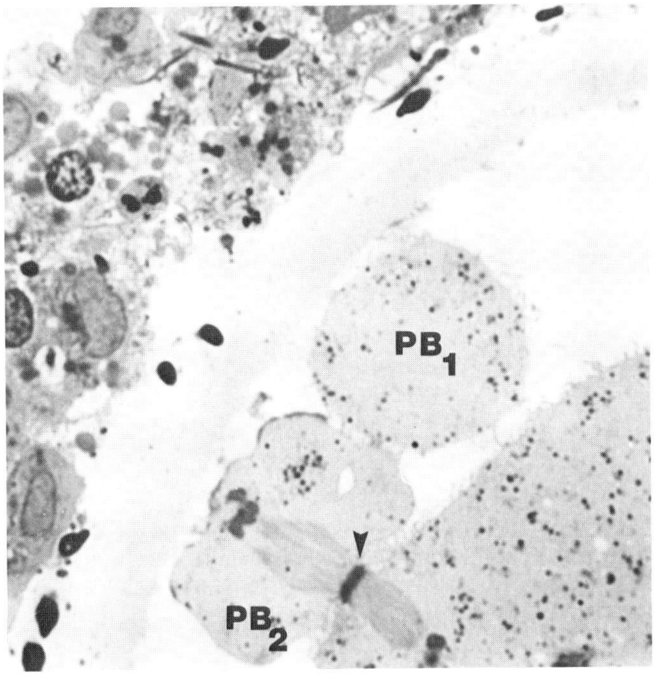

Fig. 4.6 Extrusion of the second polar body into the perivitelline space at fertilization. Chromosomes are located at each pole of the telophase II spindle, associated with an interbody (arrowhead). Supplementary sperm are seen in the outer zona. PB_1 = first polar body; PB_2 = second polar body. Light micrograph ×1500. Reproduced with permission from Sathananthan (1984).

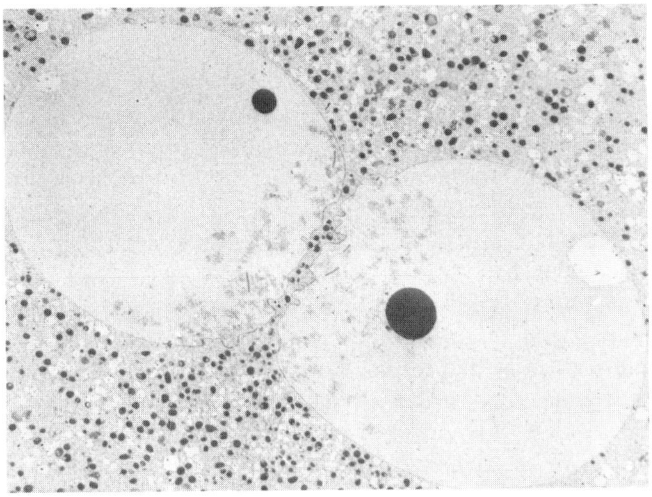

Fig. 4.7 Association of male and female pronuclei in the central ooplasm of a fertilized human ovum. Electron micrograph ×2940. Reproduced with permission from Sathananthan et al (1987).

& Chen 1986). Sperm which enter the perivitelline space through the zona are drawn close to the oolemma and held tangentially along one side of the head during the process of membrane fusion. Perpendicular entry of the apex of the sperm head is a feature of zona-denuded oocytes (Sathananthan et al 1986b) in which the forward thrust of highly motile sperm results in entry with fusion still along the mid-segment of the sperm head. There appears to be no such forward progressive momentum in sperm which enter the perivitelline space through the zona in the human. Only acrosome-reacted or reacting sperm are observed to fuse with the oolemma. The fusion of human sperm with the oolemma may be also mediated by specific glycoproteins but their exact nature is still to be elucidated. Immotile sperm from a patient with Kartagener's syndrome has also resulted in fertilization of zona-denuded human oocytes, showing that sperm motility may not be essential for sperm fusion and incorporation by the oolemma (Ng et al 1987).

The initial reaction of the oocyte to fusion with the sperm head is a rapid and progressive release of the cortical granule contents (Fig. 4.5) from under the oolemma (Sathananthan & Trounson 1982). This appears to progress from the site of sperm fusion and may be accelerated by the rapid efflux of calcium ions from the oocyte. Rapid movement of molecules between closely apposed membranes such as those surrounding the cortical granules and the plasma membrane result in their fusion, releasing cortical contents into the perivitelline space. Cortical granules may fuse with one another at the same time. The cortical contents contain a zona hardening substance which diffuses into the inner zona causing the zona reaction. Alteration occurs to the chemical structure of the inner zona which becomes more electron-dense, traps any sperm in the vicinity and prevents them from penetrating through the zona pellucida. This is the mechanism which normally blocks polyspermy and any delay of the cortical reaction or breach in the zona will usually result in fertilization by more than one sperm.

Sperm fusion with the oolemma also initiates the completion of meiosis in the oocyte (Fig. 4.6). The daughter chromatids held in the second metaphase stage are separated by the microtubules of the anaphase spindle and one complete set of chromosomes is expelled from the oocyte in the extrusion of the second polar body (Sathananthan et al 1986b). Nuclear membranes begin to form around the set of chromosomes retained by the oocyte in close proximity to the second polar body. The sperm head decondenses in the ooplasm and detaches from the flagellum. Specific cytoplasmic factors (proteins) are required for this, and are generated during oocyte maturation (Thibault 1977). A nuclear membrane is also formed around the sperm chromosomes.

Decondensing sperm heads can be located in the ooplasm within 3 hours of inseminating oocytes in vitro (McMaster et al 1978, Sathananthan et al 1986a,b). Pronuclei are visible by 6 hours and may move from peripheral locations to the centre of the oocyte by 12 hours after insemination. The male and female pronuclei in the human are of about equal size (Fig. 4.7) and remain separate but very close together until 20 to 24 hours after insemination, at which time the nuclear membranes are dismantled (Sathananthan & Trounson 1985). At the time the nuclear membrane disappears, a bipolar spindle forms with apices at opposite poles of the pronuclei. The condensing chromosomes are mixed on the metaphase plate of the first cleavage division in a stage termed syngamy. The pronuclei are no longer visible during syngamy and the time between disappearance of the pronuclei and the first cleavage division is 3–6 hours.

It is at syngamy that the maternal and paternal chromosomes are mixed for the first time, restoring the normal diploid constitution of the cell. DNA replication occurs during the pronuclear stage so that equal numbers of paternal and maternal chromosomes will be drawn into each daughter cell by the microtubules during anaphase of the first cleavage division. The cleavage furrow separates the identical components of the new embryonic genome at telophase into equal sized daughter cells or blastomeres. Cleavage is a rapid event, taking less than 10 minutes, and it is at this time that fragmentation may occur. The formation of small anucleate fragments does not normally effect embryonic viability (Killeen & Moore 1971) but severe fragmentation of many different sized anucleate bodies can be a lethal abnormality. Fragmentation occurs frequently in vitro under suboptimal culture conditions and may also be due to incomplete or abnormal oocyte maturation.

Syngamy, rapidly followed by the first cleavage division, marks the completion of fertilization. The pronuclear oocyte has been termed the zygote and initial cleavage stages have been also termed zygote or conceptus. The first cleavage stage until blastocyst stage is usually termed preimplantation embryo (pre-embryo), cleavage stage embryo or conceptus.

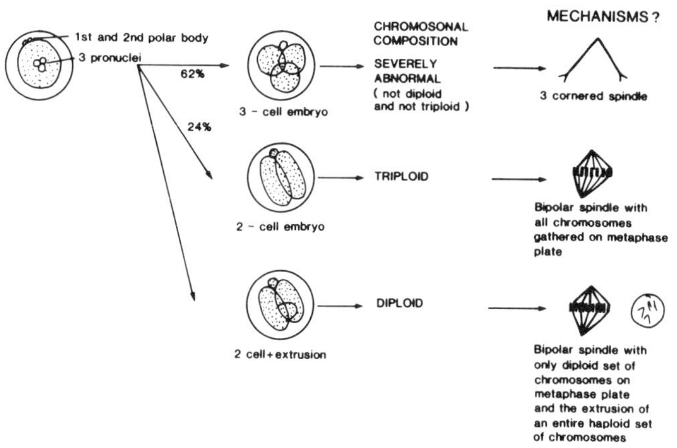

Fig. 4.8 Cleavage patterns and karyotypic analysis of tripronuclear human oocytes.

Fertilization rates

There are very few data on the failure of fertilization in vivo after natural intercourse. Factors contributing to fertilization failure may be both maternal and paternal in origin and will include reduced semen quality, intercourse at an inappropriate time relative to ovulation and factors within the female reproductive tract which reduce sperm transport and survival.

Both IVF and GIFT have been used as treatments for male factor infertility because pregnancy rates with these techniques are higher than those achieved by carefully timed intercourse and artificial insemination with the husband's semen. The probability of pregnancy in male factor infertility may be computed by life table analyses (Baker et al 1986) and compared with pregnancy success rate by IVF (Yates & de Kretser 1987). From data available in IVF, it is apparent that implantation and pregnancy rates for couples with male factor infertility are similar to those with tubal infertility if fertilization can be achieved.

Polyspermy

Multipronuclear oocytes are observed to occur in 2–10% of fertilized oocytes in IVF. The majority (>80%) are tripronuclear and are due primarily to dispermic fertilization (Sathananthan et al 1986b). This is considered the major cause of triploidy which may result in failure of preimplantation embryo development, spontaneous abortion, hydatiform moles and occasionally chorionic tumours or the birth of severely abnormal infants.

A study of tripronuclear oocytes (Kola et al 1987) has shown that the majority (62%) cleave directly to three cells rather than two cells at the first cleavage division (Fig. 4.8). Chromosome numbers in the three individual cells are variable but are never exactly diploid. This may be a lethal condition of chromosome mosaicism with severe hypoploidy and hyperploidy and development is probably limited to preimplantation cleavage. The remainder (38%) of tripronuclear oocytes cleave either to two cells (24%) which are triploid or to two cells which are diploid and an extrusion (14%) which probably contains a haploid set of chromosomes. It is possible that the diploid embryos could contain either maternal and paternal chromosomes and develop normally or contain two sets of paternal chromosomes and be androgenones which develop abnormally, including the possibility of trophoblastic disease (hydatiform moles and chorionic cancer; Patillo & Hussa 1984).

Androgenones have been made in the mouse using nuclear transplantation techniques. The maternal pronucleus is removed and a second paternal pronucleus introduced by micromanipulation. The majority of these artificial androgenones do not implant and those that do, develop abundant trophoblast whilst the embryonic component fails to develop normally (Barton et al 1984). Gynogenones made by transferring a second maternal pronucleus to an oocyte after removal of the paternal pronucleus or by parthenogenetic activation (Barton et al 1984) develop to about the 25 somite stage of embryonic development with inadequate trophoblast and other extraembryonic tissue. These experiments amply demonstrate that both maternally and paternally derived chromosomes are essential for normal embryogenesis in

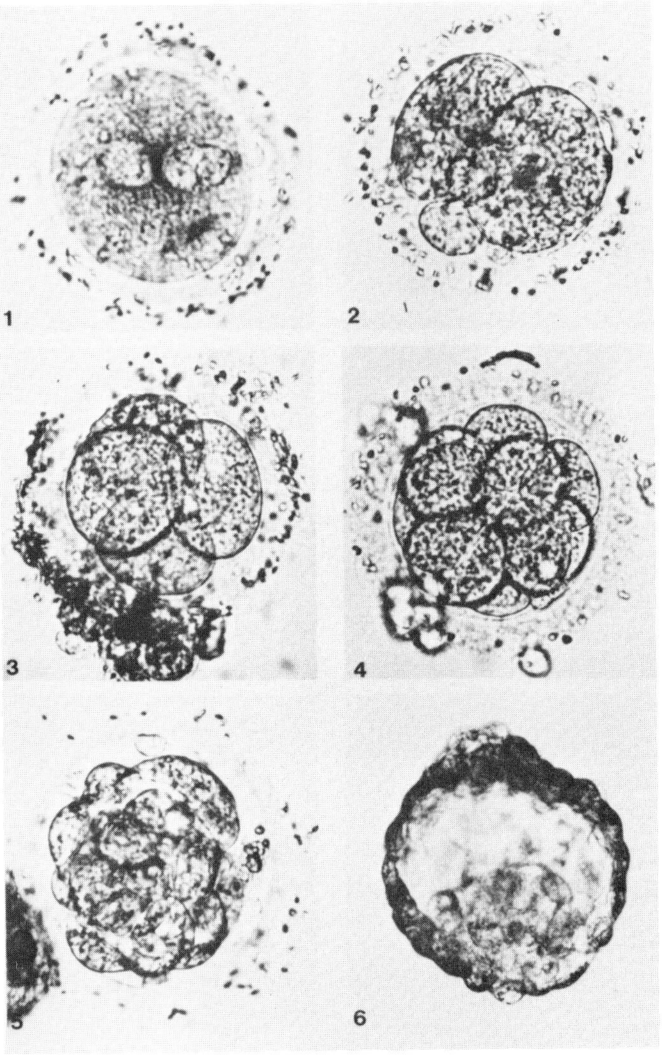

Fig. 4.9 Stages of human preimplantation development. 1. Pronuclear oocyte 16 hours after insemination. 2. Two-cell embryo. 3. Four-cell embryo. 4. Eight-cell embryo. 5. Compacted morula (16 cells). 6. Hatched blastocyst. The inner cell mass is at the lower pole surrounded by trophoblast cells and blastocoelic cavity above. Reproduced with permission from Trounson et al (1982).

mammalian species (McGrath & Solter 1984, Mann & Lovell-Badge 1984, Surani et al 1984, 1986).

EMBRYONIC DEVELOPMENT

Preimplantation embryonic cleavage

The first cleavage stage occurs about 16–22 hours after penetration of the oocyte by the fertilizing sperm (Trounson et al 1982). The second and third cleavage stages (Fig. 4.9) occur at 12–20-hour intervals (Cummins et al 1986). In the mouse the first major product of the new embryonic genome appears at the mid 2-cell stage and has been identified as heat shock protein 70 (Bensaude et al 1983). It is interesting that the embryonic genome may be activated by production

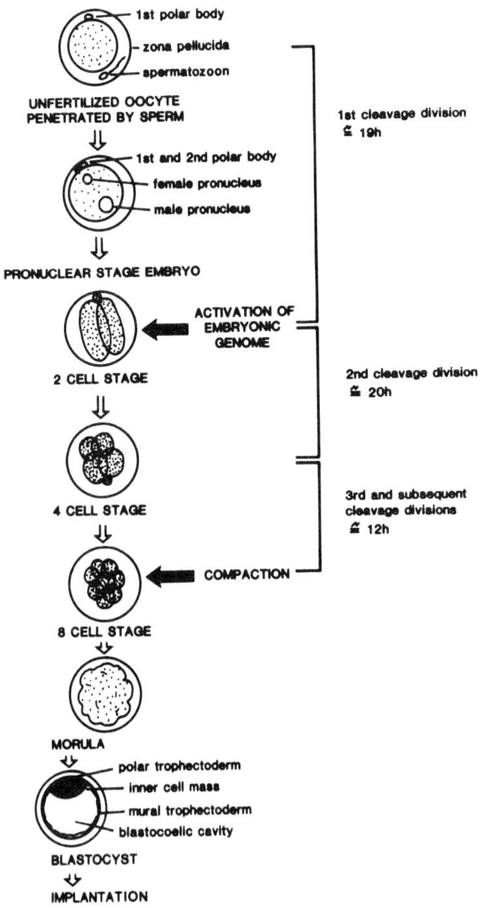

Fig. 4.10 Development of the preimplantation mouse embryo.

of a stress protein and that this occurs in the mouse at the time when many strains of mice have a block (2-cell block) of cleavage in vitro (Fig. 4.10). It is not certain when the human embryonic genome is activated but preliminary experiments suggest this may be between 4- and 8-cell stage (Tesarik et al 1986, Braude et al 1988).

In the mouse at the late 8-cell stage a process of compaction occurs when the cells flatten against each other and become firmly adherent by specific glycoproteins and focal tight junctions (Kimber et al 1982, Pratt et al 1982).

Blastomeres of the compacting 8-cell embryo become polarized (Ziomek & Johnson 1980) and give rise to a heterogeneous population of large polar cells or small non-polar cells when they divide to 16 cells (Johnson & Ziomek 1981). The small non-polar cells are completely internalized and the large polar cells form the outside cells of the morula. It can be shown that the inside or non-polar cells develop into inner cell mass cells and the outside or polar cells develop into the trophoblast lineage. An excellent review of the process of cell polarization, position within the embryo and the resulting lineage of development is given by Johnson (1986). Compaction occurs at the late 8-cell stage or during the next cleavage division in human embryos cultured in vitro (Trounson et al 1982). Figure 4.11 shows the compac-

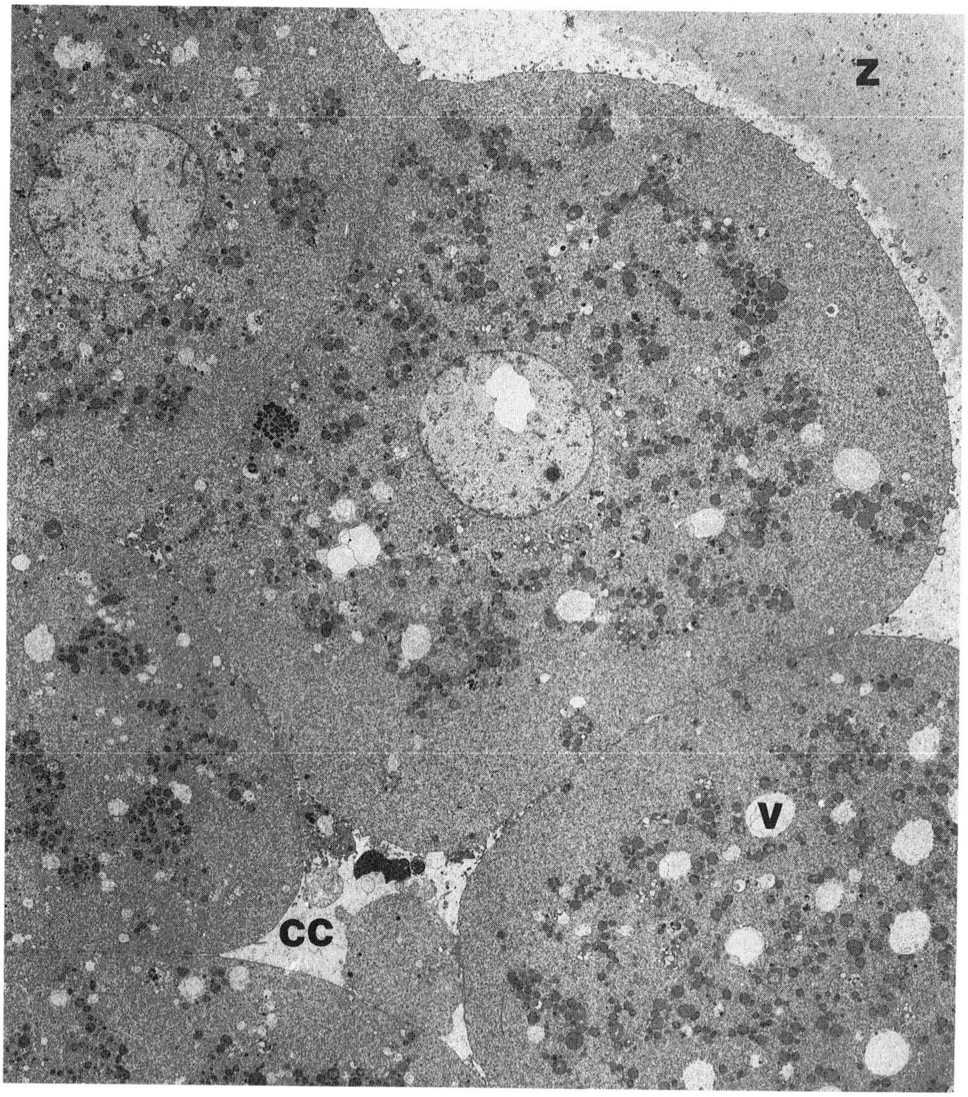

Fig. 4.11 Part of an 8-cell human embryo showing close apposition between blastomeres (early compaction). CC = cleavage cavity; V = vacuole; Z = zona pellucida. Electron micrograph ×2940. Reproduced with permission from Sathananthan et al (1982).

tion of individual blastomeres in a late 8-cell stage human embryo. It is presumed that the blastomeres of the human embryo undergo the same polarization and positioning within the morula as mouse embryos.

Individual blastomeres of the 8-cell mouse embryos lose their totipotency or capacity to form a complete embryo by themselves (Tarkowski & Wroblewska 1967). This may be due to their inability to form sufficient daughter blastomeres before blastulation rather than any intrinsic differentiation. Single blastomeres of 8-cell embryos often cleave and one daughter cell completely internalizes the other in the attempt of compaction (Johnson 1986). Division then ceases. In other species such as the sheep, totipotency still exists at the 8-cell stage; live lambs have been obtained from single blastomeres of this cleavage stage (Willadsen 1981). Compaction occurs at the 16-cell stage and blastulation at the sixth cleavage division in sheep embryos. Interestingly, Willadsen (1986) reported that even single blastomeres of 16-cell sheep embryos when fused into enucleated oocytes can develop to term, indicating that the nuclei of these late cleavage stage embryos have not differentiated and retain their totipotency if cycled through oocyte cytoplasm. In the mouse, blastulation occurs at the fifth cleavage division irrespective of the number of cells. In an intact embryo there are 32 cells with both inside (non-polar) and outside (polar) cells. Blastulation occurs by the pumping of extracellular fluid by outside cells into an intercellular space in the compacted embryo. This fluid-filled cavity, a blastocoele, increases in size, flattening the outside cells against the zona pellucida. The inside cells remain closely attached together at one pole of the blastocyst, becoming the inner cell mass. The flattened outside cells are structurally differentiated into a single layer of flattened trophoblast cells connected by tight junctions and gap junctions. Blastulation in the human occurs at the sixth cleavage division and the morphological structure of the blastocyst is similar to other species (Fig. 4.9; Mohr & Trounson 1982).

Inner cell mass cells are primarily undifferentiated cells which eventually develop into both embryonic and extra-embryonic lineages. The blastocyst emerges from the zona pellucida by the pressure of the expanding blastocoele forcing a crack in the thinned zona. The trophoblast cells emerge through the crack, giving a dumb-bell appearance to the hatching blastocyst. For the first time the cells of the embryo are able to make direct contact with the endometrial cells and it is the trophoblast cells which initiate the maternal–embryonic association necessary for continued embryonic development and the maintenance of pregnancy.

Preimplantation embryonic cleavage is relatively synchronous up to the third cleavage stage; thereafter the cell cycles are less and less synchronized and by the blastocyst stage usually only 10–20% of cells are in mitosis at the same time. From observations in IVF, embryos are 2-celled 24–36 hours after insemination, 4-celled 40–50 hours, 8-celled 52–70 hours, compact 70–86 hours and begin blastulation around 100–120 hours, hatching from the zona 110–140 hours (Trounson et al 1982, Cummins et al 1986). Implantation begins on about the sixth day after fertilization.

DNA methylation in germ cells and embryos

Interest in DNA methylation in the developing embryo is generated by its relationship to gene expression. Current data suggest that a difference exists in the DNA methylation patterns of male and female germ cells. Sanford et al (1984) have shown that the DNA of oocytes is undermethylated for the repetitive sequences, both centromeric and dispersed; it seems probable that oocytes are globally undermethylated. In contrast, the DNA of male germ cells becomes remethylated during spermatogenesis (perhaps at the stage of meiotic arrest) and remains methylated overall. It has been shown (Waalwijk & Flavell 1978) that certain structural genes in sperm are highly methylated. Centromeric sequences in sperm, however, have been shown to be undermethylated (Chapman et al 1984, Ponzetto-Zimmerman & Wolgemuth 1984). The significance of the differential pattern of DNA methylation of male and female germ cells remains to be elucidated.

In other cells a considerable body of evidence now exists which correlates the methylation status of cytosine moieties at certain sites within and near an autosomal gene with its potential to be expressed (Razin & Riggs 1980, Doerfler 1983). Thus when a gene is expressed in a particular tissue, the tendency is for it to be undermethylated and to reside in regions of chromatin more accessible to digestion by the enzyme deoxyribonuclease (Groudine et al 1980, Doerfler 1983). Chapman et al (1984) have also shown that DNA from all derivatives of the two extraembryonic mouse embryo lineages, trophectoderm and primitive endoderm, was substantially undermethylated compared with primitive ectoderm derivatives and adult somatic tissues. These same sequences, however, appear to be fully methylated at 7.5 days of development in the primitive ectoderm cell lineage, which gives rise to the embryo. It has been suggested (Chapman et al 1984) that both specific demethylation of some cytosine CpG sites and failure of de novo methylation may be occurring in preimplantation embryos.

Data on the molecular basis of X chromosome inactivation in mammals suggest that regulation is due to multiple events, one of which is DNA methylation. Holliday & Pugh (1975) proposed that methylation of the pyrimidine base cytosine in DNA might provide a molecular mechanism for X chromosome inactivation in female cells. Inactivation of the X chromosome during mouse embryonic development occurs sequentially; firstly as the extraembryonic lineages differentiate, the paternally inherited X chromosome is inactivated preferentially (Monk 1981) and secondly, just prior to gastrulation the X chromosome is randomly activated, i.e. either the maternal or paternal X chromosome is inactivated. Interestingly, when cells in which the X chromosome is inactive are treated with azacytidine (a chemical which demethylates DNA), the X chromosome is reactivated. Monk (1981) has proposed that X chromosome inactivation is coupled to cell differentiation.

Teratogens and the preimplantation embryo

Most of the research on the effects of exposure of teratogenic stimuli has been directed at the postimplantation stages of pregnancy and more specifically during the period of organogenesis. It is generally agreed that the developing embryo is most susceptible to the induction of malformations during the period of organogenesis. The preimplantation mammalian embryo however, has been shown to be relatively refractory to teratogenesis (i.e. malformations) and this has led to the wide acceptance of the all-or-none phenomenon. This has been interpreted by some teratologists as meaning that the exposure of preimplantation mammalian embryos to noxious physical and chemical stimuli may result in the death of the embryo before implantation or the embryo will survive to term without being malformed (see Spielmann et al 1981).

The effects on preimplantation mouse embryos have been investigated using the immunosuppressive and alkylating agent cyclophosphamide (a potent teratogen in animals) as a model. Cyclophosphamide was shown to have a significant effect on preimplantation embryo viability (Kola & Folb 1986). Viable cyclophosphamide-treated blastocysts were shown to have fewer cells (Eibs & Spielmann 1977, Kola & Folb 1985) and the cells displayed a significant increase in chromosomal aberrations (Kola et al 1986) and sister chromatid exchanges. Preimplantation embryo differentiation was adversely affected and a significantly higher number of embryos were resorbed during organogenesis (Kola et al 1986). However, the number of malformed embryos retrieved at term was not significantly affected. The only detectable difference at term was that the cyclophosphamide-treated fetuses were lower in weight than corresponding controls.

These data demonstrate that teratogenic exposure of preimplantation mammalian embryos induces embryo and fetal loss and that the embryos appear to be refractory to the induction of morphologically detectable abnormalities. However, caution should be exercised in drawing firm conclusions about whether or not malformations can be induced by expressing preimplantation mammalian embryos to teratogens, as Takeuchi (1984) has reported that the exposure of preimplantation mouse embryos to methylnitrosurea induced malformations in embryos retrieved at term. Iannaccone (1984) has shown that methylnitrosurea-treated neonatal mice (exposed to the drug at the blastocyst stage and then transferred into pseudopregnant recipients) had a threefold higher crude mortality rate than corresponding controls.

Nutrition and transport of the preimplantation embryo

The preimplantation cleavage stages can develop in vitro in the absence of any exogenous fixed nitrogen source (protein or amino acids) from the 1-cell to blastocyst stages (Cholewa & Whitten 1965, Caro & Trounson 1984, 1986). Essential amino acids are required for blastocyst hatching and outgrowth in vitro (Spindle & Pedersen 1973). The capacity to develop without exogenous amino acids or protein shows that the early cleavage stages are able to utilize endogenous fixed nitrogen sources for protein synthesis or they convert exogenous energy substrates (glucose, lactate and pyruvate) into amino acids (glutemate, aspartate and alanine; Wales 1975). The protein content of mouse embryos decreases by 26% during the first 3 days of embryonic development (Brinster 1967), as do some of the amino acid pools (Schultz et al 1981) and there is relatively little uptake of exogenous protein before the blastocyst stage (Pemble & Kaye 1986). These observations suggest a preferential utilization of endogenous fixed nitrogen during early cleavage development. The oocyte and preimplantation embryo can synthesize protein from radiolabelled amino acids (Levinson et al 1978) and it is apparent that both endogenous and exogenous amino acids may be used for metabolism in vivo. There is a marked increase in the utilization of exogenous amino acids and protein at the blastocyst stage.

The preimplantation embryo requires exogenous energy sources, primarily lactate and glucose (Brinster 1963). However only pyruvate can act as a single energy source for the first cleavage division (Biggers et al 1967) and the combination of pyruvate and lactate as well as glucose in culture media enables cleavage readily to occur from the 1-cell to blastocyst stage in vitro (Biggers et al 1965). These studies provided the basis for all embryo culture media presently in use.

As distinct from many other species, the human preimplantation embryo can complete development and implant in either the Fallopian tube or the uterus. In the human, ectopic or tubal pregnancy occurs quite frequently but this is exceedingly rare in other species. Fertilization and complete preimplantation development in the uterus was demonstrated by Craft et al (1982), who reported pregnancies after the transfer of sperm and oocytes into the uterus. Others had demonstrated that pronuclear and 2-cell embryos transferred to the uterus result in pregnancy (Trounson et al 1982). These observations show that human tubal and uterine secretions or even peritoneal fluid are relatively non-specific for embryonic nutrition and that embryonic transport from the Fallopian tube to the uterus is not essential for preimplantation embryonic survival, growth and development. Embryos which implant in the tube are unable to proceed to term because of space limitations. The expanding embryo may often cause rupture of the tube, resulting in serious haemorrhage. Ectopic pregnancies which do grow outside the tube or rupture the tube without causing maternal death may develop to term.

The fimbria of the Fallopian tube is responsible for removal of the ovulated oocyte–cumulus mass from the surface of the ovary. Fimbriectomy has been used as a method of sterilization and in most species ovulated oocytes remain on the surface of the ovary if the fimbria is interfered with around the time of ovulation. The oocyte is moved in ampulla by the action of cilia and slow peristaltic contractions of the ampulla. These contractions run from the fimbrial end towards the isthmus, fading at the ampulla–isthmus junction. This is the primary mechanism of oocyte and embryo transport in the Fallopian tube (Thibault 1972) and is supported by reports of fertility in women with Kartagener's syndrome where cilia are immotile (Jean et al 1979). There are strong antiperistaltic contractions in the isthmus under the control of oestrogen and progesterone. These contractions maintain the early cleavage stage embryo at the ampulla–isthmus junction for about 3 days (Croxatto et al 1978). With increasing dominance of progesterone to oestrogen, the antiperistaltic contractions weaken and the embryo passes rapidly into the uterus. It has been shown that surgical removal of the isthmus has no effect on fertility or on embryo survival and development in the pig (Paterson et al 1981).

It is also of interest to note that embryos of many species may develop for 3–4 days in the Fallopian tubes of another species. For example, cow embryos develop normally in the rabbit oviduct (Lawson et al 1972). This supports the notion that the nutritional requirements of the early cleavage stage embryo are relatively non-specific. Despite this, the cleavage rate of embryos in vitro is usually retarded (Harlow & Quinn 1982) so that prolonged culture in vitro reduces embryo viability in all species studied to date. Despite attempts to develop specific culture media based on tubal and uterine

Table 4.1 Embryonic and fetal wastage in vivo and in vitro*

Source of pregnancy, wastage and outcome	Natural conception Wastage (%)	Natural conception Cumulative survival (%)	In vitro fertilization† Wastage (%)	In vitro fertilization† Cumulative survival (%)
		100		100
Fertilization failure	16	84	14	86
Failure of preimplantation zygote development				
days 14–16 for IVF			2	84
days 14–21 for natural conception	18	69		
Implantation failure				
days 17–28 for IVF			82	15
days 22–28 for natural conception	39	42		
Pregnancy loss between weeks 5 and 40	26	31	34	9
Live births	—	31	—	9

* These estimates were of embryonic wastage following natural conception (based on Leridon 1977) and IVF (based on unpublished data from the Monash IVF programme, 1983–1986). These calculations assume that the sperm and ova are brought into contact in all cases. (This is obviously not the case under natural circumstances where a number of problems, including anovulation, reduced semen quality and intercourse at the incorrect time can interfere. Estimates of maximum human fecundability calculated to include these additional factors range from 14.4 to 31.8% for various populations and age groups of women; Leridon 1977.)
† IVF figures for fertilization, embryo development and implantation are per patient, not per embryo. Following superovulation an average of five oocytes is normally collected. The respective failure rates per oocyte or embryo are: fertilization 30%; early development 10%; implantation 90%.

secretions (Tervit et al 1972, Menezo et al 1984, Quinn et al 1985) none have prevented the retardation of cleavage in vitro and there is a growing interest in the use of physiological fluids (Gianaroli et al 1986) and media conditioned by tubal epithelial cells for culture of embryos in vitro.

Pre- and postimplantation embryonic normality and survival

Accurate figures for embryonic wastage during the first 2 weeks of development in the human are not readily available. Estimates by Leridon (1977; based on the work of Hertig et al 1956, French & Bierman 1962) calculate embryonic wastage in the first week (from fertilization to the commencement of implantation) at 18% with a further 39% of embryos failing in the second week of development (see Table 4.1). Further support for this high early embryonic wastage rate in the human compared with most other mammalian species studied comes from the work of Buster et al (1985). Of 25 preimplantation embryos flushed from the uterus between 93 and 130 hours after ovulation, only 5 (20%) were at the expected blastocyst stage of development. Studies on the chromosomal numbers of preimplantation embryos also reveal a high rate of abnormalities. In two studies on human embryos obtained either from volunteer egg donors or as spare or reject embryos from IVF, 2 out of 3 and 8 out of 22 were chromosomally abnormal (Angell et al 1983, 1986). However, these studies may not reflect the normal in vivo situation for three reasons: the high age of the maternal donors (mean 34 years); the fact that all women had undergone superovulation, and the in vitro treatment of the gametes. Karyotyping studies do not identify those embryos with normal chromosome compliments but carrying other genetic abnormalities. Although only 0.56% of liveborn babies are chromosomally abnormal (Evans 1977), over 50% of spontaneous abortions carry a lethal chromosome anomaly (Hassold et al 1980). These figures demonstrate that although there is a high incidence of chromosomal and genetic abnormality in the human preimplantation embryo, such defective embryos are usually lost by pregnancy wastage well before birth.

Surveys of in vivo conception using immunological assays and other tests for early indicators of conception, e.g. early pregnancy factor (Morton et al 1977) or platelet activating factor (O'Neil et al 1985) have not as yet been given sufficient scientific credibility for use in determining preimplantation wastage in vivo.

IMPLANTATION

Embryo implantation encompasses a complex series of events that vary quite markedly between different mammalian species. Understanding of the processes involved in implantation is poor even in the frequently studied laboratory rodents. Needless to say, morphological and physiological information on human implantation is very scarce, with most descriptions relying on a few classical publications (Hertig et al 1956, Knoth & Larsen 1972, O'Rahilly 1973).

In its broadest sense, implantation is taken to include orientation of the blastocyst within the uterus, dissolution of the zona pellucida, attachment, migration through the epithelium, localized disruption of the endometrial capillaries and the formation of trophoblastic lacunae. In the human, these processes take place during the 6th to 12th days after ovulation (ovulation is day 0) although some uncertainty exists about the exact timing of individual events.

It has been estimated that the preimplantation embryo passes through the isthmus into the uterine cavity 68–80 hours after ovulation (Croxatto et al 1978). For the next 40–76 hours the embryo is free-floating within the uterus, which at this stage has a flattened or slit-like lumen. Animal studies have demonstrated precise uterine control over blastocyst orientation and positioning within the uterus during this period (Rogers et al 1983b), and since human implantation generally occurs on the median portion of the uterine wall (equivalent to antimesometrially in a bicornuate uterus) with the embryonic disc oriented towards the endometrium, it is probable that similar mechanisms exist in the human.

In rodent blastocysts, trophoblast cells at the abembryonic pole (opposite to the inner cell mass) become sticky and contain large vesicles of unknown substances. This transfor-

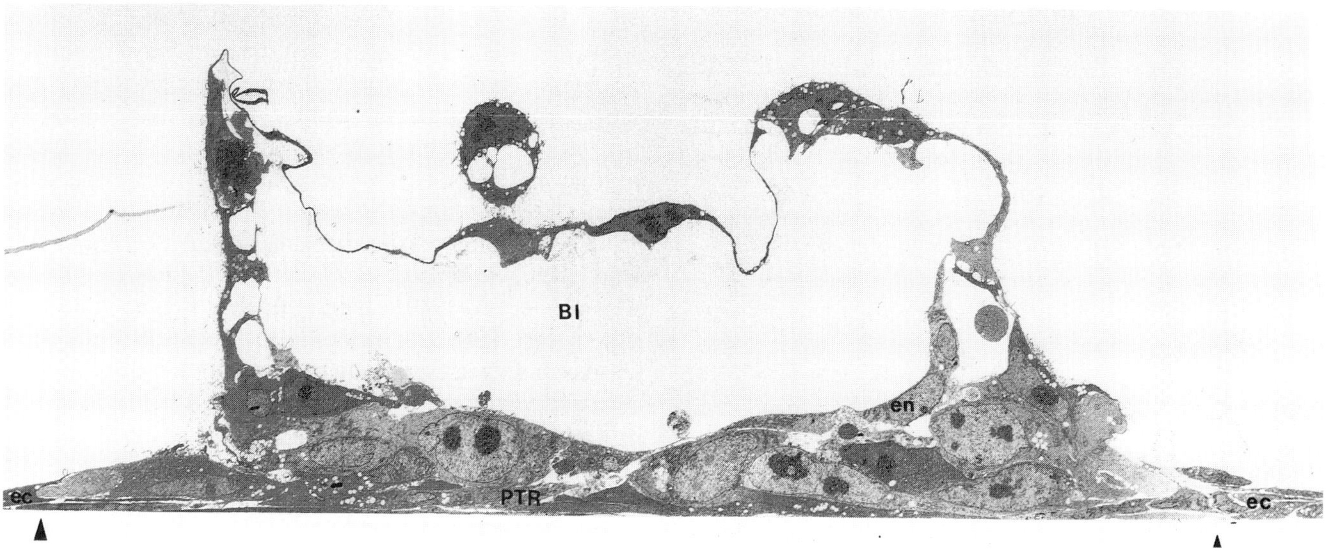

Fig. 4.12 Human blastocyst implanted in vitro with expanded blastocoele (Bl). Arrows indicate attachment to endometrial cells (ec). Inner cell mass cells, polar trophoblast cells (PTR) and endodermal cells (en) are at the pole of attachment to endometrial cells, and mural trophoblast cells are at the opposite pole. Reproduced by kind permission of Dr Svend Lindenberg.

mation at the abembryonic pole occurs within a few hours of implantation and is probably the reason why rodent embryos adhere to the endometrium and implant with the embryonic disc orientated away from the endometrium (Lindenberg et al 1988). Secretory vesicles similar to those released from mouse blastocysts can be observed bulging from the surface of human trophoblast cells allowed to implant on endometrial cells in culture (Lindenberg et al 1986, Lindenberg & Hyttel 1988).

In the human, as in the guinea-pig, lemming and chimpanzee, the blastocyst attaches to the uterine wall after escape from the zona pellucida before migrating through the epithelium into the underlying endometrial stroma (Finn & Porter 1975). Since blastocysts can be flushed from the uterine cavity 5 days after ovulation (Buster et al 1985) no firm attachment to the uterine epithelium occurs until about the sixth day. In vitro studies by Lindenberg et al (1986) with implanting human blastocysts show that the polar trophoblast cells adjacent to the inner cell mass are involved in the primary adhesion to the endometrial cells (Fig. 4.12). These in vitro studies show that initial penetration of the epithelium by the polar trophoblast is via long slender ectoplasmic protrusions which insinuate themselves between the endometrial cells (Fig. 4.13). The trophoblast cells were not phagocytotic at this stage as no degenerating epithelial cells were observed. Endometrial cells respond to the initial penetration of the cytotrophoblast by increased membrane activity which may represent either endo- or exocytosis (Fig. 4.14). In most other species similar membrane activity is endocytotic (Parr & Parr 1977). This process may be responsible for the transfer of messengers, which probably include glycoproteins such as hCG necessary for maternal recognition and the maintenance of pregnancy.

Little is known about the local endocrine requirements for human implantation. Local effects of cAMP (Holmes & Bergstrom 1975, Webb 1975) and prostaglandins, particularly PGE_2 (Holmes & Gordashko 1980), have been shown to induce implantation in diapausing mouse blastocysts. Prostaglandins also play a role in the vascular changes seen within the endometrium at the time of implantation (Kennedy & Armstrong 1981). It is likely that these substances are also involved during human implantation. In addition the production of steroids, such as the sulphated oestrogens by the pig blastocysts may be required for implantation and the maintenance of pregnancy (Perry et al 1973). Reports of plasminogen activator secretion by early embryonic trophoblast and parietal endoderm cells are consistent with the highly invasive nature of the early embryo and the major tissue reorganization that follows implantation (Strickland et al 1976). It is interesting that in the pig, where the implanting embryo does not breach the uterine epithelium, a uterine-derived progesterone-dependent inhibitor of plasminogen activator nullifies the embryonic secretion of this proteolytic activator (Mullins et al 1981). In comparison, the implantation stage pig embryo is highly invasive when placed in contact with non-uterine tissues. The role of plasminogen activator in human implantation is unknown at this time.

By 7–8 days after ovulation the embryo is fully embedded in the superficial layers of the endometrium, and the epithelium has started to migrate inwards to cover the exposed area. At this time the embryonic trophoblast begins to differentiate into syncytiotrophoblast and cytotrophoblast, with the syncytiotrophoblast forming the outermost layer between the endometrium and the invading embryo. The syncytial tissues project into the surrounding endometrium, in what appears to be an invasive growth phase. Intact mater-

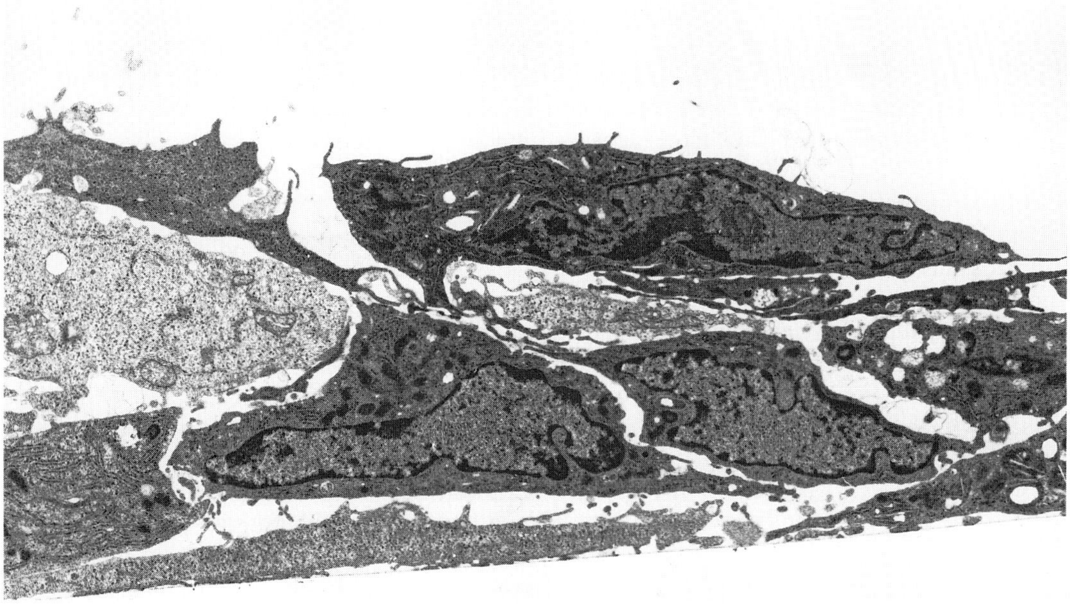

Fig. 4.13 Peripheral implantation zone of a human blastocyst in vitro. The darker cells are cells of the endometrial monolayer and the lighter cells are trophoblast cells with their long protrusions intruding between the endometrial cells. Reproduced by kind permission of Dr Svend Lindenberg.

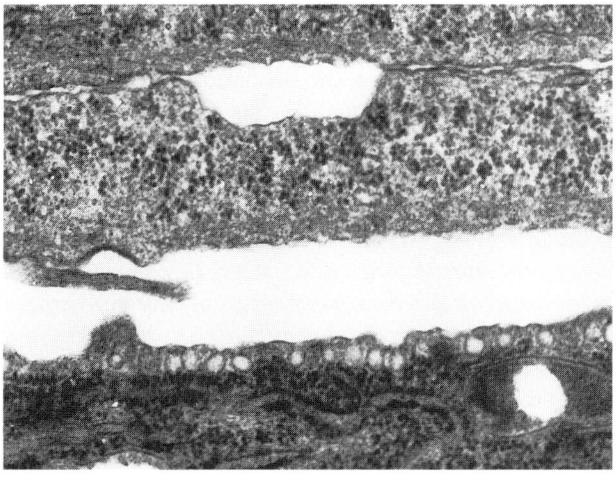

Fig. 4.14 A higher magnification electron micrograph of a trophoblastic ectoplasmic protrusion (see Fig. 4.13) between endometrial cells. Note the pinocytotic activity of closely associated endometrial cells. Reproduced by kind permission of Dr Svend Lindenberg.

nal capillaries can be traced to and from the syncytiotrophoblast, although within these areas red blood cells occupy a series of irregularly shaped spaces (Harris & Ramsey 1966). Macroscopically no congestion or haemorrhage is visible in the endometrium at this time, although microscopic examination reveals dilated capillaries and sinusoids. The embryonic disc is composed of two layers, the epiblast and the primary endoderm. The first signs of an amniotic cavity also appear, probably arising from cells of the embryonic disc (Luckett 1973), although it has been postulated that cytotrophoblastic cells are also involved in its formation.

By the ninth day after ovulation the syncytial mass surrounding the embryo is some 500–600 μm in diameter, while the embryonic disc remains at approximately 100 μm. Maternal endometrial vessels form communications with the numerous lacunae that develop within the syncytiotrophoblast at this stage, as a prelude to the placental circulation. It is not until this stage (9 days after ovulation or 23 days of a standard 28-day menstrual cycle) that predecidual cells first appear in the endometrium surrounding the embryo. Animal studies have shown a major localized increase in uterine vascular permeability around the implantation site (Rogers et al 1983a) leading to significant oedema. Oedema is also clearly seen surrounding the human implantation site at this time. It is probably this oedema, coupled with localized hyperaemia, that makes it possible to visualize human implantation sites from about this stage of development onwards using high-resolution ultrasound with a vaginal probe. The amniotic cavity has nearly developed to a fully enclosed structure by this stage, bordering on an embryonic disc that has not changed size significantly over the previous 3–4 days.

The human implantation site 11–12 days after ovulation is readily recognizable macroscopically as a 1 mm diameter red spot on the mucosal surface of the uterus. This appearance is due to maternal blood passing through the lacunar spaces within the syncytiotrophoblast. By this stage the syncytial mass surrounding the embryo is 750–1000 μm in diameter, with the syncytiotrophoblast forming about three-quarters of the whole trophoblast. Along with the developing lacunar circulation, large numbers of maternal red blood cells appear within the syncytiotrophoblast, apparently undergoing phagocytosis. Oedema around the implantation site is still present, while stromal cells show more signs of decidualization.

At this stage, cells forming the extraembryonic mesoderm, which is still lined by cytotrophoblast, begin to aggregate as precursors to chorionic villus formation. The combined syncytiotrophoblast, cytotrophoblast and extraembryonic mesoderm are collectively termed the chorion by this stage. Ultrastructural studies of an implantation site at this time (Knoth & Larsen 1972) show the syncytiotrophoblast invading maternal vessels, with the syncytium having many microvilli and pinocytotic vesicles at its surface.

Uterine factors in pregnancy wastage

Implantation failure provides the single largest contributing factor to pregnancy wastage in the human, both following natural conception (39% failure rate) and IVF (84% failure rate; see Table 4.1). While much of this failure is due to chromosomal and developmental abnormalities within the embryo, it seems certain that uterine factors must also contribute to this embryonic wastage. While it is not possible to calculate the relative contribution of embryonic and uterine factors to this high natural wastage rate in vivo, such calculations have been made using data generated by IVF programmes (Rogers et al 1986). In these calculations it was assumed that successful implantation depended on two factors: embryonic viability and uterine receptivity. For implantation to occur both a viable embryo and a receptive uterus were necessary. Using this simplified biological model in conjunction with multiple embryo transfer and pregnancy results from four large IVF programmes, it was calculated that uterine receptivity varied between 31 and 64% while embryo viability was between 21 and 32%. These figures indicate that reduced uterine receptivity may play a significant role in implantation failure following IVF. Looking at the uterine receptivity figures in more detail, it was found that patients receiving combined clomiphene citrate and human menopausal gonadotrophin (hMG) superovulation therapy had estimated uterine receptivity values of 31–42%, while those receiving hMG alone had values of 64%. These results suggest that superovulation therapy, with its resulting high oestrogen and progesterone levels, may influence the capacity of the uterus to receive implantation. It is also possible that the antioestrogen, climiphene citrate, may reduce uterine receptivity in some patients. While low uterine receptivity may reduce implantation rates following IVF it does not necessarily follow that the same is true following normal conception. Until suitable morphological or biochemical parameters are established to define uterine receptivity for implantation, the possible anti-implantation role of various superovulation drugs must remain mostly hypothetical.

Both the uterus and the blastocyst have active roles in the initiation of implantation. However, the subsequent success or otherwise of the early embryo-uterine interaction will be determined by a properly prepared uterus. When the uterus is preconditioned with the correct sequence of oestrogen and progesterone (Lutjen et al 1984) and when a blastocyst which is ready to implant is present in the uterine lumen at exactly the correct time, implantation will occur. In comparison, trophoblast cells derived from preimplantation embryos transferred to non-uterine (ectopic) sites nearly always initiate an implantation type reaction, regardless of the sex or hormonal status of the recipient (e.g. Fawcett et al 1947, Kirby 1963).

The mechanisms which control uterine receptivity or hostility to the implanting embryo are unknown. Studies in rats and mice have demonstrated the presence of embryotoxic substances in the uterine luminal fluid at times in the oestrous cycle when an embryo would not normally be present (Weitlauf 1978, Psychoyos & Casimiri 1981). However, similar experiments investigating the capacity of human uterine flushings to effect the in vitro development of mouse blastocysts failed to demonstrate any such inhibitory substance (Aitken & Maathuis 1978). There is reason to believe that the uterine luminal epithelium may play a significant role in regulating the ability of the blastocyst to implant. Cowell (1969) demonstrated that in the mouse implantation will occur in a non-progestational uterus if the epithelium is first removed. Despite the formation of some relatively normal-looking uterine decidual cells, fetal development was abnormal.

Further evidence to support the crucial role of the uterine epithelium in implantation comes from ultrastructural and molecular studies. In the rat, the luminal plasma membrane of the epithelium undergoes characteristic changes in profile depending upon the circulating levels of ovarian hormones. For most of the reproductive cycle the epithelial cells are covered by long thin regular microvilli. As the time of implantation approaches these microvilli are replaced by short flattened projections and other irregular processes (Ljungkvist 1972). These microvillar changes are accompanied by changes in membrane molecular organization, including protein density (Murphy et al 1982a), cholesterol quantity (Murphy & Martin 1985) and cell surface carbohydrate composition (Anderson & Hoffmann 1984). Changes in microvillus length and density have also been reported in ultrastructural studies on human endometrium from different stages of the menstrual cycle (Lawn 1973).

There is a large degree of variability in ultrastructural appearance between patients from similar stages of the cycle, making the correlation of such features with potential uterine receptivity for implantation difficult (Murphy et al 1987). It has also been shown that there are significant changes in uterine epithelial cell tight junction formation during the menstrual cycle (Murphy et al 1982b). This observation may prove to be important in determining whether the blastocyst is capable of intruding between the epithelial cells in vivo in a similar fashion as has been described in vitro by Lindenberg et al (1986). Further studies are required to understand better the role of the human uterine epithelium in the control of this intrusive type of implantation.

CONCLUSIONS

The knowledge which is rapidly accumulating on fertilization, preimplantation embryo development and implantation in the human from a number of new research initiatives and medical applications is providing much-needed illumination into the problems of infertility, pregnancy failure, the reasons for birth defects and fetal abnormalities. Already this information has had a profound effect on the treatment of infertility, raising great ethical and social debates; these have resulted in legislative action to regulate and control many aspects of the new reproductive technologies. It is rare that developments in medicine have such deeply felt consequences for all of us. Modern day clinicians should be well informed of the recent expansion of knowledge in the area of conception and early embryonic development in order to comprehend the clinical significance of the new reproductive technologies for their patients. This is also necessary for any reasonable discussion of the medical, social, ethical and legal issues which are raised by these new technologies. The information provided in this chapter will be helpful in this.

REFERENCES

Ahuja K K 1985a Inhibitors of glycoprotein biosynthesis block fertilization in the hamster. Gamete Research 11: 179–189

Ahuja K K 1985b Carbohydrate determinants involved in mammalian fertilization. American Journal of Anatomy 174: 207–223

Aitken R J, Maathuis J B 1978 Effect of human uterine flushings collected at various states of the menstrual cycle on mouse blastocysts in vitro. Journal of Reproduction and Fertility 53: 137–140

Anderson T L, Hoffmann L H 1984 Alterations in epithelial glycocalyx of rabbit uteri during early pseudopregnancy and pregnancy, and following ovariectomy. American Journal of Anatomy 171: 321–324

Angell R R, Aitken R J, van Look P F A, Lumsden M A, Templeton A A 1983 Chromosome abnormalities in human embryos after in vitro fertilization. Nature 303: 336–338

Angell R R, Templeton A A, Aitken R J 1986 Chromosome studies in human in vitro fertilization. Human Genetics 72: 333–339

Asch R H, Ellsworth L R, Balmaceda J P, Wong P C 1984 Pregnancy after translaparoscopic gamete intrafallopian transfer. Lancet ii: 1034–1035

Baker H W G, Burger H G, de Kretser D M, Hudson B 1986 Relative incidence of etiological disorders in male infertility. In: Santen R J, Swerdloff R S (eds) Diagnosis and management of hypogonadism, infertility and impotence. Marcel Dekker, New York, pp 341–372

Barton S C, Surani M A H, Norris M L 1984 Role of paternal and maternal genomes in mouse development. Nature 311: 374–376

Bensaude O, Babinet C, Morange M, Jacob F 1983 Heat shock proteins, first major products of zygotic gene activity in mouse embryo. Nature 305: 331–333

Biggers J D, Moore B D, Whittingham D G 1965 Development of mouse embryos in vivo after cultivation from the two-cell ova to blastocysts in vitro. Nature 206: 734–735

Biggers J D, Whittingham D G, Donahue R P 1967 The pattern of energy metabolism in the mouse oocyte and zygote. Proceedings of the National Academy of Sciences (USA) 58: 560–567

Braude P, Bolton V, Moore S 1988 Human gene expression first occurs between the four- and eight-cell stages of preimplantation development. Nature 332: 459–461

Brinster R L 1963 A method for in vitro cultivation of mouse ova from two-cell to blastocyst. Experimental Cell Research 32: 205–208

Brinster R L 1967 Protein content of the mouse embryo during the first five days of development. Journal of Reproduction and Fertility 13: 413–420

Buster J E, Bustillo M, Rodi I A et al 1985 Biologic and morphologic development of donated human ova recovered by nonsurgical uterine lavage. American Journal of Obstetrics and Gynecology 153: 211–217

Caro C M, Trounson A 1984 The effect of protein on preimplantation mouse embryo development in vitro. Journal of In Vitro Fertilization and Embryo Transfer 1: 183–187

Caro C M, Trounson A 1986 Successful fertilization, embryo development, and pregnancy in human in vitro fertilization (IVF) using chemically defined culture medium containing no protein. Journal of In Vitro Fertilization and Embryo Transfer 3: 215–217

Carson R S, Trounson A O, Findlay J K 1982 Successful fertilization of human oocytes in vitro: concentration of estradiol-17β, progesterone and androstenedione in the antral fluid of donor follicles. Journal of Clinical Endocrinology and Metabolism 55: 798–800

Chapman V, Forrester L, Sanford J, Hastie N, Rossant J 1984 Cell lineage specific undermethylation of mouse repetitive DNA. Nature 307: 284–286

Cholewa J A, Whitten W K 1965 Development of 2-cell mouse embryos in vitro. III. The effect of fixed nitrogen source. Journal of Experimental Zoology 158: 69–78

Cohen J, Fehilly C B, Walters D E 1985 Prolonged storage of human spermatozoa at room temperature or in a refrigerator. Fertility and Sterility 44: 254–262

Cowell T P 1969 Implantation and development of mouse eggs transferred to the uteri of non-progestational mice. Journal of Reproduction and Fertility 19: 239–245

Craft I L, Djahanbakheh O, McLeod F et al 1982 Human pregnancies following intrauterine transfer of preovulatory oocytes and sperm. Lancet ii: 1031–1033

Crosby I M, Osborn J C, Moor R M 1981 Follicle cell regulation of protein synthesis and developmental competance in sheep oocytes. Journal of Reproduction and Fertility 62: 575–582

Croxatto H B, Ortiz M E, Diaz S, Hess R, Balmaceda J, Croxatto H-D 1978 Studies on the duration of egg transport by the human oviduct II. Ovum locations at various intervals following luteinizing hormone peak. American Journal of Obstetrics and Gynecology 132: 629–634

Cummins J M, Breen T M, Harrison K L, Shaw J M, Wilson L M, Hennessey J F 1986 A formula for scoring human embryo growth rate in in vitro fertilization: its value in predicting pregnancy and in comparison with visual estimates of embryo quality. Journal of In Vitro Fertilization and Embryo Transfer 3: 284–295

Dekel N, Lawrence T S, Gilula N B, Beers W H 1981 Modulation of cell-to-cell communication in the cumulus–oocyte complex and the regulation of oocyte maturation by LH. Developmental Biology 86: 356–362

Doerfler W 1983 DNA methylation and gene activity. Annual Review of Biochemistry 52: 93–124

Eibs H G, Spielmann H 1977 Inhibition of postimplantation development of mouse blastocysts *in vitro* after cyclophosphamide treatment *in vivo*. Nature 270: 54–56

Eppig J J, Downs S M, Schroeder A C 1985 Perspectives of mammalian oocyte maturation in vitro and practical applications. In: Testart J, Frydman R (eds) Human in vitro fertilization. Elsevier, Amsterdam, pp 33–43

Evans H J 1977 Chromosome anomalies among live births. Journal of Medical Genetics 14: 309–312

Fawcett D W, Wioslocki G B, Waldo C M 1947 The development of mouse ova in the anterior chamber of the eye and in the abdominal cavity. American Journal of Anatomy 81: 413–443

Finn C A, Porter D G 1975 Implantation of ova. In: Finn C A (ed) The uterus. Reproductive Biology Handbooks, Elek Science, London, pp 55–73

Fishel S B, Edwards R G, Purdy J M 1984 Births after a prolonged delay between oocyte recovery and fertilization in vitro. Gamete Research 9: 175–181

French F E, Bierman J E 1962 Probabilities of fetal mortality. Public Health Report 77: 835–847

Gianaroli L, Serracchioli R, Ferraretti A P, Trounson A, Flamigni C, Bovicelli L 1986 The successful use of human amniotic fluid for mouse embryo culture and human in vitro fertilization, embryo culture and transfer. Fertility and Sterility 46: 907–913

Groudine M, Eisenmann R, Weintraub H 1980 Chromatin structure of endogenous retroviral genes and activation by an inhibitor of DNA methylation. Science 292: 311–317

Harlow G M, Quinn P 1982 Development of preimplantation mouse embryos in vivo and in vitro. Australian Journal of Biological Science 35: 187–193

Harris J W S, Ramsey E M 1966 The morphology of human uteroplacental vasculature. Carnegie Institute of Washington, Publication 625, Contributions to Embryology 33: 43–58

Hassold T, Chen N, Funkhouser J et al 1980 A cytogenetic study of 1000 spontaneous abortions. Annals of Human Genetics 44: 151–176

Hertig A T, Rock J, Adams E C 1956 A description of 34 human ova within the first 17 days of development. American Journal of Anatomy 98: 435–493

Hillier S G, Wickings E J, Afnan M, Margara R A, Harlow C R, Winston R M L 1985 Sex steroids and oocyte function. In: Rolland R, Heineman M J, Hillier S G, Vemer H (eds) Gamete quality and fertility regulation. Excerpta Medica, Amsterdam, pp 43–52

Holliday R, Pugh J E 1975 DNA modification mechanisms and gene activity during development. Science 187: 226–232

Holmes P V, Bergstrom S 1975 Induction of blastocyst implantation in mice by cyclic AMP. Journal of Reproduction and Fertility 43: 329–332

Holmes P V, Gordashko B J 1980 Evidence of prostaglandin involvement in blastocyst implantation. Journal of Embryology and Experimental Morphology 55: 109–122

Iannaccone P M 1984 Long-term effects of exposure to methylnitrosurea on blastocysts following transfer to surrogate female mice. Cancer Research 44: 2785–2789

Jean Y, Langlais J, Roberts K D, Chapdelaine A, Bleau G 1979 Fertility of a woman with nonfunctional ciliated cells in the fallopian tubes. Fertility and Sterility 31: 349–350

Johnson M H 1986 Manipulation of early mammalian development: what does it tell us about cell lineages? In: Gwatkin R B L (ed) Developmental biology, vol 4, Manipulation of mammalian development. Plenum Press, New York, pp 279–296

Johnson M H, Ziomek C A 1981 The foundation of two distinct cell lineages within the mouse morula. Cell 24: 71–80

Kennedy T G, Armstrong D T 1981 The role of prostaglandins in endometrial vascular changes at implantation In: Glasser S R, Bullock D W (eds) Cellular and molecular aspects of implantation. Plenum Press, New York, pp 349–364

Killeen I D, Moore N W 1971 The morphological appearance and development of sheep ova fertilized by surgical insemination. Journal of Reproduction and Fertility 24: 63–70

Kimber S J, Surani M A H, Barton S C 1982 Interactions of blastomeres suggest changes in cell surface adhesiveness during the formation of inner cell mass and trophectoderm in the preimplantation mouse embryo. Journal of Embryology and Experimental Morphology 70: 133–152

Kirby D R S 1963 The development of mouse blastocysts transplanted to the scrotal and cryptorchid testis. Journal of Anatomy 97: 119–130

Knoth M, Larsen J F 1972 Ultrastructure of a human implantation site. Acta Obstetricia et Gynecologica Scandinavica 51: 385–393

Koehler J K 1978 The mammalian sperm surface: studies with specific labelling techniques. International Reviews of Cytology 54: 73–105

Kola I, Folb P I 1985 The effects of cyclophosphamide on alkaline phosphatase activity and on *in vitro* postimplantation murine blastocyst development. Development Growth and Differentiation 27: 645–651

Kola I, Folb P I 1986 An assessment of the effects of cyclophosphamide and sodium valproate on the viability of preimplantation mouse embryos using the fluorescein diacetate test. Teratogenesis, Carcinogenesis and Mutagenesis 6: 23–31

Kola I, Folb P I, Parker M I 1986 Maternal administration of cyclophosphamide induces chromosomal aberrations and inhibits cell number, histone and DNA-synthesis in preimplantation mouse embryos. Teratogenesis, Carcinogenesis and Mutagenesis 6: 115–127

Kola I, Trounson A, Dawson G, Rogers P 1987 Tripronuclear human oocytes: altered cleavage patterns and subsequent karyotypic analysis of embryos. Biology of Reproduction 37: 395–401

Lawn A M 1973 The ultrastructure of the endometrium during the sexual cycle. In: Bishop M W H (ed) Advances in reproductive biology, vol 6. Elek, London, pp 61–95

Lawson R A S, Rowson L E A, Adams C E 1972 The development of cow eggs in the rabbit oviduct and their viability after retransfer to heifers. Journal of Reproduction and Fertility 28: 313–315

Leridon H 1977 Human fertility. University of Chicago Press, Chicago

Levinson J, Goodfellow P, Vadeboncoeur M, McDevitt H 1978 Identification of stage-specific polypeptide synthesis during murine preimplantation development. Proceedings of the National Academy of Sciences USA 75: 3332–3336

Lindenberg S, Hyttel P 1988 In vitro studies of the peri-implantation phase of human embryos. In: Van Blerkom J, Motta P (eds) Ultrastructure of human gametogenesis and early embryogenesis. Martinus Nijhof, Amsterdam, pp 201–211

Lindenberg S, Hyttel P, Lenz S, Holmes P V 1986 Ultrastructure of the early human implantation in vitro. Human Reproduction 1: 533–538

Lindenberg S, Hyttel P, Sjøgren A, Greve T 1988 A comparative study of attachment of human, bovine and mouse blastocysts to uterine epithelial monolayer. Biology of Reproduction (in press)

Ljungkvist M D 1972 Attachment reaction of rat uterine luminal epithelium. IV. The cellular changes in the attachment reaction and its hormonal regulation. Fertility and Sterility 23: 847–865

Luckett W P 1973 Amniogenesis in the early human and rhesus monkey embryos. Anatomical Record 175: 375 (abstract)

Lutjen P, Trounson A, Leeton J, Findlay J, Wood C, Renou P 1984 The establishment and maintenance of pregnancy using in vitro fertilization and embryo donation in a patient with primary ovarian failure. Nature 307: 174–175

Lutjen P J, Handley C J, de Witt M T, Trounson A O, McBain J C 1985 Biochemical changes in cervical mucus factor infertility. Gamete Research 12: 265–274

Mahadevan M M, Trounson A O 1985 Removal of the cumulus oophorus from the human oocyte for in vitro fertilization. Fertility and Sterility 43: 263–267

Mann J R, Lovell-Badge R H 1984 Inviability of parthenogenesis determined by pronuclei, not egg cytoplasm. Nature 310: 66–67

Martin R H 1984 A comparison of chromosomal abnormalities in hamster egg and human sperm pronuclei. Biology of Reproduction 31: 819–825

Martin R H, Mahadevan M M, Taylor P J et al 1986 Chromosomal analysis of unfertilized human oocytes. Journal of Reproduction and Fertility 78: 673–678

McGrath J, Solter D 1984 Mouse embryogenesis requires a maternal and paternal genome. Cell 37: 179–183

McMaster R, Yanagimachi R, Lopata A 1978 Pentration of human eggs by human spermatozoa in vitro. Biology of Reproduction 19: 212–216

Meizel S 1978 The mammalian sperm acrosome reaction, a biochemical approach. In: Johnson M H (ed) Development in mammals, vol 3. North Holland, Amsterdam, pp 1–64

Menezo Y, Testart J, Perrone D 1984 Serum is not necessary for human in vitro fertilization, early embryo culture and transfer. Fertility and Sterility 42: 750–755

Mohr L R, Trounson A O 1982 Comparative ultrastructure of the hatched human, mouse and bovine blastocysts. Journal of Reproduction and Fertility 66: 499–504

Monk M 1981 A stem-line model for cellular and chromosomal differentiation in early mouse development. Differentiation 19: 71–76

Moor R M, Trounson A O 1977 Hormonal and follicular factors affecting maturation of sheep oocytes in vitro and their subsequent developmental capacity. Journal of Reproduction and Fertility 49: 101–109

Moor R M, Polge C, Willadsen S M 1980 Effect of follicular steroids on the maturation and fertilization of mammalian oocytes. Journal of Embryology and Experimental Morphology 56: 319–335

Moor R M, Osborn J C, Cran D, Walters D E 1981 Selective effect of gonadotrophins on cell coupling, nuclear maturation and protein synthesis in mammalian oocytes. Journal of Embryology and Experimental Morphology 61: 347–365

Morton H, Rolfe B, Clunie G J A, Anderson M J, Morrison J 1977 An

early pregnancy factor detected in human serum by the rosette inhibition test. Lancet i: 394–397
Mullins D E, Bazer F W, Roberts R M 1981 The pig uterus secretes a progesterone-induced inhibitor of plasminogen activator In: Glasser S R, Bullock D W (eds) Cellular and molecular aspects of implantation. Plenum Press, New York, pp 420–422
Murphy C R, Martin B 1985 Cholesterol in the plasma membrane of uterine epithelial cells: a freeze-fracture cytochemical study with digitonin. Journal of Cell Science 78: 163–172
Murphy C R, Swift J G, Mukherjee T M, Rogers A W 1982a Changes in the fine structure of the apical plasma membrane of endometrial epithelial cells during implantation in the rat. Journal of Cell Science 55: 1–12
Murphy C R, Swift J G, Need J A, Mukherjee T M, Rogers A W 1982b A freeze-fracture electron microscopic study of tight junctions of epithelial cells in the human uterus. Anatomy and Embryology 163: 367–370
Murphy C R, Rogers P A W, Leeton J, Hosie M, Beaton L, Macpherson A 1987 Surface ultrastructure of uterine epithelial cells in women with premature ovarian failure following steroid hormone replacement. Acta Anatomica 130: 348–350
Ng S C, Sathananthan A H, Edirisinghe W R et al 1987 Fertilization of a human egg with sperm from a patient with immotile cilia syndrome. Case report. In: Ratnam S S, Teoh E S, Anandakumar C (eds) Advances in fertility and sterility. Parthenon, Lancaster, pp 71–76
O'Neil C, Gidley-Baird A A, Pike I L, Porter R N, Sinosich M J, Saunders D M 1985 Maternal blood platelet physiology and luteal phase endocrinology as a means of monitoring pre and post implantation embryo viability following in vitro fertilization. Journal of In Vitro Fertilization and Embryo Transfer 2: 87–93
O'Rahilly R 1973 Developmental stages in human embryos. Part A: embryos of the first 3 weeks (stages 1 to 9). Carnegie Institution of Washington, Publication 631, Washington, DC
Parr M B, Parr E L 1977 Endocytosis in the uterine epithelium of the mouse. Journal of Reproduction and Fertility 50: 151–153
Paterson P, Downing B, Trounson A O, Cumming I A 1981 Fertility and tubal morphology after microsurgical removal of segments of the porcine fallopian tube. Fertility and Sterility 35: 209–213
Patillo R A, Hussa R O 1984 Human trophoblastic neoplasms: Advances in experimental medicine and biology, vol 176. Plenum Press, New York
Pemble L B, Kaye P L 1986 Whole protein uptake and metabolism by mouse blastocysts. Journal of Reproduction and Fertility 78: 149–157
Perry F S, Heap R B, Amoroso E C 1973 Steroid hormone production by pig blastocysts. Nature 245: 45–47
Ponzetto-Zimmerman C, Wolgemuth D J 1984 Methylation of satellite sequences in mouse spermatogenic and somatic DNAs. Nucleic Acids Research 12: 2807–2822
Pratt H P M, Ziomek C A, Reeve W J D, Johnson M H 1982 Compaction of the mouse embryo: an analysis of its components. Journal of Embryology and Experimental Morphology 70: 113–132
Psychoyos A, Casimiri V 1981 Uterine blastotoxic factors. In: Glasser S R, Bullock D W (eds) Cellular and molecular aspects of implantation. Plenum Press, New York, pp 327–334
Quinn P, Kerin J F, Warnes G M 1985 Improved pregnancy rate in human in vitro fertilization with the use of a medium based on the composition of human tubal fluid. Fertility and Sterility 44: 493–498
Razin A, Riggs A D 1980 DNA methylation and gene function. Science 210: 604–610
Rogers P A W, Murphy C R, Rogers A W, Gannon B J 1983a Capillary patency and permeability in the endometrium surrounding the implanting rat blastocyst. International Journal of Microcirculation: Clinical and Experimental 2: 241–249
Rogers P A W, Murphy C R, Squires K R, MacLennan A H 1983b Effects of relaxin on the intrauterine distribution and antimesometrial positioning and orientation of rat blastocysts before implantation. Journal of Reproduction and Fertility 68: 431–435
Rogers P A W, Milne B J, Trounson A O 1986 A model to show human uterine receptivity and embryo viability following ovarian stimulation for in vitro fertilization. Journal of In Vitro Fertilization and Embryo Transfer 3: 93–98
Rudak E, Dor J, Mashiach S, Nebel L , Goldman B 1984 Chromosome analysis of multipronuclear human oocytes fertilized in vitro. Fertility and Sterility 41: 538–545
Sanford J, Forrester L, Chapman V, Chandley A, Hostie N 1984 Methylation patterns of repetitive DNA sequences in germ cells of *Mus musculus*. Nucleic Acids Research 12: 2823–2836
Sathananthan A H 1984 Ultrastructural morphology of fertilization and early cleavage in the human. In: Trounson A, Wood C (eds) In vitro fertilization and embryo transfer. Churchill Livingstone, Edinburgh, pp 131–158
Sathananthan A H, Chen C 1986 Early penetration of human sperm through the vestments of human eggs in vitro. Archives of Andrology 16: 183–197
Sathananthan A H, Trounson A O 1982 Cortical granule release and zona interaction in monospermic and polyspermic human ova fertilized in vitro. Gamete Research 6: 225–234
Sathananthan A H, Trounson A O 1985 Human pronuclear ovum: fine structure of monospermic and polyspermic fertilization in vitro. Gamete Research 12: 385–398
Sathananthan A H, Wood C, Leeton J 1982 Ultrastructural evaluation of 8–16 cell human embryos cultured in vitro. Micron 13: 193–203
Sathananthan A H, Ng S C, Edirisinghe R, Ratnam S S, Wong P C 1986a Sperm–oocyte interaction in the human during polyspermic fertilization in vitro. Gamete Research 15: 317–326
Sathananthan A H, Trounson A O, Wood C 1986b Atlas of fine structure of human sperm, eggs and embryos cultured in vitro. Praeger Scientific, Philadelphia
Sathananthan A H, Trounson A, Freemann L 1987 Morphology and fertilizability of frozen human oocytes. Gamete Research 16: 343–354
Schultz G A, Kaye P L, McKay D L, Johnson M H 1981 Endogenous amino acid pool sizes in mouse eggs and preimplantation embryos. Journal of Reproduction and Fertility 61: 387–393
Soupart P 1980 Fertilization. In: Hafez E S E (ed) Human reproduction: conception and contraception. Harper & Row, New York, pp 453–470
Spielmann H, Habernicht U, Eibs H G, Jacob-Muller U, Schimmell A 1981 Investigations on the mechanism of action and on the pharmacokinetics of cyclophosphamide treatment during the preimplantation period in the mouse. In: Neubert D, Merker J H (eds) Culture techniques: applicability for studies on prenatal differentiation and toxicity. Walter de Gruyter, Berlin, pp 436–445
Spindle A I, Pedersen R A 1973 Hatching, attachment and outgrowth of mouse blastocysts in vitro: fixed nitrogen requirement. Journal of Experimental Zoology 186: 305–318
Staigmiller R B, Moor R M 1984 Effect of follicle cells on the maturation and developmental competence of ovine oocytes matured outside the follicle. Gamete Research 9: 221–229
Strickland S, Reich E, Sherman M I 1976 Plasminogen activator in early embryogenesis: enzyme production by trophoblast and parietal endoderm. Cell 9: 231–240
Surani M A H, Barton S C, Norris M L 1984 Development of reconstituted mouse eggs suggests imprinting of the genome during gametogenesis. Nature 308: 548–550
Surani M A H, Barton S C, Norris M L 1986 Nuclear transplantation in the mouse: heritable differences between parental genomes after activation of the embryonic genome. Cell 45: 127–136
Takeuchi I K 1984 Teratogenic effects of methylnitrosurea on pregnant mice before implantation. Experientia 40: 879–881
Tarkowski A K, Wroblewska J 1967 Development of blastomeres of mouse eggs isolated at the 4- and 8-cell stage. Journal of Embryology and Experimental Morphology 18: 155–180
Templeton A A, Mortimer D 1980 Laparoscopic sperm recovery in infertile women. British Journal of Obstetrics and Gynaecology 87: 1128–1131
Tervit H R, Whittingham D G, Rowson L E A 1972 Successful culture in vitro of sheep and cattle ova. Journal of Reproduction and Fertility 30: 493–497
Tesarik J, Kopecny V, Plachot M, Mandelbaum J 1987 Activation of nucleolar and extranucleolar RNA synthesis and changes in the ribosomal content of human embryos developing in vitro. Journal of Reproduction and Fertility 78: 463–470
Thibault C 1972 Physiology and physiopathology of the fallopian tube. International Journal of Fertility 17: 1–13
Thibault C 1977 Are follicular maturation and oocyte maturation independent processes? Journal of Reproduction and Fertility 51: 1–15
Trapp M, Baukloh V, Bohnet H-G, Heeschen W 1984 Pollutants in human follicular fluid. Fertility and Sterility 42: 146–148

Trounson A O, Mohr L R, Wood C, Leeton J F 1982 Effect of delayed insemination on in vitro fertilization, culture and transfer of human embryos. Journal of Reproduction and Fertility 64: 285–294

Veeck L L, Wortham J W E, Witmyer J et al 1983 Maturation and fertilization of morphologically immature human oocytes in a program of in vitro fertilization. Fertility and Sterility 39: 594–602

Waalwijk C, Flavell R A 1978 Mspl an isoschizomer of HPA2 which cleaves both unmethylated and methylated HPA2 sites. Nucleic Acids Research 5: 3231–3236

Wales R G 1975 Maturation of the mammalian embryo: biochemical aspects. Biology of Reproduction 20: 985–990

Webb F T G 1975 Implantation on ovariectomized mice treated with dibutyryl adenosine 3′,5′-monophosphate (dibutyryl cyclic AMP). Journal of Reproduction and Fertility 42: 511–517

Weitlauf H M 1978 Factors in mouse uterine fluid that inhibit the incorporation of ^{3}H-uridine by blastocysts in vitro. Journal of Reproduction and Fertility 52: 321–325

Willadsen S M 1981 The developmental capacity of blastomeres from 4- and 8-cell sheep embryos. Journal of Embryology and Experimental Morphology 65: 165–172

Willadsen S M 1986 Nuclear transplantation in sheep embryos. Nature 320: 63–65

Wolf D P, Byrd W, Dandekar P, Quigley M M 1984 Sperm concentration and the fertilization of human eggs in vitro. Biology of Reproduction 31: 837–848

Wramsby H, Fredga K, Liedholm P 1987 Chromosome analysis of human oocytes recovered from preovulatory follicles in stimulated cycles. New England Journal of Medicine 316: 121–124

Yanagimachi R 1981 Mechanisms of fertilization in mammals. In: Mastorianni L, Biggers J D (eds) Fertilization and embryonic development in vitro. Plenum, New York, pp 81–182

Yanagimachi R 1984 Zona-free hamster eggs: their use in assessing fertilizing capacity and examining chromosomes of human spermatozoa. Gamete Research 10: 187–232

Yates C A, de Kretser D M 1987 Male-factor infertility and in vitro fertilization. Journal of In Vitro Fertilization and Embryo Transfer 4: 141–147

Ziomek C A, Johnson M H 1980 Cell surface interaction induces polarization of mouse 8-cell blastomeres at compaction. Cell 21: 935–942

5

Harold Fox

The placenta, membranes and umbilical cord

THE PLACENTA

The human placenta is a villous haemochorial structure which is of critical importance in materno–fetal transfer, has a complex synthetic capacity and plays a fundamental role in the immunological acceptance of the fetal allograft. The placenta is unique in its range of functional activities, its ability to flourish in an immunologically alien environment and, because it depends upon maternal blood for its oxygenation and nutrition, its vascular parasitism.

The placenta, as expelled from the uterus, appears to be a complete organ: this, the fetal placenta, is not the total structure, however, for there is also the maternal component of the placenta which comprises the placental bed and the uteroplacental vessels.

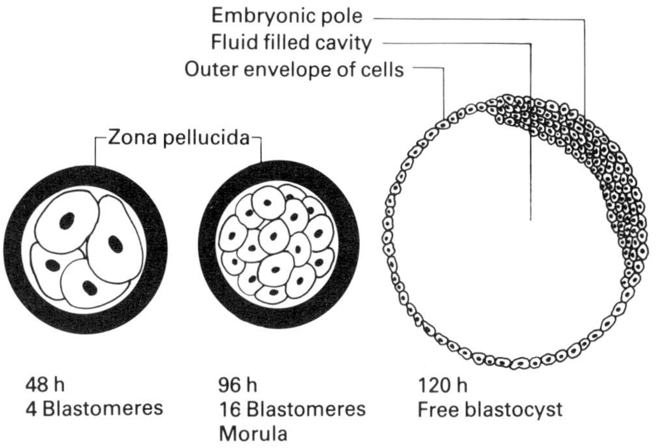

Fig. 5.1 Formation of the blastocyst. The morula sheds the zona pellucida and forms a blastocyst with an embryonic pole, or inner cell mass, and an outer envelope of cells from which the primary trophoblastic cell mass develops. Reproduced with permission from McLean (1987).

Development of the fetal placenta

The fertilized ovum enters the uterine cavity as a morula which rapidly converts into a blastocyst and loses its surrounding zona pellucida (Fig. 5.1). The outer cell layer of the blastocyst proliferates to form the primary trophoblastic cell mass from which cells infiltrate between those of the endometrial epithelium: the latter degenerate and the trophoblast thus comes into contact with the endometrial stroma; this process of implantation is complete by the 10th or 11th postovulatory day. In the 7-day ovum the trophoblast forms a peripheral circumferential plaque which rapidly differentiates into two layers, an inner layer of large, mononuclear cytotrophoblastic cells with well defined limiting membranes and an outer layer of multinucleated syncytiotrophoblast, this latter being a true syncytium (Fig. 5.2). That the syncytiotrophoblast is derived from the cytotrophoblast, not only at this early stage but throughout gestation, is now well established for even when the trophoblast is growing

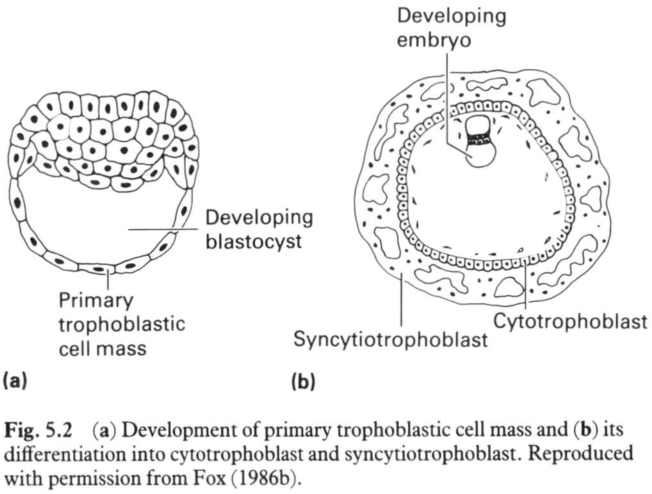

Fig. 5.2 (**a**) Development of primary trophoblastic cell mass and (**b**) its differentiation into cytotrophoblast and syncytiotrophoblast. Reproduced with permission from Fox (1986b).

rapidly DNA synthesis and mitotic activity occur only in the nuclei of the cytotrophoblastic cells (Richart 1961, Galton 1962), the syncytiotrophoblast being a postmitotic, ter-

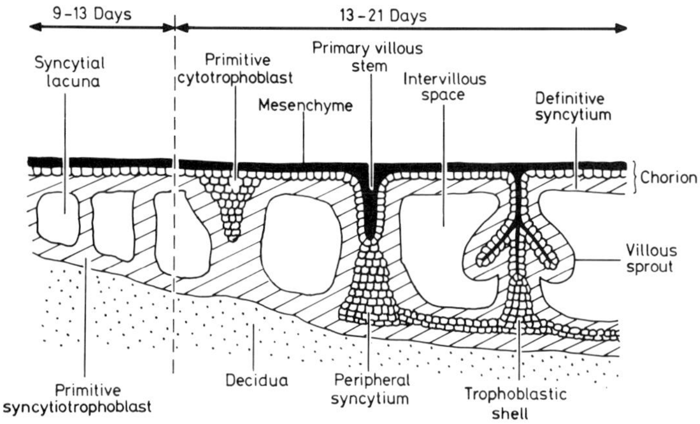

Fig. 5.3 Early development of the placenta. Reproduced with permission from Fox (1978).

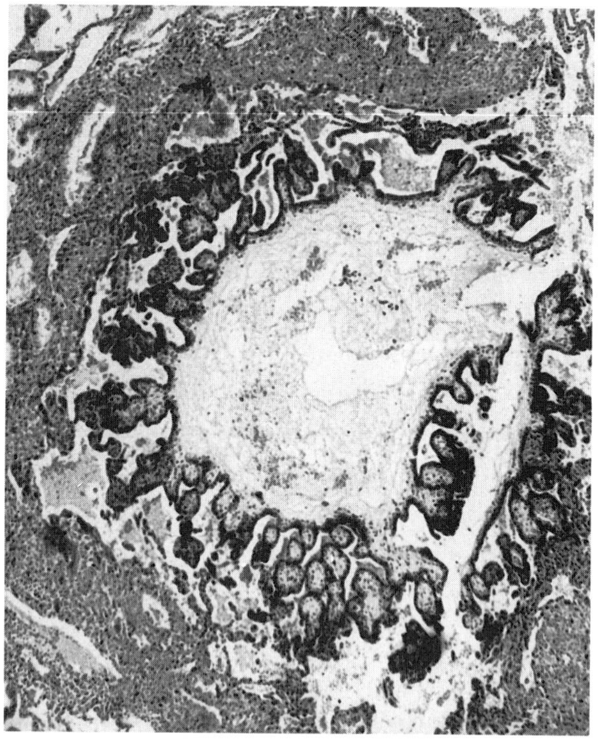

Fig. 5.4 A developing conceptus approximately 14 days after conception. Trabecular primary villous stems are arranged radially and divide the precursor of the intervillous space into a labyrinth. Haematoxylin and eosin. × 24. Reproduced with permission from Fox (1978).

minally differentiated tissue. The syncytiotrophoblast appears to be formed by a breaking down of the limiting membrane of the cytotrophoblastic cells for although no true intercellular membranes are present in the syncytial layer, remnants of such membranes can occasionally be found on electron microscopy (Enders 1965). Cells with a cytoplasmic complexity and nuclear structure intermediate between those of the trophoblastic layers can also be identified on electron microscopy and these intermediate-type cytotrophoblastic cells appear to be ones which are beginning to differentiate into syncytiotrophoblast but have not yet lost their limiting membranes. It is worth noting that the syncytiotrophoblast is the only true syncytial human tissue: this must have some currently unidentified biological advantage for the trophoblast and it has also been suggested that, in teleological terms, the lack of any necessity for the syncytiotrophoblast to synthesize DNA and undergo mitotic activity allows the full metabolic activity of the tissue to be directed towards its transfer and synthetic functions.

Between the 10th and 13th postovulatory days a series of intercommunicating clefts, or lacunae, appear in the rapidly enlarging trophoblastic cell mass (Fig. 5.3): these are probably formed as a result of engulfment of endometrial capillaries within the trophoblast. These lacunae soon become confluent to form the precursor of the intervillous space which, as maternal vessels are progressively eroded, become filled with maternal blood. At this stage the lacunae are incompletely separated from each other by trabecular columns of syncytiotrophoblast which, between the 14th and 21st postovulatory days, tend to become radially orientated (Fig. 5.4) and come to possess a central cellular core produced by proliferation of the cytotrophoblastic cells at the chorionic base. These trabeculae are not true villi but serve as the framework from which the villous tree will later develop, the placenta at this time being a labyrinthine rather than a villous structure and the trabeculae being best known as primary villous stems (Boyd & Hamilton 1970). Continued growth of the cytotrophoblast leads to its distal extension into the region of decidual attachment (Fig. 5.5) whilst, at the same time, a mesenchymal core appears within the villous stems, formed by a distal extension of the extra-embryonic mesenchyme. Later, the villous stems become vascularized; the vessels develop from mesenchyme within the core and establish, in due course, functional continuity with others differentiating in the body stalk and inner chorionic mesenchyme.

The distal part of the villous stems is now formed almost entirely by cytotrophoblastic cells which form columns anchored to the decidua of the basal plate. The cells in these cytotrophoblastic cell columns proliferate and spread laterally to form a continuous cytotrophoblastic shell which splits the syncytiotrophoblast into two layers; the definitive syncytium is on the fetal aspect of the shell and the peripheral syncytium is on the maternal side. The definitive syncytium persists as the lining of the intervillous space but the peripheral syncytium eventually degenerates and is replaced by fibrinoid material (Nitabuch's layer). The establishment of the cytotrophoblastic shell is a mechanism to allow for rapid circumferential growth of the developing placenta and this leads to an expansion of the intervillous space into which sprouts extend from the primary villous stems. These offshoots consist initially only of syncytiotrophoblast but as they enlarge they pass through the stages previously seen during the development of the primary villous stems, i.e.

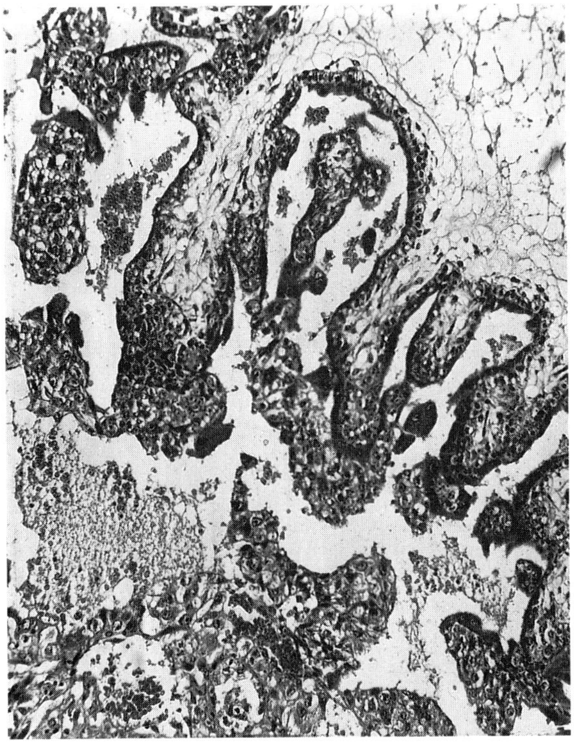

Fig. 5.5 Detail of primary villous stem in a 14-day-old conceptus. The stems have a mesenchymal core and the growing tip of each is formed by a mass of proliferating cytotrophoblastic cells. Haematoxylin and eosin. × 68. Reproduced with permission from Fox (1978).

intrusion of cytotrophoblast, formation of a mesenchymal core and eventual vascularization. These sprouts are the primary stem villi and, since they are true villous structures, the placenta is a vascularized villous organ by the 21st post-ovulatory day. The primary stem villi later grow and divide to form secondary and tertiary stem villi and these latter eventually break up into the terminal villous tree.

Between the 21st postovulatory day and the end of the fourth month of gestation there is not only continuing growth but also considerable remodelling of the placenta. The villi oriented towards the uterine cavity degenerate and form the chorion laeve whilst the thin rim of decidua covering this area gradually disappears to allow the chorion laeve to come into contact with the parietal decidua of the opposite wall of the uterus. The villi on the side of the chorion oriented towards the decidual plate proliferate and progressively arborize to form the chorion frondosum which develops into the definitive fetal placenta. During this period there is some regression of the cytotrophoblastic elements in the chorionic plate and in the trophoblastic shell, whilst the cytotrophoblastic cell columns largely degenerate and are replaced by fibrinoid material (Rohr's layer): clumps of cells persist, however, as the cytotrophoblastic cell islands.

The placental septa appear during the third month of gestation: they protrude into the intervillous space from the basal plate and divide the maternal surface of the placenta into 15–20 lobes. These septa are simply folds of the basal plate, being formed partly as a result of regional variability in placental growth and partly by the pulling up of the basal plate by the anchoring columns which have a poor growth rate (Boyd & Hamilton 1970). As the basal plate is formed principally by the remnants of the trophoblastic shell embedded in fibrinoid material it follows that the septa are similarly constituted, though some decidual cells may also be carried up into the folds. The septa are simply an incidental by-product of the architectural remodelling of the placenta and have no physiological or morphological role to play.

By the end of the fourth month of gestation the fetal placenta has achieved its definitive form and undergoes no further anatomical modification. Growth continues, however, until term and is due principally to continuing branching of the villous tree and formation of fresh villi.

Development of the maternal placenta

During the early weeks of gestation cytotrophoblastic cells stream out from the tips of the anchoring villi, penetrate the trophoblastic shell and extensively colonize the decidua and adjacent myometrium of the placental bed, these cells being known as the interstitial extravillous cytotrophoblast: in addition, trophoblastic cells stream into the lumina of the intradecidual portions of the spiral arteries of the placental bed where they form intraluminal plugs and constitute the intravascular extravillous cytotrophoblast. These endovascular trophoblastic cells destroy and replace the endothelium of the maternal vessels and then invade the media with resulting destruction of the medial elastic and muscular tissue (Brosens et al 1967): the arterial wall becomes replaced by fibrinoid material which appears to be derived partly from fibrin in the maternal blood and partly from proteins secreted by the invading trophoblastic cells (de Wolf et al 1973). This process is complete by the end of the first trimester, at which time these physiological changes within the spiral arteries of the placental bed extend to the myometrio-decidual junction.

After this there is a rest phase in this process but between the 14th and 16th week of gestation there is a resurgence of endovascular trophoblastic migration with a second wave of cells moving down into the intramyometrial segments of the spiral arteries, these cells extending as far as the origin of these vessels from the radial arteries. Within the intramyometrial portion of the spiral arteries the same process as occurs in their intradecidual portion is repeated, i.e. replacement of the endothelium, invasion and destruction of the medial musculoelastic tissue and fibrinoid change in the vessel wall. The end result of this trophoblastic invasion of, and attack on, the vessels is that the thick-walled muscular spiral arteries are converted into flaccid, sac-like uteroplacental vessels (Fig. 5.6) which can passively dilate in order to accommodate the greatly augmented blood flow through this vascular system required as pregnancy progresses.

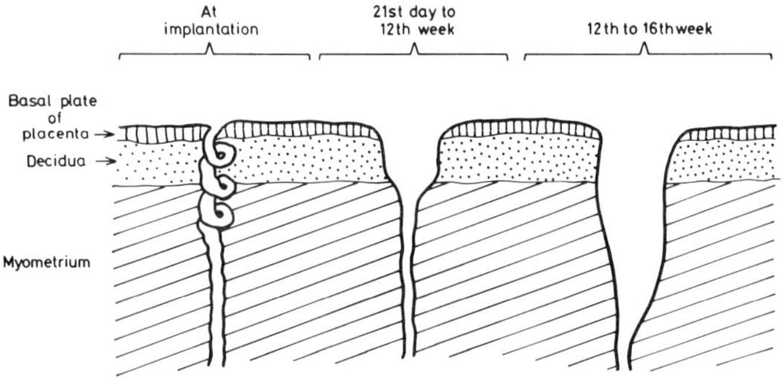

Fig. 5.6 Conversion of spiral arteries into uteroplacental vessels. Reproduced with permission from Fox (1986b).

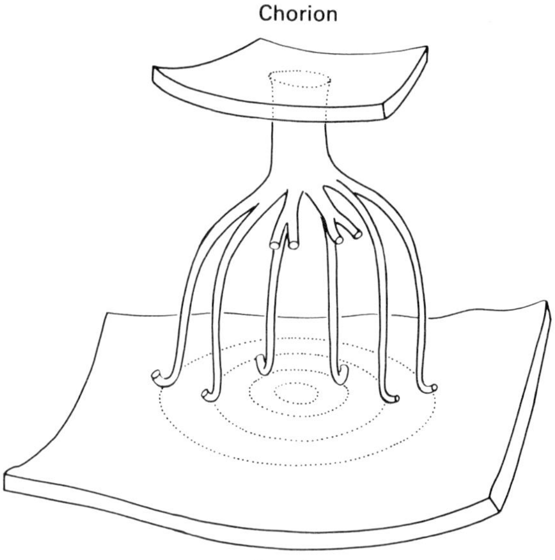

Fig. 5.7 Fetal lobule. The stem villi are arranged in a circular fashion around a central hollow core. Reproduced with permission from Fox (1978).

The extravillous population of trophoblastic cells therefore plays a key role in placentation and through these cells the placenta establishes its own low-pressure, high-conductance, vascular system, simultaneously ensuring an adequate maternal blood flow to itself and an ample supply of oxygen and nutrients to the fetus. The factors which control and limit intravascular invasion by extravillous trophoblast are unknown but the crucial importance of this process is shown by the finding that in women destined to develop pre-eclampsia in the later stages of their pregnancy there is a partial failure of placentation which results in a markedly restricted blood flow to the placenta. This failure has two components: firstly, unlike a normal pregnancy in which all the spiral arteries in the placental bed are invaded by trophoblast, this process occurs in only a proportion of these vessels in women who later develop pre-eclampsia, with a significant fraction of the placental bed arteries in such cases showing a complete absence of physiological change (Khong et al 1986). Secondly, although the first stage of the arterial invasion process occurs quite normally, with trophoblast evoking physiological changes in their intradecidual segments, there is complete failure of the second stage, with endovascular trophoblast failing to advance into the intramyometrial portion of these vessels (Robertson et al 1967, 1975). As a result, there is incomplete transformation of the spiral arteries to uteroplacental vessels and this abnormality, leading to restriction of maternal uteroplacental blood flow, accounts for all the placental abnormalities and fetal complications seen in pre-eclampsia. Pre-eclampsia is not the only serious consequence of inadequate placentation for it is now becoming clear that defective invasion of the spiral arteries by extravillous trophoblast is also a feature of many cases of intrauterine fetal growth retardation in normotensive women, the deficit in fetal growth being due to the reduced maternal supply of oxygen and nutrients (Robertson et al 1981).

Whilst the function of intravascular extravillous trophoblastic cells appears clear, that of the interstitial trophoblastic cells is obscure. The number of these cells has, in the past, been seriously underestimated for it is now known that they are a major component of the placental bed (Pijnenborg et al 1981). Interstitial trophoblastic cells tend to aggregate around spiral arteries and may prime these vessels to allow them to react to their eventual invasion by endovascular trophoblast (Pijnenborg et al 1983): if this is indeed the function of these cells, their mode of action is unknown.

Extravillous trophoblastic cells differ from villous trophoblast in their ability to express class 1 major histocompatibility antigens (Redman et al 1984) and in that their principal synthetic product is human placental lactogen rather than human chorionic gonadotrophin (Gosseye & Fox 1984, Kurman et al 1984). Studies with monoclonal antibodies have, however, shown that the morphologically homogeneous extravillous trophoblastic cells actually comprise a number of antigenically heterogeneous populations (Bulmer & Johnson 1985).

Anatomy of the fetal placenta

The fetal placenta is made up of a number of subunits, generally known as lobules. The injection studies of Wilkin (1965) have shown that the primary stem villi break up just below the chorionic plate into a number of secondary stem villi which, after running for a short distance parallel to the chorionic plate, divide into a series of tertiary stem villi. The lobules are formed by these tertiary stem villi sweeping through the intervillous space to anchor on to the basal plate. As they traverse the intervillous space, they give off multiple branches which ramify into the terminal villous network. As the tertiary stem villi pass down towards the basal plate they are arranged in a circular fashion around the periphery of an empty cylindrical space; the lobule thus forms a hollow globule (Fig. 5.7) with the bulk of the terminal villi being mainly in the outer shell and the centre relatively empty and free of villi. The lobules are separated from each other by interlobular areas which are in continuity with the subchorial space.

There has been considerable confusion as to the meaning of the term cotyledon when applied to the human placenta. This name should not be used to describe the lobes seen on the maternal surface for these are merely the areas lying between the septa and lack any other morphological significance. A cotyledon is the functional unit of the placental villous tree, which is best defined as the part derived from a single primary stem villus (Ramsey 1959). Such a villus can, however, give rise to a varying number of secondary stem villi and thus to a differing number of lobules, for there is no fixed relationship between cotyledons and lobules. Thus centrally placed cotyledons may contain as many as five lobules whilst those situated laterally may have only one or two lobules. The nomenclature has, however, been complicated because some have used the word cotyledon to describe maternal surface lobes, while others have used it to describe the lobule. In fact, the human placenta is not really a cotyledonary structure and Ramsey (1975) has suggested that the word cotyledon should be abandoned when referring to human and primate placentas.

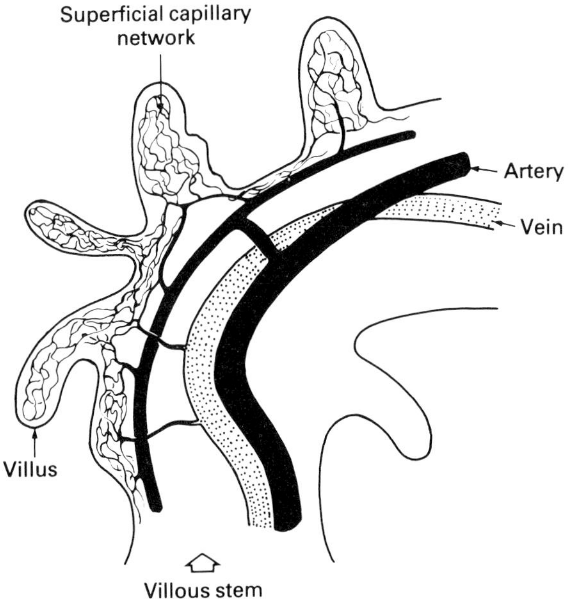

Fig. 5.8 The fetal circulation through the villi. Reproduced with permission from Fox (1978).

The fetal circulation through the placenta

Fetal blood passes to the placenta through the two umbilical arteries which spiral around the umbilical vein. Shortly before reaching the placenta the two arteries are connected by one or more anastomotic vessels and may even fuse into a single trunk which subsequently divides into two rami (Szpakowski 1974). On reaching the placenta the arteries run in the chorion, usually being of equal size and each supplying one-half of the organ. As the arteries run across the chorion they branch repeatedly, a proportion of the branches at each division entering the placental substance to run in the primary stem villi. The cotyledonary arteries soon divide into secondary stem arteries which in turn arborize into tertiary stem arteries running through the intervillous space within the tertiary stem villi giving off, throughout their course, many villous branches which eventually break up into a villous capillary system.

The villous capillary system was studied by Boe (1953) using an Indian ink injection technique (Fig. 5.8). He showed that not only is there a terminal villous network but also a paravascular capillary network, formed by branches arising directly from the main artery. Boe thought that this plexus communicated directly with the main vein, was of arteriolar rather than truly capillary nature and could serve as a shunt to buffer against focal overloading of the terminal villous circulation. Penfold et al (1981) found no evidence, however, of large-diameter vascular shunts within the lobule and Habashi et al (1983), in a scanning electron microscopic study of corrosion casts (Fig. 5.9), demonstrated that the paravascular plexus is found predominantly in those areas of the villous tree which are bathed with relatively poorly oxygenated maternal blood, prompting their suggestion that this network could be responsible for the transport of oxygen and nutrients to the stroma of larger villi. Leiser et al (1985) believe that the paravascular network plays a role in materno-fetal transfer in the earlier stage of placental development but has no functional role in the mature placenta. The terminal villi are vascularized only by capillary vessels and these are arranged in such a way that 3–5 terminal villi are supplied by the same multiply-coiled capillary loop (Kaufmann et al 1985).

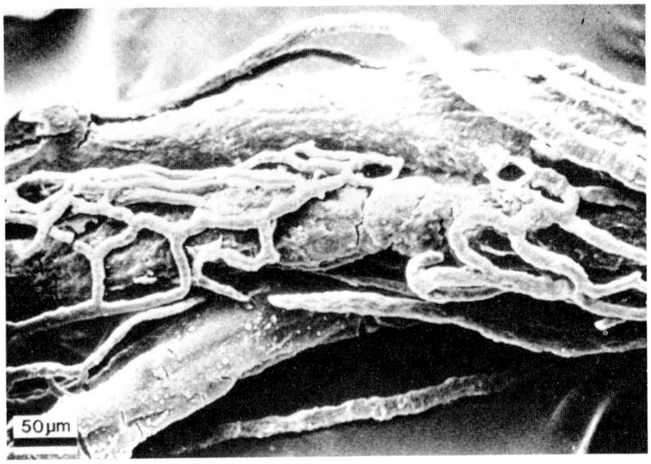

Fig. 5.9 Scanning electron micrograph of the cast of a paravascular network encircling a straight vessel of larger calibre. Reproduced with permission from Habashi et al (1983).

The fetal blood flow through the placenta is about

500 ml/min and, although the main propelling force is clearly the fetal heart, it is possible that there is also a peripheral villous pulse: smooth muscle fibres are present in the stem and anchoring villi (Krantz & Parker 1963) and it has been suggested that contraction of these fibres may help to pump blood from the placenta back to the fetus (Huszar & Bailey 1979). More recently it has been demonstrated that the fetal vessels in the placenta are ensheathed in myofibroblastic cells (Feller et al 1985), and contraction of these cells could be a more important factor in establishing the villous pulse than smooth muscle cells in stem villi.

The maternal uteroplacental circulatory system

Maternal blood enters the intervillous space via arterial inlets in the basal plate (Fig. 5.10) and is then driven by the head of maternal pressure towards the chorionic plate as a funnel-shaped stream (Ramsey & Donner 1980). The driving head of maternal pressure is gradually dissipated, a process aided by the baffling effect of the villi, and lateral dispersion of the blood occurs. This forces the blood already present in the intervillous space out through basally sited wide venous outlets into the endometrial venous network. Indian ink injection studies originally suggested that the maternal blood entered the intervillous space as a jet or spurt but cineangiography has shown that these terms give an undue impression of both speed and intermittency, the maternal blood entering the space 'much as water from an actively flowing brook penetrates a reed filled marsh' (Ramsey 1965).

The physiological basis for this circulatory system is a series of pressure differentials, the pressure in the maternal arterioles being higher than the mean intervillous space pressure which in turn exceeds that in the maternal veins during a myometrial diastole. This entire system is, however, a low-pressure one for whereas in most organs there is a progressive decrease in the diameter of the arteries as they approach their target tissues, the reverse is true for the placenta; the uteroplacental vessels assume an increasing diameter as they approach their entry into the intervillous space. There is therefore a considerable drop in pressure from the proximal to the distal portion of these vessels and the full arterial pressure is not transmitted to the intervillous space. The placenta itself offers little flow resistance to maternal blood and has a high vascular conductance: there is thus very little fall in pressure across the intervillous space and the main factor governing the rate of maternal blood flow in a normal pregnancy is the vascular resistance within the radial branches of the uterine arteries as they run through the myometrium (Moll et al 1975, Moll 1981). Despite the fact that the pressure difference between arterial and venous sides of the intervillous space is small, it is apparently sufficient to drive arterial blood towards the chorionic plate, to stop short-cutting of the stream into adjacent venous outlets and to prevent mixing of neighbouring arterial inflows.

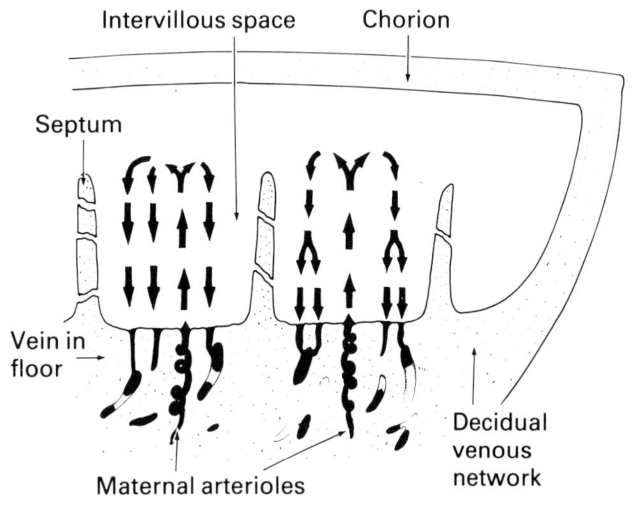

Fig. 5.10 Maternal circulation through the placenta. Reproduced with permission from Fox (1978).

Cineangiography has shown that the individual uteroplacental arteries act independently of each other and are not all patent and discharging blood simultaneously into the intervillous space. Furthermore, during myometrial contractions, the afferent blood flow through the intervillous space may be markedly reduced or can even cease. This is probably due to compression and occlusion of the veins draining the intervillous space (Adamson & Myers 1975) but ultrasonic studies have shown that during a myometrial contraction the intervillous space distends (Bleker et al 1975) and thus the fetus is not severely deprived of oxygen supply during myometrial systole.

Relationship of maternal circulatory system to fetal lobule

The haemodynamic system originally proposed by Ramsey (1965) postulated that the maternal blood flow into the intervillous space was through randomly situated arterial inlets. However, it has since become clear that a definite relationship exists between the maternal vessels and the fetal lobules, probably because the lobules tend to develop preferentially around the flow from eroded maternal vessels (Reynolds 1966). The exact nature of this relationship is still not fully determined and two contrasting schemes have been proposed. Thus, Freese (1966) and Wigglesworth (1967) thought that arterial inlets into the intervillous space are situated such that the inflow from each uteroplacental vessel is into the central villus-free space of a fetal lobule and the maternal blood then flows laterally through the lobule into the interlobular area from which it is drained by basal venous outlets (Fig. 5.11). Others (Lemtis 1970, Gruenwald 1973, Schuhmann 1981) consider that the maternal vessels open, not into the central space of a lobule, but into the interlobular spaces and that the maternal blood then encircles the lobule in streams to form a shell around them, entering and leaving

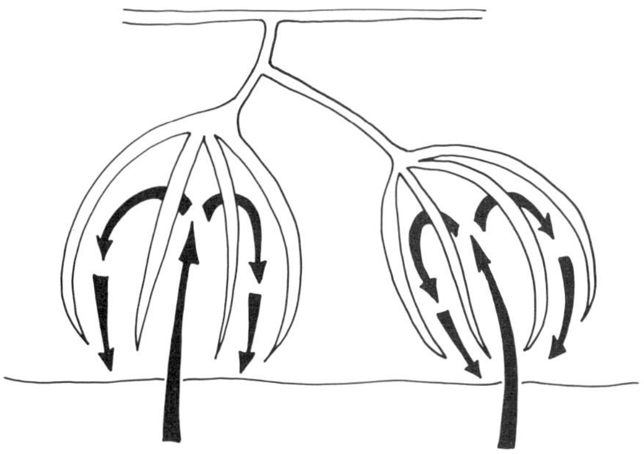

Fig. 5.11 Relationship between maternal uteroplacental blood flow and the fetal lobule, as envisaged by Freese (1966) and Wigglesworth (1967). Reproduced with permission from Fox (1986b).

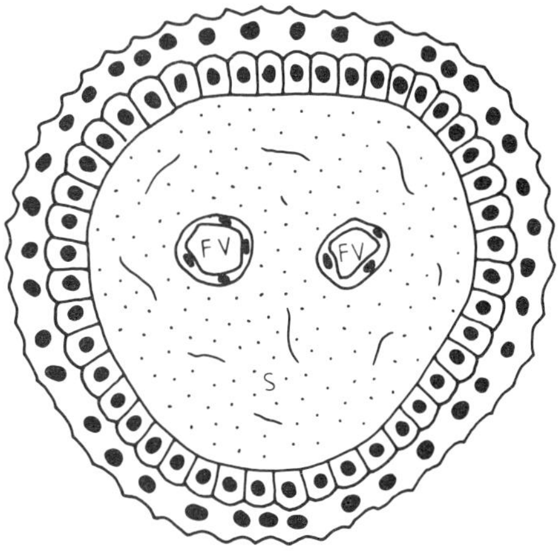

Fig. 5.13 Histological appearances of a typical first trimester villus. FV = fetal vessels; S = villous stroma. Reproduced with permission from Fox (1986b).

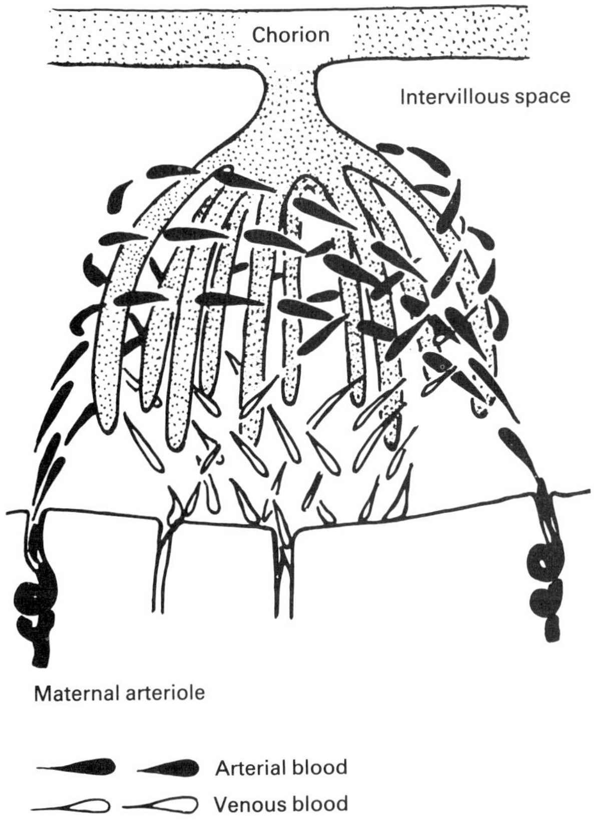

Fig. 5.12 Relationship between maternal uteroplacental blood flow and the fetal lobule, as envisaged by Lemtis (1970) and Gruenwald (1973). Reproduced with permission from Fox (1978).

the lobule whilst doing this and before draining through the basal outlets (Fig. 5.12).

Whichever of these two concepts is correct it is clear that materno-fetal exchange takes place principally in those villi that form the shell of the lobule and that it is only here that a true functional intervillous space, which is probably only of capillary calibre, exists; elsewhere, in the subchorial lake, the interlobular spaces and the central intralobular spaces, villi are either sparse or absent and these areas are in functional terms physiological dead spaces.

Histology of the placental villi

In the first two months of pregnancy the villi are relatively few in number, have a homogeneous pattern and measure approximately 170 μm in diameter (Fig. 5.13). Their outer mantle is covered by a two-layered trophoblastic mantle, an outer layer of syncytiotrophoblast and an inner layer of cytotrophoblastic cells (Langhans' cells). The latter, which form a complete layer, are cuboid, polyhedral or ovoid and have well marked cell borders: their cytoplasm is clear or slightly granular whilst the nucleus is pale staining with finely dispersed chromatin. No cell boundaries are visible between the nuclei of the syncytiotrophoblast and, indeed, microinjection studies have shown that substances flow freely through this layer and can pass from one villus to another, indicating that there is a continuous common cytoplasm over the entire surface of the placental villi (Gaunt & Ockleford 1986). The syncytiotrophoblast is of uniform thickness, whilst the syncytial nuclei are regularly spaced, smaller and more densely staining than those of the cytotrophoblast.

The syncytial cytoplasm may be homogeneous, finely granular or vacuolated. A delicate brush border is often discernible on the outer surface of the syncytium and this corresponds with the microvilli seen on electron microscopy: these probably have no absorptive function but may play a role in pinocytotic vesicle formation and could also serve to increase the density of specific surface receptor sites (Dearden & Ockleford 1983). It is worth noting that the syncytiotrophoblast lines the intervillous space and thus acts in the manner of an endothelium; since the structure of syncytiotrophoblast is quite unlike that of an endothelial cell, its

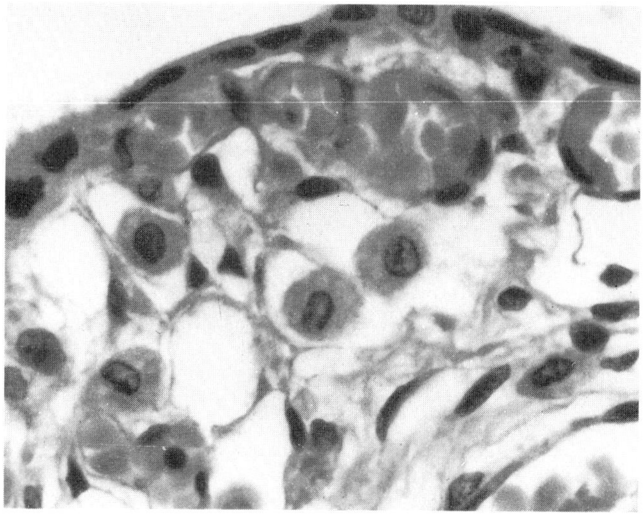

Fig. 5.14 Several typical Hofbauer cells in the stroma of a placental villus. Haematoxylin and eosin. × 840. Reproduced with permission from Fox (1967).

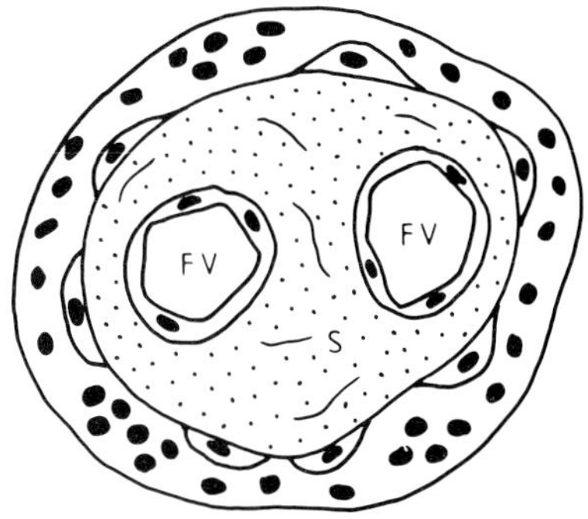

Fig. 5.15 Histological appearances of a typical second-trimester villus. FV = fetal vessels; S = villous stroma. Reproduced with permission from Fox (1986b).

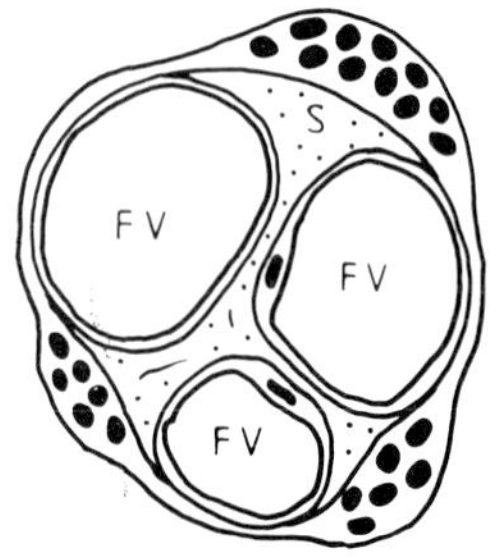

Fig. 5.16 Terminal villus — the predominant type of villus in the term placenta. FV = fetal vessels; S = villous stroma. Reproduced with permission from Fox (1986b).

ability to function in this manner is somewhat of a mystery. It is possible, however, that some of the many placental proteins secreted by the syncytiotrophoblast act to prevent coagulation. Furthermore, studies with monoclonal antibodies have shown that, despite their structural dissimilarity, syncytiotrophoblast and endothelial cells share otherwise specific antigens (Voland et al 1986).

The villous stroma is at this stage formed by loose mesenchymal tissue. The exact stage of gestation at which fetal vessels appear within the stroma is variable but by the end of 8 weeks small centrally placed vessels, lined by large immature endothelial cells, are present. Hofbauer cells are a prominent feature of the villous stroma: these cells may be round, ovoid or reniform, measure about 25 μm in diameter and have an eccentrically placed nucleus (Fig. 5.14). There is now overwhelming morphological, cytochemical and immunological evidence that the Hofbauer cells are fetal tissue macrophages (Fox & Kharkongor 1969, Moskalewski et al 1975, Castellucci et al 1980, Demir & Erbengi 1984). Their origin is obscure for they are present in the villi before they are vascularized by fetal vessels and before haematopoiesis begins in the fetus. It has recently been suggested that there are several populations of Hofbauer cells, those in early pregnancy developing from chorionic mesenchyme but later being supplemented by cells derived either from the fetal liver or bone marrow (Castellucci et al 1986). The number of Hofbauer cells has in the past been seriously underestimated (Wood 1980); they probably play a number of roles, some related to transport mechanisms and others to immunological protection of the fetus; in this latter respect their ability to trap maternal antibodies crossing over into the placental tissues is almost certainly of considerable importance.

Between the eighth and 30th weeks of gestation the villi become more numerous and the predominant form of villus has an average diameter of about 40 μm (Fig. 5.15). In these villi the cytotrophoblastic cells are less prominent whilst the syncytiotrophoblast is thinner and somewhat irregular: the syncytial nuclei are less evenly distributed than in the first trimester and often show a degree of clustering. A distinct, but thin, trophoblastic basement membrane is present, separating the trophoblast from the stroma. The stroma is more compact than is the case in the villi of early gestation and contains a variable number of fibroblasts, myofibroblasts and delicate collagen fibres. Hofbauer cells are seen in the stromal interfibrillary spaces but appear less numerous than in the villi of the early placenta. The villous fetal capillaries are quite prominent, tend to lie more towards the villous periphery and are lined by flattened, fully mature endothelial cells.

From about the 30th week of gestation small terminal villi, measuring about 40 μm in diameter, begin to appear and these are the predominant form of villi seen in the term placenta (Fig. 5.16). Their trophoblastic covering layer is irregularly thinned whilst cytotrophoblastic cells are few and inconspicuous. The cytotrophoblastic cells do however retain their proliferative capacity and represent a largely quiescent germinative zone in which a recrudescence of growth occurs, if the necessity arises, to replace damaged

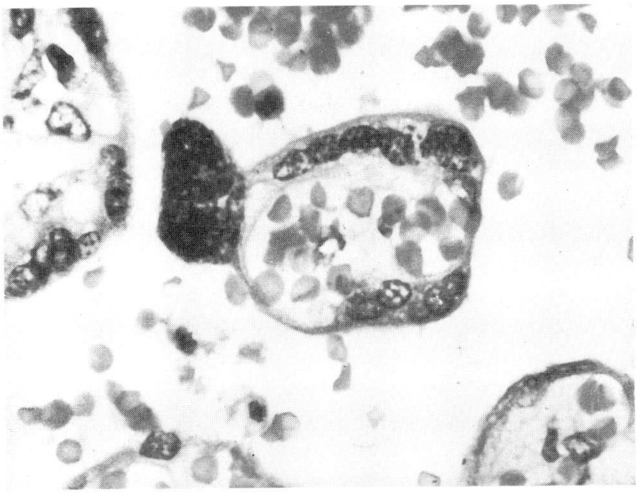

Fig. 5.17 A terminal villus bearing a syncytial knot which appears as a multinucleated protrusion from the free surface of the trophoblast. Haematoxylin and eosin. × 660. Reproduced with permission from Fox (1978).

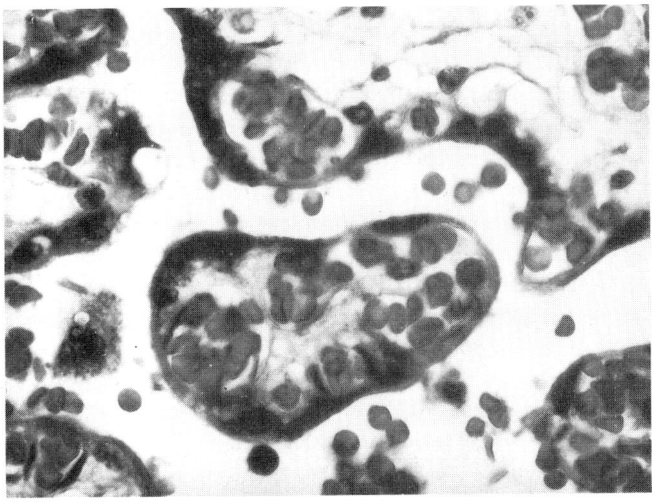

Fig. 5.18 A terminal villus with a vasculo-syncytial membrane (on the right). Haematoxylin and eosin. × 680. Reproduced with permission from Fox (1985b).

syncytiotrophoblast, e.g. in severe pre-eclampsia where ischaemically damaged syncytiotrophoblast is readily repaired by cytotrophoblastic proliferation; this phenomenon is easily recognized by the undue prominence and number of cells in which mitotic figures may be seen (Jones & Fox 1980).

In terminal villi the syncytial nuclei are irregularly distributed and are often aggregated to form multinucleated protrusions into the intervillous space (Fox 1978). It has been claimed that many — even most — of these knots (Fig. 5.17) are histological artefacts due to tangential sectioning of the villi (Küstermann 1981, Cantle et al 1986) but the nuclei within these knots differ considerably from those in the rest of the villous syncytiotrophoblast and show all the ultrastructural features of senescence. Syncytial knots are therefore seen to be formed of aged nuclei sequestrated from functional areas of the syncytium, their loss being compensated by the formation of fresh syncytial nuclei from the cytotrophoblast (Jones & Fox 1977).

In many terminal villi, the syncytiotrophoblast is focally attenuated and anuclear (Fig. 5.18): these thinned areas commonly overlie a dilated fetal capillary vessel and may, on light microscopy, appear to fuse with the vessel wall to form a vasculo-syncytial membrane (Getzowa & Sadowsky 1950). Electron microscopy shows that there is no real fusion between trophoblast and vessel wall but nevertheless these membranous areas of the syncytiotrophoblast differ markedly from the non-thinned areas of the syncytium in their content of histochemically detectable enzymes (Amstutz 1960), in their ultrastructure (Burgos & Rodriguez 1966) and in their surface characteristics (Fox & Agrofojo-Blanco 1974); it is almost certain that they are specialized zones of the placenta for the facilitation of gas transfer across the placenta. The formation of vasculo-syncytial membranes is not due simply to stretching the trophoblast by dilated fetal vessels, for scanning electron microscopy shows that they are randomly situated and very localized, often occurring along the course of a vessel; this distribution is incompatible with a purely mechanical origin (Fox & Agrofojo-Blanco 1974). Thus the functional, regional differentiation which can be detected ultrastructurally in the villous syncytiotrophoblast of the immature placenta (Dempsey & Luse 1971, Kaufmann & Stegner 1972) is sufficiently overt in the terminal villi of the mature placenta to be easily discernible on light microscopy.

The trophoblastic basement membrane of the terminal villi is well defined while the villous stromal tissue is reduced to a thin layer between the sinusoidally dilated villous capillaries. Hofbauer cells are present in the stroma but are difficult to recognize because of their compression by vessels and collagen fibres. A sprinkling of mast cells is also present in the villous stroma (Mahnke & Emmrich 1973, Durst-Zivkovic 1973); their function in this site is uncertain.

In the terminal villi there are usually 2–6 fetal capillary vessels characteristically situated towards the periphery of the villus in close approximation to the covering trophoblast. These vessels are commonly sinusoidally dilated and occupy most of the cross-sectional area of the villus (Fig. 5.19). Aherne (1975) thought that the dilatation of the fetal villous vessels was a mechanism for crowding flow lines, and hence increasing concentration gradients, for substances crossing from maternal to fetal blood and was thus a mechanism for augmenting the efficiency of placental transfer mechanisms. By contrast, Kaufmann et al (1985) considered that the sinusoidal dilatation of these vessels was a method of decreasing blood flow resistance, allowing an evenness of blood flow

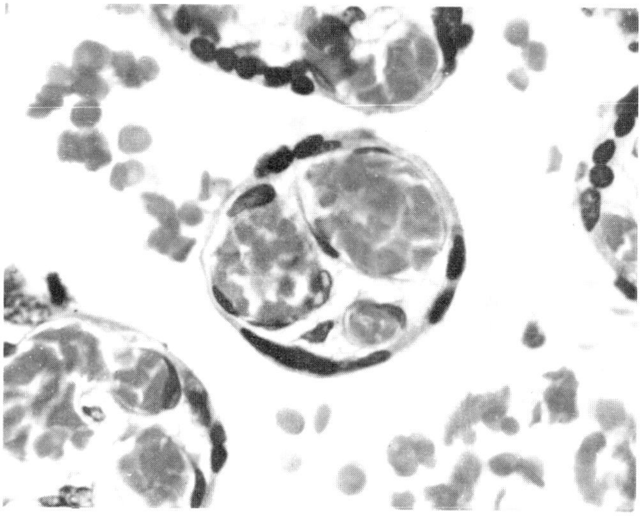

Fig. 5.19 A terminal villus with sinusoidally dilated fetal vessels. Haematoxylin and eosin. × 580. Reproduced with permission from Fox (1978).

throughout the placenta and facilitating fetal placental perfusion.

Growth, maturation and ageing of placental villi

It will be clear from the description of villous histology that the villous morphology alters considerably during pregnancy. It should not be considered that these changes occur in individual villi i.e. a first-trimester villus does not gradually transform into a third-trimester villus. The observed changes reflect the progressive growth and evolution of the villous tree (Sen et al 1979, Kaufmann et al 1979, Kaufmann 1982). The villi present in the first 2 months of pregnancy develop into stem villi, later giving off intermediate villi which represent the growth zone of the placenta; as they mature they begin to give out small outgrowths which develop into terminal villi. Thus in the second trimester the villous population consists of an admixture of immature and mature intermediate villi whilst in the term placenta nearly 60% of the villi are of the terminal type. These latter villi with their high surface area: volume ratio, their laterally placed sinusoidal vessels and with a trophoblastic layer specifically differentiated in some areas for gas transport, represent the form of villous structure which provides optimal conditions for materno-fetal transfer. The changes in villous morphology during gestation reflect a continuing process of maturation of the villous tree with a progressive increasing functional efficiency.

This maturational process within the villous tree has been widely misinterpreted as ageing; there is a tenaciously held belief that during the course of normal pregnancy the placenta progressively ages and at term is on the verge of a decline into morphological and functional senescence. An extension of this attitude is the concept of premature or accelerated ageing that used to be thought a feature of the placenta in certain complications of pregnancy, such as pre-eclampsia. In purely morphological terms there are no histological or ultrastructural changes in the villi which can be considered as indicative of an ageing process (Fox 1979) whilst the claim by Parmley et al (1981) that lipofuscin pigment accumulates in the villous syncytiotrophoblast, a change generally accepted as being a feature of ageing cells, has been shown to be erroneous (Haigh et al 1984).

It has been suggested that a sign of placental ageing is the cessation of placental DNA synthesis and growth which occurs at the 36th week of gestation (Winick et al 1967). More recent studies have however shown that total placental DNA levels continue to rise in a linear fashion until and even beyond the 40th week of gestation (Sands & Dobbing 1985). This finding is in accord with histological evidence of fresh villous growth in the term placenta (Fox 1978) and with autoradiographic and cytophotometric studies which have shown continuing DNA synthesis in the villi of the placenta at term (Geier et al 1975, Hustin et al 1984, Iversen & Farsund 1985). The continuing growth of the placenta has also been confirmed by morphometric techniques showing a continuing expansion of the villous surface area and progressive branching of the villous tree up to and past term (Boyd 1984).

Placental growth certainly slows during the last few weeks of gestation, although this decline in growth rate is neither invariable nor irreversible, for the placenta can continue to increase in size when faced with an unfavourable maternal environment (e.g. pregnancy at high altitude or severe maternal anaemia), whilst the potential for a recrudescence of growth is shown by the proliferative response mounted to repair syncytial damage in conditions such as pre-eclampsia (Jones & Fox 1980, Hustin et al 1984). Those arguing that decreased placental growth during late pregnancy is evidence of senescence often appear to be comparing the placenta to the gut; in such an organ continuing viability is dependent upon a constantly replicating stem cell layer producing short-lived postmitotic cells. A more apt comparison would be with an organ like the liver, formed principally of long-lived postmitotic cells and which, once an optimal size has been attained to meet metabolic demands, shows little evidence of cell proliferation whilst still retaining a latent capacity for growth activity. Certainly there seems to be no good reason why the placenta, having reached a size sufficient to meet its transfer function adequately, should continue to grow. The term placenta, with its considerable functional reserve capacity, more than meets this need.

Functional adequacy of the placenta

The placenta has many functions but its most important role is to transfer oxygen and nutrients from the maternal circulation to the fetal blood. Many have thought that the placenta frequently fails to meet the demands placed upon it and that this condition of placental insufficiency is responsible for many instances of fetal hypoxia, intrauterine growth retardation or death. In reality the placenta rarely becomes insufficient, for it has a considerable functional reserve capacity. Histopathological studies clearly indicate that the placenta can withstand the functional loss of 30–40% of its villous population without any evidence of a decline in its physiological capacity (Fox 1985a, 1986a). Experimental studies, involving either surgical reduction of placental mass (Robinson et al 1979) or artificially increased fetal oxygen consumption (Lorijn & Longo 1980), have confirmed the striking functional reserve of the placenta. Very few pathological lesions of the placenta are sufficiently extensive to dissipate this physiological reserve and it is difficult to accept that intrinsic placental damage is an important factor in the aetiology of inadequate materno-fetal transfer. It has become increasingly clear that the common factor in most cases of presumed placental insufficiency is reduced maternal uteroplacental blood flow which is, in turn, due to inadequate conversion of the spiral arteries into uteroplacental vessels by extravillous trophoblast during the early stages of pregnancy.

THE FETAL MEMBRANES — AMNION AND CHORION

Development of the fetal membranes

The conversion of the early morula to a blastocyst is facilitated by the formation of a central fluid-filled cavity. This separates the primary trophoblastic cell mass, which develops into the placenta and extraplacental chorion, from those cells which give rise to the embryo and contribute to the formation of the yolk sac and the amnion. The latter cells form the eccentrically situated inner cell mass which remains in contact with the cytotrophoblast on the inner aspect of the blastocyst wall.

During the 8th and 9th days postovulation the inner cell mass arranges itself into a bilaminar disc, with the inner layer, i.e. that facing the blastocyst cavity forming the primitive embryonic endoderm while the outer, in contact with cytotrophoblast, forms the primitive embryonic ectoderm. The amniotic cavity first appears as a slit-like space between embryonic ectoderm and the adjacent cytotrophoblast. This enlarges by the 12th postovulatory day to form a small cavity, of which the base is formed by embryonic ectoderm and the walls and roof by cytotrophoblast. At the same time endodermal cells migrate out from the deeper layer of the embryonic disc to line the blastocyst cavity and thus form the primary yolk sac.

Extraembryonic mesenchyme subsequently appears (Fig. 5.20), possibly derived from the trophoblast, and separates the primary yolk sac from the blastocyst wall. Extraembryonic mesenchyme also intrudes between, and largely separates off, the roof of the amniotic sac and the trophoblast of the chorion. A connection between the two is, however,

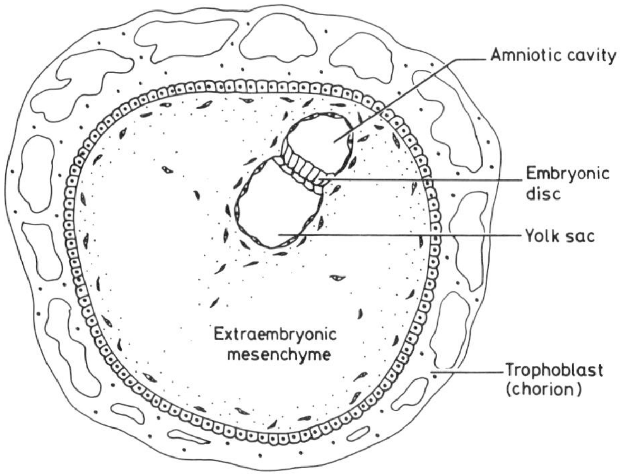

Fig. 5.20 Relationship between developing amniotic cavity and extraembryonic mesenchyme. Reproduced with permission from Fox (1986b).

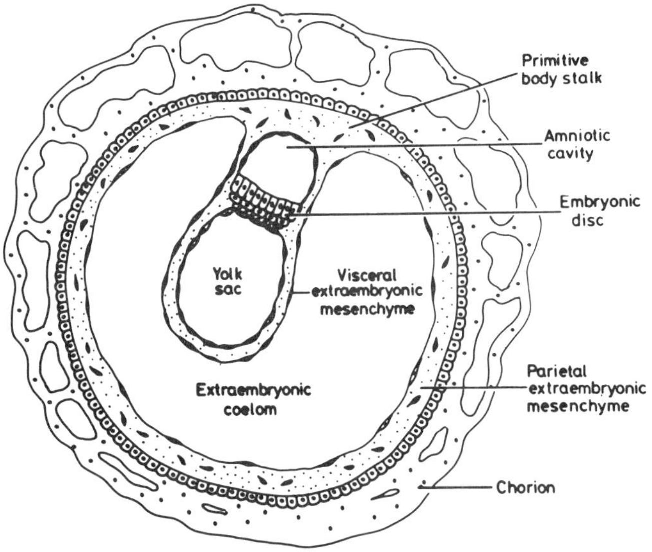

Fig. 5.21 Relationship between developing amniotic cavity, extraembryonic mesenchyme, extraembryonic coelom and primitive body stalk. Reproduced with permission from Fox (1986b).

maintained for a time by the persistence of a column of cells, the amniotic duct, which provides a pathway for continuing migration of trophoblastic cells into the amniotic epithelium. Mitotic activity at the margin of the embryonic ectodermal disc suggests that the ectoderm is also a continuing source of amniotic epithelial cells.

The extraembryonic mesenchyme forms a loose reticulum in which small cystic spaces appear. The spaces gradually enlarge and fuse to form the extraembryonic coelom which splits the extraembryonic mesenchyme into two layers (Fig. 5.21), one apposed to the trophoblast covering the amnion (the parietal extraembryonic mesenchyme) and the other covering the yolk sac (the visceral extraembryonic mesen-

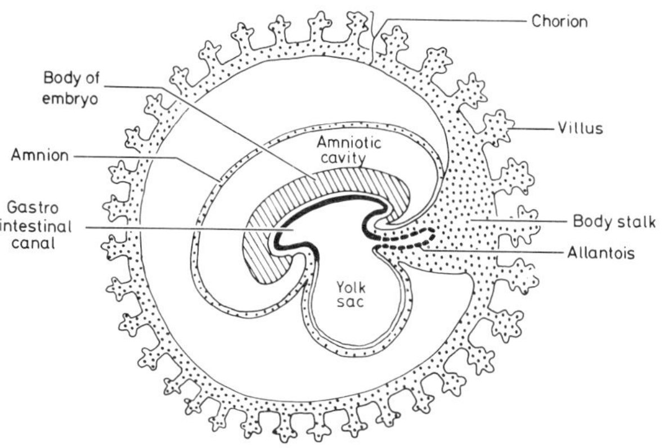

Fig. 5.22 Relationship between the expanding amniotic cavity and the developing embryo. Reproduced with permission from Fox (1986b).

chyme). The progressively enlarging extraembryonic coelom also separates the amnion from the inner aspect of the chorion, except at the caudal end of the embryo where an attachment of extraembryonic mesenchyme persists, to form the body stalk from which the umbilical cord will eventually be derived. Subsequently the amniotic space enlarges at the expense of the extraembryonic coelom and the developing embryo bulges into the expanding amniotic cavity (Fig. 5.22). Meanwhile the yolk sac becomes partially incorporated into the embryo in which it gives rise to the gut. The part of the yolk sac remaining outside the embryo communicates with the primitive gut, but this communicating channel gradually becomes elongated and attenuated to form the vitelline duct; the extraembryonic yolk sac becomes progressively removed away from the embryo, and eventually is incorporated into the lower end of the body stalk.

A further expansion of the amniotic cavity leads to more or less complete obliteration of the extraembryonic coelom with the eventual fusion of the extraembryonic mesenchyme covering the amnion with that lining the chorion. At the same time the extraplacental chorion (chorion laeve) ceases to produce syncytiotrophoblast and the cytotrophoblastic component undergoes a partial regression. The single, fused amniochorionic membrane is now fully formed.

Structure of the amnion and chorion

Bourne (1960), using a combination of light and electron microscopy, was able to define seven distinct layered components of the amniochorion but on routine histological examination of the membranes it is difficult to detect more than five histological strata (Kohler 1987). This is the number one would expect from a knowledge of the development of the amniochorion. These layers from fetal to maternal side would be:

1. Amniotic epithelium.
2. Amniotic connective tissue.
3. Spongy layer.
4. Chorionic connective tissue.
5. Trophoblast.

On embryological grounds it would be assumed that the amniotic connective tissue is derived from visceral extraembryonic mesenchyme, that the spongy layer is a vestige of the extraembryonic coelom and that the chorionic connective tissues originate from the parietal extraembryonic mesenchyme. This is probably not the entire story, however, for it is probable that the amniotic connective tissue is produced at least partly by the amniotic epithelial cells (Aplin et al 1985).

The amniotic epithelial cells are usually described as cuboidal, but there are also subpopulations of flat and columnar cells, the flattened cells being more common in the extraplacental amnion and umbilical cord and columnar cells in the placental amnion (Kohler 1987). The amniotic cells have prominent intercellular bridges near their free margins which increase the mechanical stability and coherence of the layer. It should not be thought that the amniotic cells serve only a mechanical function for they play an important role in water transport and appear to have a significant secretory capacity (Ho et al 1982). Amniotic epithelial cells do not manifest trophoblastic antigens but have a unique plasma membrane (amniotic) antigen specific to that epithelial tissue (Hsi et al 1982). The trophoblastic component of the amniochorion varies from 2 to 10 cell layers in thickness, expresses specific trophoblastic antigens and does not react with antisera to amniotic epithelium.

Macrophages, comparable in all ways with the Hofbauer cells of the chorionic villi, are present in the amniochorion: they are usually inconspicuous but can become prominent if they take up meconium. Myofibroblasts have also been described in the membranes (Wang & Schneider 1982).

UMBILICAL CORD

The umbilical cord links the fetus with the placenta. Although often regarded simply as a mechanical conduit, it also plays a role in the movement of water and other substances between the fetal circulation and the amniotic fluid.

Structure

The basic structure of the cord is simple: it consists of two arteries and a vein embedded in Wharton's jelly covered by one or more layers of amniotic epithelium. Vestigial structures are not uncommon. Remnants of the allantoic and vitelline ducts are usually lined by a simple flat or cuboidal epithelium which may differentiate into fully fledged gastrointestinal-type epithelium.

Wharton's jelly, a mucomyxoid tissue, consists of an abundant ground substance, rich in mucopolysaccharides, in which are embedded collagen fibres, mast cells and sparse large flat stellate cells arranged concentrically around the vessels. Clearly, Wharton's jelly has as its salient function a mechanical cushioning effect which protects the umbilical vessels from trauma. The tissue is metabolically very active, however, (Zawisch 1955) and it would be unwise to allot to it only a mechanistic function.

The umbilical cord arteries are unusual in lacking an internal elastic lamina. They have a well formed media zone containing both myocytes and myofibroblasts arranged in a helical fashion (Gebrane-Younes et al 1986). The arteries lack an adventitia; Zawisch (1955) pointed out that Wharton's jelly appears to substitute for this layer. The umbilical vein differs from the arteries less than is the case elsewhere in the body but has a thinner media and a better developed mural elastic component. Both arteries and veins have endothelial cells which appear to be metabolically highly active. It has been suggested that these vessels may play a role in water transfer to the amniotic fluid (Gebrane-Younes et al 1986). The umbilical vessels lack vasa vasorum and the long-standing controversy over whether or not they are innervated has still not been resolved (Reilly & Russell 1977, Bettzieche 1978).

Length of the cord

The average length of the cord is between 54 and 61 cm (Fox 1978). There is a wide variability but the minimum length of the cord which allows a normal cephalic delivery at term is 32 cm, whilst an arbitrary length of 100 cm has been accepted as the maximum which does not predispose to complications such as knotting, torsion or prolapse. Although there is a wide scatter within these extremes, Mills et al (1983) have formulated standard tables for cord length based on measurements of over 18 000 cords from babies ranging in gestational age from 34 to 43 weeks. These tables show that the cord continues to grow in length up to and beyond term and that male babies tend to have longer cords than females. This may be related to greater intrauterine movement of male fetuses, for there is both clinical and experimental evidence that restriction of fetal activity results from a short cord. Fetal movement appears to have a stimulatory effect on the longitudinal growth of the cord (Miller et al 1981, Moessinger et al 1982).

Site of cord insertion

There is a widespread impression that the cord should insert into the central portion of the placental disc. The fallacy of this belief has been admirably summarized by Kohler (1987):

> In discussing what is the normal site of insertion some authors appear to have been influenced by perfectionist idiosyncrasies: a central insertion is more gratifying, therefore it must be normal. On the other hand, the contention that eccentric insertion is more common than central and must therefore represent the norm, is also not free from fallacy. There are no natural categories of central, moderately eccentric, markedly eccentric and marginal insertions, but a continuous series and the frequency of insertion at various points within this series is, therefore, determined by the laws of probability.

This view is confirmed by the finding that the site of cord insertion into the placental disc is of no clinical significance (Fox 1978).

Velamentous insertion of the cord is not, however, a normal event. In this condition the cord does not insert into the placental surface but into the extraplacental membranes so that unprotected umbilical vessels, divested of Wharton's jelly, run for some distance between the amnion and chorion exposed to the risk of mechanical injury before reaching the placental margin. This risk is greatest when the vessels overlie the internal os (vasa praevia); as the presenting part of the fetus descends during labour it will inevitably lacerate and rupture the unprotected vessels. Bleeding from velamentously inserted vessels can occur even in sites well away from the internal os. Despite a plethora of theories, neither the aetiology nor the pathogenesis of velamentous insertion is understood (Fox 1978, Kohler 1987).

Acknowledgements

Figures 5.6, 5.13, 5.15, 5.16, 5.20, 5.21 and 5.22 were drawn by Dr Carolyn J. P. Jones. I am indebted to Dr P. Wilkin for supplying me with Figure 5.3 and to the late Dr F. Boe for Figure 5.8.

REFERENCES

Adamson K, Myers R E 1975 Circulation in the intervillous space: obstetrical considerations in fetal deprivation. In: Gruenwald P (ed) The placenta and its maternal supply line. Medical and Technical Publishing, Lancaster, pp 158–177
Aherne W 1975 Morphometry. In: Gruenwald P (ed) The placenta and its maternal supply line. Medical and Technical Publishing, Lancaster, pp 80–97
Amstutz E 1960 Beobachtungen über die Reiung der Chorionzotten in der menslichen Plazenta mit besonderer Berückichtigung der Epithelplatten. Acta Anatomica 42: 12–30
Aplin J D, Campbell S, Allen T D 1985 The extracellular matrix of human amniotic epithelium: ultrastructure, composition and deposition. Journal of Cell Science 79: 119–136
Bettzieche H 1978 Studien zur Frage der Innervation der Nabelschnur. Zentralblatt für Gynäkologie 100: 799–804
Bleker O P, Kloosterman G J, Mieras D J, Oosting J, Sallé H J A 1975 Intervillous space during uterine contractions in human subjects: an ultrasonic study. American Journal of Obstetrics and Gynecology 123: 697–699
Boe F 1953 Studies on the vascularization of the human placenta. Acta Obstetricia et Gynecologica Scandinavica 32 (suppl 5): 1–92
Bourne G L 1960 The microscopic anatomy of the human amnion and chorion. American Journal of Obstetrics and Gynecology 79: 1070–1073
Boyd J D, Hamilton W J 1970 The human placenta. Heffer, Cambridge
Boyd P A 1984 Quantitative studies of the normal human placenta from 10 weeks of gestation to term. Early Human Development 9: 297–307
Brosens I, Robertson W B, Dixon H G 1967 The physiological response of the vessels of the placental bed in normal pregnancy. Journal of Pathology and Bacteriology 93: 569–579
Bulmer J N, Johnson P M 1985 Antigen expression by trophoblast populations in the human placenta and their possible immunobiological relevance. Placenta 6: 127–140
Burgos M H, Rodriguez E M 1966 Specialized zones in the trophoblast of the human term placenta. American Journal of Obstetrics and Gynecology 96: 342–356

Cantle S J, Kaufmann P, Luckhardt M, Schweikhart G 1987 Interpretation of syncytial sprouts and bridges in the human placenta. Placenta 8: 221–234
Castellucci M, Zaccheo D, Pescetto G 1980 A three-dimensional study of the normal human placental villous core. I. The Hofbauer cells. Cell and Tissue Research 210: 235–247
Castellucci M, Celona A, Bartels H, Steininger B, Benedetto V, Kaufman P 1987 Mitoses of the Hofbauer cell: possible implications for a fetal macrophage. Placenta 8: 65–75
Dearden I, Ockleford C D 1983 Structure of human trophoblast: correlation with function. In: Loke Y W, Whyte A (eds) Biology of trophoblast. Elsevier, Amsterdam, pp 69–110
Demir R, Erbengi T 1984 Some new findings about Hofbauer cells in the chorionic villi of the human placenta. Acta Anatomica 119: 18–26
Dempsey E W, Luse S A 1971 Regional specialisations in the syncytial trophoblast of early human placenta. Journal of Anatomy 108: 545–561
de Wolf F, de Wolf-Peeters C, Brosens I 1973 Ultrastructure of the spiral arteries in the human placental bed at the end of normal pregnancy. American Journal of Obstetrics and Gynecology 117: 833–848
Durst-Zivkovic B 1973 Das Vorkommen der Mastzellen in der Nachgeburt. Anatomischer Anzeiger 134: 225–229
Enders A C 1965 A comparative study of the fine structure of the trophoblast in several hemochorial placentae. American Journal of Anatomy 116: 29–67
Feller A C, Schneider H, Schmidt D, Parwaresch M R 1985 Myofibroblast as a major cellular constituent of villous stroma in human placenta. Placenta 6: 405–415
Fox H 1967 The incidence and significance of Hofbauer cells in the mature placenta. Journal of Pathology and Bacteriology 93: 710–717
Fox H 1978 Pathology of the placenta. Saunders, London
Fox H 1979 The placenta as a model of organ ageing. In: Beaconsfield P, Villee C (eds) Placenta — a neglected experimental animal. Pergamon, Oxford, pp 351–378
Fox H 1985a Placental pathology: a contemporary approach. Obstetrics and Gynecology Annual 14: 427–440
Fox H 1985b Placental structure. In: Macdonald R R (ed) Scientific basis of obstetrics and gynaecology, 3rd edn. Churchill Livingstone, Edinburgh, pp 1–38
Fox H 1986a Pathology of the placenta. Clinics in obstetrics and gynaecology, vol 13. Churchill Livingstone, Edinburgh, pp 1–28
Fox H 1986b Development of the placenta and membranes. In: Dewhurst J, De Swiet M, Chamberlain G (eds) Basic sciences in obstetrics and gynaecology. Churchill Livingstone, Edinburgh, pp 34–41
Fox H, Agrofojo-Blanco A 1974 Scanning electron microscopy of the human placenta in normal and abnormal pregnancies. European Journal of Obstetrics, Gynecology and Reproductive Biology 4: 45–50
Fox H, Kharkongor N F 1969 Enzyme histochemistry of the Hofbauer cells of the human placenta. Journal of Obstetrics and Gynaecology of the British Commonwealth 76: 918–921
Freese U E 1966 The fetal–maternal circulation of the placenta. I. Histomorphologic, placental injection and X-ray cinematographic studies on human placenta. American Journal of Obstetrics and Gynecology 94: 354–360
Galton M 1962 DNA content of placental nuclei. Journal of Cell Biology 13: 183–203
Gaunt M, Ockleford C D 1986 Microinjection of human placenta: 2. Biological application. Placenta 7: 325–331
Gebrane-Younes J, Minh H N, Orcel O 1986 Ultrastructure of human umbilical vessels: a possible role in amniotic fluid formation. Placenta 7: 173–185
Geier G, Schuhmann R, Kraus H 1975 Regional unterschiedliche Zellproliferation innerhalb der Plazenteone reifer menschlicher Plazenten: autoradiographische Untersuchungen. Archiv für Gynäkologie 218: 31–37
Getzowa S, Sadowsky A 1950 On the structure of the human placenta with full-term and immature foetus, living or dead. Journal of Obstetrics and Gynaecology of the British Empire 57: 388–396
Gosseye S, Fox H 1984 An immunohistological comparison of the secretory capacity of villous and extravillous trophoblast in the human placenta. Placenta 5: 329–348
Gruenwald P 1973 Lobular structure of hemochorial primate placentas, and its relation to maternal vessels. American Journal of Anatomy 136: 133–152
Habashi S, Burton G J, Steven D H 1983 Morphological study of the fetal vasculature of the human term placenta: scanning electron microscopy of corrosion casts. Placenta 4: 41–56
Haigh M, Chawner L E, Fox H 1984 The human placenta does not contain lipofuscin pigment. Placenta 5: 459–464
Ho P C, Haynes W D G, Ing R M Y, Jones W R 1982 Histological, ultrastructural and immunofluorescence studies of the amniochorionic membrane. Placenta 3: 109–126
Hsi B-L, Yeh C-J G, Faulk W P 1982 Human amniochorion: tissue-specific markers, transferrin receptors and histocompatibility antigens. Placenta 3: 1–12
Hustin J, Foedart J M, Lambotte R 1984 Cellular proliferation in villi of normal and pathological pregnancies. Gynecologic and Obstetric Investigation 17: 1–9
Huszar G, Bailey P 1979 Isolation and characterization of myosin in the human term placenta. American Journal of Obstetrics and Gynecology 135: 707–712
Iversen O E, Farsund T 1985 Flow cytometry in the assessment of human placental growth. Acta Obstetricia et Gynecologica Scandinavica 64: 605–707
Jones C J P, Fox H 1977 Syncytial knots and intervillous bridges in the human placenta: an ultrastructural study. Journal of Anatomy 124: 275–286
Jones C J P, Fox H 1980 An ultrastructural and ultrahistochemical study of the human placenta in maternal pre-eclampsia. Placenta 1: 61–76
Kaufmann P 1982 Development and differentiation of the human placental villous tree. Bibliotheca Anatomica 22: 29–39
Kaufmann P, Stegner H E 1972 Uber die funktionelle Differentzeitung des Zottensyncytium in der mesnchlichen Plazenta. Zeitschrift für Zellforschung und Mikroskopische Anatomie 135: 361–382
Kaufmann P, Sen D K, Schwikhart G 1979 Classification of human placental villi. I. Histology. Cell and Tissue Research 200: 409–423
Kaufmann P, Bruns U, Leiser R, Luckhardt M, Winterhager E 1985 The fetal vascularisation of term human placental villi. II. Intermediate and terminal villi. Anatomy and Embryology 173: 203–214
Khong T Y, de Wolf F, Robertson W B, Brosens I 1986 Inadequate maternal vascular response to placentation in pregnancies complicated by preeclampsia and by small-for-gestational-age infants. British Journal of Obstetrics and Gynaecology 93: 1049–1059
Kohler H G 1987 Pathology of the umbilical cord and of the fetal membranes. In: Fox H (ed) Haines and Taylor's textbook of obstetrical and gynaecological pathology 3rd edn. Churchill Livingstone, Edinburgh, pp 1079–1116
Krantz K E, Parker J G 1963 Contractile properties of the smooth muscle in the human placenta. Clinical Obstetrics and Gynecology 6: 26–38
Kurman R J, Main C S, Chen H-H 1984 Intermediate trophoblast: a distinctive form of trophoblast with specific morphological, biochemical and functional features. Placenta 5: 349–370
Küstermann W 1981 Uber 'Proliferationsknoten' und 'Syncytialknoten' der menschlichen Plazenta. Anatomischer Anzeiger 150: 144–157
Leiser R, Luckhardt M, Kaufmann P, Winterhager E, Bruns U 1985 The fetal vascularisation of term human placental villi. I. Peripheral stem villi. Anatomy and Embryology 173: 71–80
Lemtis H 1970 Physiologie der Plazenta. Fortschritte der Geburtshilfe und Gynäkologie 41: 1–52
Lorijn R H V, Longo L D 1980 Clinical and physiologic implications of increased fetal oxygen consumption. American Journal of Obstetrics and Gynecology 136: 451–457
Mahnke P F, Emmrich P 1973 Zur Mastzellhaufigheit der menschlichen Plazentarzotte. Zentralblatt für Gynäkologie 95: 730–732
McLean J M 1987 Embryology and anatomy of the female genital tract and ovaries. In: Fox H (ed) Haines's & Taylor's textbook of gynaecological and obstetrical pathology. Churchill Livingstone, Edinburgh, pp 1–50
Miller M E, Higginbottom M, Smith D W 1981 Short umbilical cord: its origin and relevance. Pediatrics 67: 618–621
Mills J L, Harley E E, Moessinger A C 1983 Standards for measuring umbilical cord length. Placenta 4: 423–426
Moessinger A C, Blanc W A, Marone P A, Polsen D C 1982 Umbilical cord length as an index of fetal activity: experimental study and clinical implications. Pediatric Research 16: 109–112
Moll W 1981 Physiologie der maternen placentaren Durchblutung. In:

Becker V, Schiebler Th H, Kubli F (eds) Die Plazenta des Menschen. Thieme, Stuttgart, pp 172–194
Moll W, Kunzell W, Herburger J 1975 Hemodynamic implications of hemochorial placentation. European Journal of Obstetrics, Gynecology and Reproductive Biology 5: 67–74
Moskalewski S, Ptak W, Czernik Z 1975 Demonstration of cells with IgG receptor in human placenta. Biology of the Neonate 26: 268–273
Parmley T H, Gupta P K, Walker M A 1981 'Aging' pigments in term human placenta. American Journal of Obstetrics and Gynecology 139: 760–763
Penfold P, Wooten R, Hytten F E 1981 Studies of a single placental cotyledon in vitro III. The dimensions of the villous capillaries. Placenta 2: 161–168
Pijnenborg R, Bland J M, Robertson W B, Dixon G, Brosens I 1981 The pattern of interstitial trophoblastic invasion of the myometrium in early human pregnancy. Placenta 2: 303–315
Pijnenborg R, Bland J M, Robertson W B, Brosens I 1983 Uteroplacental arterial changes related to interstitial trophoblast migration in early human pregnancy. Placenta 4: 397–414
Ramsey E M 1959 Circulation in the placenta. In: Villee C A (ed) Gestation: transactions of the fifth conference. Macy Foundation, New York
Ramsey E M 1965 Circulation of the placenta. Birth Defects, Original Articles Series 1: 5–12
Ramsey E M 1975 Discussion of Gruenwald P. European Journal of Obstetrics, Gynecology and Reproductive Biology 5: 31
Ramsey E M, Donner M W 1980 Placental vasculature and circulation. Thieme, Stuttgart
Redman C W, McMichael A J, Stirrat G M, Sunderland C A, Ting A 1984 Class I major histocompatibility complex antigens on human extra-villous trophoblast. Immunology 52: 457–468
Reilly F D, Russell P T 1977 Neurohistochemical evidence supporting an absence of adrenergic and cholinergic innervation in the human placenta and umbilical cord. Anatomical Record 188: 277–285
Reynolds S R M 1966 Formation of fetal cotyledons in the hemochorial placenta: a theoretical consideration of the functional implications of such an arrangement. American Journal of Obstetrics and Gynecology 94: 425–439
Richart R 1961 Studies of placental morphogenesis I. Radiographic studies of human placenta utilizing tritiated thymidine. Proceedings of the Society for Experimental Biology and Medicine 106: 829–831
Robertson W B, Brosens I, Dixon H G 1967 The pathological response of the vessels of the placental bed in hypertensive pregnancy. Journal of Pathology and Bacteriology 93: 581–592
Robertson W B, Brosens I, Dixon H G 1975 Uteroplacental vascular pathology. European Journal of Obstetrics, Gynecology and Reproductive Biology 5: 47–65
Robertson W B, Brosens I A, Dixon H G 1981 Maternal blood supply in fetal growth retardation. In: Van Assche A, Robertson W B (eds) Fetal growth retardation. Churchill Livingstone, Edinburgh, pp 126–138
Robinson J S, Kingston E J, Jones C T, Thorburn G D 1979 Studies of experimental growth retardation in sheep: the effect of removal of endometrial caruncles on fetal size and metabolism. Journal of Developmental Physiology 1: 379–398
Sands J, Dobbing J 1985 Continuing growth and development of the third-trimester human placenta. Placenta 6: 13–22
Schuhmann R 1981 Plazenten: Begriff, Entstehung, funktionelle Anatomie. In: Becker V, Schiebler Th H, Kubli F (eds) Die Plazenta des Menschen. Thieme, Stuttgart, pp 199–207
Sen D K, Kaufmann P, Schweikhart G 1979 Classification of human placental villi. II Morphometry. Cell and Tissue Research 200: 425–434
Szpakowski M 1974 Morphology of arterial anastomoses in the human placenta. Folio Morphologica 33: 53–60
Voland J R, Frisman D M, Baird S M 1986 Presence of an endothelial antigen on the syncytiotrophoblast of human chorionic villi: detection by a monoclonal antibody. American Journal of Reproductive Immunology and Microbiology 11: 24–30
Wang T, Schneider J 1982 Myofiblasten in Bindegewebe des menschlichen Amnions. Zeitschrift für Geburtshilfe und Perinatologie 186: 164–168
Wigglesworth J S 1967 Vascular organisation of the human placenta. Nature 216: 1120–1121
Wilkin P 1965 Pathologie du placenta. Masson, Paris
Winick M, Coscia A, Noble A 1967 Cellular growth in human placenta. I. Normal cellular growth. Pediatrics 39: 248–251
Wood G W 1980 Mononuclear phagocytes in the human placenta. Placenta 1: 113–123
Zawisch C 1955 Die Whartonische Sulze und die Gefässe des Nabelstranges. Zeitschrift für Zellforschung 42: 94–133

6

Felix Beck

Structural development of the embryo and fetus

INTRODUCTION

Human implantation takes place between the sixth and eighth day after fertilization. At this stage the conceptus is in the blastocyst stage, weighs less than 1 μg and contains a few hundred cells (Fig. 6.1).

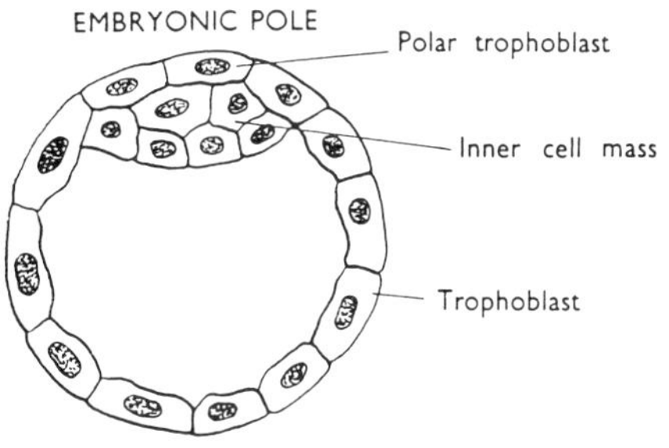

Fig. 6.1 The human blastocyst. Reproduced with permission from Beck et al (1985).

The first morphological evidence of post-implantation differentiation is manifest in the deepest cells of the inner cell mass (i.e. those facing the blastocyst cavity). They become cuboidal and form a single layer of primary embryonic endoderm. The remainder of the inner cell mass then gradually forms a layer of columnar cells which are the precursors of the embryonic ectoderm and will also give rise to the embryonic mesoderm. The amniotic cavity appears between these cells and those overlying them, which form the amniotic ectoderm derived from the deep aspects of the polar trophoblast (Fig. 6.2). At this stage (9–13 days post-fertilization) the cells of the future embryo, having been derived from the inner cell mass, form a bilaminar embryonic disc and the whole of the remainder of the conceptus goes on to form the fetal membranes.

Soon the blastocyst cavity becomes lined by squamous extraembryonic endoderm separated from the thick outer trophoblast by a loose reticular layer of extraembryonic mesoderm. The extraembryonic endoderm, in continuity with the cuboidal embryonic endoderm, forms the yolk sac (Fig. 6.3). In the future cranial area of the embryo the cuboidal cells of the yolk sac roof become columnar and form the prochordal plate which, together with overlying ectoderm, forms the buccopharyngeal membrane. Meanwhile, the extraembryonic mesoderm develops fluid-filled spaces which, becoming confluent, form the extraembryonic coelom (Fig. 6.4). Extraembryonic splanchnopleure and extraembryonic somatopleure (amnion and chorion) are therefore delineated within the structure of the chorionic vesicle about 15 days after fertilization.

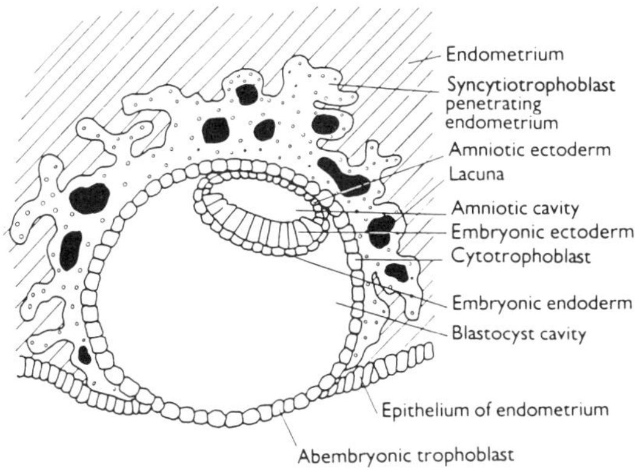

Fig. 6.2 The implanted conceptus. The embryo forms a bilaminar disc, above which the amniotic cavity lies. Reproduced with permission from Beck et al (1985).

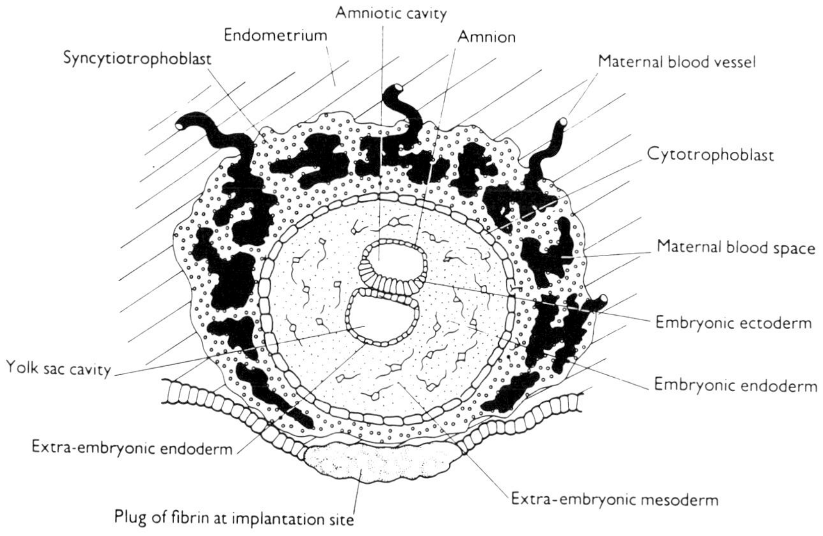

Fig. 6.3 The formation of the extraembryonic endoderm and mesoderm around the yolk sac. Reproduced with permission from Beck et al (1985).

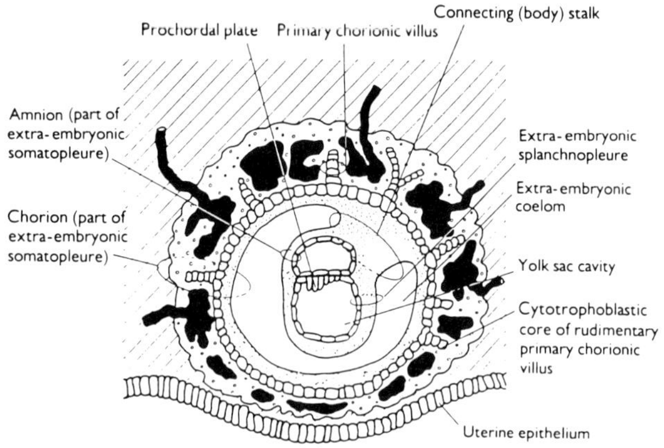

Fig. 6.4 Day 15: chorionic vesicle after the formation of the extraembryonic coelom. Reproduced with permission from Beck et al (1985).

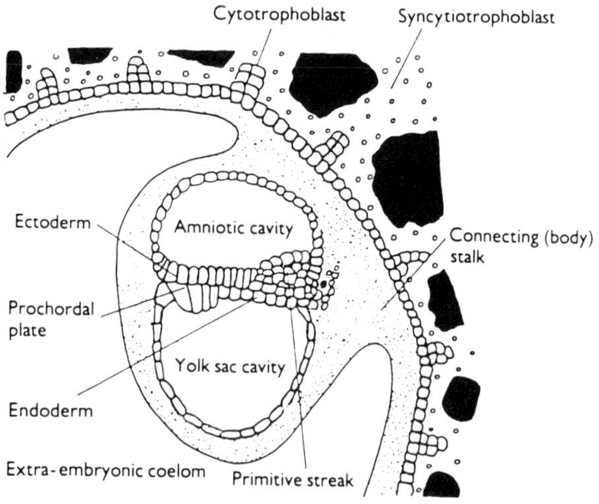

Fig. 6.5 Sagittal section of day 15 embryo within chorionic vesicle, showing formation of prochordal plate and primitive streak. Reproduced with permission from Beck et al (1985).

FORMATION OF THE TRILAMINAR DISC

Between 14 and 16 days after fertilization the trilaminar embryonic disc is formed by interposition of a notochord and mesoderm (the chordamesoderm) between embryonic ectoderm and endoderm. The cells of the upper layer of the bilaminar disc proliferate and migrate backwards and medially to amass at the posterior part of the embryonic midline to form the primitive streak (Fig. 6.5). Once within the streak the cells lose their columnar form, become rounded and spread laterally and forward between ectoderm and endoderm as intraembryonic mesoderm. At the lateral border of the embryonic disc the migrating cells become continuous with the extraembryonic mesoderm covering both yolk sac and amnion. Anteriorly the embryonic mesodermal cells of each side become continuous across the midline in front of the prochordal plate, although in the region of the plate itself ectoderm and endoderm remain in contact forming the buccopharyngeal membrane. The primitive streak elongates by addition of cells to its posterior extremity (Fig. 6.6). The endoderm in the roof of the yolk sac behind the primitive streak remains (like that of the prochordal plate) adherent to the overlying ectoderm to form the cloacal membrane but some of the embryonic mesodermal cells migrate backwards from the streak, mingling with and contributing to the extraembryonic mesoderm of the connecting

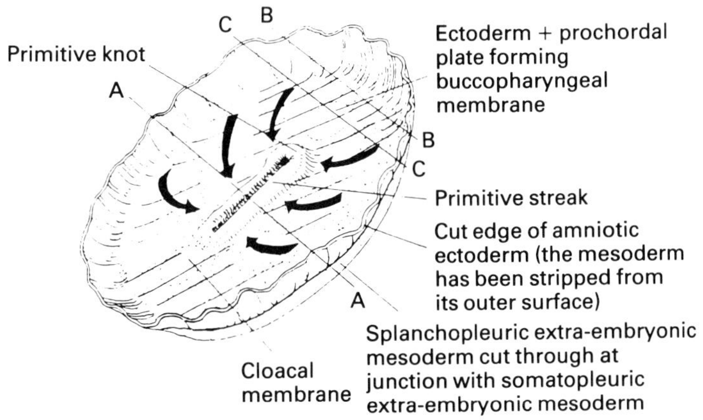

Fig. 6.6 (a) Diagram of the embryonic disc revealed by cutting away the overlying amnion. Intraembryonic ectoderm is represented as being transparent, showing the stippled intraembryonic mesoderm beneath. Note the absence of mesoderm from the region of the buccopharyngeal and cloacal membranes. Arrows indicate the direction of migration of cells towards the primitive streak.

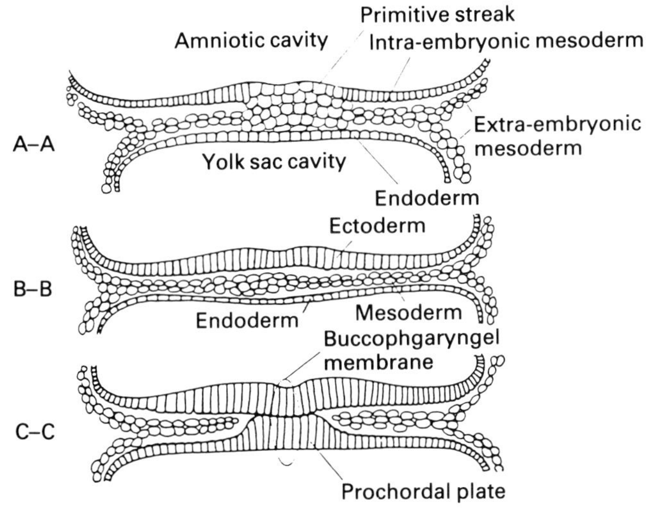

Fig. 6.6 (b) Transverse sections through the embryo shown in Fig. 6.6(a) at A–A, B–B and C–C. Reproduced with permission from Beck et al (1985).

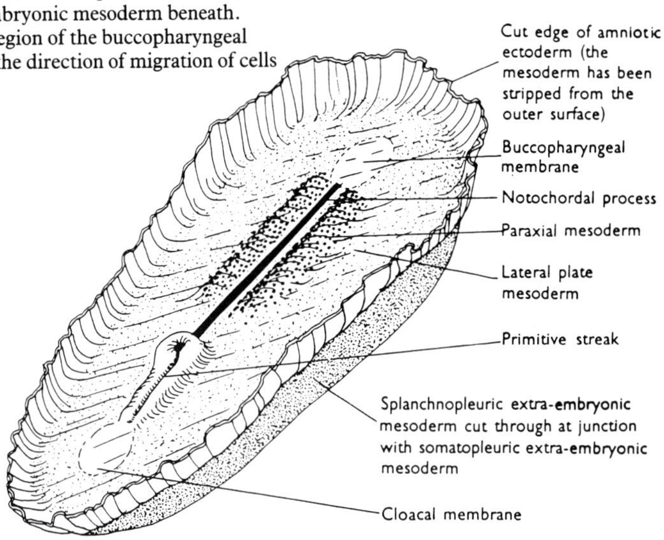

Fig. 6.7 A more advanced stage of development than that shown in Fig. 6.6(a). The notochord is elongated and the paraxial mesoderm is heaped up on either side of it as the somites begin to form. Reproduced with permission from Beck et al (1985).

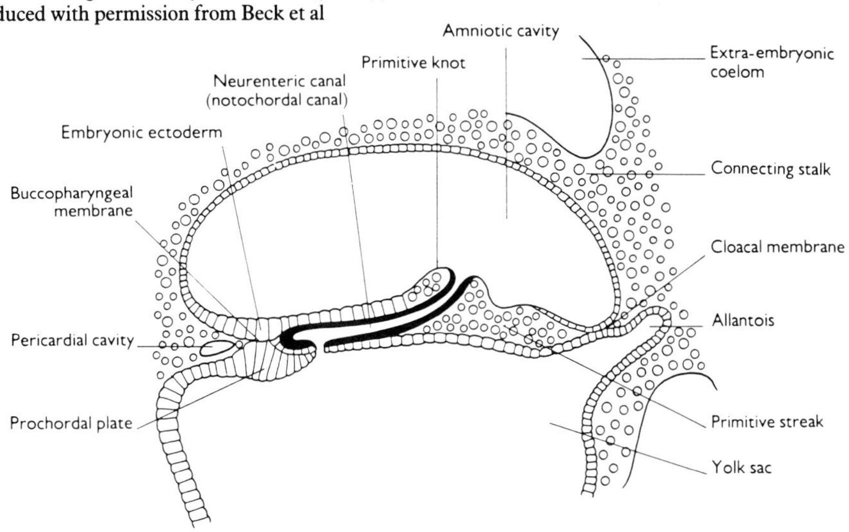

Fig. 6.8 A diagrammatic sagittal section through the embryonic disc at 16 days. Reproduced with permission from Beck et al (1985).

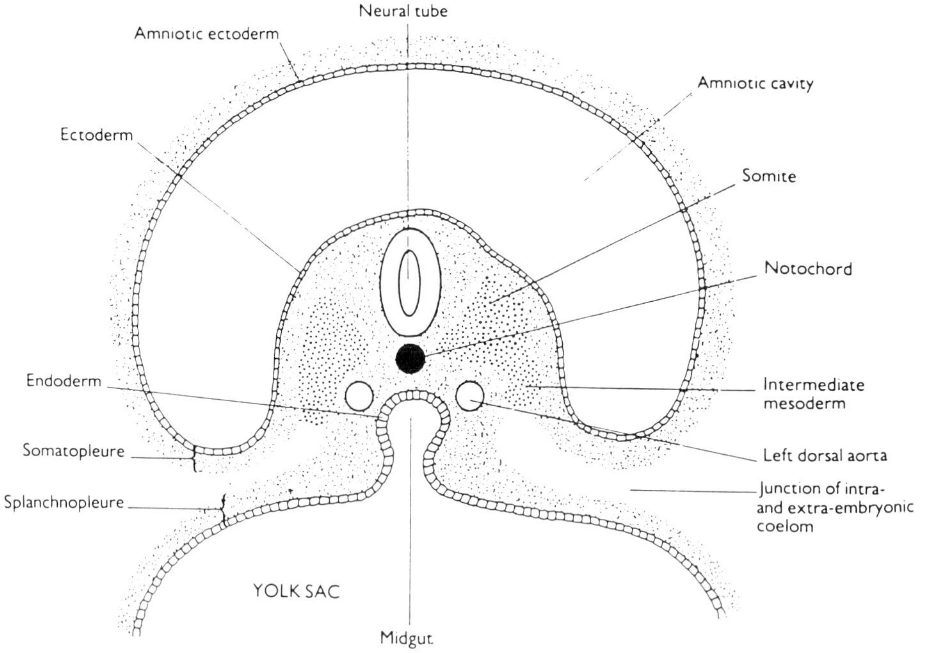

Fig. 6.9 The embryonic disc is beginning to bulge into the amniotic cavity forming lateral folds. The intraembryonic mesoderm has split to form the intraembryonic coelom which is continuous at the edges of the disc with the extraembryonic coelom (see Fig. 6.10, A–A). Reproduced with permission from Beck et al (1985).

stalk (Fig. 6.5). At 16 days a further amassing of cells takes place at the anterior extremity of the primitive streak. This is the primitive knot which will form an elongated notochordal process extending forward to the posterior edge of the prochordal plate (Fig. 6.7, 6.8). The notochordal process undergoes a series of changes, including a stage of canalization and intercalation into the yolk sac roof (Fig. 6.7), which may be of clinical importance. At 17–18 days ectoderm overlying the notochordal process and the region immediately anterior to it forms a thickened neural plate from which the neural tube arises. Mesoderm on either side of the notochord forms thickened strips of paraxial mesoderm which become segmented to form 44 somites. More anteriorly this area of thickened mesoderm remains unsegmented. Lateral to the paraxial mass the mesoderm forms lateral plate mesoderm but a longitudinal tract of intermediate mesoderm (intermediate cell mass) remains interposed between the two. This will give rise to the nephrogenic chord (Fig. 6.9). While still in the trilaminar disc stage, a small diverticulum—the allantois—grows into the connecting stalk immediately behind the cloacal membrane (Fig. 6.8).

Before leaving the subject of germ layer formation, it is worth mentioning that the phenomenon is not basically equivalent to cell determination or differentiation. In fact, the

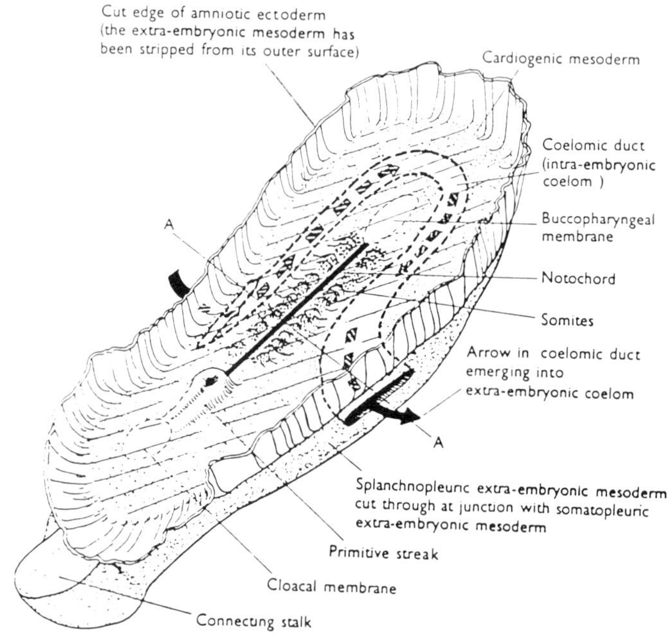

Fig. 6.10 19–20-day embryo showing the intraembryonic coelom. A section through A–A is shown in Fig. 6.9. Reproduced with permission from Beck et al (1985).

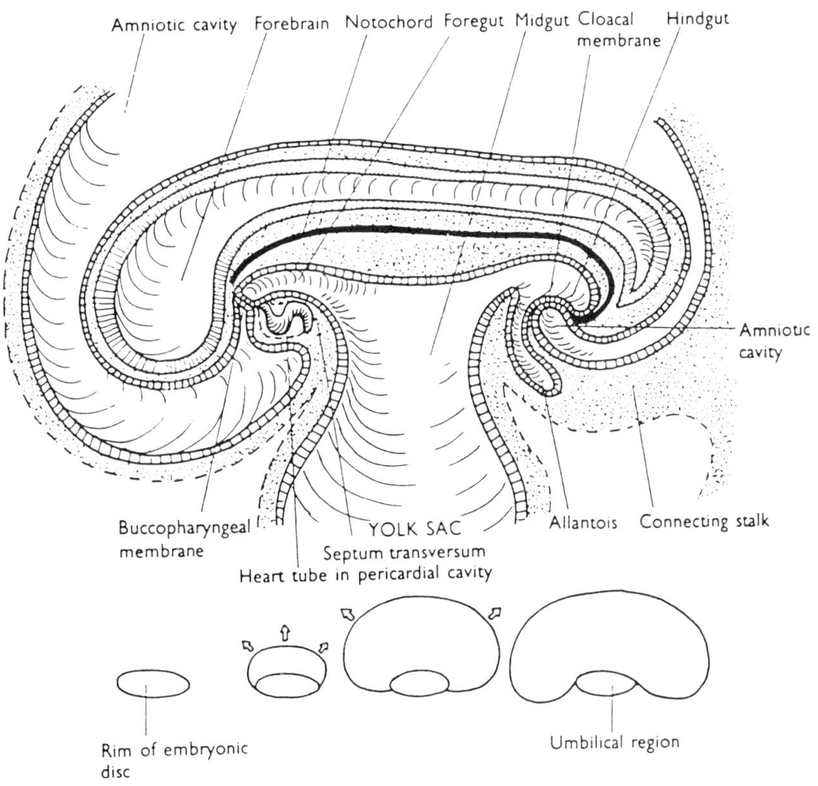

Fig. 6.11 Sagittal section through the embryo during the fourth week showing the formation of the head and tail folds. The four lower diagrams show how the head, tail and lateral folds result from the bulging upwards and outwards of the embryonic disc from its relatively fixed rim. Reproduced with permission from Beck et al (1985).

division of the early embryo into three primary germ layers is, to some extent, one of descriptive convenience.

THE INTRAEMBRYONIC COELOM AND FORMATION OF THE BODY FOLDS

A horseshoe-shaped cavity, the intraembryonic coelom, appears in the lateral plate mesoderm at 19–20 days of development (Fig. 6.10). The lateral arms of the horseshoe are connected across the midline just anterior to the buccopharyngeal membrane and this is the site of the future pericardial cavity. Caudally the horseshoe communicates with the extraembryonic coelom on either side (Fig. 6.9, 6.10) in the region of the future midgut. The embryonic splanchnopleure and somatopleure are thus formed (Fig. 6.9).

During the fourth week after fertilization the trilaminar embryonic disc bulges into the amniotic cavity. A head and tail fold are formed by folding under of the cranial and caudal parts of the disc (Fig. 6.11). Concurrently, quite marked folding takes place along the lateral margins of the embryo (Fig. 6.12). As a consequence a primitive endodermally lined foregut is formed within the head fold and a hindgut with an allantoic diverticulum is present in the tail fold. Between them the midgut is continuous inferiorly with the yolk sac (Fig. 6.11). Gradually, the lateral folds constrict the cavity of the midgut from the remainder of the yolk sac, producing an elongated vitello-intestinal duct (Fig. 6.12) which connects the midgut with a shrivelled yolk sac remnant until quite late in pregnancy.

When the head and tail folds have formed, the caudal wall of the pericardial cavity forms an important landmark called the septum transversum (Fig. 6.13). The latter is, in fact, a broad ventral mesentery for the caudal portion of the foregut and also forms the anterior extremity of the midgut. It is also the anterior limit of the connection between the intra- and extraembryonic coelom, as can be seen in Figure 6.13, and is therefore a region in which vessels can pass from the somatopleure to the splanchnopleure.

The 26-day embryo shown in Figure 6.13 illustrates the relationship between the gut and the intraembryonic coelom.

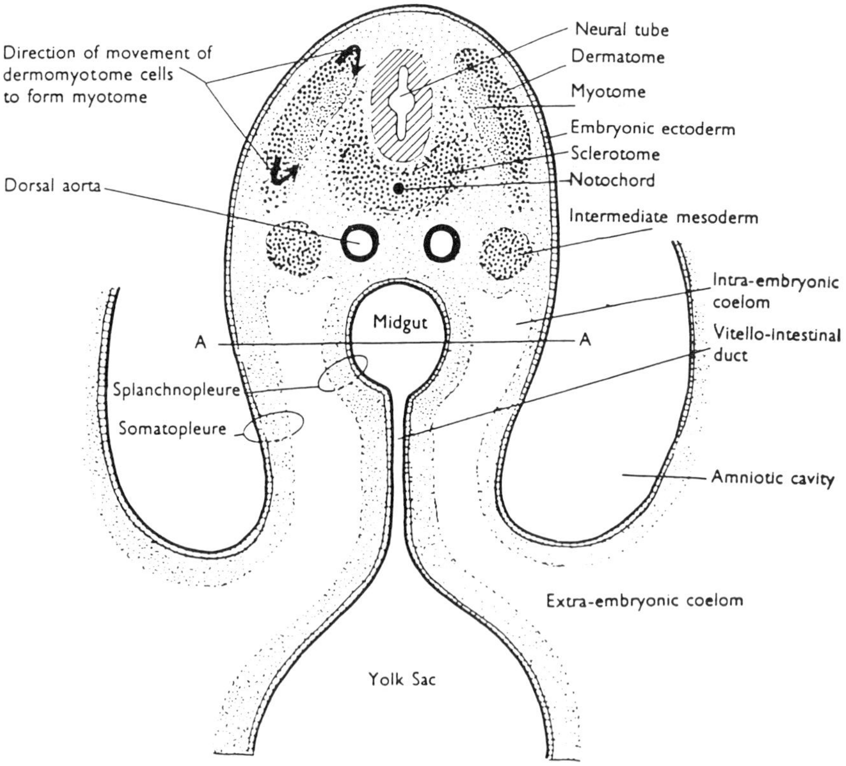

Fig. 6.12 Transverse section through the embryo after the formation of the lateral folds in the region of the midgut. Reproduced with permission from Beck et al (1985).

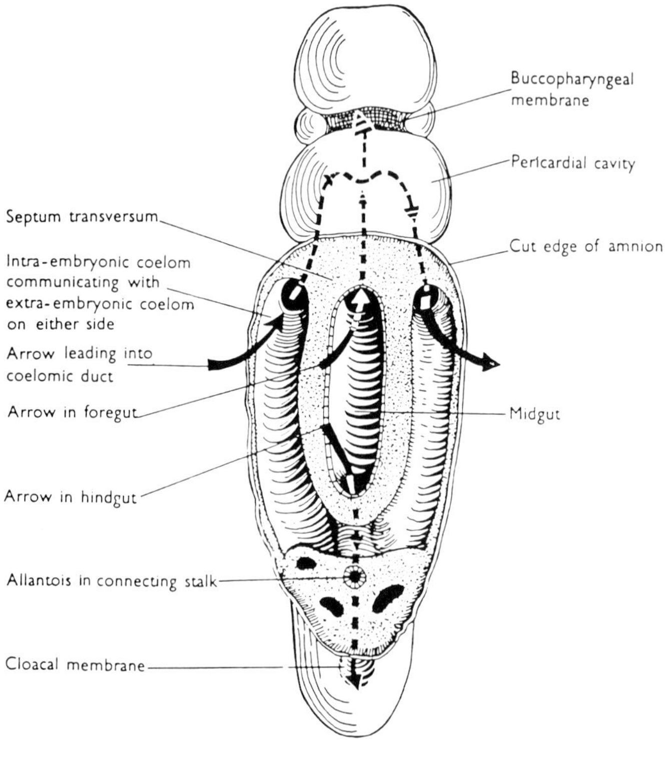

Fig. 6.13 Ventral view of a 26-day embryo in which the ventral region has been removed along the line A–A in Fig. 6.12. Reproduced with permission from Beck et al (1985).

In the tail fold region the attachment of the connecting stalk can now be seen on the ventral aspect of the embryo. The main part of the allantois has been taken into the embryo but it still extends into the stalk for a short distance. Behind the connecting stalk the cloacal membrane (see above) separates the hindgut from the amniotic cavity. The hindgut itself forms a single chamber which gives rise to the greater part of the cloaca, which will become subdivided by a septum, thus forming the primitive urogenital sinus anteriorly and the rectum posteriorly. The primitive urogenital sinus eventually forms much of the bladder and urethra (see below).

DEVELOPMENT OF THE MAJOR ORGAN SYSTEMS

In this chapter it is clearly impossible to review human organogenesis comprehensively. The approach has been, therefore, to highlight the central issues in developmental anatomy using a visual approach based upon the copious use of diagrams. These are based upon, or reproduced from, *Human Embryology* by Beck et al (1985), where there is further detail and reference to clinical significance. In the present chapter particular attention is paid to the temporal sequence of events.

The mesodermal somites

The embryo illustrated in Figure 6.13 has about 20 somites, although these are not visible in ventral view. An embryo towards the end of the somite stage (approximately 33 somites) is illustrated in Figure 6.14. The somites have developed from the parachordal mesoderm (see above) and at this stage have the appearance of square opacities in the rather transparent tissues of the embryo. They form the basic segmental structure of the body and somite-derived tissue will spread medially to form vertebrae, dorsally to form the extensor musculature of the back and ventrally into the body wall to form ribs, intercostal muscles and abdominal muscles. The dermis of the skin is also of somite origin; without it the skin would remain a thin and semi-transparent somatopleure and eventually would lose its viability. The somites form a craniocaudal gradient of maturity, the first appearing in the future occipital region at about 21 days after fertilization. Caudal somites remain visible until 40–45 days but after the first month (26 somites) it is usual to stage embryos by reference to the crown–rump length rather than by somite number.

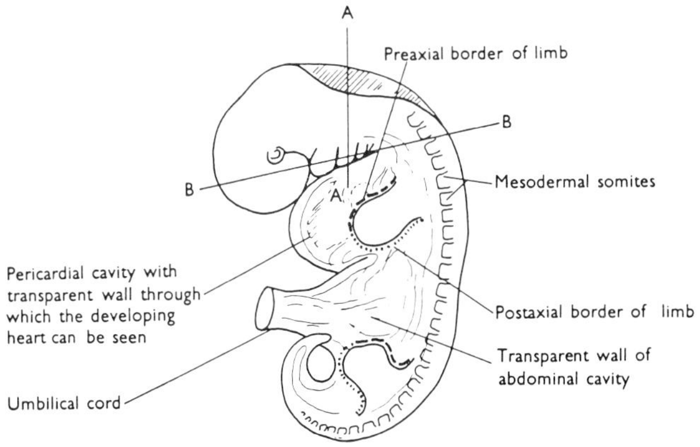

Fig. 6.14 An embryo in the somite stage of development (about 33 days) before invasion of the body wall by cells from the somites. The limb buds have just begun to develop. Reproduced with permission from Beck et al (1985).

In total, about 44 somites develop in the human although the most cranial ones begin to break up before the caudal ones are completed. There are 4 occipital, 8 cervical, 12 thoracic, 5 lumbar, 5 sacral and 8–10 coccygeal somites.

The ventro-medial part of each somite forms the sclerotome (Sensenig 1949) and its cells stream medially to surround the neural tube (Fig. 6.9, 6.12). The largest accumulation of cells surrounds the notochord. At 4 weeks the caudal portion of each sclerotome begins to unite with the cranial portion of the next to form the vertebral body which is, therefore, an *intersegmental structure* so that the nerves which originally innervated each of the somites now lie between the vertebrae, while the arteries which originally passed between the somites now lie close to the vertebral bodies (Fig. 6.15). Each sclerotome, in addition to forming

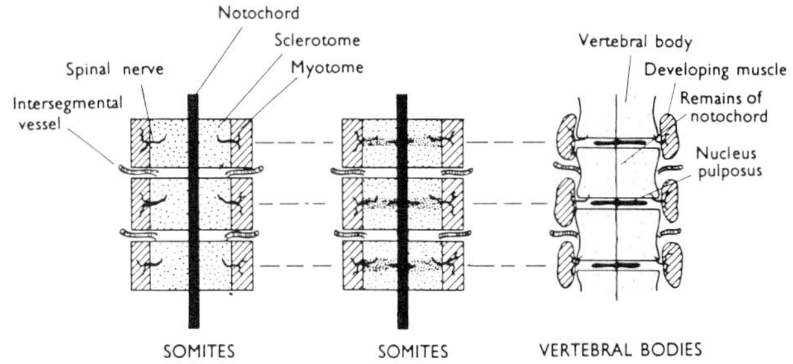

Fig. 6.15 Each vertebral body is formed from the adjacent halves of two somites. A segmental nerve supplies the myotome of each somite and an intersegmental artery passes between each somite pair. With the formation of the vertebral bodies the nerves become intervertebral in position and the arteries run in relation to the vertebral bodies. Reproduced with permission from Beck et al (1985).

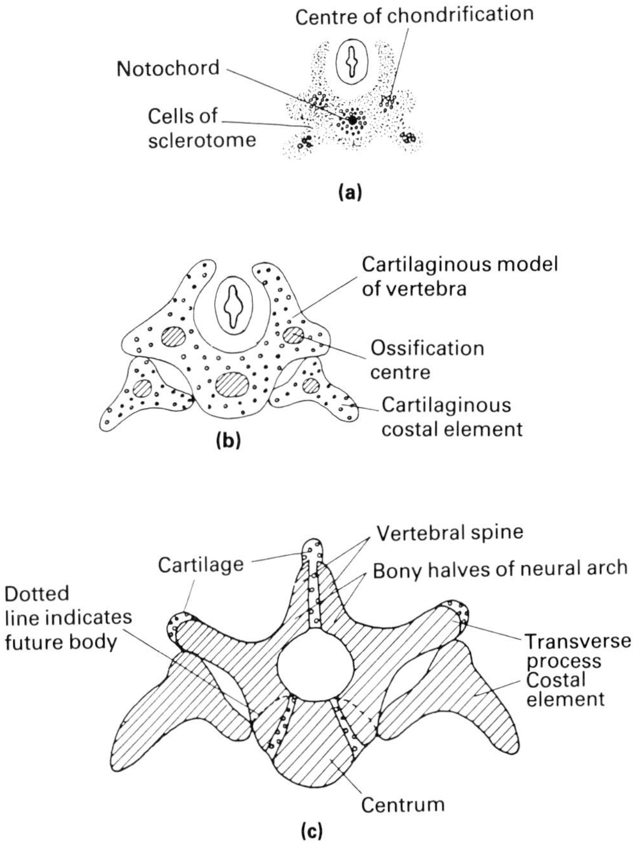

Fig. 6.16 (a) The cells of the sclerotome migrate towards the neural tube and form the rough shape of a vertebra. (**b**) Cartilaginous models of vertebrae and costal elements develop, with centres of ossification for the centrum, for each half of the neural arch and for each rib. (**c**) The vertebra and costal elements are almost completely ossified but some cartilage remains so that at birth each bony vertebra is in three pieces. Reproduced with permission from Beck et al (1985).

the vertebral centrum, also forms a neural arch and transverse processes and these elements begin to chondrify in the cervical region in the seventh week. Ossification begins between T5 and S2 in the eighth week, between C5 and T4 and L5 and S2 after 12 weeks, in C2 and C4 and S3 by about 16 weeks, at C1 and S4 after 20 weeks and at S5 at about 28 weeks. At birth the vertebrae have three ossific centres—one in the centrum and one on each side of the neural arch. Costal elements develop in close relation to the transverse processes and their ultimate fate varies in different regions of the spine (Fig. 6.16, 6.17).

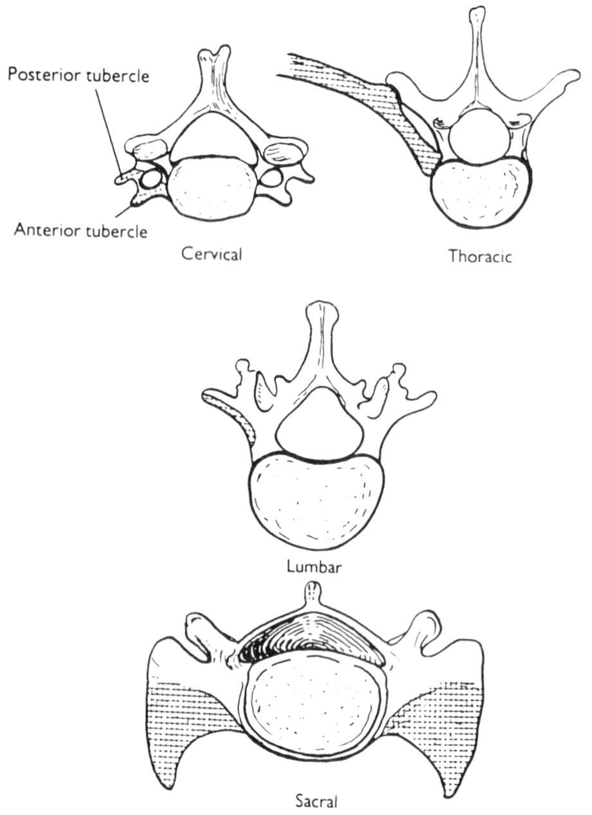

Fig. 6.17 Cervical, thoracic, lumbar and sacral vertebrae. The costal element is shaded. Reproduced with permission from Beck et al (1985).

The tissue remaining after segregation of the sclerotome (Fig. 6.12) differentiates into an inner myotome and an outer dermatome. The spindle-shaped myoblasts of the myotome form the epaxial and hypaxial skeletal musculature, the former by moving into a position between the transverse processes and the spines of the vertebrae, while the latter moves into the body wall which thus becomes thicker and less transparent. The myotomes of certain somites adopt an atypical location giving rise, for example, to tongue, diaphragmatic and pelvic floor musculature. In the whole of the trunk (including the pectoral and pelvic girdles) migrating myoblasts are followed by their nerves so that it becomes a simple matter to deduce the origin of any trunk muscle. Even though the subjective sensation of quickening is not appreciated until about 20 weeks, the first local reflexes, i.e. mouth-opening after stimulation of the facial skin, are present at 8 weeks and motor end-plates are well developed by the 12th week. Motor responses to cutaneous stimulation thus occur in the hands by 12 weeks and in the feet by 16 weeks. The definitive body wall is complete by 12 weeks.

Like the myotomes, the dermatomes take their nerve supply with them and the dermis is established by 12 weeks.

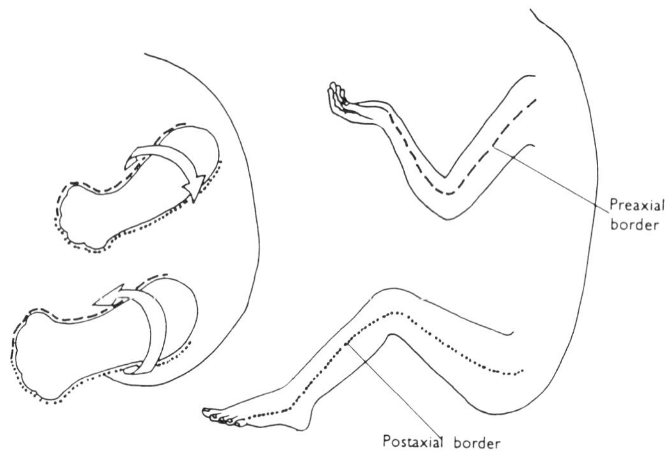

Fig. 6.18 Stages in the development of the limbs to show their changes in position. Reproduced with permission from Beck et al (1985).

By 10 weeks the nail anlages appear, as do lanugo hairs. By 20 weeks the vernix caseosa is present and at around 28 weeks of gestation the scalp and eyebrow hairs develop. At birth the nails reach the end of the fingers and the nipples are everted.

As in birds, the limb musculature of mammals probably develops in situ rather than from the somites. Limb buds appear at the somite stage of development (Fig. 6.14) and at about 5 weeks the prominences of the future knee and elbow region can be recognized, projecting both laterally and backwards. Hand and foot plates appear as flattened expansions and between 36 and 38 days the digital rays become apparent. The limb bones differentiate from the mesenchyme of the limb bud. The limb buds grow in such a way that they appear to rotate in different directions (Fig. 6.18) so that the preaxial border of the hand is located laterally and that of the foot medially.

The nervous system

The development of the primitive neural tube from the neural groove overlying the notochord is illustrated in Figure

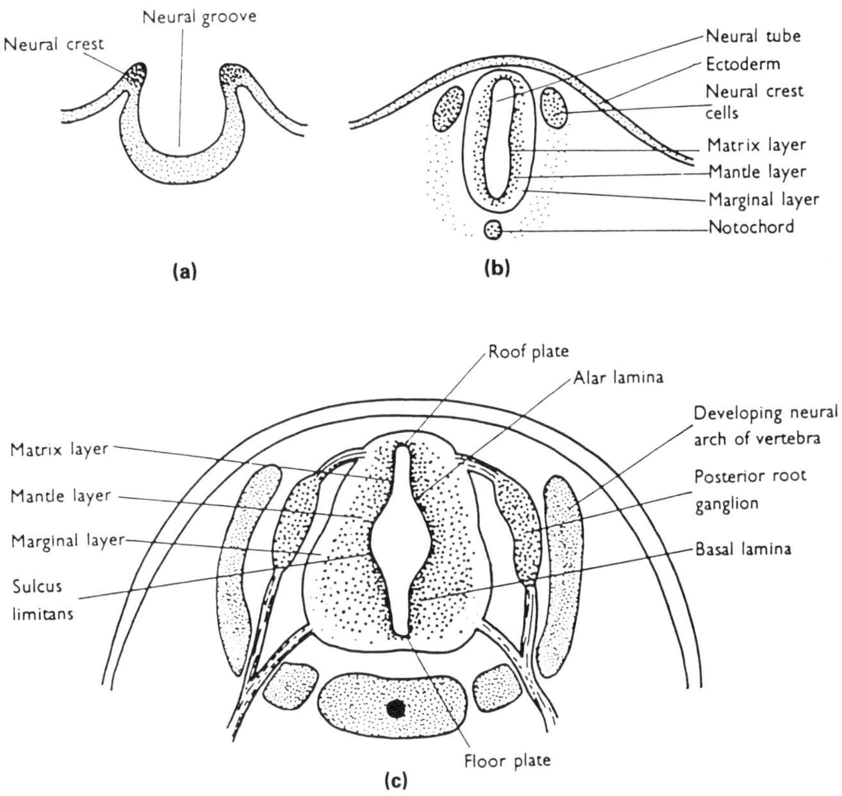

Fig. 6.19 (a) The neural groove and neural crest. (b) and (c) The neural crest cells form inter alia the posterior root ganglia. The three layers of the neural tube can be distinguished. Reproduced with permission from Beck et al (1985).

6.19. Excellent reviews of the histogenesis and general development of the central nervous system are available (Langman 1968, O'Rahilly & Gardner 1971, S. Jacobson 1972, M. Jacobson 1978, Lemire et al 1975) and the afferent and efferent columns of grey matter which develop in the alar (sensory) and basal (motor) laminae of the spinal cord are illustrated in Figure 6.20. It will be appreciated that the visceral afferent and efferent columns are restricted to the thoraco-lumbar and sacral outflow regions. In the brain stem additional special visceral afferent (gustatory) and special visceral efferent (branchial) columns appear in connection with the special sense of taste and the voluntary muscles associated with the branchial arches. This is illustrated in a diagrammatic transverse section through the fourth ventricle (Fig. 6.21).

At 21 days the neural groove begins to form the neural tube at the level of somites 4–6; by 25 days the groove is closed except for its anterior and posterior ends (neuropores) and by day 30 closure is complete. By this time it is possible to recognize three well defined subdivisions of

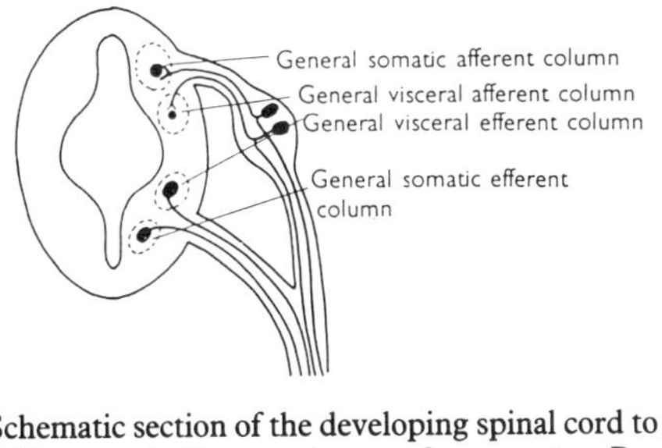

Fig. 6.20 Schematic section of the developing spinal cord to show the two types of efferent and afferent columns of grey matter. Reproduced with permission from Beck et al (1985).

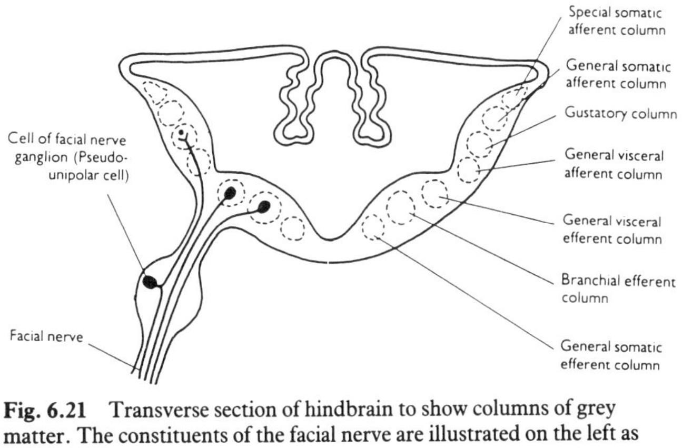

Fig. 6.21 Transverse section of hindbrain to show columns of grey matter. The constituents of the facial nerve are illustrated on the left as an example of the connections of a cranial nerve. Reproduced with permission from Beck et al (1985).

the brain — the forebrain (prosencephalon), midbrain (mesencephalon) and hindbrain (rhombencephalon; Fig. 6.22). The cervical and midbrain flexures have formed. By 35 days the pontine flexure forms as a corollary to a thinning

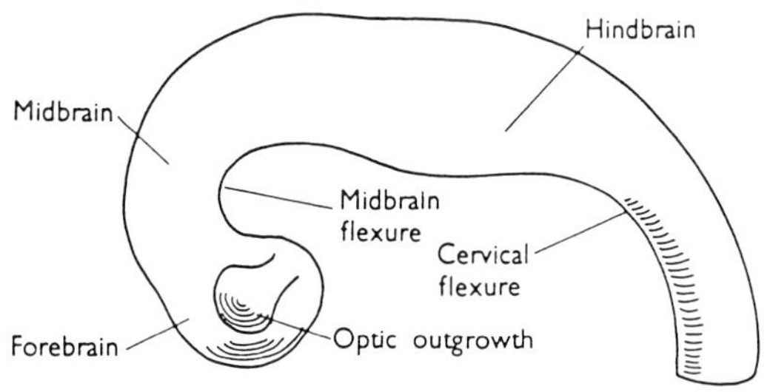

Fig. 6.22 The cranial end of the neural tube at 28 days showing the primitive forebrain, midbrain and hindbrain. Reproduced with permission from Beck et al (1985).

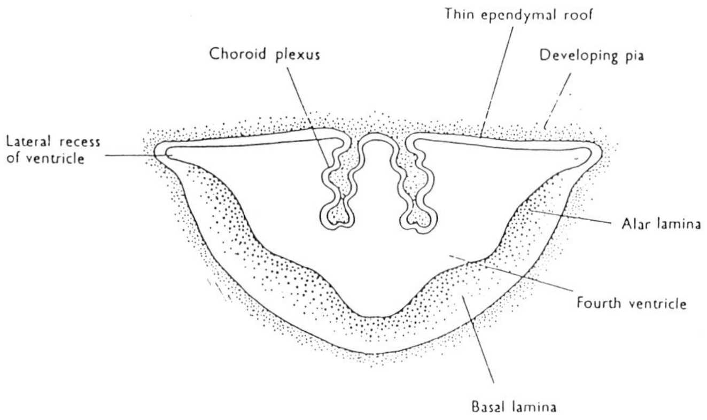

Fig. 6.24 The pontine flexure causes the lateral walls of the hindbrain to spread out so that the roof plate is thinned. Note its invagination by the choroid plexus. Reproduced with permission from Beck et al (1985).

of the roof of the hindbrain in the region of the fourth ventricle (Fig. 6.23, 6.24). Within the fifth week the optic vesicles become invaginated and the lens of the eye is formed from an ectodermal placode. By this time the otic vesicles,

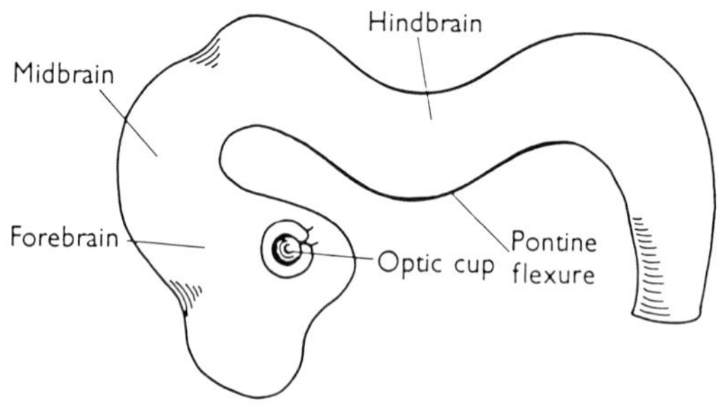

Fig. 6.23 The development of the pontine flexure at approximately 35 days. Reproduced with permission from Beck et al (1985).

which will develop into the inner ear, have formed from ectodermal placodes situated in the rhombencephalic region. Meanwhile the forebrain shows signs of increasing complexity with the formation of the telencephalic vesicles (Fig. 6.25). The two vesicles and the intervening part of the forebrain together form the telencephalon while the posterior part of the forebrain forms the diencephalon (Fig. 6.26). The telencephalic vesicles increase rapidly in size and soon hide the diencephalon completely. Their walls remain relatively thin except in the floor and lateral walls where the corpus striatum develops. A further thickening, the thalamus, appears in the lateral wall of the diencephalon. The original cranial end of the neural tube — the lamina terminalis — is a region in which commissural fibres develop and the corpus callosum begins to develop here (Fig. 6.27). Projection fibres develop and fill up the space between the telencephalon and diencephalon until eventually these two parts of the forebrain

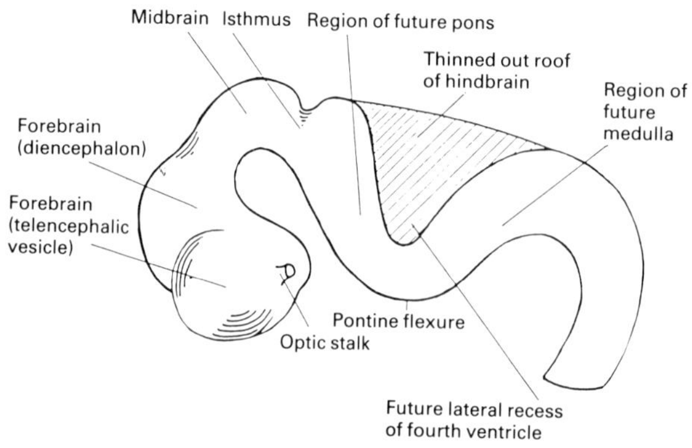

Fig. 6.25 The brain at 37 days. The pontine flexure is further developed and the telencephalic vesicles are forming. Reproduced with permission from Beck et al (1985).

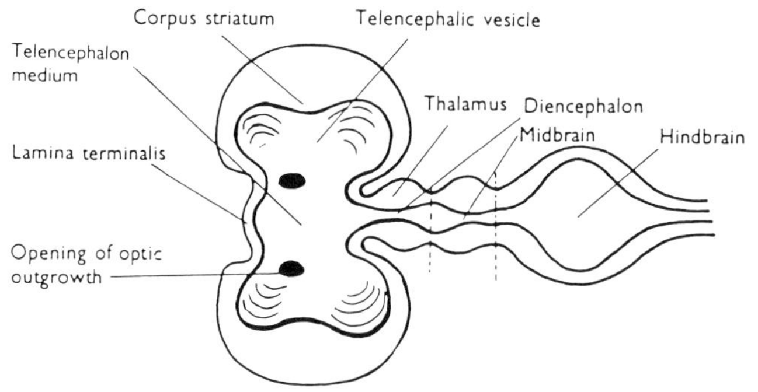

Fig. 6.26 Diagrammatic horizontal section through the developing brain. Reproduced with permission from Beck et al (1985).

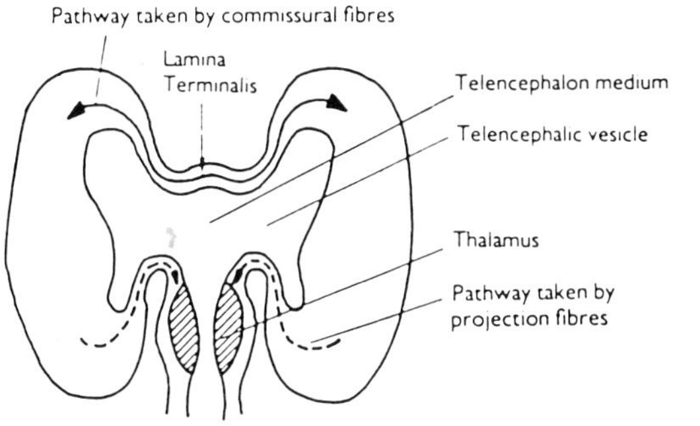

Fig. 6.27 Diagrammatic horizontal section through the developing forebrain to show how the commissural fibres use the lamina terminalis as a pathway while the projection fibres bend sharply round into the diencephalon. Reproduced with permission from Beck et al (1985).

fuse so that the projection fibres and the developing corpus striatum lie immediately lateral to the thalamus (Fig. 6.28).

Around the developing brain a condensation of vascular mesenchyme, the meninx primitiva, gives rise to the membranous neurocranium and to the three layers of the meninges. The choroid plexuses are formed because the medial wall of the telencephalic vesicle remains very thin in one region and the vascular pia, together with the ependyma, becomes invaginated into the medial walls of the lateral ventricle and also forms the roof of the third ventricle (Fig. 6.28). A slight longitudinal swelling above the thin part of the medial wall of the telencephalon develops into the hippocampus. A bundle of nerve fibres of hippocampal origin decussate in the fornix, and the choroid fissure through which the choroid plexuses invaginate the ventricle lies immediately below this (Fig. 6.28). The cerebral hemispheres grow caudally and the caudal pole folds over to form the temporal lobe in which lies the inferior horn of the lateral ventricle. As a result the choroid fissure, fornix and hippocampus become reversed in position in the temporal lobe. This is illustrated in Figure 6.29, which also shows the development of the corpus callosum from the region of the lamina terminalis. The events described above happen early in gestation. At 7 weeks there is already a large corpus striatum and thalamus and at 8 weeks, the meninges have formed and the cerebral cortex is differentiating. At this stage the downgrowth of the forebrain, which will form the posterior lobe of the pituitary, fuses with an upgrowth from the primitive mouth (Rathke's pouch) to form the pituitary gland (Fig. 6.30). Gonadotrophs are immunocytochemically identifiable in the pars distalis at the beginning of the fourth month and gradually other cell types differentiate, ending with follicle-stimulating hormone-secreting cells at about 30 weeks.

By 12–16 weeks the brain begins to resemble that of the adult and the corpus callosum together with the other commissures are formed. From 16 weeks to full term, the cerebral gyri and sulci appear, the insula sinks below the surface

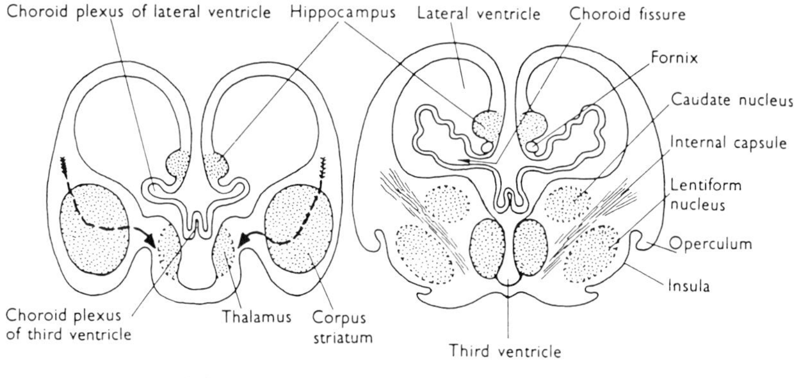

Fig. 6.28 Frontal section through the forebrain. (**a**) Arrows show the pathway taken by projection fibres through the corpus striatum and into the diencephalon. (**b**) Fusion has taken place between the lateral sides of the diencephalon and the medial side of the telencephalon lateral to the thalamus. The corpus striatum is divided into lentiform and caudate nuclei. The choroid fissure is developing in relation to the hippocampus and fornix. Reproduced with permission from Beck et al (1985).

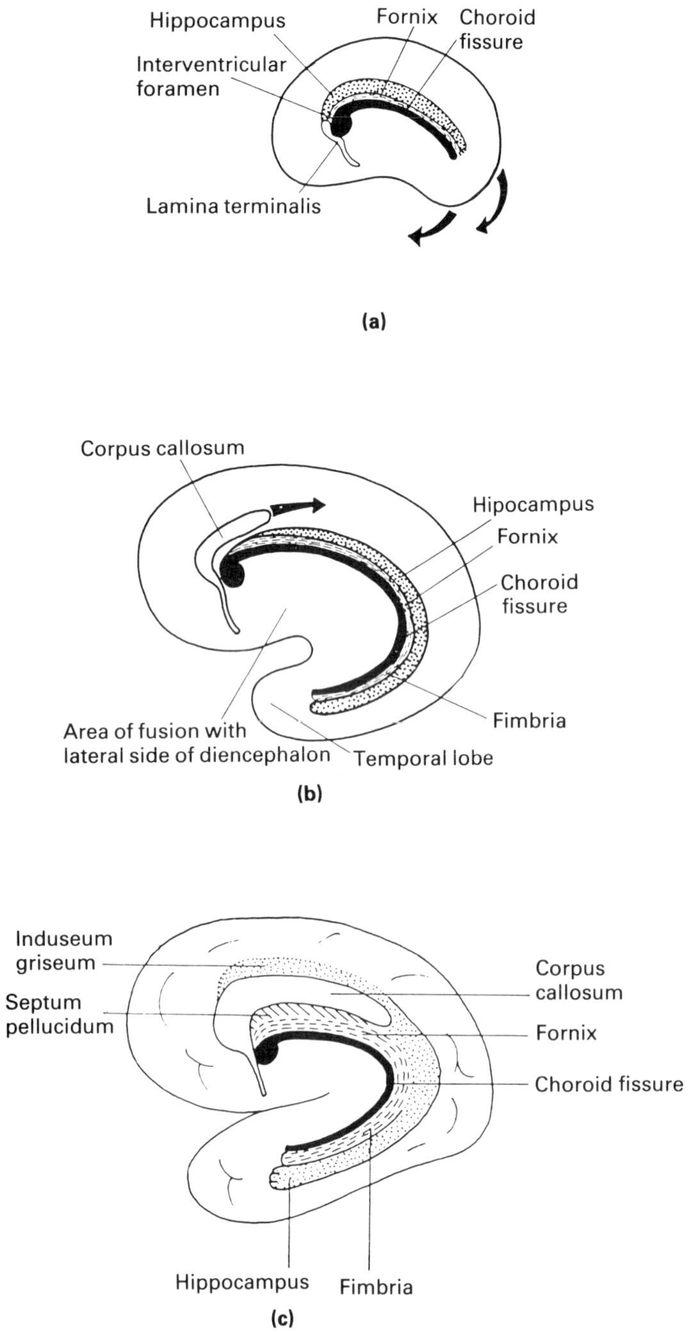

Fig. 6.29 Diagram of the medial side of the telencephalic vesicle detached from the mesencephalon. (**a**) Arrows show the main direction of growth. (**b**) Growth of the caudal part of the telencephalic vesicle has formed the temporal lobe. The fornix lies above the choroid fissure but its continuation, the fimbria, lies *below* the choroid fissure in the *temporal* lobe. (**c**) The corpus callosum has grown caudally and the upper part of the hippocampus is represented only by the indusium griseum. Reproduced with permission from Beck et al (1985).

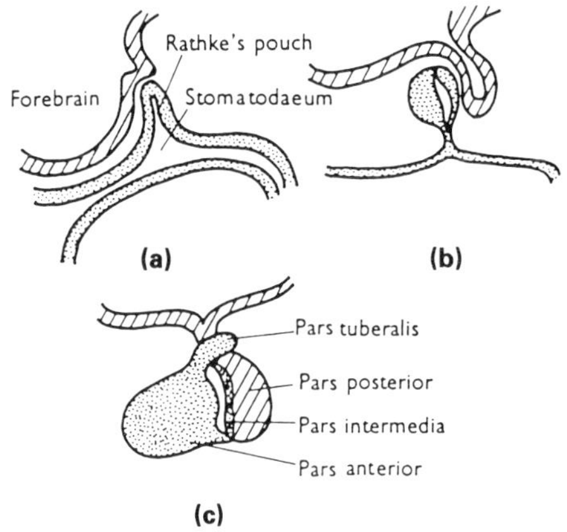

Fig. 6.30 The development of the pituitary gland. (**a**) An upgrowth (Rathke's pouch) from the stomatodaeum meets a downgrowth from the forebrain. (**b**) The walls of Rathke's pouch become thicker, particularly the anterior wall, and the pouch separates from the stomatodaeum. (**c**) The mature pituitary gland. Reproduced with permission from Beck et al (1985).

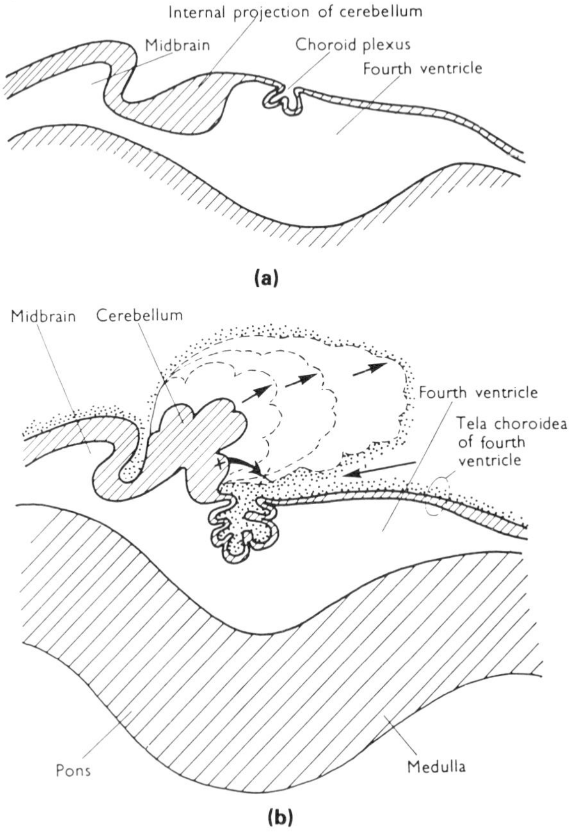

Fig. 6.31 (**a**) The cerebellum begins to grow into the fourth ventricle. (**b**) It then becomes everted to overhang the thin roof of the fourth ventricle. The small arrows indicate the backward growth of the neocerebellum. The long arrow indicates the cerebello-medullary subarachnoid cistern of the adult. Reproduced with permission from Beck et al (1985).

and considerable myelinization takes place though, as is well known, this is not complete until well after birth. By about 16 weeks the neuronal cell complement of the brain is almost complete. There follows a phase of brain growth spurt beginning at 20 weeks of gestation, reaching a maximum at 40 weeks, completed by about the fifth year after conception. The growth spurt involves multiplication of glia and increasing myelinization. Figure 6.31 illustrates the formation of the cerebellum which first grows into the fourth ventricle (contained in the hindbrain) and then evaginates to its adult position. Its relationship to the choroid plexus of the fourth ventricle should be noted. The cerebellum begins to develop at 6 weeks and its main lobes are large and clearly delineated by the fourth month.

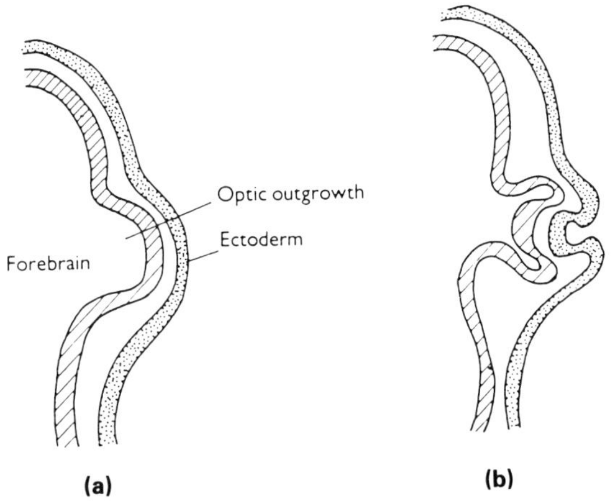

Fig. 6.32 (a) The optic outgrowth from the forebrain. (b) The formation of the lens vesicle and the optic cup. Reproduced with permission from Beck et al (1985).

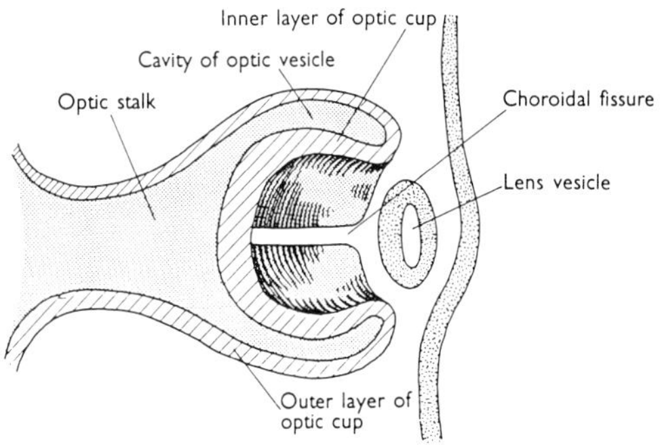

Fig. 6.33 Horizontal section through the optic cup viewed from above. The lens vesicle has detached itself from the surface ectoderm. Reproduced with permission from Beck et al (1985).

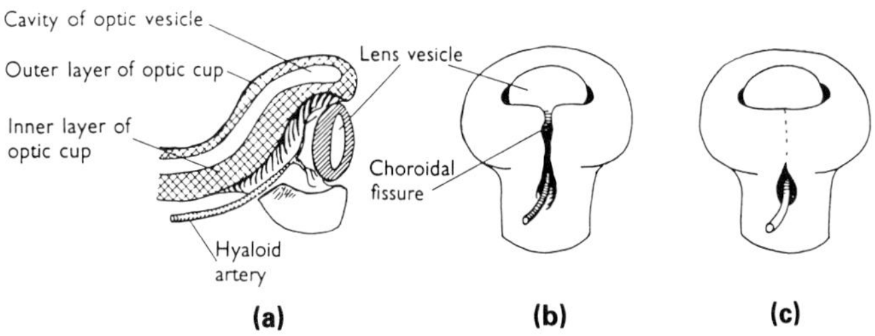

Fig. 6.34 (a) Midline section through the developing eye. The section passes through the choroidal fissure. (b) The optic vesicle seen from below. The hyaloid artery enters through the choroidal fissure. (c) Closure of the choroidal fissure. Reproduced with permission from Beck et al (1985).

Detailed consideration of the special senses is beyond the scope of this review; Figures 6.32–6.35 illustrate the basic development of the eye. Optic pits appear in the floor of the neural plate as early as 4 weeks; the optic cup is formed

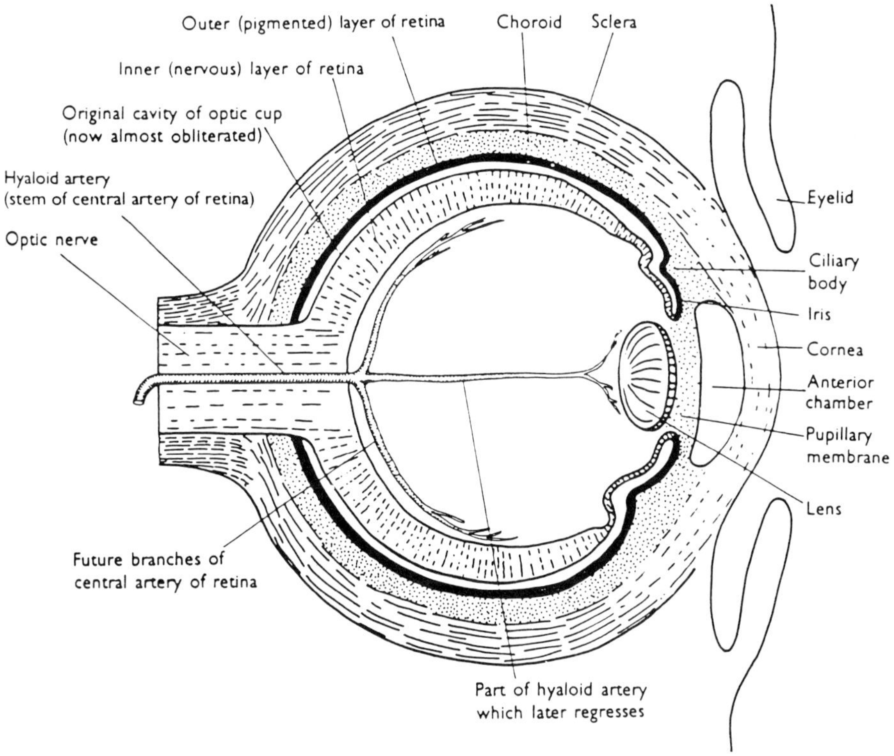

Fig. 6.35 Vertical section through the developing eye. Reproduced with permission from Beck et al (1985).

in the fifth week, the lens vesicle in the sixth, the cornea and sclera in the seventh. By the eighth week the retina has eight layers and optic nerve fibres are well established. By 12 weeks the eyelids have fused and the ciliary muscles of the eye have developed, while by 24 weeks myelination is present in the optic tract and a few weeks later separation of the eyelids is complete. The maculae differentiate late by about 32 weeks and, at this stage, the pupillary light response appears. At full term myelination of the optic nerve — which is proceeding distally — reaches the lamina cribrosa sclerae.

The face, mouth, palate and branchial region

At about the 20-somite stage (Fig. 6.13) the stomatodaeum, or primitive mouth, has been delineated. The mesenchyme covering the forebrain is seen to form its cranial boundary, the mandibular arches are lateral and the pericardial cavity is placed inferiorly. These topographical relations can be seen in sagittal section in Figure 6.11. With the breakdown of the buccopharyngeal membrane the ectodermally derived stomatodaeum becomes continuous with the endodermally lined foregut. The transition occurs at the level of Rathke's pouch but leaves no visible sign after the disappearance of the buccopharyngeal membrane.

Figure 6.36 illustrates the subsequent development of the face (Slarkin 1979). The mandibular arches fuse below the stomatodeal opening and a dorsal wing from each mandibular arch gives rise to the maxillary process on that side. Bilateral thickenings in the ectoderm, the olfactory placodes, sink beneath the surface each to lie in the floor of a nasal sac. The external opening of the sac forms the external nares with mesodermal thickenings — the medial and lateral nasal processes — on each side of it. The mesoderm of the lateral nasal process soon becomes continuous with the maxillary processes and the line of junction between them runs up to the eye. The two medial nasal processes together form the frontonasal process, and the maxillary processes growing further medially fuse with each other and with the frontonasal process in the midline. The embryological basis of hare lip and oblique facial cleft is therefore clear.

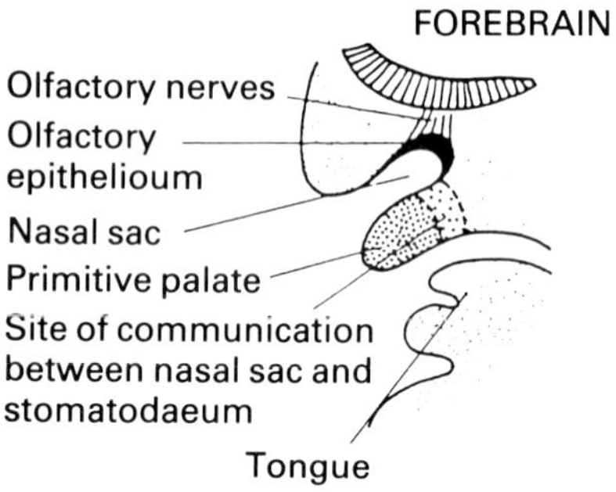

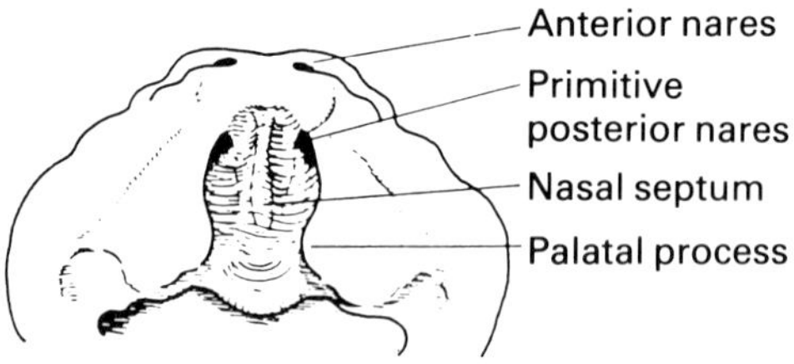

Fig. 6.37 Parasagittal section through the head of an embryo passing through the nasal sac. The sparsely dotted area will later break down to form a communication between nasal sac and stomatodaeum (the primitive posterior nares). Reproduced with permission from Beck et al (1985).

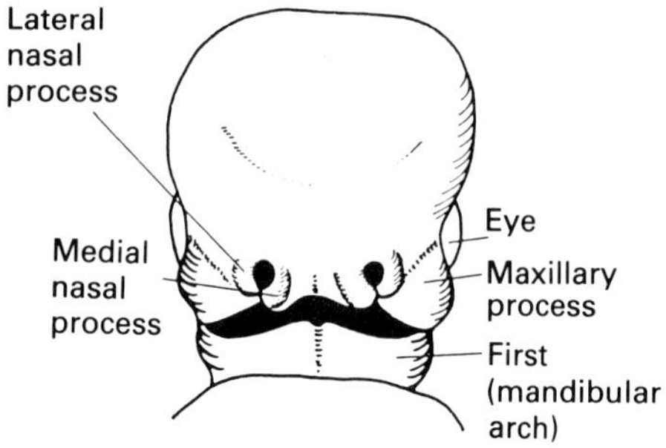

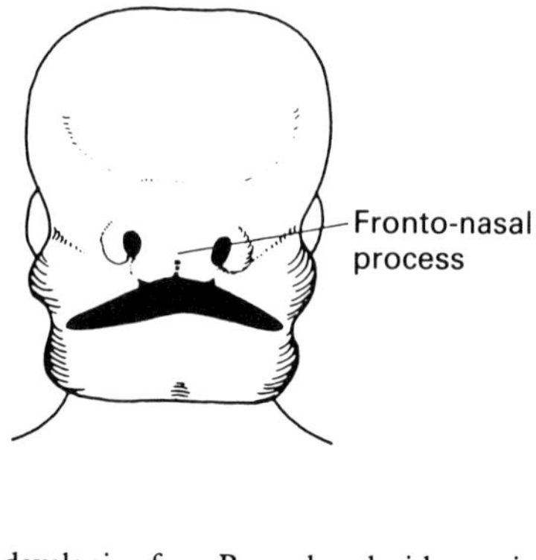

Fig. 6.36 The developing face. Reproduced with permission from Beck et al (1985).

The nasal sac establishes continuity with the stomatodaeum posteriorly to form the primitive posterior nares (Fig. 6.37) and the mesoderm of the maxillary processes becomes continuous with that of the frontonasal process to form the upper lip. The primitive palate is thus established but the greater part of the definitive palate is formed behind this when the palatal processes on each side grow medially from the inner surface of the maxillary processes (Fig. 6.38). At first the palatal processes hang down on either side of the tongue but they eventually rise to meet and fuse with each other and with the edge of the nasal septum. The adoption of the horizontal attitude by the palatal processes is multifactorial, including an increased turgor due to water imbibition, extension of the embryonic head, movements of the tongue etc.

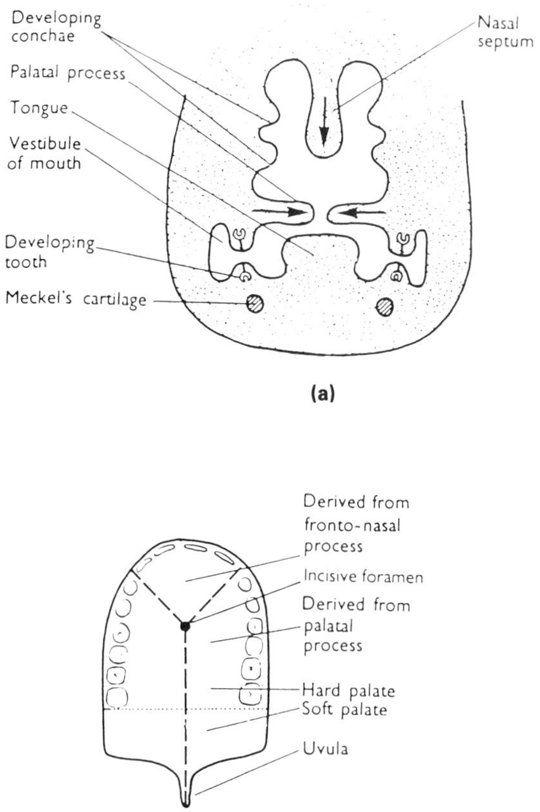

Fig. 6.38 (**a**) Coronal section through the head to show the formation of the palate and nasal septum. The diagram is simplified — in a real embryo the tongue at first lies between the palatal processes so that its dorsum is in contact with the free border of the nasal septum. (**b**) The origin of the constituents of the adult palate. Reproduced with permission from Beck et al (1985).

The maxillary processes appear and the buccopharyngeal membrane ruptures at about 4 weeks. The upper lip is completed in the seventh week though it does not separate from the gums until about 12 weeks. The face is recognizably human at 8 weeks and palatal fusion is complete at 11 weeks. This marks one of the final events of organogenesis of the human embryo.

Figure 6.14 is a lateral view of a somite stage (33 days) embryo. The developing face is seen to be pressed against the pericardium and a little more caudally the lateral surface of the embryo shows a series of elevations, the branchial (or pharyngeal) arches. The two most cranial are clearly marked but, behind these, the arches are progressively smaller and, at about 40 days, they are completely overgrown by the second arch so that the smooth surface of the neck is established (Fig. 6.39). The external groove between the first and second arches forms the external auditory meatus.

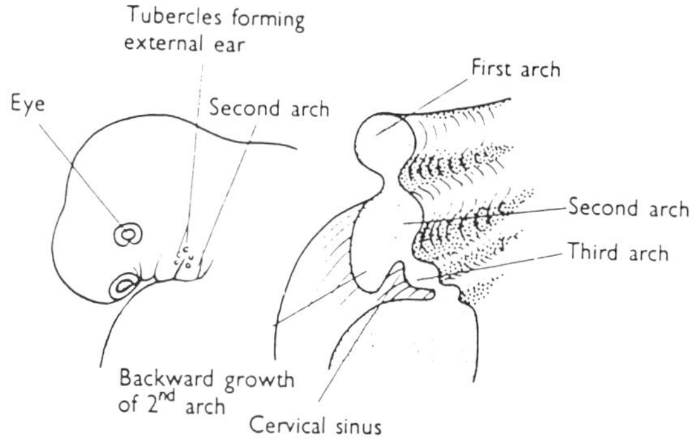

Fig. 6.39 Diagram to show how backward growth of the second arch forms the cervical sinus. Its obliteration will form the smooth line of the neck. Reproduced with permission from Beck et al (1985).

The relationship of the branchial arches and the brain is illustrated by Figure 6.40, which passes through the second arch. The arch consists of a thickening of the mesoderm on each side of the pharynx. This mesoderm blends with mesoderm in the roof and floor of the pharynx. In the floor lies the aortic sac which is the cranial end of the heart tube. From the sac an artery passes dorsally through

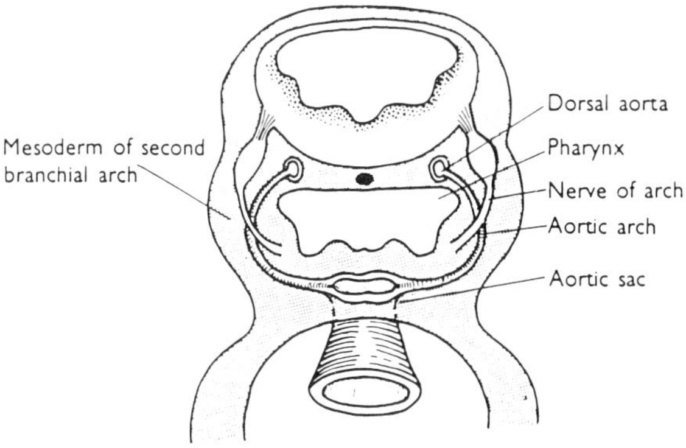

Fig. 6.40 A section through the pharynx at the level of the second branchial arch (A–A in Fig. 6.14), seen from the front. Each arch contains a nerve and an artery. Reproduced with permission from Beck et al (1985).

the arch substance to join one of the paired dorsal aortae which further caudally fuse to form a midline vessel. From the brain one of the cranial nerves (in this case, the seventh) passes ventrally into the arch eventually to supply skeletal muscle of branchial arch origin. Some of the arch mesoderm will also differentiate into skeletal tissue (cartilage, bone). The other branchial arches are very similar, each containing an aortic arch artery, a nerve, muscle and skeletal tissue. Altogether there are six branchial arches; the first gives rise to the muscles of mastication (V); the second the muscles of facial expression (VII); the third to the stylopharyngeus muscle (IX); and the fourth and sixth to the pharyngeal and laryngeal muscles (X). The fifth arch has never developed in mammals. Skeletal elements of branchial arch origin are depicted in Figure 6.41 and the arch arteries are discussed below in connection with the cardiovascular system.

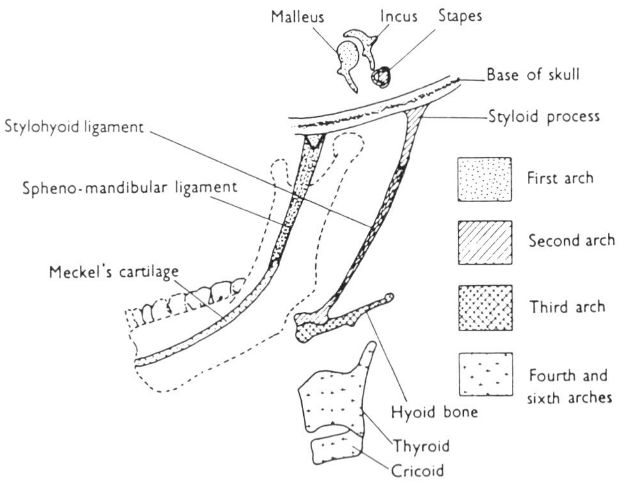

Fig. 6.41 The derivatives of the skeletal elements of the branchial arches. Reproduced with permission from Beck et al (1985).

Between the branchial arches lie the endodermally lined branchial pouches which at first are continuous with the cavity of the pharynx (Fig. 6.42). The endodermal lining of these pouches differentiates into various important structures situated chiefly in the neck and these are illustrated

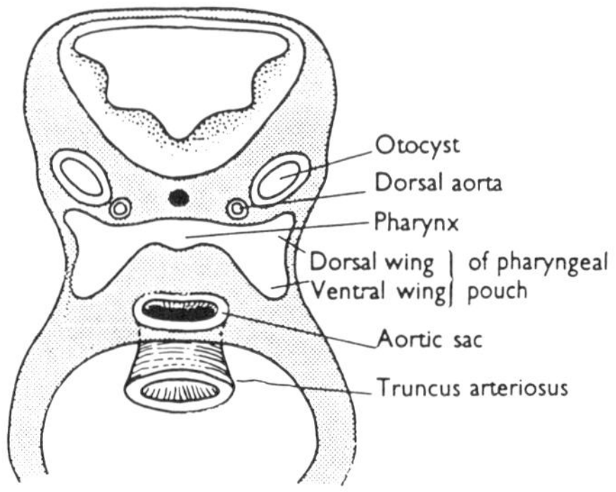

Fig. 6.42 Vertical section through the pharyngeal region (just posterior to Fig. 6.40) passing through the second pharyngeal pouch on each side. Reproduced with permission from Beck et al (1985).

in Figure 6.43. Of particular note is the position of the inferior parathyroid gland which, although derived from a more anterior arch than the superior gland, is nevertheless dragged to its final position by the descent of the inferior part of the pouch (which gives rise to the thymus) into the thorax. Figure 6.43 also illustrates the development of the pituitary and thyroid glands (see also Fig. 6.44). The pharyngeal

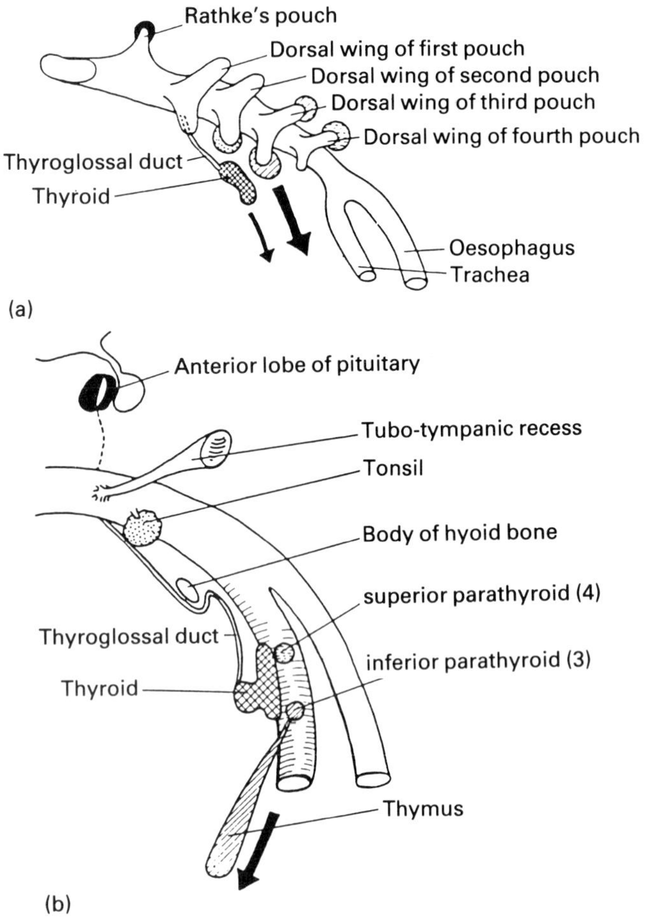

Fig. 6.43 Side view of the pharynx to show: **(a)** the origin of the endodermal proliferations giving rise to the pharyngeal pouch derivatives. Also shown is Rathke's pouch and the thyroid outgrowth; **(b)** the fate of the structures depicted in (a). Reproduced with permission from Beck et al (1985).

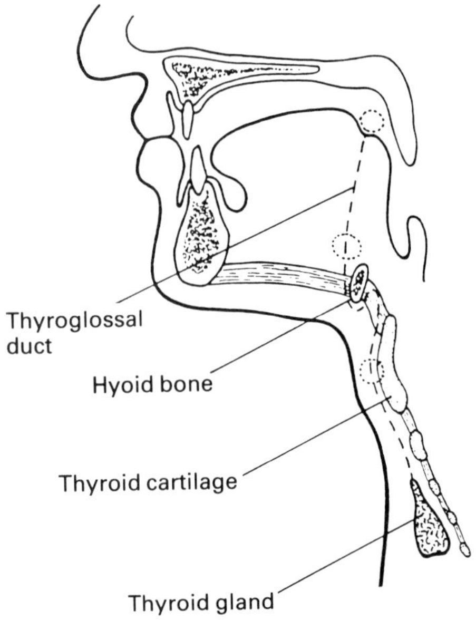

Fig. 6.44 The path of the thyroglossal duct, indicating the possible sites of aberrant thyroid tissue or thyroglossal cysts. Reproduced with permission from Beck et al (1985).

arches and hyoid rudiment are first recognizable at 4 weeks and their derivatives become functional at various stages of gestation, thus parathormone is demonstrable by 12 weeks and T3 by the 20th week of gestation. It will be seen that the thyroid anlage becomes attached to the ventral part of pouch 4. Here its cells are joined by cells which have migrated from the neural crest via the more caudal pouches (the ultimobranchial body). These will form the calcitonin-secreting C cells of the gland.

The floor of the pharynx at the end of the somite period is illustrated in Figure 6.45. From its lining the mucous membrane of the tongue will develop by overgrowth of the second arch mesoderm by that of the third (Fig. 6.46). The musculature of the tongue, however, is of occipital somite origin. Tongue development is reflected in its nerve supply both for taste and general sensation as well as for the musculature. The tongue primordia (Fig. 6.46) are first recognizable at 5 weeks of development.

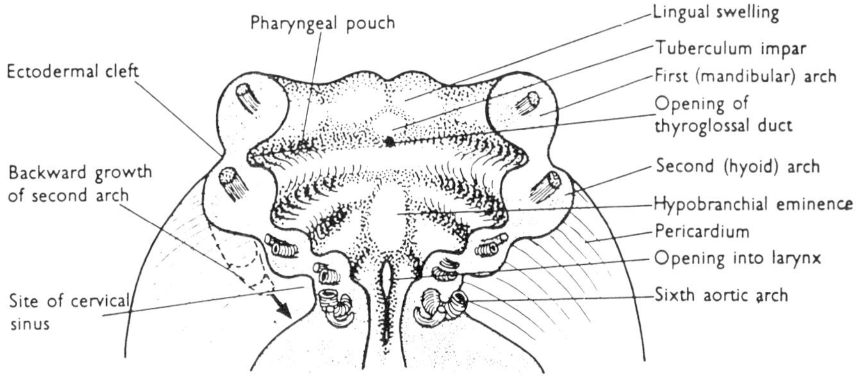

Fig. 6.45 Horizontal section through the pharyngeal region (B–B in Fig. 6.14) viewed from above. The first and second aortic arch arteries have already regressed. Reproduced with permission from Beck et al (1985).

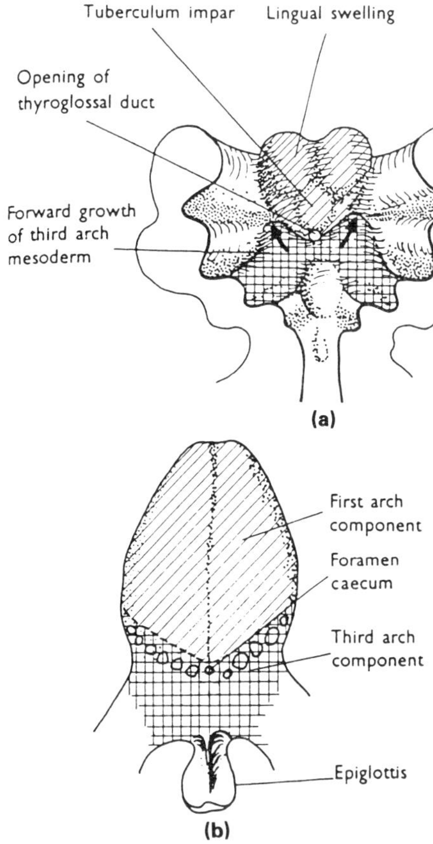

Fig. 6.46 (a) The tongue, with the exception of its muscles, develops from the first and third arches in the floor of the embryonic pharynx. (b) Adult tongue showing first and third arch components. Reproduced with permission from Beck et al (1985).

The cardiovascular system

The blood vascular system, including the heart, is formed initially from endothelial tubes which develop in mesenchyme both within the embryo and in the extraembryonic tissues. Blood islets first appear in the yolk sac, although some authorities have recently suggested that haematopoietic stem cells originate in the embryo itself (Le Dourain 1982). The scattered endothelial tubes link up to form a primitive circulatory system in which the first peristalsis-like heart beats begin on day 21. At this stage a single heart tube which has formed by fusion of right and left tubes (Fig. 6.47) lies

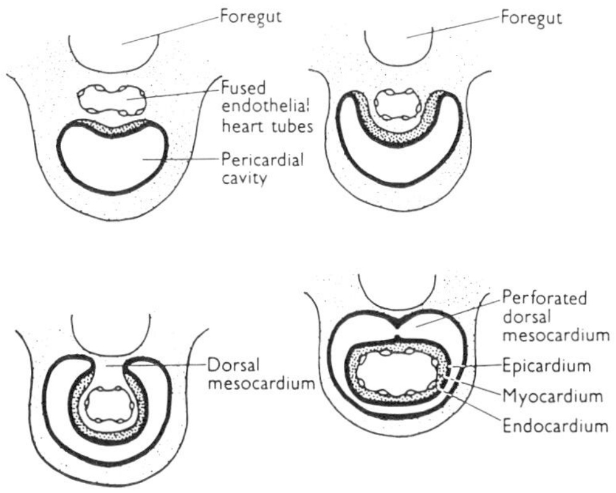

Fig. 6.47 The heart develops from a pair of endothelial tubes which fuse and invaginate the pericardial cavity. The dorsal mesocardium, which is thus formed, becomes perforated so that the heart tube runs freely through the pericardial cavity. Reproduced with permission from Beck et al (1985).

in the pericardium ventral to the foregut and delineated posteriorly by the septum transversum (Fig. 6.48). The heart tube is divided into four primitive chambers of which the most caudal (the sinus venosus) is still embedded in the septum. The cranially situated bulbus cordis leads into a short wide segment, the truncus arteriosus, which, further forward, runs into an aortic sac. Two vessels pass dorsally from the sac on either side of the foregut in the mesenchyme of the first branchial arch. These are the first aortic arch arteries and they join the corresponding dorsal aortae in the roof of the pharynx (O'Rahilly 1971).

A cranial prolongation of each dorsal aorta (the future internal carotid artery) supplies the forebrain. Caudal to the branchial region the paired dorsal aortae eventually fuse to form a single midline vessel. At about 28–30 days the first aortic arch arteries are followed by second and third arch arteries which lie in the succeeding branchial arches. By the time the third arch has formed, the first aortic arch artery has begun to break up (about 30 days) and, a short time later, the fourth develops and the second disappears. Finally, at about 37–39 days, the sixth aortic arch artery forms (it will be remembered that there is no fifth arch in the human embryo); Figures 6.49a and 6.50a illustrate this stage. The further development of the aortic arch arteries is illustrated in Figures 6.49b and 6.50b. From the ventral end of the

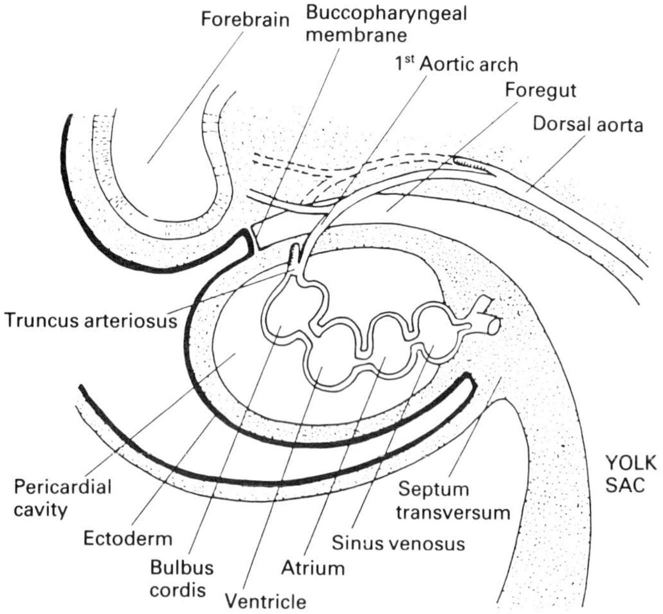

Fig. 6.48 The heart tube consists of four chambers. The first aortic arch arteries only have developed at this stage. Reproduced with permission from Beck et al (1985).

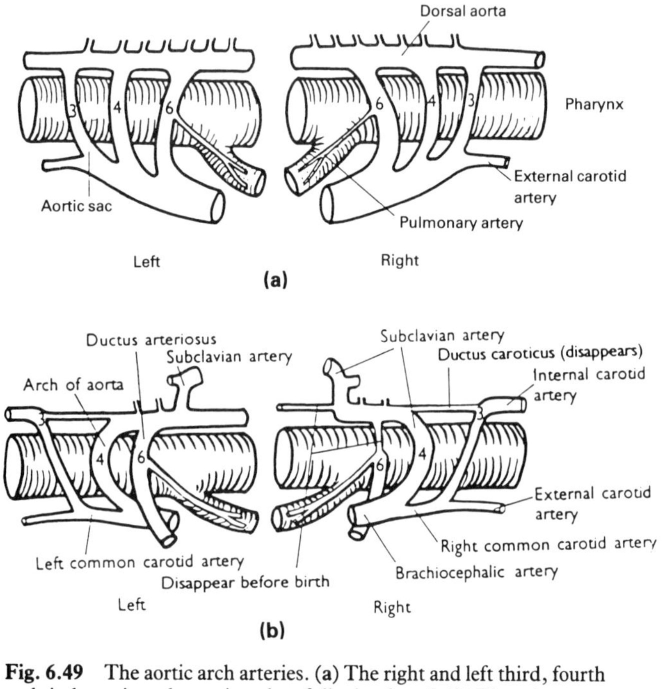

Fig. 6.49 The aortic arch arteries. (**a**) The right and left third, fourth and sixth aortic arch arteries when fully developed. (**b**) The subsequent fate of these arteries. Reproduced with permission from Beck et al (1985).

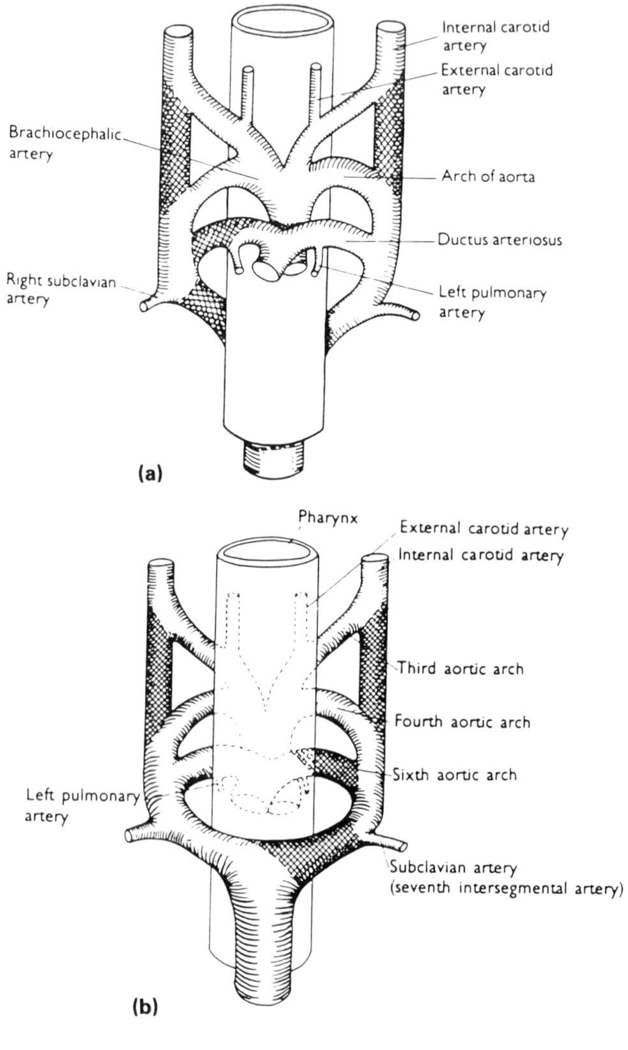

Fig. 6.50 The relation of the aortic arch arteries to the pharynx (**a**) viewed from in front and (**b**) from behind. The cross-hatched vessels will later disappear. Reproduced with permission from Beck et al (1985).

third arch the external carotid artery grows forward to the face. From the middle of the sixth arch another vessel grows down to the developing lung. The dorsal aorta between the third and fourth arches (ductus caroticus) disappears and the third arch, together with the cranial part of the dorsal aorta, thus forms the internal carotid artery while the common carotid results from the elongation of the aortic sac proximal to the junction of the internal and external carotids.

On the left side the fourth arch artery forms the arch of the aorta from which the left common carotid may now be said to arise. The sixth arch artery, together with the vessel that passes down to the lung, forms the left pulmonary artery while the distal part of the sixth arch artery becomes the ductus arteriosus. The seventh intersegmental artery forms the subclavian artery and the subsequent relative descent of the heart causes it to adopt its adult position. On the right side the fourth arch artery, together with a part of the right dorsal aorta and the seventh intersegmental artery, forms the right subclavian artery. The proximal part of the right sixth aortic arch artery, together with its branch to the lung, forms the right pulmonary artery but the distal part of the sixth arch and the dorsal aorta caudal to the seventh intersegmental artery disappear at about 45 days of development.

From its inception the heart tube (Fig. 6.48) grows faster than the pericardium. Since it is fixed both cranially and caudally it becomes kinked and this occurs in both the anteroposterior and the transverse planes. These acute bends of the heart tube are shown in Figure 6.51. In a lateral view (Fig. 6.51a) at about 25–26 days it will be seen that the bulbus cordis and ventricle lie ventral to the atrium and sinus venosus. Endocardial cushions have begun to form in the atrioventricular canals. Figure 6.51b (at about 32 days) indicates how a further lateral twist of the tube brings the bulbus cordis to lie to the right of the ventricle so that the two form a common chamber in which a depression corresponding to the interventricular septum can already be seen. The thin-walled atrium is clearly bulging forward on either side of the truncus arteriosus.

At this stage the sinus venosus has become asymmetrical due to shunting of the venous return from the head and neck to the right by development of the brachiocephalic vein (Fig. 6.52). As a result of the relative decrease in size of the left horn it is now the right horn of the sinus venosus that opens into the posterior wall of the common atrial cavity, rather to the right side, by a slit which is guarded by two venous valves. This is shown at a slightly later stage of development in Figure 6.53 which also indicates that the atrioventricular cushions have fused across the atrioventricular canal which thus becomes divided into right and left canals.

At about 32 days or so the growth of the septum primum begins the formation of the interatrial septum, illustrated

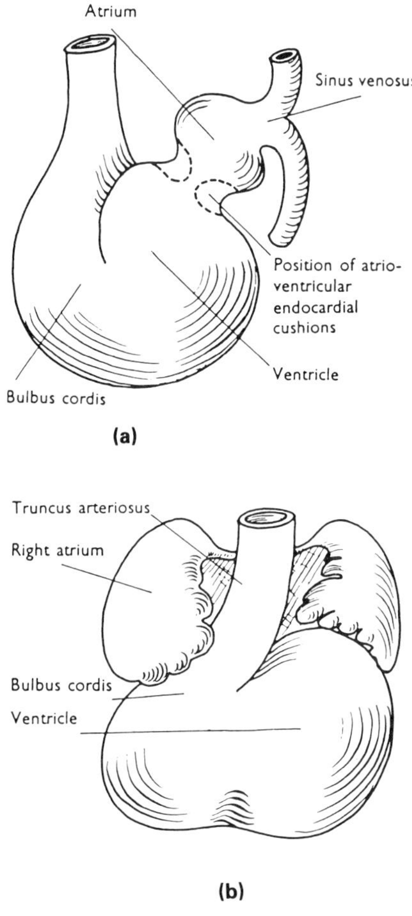

Fig. 6.51 (**a**) Lateral and (**b**) anterior views of the developing heart after the formation of the acute bends in the heart tube. (**a**) is at a slightly earlier stage of development than (**b**). Reproduced with permission from Beck et al (1985).

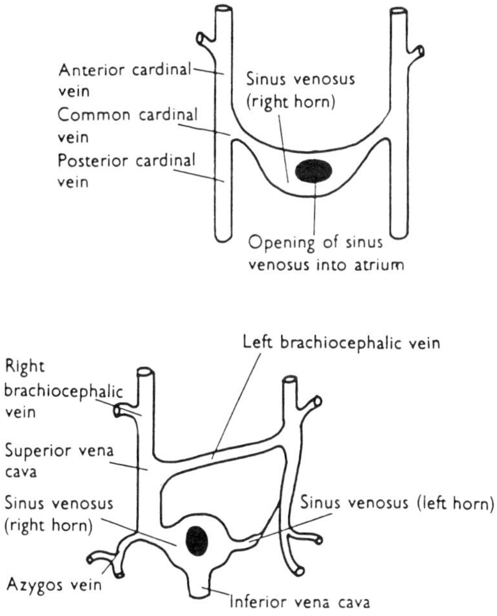

Fig. 6.52 The shunting of blood from left to right by the development of the brachiocephalic vein causes the right horn of the sinus venosus to enlarge at the expense of the left. Reproduced with permission from Beck et al (1985).

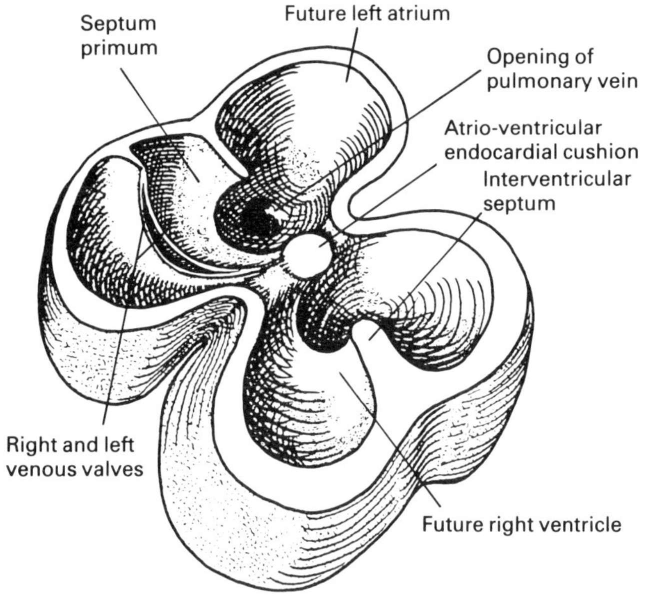

Fig. 6.53 Coronal section through the plane of the developing heart at about 37 days. Reproduced with permission from Beck et al (1985).

in Figure 6.54. The fully functional foramen ovale is present towards the end of the organogenetic period, though the septum secundum is quite well developed by about 46 days. Two other changes take place in the atria; on the left the walls of the pulmonary vein become incorporated into the atrial wall to form its smooth-walled part and on the right the sinus venosus is incorporated into the right atrium. The left venous valve disappears, the right horn of the sinus venosus forms the smooth posterior portion of the right atrium and into it opens the coronary sinus which is the original left horn of the sinus venosus. The embryology of the interior of the right atrium (Fig. 6.55) is thus clear.

Septation of the bulbo-ventricular cavity is illustrated in Figure 6.56. It will be seen that the common outflow tract (truncus arteriosus) becomes divided into two at about 42 days of development by a spiral aorticopulmonary septum formed by fusion of bulbar ridges developed in its walls. The lower ends of these bulbar ridges, together with a contribution from the atrioventricular cushion, fuse with the crescentic upper edge of the muscular interventricular septum. The result is the formation of the membranous part of the

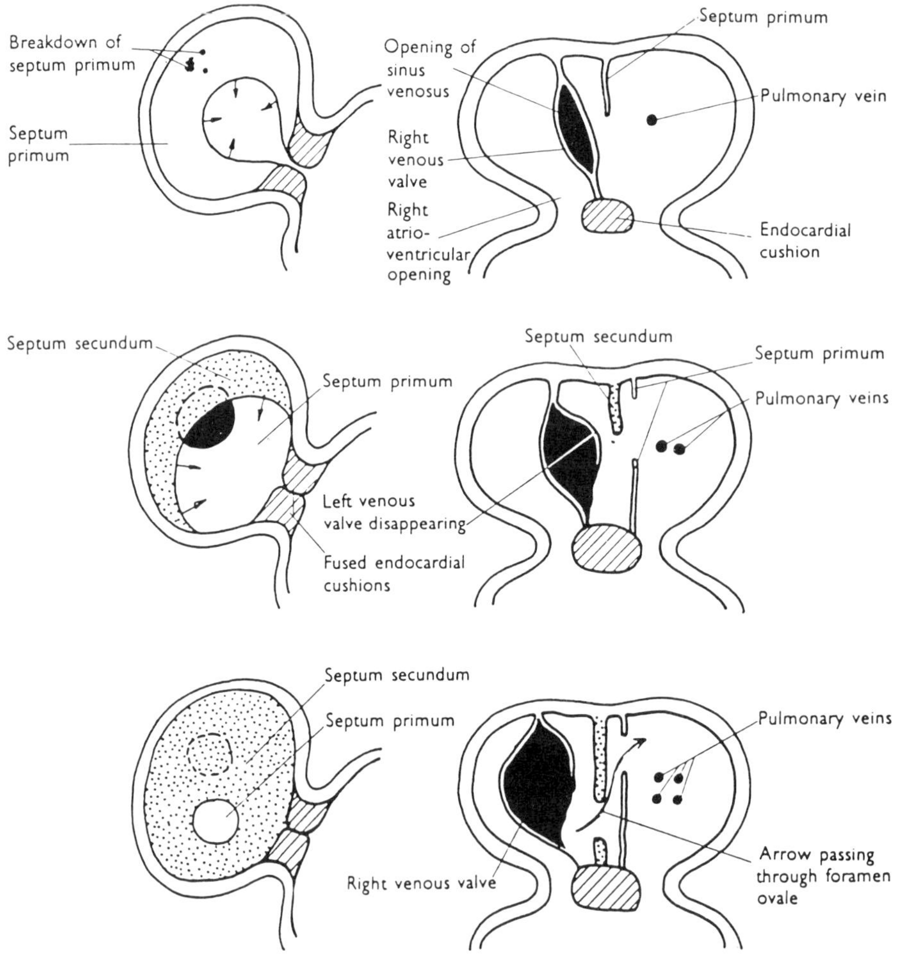

Fig. 6.54 Three stages in the development of the atrial septum. The left-hand diagrams show the right side of the developing septum and the right-hand diagrams show a coronal section in the plane of the atria. The septum secundum is stippled. Reproduced with permission from Beck et al (1985).

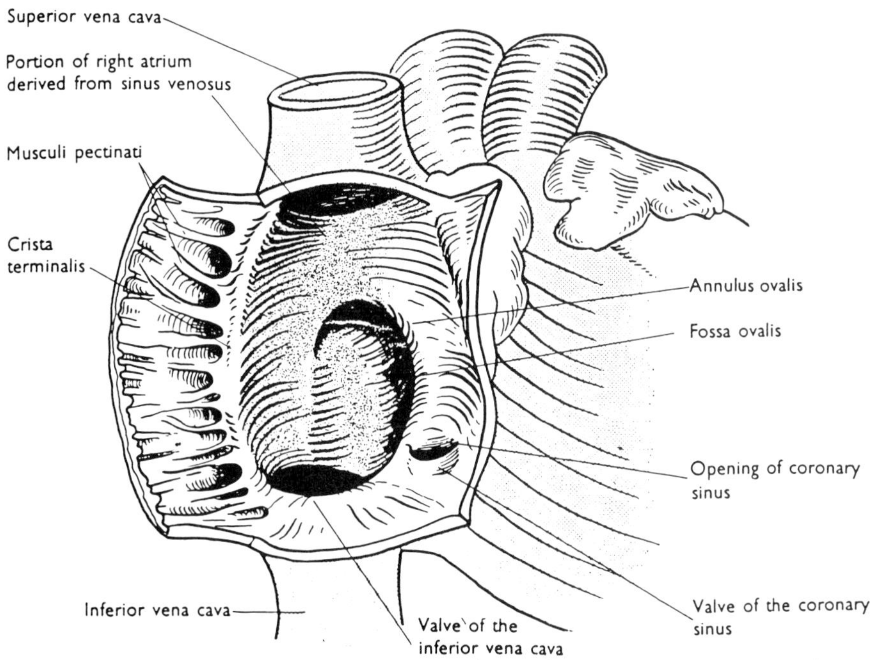

Fig. 6.55 The interior of the adult right atrium seen from in front. Reproduced with permission from Beck et al (1985).

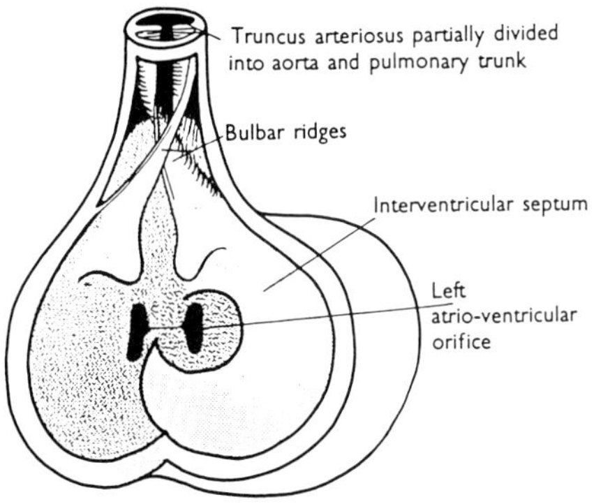

Fig. 6.56(a) The heart viewed open from the front to show the spiral bulbar ridges.

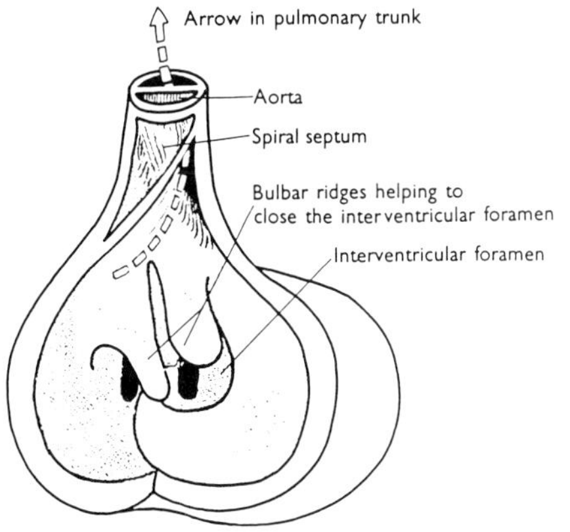

Fig. 6.56(b) Fusion of the right and left bulbar ridges has formed a separate aorta and pulmonary trunk. The interventricular foramen is partly closed and will later completely close by further development of the bulbar ridges and by proliferation of the tissues of the atrioventricular cushions. After closure of the interventricular septum the right atrioventricular orifice will open exclusively into the right ventricle and the left orifice into the left ventricle. Reproduced with permission from Beck et al (1985).

interventricular septum which causes blood from the left ventricle to empty exclusively into the aorta and from the right into the pulmonary trunk. Septation of the ventricles is complete at about 46 days of development. The fetal circulation is depicted in Figure 6.57 and the changes occurring at birth are discussed in Chapter 8.

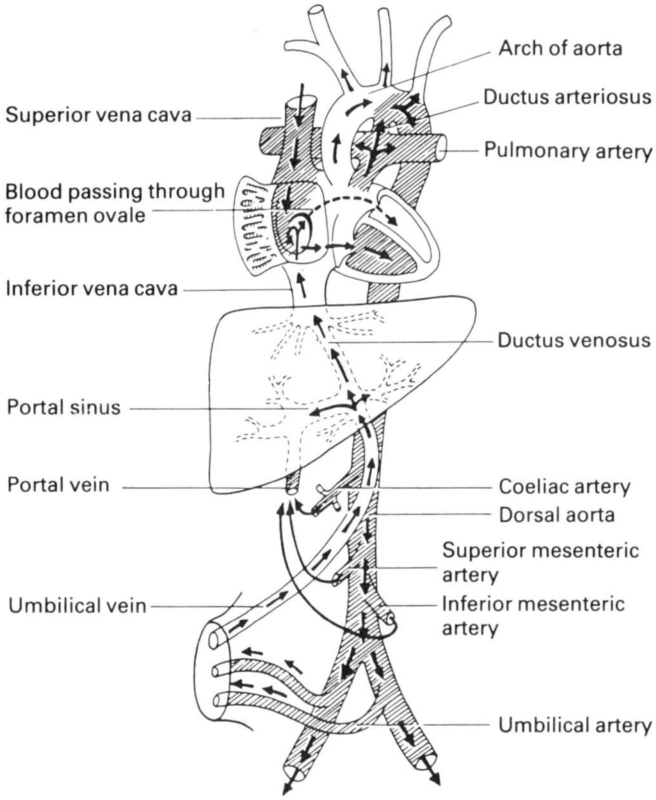

Fig. 6.57 Diagram of the fetal circulation. The cross-hatching represents deoxygenated or mixed blood. Reproduced with permission from Beck et al (1985).

The development of the aortic and pulmonary valves is shown in Figure 6.58, while a summary diagram of the development of the inferior vena cava is given in Figure 6.59.

ment. Figure 6.64 shows how the right lung bud (developed from a midline ventral foregut diverticulum at the caudal extremity of the pharynx) grows into the coelomic cavity.

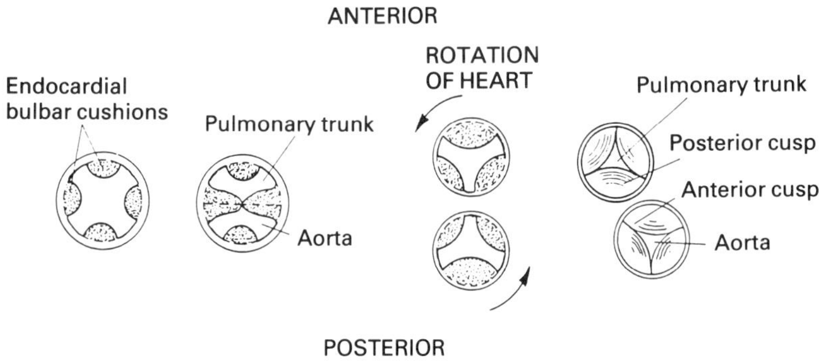

Fig. 6.58 The development of the aortic and pulmonary valves viewed from above. Reproduced with permission from Beck et al (1985).

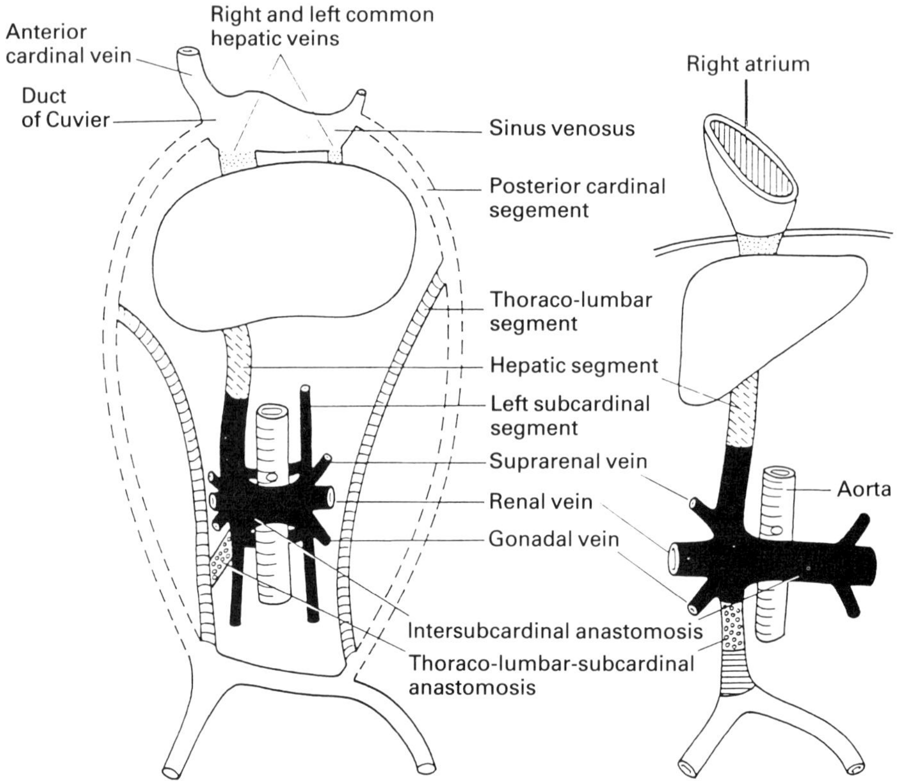

Fig. 6.59 Development of the inferior vena cava. The segments which make up the adult vessel are shown in the right-hand diagram. Reproduced with permission from Beck et al (1985).

The coelom, lungs and diaphragm

The early development of the coelom is illustrated by reference to Figures 6.10 and 6.11. Figures 6.60–6.63 illustrate the detailed relationship of the coelomic cavity to the foregut and midgut in the middle of the somite period of develop-

This section of the coelom now becomes the pleural cavity because, as the heart descends relatively, the common cardinal veins become increasingly vertical and raise prominent ridges which eventually fuse with the mesoderm covering the front of the oesophagus. Figures 6.65a and b illustrate this process; Figure 6.65c shows the further growth of the

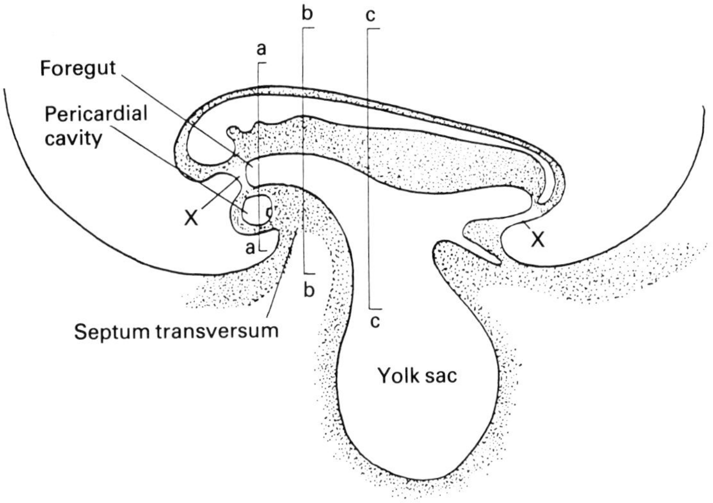

Fig. 6.60 Sagittal section through an embryo to show the planes of Figures 6.61, 6.62 and 6.63. Reproduced with permission from Beck et al (1985).

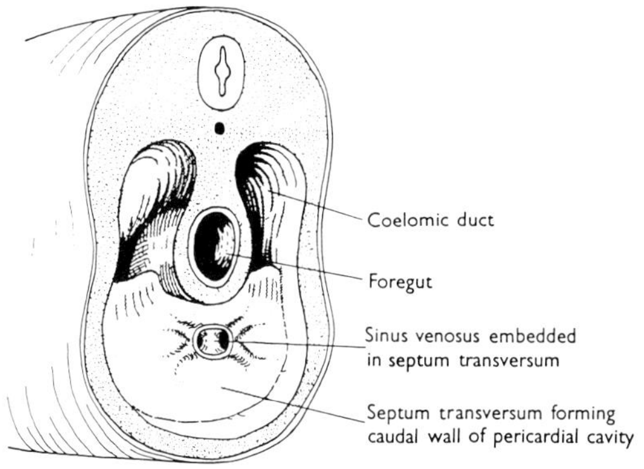

Fig. 6.61 Section through a–a in Figure 6.60 seen from in front. Reproduced with permission from Beck et al (1985).

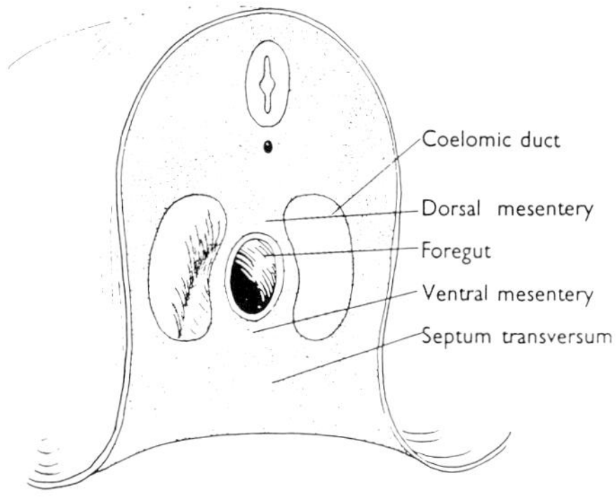

Fig. 6.62 Section through b–b in Figure 6.60 seen from in front. Reproduced with permission from Beck et al (1985).

lungs around the heart by burrowing into the body wall. The growing lungs raise a septum (the pleuroperitoneal membrane) situated on their caudal aspect and eventually the adult diaphragm is formed as shown in Figure 6.66.

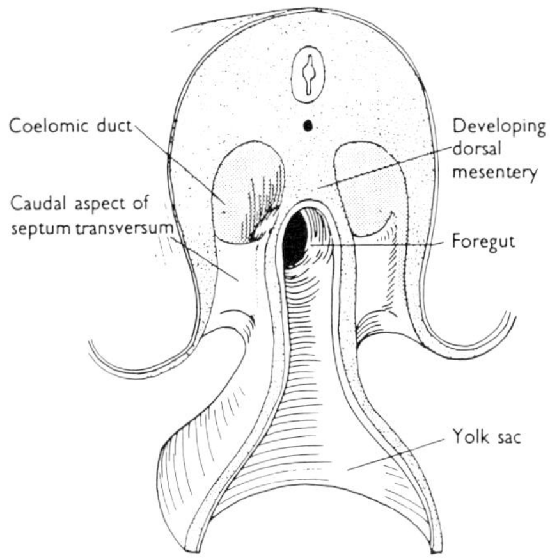

Fig. 6.63 Section through c–c in Figure 6.60 seen from behind. Reproduced with permission from Beck et al (1985).

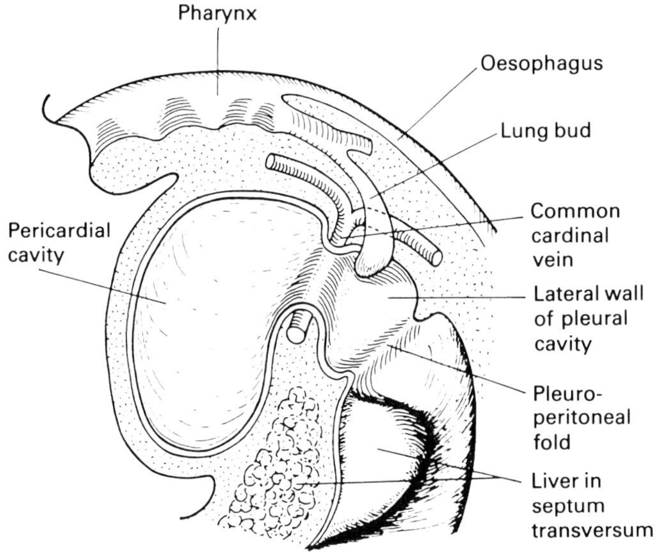

Fig. 6.64 Parasagittal section through the region of the septum transversum to show the right lateral wall of the pericardial cavity and the right coelomic duct (pleural cavity). Reproduced with permission from Beck et al (1985).

The small remaining pleuroperitoneal opening is crowded out as a result of invasion of the diaphragm by myotomes from C3–C5 and by growth of the subjacent liver and suprarenal glands. The derivation of the trachea is shown in Figures 6.45 and 6.67. The laryngotracheal groove (Fig. 6.45) appears at 22 days but the trachea does not fully separate from the oesophagus until 4–5 weeks. At this stage the lobar bronchi are recognizable. At 5 weeks the pericardium and pleura separate and at 7 weeks pleura and peritoneum separate. The *glandular* stage of lung development is present at 4 months, giving rise to a *canalicular* stage at 4–6 months and an alveolar stage beginning at 6 months. New alveoli form as the lungs grow until the eighth year of life. The

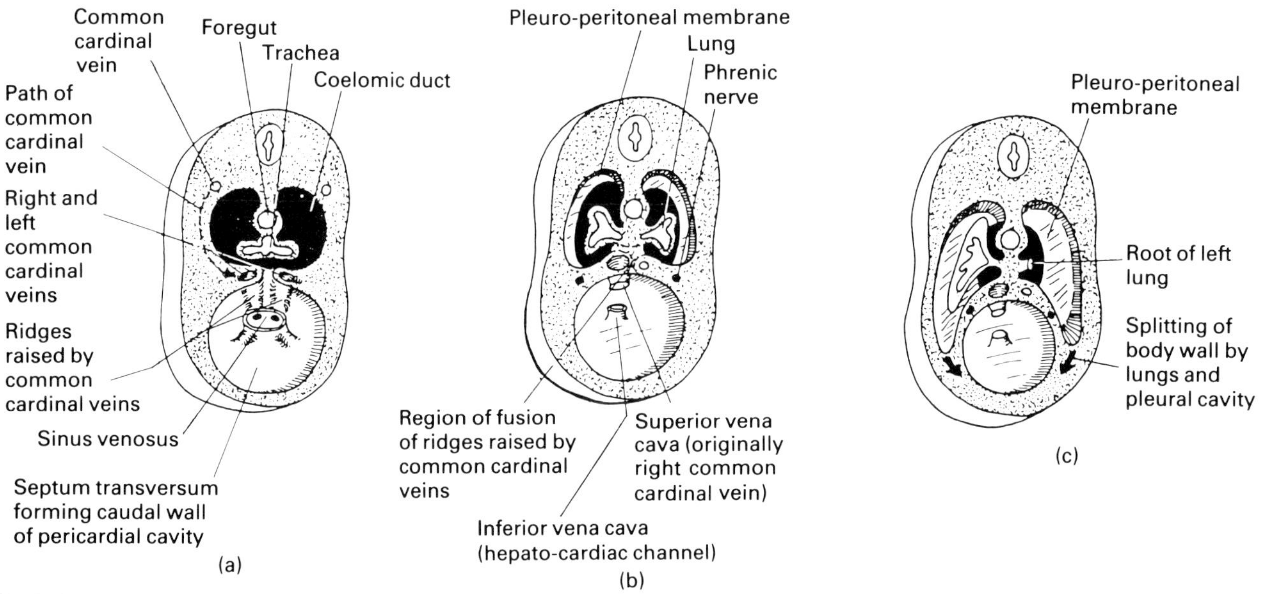

Fig. 6.65 Three sections showing the development of the lungs and the pleuroperitoneal membranes. The lungs grow ventrally in the direction of the arrows in (**c**). Reproduced with permission from Beck et al (1985).

development and significance of surfactant is discussed in Chapter 70.

The urogenital system

Reference to Figures 6.10 and 6.11 will remind the reader of the cloacal membrane lying behind the remnants of the primitive streak. When the tail fold is formed the cloacal membrane comes to lie on the ventral aspect of the embryo (Fig. 6.68). The proximal end of the allantois now opens into the cloaca just anterior to the cloacal membrane and takes part in the formation of the apex of the adult bladder. The cloaca is thus common to the hindgut and a portion of the allantois. Later in development the urinary system establishes an opening into the cloaca which becomes split into a urinary and rectal part by the development of the urorectal septum (Fig. 6.68).

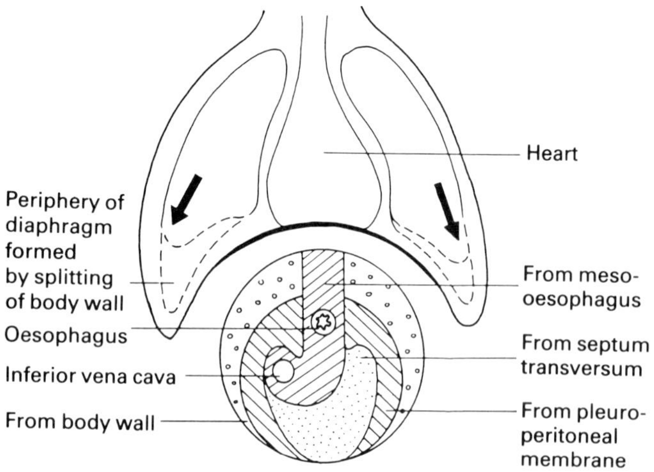

Fig. 6.66 Coronal section (above) showing how the lungs split the body wall to form the peripheral portion of the diaphragm. The arrows show the direction of lung growth in this plane. The lower diagram shows the embryonic constituents of the adult diaphragm viewed from above. Reproduced with permission from Beck et al (1985).

At 23–24 days of development the intermediate cell mass (Fig. 6.9, 6.12) proliferates to give rise to two long nephrogenic ridges lying one on either side of the midline from the cervical region to the caudal end of the coelomic cavity. From it will develop the mesonephros as well as the stroma of the gonads and their associated ducts (Fig. 6.69). On the ventrolateral aspect of the ridge the mesonephric (Wolffian) duct develops and grows caudally to open into the ventral (urinary) region of the cloaca (Fig. 6.68). The mesonephros consists of a series of glomeruli and tubules which are similar to, but less complicated than, those of the adult kidney and develop in a craniocaudal direction between days 24 and 28. It functions as an excretory organ during embryonic life. A second longitudinal duct (Fig. 6.69) develops at between 5 and 6 weeks lateral to the mesonephric duct. This is the paramesonephric (Müllerian) duct which will form much of the reproductive system in the female.

The urorectal septum divides the cloaca into a dorsal region, which forms part of the hindgut, and a ventral primitive urogenital sinus (Fig. 6.68, 6.70). The primitive uro-

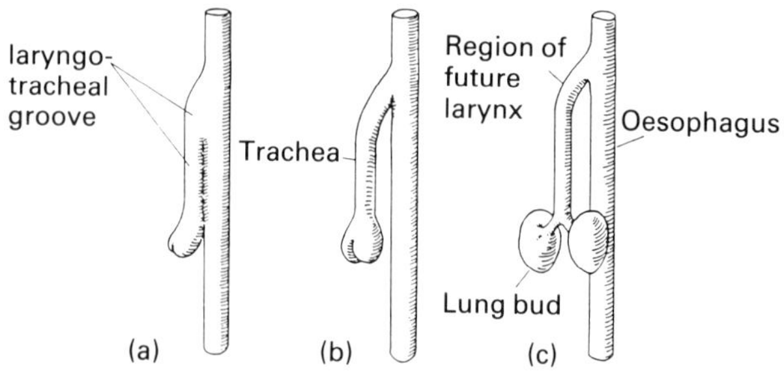

Fig. 6.67 Three stages in the development of the trachea. Reproduced with permission from Beck et al (1985).

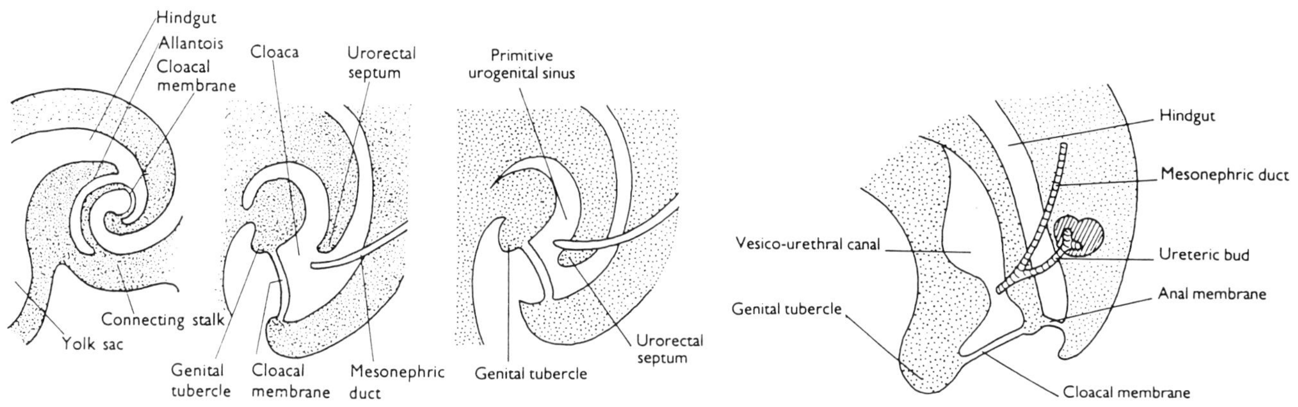

Fig. 6.68 The splitting of the cloaca by the urorectal septum to form the primitive urogenital sinus; also shown is the ureteric bud. Reproduced with permission from Beck et al (1985).

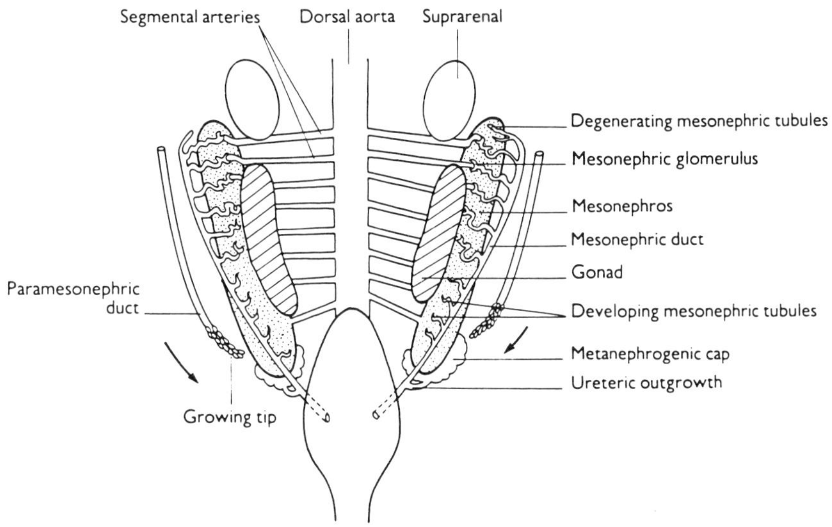

Fig. 6.69 The mesonephros and its relations. The glomeruli are functional at this stage but will disappear later. Reproduced with permission from Beck et al (1985).

genital sinus then becomes further subdivided by the entrance of the mesonephric ducts at about 28 days into an upper portion (the vesico-urethral canal) from which the bladder and part of the urethra develop and a lower definitive urogenital sinus. The lower part has a short, narrow cylindrical pelvic portion lying above a laterally compressed phallic portion (Fig. 6.70). The phallic portion extends forwards on to the ventral surface of a midline mesodermal swelling covered by ectoderm called the genital tubercle which develops at about 5 weeks. At first this is similar in both males and females (Fig. 6.71). On either side of the urogenital membrane a ridge of ectoderm-covered mesoderm forms the urethral folds. Outside this lies a less well defined elevation, the genital swelling. Further growth in the region between the genital tubercle and the umbilicus leads to the development of the infraumbilical abdominal wall which will become invaded by tissues of dermatomyotome origin. From the lower end of the mesonephric duct at about 5 weeks of development a diverticulum grows dorsally and cranially to meet the lower end of the nephrogenic ridge. This is the ureteric bud and a slightly dilated ampulla at its upper end becomes surrounded by a mass of cells from the ridge (Fig. 6.70). These cells form the greater part of the permanent kidney (the metanephros) which begins to function as an excretory organ at the end of embryonic and the beginning of fetal life (8 weeks). At this stage the cells form the metanephrogenic cap. A complex pattern of branching of the ureteric bud results in the establishment of the renal pelvis. Junction of the portion of the kidney derived from the metanephrogenic cap and that from the ureteric bud occurs just distal to the distal convoluted tubule of the nephron. The kidneys undergo relative ascent during development and rotate so

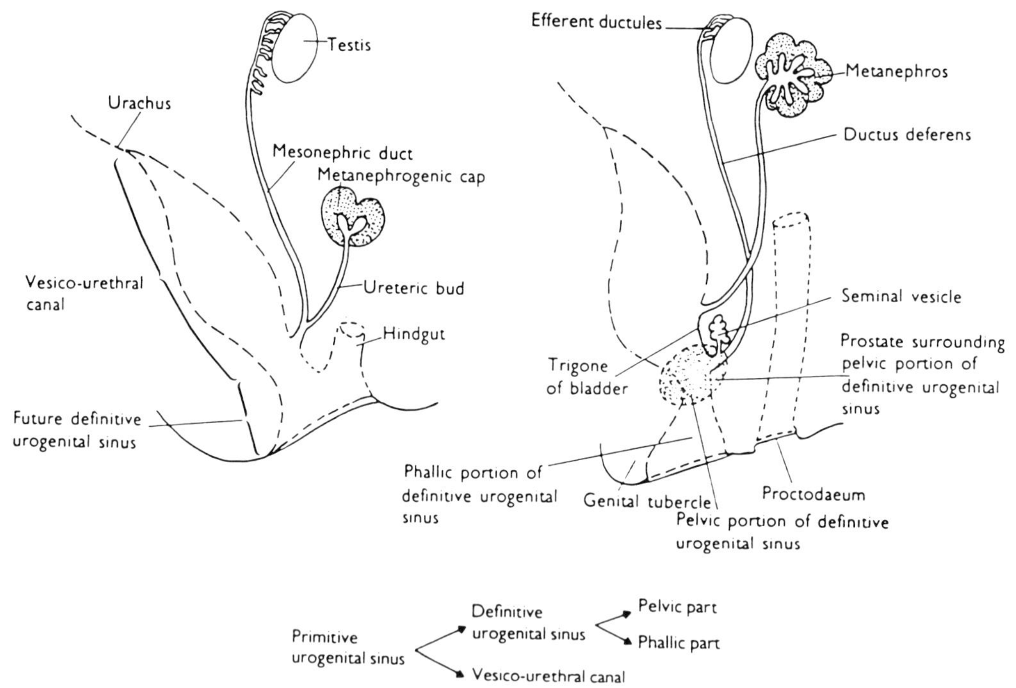

Fig. 6.70 The development of the bladder and internal genitalia. The endodermal derivatives are dotted. The flow chart shows how the primitive urogenital sinus becomes divided. Reproduced with permission from Beck et al (1985).

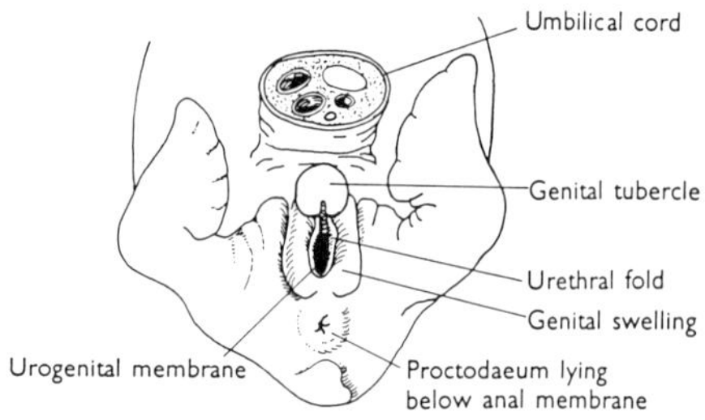

Fig. 6.71 The external genitalia at the end of the second month. There is little development of the infraumbilical abdominal wall at this stage; the genital tubercle reaches up as far as the umbilicus. Reproduced with permission from Beck et al (1985).

that the hilum faces medially instead of forwards. Figure 6.70 illustrates that the lower ends of the mesonephric ducts up to and beyond the ureteric buds become taken into the endodermal vesico-urethral canal so that part of the wall of the canal becomes mesodermal. At the same time complicated growth changes occur so that the ureters finally open into the definitive bladder while the mesonephric ducts open lower down into the pelvic part of the definitive urogenital sinus. This results in the formation of the trigone of the bladder. The bladder is therefore derived mainly from the vesico-urethral canal and from the lower ends of the mesonephric ducts. The allantois makes a small contribution to its apex but largely regresses to form the urachus.

The gonads, which at first have a similar appearance in both sexes, are first seen as thickenings along the middle two quarters of the medial aspect of the nephrogenic ridge (Fig. 6.69, 6.72). They first appear during the fifth week of development and become colonized by primordial germ cells which originate in the yolk sac wall, having segregated there at an early stage of development. At 7–8 weeks (but not earlier) it becomes possible to determine sex by the histology of the gonad. Prior to this cytogenetic techniques are required to establish sex. The histological differentiation of the gonads has been well documented (Gillman 1948, Pinkerton et al 1961, Zuckerman & Weir 1977, Guraya 1980, Steinberger & Steinberger 1980) and good reviews concerning the genetic and endocrinological basis of sexual differentiation are available (Visser 1974, Short 1979).

In the male the mesonephric duct, after the mesonephros has ceased to function, becomes taken over by the genital system. Mesonephric tubules in the region of the testis link up with the rete testis to become the efferent ductules which constitute much of the caput epididymis and are continued into the mesonephric duct which becomes tightly coiled to form the body and tail of the epididymis followed by the ductus deferens (Fig. 6.73). Atavistic mesonephric tubules form various remnants around the testis and epididymis which can give rise to cysts in later life.

As the testis and epididymis form, a thick column of mesodermal tissue, called the gubernaculum, is separated from the dorsal body wall. This structure remains attached to the lower pole of the testis and, passing through the tissues around which the abdominal muscles will develop, ends in

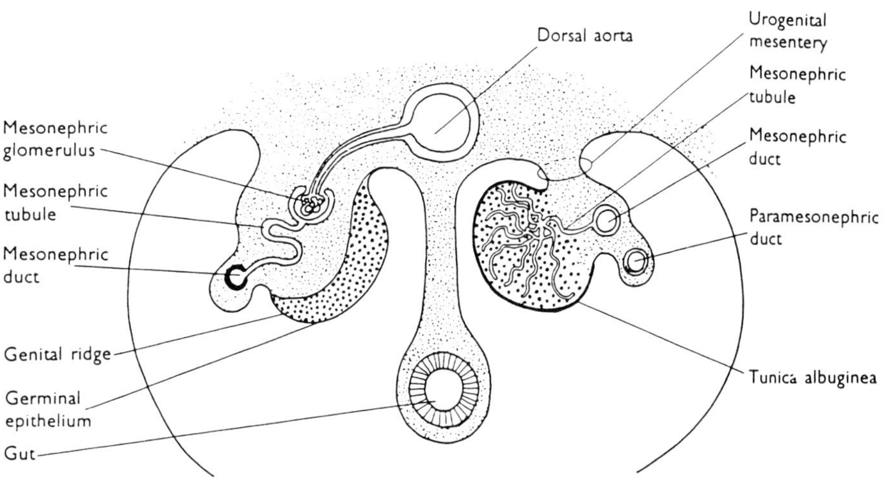

Fig. 6.72 Transverse section through the abdomen. The right side of the diagram shows a more advanced stage of development than the left. Reproduced with permission from Beck et al (1985).

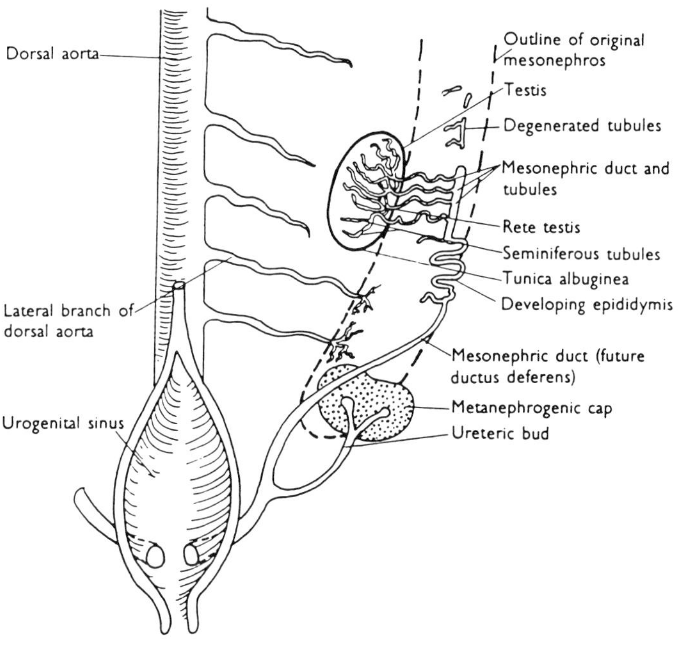

Fig. 6.73 Diagram to show the takeover of the mesonephric duct by the testis and the development of the metanephros. Reproduced with permission from Beck et al (1985).

from the general peritoneal cavity shortly after birth (Fig. 6.74). Prostatic buds begin to proliferate from the urethral epithelium at about 12 weeks and a diverticulum of the lower end of each ductus deferens grows out to form the seminal vesicles.

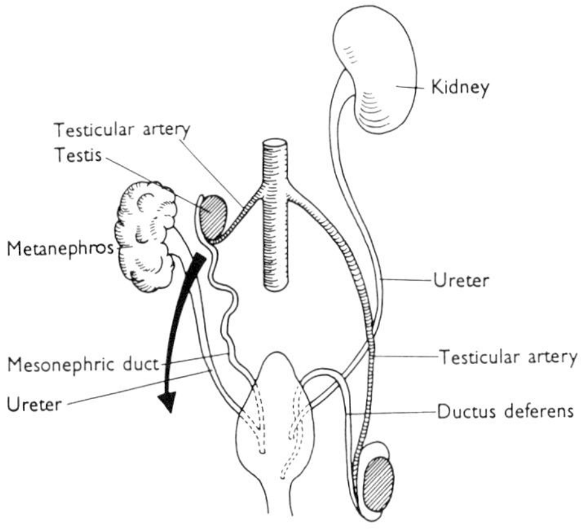

Fig. 6.74 Diagram to explain the adult relations of the testicular artery and ductus deferens to the ureter. The arrow shows the path of testicular descent. Reproduced with permission from Beck et al (1985).

the genital swelling, which will eventually form the scrotum. By a complex series of morphological changes which are not completely understood in mechanical terms but are known to include differential growth and swelling of the gubernaculum to dilate the inguinal canal, the testis— together with its vessels, nerves and lymphatics as well as the tunica vaginalis—is guided into the scrotum. True testicular descent, i.e. from the region of the internal ring to the scrotum, usually takes place during the last weeks (32–36) of intrauterine life and the tunica vaginalis is separated

The ovary remains histologically undifferentiated until 16 weeks; like the testis, it undergoes a relative descent but remains in the pelvis. The paramesonephric ducts lie laterally at the cranial end of the nephrogenic ridge but caudally they meet in the midline. Their fused lower portions are closely related to the dorsal wall of the urogenital sinus (Fig. 6.75) where, by 15 weeks, they produce an elevation, the Müllerian tubercle. The fused portions of the ducts, known as the uterovaginal canal, form the uterus and probably a part of the vagina. The original urogenital mesentery will

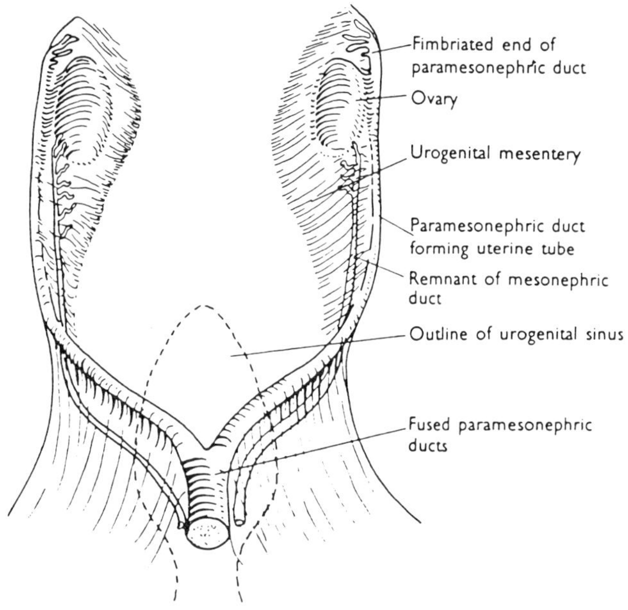

Fig. 6.75 Development of the urogenital mesentery into the broad ligament of the uterus. The mesonephros, together with its ducts and tubules, has almost completely disappeared. Reproduced with permission from Beck et al (1985).

form the broad ligament of the uterus and the gubernaculum develops in it. The latter gains a secondary attachment to the uterus and there becomes converted into a fibrous cord. It thus becomes converted into two ligaments — the ligament of the ovary and the round ligament of the uterus (Fig. 6.76). The Müllerian tubercles now become pushed away from the urogenital sinus by a solid mass of cells growing posteriorly from the sinus, known as the sinus upgrowth. The sinus upgrowth and Müllerian tubercles together form the vagina, and much of the pars phallica of the definitive urogenital

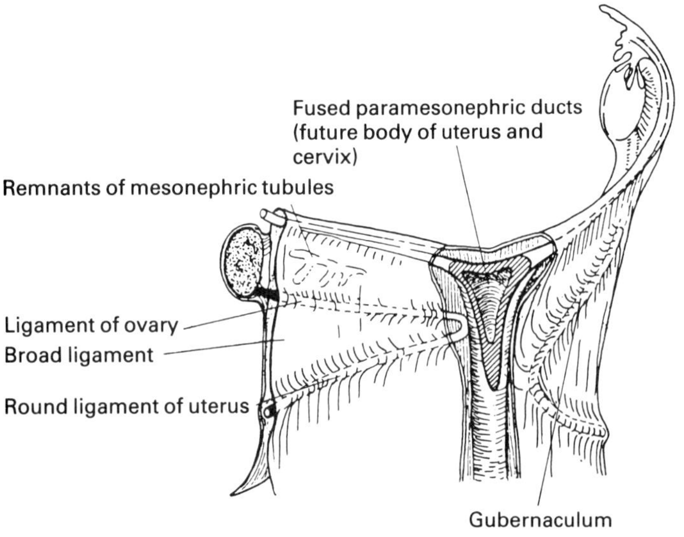

Fig. 6.76 Diagram to show how the gubernaculum becomes the round ligaments of the uterus and the ligament of the ovary. Reproduced with permission from Beck et al (1985).

sinus forms the vestibule (Fig. 6.77). Reference to Figures 6.71 and 6.77 explains the development of the female external genitalia.

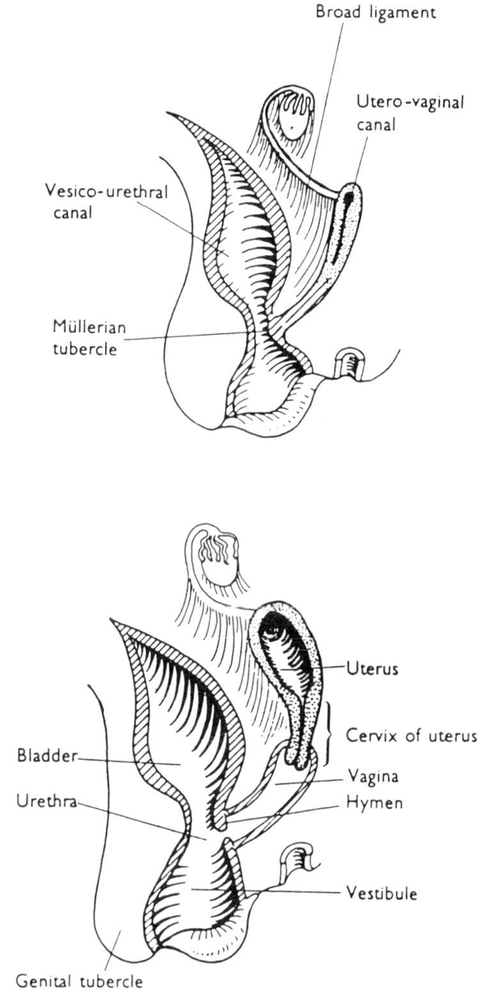

Fig. 6.77 Development of the female internal genitalia. Reproduced with permission from Beck et al (1985).

The male phallus is developed from the genital tubercle, which enlarges greatly. A proliferation of endodermal cells from the anterior extremity of the phallic part of the urogenital sinus extends forwards into it to form the urethral plate. From this the penile urethra will develop, as shown in Figure 6.78. After dissolution of the urogenital membrane, the urethral folds begin to fuse with each other from behind

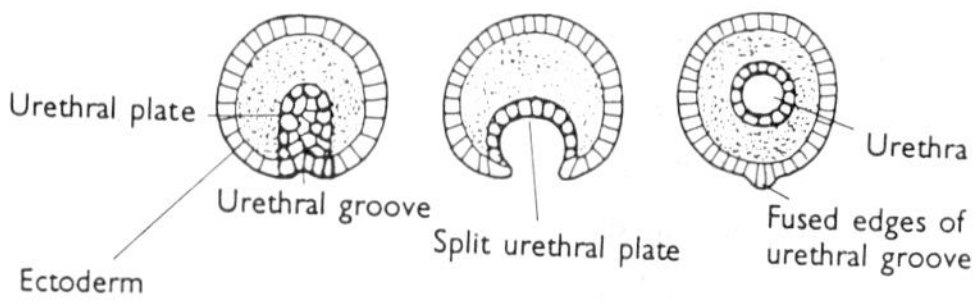

Fig. 6.78 Transverse sections through the phallus of a male embryo to show the development of the urethra from the urethral plate. Reproduced with permission from Beck et al (1985).

forwards (Fig. 6.79). This process involves the urethral plate and the development of the male external genitalia may therefore be understood by reference to Figures 6.71, 6.78 and 6.79. In Figure 6.79 the completion of the penile urethra by an ectodermal plate which canalizes the glans is shown.

It becomes possible to distinguish the sexes by examination of the external genitalia at 12–16 weeks of development.

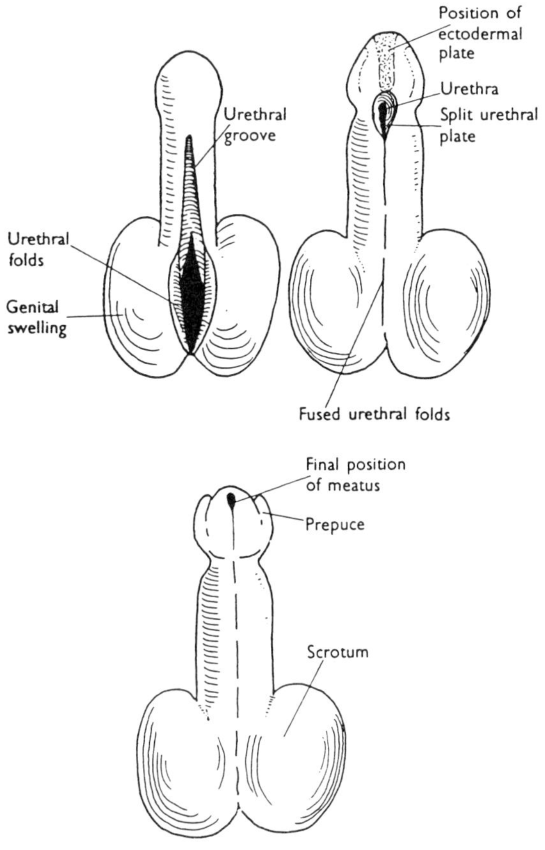

Fig. 6.79 Development of the male external genitalia. Reproduced with permission from Beck et al (1985).

The digestive system

The division of the primitive gut into foregut, midgut and hindgut, which begins to be apparent at 21–22 days of development, is shown in Figure 6.13. Histogenesis of the gut has been extensively reviewed (Trier & Moxey 1979, Tench 1936, Salenius 1962, Deren 1968, Severn 1971, 1972, Grand et al 1976, McLean 1979).

As development proceeds the gut pulls away from the dorsal body wall mesoderm to form a dorsal mesentery and from the septum transversum to form a ventral mesentery (Fig. 6.80). The liver bud grows into the ventral mesentery between 24 and 26 days at the junction of the foregut and midgut (Fig. 6.81) and a ventral division of this outgrowth forms the gallbladder. The liver is gradually everted from its intraseptal position and, in the adult, remains attached to the diaphragm only by its base area (Fig. 6.82). The lesser

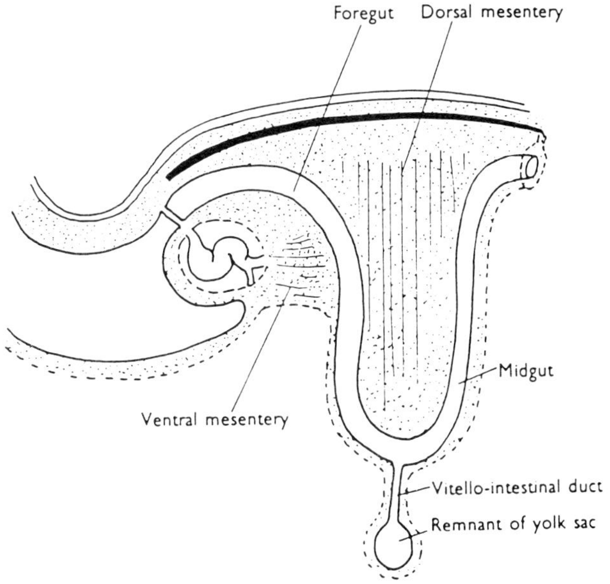

Fig. 6.80 Formation of the dorsal and ventral mesenteries of the gut. Reproduced with permission from Beck et al (1985).

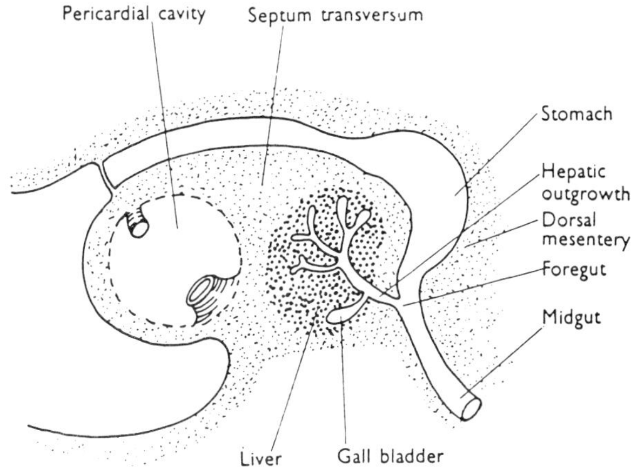

Fig. 6.81 The hepatic outgrowth grows into the ventral mesentery from the end of the foregut. Liver cells invade the septum transversum. Reproduced with permission from Beck et al (1985).

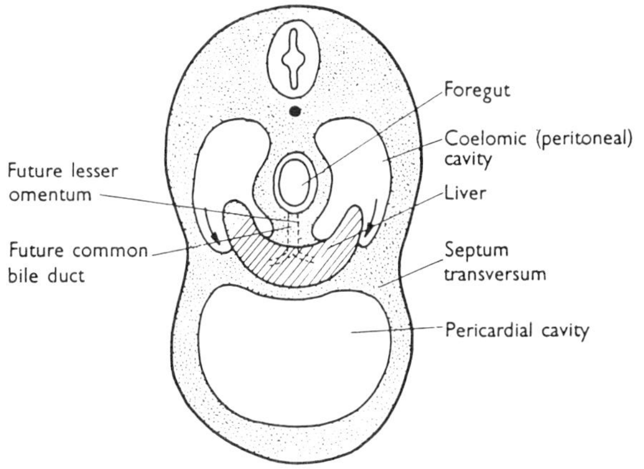

Fig. 6.82 Transverse section through the peritoneal and pericardial cavities to show the position of the liver within the septum transversum. To a large extent the liver becomes separated from the diaphragm except for the region lying between the arrows (the bare area). Reproduced with permission from Beck et al (1985).

sac is formed by an erosion of the dorsal mesentery (the bursa omentalis; Fig. 6.83), followed by rotation of the stomach so that its left surface comes to face anteriorly (Fig. 6.84). Finally, the portion of the mesentery lying between the aorta and kidney fuses with the posterior abdominal wall; the spleen develops at about 6 weeks (Fig. 6.85) and the inferior wall of the sac is extended downwards to form the greater omentum and to fuse with the transverse mesocolon (Fig. 6.86). The pancreas also develops (24–26 days) at the junction of the foregut and midgut (Fig. 6.87). This figure also explains the retroperitoneal position of both the duodenum and the pancreas. The development of the portal vein is shown in Figure 6.88. The ductus venosus is occluded at birth to form the ligamentum venosum and the position of the terminal part of the inferior vena cava is apparent from reference to Figure 6.59.

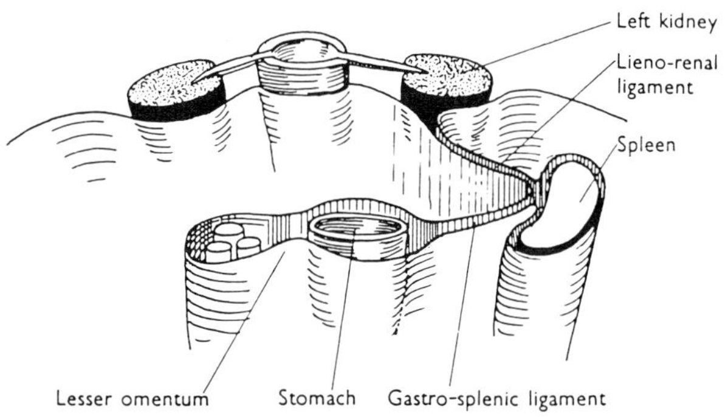

Fig. 6.85 Similar view to Figure 6.84 after fusion of part of the dorsal mesentery to the dorsal body wall. Reproduced with permission from Beck et al (1985).

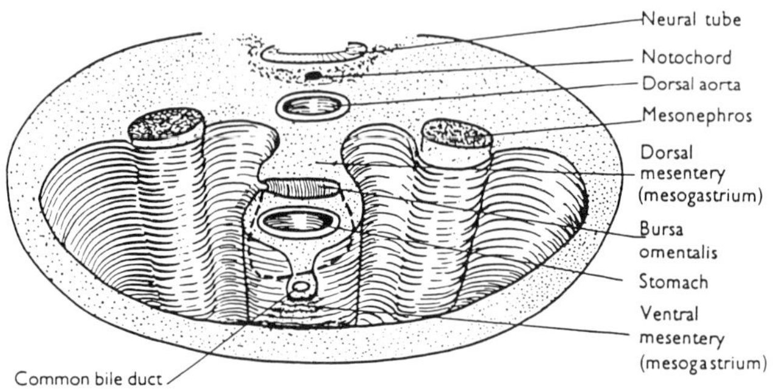

Fig. 6.83 The bursa omentalis grows into the mesentery from the (embryo's) right. Its lower part is indicated by a dashed line. Reproduced with permission from Beck et al (1985).

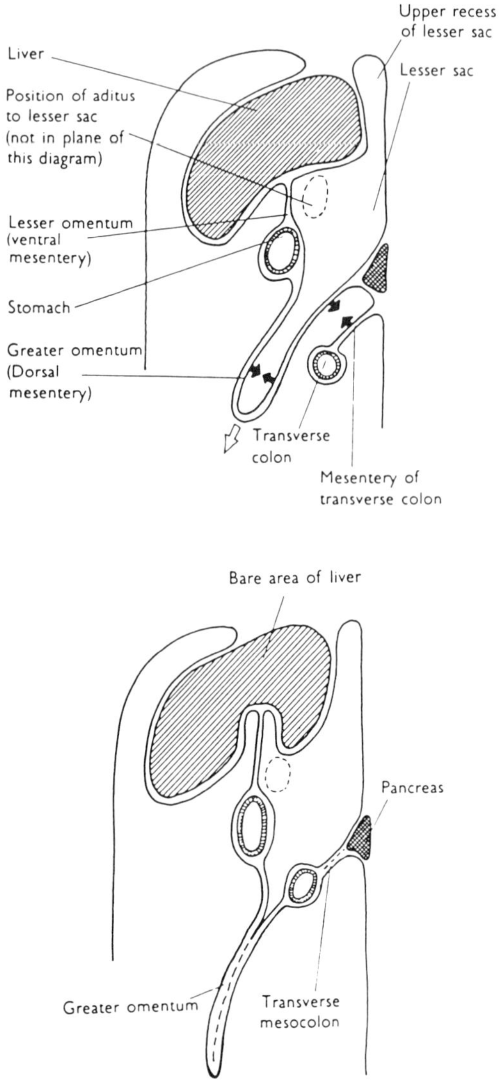

Fig. 6.86 Midline sagittal sections to show the formation of the lesser sac. Reproduced with permission from Beck et al (1985).

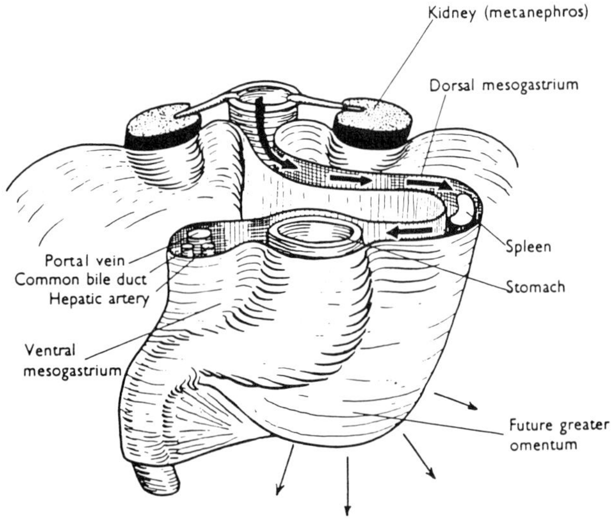

Fig. 6.84 Rotation of the stomach causes the dorsal mesentery to be diverted to the left. It also grows in the direction of the thin arrows. The darker arrows show the course of the arteries to the spleen and stomach. Reproduced with permission from Beck et al (1985).

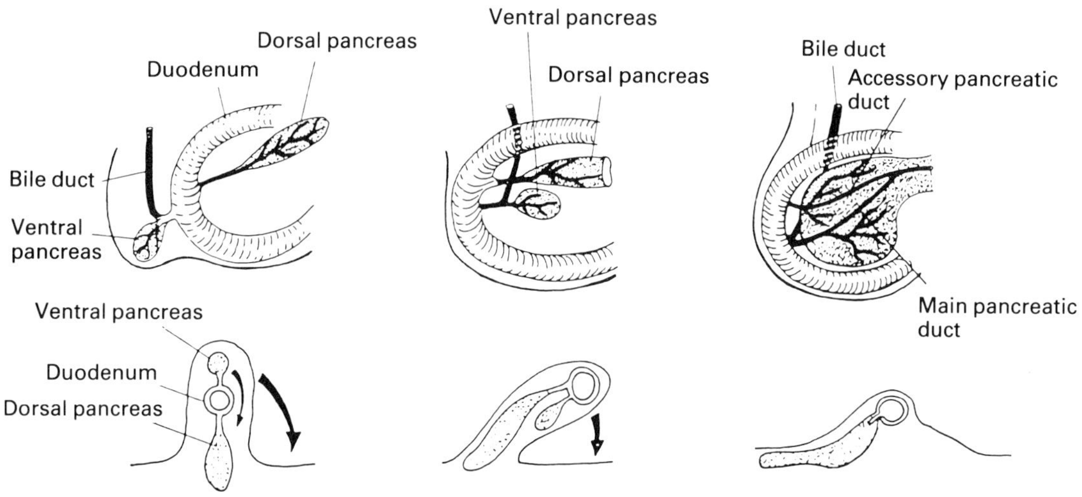

Fig. 6.87 The development of the pancreas. Upper diagrams show the pancreas and bile duct seen from in front; the lower row is a series of cross-sections seen from above. Reproduced with permission from Beck et al (1985).

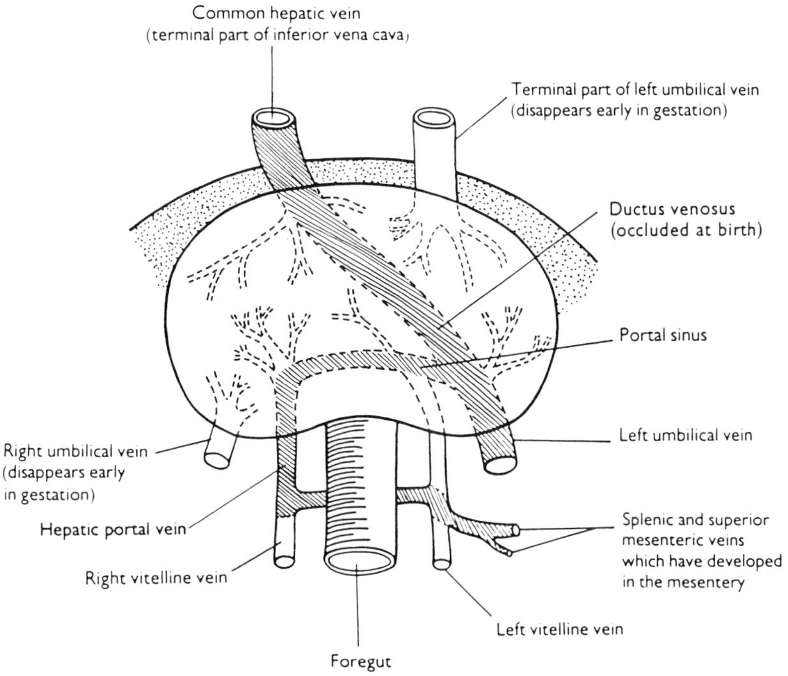

Fig. 6.88 The vessels in the region of the liver. The cross-hatched vessels persist at least until birth, while the others disappear. Reproduced with permission from Beck et al (1985).

The large size of the liver at 5 weeks causes most of the midgut, which has an extensive dorsal mesentery (Fig. 6.80), to be forced into the extraembryonic coelom (Fig. 6.89). At 6 weeks external inspection of the embryo demonstrates that the liver is large enough to produce an external bulge above the midgut hernia. While in the extraembryonic situation the midgut loop forms a caecal swelling and undergoes rotation through 90° (Fig. 6.90). Between 8 and 9 weeks the relative size of the liver allows the herniated gut to return to the abdominal cavity; the proximal part of the midgut

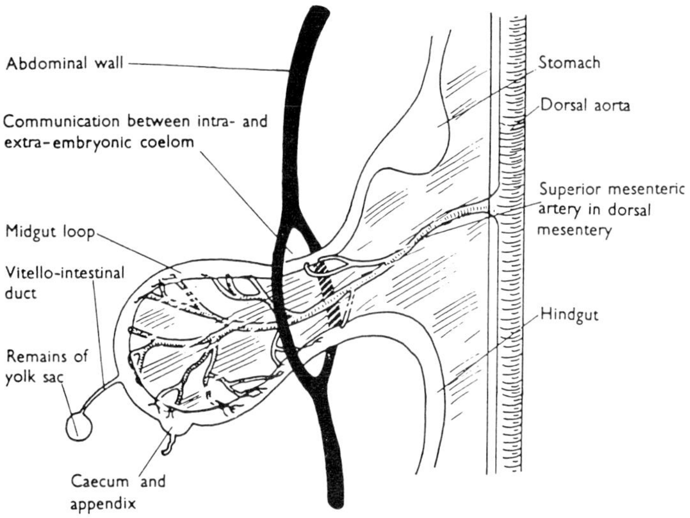

Fig. 6.89 Side view of the midgut loop herniated out into the extraembryonic coelom. Reproduced with permission from Beck et al (1985).

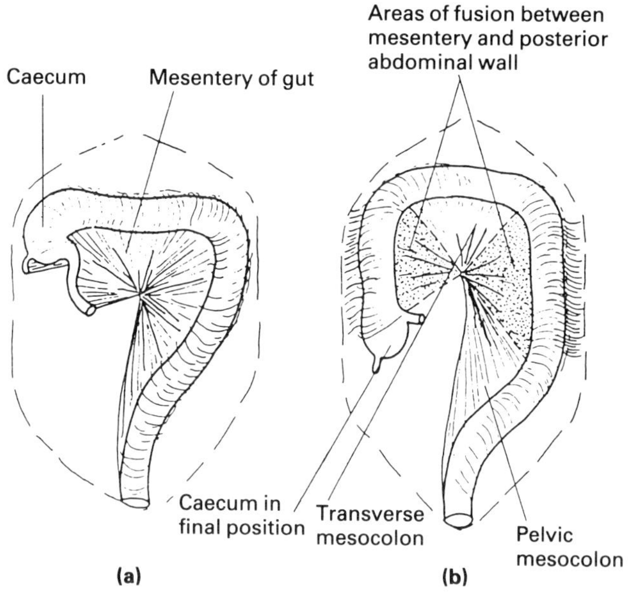

Fig. 6.91 (**a**) The colon and its mesentery immediately after the return of the midgut loop. (**b**) The final stage of rotation of the gut. The caecum has attained its final position and the ascending and descending colon have become retroperitoneal. Reproduced with permission from Beck et al (1985).

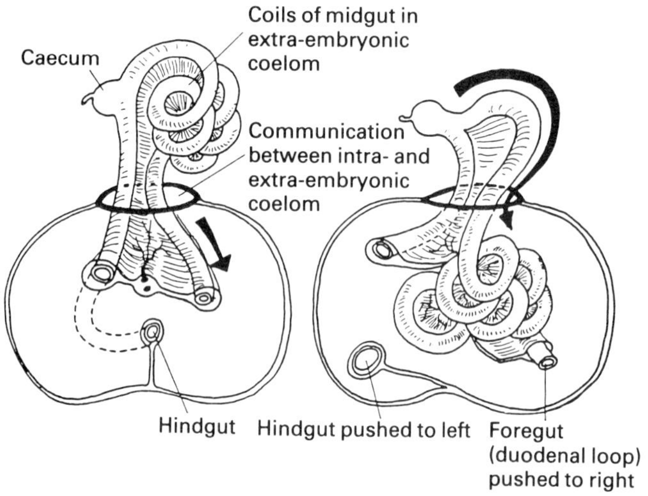

Fig. 6.90 The return of the midgut loop into the abdomen, seen from above. The right (proximal) limb returns first; the caecum is the last to return and comes to lie high in the abdomen on the right side. Reproduced with permission from Beck et al (1985).

loop returns first (because of the caecal swelling) and this results in a further rotation of 90°. On return the gut lies in the position it will occupy in the adult. The remaining development concerns the formation of the ascending colon and the fixation of the descending colon (Fig. 6.91). Peristalsis begins at about the tenth week. It is interesting to note that, while the buccopharyngeal membrane disappears between 24 and 26 days, the cloacal membrane persists until 7–8 weeks.

EXTERNAL FEATURES DURING THE EMBRYONIC AND EARLY FETAL PERIOD (Fig. 6.92)

The embryonic period of development extends from conception to 8 weeks and the post-implantation formation of the germ layers has been described in the introduction to this chapter. The crown–rump length (4 mm) can first be measured at 28 days when the embryo has between 28 and 30 somites. At this stage there is a large pericardial cavity which forms a bulge below the developing facial and pharyngeal regions, although the branchial arches are not yet all present. The neural tube is completely closed and the mesodermal somites are a prominent feature. Shortly thereafter the limb buds appear. The embryo is growing in length at about 1 mm/day and by the end of the embryonic period has reached a length of 30 mm. Thereafter, during the early fetal period, the rate of growth increases to 1.5 mm per day.

The early fetal period lasts from 8–28 weeks (Fig. 6.93). There is very rapid growth of the body, together with maturation of tissues and organs. The average crown–rump length at 8 weeks is 29 mm whilst, at 28 weeks, measurement of 28 cm and weight of 1000 g are recorded. Accompanying this growth there are profound changes in external form. At 12 weeks the embryo has a disproportionately large head and the physiological hernia has just re-entered the abdominal cavity. Sex is easily identified. At 16 weeks the human appearance is even clearer, with the eyes looking forward

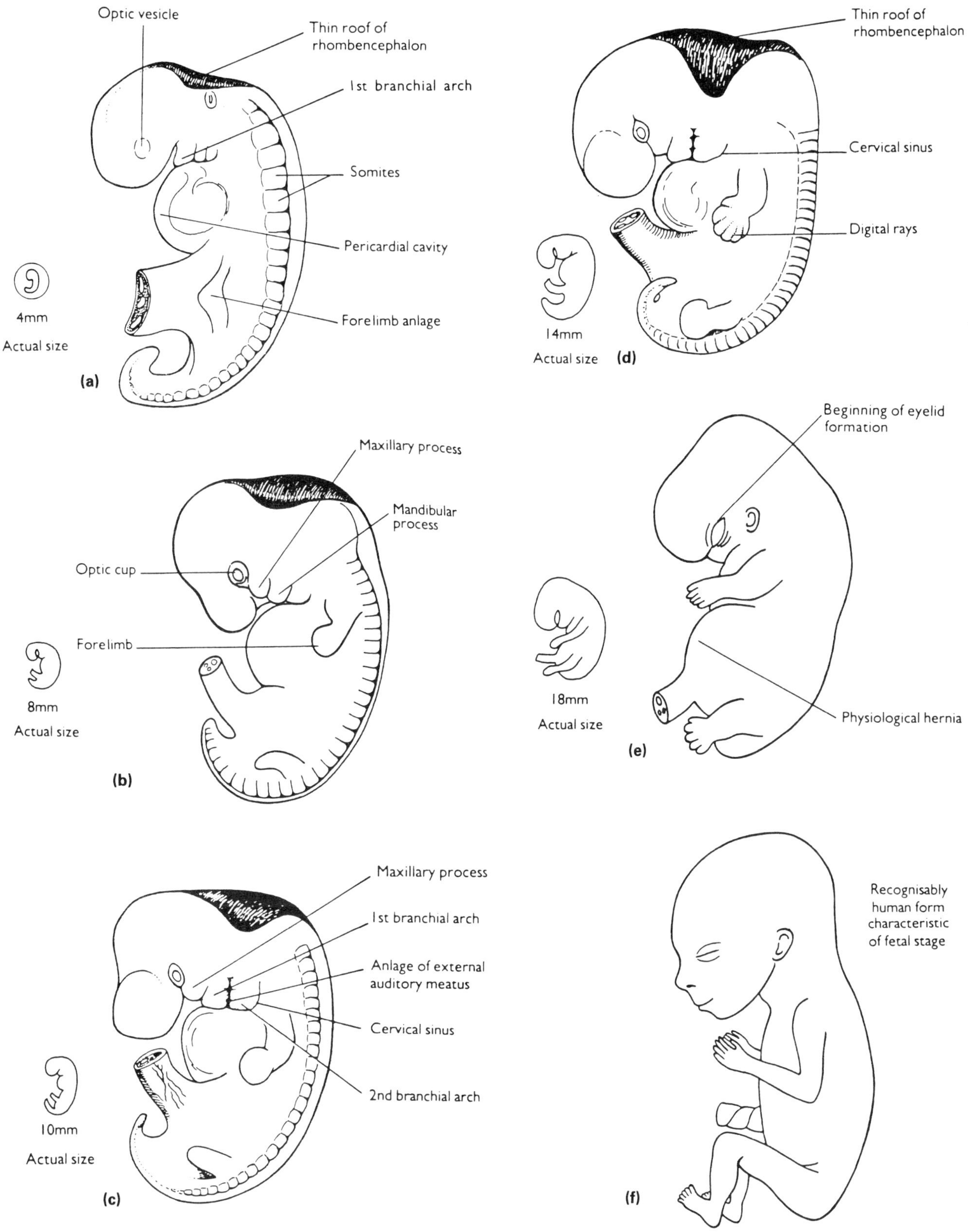

Fig. 6.92 Human embryos and fetuses at different stages of development. These are not to scale but the approximate actual size of the embryo is shown in the insets: **a** 28 days 4 mm O'Rahilly (1979) stage 13; **b** 35 days 8 mm O'Rahilly (1979) stage 15; **c** 37 days 10 mm O'Rahilly (1979) stage 16; **d** 40 days 13.5 mm O'Rahilly (1979) stage 16/17; **e** 47 days 18 mm O'Rahilly (1979) stage 19; **f** 100 days 100 mm. Reproduced with permission from Beck et al (1985).

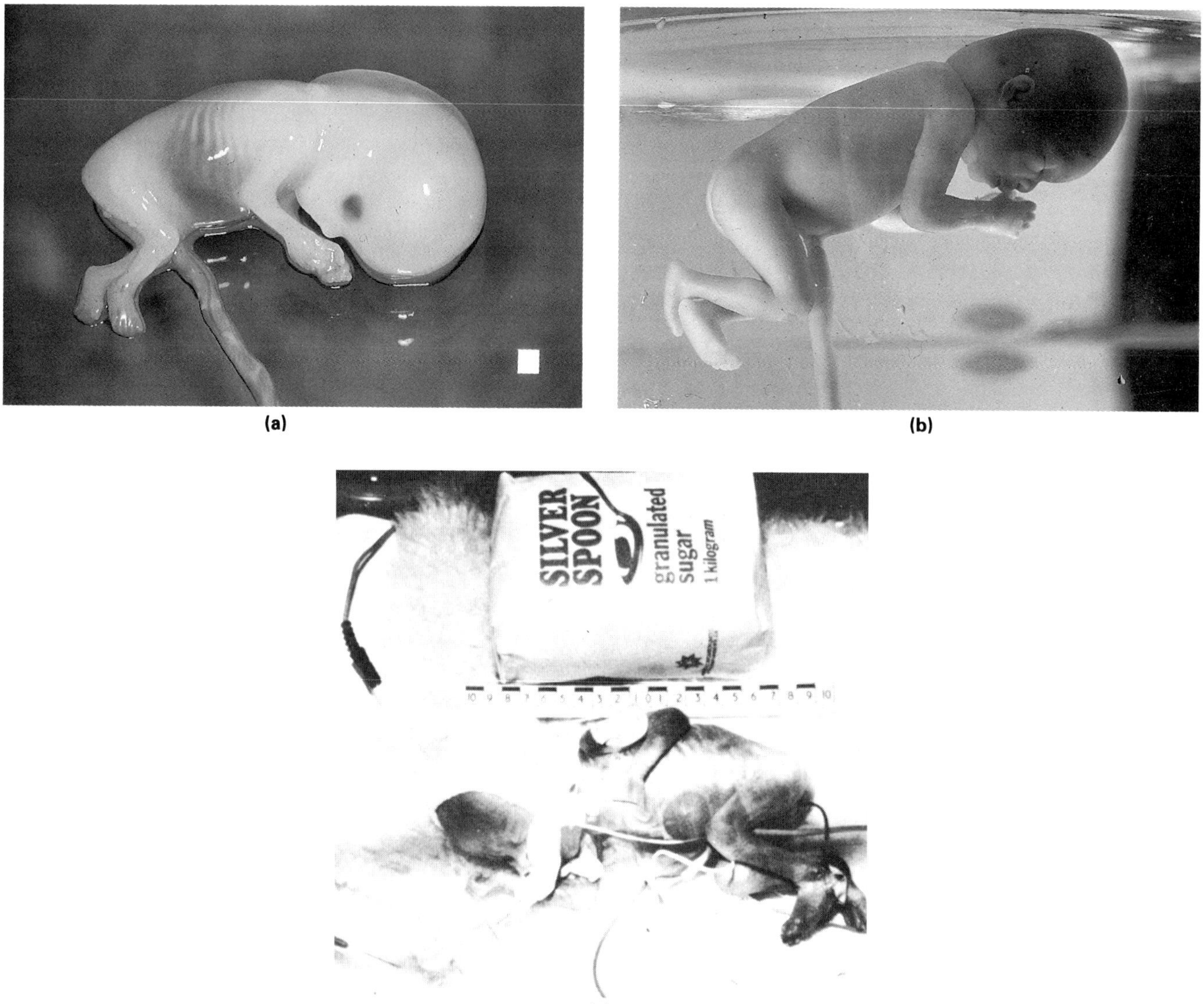

(a) (b) (c)

Fig. 6.93 The fetus at (**a**) 8 weeks; (**b**) 18 weeks; (**c**) 27 weeks.

rather than laterally, the ears much closer to their definitive positions and the infraumbilical region of the abdominal wall beginning to expand so that the umbilicus lies relatively higher in the abdomen. At 20 weeks lanugo hair covers the whole body, including the head. Between 24 and 28 weeks there is still almost complete absence of subcutaneous fat. Extensive documentation of timed stages in human development were first produced by Streeter (1942, 1945, 1948, 1951) and have been added to and improved by O'Rahilly & Müller (1987).

REFERENCES

Beck F, Moffat D B, Davies D P 1985 Human embryology, 2nd edn. Blackwell, Oxford

Deren J J 1968 Development of intestinal structure and function. In: Cook C F (ed) Handbook of physiology, vol 3. American Physiological Society, Bethesda, Maryland, p 1099

Gillman J 1948 The development of the gonads in man with a consideration of the role of fetal endocrines and histogenesis of ovarian tumours. Contributions to Embryology, Carnegie Institute 32: 81

Grand R J, Watkins J B, Troti F M 1976 Progress in gastroenterology. Development of the human gastrointestinal tract. A review. Gastroenterology 70: 790

Guraya S S 1980 Recent progress in morphology, histochemistry, biochemistry and physiology of developing and maturing human testes. International Review of Cytology 62: 187–309

Jacobson M 1978 Developmental neurobiology. Plenum Press, New York

Jacobson S 1972 Neuroembryology. In: Curtis B H, Jacobson S (eds) An introduction to neurosciences. Saunders, Philadelphia

Langman J 1968 Histogenesis of the central nervous system. In: Bourne G H (ed) The structure and function of nervous tissues. Academic Press, New York

Le Dourain 1982 In: Cohen N, Segal M M (eds) The reticulo endothelial system 3. Phylogeny and ontogeny. Plenum Press, New York

Lemire R J, Loeser J D, Leech R W, Alvord E C 1975 Normal and abnormal development of the human nervous system. Harper & Row, Hagerstown
McLean J M 1979 Embryology of the pancreas. In: Howart H T, Sarles H (eds) The exocrine pancreas. Saunders, London, p 3
O'Rahilly R 1971 The timing and sequence of events in human cardiogenesis. Acta Anatomica 79: 70
O'Rahilly R 1979 Developmental stages in human embryos. European Journal of Obstetrics, Gynecology and Reproductive Biology 9: 273
O'Rahilly R, Gardner E 1971 The timing and sequence of events in the development of the human nervous system during the embryonic period proper. Zeitschrift vür Anatomie und Entwicklungsgeschichte 134: 1
O'Rahilly R, Müller K 1987 Developmental stages in human embryos. Carnegie Institute of Washington, Publication 637
Pinkerton J H M, McKay D G, Adams C, Hertig A T 1961 Development of the human ovary — a study using histochemical techniques. Obstetrics and Gynecology 18: 152
Salenius P 1962 On the ontogenesis of the human gastric epithelial cells. A histologic and histochemical study. Acta Anatomica 50 (suppl 46): 1
Sensenig E C 1949 The early development of the human vertebral column. Contributions to Embryology, Carnegie Institute 33: 23
Severn C B 1971 A morphological study of the development of the human liver. I. Development of the hepatic diverticulum. American Journal of Anatomy 131: 133
Severn C B 1972 A morphological study of the development of the human liver. II. Establishment of liver parenchyma, extrahepatic ducts and associated venous channels. American Journal of Anatomy 133: 85
Short R V 1979 Sex determination and differentiation. British Medical Bulletin 35: 121
Slarkin H C 1979 Developmental craniofacial biology. Lea & Febiger, Philadelphia
Steinberger H, Steinberger E 1980 Testicular development structure and function. Raven Press, New York
Streeter G L 1942 Developmental horizons in human embryos, description of age group XI, 13–20 somites and age group XII 21–29 somites. Contributions to Embryology, Carnegie Institute 30: 211
Streeter G L 1945 Developmental horizons in human embryos, description of age group XIII embryo of about 4 or 5 mm long and age group XIV period of indentation of lens vesicle. Contributions to Embryology, Carnegie Institute 31: 27
Streeter G L 1948 Developmental horizons in human embryos, description of age groups XV. Being the 3rd issue of a survey of the Carnegie Collection XVI, XVII and XVIII. Contributions to Embryology, Carnegie Institute 32: 133
Streeter G L 1951 Developmental horizons in human embryos, description of age groups XIX, XX, XXI, XXII and XXIII. Being the 5th issue of a survey of the Carnegie Collection. Contributions to Embryology, Carnegie Institute 34: 165
Tench E M 1936 Development of the anus in the human embryo. American Journal of Anatomy 59: 333
Trier J S, Moxey P C 1979 Morphogenesis of the small intestine during fetal development. Ciba Foundation Symposium 70: 3
Visser H K A 1974 Sexual differentiation in the fetus and newborn. In: Davies J A, Dobbing J (eds) Scientific foundation of paediatrics. Saunders, Philadelphia, p 455
Zuckerman S, Weir B J 1977 The ovary (2nd edn). Academic Press, New York

7

Colin T. Jones

Fetal maturation in late pregnancy

INTRODUCTION

The development of the fetus in the last third of pregnancy occurs against a background of linear growth rate and largely involves the maturation of fetal organ systems, the preparation of energy stores and the establishment of reflexes essential for survival in the immediate postnatal period. Hence there is growth and distension of the lung and appearance of its surfactant system (Possmayer 1982, Ballard 1986). The liver increasingly takes over the function of regulating blood glucose (Girard & Ferre 1982, Jones & Rolph 1985). Voluntary muscle acquires the myofibrillar structures and innervation essential for motor activity (Curless 1977, Rubenstein & Kelly 1978). The intestinal tract becomes competent to secrete acid and digestive enzymes and to absorb foodstuffs (Hamosh 1982, Larsson 1988). The brain, which has already experienced its main phase of neuronal growth, undergoes myelination (Prestige 1974, Ramsay & Nicholas 1972).

In addition to these events, structures appear that have a minor role in adult life. For example, the fetus develops a particularly extensive brown adipose system (Alexander 1979, Cannon & Nedergaard 1982), its gastrointestinal tract has the ability briefly to absorb intact proteins (Hamosh 1982) and it possesses a diffuse distribution of chromaffin tissues containing biogenic amines (Coupland 1980, Jones et al 1987). In most instances these aid neonatal survival.

This phase of fetal development is characterized by high rates of linear growth and hence of accretion of protein, lipid and carbohydrate. Despite this there is substantial metabolic turnover, much of which leads to heat production (Jones & Rolph 1985). Consequently, even though the fetus is in an essentially thermoneutral environment, it is constantly producing heat to be extracted by the placenta. Cooling of the fetus activates pathways that normally lead to increased heat production, but little or no non-shivering thermogenesis occurs. The pathways activated are those involved in neonatal heat production and not those primarily responsible for the normally high rates of heat generation in the fetus (Jones & Rolph 1985, Alexander 1979, Cannon & Nedergaard 1982, Gunn et al 1986).

The late phase of fetal development therefore is preoccupied with tissue maturation essential to postnatal survival, and with rapid increase in bodyweight. These necessitate high rates of anabolism and catabolism, a uniquely prenatal circumstance. The endocrine background against which this development occurs is fairly well understood. The fetus has relatively high plasma levels of insulin and insulin-like growth factor II (IGF II), and low values of plasma T_3 but not T_4 (Nathanielsz 1976, Gluckman 1986). Then, relatively late in gestation, there are large changes in fetal plasma glucocorticoid levels that provide the signal for many of the late maturational changes in fetal tissues (Nathanielsz 1976).

Although the normal progressive and slow changes in fetal plasma hormone concentration are essential for ordered maturation, much more dramatic endocrine responses are essential to ensure survival. For instance in the course of labour the fetus may experience severe asphyxia, during which time there are hormone-driven mechanisms essential to ensure adequate maintenance of the fetal heart and brain. Hence the objective of this review is to outline the important maturational events late in fetal life and to review the various endocrine responses that protect the fetus during times of stress and that enable the birth of a healthy newborn.

ORGAN MATURATION

Hepatic development

In the latter half of gestation dramatic metabolic changes take place in the fetal liver; it shows at first high then comparatively low rates of lipid, nucleic acid and protein synthesis (Jones & Rolph 1985, Jones 1982). However, by far the most important changes for neonatal survival are those in carbohydrate metabolism. Over the last 10–25% of gestation

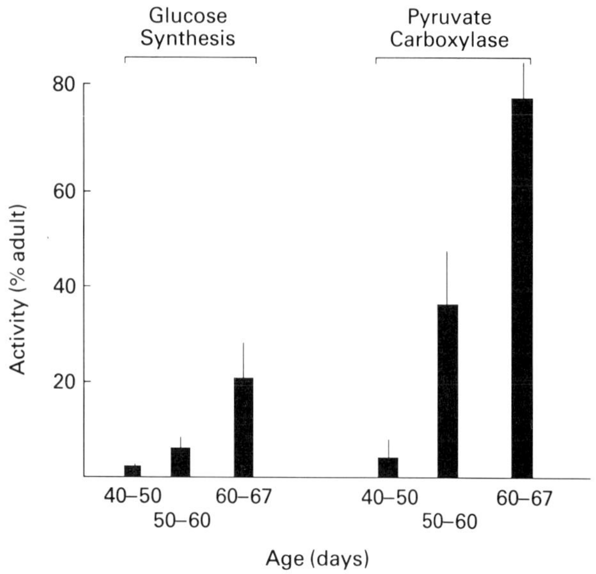

Fig. 7.1 Changes in the capacity of the liver to synthesize glucose and the activity of hepatic pyruvate carboxylase in fetal guinea pigs. Glucose synthesis was measured from lactate in liver perfused with medium containing 10 ng/ml of glucagon.

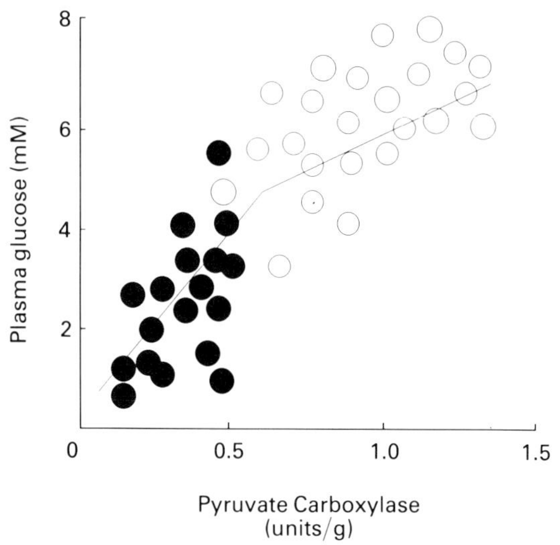

Fig. 7.2 The relationship between plasma glucose and hepatic pyruvate carboxylase activity in newborn guinea pigs 40–48 hours old. Normal guinea pigs of 100–120 g (○), growth-retarded guinea pigs of <50 g (●).

glycogen is deposited in substantial quantities (Jones & Rolph 1985, Jones 1982), much arising from the conversion of lactate into glucose, although glucose is also an important source. The glycogen is essential for normal postnatal survival for the first 24 hours after birth and its deposition is maintained even when intrauterine growth retardation and severe fetal hypoglycaemia is present (Lafeber et al 1984, Jones et al 1988a).

The second important hepatic event late in gestation is the development of the pathway for glucose synthesis (Fig. 7.1). In some species, such as rat and rabbit this pathway is virtually absent from the fetal liver (Girard & Ferre 1982, Jones & Rolph 1985, Jones 1982), while in others, such as guinea pig, sheep and man, it appears late in gestation. There is much controversy over whether it functions to a significant extent in the fetus. The balance of the evidence suggests that it does not, as relatively high glucagon : insulin ratios are required to activate it (Girard & Ferre 1982, Jones & Rolph 1985, Jones 1982). Its late development serves two functions, to be available for immediate postnatal use and to provide an additional pathway for glycogen deposition before birth (Jones & Rolph 1981). When the development of the pathway for hepatic gluconeogenesis is impaired, as in intrauterine growth retardation, neonatal hypoglycaemia ensues until the postnatal pathway developes adequately (Fig. 7.2, Rolph & Jones 1982).

The other event that occurs late in fetal liver development that is important for postnatal survival is the development of the pathways for detoxification and inactivation. The capacity of the fetal liver to metabolize hormones and peptides is limited until late in fetal life. The fetus takes up drugs rapidly and clears them slowly because the hepatic pathways for drug metabolism are poorly developed (Yaffe & Danish 1978, Dutton & Leakey 1981, Bernstein et al 1969). Hence for much of fetal life hepatic mono-oxygenase, epoxide hydratase, glucuronidation and sulphation activities are low and increase late in gestation (Neims et al 1976, Short et al 1976, Leakey et al 1983, Dancis et al 1967). The activities continue to rise after birth and can achieve high levels. Hence, in many species, the fetus near to term has a significant capacity for detoxification and inactivation that is absent for much of fetal life.

Brain development

The timing of development of the fetal brain shows more variation across the species than do most other organs. Hence in the rhesus monkey, guinea pig and sheep brains neurogenesis is essentially complete and myelination virtually complete by birth (Jones & Rolph 1985, Dobbing 1972, Berry et al 1980, Balasz 1974). In human brains neuroblast differentiation occurs before birth and continues after, with neuronal development in some structures such as the cerebellum, being postnatal events (Table 7.1, Jones & Rolph 1985, Dobbing 1972, Meisami & Timiras 1982). Myelination in the human brain occurs substantially between 22 and 36 weeks and continues extensively after birth. It occurs first in the phylogenetically older parts of the brain (Berry et al 1980, Balazs 1974, Meisami & Timiras 1982). Hence the corpus callosum is essentially unmyelinated at birth. Myelination occurs up to the second year of postnatal life. In the rat, by comparison, much of the major phase of brain development occurs after birth and is complete by about 30 days.

Development of neurotransmitter systems generally mimics the phase of neurogenesis with some important variations. Aminergic neurones appear early in gestation but show

Table 7.1 Main events in brain development in man and rat

Event	Structures involved	Timing	
		Man	Rat
Cell proliferation	Macroneurones	<20 weeks (f)	Prenatal
	Microneurones	Late fetal & postnatal	Late fetal & postnatal
	Glial cells	Late fetal & postnatal	Postnatal
Growth and differentation	Axon growth	Fetal	Fetal to 21 days (n)
	Dendrite proliferation	Late fetal & postnatal	2–3 weeks (n)
	Axon collaterals	Late fetal & postnatal	2–3 weeks (n)
	Synaptogenesis	Late fetal & postnatal	2–3 weeks (n)
	Electrical activity	Late fetal & postnatal	2–3 weeks (n)
Myelination	Phylogenetically older structures	Third trimester to late childhood up to 20 years	10–90 days postnatal

f = fetal; n = neonatal
Adapted from Meisami & Timiras 1982

a late spurt associated with the phases of high rates of neurogenesis (Coyle & Axelrod 1972, Coyle & Henry 1973). However beta-adrenergic receptors are present at very low levels throughout much of fetal life (Perlins & Moore 1973). The development of cholinergic systems is also a late event, with choline acetyl transferase appearing during the major phases of cerebral and cerebellar development (Meisami 1979, McCammon & Aprison 1964). Similarly, muscarinic receptors are at very low density throughout much of prenatal brain development and rise sharply after birth in those species in which CNS maturation is mostly postnatal.

Little is known about the factors controlling prenatal brain development, but it is clear that it is substantially, but not completely, resistant to the effects of nutritional deprivation (Jones & Rolph 1985, Meisami & Timiras 1982, McCammon & Aprison 1964). Development after birth requires normal thyroid activity and excess glucocorticoid decreases neuronal growth and brain size (Jones & Rolph 1985, Meisami & Timiras 1982, Balasz et al 1975, Cotterell et al 1972). Gonadal steroids are major determinants of the development of sexual behaviour (Ehrhart & Meyer-Bahlburg 1979).

Because the late fetal brain is still undergoing maturation in most species and because its electrical activity is low relative to postnatal life, energy demand is low. This is reflected in low ATPase activity (Tahagai 1974). It is the most likely explanation for the relative resistance of the immature brain to hypoxia (Jones & Rolph 1985, Meisami & Timiras 1982, Dawes 1968). Although the brain takes a substantial proportion of the cardiac output in the fetus, and late in gestation contributes significantly to total body oxygen consumption, this proportion is small by comparison with the adult. Nevertheless fetal cardiovascular reflexes operate to ensure that during asphyxia, induced for instance by uterine blood flow reduction, blood flow to the brain is increased to maintain oxygen and glucose delivery. The fetal brain depends largely on glucose as its metabolic substrate, but at times of possible limitation of supply, such as in the late fetal guinea pig or newborn human or rat, the ability to oxidize ketone bodies and to convert them into lipid appears (Jones & Rolph 1985, Meisami & Timiras 1982, Robinson & Williamson 1980, Rudolph & Sherwin 1983). This latter pathway protects brain development from the effects of insults such as maternal starvation. Similarly the fetal and neonatal brains of many species have the ability to oxidize fatty acids, a pathway lost in the adult (Yoshiolia & Roux 1972).

Lung development

There are two major cell types in the lung, squamous epithelial type I cells that cover most of the alveolar surface and the highly active type II cells that become apparent immediately before lung viability (Possmayer 1982, Ballard 1986, Jones & Rolph 1985, Thurlbech 1975). The type II cells are the site of surfactant production and in addition to large numbers of mitochondria they contain membranous lamellar bodies, the storage form of surfactant. The development of gas exchange in the perinatal lung, which has a much smaller surface area than in the adult, is associated with a sharp increase in the number of lamellar bodies in alveolar type II cells (Ballard 1986, Jones & Rolph 1985).

Although the changes in lung distensibility during late development are important in preparing the lung for postnatal life (Liggins & Schellenberg 1985) most attention has focused on the development of surfactant production, which, if impaired, leads to the onset of respiratory distress syndrome (Possmayer 1982, Ballard 1986). Surfactant is composed mostly of disaturated phosphatidylcholine and small percentages of phosphatidylglycerol, phosphatidylinositol, phosphatidylethanolamine and lipid and protein (Table 7.2). Reduced surface tension allowing inflation of the lungs at low tracheal pressures is caused largely by phosphatidylcholine spreading over the alveolar surface. The minor constituents aid the phospholipid packing and unpacking in lamellar bodies and the formation of a monolayer over the alveolar surface (Possmayer 1982, Ballard 1986).

Maturation of the fetal lung coincides with a sharp increase in lung concentrations of surfactant phospholipid and protein in the last few days before birth in many species (Possmayer 1982, Ballard 1986, Jones & Rolph 1985), although in the human fetus this change starts earlier and is much

Table 7.2 Composition of lung-wash surfactant

Constituent	Mol %
Phospholipids	
Disaturated phosphatidylcholine	40
Other phosphatidylcholines	21
Phosphatidylglycerol	8
Phosphatidylinositol	5
Phosphatidylethanolamine	5
Other phospholipids	4
Neutral lipids	
Glycerides	6
Cholesterol	2
Cholesterol esters	1
Fatty acids	1
Protein	7

Taken from data for the dog (Metcalf et al 1980)

Table 7.3 Development of adrenergic innervation in the mouse heart as indicated by noradrenaline content

Time of development (days)	% adult value
Fetal	
17	4.2
19	14.8
20	18.7
Postnatal	
1	13.2
2	15.9
6	21.8
14	131
21	110
40	108

more progressive. The fact that this increase in synthesis occurs at the same time as rising fetal plasma cortisol concentrations suggests that glucocorticoids play a role in the induction of lung maturation (Possmayer 1982, Ballard 1986, Jones & Rolph 1985, Batenberg & Van Golde 1979, Smith et al 1974, Van Golde et al 1985). Such a role has been confirmed by studies on the effects of adrenalectomy or steroid administration. However, steroids do not activate alveolar type II cells directly but induce fibroblasts to produce a protein factor that produces this effect (Smith et al 1974). The fact that steroids frequently do not induce lung maturation in utero has led to the search for other modulating agents. Hence thyroid hormones, TRH, oestrogens, prolactin and insulin have all been implicated to be involved at various steps in the pathway (Possmayer 1982, Ballard 1986, Jones & Rolph 1985). However, of all of these, only for thyroid hormones has the effect been shown clearly to have specific actions, where they are required to maintain phospholipid synthesis (Smith 1979). Another interesting hormonal effect on lung development is the clearance of lung liquid at birth by activation of beta-receptors by the large rise in plasma adrenaline that occurs (Ballard 1986).

Heart development

The heart develops early in fetal life and in man can be observed to contract after about 8% of gestation. Its primary function as a pump determines that it grows in close proportion to body weight, but at a systolic pressure of about 50% of that of the adult. However, its relative combined ventricular output is up to 10-fold above that of the adult heart (Anderson et al 1981). Cardiac growth throughout most of fetal life is by hyperplasia, but shortly after birth mitotic activity declines sharply and most of the further growth results from hypertrophy (Jones & Rolph 1985).

The most striking changes in the late maturation of the heart are sharp increases in numbers of mitochondria and transverse tubules (Jones & Rolph 1985, Rolph et al 1982, Hirakow & Gotoh 1976) which continue after birth. In addition there are increases in the number, but particularly in the composition, of contractile proteins (Jones & Rolph 1985, Hoh et al 1977, Lompre et al 1981). Hence, in fetal ventricles, the dominant myosin isoenzyme is largely V_3 which is replaced by V_1 after birth, a change which coincides with an increase in myosin Ca^{2+}-ATPase activity and work load (Schwartz et al 1981).

Neural control of the heart is a postnatal event in rat and mouse (Table 7.3), but occurs at about mid-gestation in sheep and guinea pig (Jones & Rolph 1985). Beta-receptor sensitivity increases in the late fetal heart and after birth, set against a background of increasing, or, in some instances, increasing then falling, adenylate cyclase activity (Clark et al 1980). This increase in sensitivity is associated with rising ionotropic responsiveness (Cohen 1986).

One of the striking features of the fetal heart is its much greater resistance to oxygen lack than in the adult. Metabolism in the fetal heart is largely sustained by glucose oxidation with a small amount of fatty acid utilization (Jones & Rolph 1985, Rolph et al 1982, Hoerter & Opre 1978). Hence the fetal heart has a significantly greater glycolytic capacity than that of the adult, although its oxidative capacity is smaller (Jones & Rolph 1985). The lower oxygen consumption determines that, in hypoxia, glycolytic flux is able to sustain energy needs much better than in the adult (Jones & Rolph 1985, Rolph et al 1982, Hoerter & Opre 1978). Under such conditions endogenous glycogen is an important fuel source. Glycogen levels are high at the start of the last third of gestation but fall as term approaches and the fetal heart gradually begins to shift to a more adult type metabolism (Jones & Rolph 1985).

Skeletal muscle development

Unlike the fetal heart, where major developmental changes take place well before the last third of gestation, in skeletal muscle this period and immediately after birth is a time of major differentiation and maturation. In species that are mobile at birth there is much prenatal development of limb muscles, whose fibres by birth are well differentiated both metabolically and electrophysiologically (Jones & Rolph 1985). In species that are immobile at birth all functional development is postnatal (Jones & Rolph 1985, Curless 1977). After the formation of the myotubes, the contractile proteins that appear in fetal muscle are mostly, if not exclusively, of the slow twitch type (Buller & Lewis 1965). Many of these proteins have isoenzyme forms specific to the fetus (Whalen et al 1981). The slow twitch nature of the fetal muscles is confirmed by isometric-twitch/contraction studies, but not always by histological analysis (Buller & Lewis 1965). Subsequent postnatal maturation of the skeletal muscle type is largely determined by the nature of the innervation (Jones & Rolph 1985, Dhoot et al 1981).

Prior to formation of myotubes, muscle is metabolically fairly inactive (Jones & Rolph 1985). Subsequently, in those species born mobile, there is a substantial increase in mitochondrial number and glycolytic enzyme activity (Jones & Rolph 1985, Rolph et al 1982), presumably in preparation for the major surge in physical activity after birth. There is limited activity in muscle before birth (Natale et al 1981). Skeletal muscle is also the site of the major store of glycogen deposition before birth, representing about one-half of the fetal pool (Jones & Rolph 1985). One of the factors contributing to the maintained skeletal muscle glycogen store in the fetus, ensuring postnatal use, is limited ability of beta-receptor stimulation to activate adenylate cyclase at this time (Jones & Rolph 1985).

In the adult, the muscle mass makes a major quantitative contribution to body metabolism. Whether this applies to the mature fetus is unclear. The limited metabolic capacity of fetal muscle suggests not, but theoretical analysis suggests otherwise (Jones & Rolph 1985).

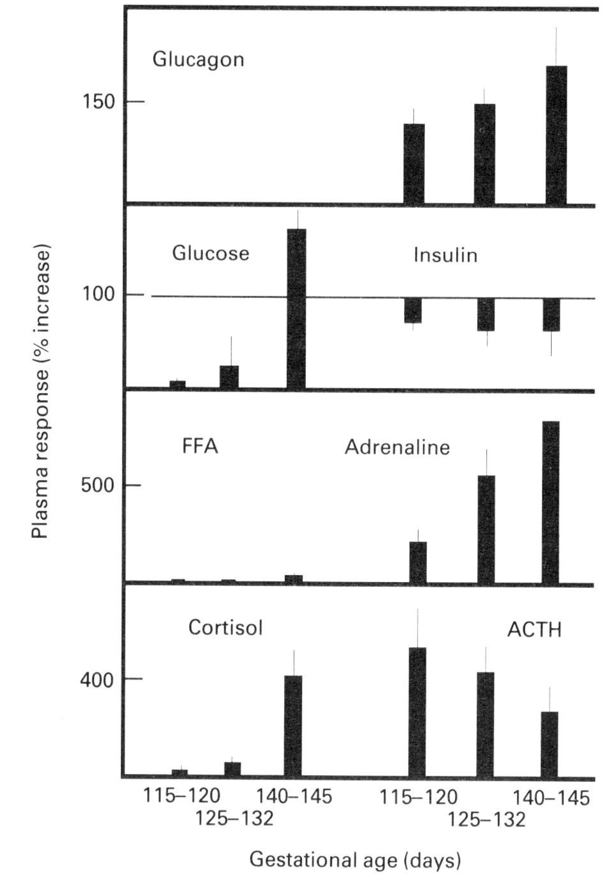

Fig. 7.3 Fetal plasma hormone and metabolite responses to hypoxia caused by pregnant sheep breathing 9% O_2 + 3% CO_2 for 60 minutes. Fetal PO_2 was depressed by about 40%.

INTEGRATED RESPONSES

The clearest insight into the late maturation of fetal organ and endocrine systems is provided by analysis of the integrated responses to physiological insult. The commonest forms of insult in the late fetus, and particularly during birth, are hypoxia and asphyxia, caused, amongst other things, by compression of the umbilical cord and reduction of uterine blood flow. Hence experimental studies using such insults are used as models to define the nature of integrated responses of the fetus. Consideration of the physiological responses of the mature fetus will be restricted to analysis of the observations from studies using such models.

Fetal responses to hypoxia and reduced uterine blood flow

Before about the third trimester in many species reduced availability of oxygen is well tolerated. This presumably reflects the limited development of the fetal heart and the relatively low metabolic demands of the fetal brain at this time. Hence the endocrine and metabolic responses of the fetus to hypoxia at the beginning of the third trimester are small with little change in plasma glucose, fatty acid or amino acid concentrations and particularly modest changes in plasma insulin, glucagon, adrenaline, noradrenaline, T_4 and growth hormone are seen (Fig. 7.3; Jones et al 1977, 1988b, Jones 1977). In contrast plasma adrenocorticotrophic hormone (ACTH) concentration shows a sharp increase which is not reflected in a comparably large rise in plasma cortisol (Fig. 7.3, Jones 1977). This illustrates that the hormones involved in initiation of acute mobilization of metabolic stores are little activated at about two-thirds of the way through fetal development. This relatively quiescent state is not necessarily the result of passive inactivity of endocrine glands as, at least in some instances, endocrine activity is actively suppressed. For instance, the poor response of the fetal adrenal to elevation of plasma ACTH is at least in part the result of relatively high levels of pro-opiomelanocortin, which is inhibitory to the steroidogenic action of ACTH (Roebuck et al 1980). This peptide is produced both by the placenta and the pituitary and ensures that maternal and hence fetal stress does not precociously induce premature birth (Jones 1988a).

During the third trimester the endocrine responses to hypoxia and reduced uterine blood flow increase sharply, but the timing of the increased response varies substantially between endocrine systems. Hence the increased adrenocortical activity usually occurs very late in gestation, whilst adrenal medullary activity, as reflected in catecholamine and enkephalin release develops very quickly (Jones et al 1977, 1988b; Jones 1977, 1988a, Roebuck et al 1980).

The endocrine responses to hypoxia and reduced uterine blood flow may be divided into the following: those of the pituitary–thyroid axis, those of the pituitary–adrenal axis, adrenal medullary activity, pancreatic hormone changes and placental peptide production and hormone clearance.

Pituitary–thyroid–placental axis

In response to maternally-induced hypoxia there are no detectable changes in fetal plasma level of T_4 or of rT_3 or T_3, but plasma thyroid-stimulating hormone (TSH) concentration rises (Fisher 1986). This is consistent with the role of this axis in responding to relatively long-term changes in nutritional state. In contrast if uterine blood flow is reduced, particularly by infusion of adrenaline into the maternal circulation, there is a sharp reduction in the fetal plasma level of T_3. An important contribution to this is a reduction in placental conversion of T_4 to T_3. As this is probably a mostly placental effect there are no apparent changes in the extent of the T_3 response during the third trimester (Fisher 1986). Such a placentally initiated fall in circulating T_3 concentration in the fetus does provide a potential mechanism for communication of changes in perfusion of the maternal placenta to the fetus.

Pituitary–adrenal–placental axis

In contrast to the changes in the activity of the pituitary–thyroid–placental axis, activation of the pituitary adrenal axis causes substantial changes in the circulating concentrations of both ACTH and cortisol, the responses of which increase progressively as term approaches (Jones et al 1977, Roebuck 1980, Jones 1988a, Challis et al 1984). These responses are complex, with pro-opiomelanocortin being the predominant ACTH-containing peptide to be released early in the third trimester; then, towards term, ACTH rather than pro-opiomelanocortin is the primary secretion product. This maturation of the pituitary corticotrophs from mid to late in gestation shows the capacity to enhance processing of pro-opiomelanocortin and increase ACTH output. This ensures that hypoxia or reduced uterine blood flow does not prematurely induce adrenal maturation and birth (Jones 1977, Jones & Roebuck 1980). Hence the fetal adrenocortical responses to these stimuli are relatively small until just before birth when the fetal pituitary is releasing predominantly ACTH (Fig. 7.4; Jones 1977, 1988a, Roebuck et al 1980, Challis et al 1984).

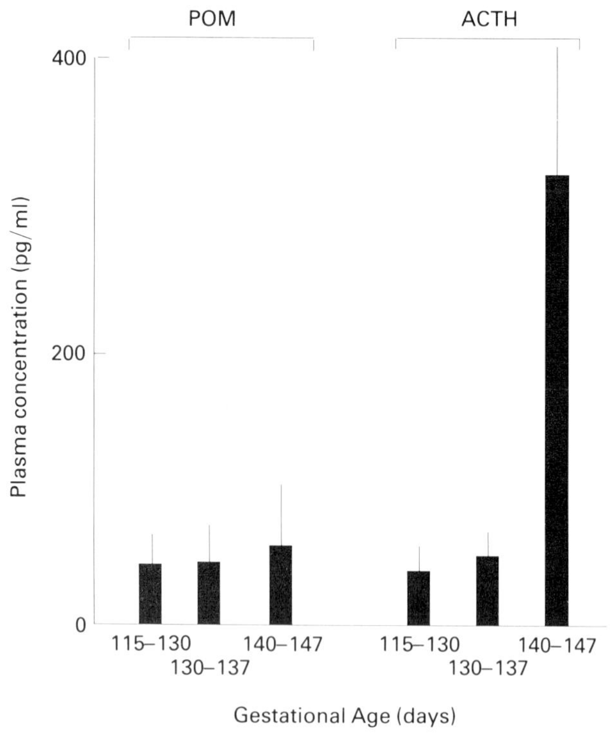

Fig. 7.4 Changes in basal plasma concentrations of pro-opiomelanocortin and $_{1-39}$ACTH in fetal sheep over the last third of pregnancy.

The fetal pituitary is not the only source of ACTH and pro-opiomelanocortin, the placenta is also rich in both peptides and they are released particularly in response to reduced uterine blood flow. However, it is pro-opiomelanocortin release that predominates and therefore manipulation of uterine blood flow has little effect upon the glucocorticoid concentration in the fetal circulation. Why ACTH-containing peptides should be released from the placenta is unclear. They may function to maintain suppression of adrenocortical activity (Jones 1988a). However, in adult life, such peptides are found at many sites; hence other functions are suggested. In primates, although ACTH, which probably shows the above changes in nature during fetal development, stimulates adrenal cortisol production, its primary role is probably to enhance dehydroepiandrosterone (DHEA) production from the adrenal.

In addition to the release of ACTH peptides the placenta also secretes large quantities of corticotrophin-releasing factor (CRF) into the fetal and maternal circulations, achieving high concentrations late in pregnancy (Jones 1988a). Even though the levels are high, it is unlikely they are sufficiently high to stimulate substantially the pituitary release of ACTH. A more probable role is a contribution to the low vascular resistance in the placental circulations as CRF is a powerful vasodilator (Edwards & Jones 1988). It may, however, regulate the release of ACTH from trophoblastic tissue. Whether the placenta contains an autonomous CRF-ACTH regulatory system is less clear. CRF infusion into

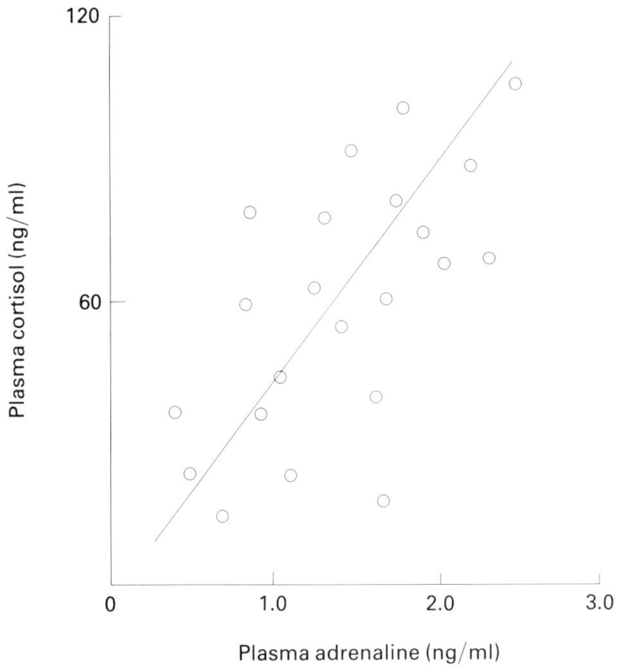

Fig. 7.5 The relationship between changes in plasma adrenaline and cortisol in response to fetal hypoxia in sheep over the last third of gestation.

the fetal circulation, at rates comparable to the output from the placenta at any time except close to term, does lead to the release of ACTH.

Adrenal medullary activity and catecholamine release

In the adult, the adrenal medulla secretes large quantities of adrenaline, noradrenaline, CRF and enkephalins at rates that are determined by the pattern of stimulation and usually in response to hypoxia, haemorrhage or hypoglycaemia (Edwards & Jones 1988, Bloom et al 1987). In the fetus the capacity to secrete catecholamines in relatively large quantities first appears around the beginning of the third trimester when splanchnic innervation takes place (Jones 1980, Slotlin 1986). Before then there is a relatively small response to hypoxia which is thought to be mediated by a non-neural pathway (Jones 1980). In species that are immature at birth, such as the rat, the neural pathway develops after birth, hence fetal activation of the adrenal medulla appears to be entirely non-neurogenic (Jones 1980).

The fetal adrenal output of catecholamines at the start of the third trimester is largely of noradrenaline, and this response increases as term approaches. Simultaneous with this, adrenaline is found in increasing quantities so that by term it makes the major contribution to total catecholamine output (Jones 1980, Slotlin 1986, Jones & Wei 1985). These changes in the noradrenaline : adrenaline ratio correlate with those in the composition of the adrenal gland and with the increasing capacity for glucocorticoid production (Fig. 7.5).

From a functional standpoint, the increasing output of adrenaline in response to stimulation correlates with the development of important metabolic responses such as glycogen mobilization (Jones et al 1977, Jones & Wei 1985). This is particularly important for neonatal survival in the first few hours of life as is probably the adrenaline-induced activation of lipolysis and thermogenesis in brown adipose.

Table 7.4 Developmental changes in the sensitivity of the heart to catecholamines

	Noradrenaline (ng/ml)	
	Fetus	Adult
Plasma concentration		
Resting	0.1–0.25	0.03–0.1
Hypoxia	0.75–10	0.1–0.5
Level causing positive ionotropic response		
Lower limit	0.04–0.08	0.75–0.15
50% maximum response	10–20	75–150
Maximum response	1000–2000	>2000

The cardiovascular responses of the fetus to insults such as hypoxia also show a marked change with increased output of adrenaline, the hypertensive effects being progressively more apparent (Jones & Wei 1985). Also the heart rate response, which changes from a sustained rise to a prolonged fall during hypoxia, correlates with the magnitude of the increase in adrenaline output, as does the extent to which heart rate recovers during hypoxia it being greatest when adrenaline shows large increases. This relationship between changes in plasma adrenaline concentration and heart rate is in part explained by the much higher sensitivity of the fetal than the adult heart to the ionotropic effects of adrenaline stimulation. Hence, whilst adrenaline has marked ionotropic effects upon the fetal heart at physiological plasma concentrations this is not so for the adult (Table 7.4; Jones & Wei 1985).

Clearly the secretion of adrenaline from the adrenal medulla is required close to term and during labour for activation of lung fluid reabsorption (Ballard 1986). Hence the maturation of the adrenal is particularly important in recruiting responses essential to postnatal survival from the liver, lung and cardiovascular system.

Changes in circulating concentrations of catecholamines are not only brought about in the fetus by variations in secretion from the adrenal medulla and release from sympathetic terminals. Alteration in clearance is an important mechanism of causing fluctuations in plasma concentration. In the fetus the placenta is a major site of clearance, with catecholamines being removed almost completely in one passage through the umbilical circulation (Jones & Wei 1985). However, the rate of clearance is influenced by uterine perfusion and as that falls umbilical extraction declines and fetal plasma concentration rises (Jones 1988a, Jones & Wei 1985). For instance a 30–50% fall in uterine perfusion will increase fetal plasma catecholamine concentrations two- to six-fold (Jones 1988a, Jones & Wei 1985). The clearance of catecholamines is also the mechanism of maintaining a placental barrier. Hence if uterine perfusion is reduced to lower placental oxygen consumption the permeability barrier breaks down and catecholamines pass freely across both sides of the placenta. Such changes in placental clearance provide one means by which alterations in uterine perfusion can be communicated to the fetus (Jones 1988a).

Pancreatic activity

Hypoxia and reduced uterine blood flow cause a fall in fetal plasma insulin and a rise in glucagon (Jones et al 1988b). The magnitude of these changes does not vary over the last third of gestation. Their function is predominantly to depress fetal utilization of glucose and enhance output by the fetus, both through glycogen mobilization and to a lesser extent by glucose synthesis (Jones et al 1983). The obvious function of such changes is to ensure that glucose supply to the fetal brain and heart are maintained, particularly during events such as labour. However, this pathway is also important in ensuring that glucose supply to the placenta is sustained when that from the uterine circulation is reduced, a mechanism illustrated by the relatively large proportion of glucose supplied to the placenta from the fetal circulation (Jones 1988b).

REFERENCES

Alexander G 1979 Thermogenesis. In: Robertshaw D (ed) Environmental physiology III, vol 20. University Park Press, Baltimore, pp 43–155

Anderson D F, Bissonette J M, Faber J J, Thornburg K L 1981 Central shunt flows and pressures in mature fetal lamb. American Journal of Physiology 241: H60

Balazs R 1974 Influence of metabolic factors on brain development. British Medical Bulletin 30: 126

Balasz R, Lewis P D, Patel A J 1975 In: Brazier M A B (ed) Growth and development of the brain. Raven Press, New York, pp 83–115

Ballard P 1986 Hormones and lung maturation. Springer-Verlag, Heidelberg

Batenberg J J, Van Golde L M G 1979 Formation of pulmonary surfactant in the whole lung and isolated type III alveolar cells. Review of Perinatal Medicine 3: 71

Bernstein R B, Novy M J, Piasecki G J, Lester, R, Jackson B T 1969 Bilirubin metabolism in the fetus. Journal of Clinical Investigation 48: 1678

Berry M, McConnell P, Sievers J 1980 Dendritic growth and control of neuronal form. Current Topics in Developmental Biology 15: 67

Bloom S R, Edwards A V, Jones C T 1987 The release of certain neuropeptides in response to splanchnic nerve stimulation in conscious calves. Journal of Physiology 384: 29P

Buller A J, Lewis D M 1965 Further observations on the differentiation of skeletal muscles in the kitten hindlimb. Journal of Physiology, 176: 355

Cannon B, Nedergaard J 1982 The function and properties of brown adipose tissue in the newborn. In: Jones C T (ed) Biochemical development of the fetus and neonate. Elsevier Biomedical Press, Amsterdam, pp 697–730

Challis J R G, Mitchell B F, Lye S J 1984 Activation of fetal adrenal function. Journal of Developmental Physiology 6: 93

Clark J B, Vinicor F, Carr L, Clark C M 1980 Adenyl cyclase responsiveness to guanyl nucleotides in the developing rat heart. Pediatric Research 14: 291

Cohen H L 1986 Development of autonomic innervation in the mammalian myocardium. In: Gootman P M (ed) Developmental neurobiology of the autonomic nervous system. Humana Press, New Jersey, pp 159–192

Cotterell M, Balasz R, Johnson A L 1972 Effects of corticosteroids on the biochemical maturation of rat brain: postnatal cell formation. Journal of Neurochemistry 19: 2151

Coupland R E 1980 The development and fate of catecholamine secreting endocrine cells. In: Parvez H, Parvez S (eds) Biogenic amines in development. North-Holland Biomedical Press, Amsterdam, pp 3–28

Coyle J T, Axelrod J 1972 Dopamine-beta-hydroxylase in rat brain: developmental characterization. Journal of Neurochemistry 19: 449

Coyle J T, Henry D 1973 Catecholamines in fetal and neonatal rat brain. Journal of Neurochemistry 21: 61

Curless R G 1977 Developmental patterns of peripheral nerve, myoneural junction and muscle: a review. Progress in Neurobiology 9: 197

Dancis J, Hutzler J, Rokkones T 1967 Intermittent branched-chain ketonuria-variant of maple-syrup-urine disease. New England Journal of Medicine 267: 84

Dawes G S 1968 Fetal and neonatal physiology. Year Book, Chicago

Dhoot G S, Perry S V, Vrbova G 1981 Changes in the distribution of the components of the troponin complex in muscle fibres after cross-reinnervation. Experimental Neurology 72: 513

Dobbing J 1972 Vulnerable periods of brain development. In: Lipids, malnutrition and the developing brain. CIBA Foundation Symposium. Associated Scientific Publishers, Amsterdam, pp 9–20

Dutton G J, Leakey J E A 1981 Progress in Drug Research 25: 189

Edwards A V, Jones C T 1988 Secretion of corticotrophin releasing factor from the adrenal during splanchnic nerve stimulation in conscious calves. Journal of Physiology 400: 89

Ehrhart A A, Meyer-Bahlburg H F L 1979 Prenatal sex hormones and the developing brain: effects on psychosexual differentiation and cognitive function. Annual Review of Medicine 30: 417

Fisher D A 1986 The unique endocrine milieu of the fetus. Journal of Clinical Investigation 78: 603

Girard J, Ferre P 1982 Metabolic and hormonal changes around the time of birth. In: Jones C T (ed) Biochemical development of the fetus and neonate. Elsevier Biomedical Press, Amsterdam, pp 517–551

Gluckman P D 1986 Hormones and fetal growth. Oxford Review of Reproductive Biology 8: 1

Gunn T R, Butler J, Gluckman P 1986 Metabolic and hormonal responses to cooling the fetal sheep in utero. Journal of Developmental Physiology 8: 55–66

Hamosh M 1982 The development of the metabolic and transport function of the gastrointestinal tract. In: Jones C T (ed) Biochemical development of the fetus and neonate. Elsevier Biomedical Press, Amsterdam, pp 591–619

Hirakow R, Gotoh J 1976 A quantitative ultrastructural study on the developing rat heart. In: Lieberman M, Sano T (eds) Developmental and physiological correlates of cardiac muscle. Raven, New York, pp 37–49

Hoerter J A, Opie L H 1978 Perinatal changes in glycolytic function in response to hypoxia in the incubated perfused rat heart. Biology of the Neonate 33: 144

Hoh J F Y, McGrath P A, Hale P T 1977 Electrophoretic analysis of multiple forms of rat cardiac myosin: effects of hypophysectomy and thyroxine replacement. Journal of Molecular and Cellular Cardiology 10: 1053

Jones C T 1977 The development of some metabolic responses to hypoxia in the fetal sheep. Journal of Physiology 266: 743

Jones C T 1980 Circulating catecholamines in the fetus, their origin, actions and significance. In: Parvez H, Parvez S (eds) Biogenic amines in development. Elsevier/North-Holland, Amsterdam, pp 63–85

Jones C T 1982 The development of metabolism in fetal liver. In: Jones C T (ed) Biochemical development of the fetus and neonate. Elsevier Biomedical Press, Amsterdam, pp 249–286

Jones C T 1988a Pathways of communication between the placenta and fetus, potentially important in the regulation of growth and state. In: Jones C T (ed) Fetal and neonatal development. Perinatology Press, Ithaca, pp 68–78

Jones C T 1988b Relationship between alterations in uterine blood flow and the handling of glucose by fetus and placenta. In: Jensen A, Kunzel W (eds) The endocrine control of the fetus. Physiologic and pathophysiologic aspects. Springer-Verlag, Berlin, pp 333–342

Jones C T, Roebuck M M 1980 ACTH peptides and the development of the fetal adrenal. Journal of Steroid Biochemistry 12: 77

Jones C T, Rolph T P 1981 Metabolic events associated with the preparation of the fetus for independent life. CIBA Symposium 86: 214

Jones C T, Rolph T P 1985 Metabolism during fetal life: a functional assessment of metabolic development. Physiological Reviews 65: 357

Jones C T, Wei G 1985 Adrenal-medullary activity and cardiovascular control in the fetal sheep. In: Kunzel W (ed) Fetal heart rate monitoring. Springer-Verlag, Heidelberg, pp 127–135

Jones C T, Boddy K, Robinson J S, Ratcliffe J G 1977 Developmental changes in the responses of the adrenal glands of fetal sheep to endogenous adrenocorticotrophin, as indicated by hormone responses to hypoxia. Journal of Endocrinology 72: 279

Jones C T, Ritchie J W K, Walker D W 1983 The effects of hypoxia on glucose turnover in the fetal sheep. Journal of Developmental Physiology 5: 223

Jones C T, Roebuck M M, Walker D W, Lagercrantz H, Johnston B M 1987 Cardiovascular, metabolic and endocrine effects of chemical sympathectomy and adrenal demedullation in fetal sheep. Journal of Developmental Physiology 9: 347

Jones C T, Harding J E, Gu W, Lafeber H N 1988a Placental metabolism and endocrine effects in relation to the control of fetal and placental growth. In: Jensen A, Kunzel W (eds) The endocrine control of the fetus. Physiologic and pathophysiologic aspects. Springer-Verlag, Berlin, pp 213–222

Jones C T, Roebuck M M, Walker D W, Johnston B M 1988b The role of the adrenal medulla and peripheral sympathetic nerves in the physiological responses of the fetal sheep to hypoxia. Journal of Developmental Physiology 10: 17

Lafeber H N, Rolph T P, Jones C T 1984 Studies on the growth of the fetal guinea pig. The effects of ligation of the uterine artery on organ growth and development. Journal of Developmental Physiology 6: 440

Larsson L I 1988 Endocrine development of gut in relation to function. In: Jones C T (ed) Fetal and neonatal development. Perinatology Press, Ithaca, pp 457–462

Leaky J E A, Althaus Z R, Bailey J R, Slikker W 1983 UDP-glucuronyl-transferase activity exhibits two developmental groups in liver from foetal rhesus monkeys. Biochemical Journal 214: 1007

Liggins G C, Schellenberg J C 1985 Aspects of fetal lung development. In: Jones C T (ed) The physiological development of the fetus and newborn. Academic Press, London, pp 179–189

Lompre A M, Mercadier J C, Wisnewsky C, Bouveret P, Pantaloni C, D'Albis A, Schwartz K 1981 Species and age-dependent changes in the relative amounts of cardiac myosin isoenzymes — mammals. Developmental Biology 84: 286

McCammon R E, Aprison M H 1964 Progress in Brain Research 9: 220

Meisami E 1979 In: Meisami E, Brazier M A B (eds) Neural growth and differentiation. Raven Press, New York, pp 183–206

Meisami E, Timiras P 1982 Normal and abnormal biochemical development of the brain after birth. In: Jones C T (ed) Biochemical development of the fetus and neonate. Elsevier Biomedical Press, Amsterdam, pp 759–821

Metcalf I R, Enhorning G, Possmayer F 1980 Pulmonary surfactant-associated proteins: their role in the expression of surface activity. Journal of Applied Physiology 49: 34

Natale R, Clewlow F, Dawes G S 1981 Measurement of fetal forelimb movements in the lamb in utero. American Journal of Physiology 140: 545

Nathanielsz P W 1976 Fetal endocrinology: an experimental approach. North-Holland, Amsterdam

Neims A H, Warner M, Loughnan P M, Aranda J V 1976 Developmental aspects of the hepatic cytochrome P450 monooxygenase system. Annual Review of Pharmacology and Toxicology 16: 427

Perkins J P, Moore M M 1973 Regulation of the adenosine cyclic 3′5′-monophosphate content of rat cerebral cortex: ontogenic development of the responsiveness to catecholamines and adenosine. Molecular Pharmacology 9: 774

Possmayer F 1982 In: Jones C T (ed) Biochemical development of the fetus and neonate. Elsevier Biomedical Press, Amsterdam, pp 337–391

Prestige M C 1974 Axon and cell numbers in the developing nervous system. British Medical Bulletin 30: 107

Robinson A M, Williamson D H 1980 Physiological roles of ketone bodies as substrates and signals in mammalian tissues. Physiological Reviews 60: 143

Roebuck M M, Jones C T, Holland D, Silman R B 1980 The effects of large-molecular-weight forms of ACTH on the fetal sheep adrenal in vitro. Nature 284: 616

Rolph T P, Jones C T 1982 Delayed development of gluconeogenic capacity and the appearance of hypoglycaemia in the newborn guinea pig after intrauterine growth restriction. Developmental Physiology 4: 1

Rolph T P, Jones C T, Parry D 1982 Ultrastructural and enzymatic development of fetal guinea pig heart. American Journal of Physiology 243: H87

Ramsay R B, Nicholas H J 1972 Brain lipids. Advances in Lipid Research 10: 143

Rubenstein N A F, Kelly A M 1978 Myogenic and neurogenic contributions to the development of fast and slow twitch muscles in rat. Developmental Biology 62: 473

Rudolph M C J, Sherwin R S 1983 Metabolic ketosis and its effects on the fetus. Clinical Endocrinology and Metabolism 12: 413

Schwartz K, Lecarpentier Y, Martin J L, Lompre A M, Mercadier J J, Swynghedauw B 1981 Myosin isoenzymic distribution correlates with speed of myocardial contraction. Journal of Molecular and Cellular Cardiology 13: 1071

Short C R, Kinden D A, Stith R 1976 Drug Metabolism Review 5: 1

Slotkin T A 1986 Development of the sympathoadrenal axis. In: Gootman P M (ed) Developmental neurobiology of the autonomic nervous system. Humana Press, New Jersey, pp 69–96

Smith B T 1979 Lung maturation in the fetal rat: acceleration by injection of fibroblast-pneumocyte factor. Science 204: 1094

Smith B T, Torday J S, Giroud C J P 1974 Evidence for different gestation-dependent effects of cortisol on cultured fetal lung cells. Journal of Clinical Investigation 53: 1518

Takagai G 1974 Developmental changes in glycolysis in rat cerebral cortex. Journal of Neurochemistry 23: 479

Thurlbeck W M 1975 Postnatal growth and development of the lung. American Review of Respiratory Diseases 111: 803

Van Golde L M G, Batenburgh J J, Post M, De Vries A C J, Smith B T 1985 Synthesis of surfactant lipids in the developing lung. In: Jones C T (ed) The physiological development of the fetus and newborn. Academic Press, London, pp 191–200

Whalen R G, Sell S M, Butler-Browne G S, Schwartz K, Boiuveret P, Pinset-Harstrom I 1981 Three myosin heavy-chain isozymes appear sequentially in rat muscle development. Nature 292: 805

Winick M 1976 Malnutrition and brain development. Oxford University Press, Oxford

Yaffe S J, Danish M 1978 Problems of drug administration in the paediatric patient. Drug Metabolism Review 8: 303

Yoshioka T, Roux J F 1972 In vitro metabolism of palmitic acid in human fetal tissue. Pediatric Research 6: 675

8

G. S. Dawes

Cardiovascular fetal function

INTRODUCTION

During the past few years extensive reviews of the fetal circulation have appeared dealing with the whole system (e.g. Mott & Walker 1983) or some of its parts (Mott 1982, Rudolph 1985). The main features are well known. Briefly, in the fetus both sides of the heart work in parallel to pump the blood returning to the heart from the great veins (including that from the placenta) to the aorta (Fig. 8.1). Only a small proportion of the right ventricular output reaches the lungs, varying from 6% of total cardiac output in sheep to 16–26% in pigs (Macdonald et al 1985). The remainder passes through the ductus arteriosus to reach the descending aorta.

In all mammalian species studied the venous return from the lower part of the body is split by the crista dividens, a sharp projection of the atria into the inferior vena cava, into a smaller part which passes directly into the left atrium, and a larger fraction which mixes in the right atrium with blood returning from the superior vena cava. In many species, but not all, some of the blood returning from the placenta bypasses the liver through a vessel, the ductus venosus, which like the ductus arteriosus disappears postnatally. Whereas the functional importance of the foramen ovale and ductus arteriosus to the fetal circulation, in their task of distributing oxygen and otherwise, is not in doubt, that of the ductus venosus is uncertain.

In those species studied experimentally, especially sheep, pig, goat and to some extent man, the fetal cardiovascular systems have many features in common but there are also quantitative differences. Arterial blood pressure is relatively low compared with adults of the same species, rising during pregnancy to reach values of about 55–65 mmHg near term in large domestic animals and the rhesus monkey. Heart rate is high in mid-gestation, falling towards term. Near term cardiac output, measured as the combined output of both ventricles, is very high: 450 ml/kg/min in the rhesus monkey, 548 ml/kg/min in the sheep and 615 ml/kg/min in the pig (mean values from Mott & Walker 1983 and Macdonald et al 1985). Such estimates as have been made in the human fetus in utero of pulse volume, based on measurements of ventricular dimensions in diastole and systole using ultrasound, also accord with a high cardiac output. Consequently the conductance of the fetal tissues (and of the placenta) must be very high — higher than in adults — since pressure is low and flow is large.

A large proportion of cardiac output passes through the placenta. In sheep this has been estimated as 160–220 ml/kg/min using the isotope-labelled microsphere method, introduced by Rudolph & Heymann in 1967; this amounts to between 40 and 45% of cardiac output in normal conditions. In the pig umbilical flow is less, about 168 ml/kg/min; 22–33% of total cardiac output. In man, measurements using Doppler ultrasound to estimate mean velocity in the umbilical cord vessels and real-time ultrasound scan to measure diameter (and hence calculate the area of cross-section) have given values of about 115 ml/kg/min. This type of measurement has a large potential error due to the inaccuracy of measuring small diameters, squared to calculate the cross-sectional area; of measuring fetal weight in utero, and of estimating the distribution of velocities across the vessel. However the values now reported in the literature agree well.

We should not be surprised that umbilical flow in man may turn out to be rather less than in some large animal species near term; the minimum umbilical blood flow required to maintain oxygen uptake in man was calculated as 90 ml/kg/min (Dawes 1968). This was based on an estimated oxygen consumption of 4.5 ml/kg/min at birth, while that of fetal lambs is 8–10 ml/kg/min, consistent with their precocial development: lambs have to rise to their feet and find their mother's teat soon after birth. The fetal lamb also

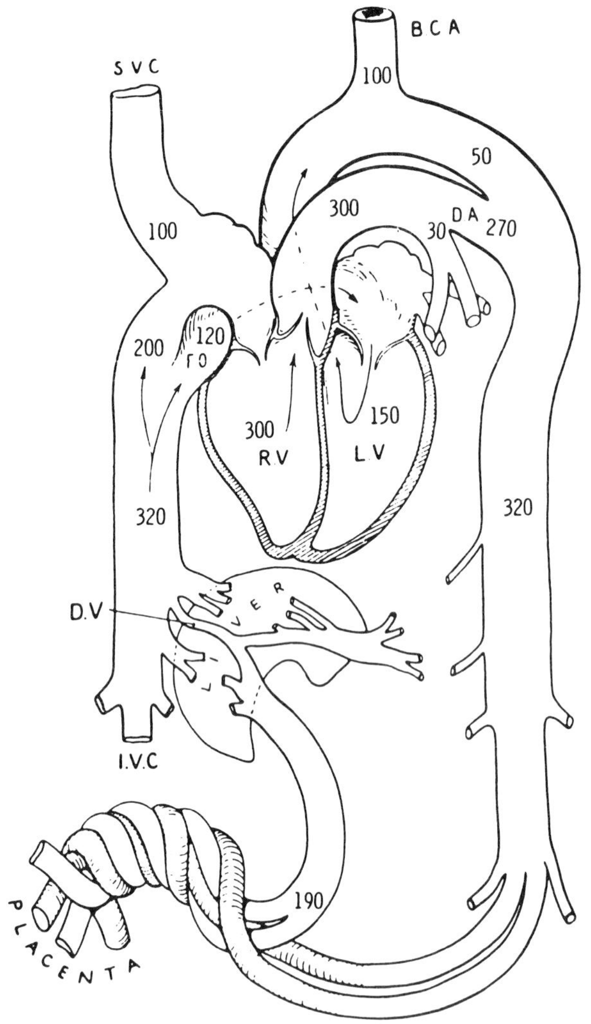

Fig. 8.1 The distribution of blood flow (ml/kg/min) in a fetal lamb in utero near term. Note that the output of the right ventricle (RV) is greater than that of the left (LV); that only a third of left ventricular output passes through the aortic isthmus, while the remainder supplies the head and upper limbs through the brachiocephalic artery (BCA); and that 0.9 of right ventricular output flows through the ductus arteriosus (DA) into the descending aorta. Umbilical flow is high (190 ml/kg/min) and an unknown proportion bypasses the liver through the ductus venosus (DV). A small proportion of inferior vena caval (IVC) flow passes directly into the left atrium through the foramen ovale (FO). SVC = superior vena cava. Redrawn from Dawes (1968).

usually has a low haematocrit (30–32%) near term, so the quantitative difference, so far established, may have a sound physiological reason.

It would be absurd to suppose that the sheep fetus is identical in all important respects to man; those who speak of it as a model for the human fetus are misleading themselves and others by implying an identity of function which would not be expected and does not exist. They are using language to confuse rather than clarify, to suggest an importance for their biological studies which do not require such justification.

Another interesting feature of the fetal circulation deserves notice at this point. Since the two fetal cardiac ventricles work in parallel, their outputs need not be identical. This contrasts with the postnatal situation where the outputs are closely related, beat by beat. Rudolph & Heymann (1973), using an isotope-labelled microsphere method, showed that the output of the fetal right heart was nearly double that of the left heart in the normoxic lamb in utero. Subsequent measurements with electromagnetic flowmeters on the ascending aorta and pulmonary trunk confirmed this conclusion.

In man, measurements of ventricular dimensions in systole and diastole also suggest that the output of the right fetal heart is greater than that of the left, though the difference is less dramatic than in sheep. This is perhaps not surprising since the sheep's brain at birth only weighs about 1.3% of body mass, while that of the human infant is 10–13%. We also have to take into account the probability that human umbilical blood flow is relatively less (per kg body weight) than that of the sheep. In any event the proportions of right and left ventricular output are likely to change with circumstances. We noted, using cineangiographic methods, that slowing of the heart was accompanied by intermittent flow of contrast medium from the superior vena cava through the foramen ovale into the left atrium (Dawes 1968). Hypoxia also resulted in a relative fall in right compared with left ventricular output. The possibility that the distribution of blood flow into and through the cardiac ventricles may change with different physiological circumstances, different species or gestational age, will be worth further study.

FETAL BEHAVIOUR: SLEEP STATES AND GESTATIONAL AGE

Until the mid 1960s, almost all experiments on fetal goats or sheep were done under general, local or maternal spinal anaesthesia, with the fetus partly or wholly exteriorized. The effects of general anaesthesia on the changing physiological responses were already recognized, although even in adult animals, experiments without anaesthesia, e.g. on trained dogs, were uncommon. The primary objective was to establish the existence of physiological mechanisms in the fetus and to study their integration against the consistent background ensured by anaesthesia, rather than to examine the natural physiological variables in utero. As soon as it was shown it was possible to measure such variables continuously in utero by the implantation of catheters, electrodes or other transducers, there was a rush to exploit the possibilities, and the danger of making measurements before thoroughly investigating natural behavioural fetal changes was not widely appreciated. The situation is now gradually being redressed.

At least four natural phenomena must be taken into account in designing experiments on unanaesthetized fetuses in utero because these phenomena — fetal sleep state, uterine contractions, diurnal variations and maternal food intake — may affect cardiovascular function. Between the age of 110 and 130 days' gestation in sheep, and from 28 to 36 weeks' in man, the fetus develops episodic behavioural patterns, accompanied in sheep by gross changes in electrocortical activity, which correspond either to active rapid eye movement (REM) sleep or quiet non-REM sleep. Direct evidence of fetal wakefulness in utero has not been produced. In sheep near term, when this episodic behaviour is well developed, heart rate and its short-term variation are raised during episodes of high-voltage electrocortical activity, while arterial pressure is increased. After section of the brain stem above the pons there is no longer an association between electrocortical state of activity and heart rate or its variation. Episodes of breathing are associated with a larger heart rate variation, whether or not the brain stem is intact (Hofmeyr et al 1985a). Other studies showed that during low-voltage electrocortical activity there were increases in blood flow to the stomach, small bowel and pancreas (25–36%) and to many parts of the brain (22–38%) excluding the cerebrum and cerebellum. Since arterial pressure fell these increases were due to vasodilatation. The cerebral regions involved correspond to the area of distribution of the reticular formation (Jensen et al 1986).

In 1980 Nathanielsz et al described an association between non-labour uterine contractions, change in fetal electrocortical state, arrest of breathing and a small fall in fetal PaO_2. These contractions last 6–8 minutes and occur 2–3 times an hour, so they are likely to be present up to one-third of the time. It is now believed that the association is only partial, that it occurs from time to time in any one fetus (Hofmeyr et al 1985b), and the effects are liable to be only marginal on the cardiovascular system except for unusual instances when the umbilical cord is compressed, possibly against a fetal limb. Experiments designed to detect such an association with Braxton Hicks contractions in man have proved negative so far.

In contrast there is good evidence of diurnal variation in fetal heart rate and its variability both in sheep (Dalton et al 1977) and in man (Visser et al 1982). Towards the late evening and for 5–7 hours, heart rate and its variation are much increased. Patrick et al (1980) raised the question whether these diurnal rhythms, and that of fetal breathing in man might be associated with diurnal variations in maternal plasma cortisol levels. Arduini et al (1986) tested this hypothesis by giving triamcinolone to healthy pregnant volunteers for 3 days at 35 weeks' gestation; this suppressed the diurnal rhythms of three hormones—cortisol, adrenocorticotrophic hormone and unconjugated oestriol — and also of the fetal heart rate, compared with controls. After a further 3 weeks (i.e. by 38 weeks' gestation) the diurnal rhythms of hormones and heart rate had returned.

Finally there is the question whether maternal food intake modifies fetal behaviour. It does in man, where meals are followed by a period of 1–3 hours during which maternal plasma glucose rises and there is an increase in the time spent by the fetus in breathing. This undoubtedly induces a high-frequency variation in fetal heart rate. This phenomenon is not seen in sheep, probably because digestion is almost continuous owing to ruminal activity.

These four phenomena — sleep state, uterine activity, diurnal variation and maternal food intake — have been selected as examples of physiological traps for the unwary who may think that studying unanaesthetized fetuses in utero is closest to a normal state. They may be right, but need to beware of the natural variations that are largely eliminated by general anaesthesia. And indeed on ethical grounds experiments without anaesthesia should be designed as precisely and economically as possible. The decision to study fetuses in utero without anaesthesia carries with it great difficulties, not only because of the natural variations outlined above, but also because relative inaccessibility makes it difficult to analyse mechanisms by longitudinal studies, as for instance by examining the response to a stimulus before and after section of the afferent or efferent limb of a suspected reflex pathway in a single animal. Yet progress is only possible and rapid by the identification of mechanisms at the system and cellular level.

There are other perplexing difficulties in studying the circulation, especially in respect of the venous return from the lower body and the placenta. Rudolph (1985) reviewed this subject, to which he and his colleagues have made considerable contributions. Yet their experiments on sheep took no account of electrocortical or sleep state, and we know that fetal breathing movements (normally present only in low-voltage electrocortical activity, REM sleep) are associated with partial arrest of umbilical blood flow and a great increase in the velocity of inferior vena caval flow, attributed to the large transdiaphragmatic pressure gradient (and perhaps to some compression of the vessel). These authors demonstrated an uneven distribution of blood flow by the streamlining of the mainly umbilical flow through the ductus venosus to reach the left side of the heart via the foramen ovale. This would have the effect of maintaining the oxygen saturation in the ascending aorta above that in the descending aorta and hence favour oxygen supply to the heart and brain. It is a half-step towards the hypothesis of Sabatier (1778), who suggested that the fetal circulation was arranged in a figure-of-eight, so that all the well oxygenated blood was directed to the head and the least well oxygenated to the placenta. As is well known, there is considerable admixture of blood streams in the heart and great vessels, so that the oxygen content of ascending aortic blood is only a little greater than of the descending aorta.

One factor in these calculations is admixture of blood streams in the liver. Rudolph and his colleagues injected isotope-labelled microspheres into one of the two umbilical veins in sheep, and assumed there was even mixing in order to measure the distribution of blood flow to the hepatic sinusoids or ductus venosus. Their results showed a very large range of variation in the distribution of flow (Edelstone et al 1978) which may be attributed to failure of adequate mixing in the short distance between the junction of the two umbilical veins within the abdomen and the origin of the ductus venosus. You cannot have it both ways; either flow is turbulent and mixture is adequate or it is laminar and stream-lined flow is likely. There is no doubt from calculation of flow velocity in the umbilical veins that flow is relatively non-pulsatile (in the absence of fetal breathing) and well below the critical Reynold's number for turbulence. We do not yet have reliable measurements of the distribution of hepatic flows in the fetal lamb since the microsphere method is not reliable in this location. In some species, e.g. the horse, the ductus venosus is not present and therefore is unlikely to be of general importance.

According to Rudolph (1985), cardiac output is similar at all ages in the latter half of gestation, though study of the same data by Mott & Walker (1983) suggested that it was less before 100 days. Alternatively we may suspect that the variation in interpretation of the microsphere method may be responsible for the large variations documented in the literature—from 377 to 680 ml/kg/min in sheep. Macdonald et al (1985) suggest that further studies are required in the pig to confirm the large increase in pulmonary flow, from 16% of combined ventricular output to 26% shortly before birth. It would not be surprising if there were changes in cardiac output per unit fetal body mass, and in its distribution, with gestational age, irrespective of pathophysiological variations. But in the future such measurements need to take account of episodic behavioural changes near term.

REGULATION OF THE FETAL CIRCULATION, BARORECEPTORS AND CHEMORECEPTORS

It is now known that in the fetal lamb, the systemic arterial baroreceptors and chemoreceptors (aortic and carotid) are active over the normal fetal arterial pressure and blood gas ranges from as early as 90 days' gestation (Blanco et al 1984, 1985). Considering the chemoreceptors first, they respond to both a fall in PaO_2 and a rise in $PaCO_2$. There is good evidence from observations on exteriorized fetal lambs under general anaesthesia that circulatory responses to asphyxia (e.g. reflex hindlimb vasoconstriction) are determined wholly by the aortic chemoreceptors (Dawes et al 1968). In these experiments the reflex component was separated from the release of catecholamines and vasopressin by introducing a delay loop into the arterial blood supply to the hindlimbs. Such arrangements are more difficult in unanaesthetized chronic experiments in utero, which may perhaps explain why they have not yet been attempted. Nevertheless it would be desirable to test the hypothesis that the aortic chemoreceptors are of such predominant importance in the circulatory responses to hypoxia or asphyxia by methods which avoid fetal anaesthesia and exposure. The reflex vasoconstriction in the hindlimbs (presumably in the skin and muscle, altogether about 35% of total body weight) is only part of the response to asphyxia. Elsewhere, there is vasodilatation in the heart and brain, and vasoconstriction in the lungs, of which only the latter is only partly under reflex control.

The circulatory response is complex. The reflex and hormonal agents which cause vasoconstriction in the peripheral vascular beds of skin, muscle or kidney do so in spite of local vasodilatation caused by perfusion with asphyxial blood (i.e. blood with a reduced oxygen and raised carbon dioxide content). The effects are greatly influenced by gestational age. The reflex vasoconstriction of the hindlimbs is less at 95 days' gestation than at term (147 days) in sheep (Dawes et al 1968); stimulation of the peripheral vagi or sympathetic system caused no change in heart rate before 60 days' gestation. Whereas isocapnic hypoxia in unanaesthetized fetal lambs in utero causes an immediate rise in arterial pressure and fall in heart rate near term, it caused no change in pressure and a rise in heart rate at 95–110 days' gestation (Dawes 1985). This may be important when considering the responses to hypoxaemia in young human fetuses of less than 28 weeks' gestation.

Studies of single carotid baroreceptors suggest, from both dynamic and steady-state curves relating discharge frequency to pressure, that they are as much as four times more sensitive in younger (88–113 days' gestation) than in older or newborn lambs (Blanco et al 1985). This may be due to the small quantity of collagen in immature vessels. With regard to the baroreflex, the balance of evidence suggests that it becomes more sensitive with age when elicited by means (e.g. an inflatable balloon in the descending aorta) which avoid the access of drugs, such as phenylephrine to the medulla. Hence the sensitivity of the efferent limb of the baroreflex, and perhaps of its central control, must increase greatly during the latter half of gestation.

The reflex pathway involves only the medulla, since it is unaffected by section of the brain stem above the pons, but is abolished by destruction of the brain above the cervical cord (Dawes et al 1983). Its sensitivity is increased by more rostral transection of the brain, therefore central control is complex. Baroreflex sensitivity is unaffected by changes in fetal sleep state.

Control of fetal heart rate in response to hypoxia or asphyxia is complex. A rise in arterial pressure, consequent on vasoconstriction in the skeletal muscles, skin and kidneys for example, is liable to cause a baroreflex fall of heart rate near term, as is direct excitation of the carotid bodies. The release into the circulation of catecholamines tends to cause tachycardia. We also have to take into account the fact that the baroreceptors adapt more quickly—within minutes—while the arterial chemoreceptors appear to take many hours to reset. This helps to explain the fact that, near term, prolonged isocapnic hypoxia in the fetal lamb causes an immediate rise in arterial pressure and bradycardia, followed after 30 minutes by tachycardia which is raised even further on reoxygenation. When isocapnic hypoxia is maintained over days, not only do the chemoreceptors reset but plasma erythropoietin concentration is increased, red cells are produced more rapidly, the blood haemoglobin concentration is increased and more oxygen is carried at reduced PaO_2 rate. This is a slower process which takes several days. These processes of fetal adaptation to diminished oxygen availability should not be overlooked.

Finally we may consider the evidence of Itskovitz et al (1983) and Yardley et al (1983) who denervated the baroreceptors by cutting the carotid and aortic nerves or vagi in fetal lambs near term. Both groups observed a large increase in arterial pressure variation. Itskovitz et al also recorded an increase in fetal heart rate variation. Both groups ascribed their results to section of the baroreceptors, although it is likely that they also cut all the systemic arterial chemoreceptor nerves. Their results are consistent with the proposition that in late fetal life the fine rapid regulation of arterial pressure and heart rate is dependent on the integrity of the baroreflex mechanism (including, possibly, peripheral circulatory changes). However the results do not prove the hypothesis because the authors did not consider or investigate the possible effects of chemoreceptor denervation, e.g. greater variability in fetal PaO_2 or $PaCO_2$.

The slower, coarse regulation of arterial pressure is probably dependent on the principles enunciated by Faber et al (1974), who pointed out that the osmotic and hydrostatic pressures across the maternal and fetal sides of the placenta must eventually reach equilibrium, according to Starling's law, by water and electrolyte exchange, which would favour an increased flow from mother to fetus if fetal hydrostatic pressure fell — an exchange which should ultimately stabilize fetal in relation to maternal arterial pressure. Other factors should be mentioned, e.g. the ability of the fetal heart to hypertrophy rapidly within a few days, in response to hypertension. This raises the question of fetal cardiac performance.

The fetal heart

Much has been made of the fact that when the performance of the lamb fetal heart is examined using the tests considered appropriate in adults, the active tension developed is less than in adults; this fact has been attributed to a lower myofibrillar content and a poorly developed T-tubular system (Friedman 1973). The increase in cytosolic calcium after excitation may be provided in the fetus or newborn by mechanisms which are quantitatively different from those in the adult (Boucek et al 1984). Certainly, ventricular function curves in chronic fetal lamb preparations reach a plateau above filling pressures of 3–4 mmHg (e.g. Gilbert 1982, Thornburg & Morton 1983). Postnatally output doubles, and Rudolph (1985) has described the situation as shown in Figure 8.2. Evidently there is the possibility of several factors operating slowly or more rapidly after delivery. Morton et al (1987) have shown a rapid upward shift of left ventricular function curves on ventilating fetal lambs in utero to cause a rise in PaO_2 to or above neonatal levels. This interesting observation shows that there is more to be learnt about the mechanism involved.

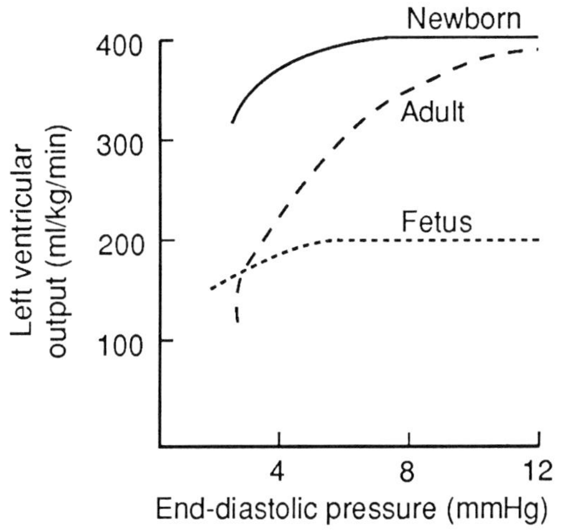

Fig. 8.2 Ventricular function changes after birth, as proposed by Rudolph (1985). It was suggested that the fetus has poor myocardial function, with little reserves; output is doubled in the newborn, but there is only a small reserve because of high resting demand. See text for critical discussion.

The human fetus survives after birth with a large range of congenital malformations. The Frank–Starling cardiac function relationship, by which increased stretch leads to greater output, is already established at an early embryonic stage (at septation in the embryonic chick) and it is evident that the fetal heart is well adapted to its normal physiological requirements. However obstetricians need to consider carefully the effects of new drugs used in the treatment of maternal hypertension; these drugs cross to the fetus and may affect some aspect of fetal cardiac physiology (e.g. by catecholamine or calcium channel blockade).

Placental circulation

The possibility has often been considered that the maternal and fetal placental circulations (umbilical and uterine) may interact, at least to improve flow relationships on both sides, to maintain an efficient or best possible perfusion : perfusion ratio, i.e. the ratio between maternal and fetal flows within the placenta, comparable to the ventilation : perfusion ratio of the adult lung (Dawes 1968). There appears to be no evidence of vascular pressure interaction analogous to the waterfall phenomenon in the adult lung. Trudinger (1986) embolized the umbilical arteries in fetal lambs and showed that the maternal uteroplacental blood flow fell in parallel with the fall in umbilical flow; both were measured with radio-labelled microspheres. Placental morphology varies so greatly with species that it would be unwise to extrapolate this work to man. However the proposition could be tested in rhesus monkeys or baboons. The principle is important.

It is well known that isocapnic hypoxia causes a rise in fetal arterial pressure near term, with a redistribution of cardiac output but maintenance of umbilical flow. So there is clearly some degree of umbilical vasoconstriction (Dawes 1968). Blanco et al (1986) have shown that raising the fetal PaO_2 by ventilation in utero causes a fall in umbilical flow proportional to the rise in PaO_2 above 40 mmHg, with no change in arterial pressure. Incidentally, blood flow to the various parts of the brain was much decreased, also by up to 75%. So it would seem that normal fetal PaO_2 is related to maximal umbilical vasodilatation. In comparison with the other fetal vascular beds, the umbilical circulation normally responds only to a small extent to normal physiological changes, hypoxia or asphyxia, as appropriate to an organ of gas exchange.

Berman et al (1978) proposed that various drugs, including noradrenaline, might decrease umbilical flow in the sheep fetus near term by lowering heart rate, rather than by affecting the umbilical resistance vessels. No explanation in terms of the transplacental pressure gradient was offered. This is physiologically incomprehensible, since heart rate must affect umbilical flow solely by its effect on arterial, and to a lesser extent venous, pressure. Rankin et al (1980), by measuring transplacental resistance in fetal lambs have shown that heart rate is not a direct determinant of umbilical blood flow; large changes in heart rate were not directly associated with changes in resistance.

Observations on man by Giles et al (1985), for example, and by others in Europe and the USA, have established a prima facie case for concluding that measurement of the pulsatility index of the fetal aortic or umbilical, or indeed the maternal uterine, waveform velocity profile provides an empirical association with intrauterine growth retardation. The index is the peak or mean systolic–diastolic velocity, divided by the mean value for the cardiac cycle; it is independent of the angle of insonation of the Doppler beam, and has been considered a measure of placental vascular resistance. An increase in the index has been associated with pathological changes in the uterine vasculature determined after delivery. It seems to be a useful measure for identifying high-risk pregnancies before 28 weeks' gestation, and in skilled hands (e.g. a nurse-technician) is rapid. Its relationship to vascular resistance, measured directly by blood flow and arteriovenous pressure difference, is still uncertain, even in animals. It could well be non-linear and vary with the vascular location, morphology, heart rate and cardiac status of the fetus, since such a high proportion of the cardiac output flows through the placenta. From a practical point of view this measure appears to have much to offer, but its theoretical basis is uncertain.

Fetal heart rate variation

Too much has been written about fetal heart rate (FHR) and too little has been measured. The FHR varies diurnally and with fetal sleep state and its variation increases greatly with gestational age. Indeed in more than 15% of normal pregnancies at 28–33 weeks' gestation there are less than 2 accelerations (>10 b.p.m. above baseline and >15 s) in each hour. The mean number of accelerations per hour rises in normal pregnancies, from 3.8 ± 0.4 (SEM) at 28 weeks to 8.4 ± 0.7 at 40 weeks (Dawes et al 1985). But even at term a few normal fetuses have less than 2 accelerations per hour (Dawes et al 1982). For clinical purposes, a more accurate antenatal measure of FHR variation was needed, and one has been provided by computer analysis (Dawes et al 1985). A medium-term measure of FHR variation (within the range 16–0.1 cycles/min) provided a wide discrimination between normal and pathological FHR traces associated with chronic fetal hypoxaemia antenatally (mean umbilical PaO_2 6 mmHg on delivery by Caesarean section; the normal value is 13 mmHg). This is the only measure of FHR variation which has been tested in practice for the best use of the filter characteristics: that is, it has been shown to be superior to indices which select shorter or longer components of FHR variation. Indeed there are solid grounds for rejecting beat-to-beat variation based on sequential pulse intervals for its mean value (2.3 ms near term) is too close to the limit of pulse interval measurement (1 ms).

Computerization of the record permits its display (Fig. 8.3, 8.4) by the hour; accelerations (or if required, decelerations of different categories) may be identified by symbols. It is a bad feature of strip-chart design that conventional monitors produce 2–3 cm/min, much more than can be contained in one field of vision. Printers use the phrase—*an eyeful*—to describe the maximum width of a page of type which can be taken in without unnecessary effort and this corresponds to one computer display. An important feature of this system also has been the capacity to identify signal loss, which has been reduced from a mean value in excess of 20% near term to 2.5% by using improved transducers and autocorrelation (Hewlett-Packard and Sonicaid).

Much interest has been expressed in the use of FHR as a diagnostic aid in identifying hypoxia or, especially, metabolic acidaemia in labour. The principal weakness in the conventional approach has been to attempt to understand the complex patterns by visual analysis without thorough analysis of antenatal records. Conventional wisdom is dependent on opinions rather than measurements, and is liable to upset. Animal experiments, except in that they have shown that brief abrupt episodes of hypoxia initially cause cardiac slowing near term, have not been helpful. What is required is a thorough analysis of the frequency distribution of FHR

HOSPITAL No. RECORD
DATE 8—Aug-1984 No. 5 Z
Time of recording 1450 Gestation 40 weeks

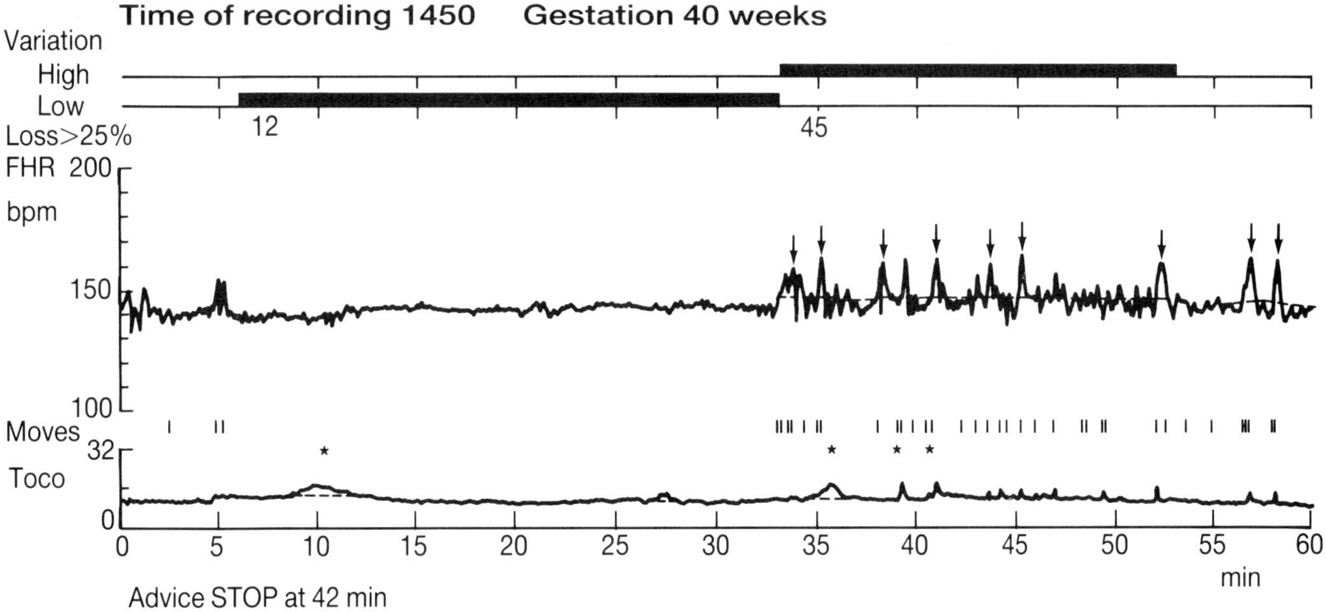

Advice STOP at 42 min

Normal Values	ANALYSIS at 60 min.	
(0)	1. SIGNAL LOSS (%)	0.0
	2. CONTRACTION PEAKS	4
(>12)	3. FETAL MOVEMENTS (per hour)	55
	per min in High 2.10 in Low 0.04	
(<160)	4. BASAL HEART RATE (bpm)	142
(>8/hr)	5. ACCELERATIONS >10 bpm & 15 sec	10
(0)	6. DECELERATIONS > 20 lost beats	0
(>4)	7. HIGH EPISODES (min) : Threshold 32 msec	20
	LOW EPISODES (min)	27 *
	8. **VARIATION** OVERALL (Mean range : msec)	28.0 *

INTERPRETATION OF VARIATION

Normal		> 30 msec
Questionable	20 –	30 msec
Abnormal		< 20 msec

HOWEVER – note High episodes of 20 minutes with 2.10 moves/minute

Fig. 8.3 Example of a normal fetal heart rate (FHR) record at term illustrating an unusually long episode of low heart rate variation (attributed to quiet sleep) during the first 33 min. Thereafter an episode of high variation began, accompanied by fetal movements and identified by the computer, which advised the nurse to stop recording 7 min later (after 40 min).

The average length of such computerized records, required to identify normal episodes of high variation in frequency, was 15 min (Dawes et al 1985). Note the absence of signal loss; the monitor was Hewlett-Packard 8040 using autocorrelation and interfaced to a small microprocessor. The range of FHR variation is derived from the pulse intervals in ms (e.g. 11.5 ms in low episodes; 48.7 ms in high episodes).

patterns in normal labour and in those few (perhaps <1%) which result in asphyxia and metabolic acidaemia. The present view is that the only truly sinister patterns are flat traces with persistent tachycardia and prolonged variable decelerations lasting for more than 3 minutes. This can be tested by persistent objective measurement. It is evident that FHR

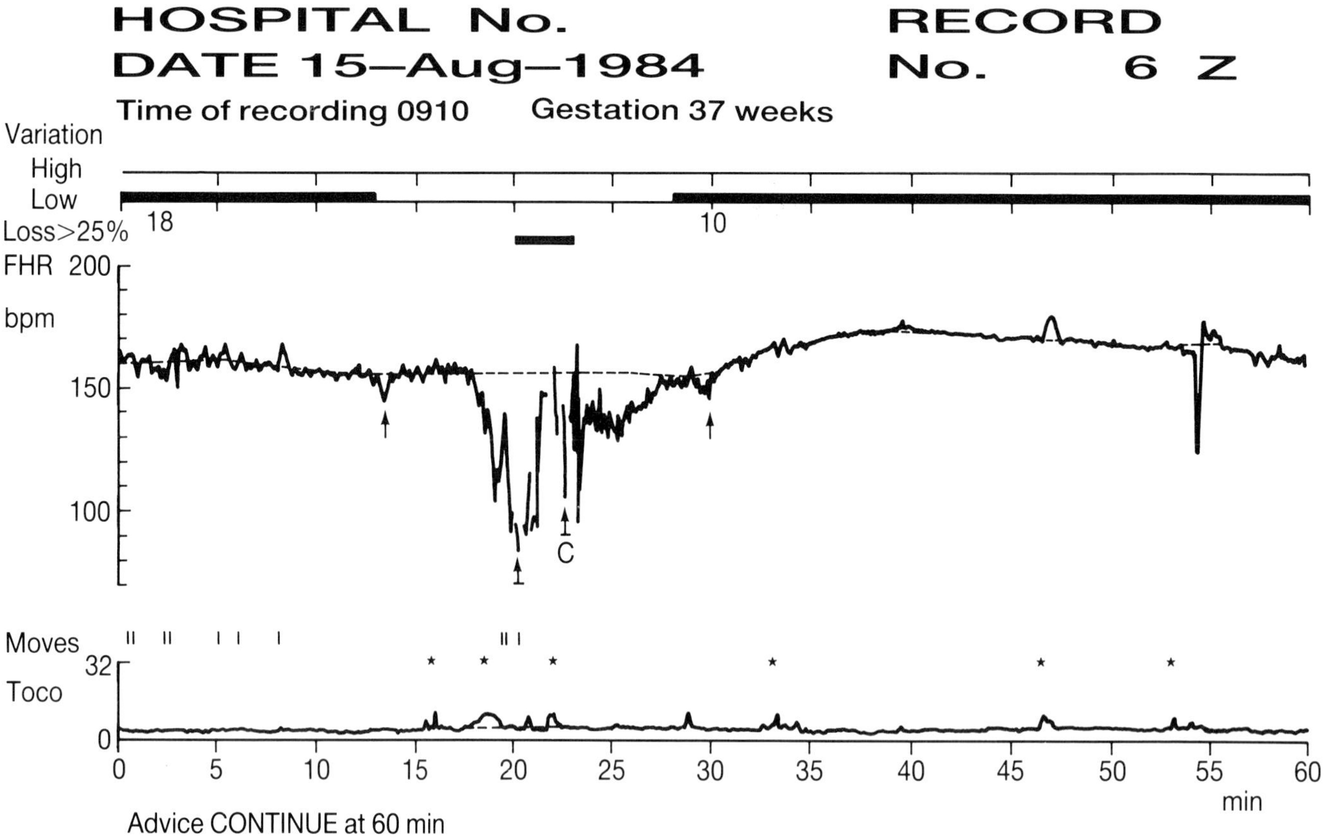

Advice CONTINUE at 60 min

Normal Values

ANALYSIS at 60 min.

Normal Values		
(0)	1. SIGNAL LOSS (%)	2.3
	2. CONTRACTION PEAKS	6
(>12)	3. FETAL MOVEMENTS (per hour)	11 *
	per min in Low 0.16	
(<160)	4. BASAL HEART RATE (bpm)	164 *
(>8/hr)	5. ACCELERATIONS >10 bpm & 15 sec	0 *
(0)	6. DECELERATIONS > 20 lost beats	2 *

Time (min)	Lost beats	Length (min)	Trough (bpm)	Variation msec 3′ before	Variation msec after	Signal loss %
20.2	139	4.3	74	17.7	10.0	19 *
22.6	97	6.7	51	17.7	10.0	6 *

(>4)	7. HIGH EPISODES (min) : Threshold 24 msec	0 *
	LOW EPISODES (min)	45 *
	8. **VARIATION** OVERALL (Mean range : msec)	12.3 **

INTERPRETATION OF VARIATION

Normal	> 30 msec
Questionable	20 – 30 msec
Abnormal	< 20 msec

* **FLAT DECELERATIVE TRACE WITH CONTRACTIONS**

Fig. 8.4 Example of an abnormal fetal heart rate (FHR) record at 37 weeks' gestation in which a contraction was followed by transient fetal movements accompanied by a large (interrupted) deceleration with continued flattening of the FHR trace, so generating two successive episodes of low variation (14 and 13 ms respectively). For definitions of FHR variation, and in low and high episodes, see Dawes et al (1985).

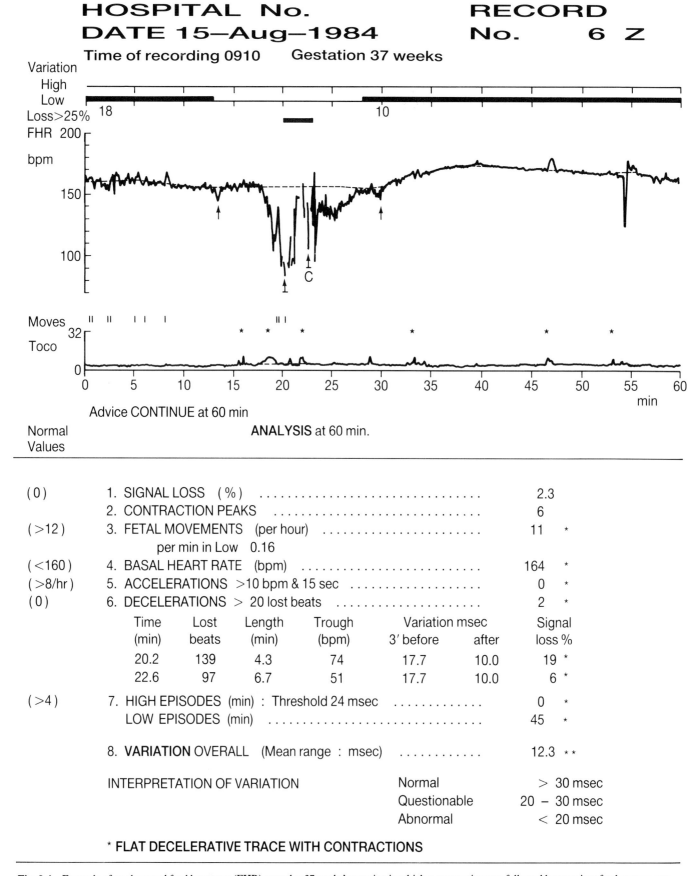

patterns in normal labour are highly variable, especially after the end of the first stage.

Accelerations in FHR are associated with fetal movements, but the association is not causal since neuromuscular paralysis with gallamine in sheep abolishes the movements but only slightly reduces the FHR accelerations (Bocking et al 1985, Clewlow & Dawes 1985). The reduction is, in part at least, due to the abolition of fetal breathing movements which imposes a high frequency variation. The mean FHR variation is scarcely affected by section of the brain stem above the pons (Dawes et al 1983), but is abolished by destruction of the medulla. It was unaffected by a localized medullary lesion which abolishes fetal breathing movements.

The modulation of FHR variation in association with sleep state is dramatic in man, with episodes of flat heart rate (as low as a mean range of 11 ms pulse interval variation) near term lasting up to 40 minutes and interpolated between episodes of high variation (see Fig. 8.3). This episodic variation persists in early labour, and is often discernible until the onset of the second stage.

In sheep acute, or indeed chronic, hypoxaemia induced by partial destruction of uterine caruncles before conception is normally associated with an increase in FHR variation. Attempts to reproduce the pathological flattening of the heart rate seen antenatally in man have so far proved unsuccessful. However, clonidine (a powerful synthetic alpha$_2$-agonist) administered to fetal lambs causes a remarkable flattening of FHR, with arrest of breathing and limb movements, by a direct action, probably on the medulla, since it is seen after section of the brain stem (Bamford et al 1986). It is a striking feature of the reduction in human FHR variation associated with chronic hypoxaemia and growth retardation that it is accompanied by no change in mean heart rate. Blockade of the sympathetics or parasympathetics with propranolol and atropine respectively causes large changes in mean rate. An explanation for the natural phenomenon other than simple autonomic blockade must be sought; a central alpha$_2$-agonist action may be the answer.

Hypoxia and asphyxia

It is not surprising that much attention has been paid to the effects of isocapnic hypoxia or asphyxia on the fetus. As might be expected from general physiological principles and from practical experience, the normal fetus has a wide margin of safety. Blood flow to the maternal side of the placenta must be reduced by almost 50% before there is a small fall in fetal PaO_2 or rise in $PaCO_2$. In adults subjected to progressive hypoxia, oxygen uptake is maintained in a neutral thermal environment until circulatory collapse is imminent. The fetus subjected to acute hypoxia however not only centralizes its circulation, maintaining that to the placenta (the organ of gas exchange) and to the vital organs (heart and brain) at the expense of other tissues (lung, skin, muscle, kidney and gut), but it also reduces its oxygen uptake to make the best use of available oxygen. In part this is due to the arrest of breathing and fetal movements, and the blockade of spinal motor reflexes (Dawes 1984). The arrest of breathing by hypoxia is dependent on the integrity of centres above the pons (Dawes et al 1983), while the abolition of the spinal flexor reflex is dependent on centres at or below the pons. Yet two cerebral reflexes, the digastric and thyroarytenoid, are not inhibited by an abrupt fall in PaO_2 down to 12 mmHg in lambs near term (Walker & Harding 1984). The abrupt fall in PaO_2 has only a transient effect on fetal electrocortical state, which, if in low voltage, usually switches to high-voltage activity for only a short period of time. Even when PaO_2 is reduced to 10–12 mmHg the fetus responds selectively and apparently purposefully.

Acute isocapnic hypoxia induces a very large increase in the plasma concentrations of catecholamines (Jones & Robinson 1975) by 5–100-fold to reach levels seen in phaeochromocytoma in adults. Early in gestation the predominant amine is noradrenaline; the proportion of adrenaline increases near term. The placenta accounts for about half the clearance rate of catecholamines from the circulation in the fetal lamb (Jones & Rurak 1976). The plasma levels of vasopressin are also greatly increased during hypoxia in fetal lambs, when the hypertensive effect is greater than in adults (Rurak 1978). Although renin angiotensin is active in the fetus early in gestation, it does not seem to be involved in the response to hypoxia. It is curious that, in spite of the large volume of work on the atrial natriuretic factor in adults, few publications have appeared on its fetal physiological role, e.g. in regulating blood or amniotic fluid volume. First reports suggest that its concentration in fetal lamb plasma may be five times greater than in maternal plasma (Cheung et al 1987).

A word of warning should also be given on the use of blocking agents. Neither propranolol, an effective beta-adrenergic antagonist, nor nifedipine, a calcium channel blocker, affects the PaO_2 of fetal lambs in utero when given separately (Roebuck et al 1985); however, when given together PaO_2 falls. It is also not uncommon to observe fetal distress in women whose hypertension was treated with labetalol and who then received nifedipine in an attempt to arrest premature labour. The fact that a drug has not produced fetal hypoxia does not mean that it is safe to use in all circumstances. The fetus may be able to withstand blockade of one physiological system. Indeed, lambs have survived delivery after the sympathetic nervous system has been largely destroyed by 6-hydroxydopamine, presumably because other control systems adapted to maintain homeostasis (Lumbers et al 1980). But to attack two of the control systems is asking too much.

Changes at birth

There are three primary changes at birth:

1. Delivery of the fetus into a relatively cool environment;
2. Separation of the placenta at the tying of the umbilical cord;
3. Establishment of continued pulmonary ventilation.

To what extent the last change depends on the first two is still uncertain. Continued breathing movements can be established by tying the cord of a fetus exteriorized into a warm saline bath (Johnson et al 1973) or in utero (Adamson et al 1987), when the tracheobronchial tree is cleared of fluid and oxygen-enriched gas is made available. Breathing is arrested when the cord is released, which suggests that the placenta may release a substance, possibly prostaglandin E_2, which normally arrests or decreases the incidence of breathing before birth. Continued breathing can also be established for some hours by cooling the surface of a fetus in utero by circulating cool water through a coil around its thorax, but not by cooling its core (Gluckman et al 1983). There remains doubt as to whether either of these manoeuvres alone establishes normal breathing, i.e. with normal responsiveness to small changes in $PaCO_2$. Continued breathing has been established normally after delivery of fetal lambs in which the carotid nerves had been cut some days previously.

The immediate consequence of effective gaseous pulmonary ventilation is to cause a great fall in pulmonary vascular resistance, with a 7- to 10-fold increase in pulmonary blood flow and a decrease in pulmonary arterial pressure below that in the descending aorta. The direction of blood flow through the ductus arteriosus reverses and, because of the changes in central venous pressure, the valve of the foramen ovale closes permanently and eventually adheres to the wall of the left atrium. The principal mechanisms responsible for the pulmonary vasodilatation are gaseous expansion of the lungs, rise of alveolar PO_2 and fall in PCO_2; these mechanisms were identified by the mid-1960s (Dawes 1968), but the cellular mechanisms responsible for them and for hypoxic vasoconstriction in adult lungs remain obscure. They are not related to leukotrienes (S. Cassin, personal communication).

The mechanism of closure of the ductus arteriosus also appears to be dependent on prostaglandins (Cocceani & Olley 1980), since prostaglandins E and I_2 dilate the vessel. Conversely, inhibitors of prostaglandin synthesis cause constriction in fetuses near term; at an early gestational age the muscle wall is inadequately developed. However in vivo there is no doubt that the normal stimulus is a rise in PO_2; the relation between this and prostaglandin metabolism is obscure. Alternatively it has been proposed that prostaglandin E_2 may be acting as a circulating rather than a local hormone; the fetus has a high circulating concentration of this, probably derived from the placenta.

Birth is normally followed by many readjustments; for example, by the thyroid to the new environmental temperature; by the gut to feeding, and by the systemic arterial chemoreceptors to the new gaseous environment. The aortic and carotid chemoreceptors reset over a period of many days in lambs delivered at term (Blanco et al 1984). It is not known whether resetting is less rapid after premature birth, though this would help explain intermittent apnoea in such babies. The consequences for control of the cardiovascular system postnatally do not seem to have been explored. We wonder also whether the relation between vascular resistance and PaO_2 in the coronary and cerebral circulation of the fetus are appropriate to neonatal life, or whether progressive adaptation is also required in these organs.

After the carotid bodies adapted to the new environment, and reset to operate over the normal neonatal blood gas range, isocapnic hypoxia no longer caused a reduction in the hindlimb flexor reflex. This was due to the activity of the carotid nerves, since after their section hypoxia had its former effect and reflex amplitude fell by 77% at a PaO_2 of 22 mmHg (Blanco et al 1983). Hence progress from fetal to neonatal life is not a simple smooth transition. New systems and behavioural patterns, such as wakefulness, are established. In those fetuses which have low FHR variation (in the absence of hypoxaemia, growth retardation or other possible causes) the variation rises to or above the normal mean value within 24 hours of birth (Smith et al 1987).

CONCLUSIONS

The introduction and progressive improvement of real-time ultrasound methods have revolutionized our approach to human fetal cardiovascular function. It has already enabled us to make high-quality recordings of FHR early in gestation; to analyse fetal movements and behavioural patterns from 8 weeks; to measure the velocities of blood flow and the pulsation of fetal blood vessels in utero; to guide needles into fetal blood vessels to withdraw arterial samples; and to measure the dimensions of the fetal heart in diastole and systole.

To measure flow per kg fetal body weight is more difficult. But there is little doubt that Figure 8.1, which has graced textbooks of physiology and obstetrics in one form or another for the past 25 years, illustrating the distribution of oxygenated blood and cardiac output in fetal lamb, will soon be replaced by values derived from human measurements; the sooner the better, so long as they are accurate.

We are less well placed as regards the measurement of venous or arterial pressure. It is difficult to understand how it is that while obstetricians have seized the opportunity to take a little more fetal blood for safety, leading to useful additional hormonal or blood gas measurements, they have failed to measure amniotic and intravascular pressures. All they needed was a flexible tube attached to a calibrated sterile manometer, available in every fetal sheep laboratory and most anaesthetic departments.

Since fetal scalp sampling in labour and diagnostic ultrasound became available, a new era of fetal measurement has begun. It has become possible to study the range of normal human fetal variation, although old habits die hard and it is hard to accept that a computer can enable a new house officer to interpret an FHR trace as well as a doctor of the older generation could.

Already fetal medicine has been recognized as a new area for exploration. It is something of a relief to find that the first tentative essays in fetal surgery are now reviewed with conservative criticism. There are so many things which can unexpectedly go wrong in fetal surgery, such as infection. The idea that the fetus is simpler than the adult, that it is less adaptable and has few reserves, has been repeatedly and successfully challenged. The problems posed by its unusual environment have been admirably met; the fetus has an elevated body temperature; lower PaO_2; extremely rapid body and organ growth and, even in man, some hormonal control of parturition. The last resort is, of course, escape from the intrauterine environment.

The fetal cardiovascular system is just a small part of the whole. The experience of the past 25 years has shown that, in this field of physiology and medicine, discoveries in what Sir Joseph Barcroft (1934) called the architecture of physiological function are still being made. The last word has yet to be said on fetal circulation and its control.

REFERENCES

Adamson S L, Richardson B S, Homan J 1987 Initiation of pulmonary gas exchange by fetal sheep in utero. Journal of Applied Physiology: Respiratory, Environmental and Exercise Physiology 62: 989–998

Arduini D, Rizzo G, Giorlandino G, Valensisse H, Dell'Acqua S, Romanini C 1986 Modifications of ultradian and circadian rhythms of fetal heart rate after fetal maternal adrenal gland suppression: a double-blind study. Prenatal Diagnosis 6: 409–417

Bamford O S, Dawes G S, Denny R, Ward R A 1986 Effects of the α_2-adrenergic agonist clonidine and its antagonist idazoxan on the fetal lamb. Journal of Physiology 381: 29–37

Barcroft J 1934 Lectures in the architecture of physiological function. Cambridge University Press, Cambridge

Berman W, Goodlin C, Heymann M A, Rudolph A M 1978 Effects of pharmacologic agents on umbilical blood flow in fetal lambs in utero. Biology of the Neonate 33: 225–235

Blanco C E, Dawes G S, Walker D W 1983 Effects of hypoxia on polysynaptic hind-limb reflexes in new-born lambs before and after carotid denervation. Journal of Physiology 339: 467–474

Blanco C E, Dawes G S, Hanson M A, McCooke H B 1984 The response to hypoxia of arterial chemoreceptors in fetal sheep and new-born lambs. Journal of Physiology 351: 25–37

Blanco C E, Dawes G S, Hanson M A, McCooke H B 1985 Studies of carotid baroreceptor afferents in fetal and newborn lambs. In: Jones C T (ed.) The physiological development of the fetus and newborn. Academic Press, London, pp 595–598

Blanco C E, Martin C B, Rankin J, Landauer M, Pherneton T 1986 Changes in fetal organ blood flow during hyperoxia. Thirteenth annual conference of the society for the study of fetal physiology. University of Calgary, Calgary, p 22

Bocking A D, Harding R, Wickham P J D 1983 Relationship between accelerations and decelerations in heart rate and skeletal muscle activity in fetal sheep. Journal of Developmental Physiology 7: 47–54

Boucek R J, Shelton M, Artman M, Mushlin P S, Starnes V A, Olson R D 1984 Comparative effects of verapamil, nifedipine and diltiazem on contractile function in the isolated immature and adult rabbit heart. Pediatric Research 18: 948–952

Cheung C Y, Gibbs D M, Brace R A 1987 Atrial natriuretic factor in maternal and fetal sheep. American Journal of Physiology 252: E279–282

Clewlow F, Dawes G S 1985 The association between cardiac accelerations and movements in fetal sheep. Journal of Developmental Physiology 7: 281–287

Cocceani F, Olley P M 1980 Role of prostaglandins, prostacyclin and thromboxanes in the control of prenatal patency and postnatal closure of the ductus arteriosus. Seminars in Perinatology 4: 109–113

Dalton K J, Dawes G S, Patrick J E 1977 Diurnal, respiratory and other rhythms of fetal heart rate in lambs. American Journal of Obstetrics and Gynecology 127: 414–424

Dawes G S 1968 Foetal and neonatal physiology. Year Book Medical Publishers, Chicago

Dawes G S 1984 The central control of fetal breathing and skeletal muscle movements. Journal of Physiology 346: 1–18

Dawes G S 1985 The control of fetal heart rate and its variability in lamb. In: Kunzel W (ed) Fetal heart rate monitoring. Springer-Verlag, Berlin, pp 187–190

Dawes G S, Lewis B V, Milligan J E, Roach M R, Talner N S 1968 Vasomotor responses in the hind limbs of fetal and new-born lambs to asphyxia and aortic chemoreceptor stimulation. Journal of Physiology 195: 55–81

Dawes G S, Houghton C R S, Redman C W G, Visser G H A 1982 Pattern of the normal human fetal heart rate. British Journal of Obstetrics and Gynaecology 89: 276–284

Dawes G S, Gardner W N, Johnston B M, Walker D W 1983 Breathing in fetal lambs: the effect of brain stem section. Journal of Physiology 335: 525–553

Dawes G S, Redman C W G, Smith J 1985 Improvements in the registration and analysis of fetal heart rate records at the bedside. British Journal of Obstetrics and Gynaecology 92: 317–325

Edelstone D I, Rudolph A M, Heymann M A 1978 Liver and ductus venosus blood flows in fetal lambs in utero. Circulation Research 42: 426–433

Faber J J, Green T J, Thornburg K L 1974 Arterial blood pressure in the unanesthetized fetal lamb after changes in fetal blood volume and haematocrit. Quarterly Journal of Experimental Physiology 59: 241–255

Friedman W F 1973 The intrinsic properties of the developing heart. In: Friedman W F et al (eds) Neonatal heart disease. Grune & Stratton, New York, pp 21–49

Gilbert R D 1982 Effects of afterload and baroreceptors on cardiac function in fetal sheep. Journal of Developmental Physiology 4: 299–309

Giles W B, Trudinger B J, Baird P J 1985 Fetal umbilical artery velocity wave forms and placental resistance: pathological correlation. British Journal of Obstetrics and Gynaecology 92: 31–38

Gluckman P D, Gunn T R, Johnston B M 1983 The effect of cooling on breathing and shivering in unanaesthetized fetal lambs in utero. Journal of Physiology 343: 495–506

Hofmeyr G J, Bamford O S, Dawes G S, Parkes M J 1985a High frequency heart rate variability in the fetal lamb. In: Jones C T, Nathanielsz P W (eds) The physiological development of the fetus and newborn. Academic Press, London, pp 439–444

Hofmeyr G J, Bamford O S, Gianapoulos J G, Parkes M J, Dawes G S 1985b The partial association of uterine contractions with changes in electrocortical activity, breathing and PaO_2 in the fetal lamb: effects of brain stem section. American Journal of Obstetrics and Gynecology 152: 905–910

Itskovitz J, LaGamma E F, Rudolph E M 1983 Baroreflex control of the circulation in chronically instrumented fetal lambs. Circulation Research 52: 589–596

Jensen A, Bamford O S, Dawes G S, Hofmeyr G, Parkes M J 1986 Changes in organ blood flow between high and low voltage electrocortical activity in fetal sheep. Journal of Developmental Physiology 8: 187–194

Johnson P, Robinson J S, Salisbury D 1973 The onset and control of breathing after birth. In: Foetal and neonatal physiology. Cambridge University Press, Cambridge, pp 217–222

Jones C T, Robinson R O 1975 Plasma catecholamines in foetal and adult sheep. Journal of Physiology 248: 15–53
Jones C T, Rurak D W 1976 The distribution and clearance of hormones and metabolites in the circulation of the fetal sheep. Quarterly Journal of Experimental Physiology 61: 287–295
Lumbers E R, Stevens A D, Alexander G, Stevens A 1980 The cardiovascular responses of conscious newborn lambs treated in utero with 6-hydroxydopamine. Journal of Developmental Physiology 2: 139–149
Macdonald A A, Heymann M A, Llanos A J, Personen E, Rudolph A M 1985 Distribution of cardiac output in the fetal pig during late gestation. In: Jones C T, Nathanielsz P W (eds) The physiological development of the fetus and newborn. Academic Press, London, pp 402–404
Morton M J, Pinson C W, Thornburg K L 1987 In utero ventilation with oxygen augments left ventricular stroke volume in lambs. Journal of Physiology 383: 413–424
Mott J C 1982 Control of the foetal circulation. Journal of Experimental Biology 100: 129–146
Mott J C, Walker D W 1983 Neural and endocrine regulation of circulation in the fetus and newborn. Handbook of physiology — The cardiovascular system III. American Physiological Society, Bethesda, pp 837–883
Nathanielsz P W, Bailey A A, Poore E R, Thorburn G D, Harding R 1980 The relationship between myometrial activity and sleep state and breathing in fetal sheep throughout the last third of gestation. American Journal of Obstetrics and Gynecology 138: 653–659
Patrick J, Campbell K, Carmichael L, Natale R, Richardson B 1980 Patterns of human fetal breathing movements during the last 10 weeks of pregnancy. Obstetrics and Gynecology 58: 24–30
Rankin J H G, Stock M K, Anderson D F 1980 Fetal heart rate and umbilical blood flow. Journal of Developmental Physiology 2: 11–16
Roebuck M M, Castle B M, Vojcek L, Weingold A, Dawes G S, Turnbull A C 1985 The effect of nifedipine administration on the fetus and the myometrium of pregnant sheep during oxytocin induced contractions. In: Jones C T (ed) The physiological development of the fetus and newborn. Academic Press, London, pp 499–503
Rudolph A M 1985 Organization and control of the fetal circulation. In: Jones C T, Nathanielsz P W (eds) The physiological development of the fetus and newborn. Academic Press, London, pp 343–353
Rudolph A M, Heymann M A 1967 The circulation of the fetus in utero: methods for studying distribution of blood flow. Circulation Research 21: 163–184
Rudolph A M, Heymann M A 1973 Control of the foetal circulation. In: Comline K S, Cross K W, Nathanielsz P W (eds) Foetal and neonatal physiology. Cambridge University Press, Cambridge, pp 89–111
Rurak D W 1978 Plasma vasopressin levels during hypoxaemia and the cardiovascular effects of exogenous vasopressin in fetal and adult sheep. Journal of Physiology 277: 341–357
Sabatier R B 1778 Mémoire sur les organes de la circulation du sang du foetus. Memoires de L'Académie Royale de Société de Paris 198: 778
Smith J H, Dawes G S, Redman C W G 1987 Low human fetal heart rate variation in normal pregnancy. British Journal of Obstetrics and Gynaecology 94: 656–664
Thornburg K L, Morton M J 1983 Filling and arterial pressures as determinants of RV stroke volume in the sheep fetus. American Journal of Physiology 244: H656–663
Trudinger B 1986 The effects of umbilical artery embolization on the flow velocity waveforms and resistance. IUPS. 1986 Satellite symposium, fetal physiology — Cellular and systems approaches, p 30
Visser G, Goodman J D S, Levine D H, Dawes G S 1982 Diurnal and other cyclic variations in human fetal heart rate near term. American Journal of Obstetrics and Gynecology 142: 535–544
Walker D W, Harding R 1984 Effect of hypoxia on the excitability of two cranial reflexes in unanaesthetized fetal sheep. Journal of Developmental Physiology 6: 387–400
Yardley R W, Bowes G, Wilkinson M et al 1983 Increased arterial pressure variability after arterial baroreceptor denervation in fetal lambs. Circulation Research 52: 580–588

9

J. S. Robinson

Fetal growth

INTRODUCTION

Although the phenomenon of runting has been recognized in many species for a long time, it is only 40 years since it was suggested that some human babies had grown slowly, rather than being small because they were premature (McBurney 1947). The formal definition of preterm babies came in 1961 (World Health Organization 1961) and soon afterwards the morphological characteristics of the small-for-dates baby dying in the perinatal period were described (Gruendwald 1963, Naeye 1965). Perinatal mortality correlates closely with birthweight and is higher in small-for-dates or growth-retarded fetuses. These fetuses are also likely to be delivered prematurely, to suffer from fetal distress or perinatal asphyxia. The neonate who is growth-retarded may also have significant morbidity due to hypoglycaemia, polycythaemia, hyperbilirubinaemia or the asphyxia which began before birth (see Robinson 1979). Perhaps of greater concern is the comparatively slow decline in the rate of unexplained stillbirths, many of whom are normally formed but growth-retarded (Northern Region 1984). Unexplained stillbirths now account for about a quarter of all perinatal deaths. Further, unlike most other causes of perinatal death, these increase in frequency with gestational age, particularly when the rate is calculated as the number of deaths related to the number of undelivered babies (Yudkin et al 1987b).

Long-term follow-up studies have shown that growth-retarded babies, especially if born prematurely, are more frequently handicapped either physically or neurologically (Comney & Fitzhardinge 1979, Ounsted et al 1982, 1984, Rantakallio 1985). The risk of a poor developmental outcome for infants relates to the time when failure of fetal growth was estimated to have begun, by extrapolation from ultrasound scans (Harvey et al 1982). However, not all authors agree that the risk of handicap is increased in growth-retarded babies born at term (Low et al 1982). Perhaps these different views may be accounted for by the presence or absence of catch-up growth in the first few months after birth (Hack et al 1982).

There have been a number of advances in the last decade which have made it possible to recognize deviations from normal fetal growth on most if not all occasions, enabling selective early delivery of compromised fetuses. New interventions, such as maternal hyperoxia to gain more time in utero, have been proposed when the alternative of early delivery offers only a very poor prognosis for the neonate (Nicolaides et al 1987). The purpose of this chapter is to provide an account of the factors associated with abnormal fetal growth and its management when it is diagnosed. In addition, the physiological changes which have been observed in experimental growth retardation will be outlined. These provide the necessary scientific base for new interventions which at present are being subjected to clinical trial.

DEFINITIONS

A number of criteria have been used to define intrauterine growth retardation, small-for-dates and large-for-dates. Small-for-dates is easier to define than growth retardation. The most commonly used definition is a baby whose birthweight is below the 10th percentile allowing for both age and sex. Additional criteria such as maternal size (weight, height or weight-for-height) and parity may also be used to determine centiles for birthweight within subpopulations. Since these definitions include many healthy but genetically small fetuses, more extreme limits — less than the third percentile or more than two standard deviations below the mean

Table 9.1 Factors associated with intrauterine growth retardation (adapted from Miller & Merritt 1979)

Medical complications	Maternal behavioural conditions	Fetal problems	Environmental problems	Abnormalities of the placenta
Pre-eclampsia Acute or chronic hypertension Antepartum haemorrhage Severe chronic disease Severe chronic infections Disseminated lupus erythematosus Lupus obstetric syndrome Anaemia Malignancy Abnormalities of the uterus Uterine fibroids	Malnutrition Low prepregnancy weight-for-height Low maternal weight gain Delivery at age <16 or >35 years Drug use: smoking, alcohol, hard drugs Low socioeconomic status	Multiple births Malformation Chromosomal anomalies Inborn errors of metabolism Intrauterine infections	High altitude Toxic substances	Reduced blood flow Reduced area for exchange Focal lesions: infarcts haematomas Partial abruption Placental praevia Placenta membranacae Extrachorial placenta Circumvallate placenta

weight-for-age and sex — are also used. Large-for-dates is categorized in an analogous fashion as more than the 90th or 97th percentiles or more than two standard deviations above the mean. Since small-for-dates presents the greater clinical problem, emphasis will be given to it in this chapter.

Many charts of centiles for birthweight for gestational age have been produced. In the USA, the chart prepared by Lubchencho et al (1963) was widely used before others became available but suffered the disadvantage of being derived from a population which lives at altitude. Accurate assessment of gestational age remained a problem and was addressed statistically by Milner & Richards (1974). More recently it was proposed that an international reference chart should be made available (Dunn 1985). Factors adversely affecting fetal growth are more likely to be present when preterm delivery is undertaken electively for maternal or fetal reasons (Yudkin et al 1987a). These authors noticed that this can have a major effect on the mean weight for gestation since as many as 28% were delivered before 34 weeks for fetal problems. The difference in mean birthweight for spontaneous compared with elective preterm birth ranged from 169 to 569 g and was significant at all weeks from 27 to 34 except for 28 weeks. If these birthweight charts are supposed to reflect normal growth then it would be useful to compare growth of the fetus for some weeks before preterm birth with that for fetuses delivering normally at term (Persson et al 1978).

Normal growth is the expression of the genetic potential to grow which is neither abnormally constrained nor promoted by internal or external factors. This is a nebulous concept for clinical purposes and it may be difficult to identify real or true variations from normal growth in a particular fetus. Intrauterine growth retardation is often loosely defined as being the same as small-for-dates but it should also include fetuses which remain within normal limits but which fail to maintain growth. This is sometimes recognized by ultrasound with measurements showing that the fetus is crossing to lower centiles as pregnancy proceeds. Whenever possible, it is better to define the factors constraining or promoting growth and causing the fetus to be growth-retarded or large-for-dates respectively. Thus, intrauterine growth retardation can be caused by fetal malnutrition and hypoxia, or by problems such as congenital viral infections or chromosome anomalies. It is obvious that each of these has a different prognosis for the fetus during pregnancy and parturition and for its subsequent development. Furthermore, fetal malnutrition and hypoxia may result from many different aetiological factors, e.g. starvation or living at altitude. In affluent societies, pre-existing or pregnancy-induced disease may play a more significant role but socioeconomic circumstances still remain very important.

PREVENTION AND PREPREGNANCY COUNSELLING

Successful management of abnormal intrauterine growth has to begin with knowledge of the factors which may alter fetal growth. When these (Table 9.1) have been defined, education to avoid their consequences must begin in the community. For example, most of the community is aware of the adverse effects of alcohol and smoking on growth and development of the fetus. However, few strategies are successful in altering long-standing habits. Programmes which alter community attitudes may have greater effects on fetal growth than trying to persuade or bully an addict into giving up drug use during pregnancy (Bryce & Enkin 1984, Lumley 1987a). Since reproduction can begin in the young teenager, school children need to be informed of some of the common factors adversely affecting prenatal growth.

Prepregnancy counselling may identify significant factors in previous pregnancies, family or medical history which may increase the risk of either a growth-retarded or large-for-dates fetus. However, it must be acknowledged that often the causes of growth retardation remain obscure. Despite this, identification of putative factors before pregnancy enables counselling of the woman and her partner so that risks of factors constraining or promoting growth can be minimized.

FACTORS ASSOCIATED WITH GROWTH RETARDATION

Low birthweight is a weight at birth of less than 2500 g. The percentage of babies with low birthweight varies widely in different communities. In some, the incidence is more than 30% and even in affluent communities with well developed community services, including those for health and welfare, the rate is usually between 5 and 10% (Ebrahim 1984). Communities with a high proportion of low birthweight babies have a high percentage of these babies born at term, suggesting that growth retardation is common, although genetic effects on size at birth could not be excluded by this analysis (Vilar & Belizan 1982). Later studies in Indian communities show close relationship between low birthweight and social class. However, nutritional problems, recognized by low fasting glucose (less than 50 mg per 100 ml) or low maternal weight-for-height, can identify a group of women across the social classes who are at risk of having a low birthweight baby (Raman 1987).

Failure of normal fetal growth is common in preterm babies. This was recognized by analysis of the fetal growth curves, where it was shown that the coefficient of birthweight around the mean weight-for-age increased with prematurity (Dunn 1981). Ultrasonic measurements indicated that growth may decelerate but remain within normal limits some weeks before women go into unexplained premature labour (Persson et al 1978). Others have observed that elective preterm delivery for maternal or fetal indications is associated with significantly lower mean birthweight than that for babies born after spontaneous preterm labour (Yudkin et al 1987a).

Surveys conducted in Britain at different times have highlighted a small number of factors which have a strong association with low birthweight (Peters et al 1983). Smoking, maternal size, low parity and pre-eclampsia were identified by both the 1958 (Butler & Bonham 1963, Butler & Alberman 1969) and 1970 (Chamberlain et al 1975, 1978) British Births Surveys despite substantial changes in the obstetric population and in the obstetric services, promoting the comment: *plus ça change*. Lower mean birthweight is found in primigravidae and can be considered an unavoidable biological factor. Many other factors have been identified as adversely affecting fetal growth and will be divided into behavioural, medical, fetal and environmental factors and abnormalities of the placenta (Table 9.1).

Maternal behavioural factors

Another facet of education of the school child is the benefit of delaying pregnancy until at least the later teens. Pregnancy in the under 16-year-old is more often complicated by poor fetal growth, even after social circumstances have been taken into account (Russell 1982). It is more difficult to alleviate the effects of poor social circumstances, but in at least one affluent society the differences in birthweight in different socioeconomic groups could be largely ascribed to differences in the incidence of smoking across the groups (Lumley et al 1985). In poorer communities other factors obviously play a more significant role, e.g. nutrition, poor housing and heavy maternal work. Pressure to improve these must come from many parts of the community and will often be political in nature.

Maternal smoking remains a major factor constraining the growth of the fetus. On average, smoking reduces birthweight by 13 g per cigarette smoked daily (Anderson et al 1984). Numerous studies have shown a similar effect of smoking on the growth of the fetus, but few interventions have been successful in reducing or stopping smoking by women during pregnancy, if they present for antenatal care and are still smoking (Bryce & Enkin 1984, Lumley 1987). Lumley noted that it was ineffective to tell the smoker about carbon monoxide but that it was effective to discuss the effects of smoking on the fetus while the fetus was being scanned. Similarly, smokers reduced or stopped smoking after discovering that it caused a fetal tachycardia (Kelly & O'Connor 1984). However, problems with staff attitudes about giving information to smokers remain. Many midwives and doctors remain reluctant to tell women about smoking and implementation of programmes to stop smoking may fail for this reason (MacArthur et al 1987). Many of the same problems may emerge when programmes to reduce alcohol consumption are assessed, although the majority of social drinkers reduce or stop drinking alcohol in pregnancy.

DETECTION OF THE GROWTH-RETARDED FETUS

Detection of the woman who is at risk for growth retardation should begin at the first antenatal visit. Detailed history should be obtained about her family history. For example, a strong family history for pre-eclampsia may indicate that the woman may have a 25% chance of this condition (Chesley & Cooper 1986). Previous obstetric history of a growth-retarded fetus would be a strong indicator to seek recurrent causes of growth retardation or to ensure that increased monitoring of fetal growth occurs in the current pregnancy. Previous studies from Aberdeen (Hall & Chng 1982) suggest that history of growth retardation in previous pregnancies is often overlooked, although previous stillbirth is not. Indeed only 32% of previous children who were growth-retarded were clearly identified.

The traditional method of palpation of the maternal abdomen is not effective in detecting growth-retarded fetuses. The success rate is low and many fetuses are considered to be small but subsequently shown to be normally grown. Re-introduction of the technique of symphysial–fundal height improves the detection rates for growth-retarded fetuses but the sensitivity (70–88%) and specificity, although better than for palpation, are still not good enough (Belizan et al 1978, Quaranta et al 1981, Calvert et al 1982, Taylor et al 1984). Even so, it provides a useful predictor of fetal size and should be part of the normal assessment of uterine and fetal size. In addition to detecting the growth-retarded fetus, multiple pregnancy (Westin 1977) and a group of women at high risk for problems in labour can be identified (Hughes et al 1987). Women with symphysial–fundal heights above the 90th centile are at risk of abnormal labour and operative delivery. Fetal distress is more common in women with symphysial–fundal heights below the 10th centile and should be an indication or continuous monitoring in labour (Hughes et al 1987).

Ultrasound scanning programmes which include a dating scan combined with an assessment of fetal morphology, followed later by a second scan in the third trimester, offer the highest detection rates for growth-retarded fetuses (Neilson et al 1980). In addition, only about 2% of multiple pregnancies are missed at the first scan (Persson & Kullander 1983). In the same community, where the prevalence of growth retardation is 3%, the predictive value of a positive scan for growth retardation was 0.57 and of a negative test was 0.99 (Gennser & Persson 1986). Calculation of the kappa statistic (0.63) indicated that there is still much room for improvement in the detection of the growth-retarded fetus (Grant & Mohide 1982).

An audit in a unit where an ultrasound screening programme has been recommended found a disappointingly low detection rate for growth retardation (Hepburn & Rosenberg 1986). Mortality and morbidity remained higher in the growth-retarded babies. More disturbingly, the management of women with suspected growth retardation sometimes bore no relationship to the test results.

Detection of a growth-retarded fetus should prompt a repeat careful anatomical survey, particularly if polyhydramnios is present since some malformations, for example, microcephaly or hydrocephaly, may only become apparent later than the normal time of a first dating and morphology ultrasound scan (about 18 weeks). Recognition of these may add to the indications for late chorion villus biopsy or cordocentesis.

Separation of the normally grown but premature fetus from the growth-retarded one continues to be a problem if the woman presents late in pregnancy with uncertain dates. If circumstances allow it, then assessment of the growth rate of the abdominal circumference or length of the femur over a period of at least 14 days will identify most of the small-for-dates fetuses. Indeed wasting or reduction in the abdominal circumference has been observed in a few small fetuses (Divon et al 1986). Since the publication of this report, anecdotal comment suggests that this may not be too rare a finding on ultrasound examination of the growth-retarded fetus. Without an obvious cause (e.g. renal agenesis), oligohydramnios identified by the absence of a pocket of amniotic fluid of more than 2 cm adds further evidence supporting a diagnosis of a growth-retarded fetus (Divon et al 1986). Further, a high perinatal mortality was found in women whose pregnancies were complicated by oligohydramnios (Chamberlain et al 1984). Oligohydramnios should lead to a careful assessment of the fetal urinary tract and this should include determination of the rate of urine production (Wladmiroff & Campbell 1974). In the presence of obstruction, urine may have to be aspirated before this evaluation can be made.

Assessment of the appearance of the placenta on ultrasound is another means of identifying the growth-retarded fetus (Fisher et al 1967) but is subject to observer error or bias. This bias may be removed by quantitation of the returning signal before picture quality is adjusted to suit the observing ultrasonologist. Despite this present limitation some interesting findings have been recorded. First, a grading system for the maturation in the appearance of the placenta has been devised (Grannum et al 1979). Confirmation of the appearance of the placenta on ultrasound examination, together with inspection of the fixed placenta after delivery, showed that the transonic or fallout areas corresponded to spaces in which spiral arteries ended (Vermeulen et al 1985). Early placental maturation identifies a group of women with a high incidence of growth-retarded fetuses and, in contrast, a low incidence when this early maturation is absent (Patterson et al 1983). The grade III (the most mature placenta) also helps to separate the growth-retarded fetus from others of relatively low birthweight (Kazzi et al 1983). The usefulness of this test has recently been subjected to clinical trial with randomization to report and non-report groups (Proud & Grant 1987). In the first phase of the study it was found that a grade III placenta was found in 15% of pregnancies at 34 to 36 weeks and was significantly associated with teenage mothers, nulliparity, maternal smoking, meconium staining of amniotic fluid, fetal distress in labour, low Apgar, low birthweight and perinatal death. In the second phase, reporting of the results was associated with a significant decrease in the risk of perinatal death. Proud & Grant (1987) noted that the predictive value of positive results was low but led to increased surveillance and supplementary testing of fetal well-being and reduced the risk of death of a normally formed infant. A disappointing feature of the study was the subjective element of the test, readily acknowledged by the authors and demonstrated when a new ultrasonographer was unable to grade placentas.

Morphological examination of the placenta has shown that the surface area for exchange is substantially reduced in pregnancies complicated by growth retardation (Aherne & Dunhill 1966). This has recently been confirmed when it was shown that placental volume was substantially reduced when the fetus was small-for-dates in the presence or absence of hypertensive disorders. Villous surface area was related to both gestational age and fetal weight (Boyd & Scott 1985). Attempts have been made to assess placental size from linear

Table 9.2 Management of intrauterine growth retardation

Prevention:
Education
Prepregnancy counselling
Minimize the effects of medical conditions
Early confirmation of pregnancy
Dating and morphology scan
Serum alpha-fetoprotein
Monitor fetal growth:
Symphysial–fundal height
Ultrasound
Modification of lifestyle:
Stopping work
Bedrest
Monitor fetal well-being:
Fetal movement counting (hormonal tests of fetoplacental function)
Cardiotocography
Umbilical flow velocity waveforms
Uterine flow velocity waveforms
Umbilical blood flow
Cordocentesis
Timing of delivery:
Well-being judged from monitoring
Growth versus prematurity
Method of delivery:
Spontaneous
Induction
Elective Caesarean section
Assessment of the infant
Follow-up of the child

measurements made using ultrasound and an association of a small placenta with small-for-dates baby was found (Hoogland et al 1980). Recently a compound B-scan has been used to obtain parallel transverse scans of the uterus at intervals of 2 cm. When the placenta was oblique to the horizontal plane 1-cm intervals were used. Computer reconstructions were made and placental volume determined. There was a large difference between antepartum placental volume and postpartum placental weight: volume : weight ratio 1.6 : 1 (Wolf et al 1987). This interesting approach is worthy of further development, particularly since a high fetal : placental weight ratio identifies a group which is at risk for fetal distress even in the absence of growth retardation.

MANAGEMENT OF INTRAUTERINE GROWTH RETARDATION

It has already been emphasized that it is better to attempt to prevent growth retardation by education or counselling before pregnancy (Table 9.2). Management after growth retardation has been detected should include attempts to modify factors which may compromise the fetus. In the past much importance was given to hormonal measurements such as oestriol and placental lactogen but in recent years these have largely been abandoned in favour of dynamic or biophysical measurements, especially cardiotocography, biophysical profile or Doppler measurements of velocity waveforms. These may be used in conjunction with maternal movement counting. Indeed the latter was found to be effective in reducing perinatal mortality (Neldham 1980) and is currently being subjected to more extensive testing in a large randomized trial (British Fetal Movement Trial). Pending the result of that trial it seems prudent to encourage all pregnant women to note the movements of their fetus and to report promptly any substantial change in movements. Preferably, this should be done using a fetal movement chart such as the Cardiff Count-to-Ten method, but it has also been suggested that each women should determine the normal pattern of movements for her fetus (Grant & Hepburn 1984). The advantage of this approach is that the individualized hourly counting rate is determined first and then time to count this number of movements is recorded each day for the remainder of pregnancy. It was claimed that this method was associated with fewer false alarms and that the amount of time spent counting movements was halved overall when compared with the Cardiff Count-to-Ten method (Pearson & Weaver 1976). No matter which method is used, a reduction in fetal movements should lead to more detailed assessment of the fetus by cardiotocography.

Asking women to count their baby's movements each day creates anxiety in about 23% of women in filling fetal movement charts. A more adequate explanation for keeping the chart or the possible importance of a reduction in fetal activity may help to allay some of this anxiety. However, it should be noted that more than 50% of women were reassured by filling the chart. Unfavourable comments related to the difficulty of counting movements by busy women, particularly mothers with older children. Others were discouraged by the fact that none of their medical attendants asked about or looked at their charts (Draper et al 1986).

Antenatal cardiotocography was not found to be of value when used as a screening test at 32 weeks or regularly in late pregnancy (Lawson et al 1984, Lumley et al 1983). The only conclusion that can be drawn from the randomized trials concerned with antenatal cardiotocography is that a much larger trial would be required to determine the efficacy of cardiotocography (Brown et al 1982, Flynn et al 1982, Lumley et al 1983, Kidd et al 1985). However, Lumley (1987b) has drawn attention to the relevance of the hypothesis being tested to the clinicians concerned with clinical management. It was clear that the outcome of the trial would not greatly alter clinical management; in other words, the trial seemed not to be relevant to the practising clinician. She considered that the likely reason for this was that, in practice, obstetricians were not using cardiotocography to reduce perinatal mortality but rather to seek reassurance of the health of the fetus. The wide adoption of antenatal cardiotocography (Humphrey et al 1987, Oats et al 1987) is not universally accepted (Thacker & Berkelman 1986).

Dynamic measurements obtained by ultrasound may add to the management of the woman whose pregnancy is complicated with maternal or fetal problems. Abnormal flow velocity waveforms are found in the umbilical arteries of growth-retarded fetuses (Erskine & Ritchie 1985, Trudinger et al

1985). It has also been suggested that these abnormal waveforms are associated with obliteration of small arteries (the resistance vessels) of the tertiary villi of the placenta (Giles et al 1985). Umbilical arterial waveforms have been subjected to prospective clinical trial with randomization to report and non-report groups. Knowledge of the test resulted in fewer cases of fetal distress in labour and to fewer Caesarean sections, indicating better selection of patients for labour or operative delivery (Trudinger et al 1987). Further trials of a similar nature are required to test whether the correct pregnancies are allowed to continue longer without increasing perinatal mortality. Such trials are likely to pose difficult ethical problems since many will argue that non-report groups may include fetuses with unacceptable risks for necrotizing enterocolitis, haemorrhage or a more complicated neonatal period (Hackett et al 1987). Problems of the acceptance of clinical trials in perinatal medicine have been highlighted recently (Lumley 1987b, Silverman 1987). Public awareness of the relevance of these studies unfortunately remains a major task. Given these remarks it need hardly be added that other methods such as uterine artery waveforms (Campbell et al 1983, Trudinger & Cook 1985, Schulman et al 1986) or cerebral artery waveforms (Wladmiroff et al 1987) must be evaluated in well designed clinical trials.

Placenta and intrauterine growth retardation

The importance of the placenta to the development of intrauterine growth retardation has been alluded to. Morphological examination of the placenta has shown reduction in the area available for exchange, lower volume of parenchymal tissue and total volume (Aherne & Dunhill 1966, Boyd & Scott 1985). A common pathogenesis may exist for preeclampsia and for at least a proportion of growth-retarded fetuses. Normally, the spiral arterioles in the placental bed lose their muscular and elastic layers and these are replaced by a fibrinoid layer in which trophoblast cells are embedded. The vessels become greatly distended. This vascular development probably occurs in two stages with invasion of the decidual portion of the vessels in the first trimester and the myometrial portions in the second (Robertson et al 1975, Pijnenborg et al 1983). These changes, extending from the decidua to the inner myometrium, fail to occur in preeclampsia and in some pregnancies complicated by growth retardation. Intraluminal endovascular trophoblast may be seen in the spiral arterioles in the third trimester whereas this is not normally seen after the second trimester (Khong et al 1986). It is interesting to note that the timing of the normal vascular response to pregnancy is similar to the timing of the major changes in uterine vascular compliance as measured by Doppler ultrasound (Schulman et al 1986).

Relative failure of placental growth may also present problems for the fetus during labour and delivery. In order to investigate this, the placenta needs to be weighed after removal of the membranes, blood clots, draining blood from the fetal surface vessels and after blotting dry. When this has been done, it has been shown in cross-sectional studies that placental weight did not increase after 36 weeks in pregnancies with growth-retarded fetuses. However, the fetoplacental weight ratio continued to increase, reaching values similar to those for appropriate-for-dates or large-for-dates fetuses. Plotting fetoplacental weight ratios against placental weight segregated babies into three distinct curves depending on their growth. In each group low Apgar scores were more common when the fetoplacental weight ratio exceeded 10 (Molteni et al 1978). These findings have been confirmed and extended: high fetoplacental weight ratios are associated with fetal distress and meconium staining of amniotic fluid in addition to low Apgar scores (Bonds et al 1984).

All these findings place great emphasis on the need to define the effects of failure of placental development on the fetus. A number of experimental approaches have been devised to restrict placental growth and most are designed to alter or prevent the normal development of the maternal vasculature (Owens & Robinson 1987). A few will be mentioned since they provide a basis for interpretation of recently acquired data from human pregnancy. Excision of endometrial caruncles from the uterus of the non-pregnant sheep restricts placental growth in subsequent pregnancies (Alexander 1964, Robinson et al 1979). If the growth of the placenta is not too severely restricted, the fetal weight can remain within normal limits (within 2 standard deviations of the mean weight for control fetuses) but is accompanied by higher fetoplacental weight ratios, altered body proportions (similar to those seen in growth retardation), chronic hypoglycaemia and hypoxaemia. The latter develops progressively in late pregnancy to values comparable to those found at younger ages in more severely growth-retarded fetuses. More severe restriction of placental growth is associated with growth retardation (>2 standard deviations below mean for controls), high fetoplacental weight ratio, prolonged chronic hypoxaemia and hypoglycaemia. The altered body proportions are likely to be due, in part, to circulatory changes similar to those found when fetal growth was restricted by embolization of the maternal side of the placenta (Creasy et al 1973). Endocrine responses to the hypoxaemia and hypoglycaemia would alter the distribution of nutrients in addition to orchestrating or augmenting the cardiovascular response (Robinson et al 1985). However, changes in nutrient supply following restriction of placental growth are more likely to account for the reduction in fetal weight since prolonged hypobaric hypoxaemia only causes a moderate impairment of fetal growth (Jacobs et al 1988).

In our experiments we assessed the adequacy of the supply of oxygen and glucose by calculating the margin of safety which was defined as the ratio of the delivery (umbilical vein content × umbilical blood flow) to consumption (umbilical venoarterial concentration difference × blood flow). There is a progressive decrease in the margin of safety for the supply of both oxygen and glucose, with both decreasing placental and fetal weight despite a relative increase in the efficiency of placental transport of these two substances in the smallest placentas (Owens et al 1986, 1987a,b). This occurred even though the placenta consumed less of each per unit mass of placenta and there was a redistribution within the uterus favouring the fetus. Indeed there was no evidence that the fetus can reduce its consumption of these substances per unit mass of fetus. Expressed in another way, fetal growth was limited by supply and the fetus was not able to alter consumption, in contrast to the placenta, which may have had to in part because it derives a significant part of its supply from the fetal circulation.

Although glucose consumption by the small placenta was reduced it continued to secrete lactate into the fetal but not maternal circulation at a rate similar to that of a normal placenta. This output of lactate could not be sustained by placental glucose consumption, but is probably met by the fetus releasing amino acids to the placenta, perhaps subsequent to net protein breakdown. Indeed the consumption of amino acids by the small placenta per gram of tissue was increased several-fold and was mostly met by supply of alanine and branched chain amino acids from the fetus as well as the mother (Kind & Owens, unpublished observation). Thus we may have identified an analogous situation to the human fetus whose abdominal circumference is shrinking (Divon et al 1986).

Supplementation by giving the mother oxygen, glucose or other nutrients seems an attractive way to attempt to overcome the restriction of placental growth. Maternal hyperoxia achieved by giving the mother 50% oxygen to breathe for 4 hours increases the margin of safety and oxygen tension in the fetus but does not increase oxygen consumption (Owens et al 1985). Somewhat disturbingly, when hyperoxia ceased there was a significant reduction in oxygen consumption to values below those observed in the control period before hyperoxia. Thus it might be suggested that reduction in oxygenation in the post-hyperoxic period could harm the fetus.

Long-term nutrient supplementation has been given to fetuses whose placentas were embolized at the same time (Charlton & Johengen 1987). The fetuses were infused with 5% glucose and 6.8% amino acids. The supplemented fetuses maintained normal growth without development of hypoxaemia. This may have been achieved by stimulation of placental growth which exceeded that of control fetuses.

An exciting picture is beginning to emerge of the growth-retarded human fetus, with a proportion of the fetuses having features remarkably similar to those characterized in the experimental work described above. It has only been possible to obtain this information since the development of ultrasound-guided sampling of umbilical cord and placental blood — cordocentesis or percutaneous umbilical blood sampling (Daffos et al 1983, Hobbins et al 1985, Nicolaides et al 1986). The growth-retarded human fetus, like its animal counterpart, can have chronic hypoxaemia and hypoglycaemia but may also have severe acidaemia and high concentrations of lactate (Soothill et al 1987). The latter two have only been found in sheep fetuses shortly before fetal demise. Not surprisingly, when acidaemia has been found in human fetuses, prompt delivery by Caesarean section has been undertaken (Pearce & Chamberlain 1987). Mothers with severely growth-retarded and hypoxaemic fetuses have been given supplemental oxygen (55%) for prolonged periods in a preliminary study (Nicolaides et al 1987). This hyperoxia was sufficient to restore oxygen tension to the normal range and presumably increased the margin of safety for the supply of oxygen for the fetus. It may also have increased oxygen consumption since mean blood velocity in the fetal aorta increased. Since there were no measurements of extraction of oxygen across the umbilical circulation (Rurak et al 1987), this would need to be the subject of further study. Even though oxygen tension was increased, there was no clear evidence of improved growth rate, as might have been anticipated from animal studies (Jacobs et al 1988). One important consequence of this work is reinforcement of the view that, most often, perinatal brain damage has its origins long before labour or delivery (Symonds 1987); these results add weight to earlier epidemiological studies (Illingworth 1979, Nelson & Ellenberg 1986).

LATE GENETIC DIAGNOSIS

Management of severe intrauterine growth retardation should include utilization of techniques for late genetic or chromosome analysis and for detection of intrauterine infection. Chorionic villus (placental) biopsy can be undertaken in the second and third trimesters (Nicolaides et al 1986). However, the technique of cordocentesis (percutaneous umbilical blood sampling) probably offers greater potential for diagnosis of problems which affect fetal growth. For some women, recognition that a fetus has a lethal trisomy would alter management of the remainder of pregnancy and delivery. This would also include counselling of the women and her partner about the prognosis for their child. Others may avoid unnecessary termination when the mother has had infections such as rubella when direct evidence is obtained that the fetus was not infected.

TIMING AND MODE OF DELIVERY

There are still many unresolved issues concerning the best time to deliver the growth-retarded fetus. Where extreme prematurity offers a dismal prognosis then it is appropriate to test new and expensive interventions which may prolong pregnancy. For most, a balance between the fetal and maternal conditions and fetal maturity remains the cornerstone of timing of delivery. Improvements in neonatal care and the introduction of corticosteroids to enhance maturity over the last 10–15 years have encouraged perinatologists to deliver the fetus earlier, before there is evidence of impending fetal death. Waiting for evidence of compromise of the severely growth-retarded fetus, as obtained by maternal fetal movement counting or on cardiotocography, certainly has little place after 36 weeks, but timing of delivery of the severely growth-retarded fetus between 28 and 36 weeks is more difficult. If waveform analysis can provide an earlier indication of fetal compromise, then long-term studies of the outcome for infants delivered on this basis, compared to current conventional methods, will have to be completed. Similarly, identification of the hypoxaemic fetus, with evidence of long-term compensation, should lead to studies testing early delivery before evidence of compromise, apart from growth rate, becomes apparent.

LONG-TERM FOLLOW-UP

No discussion of growth retardation is complete without emphasizing the continuing need for long-term follow-up studies. Many of these will have to be continued until early adult life. Some of the early studies have been referred to in this chapter (Hack et al 1982, Harvey et al 1982, Low et al 1982) but additional studies comparing pre- and postnatal growth problems for each identified cause of growth retardation will need to be undertaken, particularly if new interventions, such as supplementation with oxygen or nutrients in response to a defined deficit, are undertaken.

Acknowledgements

I wish to thank Dr Julie Owens for critical comment and G. Perrotta for typing the manuscript. The experimental work described was generously supported by NH & MRC and the Ramaciotti Foundation.

REFERENCES

Aherne W, Dunhill M S 1966 Quantitative aspects of placental structure. Journal of Pathology and Bacteriology 91: 123
Alexander G 1964 Studies on the placenta of the sheep (*Ovis aries* L.): effect of reduction in the number of caruncles. Journal of Reproduction and Fertility 7: 307
Anderson G D, Blidner I N, McClemont S, Sinclair J C 1984 Determinants of size at birth in a Canadian population. American Journal of Obstetrics and Gynecology 150: 236
Belizan J M, Vilar J, Nardin J C, Malmud J, de Vinca L S 1978 Diagnosis of intrauterine growth retardation by a simple clinical method: measurement of uterine height. American Journal of Obstetrics and Gynecology 131: 643
Bonds D R, Gabbe S G, Kumar S 1984 Fetal weight/placental weight ratios and perinatal outcome. American Journal of Obstetrics and Gynecology 149: 195
Boyd P A, Scott A 1985 Quantitative structural studies on human placentas associated with pre-eclampsia, essential hypertension and intrauterine growth retardation. British Journal of Obstetrics and Gynaecology 92: 714
Brown V A, Sawers R S, Parsons R J, Duncan S L B, Cooke I D 1982 The value of antenatal cardiotocography in the management of high-risk pregnancy: a randomised controlled trial. British Journal of Obstetrics and Gynaecology 89: 716
Bryce R L, Enkin M W 1984 Lifestyle in pregnancy. Canadian Family Physician 30: 2127
Butler N R, Alberman E D 1969 Perinatal mortality: the second report of the 1958 British Perinatal Mortality Survey. Livingstone, Edinburgh
Butler N R, Bonham 1963 Perinatal problems: the first report of the 1958 British Perinatal Mortality Survey. Livingstone, Edinburgh
Calvert J P, Crean E E, Newcombe R G, Pearson J F 1982 Antenatal screening by measurement of fundal height. British Medical Journal 285: 846
Campbell S, Griffin D R, Pearce J M et al 1983 New Doppler technique for assessing uteroplacental blood flow. Lancet i: 675
Chamberlain R, Chamberlain G, Howlett B, Claireaux A 1975 British births 1970 vol 1: The first week of life. Heinemann Medical, London
Chamberlain G, Phillip E, Howlett B, Masters K 1978 British births 1970 vol 2: Obstetric care. Heinemann Medical, London
Chamberlain P F, Manning F A, Morrison I, Harman C R, Lange I R 1984 Ultrasonic evaluation of amniotic fluid volume II. The relationship of marginal or decreased amniotic fluid volume to perinatal outcome. American Journal of Obstetrics and Gynecology 150: 245
Charlton V, Johengen M 1987 Fetal intravenous nutritional supplementation ameliorates the development of embolization-induced growth retardation in sheep. Pediatric Research 22: 55
Chesley L C, Cooper D W 1986 Genetics of hypertension in pregnancy: possible single gene control of pre-eclampsia and eclampsia in the descendants of eclamptic women. British Journal of Obstetrics and Gynaecology 93: 898
Comney J O O, Fitzhardinge P M 1979 Handicap in the preterm small-for-gestational age infant. Journal of Pediatrics 94: 779
Creasy R K, de Swiet M, Kahanpää K V, Young W P, Rudolph A M 1973 Pathophysiological changes in the foetal lamb with growth retardation. In: Comline R S, Cross K W, Dawes G S, Nathaniels P W (eds) Foetal and neonatal physiology. Cambridge University Press, Cambridge p 398
Daffos F, Capell-Pavlosky M, Forstier F 1983 Fetal blood sampling via the umbilical cord using a needle guided by ultrasound. Report of 66 cases. Prenatal Diagnosis 3: 271
Divon M Y, Chamberlain P F, Sipos L, Manning F A, Platt L D 1986 Identification of the small for gestational age fetus with the use of gestational age-independent indices of fetal growth. American Journal of Obstetrics and Gynecology 155: 1197
Draper J, Feild S, Thomas H 1986 Women's views on keeping fetal movement charts. British Journal of Obstetrics and Gynaecology 93: 334
Dunn P M 1981 Variations of fetal growth: some causes and effects. In: van Assche F A, Robertson W B (eds) Fetal growth retardation. Churchill Livingstone, Edinburgh, p 79
Dunn P 1985 A perinatal growth chart for international reference. Acta Paediatrica Scandinavica (suppl) 319: 180
Ebrahim G J 1984 Care of the newborn. British Medical Journal 289: 899
Erskine R L A, Ritchie J W K 1985 Umbilical artery blood flow characteristics in normal and growth retarded fetuses. British Journal of Obstetrics and Gynaecology 92: 605
Fisher C C, Garrett W, Kossoff M E 1976 Placental aging monitored by gray scale echography. American Journal of Obstetrics and Gynecology 124: 483
Flynn A M, Kelly J, Mansfield H, Needham P, O'Conor M, Viegas O 1982 A randomised trial of non-stress antepartum cardiotocography. British Journal of Obstetrics and Gynaecology 89: 427
Gennser G, Persson P-H 1986 Biophysical assessment of placental function. Clinics in Obstetrics and Gynaecology 13: 521
Giles W B, Trudinger B J, Baird P J 1985 Fetal umbilical artery velocity waveforms and placental resistance: pathological correlations. British Journal of Obstetrics and Gynaecology 92: 31
Grannum P A T, Berkowitz R L, Hobbins J C 1979 The ultrasonic changes in the maturing placenta. American Journal of Obstetrics and Gynecology 133: 915
Grant A, Hepburn M 1984 Merits of an individualised approach to fetal movement counting compared with fixed-time and fixed-number methods. British Journal of Obstetrics and Gynaecology 91: 1087
Grant A, Mohide P 1982 Screening and diagnostic tests in antenatal care.

In: Enkin M W, Chalmers I (eds) Effectiveness and satisfaction in antenatal care. Heinemann, London, pp 22–59
Gruendwald P 1963 Chronic fetal distress and placental insufficiency. Biology of the Neonate 5: 215
Hack M, Merkatz I R, Gordon D, Jones P K, Fanaroff A A 1982 The significance of postnatal growth in very low-birth weight infants. American Journal of Obstetrics and Gynecology 143: 693
Hackett G A, Campbell S, Gamsu H, Cohen-Overbeek T, Pearce J M 1987 Doppler studies in the growth retarded fetus and prediction of neonatal necrotising enterocolitis, haemorrhage, and neonatal morbidity. British Medical Journal 294: 13
Hall, M, Chng P K 1982 Antenatal care in practice. In: Enkin M W, Chalmers I (eds) Effectiveness and satisfaction in antenatal care. Heinemann, London, pp 60–68
Harvey D, Prince J, Bunton J, Parkinson C, Campbell S 1982 Abilities of children who were small-for-gestational age babies. Pediatrics 69: 296
Hepburn M, Rosenberg K 1986 An audit of the detection and management of small-for-gestational age babies. British Journal of Obstetrics and Gynaecology 93: 212
Hobbins J C, Grannum P A, Romero R R, Reece E A, Mahoney M J 1985 Percutaneous umbilical blood sampling. American Journal of Obstetrics and Gynecology 152: 1
Hoogland H J, De Haan J, Martin C B 1980 Placental size during early pregnancy and fetal outcome: a preliminary report of a sequential ultrasonographic study. American Journal of Obstetrics and Gynecology 138: 441
Hughes A B, Jenkins D A, Newcombe R G, Pearson J F 1987 Symphysis–fundus height, maternal height, labor pattern, and mode of delivery. American Journal of Obstetrics and Gynecology 156: 644
Humphrey M D, Dosser S L, Trickey D J et al 1987 The relevance of antenatal cardiotocography. Australian and New Zealand Journal of Obstetrics and Gynaecology 27: 87
Illingworth R S 1979 Why blame the obstetrician? A review. British Medical Journal 1: 797
Jacobs R, Robinson J S, Owens J A, Falconer J, Webster M E D 1988 The effect of prolonged hypobaric hypoxia on growth of fetal sheep. Journal of Developmental Physiology 10: 97–112
Kazzi G M, Gross T L, Sokol R J, Kazzi N J 1983 Detection of intrauterine growth retardation: a new use for sonographic placental grading. American Journal of Obstetrics and Gynecology 145: 733
Kelly J, O'Connor M 1984 Smoking in pregnancy: effects on the fetus. British Journal of Obstetrics and Gynaecology 91: 111
Khong T Y, de Wolf F, Robertson W B, Brosens I 1986 Inadequate maternal vascular response to placentation in pregnancies complicated by pre-eclampsia and by small-for-gestational age infants. British Journal of Obstetrics and Gynaecology 93: 1049
Kidd L C, Patel N B, Smith R 1985 Non-stress antenatal cardiotocography — prospective randomised clinical trial. British Journal of Obstetrics and Gynaecology 92: 1156
Lawson G W, Dawes G S, Redman C W G 1984 Analysis of fetal heart rate at 32 weeks gestation. British Journal of Obstetrics and Gynaecology 91: 542
Low J A, Galbraith R S, Muir D, Killen H, Pater B, Karchmar J 1982 Intrauterine growth retardation: a study of long-term morbidity. American Journal of Obstetrics and Gynecology 142: 670
Lubchencho L O, Hansman C, Dressler M, Boyd B 1963 Intrauterine growth as estimated from liveborn birthweight data at 24 to 42 weeks of gestation. Pediatrics 32: 793
Lumley J 1987a Stopping smoking. British Journal of Obstetrics and Gynaecology 94: 289
Lumley J 1987b Does this work? Pediatrics 79: 1040
Lumley J, Lester A, Anderson I, Renou P, Wood C 1983 A randomised trial of weekly cardiotocography in high-risk obstetric patients. British Journal of Obstetrics and Gynaecology 90: 1018
Lumley J, Correy J, Newman N, Curran J 1985 Cigarette smoking, alcohol consumption in Tasmania 1981–2. Australian and New Zealand Journal of Obstetrics and Gynaecology 25: 33
MacArthur C, Newton J R, Knox E G 1987 Effect of anti-smoking health education on infant size: a randomised controlled trial. British Journal of Obstetrics and Gynaecology 94: 295
McBurney R D 1947 Undernourished full-term infant: case report. Western Journal of Surgery, Obstetrics and Gynecology 55: 363–370
Miller H C, Merriott T A 1979 Fetal growth in humans. Year Book Publishing, New York, p 26
Milner R D G, Richards B 1974 An analysis of birthweight by gestational age in infants born in England and Wales. Journal of Obstetrics and Gynaecology of the British Commonwealth 81: 956
Molteni R A, Stys S J, Battaglia F C 1978 Relationship of fetal and placental weight in human beings: fetal/placental weight ratios at various gestational ages and birthweight distributions. Journal of Reproductive Medicine 21: 327
Naeye R L 1965 Malnutrition: probable cause of fetal growth retardation. Archives of Pathology 79: 284
Neilson J P, Whitfield C R, Aitchison T C 1980 Screening of the small-for-dates fetus: a two stage ultrasonic examination. British Medical Journal 1: 1203
Neldham S 1980 Fetal movements as an indicator of fetal wellbeing. Lancet i: 1222
Nelson K B, Ellenberg J H 1986 Antecedents of cerebral palsy. A multivariate analysis. New England Journal of Medicine 315: 81
Nicolaides K H, Soothill P W, Rodeck C H, Campbell S 1986 Ultrasound-guided sampling of umbilical cord and placental blood to assess fetal wellbeing. Lancet i: 1065
Nicolaides K H, Campbell S, Bradley R J, Bilardo C M, Soothill P W, Gibb D 1987 Maternal oxygen therapy for intrauterine growth retardation. Lancet i: 942
Northern Region 1984 Collaborative survey of perinatal mortality report, 1982. Newcastle upon Tyne, Northern Regional Health Authority
Oats J N, Chew F T K, Ratten V J 1987 Antepartum cardiotocography — an audit. Australian and New Zealand Journal of Obstetrics and Gynaecology 27: 82
Ounsted M, Moar V, Scott A 1982 Growth in the first four years: III. The effects of maternal factors associated with small-for-dates and large-for-dates pregnancies. Early Human Development 7: 347
Ounsted M, Moar V A, Cockburn J, Redman C W G 1984 Factors associated with the intellectual ability of children born to mothers with high risk pregnancies. British Medical Journal 288: 1038
Owens J A, Robinson J S 1987 The effect of experimental manipulation of placental growth and development. In: Coburn F (ed) Fetal and neonatal growth. Wiley, Chichester, p 49
Owens J A, Falconer J, Robinson J S 1985 Effect of maternal hyperoxia on fetal metabolism in experimental intrauterine growth retardation. Journal of Australian Perinatal Society 3: 122
Owens J A, Falconer J, Robinson J S 1986 Effect of restriction of placental growth on umbilical and uterine blood flows. American Journal of Physiology 250: R427
Owens J A, Falconer J, Robinson J S 1987a Effect of restriction of placental growth on oxygen delivery to and consumption by the pregnant uterus and fetus. Journal of Developmental Physiology 9: 137
Owens J A, Falconer J, Robinson J S 1987b Effect of restriction of placental growth on fetal and utero-placental metabolism. Journal of Developmental Physiology 9: 225
Patterson R M, Hayashi R H, Cavazos D 1983 Ultrasonically observed early placental maturation and perinatal outcome. American Journal of Obstetrics and Gynecology 147: 773
Pearce J M, Chamberlain G V P 1987 Ultrasonically guided percutaneous umbilical blood sampling in the management of intrauterine growth retardation. British Journal of Obstetrics and Gynaecology 94: 318
Pearson J E, Weaver 1976 Fetal activity and fetal wellbeing: an evaluation. British Medical Journal 1: 1305–1307
Persson P-H, Kullander S 1983 Long-term experience of general ultrasound screening in pregnancy. American Journal of Obstetrics and Gynecology 146: 942
Persson P-H, Grennert L, Gennser G 1978 Impact of maternal and fetal factors on the normal growth of the biparietal diameter. Acta Obstetricia et Gynecologica Scandinavica (suppl) 78: 21
Peters T J, Golding J, Butler N R, Fryer J G, Lawrence C J, Chamberlain G V P 1983 *Plus ça change:* predictors of birthweight in two national studies. British Journal of Obstetrics and Gynaecology 90: 1040
Pijnenborg R, Bland J M, Robertson W B, Brosens I 1983 Uteroplacental arterial changes related to interstitial trophoblast migration in early pregnancy. Placenta 4: 387
Proud J, Grant A M 1987 Third trimester placental grading by ultrasonography as a test of fetal wellbeing. British Medical Journal 294: 1641

Quaranta P, Currell R, Redman C W G, Robinson J S 1981 Prediction of small-for-dates by measurement of symphysial–fundal height. British Journal of Obstetrics and Gynaecology 88: 115
Raman L 1987 Maternal nutritional status influencing intrauterine growth. In: Maeda K (ed) The fetus as a patient. Elsevier, Amsterdam, pp 221–229
Rantakallio P 1985 A 14-year follow-up of children with normal and abnormal birth weight for their gestational age. Acta Paediatrica Scandinavica 74: 62
Robertson W B, Brosens I, Dixon G 1975 Uteroplacental vascular pathology. European Journal of Obstetrics and Gynecological Reproductive Biology 5: 581
Robinson J S 1979 Growth of the fetus. British Medical Bulletin 35: 137
Robinson J S, Kingston E J, Jones C T, Thorburn G D 1979 Studies on experimental growth retardation in sheep. The effect of removal of endometrial caruncles on fetal size and metabolism. Journal of Developmental Physiology 1: 379
Robinson J S, Falconer J Owens J A 1985 Intrauterine growth retardation: clinical and experimental. Acta Paediatrica Scandinavica (suppl) 319: 135
Rurak D, Selke P, Fisher M, Taylor S, Wittman B 1987 Fetal oxygen extraction: comparision of the human and sheep. American Journal of Obstetrics and Gynecology 156: 360
Russell J K 1982 Early teenage pregnancy. Churchill Livingstone, Edinburgh
Schulman H, Fleischer A, Famakides G, Bracero L, Rochelson B, Grunfeld L 1986 Development of uterine artery compliance in pregnancy as detected by Doppler ultrasound. American Journal of Obstetrics and Gynecology 155: 1031
Silverman W A 1987 Sample size, representativeness, and credibility in pragmatic neonatal trials. American Journal of Perinatology 4: 129
Soothill P W, Nicolaides K H, Campbell S 1987 Prenatal asphyxia, hyperlacticaemia, hypoglycaemia in growth retarded fetuses. British Medical Journal 294: 1051
Symonds E M 1987 Antenatal, perinatal or postnatal brain damage. British Medical Journal 294: 1046
Taylor P, Coulthard A C, Robinson J S 1984 Symphysial–fundal height from 12 weeks' gestation. Australian and New Zealand Journal of Obstetrics and Gynaecology 24: 189
Thacker S B, Berkelman R L 1986 Assessing the diagnostic accuracy and efficacy of selected antepartum fetal surveillance techniques. Obstetrics and Gynecology Survey 41: 121
Trudinger B J, Cook C M 1985 Umbilical and uterine artery flow velocity waveforms in pregnancy associated with major fetal abnormality. British Journal of Obstetrics and Gynaecology 92: 666
Trudinger B J, Giles W B, Cook C M, Bombardieri J, Collins L 1985 Fetal umbilical artery flow velocity waveforms and placental resistance: clinical correlations. British Journal of Obstetrics and Gynaecology 92: 23
Trudinger B J, Cook C M, Giles W B, Connelly A, Thompson R S 1987 Umbilical artery velocity waveforms in high risk pregnancies. Randomised controlled trial. Lancet i: 188
Vermeulen R C W, Lambalk N B, Exalto N, Arts N F T 1985 An anatomic basis for ultrasound images of the human placenta. American Journal of Obstetrics and Gynecology 153: 806
Vilar J, Belizan J M 1982 The relative contribution of prematurity and fetal growth retardation to low birthweight in developing and developed societies. American Journal of Obstetrics and Gynecology 143: 793
Westin B 1977 Gravidogram and fetal growth. Acta Obstetricia et Gynecologica Scandinavica 56: 273
Wladmiroff J W, Campbell S 1974 Fetal urine production rates in normal and complicated pregnancies. Lancet i: 151
Wladmiroff J W, v.d. Wijngaard J A G W, Degeni S, Noordam M J, v. Eyck J, Tonge H M 1987 Cerebral and umbilical arterial blood flow velocity waveforms in normal and growth retarded pregnancies. Obstetrics and Gynecology 69: 705
Wolf H, Oosting H, Treffers P E 1987 Placental volume measurement by ultrasonography: evaluation of the method. American Journal of Obstetrics and Gynecology 156: 1191
World Health Organization 1961 Public health aspects of low birthweight. Technical Report Series No 217. Geneva, World Health Organization
Yudkin P L, Aboualfa M, Eyre J A, Redman C W G, Wilkinson A R 1987a Influence of elective preterm delivery on birthweight and head circumference standards. Archives of Disease in Childhood 62: 24
Yudkin P L, Wood L, Redman C W G 1987b Risk of unexplained stillbirth at different gestational ages. Lancet i: 1192

10

I. R. McFadyen

Maternal changes in normal pregnancy

Maternal adaptation to conception starts early in pregnancy. Every system is affected progressively but the changes occur at different rates throughout the body; they do not peak at the same time. Similarly, recovery from the pregnancy does not take place at one speed and some organs never return to their nulliparous state. The quality and degree of adaptation varies from one individual to another, being affected by factors such as maternal age. If adaptation is not wholly physiological it may lead to overt pathology; even if physiological, the changes produced may be interpreted as pathological by the mother or her attendants. The proper practice of obstetrics requires knowledge of the whole range of normality and of the consequences of physiological adaptation.

MATERNAL CHARACTERISTICS WHICH AFFECT ADAPTATION

Maternal adaptation to pregnancy may be physiologically complete or incomplete. Inadequate physiological changes are most likely to occur in first pregnancies, but the mother's physical reaction to pregnancy may also be influenced by maternal age, previous obstetric history, overt or covert illness and present or previous environment. A previous normal pregnancy is the factor most likely to ensure that maternal adaptation in the current pregnancy will be normal and complete. Many of the changes of pregnancy disappear after delivery but reappear during subsequent pregnancies. Others do not and they may be important determinants in the response to the conceptus. Changes in uterine vessels and possibly in the maternal immune response are permanent and help to ensure satisfactory adaptation. First pregnancies are less physiological than subsequent ones; this is suggested by the reduced mean birthweight (Thomson et al 1968), increased rate of complications and raised perinatal mortality in primigravidae.

A first pregnancy need not go to term to have a helpful effect: spontaneous abortion of the first pregnancy ensures that mean birthweight in subsequent pregnancies is similar to that of other multiparous women (Billewicz & Thomson 1973, Alberman et al 1980). Therapeutic termination has a similar effect (WHO Task Force 1979). A previous spontaneous abortion also protects against pregnancy-induced hypertension but, paradoxically, not as completely as one which is therapeutically aborted or which reaches viability (MacGillivray 1958, Beck 1985, Strickland et al 1986). More abortions do not confer additional protection. Curiously, however, increasing gravidity increases the risk of spontaneous abortion (Naylor & Warburton 1979).

Maternal age influences adaptation to pregnancy. Women can conceive in any decade from the first to the sixth; it may not be calendar age so much as the number of years following menarche or even those preceding the menopause which is important. The probability of conceiving an aneuploid fetus is possibly determined by the interval between conception and the menopause (Brook et al 1984). Spontaneous abortion and an empty gestation sac are both more frequent at the extremes of reproductive age (McFadyen 1985). Before the menarche, increase in pelvic size is slower than increase in height. After the menarche growth in height continues for only 2 years whereas pelvic diameter continues to enlarge for 5–12 years (Moerman 1982). By the time women reach 18, the age of the menarche and pelvic capacity are not well related, but among younger girls those who have an early menarche are shorter and have a smaller pelvis than those who start to menstruate when they are older. This difference is not of great clinical significance in most societies but if a girl conceives when she is in her early teens she is not only small but her pelvis will be even less capacious than would be expected from her height so that if she survives the pregnancy the chances of her sustaining a vesicovaginal fistula are high (McFadyen 1962, Tahzib 1983). Nature may be partly on her side, however, for among a group of Nigerian girls who were pregnant at 13–16 years, more than half grew 2–16 cm in height during the pregnancy; this reduced the proportion who had mechanical problems in labour (Harrison 1985). The rest of her body is less likely to adapt satisfactorily to the pregnancy. In every society, pregnancy-induced hypertension is commoner in young mothers (Stearn 1963, Harrison 1985). It is not a situation in which youngest is best: 18–25 years of age is probably the period for optimal physiological adaptation (Baird & Thomson 1969).

The older woman has other problems. Her development is complete but the physiological changes of ageing or concurrent disease may prevent the development of a totally healthy pregnancy although only a minority exhibit frank pathology. She may have developed habits with cumulative effects; for example, the higher risk of retarded fetal growth in women of 35 or more who smoke (Chattinguis et al 1985) may be a consequence of the effects of tobacco on her cardiovascular system. Increasing age raises the possibility of fetal chromosome anomalies and of dizygotic twins (Campbell et al 1974). After the age of 35 blood vessels become less flexible (Roach & Burton 1957) and with increasing age both systolic and diastolic blood pressures rise (MacGillivray et al 1969). In the childbearing age group this is rarely of clinical significance but it is worth remembering that at any age a primigravida with a normal pregnancy has a higher blood pressure than a multigravida (Christianson 1976).

Many diseases are covert in the childbearing ages; abnormalities of carbohydrate metabolism, bacteriuria, chronic renal disease, hypertension and many other disorders may be undetected before conception, yet affect the mother's reaction to pregnancy. Treatment of disease may also modify reactions. Many women are on long-term treatment with steroids, non-steroidal analgesics, drugs affecting the adrenergic system or other drugs which can affect their mechanisms of adaptation. Treatment of involuntary infertility with gonadotrophins or other drugs may have an effect, but little is known about this apart from an increased rate of abortion (Australian In Vitro Fertilisation Collaborative Group 1985). Many of these women are however poor reproducers who can be recognized by their history of recurrent abortion or other obstetric problems as being less likely to respond physiologically to the stimulus of pregnancy (Gibson 1973).

Social class and reproductive performance are related for the lower the social class the worse is pregnancy outcome. Since adaptation and outcome are also related, it is likely that social class does affect how well the mother adapts, but there is little direct evidence for this. Physiological investigations and reference ranges of normality do not often define the social class of the population on which they are based. Young age at first conception, high parity which depletes stores, smoking, inappropriate diet, not knowing what care and advice is available — all are associated with lower social class and may affect adaptation. Even the effect of smoking is social class-related (Rush & Cassano 1983). While reduced birthweight is found in smokers of all classes, increased perinatal mortality is present only in smokers of classes III, IV and V. Studies of the non-pregnant may, however, be relevant to the mechanism of the effects of social class on maternal adaptation. Iron stores are frequently low in lower social class women, and cell-mediated immune responses are less effective in iron deficiency (Jacobs 1977). Other less well defined deficiencies may also affect adaptation. Fibrinogen levels in the blood are raised in lower social class men and women (Markowe et al 1985). Raised fibrinogen increases viscosity which in pregnancy is associated with poor results. More observations such as these could be illuminating but would be better done during pregnancy.

Heavy work may also affect adaptation. Certainly in pregnancy the respiratory system does not respond to increasing workloads as well as in the non-pregnant (Artal et al 1986), but in both pregnant sheep and women training increases physical work capacity (Errkkola 1976) and uterine blood flow during exercise (Curet et al 1976). Africans who work hard adopt methods which are economical in energy use (Thomson & Baird 1967, Maloiy et al 1986). Such satisfactory dynamic adaptation may reflect good physiological adjustment to pregnancy, but only indirectly. Raised blood pressure at conception affects adaptation and at age 36 (an age relevant to childbearing) hypertension is more common in lower than upper social classes (Wadsworth et al 1985). Although many data such as these suggest that there is a social class effect on maternal adaptation to pregnancy, accurate and specific information is incomplete.

The effects of social class and of ethnic origin are not always clearly differentiated. In part this is due to the difficulty of allocating one ethnic group to another's social classification. If an Asian husband was a qualified accountant before moving to the UK where he runs a shop, what is his real social class? Religion may also be associated with differences in traditions and practices; in diet there are variations which could affect birthweight and other measures of adaptation. Intermarriage between close relatives reduces mean birthweight (Rao & Imbarj 1977). Hindus have lighter babies than Europeans, even when the weights are adjusted for maternal size and the other variables relevant to birthweight (McFadyen et al 1984). This is not due to calorie deficiency as both groups have equal intake from different diets. Essential nutrients can be in short supply or the balance of constituents may be relevant. High fibre content reduces blood oestrogen (Hughes 1986), which is associated with delay in sexual maturation. Dietary differences may also account for the wide range of twinning rates among neighbouring rural Africans (Nylander 1978). Migration unavoidably alters factors such as the hardness of water, which is relevant to maternal health and usually leads to gradual alteration in diet and social patterns. Whatever the mechanism, migration appears also to affect maternal adaptation. For example, mean birthweight falls in Jewish women who move from North Africa to Israel; the longer they live in Israel the more it falls (Yudkin et al 1983).

Ethnic variations also influence some basic physiological differences. Nigerians have a smaller non-pregnant blood volume than Europeans, so that while an increase of 1270 ml during pregnancy is a 55% increase (Harrison 1966), it is considerably less than occurs in Europeans. Negroid peoples may not have a developed renal dopamine response to sodium as it is not required in warm and humid climates (Lee 1981) but the relevance of this and other differences to pregnancy has not been fully explored. Some features of other communities have however been examined in detail. While Indian Asians have lipid changes in pregnancy which are almost identical with those of whites (Rouse et al 1985a), the Asians require a higher level of insulin in the blood to maintain the same blood sugar (Rouse et al 1985b). Asians have a lower blood pressure but a similar pattern of change during pregnancy to Europeans (McFadyen et al 1989). Vegetarian Asians have low serum vitamin B_{12} levels without suffering ill effects from it possibly because of an effective enterohepatic circulation of the vitamin (Abraham et al 1985). This wide range of ethnic similarities and differences is relevant to the construction of reference ranges and to the recognition that normality is not the same for each race or even for racial subgroups.

The number of fetuses in the uterus determines the extent of many adaptive changes. While electrolyte concentrations, osmolality and other indices of the *milieu intérieur* are the same in single and multiple pregnancy, the increase in blood volume is 30% greater with twins and 50% greater with quadruplets. Plasma volume increases proportionately more with twins than singletons so haemodilution is greater (Rovinsky & Jaffin 1965, MacGillivray et al 1971, Fullerton et al 1965). Total body water increase is greater in twins, even in the first trimester, so that weight gain is increased by more than that of the additional conceptus. Cardiac output, glomerular filtration rate, uterine blood flow and tidal volume increases are greater than in singletons. Mothers carrying twins have more potential stresses on almost all of their systems than mothers of singletons.

GENERAL EFFECTS OF PREGNANCY ON THE MOTHER

Pregnancy affects each system, and some in several ways. The substance common to every system is water and this increases from early pregnancy. The mean total increase is about 8.5 litres although there is wide individual variation. It is one of the few adaptations in which there is no difference between primigravid and multiparous women (Hytten et al 1966). The greater the increase in total body water, the more likely is the mother to become oedematous and clinically detectable oedema appears in half of all pregnancies. Since oedema in otherwise normal pregnancies is associated with increased birthweight and reduced perinatal mortality (Thomson et al 1967) it is an index of good physiological adaptation. The increase in body water deduced from the amount calculated to be present in the fetus, amniotic fluid, placenta and maternal tissues is 2.5–3 litres short of the actual increase. The deficit is due partly to oedema fluid and partly to increased hydration of the connective tissue ground substance. This leads to laxity and swelling of connective tissue and consequent changes in joints which occur mainly in the last trimester and are not related to maternal age. It is, however, more marked in those having second than first babies (Calguneri et al 1982). These joint changes, together with the postural changes consequent on the alteration in the centre of gravity, produce much of the backache and other aches which are so common in pregnancy. The symphysis pubis may become very lax and extremely painful (especially during walking) but this has physiological benefit, because as it occurs the capacity of the pelvis increases (Abramson et al 1934). Generalized tissue swelling produces corneal swelling and intraocular pressure changes, gingival oedema and the common and persistent symptons arising in the cranial sinuses resulting from their increased vascularity (Fabricant 1960). It may also produce tracheal oedema which can lead to problems with anaesthesia if intubation is required and the carpal tunnel syndrome often develops.

Extra energy is required during pregnancy to fuel the growth of the conceptus and for the increased work which the mother must do because she is pregnant. The total requirement has been calculcated to be 80 000 kcal, of which 36 000 is for maintenance metabolism (Hytten & Leitch 1971). This estimate may be too high. Studies in the Gambia (Lawrence et al 1984) and in Glasgow (Durnin 1985) suggest that the additional energy required for a successful pregnancy is 13 000–20 000 kcal. The difference between the calculated and observed requirements arises because the calculation assumes a steady increase in resting metabolic rate which does not occur. Among the well nourished, or those whose diet has been supplemented, there is little change in the first 10 weeks of pregnancy; a gradual rise from then until 36 weeks of 50–100 kcal/day and an increase of 200–300 kcal/day in the final 4 weeks. All this occurs with no change in maternal activity, or at most a slight reduction close to term (Durnin 1985). In rural Africans with a low food intake, resting metabolism falls in the first 2 weeks and may not return to prepregnancy levels until 25–30 weeks. In these women, the total energy cost of pregnancy may be as little as 1000 kcal but this is associated with low birthweight (Lawrence et al 1984).

Weight gain in pregnancy is usually in the range of 10–12 kg. It comprises increases in maternal body water, fat and other tissues but at term 40% of the weight gained is in the fetus, amniotic fluid, placenta and uterus (Hytten 1980). The rate of weight gain is fairly steady throughout pregnancy and in the last trimester the mean is about

0.4 kg/week. The total gained during pregnancy is slightly greater in younger women, and possibly in primigravidae than in multigravidae but the difference is not large enough to affect the clinical significance of weekly weight gain. Overall weight gain has a positive association with birthweight (Simpson et al 1965), with low weight gain being associated with light babies. There may be a fall in weight during the first trimester because of nausea and vomiting, but this is usually made up quickly from about 15 weeks.

While the physiology of early morning sickness is uncertain it is associated with a satisfactory outcome for the pregnancy. Those who report vomiting to their doctor are less likely to abort or have a preterm or stillborn child (Klebanoff et al 1985). Other common reasons for failure to gain weight in physiological amounts are dieting, vomiting due to oesophageal reflux or diarrhoea. Excessive weight gain is sometimes a consequence of reducing or stopping smoking (Hofstetter et al 1986).

Fat deposition accounts for about 3.5 kg of weight gain. It accumulates in the abdominal wall, upper back, hips and thighs. Fat deposition is most rapid between 20 and 30 weeks (Taggart et al 1967) and is possibly less in those who have generalized oedema. The other tissues which contribute to weight gain are shown in Figure 10.1.

Diurnal, circadian and other rhythms change but there is no consistent pattern. In normotensive pregnancy the blood pressure has a 24-hour periodicity initially but after 30 weeks this shortens to 20 hours (Ruff et al 1982). Sodium excretion shows two patterns: in the ambulant, it peaks at night (Kalousek et al 1969) whereas in the recumbent, it peaks near the middle of the day (Lindheimer et al 1973). Another rhythm which changes in many women is sleep. Insomnia is common but there are often good reasons for this, including nocturia, excessive fetal movements or feeling too hot because of peripheral vasodilatation. Insomnia can also be a sign of depression.

Baroreceptors and other sensing mechanisms are reset to aid physiological adaptation. Osmoregulation uses the same arginine vasopressor (AVP) mechanism as in the non-pregnant woman but the threshold for AVP secretion and thirst is set 6–8 mosmol/kg lower (Davison et al 1984). The volume-sensing mechanism is also reset (Davison 1984), as is that for respiratory regulation.

Adrenoceptors may increase in number during pregnancy. Animal experiments suggest that α-receptor responsiveness increases with oestrogens and β-receptor with progesterone (Roberts et al 1977). While this occurs in the human uterus it does not occur in all tissues, for example in human platelets (Roberts et al 1986).

The fetoplacental unit produces hormones which affect the mother. Renin, human placental lactogen, oestrogens, progesterone and others pass into the maternal circulation and exert their activity. Fetal excretion across the placenta may contribute to serum levels in the mother's blood. Some of the plasma proteins which bind and transport hormones,

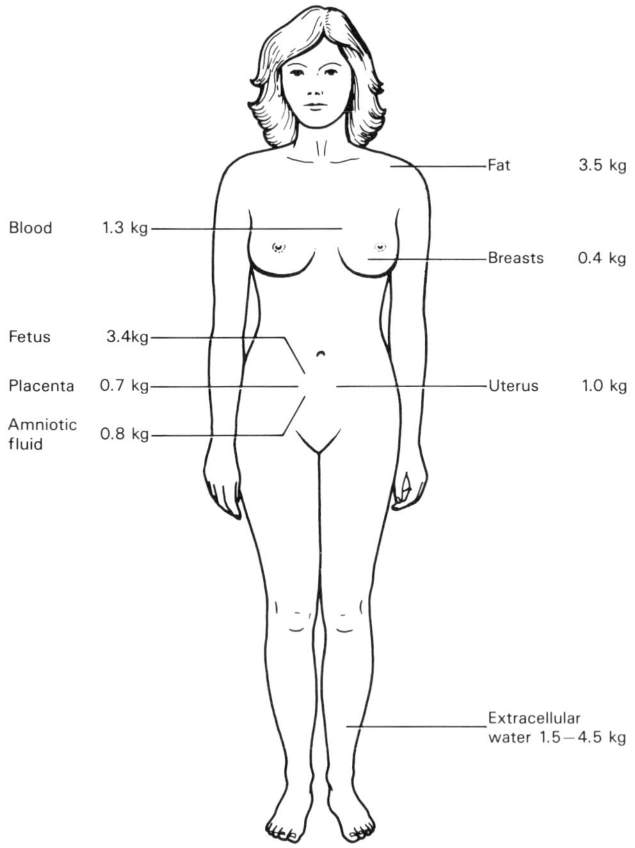

Fig. 10.1 The tissues which form the major part of weight gain in pregnancy (after Hytten 1980). There is considerable variation; the range in normal pregnancy is from 0 to 23 kg. Mean weight gain in primigravidae is 12.5 kg.

drugs and other substances in the circulation increase during pregnancy. For example, total globulin increases but albumin remains unchanged. Thyroxine-binding globulin increases from increased hepatic synthesis (Dowling et al 1960). Hormone binding also varies. For example, aldosterone is not tightly bound, so its rising concentration in plasma during pregnancy probably implies increasing biological activity. Desoxycorticosterone levels are also raised in the plasma but the compound binds avidly to globulin. Nevertheless, secretion is increased enough to produce normal free desoxycorticosterone levels in plasma which will be metabolically active (Nolten et al 1979).

Plasma aldosterone rises within 2 weeks of conception; by mid-pregnancy it is 3–5 times the non-pregnant level and by 36 weeks it is 8–10 times that level (Weir et al 1975). This balances the rise in plasma progesterone from the placenta and the normal pregnancy increase in glomerular filtration rate, both of which promote sodium loss and potassium retention (Sundsfjord 1971). Both progesterone and oestrogen increase plasma renin substrate, which reaches 2–3 times the non-pregnant level at 30 weeks, so that the renin–angiotensin–aldosterone activation balances the sodium-losing volume-reducing effect of progesterone.

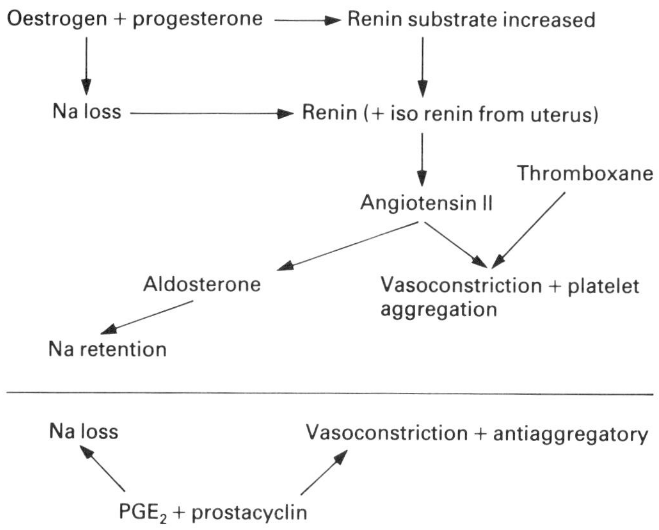

Fig. 10.2 Blood pressure in pregnancy is maintained within the normal range by a balance between mechanisms which affect the circulation. This scheme helps to explain why aspirin is effective in preventing low birthweight in pre-eclampsia, but it is incomplete. Plasma α-natriuretic peptide, calcitonin gene-related peptide and other physiological substances are also relevant to cardiovascular control.

Plasma angiotensin II increases to twice normal non-pregnant levels within 2 weeks of conception (Weir et al 1975). If this very active vasopressor compound was not antagonized the maternal blood pressure would rise quickly. It does not in normal pregnancy, due to increased synthesis of the vasodilators prostaglandin E_2 (PGE_2) and prostacyclin (PGI_2), which also have an antiaggregatory effect on platelets (Bolton et al 1981, Broughton Pipkin et al 1982). The effects of PGI_2 are balanced by the vasoconstrictor and aggregatory thromboxane. It is by the maintenance of equilibrium between changes such as these that the physiology of normal pregnancy is maintained (Fig. 10.2). If equilibria are upset pathology appears. Pathological processes are complex: reduction in production of PGE_2 and PGI_2 would lead not only to vasoconstriction and increased platelet aggregation but because their vasodilator and natriuretic effects on the kidney would also be reduced, glomerular filtration would be reduced and sodium retained. Fortunately, most systems have a large reserve of normal function and can maintain the correct balance of adaptive changes necessary for a healthy normal pregnancy.

INDIVIDUAL SYSTEMS

Cardiovascular

Cardiac output increased by 1.5 l/min to 6.5–7 l/min in the first 10 weeks of pregnancy and is maintained at that level to term (Walters et al 1966). Pulse rate rises by about 15 beats/min and stroke volume also rises by about 10%. In labour, cardiac output rises by 30% during each contraction with an increase in stroke volume but no rise in heart rate (Hendricks 1958). The increase is less in the lateral than in the supine position because the supine position interferes less with flow to the heart between contractions for the uterus is not compressing the inferior vena cava (Lees et al 1967). Blood expressed from the uterus by each contraction produces a rise in central venous pressure of 3–5 mmHg and largely accounts for the increase in cardiac output. Arterial pressure increases by 10–20 mmHg following this increase in central venous pressure and with the peripheral vasoconstriction which starts with every contraction (Herbert et al 1958). The effort of pushing in the second stage raises both cardiac output and blood pressure even higher in many women. The normotensive healthy cardiovascular system can cope with these changes but cardiac disease or hypertensive disease in addition may produce progressive or sudden deterioration.

Severe illness may be mimicked by these physiological changes. Early or mid-systolic functional murmurs develop in many women; these cannot be differentiated during pregnancy from those due to significant cardiac or valvular pathology. They may be very loud along the left edge of the sternum, develop during mid-pregnancy and disappear a few days after delivery. Some of these arise in the mammary vessels (Tabatznik et al 1960) and others are functional (Cutforth & MacDonald 1966). Their importance is that healthy women have been treated as potential cardiac problems during pregnancy and the puerperium until these functional murmurs disappear as the cardiovascular system returns to normal. They are due not only to the increased cardiac output and change in configuration of the heart but also to the physiological haemodilution which occurs in pregnancy.

Haemodilution is not due to a fall in total circulating haemoglobin because the red cell mass increases progressively during pregnancy by about 18% in women not given iron supplements and by 30% in those who are supplemented (Hytten & Leitch 1971). The plasma volume, however, increases by almost 50% in healthy women (Pirani et al 1973) so that there is an apparent haemodilution. This is greater in multigravid than in primigravid women and in multiple than in single pregnancies (Fig. 10.2). It is positively associated with birthweight (Hytten & Paintin 1963) and the increase is less marked in poor reproducers who recurrently abort or have low birthweight children (Gibson 1973). The advantages of the increase in circulating volume are that it helps to compensate for the increased blood flow to the uterus and other organs and it reduces the viscosity of the blood (Baum 1966) which improves capillary flow. Apparent anaemia may therefore be a sign of excellent physiological adjustment to pregnancy while a high haemoglobin may be a sign of pathology.

Measurement of the circulating blood volume is not practical clinically, but a useful assessment can be made from Coulter counter measurements. In this context, the most important are the packed cell volume (PCV) and the mean

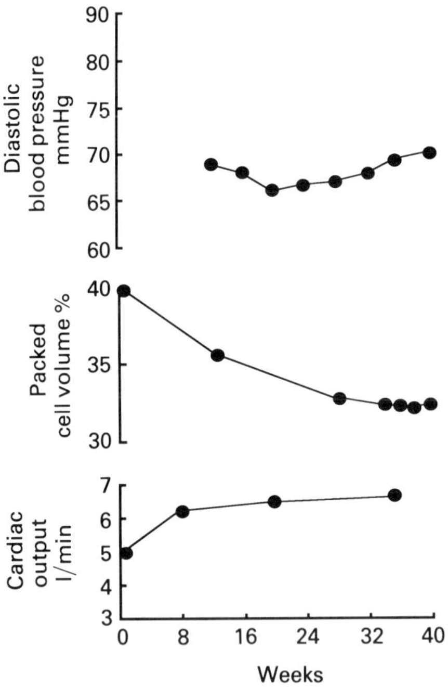

Fig. 10.3a *Cardiac output* is related to body size so there is wide variation at the beginning of pregnancy but in the average woman it is 5 l/min. During pregnancy cardiac output increases by 1.5–3 l/min, most of this occurring in the first trimester. Changes in cardiac output are independent of changes in blood volume (Rovinsky & Jaffin 1965).

Packed cell volume: with haemodilution the packed cell volume decreases progressively in normal pregnancy until around 34 weeks, and then rises slightly. If the woman takes oral iron during the pregnancy the packed cell volume is 0.5–3% higher.

Diastolic blood pressure falls early in pregnancy, the lowest levels being at 16–20 weeks, then rising to term. The values shown here are for multigravid women with singleton pregnancies: in primigravid mothers mean diastolic pressure is 1–3 mmHg higher at all gestational ages (Christianson 1976). Systolic pressure shows a similar pattern but the later increase is less.

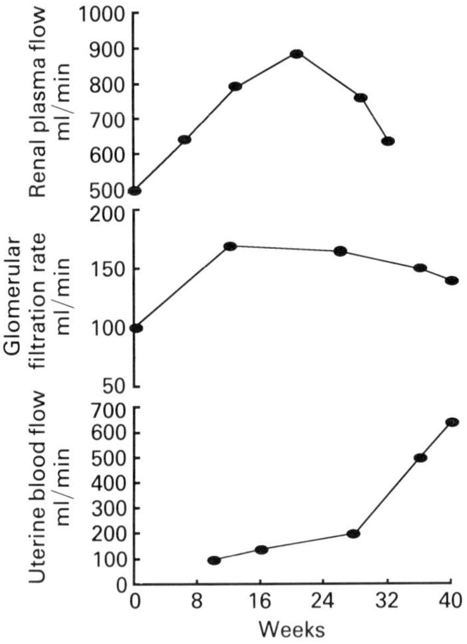

Fig. 10.3b *Uterine blood flow* is 12–15 ml/100 g conceptus throughout pregnancy. As the myometrium and its contents enlarge total flow increases. Intervillous flow near term is 65–120 ml/100 g placenta/min.

Glomerular filtration rate and renal plasma flow: both increase during pregnancy but while the glomerular filtration rate remains raised for the whole of the pregnancy renal plasma flow falls in the third trimester.

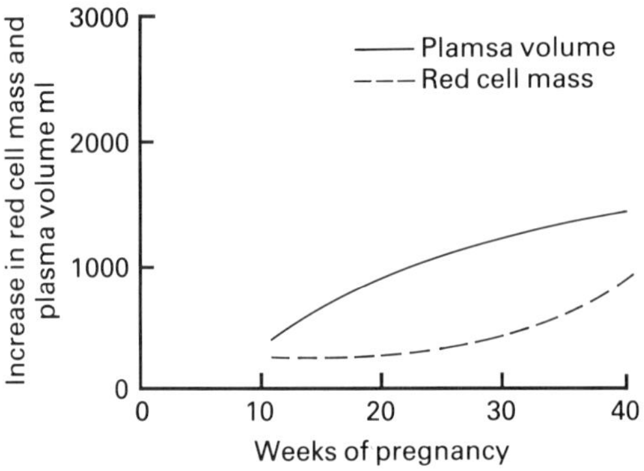

Fig. 10.4 The increase in plasma volume is greater in multigravid than in primigravid mothers, and greater in multiple than singleton pregnancies. The red cell mass shows a similar pattern of increase but is proportionately less, so haemoglobin levels in the blood are reduced.

cell volume (MCV). The MCV is steady or rises in normal pregnancy from 82–84 fl in the first trimester to 86–100 fl or more at term (Taylor & Lind 1976, Chanarin et al 1977), being greatest in those who are iron-supplemented. Thus in those who have a normal MCV at the start of pregnancy and a normal increase during it, a PCV of 36 or less early in pregnancy, falling to 32 in the third trimester is a sign of normality and a haemoglobin of 9 g/dl in these circumstances would be within normal limits. On the other hand, a PCV of 40 early in pregnancy which does not fall below 38 is likely to be a sign of unsatisfactory physiological change and a haemoglobin of 14.5 g/dl would actually represent a warning signal of risk pregnancy with a reduced plasma value. Both the actual values and the pattern of change are significant in this assessment (Fig. 10.3, 10.4).

The output from the heart is not distributed in the same way in the pregnant woman as in the non-pregnant woman. There is peripheral vasodilatation, with a rise in temperature of the hands and feet which is greater in smokers than non-smokers (Ashton 1975). While flow to the uterus and kidneys also rises, that to the brain does not (McCall 1949) nor does flow to the liver (Munnell & Taylor 1947, Laaks et al 1971).

Blood pressure does not rise with the increase in cardiac output. While the systolic pressure remains almost constant, the diastolic pressure falls during the first trimester and reaches its lowest level at 16–20 weeks, the mean fall being 15 mmHg or possibly more; after that it rises again to reach its early pregnancy level by term (MacGillivray et al 1969). These observations were made on women who were sitting. If the blood pressure is taken with the mother supine, 70% have a fall in blood pressure of at least 10% and in 8%

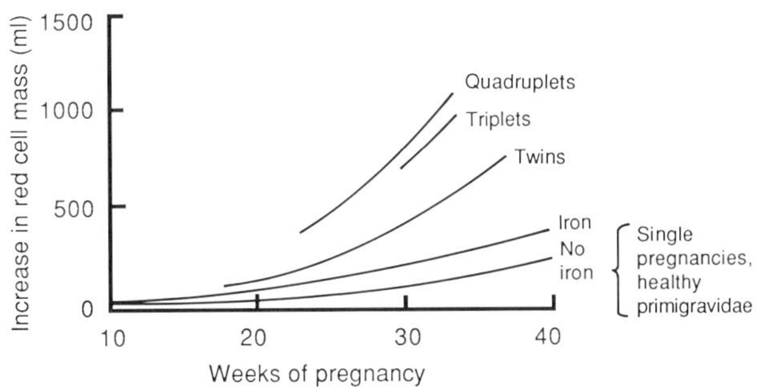

Fig. 10.5a Red cell mass in single and multiple pregnancies.

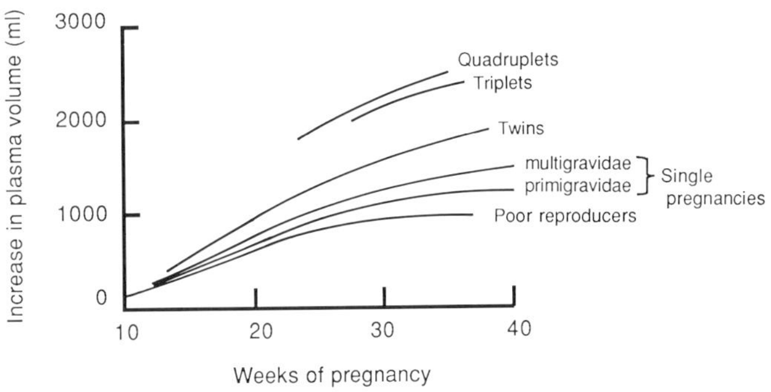

Fig. 10.5b Plasma volume in single and multiple pregnancies.

it falls by 30–50% (Holmes 1960). The supine position leads to compression of the inferior vena cava at its bifurcation (Lees et al 1967) and of the aorta from the level of the first lumbar vertebra to its bifurcation (Bieniarz et al 1968) by the uterus once it has enlarged sufficiently to do so.

Late in pregnancy the uterus may completely obliterate the lumen at the level of the bifurcation. This reduces flow to the right heart which is partly compensated for by increased systemic vascular resistance. If this compensatory mechanism is inadequate, blood pressure falls. This fall is less marked once the fetal head engages (Holmes 1960, Lees et al 1967). That most women show only a fall in blood pressure and do not develop the supine hypotensive syndrome is due to collateral venous return to the heart via the paravertebral veins and azygos vessels (Kerr et al 1964) and to the uterine venous return via the ovarian veins, also bypassing the constricted inferior vena cava (Bieniarz et al 1969). The fall in blood pressure in the remainder of women is not consistent: it may be marked if they have an illness and is particularly important if there is a shock. Obstetric intervention may unintentionally have a similar effect: placing a pregnant woman in the lithotomy position may reduce her cardiac output by 17% (Vorys et al 1961). These postural effects emphasize the necessity for standardizing the technique of measuring blood pressure in the management of individual patients or in epidemiological comparisons. Not only must the mother be relaxed at rest with the correct size of cuff properly placed on her arm, but she should be sitting or semi-recumbent with the cuff at the level of the left atrium. A standardized technique produces consistent clinically useful information.

The structure of the vessels of the uterus undergoes considerable modification during pregnancy, influencing the distribution of blood flow. Before conception, flow to the uterus is almost completely via the uterine arteries, but during pregnancy the ovarian arteries make a significant contribution in 70% of women and are particularly likely to do so if the pregnancy is multiple (Bieniarz et al 1969). In a few mothers, arteries in the round ligaments which flow from the external iliacs supply the myometrium and may join the uteroovarian anastomosis. During pregnancy, the uterine arteries dilate so that their diameter is 1.5 times that in the non-pregnant woman; the arteries which stem from them become three times as wide and the arcuate arteries which supply the placenta become 10 times as wide (Bieniarz et al 1969). The spiral arteries supplying the placenta also dilate due to physiological alterations in their structure and can reach 30 times their prepregnancy diameter.

A total of 100–150 spiral arteries supply the intervillous space. On average, there is one per 2 cm^2 of the placental bed, but they cluster so distribution is uneven (Brosens & Dixon 1966). Each placental cotyledon is supplied by at least one spiral artery. Two or three of these rise from each radial artery. Before conception they lie coiled in the myometrium and basal layers of the endometrium which are not shed at menstruation. They are muscular vessels, well able to respond to vasoactive stimuli. During pregnancy the majority of the spiral arteries in the placental bed lose this ability and dilate as a consequence of trophoblastic invasion, dilation being progressive as they approach the placenta (Ramsey et al 1976). Non-villous trophoblast invades the interstitial tissues of the decidua and myometrium in the first 10 weeks of the pregnancy (Robertson et al 1975, Pijnenborg et al 1983; Fig. 10.5). This trophoblast extends from the decidua into the walls of the spiral arteries producing distintegration of the smooth muscle. A wave of trophoblastic invasion starts at 10 weeks and is complete by 16 weeks. It is villous trophoblast and extends down the lumen of the decidual portion of the vessel (Robertson et al 1975). A second wave of endovascular trophoblastic invasion occurs at 16–22 weeks and extends more deeply to involve the myometrial portions of the spiral (but not the basal) arteries. This increases the capacity of the spiral arteries and reduces or abolishes their capacity to respond to vasoactive stimuli (Robertson et al 1967, Moll et al 1975, Zuspan et al 1981). A small proportion of arteries do not undergo these physiological changes, particularly at the periphery of the placental bed (Pijnenborg et al 1981, Khong et al 1987).

Failure of physiological change is found in the myometrial segments of the spiral arteries in pre-eclampsia and intrauterine growth retardation, which means that in these abnormal states these vessels can still respond to vasoactive stimuli and reduce flow to the intervillous space. This failure of normal adaptation is associated with maternal serum uric acid levels of 300 μmol/l or more (McFadyen et al 1986) which helps to explain the clinical value of this measurement.

Uterine blood flow increases progressively during pregnancy. At 34–40 weeks mean uterine flow in a singleton pregnancy is 500–600 ml/min but there is a wide range which is partly dependent on the method of measurement used (Assali et al 1953, Browne 1954, Blechner et al 1974). Variation is also due to gestational age and to birthweight; flow is directly proportional to birthweight (Wootton et al 1977). The intervillous space receives 84–90% of the uterine flow near term; the myometrium and decidua receive the remainder (Makowski et al 1968, Lees et al 1971). The myometrium underlying the placenta has a flow 2.5 times as great as that of the rest of the myometrium and this does not change between mid and late pregnancy (Jansson 1969).

Flow in the arcuate and radial arteries during normal pregnancy is high with low resistance. There is a considerable fall in resistance after 20 weeks, although later in pregnancy this falls only slowly (Trudinger et al 1985). In abnormal pregnancies in which the spiral arteries show unsatisfactory or incomplete physiological changes, resistance remains relatively high and flow remains low.

Flow into the intervillous space is from the openings of the spiral arteries situated under the centre of the placental cotyledons (Freese 1968). A bolus of blood emerges and spreads through the spaces between the villi. Some passes into the intervillous space of adjacent cotyledons but most leaves through veins around the artery. In the monkey (whose uterine blood supply is similar to the human) not all spiral arteries supply blood at the same time so that blood flow through them is intermittent (Martin et al 1964). Closure of these vessels may be due to myometrial contraction, but contraction of the vessel itself at the endometrial–myometrial junction is probably the commoner explanation.

Monkey spiral arteries do not undergo the physiological changes found in human pregnancy; this makes such intermittence in the human unlikely, although possible in pregnancies with incomplete physiological vascular changes. Pressure and oxygen content are highest at the centre of the cotyledonary intervillous space and fall towards its periphery (Reynolds et al 1968). In the human, mean intervillous flow at 35–42 weeks is 140 ml/100 ml intervillous blood/min (Kaur et al, 1980).

The pressure within the spiral arteries is 70–80 mmHg; in the intervillous space 5–10 mmHg and in the veins draining placenta and uterine wall 6–8 mmHg (Brown 1954, Boyd & Hamilton 1970). During labour, the pressure within the intervillous space rises to four times its resting level (Eastman 1958) so arterial flow to it slows. At the beginning of a contraction blood is expelled from the uterus but the rise in intramyometrial pressure then closes the veins. Arterial flow continues and the volume of the intervillous space may be increased (Borell et al 1965).

The vascular system of the placental bed is less well developed in first pregnancies than in later pregnancies, so flow is less in first than in subsequent pregnancies (Becker 1948). In some women, one or both ascending uterine arteries divides into two branches so that the anterior and posterior arcuate arteries arise from separate vessels. This may reduce uterine blood flow for it is certainly associated with an increased rate of abortion and unsuccessful pregnancy (Burchell et al 1978).

Compression and displacement of the aorta by the pregnant uterus diminishes placental perfusion, but this returns to normal if the mother lies on her side (Abitbol 1976). The diminution is in intervillous rather than in myometrial flow (Kauppila et al 1980). The myometrium normally receives about 10% of uterine blood flow and this is not affected by the mother's position. If she lies supine, however, intervillous flow falls by 20%. This suggests that there is a regulatory mechanism whereby the myometrium can respond to reduced perfusion.

The kidney can maintain its blood flow despite changes in perfusion pressure, probably by altering the tone of afferent and efferent arterioles. Whether or not the uterus can do the same is uncertain. Certainly in anaesthetized sheep (Greiss 1966, Ladner et al 1970) or rats (Bruce 1973) uterine blood flow is directly related to cardiac output but if this falls below a critical pressure (25–40 mmHg in sheep), uterine flow is reduced considerably more than is cardiac output. In sheep which are not anaesthetized and have been made hypertensive, the uterus may be able to autoregulate its flow (Brinkman 1975). The sheep uterus and placenta are different from the human while the rabbit has a haemochorial circulation similar to the human. The rabbit can autoregulate uterine flow in response to hypertension or hypotension provided the blood pressure does not fall below a mean arterial pressure of 40 mmHg: if this occurs renal flow is maintained but uterine flow falls (Venuto et al 1976). Human myometrial flow falls if the mother is alarmed but quickly recovers (Brown 1954), a response which protects the placenta.

In animals, myometrial flow is maintained even if placental flow is reduced by hypotension (Novy et al 1975). In hyperoxia, however, both flows are reduced, protecting the fetus against unduly high levels of oxygen (Karlsson & Kjellmer 1974). Whether or not human pregnancy possesses a similar differential response by the myometrium and placental bed is not known. While intervillous flow is dependent on a balance between prostacyclin and thromboxane (Makila et al 1986), more peripheral vessels are controlled by a combination of humoral and nervous influences. Their site may affect their response. Uterine arteries contract more strongly than myometrial when stimulated by prostaglandins but both respond equally to noradrenaline and vasopressin (Maigaard et al 1985). It is therefore possible that different vessels respond differently to stress. The extent to which physiological changes in the spiral arteries are essential for alteration in the uterine circulation is not known. Possibly in those without physiological changes the spiral vessels contract when blood pressure rises but whether or not they relax when blood pressure falls, and so help to maintain placental perfusion, remains to be established.

The venous system gradually becomes more distensible as pregnancy progresses. The mean increase is 50% (McCauseland et al 1961) but there is considerable variation. Some women have an inherited predisposition to venous laxity and are more likely to develop varicose veins in pregnancy (Reagan & Folse 1971). Those with varicose veins in pregnancy have more distensible veins than those who do not (McCauseland et al 1961). The pressure within leg veins also rises. In the legs, venous pressure rises from 9 cmH_2O early in pregnancy to 24 cmH_2O at term (McLennan 1943). Flow through the veins slows as the pressure rises, being halved by term (Wright et al 1950). The increase in pressure is due to mechanical obstruction of venous return by the pressure of the uterus on the iliac veins and inferior vena cava. The intervillous pressure is 10 mmHg and that at the confluence of the iliac veins is 16 mmHg. Venous flow from the uterine veins which occurs maximally during a uterine contraction (Bieniarz et al 1969), intermittently reduces flow in the legs. This also produces intermittent rises in central venous pressure of 2.0–4.6 mmHg (Colditz & Josey 1970) with rises during Braxton Hicks contractions being 4–10 cm saline (Palmer & Walker 1949).

The predisposition of pregnant women to varicose veins of the legs, vulva, rectum and pelvis is a consequence of their increased distensibility and pressure; this is compounded by their changed anatomy. The plexuses of veins around the vagina, uterus, bladder and rectum anastomose with each other. The superior rectal vein is part of the portal system but has no valves, so the increased pressure is communicated to all of its venous drainage and to the anastomosing plexuses.

The behaviour of the veins in the arm is not so uniform. The increase in distensibility of finger veins is greater in women who have varicose veins in their legs than in those who do not (McCauseland et al 1961) but there is disagreement between those who found a general increase (Goodrich & Wood 1964) and those who found little or none (Duncan 1967). Perhaps in the absence of the back pressure affecting the lower half of the body, inherited differences in veins may determine their behaviour in pregnancy.

The peripheral resistance of the circulation (mean arterial pressure/cardiac output) falls during pregnancy due to the general relaxation in arterial and venous tone and to the changes in the uterine vessels. In the non-pregnant woman it is 1700 $dyn/s/cm^{-5}$ but falls in the middle trimester to 980 $dyn/s/cm^{-5}$ then rises toward term to 1200–1300 $dyn/s/cm^{-5}$ (Pyorala 1966).

Respiratory system

While the lungs effect gas exchange for the mother, the placenta does it for the fetus. Effective exchange of CO_2 from fetus to mother requires the PCO_2 to be higher in the fetus than in the mother. Resetting the maternal respiratory centre achieves this. During pregnancy the threshold at which the respiratory centre is stimulated is reduced. A rise of 1 mmHg in maternal PCO_2 increases the mother's ventilation by 6 l/min instead of by the 1.5 l/min this would produce when she is not pregnant (Prowse & Gaensler 1965). This change depends on increased tidal volume but not on increased respiratory rate. The mechanics of breathing also change in pregnancy. The shape of the chest changes, with the lower ribs flaring outwards and the level of the diaphragm rising by 4 cm (Thomson & Cohen 1938). Diaphragmatic movement is increased and costal breathing reduced in pregnancy (McGinty 1938). These changes rotate the heart forwards and alter the electrocardiogram signal; this must be taken into account in pregnancy.

The pulmonary alterations in pregnancy increase tidal volume by 200 ml and vital capacity by 100–200 ml (Eng et al 1975). Thus less air is left in the lungs at the end of expiration, so less expired air is mixed with the next inspiration and the CO_2 gradient favourable for the fetus is maintained. The maternal PCO_2 is reduced to 4 kPa or lower, while fetal PCO_2 is 6 kPa. The reduction in threshold of the respiratory centre is probably a progesterone effect (a similar pattern of increased respiration is found in women treated with large doses of progestogens for endometrial carcinoma), with the raised level of oestrogen increasing the centre's sensitivity (Wilbrand et al 1959). These influences combine to make the pregnant woman prone to dyspnoea and dizzy spells (Gilbert & Auchincloss 1966). The woman whose respiratory centre is set to an alveolar PCO_2 of 4.7 kPa when she is not pregnant may well become dyspnoeic when alveolar PCO_2 falls to 4 kPa during pregnancy. The higher her normal PCO_2, the more likely she is to develop dyspnoea at rest when pregnant. Exercise has an exaggerated effect on such dyspnoeic women. The PCO_2 can be reduced to 2 kPa or lower, producing cerebral arteriospasm and dizziness. Even without such extreme changes, pregnant women produce a less effective response than non-pregnant women to work (Artal et al 1986). Anaesthesia is affected by these physiological changes. If the normally hyperventilating pregnant patient hypoventilates under general anaesthesia, she requires less inhalational agents than are required by a woman who is not pregnant (Schnider 1981). The cardiovascular and respiratory changes of pregnancy do not have deleterious effects during air travel (Huch et al 1986).

Genital tract

The uterus consists of smooth muscle arranged in bundles which are 100 μm in diameter. Before conception the uterus weighs about 100 g and is pear-shaped, measuring 10 × 5 × 2.5 cm. During pregnancy, it grows initially by hyperplasia of the myometrium and later by hypertrophy and stretching of the cells (Csapo et al 1965, Marshall 1973). By 20 weeks it weighs 300–400 g and by term 1100 g, almost

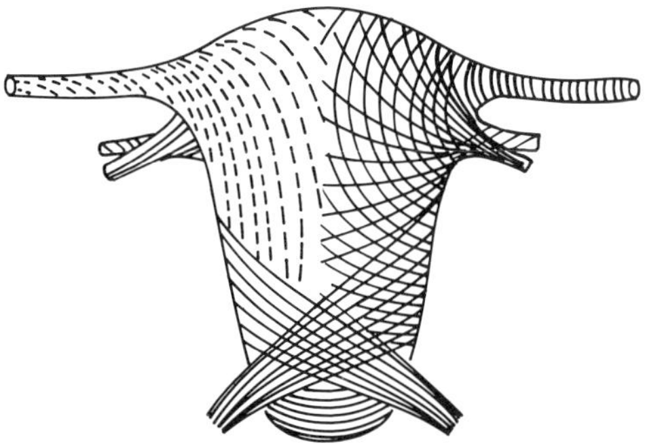

Fig. 10.6 The innermost longitudinal layer of muscle fibres is shown on the left and the outer circular layers on the right. These layers extend into the Fallopian tube, round ligament, and supporting structures of the uterus.

completely filling the abdominal cavity (Hytten & Cheyne 1969). The individual cells lengthen from 50 μm in their non-pregnant state to 200–600 μm at term. In the first half of pregnancy, the muscle cells in the fundus are stretched to 70–90% of the optimal length for contraction. By term they have reached 90–100% of the optimal length and those in the lower segment are also close to their optimal length for isometric contraction (Wood 1964). The connective, elastic, and other tissue components of the uterus also grow during pregnancy. The cervix contains more fibrous and less muscular tissue than the body of the uterus. Only 10% of uterine muscle fibres are in the cervix (Danforth 1954, Schwalm & Dubrawsky 1966). This helps to explain the fundal dominance of uterine contraction. The uterine body and the cervix also differ in their content of glycogen, actomyosin, prostaglandins and other substances related to their activity.

The myometrium is a functional syncytium. In labour myometrial cells are coupled by low resistance pathways (gap junctions) so that the wave of contraction can pass rapidly through the organ (Marshall 1973). The myometrium is arranged in three layers which interdigitate and interconnect with a characteristic pattern. The external layer is thin and passes longitudinally over the fundus, extending into the round and transverse cervical ligaments and into the vault of the vagina (Fig. 10.6). The middle layer is thick; it runs downwards and inwards from the fundus interlacing with muscle bundles from the other side and is the main muscle mass involved with parturient uterine contractions. The internal layer is thin and runs obliquely under the endometrium, forming sphincters around the openings of the Fallopian tubes and the cervix (Youssef 1958). The muscular spirals of the uterine vessels tend to uncoil as pregnancy progresses. The shape of the uterine cavity changes during pregnancy. Initially pear-shaped, it becomes spherical at about 20 weeks and elongates thereafter to term, although more slowly after 32 weeks (Gillespie 1950). Not only does this alter the shape of the cavity but it reduces the tension in the uterine wall, which becomes thinner towards term.

Spontaneous contractions of the myometrium occur from 20 weeks. They increase intrauterine pressure by 10–15 cm H_2O and may improve the circulation within the uterus. Such spontaneous uterine activity is greater in multiple than in singleton pregnancies (Newman et al 1986) and increases in strength and frequency up to term. It also facilitates the formation of the lower uterine segment by stretching and thinning the cervix between the anatomical and the histological internal os (Danforth 1947). There may also be dilatation of the cervix, the degree of which is related to the time of onset of labour, although this is far from absolute. If the cervix is completely uneffaced and closed at 42 weeks it may indicate a degree of uterine dysfunction or doubt about the calculated gestational age.

Although the uterus can function in a partially or totally denervated state, it does have afferent and efferent nerve supplies. There is an afferent pathway from uterus to hypothalamus (Ferguson 1941). Cervical cerclage may interrupt this reflex and so prevent abortion. Ferguson's reflex, by which distension of the cervix and vagina stimulates release of oxytocin (Fitzpatrick 1961, Dawood et al 1978), may in turn stimulate prostaglandin production in the myometrium (Flint et al 1975). Epidural analgesia, by blocking this reflex and preventing oxytocin release, will prolong the second stage of labour (Bates et al 1985). The cervix (internal os and isthmus) and uterine vessels are well supplied with adrenergic nerves (Owman et al 1967) while cholinergic nerves are confined to the blood vessels of the cervix (Coupland 1962). Adrenergic receptors in the myometrium have both α and β activity but near term the β activity is dominant.

The cervix undergoes characteristic changes both in early and late pregnancy. Early in the first trimester, the squamous epithelium of the ectocervix becomes hyperactive and occasionally the changes are so marked as to mimic carcinoma in situ. The endocervical epithelium also proliferates and grows out over the ectocervix. Being vascular, this tissue produces the clinical appearance of cervical erosion, a normal physiological response to the hormonal changes in pregnancy. Being mucus-secreting tissue, this proliferation adds to the physiological vaginal discharge which may become heavy enough to be noticed by the mother. These secretions within the endocervical canal produce the antibacterial mucus plug of the cervix.

Towards the end of the pregnancy, the cervical collagen network is disorganized and the amount of collagen within the cervix is reduced to one-third of the non-pregnant amount. The quantity of elastin is unchanged but there is marked accumulation of glycosaminoglycans and water (Buckingham et al 1962). These factors bring about the changes of cervical ripening. The duration of spontaneous labour is inversely proportionate to the concentration of collagen in the cervix at the beginning of dilation (Uldbjerg et al 1983). The cervix contains prostaglandin receptors, more for PGE_2 than for $PGF_{2\alpha}$. These do not appear to increase during pregnancy. The cervical stroma can synthesize eicosanoids but the relationship between these and the outcome of pregnancy or labour has yet to be established.

The round ligaments increase in length, muscular content and diameter during pregnancy. In labour contraction of the ligaments pulls the uterus forward so that the expulsive force is directed as much into the pelvis as possible. During pregnancy the ligaments may contract spontaneously or in response to movement of the uterus (Mahran & Ghaleb 1964). This may produce pain in either iliac fossa, close to the site of insertion of the ligament into the uterus where it enters the internal inguinal ring or between these two points.

The vaginal epithelium also hypertrophies and its connective tissues undergoes changes similar to those in the cervix. With this hypertrophy, the quantity of glycogen-containing cells shed into the vagina increases. Doderlein's bacilli convert this into lactic acid which produces an acid environment of pH 4.0–5.0 (Hanna et al 1985). This discourages the growth of most pathogens but yeasts thrive in it.

Endocrine system

The maternal endocrine system is modified during pregnancy by the addition of the fetoplacental unit. This produces human chorionic gonadotrophin, human placental lactogen and other unique hormones which affect the mother's endocrine organs directly or indirectly. The placenta also contains steroid metabolic pathways which are absent in the non-pregnant woman, but the capacity for the production of oestrogens and other hormones is underused before conception and can cope with the revised demands of pregnancy (Slaunwhite et al 1973). Raised oestrogen levels increase the production of the globulins which bind thyroxine, corticosteroids and the sex steroids. This increases the total plasma content of these hormones but does not necessarily raise the amount which is free in the plasma and is physiologically active. It may however be a readily available store and a protective mechanism which prevents exposure of the fetus to harmful quantities of hormones (Soloff et al 1974). Raised levels would also be required if binding sites on target organs were increased.

The psyche alters during pregnancy and, at least in part, this is a hormonal effect. Progesterone produces tiredness and dyspnoea and can also produce depression. Many pregnant women, however, are almost euphoric — a side-effect of corticosteroids. The changing balance of hormones may affect the function of the hypothalamus and higher centres. Some hypothalamic functions continue normally but the level at which feedback control is set can alter. Dexamethasone does not suppress adrenocorticotrophic hormone (ACTH) secretion as effectively as in the non-pregnant woman (Nolton & Rueckert 1981), which results from the control being set at a higher level. It may also be due to the secretion of placental ACTH (Genazzani et al 1975), to a fetal contribution to the level of maternal cortisol which

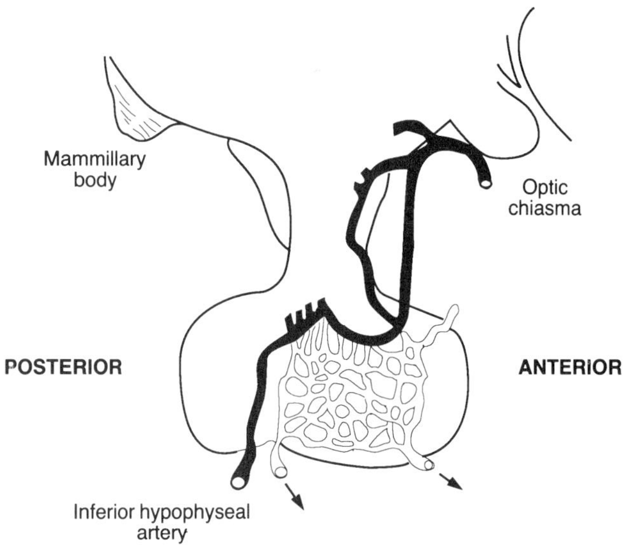

Fig. 10.7 The posterior pituitary has a direct arterial blood supply from the inferior hypophyseal artery. The anterior pituitary has no direct arterial supply. Blood reaches the anterior pituitary only after it has passed through the hypothalamus. The superior hypophyseal arteries divide into capillaries in the hypothalamus which drain directly into vessels in the anterior pituitary, where they become vascular sinusoids among the secretory cells of the anterior pituitary. There is also an anastomosis between the superior and inferior hypophyseal arteries from which vessels pass into the anterior pituitary. These portal systems are the route for hypothalamic-releasing factors to reach the anterior pituitary. Its trophic hormones enter the general circulation by veins which pass from the gland into the dural venous sinuses.

regulates the hypothalamic response (Fenel et al 1980), or to suppression of pituitary ACTH secretion by progesterone or oestrogen (Carr et al 1979). Not only is the psyche affected by pregnancy, the whole system of endocrine control undergoes perturbation.

Pituitary gland

The pituitary gland increases in weight by 30% in first pregnancies and by 50% in subsequent conceptions (Rasmussen 1934). Even this normal increase can produce headache. It also increases the gland's sensitivity to haemorrhage, a feature which is accentuated by the lack of a direct arterial supply to the anterior pituitary (Fig. 10.7). Since blood is delivered via a portal system, in which the pressure is lower than the systemic arterial pressure, the effects of any hypotension will be greater in the anterior pituitary circulation; hypotension may be aggravated by thrombotic tendencies or necrotic swelling (Sheehan & Stanfield 1961). Since the posterior pituitary has a direct arterial supply, its function is rarely permanently affected by hypotension.

The increase in weight of the pituitary is not due to an increase in the number or size of all cells. While the prolactin-secreting cells do increase, the number of growth hormone-secreting cells is reduced (Golubuff & Ezrin 1969), their secretion possibly being suppressed by high levels of cortisol or human placental lactogen. Plasma prolactin begins to rise within a few days of conception and by term may be 10–20 times as high as in the non-pregnant woman (see Chapter 25). The secretion of other anterior pituitary hormones may be unchanged or reduced. Thyroid-stimulating hormone secretion is not different from that in the non-pregnant woman (except that it is possibly lower in the first trimester) and it responds normally to thyrotropin-releasing hormone from the hypothalamus (Kannan 1973). There is, however, a blunted response of follicle-stimulating hormone to gonadotrophin-releasing hormone (GnRH). This shows a progressive decrease, finally leading to no response, 3 weeks after ovulation (Jeppsson et al 1977). The luteinizing hormone response also disappears but not until some weeks after the loss of GnRH response (Miyake et al 1977). This blunting of GnRH response may be due to human chorionic gonadotrophin, as it starts to rise before oestrogen levels rise, and before progesterone or prolactin rises significantly (Miyake et al 1977). ACTH also shows a subnormal response to glucocorticoid deprivation and metyrapone and to ACTH produced by the placenta (Genazzani et al 1975). A reduced rate of cortisol clearance (Migeon et al 1957, Beitins et al 1973) would also account for the increased response of cortisol and 17-hydroxycorticosterone (17-OHCS) to ACTH while urinary 17-OHCS and ketosteroid are unchanged (Jailer et al 1959). ACTH does not cross the placenta.

The posterior pituitary hormone oxytocin is discussed in Chapters 25 and 62. Vasopressin (ADH) is discussed in Chapter 25.

Adrenal gland

Adrenal cortical metabolism in pregnancy is closely related to the fetoplacental unit. The placenta passes oestrogens and other hormones into the maternal circulation; the cortisol which passes from fetus to mother may affect her blood levels and their rate of change. The kidneys may produce DOC (deoxycorticosterone) (Winkel et al 1980).

The maternal adrenal glands do not enlarge during pregnancy but there is an increase in width of the zona fasciculata, with histological changes there suggesting increased secretion (Whiteley & Stoner 1957). Plasma cortisol and other corticosteroids increase progressively from 12 weeks to term, reaching 3–5 times their non-pregnant levels (Gemzell 1953, Wintour et al 1978). The half-life of cortisol in the plasma is prolonged (Migeon et al 1957) and its metabolic clearance rate is reduced. This is associated with a rise in transcortin levels to 2–3 times above the non-pregnant level at term. The proportion of unbound cortisol does not change significantly during pregnancy, partly because the rising concentration of progesterone fills 10% of binding sites (Dunn et al 1981). There is no change in glucocorticoid receptor numbers in the cells during pregnancy (Nolten et al 1981) but again the high levels of progesterone may compete for binding sites. Other corticosteroids show similar patterns during normal pregnancy (Wintour et al 1978).

Thyroid

The thyroid increases in size during pregnancy. A frank goitre may develop due to increased blood flow and hyperplasia of the follicular tissue (Stoffer et al 1957). Clearance of iodide from the plasma by the thyroid increases (Aboul-Khair et al 1964) unless the diet has a high iodine content (Dworkin et al 1966). Renal clearance of iodine doubles by the end of the first trimester and then remains constant for the rest of the pregnancy (Man et al 1969). During pregnancy, thyroid-binding globulin levels also double but other thyroid-binding proteins do not increase. The result of these changes is that while free plasma triiodothyronine (T3) and thyroxine (T4) remain at the non-pregnant level or fall (Franklyn et al 1983), the mother remains euthyroid.

Long-acting thyroid-stimulating hormone, human thyroid-stimulating immunoglobulin and T4 all cross the placenta but in normal pregnancy the quantities are not sufficient to produce ill effects on the fetus. Iodide crosses the placenta and satisfies fetal requirements. Thyrotrophin-releasing hormone also crosses the placenta but thyroid-stimulating hormone does not.

Parathyroid

Parathormone levels are raised in pregnancy (Pitkin 1975), increasing calcium absorption by the mother and thus offsetting loss across the placenta to the fetus. Neither calcitonin nor parathormone cross from mother to fetus. By term, serum parathormone is higher in the mother but calcitonin is higher in the fetus (Somaan et al 1975), encouraging the deposition of bone in the fetus.

Pancreas

The size of the islets of Langerhans and the number of β cells increase during pregnancy, as does the number of receptor sites for insulin (Puavilai et al 1982). The serum level of insulin rises during the second half of pregnancy; its response to a glucose load is a greater increase than in the non-pregnant woman but blood sugar does not fall in proportion — it is less (Spellacy et al 1965, Lind et al 1968). This resistance to the action of insulin which appears during normal pregnancy may be due to the presence of human placental lactogen, prolactin, or other pregnancy hormones; it is not a consequence of changes in hepatic utilization or in peripheral sensitivity to insulin, which remain at non-pregnant levels (Kuhl et al 1981, Cowett 1985). As pregnancy advances the resistance increases. One practical effect of this and other physiological changes in pregnancy is that the upper limit of normal blood sugar in a glucose tolerance test increases from 7.5 mmol/l in the second trimester to 9.6 mmol/l in the third trimester (Hatem et al 1988).

Glucagon levels are slightly raised during pregnancy, but not to the same extent as insulin. A glucose load suppresses glucagon further in pregnant than in non-pregnant women (Metzger et al 1973).

The cells in the blood

The circulating red cell mass increases by 20–30% during pregnancy; the maximum rise occurs in those who take oral iron. From the non-pregnant level of 1400 ml it can rise in singleton pregnancy by 240 ml in those who do not take iron supplements and by 400 ml in those who do (Pritchard et al 1960). In women expecting twins the increase is about 680 ml and in triplets 900 ml. The rise is due to an increase in the number and size of red cells, which have a normal 120-day lifespan (Pritchard and Adams 1960). It is accompanied by an increase in the reticulocyte count to 2% or more (Pritchard & Adams 1960; Trail 1975). In pregnant women not taking iron, red cell volume shows an increase from 82–85 to 87–88 fl, whereas in those supplemented with iron, with or without folic acid, it rises to 88–90 fl (Taylor & Lind 1976, Chanarin et al 1977). These are mean changes, but by the third trimester some individuals may have red cells of 100 fl or more yet no abnormality in their bone marrow. A possible advantage of these large red cells would be better transport of oxygen and carbon dioxide. A disadvantage would be reduced deformability of the cells in the capillary circulation although the raised fibrinogen concentration in pregnancy may counteract this tendency (Rampling & Sirs 1972).

The increased size of the red cells could be due in part to the fall in plasma oncotic pressure leading to increased red cell uptake of water. It could also be due to release of relatively immature cells from the marrow, which tend to be large. The marrow is hyperplastic with an increase in immature erythyroid precursors (De Leeuw et al 1966). The concentration of fetal haemoglobin (HbF) increases by 1–2% during pregnancy, due to an increase in the number of red cells containing HbF which are also large (Popat et al 1977). Iron is incorporated more quickly into pregnancy cells than it is in the non-pregnant woman (Pritchard & Adams 1960). The physiological mechanisms producing the increase in circulating haemoglobin are not yet clear. Although plasma erythropoietin rises during pregnancy the reticulocyte count increases and the iron stores decrease before this rise occurs (Howells et al 1986). Human placental lactogen and other hormones which increase early in pregnancy probably have erythropoietic actions.

That the marrow is able to respond so actively in normal pregnancy is surprising. While the 10 or more periods of menstruation which are suppressed contribute 250 mg of iron saved toward the cost of conception, this does not balance the 300–500 mg required for the increase in maternal haemoglobin or the 500 mg required for fetus and placenta (Scott 1962). This deficit could be compounded by reduction in iron absorption and by the loss of folic acid and other nutrients in the urine. Maternal stores of these are, however usually adequate for normal adaptation to pregnancy. Some of these are quickly replenished after delivery, but it may take months for iron stores to return to normal. Frequent pregnancies can prevent this replenishment, especially if diet is inadequate; this may produce anaemia in multigravida.

If the mother has a haemoglobinopathy, her haematological responses to pregnancy may be modified. Those with beta-thalassaemia trait have a smaller increase in their red cell mass because of the disorder of haemoglobin synthesis (Schuman et al 1973). This is not improved by iron supplementation unless there are other signs of iron deficiency.

The white cells do not show a uniform pattern of change during pregnancy. The number of eosinophils, basophils, and monocytes in each millilitre of blood does not change significantly during pregnancy (Cruikshank 1970, Pitkin & Witte 1979), but with the increase in circulating volume the total numbers of these cells are increased. Neutrophil numbers rise in the first trimester and continue to do so until about 30 weeks, after which their count remains steady: the mean value they reach is 6.8×10^9/l, but there is a wide range which may reach 20×10^9/l in normal pregnancy. Neutrophil metabolic activity increases (Poloshuk et al 1970), as does phagocytic function (Mitchell 1966). Lymphocyte counts do not change but their function is suppressed. This renders the pregnant woman more susceptible to viral infections, malaria, and leprosy (Duncan 1980).

Platelet counts decrease slightly during pregnancy but remain above 200×10^9/l in normal pregnancy (Pitkin & Witte 1979). The erythrocyte sedimentation rate rises early in pregnancy due to the increase in fibrinogen and plasma proteins; 100 mm in an hour is not uncommon in a normal pregnant woman.

The kidney and urinary tract

Early in pregnancy the mother is aware of changes in her urinary tract. Increased frequency of micturition is one of the commonest symptoms in the first trimester and frequently persists for the remainder of the pregnancy. Nocturia is physiological later in pregnancy. Passing urine even 4 times during the night is within normal limits (McFadyen et al 1973). Polydypsia by day aggravates the tendency to nocturia, as does the transfer of fluid from oedematous tissue into the general circulation when lying recumbent in bed. Fetal movements and the insomnia which is so common in pregnancy also contribute to nocturia. Stress incontinence occurs frequently during normal pregnancy, resulting from relaxation of the bladder supports (Francis 1960). The urethra normally elongates during pregnancy but this does not occur in those who develop stress incontinence (Iosif & Uemsten 1981). Bladder tone decreases and its capacity increases progressively during pregnancy but there is no residual urine after micturition (Muellner 1939). Despite the relaxation of ureters and bladder, ureteric reflux is very uncommon in normal pregnancy (Mattingly & Borkowf 1978), although it may appear during an episode of urinary tract infection (Bumpus 1924). The protection against ureteric reflux is proliferation of Waldeyer's sheath around the ureter where it passes through the bladder wall (Baird 1935).

Progressive dilatation and kinking of the ureters is found in over 90% of pregnant women and may appear as early as 6 weeks (Baird 1935). It is more marked in multiparous than primigravid women and is accompanied by a slowing of flow of urine down the ureter, perhaps by 4–6 times (Baird 1935). It is not accompanied by a decrease in ureteric tone or contractions (Rubi & Sala 1968, Mattingly & Borkowf 1978). Dilatation is greater on the right than the left due to dextrorotation of the uterus and does not extend below the pelvic brim (Dure-Smith 1970); it is due to a combination of physical obstruction by the pregnant uterus (as may occur with other large masses rising out of the pelvis) and the effects of pregnancy hormones (Hundley et al 1935, Van Wagenen & Jenkins 1948). Ureteric dilatation extends up to the calyces. Kidneys are enlarged by this, by increased glomerular size, and by increased interstitial fluid. Their length increases by 1 cm (Bailey & Rolleston 1971) and their weight by 20% (Sheehan & Lynch 1973).

Renal function changes early in pregnancy. Renal plasma flow increases from early in the first trimester, reaching 30–50% above non-pregnant levels by 20 weeks and remaining at that level until 30 weeks, when it starts to decline slowly although at term it is still above non-pregnant levels (Davison & Dunlop 1980). The glomerular filtration rate (GFR) also begins to increase soon after conception, reaching 60% above non-pregnant levels by the 16th week of gestation and remaining there for the remainder of the pregnancy (Davison 1974, 1978). The initial rise in GFR appears to be due to the rise in cardiac output but subsequently there is a fall in the resistance of the efferent glomerular arteriole (Dal Canton et al 1982). The agents which effect these changes may be intrarenal prostacyclin, angiotensin II, parathyroid hormone or prolactin. The reduction in plasma albumin which occurs early in pregnancy and remains until term tends to increase GFR by reducing the oncotic pressure within the glomerular capillaries.

Tubular function also changes during pregnancy. While the tubules are presented with increased quantities of urine because of the increased GFR, they also lose some of their reabsorptive capacity. Glucose (Davison & Hytten 1974), uric acid (Dunlop & Davison 1977), amino acids (Hytten & Cheyne 1969) and other substances are not so completely reabsorbed as in the non-pregnant woman. There is an increase in protein loss (possibly due to increased GFR) of up to 300 mg in a 24-hour period.

The plasma osmolality at which arginine vasopressor secretion is stimulated falls by 10 mosmol during pregnancy (Davison et al 1984). Renal handling of water is otherwise similar to that in the non-pregnant state, although more sensitive to maternal posture. The excretion of water in the upright position is reduced more in the pregnant than the non-pregnant woman and is also reduced by moving from lateral recumbent to supine position (Lindheimer & Weston 1969). Women who had prolonged lateral recumbency and then changed to upright had retention of sodium for 72 hours (Lindheimer et al 1973). Sitting also affects excretion of water load. In this position pregnant women have greater diuretic response than the non-pregnant and this difference is greater early in pregnancy than it is toward term (Hytten & Klopper 1963). Posture also affects circadian rhythms of sodium excretion. Recumbent pregnant women have maximal excretion in the middle of the day whereas women who are active tend to have maximum excretion at night (Kalousek et al 1969), which tends to aggravate nocturia.

Renal retention of sodium is the factor determining increased water retention in pregnancy. The mother and conceptus increase their sodium content by 500–900 nmol due to increased reabsorption by the renal tubules. Progesterone increases sodium excretion but its increase during pregnancy is balanced by the effects of increased aldosterone, mineralocorticoids and prostaglandins. It may be the increased progesterone which helps to conserve 350 nmol potassium during pregnancy.

The hyperventilation of pregnant women produces a mild alkalaemia (arterial pH 7.44) with a decrease in plasma bicarbonate. Renal bicarbonate absorption and hydrogen ion excretion are unchanged in pregnancy so that pregnant women are at a disadvantage if there is a sudden metabolic acidosis.

These changes in renal function may be beneficial in a healthy pregnancy, but the alterations in normal values in blood and urine which they produce must be recognized as part of the physiological adaptation to normal pregnancy if clinical care is to be based on a clear understanding of what is, and is not, normal.

Gastrointestinal system

Taste often alters early in pregnancy and the change can occur even before a period has been missed. It may be a metallic taste, similar to that experienced in liver disease, a loss of taste for something usually enjoyed or a craving for a food or other substance not normally eaten, such as wall plaster. Such cravings (pica) may be an expression of nutritional lack but many have no such potentially therapeutic effect. Some are potentially hazardous. Eating mothballs is not uncommon; this may produce a fetal haemolytic anaemia. Many cravings are concealed by the mother and may be discovered only after delivery.

Salivary secretion is usually within the normal non-pregnant range (Marder et al 1972) but is occasionally excessive although it is more of a nuisance to the mother than a threat to her fluid balance. Gastric secretion is reduced (Murray et al 1957). So is the motility of the stomach and it used to be considered to cause delayed emptying, particularly in labour (Davison et al 1970) with the risk of regurgitation during the induction of anaesthesia. It is now widely recognized that intrapartum changes in gastric emptying are entirely the result of analgesic drug administration. Nevertheless, the whole intestinal tract has decreased motility: this may be the explanation for increased absorption of water and salt (Parry et al 1970) and other substances. Gut transit time returns to non-pregnant levels in the third trimester (O'Sullivan & Bullingham 1984). The increase in water absorption produces a tendency to constipation, although oral iron may also contribute. Another symptom, so common that many mothers do not complain of it, is heartburn — reflux, producing regurgitation of acid mouthfuls with retrosternal or epigastric pain. This is a consequence of increased intragastric pressure without concomitant increase in tone of the oesophageal cardiac sphincter (Lind et al 1968). It is greater in heavier patients (Brock-Utne et al 1981). There may also be reflux of bile into the stomach due to pyloric incompetence (Atlay et al 1978) which responds to treatment with aluminium hydroxide rather than magnesium sulphate. The underlying mechanism may be increased progesterone or decreased concentrations of the hormonal peptide motilin (Christofides et al 1982).

Although the gallbladder empties more slowly during pregnancy (Gerdes & Boyden 1938), there is no change in the constitution of bile. Some hepatic functions do change. Albumin concentration in the plasma falls but the total amount circulating is the same as in the non-pregnant woman so that binding capacity is not affected. Globulin concentration does rise. Cholestasis is almost physiological in pregnancy. There is stasis of bile in dilated biliary canaliculi but no cellular necrosis or alteration in the secretion of bile (Adlercreutz et al 1967). This can produce generalized pruritus which responds to cholestyramine. Only rarely does it lead to jaundice. Frequently it recurs in subsequent pregnancies or if the mother uses a combined oral contraceptive or hormone replacement therapy. Hepatic malfunction during pregnancy may be suggested by the appearance of reddening of the palms or spider naevi. Alkaline phosphatase levels rise but this is largely due to placental production of the heat stable enzyme. The results of tests of liver function must be treated with caution during pregnancy.

Maternal handling of many drugs alters during pregnancy (Cummings 1983). Renal clearance is speeded up, reducing the effective dose of many antibiotics elsewhere in the body. Plasma binding may change, as may intestinal absorption. Hepatic metabolism is not usually affected. The mechanisms for the fall in plasma levels of phenytoin of those on treatment or the doubling of the half-life of caffeine, have not been established. Whatever the reason for these differences they are very relevant to treatment with phenytoin during pregnancy or in advising about coffee drinking.

Skin

The most obvious change in the skin is pigmentation in some areas. The development of a linea nigra and darkening of the nipple and areola are almost universal, although the depth of pigmentation varies in different people and different races. Facial chloasma is almost as common. All are due to increased secretion of pituitary melanocyte-stimulating hormone (Ances & Pomerantz 1974). A suntan acquired during pregnancy lasts longer than any other. Spider naevi are also common and some reddening of the palms is found in most mothers. Both are oestrogen effects. The striae which develop on the abdomen, breasts and elsewhere are a response to increased circulating corticosteroids (Poidevin 1959). There is generalized vasodilatation to assist in losing the extra heat produced by maternal, placental and fetal metabolism.

Fingernails grow more quickly during pregnancy (Hillman 1960). Hair does not but the rate at which hair is shed is reduced (Lynfield 1960). The excess which is retained is lost in the puerperium, to the consternation of many mothers who worry that they may be going bald. Subcutaneous fat increases but the generalized increase in skinfold thickness is due to oedema and increased vascularity (Taggart et al 1967). Intensely itchy papules sometimes appear during normal pregnancy — pregnancy prurigo — and disappear spontaneously either before or after delivery (Nurse 1968); there does not appear to be underlying pathology.

AFTER DELIVERY

Maternal metabolism and anatomy do not necessarily return to their nulliparous state even after a normal first pregnancy and delivery. Skin striae and pigmentation become less obvious but persist. Maternal weight often remains 1 kg or more above the preconception weight — more if the woman does not breastfeed (Stallabrass & Huntingford, personal communication). Menstruation may be longer or heavier; uterine vascularization frequently is permanently increased. Sensing system settings may be permanently altered; if the osmoreceptors return to a higher level than before pregnancy this may account for the greater increase in circulating volume found in later pregnancies (Davison et al 1981). Most systems of the body do however return close to their prepregnancy state.

The rate of return is not uniform. Carbohydrate metabolism is close to prepregnant levels within 24 hours of delivery but it may take months for iron stores to recover. Cardiac output is back to normal within 2 weeks, venous distensibility within 3–12 weeks but stroke volume not until 24 weeks after delivery (McCauseland et al 1961, Robson et al 1987). Cervical erosions may persist for a year (McLaren 1952) while circulating volume reverts within days. These data are not academic since a cervical erosion found at the 6-week postnatal visit is not abnormal and a haemoglobin estimation the day after delivery is an accurate reflection of the maternal situation (Taylor et al 1981). Joint changes may take 3–5 months to return to normal (Abramson et al 1934). The rate of involution is dependent on whether or not the mother is breastfeeding.

Some changes are peculiar to this period rather than a loss of adaptation. In one-third of women who have had normotensive pregnancies, diastolic blood pressure rises to 90 mmHg or more 48 hours after delivery (Brown 1958). Oestrogen formation falls, remaining low during breastfeeding (Bonnar et al 1975), and may produce vaginal atrophy (Hytten & Lind 1973). White cell count rises to 20×10^9 or more (Gibson 1937, Taylor et al 1981). Thyroid function is frequently altered, possibly in as many as one-fifth of mothers. This may be asymptomatic or produce overt hyperthyroidism or hypothyroidism, but often only lassitude (Fung et al 1988, How & Bewsher 1978). Almost always function returns to normal spontaneously, but this may take 6 months. Although the puerperium is defined as the 6 weeks which follow delivery it takes considerably longer than this for all the physical and psychological changes of pregnancy to return as close to their previous state as they will do. Repeated childbearing at short intervals may prevent this ever happening.

CONCLUSIONS

Maternal adaptations to pregnancy occur before they appear to be necessary. Reduction in maternal PCO_2 occurs in the luteal phase of the menstrual cycle before the fertilized ovum has embedded (Goodland & Romerrenke 1952). Cardiovascular and renal changes are apparent in the first trimester when fetus and placenta are still small, although their rate of growth is rapid. Such modification of physiology may however be necessary for implantation and healthy growth in early pregnancy. A thorough understanding of the wide range in degree, rates and consequences of adaptation is necessary before the possibility of pathology can be assessed. The influence of parity, age, race and other relevant variables must always be taken into account; multiple pregnancy adds another dimension. There remain many unexplained data. Fresh observations will continue and new knowledge be gained. But three generalizations are likely to remain true. Firstly, the initial conception is the one which starts the process of adaptation of the mother for reproduction; adaptation is generally not so effective in the first as in subsequent pregnancies. Secondly, not all adaptation is obviously advantageous to the mother. Thirdly, the passenger is a benign parasite and in nature the severely stressed fetus is not preferred to the mother.

REFERENCES

Abitbol M M 1976 Aortic compression by the pregnant uterus. New York State Journal of Medicine 76: 1470–1475

Aboul-Khair S A, Crooks J, Turnbull A C, Hytten F E 1964 The physiological changes in thyroid function during pregnancy. Clinical Science 27: 195–207

Abraham R, Campbell Brown M, Haines A P et al 1985 Diet during pregnancy in an Asian community in Britain — energy, protein, zinc, copper, fibre and calcium. Human Nutrition: Applied Nutrition 39a: 23–35

Abramson D, Roberts S M, Wilson P D 1934 Relaxation of the pelvic joints in pregnancy. Surgery, Gynecology and Obstetrics 58: 595–613

Adlercreutz H, Svanborg A, Anberg A 1967 Recurrent jaundice in pregnancy. I A clinical and ultrastructural study. American Journal of Medicine 42: 335–340

Alberman E, Roman E, Pharoah P O D, Chamberlain G 1980 Birth weight before and after a spontaneous abortion. British Journal of Obstetrics and Gynaecology 87: 275–280

Ances I G, Pomerantz S H 1974 Serum concentrations of B-melanocyte-stimulating hormone in human pregnancy. American Journal of Obstetrics and Gynecology 119: 1062–1065

Artal R, Wiswell R, Roman Y, Dorey F 1986 Pulmonary responses to exercise in pregnancy. American Journal of Obstetrics and Gynecology 154: 378–383

Ashton H 1975 Cigarette smoking in pregnancy — differences in circulation between smokers and non-smokers. British Journal of Obstetrics and Gynaecology 82: 868–881

Assali N S, Douglas R A, Baird W W et al 1953 Measurement of uterine blood flow and uterine metabolism: IV Results in normal pregnancy. American Journal of Obstetrics and Gynecology 66: 248–253

Atlay R D, Weekes A R L, Entwistle G D, Parkinson D J 1978 Treating heartburn in pregnancy: comparison of acid and alkali mixtures. British Medical Journal 2: 919–920

Australian In Vitro Fertilisation Collaborative Group 1985 High incidence of preterm births and early losses in pregnancy after in vitro fertilisation. British Medical Journal 291: 1160–1163

Bailey R R, Rolleston G L 1971 Kidney length and ureteric dilatation in the puerperium. Journal of Obstetrics and Gynaecology of the British Commonwealth 78: 55–61

Baird D 1935 The upper urinary tract in pregnancy and puerperium, with special reference to pyelitis of pregnancy. Journal of Obstetrics and Gynaecology of the British Empire 42: 733–774

Baird D, Thomson A M 1969 General factors underlying perinatal mortality rates. In: Butler M R, Alberman E D (eds) Perinatal problems. Livingstone, Edinburgh, pp 16–35

Bates R G, Helm C W, Duncan A, Edmonds D K 1985 Uterine activity in the second stage of labour and the effect of epidural analgesia. British Journal of Obstetrics and Gynaecology 92: 1246–1250

Baum R S 1966 Viscous forces in neonatal polycythemia. Journal of Pediatrics 69: 975

Beck I 1985 Incidence of pre-eclampsia in first full-term pregnancies preceded by abortion. Journal of Obstetrics and Gynaecology 6: 82–84

Becker J G 1948 Aetiology of eclampsia. Journal of Obstetrics and Gynaecology of the British Empire 55: 756–765

Beitins I Z, Bayard F, Angus J G et al 1973 The metabolic clearance rate, blood production, interconversion and transplacental passage of cortisol and cortisone in pregnancy near term. Pediatric Research 7: 509–519

Bieniarz J, Crottogini J J, Curuchet E et al 1968 Aortocaval compression by the uterus in late human pregnancy. American Journal of Obstetrics and Gynecology 100: 203–217

Bieniarz J, Yoshida T, Romero-Salinas G et al 1969 Aortocaval compression by the uterus in late human pregnancy. IV Circulatory homeostasis by preferential perfusion of the placenta. American Journal of Obstetrics and Gynecology 103: 19–31

Billewicz W Z, Thomson A M 1973 Birthweights in consecutive pregnancies. Journal of Obstetrics and Gynaecology of the British Commonwealth 80: 491–498

Blechner J N, Stenger V G, Prystowsky H 1974 Uterine blood flow in women at term. American Journal of Obstetrics and Gynecology 120: 633–638

Bolton P J, Jogee M, Myatt L, Elder M G 1981 Maternal plasma 6-oxo-prostaglandin F1 alpha levels throughout pregnancy: a longitudinal study. British Journal of Obstetrics and Gynaecology 88: 1101–1103

Bonnar J, Franklin M, Nott P N, McNeilly A S 1975 Effect of breast-feeding on pituitary–ovarian function after childbirth. British Medical Journal 4: 82–84

Borell U L F, Fernstrom I, Ohlson L, Wiquist N 1965 Influence of uterine contractions on the utero-placental blood flow at term. American Journal of Obstetrics and Gynecology 93: 44–57
Boyd J D, Hamilton W J 1970 In: The human placenta. Heffer, Cambridge, p 271
Brinkman C R 1975 Renal hypertension and pregnancy in the sheep. I. Behaviour of uteroplacental vasomotor tone during mild hypertension. American Journal of Obstetrics and Gynecology 121: 931–937
Brock-Utne J G, Dow T G B, Dimopoulos G E et al 1981 Gastric and lower oesophageal sphincter (LOS) pressures in early pregnancy. British Journal of Anaesthesia 53: 381–384
Brook J D, Gosden R G, Chandley A C 1984 Maternal ageing and aneuploid embryos — evidence from the mouse that biological and not chronological age is the important factor. Human Genetics 66: 41–45
Brosens I, Dixon H G 1966 The anatomy of the maternal side of the placenta. Journal of Obstetrics and Gynaecology of the British Commonwealth 73: 357–363
Broughton Pipkin F, Hunter J C, Turner S R, O'Brien P M S 1982 Prostaglandin E_2 attenuates the pressor response to angiotensin II in pregnant subjects but not in non-pregnant subjects. American Journal of Obstetrics and Gynecology 142: 166–176
Brown F J 1958 Aetiology of pre-eclamptic toxaemia and eclampsia. Fact and theory. Lancet i: 115–120
Browne J C M 1954 Utero-placental circulation. Cold Spring Harbor Symposia on Quantitative Biology, vol XIX. Long Island Biological Association, New York
Bruce N W 1973 The distribution of blood flow to the reproductive organs of rats near term. Journal of Reproduction and Fertility 46: 359–362
Buckingham J C, Selden R, Danforth D 1962 Connective tissue changes in the cervix during pregnancy and labour. Annals of the New York Academy of Sciences 97: 733–741
Bumpus H C 1924 Urinary reflux. Journal of Urology 12: 341–346
Burchell R C, Creed F, Rasoulpour M, Whitcomb B 1978 Vascular anatomy of the human uterus and pregnancy wastage. British Journal of Obstetrics and Gynaecology 85: 698–706
Calguneri M, Bird H A, Wright V 1982 Changes in joint laxity occurring during pregnancy. Annals of Rheumatic Disease 41: 126–128
Campbell D M, Campbell A J, MacGillivray I 1974 Maternal characteristics of women having twin pregnancies. Journal of Biosocial Science 6: 463–470
Carr B R, Parker C R, Madden J D et al 1979 Plasma levels of adrenocorticotropin and cortisol in women receiving oral contraceptive steroid treatment. Journal of Clinical Endocrinology and Metabolism 49: 346–349
Chanarin I, McFadyen I R, Kyle R 1977 The physiological macrocytosis of pregnancy. British Journal of Obstetrics and Gynaecology 84: 504–508
Chattinguis S, Axelsson O, Eklund G, Lindmark G 1985 Smoking, maternal age and fetal growth. Obstetrics and Gynecology 66: 449–452
Christianson R E 1976 Studies on blood pressure during pregnancy. I Influence of parity and age. American Journal of Obstetrics and Gynecology 125: 509–513
Christofides N D, Ghatei M A, Bloom S R, Borberg C, Gillmer M D G 1982 Decreased plasma motilin concentrations in pregnancy. British Medical Journal 285: 1453–1454
Colditz R B, Josey W E 1970 Central venous pressure in supine position during normal pregnancy. Obstetrics and Gynecology 36: 759–772
Coupland R E 1962 Histochemical observations on the distribution of cholinesterase in the human uterus. Journal of Obstetrics and Gynaecology of the British Commonwealth 69: 1041–1043
Cowett R M 1985 Hepatic and peripheral responsiveness to a glucose infusion in pregnancy. American Journal of Obstetrics and Gynecology 153: 272–279
Cruikshank J M 1970 The effects of parity on the leucocyte count in pregnant and non-pregnant women. British Journal of Haematology 18: 531–537
Csapo A, Erdos T, De Mattos C R et al 1965 Stretch-induced uterine growth, protein synthesis and function. Nature 207: 1378–1379
Cummings A J 1983 A survey of pharmacokinetic data from pregnant women. Clinical Pharmacokinetics 8: 344–354
Curet L B, Orr J A, Raukin J H G, Ilugloed T 1976 Effect of exercise on cardiac output and distribution of uterine blood flow in pregnant ewes. Journal of Applied Physiology 40: 725–728
Cutforth R, MacDonald C B 1966 Heart sounds and murmurs during pregnancy. American Heart Journal 71: 741–747
Dal Canton A, Conte G, Esposito C et al 1982 Effects of pregnancy on glomerular dynamics: micropuncture study in the rat. Kidney International 22: 608–612
Danforth D N 1947 The fibrous nature of the uterine cervix, and its relation to the isthmic segment in gravid and non-gravid uteri. American Journal of Obstetrics and Gynecology 53: 541–560
Danforth D N 1954 The distribution and functional activity of the cervical musculature. American Journal of Obstetrics and Gynecology 68: 1261–1270
Davison J M 1974 Changes in renal function and other aspects of homeostasis in early pregnancy. Journal of Obstetrics and Gynaecology of the British Commonwealth 81: 1003
Davison J M 1978 Changes in renal function in early pregnancy in women with one kidney. Yale Journal of Biology and Medicine 51: 347–352
Davison J M 1984 Renal haemodynamics and volume homeostasis in pregnancy. Scandinavian Journal of Clinical and Laboratory Investigation 44: 15–27
Davison J M, Dunlop W 1980 Renal hemodynamics and tubular function in normal human pregnancy. Kidney International 18: 152–161
Davison J M, Hytten F E 1974 Glomerular filtration during and after pregnancy. Journal of Obstetrics and Gynaecology of the British Commonwealth 81: 588–595
Davison J S, Davison M C, Hay D M 1970 Gastric emptying time in late pregnancy and labour. Journal of Obstetrics and Gynaecology of the British Commonwealth 77: 37–41
Davison J M, Vallotton M B, Lindheimer M D 1981 Plasma osmolality and urinary concentration and dilution during and after pregnancy: evidence that lateral recumbency inhibits maximal urinary concentrating ability. British Journal of Obstetrics and Gynaecology 88: 472–479
Davison J M, Gilmore E A, Durr J, Robertson G L, Lindheimer M D 1984 Altered osmotic thresholds for vasopressin secretion and thirst in human pregnancy. American Journal of Physiology 246: F105–F109
Dawood M Y, Raghavan K S, Pociask C, Fuchs F 1978 Oxytocin in human pregnancy and parturition. Obstetrics and Gynecology 51: 138–143
DeLeeuw N K M, Loevenstein L, Hsieh Y S 1966 Iron deficiency and hydremia in normal pregnancy. Medicine (Baltimore) 45: 291–315
Dowling J T, Freinkel N, Ingbar S H 1960 The effect of oestrogens upon the peripheral metabolism of thyroxine. Journal of Clinical Investigation 39: 1119–1123
Duncan D L 1967 Some aspects of the interpretation of mineral balances. Proceedings of the Nutrition Society 26: 102
Duncan M E 1980 Babies of mothers with leprosy have small placentae, low birthweight and grow slowly. British Journal of Obstetrics and Gynaecology 87: 471–476
Dunlop W, Davison J M 1977 The effect of normal pregnancy upon the renal handling of uric acid. British Journal of Obstetrics and Gynaecology 84: 13–21
Dunn J F, Nisula B C, Robard D 1981 Transport of steroid hormone: binding of 21 endogenous steroids to both testosterone-binding globulin and corticosteroid-binding globulin in human plasma. Journal of Clinical Endocrinology and Metabolism 53: 58–68
Dure-Smith P 1970 Pregnancy dilatation of the urinary tract: the iliac sign and its significance. Radiology 96: 545–549
Durnin J V G A 1985 Is nutritional status endangered by virtually no extra intake during pregnancy? Lancet ii: 823–825
Dworkin H J, Jacquez J A, Beierwaltes W H 1966 Relationship of iodine ingestion to iodine excretion in pregnancy. Journal of Clinical Endocrinology and Metabolism 26: 1329–1342
Eastman N J 1958 Hemodynamics of uterine contraction. American Journal of Obstetrics and Gynecology 76: 981–982
Eng M, Butler J, Bonica J J 1975 Respiratory function in pregnant obese women. American Journal of Obstetrics and Gynecology 123: 241–245
Errkkola R 1976 The influence of physical training during pregnancy on physical work capacity and circulatory parameters. Scandinavian Journal of Clinical and Laboratory Investigation 36: 747–754
Fabricant N D 1960 Sexual functions and the nose. American Journal of Medical Science 239: 498–502
Fencl M de M, Stillman R J, Cohen J, Tulchinsky D 1980 Direct evidence of sudden rise in fetal corticoids late in human gestation. Nature 287: 225–226

Ferguson J K W 1941 A study of the motility of the intact uterus at term. Surgery, Gynecology and Obstetrics 73: 359–366

Fitzpatrick R J 1961 Blood concentration of oxytocin in labour. Journal of Endocrinology 22: XIX–XX

Flint A P F, Forsling M L, Mitchell M D, Turnbull A C 1975 Temporal relationship between changes in oxytocin and prostaglandin F levels in response to vaginal distension in the pregnant and puerperal ewe. Journal of Reproduction and Fertility 43: 551–554

Francis W J A 1960 The onset of stress incontinence. Journal of Obstetrics and Gynaecology of the British Commonwealth 67: 899–903

Franklyn J A, Sheppard M C, Ramsden D B 1983 Serum free thyroxine and free triodothyronine concentrations in pregnancy. British Medical Journal 287: 394

Freese U E 1968 The uteroplacental vascular relationship in the human. American Journal of Obstetrics and Gynecology 101: 8–16

Fullerton W T, Hytten F E, Klopper A I, McKay E 1965 A case of quadruplet pregnancy. Journal of Obstetrics and Gynaecology of the British Commonwealth 72: 791–796

Fung H Y M, Kologlu M, Collinson K et al 1988. Postpartum thyroid dysfunction in Mid Glamorgan. British Medical Journal 296: 241–244

Gemzell C A 1953 Blood levels of 17 hydroxycorticosteroids in normal pregnancy. Journal of Clinical Endocrinology 13: 898–901

Genazzani A R, Fraioli F, Hierlimann J et al 1975 Immunoreactive ACTH and cortisol plasma levels during pregnancy. Detection and partial purification of corticotropin-like placental hormone: the human chorionic corticotropin (hCC). Clinical Endocrinology 4: 1–14

Gerdes M M, Boyden E A 1938 The rate of emptying of the human gall-bladder in pregnancy. Surgery, Gynecology and Obstetrics 66: 145–149

Gibson A 1937 On leucocyte changes during labour and the puerperium. Journal of Obstetrics and Gynaecology of the British Empire 44: 500–509

Gibson H M 1973 Plasma volume and glomerular filtration rate in pregnancy and their relation to differences in fetal growth. Journal of Obstetrics and Gynaecology of the British Commonwealth 80: 1067–1074

Gilbert R, Auchincloss J H 1966 Dyspnea of pregnancy — clinical and physiological observations. American Journal of Medical Science 252: 270–276

Gillespie E C 1950 Principles of uterine growth in pregnancy. American Journal of Obstetrics and Gynecology 59: 949–959

Goluboff L G, Ezrin C 1969 The effect of pregnancy on the somatotroph and the prolactin cell of the human adenohypophysis. Journal of Clinical Endocrinology 29: 1533–1538

Goodland R L, Rommerenke W T 1952 Cyclic fluctuations of the alveolar carbon dioxide tension during the normal menstrual cycle. Fertility and Sterility 3: 394–399

Goodrich S M, Wood J E 1964 Peripheral venous distensibility and velocity of venous blood flow during pregnancy and during oral contraceptive therapy. American Journal of Obstetrics and Gynecology 90: 740–744

Greiss F C 1966 Pressure-flow relationship in the gravid uterine vascular bed. American Journal of Obstetrics and Gynecology 96: 41–46

Hanna N F, Taylor-Robinson D, Kalodiki-Karamanoli M, Harris J R, McFadyen I R 1985 The relation between vaginal pH and the microbiological status in vaginitis. British Journal of Obstetrics and Gynaecology 92: 1267–1271

Harrison K A 1966 Blood volume changes in normal pregnant Nigerian women. Journal of Obstetrics and Gynaecology of the British Commonwealth 73: 717–721

Harrison K A 1985 Childbearing, health and social priorities: a survey of 22 774 consecutive hospital births in Zaria, Northern Nigeria. British Journal of Obstetrics and Gynaecology (suppl 5): 1–119

Hatem M, Anthony F, Hogston P, Rowe D J F, Dennis K J 1988 Reference values for 75 g oral glucose tolerance test in pregnancy. British Medical Journal 296: 676–678

Hendricks C H 1958 The hemodynamics of a uterine contraction. American Journal of Obstetrics and Gynecology 76: 969–974

Herbert C N, Banner E A, Watkin K G 1958 Variations in the peripheral circulation during pregnancy. American Journal of Obstetrics and Gynecology 76: 742–744

Hillman R W 1960 Fingernail growth in pregnancy. Relations to some common parameters of the reproductive process. Human Biology 32: 119–124

Hofstetter A, Schutz Y, Jequier E, Wahren J 1986 Increased 24-hour energy expenditure in cigarette smokers. New England Journal of Medicine 314: 79–82

Holmes F 1960 Incidence of the supine hypotensive syndrome in late pregnancy. Journal of Obstetrics and Gynaecology of the British Empire 67: 254–258

How J, Bewsher P D 1978 Thyroid disease and pregnancy. British Medical Journal 2: 1568–1569

Howells M R, Jones S E, Napier J A F, Saunders K, Cavill I 1986 Erythropoiesis in pregnancy. British Journal of Haematology 64: 595–599

Huch R, Baumann H, Fallenstein G, Schneider K T M, Holdener F, Huch A 1986 Physiologic changes in pregnant women and their fetuses during jet air travel. American Journal of Obstetrics and Gynecology 154: 996–1000

Hughes R E 1986 Dietary fibre may retard uterus development. Human Nutrition: Clinical Nutrition 40C: 81–86

Hundley W P, Walton J M, Hibbits J T et al 1935 Physiologic changes occurring in the urinary tract during pregnancy. American Journal of Obstetrics and Gynecology 30: 625–649

Hytten F E 1980 Weight gain in pregnancy. In: Hytten F E, Chamberlain G V P (eds) Clinical physiology in obstetrics. Blackwell, Oxford, pp 193–233

Hytten F E, Cheyne G A 1969 The size and composition of the human pregnant uterus. Journal of Obstetrics and Gynaecology of the British Commonwealth 76: 400–403

Hytten F E, Klopper A I 1963 Response to a water load in pregnancy. Journal of Obstetrics and Gynaecology of the British Commonwealth 70: 811–816

Hytten F E, Leitch I 1971 The physiology of human pregnancy, 2nd edn. Blackwell Scientific Publications, Oxford

Hytten F E, Lind T 1973 Diagnostic indices in pregnancy. CIBA-Geigy, Basle

Hytten F E, Paintin D B 1963 Increase in plasma volume during normal pregnancy. Journal of Obstetrics and Gynaecology of the British Commonwealth 70: 402–407

Hytten F E, Thomson A M, Taggart N 1966 Total body water in normal pregnancy. Journal of Obstetrics and Gynaecology of the British Commonwealth 73: 553–561

Iosif S, Uemsten U 1981 Comparative urodynamic studies of continent and stress incontinent women in pregnancy and in the puerperium. American Journal of Obstetrics and Gynecology 140: 645–650

Jacobs A 1977 Disorders of iron metabolism. In: Hoffbrand A V, Brain M E, Hirsh J (eds) Recent advances in haematology, vol 2. Churchill Livingstone, Edinburgh, pp 1–26

Jailer J W, Christy N P, Longson D et al 1959 Further observations on adrenal cortical function during pregnancy. American Journal of Obstetrics and Gynecology 78: 1–10

Jansson I 1969 ^{133}Xenon clearance in the myometrium of pregnant and non-pregnant women. Acta Obstetricia et Gynecologica Scandinavica 48: 302–321

Jeppsson S, Rennevik G, Thorell J I 1977 Pituitary gonadotrophin secretion during the first weeks of pregnancy. Acta Endocrinologica 85: 177–188

Kalousek G, Hlavacek C, Nedoss B, Pollek V E 1969 Circadian rhythms of creatinine and electrolyte excretion in healthy pregnant women. American Journal of Obstetrics and Gynecology 103: 856–867

Kannan V 1973 Plasma thyrotropin and its response to thyrotropin releasing hormone in normal pregnancy. Obstetrics and Gynecology 42: 547–549

Karlsson K, Kjellmer I 1974 The influence of asphyxia on uterine blood flow. Journal of Perinatal Medicine 2: 170–176

Kauppila A, Koskinen M, Puolakka J, Twimala R, Kuikka J 1980 Decreased intervillous and unchanged myometrial blood flow in supine recumbency. Obstetrics and Gynecology 55: 203–205

Kaur K, Joppila P, Kuikka J, Luotola H, Ioivanen J, Rekonen A 1980 Intervillous blood flow in normal and complicated late pregnancy measured by means of an intravenous ^{133}Xe method. Acta Obstetricia et Gynecologica Scandinavica 59: 7–10

Kerr M G, Scott D B, Samuel E 1964 Studies of the inferior vena cava in late pregnancy. British Medical Journal 1: 532–533

Khong T Y, Liddell H S, Robertson W B 1987 Defective haemochorial placentation as a cause of miscarriage: a preliminary study. British Journal of Obstetrics and Gynaecology 94: 649–655

Klebanoff M A, Koslowe P A, Kaslow R, Rhoads G G 1985 Epidemiology of vomiting in early pregnancy. Obstetrics and Gynecology 66: 612–616
Kuhl C, Holmes P J, Faber P K 1981 Hepatic insulin extraction in human pregnancy. Hormonal Metabolism Research 13: 71–72
Laaks L, Ruotsalainen P, Punnonen R, Maatela J 1971 Hepatic blood flow during late pregnancy. Acta Obstetricia et Gynecologica Scandinavica 50: 175–178
Ladner C, Brinkman C R, Weston P, Assali N S 1970 Dynamics of uterine circulation in pregnant and non-pregnant sheep. American Journal of Physiology 218: 257–263
Lawrence M, Lawrence F, Lamb W H, Whitehead R G 1984 Maintenance energy cost of pregnancy in rural Gambian women and influence of dietary status. Lancet ii: 363–365
Lee M R 1981 The kidney fault in essential hypertension may be a failure to mobilize renal dopamine adequately when dietary sodium chloride is increased. Cardiovascular Reviews and Reports 2: 785–789
Lees M H, Hill J D, Ochsner A J, Thomas C L, Novy M J 1971 Maternal placental and myometrial blood flow of the rhesus monkey during uterine contractions. American Journal of Obstetrics and Gynecology 110: 68–81
Lees M M, Scott D B, Kerr M G, Taylor S H 1967 The circulatory effects of recumbent postural change in late pregnancy. Clinical Science 32: 453–465
Lind J F, Smith A M, McIver D K et al 1968 Heartburn in pregnancy — a manometric study. Canadian Medical Association Journal 98: 571–575
Lindheimer M D, Weston P V 1969 Effects of hypotonic expansion on sodium, water and urea excretion in late pregnancy: the influence of posture on these results. Journal of Clinical Investigations 48: 947–950
Lindheimer M D, DelGreco F, Ehrlich E N 1973 Postural effects on Na and steroid excretion and serum renin activity during pregnancy. Journal of Applied Physiology 35: 343–348
Lynfield Y L 1960 Effect of pregnancy on the human hair cycle. Journal of Investigative Dermatology 35: 323–327
MacGillivray I 1958 Some observations on the incidence of pre-eclampsia. Journal of Obstetrics and Gynaecology of the British Empire 65: 536–539
MacGillivray I, Rose G A, Rowe B 1969 Blood pressure survey in pregnancy. Clinical Science 37: 395–407
MacGillivray I, Campbell D M, Duffus G M 1971 Maternal metabolic response to twin pregnancy in primigravidae. Journal of Obstetrics and Gynaecology of the British Commonwealth 78: 530–536
Mahran M, Ghaleb H A 1964 The physiology of the human round ligament. Journal of Obstetrics and Gynaecology of the British Commonwealth 71: 374–378
Maigaard S, Forman A, Anderson K E 1985 Different responses to prostaglandin $F_{2\alpha}$ and E_2 in human extra- and intramyometrial arteries. Prostaglandins 30: 599–607
Makila U M, Jouppila P, Kirkinen P, Viinikka L, Ylikorkala O 1986 Placental thromboxane and prostacyclin in the regulation of placental blood flow. Obstetrics and Gynecology 68: 537–540
Makowski E L, Meschia G, Droegemudler W, Battaglia F C 1968 Distribution of uterine blood flow in the pregnant sheep. American Journal of Obstetrics and Gynecology 101: 409–412
Maloiy G M O, Heglund N C, Prager L M, Cavagna G A, Taylor C R 1986 Energetic cost of carrying loads: have African women discovered an economic way? Nature 319: 668–669
Man E B, Reid W A, Hellegers A E, Jones W S 1969 Thyroid function in human pregnancy. III. Serum thyroxine-binding pre-albumin (TBPAT) and thyroxine-binding globulin (TBG) of pregnant women aged 14 through 43 years. American Journal of Obstetrics and Gynecology 103: 328–347
Marder M Z, Wotman S, Mandel I D 1972 Salivary electrolyte changes during pregnancy. I. Normal pregnancy. American Journal of Obstetrics and Gynecology 112: 233–236
Markowe H L J, Marmot M G, Shipley M J et al 1985 Fibrinogen: a possible link between social class and coronary heart disease. British Medical Journal 291: 1312–1314
Marshall J M 1973 In: Morris H J, Hertig A T, Abell M R (eds) The physiology of the myometrium in the uterus. Williams & Wilkins, Baltimore, pp 89–109
Martin C B, McGaughey H S, Kaiser I H, Donner M W, Ramsey E M 1964 Intermittent functioning of the uteroplacental arteries. American Journal of Obstetrics and Gynecology 90: 819–823
Mattingly R F, Borkowf H I 1978 Clinical implications of ureteric reflux in pregnancy. Clinics in Obstetrics and Gynaecology 21: 863–873
McCall M L 1949 Cerebral blood flow and metabolism in toxemias of pregnancy. Surgery, Gynecology and Obstetrics 89: 715–720
McCauseland A M, Hyman C, Winsor T, Trotter A D 1961 Venous distensibility during pregnancy. American Journal of Obstetrics and Gynecology 81: 472–478.
McFadyen I R 1962 Vesico-vaginal fistula. A series of 27 cases. British Medical Journal ii: 1717–1720
McFadyen I R 1985 Missed abortion, and later spontaneous abortion, in pregnancies clinically normal at 7–12 weeks. European Journal of Obstetrics and Gynecology and Reproductive Biology 20: 381–384
McFadyen I R, Eykyn S J, Gardner N H N et al 1973 Bacteriuria in pregnancy. Journal of Obstetrics and Gynaecology of the British Commonwealth 80: 385–405
McFadyen I R, Campbell Brown M, Abraham R, North W R S, Harris A P 1984 Factors affecting birthweight in Hindus, Moslems and Europeans. British Journal of Obstetrics and Gynaecology 91: 968–972
McFadyen I R, Price A B, Geirsson R T 1986 The relation of birth weight to histological appearances in vessels of the placental bed. British Journal of Obstetrics and Gynaecology 93: 476–481
McFadyen I R, Duffy S, De Chazal R C S et al 1989 The relationship of birth weight to the adaptation of maternal placental bed vessels to pregnancy changes in packed cell volume, and mean arterial pressure (submitted for publication)
McGinty A P 1938 The comparative effect of pregnancy and phrenic nerve interruption on the diaphragm and their relation to pulmonary tuberculosis. American Journal of Obstetrics and Gynecology 35: 237–241
McLaren H C 1952 The involution of the cervix. British Medical Journal 1: 347–352
McLennan C 1943 Antecubital and femoral venous pressure in normal and toxemic pregnancy. American Journal of Obstetrics and Gynecology 45: 568–591
Metzger B E, Daniel R R, Frienkel N et al 1973 The role of glucagon in gestational diabetogenesis. Clinical Research 21: 887–891
Migeon C J, Bertrand J, Wall P E 1957 Physiological disposition of 4-C-14 cortisol during late pregnancy. Journal of Clinical Investigation 36: 1350–1362
Mitchel G W 1966 The role of the phagocyte in host–parasite interactions. IV. The phagocytic activity of leucocytes in pregnancy and its relationship to urinary tract infections. American Journal of Obstetrics and Gynecology 96: 687–695
Miyake A, Tanizawa O, Toshihiro A, Kurachi K 1977 Pituitary responses in LH secretion to LHRH during pregnancy. Obstetrics and Gynecology 49: 549–551
Moerman M L 1982 Growth of the birth canal in adolescent girls. American Journal of Obstetrics and Gynecology 143: 528–532
Moll W, Kunzel W, Herberger J 1975 The haemodynamic implications of hemochorial placentation. European Journal of Obstetrics, Gynecology and Reproductive Biology 5: 67–71
Muellner S R 1939 Physiological bladder changes during pregnancy and the puerperium. Journal of Urology 41: 691–695
Munnell G W, Taylor H C 1947 Liver blood flow in pregnancy — hepatic vein catheterization. Journal of Clinical Investigation 26: 952–955
Murray F A, Erskine J P, Fielding J 1957 Gastric secretion in pregnancy. Journal of Obstetrics and Gynaecology of the British Empire 64: 373–378
Naylor A F, Warburton D 1979 Sequential analysis of spontaneous abortion. II. Collaborative study data show that gravidity determines a very substantial rise in risk. Fertility and Sterility 31: 282–286
Newman R B, Gill P J, Katz M 1986 Uterine activity during pregnancy in ambulatory patients: comparison of singleton and twin gestations. American Journal of Obstetrics and Gynecology 154: 530–531
Nolten W E, Rueckert P A 1981 Elevated free cortisol level in pregnancy: possible regulatory mechanisms. American Journal of Obstetrics and Gynecology 139: 492–498
Nolten W E, Lindheimer M D, Oparil S et al 1979 Desoxycorticosterone in normal pregnancy. II. Cortisol-dependent fluctuations in free plasma desoxycorticosterone. American Journal of Obstetrics and Gynecology 133: 644–648
Nolten W E, McKenna M V, Rueckert P A, Ehrlich E N 1981 Inhibition of 3H-dexamethasone binding to lymphocytes in vitro: relevance to the

apparent development of refractoriness to cortisol in pregnancy. Clinical Research 29: 760a
Novy M J, Thomas C L, Lees M H 1975 Uterine contractility and regional blood flow responses to oxytocin and prostaglandin E_2 in pregnant rhesus monkeys. American Journal of Obstetrics and Gynecology 122: 419–433
Nurse D S 1968 Pregnancy prurigo: a study of 40 cases. Australian Journal of Dermatology 9: 258–261
Nylander P P S 1978 Causes of high twinning frequencies in Nigeria. Proceedings of Clinical and Biological Research 246: 35–43
O'Sullivan G M, Bullingham R E S 1984 The assessment of gastric acidity and antacid effect in pregnant women by a non-invasive radiotelemetry technique. British Journal of Obstetrics and Gynaecology 91: 973–978
Owman C, Rosenbren E, Sjoberg N O 1967 Adrenergic innervation of the human female reproductive organs: a histochemical and chemical investigation. Obstetrics and Gynecology 30: 763–773
Palmer A J, Walker A H C 1949 The maternal circulation in normal pregnancy. Journal of Obstetrics and Gynaecology of the British Empire 56: 537–547
Parry E, Shields R, Turnbull A C 1970 The effect of pregnancy on the colonic absorption of sodium, potassium and water. Journal of Obstetrics and Gynaecology of the British Commonwealth 77: 616–619
Pijnenborg R, Bland J M, Robertson W B, Dixon G, Brosens I 1981 The pattern of interstitial trophoblast invasion of the myometrium in early human pregnancy. Placenta 2: 303–316
Pijnenborg R, Bland J M, Robertson W B, Brosens I 1983 Uteroplacental arterial changes related to interstitial trophoblast migration in early human pregnancy. Placenta 4: 397–414
Pirani B B K, Campbell D M, MacGillivray I 1973 Plasma volume in normal first pregnancy. Journal of Obstetrics and Gynaecology of the British Commonwealth 80: 884–887
Pitkin R M 1975 Calcium metabolism in pregnancy: a review. American Journal of Obstetrics and Gynecology 121: 724
Pitkin R M, Witte D L 1979 Platelet and leukocyte counts in pregnancy. Journal of the American Medical Association 242: 2696–2699
Poidevin L O S 1959 Striae gravidarum. Their relation to adrenal cortical hyperfunction. Lancet ii: 436–439
Poloshuk W Z, Diamant Y Z, Zuckerman H, Sadousky E 1970 Leukocyte alkaline phosphatase in pregnancy and the puerperium. American Journal of Obstetrics and Gynecology 107: 604–609
Popat N, Wood W G, Weatherall D J, Turnbull A C 1977 Pattern of maternal F-cell production during pregnancy. Lancet ii: 377
Pritchard J A, Adams R H 1960 Erythrocyte production and destruction during pregnancy. American Journal of Obstetrics and Gynecology 79: 750–755
Pritchard J A, Wiggins K M, Dickey J C 1960 Blood volume changes in pregnancy and the puerperium. I. Does sequestration of red blood cells accompany parturition? American Journal of Obstetrics and Gynecology 80: 956–963
Prowse C M, Gaensler E A 1965 Respiratory and acid base changes during pregnancy. Anaesthesiology 26: 381–392
Puavilai G, Drogny E C, Domont L A, Bauma G 1982 Insulin receptors and insulin resistance in human pregnancy: evidence for a post receptor defect in insulin action. Journal of Clinical Endocrinological Metabolism 54: 247–253
Pyorala T 1966 Cardiovascular response to the upright position during pregnancy. Acta Obstetricia et Gynecologica Scandinavica 45 (suppl 5): 1–116
Rampling M, Sirs J A 1972 The interactions of fibrinogen and dextrans with erythrocytes. Journal of Physiology (London) 223: 199–212
Ramsey E M, Houston M L, Harris J W S 1976 Interactions of the trophoblast and maternal tissues in three closely related primate species. American Journal of Obstetrics and Gynecology 124: 647–652
Rao P S S, Inbergi S G 1977 Inbreeding effects on human reproduction in Tamil Kadu of South India. Annals of Human Genetics 41: 87–98
Rasmussen A T 1934 The weight of the principal components of the normal hypophysis cerebri of the adult human female. American Journal of Anatomy 55: 253–275
Reagan B, Folse R 1971 Lower limb venous dynamics in normal persons and children of patients with varicose veins. Surgery, Gynecology and Obstetrics 132: 15–18
Reynolds S R M, Freese U E, Bieniarz J, Caldeyro-Barcia R, Mendez-Bauer C, Escarcena L 1968 Multiple simultaneous intervillous space pressures recorded in several regions of the hemochorial placenta in relation to functional anatomy of the fetal cotyledon. American Journal of Obstetrics and Gynecology 102: 1128–1134
Roach M R, Burton A C 1957 The reason for the shape of the distensibility curves of arteries. Canadian Journal of Biochemistry and Physiology 35: 681–687
Roberts J M, Insel P A, Goldflien R, Goldflien A 1977 The effect of progesterone and/or estradiol on uterine contractility and β-adrenergic receptor number. Gynecologic Investigation 8: 56
Roberts J M, Lewis V, Mize N, Tsuchiya A, Starr J 1986 Human platelet α-adrenergic receptors and responses during pregnancy: no change except that with differing hematocrit. American Journal of Obstetrics and Gynecology 154: 206–210
Robertson W B, Brosens I, Dixon H G 1967 The pathological response of the vessels of the placental bed to hypertensive pregnancy. Journal of Pathology and Bacteriology 93: 481–592
Robertson W B, Brosens I, Dixon G 1975 Uteroplacental vascular pathology. European Journal of Obstetrics, Gynecology and Reproductive Biology 5: 47–65
Robson S C, Hunter S, Moore M, Dunlop W 1987 Haemodynamic changes during the puerperium: a Doppler and M-mode echo cardiographic study. British Journal of Obstetrics and Gynaecology 94: 1028–1039
Rouse K A, Montague W, MacVicar J 1985a Carbohydrate metabolism during pregnancy in groups of women with differing perinatal mortality rates. Journal of Obstetrics and Gynaecology 6: 24–27
Rouse K A, Montague W, MacVicar J 1985b Cholesterol and triglyceride metabolism during pregnancy in women of different ethnic origins and dietary habits. Journal of Obstetrics and Gynaecology 6: 28–31
Rovinsky J J, Jaffin H 1965 Cardiovascular hemodynamics in pregnancy. I. Blood and plasma volumes in multiple pregnancy. American Journal of Obstetrics and Gynecology 93: 1–13
Rubi R A, Sala N L 1968 Ureteral function in pregnant women. III. Effect of different positions and fetal delivery upon uterine tonus. American Journal of Obstetrics and Gynecology 101: 230–237
Ruff S C, Mitchell R H, Murnaghan G A 1982 Long term variations of blood pressure rhythms in normotensive pregnancy and pre-eclampsia. In: Sammour M, Symonds M, Zuspan F, El-Tomi N (eds) Pregnancy hypertension. Ain Shams University Press, Cairo, pp 129–143
Rush D, Cassano P 1983 Relationship of cigarette smoking and social class to birth weight and perinatal mortality among all births in Britain, 5–11 April 1970. Journal of Epidemiology and Community Health 37: 249–255
Schnider S M 1981 Choice of anaesthesia for labour and delivery. Obstetrics and Gynecology 58: 245–345
Schuman J E, Tanser C L, Peloquin R, De Leeuw N K M 1973 The erythropoietic response to pregnancy in B-thalassaemia minor. British Journal of Haematology 25: 249–260
Schwalm H, Dubrawsky V 1966 The structure of the musculature of the human uterus — muscles and connective tissue. American Journal of Obstetrics and Gynecology 94: 391–404
Scott J M 1962 Anaemia in pregnancy. Postgraduate Medical Journal 38: 202–213
Sheehan H L, Lynch J B 1973 In: Pathology of toxaemia of pregnancy. Churchill Livingstone, Edinburgh, p 47
Sheehan H L, Stanfield J P 1961 The pathogenesis of postpartum necrosis of the anterior lobe of the pituitary gland. Acta Endocrinologica 37: 479–510
Simpson J, Jameson E, Dickhams D, Glover R 1965 Effect of size of cuff bladder on accuracy of measurement of indirect blood pressure. American Heart Journal 70: 208–215
Slaunwhite W R Jr, Kirdani R Y, Sandberg A A 1973 Metabolic aspects of oestrogens in man. In Magoun H W, Hall V E (eds) Handbook of Physiology, vol II. American Physiology Society, Washington DC, p 485
Soloff M S, Swartz T L, Steinberg A H 1974 Oxytocin receptors in the human uterus. Journal of Clinical Endocrinology and Metabolism 38: 1052–1056
Somaan N A, Anderson G D, Adam-Mayne M E 1975 Immunoreactive calcitonin in the mother, neonate, child and adult. American Journal of Obstetrics and Gynecology 121: 622
Stearn R H 1963 The adolescent primigravida. Lancet ii: 1083–1085

Stoffer R P, Koeneke I A, Chesky V E, Hellwig C A 1957 The thyroid in pregnancy. American Journal of Obstetrics and Gynecology 74: 300–308
Strictland D M, Guzick D S, Cox K, Gant N F, Rosenfield C R 1986 The relationship between abortion in the first pregnancy and development of pregnancy-induced hypertension in the subsequent pregnancy. American Journal of Obstetrics and Gynecology 154: 146–148
Sundsfjord J A 1971 Plasma renin activity and aldosterone excretion during prolonged progesterone administration. Acta Endocrinologica 67: 483–490
Tabatznik B, Randall T W, Hearsch C 1960 The mammary souffle in pregnancy and lactation. Circulation 22: 1069
Taggart N R, Holliday R M, Billewicz W Z, Hytten F E, Thomson A M 1967 Changes in skinfolds during pregnancy. British Journal of Nutrition 21: 439–444
Taylor D J, Lind T 1976 Haematological changes during normal pregnancy: iron induced macrocytosis. British Journal of Obstetrics and Gynaecology 83: 760–767
Taylor D J, Phillips P, Lind T 1981 Puerperal haematological indices. British Journal of Obstetrics and Gynaecology 88: 601–606
Tahzib F 1983 Epidemiological determinants of vesico-vaginal fistulas. British Journal of Obstetrics and Gynaecology 90: 387–391
Thomson B, Baird D 1967 Some impressions of child-bearing in a tropical area. Part II. Pre-eclampsia and low birth weight. Journal of Obstetrics and Gynaecology of the British Commonwealth 74: 499–509
Thomson K J, Cohen M E 1938 Studies on the circulation in pregnancy. II. Vital capacity observations in normal pregnant women. Surgery, Gynecology and Obstetrics 66: 591–597
Thomson A M, Hytten F E, Billewicz W Z 1967 The epidemiology of oedema during pregnancy. Journal of Obstetrics and Gynaecology of the British Commonwealth 74: 1–10
Thomson A M, Billewicz W Z, Hytten F E 1968 The assessment of fetal growth. Journal of Obstetrics and Gynaecology of the British Commonwealth 75: 903–916
Trail L M 1975 Reticulocytes in healthy pregnancy. Medical Journal of Australia 2: 205–206
Trudinger B J, Giles W B, Cook C M 1985 Uteroplacental blood flow velocity-time waveforms in normal and complicated pregnancy. British Journal of Obstetrics and Gynaecology 92: 39–45
Uldbjerg N, Ekman G, Malmstrom A, Olsson K, Ulmsten U 1983 Ripening of the human uterine cervix related to changes in collagen, glycosaminoglycans, and collagenolytic activity. American Journal of Obstetrics and Gynecology 147: 662–666
Van Wagenen G, Jenkins R H 1948 Pyeloureteral dilatation or pregnancy after death of the fetus: an experimental study. American Journal of Obstetrics and Gynecology 56: 1146–1151
Venuto R C, Cox J W, Stein J H, Ferris T F 1976 The effect of changes in perfusion pressure on uteroplacental blood flow in the pregnant rabbit. Journal of Clinical Investigation 57: 938–944
Vorys N, Ulberg J C, Hanusek G E 1961 The cardiac output changes in various positions in pregnancy. American Journal of Obstetrics and Gynecology 82: 1312–1321
Wadsworth M E J, Cripps H A, Midwinter R E, Colley J R T 1985 Blood pressure in a national birth cohort at the age of 36 related to social and familial factors, smoking, and body mass. British Medical Journal 291: 1534–1538
Walters W A W, MacGregor W G, Hills M 1966 Cardiac output at rest during pregnancy and the puerperium. Clinical Science 30: 1–11
Weir R J, Brown J J, Fraser et al 1975 Relationship between plasma renin substrate, angiotensin II, aldosterone, and electrolytes in normal pregnancy. Journal of Clinical Endocrinology 40: 108–115
Whiteley H J, Stoner H B 1957 The effect of pregnancy on the human adrenal cortex. Journal of Endocrinology 14: 325–334
WHO Task Force 1970 Spontaneous and induced abortion. Technical Report Series 110, 461. WHO, Geneva
Wilbrand U, Porath C H, Mathaes P, Jaster R 1959 Der Einfluss der Ovariaesteroide auf die Funktion des Atemzentrums. Archiv für Gynäkologie 191: 507–511
Winkel C A, Simpson E R, Milewich L, MacDonald P C 1980 Deoxycorticosterone biosynthesis in human kidney: potential for formation of a potent mineralo-corticosteroid in its site of action. Proceedings of the National Academy of Sciences (USA) 77: 7069–7073
Wintour E M, Coghlan J P, Oddie C J, Scoggins B A, Walters W A W 1978 A sequential study of adrenocorticosteroid level in human pregnancy. Clinical Experience of Pharmacology and Physiology 5: 399–403
Wood C 1964 Physiology of uterine contractions. Journal of Obstetrics and Gynaecology of the British Commonwealth 71: 360–373
Wootton R, McFadyen I R, Cooper J E 1977 Measurement of placental blood flow in the pig and its relation to placental and fetal weight. Biology of the Neonate 31: 333–338
Wright H P, Osborn S B, Edmonds D G 1950 Changes in the rate of flow of venous blood in the leg during pregnancy measured with radio-active sodium. Surgery, Gynecology and Obstetrics 90: 481–486
Youssef A F 1958 The uterine isthmus and its sphincter mechanism, a radiographic study. American Journal of Obstetrics and Gynecology 75: 1305–1332
Yudkin P K, Harlap S, Baras M 1983 High birth weight in an ethnic group of low socio-economic status. British Journal of Obstetrics and Gynaecology 90: 291–296
Zuspan F P, O'Shaughnessy R W, Vinsel J, Zuspan M 1981 Adrenergic innervation of uteric vasculature in human term pregnancy. American Journal of Obstetrics and Gynecology 139: 678–680

11

P. M. Johnson

Immunology of pregnancy

INTRODUCTION

Immunology is still considered a young discipline, although it originates essentially from the first effective immunization performed by Edward Jenner in 1796 with cowpox vaccination for protection against smallpox. It has since consistently attracted a small band of talented scientists, many of whom are among the best known names in medicine — including Pasteur, Metchnikoff, von Behring, Ehrlich, Bordet, Landsteiner, Medawar, Burnet, Jerne, Dausset and Milstein to name only a few from the roll-call along this historic road. Indeed, immunology has gained a lion's share of Nobel prizes (a total of 19 from 1901 to 1987) and yet, paradoxically, many medical schools do not even now include a separate department for immunology. To some extent, this has resulted from the topic rapidly spreading its wings to encompass a wide spectrum from basic science to applied medicine as well as sending its tentacles into virtually every medical subdiscipline.

Against this historical backdrop, there has been a tremendous explosion of advances in immunology over the past 30 years, seemingly at an ever-increasing pace. The subject has become diversified into specialized fields (immunohistochemistry, immunogenetics, immunopathology and immunotherapy), each now including detail that would have daunted the pioneers of the 19th and early 20th centuries. For example, it is pertinent to remember that separate identification of T and B lymphocytes only became established 20 years ago, since when an ever-increasing complexity of lymphocyte subsets has been characterized using cell marker or cell function analyses. Many of the recent exciting observations in immunology need time to be distilled into simple cogent dogma before being applied to relevant allied areas, such as pregnancy.

The immunology of pregnancy, although potentially a vast topic, thus still remains somewhat of an outsider. With the one remarkable exception of immunoprophylaxis for rhesus haemolytic disease of the newborn (see Chapter 35), it is only in the past 15 years that relevant factual information has accumulated (Crighton 1984, Clark & Croy 1986, Chaouat 1987, Gill & Wegmann 1987). Because concepts and technical capabilities in immunology are now so fast-moving, our scope of application will certainly accelerate in the coming years. At present, there is both awareness and speculation of immunological involvement in clinical and pathological events associated with pregnancy, although the foundations rest with the body of knowledge gained in studying essential immunobiological events in normal pregnancy. Two broad areas can be identified:

1. The embryo acquires its genetic information equally from both parents and hence, in outbred populations such as man, represents a foreign tissue graft (allograft), known colloquially as *Nature's transplant*. Immunologists have been intrigued to identify the multifactorial immunoregulatory mechanisms contributing normally to successful evasion of any maternal immune rejection in utero, hence allowing viviparous reproduction.
2. The fetus, and indeed neonate, develop facets of the immune system progressively to achieve full immunocompetence. Various interactions occur between the maternal and fetal immune systems within the intrauterine environment, including essential selective transfer of maternal IgG across the placenta, whereby the fetus passively acquires antibody immunity prior to exposure to the non-sterile extrauterine environment at parturition. In specific instances, unusual maternal–fetal immunological interactions may lead to a disorder of pregnancy itself with possible effects on the pregnant woman or her baby. Alternatively, since an immunological component is apparent in many, if not most, disease

states, in certain situations this can influence outcome in any concomitant pregnancy.

This chapter attempts to develop basic and clinical feto-maternal immunobiology, but first an introductory outline of the essential elements of the immune system is presented (see also Roitt et al 1985, Stites et al 1987).

BASIC IMMUNOLOGY

Leukocytic cells

The average adult has about 10^{12} lymphoid cells; the lymphoid system as a whole represents 2% of total body weight. Lymphocytes can be divided into two major groups:

1. *B cells* express surface immunoglobulins acting as specific antigen receptors and are the precursors of plasma cells which secrete immunoglobulins (antibodies), they constitute 5–20% of the circulating lymphoid pool.
2. *T cells* differentiate in the thymus and include many important subpopulations, defined either functionally or by cell surface marker analysis, such as *helper*, *suppressor*, *cytotoxic* and *memory* T cells, whose functions in orchestrating the immune response by direct action or controlling mechanisms are synonymous with their generic name. All mature T cells express a specific cell surface dimeric molecule that, like an immunoglobulin molecule, has both a constant and a variable region and acts as a specific antigen receptor.

During early maturation, both B and T lymphocytes develop their cell surface receptor for antigen so that each cell is then committed to a single antigenic specificity for its entire lifespan. A third group of lymphocytes, less well defined, does not express specific antigen receptors or markers of either B or T cells. These *null* cells are of bone marrow origin, are usually granulated and may express cell surface receptors for the Fc region of IgG. They include antibody-dependent cellular cytotoxic (ADCC) cells which can lyse cells via antibodies bound to the target surface, and also the majority of *natural killer* (NK) cells which lyse various tumour or virally infected cell targets in an antigen non-specific manner. Recent observations suggest that this third population may also include cells with other, less overt, biological properties — possibly including cells with a natural suppressor function (Maier et al 1986), whose relationship to suppressor T cells may be analogous to that between NK and cytotoxic T cells. Indeed, the granulated lymphoid cell population may play a particularly important role in regulating immune responses.

Finally, macrophages and other phagocytic cells are also important because they act both as antigen-presenting cells (APC) processing antigens for presentation to specific antigen-sensitive lymphocytes and also in a phagocytic capacity removing debris following local immunological or inflammatory reactions.

Cytokines

The cellular release of soluble factors (cytokines) can dramatically influence lymphocytes and macrophages. There are many different cytokines, including lymphocyte-derived mediators (lymphokines), and their individual contribution to the growth, differentiation or function of separate leukocytic cell populations is complex. Of particular note, however, are the following antigen-nonspecific cytokines:

1. *Interleukin-1* (IL-1), a lymphocyte-activating factor produced by macrophages, which also promotes a variety of other pyrogenic and cell proliferative sequelae.
2. *Interleukin-2* (IL-2), a polypeptide hormone produced by activated T cells and essential for long-term lymphocyte growth.
3. *Interferons* (IFN), a family of related glycoproteins produced by many cell types following activation or infection which may act on neighbouring cells to inhibit cell or viral growth, increase expression of human leukocyte antigens (HLA), activate macrophages and NK cells, as well as having an immunoregulatory role that can result in either enhancement or suppression of immune responses.
4. *Colony-stimulating factors* (CSF), leukocyte-derived glycoproteins which regulate the bone marrow production and proliferation of cells along the mononuclear phagocyte pathway.
5. *Tumour necrosis factor/lymphotoxin* (TNF α and β), factors produced by macrophages or activated lymphocytes respectively, which can directly lyse some tumour cells as well as also be toxic and partake in inflammatory responses.

Major histocompatibility complex (MHC)

The MHC complex is located on the short arm of chromosome 6 and represents a gene cluster occupying about 1/3000th of the total genome (Roitt et al 1985, Stites et al 1987). It was originally identified because cell surface histocompatibility antigens (HLA antigens) encoded within the MHC genetic region play a central role in transplantation rejection. It is now also recognized that MHC proteins direct fundamental cellular interactions in the immune response, and also that the genes for several other biologically important proteins lie within this region (Fig. 11.1). HLA antigens are encoded by multiple loci within MHC and express a remarkable degree of genetic polymorphism, with between three and 45 closely related alternative genes (alleles) that may be inherited at any individual HLA gene locus. This pool of multiple alleles creates a vast genetic variability and, although some HLA alleles are more common than others, the likelihood of any two unrelated individuals being HLA-

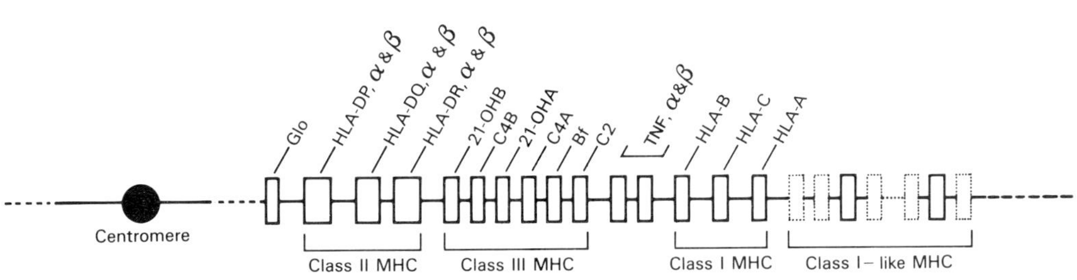

Fig. 11.1 Schematic representation of the human major histocompatibility gene complex on the short arm of chromosome 6.

identical is extremely remote. HLA alleles are inherited within intact sets (haplotypes) containing all the MHC genes, one from each parent in an orderly Mendelian fashion. There is codominant expression of maternally and paternally inherited HLA antigens.

It has been convenient to divide HLA antigens into two broad classes based on biochemical and functional similarities. Thus, the products of the HLA-A, -B and -C loci are called class I MHC antigens, each is a 43–46 000 dalton glycoprotein associated non-covalently at the cell surface with a non-polymorphic polypeptide called β_2-microglobulin (12 000 daltons) encoded by a gene on chromosome 15. These class I MHC antigens are carried by nearly all nucleated cells in varying amounts, and are essential cell surface recognition molecules identified by cytotoxic T cells. There are also numerous MHC gene loci distal to HLA-A that have been termed class I-like or, sometimes, class IV (Jordan et al 1985). There are at least 17 such loci and, although the majority are pseudogenes or fragments, a small number may be intact genes capable of translation into protein. It is thought that the human class I-like MHC genes are analogous to a region defined for the murine MHC and termed *Qa/Tl* genes; these have a gene structure and association with β_2-microglobulin similar to regular class I MHC genes, but express much less genetic polymorphism and have a restricted tissue distribution; their biological functions are unknown.

Class II MHC antigens (HLA-DP, -DQ and -DR) are cell surface glycoproteins composed of a 32–35 000 dalton (α) chain together with a related 27–30 000 dalton (β) chain; both are encoded within the MHC and both may carry allelic determinants. Class II MHC antigens display a restricted tissue expression (B cells, monocytes and macrophages, activated T cells and certain epithelia) and are essential as cell surface recognition molecules presenting antigen to helper T cells. The concept that cytotoxic and helper T cells do not bind free antigen but only recognize antigen in association with class I or II MHC antigens, respectively, on cell surfaces has become a central dogma in modern immunology (Zinkernagel & Doherty 1979).

The genetic region between class I and II encodes a closely knit group of genes for certain of the complement proteins — those for factor B (Bf), the complement protein C2 and the tandem genes for the complement protein C4 (C4A and C4B). This region is sometimes known as the class III MHC region. Other genes, not necessarily of direct immunological interest, are also found in this area; these include the tandem genes for the enzyme 21-hydroxylase (21-OHA and 21-OHB) as well as the genes for TNF. Finally, the gene for the enzyme glyoxylase (Glo) is located immediately adjacent to the MHC region (Fig. 11.1).

CELLULAR AND ANTIBODY TRANSFER BETWEEN MOTHER AND FETUS

It is well established that fetal red cells can be detected in maternal blood, particularly after delivery, but there is also a progressive rise in fetal red cells entering maternal circulation during the third trimester (Woodrow & Finn 1968). Transplacental haemorrhage can result in rhesus isoimmunization and, more rarely, immunological sensitization to other blood group antigens or platelet antigens has been described. Similarly, some passage of leukocytes into maternal blood occurs, which may sensitize the mother to fetal (paternally inherited) HLA. The prevalence of detection of antibodies against paternal leukocytes will depend on the specificity and sensitivity of assay technique, although 10–20% of women may develop cytotoxic antibody in primiparous pregnancy and up to 50% of women in multiparous pregnancy (Ahrons 1971). Indeed, multiparous sera are the usual source for serological tissue typing reagents. It is known that the presence of these HLA antibodies from previous pregnancies or prior blood transfusions (or, indeed their absence) does not prejudice the immunological viability of the pregnancy (Jazwinska et al 1987). However, the nature of the fetal leukocytes which sensitize the mother is unknown; these could be Hofbauer cells, other tissue cells or blood leukocytes from fetomaternal haemorrhage.

Transplacental trafficking of sensitized lymphocytes from mother to fetus has been difficult to assess other than when associated with a subsequent abnormality. For example, chimerism has been found in occasional children with severe combined immunodeficiency and runting shown in experimental animals following adoptive transfer to the mother of hyperimmune cells specific for the fetal MHC antigens (Hunziker & Wegmann 1986). The conclusion from studies to date using cell labelling techniques is that small numbers of maternal erythrocytes may enter the fetus but that leukocytes are generally excluded (Hunziker et al 1984).

Immunoglobulins of the IgG class are selectively transported across the human placenta from maternal blood within the intervillous spaces. The initial molecular event is specific recognition by receptors on the surface of placental syncytiotrophoblast microvilli that bind the Fc region of IgG — Fcγ receptors (Johnson & Brown 1981). Protected cellular transfer of IgG then occurs within intracellular endocytotic vesicles prior to release into placental tissue and subsequent movement into the lumen of fetal stem vessels to confer passive immunity to the fetus. Significant transplacental passage of maternal IgG to fetal circulation commences around the 20th to 22nd week of gestation and all four subclasses of IgG (IgG1, 2, 3 and 4) are actively transferred from mother to fetus, although it has occasionally been suggested that IgG2 transfer may lag very slightly behind the others; there is no selective transport of any other immunoglobulin class or plasma protein.

THE SURVIVAL OF THE FETAL ALLOGRAFT

Background

Medawar (1953) proposed various hypotheses to account for mammalian viviparity as a unique example of successful transplantation; these theories created a fundamental basis from which most modern investigations have been derived. Medawar's hypotheses included the following:

1. The conceptus is not immunogenic and therefore does not evoke an immunologic response. However, it is now known that the conceptus itself does express MHC antigens in pregnancy and, for example, that maternal anti-fetal HLA antibodies are a common occurrence.
2. Pregnancy alters the immune response. It is now accepted that pregnant women are not non-specifically immunosuppressed since normally they neither succumb to systemic or local infection in pregnancy nor, in experimental animals, do they accept mismatched tissue allografts (including, for example, paternal skin grafts or ectopic fetal tissue grafts). Nevertheless, more subtle alterations to antigen-specific responses remain possible.
3. The uterus is an immunologically privileged site. However, other foreign tissue allografts placed within the uterus will be rejected, even in hormonally primed animals, albeit often after a longer time than tissue grafts at other sites. This emphasizes the unique status of the fetal graft, as do observations in experimental animals that grafts placed at other privileged sites, such as the brain, anterior chamber of the eye or the testis, do not induce transplantation immunity yet are nevertheless rejected if the host has been pre-immunized — unlike the situation for intrauterine pregnancy (Beer & Billingham 1976). However, the response to paternal tissue grafts placed directly at the chorio-decidual junction is uncertain and difficult to ascertain because of anatomical as well as immunological considerations.
4. The placenta is an effective immunological barrier between mother and fetus. This has been discussed above, and it is also pertinent to remember that both the lymphatic and vascular systems remain essentially distinct for both mother and fetus, in contrast to the direct contact in most examples of clinical transplantation. Together with the effect of endometrial decidualization, this may lead to a slight immunological quarantining effect.

Current concepts on the riddle of the fetal allograft acknowledge multifactorial mechanisms, discussed below.

HLA expression at fetomaternal interfaces

Because of the extensive genetic polymorphism, nearly all human pregnancies involve fetomaternal MHC disparity. Since HLA molecules are the focus of both regulatory and cytotoxic immune responses, the maternal–fetal immunogenetic enigma is central to our understanding of the immunology of pregnancy. Faulk & McIntyre (1983) highlighted the fact that it is trophoblast in its various differentiated forms which forms the sole and continuous fetal tissue interface with both maternal blood and decidual tissue. The extensive interfaces between fetal trophoblast and maternal tissues are anatomically complex (see Chapter 5), and it is important to view trophoblast as acting in response to a variety of differentiation signals at these sites. Hence, anatomically defined trophoblast subpopulations may express distinct cell surface antigen phenotypes (Bulmer & Johnson 1985).

It has been consistently established that there is no detectable expression of either classical class I (HLA-A, -B, -C) or class II (HLA-DP, -DQ, -DR) MHC antigens by human chorionic villous trophoblast throughout gestation (Faulk & McIntyre 1983, Bulmer & Johnson 1985, Hunt et al 1987). However, there is normal development of class I and, more latterly in gestation, class II MHC antigens on non-trophoblastic cells in extraembryonic tissues. The remarkable absence of regular HLA transplantation antigen expression on trophoblast is undoubtedly of pivotal significance in protecting this vital tissue from effective maternal immune recognition or cytotoxic cell attack.

This observation explains why there is no rejection response to trophoblast placed under the kidney capsule in experimental animals, unlike for other foreign tissues placed adjacent to trophoblast at this ectopic site (Simmons & Russell 1967). Also, trophoblastic cellular elements continuously break away from the implantation site during human pregnancy, pass into the uterine vein, lodge eventually in the lung and mostly degrade (Thomas et al 1959, Attwood & Park 1961, Kozma et al 1986); this process occurs without provoking any inflammatory or immunological rejection response. It is unknown whether the continuous deportation of villous trophoblastic elements into maternal blood induces a form of systemic immunological tolerance to fetal trophoblast antigens in the mother. However, during the second half of pregnancy, these exfoliated elements will carry the heat-stable placental-type alkaline phosphatase (PLAP) isoenzyme which itself expresses significant genetic polymorphism (McLaughlin & Johnson 1984, Webb et al 1985). Maternal immunity to paternally inherited fetal PLAP alleles has never been described in pregnancy and hence unidentified mechanisms may exist to enable the mother to tolerate these fetal trophoblast antigens but not other polymorphic antigens expressed by non-trophoblastic fetal cells, such as HLA-A, -B or -DR.

Since MHC molecules regulate the T cell immune response, HLA-negative villous trophoblast also may not be recognized by cellular antiviral or other foreign antigen responses. There is some attraction for this concept. Thus, trophoblast in cell culture may have an unusual resistance to cytotoxic effector cells (Clark & Chaouat 1986). In addition, human trophoblast has been shown to contain both retrovirus-like particles and antigenic activity, to express retrovirus-like RNA-directed DNA polymerase activity; also it may be involved in the antibody response to retroviruses observed in some pregnancy sera (Suni et al 1984, Wahlstrom et al 1984, Risk & Johnson 1985).

Our understanding of the molecular genetics of how fetal trophoblast exceptionally fails to transcribe regular HLA molecules is much in its infancy, as is the determination of factors that might influence this unusual example of gene regulation (Head et al 1987, Hunt et al 1987). It may require the development of uncontaminated homogeneous trophoblast cell lines to test mechanistic models, although this approach has not yet achieved full success (Loke et al 1986). Thus, at present, it is unknown whether normal human trophoblast can be induced to express such transplantation target antigens, or whether this might abnormally occur in occasional examples of spontaneous abortion.

Although trophoblast does not express regular class I MHC antigens, extravillous cytotrophoblast populations do express an antigenically related molecule that appears not to be a classical HLA-A or -B antigen (Redman et al 1984, Hsi et al 1984, Bulmer & Johnson 1985). It has been suggested that this is a class I-like MHC molecule; this is further discussed below in the section on immunoregulation in pregnancy.

Fetal protection from maternal IgG antibody

Fcγ receptors are also abundant on non-trophoblastic cells within the placental villous stroma, notably macrophages (Hofbauer cells) and fetal stem vessel endothelium. Unlike syncytiotrophoblast Fcγ receptors, the non-trophoblastic placental Fcγ receptors do not bind native IgG but instead have specificity for aggregated or antigen-complexed IgG (Johnson & Brown 1981). This selective binding has been termed the placental sink, since these high avidity Fcγ receptors are thought to act as an extensive filter, sequestering soluble immune complexes formed locally between fetal antigens and any corresponding maternal IgG antibody transported across trophoblastic tissue (Johnson et al 1980). This protective mechanism may be expected to be essential since any such deleterious IgG antibodies and immune complexes, if allowed to penetrate further than extraembryonic tissue, could potentially have catastrophic consequences on the fetus for the development of its own immunological capacity. The trapping of a significant amount of maternal IgG as immune complexes within placental tissue is evident from the extensive immunopathology involving immunoglobulin and complement deposition within normal term placentae (Faulk & Johnson 1977, Johnson et al 1977).

Several situations involving specific antibodies illustrate this phenomenon. Firstly, maternal IgG autoantibodies that are organ-specific and do not have their corresponding autoantigen accessible within the placenta, such as in Graves' thyrotoxicosis or myasthenia gravis, would not form immune complexes and be retained within placental tissue. These IgG antibodies would be expected to reach the fetus; that this does indeed occur is shown by clinical reports of transient neonatal manifestations of the corresponding autoimmune disease (Scott 1976). Secondly, maternal IgG antibodies to fetal HLA are not uncommon in pregnancy and, following transfer across HLA-negative syncytiotrophoblast, these antibodies would then bind to HLA-positive non-trophoblastic cells within chorionic villi; soluble complexes would be removed on to the macrophage and endothelial Fcγ receptors. This process is remarkably efficient in negating maternal antifetal HLA antibodies access to cord blood. Thus, such antibodies with specificity for the present pregnancy are detected in placental eluates but not in neonatal sera (Jeannet et al 1977), whereas the converse is the case for any maternal anti-HLA antibody without specificity for the present pregnancy that may have arisen from a previous pregnancy or blood transfusion (Doughty & Gelsthorpe 1976). Finally, this concept cannot be directly applied to rhesus antigens because these are not expressed in the placenta other than on erythrocytes. Thus, fetal red cell haemolysis by native maternal IgG antibody will occur prior to retention of any antibody on endothelial Fcγ receptors for immune complexes; nevertheless, it is of interest that endothelial cell damage can occur in placentae from cases of maternal–fetal rhesus incompatibility (Jones & Fox 1978).

Immunoregulation in pregnancy

The discussion above describes passive mechanisms for protection of the fetal graft. Current concepts also emphasize a variety of active mechanisms induced by pregnancy-associated events involving production of specific immunological factors or immunoregulatory proteins.

Trophoblast membrane antigens

Immunohistochemical studies have shown that human cytotrophoblast populations in the placental bed and chorion leave express class I MHC-type molecules that are unreactive with antibodies to the relevant fetal HLA-A or -B polymorphic tissue-type expected from the paternal genotype (Redman et al 1984). The general rule in normal pregnancy of complete HLA-negativity for all syncytial and villous trophoblast, and expression only of an unusual class I-type MHC molecule by extravillous cytotrophoblast, appears also to hold for pregnancy disorders such as ectopic pregnancy, hydatidiform mole and choriocarcinoma (Earl et al 1985, Bulmer et al 1988). Difficulties in separation of invasive fetal extravillous trophoblast from the complex cellular constitution of HLA-positive maternal decidual tissues has hindered more precise biochemical studies. However, observations from choriocarcinoma cell lines and from baboon placentae have indicated the unusual class I-type MHC antigen to be a 40–41 000 dalton molecule associated with β_2-microglobulin and of limited polymorphism (Ellis et al 1986, Stern et al 1987).

Current thought favours this molecule to be closely related to HLA-C and may be an unusual class I-like MHC antigen (Johnson & Stern 1986). Since it is expressed at maternal-facing surfaces prior to full establishment of fetal T cell immunocompetence, the biological drive for its expression may be in the context of a meaningful dialogue with the maternal immune system, either to provide T cell surveillance of fetal tissue at risk of viral infection or, more likely, for fetal signalling of maternal immunoregulatory responses. This unusual class I MHC-like trophoblastic antigen is expressed within first-trimester human uteroplacental tissues, although any expression during the important peri-implantation and early post-implantation events is unknown. Because of the genetic similarity of class I-type MHC gene products, elucidation of the exact nature of this intriguing trophoblastic antigen awaits current research on its identification and characterization using molecular biological techniques.

A separate molecular system expressed by both trophoblast and leukocytes was originally identified using rabbit antisera and termed the trophoblast–leukocyte common (TLX) antigen system (Faulk & McIntyre 1983); these antisera exhibit HLA-independent inhibition of lymphocyte stimulation in mixed lymphocyte culture reactions (MLR). Monoclonal antibodies have been produced that may recognize molecules of the TLX family, and the corresponding protein antigens identified which exhibit a size heterogeneity between individuals (Johnson et al 1981, Stern et al 1986). These TLX molecules are thought to be encoded on chromosome 1, and are expressed by all human trophoblast and peripheral blood leukocyte populations, as well as a variety of other cell types including endometrial glandular epithelium and capacitated sperm (Johnson & Stern 1986, Stern et al 1986).

The unusual class I-like MHC antigen and the TLX antigen expressed by trophoblast are both strong candidates to influence maternal humoral or cellular immunoregulatory mechanisms. Those responses whose biological significance is in the content of immune suppression will be more elusive to identify than cytotoxic responses and require the development of relevant assay systems. Current information is reviewed below.

Maternal antibody responses

Pregnancy sera have been reported to contain molecules, including many pregnancy-associated proteins and steroidal hormones, which non-specifically inhibit a wide variety of in vitro assays of T lymphocyte proliferation or function (Rocklin et al 1976, Bissenden et al 1980, Stimson 1983, Stites et al 1983). Since extrauterine immunocompetence is not extensively prejudiced in pregnancy, attention has focused on pregnancy-induced maternal antibodies that may serve a more specific blocking function (Lancet Editorial 1983). It is an attractive concept that such blocking antibodies could influence maternal cell-mediated immunity to the fetus. There are several candidates that, individually or together, may contribute to blocking antibody activity in pregnancy.

Although anti-HLA-A and -B antibodies can be detected in many multiparous sera, recent serological data have shown the majority of reactivity to be directed against broadly shared class I MHC antigenic determinants rather than single specific HLA tissue-type antigens (Konoeda et al 1986). Furthermore, up to 20% of multiparous sera contains antibodies reactive only with activated T cells and not ascribable to classical class I or II MHC antigen specificities (Johnson & Stern 1986). Any inter-relationship of these pregnancy-induced antibody activities with class I-like MHC antigens expressed on extravillous cytotrophoblast remains to be explored. Antibodies to class II MHC antigens can block stimulator function in MLR assays; however, they are infrequent in pregnancy and may not arise until late in gestation when class II MHC antigens are eventually expressed in extraembryonic tissues (Redman et al 1984).

Other pregnancy-induced antibodies that could contribute to an immunoregulatory function include several less well defined systems, such as non-cytotoxic antibodies that block Fcγ receptors of B cells (Power et al 1986) and also autoanti-idiotypic antibodies reactive with maternal T cell receptors for paternal HLA (Suciu-Foca et al 1983); idiotypic determinants are unique antigenic determinants characteristic of the specific variable region of individual immunoglobulin or T cell receptor molecules (Roitt et al 1985). It should be borne in mind, however, that laboratory procedures for these in vitro blocking antibody assays are technically complex and difficult to repeat. Furthermore, results with pregnancy sera in any one assay system will not necessarily be of clinical usefulness. For example, it is attractive to postulate an anti-trophoblast, and specifically anti-TLX, antibody response in normal pregnancy, although this has not yet been convincingly demonstrated by laboratory assay and remains a matter of some controversy. Thus, the relative importance of blocking antibody to the immunological viability of an on-going pregnancy remains to be defined, and it is still possible that this may be no more than a consequence of pregnancy rather than of fundamental biological importance for the maintenance of that pregnancy.

Maternal cellular responses

There is little consistent evidence for intrinsic non-specific depression for in vitro responses of maternal peripheral blood lymphocytes to foreign antigens or mitogens (Gusdon 1976, Loke 1978), although there have been reports of impaired specific lymphocyte blastogenic responses to various micro-organisms, including cytomegalovirus (Gehrz et al 1981a,b); this could be due to increased environmental exposure or an inadequate immune response associated with hormonal changes in pregnancy. Most studies agree that there is no significant change in the balance between helper and suppressor T cells in peripheral blood (Moore et al 1983). More important is whether maternal cell-mediated sensitization to paternally inherited fetal antigens commonly occurs in a manner analogous to maternal anti-HLA antibody production. Recent work has shown that circulating cytotoxic effector T cells specific for paternal lymphocytes may occur only rarely in normal pregnancy (Sargent et al 1987).

Events at maternal–fetal interfaces may be of particular importance in controlling maternal cellular or humoral sensitization to fetal antigens. Endometrial tissue undergoes cellular changes in pregnancy with hormonal alterations leading to the decidual reaction and with invasion by fetal trophoblast. Extensive numbers of leukocytes can also be highlighted in decidua (Bulmer & Sunderland 1984). A proportion are class II MHC-positive macrophages, often found closely associated with extravillous cytotrophoblast; these may serve essential phagocytic functions and provide a defence to infection in the presence of local immunosuppression, allowing fetal graft survival (Bulmer & Johnson 1984). However, a major leukocytic component in early pregnancy decidua has been characterized as unusual lymphoid cells which, intriguingly despite the potential of activated macrophages to act as fetal antigen-presenting cells and to prime T cell responses by release of IL-1, do not express any immunological activation markers such as the IL-2 receptor (Bulmer & Johnson 1986).

Local cellular production within uteroplacental tissues of various factors shown to have immunomodulatory properties, albeit sometimes only at supraphysiological levels, may together give some bias towards non-specific immunosuppression at maternal–fetal interfaces (Stimson 1983, Stites et al 1983, Anderson & Yunis 1985); these would include progesterone and other steroids, pregnancy-associated proteins, prostaglandins, polyamines, interferons and, possibly, soluble HLA molecules. There is also evidence that some decidual leukocytes may act as suppressor cells through the generation of a soluble factor which impairs IL-2-dependent lymphocyte responses (Clark et al 1985, Daya et al 1985). However, investigations with heterogeneous decidual or placental cell populations can be difficult to interpret, and the exact nature and cellular sources(s) of decidual suppressor factors await clarification by functional studies with homogeneous cell preparations (Nakayama et al 1985). Nevertheless, there is general support favouring local decidual production of potent factors which inhibit IL-2 activity (Nicholas & Panayi 1986, Bulmer & Johnson 1986). This could provide a cocoon of an appropriate form of non-specific immunosuppression in the pregnant uterus since a requirement for IL-2 is a common denominator for the generation of cytotoxic T cell or NK cell responses; any failure of this mechanism could potentially lead to an IL-2-dependent cytotoxic attack against fetal tissue.

Two additional concepts are also worth mentioning. Firstly, the placental syncytiotrophoblastic surface is rich in a specific receptor for the iron-transport plasma protein, transferrin, which effectively lines the intervillous blood space and acts as the initial molecular recognition step in the transfer of iron from mother to fetus (Webb et al 1985). However, since transferrin-bound iron is also an essential growth factor for lymphocyte proliferation, any rapidly dividing lymphocyte within intervillous spaces would need to compete for binding transferrin with the excess expression of transferrin receptors on the surrounding syncytiotrophoblastic tissue (Johnson et al 1980). Secondly, an alternative biological role for decidual leukocytes has been considered — that fetal trophoblast may be dependent on leukocyte-derived growth factors (lymphokines) for its development (Athannasakis et al 1987, Wegmann 1987). Thus, local maternal leukocyte activity could be beneficial to trophoblastic growth and function by a paraimmunological mechanism. CSF is the cytokine which has attracted most interest in this role, and it is of note that syncytiotrophoblast unusually expresses the specific receptor for M-CSF on its surface (Adamson 1987, Webb & Johnson, unpublished observations); the M-CSF receptor is otherwise found only on cells of the monocyte–macrophage lineage. The M-CSF receptor is the protein product of the c-fms proto-oncogene and, indeed, all proto-oncogene proteins so far identified are expressed in the placenta (Adamson 1987). This reflects its rapid controlled growth and development, and hence this organ is a plentiful source of growth factors, hormones and growth factor receptors.

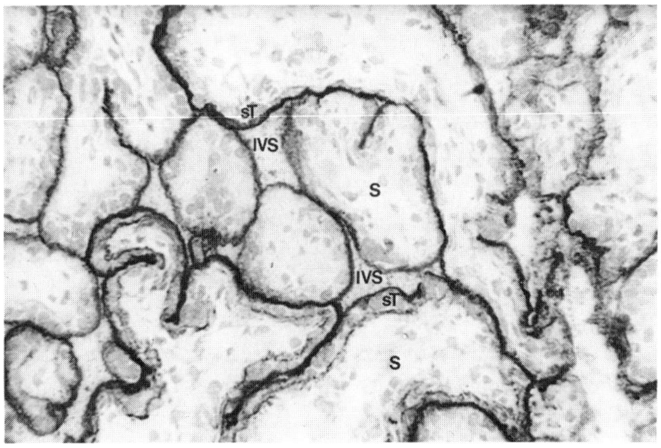

Fig. 11.2 Indirect immunoperoxidase staining of a cryostat section of normal term chorionic villous tissue using the murine H317 monoclonal antibody to placenta-like alkaline phosphatase (PLAP) followed by peroxidase-conjugated anti-mouse immunoglobulin. Note the intense staining for PLAP on the apical surface of syncytiotrophoblast. sT = syncytiotrophoblast; S = villous stroma; IVS = intervillous space.

IMMUNOLOGICAL IDENTIFICATION OF TROPHOBLAST

The syncytiotrophoblast plasma membrane expresses numerous protein components (Webb et al 1985), although much less detail is known about the surface of cytotrophoblast populations. However, the development and application of monoclonal antibodies has identified many cellular antigens that, taken together, constitute the characteristic cellular antigenic phenotype of different trophoblast populations in the chorionic villous tissue (Fig. 11.2), placental bed and surrounding chorion laeve (Bulmer & Johnson 1985). This approach, based on a panel of monoclonal antibodies, has been useful for the immunohistological identification of trophoblast and non-trophoblastic cell types in abnormal pregnancies (Earl et al 1985, Bulmer et al 1988) as well as for identification of cell types within isolated placental cell cultures (Loke et al 1986).

Certain monoclonal antibodies recognize cell surface antigens with a relatively restricted tissue distribution other than expression by trophoblast; several are also abnormally expressed by various tumour cells and can be described under a generic term of oncotrophoblast antigens, e.g. PLAP, which has proven to be of some value as a tumour marker in ovarian carcinoma and seminoma (McLaughlin & Johnson 1984). However, a recent workshop screened 45 selected monoclonal antibodies and confirmed the elusive nature of an entirely trophoblast-specific membrane antigen represented on all human trophoblast populations (Anderson et al 1987), although further monoclonal antibodies are continuously being added to the available panel of interesting candidates (see Hsi et al 1987).

There are two major thrusts for this line of research. Firstly, a monoclonal antibody recognizing a cell surface antigen entirely specific for fetal trophoblast, in concert with a fluorescence-activated cell sorter, could potentially provide a means for isolating from peripheral blood any trace numbers of the extensive amount of fetal trophoblastic cells that are detached from the implantation site and enter the uterine vein (100–200 000 cells per day are oft-quoted figures). This would enable prenatal genetic diagnosis of inherited disease by a minimally invasive technique in situations where there was a sensitive probe analysis available for the disease gene. However, this approach has yet to reach maturity because the numbers of fetal trophoblastic cells that cross the lung barrier into peripheral blood may be infinitesimally small and also there may be intravascular uptake of trophoblastic cell membrane fragments by maternal cells which would then contaminate any subsequent separation of fetal cells.

Secondly, a specific trophoblast cell surface antigen, expressed very early in gestation but not represented in any other normal adult or fetal tissue, could be engineered to form the basis for future development of a birth control (contragestational) vaccine. Such a target antigen would only be expressed at a defined anatomic site, initially in small amounts and exclusively following conception. The approach fits into a wider development programme for birth control vaccines aimed primarily to meet a developing world requirement and is analogous to that established for very early interruption of pregnancy by prior vaccination against a synthetic peptide representing the C-terminal portion of the β-chain of human chorionic gonadotrophin, a secreted protein hormone of trophoblast. This strategy has achieved an effective repeatable contragestational effect of limited duration in baboons (Stevens 1986), and a World Health Organization-sponsored clinical trial to assess safety and immunogenicity in sterilized women is currently in progress.

CLINICAL ASPECTS OF PREGNANCY IMMUNOLOGY

Recurrent spontaneous abortion (RSA)

Recent evidence has focused attention towards a possible immunological background for a proportion of patients suffering repeated early fetal loss. This is usually identified by three or more consecutive confirmed unexplained first-trimester spontaneous abortions and sometimes divided into two groups:

1. No live births or pregnancy exceeding 28 weeks' gestation (primary abortion);
2. A single live birth or pregnancy of at least 28 weeks' gestation preceding the unbroken series of pregnancy losses (secondary abortion).

Cytogenetic, anatomical endocrinological, infectious and other medical causes (e.g. diabetes) that could contribute to recurring fetal loss will have been ruled out by both clinical and laboratory investigation, including karyotypic analyses, hysterosalpingogram, thyroid function tests and cervical cultures. Immunotherapeutic studies would exclude women with a history of aneuploidic pregnancy loss, detectable serum antinuclear or lupus anticoagulant autoantibody (see later section), clinical evidence of autoimmune disease or an abnormal full blood count. Thus, these women fall into an, as yet, unexplained group of RSA patients. Their selection is essentially one of exclusion of other causes and clearly it is unjustified to assume a single common mechanism for all cases of unexplained RSA.

Investigation

Whilst animal models of recurrent fetal loss have been described which are responsive to immunotherapeutic procedures (Clark et al 1987), there is little histopathological evidence in humans of immune-mediated attack in the placenta of an abortus (Fox 1978). Nevertheless, it has been proposed that defects within immunoregulatory responses normally resultant from fetomaternal immunological interactions might lead to occasional women suffering RSA because of failure in immune adaptation in early pregnancy (Faulk & McIntyre 1983, Mowbray & Underwood 1985, Johnson et al 1986, Clark et al 1987). This could involve either intrinsic maternal hyporesponsiveness (which would be partner-non-specific) or absent maternal recognition due to repeated maternal–fetal allelic identity of a relevant genetically polymorphic antigen (which would be partner-specific).

What evidence in man is there to support this conjecture? Some work has pointed towards greater parental HLA sharing than expected by chance (Thomas et al 1985, McIntyre et al 1986), although this does not achieve statistical significance at all centres (Johnson et al 1986, 1988b). Healthy neonates can be completely HLA-identical with their mother (Jazwinska et al 1987) and, conversely, completely HLA-mismatched pregnancies often occur in donor oocyte motherhood; hence there is no gross correlation between fetomaternal HLA disparity and pregnancy outcome. In addition, a significant trend towards increased female HLA-B and C4 locus homozygosity has been described in RSA women, as well as increased prevalence of certain unusual HLA haplotypes, although this does not necessarily involve the majority of patients (Johnson & Ramsden 1988, Johnson et al 1988b). The cumulative immunogenetic data in RSA, although fragmentary and inconsistent between centres, could nonetheless reflect a subtle genetic variation within MHC or the presence of an MHC-linked gene which influences intrauterine prenatal selection. Other studies of serum lymphocytotoxic antibodies, tissue-reactive autoantibodies, total serum IgE levels and circulating T cell populations also have not identified a major subgroup of unexplained RSA patients that clearly correlates with either the previous clinical history (primary or secondary RSA) or outcome in a subsequent pregnancy (Johnson & Ramsden 1988, Johnson et al 1988b). Thus, these parameters do not presently appear to assist prediction of clinical behaviour.

There are indications that other pregnancy-induced lymphocyte-reactive antibodies, detected by functional blocking activity in various laboratory assays, are absent in RSA women during pregnancies which abort (Rocklin et al 1976, Beer et al 1985, Power et al 1986, Takakuwa et al 1986). In addition, hyporesponsiveness of maternal lymphocytes reacting to paternal cells has been described in RSA (Beer et al 1985, McIntyre et al 1986), although it is unclear whether this inconsistent observation identifies an intrinsic cellular hyporesponsiveness or action of serum factors within the cell culture assay. Nevertheless, these findings formed the original basis for immunization with paternal or third-party unmatched leukocytes as immunotherapy in unexplained RSA (Beer et al 1985, McIntyre et al 1986).

Immunotherapy

Although the cell source (paternal or third-party leukocytes), dose (up to 5×10^8 cells) and route of administration (intravenous, intradermal, subcutaneous) has varied between centres, initial studies have indicated favourable reproductive outcome following leukocyte immunization and describe successful pregnancies occurring in 70–90% of cases. Patient referral and selection will vary between centres, some of which exclude lymphocytotoxic antibody-positive patients partly because of a risk of anaphylactic reaction and also because its presence indicates that at least one particular maternal–fetal immunological interaction has occurred. Only one controlled trial has been completed (Mowbray et al 1985) and the strength of undoubted placebo effect remains to be fully assessed.

Although convenient, repeated immunization of healthy immunocompetent women with viable leukocytes should be approached with extreme clinical caution and considered at present only within research centres with appropriate multidisciplinary interests. Thus, concomitant sensitization to fetal HLA or other leukocyte antigens may occur and could be associated with an increased risk of intrauterine growth retardation and, at least theoretically, entry of any maternal immune cells could cause fetal engraftment in rare cases, leading to graft-versus-host disease (Lancet Editorial 1983, Beer et al 1985, Johnson & Ramsden 1988). Concomitant sensitization to blood group or platelet antigens may also compromise a subsequent pregnancy, although leukocyte immunization can be given with anti-Rh(D) immunoglobulin cover. In addition, transfusion-related risks have to be considered, including viral (e.g. cytomegalovirus or human immunodeficiency virus) transmission by viable leukocytes. Congenital cytomegalovirus is the commonest infective cause of fetal malformation and hence the cytomegalovirus immune status of RSA couples is relevant when considering leukocyte immunization during the periconception period (Radcliffe et al 1988). Finally, some genetic developmental abnormalities may occasionally be associated with parental HLA sharing (Beer et al 1985). Thus, although an attractive approach, it is imperative to remember that it is quicker to identify successful outcome than risk factors in this area with substantial emotive pressure. Detailed assessment, particularly for intrauterine growth retardation and neonatal congenital abnormalities, as well as long-term follow-up of RSA patients following leukocyte immunization is required before these controversial issues are finally settled.

Alternative approaches may also require further exploration, such as intravenous infusion with isolated sterile (non-nucleated) syncytiotrophoblast microvillous plasma membrane preparations which, although less convenient, have the advantage of being HLA-negative and mimic one example of fetal cellular contact with the maternal immune system in normal pregnancy; initial results have shown promise in unexplained RSA (Johnson et al 1988a). Indeed, central questions focus on the most rational and safe approach to immunotherapy. Further placebo-controlled or comparative studies need to be undertaken to assess accurately the efficacy of active immunotherapy, particularly since similar claims have been made in favour of supportive psychotherapy (Stray-Pedersen & Stray-Pedersen 1984). Equally, attention needs to be directed towards improvements in laboratory identification of women from within the undoubted clinical heterogeneity of unexplained RSA who may benefit from an immunotherapeutic approach. Since immunization is not an insignificant procedure, this is urgently required to improve patient selection and to avoid unnecessarily offering false hope. At present, active immunotherapy presupposes the development of a relevant immunoregulatory response — which has been elusive to identification by laboratory assays (as indeed has been the consistent identification of laboratory parameters characteristic of trophoblast survival in normal pregnancy). Thus, the exact mechanism of action could involve direct cellular, antibody or cytokine stimulation effects.

Leukocyte immunization may increase apparent fertility and twinning rates (Mowbray, personal communication), hence introducing the question whether immunotherapy could influence very early pregnancy events. More than 30% of all conceptions are lost during the peri-implantation period, many of which are due to cytogenetic or implantation defects. It is difficult to envisage immunological (as distinct, for example, from hormonal) events acting so immediately in response to pregnancy, although factors have been described in very early pregnancy with apparent in vitro immunoregulatory properties (such as early pregnancy factor). Antisperm antibodies have been reported in unexplained infertility and contrasting results may depend on the precise assay procedure employed (Haas 1987); there is some doubt, however, as to the strength of their biological effect in vivo other than in extreme cases of immunological infertility. Nevertheless, since the early embryo might express some of the same surface antigens as spermatozoa, there could be an inter-relationship between embryotoxic and antisperm antibodies in certain cases of recurring occult or early fetal loss (Haas et al 1986). This may be more pronounced in a subgroup of secondary RSA women associated with the development of antibody responses, including lymphocytotoxic and trophoblast-reactive antibodies (McIntyre et al 1986).

Autoimmunity and pregnancy

Childbearing women may be affected by various connective tissue diseases which are themselves linked with particular antibody or HLA patterns, as well as a multifactorial background including genetic and environmental factors (Scott 1984). Some correlation is emerging between fetal and neonatal effects and particular types of maternal autoantibody.

Antiphospholipid antibodies (APA)

These are autoantibodies directed against negatively charged phospholipids and are found in various myeloproliferative disorders, acute infections and connective tissue disease, including 15–20% of systemic lupus erythematosus patients; APA can occur as IgM or IgG, or both. They are associated with a syndrome that may involve a history of thrombotic episodes, thrombocytopenia and intrauterine fetal death, although additional features can include neurological complaints and livedo reticularis. However, only a small fraction (no more than 5%) of all RSA patients will have significant APA levels. Women with APA need not necessarily have clinical evidence of connective tissue disease at the time of investigation (Scott 1984, Lubbe & Liggins 1985).

APA exert a complicated effect on the coagulation system which led to a rather enigmatic definition as lupus anticoagulant antibody. Thus, in contrast to an association with thromboembolic events in vivo, APA in fresh plasma paradoxically prolong phospholipid-dependent coagulation times in vitro (including the activated partial thromboplastin or kaolin-cephalin clotting times) even when the plasma is mixed with an equal quantity of normal plasma (Scott 1984). APA are also frequently associated with a biologically false positive Venereal Disease Research Laboratories serological test for syphilis. There has been a drive to identify a specific immunological test for APA and the most promising has been immunoassay of antibody reactive with cardiolipin, a particular mixture of negatively charged phospholipids. Although there is some uncertainty about clinically significant cut-offs in cardiolipin antibody assays, this has proved to be a sensitive, if not entirely specific, method for APA detection applied to pregnancy monitoring (Lockshin et al 1985). Low transient levels of anticardiolipin antibodies can occur in many asymptomatic women, although screening in pregnancy is also advised for APA-negative women with a history of thrombotic episodes and fetal loss. The conclusions from application of these various assays point to an overlapping family of antiphospholipid autoantibodies, including lupus anticoagulant; these are actively acquired and it is unknown whether they can result from a form of immunological autosensitization in a previous pregnancy.

There is a correlation between maternal APA and recurrent intrauterine death in all three trimesters of pregnancy. APA can bind to cell surface phospholipids of a variety of cell types, including platelets, vascular endothelial cells and, possibly, trophoblastic cells. There may also be an overlap between APA and lymphocytotoxic antibodies found in systemic lupus erythematosus or subgroups of secondary RSA patients (McIntyre et al 1986). The possible mechanism of action of APA in recurring fetal death might include platelet damage with increased adhesiveness, interference with the phospholipid part of the prothrombin activator complex and inhibition of prostacyclin (PGI_2) production by vascular tissues leading to decidual vasculopathy and placental infarction; prostacyclin is a potent vasodilator and inhibitor of platelet aggregation (Branch et al 1985). Therapeutic doses of heparin anticoagulation, or prednisone with low-dose aspirin, compatible with maintaining maternal health in pregnancy have been reported to correct the serological detection of APA with subsequent successful achievement of healthy offspring in many but not all pregnancies (Lubbe & Liggins 1985, McIntyre et al 1986). However, no controlled clinical studies have been reported to date. Treatment with prednisone and low-dose aspirin may not completely alleviate the underlying pathophysiology, and a high incidence of pre-eclamptic toxaemia and intrauterine growth retardation has been observed (Branch et al 1985). In addition, a postpartum maternal syndrome of pleuropulmonary disease, fever and cardiac manifestation has been described (Kochenour et al 1987).

Anti-Ro(SS-A) antibodies

Systemic lupus erythematosus sera may contain a bewildering array of autoantibodies against nucleic acids, nucleoproteins, cell surface antigens and phospholipids. The detection of a serum autoantibody in an individual in the general population, however, does not necessarily imply a pathological process. One particular IgG autoantibody to a soluble ribonucleoprotein, anti-Ro(SS-A), is found in approximately 25% of systemic lupus erythematosus patients and 50% of patients with Sjögren's syndrome (Scott 1984). Anti-Ro(SS-A) antibodies are associated with photosensitive cutaneous lesions and renal damage, usually in mild systemic lupus erythematosus; they have also been reported in asymptomatic ANA-negative women. Similar neonatal lupus-like skin lesions may occur in offspring of systemic lupus erythematosus mothers due to passively acquired maternal autoantibody. There can also be haemolytic anaemia and thrombocytopenia, although the most dramatic association of anti-Ro(SS-A) antibodies is with congenital complete heart block (Scott et al 1983). This lesion is permanent, whilst other neonatal symptoms are short-lived. The strong association suggests that transplacental passage of maternal anti-Ro(SS-A) or related antibodies is involved in pathological events causing this permanent sequela for the fetus in utero, whilst there is no evidence of a related pathological effect in the mother herself; this could involve either direct action on fetal cardiac tissues or the IgG anti-Ro(SS-A) autoantibody being a marker of a coincidental pathogenetic agent that is transferred to the fetus in pregnancy.

Immune thrombocytopenic purpura (ITP)

ITP can have an insidious onset and may only be diagnosed following exclusion of other possible causes for thrombocytopenia. The maternal disease is characterized by destruction of circulating platelets by *autoantibodies*, although these IgG antibodies can also cross the placenta and cause transitory neonatal thrombocytopenia in around 45% of cases. Maternal risk is mainly from bleeding at the time of parturition. It should be distinguished from the rarer *isoimmune* neonatal thrombocytopenia, which follows placental transfer of maternal IgG antibody resultant from isoimmunization with fetal platelets; the platelet antigen to which these antibodies are directed (PLA-1) is common in the general population, and hence the majority of mothers are positive for this antigen and do not produce antibodies. Testing of maternal and neonatal platelets will determine whether the maternal antibody is reactive with platelets from both individuals (due to autoimmunity) or only the neonate (due to isoimmunization).

Maternal therapy for ITP may involve corticosteroids to reduce the antibody level. Plasmapheresis and, latterly, high doses of intravenous immunoglobulin have also been used in extreme cases with some success. Several mechanisms, which may act singly or in concert, have been proposed to explain the effect of high-dose intravenous immunoglobulin: these include transient blockade of $Fc\gamma$ receptors on cells in the reticuloendothelial system, protection of platelets by non-specific coating with IgG, antiviral therapy, suppression of antibody production and anti-idiotypic immunoregulatory effects.

Pemphigoid gestationis

Pemphigoid gestationis is an uncommon bullous skin disorder induced only by pregnancy, including molar pregnancies with no fetus or fetal circulation. The diagnosis of pemphigoid gestationis (previously termed herpes gestationis) centres on immunopathological demonstration of C3 complement component deposition at the basement membrane zone of skin. A complement-fixing autoantibody which binds to this site is also found in pemphigoid gestationis sera; it is thought that this may be induced by placental antigens abnormally provoking an immune response which is cross-reactive with skin (Holmes et al 1983). There is a strong association with HLA-DR3 and -DR4, as well as with the HLA-A1, B8, DR3 haplotype, which could reflect an immunogenetic susceptibility to autoimmune reactions. Pemphigoid gestationis usually recurs with subsequent pregnancies; occasional subsequent unaffected pregnancies are associated either with a change of sexual partner or complete HLA-DR compatibility between mother and fetus, indicative of the importance of a paternal genetic component (Holmes et al 1983). The nature of the provoking placental antigen is unknown; nevertheless, pemphigoid gestationis appears to be a rare but fascinating example of a detectable immune response to a placental antigen associated with subsequent pathology.

Blood group incompatibilities

Blood group incompatibility is the most clinically significant isoimmunization that can occur in pregnancy and results from leakage of fetal cells into maternal circulation, mostly at parturition. Any maternal IgG antibody can cross into the fetus in a subsequent pregnancy and provoke haemolysis which may result in severe anaemia, jaundice, hydrops and fetal death. Rhesus isoimmunization is discussed in depth in Chapter 35. The use of anti-Rh(D) to prevent sensitization demonstrates specific antibody-mediated immune suppression, probably by accelerating removal of fetal Rh(D)-positive erythrocytes in the spleen before the maternal immune system becomes sensitized. Antibodies in the ABO system are nearly always of the IgM type and hence do not cross into the fetal compartment. However, other blood group incompatibilities, notably of the Kell system, can occasionally cause neonatal haemolysis (Beal 1979). Maternal isoantibodies to Lewis and other blood group antigens may also develop in pregnancy, although these do not cause haemolytic disease of the newborn because fetal red cells express insufficient antigen on their surface (Beal 1979). Maternal antineutrophil antibodies, resulting from isoimmunization, and which may cause a neonatal neutropenia, have also been described but are extremely rare.

Pre-eclamptic toxaemia (PET)

Numerous concepts have been proposed to account for the pathogenesis of PET, and further consideration of hypertension in pregnancy is given in Chapter 36. An immunological explanation based on fetomaternal compatibility has gained particular attention since the clinical picture may fit with that expected in an immune response. Thus, PET is a disorder of the second half of pregnancy, more common in primigravidae, and previous pregnancy or pre-immunization may be protective; hence, there could be an impaired or absent beneficial maternal immunoregulatory response in primigravidae that is counteracted by prior blood transfusion or more frequent exposure to sperm or seminal antigens prior to conception (Redman 1980, Need et al 1983). However, available immunological data now give, at best, tenuous and tantalizingly inconclusive support.

The placenta is of central importance, since PET can occur in molar pregnancy in the absence of fetal tissue or circulation and it regresses immediately on placental removal. Endovascular cytotrophoblast invasion into spiral arteries in the placental bed is decreased in PET, resulting in inadequate physiological changes and failure to form uteroplacental arteries. These histopathological changes do not show evidence of cellular immune attack on trophoblast or appear to involve a contribution from the decidual leukocyte component (Fox 1978, Khong 1987). Immunoglobulin, complement and fibrin deposits in decidual vessels (Kitzmiller & Benirschke 1973) may be the effect of occluded blood flow, rather than the cause; analogous results have been described in chorionic villous tissue (Sinha et al 1984) that may have resulted from placental ischaemia, and similar necrotic foci have also been identified in placentae from insulin-dependent diabetic and healthy mothers. Hence, there are no sustained data favouring an immune response to fetal trophoblast antigens in PET. Conversely, several wisps of evidence have been put forward to support a reduced maternal response in PET. Thus, a decreased prevalence of pregnancy-induced antibodies to paternal HLA (Jenkins et al 1977) and an abnormal mixed lymphocyte reaction between parents in pre-eclamptic pregnancy (Sargent et al 1982) have been claimed. However, other studies have shown no difference for antigen- or mitogen-stimulated lymphocyte responses between PET and uncomplicated pregnancy (Alanen & Lassila 1982) and there appears to be little concordance of information in the literature on cell-mediated immunity in PET.

There is evidence that PET is a familial disorder with a possible single recessive gene determination (Chesley & Cooper 1986). It is not associated with any particular HLA or blood group antigens, although a weak association with maternal HLA homozygosity has been reported (Redman 1980). A putative role for an as yet ill defined maternal–fetal genetic interaction is supported by other observations: thus, PET occurs more frequently in situations with increased placental mass (including multiple gestation) and in fetal triploidy, notably trisomy-13 (Redman 1980, Boyd et al 1987). The relevance of a male genetic factor in PET merits further investigation since it has now been shown that heritable paternal rather than maternal imprinting of the genome is necessary for the normal development of trophoblast and extraembryonic membranes (Reik et al 1987). Hence, this could also be related to unusual presentations of PET occurring with hydatidiform mole. Opinion on whether placental antigens or the fetal genetic component appears to be more relevant in the pathogenesis of PET may be moving towards genetic rather than immunological interpretation.

Gestational trophoblastic disease

Complete hydatidiform moles lack a fetus and have a diploid nuclear genome entirely of paternal genetic (androgenetic) origin; hence, they are completely mismatched with the maternal host (Kajii & Ohama 1977). Partial moles are associated with the presence of a fetus and are usually triploid, the extra haploid component being paternal (Lawler & Fisher 1987a). Choriocarcinoma may follow normal term delivery, molar pregnancy or non-molar abortion; it can often be associated with a local mononuclear cell response (Fox 1978). Both hydatidiform mole and choriocarcinoma are discussed in detail in Chapter 31, although points of immunological relevance are highlighted here.

Because trophoblast may be both proliferative and invasive in normal early pregnancy, the distinction between normal and malignant trophoblast can be unclear; nevertheless, trophoblastic neoplasms are of interest because they represent the only naturally occurring examples of genetically foreign (allogeneic) tumours (Loke 1978). Fetal trophoblast antigen expression in both molar pregnancy and choriocarcinoma obeys the same general principles according to morphological and anatomical classification as for normal pregnancy (Bulmer et al 1988). This phenotypic heterogeneity in choriocarcinoma highlights the extensive differentiation into cellular subgroups that occurs for malignant trophoblast. The unusual granulated lymphoid cells found in normal pregnancy decidua are also found in molar pregnancy but not in uterine tissue in choriocarcinoma, suggesting that these cells are associated with decidualization rather than presence of fetal trophoblast (Bulmer et al 1988).

High serum levels of antipaternal HLA antibodies may be found in trophoblastic neoplasia (Shaw et al 1979, Lawler & Fisher 1987b). This introduces the question as to how these women may become sensitized, since trophoblast lacks classical HLA-A or -B antigens. In the case of a complete mole lacking a fetus or fetal blood cells, it appears that the immunogenic source may be stromal cells of the chorionic villi (Lawler & Fisher 1987b).

Choriocarcinoma may be associated with a small increase in HLA compatibility between patient and spouse although a higher risk depends on the ABO system. Thus, there is an increased preponderance in group A women, particularly with a group O partner, and women with ABO-compatible partners appear to be protected from subsequent development of a trophoblastic tumour following evacuation of a mole (Bagshawe et al 1971, Lawler & Fisher 1987b). How ABO antigens could influence postmolar trophoblastic proliferation is immunologically obscure, since trophoblast does not express ABO blood group antigens, and direct immunological sensitization is clearly not involved, but could instead include the action of a separate gene linked to the ABO system.

REFERENCES

Adamson E D 1987 Expression of proto-oncogenes in the placenta. Placenta 8: 449–466

Ahrons S 1971 HL-A antibodies: influence on the human foetus. Tissue Antigens 1: 121–128

Alanen A, Lassila O 1982 Cell-mediated immunity in normal pregnancy and pre-eclampsia. Journal of Reproductive Immunology 4: 349–354

Anderson D J, Yunis E J 1985 The elusive immunosuppressive factors of pregnancy. American Journal of Reproductive Immunology and Microbiology 9: 91–92

Anderson D J, Johnson P M, Alexander N J, Jones W R, Griffin P D 1987 Monoclonal antibodies to human trophoblast and sperm antigens: report of two WHO-sponsored workshops. Journal of Reproductive Immunology 10: 231–257

Athannasakis A, Bleachley R C, Paetkau V, Guilbert L, Barr P J, Wegmann T G 1987 The immunostimulatory effect of T cells and T cell lymphokines on murine fetally-derived placental cells. Journal of Immunology 138: 37–44

Attwood H O, Park W O 1961 Embolism to the lungs by trophoblast. Journal of Obstetrics and Gynaecology of the British Commonwealth 68: 611–617

Bagshawe K D, Rawlins G, Pike M, Lawler S D 1971 ABO blood-groups in trophoblastic neoplasia. Lancet i: 553–557

Beal R W 1979 Non-rhesus (D) blood group isoimmunisation in obstetrics. Clinics in Obstetrics and Gynaecology 6: 493–508

Beer A E, Billingham R E 1976 The immunobiology of mammalian reproduction. Prentice-Hall, New Jersey

Beer A E, Semprini A E, Xiaoyn Z, Quebbeman J F 1985 Pregnancy outcome in human couples with recurrent spontaneous abortion: HLA antigen profiles, HLA antigen sharing, female serum MLR blocking factors and paternal leucocyte immunization. Experimental and Clinical Immunogenetics 2: 137–153

Bissenden J G, Ling N R, MacKintosh P 1980 Suppression of mixed lymphocyte reactions by pregnancy serum. Clinical and Experimental Immunology 39: 195–202

Boyd P A, Lindenbaum R H, Redman C W G 1987 Pre-eclampsia and trisomy 13: a possible association. Lancet ii: 425–427

Branch W B, Scott J R, Kochenour N K, Hershgold E 1985 Obstetric complications associated with the lupus anticoagulant. New England Journal of Medicine 313: 1322–1326

Bulmer J N, Johnson P M 1984 Macrophage populations in the human placenta and amniochorion. Clinical and Experimental Immunology 57: 393–403

Bulmer J N, Johnson P M 1985 Antigen expression by trophoblast populations in the human placenta and their possible immunobiological relevance. Placenta 6: 127–140

Bulmer J N, Johnson P M 1986 The T-lymphocyte population in first-trimester human decidua does not express the interleukin-2 receptor. Immunology 58: 685–687

Bulmer J N, Sunderland C A 1984 Immunohistological characterisation of lymphoid cell populations in the early human placental bed. Immunology 52: 349–357

Bulmer J N, Johnson P M, Sasagawa M, Takeuchi S 1988 Immunohistochemical studies of fetal trophoblast and maternal decidua in hydatiform mole and choriocarcinoma. Placenta 9: 183–200

Chaouat G (ed) 1987 Reproductive immunology: materno–fetal relationship. INSERM Colloque 154. Editions INSERM, Paris

Chesley L C, Cooper D W 1986 Genetics of hypertension in pregnancy: possible single gene control of pre-eclampsia and eclampsia in the descendants of eclamptic women. British Journal of Obstetrics and Gynaecology 93: 898–908

Clark D A, Chaouat G 1986 Characterisation of the cellular basis for the inhibition of cytotoxic cells by murine placenta. Cellular Immunology 102: 43–51

Clark D A, Croy B A (eds) 1986 Reproductive immunology 1986. Elsevier Biomedical, Amsterdam

Clark D A, Chaput A, Walker C, Rosenthal K L 1985. Active suppression of host-vs-graft reaction in pregnant mice. VI Soluble suppressor activity obtained from decidua of allopregnant mice blocks the response to IL 2. Journal of Immunology 134: 1659–1664

Clark D A, Croy B A, Wegmann T G, Chaouat G 1987 Immunological and para-immunological mechanisms in spontaneous abortion: recent

insights and future directions. Journal of Reproductive Immunology 12: 1–12
Crighton D B (ed) 1984 Immunological aspects of reproduction in mammals. Butterworths, London
Daya S, Clark D A, Devlin C, Jarrell J, Chaput A 1985 Suppressor cells in human decidua. American Journal of Obstetrics and Gynecology 151: 267–270
Doughty R W, Gelsthrope K 1976 Some parameters of lymphocyte antibody activity through pregnancy and further eluates of placental material. Tissue Antigens 8: 43–48
Earl U, Wells M, Bulmer J N 1985 The expression of major histocompatibility complex antigens by trophoblast in ectopic tubal pregnancy. Journal of Reproductive Immunology 8: 13–24
Ellis S A, Sargent I L, Redman C W G, McMichael A J 1986 Evidence for a novel HLA antigen found on human extravillous trophoblast and a choriocarcinoma cell line. Immunology 59: 595–601
Faulk W P, Johnson P M 1977 Immunological studies of human placentae: identification and distribution of proteins in mature chorionic villi. Clinical and Experimental Immunology 27: 365–375
Faulk W P, McIntyre J A 1983 Immunological studies of human trophoblast: markers, subsets and functions. Immunological Reviews 75: 139–175
Fox H 1978 Pathology of the placenta. Saunders, London
Gehrz R C, Christianson W R, Linner K M, Conroy M M, McCue S A, Balfour H H 1981a Cytomegalovirus-specific humoral and cellular immune responses in human pregnancy. Journal of Infectious Diseases 143: 391–395
Gehrz R C, Christianson W R, Linner K M, Conroy M M, McCue S A, Balfour H H 1981b A longitudinal analysis of lymphocyte proliferative responses to mitogens and antigens during human pregnancy. American Journal of Obstetrics and Gynecology 140: 665–670
Gill T J III, Wegmann T G (eds) 1987 Immunoregulation and fetal survival. Oxford University Press, New York
Gusdon J P 1976 Maternal immune responses in pregnancy. In: Scott J S, Jones W R (eds) Immunology of human reproduction. Academic Press, London, pp 103–125
Haas G G 1987 How should sperm antibody tests be used clinically? American Journal of Reproductive Immunology and Microbiology 15: 106–111
Haas G G, Kubota K, Quebbeman J F, Jijon A, Menge A C, Beer A E 1986 Circulating anti-sperm antibodies in recurrently aborting women. Fertility and Sterility 45: 209–215
Head J R, Drake B L, Zuckermann F A 1987 Major histocompatibility antigens on trophoblast and their regulation: implications in the maternal–fetal relationship. American Journal of Reproductive Immunology and Microbiology 15: 12–18
Holmes R C, Black M M, Jurecka W et al 1983 Clues to the aetiology and pathogenesis of herpes gestationis. British Journal of Dermatology 109: 131–139
Hsi B-L, Yeh C-J G, Faulk W P 1984 Class I antigens of the major histocompatibility complex on cytotrophoblast of human chorion laeve. Immunology 52: 621–629
Hsi B-L, Yeh C-J G, Johnson P M, Beresford N, Stern P L 1987 Monoclonal antibody GB17 recognizes human syncytiotrophoblast. Journal of Reproductive Immunology 12: 235–244
Hunt J S, Andrews G K, Wood G W 1987 Normal trophoblasts resist induction of class I HLA. Journal of Immunology 138: 2481–2487
Hunziker R D, Wegmann T G 1986 Placental immunoregulation. CRC Critical Reviews in Immunology 6: 245–285
Hunziker R D, Gambel P, Wegmann T G 1984 Placenta as a selective barrier to cellular traffic. Journal of Immunology 133: 667–671
Jazwinska E C, Kilpatrick D C, Smart G E, Liston W A 1987 Feto-maternal HLA compatibility does not have a major influence on human pregnancy except for lymphocytotoxin production. Clinical and Experimental Immunology 68: 116–122
Jeannet M, Werner C, Ramirez E, Vassalli P, Faulk W P 1977 Anti-HLA, anti-human 'Ia-like' and MLC blocking activity of human placental IgG. Transplantation Proceedings 9: 1417–1422
Jenkins D M, Need J, Rajah S M 1977 Deficiency of specific HLA antibodies in severe pregnancy pre-eclampsia/eclampsia. Clinical and Experimental Immunology 27: 485–486
Johnson P M, Brown P J 1981 Fcγ receptors in the human placenta. Placenta 2: 355–370
Johnson P M, Ramsden G H 1988 Immunology of recurrent miscarriage. In: Johnson P M (ed) Baillière's clinical immunology and allergy. Ballière Tindall, London 2(3): in press
Johnson P M, Stern P L 1986 Antigen expression at human maternal–fetal interfaces. In: Cinader B, Miller R G (eds) Progress in immunology VI. Academic Press, Orlando, pp 1056–1069
Johnson P M, Natvig J B, Ystehede U A, Faulk W P 1977 Immunological studies of human placentae: the distribution and character of immunoglobulins in chorionic villi. Cilinical and Experimental Immunology 30: 145–153
Johnson P M, Brown P J, Faulk W P 1980 Immunobiological aspects of the human placenta. In: Finn C A (ed) Oxford reviews in reproductive biology, vol 2. Oxford University Press, Oxford, pp 1–40
Johnson P M, Cheng H M, Molloy C M, Stern C M M, Slade M B 1981 Human trophoblast-specific surface antigens identified using monoclonal antibodies. American Journal of Reproductive Immunology 1: 246–254
Johnson P M, Chia K V, Risk J M 1986 Immunological question marks in recurrent spontaneous abortion. In: Clark D A, Croy B A (eds) Reproductive immunology 1986. Elsevier Biomedical, Amsterdam, pp 239–246
Johnson P M, Chia K V, Hart C A, Griffith H B, Francis W J A 1988a Trophoblast membrane infusion for unexplained recurrent miscarriage. British Journal of Obstetrics and Gynaecology 95: 342–347
Johnson P M, Chia K V, Risk J M, Barnes R M R, Woodrow J C 1988b Immunological and immunogenetic investigation of recurrent spontaneous abortion. Disease Markers 6: 163–171
Jones C J P, Fox H 1978 An ultrastructural study of the placenta in materno–fetal rhesus incompatibility. Virchows Archiv Pathologische Anatomie und Histologie 379: 229–241
Jordan B R, Caillol D, Damotte M et al 1985 HLA class I genes: from structure to expression, serology and function. Immunological Reviews 85: 73–92
Kajii T, Ohama K 1977 Androgenetic origin of hydatidiform mole. Nature 268: 633–634
Khong T Y 1987 Immunohistologic study of the leukocytic infiltrate in maternal uterine tissues in normal and pre-eclamptic pregnancies at term. American Journal of Reproductive Immunology and Microbiology 15: 1–8
Kitzmiller J L, Benirschke K 1973 Immunofluorescent study of placental bed vessels in pre-eclampsia of pregnancy. American Journal of Obstetrics and Gynecology 115: 248–251
Kochenour N K, Branch D W, Rote N S, Scott J R 1987 A new postpartum syndrome associated with antiphospholipid antibodies. Obstetrics and Gynecology 69: 460–468
Konoeda Y, Terasaki P I, Wakisaka A, Park M S, Mickey M R 1986 Public determinants of HLA indicated by pregnancy antibodies. Transplantation 41: 253–259
Kozma R, Spring J, Johnson P M, Adinolfi M 1986 Detection of syncytiotrophoblast in maternal peripheral and uterine veins using a monoclonal antibody and flow cytometry. Human Reproduction 5: 335–336
Lancet Editorial 1983 Maternal blocking antibodies, the fetal allograft, and recurrent abortion. Lancet ii: 1175–1176
Lawler S D, Fisher R A 1987a Genetic studies in hydatidiform mole with clinical correlations. Placenta 8: 77–88
Lawler S D, Fisher R A 1987b Immunogenicity of hydatidiform mole. Placenta 8: 195–199
Lockshin M D, Druzin M L, Goei S et al 1985 Antibody to cardiolipin as a predictor of fetal distress or death in pregnant patients with systemic lupus erythematosus. New England Journal of Medicine 313: 152–156
Loke Y W 1978 Immunology and immunopathology of the human foetal–maternal interaction. Elsevier/North Holland, Amsterdam
Loke Y W, Butterworth B H, Margetts J J, Burland K 1986 Identification of cytotrophoblast colonies in cultures of human placental cells using monoclonal antibodies. Placenta 7: 221–231
Lubbe W F, Liggins G C 1985 Lupus anticoagulant and pregnancy. American Journal of Obstetrics and Gynecology 153: 322–327
Maier T, Holda J H, Claman H N 1986 Natural suppressor (NS) cells: member of the LGL regulatory family. Immunology Today 7: 312–315
McIntyre J A, Faulk W P, Nichols-Johnson V R, Taylor C G 1986

Immunologic testing and immunotherapy in recurrent spontaneous abortion. Obstetrics and Gynecology 67: 169–175
McLaughlin P J, Johnson P M 1984 A search for human placental-type alkaline phosphatases using monoclonal antibodies. In: Stigbrand T, Fishman W H (eds) Human alkaline phosphatases. Alan R Liss, New York, pp 67–75
Medawar P B 1953 Some immunological and endocrinological problems raised by the evolution of viviparity in vertebrates. Symposium of the Society of Experimental Biology 7: 320–328
Moore M P, Carter N P, Redman C W G 1983 Lymphocyte subsets defined by monoclonal antibodies in human pregnancy. American Journal of Reproductive Immunology 3: 161–164
Mowbray J F, Underwood J L 1985 Immunology of abortion. Clinical and Experimental Immunology 60: 1–7
Mowbray J F, Gibbings C, Liddell H, Reginald P W, Underwood J L, Beard R W 1985 Controlled trial of treatment of recurrent spontaneous abortion by immunisation with paternal cells. Lancet i: 941–943
Nakayama E, Asano S, Kodo H, Miwa S 1985 Suppression of mixed lymphocyte reaction by cells of human first trimester pregnancy endometrium. Journal of Reproductive Immunology 8: 25–31
Need J A, Bell B, Meffin E, Jones W R 1983 Pre-eclampsia in pregnancies from donor inseminations. Journal of Reproductive Immunology 5: 329–338
Nicholas N S, Panayi G S 1986 Inhibition of interleukin-2 production by retroplacental sera; a possible mechanism for human fetal allograft survival. American Journal of Reproductive Immunology and Microbiology 9: 6–11
Power D A, Mather A J, MacLeod A M, Lind T, Catto G R D 1986 Maternal antibodies to paternal B lymphocytes in normal and abnormal pregnancy. American Journal of Reproductive Immunology and Microbiology 10: 10–13
Radcliffe J J, Hart C A, Francis W J A, Johnson P M 1986 Immunity to cytomegalovirus in women with unexplained recurrent spontaneous abortion. American Journal of Reproductive Immunology and Microbiology 12: 103–105
Redman C W G 1980 Immunological aspects of eclampsia and pre-eclampsia. In: Hearn J P (ed) Immunological aspects of reproduction and fertility control. MTP Press, Lancaster, pp 83–103
Redman C W G, McMichael A J, Stirrat G M, Sunderland C A, Ting L A 1984 Class I major histocompatibility antigens on human extravillous cytotrophoblast. Immunology 52: 457–468
Reik W, Collick A, Norris M L, Barton S C, Surani M A 1987 Genomic imprinting determines methylation of parental alleles in transgenic mice. Nature 328: 248–251
Risk J M, Johnson P M 1985 Antigen expression by human trophoblast and tumour cells: models for gene regulation? Contributions to Gynecology and Obstetrics 14: 74–82
Rocklin R E, Kitzmiller J L, Carpenter C B, Garovoy M R, David J R 1976 Maternal–fetal relation: absence of an immunologic blocking factor from the serum of women with chronic abortions. New England Journal of Medicine 295: 1209–1213
Roitt I M, Brostoff J, Male D K 1985 Immunology. Churchill Livingstone, Edinburgh/Gower Medical Publishing, London
Sargent I L, Redman C W G, Stirrat G M 1982 Maternal cell-mediated immunity in normal and pre-eclamptic pregnancy. Clinical and Experimental Immunology 50: 601–609
Sargent I L, Arenas J, Redman C W G 1987 Maternal cell-mediated sensitisation to paternal HLA may occur, but is not a regular event in normal human pregnancy. Journal of Reproductive Immunology 10: 111–120
Scott J S 1976 Pregnancy: nature's experimental system. Transient manifestations of immunological disease in the child. Lancet i: 704–706
Scott J S 1984 Connective tissue disease antibodies and pregnancy. American Journal of Reproductive Immunology 6: 19–24
Scott J S, Maddison P J, Taylor P V, Esscher E, Scott O, Skinner R P 1983 Connective-tissue disease, antibodies to ribonucleoprotein, and congenital heart block. New England Journal of Medicine 309: 209–212
Shaw A R E, Dasgupta M K, Kovithavongs T et al 1979 Humoral and cellular immunity to paternal antigens in trophoblastic neoplasia. International Journal of Cancer 24: 586–593
Simmons R L, Russell P S 1967 Immunologic interactions between mother and fetus. Advances in Obstetrics and Gynecology 1: 38–58
Sinha D, Wells M, Faulk W P 1984 Immunological studies of human placentae: complement components in pre-eclamptic chorionic villi. Clinical and Experimental Immunology 56: 175–184
Stern P L, Beresford N, Thompson S, Johnson P M, Webb P D, Hole N 1986 Characterization of the human trophoblast-leukocyte antigenic molecules defined by a monoclonal antibody. Journal of Immunology 137: 1604–1609
Stern P L, Beresford N, Friedman C I, Stevens V C, Risk J M, Johnson P M 1987 Class I-like M H C molecules expressed by baboon placental syncytiotrophoblast. Journal of Immunology 138: 1088–1091
Stevens V C 1986 Current status of anti-fertility vaccines using gonadotrophin immunogens. Immunology Today 7: 369–374
Stimson W H 1983 The influence of pregnancy-associated serum proteins and steroids on the maternal immune response. In: Wegmann T G, Gill T J III (eds) Immunology of reproduction. Oxford University Press, New York, pp 281–301
Stites D P, Bugbee S, Siiteri P K 1983 Differential actions of progesterone and cortisol on lymphocyte and monocyte interaction during lymphocyte activation — relevance to immunosuppression in pregnancy. Journal of Reproductive Immunology 5: 215–228
Stites D P, Stobo J D, Wells J V (eds) 1987 Basic and clinical immunology, 6th edn. Appleton & Lange, Norwalk, Connecticut
Stray-Pedersen B, Stray-Pedersen S 1984 Etiologic factors and subsequent reproductive performance in 195 couples with a prior history of habitual abortion. American Journal of Obstetrics and Gynecology 148: 140–146
Suciu-Foca N, Reed E, Rohowsky C, Kung P, King D W 1983 Anti-idiotypic antibodies to anti-HLA receptors induced by pregnancy. Proceedings of the National Academy of Sciences (USA) 80: 830–831
Suni J, Narvanen A, Wahlstrom T et al 1984 Human placental syncytiotrophoblastic Mr 75 000 polypeptide defined by antibodies to a synthetic peptide based on a cloned human endogenous retroviral DNA sequence. Proceedings of the National Academy of Sciences (USA) 81: 6197–6201
Takakuwa K, Kanazawa K, Takeuchi S 1986 Production of blocking antibodies by vaccination with husband's lymphocytes in unexplained recurrent aborters: the role in successful pregnancy. American Journal of Reproductive Immunology and Microbiology 10: 1–9
Thomas L, Douglas G W, Carr M C 1959 The continual migration of syncytial trophoblast from the fetal placenta into the maternal circulation. Transactions of the Association of American Physicians 72: 140–148
Thomas M L, Harger J H, Wagener D K, Rabin B S, Gill T J III 1985 HLA sharing and spontaneous abortion in humans. American Journal of Obstetrics and Gynecology 151: 1053–1058
Wahlstrom T, Nieminen P, Narvanen A et al 1984 Monoclonal antibody defining a human syncytiotrophoblastic polypeptide immunologically related to mammalian retrovirus structural protein p30. Placenta 5: 465–474
Webb P D, Evans, P W, Molloy C M, Johnson P M 1985 Biochemical studies of human placental microvillous plasma membrane proteins. American Journal of Reproductive Immunology and Microbiology 8: 113–117
Wegmann T G 1987 Placental immunotrophism; maternal T cells enhance placental growth and function. American Journal of Reproductive Immunology and Microbiology 15: 67–70
Woodrow J C, Finn R 1968 Transplacental haemorrhage. British Journal of Haematology 12: 297–309
Zinkernagel R M, Doherty P C 1979 MHC-restricted cytotoxic cell studies on the biological role of polymorphism restriction, specificity, function and responsiveness. Advances in Immunology 27: 51–70

12

Alec Turnbull

The endocrine control of labour

The birth of a mature and healthy infant depends on the mechanism which ensures that the uterus stays quiescent during pregnancy while the fetus is developing and then at the appropriate time initiates the powerful and co-ordinated uterine activity and the softening of the cervix which cause cervical dilatation and ultimately delivery of the mature infant. The vital importance of this control mechanism working as reliably as it does is illustrated by the fact that 95% of human infants are born at term. Although only 5% are born preterm, they account for 85% of early neonatal deaths not due to lethal deformity (Rush et al 1976).

It is remarkable how, in each species, the uterus remains quiescent throughout a pregnancy of whatever duration is necessary for the full development of the fetus. Then, and normally only when the fetus is fully mature, the quiescent uterus becomes contractile, the cervix softens and dilates and the transition from an intrauterine to an extrauterine existence is completed by the expulsion of a fetus capable of maintaining its own existence.

There is substantial evidence in many animals implicating the fetus in the timing of the onset of labour (Thorburn et al 1977) and this applies whether pregnancy is maintained by the placenta, as in the sheep, or by the corpus luteum, as in the goat. In the human it is difficult to obtain direct evidence because of the inaccessibility of the normal intrauterine fetus in late pregnancy. In the first instance, therefore, it seems helpful to review the now well known cascade of hormonal events associated with the initiation of labour in the sheep and then proceed to consider the evidence for and against a similar control mechanism in man.

PARTURITION IN THE SHEEP

The earliest well defined event in ovine parturition is a sharp rise in the concentration of cortisol in the fetal circulation 7–10 days before delivery (Bassett & Thorburn 1969), due mainly to an increase in cortisol secretion (Liggins et al 1973). The increased cortisol secretion probably reflects an increased adrenocortical sensitivity to adrenocorticotrophin (ACTH), since fetal ACTH levels rise at the same time, rather than before the levels of cortisol (Liggins et al 1977a). The increased cortisol secretion may also depend on the process of maturation in the character of fetal pituitary ACTH secretion. Silman et al (1976) have demonstrated quality of difference between fetal and adult sheep which may develop to some extent before birth.

The importance of fetal adrenal activity in the sheep rests, of course, on the original observation that fetal hypophysectomy prevents the onset of labour (Liggins et al 1967), while intrafetal infusion of ACTH, cortisol or dexamethasone all induce labour, bringing about the endocrine changes found in the spontaneous onset of labour in this species (Liggins 1969a,b). Figure 12.1, taken from studies published by Flint et al (1975a), demonstrates that following the intrafetal injection of dexamethasone, measurements in serial blood samples from the uteroovarian vein show a marked fall in progesterone concentration, followed by an increase in oestrogen and then a sharp increase in prostaglandin F, which reaches a peak with delivery of the fetus.

The mechanism by which increased levels of glucocorticoids in the sheep fetus bring about changes in placental steroids and prostaglandin F was clarified by Anderson et al (1975) and Steele et al (1976) when they showed that fetal cortisol induced increased activity of the enzymes 17α-hydroxylase and $C_{17,20}$-lyase in the fetal placenta. With the progesterone being metabolized its level falls, while that of 17α-hydroxyprogesterone, androstenedione, oestrone and oestrone sulphate all increase. Figure 12.2 shows the enzymatic steps in which fetal cortisol can apparently increase activity and thus bring about the synthesis of oestrogens from C_{21} precursors.

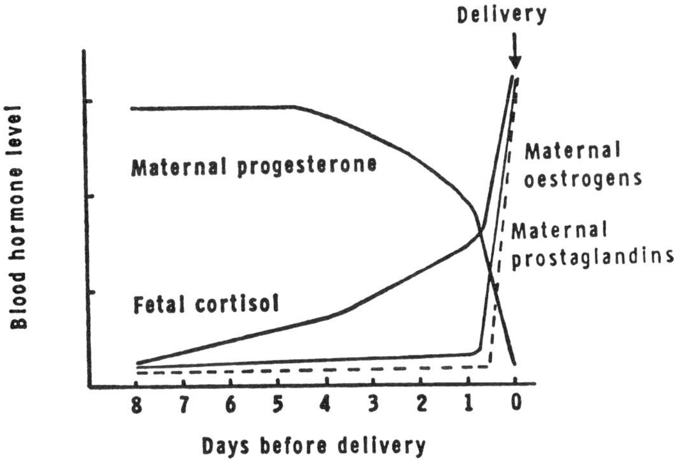

Fig. 12.1 Diagrammatic representation of the hormonal changes in the fetal and maternal circulation associated with parturition in the sheep. After Flint et al (1975a).

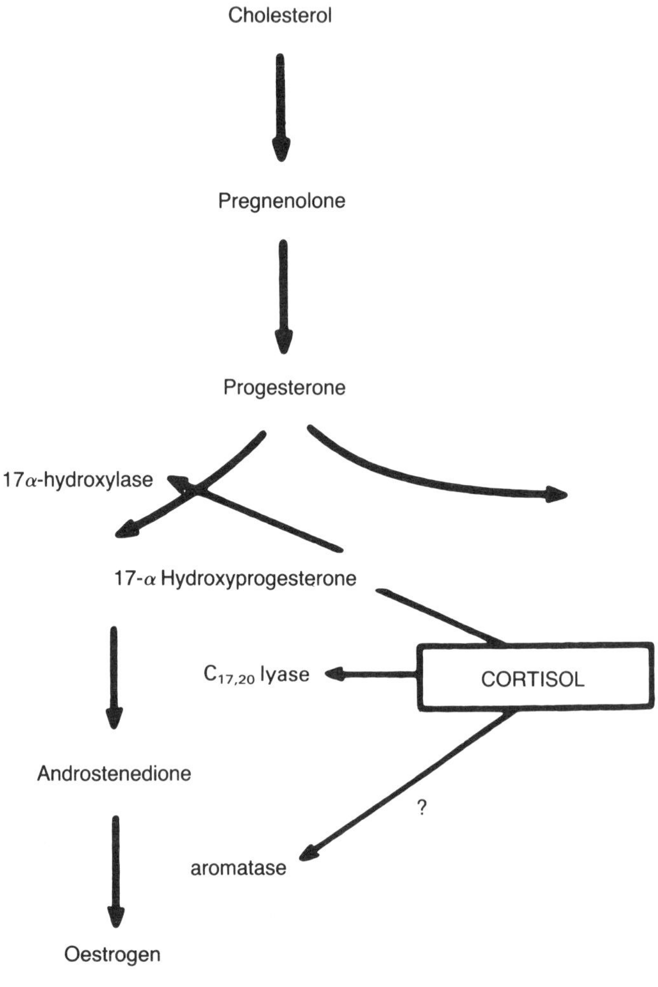

Fig. 12.2 Pathway of biosynthesis of progesterone and oestrogen in sheep placenta, indicating the possible sites of action of fetal cortisol on 17α-hydroxylase, $C_{17,20}$-lyase and aromatase. From Liggins et al (1977a).

Placental steroids and prostaglandin F (PGF)

Figure 12.1 shows how in sheep parturition increased synthesis of PGF immediately follows the sharp increase in oestrogen level in the uteroovarian vein. Liggins et al (1977a) showed that PGF synthesis may be stimulated by the raised oestrogens, but PGF can also be released and parturition induced without an increase in oestrogen levels by administering inhibitors of 3β-hydroxysteroid dehydrogenase, such as cyanoketone (Mitchell & Flint 1977), trilostane (Taylor et al 1982) or epostane (Ledger et al 1985a) which all reduce the blood level of progesterone.

Oxytocin, prostaglandins and the Ferguson reflex

As labour progresses, pressure of the fetal presenting part on the cervix and vagina activates a neurohumoral reflex (Ferguson reflex) by which a neural afferent pathway from the dilating cervix or the distending vagina reaches the hypothalamus via the spinal cord, and results in a humoral efferent, the secretion of oxytocin from the posterior pituitary (Flint et al 1975b). As well as stimulating uterine contractility, oxytocin also causes a release of PGF from uterine tissues (Mitchell et al 1976) which in turn stimulates more uterine contractions and thus further oxytocin release, so that the process of parturition, once established, accelerates until the fetus is delivered.

Local prostaglandin production, cervical softening and dilatation

Prostaglandin production within the uterine cervix itself appears to play an important part in the process of cervical softening, dilatation and effacement (Ellwood et al 1979, 1981). The studies by Ellwood et al suggest that in the sheep cervix, increased prostaglandin E (PGE) and prostacyclin synthesis in the cervix may be more important than PGF in bringing about the remarkably rapid connective tissue changes in the cervix associated with parturition (Fig. 12.3) with breakdown of collagen fibres into fibrils, activation of fibrocytes and increased tissue fluid, all predisposing to greater extensibility. The sheep cervix changes from being long, hard and tightly closed, to being fully dilated with a few hours of a labour in which amniotic fluid pressure changes are much less marked than in human labour (Ellwood et al 1980a). The possibility that these changes depend more on the effects of local prostaglandins on the cervical tissues than on traction on the cervix from myometrial contractions is supported by the findings of Ledger et al (1985b) who found that the usual changes in cervical extensibility occurred during labour in sheep even when the cervix was surgically isolated from the uterus.

Thus, the process of parturition in the sheep is initiated by a maturational process in the fetus leading to activation of the pituitary–adrenal axis and increasing cortisol in the fetal circulation. This initiates the whole cascade of hormonal

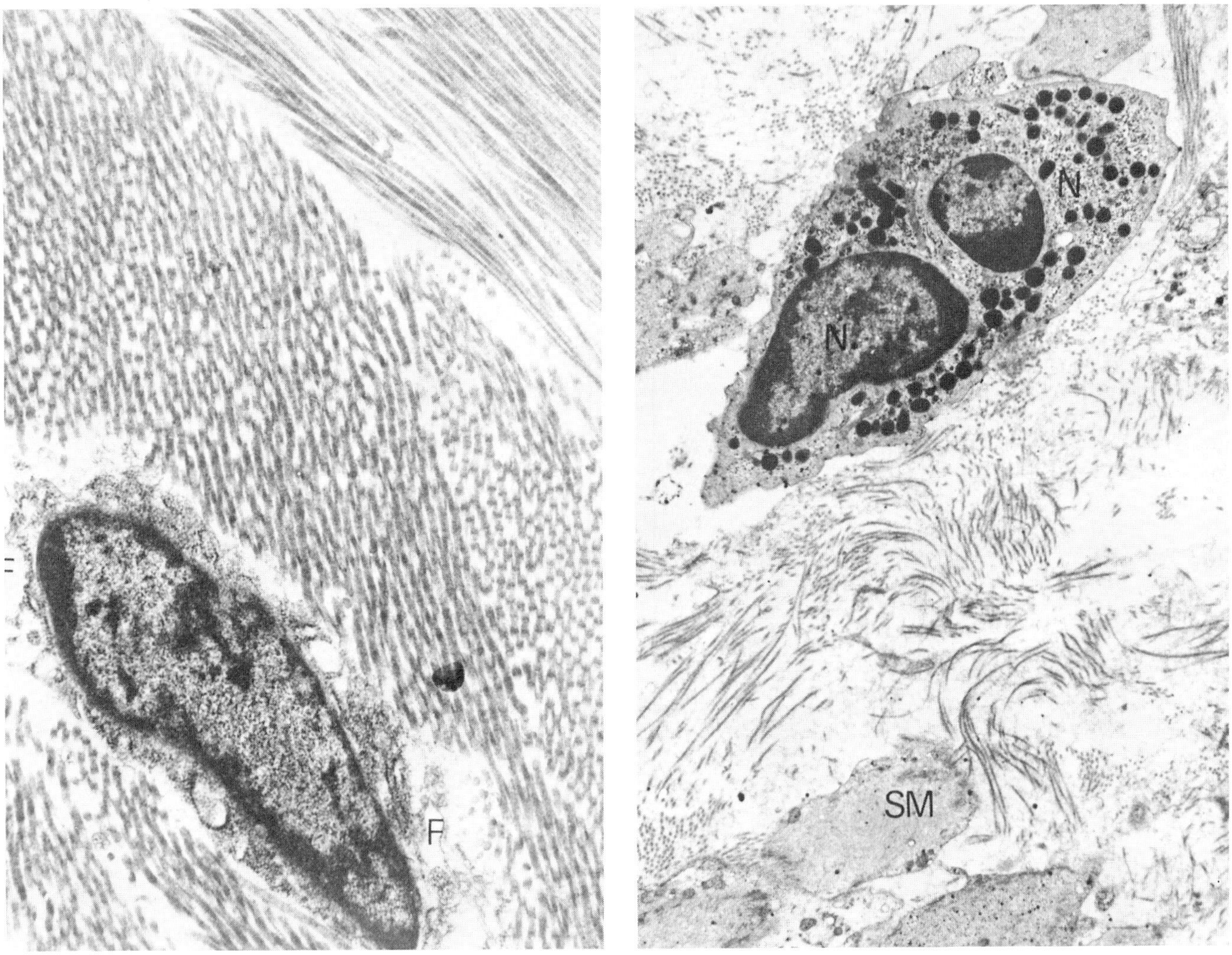

Fig. 12.3 (**a**) High power micrograph of tissue from a sheep cervix in late pregnancy (105 days' gestation) showing the highly organized collagen fibrils arranged in dense bundles running in a number of directions. Fibroblast cells (F) are found within and between fibril bundles (×26 000). (**b**) Micrograph of tissue from a sheep cervix immediately after spontaneous vaginal delivery at 140 days' gestation. Collagen fibrils are no longer arranged in compact bundles and the arrangement of the extracellular materials is now apparently random. Increased tissue fluid spaces are present. A polymorphonuclear leukocyte (N) has invaded the tissue. A group of smooth muscle cells are also visible (SM) (×11 480). From Ellwood (1981).

events involving changes in the secretion of placental steroid hormones, PGF, oxytocin activation of the Ferguson reflex and softening and dilatation of the uterine cervix.

Although pregnancy maintenance in other ruminants such as the goat and the cow depends on the corpus luteum, parturition is also controlled by a mechanism similar to that in the sheep, in which fetal cortisol acts as a trigger. On the other hand, different mechanisms control parturition in small mammals and the fetus does not seem to play a critical role. In the rat, removing the fetus or aspirating the fetal brain during pregnancy has no effect on the duration of pregnancy, at which the uterus empties its remaining contents, although labour may be protracted (Challis & Nathanielsz 1979). While the monkey fetus may play a small part in controlling the time of its own birth (Kittinger 1977, Novy 1977), Challis et al (1977) could find no progesterone withdrawal before labour in this species. The main factor in common with sheep labour was increased PGF in amniotic fluid and unconjugated oestrogens in maternal venous blood.

What mechanisms control human parturition?

INITIATION OF PARTURITION IN HUMAN PREGNANCY

Fetal pituitary–adrenal activity

In the absence of uterine distension by polyhydramnios, anencephaly of the human fetus with absence of the cerebrum, malformation of the pituitary and hypoplasia of the adrenal glands is associated with an increased range of gestation at delivery following spontaneous onset of labour, compared with pregnancies with a normal fetus (Fig. 12.4).

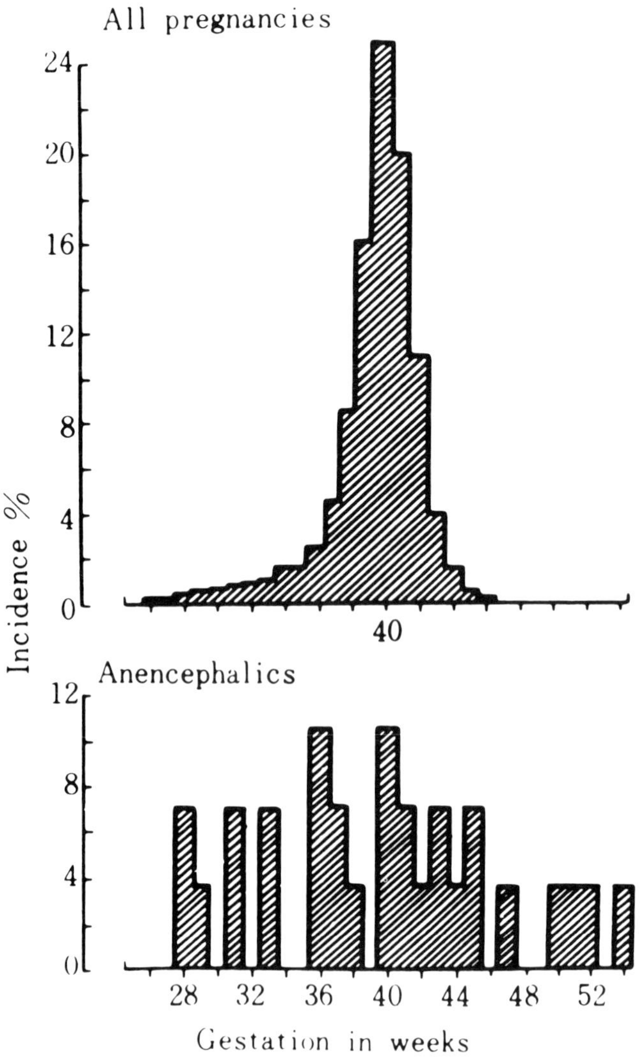

Fig. 12.4 Distribution of gestational age at delivery in human pregnancy comparing all pregnancies with those complicated by an anencephalic fetus without hydramnios. Adapted from Honnebier & Swaab (1973).

About one-third delivered preterm, one-third at term and one third past term. Although most other studies of pregnancy complicated by anencephaly without hydramnios have reported an increased proportion with extreme prolongation of gestation, the study of Honnebier & Swaab (1973) was by far the largest and their findings imply that in man the fetal pituitary–adrenal axis acts as a fine tuner of the time of onset of labour, rather than acting as the on/off switch as it does for sheep parturition.

Silman et al (1976) have demonstrated maturational changes in the function of the human fetal anterior pituitary during the last few weeks of gestation, when secretion of real ACTH 1–39 apparently supersedes that of fragments similar to α-melanotrophin (α-MSH) and corticotrophin-like intermediate peptide (CLIP). Rising concentrations of cortisol have been demonstrated in amniotic fluid during late pregnancy (Gautray et al 1974, Fencl & Tulchinsky 1975, Murphy et al 1975, Turnbull et al 1977) and cortisol levels are higher in cord blood from infants born following the spontaneous onset of labour than in infants delivered following induced labour or elective Caesarean section (Cawson et al 1974, Murphy 1975, Leong & Murphy 1976). Such findings suggest that fetal cortisol secretion increases before the spontaneous onset of human labour but in a critically important study, Gennser et al (1977) found no difference between the levels of cortisol in human fetal blood samples obtained before and soon after spontaneous onset of labour at term, disproving any surge of fetal cortisol secretion before the onset of human labour.

There is no 17α-hydroxylation in the human placenta delivered following spontaneous onset labour (A. P. F. Flint, unpublished observations). Administration of potent synthetic glucocorticoids to the mother in late human pregnancy simply suppresses maternal and fetal adrenal activity and reduces maternal levels of cortisol, dehydroepiandrosterone (DHEA) and oestriol (Anderson 1976).

Cortisol crosses the human placenta more readily than it does that of the sheep. High cortisol levels in the human fetus after delivery seem to have resulted from transfer from the high levels in the mother during labour. When the pain of labour is prevented by lumbar epidural block in human labour, neither maternal nor fetal cortisol levels increase (Thornton et al 1976, Cawson et al 1974). Glucocorticoid administration to human mothers does not reduce progesterone or increase oestrogen levels as it does in the sheep.

If increased fetal adrenal activity has any role in human parturition, its mechanism of action remains unknown. DHEA sulphate (DHEAS) is a fetal adrenal steroid of major importance which could have a potential role in human labour as an oestrogen precursor. DHEAS of both maternal and fetal origin contributes equally to placental oestradiol-17β synthesis, whereas the contribution of maternal DHEAS to oestriol production is less than 10% (Siiteri & Macdonald 1966). During pregnancy, maternal metabolic clearance of DHEAS increases (Gant et al 1971) with a progressive fall in maternal plasma DHEAS, although the level in amniotic fluid tends to increase (Turnbull et al 1977). Mochizuki & Tojo (1980) have demonstrated that intravenous injection of DHEAS in late human pregnancy seems to accelerate softening and dilatation of the cervix in comparison with controls, probably by causing increased concentrations of oestradiol-17β in the maternal serum, myometrium and cervix, and perhaps also by activating collagenolytic activity in the cervix.

These findings suggest gradually increasing fetal adrenal activity with effects on placental biosynthesis over the last few weeks of human pregnancy, rather than a relatively sudden change like that in sheep pregnancy. Decreased maternal levels of progesterone before human labour have been reported in only two studies (Caspo et al 1971, Turnbull et al 1974), both conducted serially in primigravidae and collected with the strictest possible criteria of normality. Pro-

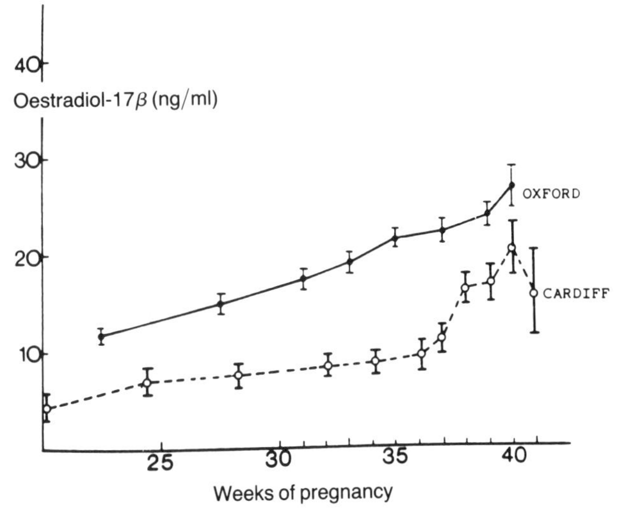

Fig. 12.5 Mean (± SEM) of peripheral plasma oestradiol-17β measured serially during pregnancy in 23 normal women of mixed parity in Oxford and 33 normal Cardiff primigravidae, from 20 weeks until the spontaneous onset of labour. Oxford women were investigated by Bibby (1980); Cardiff women were investigated by Turnbull et al (1974).

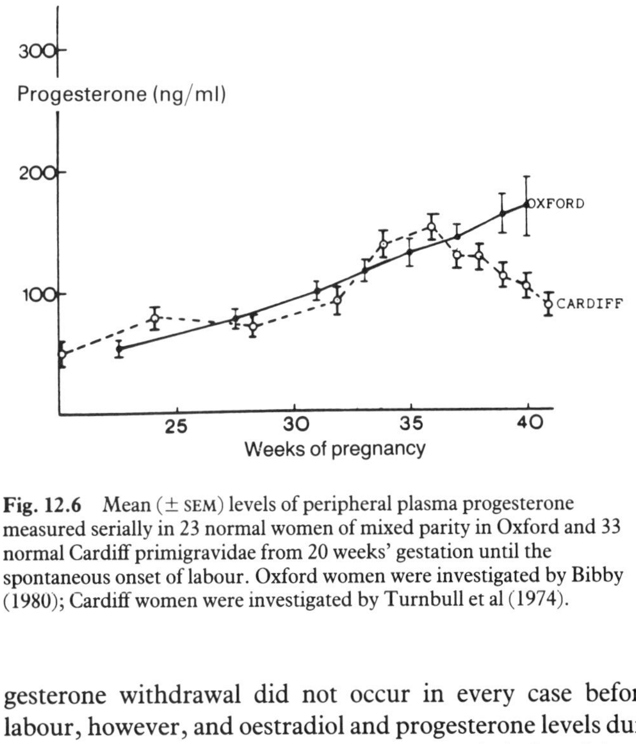

Fig. 12.6 Mean (± SEM) levels of peripheral plasma progesterone measured serially in 23 normal women of mixed parity in Oxford and 33 normal Cardiff primigravidae from 20 weeks' gestation until the spontaneous onset of labour. Oxford women were investigated by Bibby (1980); Cardiff women were investigated by Turnbull et al (1974).

gesterone withdrawal did not occur in every case before labour, however, and oestradiol and progesterone levels during labour were the same as those 1 week before labour (Turnbull et al 1974). Further studies by Bibby (1980) demonstrated the same continuing increase in progesterone and oestradiol in late human pregnancy found in most other studies. Figures 12.5 and 12.6 show how the findings in his cases compared with those of Turnbull et al (1974). In human peripheral venous blood, the levels of both oestrogens and progesterone seem to increase up to the onset of term and preterm labour. Salivary steroid concentrations are thought to reflect the circulating concentrations of the free hormone and hence may be more biologically relevant than the total plasma concentration or the urinary excretion of a metabolite. Recently, Darne et al (1987) reported an increase in the salivary oestriol:progesterone ratio most marked in the 5 weeks before spontaneous human labour. However, these findings were not confirmed in another study in Australian women by Lewis et al (1987).

These findings do not exclude the possibility that changes in oestrogens or progesterone in target tissues may play a crucial role in the initiation of labour. As will be described later, increased prostaglandin secretion plays a key role in the initiation of parturition. Prostaglandins are synthesized in the amnion, chorion and decidua; Mitchell et al (1982) have shown that unconjugated oestrogens and DHEA may be capable both of stimulating the synthesis of prostaglandins in dispersed cell preparations of fetal membranes and also of inhibiting progesterone synthesis in the decidua and chorion. Thus, these tissues could be subjected to local progesterone withdrawal and increased oestrogen action great enough to initiate labour without any detectable change in peripheral hormone levels. Lopez-Bernal et al (1986b) demonstrated that Epostane, which inhibits the conversion of pregnenolone to progesterone, will almost completely inhibit progesterone synthesis both by the human placenta and the choriodecidua. Tissues obtained at term are more sensitive than those obtained early in pregnancy. In adequate dosage, Epostane can induce abortion or facilitate the effect of prostaglandins (Pattison et al 1985, Webster et al 1985, Selinger et al 1987). However, no reduction in progesterone production by the chorion or decidua was demonstrated in relation to the spontaneous onset of human labour by Lopez-Bernal et al (1987b). Nevertheless, progesterone withdrawal is such an important feature of the initiation of labour in so many species that local progesterone inhibition and its release remain a regulatory option for human pregnancy maintenance and the initiation of labour. This possible mechanism has not been finally excluded although it is now largely discounted. It appears that progesterone is essential for the maintenance of human pregnancy but that human parturition begins and progresses to the birth of the fetus without progesterone being withdrawn as occurs in some other species.

MYOMETRIAL GAP JUNCTIONS

Garfield et al (1979) demonstrated myometrial cell contacts termed gap junctions, which are thought to represent low-resistance pathways to the flow of excitation, in uterine muscle obtained from guinea-pigs and sheep at delivery or postpartum. In human tissues, they were also present in a much higher proportion of samples after the onset of spontaneous labour than before it. Gap junctions are composed of sym-

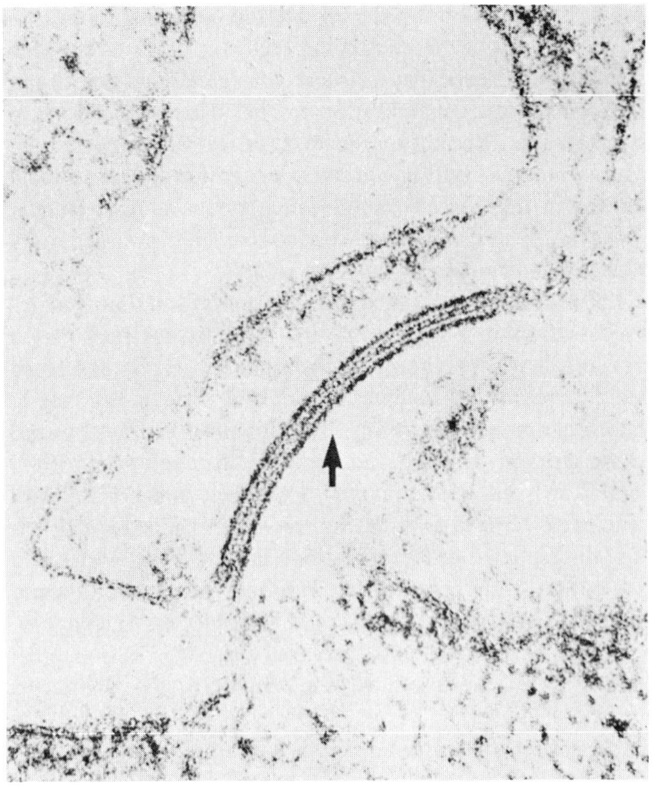

Fig. 12.7 Gap junction (arrow) between two muscle cells from the myometrium of a ewe obtained during parturition (thin section ×200 000). From Verhoeff & Garfield (1986).

metrical portions of the plasma membrane from two opposing cells; intermembranous protein particles protrude through each membrane to span the gap between the membranes. The structure of myometrial gap junctions is similar to that described in other cells (Fig. 12.7).

Garfield et al (1979) proposed that gap junctions between myometrial cells were essential for the development of the effective uterine muscle contractility which leads to the expulsion of the uterine contents in pregnancy in all animals, including man. In rats and sheep, progesterone withdrawal appears necessary for their formation, again raising the possibility that in some subtle way progesterone withdrawal may initiate human labour. Alternatively, and probably more likely with human parturition, prostaglandins can stimulate gap junction formation, according to Garfield et al (1979). The authors claim that oxytocin does not possess this ability and cannot stimulate myometrium in the absence of gap junctions. Additional support for the hypothesis of increased prostaglandin alone being enough to activate the uterus and expel its contents is provided by the work of Manabe et al (1981) who investigated the Japanese method for inducing mid-trimester abortion — inserting a balloon catheter into the lower uterine cavity through the cervix and applying prolonged traction. This method, which reliably causes abortion, often of a live fetus, has no effect on plasma levels of oestradiol, oestriol or progesterone. Although Manabe et al (1981) did not measure prostaglandin levels in their cases, studies by Mitchell et al (1977b) and by Keirse et al (1983), which demonstrated that cervical manipulation increases levels of prostaglandin metabolites in peripheral blood, suggest that the Japanese technique probably induces abortion by causing prolonged or repeated release of PGF, which must also lead to the formation of gap junctions, since abortion occurs.

Prostaglandins

The mechanism which controls prostaglandin synthesis in the pregnant human uterus and initiates the onset of labour remains unknown. This may seem surprising, considering how much the phenomenon has been investigated and the importance of prostaglandins in labour in most species (Liggins 1979). The difficulty in elucidating the regulation of human labour is that it seems to be of a paracrine nature; that is, it resides largely within the uterus and is determined by interactions between contiguous cells (Liggins 1981) rather than by changes in circulating levels of hormones. It is therefore a paracrine rather than an endocrine control system, and shares with other paracrine systems the problems of complexity and inaccessibility.

Biosynthesis of prostaglandins

Figure 12.8 illustrates the main pathways of synthesis and metabolism of prostanoids from arachidonic acid — the arachidonic acid cascade. Measurement of PGE and PGF in peripheral plasma is hampered by their low concentrations, due to their rapid clearance, especially in the lungs. Measurement of the main, stable PGF metabolite, 13,14-dihydro-15-keto-PGF (PGFM) in peripheral plasma is a better measurement of PGF production. Measurement of the same PGE metabolite (PGEM) is hindered by its instability. While the 11–16 bicyclo-PGEM metabolite is stable, its concentration does not change significantly during pregnancy or with the onset of progression of labour to delivery, in contrast to the several-fold increase in the plasma concentration of PGFM during human labour (Demers et al 1983). However, bicyclo-PGEM assay can be reliably used to detect and measure increases in plasma following administration of exogenous prostaglandins (Brennecke et al 1985).

Arachidonic acid is converted into prostaglandin endoperoxides, from which are formed all the prostaglandins of the 2 series, as well as thromboxane A_2. Cyclo-oxygenase, the enzyme catalysing the formation of prostaglandins from arachidonic acid, is present in cells either in an active form, or is readily activated. The rate of prostaglandin synthesis is controlled more by the rate of release of arachidonic acid than the activity of cyclo-oxygenase. Factors which activate phospholipase A_2 are therefore likely to be of greater importance in stimulating the increased prostaglandin which initiates labour than those which activate cyclo-oxygenase.

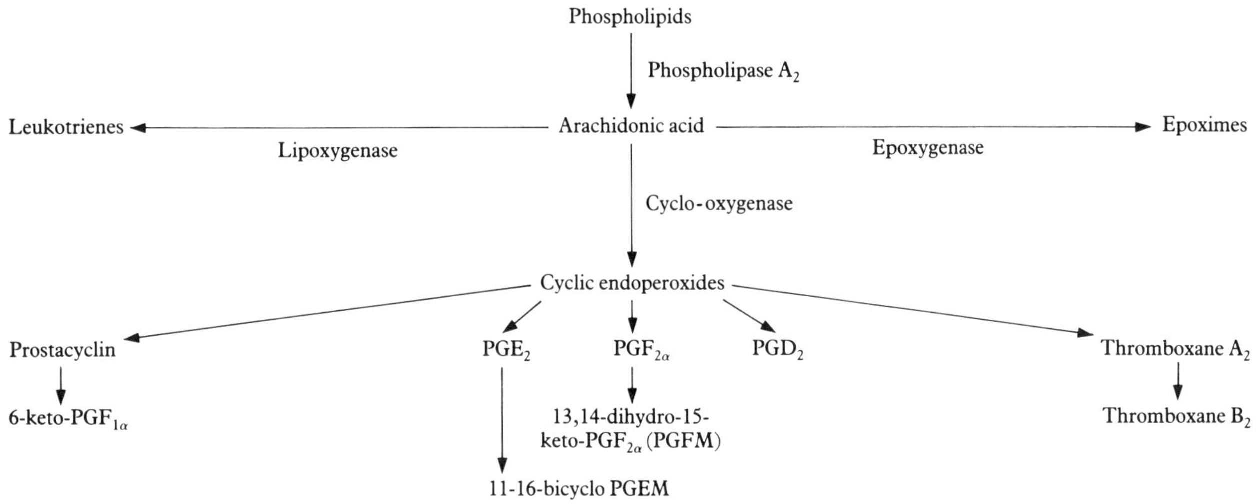

Fig. 12.8 Pathways from phospholipids to prostaglandins, prostacyclin, thromboxane, and their major metabolites and to leukotrienes and epoximes.

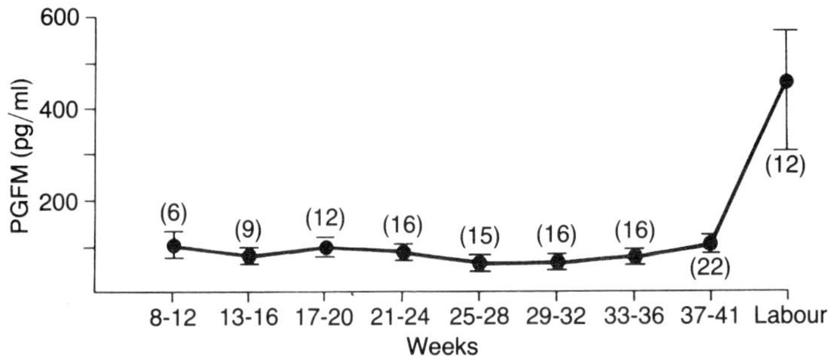

Fig. 12.9 Peripheral plasma concentrations (mean ± SEM) number of samples (in parentheses) of 13,14-dihydro-15-keto-PGF (PGFM) in 16 women throughout pregnancy and labour. From Mitchell (1984).

Little is so far known of the factors which determine the extent to which free arachidonic acid is metabolized via cyclo-oxygenase to prostaglandin or by lipoxygenase to leukotrienes.

During pregnancy, peripheral blood levels of PGFM show little change but increase massively during labour (Fig. 12.9; Sellers et al 1981a, Mitchell 1984). This demonstrates the importance of metabolite assays in revealing prostaglandin production in labour. By contrast, there were no significant increases in peripheral plasma concentrations of PGE or PGF during labour (Mitchell et al 1978a).

Measurements made in amniotic fluid first demonstrated the increase in prostaglandins during labour. Since none of the tissues which surround it contain prostaglandin-metabolizing enzymes, amniotic fluid concentrations of prostaglandins are high and increase rapidly as labour progresses. The concentration of PGF increases more rapidly than that of PGE (Fig. 12.10).

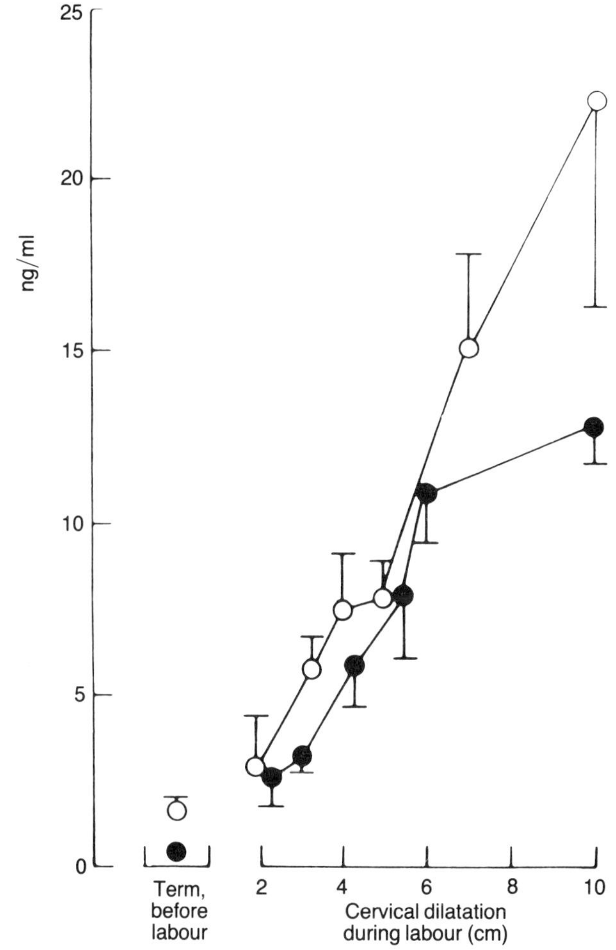

Fig. 12.10 Mean concentrations (± SEM) of PGE_2 (●) and $PGF_{2\alpha}$ (○) in amniotic fluid during late pregnancy and labour at term. After data from Keirse & Turnbull (1973) and Keirse et al (1974).

An early publication (Hibbard et al 1974) suggested that prostaglandin levels in amniotic fluid increased progressively from 36 weeks towards term. We could not demonstrate this trend when samples obtained by amniotomy at rupture of the membranes were separated from those obtained by amniocentesis (Fig. 12.11).

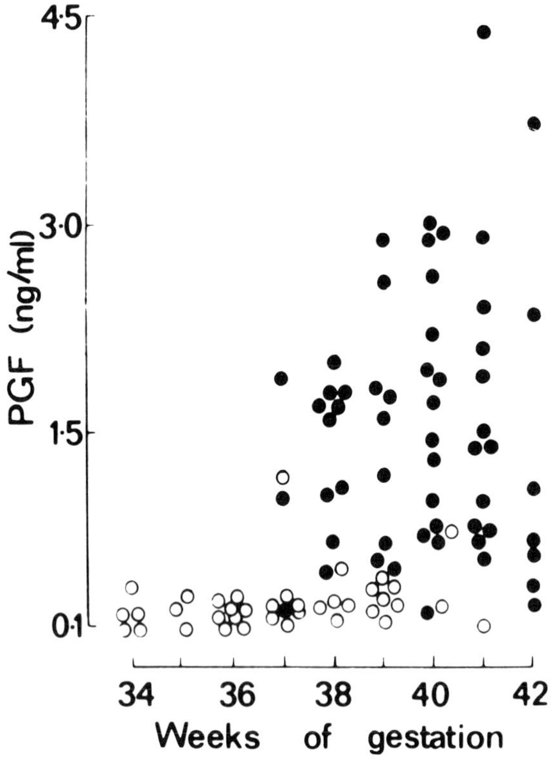

Fig. 12.11 Concentrations of PGF in amniotic fluid obtained by amniocentesis (○) and by amniotomy (●) before the onset of labour. Adapted from Mitchell et al (1977a).

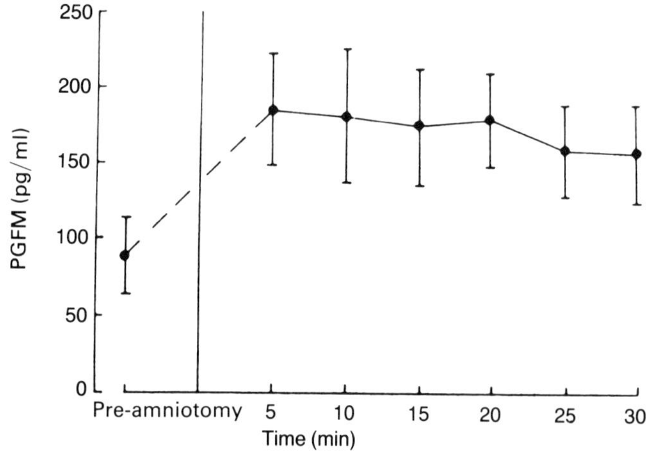

Fig. 12.12 Peripheral plasma concentrations of PGFM (mean ± SEM) before and for 30 min after amniotomy. Adapted from Sellers et al (1980).

The raised levels of PGF in amniotic fluid obtained by amniotomy in comparison with amniocentesis were among the first observations to suggest a local intrauterine control of prostaglandin biosynthesis. This concept was also favoured by subsequent findings that peripheral plasma levels of PGFM were elevated within 5 minutes of amniotomy and remained high for at least 30 minutes thereafter (Fig. 12.12). This initial increase in PGFM is not associated with the onset of labour, which seems to depend on a secondary and continuing increase in PGFM (Sellers et al 1981c).

Regulation of prostaglandins for the initiation of human labour

At present, the mechanism which brings about the increased levels of prostaglandins found in association with human labour remains unknown. Even the source of the increased prostaglandins is not entirely resolved. In reviewing the whole field, however, Casey & MacDonald (1986) concluded: 'increased synthesis of PGE_2 in amnion is the key event in the onset of labour'. The authors suggest that increased prostaglandin synthesis in the amnion results either from an increase in the rate of release of arachidonic acid from glycerophospholipids, or an increase in the activity of the prostaglandin synthetase in amnion, or from both. They believed that these changes depended on a fetal signal, possibly reaching the amnion through fetal urine which stimulates increased PGE_2 synthesis by amnion (Casey et al 1983). Since fetal urine samples obtained before labour also exert this effect, other regulatory mechanisms must be involved. More recently, Casey & MacDonald (1988) have suggested that human pregnancy maintenance depends on the inhibition of $PGF_{2\alpha}$ formation in decidua, and that the onset of labour therefore results from release of inhibition of decidual $PGF_{2\alpha}$ synthesis.

Sites of prostaglandin synthesis

Early studies of prostaglandin production from the uterus usually assumed that the main source of $PGF_{2\alpha}$ was the myometrium. However, early studies in the pregnant sheep by Liggins & Greaves (1971) showed that at the onset of parturition when the concentration of $PGF_{2\alpha}$ was rising in the uterine vein, the concentration of $PGF_{2\alpha}$ was elevated in the maternal component of the placental cotyledon but only later in the myometrium. This suggested that the prostaglandin in the myometrium had diffused there from the uterine epithelium. Both in the pregnant sheep uterus (Campos et al 1980) and in the non-pregnant human uterus (Abel et al 1980) the uterine epithelium or endometrium predominantly converts arachidonic acid to $PGF_{2\alpha}$ and PGE_2, whereas the myometrium produces mainly prostacyclin (PGI_2). An additional site of prostaglandin synthesis is the cervix. During incubation of sheep cervical tissues, substantial quantities of prostanoids are released into the medium, predominantly PGE_2 and PGI_2 (Ellwood et al 1981). The parturient cervix releases greater quantities than the non-parturient. The concentration of PGE_2 and PGI_2 in the cervical vein of sheep increases sharply at the time when cervical ripening begins. Ellwood et al (1980b) also investigated the potential of the pregnant human cervix to produce prostaglandins. Tissues obtained during the first trimester of pregnancy produced PGE, PGF, PGFM and 6-keto-$PGF_{1\alpha}$ when

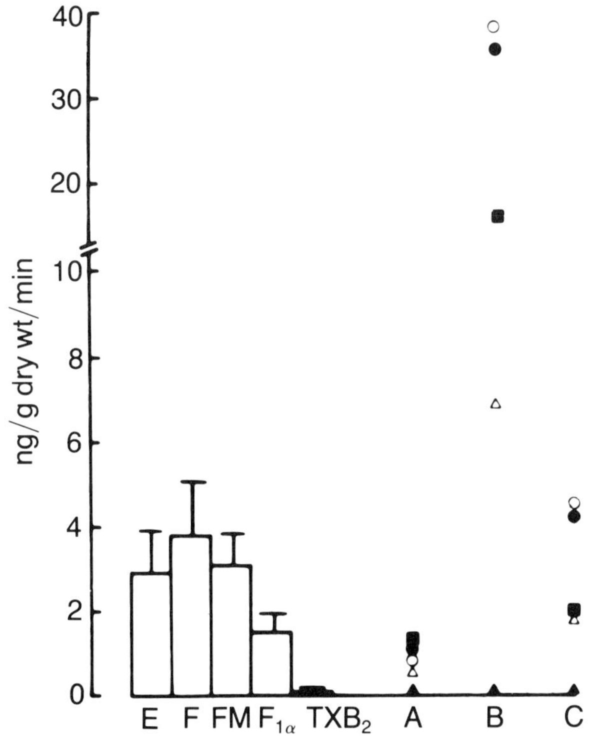

Fig. 12.13 Prostanoid production rates in cervical tissues obtained from three women in the third trimester of pregnancy are shown in comparison with the mean rates found in cervical tissues from women in the first trimester. Patient A: elective Caesarean section at 37 weeks; patient B: emergency Caesarean section at 34 weeks, 6–7 cm dilatation; patient C: emergency Caesarean section at 40 weeks, full dilatation. For each patient, the production rates are shown for PGE (●), PGF (○), PGFM (△), 6-oxo-$PGF_{1\alpha}$ (■) and TBX_2 (▲). Each point represents the mean of between four and six measurements. Adapted from Ellwood et al (1980b).

superfused in vitro. Thromboxane B_2 (TXB_2) production was minimal. Preliminary evidence from tissues taken at Caesarean hysterectomy during the third trimester of human pregnancy suggested that at this stage the cervix may exhibit greater production of prostaglandin production (Fig. 12.13). Hence, the human cervix may produce prostaglandins in vivo which could act locally during pregnancy and contribute to cervical softening and dilatation over the last few weeks of pregnancy — unlike the sheep — as well as contributing to the accelerating dilatation which characterizes labour.

In reviewing prostaglandin synthesis in human parturition, Casey & MacDonald (1986) agree that prostaglandin synthesis in the fetal membranes and decidua plays a central role in the initiation of labour. In the amnion, PGE_2 is by far the most important prostaglandin produced and since there is little or no 15-keto-prostaglandin dehydrogenase (PGDH) in amnion, the large quantities of PGE_2 formed are not metabolized. However, the human myometrium is capable of actively metabolizing PGE_2 to $PGF_{2\alpha}$ because it is an important source of PG-9-oxo-reductase activity (Canete Soler et al 1987). While the chorion also synthesizes PGE_2 and the decidua synthesizes PGE_2 and $PGF_{2\alpha}$, both tissues show considerable prostaglandin dehydrogenase

Table 12.1 Prostaglandin E production by collagenase-dispersed amnion cells (pmol/10^6 cells/3 h)

	Spontaneous labour ($n = 14$)	Elective Caesarean section ($n = 9$)	Induced labour ($n = 6$)
Basal	27.5 ± 5.5	13.6 ± 2.7	10 ± 3.1
	└── $P = 0.05$ ──┘ (spontaneous vs elective)		
	└── $P = 0.02$ ──┘ (spontaneous vs induced)		
+ 10 μmol/l Arachidonic acid	46.6 ± 5.8	39.3 ± 7.8	32.9 ± 6.5

Mean ± SEM
From Lopez Bernal et al (1987a).

activity which tends quickly to inactivate the prostaglandins synthesized.

The availability of free arachidonic acid also appears to be an important rate-limiting factor in the synthesis of prostaglandins. Table 12.1 shows the result of studies of PGE_2 synthesis of collagenase-dispersed amnion cells in culture, comparing samples obtained from women during continuing pregnancy and those during labour at delivery (Lopez-Bernal et al 1987a). The rate of PGE_2 synthesis is greater in the amnion samples obtained from women in labour. When arachidonic acid is added to these cultures, however, the differences between samples obtained from continuing late pregnancy and labour almost disappear, indicating that the previous difference simply depended on the greater availability of arachidonic acid during labour.

Regulation of increased prostaglandin biosynthesis in labour

Gustavii (1978) suggested that phospholipase A_2 was released from decidual lysosomes destabilized by the local withdrawal of progesterone and increase of oestrogens. Increased phospholipase A_2 activity would stimulate the release of free arachidonic acid from membranes as well as phospholipids. In fact, human amniotic fluid contains much more arachidonic acid than is required for the amount of prostaglandin synthesized in labour and the same is true of uterine muscle (Keirse et al 1977). However, as these workers point out, the intracellular availability of arachidonic acid for prostaglandin-synthesizing enzymes is unknown and could be an important regulatory factor.

Inhibition of prostaglandin biosynthesis during pregnancy

Maathius & Kelly (1978) demonstrated that the concentration of prostaglandins in human pregnancy decidua is lower in pregnancy than that in the endometrium at any stage of the normal menstrual cycle. Apparently the human conceptus somehow interferes with endometrial synthesis or metabolism of PGE and PGF soon after plantation. There were extremely low levels of both PGF and PGE in endometrium early in pregnancy at a conceptual age of about 17 days. The prostaglandin levels in normal late secretory endo-

Table 12.2 Prostaglandins in maternal and umbilical circulation at term (pg/ml)

	Maternal circulation		Umbilical (spontaneous labour)	
	Late pregnancy ($n = 13$)	Late labour (cervix 5–8 cm) ($n = 5$)	Artery ($n = 12$)	Vein ($n = 12$)
PGE	4.8 + 1.0	5.4 ± 2.2	109.3 ± 26.9	241.9 ± 24.9
PGF	6.2 ± 0.5	12.4 ± 3.5	79.7 ± 10.4	87.8 ± 11.1
PGFM	59.0 ± 6.7	282.7 ± 55.3	639.9 ± 180.2	630.8 ± 107.3

Mean ± SEM.
After Mitchell et al (1978a,b).

metrium were about 200 times greater than in early pregnancy. Increased oestrogen and progesterone levels do not suppress prostaglandin synthesis, for in non-pregnant endometrium, high levels of oestradiol and progesterone are associated with high prostaglandin levels.

These findings, coupled with the great excess of arachidonic acid over PGE and PGF in amniotic fluid and uterine tissues in late human pregnancy (Keirse et al 1977), suggest that human pregnancy maintenance may depend on inhibition of prostaglandin synthesis in intrauterine tissues, particularly decidua. The fact that decidual prostaglandins are suppressed even when the pregnancy is extrauterine (Abel et al 1980) suggests that the factors may have a systemic rather than a local action.

Saeed et al (1977) discovered that mammalian plasma inhibited bovine seminal vesical prostaglandin synthase because it contained endogenous inhibitors of prostaglandin synthesis (EIPS) in blood protein fractions rich in haptoglobin and albumin, respectively. Brennecke et al (1982, 1985) investigated EIPS in human pregnancy but found similar activities in the plasma of non-pregnant women; men; women in the first and second trimesters of pregnancy, and at full term and postpartum. There appeared to be a small but significant decrease in EIPS activities in plasma samples obtained from women in the third trimester and from those at full term, but since this was not maintained in labour or the puerperium, a decrease in EIPS is not the cause of the increased prostaglandin formation during labour.

Although measurement of EIPS activity has not clarified the mechanism which inhibits prostaglandin synthesis effectively in human pregnancy, Mortimer et al (1985) demonstrated that amnion obtained from pregnant women could contain an endogenous prostaglandin synthetase inhibitor which was no longer present in amnion obtained from women during labour. Wilson et al (1985) have demonstrated in amniotic fluid two proteins which can inhibit PGF synthesis in human endometrial cells. These proved to be novel endogenous proteins which inhibited endometrial cell phospholipase A_2. These inhibitors could be identified in amniotic fluid from women with continuing pregnancy but not from fluid obtained in labour. Wilson (1988) has recently reviewed progress in this field. One of the proteins is a dimer of the other and had been called chorionic inhibitor of phospholipase. It resembles lipocortin in many ways and is not glucocorticoid-dependent. Work continues in this exciting area.

Prostanoids in the fetal and neonatal circulation

This topic has been reviewed by Turnbull et al (1981). Table 12.2 shows the levels of prostaglandins in the maternal circulation in late pregnancy and late labour and in the umbilical circulation after spontaneous delivery. The concentrations of PGE, PGF and PGFM are much higher in the umbilical than in the maternal circulation in either pregnancy or labour. Prostaglandin levels are higher in the umbilical vein than in the artery, indicating that the increased PGE must be of maternal rather than fetal origin.

Prostaglandins have a role in the control of fetal and placental haemodynamics and influence the fetal circulation. Respiratory distress syndrome is associated with high levels of PGF in the infant's circulation, and patent ductus arteriosus with high levels of PGE (Turnbull et al 1981). The fact that PGE can open the ductus and that inhibitors of PG synthesis (PGSI) can close the ductus indicates the importance of prostaglandins in the fetus and also shows that use of PGSI in pregnancy or labour can lead to potentially dangerous intrauterine ductal closure. This may occur if PGSI are given to treat preterm labour. They could cross the placenta, cause in utero closure of the ductus arteriosus and lead to increased pulmonary arterial pressure, associated with hyperplasia of the fetal pulmonary vascular smooth muscle and leading eventually to persistent pulmonary hypertension of the newborn (Wilkinson et al 1979). This complication can result from unusually low circulating levels of PGE in the neonate caused by excessive levels of PGSI (Wilkinson et al 1979). Great caution must therefore be exercised before prescribing treatment with PGSI during pregnancy. Nowadays, however, the benefit of prolonging intrauterine existence for even a few days more may be vital when preterm delivery threatens at 25–26 weeks. The benefits may outweigh the potential hazards of PGSI as additional tocolytics. The human ductus arteriosus does not contain prostaglandin receptors before 21 weeks and the gestational age at which these receptors develop is not known, but probably varies to some extent from one fetus to another (Lopez-Bernal et al 1986a).

OXYTOCIN

Although oxytocin has been extensively used for the induction and augmentation of labour, there has been much uncertainty about its importance in the normal physiological onset and maintenance of human labour. Maternal oxytocin levels are only of the order of a few microunits and shows little or no change before labour. Fetal oxytocin by comparison increases significantly in association with spontaneous labour (Chard et al 1971). Since the increase is greater in umbilical arterial than venous plasma (Chard 1977), oxytocin must be synthesized by the fetus and seems to be transferred from fetus to mother (Dawood et al 1978a).

Of critical importance has been the discovery that the concentration of oxytocin receptors in human myometrium and decidua increases during late pregnancy and also considerably in relation to labour, indicating that labour results from increasing sensitivity of the uterus to oxytocin, so that the uterus can be stimulated by an oxytocin level in maternal blood which would have had no effect previously when the concentration of myometrial oxytocin receptors was low (Fuchs et al 1982, Husslein 1985).

Maternal oxytocin

Oxytocin levels have been investigated increasingly in recent years, with the development of sensitive radioimmunoassays. The earlier data were reported by Chard et al (1970), who were initially unable to detect oxytocin in maternal plasma during pregnancy or labour, but found measurable amounts in 40% of mixed umbilical cord plasma samples. Subsequently, Chard et al (1971) identified oxytocin in the peripheral circulation of some women during labour. The frequency of positive values gradually increased during the first stage and reached a maximum of 60% of positive values during delivery, implying spurt release of oxytocin from the posterior pituitary gland (Gibbens et al 1972). Several recent studies have detected oxytocin in maternal plasma throughout pregnancy and labour (Kumaresan et al 1974, Dawood et al 1978b, Vasicka et al 1978, Leake et al 1979). The studies in Oxford by Sellers et al (1981b) showed measurable concentrations of oxytocin in 93% of maternal plasma samples during pregnancy (Fig. 12.14). Values varied widely between patients throughout pregnancy, ranging from less than 1 to 27 pg/ml. There was no change in maternal plasma oxytocin concentration during early or late labour. These findings agreed with those of Kumaresan et al (1974), Gazárek et al (1976) and Vasicka et al (1978). However, Dawood et al (1978b) found higher levels in second-stage labour and Leake et al (1979) found high levels at delivery of the fetal head. Disparity in the results may be due to the spurt release of oxytocin; blood may not have been sampled frequently enough during labour to demonstrate a change in levels.

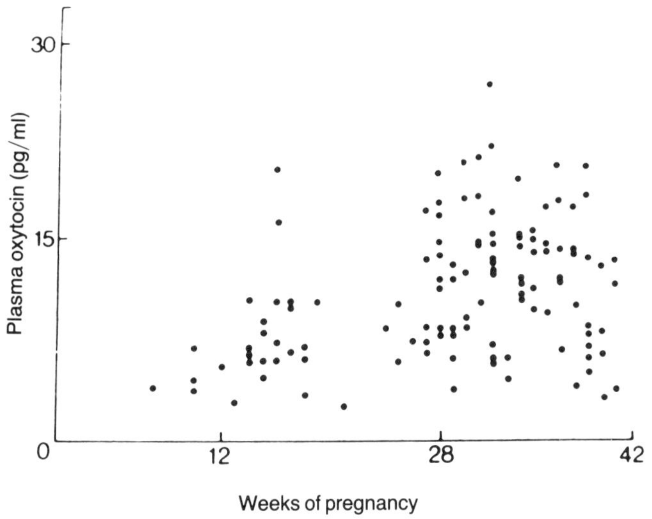

Fig. 12.14 Maternal plasma oxytocin concentrations during pregnancy. From Sellers et al (1981b).

Table 12.3 Oxytocin receptors in the myometrium and decidua (fmol/ng DNA)

	Myometrium		Decidua	
	n	Receptor concentration	*n*	Receptor concentration
Non-pregnant: menstruating	14	27.6 ± 7.97	6	24.9 ± 5.59
Pregnant: 13–17 weeks	5	171.6 ± 67.4	1	629
Pre-term labour: 28–36 weeks	8	2353 ± 358	8	3673 ± 947
Before labour: 37–43 weeks	6	1391 ± 180	6	1510 ± 302
Early labour: 37–43 weeks	5	3458 ± 886	3	3177 ± 1426
Advanced labour*: 37–43 weeks	7	257 ± 104	2	786

*Samples taken from lower uterine segment.
Mean ± SEM
From Fuchs et al (1982).

Oxytocin receptors

The concentration of oxytocin receptors in the myometrium correlates well with the sensitivity of the uterus to oxytocin. Table 12.3 shows the concentration of oxytocin receptors in the human myometrium in the non-pregnant state, during early and late pregnancy and in early labour, and demonstrates the dramatic increase in labour found by Fuchs et al (1982). There are also marked increases in oxytocin receptors in the decidua. Treating decidual cells with oxytocin causes release of prostaglandins (Fuchs et al 1981), confirming the mechanism which had earlier been demonstrated by Mitchell et al (1977b) that vaginal examination in late human pregnancy causes increased blood levels of prostaglandins in maternal blood, reaching a peak 5 minutes after examination. Examination stimulates the Ferguson reflex, by which a neural afferent from the cervix causes oxytocin release from the posterior pituitary. The humoral effect depends on the oxytocin being taken up by decidual oxytocin receptors which promote decidual prostaglandin release.

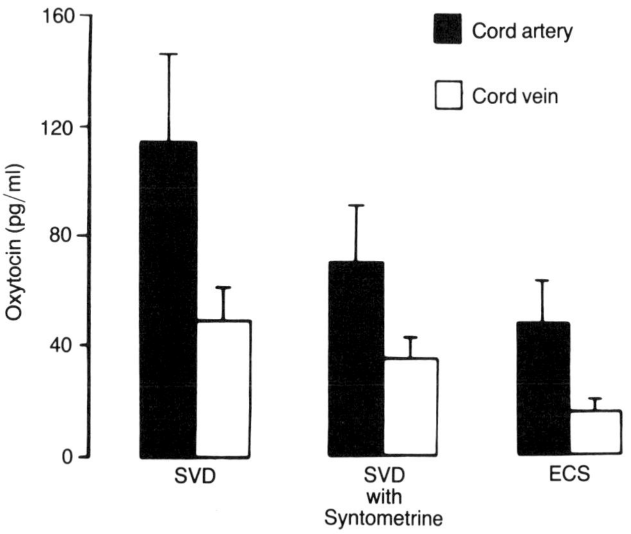

Fig. 12.15 Umbilical cord plasma oxytocin concentration. Mean ± SEM. SVD = spontaneous vaginal delivery; ECS = elective Caesarean section. From Sellers et al (1981b).

Clearly, the initiation of labour depends not so much on the oxytocin level itself as on the mechanism which induces oxytocin receptors in the myometrium. Liggins (1973) showed in the sheep that continuous intravenous infusion of relatively small doses of prostaglandins in late pregnancy caused increasing myometrial responsiveness both to prostaglandins and to oxytocin after several hours. A similar response has been observed in human pregnancy (Liggins et al 1977b). The basis of this sensitization is unknown, but could result from the formation of gap junctions. Liggins' observations suggest that gap junctions could be formed by continuous myometrial stimulation with low levels of prostaglandins. Indomethacin, a prostaglandin synthase inhibitor, partly inhibits gap junction formation in vitro (Garfield et al 1980).

Fetal oxytocin

Fetal oxytocin has been investigated by Chard et al (1970, 1971) and more recently by Dawood et al (1978a) and Sellers et al (1981b). The mean oxytocin concentrations in umbilical arterial and venous plasma collected after labour following spontaneous vaginal delivery, and before labour at elective Caesarean section, reported by Sellers et al (1981b) are shown in Figure 12.15. These levels are very similar to those found both by Dawood et al (1978a) and Chard et al (1971), with a significant arteriovenous oxytocin difference in samples obtained before and after labour. Umbilical arterial plasma oxytocin levels are consistently higher than umbilical venous levels. The levels in both fetal umbilical arterial and venous plasma are significantly higher than in maternal plasma. Initiation and maintenance of human labour may therefore be influenced by fetal oxytocin. Dawood et al (1978a) calculated that the fetal oxytocin secretion rate could be as high as 2.75 ± 0.5 mu/min (mean ± SEM) in infants delivered by Caesarean section after the spontaneous onset of labour. By contrast, in infants delivered by elective Caesarean section before labour, the calculated oxytocin secretion rate was only 1.0 ± 0.2 mu/min. Fetal oxytocin secretion rates in infants delivered after spontaneous labour were around 3 mu/min, similar to the dose of oxytocin of around 2–8 mu/min, which is normally administered to women to induce labour at term.

The situation should not be over-simplified. Chard et al (1971) showed that spontaneous labour was also associated with an even greater increase in vasopressin than oxytocin in the fetal circulation. Furthermore, the possible influence of low and unchanging maternal oxytocin levels on human uterine contractility may be of primary importance in initiating labour, since the uterus will become increasingly sensitive to its potential effects as the concentration of myometrial oxytocin receptors increases.

Relaxin, prolactin and prostaglandins

Relaxin, prolactin and prostaglandins all appear to be paracrine hormones of the human amnion, chorion and decidua and to be involved in parturition. While the role of prostaglandins is well established, the specific effects of relaxin and prolactin remain to be established (Bryant-Greenwood et al 1987). According to MacLennan (1983), the polypeptide hormone relaxin is thought in mammals to promote connective tissue remodelling during reproduction, inhibition of myometrial contractility until late pregnancy and cervical ripening at parturition. In fact, little is known about the actions of relaxin and it is only recently that an analogue of human relaxin has been synthesized and used to develop a radioimmunoassay with which Eddie et al (1986) measured blood levels of relaxin in human pregnancy. Relaxin was not detectable in men or in non-pregnant women, but was present in all serial blood samples collected from three pregnant women. Concentrations ranged from 0.9 to 1.18 mg/ml; the highest levels were in the first trimester and almost all the readings after 24 weeks were under 0.5 mg/ml and showed no consistent rising or falling trend. MacLennan et al (1986) measured relaxin blood levels in 368 samples from 302 pregnant women between 6 and 41 weeks' gestation, using a guinea-pig relaxin antiserum utilizing a porcine label and a porcine standard. The levels they found were similar to those of Eddie et al (1986) and significantly lower levels were also found in the third trimester than in the first or second. In one woman in whom the subsequent onset of labour was preterm, relaxin levels fell steadily, below the 95% confidence levels for normal pregnancy.

Relaxin appears to be produced particularly by the cells of the chorionic cytotrophoblast (Bryant-Greenwood et al 1987) and only half the tissues after spontaneous delivery contained positive relaxin-stained cells, whereas all the tissues from elective Caesarean section contained cells positively stained with antiserum to relaxin.

Prolactin was positively localized in the decidua and occasionally also in the amnion (Bryant-Greenwood et al 1987). Prostaglandin synthase was previously localized in the amnion and chorion. Recently Lopez-Bernal et al (1987b) have demonstrated that relaxin, present in the chorion laeve and decidua at term, may have a paracrine effect on the amnion, inhibiting PGE production during continuing pregnancy but favouring its production during spontaneous labour. These findings may help to explain the mechanism by which local vaginal application of purified porcine relaxin facilitates cervical ripening and induction of labour (MacLennan et al 1980).

CONCLUSIONS

Parturition in human pregnancy, unlike that in the sheep and some other species, is not preceded by dramatic changes in maternal peripheral plasma levels of oestradiol or progesterone. Fetal cortisol secretion does not suddenly increase before labour, nor does it have any effects on the endocrine function of the fetal placenta as it does in the sheep. Maternal administration of corticosteroids in human pregnancy simply suppresses maternal and fetal adrenocortical function, causing a fall in maternal oestrogen levels.

The maintenance of human pregnancy may depend on a mechanism which tonically inhibits prostaglandin synthesis in uterine tissues. Unlike the sheep, human myometrium is relatively sensitive to prostaglandins throughout pregnancy. Human amnion and decidua are capable of synthesizing prostaglandins in vitro at any stage of pregnancy and labour may depend on the withdrawal of potent inhibitors of prostaglandin synthesis from these tissues. The inhibitory process normally seems to be particularly effective in early pregnancy and may lessen as pregnancy advances. It may involve the presence in intrauterine tissues of lipocortins capable of synthesizing prostaglandins. We have been unable to demonstrate obvious effects of oestrogen or progesterone on PGE production by fetal membranes or decidua (Lopez-Bernal et al 1987c).

In late human pregnancy, the prostaglandin-synthesizing mechanism seems to be readily, if transiently, activated by minor local stimuli such as vaginal examination, sweeping the membranes or amniotomy. The stable PGFM increases markedly within 5 minutes of amniotomy and the increase persists for 30 minutes afterwards. While Sellers et al (1980) could not show this increase to be associated with oxytocin release, as in the sheep, Chard & Gibbens (1983) demonstrated that amniotomy does cause a transient increase in maternal plasma oxytocin levels, indicating that the Ferguson reflex may be involved in human as well as in sheep pregnancy.

It has been shown (Sellers et al 1981c) that an increase in maternal PGFM levels occurs in all patients immediately following amniotomy, but that this increase is transient. The onset of progressive labour depends on a subsequent continuing increase in PGFM, usually associated with a steady increase in uterine contractility.

It has proved difficult to measure the changes in PGE at the onset of labour in human pregnancy. PGEM proved to be unstable (Granström et al 1980). Radioimmunoassay of a stable metabolite (biocyclo-PGEM) was developed (Demers et al 1983). Although this effectively measured increased blood levels when exogenous PGE was administered, it showed no change in level during human pregnancy, labour or the puerperium, implying that if increased PGE_2 is secreted by uterine tissues during labour, it must somehow be retained with the uterus. There is, however, indirect evidence that PGE_2 increases in the fetal circulation in the 48–72 hours before the onset of labour. Boddy et al (1974) showed that fetal breathing movements ceased during that period and Castle & Turnbull (1983) have reviewed the evidence that in man and animals, increasing the level of PGE in the fetal circulation inhibits fetal breathing, while intrafetal infusion of a prostaglandin synthetase inhibitor stimulates breathing. It is possible that a local increase in PGE levels occurring in uterine tissues 48–72 hours before labour may therefore initiate the whole process of human parturition.

The increasing synthesis of PGE and PGF in the human uterus at term can undoubtedly bring about all the features of progressive labour — in the uterine muscle, powerful coordinated contractions; in the cervix, breakdown and fibrillation of collagen fibres and other connective tissue changes associated with cervical softening and increased extensibility (Ellwood et al 1979, 1980b, Ellwood 1981). Working together, these factors can bring about dilatation and effacement of the cervix, formation of the lower uterine segment, rupture of the membranes and the whole process of labour and parturition, culminating in the safe and effective delivery of the infant and placenta.

The action of oxytocin has, in recent years, been shown to play an important role in human labour. This is not due to elevation of the oxytocin level in the maternal circulation but to a large increase in the concentration of oxytocin receptors in the myometrium and in the decidua, sensitizing the uterus to the effects of oxytocin already present in maternal blood. Stimulating decidual cells with oxytocin causes prostaglandin release. In labour, dilatation of the cervix and vagina can stimulate oxytocin secretion through the Ferguson reflex, causing increased prostaglandin release from the decidua. Once the excitation system has been activated, it therefore leads to accelerating labour progress as in other species.

In the human fetus, high levels of oxytocin are found in the umbilical arterial blood after vaginal delivery — higher than in the umbilical vein blood — indicating a fetal origin for the oxytocin. Cord blood oxytocin levels are much lower before the onset of labour but it is not known if the increased fetal production of oxytocin (and vasopressin) plays a part in the initiation or maintenance of human labour.

Prostaglandins are also involved in the third stage of labour. PGFM levels in the maternal circulation rise in the first and second stages of labour but much more after delivery of the baby, reaching their highest levels 5 min after delivery (Sellers et al 1982). While these prostaglandins probably originate in the uterus, the factors controlling their release are unknown. The surge of prostaglandins after delivery of the fetus is likely to influence expulsion of the placenta and fetal membranes.

Although intramuscular administration of a mixture of ergometrine and oxytocin (Syntometrine) has been used in the UK for many years to facilitate delivery of the placenta by controlled traction and to reduce postpartum haemorrhage, there have been several reports in which severe postpartum haemorrhage could not be controlled until PGF or PGE was administered by intravenous or intramyometrial injection (Henson et al 1983).

While there is increased understanding of the factors which maintain human pregnancy and initiate labour at term, much remains to be done before full understanding is achieved.

REFERENCES

Abel M H, Smith S K, Baird D T 1980 Suppression of concentration of endometrial prostaglandin in early intrauterine and ectopic pregnancy in women. Journal of Endocrinology 85: 379–386

Anderson A B M 1976 Hormone changes preceding premature labour. In: Turnbull A C, Woodford F P (eds) Prevention of fetal handicap through antenatal care, vol 3. Associated Scientific Publishers, Amsterdam, pp 137–148

Anderson A B M, Flint A P F, Turnbull A C 1975 Mechanism of action of glucocorticoids in induction of ovine parturition: effect on placental steroid metabolism. Journal of Endocrinology 66: 61–70

Bassett J M, Thorburn G D 1969 Fetal plasma corticosteroids and the initiation of parturition in sheep. Journal of Endocrinology 44: 285–288

Bibby J G 1980 Studies in human pregnancy and parturition with particular reference to the role of prostaglandins and steroid hormones. Thesis for MD, University of Otago, Dunedin, New Zealand

Boddy K, Dawes G S, Robinson J 1974 Intra uterine fetal breathing movements. In: Gluck L (ed) Modern perinatal medicine. Year Book Publishers, Chicago, pp 381–390

Brennecke S P, Bryce R L, Turnbull A C 1982 The prostaglandin synthase inhibiting ability of maternal plasma and the onset of human labour. European Journal of Obstetrics and Gynecology and Reproductive Biology 14: 81–88

Brennecke S P, Castle B M, Demers L M, Turnbull A C 1985 Maternal plasma prostaglandin E_2 metabolite levels during human pregnancy and parturition. British Journal of Obstetrics and Gynaecology 92: 345–349

Bryant-Greenwood G D, Rees M C P, Turnbull A C 1987 Immunohistochemical localisation of relaxin, prolactin and prostaglandin synthase in human amnion, chorion and decidua. Journal of Endocrinology 114: 491–496

Campos G A, Liggins G C, Seamark R F 1980 Differential production of PGF and 6-keto-$PGF_{1\alpha}$ by the rat endometrium and myometrium in response to oxytocin, catecholamines and calcium ionophore. Prostaglandins 20: 297–310

Canete Soler R, Lopez-Bernal A, Turnbull A C 1987 Conversion of prostaglandin E_2 to prostaglandin $F_{2\alpha}$ by human myometrium. Hormone and Metabolism Research 19: 515–516

Casey M L, MacDonald P C 1986 Initiation of labor in women. In: Huszar G (ed) The physiology and biochemistry of the uterus in pregnancy and labor. CRC Press, Boca Raton, Florida, pp 155–161

Casey M L, MacDonald P C 1988 The role of a fetal–maternal paracrine system in the maintenance of pregnancy and the initiation of parturition. In: Jones C T (ed.) Fetal and neonatal development. Perinatology Press, Ithaca, New York

Casey M L, MacDonald P C, Mitchell M D 1983 Stimulation of prostaglandin E_2 production in amnion cells in culture by a substance(s) in human fetal and adult urine. Biochemical and Biophysical Research Communications 114: 1056–1063

Castle B M, Turnbull A C 1983 The presence or absence of fetal breathing movements predicts the outcome of preterm labour. Lancet ii: 471–472

Cawson M J, Anderson A B M, Turnbull A C, Lampe L 1974 Cortisol, cortisone and 11-deoxycortisol levels in human umbilical and maternal plasma in relation to the onset of labour. Journal of Obstetrics and Gynaecology of the British Commonwealth 81: 737–745

Challis J R G, Nathanielsz P W 1979 Parturition in small mammals. In: Keirse M J N C, Anderson A B M, Bennebroek Gravenhorst (eds) Human parturition. Leiden University Press, Leiden, pp 1–10

Challis J R G, Robinson J S, Thorburn G D 1977 Fetal and maternal endocrine changes during pregnancy and parturition in the Rhesus monkey. In: Knight J, O'Connor M (eds) The fetus and birth vol 47. Ciba Foundation Symposium. Elsevier/Excerpta Medica/North Holland, Amsterdam, pp 211–228

Chard T 1977 The posterior pituitary gland. In: Fuchs F, Klopper A (eds) Endocrinology of pregnancy. Harper & Row, New York, pp 271–290

Chard T, Gibbens G L D 1983 Spurt release of oxytocin during surgical induction of labor in women. American Journal of Obstetrics and Gynecology 147: 678–680

Chard T, Boyd N R H, Forsling M L, McNeilly A S, London J 1970 The development of a radioimmunoassay for oxytocin: the extraction of oxytocin from plasma and its measurement during parturition in human and goat blood. Journal of Endocrinology 48: 223–234

Chard T, Hudson C N, Edwards C R N 1971 Release of oxytocin and vasopressin by the human fetus during labour. Nature 234: 352–354

Caspo A I, Knobil E, van der Molan H J, Wiest W G 1971 Peripheral plasma progesterone levels during human pregnancy and labor. American Journal of Obstetrics and Gynecology 110: 630–632

Darne J, McGarrigle H H G, Lachelin G C L 1987 Saliva oestriol, oestradiol, oestrone and progesterone levels in pregnancy: spontaneous labour at term is preceded by a rise in the saliva oestriol: progesterone ratio. British Journal of Obstetrics and Gynaecology 94: 227–235

Dawood M Y, Wang C F, Gupta R, Fuchs F 1978a Fetal contribution to oxytocin in human labor. Obstetrics and Gynecology 52: 205–209

Dawood M Y, Raghavan K S, Pociask C, Fuchs F 1978b Oxytocin in human pregnancy and parturition. Obstetrics and Gynecology 51: 138–143

Demers L M, Brennecke S P, Mountford L A, Brunt J D, Turnbull A C 1983 Development and validation of a radioimmunoassay for prostaglandin E_2 metabolite levels in plasma. Journal of Clinical Endocrinology and Metabolism 57: 101–106

Eddie L N, Bell R J, Lester A et al 1986 Radioimmunoassay of relaxin in pregnancy with an analogue of human relaxin. Lancet i: 1344–1346

Ellwood D A 1981 The uterine cervix in pregnancy and at parturition. DPhil Thesis, University of Oxford

Ellwood D A, Anderson A B M, Mitchell M D, Turnbull A C 1979 A significant increase in the in-vitro production of prostaglandin E by ovine cervical tissue at delivery. Journal of Endocriology 81: 133P–134P

Ellwood D A, Mitchell M D, Anderson A B M, Turnbull A C 1980a Specific changes in the in vitro production of prostanoids by the ovine cervix at parturition. Prostaglandins 19: 479–488

Ellwood D A, Mitchell M D, Anderson A B M, Turnbull A C 1980b The in vitro production of prostanoids by the human cervix during pregnancy; preliminary observations. British Journal of Obstetrics and Gynaecology 87: 210–214

Ellwood D A, Anderson A B M, Mitchell M D, Turnbull A C 1981 Prostanoids, collagenase and cervical softening in the sheep. In: Ellwood D A, Anderson A B M (eds) The cervix in pregnancy and labour. Churchill Livingstone, Edinburgh, pp 57–73

Fencl M, Tulchinsky D 1975 Total cortisol in amniotic fluid and fetal lung maturation. New England Journal of Medicine 292: 133–136

Flint A P F, Anderson A B M, Steele P A, Turnbull A C 1975a The

mechanism by which fetal cortisol controls the onset of parturition in the sheep. Biochemical Society Transactions 3: 1189–1194
Flint A P F, Forsling M L, Mitchell M D, Turnbull A C 1975b Temporal relationship between changes in oxytocin and prostaglandin F levels in response to vaginal distension in the pregnant and puerperal ewe. Journal of Reproduction and Fertility 43: 551–554
Fuchs A R, Husslein P, Fuchs F 1981 Oxytocin and the initiation of human parturition. II. Stimulation of prostaglandin production in human decidua by oxytocin. American Journal of Obstetrics and Gynecology 141: 694–697
Fuchs A R, Fuchs F, Husslein P, Soloff M S, Fernstrom M J 1982 Oxytocin receptors and parturition, a dual role for oxytocin in the initiation of labor. Science 215: 1396–1398
Gant N F, Hutchinson H T, Siiteri P K, MacDonald P C 1971 Study of the metabolic clearance rate of dehydroisoandrosterone sulfate in pregnancy. American Journal of Obstetrics and Gynecology 111: 555–563
Garfield R E, Rabidean S, Challis J R G, Daniel E E 1979 Ultrastructural basis for maintenance and termination of pregnancy. American Journal of Obstetrics and Gynecology 133: 308–315
Garfield R E, Kannan M S, Daniel E E 1980 Gap junction formation in myometrium; control by oestrogens, progesterone and prostaglandins. American Journal of Physiology 238: C81–C89
Gautray J-P, Jolivet A, Dhem N, Vielk J-P, Tajchner G 1974 Reflexion sur le rôle du foetus dans le déclenchement du travail à terme: exploration du liquide amniotique. In: Bose M J, Palmer R, Savean Cl (eds) Avortement et parturition provoqués. Masson, Paris, pp 227–238
Gazárek F, Polanka J, Talaš M et al 1976 Plasma oxytocin and oxytocinase levels in third trimester of pregnancy and at labour. Endocrinologia Experimentalis 10: 283–287
Gennser G, Ohrlander S, Eneroth P 1977 Fetal cortisol and the initiation of labour in the human. In: Knight J, O'Connor M (eds) The fetus and birth. Elsevier/Excerpta Medica/North Holland, Amsterdam, pp 401–420
Gibbens D, Boyd N R H, Chard T 1972 Spurt release of oxytocin during human labour. Journal of Endocrinology 53: LIV–LV
Granström E, Hamberg M, Hamsson C, Kindhal H 1980 Chemical instability of 15-keto-13,14-dihydro-PGE_2. The reason for low assay reliability. Prostaglandins 19: 933–957
Gustavii B 1978 Local membrane mechanism in the onset of labor in humans. In: Prenatal endocrinology and parturition. Inserm Symposium, INSERM, Paris, p 93
Henson G, Gough J D, Gillmer M D G 1983 The control of persistent primary post-partum haemorrhage due to uterine atony with intravenous prostaglandin E_2. British Journal of Obstetrics and Gynaecology 90: 280–282
Hibbard B M, Sharma S C, Fitzpatrick R J, Hamlett J D 1974 Prostaglandin $F_{2\alpha}$ concentrations in amniotic fluid in late pregnancy. Journal of Obstetrics and Gynaecology of the British Commonwealth 81: 35–38
Honnebier W J, Swaab D F 1973 The influence of anencephaly upon intrauterine growth of fetus and placenta and upon gestation length. Journal of Obstetrics and Gynaecology of the British Commonwealth 80: 577–588
Husslein P 1985 Mode of action of oxytocin and the role of its receptor in the production of prostaglandins. In: Wood C (ed.) The role of prostaglandins in labour. Royal Society of Medicine Services, International Congress and Symposium Series, London, no. 92, pp 15– 23
Keirse M J N C, Turnbull A C 1973 Prostaglandins in amniotic fluid during late pregnancy and labour. Journal of Obstetrics and Gynaecology of the British Commonwealth 80: 970–973
Keirse M J N C, Flint A P F, Turnbull A C 1974 Prostaglandins in amniotic fluid during pregnancy and labour. Journal of Obstetrics and Gynaecology of the British Commonwealth 81: 131–135
Keirse M J N C, Hicks B R, Mitchell M D, Turnbull A C 1977 Increase of the prostaglandin precursor, arachidonic acid, in amniotic fluid during spontaneous labour. British Journal of Obstetrics and Gynaecology 84: 937–940
Keirse M J N C, Thiery M, Parevijck W, Mitchell M D 1983 Chronic stimulation of uterine prostaglandin synthesis during cervical ripening before the onset of labour. Prostaglandins 25: 671–682
Kittinger G W 1977 Endocrine regulation of fetal development and its relation to parturition in the rhesus monkey. In: Knight J, O'Connor M (eds) The fetus and birth. Ciba Foundation Symposium 47, Elsevier/Excerpta Medica/North Holland, Amsterdam, pp 235–249
Kumaresan P, Anandagarangam P B, Dianzon W, Vasicka A 1974 Plasma oxytocin levels during human pregnancy and labor as determined by radioimmunoassay. American Journal of Obstetrics and Gynecology 119: 215–223
Leake R D, Weitsman R E, Glatz T H, Fisher D A 1979 Stimulation of oxytocin secretion in the human. Clinical Research 27: 99A
Ledger W L, Webster M A, Anderson A B M, Turnbull A C 1985a Effect of inhibition of prostaglandin synthesis on cervical softening and uterine activity during ovine parturition resulting from progesterone withdrawal induced by epostane. Journal of Endocrinology 105: 227–233
Ledger W L, Webster M, Harrison L P, Anderson A B M, Turnbull A C 1985b Increase in cervical extensibility during labor induced after isolation of the cervix from the uterus in pregnant ewes. American Journal of Obstetrics and Gynecology 151: 397–402
Leong M K H, Murphy B E P 1976 Cortisol levels in maternal venous and umbilical cord arterial and venous serum at vaginal delivery. American Journal of Obstetrics and Gynecology 124: 471–473
Lewis P R, Galvin P M, Short R V 1987 Salivary oestriol and progesterone concentrations in women during late pregnancy, parturition and the puerperium. Journal of Endocrinology 115: 177–181
Liggins G C 1969a Premature parturition after infusion of corticotrophin or cortisol into fetal lambs. Journal of Endocrinology 42: 323–329
Liggins G C 1969b The fetal role in the initiation of parturition in the ewe. In: Foetal autonomy. Ciba Foundation Symposium 14, Associated Scientific Publishers, Amsterdam, pp 218–231
Liggins G C 1973 Hormonal interactions in the mechanisms of parturition. Memoirs of the Society of Endocrinology 20: 119–139
Liggins G C 1979 Initiation of parturition. British Medical Bulletin 35: 145–150
Liggins G C 1981 Initiation of parturition. In: Novy M J, Resko J A (eds) Fetal endocrinology. Academic Press, New York, pp 211–238
Liggins G C, Grieves S A 1971 Possible role for prostaglandin $F_{2\alpha}$ in parturition in sheep. Nature, London 232: 629–631
Liggins G C, Kennedy P C, Holen L W 1967 Failure of initiation of parturition after electrocoagulation of the pituitary of the fetal lamb. American Journal of Obstetrics and Gynecology 98: 1080–1086
Liggins G C, Fairclough R J, Grieves S A, Kendall J Z, Knox B S 1973 The mechanism of parturition in the ewe. Recent Progress in Hormone Research 29: 111–150
Liggins G C, Fairclough R J, Grieves S A, Forster C S, Knox B S 1977a Parturition in the sheep. In: Knight J, O'Connor M (eds) The fetus and birth. Elsevier/Excerpta Medica/North Holland, Amsterdam, pp 5–25
Liggins G C, Forster C S, Grieves S A, Schwarz A L 1977b Control of parturition in man. Biology and Reproduction 16: 39–56
Lopez-Bernal A, Castle B, Turnbull A C 1986a Prostaglandin binding by human fetal ducts arteriosus at mid gestation. Hormone and Metabolic Research 18: 214–215
Lopez-Bernal A, Tindell D J, Selinger M, Turnbull A C 1986b Local inhibition of progesterone production in human chorio-decidua by Epostane. Hormone and Metabolic Research 18: 503
Lopez-Bernal A, Hansell D J, Alexander S, Turnbull A C 1987a Prostaglandin E production by amniotic cells in relation to term and pre-term labour. British Journal of Obstetrics and Gynaecology 94: 864–869
Lopez-Bernal A, Gryant-Greenwood G D, Hansell D J, Hicks B R, Greenwood F C, Turnbull A C 1987b Effect of relaxin on prostaglandin E production by human amnion: changes in relation to the onset of labour. British Journal of Obstetrics and Gynaecology 94: 1045–1051
Lopez-Bernal A, Hansell D J, Alexander S, Turnbull A C 1987c Steroid conversion and prostaglandin production by chorionic and decidual cells in relation to term and pre-term labour. British Journal of Obstetrics and Gynaecology 94: 1052–1058
Maathius J B, Kelly R W 1978 Concentrations of prostaglandins $F_{2\alpha}$ and E_2 in the endometrium throughout the human menstrual cycle after the administration of clomiphene or an oestrogen–progesterone pill and in early pregnancy. Journal of Endocrinology 77: 361–371
MacLennan A H 1983 The role of relaxin in human reproduction. Clinics in Reproduction and Fertility 2: 77–95

MacLennan A H, Green R C, Bryant-Greenwood G D, Greenwood F C, Seamark R F 1980 Ripening of the human cervix and induction of labour with purified relaxin. Lancet i: 220–223
MacLennan A H, Nicholson R, Green R C 1986 Serum relaxin in pregnancy. Lancet ii: 241–243
Manabe Y, Manabe A, Aso T 1981 Plasma concentrations of oestrone, oestradiol, oestriol and progesterone during mechanical stretch-induced abortion at mid-trimester. Journal of Endocrinology 91: 385–389
Mitchell B, Cruikshank B, McLean D, Challis J R G 1982 Local modulation of progesterone production in human fetal membranes. Journal of Clinical Endocrinology and Metabolism 55: 1237–1239
Mitchell M D 1984 Role of prostaglandins in parturition. In: Ridge J, Freedman P S, Brierly C A (eds) Prostaglandin perspectives. Media Medica, Wiley, Chichester, pp 1–4
Mitchell M D, Flint A P F 1977 Progesterone withdrawal: effects on prostaglandins and parturition. Prostaglandins 14: 611–614
Mitchell M D, Flint A P F, Turnbull A C 1976 Stimulation by oxytocin of prostaglandin F levels in uterine venous effluent in pregnant and puerperal sheep. Prostaglandins 9: 47–56
Mitchell M D, Keirse M J N C, Anderson A B M, Turnbull A C 1977a Evidence for local control of prostaglandins within the human uterus. British Journal of Obstetrics and Gynaecology 84: 35–38
Mitchell M D, Flint A P F, Bibby J, Brunt J, Arnold J M, Anderson A B M, Turnbull A C 1977b Rapid increases in plasma prostaglandin concentrations after vaginal examination and amniotomy. British Medical Journal ii: 1183–1185
Mitchell M D, Flint A P F, Bibby et al 1978a Plasma concentrations of prostaglandins during late human pregnancy: influence of normal and pre-term labor. Journal of Clinical Endocrinology and Metabolism 46: 947–951
Mitchell M D, Brunt J, Bibby J, Flint A P F, Anderson A B M, Turnbull A C 1978b Prostaglandins in the human umbilical circulation at birth. British Journal of Obstetrics and Gynaecology 85: 114–118
Mochizuki M, Tojo S 1980 Effects of dehydroepiandrosterone sulfate on softening and dilatation of the uterine cervix in pregnant women. In: Naftolin F, Stubblefield P G (eds) Dilatation of the uterine cervix. Raven Press, New York, pp 267–286
Mortimer G, Stimson W H, Hunter I C, Govan A D T 1985 A role for amniotic epithelium in the control of human parturition. Lancet i: 1074–1075
Murphy B E P 1975 Does the human fetal adrenal play a role in parturition? American Journal of Obstetrics and Gynecology 115: 521–525
Murphy B E P, Patrick J, Denton R L 1975 Cortisol in amniotic fluid during human gestation. Journal of Clinical Endocrinology and Metabolism 40: 164–167
Novy M J 1977 Endocrine and pharmacological factors which influence the onset of labour in rhesus monkeys. In: Knight J, O'Connor M (eds) The fetus and birth. Ciba Foundation Symposium 47, Elsevier/Excerpta Medica/North Holland, Amsterdam, pp 259–288
Pattison N S, Webster M A, Phipps S L, Anderson A B M, Gillmer M D G 1985 Inhibition of 3β-hydroxysteroid dehydrogenase activity in first and second trimester human pregnancy and the luteal phase using Epostane. Fertility and Sterility 42: 875–881
Rush R W, Keirse M J N C, Howat P, Baum J D, Anderson A B M, Turnbull A C 1976 Contribution of pre-term delivery to perinatal mortality. British Medical Journal 2: 965–968
Saeed S A, McDonald Gibson W J, Cuthbert J et al 1977 Endogenous inhibitor of prostaglandin synthetase. Nature (London) 270: 32–36
Selinger M, MacKenzie I Z, Gillmer M D G, Phipps S L, Ferguson J 1987 Progesterone inhibition in mid-trimester termination of pregnancy: physiological and clinical effects. British Journal of Obstetrics and Gynaecology 94: 1218–1222
Sellers S M, Hodgson H T, Mitchell M D, Anderson A B M, Turnbull A C 1980 Release of prostaglandins following amniotomy is not mediated by oxytocin. British Journal of Obstetrics and Gynaecology 87: 43–46
Sellers S M, Mitchell M D, Bibby J G, Anderson A B M, Turnbull A C 1981a A comparison of plasma prostaglandin levels in term and pre-term labour. British Journal of Obstetrics and Gynaecology 88: 362–366
Sellers S M, Hodgson H T, Mountford L A, Mitchell M D, Anderson A B M, Turnbull A C 1981b Is oxytocin involved in parturition? British Journal of Obstetrics and Gynaecology 88: 725–729
Sellers S M, Mitchell M D, Anderson A B M, Turnbull A C 1981c The relation between the release of prostaglandins at amniotomy and the subsequent onset of labour. British Journal of Obstetrics and Gynaecology 88: 1211–1216
Sellers S M, Hodgson H T, Mitchell M D, Anderson A B M, Turnbull A C 1982 Raised prostaglandin levels in the third stage of labor. American Journal of Obstetrics and Gynecology 144: 209–212
Siiteri P K, MacDonald P C 1966 Placental oestrogen biosynthesis during human pregnancy. Journal of Clinical Endocrinology 26: 751–761
Silman R E, Chard T, Lowry P J, Smith I, Young I M 1976 Human foetal pituitary peptides and parturition. Nature (London) 260L: 716–718
Steele P A, Flint A P F, Turnbull A C 1976 Activity of steroid C17,20 lyase in the ovine placenta: effect of exposure to foetal glucocorticoid. Journal of Endocrinology 69: 239–246
Taylor M J, Webb R, Mitchell M D, Robinson J S 1982 Effect of progesterone withdrawal in sheep during late pregnancy. Journal of Endocrinology 92: 85–93
Thorburn G D, Challis J R G, Robinson J S 1977 The endocrinology of parturition. In: Wynn R M (ed) Cellular biology of the uterus. Plenum Press, New York, pp 653–732
Thornton C A, Carrie L E S, Sayers L, Anderson A B M, Turnbull A C 1976 A comparison of the effect of extradural and parenteral analgesia on maternal plasma cortisol concentrations during labour and the puerperium. British Journal of Obstetrics and Gynaecology 83: 631–635
Turnbull A C, Patten P T, Flint A P F, Keirse M J N C, Jeremy J Y, Anderson A B M 1974 Significant fall in progesterone and rise in oestradiol levels in human peripheral plasma before the onset of labour. Lancet i: 101–104
Turnbull A C, Anderson A B M, Flint A P F, Jeremy J Y, Keirse M J N C, Mitchell M D 1977 Human parturition. In: Knight J, O'Connor M (eds) The fetus and birth. Elsevier/Excerpta Medica/North Holland, Amsterdam, 427–452
Turnbull A C, Lucas A, Mitchell M D 1981 Prostaglandins in the perinatal period. In: Scarpelli E M, Cosmi E V (eds) Reviews in perinatal medicine, vol 4. Raven Press, New York, pp 273–297
Vasicka A, Kumaresan P, Han G S, Kumaresan M 1978 Plasma oxytocin in initiation of labor. American Journal of Obstetrics and Gynecology 130: 263–273
Verhoeff A, Garfield R A 1986 Ultrastructure of the myometrium and the role of gap junctions in myometrial function. In: Huszar G (ed.) The physiology and biochemistry of the uterus. CRC Press, Boca Raton, pp 73–91
Webster M A, Phipps S L, Gillmer M D G 1985 Interruption of first trimester human pregnancy following Epostane therapy. Effect of prostaglandin E_2 pessaries. British Journal of Obstetics and Gynaecology 92: 963–968
Wilkinson A R, Aynsley-Green A, Mitchell M D 1979 Persistent pulmonary hypertension with abnormal prostaglandin E levels in pre-term infants after maternal treatment with naproxan. Archives of Disease in Childhood 54: 942–945
Wilson T 1988 Lipocortins and their possible role in the onset of labour. In: Brierley C A (ed.) Prostaglandin perspectives. Media Medica, Wiley, Chichester, pp 1–3
Wilson T, Liggins G C, Aimer G P, Skinner S J M 1985 Partial purification and characterisation of two compounds from amniotic fluid which inhibit phospholipase activity in human endometrial cells. Biochemical and Biophysical Research Communications 131: 22–29

SECTION 2

Care in Pregnancy

13

Geoffrey Chamberlain

Prepregnancy care

Antenatal care is now a well established feature of all maternity services. Both consumers and professionals see the advantage of such services and in 80 years the system has been modified many times to include advances in knowledge about mother and baby. When regular antenatal examinations were suggested in 1901, however, this was thought a strange innovation. Why should normal pregnant women subject themselves to scrutiny and examination by doctors and midwives? Surely this was an intrusion upon the freedom of women and an unnecessary use of professional time. It was further argued that since having a baby was a natural event, there should be no need to interfere in pregnancy—although, somewhat illogically, it has been recognized for some years that obstetricians and midwives often had to interfere in labour. During the 20th century antenatal care slowly became accepted so that by 1925, 30% of women who delivered in England and Wales were going to such clinics and 95% by 1945. Now, less than 2% of women who deliver have not had some antenatal care and the system has been accepted as the norm.

Similar arguments are now being advanced against prepregnancy care which has been in existence for less than 20 years. The concept was not codified until the late 1970s, when workers in the UK and USA began to suggest guidelines and establish special clinics to see women who wanted advice and occasionally treatment before embarking on pregnancy.

THE EXTENSION OF ANTENATAL CARE

Prepreganancy care is the logical precursor to antenatal care. Since it occurs before pregnancy, it allows a wider series of choices for the couple than may be available once pregnancy begins.

For early pregnancy problems, there are only two options: to continue the pregnancy or to terminate it. Pregnancy termination is a profound step for any couple and for many it is unacceptable; for them there is no alternative to continuing with the pregnancy, whatever the problem and its risks.

For the same couple attending in the prepregnancy stage, a series of options can be offered. In some cases, the effects on the mother and fetus of her chronic disease or the drugs used to treat this disease can be more precisely delineated and the exact risks calculated and explained. Although the drug regimen may be teratogenic, it may be possible, in consultation with her physician, temporarily to discontinue medication to allow an interval when pregnancy can be achieved and the embryo established safely; after the first trimester of pregnancy drug therapy could be restarted, since by this time the risk of teratogenesis would be greatly reduced.

In many countries, adoption is still a possibility and may be one option.

If there is a problem with the woman's partner being somehow incompatible with the chances of a successful outcome to pregnancy, as in severe rhesus sensitization, a decision could be made to use semen from a rhesus-negative donor (artificial insemination by donor) if the partner is homozygous rhesus-positive and if there is otherwise little chance of the woman producing a healthy infant.

In the near future, extracorporeal fertilization of donor oocytes may be considered an acceptable alternative by society.

After full discussion, a couple can be advised of the risks of the mother or child being affected by an inherited disorder in the next pregnancy. The couple may consider these odds to be so high they do not wish to start a pregnancy and therefore will continue with effective contraception or even decide on male or female sterilization.

All these options are available at discussion in the prepregnancy clinic; it is too late to consider them once pregnancy has started.

The first visit of a pregnant woman for early antenatal care is stressed but this actually happens rarely in the UK. A few women with previous problems may see an obstetrician at 6 or 7 weeks' gestation, but the vast majority do not attend a booking clinic until 11–13 weeks of pregnancy. The avowed purposes of early antenatal care are:

1. To ensure that the mother avoids exposure to teratogens in early pregnancy;
2. To check basic measurements such as maternal blood pressure and weight before pregnancy;
3. To introduce the pregnant mother to the system of medical and social benefits sufficiently early for her to receive most help from them.

All these aspects are better done in the prepregnancy phase. In most instances, by the time a pregnant woman arrives at a booking clinic for antenatal care, fetal organogenesis is complete and it is too late to give advice about avoiding teratogens. The woman's blood pressure may not be basal if the booking visit is in the second trimester, since many women will have reduced their normal diastolic pressure by 5–10 mmHg. Advice about the obstetric future and measures to be taken is better given at a prepregnancy clinic.

It was with these ideas in mind that the author started one of the first hospital-based prepregnancy clinics at Queen Charlotte's Hospital on 9 January 1978 (Chamberlain 1980). Since then, many of the aims of prepregnancy care have changed and the subject is now quite properly generally considered to be one of general health education.

ASPECTS OF PREPREGNANCY CARE

When a couple consult a doctor for prepregnancy care, he or she can be helpful to them in a very short time if properly prepared. To do this most effectively, the tangled skein of threads affecting mother and baby in pregnancy must be unravelled. The doctor must distinguish clearly between those aspects which are unchangeable and those which can be modified; he or she must explain this clearly to the couple, pointing out those factors which are already fixed and cannot be altered.

Fixed features include:

1. The *age* of the woman and sometimes that of her partner.
2. The woman's *parity*.
3. If parous, her *past obstetric performance*.
4. The couple's *socioeconomic class*.
5. The *race* of each partner.
6. The *genetic* and *biological background* of both.

Other influences affecting the fetus or pregnant woman are variable; these are the ones for which prepregnancy counselling can be most effective. Features which might be changed include:

Table 13.1 The proportion of anovular and normal cycles at different quinquennia of reproductive life

Age group (years)	Number of cycles studied	Anovular cycles (%)	Normal cycles (%)
<15	268	52	16
16–20	495	34	28
21–25	287	17	60
26–30	418	6	85
31–35	822	7	87
36–40	640	4	83
41–45	275	11	70
46–50	67	13	50

Data do not add up to 100% because the variable proportion of cycles with ovulation but with a short luteal phase are not in either column.

1. *Tobacco* and *alcohol* consumption — the twin scourges of modern society.
2. *Nutrition* before and in very early pregnancy.
3. *Maternal diseases*, existing before the pregnancy.
4. *Drug treatments* being given for pre-existing disease.
5. The levels of *exercise* and *stress* during pregnancy.

Another important feature of prepregnancy consultations is recognizing complications arising from a previous pregnancy or delivery and advising about the risk of recurrence in the present pregnancy. Many obstetricians consider this part of postnatal clinic care. After the previous pregnancy, those who looked after the woman may have considered all the data about any problems that had occurred and discussed with the woman and her partner the risk of further problems in future pregnancies. However, hospital postnatal clinics are rapidly diminishing and postnatal care is being passed to general practitioners who may not have either all the information about what happened or the expertise to advise about the implications. In any case, the fact that people tend to erase unhappy events from their memories reduces the potential benefit of postnatal discussion. It is therefore of great value to reconsider the previous pregnancy problem at some later time. In practice, this forms the basis of prepregnancy counselling in hospital clinics.

FIXED FACTORS IN PREPREGNANCY CARE

Age

Maternal age has a distinct influence on outcome. For a few years after the menarche, and before menopause, ovulation is irregular, probably because of fluctuations in hormone secretion (Table 13.1). In the premenopausal phase, in the latter part of reproductive life, intercourse tends to be less frequent and this, combined with irregular ovulation, leads to the low fertility rate characteristic of the climacteric.

In addition, in the older woman oocytes, which have been present since birth, are ageing and there is an increase in chromosomal abnormalities such as Down's syndrome. The incidence increases after the age of 35 and especially so after

40 years. Other variations or abnormalities are commoner in the older mother, such as monozygotic twins, hydatidiform moles and the presence of a single umbilical artery.

A further feature of increased maternal age is diminished flexibility of the ligamentous and muscular system. In such women, in consequence, pregnancy is a greater burden than in younger women and increased rest is needed earlier in pregnancy. If warned before pregnancy, the woman can make plans to adjust her lifestyle at home and at work; being forewarned, arrangements can often be made more easily than in mid-pregnancy.

States associated with the increased ageing processes of life will obviously have a higher incidence in the later reproductive years. Hence, conditions such as essential hypertension and diabetes increase in relative frequency. It is wise to warn the prospective mother aged over 35 years that she may have to think of reducing or even giving up paid employment at an earlier stage than her younger contemporaries. If this advice is given at a prepregnancy clinic the mother is less disappointed than if she first hears of this during pregnancy. There is a sliding scale of probable complications which are worse after the age of 40 and these have to be freely discussed at the prepregnancy clinic.

Parity

In many ways the effects of parity on pregnancy are similar to those of age. The relationship is obvious, for a woman will obviously be older when she delivers her third child than when she had her second. However, some aspects are associated mainly with increased parity alone. In most societies the risks of increasing parity do not appear until three or four children have been born. In subsequent pregnancies there are increased risks of uterine laxity, fetal malpresentation and postpartum haemorrhage for the mother and accidents of birth, such as cord prolapse, for the fetus.

Past obstetric history

Many women attending a prepregnancy clinic who have had problems in their previous obstetrical experience want information about the chances of recurrence and must be accurately informed by the prepregnancy counsellor.

The progress and outcome of any previous pregnancy must be obtained in some detail. If the woman is attending the same hospital the information should be in the hospital records but if she attends another unit, it is wise to write to the hospital where she was previously confined to obtain details from her records, unless a very full summary is available. Again, it would be best if the advice was given by her previous obstetrician at the time of postnatal examination but this is often not done.

Prepregnancy counsellors must be willing to listen to much irrelevant material. It is essential to allow the couple to talk about what is central to their anxiety. They have normally mulled the problem over in their minds so that it may have been exaggerated and had additional blemishes added. The counsellor should dissect out enough to know what actually happened in pregnancy or labour and offer helpful, prospective advice. The chances of a problem recurring should be based on data relevant to the couple. There is little point referring to publications, however well written and statistically sound, which are concerned with different populations. A good example is the problem of fibroids in pregnancy. Much of the literature refers to American black women, who often develop fibroids at an earlier age than do white women. In most published series, women were dealt with under the American medical system which has very different treatment approaches from the National Health Service.

Table 13.2 Risk of recurrent abortion in relation to number of previous abortions

Number of previous abortions	Number of succeeding pregnancies examined	Abortions (%)
0	5432	12.3
1	1403	23.7
2	385	36.2
3	121	32.2
4	58	25.9

The recurrent risk rates of common conditions should be known. Some of them are more reassuring once looked at fully. For example, a common problem is a series of previous spontaneous abortions. On the whole, textbooks and conventional wisdom imply a steeply increasing risk of recurrence as the number of previous abortions inveighs but data produced by Warburton & Fraser (1964; Table 13.2) indicate that, in general, the risk of recurrent abortion does not increase greatly after the first. Although the studied number of women having three or four abortions is small, the chances of successful pregnancy seem to be good and a reasonably optimistic assessment can be given. Women who have had more than one previous abortion can be told genuinely that if there was no obvious cause for the spontaneous abortion, the chances of a normal term pregnancy are about two in three.

Nayler & Warburton (1979) have further fractionated the risk of spontaneous abortion in relation to live pregnancies in multiparae (Table 13.3) among 14 000 reproductive histories. These data show that the risk of a repeated abortion relates not just to the number of previous abortions but to the closeness of any previous abortions in pregnancy order.

Similar data can be obtained by the prepregnancy doctor about the major forms of congenital abnormalities, problems associated with cervical incompetence, preterm delivery, polyhydramnios, multiple pregnancy, pre-eclampsia and intrauterine growth retardation. A review of many of these is given by Howie (1986).

The best advice to give a woman with a previous obstetric

Table 13.3 Risk of spontaneous abortion in relation to past obstetrical history

Past obstetric history	Risk of spontaneous abortion (%)
L	13
LL	14
LLL	14
A	23
AA	36
AAA	33
AL	19
LA	27
ALL	21
LAL	23
LLA	29
AAL	36
ALA	18
LAA	27
ALLL	19
LALL	19
LLAL	34

L = live birth; A = abortion.
Adapted from Nayler & Warburton (1974).

problem is to discuss the problem with the obstetrician who will be supervising her next pregnancy. There is much variation in obstetricians' opinions and in their intervention rates after previous events; the couple should consult him or her and feel happy about the proposed management. However, a general indication can be given at the prepregnancy clinic and the doctor there may act as a catalyst or mediator, stimulating the woman to approach her obstetrician, or helping her do so if she is hesitating. It is important at the prepregnancy clinic that no firm rules should be laid down which might clash later with other ideas on treatment. One should avoid giving absolute answers because unforeseen circumstances in later pregnancy may completely alter management.

Socioeconomic class

In the UK socioeconomic class is assessed from the Registrar General's classification of male occupations. The use of the husband's occupation to label socioeconomic class may seem chauvinistic but it is not just hallowed by tradition. Male occupations still offer a wider range of gradation than do female activities and the varieties of male job classifications provide a wider spectrum. Female employment tends to group round the home (housewife) and posts connected with secretarial work. In most epidemiological studies nowadays, the partner's post is accepted for a husband or for a permanent partner who has a job which can be used for classification. When women marry out of their social class, a few at the upper boundaries of a socioeconomic class group — the more intelligent and the taller — may migrate upwards at marriage but fewer marry into a lower class. Hence the partner's socioeconomic class is a good approximation of the woman's status.

Socioeconomic class represents a marker indicating a most important group of aspects of the woman's youth such as nutrition, diseases, education, attitudes to medical care and genetic inheritance. All these factors influence the woman's obstetric performance. Good correlation and gradients exist between socioeconomic groups and the incidence of many types of congenital abnormality, and reduced birthweight. Both preterm labour and intrauterine growth retardation are measures of fetal and neonatal outcome and are increased with socioeconomic deprivation. Many of the differences between perinatal mortality rates in different regions of the country are influenced more by the socioeconomic structure of the population than by the provision of medical care and facilities.

Some personal habits are related to socioeconomic status. Cigarette smoking in excess occurs in the same lower socioeconomic groups who have higher rates of preterm labour and intrauterine growth retardation. It may not therefore be correct to say that cigarette smoking causes low birthweight babies; it may be causal, but could very well simply be an associated factor.

No woman can resign from her assigned socioeconomic class, but she can overcome adverse influences. She can, for example, reduce or stop smoking or alcohol consumption, and improve her diet and approach to exercise.

Race

Race again is a marker of a couple's genetic background and may include factors of varying relevance in differing countries of the world. The differences may be:

1. In the genetics of their race.
2. In the upbringing of the woman or her partner in their youth in another country.
3. In the nutrition of that country.
4. In the schooling and educational standards.
5. In the diseases endemic to that country.

Many immigrants from the West Indies and the Indian subcontinent lived in a very different environment during the earlier years of their lives. Conversely, a black woman born in Tooting, London, and living there all her life may suffer problems relating to the genetics of her race but her pregnancy outcome will be similar to those of any other women brought up in the environment of south London. Many immigrant families such as West Indians integrate well with their host communities and share their background. Other groups, such as those from Pakistan, tend to live in close communities which reduce the influence of surrounding communities; here, the original nutritional, educational and attitudinal influences may be strong, even when the woman has been born in this country.

Thalassaemia and certain haemoglobinopathies are well known to be associated with race (see Chapter 23). Inherited haemoglobin defects can cause problems for the mother because of increased haemopoiesis in pregnancy, even in those women who are heterozygous or carriers. Prenatal diagnosis of whether or not the fetus is affected may be of vital importance in deciding on further management. It is therefore important to check before pregnancy both for the thalassaemia status and for the presence of abnormal haemoglobins in those who come from races at high risk; this can lead to proper advice for couples on the chances of the problems affecting their potential offspring, and how to predict these problems in future pregnancies.

Genetic background

Some couples are already aware of familial or medical histories which raise worries about the health of their future children. If any condition discussed at a prepregnancy clinic has an obvious genetic background, it is wise to seek the help of a clinical geneticist. In most parts of the UK there is a regional genetic centre providing a service for counselling and risk assessment for families with known genetic disease. The prepregnancy adviser will be wise to consult early. Clinical genetics is a rapidly expanding subject; those who are experts at genetics can give correct authoritative advice at once. This avoids the series of conflicts and doubts sometimes set up in the minds of the couple following incorrect advice given earlier by well meaning but less well informed doctors.

Many conditions not previously considered to have a genetic component can now be shown to have a chromosomal element amongst the multifactorial modes of inheritance. For example, asthma and pre-eclampsia may be shown to fall into this category in the near future. In consequence, the larger prepregnancy clinics should have easy access to genetic counselling and do some work in parallel, with the geneticist attending the prepregnancy consultation clinics.

The geneticist may wish to perform karyotyping of potential parents. This will be useful if a potential or known medical condition with chromosome flagging is present in either parent, in the family, or if a previous baby has been shown to have a chromosomal abnormality. Otherwise it may be necessary to karyotype the fetus in the next pregnancy. This may be performed in cells obtained by transcervical chorionic villus sampling (CVS) at 8–10 weeks, at transabdominal CVS at 12–14 weeks or by amniocentesis at 16–18 weeks with culture of amnion cells of fetal origin. As well as the simple light microscopic examination of chromosomes on which karyometric studies have been based for 30 years, the new potential of DNA recombinant technology is allowing many more diagnoses to be made; this subject is well reviewed by Weatherall & Higgs (1982).

At the prepregnancy clinic it is wise to advise couples with chromosomally based problems which are not currently capable of being treated against undergoing irrevocable sterilization of either partner. The surge of advance in DNA technology is so rapid that treatments may well be available in 5 years' time which will effectively treat conditions which we can at present only diagnose and cannot treat. The subject is dealt with in detail in Chapter 22.

VARIABLE FACTORS IN PREPREGNANCY CARE

Cigarette smoking

One of the important contributions which prepregnancy counselling can make to pregnancy relates to the effects of cigarette smoking. In the UK, 37% of women were smoking in pregnancy (Office of Population and Census Surveys 1981) whilst about 30% of the women of the same age group in the USA smoked (Moore 1980); in Australia and New Zealand the proportion was also about 30% (Hill & Gray 1982). The potential effects of prepregnancy advice were shown when Sexton & Hebel (1984) found that 11% of pregnant women who had previously smoked stopped before becoming pregnant following counselling. In the British Births 1970 study (Chamberlain et al 1975), 42% of women were still smoking at the end of pregnancy, but 59% had been smoking before pregnancy; therefore 17% of the 17 000 women had given up during or before pregnancy.

Effects of smoking

Cigarette smoking can affect fertility by decreasing ovulation (Vessey et al 1978); Mattison (1982) showed that smoking diminished male sperm penetrating capacity and was associated with a higher percentage of abnormal sperms than in non-smokers. The risk of spontaneous abortion in early pregnancy is about twice as high in smokers as among non-smokers (Kline et al 1983). This may result partly from an increased number of abnormal embryos, with which smoking is associated.

Meyer et al (1976) showed a relative risk of preterm labour of 1.5 times greater for smokers than for non-smokers. The same authors assessed the perinatal deaths in their series and considered that about 10% of all such deaths could be attributed to maternal smoking.

As with all findings in the perinatal mortality field, there are no simple straightforward cause-and-effect relationships, but smoking may be associated with other variables such as anaemia, previous low birthweight, high parity and low socioeconomic status. Moore (1980) found the risk ratio for babies born with a birthweight below 2500 g to be 1.9 times greater for smokers than for non-smokers. His analysis in *Public Health Reports* also showed increased risks of spontaneous abortion of 1.7 times and perinatal deaths of 1.2 times greater.

The relationship between congenital abnormalities and smoking is complex. Butler & Alberman (1969) found no difference in the incidence of congenital abnormalities amongst the smoking population of the National Birthday Trust Perinatal Mortality Survey. Most studies, however, have shown a relative risk of abnormalities—some are as high as 2.3 times greater for the smoker than for the non-smoker (Himmelberger et al 1978). These were also related to other factors such as pregnancy history and maternal age. There was in addition a firm association with preterm labour.

Perhaps the most marked associations with cigarette smoking are reduced length of pregnancy and low birthweight. The birthweight effect can be seen in the National Birthday Trust study, British Births 1970 (Chamberlain et al 1975). The mean birthweight of infants born to smokers was 3200 g, while those babies of mothers who had never smoked weighed on average 3376 g—a difference of birthweight of 170 g at term. While babies seemed to be small for dates whatever the length of pregnancy at birth, the effect was greatest after 36 weeks.

Superficially, some women might think that a baby of slightly reduced birthweight would ensure an easier labour. Reduced birthweight is not the only fetal effect of tobacco. There is also delay in maturation which may be serious for the child's future development. Children of mothers who smoke cigarettes in pregnancy have a deficit in reading ability and educational testing standards up to the age of 11. Persuading a potential mother to stop smoking before pregnancy starts is perhaps the best present she can give her future child.

Mechanism

The cause of deficient birthweight among smoking mothers is unknown. It may be due to the action of nicotine constricting the placental bed blood vessel flow. Secondly, since carbon monoxide (found in tobacco smoke) binds preferentially to fetal haemoglobin excluding oxygen, the higher fetal carboxyhaemoglobin levels probably reduce oxygen delivery to fetal tissues. Thirdly, smoking may have a direct toxic effect on the syncytiotrophoblast, reducing the transfer of amino acids and other nutrients (Browne 1989).

Prepregnancy care

Prepregnancy advisers should warn women about the increased risks of smoking in pregnancy. There is a graduated fetal response to maternal inhaled cigarette smoke and there is no cutoff point below which it can be said not to affect the fetus. The only advice is no smoking in the lead-up time to pregnancy.

More difficult is the problem of passive smoking. In theory, if a non-smoking woman lives in the atmosphere of her husband's cigarette smoke, the fetus could receive a tertiary effect of the smoke. But concentrations are very low and firm evidence on this is not yet clear.

Alcohol

Alcohol is a fetal teratogen in early gestation and also has subtle effects on fetal growth throughout the whole of pregnancy. Like cigarette smoking, there seems to be no critical dose and if a woman seeking pregnancy is already concerned, she should be advised not to drink any alcohol at all. At the other end of the scale is binge drinking, with a large amount of alcohol being consumed on one occasion. These are two different alcohol-related problems to pregnancy and prepregnancy counsellors should be prepared to address themselves to either.

Extent of the problem

The extent of women's drinking in the prepregnancy age group is difficult to assess. Little (1976) reported a poor correlation between questions about alcohol intake asked by the obstetrician at the antenatal clinic and answers obtained by skilled interviewers. In consequence, estimates obtained by questioning at antenatal clinics may under-represent the problem. Wright et al (1983) found 44% of a west London population of women attending for antenatal care admitted taking alcohol. Newman (1986) reported 54% of a Tasmanian population drinking, while even higher levels were found in Scotland where a recent study in Dundee examined a population of women attending for antenatal care (Sulaiman et al 1988). Using questionnaires and gamma glutamine transferase activity, they showed that, before realizing they were pregnant, more than 90% of the women drank alcohol. In the first 4 months of pregnancy the proportion consuming alcohol reduced by 56%; 58% of women who drank were consuming less than 50 g of alcohol a week before pregnancy while 19% took over 100 g a week. In the Dundee study, after adjustment for the effects of the other variables, an alcohol intake of more than 120 g per week was significantly related to a shorter gestational age and a lower Apgar score at 5 minutes. The Dundee study was unable to show a detectable effect on fetus or neonate of a maternal alcohol consumption below 100 g a week.

Mechanism

Alcohol is a tissue poison and probably affects the growing fetus at the time of maximum cell division. However, for many years the effects have been so gradual that people have not noticed. Smoking has received its reprobation because of the very obvious effects on the lung where most of the tobacco smoke goes. If alcohol ingestion produced cancer of the stomach, people would be much more willing to believe that it was a major problem. Its effect on organs like the brain is gradual and long-term; this allows doubt about the effects of alcohol taken in pregnancy to develop in the minds of the observers.

The effect of maternal alcohol on an unborn child is even more remote. It has been known for many years that alcohol can affect the fetus and that the placenta is no barrier to alcohol; it is distributed in the fetus in direct proportion to the water content of the tissues so that organs with a

Table 13.4 Characteristics of the fetal alcohol syndrome

Characteristic facial features	
	Microcephaly
	Microphothalmia
	Short palpebral fissures
	Poorly developed philtrum
	Narrow vermilion border of upper lip
Central nervous system involvement	
	Mental retardation
	Developmental delay
	Hyperactivity
	Neurological abnormality
Intrauterine growth retardation	
	Less than tenth percentile for gestational age of:
	Birthweight
	Length
	Head circumference

high proportion of water, such as the fetal brain, are particularly exposed to the potentially harmful effects of alcohol. Since the blood alcohol clearance rate of the fetus at term is only half that of the mother, the fetal compartments maintain higher levels for longer than do the maternal compartments. Lemoine et al (1968) showed that among infants born to alcoholic mothers, the effect on the fetus relates to the maturation of fetal liver enzymes in the second trimester of pregnancy. In the first trimester, alcohol is handled as though the fetus is another body compartment of the mother while in the second trimester, alcohol effects may be modified by maturing fetal liver enzymes.

Many women reduce alcohol intake spontaneously when they realize they are pregnant, possibly because of a fear of affecting the baby. Raised oestrogen levels may play a part by removing the desire to drink alcohol, a phenomenon noted amongst women taking combined oral contraception as well as those in early pregnancy.

Fetal alcohol syndrome

The fetal alcohol syndrome is a group of neonatal features characterized in association with higher alcohol drinking. On the basis of 245 cases, the Fetal Alcohol Study Group (Majewski 1981) has defined the criteria outlined in Table 13.4.

Growth retardation is symmetrical, indicating an early intrauterine influence rather than late malnutrition. There is a lack of catch-up growth after delivery.

The face is used as a characteristic area by those who diagnose the condition. In many ways it is reminiscent of those in children born with Cornelia Lang syndrome, or of babies of mothers with phenylketonuria. The diagnosis is not very specific but the baby with true fetal alcohol syndrome has microphthalmia with short palpebral features, prominent epicanthic folds and often a squint. There is a short, retroussé nose and the whole mid-face seems squashed or frog-like. The philtrum is not well formed and the upper lip is thin. Ears may be low-set (as they are in so many conditions) and rotated posteriorly.

Milder degrees of alcohol consumption may produce more subtle effects on the fetus. About 20% of children born to mothers who had drunk heavily in pregnancy but did not have the full diagnostic criteria of a fetal alcohol syndrome have been shown by Shawitz et al (1980) to be generally small, with a low IQ, hyperactive behaviour and failing to progress at school.

Other hazards

Alcohol consumption in early pregnancy relates to embryonic morbidity. Moderate alcohol intake has been associated with increased spontaneous abortion rates, even adjusting for maternal age, previous abortions, the stage of gestation and smoking habits. It has been reported that there is a two-times increased risk of spontaneous abortion with as little as two drinks a week (Kline et al 1980). Wright et al (1983) examined 900 pregnancies in London. Women were classified as heavy drinkers (more than 10 drinks a week), moderate drinkers (5–10 drinks a week) or light drinkers (less than 5 drinks a week). The heavy drinking group had a two times greater risk factor of having a low birthweight baby, compared with those in the light-risk group.

Binge drinking

Binge drinking is harder to document but may be the real associate of the fetal alcohol syndrome, as excessive alcohol intake may impair the transfer of nutrients across the placenta at crucial stages in the development of the fetus.

Other variables such as caffeine and nicotine need to be assessed separately from alcohol intake, for high consumption of these three drugs commonly goes together.

Advice

Prepregnancy advice is difficult in this field. On the one hand, there are authoritative groups such as the Royal College of Psychiatrists (1982) who advised no alcohol intake in the prepregnancy phase or during pregnancy. This measure is Draconian and may drive women who are used to alcohol into other abuses. The Dundee study indicated that moderate to light drinking had little effect on fetal health (Sulaiman et al 1988). The more studies produced, the more difficult it is to be dogmatic, but it may be that a high blood alcohol concentration achieved in a given episode of binge drinking has more serious effects on the fetus than the background daily average. If one of these peaks of alcohol consumption happened to correspond with a critical time of embryo development, it could be important. The detrimental effect of binge drinking may be more important than a constant low rate of social drinking.

Nutrition

If we believe that *we are what we eat* then we should logically concur that *the fetus is what its mother eats*. Generally, what people eat is decided by their appetite more than any other single factor. In pregnancy itself, many myths exist about the amount that should be eaten. The Victorian idea of eating for two has probably been overcome in the western world but it still exists in many developing countries. In its place has come the myth of supplementation with vitamin and trace elements, an idea of the 1930s which still persists in some western societies.

If a woman is eating a normal diet, she is almost certainly providing enough of all nutrients for her fetus to develop and grow normally. A major aspect of nutrition is the energy balance. During pregnancy a woman takes in about 2400 kcal/day in order to satisfy her energy needs. Assuming this comes from a mixed diet, it will contain more than enough of all the other constituents required in nutrition. For instance, there will be more than 10 g of protein a day; most of the vitamin and all the mineral requirements will be provided. Hence, if a good mixed diet is taken to the level at which a woman feels she needs it, there is no need for any supplementation or manipulation of the diet. This obviously does not apply to women who are having unusual diets, such as vegans or those with intestinal absorption diseases, but they are a small minority.

Different nutrients are handled in different ways and the nutritional needs of pregnancy should be seen to be aimed at a common purpose rather than manipulated by a common mechanism. Hence, it is meddlesome for us to interfere, changing complex patterns by supplementing perceived needs such as certain vitamins, proteins or even iron and folate. In the prepregnancy period, general advice is that a diet should contain less fatty meats, sugar and salt and more proteins, vegetables, cereals and fibre. This would provide most of the protein need, the energy requirements and more vitamins and minerals than women require. In the western world, nutrition is rarely deficient in a person taking a non-fad diet.

Nutritional status does have an effect upon ovulation and readers are referred to a good review by Warren (1983). If fat stores are low, menarche is delayed, ovulation is infrequent and may even stop. When fat stores are replaced in normal women, there is usually a return of normal pituitary ovarian activity. When consulting a prepregnancy counsellor, a couple's diet should be reviewed to ensure that it provides adequate amounts of protein, vitamins and mineral-containing foods. There is little point in supplementing vitamins if the diet is normal; additional minerals are rarely needed.

There are organizations which believe that many pregnancy problems are due to lack of vitamins or minerals. They place much emphasis on the international standards of requirements for pregnant women. Such recommendations are very suspect. They usually advise quantities greatly in excess of the needs of the body, even in pregnancy. To compare this poor database with measurements of the mineral content of various body fluids or hair merely compounds confusion. There is little evidence that the mineral content of any of these fluids or tissues relates to the correct tissue content, except in severe deficiencies. Further, to add extra minerals to the diet does not of necessity mean they will be absorbed, and even if they are, they may not be metabolized along usual pathways. Finally, there is little evidence that exogenous administration of minerals to correct levels in peripheral tissues is of help in prepregnancy care, or improves fetal or neonatal outcome; such attempts are generally dismissed by recognized nutritionists.

One aspect of a potential vitamin deficiency has received much publicity in the prepregnancy sphere. Several reports have been published about women who, having previously had a baby with a neural tube defect, have taken mixed vitamin supplements in early pregnancy and are claimed to have a lower risk of having a subsequent baby born with central nervous system abnormalities (Smithells et al 1983). In order to ensure the availability of these vitamins in very early pregnancy, the vitamin supplements had to be started in the prepregnancy time. These studies were not designed to distinguish which of the micronutrients were effective; in some cases the doses used were higher than physiological. Such has been the concern that the Medical Research Council has mounted a multicentre randomized controlled trial to test the potential benefit of folate and multivitamins independently; this is proceeding at the moment and should be finished in the early years of the next decade. Even if the study does show improvement and a lowering of risk amongst those women in the trial, it does not automatically mean that normal women who have never given birth to a baby with a neural tube defect would also benefit from receiving vitamins. It is important that the prepregnancy counsellor advises couples that there is no proven benefit from taking vitamins unless there is a need for them. The argument that vitamins can do no harm but might do some good is a false one. Clinical syndromes of hypervitaminosis have been described for most vitamins.

At the prepregnancy clinic, advisers can persuade individuals to avoid any persistent dietary excesses so that when they do become pregnant, they can easily adopt a healthy diet and provide all the appropriate nutrition for the growing fetus.

Pre-existing medical diseases

Women who have chronic disease from their youth are often anxious about the possible effects of the disease on preg-

Table 13.5 Some long-term medical conditions in women attending the prepregnancy clinic at St George's Hospital from 1985 to 1987

Cardiac diseases
Rheumatic mitral stenosis
Rheumatic aortic incompetence
Congenital diseases
Eisenmenger's syndrome
Fallot's tetralogy
Aortic coarctation
Women with artificial heart valves
Supraventricular tachycardia
Hypertension
Essential hypertension
Renal hypertension
Respiratory diseases
Asthma
Sarcoidosis
Cystic fibrosis
Bronchiectasis
Haemorrhagic diseases
Thrombocytopenia purpura
von Willebrand's disease
Leukaemia
Deep vein thrombosis
Pulmonary embolism
Urinary diseases
Renal stone
Renal failure
Acute nephritis
Chronic nephritis
Stress incontinence
Time incontinence
Connective tissue diseases
Lupus erythematosus
Rheumatoid arthritis
Endocrine problems
Diabetes
Hyperthyroidism
Hypothyroidism
Addison's disease
Congenital adrenal hyperplasia
Carcinoma of the breast
Neurological conditions
Epilepsy
Multiple sclerosis
Peripheral neuritis

nancy. Mostly, the fears are about the effects of the disease on the fetus but the prepregnancy counsellor should also remember the potential effects of the pregnancy on the disease. Women may consult the physician who is in charge of their particular disease but he or she may not be very experienced about its management in pregnancy. It therefore needs an obstetrician or physician who has looked after this condition in pregnancy to give advice at a prepregnancy clinic on the dual aspects of the disease affecting the pregnancy, and of pregnancy affecting the disease. A further aspect is the pharmacological therapy of any disease, which can be of more serious import to the fetus than the condition itself; this should be carefully considered.

Generally, women in the childbearing years are fit and only a few have any long-term illnesses. Table 13.5 shows the conditions present in women who have attended the author's prepregnancy clinic in the last 2 years.

The prepregnancy advice for women whith these conditions is well reviewed by de Swiet (1986) who considers all the diseases occurring in this age group and their therapies.

Stress

This word is one of the four hangovers left in modern medicine from Victorian times when doctors were mainly concerned with symptoms. Words such as shock, miasma, pyrexia or toxaemia have been replaced by terms based more scientifically on the underlying pathophysiology of the various disorders. Stress is still recognized in modern medicine, however, having effects at most times of life. It would be surprising therefore if it did not affect early pregnancy, but its effects remain difficult to quantify.

In the prepregnancy clinic, the subject of stress is often raised by couples as a potential cause of problems. They see the economic and work stresses to which women are subjected in the 1980s as a potential cause of problems and expect doctors to understand what they are talking about. Sometimes the questions relate to specific stresses such as previous pregnancy loss in relation to future pregnancies (Barnett et al 1983). Unfortunately they are usually much more general and vague and the importance of psychosocial stress as a cause of pregnancy pathology has now become inflated to an entirely unrealistic level in the minds of many lay people. The *Schedule of Recent Experiences* is a commonly used questionnaire to measure stress but its questions are very tightly phrased and do not allow much variation within the experience expressed. *Life Event Scales* may be useful for acute phenomena but are poor at measuring more chronic problems such as an unsatisfactory marriage or living beyond available means.

The prepregnancy counsellor's advice should avoid adding to stress. For example, if a woman has for many years had a glass of sherry before dinner or a glass of wine with her meals, unnecessary stress might be induced by advising her to cut out all alcohol to achieve a normal pregnancy result. Prepregnancy care is a sensitive area; badly done it can cause more harm than good.

Najman et al (1983) consider that altered neuroendocrine functions resulting from stress may influence fertility. Norbeck & Tilden (1983) have reported increased pregnancy complications after life stresses in the year preceding pregnancy. In such women, continuing stress may be associated with preterm delivery and with increased need for analgesia in labour. A comprehensive review has been written by Haddad (1989), while the lasting influence of women's emotions in pregnancy on the subsequent development of the child is addressed by Wolkind (1981). The fact that there is still too little evidence in the field to answer these questions should be borne in mind when giving advice in the prepregnancy period.

Work

Couples attending a prepregnancy clinic are often concerned about the potential effect of work done by the female partner on future pregnancy. This problem has increased in the last decade because more women are working out of the home and more women are working later in pregnancy. There is no barrier at 28 weeks of pregnancy and many women work up to even 38 or 39 weeks.

There are two main reasons for this. First, many women, particularly in social classes I and II, wish to advance their careers by promotion and this is best done between the ages of 25 and 35, which are also the childbearing years. In consequence, career and childbearing may compete. Secondly, most young couples nowadays entering marriage have a double income and their whole lifestyle depends upon this. With the poor maternity allowances in this country, giving up work because of pregnancy carries an almost unacceptable financial penalty.

When discussing the problems of women's work, couples must appreciate early that every woman works at home and although there may be fewer hazards there, the physical work is as great or greater than when working outside. There are no rest rooms or facilities for days off; often there are other children or the couple's parents to be looked after.

As well as doing their own housework, many women take on additional paid work outside the house. In only a small proportion does this involve specific environmental hazards of a chemical, physical or biological nature. For example, female anaesthetists, radiologists and teachers are at higher risk, respectively, from contact with inhalant gases, from X-rays or from children with rubella. Any known hazards should be identified and avoided. A careful history must be taken about the mother's work and if the counsellor is uncertain about any risk, enquiries should be made through the health and safety officers or the relevant trade union. A good introduction to the problem of chemical hazards is the comprehensive review by Barlow & Sullivan (1982).

From time to time, particular aspects become a source of many questions and public interest increases. Working during pregnancy at visual display units was a source of anxiety for five years. Whilst it is hard to prove a negative, so many studies have now indicated they are associated with no harm to pregnant women that 'statements to the contrary are not soundly based'. This quotation and a good review of the whole subject is provided by Blackwell & Chang (1988).

As well as specific hazards that cause anxiety, many couples need to be reminded that the effects of fatigue and boredom at work — whether paid or unpaid — are important. The best studies so far performed have been by Mamelle et al (1984). They looked at the harder-to-measure indices of boredom, noise and the effects of standing jobs, and also examined physical work in the open air, as opposed to that done sitting at desks. They were able to correlate low birthweight and preterm labour with an increasing number of fatigue measures. Because of the difficult nature of isolating any one factor, particularly those relating to socioeconomic class and age, regression analysis was carried out for these and for parity, ethnic origin, past obstetric history and pathology in the current pregnancy. The various factors found at work, especially mental stress and environmental conditions leading to boredom and tiredness, still showed an association with a bad obstetric outcome.

In giving advice at the prepregnancy clinic, the obstetrician must be careful to avoid causing undue worry. A balance is needed in deciding between the hazards that might exist at work compared with the boredom or dissatisfaction which could result from stopping work. For many women, getting out of the house during the day is important; they enjoy meeting others at work and doing non-stressful work. It is inadvisable for prepregnancy counsellors to be too didactic. It is probably safest to concentrate on women with previous obstetric problems such as preterm labour or low birthweight babies to try to ensure that they are not subjecting themselves to inadvisable levels to work, travel or stress. There is a little evidence that if such women did less strenuous work in late pregnancy they would have a better chance of continuing pregnancy for longer and having a baby of a reasonable size. It is less sure however that if the baby's birthweight is increased or the length of gestation prolonged the infant will automatically enter the level of perinatal mortality or morbidity of the heavier or longer pregnancy group, independent of the condition causing the hazard.

WIDER PREPREGNANCY CARE

Full prepregnancy care should be set out like an archery target. In the centre is the prepregnancy clinic acting as the apex of a series of levels of prepregnancy care. It is staffed by an obstetrician, considering precise medical conditions or past obstetric problems, and is essential for those who have such problems. The next ring of the target is a slightly less intense level where prepregnancy care can be given in groups. Advice can be given to five or six couples who attend the contraceptive clinic, for example, and who may wish to ask questions or develop further consultations from this. The prepregnancy workers on this level answer general questions about health and diet and perform checks on haemoglobin, rhesus or rubella status and haemoglobinopathies. Such a clinic is well run by a trained nurse or midwife who can deal with six to eight couples in the course of an evening, referring to the specialist clinic problems which she feels need more consultation.

In the outer zone of the target of prepregnancy care, personnel may go out to youth clubs and schools to talk to young people before pregnancy is imminent. This may influence them and also allows them to consider their reproductive future. Such dissemination of simple information about functions can also be helped by the use of the mass media, including radio and television, for these have more influence than the written word in some segments of the population.

All this is prepregnancy care; whilst consultant obstetricians may see the obvious advantages of the formal clinic setting to which they are used, they must also be prepared to take themselves out to the community and to the public, so influencing attitudes at the times when they are being formed.

REFERENCES

Barlow S, Sullivan F 1982 Reproductive hazards of industrial chemicals. Academic Press, London
Barnett B, Harma B, Parker G. 1983 Life event scales for obstetric groups. Psychosomatic Research 27: 313–320
Blackwell R, Chang A 1988 Visual display units and pregnancy. British Journal of Obstetrics and Gynaecology 95: 446–453
Browne A 1989 Placental transfer of amino acids. Contemporary Reviews in Obstetrics and Gynaecology 1: 22–28
Butler N, Alberman E 1969 Perinatal problems. Livingstone, London
Chamberlain G, 1980 The prepregnancy clinic. British Medical Journal 281: 29–30
Chamberlain R, Chamberlain G, Haslett B, Claireaux A 1975 British births 1970. Heinemann Medical, London, p 19
de Swiet M 1984 Medical disorders in obstetrical practice. Blackwell Scientific, Oxford
de Swiet M 1986 Pre-existing medical disease In: Chamberlain G, Lumley J (eds) Prepregnancy care. John Wiley, Chichester
Haddad A 1989 Anxiety in pregnancy. Contemporary Reviews in Obstetrics and Gynaecology 2: 123–133
Hill D J, Gray N 1982 Patterns of tobacco smoking in Australia. Medical Journal of Australia 1: 23–25
Himmelberger D, Brown B, Cohen E 1978 Cigarette smoking during pregnancy. American Journal of Epidemiology 108: 470–479
Howie P 1986 Past obstetrical performance. In: Chamberlain G, Lumley J (eds) Prepregnancy care. John Wiley, Chichester
Kline J, Shrout P, Stein Z, Zusser M, Warburton D 1980 Drinking during pregnancy and spontaneous abortion. Lancet ii: 176–179
Kline J, Levine B, Shrout P, Steil L, Susser M, Warburton D 1983 Maternal smoking and trisomy among spontaneously aborted conceptions. American Journal of Human Genetics 35: 421–431
Lemoine P et al 1968 Les enfants de parents alcooliques. Ouest Medicine 21: 476–482
Little R 1976 Alcohol consumption during pregnancy. Annals of the New York Academy of Sciences (USA) 273: 588–592
Majewski F 1981 Alcohol embryopathy. Neurobehavioral Toxicology and Teratology 3: 129–144
Mamelle N, Lauarmon B, Lazer P 1984 Prematurity and occupational activity during pregnancy. American Journal of Epidemiology 19: 309–322
Mattison D 1982 The effects of smoking on fertility. Environmental Research 28: 410–433
Meyer M B, Jones B, Jonassen J 1976 Perinatal events and maternal smoking in pregnancy. American Journal of Epidemiology 103: 464–476
Moore E 1980 Women and Health. Public Health Reports
Najman J, Keepling J, Chang A, Morrison J, Western P 1983 Employment, unemployment and the health of pregnant women. New Doctor 8: 8
Nayler A, Warburton D 1979 Segmented analysis of spontaneous abortion. Fertility and Sterility 31: 282–286
Newman N 1986 In: Chamberlain G, Lumley J (eds) Prepregnancy care. John Wiley, Chichester
Norbeck J, Tilden V 1983 Life stress, social support and emotional disequilibrium in complications of pregnancy. Health, Society and Behaviour 24: 30–46
Office of Population and Census Surveys 1981 General household survey 81/1. HMSO, London
Royal College of Psychiatrists 1982 Alcohol and alcoholism. Bulletin of the Royal College of Psychiatrists of London 6: 69
Sexton M, Hebel J 1984 A clinical trial of change of maternal smoking. Journal of the American Medical Association 251: 911–915
Shawitz S, Cohen D, Shawitz B 1980 Behaviour and learning defects in children born to alcoholic mothers. Journal of Pediatrics 96: 972–982
Smithells et al 1983 Further experiences in vitamin supplementation for prevention of neural tube defect recurrences. Lancet i: 1027–1031
Steel J, Johnston F 1986 Prepregnancy management of the diabetic. In: Chamberlain G, Lumley J (eds) Prepregnancy care. John Wiley, Chichester
Sulaiman N, Florey C, Taylor D, Ogston S 1988 Alcohol consumption in Dundee primigravidas. British Medical Journal 296: 1500–1503
Vessey M, Weight N, McPherson K, Wiggins P 1978 Fertility after stopping different methods of contraception. Bristish Medical Journal 1: 265–267
Warburton D, Fraser F 1964 Spontaneous abortion risks in man. American Journal of Human Genetics 16: 1–25
Warren M 1983 Effects of undernutrition on reproductive function. Endocrinology Review 4: 363–377
Weatherall D, Higgs J 1982 Application of genetic engineering techniques to the study of haemoglobinopathies. Hospital Update 8: 927–933
Wolkind S 1981 Prepregnancy emotional stress — effects on the fetus. Psychological and social study. Academic Press, London, pp 177–194
Wright J T et al 1983 Alcohol consumption, pregnancy and low birthweight. Lancet i: 663–665

14

Geoffrey Chamberlain

Diagnosis of pregnancy

Given time, the diagnosis of pregnancy is easy. The abdomen swells, the woman feels fetal movements and eventually a child is born. However, for a variety of reasons the diagnosis often has to be made much earlier, before any of these simple physical signs appear. It is obviously convenient for the woman to know that she is pregnant sooner rather than later, so she may arrange her life. She may need to make early booking arrangements for delivery. Conversely, she may wish for a termination of pregnancy; earlier confirmation of her diagnosis may bring her to the gynaecological clinic sooner and so lead to an easier procedure. Occasionally it may be important to confirm a very early pregnancy as in the differential diagnosis of unruptured ectopic pregnancy.

The various methods of diagnosis have differing strengths. Some of the symptoms can be produced by other conditions and even the signs of earlier pregnancy can be confused with other findings. The investigations are usually more specific but in all cases, if circumstances allow, waiting a little will help to strengthen the validity of any symptom, sign or investigation.

CLINICAL DIAGNOSIS

Symptoms

Amenorrhoea is an obvious and expected symptom of pregnancy. Once the implantation of a blastocyst has occurred, there are usually no more periods. This symptom develops some 14 days after fertilization or about 4 days after implantation. In many women, it is the first symptom of pregnancy.

Amenorrhoea is not very specific. It can be caused by a series of physical diseases but perhaps more important in this context, it can also be affected greatly by hypothalamic activity when a woman strongly wants or does not want to be pregnant; the fear of pregnancy or a great desire for pregnancy can be associated with amenorrhoea.

Table 14.1 Responses of 200 primigravidae and 197 multigravidae to questioning about when they first thought they were pregnant in weeks from LMP

	Mean ($\bar{x}$)	Range (±2 SD)
Primigravida	6.4	3.5–16.3
Multigravida	4.7	2.1–20.6

Conversely, there may be a little bleeding after normal implantation of pregnancy. This is probably from the decidua parietalis, the lining of the pregnant uterus away from the site of implantation. Slowly in pregnancy, the growing embryo sac, covered by decidua capsularis, covers the whole surface of the inside of the uterine cavity. Until that happens by about 12 weeks, bleeding can come from the decidua parietalis. This is not regular and is of less significance than bleeding occurring later in pregnancy (see Chapter 28).

Amenorrhoea is a much sought for symptom by the public and the profession. Its relationship to the time when the woman first thought she was pregnant however is more variable. At a study at Queen Charlotte's Hospital, the author showed that among 397 primiparous and multiparous women, the mean age when the former thought they were pregnant was 6.4 weeks from the last menstrual period, while among the latter it was 4.7 weeks. However, the ranges given in Table 14.1 show that many women in both groups considered they were pregnant before amenorrhoea could have occurred, i.e. before the first missed period.

Nausea and vomiting are other well known symptoms of pregnancy, previously called morning sickness. It is well recognized that such sickness occurs any time of the day. In a recent study, 29% of women had their regular sickness in the afternoon or evening (Chamberlain & Whitehead, unpublished data). The problem commonly starts after amenorrhoea is noticed but can occasionally precede it.

The nausea and vomiting of pregnancy differ from that of seasickness or vomiting following the ingestion of toxins;

the woman does not usually feel ill but commonly the feeling of sickness wells up suddenly. The woman vomits a small amount of fluid and then returns to her everyday life. She is usually not upset by this, nor is she affected metabolically.

Breast symptoms are very common and are noted particularly by those who have never had a pregnancy before. First to be noticed are tingling and irritability of the breasts against the woman's bra. This follows the increased blood supply of the skin of the breast due to increased oestrogen levels.

This symptom is noted from 6 weeks of pregnancy and soon afterwards, breast enlargement makes itself noticeable by the bra appearing to be too tight. Later still, at about 8 weeks of gestation, the nipple becomes darker and the areola appears to spread. This is most noticeable in blonde women. By 8–10 weeks, Montgomery's tubercles appear around the nipple.

Urinary symptoms are often present. The first symptom is usually increased frequency of micturition, which starts long before the size of the increasing uterus could be responsible and is probably due to a higher progesterone level. The woman notices this at 8–10 weeks of pregnancy and it can be very disturbing. There is little that can be done about it and there is no point in recommending restriction of fluids; this merely makes the woman thirsty but she still has increased frequency of micturition.

Many women notice a feeling of well-being in pregnancy. This is sometimes hard to describe but is a symptom which is extremely well known to women — the pride of pregnancy. If a woman who has had a baby before tells her doctor she is pregnant, he would do well to consider her assertion high amongst the diagnosis. Women know their own bodies and can often make the diagnosis correctly.

Other symptoms of pregnancy do occur in varying degrees. Increased salivation can be troublesome and may appear any time fter the eighth week of pregnancy. Sometimes unusual articles of food are desired. These *pica* usually come later on in pregnancy, after about 12 weeks, when a woman knows she is pregnant. A few women feel particularly tired in early pregnancy; this may be due to a redistribution of the blood supply to the components of the body.

Signs

The examination of the breasts usually reveals the first sign of pregnancy. The darkening of the areolae and nipples with the presence of Montgomery's tubercles has already been mentioned and these can be seen by the observer. In addition, the breast feels globular and warm with veins apparent just under the surface of the skin. The signs are best seen in the primigravida. Some clinicians would consider they are always present in pregnancy and thus would not diagnose an ectopic pregnancy unless the breasts were warm and showing early signs. Such an interpolation would be open to a high false negative rate.

Abdominal examination is usually unhelpful in early pregnancy. By the time the uterus can be convincingly felt above the symphysis pubis, usually the pregnancy has advanced 12 or 14 weeks. By then the diagnosis is usually made by other means; however, examination is helpful in a woman who has not thought of the diagnosis and presents after 12 weeks of gestation. If she presents even later, the growth of the uterus becomes more obvious and indeed by 22–24 weeks of pregnancy, fetal parts can be palpated and fetal movements felt.

From about 12 weeks of pregnancy, the fetal heart can be detected with a small portable ultrasound machine (Doptone); this is a good positive sign of pregnancy for the pulse rate generated by the fetal heart is usually about 140 beats/min while the maternal heart rate is about 80 beats/min. These two can be easily differentiated and the sounds make a convincing sign to both the mother and the examining physician.

Vaginal examination is a most useful method of checking for early pregnancy. A gentle bimanual examination can detect the softness and fullness of the uterus by 6–8 weeks of pregnancy. The uterus may not be very enlarged but it feels much broader and globular. The cervix becomes very soft, changing in consistency from the fibrous feel of the non-pregnant uterus and cervix. The variation is equal to the difference in palpation of the end of the nose with its underlying cartilage and the upper lip with its absence of any firmness. If a speculum is passed, the cervix may appear pigeon-blue rather than its more usual pink. However, there is no reason for speculum examination at this stage and this sign is very unspecific.

There is no merit in attempting to assess uterine softness by Hegar's sign. Reference to this may be found in old textbooks; the examiner aims to appreciate the softness and emptiness of the isthmus of the uterus so that the fundus of the uterus with the growing embryo appears to be entirely separate from the cervix. In order to detect this sign, firm pressure must be used by the examining fingers on the abdomen and in the vagina; if a miscarriage occurs after this, the vaginal examination would be considered to be responsible. Those who used to use this examination claimed Hegar's sign was present in about 60% of pregnant women by 8 weeks of gestation; the method is not recommended.

INVESTIGATIONS

Pregnancy tests

Not long ago, investigations used to be done in medicine only to confirm a clinical diagnosis made from the assessment of symptoms and signs. More recently, tests have been used to screen asymptomatic populations and make the diagnosis de novo. This system produces a diagnosis before symptoms or signs are produced. Pregnancy testing seems to have

Table 14.2 Pregnancy testing by region in Great Britain (1982)

	Health region	Number of requests (T)	Number of births (B)	T/B Ratio
England				
North	Northern	73 652	40 166	1.83
	Yorkshire	80 333	46 827	1.72
	North West	76 870	53 258	1.44
	Mersey	45 963	32 049	1.43
Mid	East Anglia	42 283	23 819	1.78
	West Midlands	108 608	67 933	1.60
	Trent	86 417	58 470	1.48
South	South West	61 155	37 848	1.62
	Wessex	50 178	33 395	1.50
	South West Thames	53 765	34 718	1.55
	South East Thames	67 144	44 805	1.50
	North East Thames	83 698	50 339	1.66
	North West Thames	64 363	46 667	1.38
	Oxford	30 947	31 809	0.97
		925 376	602 098	1.54
Wales		46 941	36 107	1.30
Scotland		105 287	75 590	1.39
Total		1 077 604	713 795	1.51

Requests are less than numbers of tests used, for a given sample may be tested several times.

moved from the first category of tests into the second in the last few years.

Twenty years ago, the only tests available were the biological ones — the Aschheim–Zondek and the Bufo-Bufo tests which involved laboratory animals. These tests were moderately expensive and required special skills. In consequence, they were not used often unless there was a medical indication. With the advent of the immunological test and later radioimmunoassays, human chorionic gonadotrophin (hCG) can now be detected at much lower concentrations and more cheaply, so pregnancy testing has entered the market for use of the screening test. A measure of this change can be seen in recent data. In 1983, hospital laboratories in the United Kingdom performed approximately 1 300 000 tests and non-hospital laboratories did another 178 000 tests. Pharmacists offering a testing service carried out about 180 000 tests while approximately 400 000 self-read tests were sold to the public. Thus, about 2 million tests were performed in a year when about 700 000 births occurred; probably the number of tests is higher now.

Among the hospital laboratory tests, 79.5% were requested by general practitioners while 19.5% came from other departments of the hospital, mostly from the obstetrical unit. Slide tests were used in 72%, tube tests in 27% and the radioimmunoassay test in less than 1% in 1983.

The evolution of the service of pregnancy testing in hospitals has been piecemeal and owes much to history. Table 14.2 shows the distribution of hospital laboratories in which the tests were performed. There is no logic in the microbiology laboratory doing over half the pregnancy tests but originally that is where animals were kept so animal-based pregnancy tests started there. Such is inertia that they have stayed there in most cases.

A distribution of the hospital laboratory tests done in the health regions of Britain in 1982 is shown in Table 14.2. The number of requests is collated with the number of births to produce a test:birth ratio, to indicate the load of requests compared with actual pregnancies. The ratio seems to be lowest in the Oxfordshire Regional Health Authority and generally higher in the Northern and Yorkshire Regions. There is no significant correlation between these ratios and the perinatal mortality rate in each region.

Basis of pregnancy tests

All pregnancy tests depend upon the detection of hCG in either urine or the blood. The usefulness of the test depends upon:

1. The stage of development of the chorionic tissue and hence the amount of hCG in the body fluids.
2. The sensitivity of the test to detect lower concentrations of hCG.
3. The specificity of the test, particularly in relation to cross-reaction with pituitary gonadotrophins (luteinizing hormone and follicle-stimulating hormone). A luteinizing hormone peak may occur at the time of ovulation, while pituitary gonadotrophins are often increased in later reproductive life in an effort to stimulate ovulation in an ageing ovary.

The biological, animal-based pregnancy tests are not used in pregnancy testing now. Aschheim and Zondek, in 1928, first showed the induction of ovulation in immature mice stimulated with hCG. This was followed by the Friedman test in rats and then the Bufo-Bufo test, inducing spermatogenesis with hCG in frogs. These investigations were all highly labour-intensive, requiring laboratories to keep large stocks of appropriate animals and it often took a long time to get a result back. In the 1960s, Wide & Gemzel introduced the immunochemical test which depends on the agglutination inhibition reaction of hCG-coated red cells and antiserum to hCG. From this, the agglutination inhibition tests and radioimmunoassays were developed.

The gonadotrophin molecule is made up of two subunits — the alpha and the beta. The alpha subunits are similar throughout all gonadotrophins while the beta subunits are individually different. Antibodies have been raised to the beta subunit of hCG in order to increase specificity. Another advance came in the mid 1970s when the preparation of monoclonal antibodies artificially enabled specific antibodies to the beta unit of hCG to be produced cheaply and cross-reaction with the beta unit of pituitary gonadotrophins was excluded. This allowed not just a more precise result but the test was applicable earlier in pregnancy, since a positive result could occur at a lower concentration of hCG.

Mechanism of action of pregnancy tests

The reaction of hCG antigen with the antibody is made obvious by attaching one or the other to either latex particles or sheep red blood cells; latex particles are commonly used for slide tests and red blood cells for tube tests. When agglutination occurs, clumps of particles adhere to each other, making visible masses which precipitate and can be seen with the naked eye.

If the latex particles or the red blood cells coated with antigen are added to hCG antibody, agglutination results. If the test urine (which, if the woman is pregnant, will contain hCG) is added before this, it blocks the antibodies so that they are not agglutinated and do not produce a visible precipitate. Hence the presence of hCG in a positive pregnancy test is indicated by the agglutination inhibition provided to the latex particles (latex agglutination inhibition, LAI) or the red blood cells (haemoagglutination inhibition, HAI).

Different results are obtained if the inert particles are coated with anti-hCG. In this case the addition of the woman's urine, containing hCG, results in agglutination. This is the reversed agglutination test (rLA for latex particles or rHA for red blood cells). It is important to remember that these opposite end-points are used as a measure of a positive result in pregnancy tests; the end-point depends upon whether it is an agglutination inhibition or a reversed agglutination reaction.

The addition of monoclonal antibodies has increased the sensitivity and specificity of pregnancy testing but does not alter this basic point. Further precision has been made possible in the last few years by the use of a double antibody—one specific for intact hCG (alpha and beta units) and one specific for the beta unit of hCG only, a reversed agglutination reaction. The hCG is sandwiched between the two antibodies. Then two antibodies produce agglutination with hCG only, giving greater precision.

The radioimmunoassays are fast being rivalled by the enzyme-linked immunosorbent assays (ELISA), which involve a double reaction; the test shows a positive result on much lower levels of hCG. The ELISA tests use hCG which is sandwiched between the standard-phase antibody and enzyme-labelled antibody. Urine containing hCG is added to a tube which is already coated with the double antibody; binding occurs and after washing, the enzyme, which is alkaline phosphatase-linked antibody, is added. This becomes bound to the already captured hCG. A second wash is followed by enzyme substrate which is broken down by the bound enzyme, resulting in a blue coloration. Hence, a pregnant woman will have as a positive end-point a blue solution in the tube.

Commercial tests

There are many pregnancy tests on the market. Most of them are for laboratory use but a few can be purchased over the counter for home use. The red blood cell inhibition tests (rHA and HAI) are not very sensitive to less than 100 units of hCG per litre, hence they are best used later than 14 days after fertilization. The end-result depends upon the formation of a brown ring of precipitated particles for HAI tests and no brown ring for the rHA tests.

The LAI tests are slightly less sensitive and usually need between 500 and 2000 units of hCG per litre and so are best used after 18 days from fertilization. They are much swifter than the haemoagglutination tests, being ready in minutes rather than hours. Again, it must be remembered that the end-result for the rLA test is agglutination but most of the tests on the market are LAI, for which the positive end-result is no agglutination.

The ELISA test is sensitive to much lower concentrations of hCG (25–50 u/l) and in consequence can give a positive result as early as 8–10 days after fertilization. They all depend upon a blue colour and one of them (Clear Blue) shows the blue colour change on a dipstick.

Of the tests available to women over the counter, costs are very similar. With the ring tests, most manufacturers produce two test kits in one pack to allow the woman to check a negative result a few days later. A problem is that the ring tests are very sensitive to vibration; reports have been received of women having false negative tests because they have set up the test on top of electric equipment such as a refrigerator, not realizing that the vibration from the motor can break up the ring. If the fluid in the tube is warmed while the test is going on, convection currents may disturb the settling of the ring. This happens if the test is set up on top of a central heating radiator. This seems an unusual thing to do but it has been reported in several instances. Further, the reading must be made fairly quickly and if the test is left for rather longer than the manufacturer's instruction before reading, it can be falsely positive. In most cases, one has to wait about an hour for results and this is sometimes inconvenient.

The blue tests are becoming more popular now. Clear Blue is available to the public and there are two tests in the pack. The procedure has two stages, which doubles the potential for mistakes, but this is compensated by the result being available in a matter of minutes. The waiting time as given in the instructions can be a nuisance for it is not long enough for the woman to do something else in between stages but is not short enough not to matter.

False results

In the laboratory, tests are usually done under standard and uniform conditions by a technician who has done them before. In consequence, he or she follows the manufacturer's exact instructions and usually performs a valid test. At home, however, the woman is not experienced and not used to laboratory techniques; she may be doing the test for the

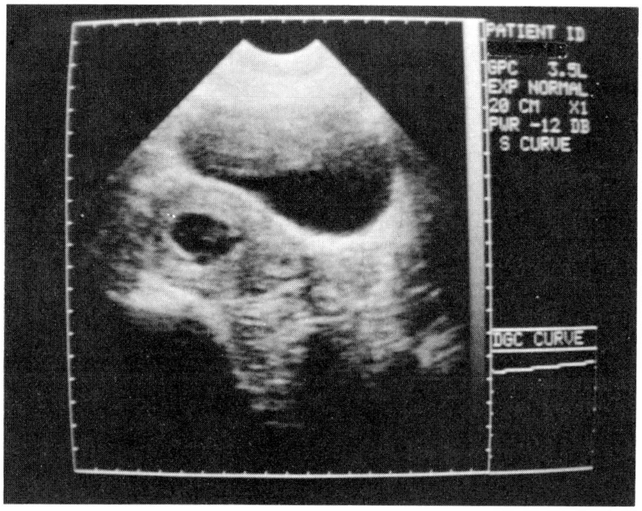

Fig. 14.1 An ultrasound taken 6 weeks after the last menstrual period shows a gestation sac but no fetal echoes yet. Ultrasound kindly provided by Dr R. Patel.

first time, so errors can creep in. However, the manufacturer's instructions are clear and precise. If followed, the test should work.

As well as procedure failures, there may be false negative results if there is too little hCG present in the urine; either an early morning specimen is not used or the urine is too dilute because the woman has been drinking a lot of fluid. Possibly the test is being tried too early in pregnancy to expect a reasonable level of hCG for that test. Other products in the urine can affect the test, such as bacteria or other proteinuria.

False positive tests are rarer but they can occur in the polyclonal tests if there are high luteinizing hormone levels for other reasons or if the woman is taking treatments with hCG or luteinizing hormone-releasing hormone.

Ultrasound

With a high-resolution machine and competent ultrasonographer, a sac can be detected in the uterus at about 6 weeks' gestation (Fig. 14.1) and fetal tissue by 7–8 weeks (Fig. 14.2). The fetal heart beat can often be seen by 7 weeks and fetal movements by 8 or 9 weeks.

These are good discriminatory tests for they can be seen and comprehended by both the physician and the woman. However, at the crucial time of 5–6 weeks, it must be stressed that the equipment and the user should not be stretched beyond their capacity.

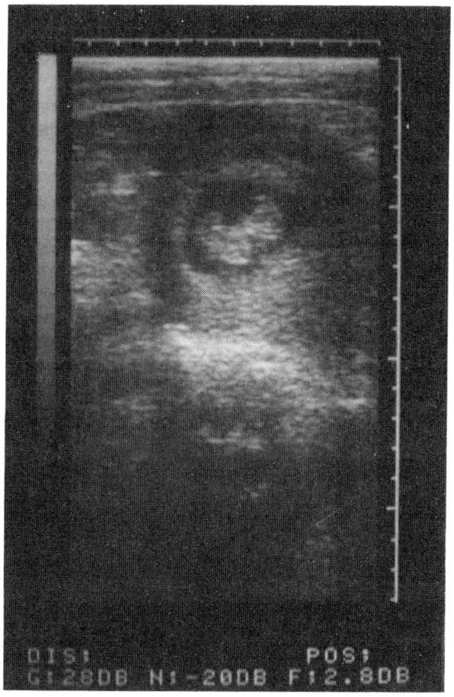

Fig. 14.2 By 7 weeks from the last menstrual period, fetal tissue can be distinguished. Ultrasound kindly provided by Dr R. Patel.

X-rays

An X-ray can only detect a fetus when there is sufficient calcification in the bones to block X-rays. This is unusual before 16 weeks. By this time other tests have usually confirmed the pregnancy. Further, the dangers of irradiation in pregnancy make X-rays an unusual pregnancy test but they may still be used when ultrasound equipment is not available and a very obese woman presents with a pelvic tumour rising up to the umbilicus.

CONCLUSIONS

For most women, pregnancy is a desired event. The symptoms gradually evolve in her consciousness and she is perfectly happy to let time tell the diagnosis. For a few, there is a medical or social need for an early diagnosis and for these the various tests for hCG are useful. However, in the West, it is becoming an increasingly commonly held belief that every normal woman should have a pregnancy test as soon as she thinks she is pregnant. This is usually unnecessary and is grossly expensive on resources. Pressure to test should be resisted if there is any limitation of funding for other more essential services.

15

Marion H. Hall

Critique of antenatal care

INTRODUCTION

In many parts of the world, a great many women deliver their babies without any professional antenatal care at all. In the developed world, however, professional expertise is widely available in the form of specialist obstetricians, general practitioners or primary care doctors, and midwives (and/or nurses). There can be no doubt that the practice of antenatal care is one factor in the very low maternal and perinatal mortality and morbidity rates prevailing in western countries compared with those in developing areas. However, demographic differences, higher standards of living, better general health of the population, availability of expertise and sophisticated equipment for delivery and of course, neonatal care, are also factors, and the precise contribution of antenatal care can be determined only after more careful scrutiny and analysis than it has had hitherto.

The history of the introduction of antenatal care in Britain has been reviewed by Oakley (1982). She makes it clear that the 1929 standard pattern of monthly visits until 28–30 weeks, fortnightly until 36 weeks then weekly until delivery was not based on a systematic analysis of risks, problems and appropriate interventions at any particular gestation, but on an inquiry into what doctors seemed to be doing. There was initially divided opinion as to whether the results of antenatal care were uniformly good, but after the Second World War the standard pattern was more and more widely advocated and practised. It had reached the stage in the career of a medical innovation that McKinlay (1981) describes as 'standard procedure', having passed from 'promising report' without formal evaluation.

It is perhaps not surprising that there was so little criticism or scepticism in the field of antenatal care, since virtually all studies, including the major national surveys (Douglas 1948, Butler & Bonham 1963, Butler & Alberman 1969, Chamberlain et al 1975, Chamberlain 1978) documented that women who received no antenatal care at all experienced very high perinatal mortality, and on the whole, perinatal mortality showed an inverse relationship to the number of antenatal visits. Although a causal relationship was not explicitly claimed by any of the above authors, these findings were widely believed to prove firstly that antenatal care was beneficial, and secondly that the more of it the women had, the better.

A great many problems and reservations surround this simplistic conclusion. Firstly women who book early will have more visits than those who book late and the possible effect of booking early must be separated from the possible effect of frequent visits. Next, women who deliver preterm (either because of spontaneous preterm labour or a major complication requiring induction) are bound to show higher perinatal mortality rates and to experience fewer visits than their sisters who have reached full term and are still attending clinics weekly. Thus, cause and effect are confused: the preterm delivery is actually the cause of the small number of antenatal visits, not the effect of a paucity of visits (even if antenatal care is beneficial). This problem has been addressed by the use of an index (Kessner 1973) which is popular in the American literature on this subject, and a similar strategy was used by Hall et al (1985a) when the average time interval between visits was used as an index of the frequency of visits, independent of gestation at booking and gestation at delivery. However, these manoeuvres solve only one of the problems associated with the 'more is always better' fallacy.

Another important aspect is that women who attend early and often are on average healthier, taller, better educated, more likely to be married or supported, more likely to be in a favoured socioeconomic group and more likely to value medical advice than those who attend late or not at all or default from visits. (There are of course some exceptions—very high-risk women with previous complications who attend very early and often.) Many authors have tried to make allowances for these confounding variables by standardizing for socioeconomic group etc., but controlling in this way can never be completely successful and so far unidentified risk factors remain associated with women who do not comply with treatment or care (Coronary Drug Project Research Group 1980) or those whose care is poorly documented (Buekens et al 1984, Hall & Carr-Hill 1985). Thus, negative correlations between total visits, or the Kessner index and any form of morbidity, cannot be taken at face value.

These problems could theoretically be resolved by a prospective randomized controlled trial of care versus no care, or less care versus more care, but researchers have usually been deterred by the variety and complexity of the components of antenatal care. Randomized controlled trials are most easily conducted for individual circumscribed interventions which can be applied to selected or unselected groups of women. A great many new tests and treatments have been introduced in antenatal care, not always adequately evaluated with regards to their practical benefit or cost-effectiveness. However, they are invariably added to the traditional package of care, without replacing any of its components and they generally have to be administered by specialists, thus contributing to the centralization of care.

To the uncertainty (expressed later in the Short Report 1980) as to 'what exactly antenatal care consists of and how it works' may be added another factor which obliged obstetricians and midwives to reflect upon their practice. This was the consumer movement which channelled and focused a great deal of criticism by pregnant women of antenatal care, especially as they experienced it in hospital (Graham & McKee 1979, Reid & McIlwaine 1980, McIntyre 1981, Garcia 1982). Among the subjects of complaint were long waiting times, lack of continuity, lack of information and depersonalized care. The Short Report (1980) suggests that these problems, and those of non-compliance, might be solved by expanding the staff of clinics, improving premises, adjusting the times and venues of clinics etc.

But the criticisms also led some obstetricians to consider just how essential it was for women to attend so frequently. Their scepticism was fuelled by the experience of scrutinizing many case records and annotating up to 20 visits per pregnancy with no detection of any problem. Research was carried out on all Aberdeen women delivered in 1975, to determine the following:

1. To what extent were high-risk (and indeed low-risk) cases identified at the booking visit?
2. Which abnormal conditions of mother or baby were detected by routine care, when, and with what false positive rates?
3. Which problems occurred in spite of antenatal care?

The conclusions from this study led to a decision to recommend and introduce a new plan for antenatal care of which the main features were a minimum skeleton of care for normal women — modified as to whether it was a first or subsequent pregnancy, with an individual prescription of additional care for women with problems. The main objectives of each visit would be specified, and a bigger proportion of the care would be given by general practitioners and midwives. Anticipated improvements from these innovations were firstly, an increase in the productivity of antenatal care (defined as the proportion of visits which resulted in the detection of a previously unsuspected problem) and in detection rates of problems. Secondly, it was hoped that the elimination of unproductive, unnecessary visits would be appreciated by women and would free resources for more relaxed and unhurried discussions at the remaining visits. Thirdly, the satisfaction of health professionals was expected to increase with the reduction in routine work.

Because of the radical nature of the proposed schedules of care (offering considerably fewer routine visits than traditional care) there was some concern whether health providers would be willing or able to adhere to them; the evaluation of the effects of the new system on women delivering in 1981–1982 included an assessment of the extent to which the planned changes had actually occurred, as well as whether they achieved their aims, and what the pregnant women and the health providers thought about the changes. It is important to emphasize that the views of women and health providers were objectively ascertained by research sociologists who had no responsibility for providing care. (Innovations tend to be judged successful and popular by those who originate them.)

Attention needs to be given not just to the theoretical basis for the timing of antenatal visits, and to the potential for identification of high-risk groups to whom interventions may be offered, but to how these strategies work in practice when applied to a total population, not just a select band of research volunteers. If a women with a concealed pregnancy presents with an eclamptic fit, it is certainly reasonable to suppose that antenatal care might have prevented this; but if the care offered is inconvenient and alienating, it will be less likely to reach all women. Concealed pregnancy was found in only 5 per 1000 women in Aberdeen (Hall et al 1985a) but in as many as 55 per 1000 in Kentucky (Kentucky Coalition for Maternal and Child Health 1983). There appear to be major financial barriers preventing women from obtaining antenatal care in the USA, where it is reported that many obstetricians refuse to accept Medicaid patients (Preventing Low Birthweight 1985).

The results of these research studies will be discussed together with other relevant work in the field in two sections — booking visit and routine investigations.

BOOKING VISIT

The three areas for discussion here are gestation at booking; identification of high-risk and low-risk women and routine investigations.

Gestation at booking

This denotes the consultation at which antenatal care by the midwife, family doctor or obstetrician may be considered to have started. Usually when a full medical and obstetrical history is taken, physical examination is made and plans are made for care for the rest of the pregnancy and for the venue and sometimes the mode of delivery. In studies comparing different centres or countries it may be difficult to ascertain exactly when care does start as this is not always well documented (Morehead et al 1971).

A frequent subject for concern is the gestation at which care does start. This is logical as early consultation allows the earliest possible advice about abstaining from or reducing consumption of harmful substances such as nicotine and alcohol, discussion on the taking of medicines and attention to good dietary practices. This advice should ideally be given before pregnancy at a prepregnancy clinic (Chamberlain 1980a) or in health education to the whole population, as organogenesis may be largely complete by the time most women receive advice. Clarification of uncertain gestation, by a careful menstrual history, by abdominal and pelvic examination and sometimes by ultrasonic scan, is another rationale for advocating early attendance. An accurate estimate of the expected date of delivery is essential for the management of any pregnancy complications which may arise later.

Increasingly, screening for fetal malformation is offered to pregnant women. If this is to be a serum alpha-fetoprotein assay, attendance by 16–18 weeks is sufficient, as it is for amniocentesis for karyotyping or for enzyme tests. However, it is important to remember that a proportion of women are mistaken about gestation, and in order to screen everyone at 16 weeks it would be necessary to request attendance by about 12 weeks' gestation. Furthermore, if chorion biopsy is available, this can and should be done in the first trimester; this has the great advantage of permitting earlier and safer pregnancy termination. However, this would apply only to high-risk women (older women or those with a previous history of a detectable malformation) and can hardly be used as an argument for obliging all women to attend so early. There are some other interventions of unproven value, such as cerclage, which are sometimes done at 12–14 weeks, but again only on high-risk women.

Many studies (Simpson & Walker 1980, Chng et al 1980, O'Brien & Smith 1981, Lewis 1982, Clarke & Clayton 1983) have shown that in Britain disadvantaged women more often attend late (variously defined as after 16–20 weeks' gestation) and many studies in the USA have also found that single women, black women, or those on Medicaid were less likely to have attended during the first trimester. However, delays in attendance may not always be due to ignorance or lack of motivation on the woman's part.

Chamberlain (1980b) reported that London primigravidae knew they were pregnant by 5 weeks on average, and attended their family doctor within 3 weeks of that date. In Aberdeen (Hall et al 1985a) the interval between attending the general practitioner and attendance at hospital was usually 2–3 weeks for primigravidae, though a little longer for multigravidae. Much longer delays in obtaining a hospital appointment in a health district in Liverpool were reported by Gilligan (1980). In the Aberdeen studies, the clinicians were disappointed that a letter exhorting family doctors to refer women earlier seemed to have had no effect, perhaps because family doctors could themselves take responsibility for alpha-fetoprotein screening and may have seen no need for earlier referral. One way of solving this problem is to take specialist care into the community, as described in Sighthill (McKee 1984), where a big improvement in the proportion of women attending before 16 weeks' gestation has been reported.

However, the importance of early attendance should not be overestimated since the good results associated with early booking may be due rather to the type of woman who books early than to early booking itself (selection bias). Furthermore, as pointed out by Pearson (1982), ultrasonic scanning to detect fetal malformation and twins may be more appropriate from 16 to 18 weeks' gestation than in the first trimester and it would be inconvenient and expensive to require women to attend hospital twice at this stage. The whole subject of dietary advice in pregnancy is not one in which there is scientific certainty (Campbell & Gillmer 1982, Durnin et al 1985) and antismoking interventions can successfully be undertaken later (Sexton & Hebel 1984).

One last area for which early attendance might be recommended is discussion of work hazards. Possible harmful substances are discussed by Abdul-Karim (1984) but if there is known to be a definite risk, exposure should cease before pregnancy. However, there is no evidence that work as such is harmful (Murphy et al 1984). There is some evidence of an increase in preterm labour in certain boring or fatiguing occupations (Mamelle 1983) but preventive interventions have not yet been fully evaluated and would usually be advocated during the middle and last rather than the first trimester.

Identification of high-risk women

Medical history

It is usually taken for granted that women with a serious medical problem, such as diabetes, cardiac disease, thyroid disease or pyelonephritis, would constitute an at-risk group, though the extent of the risk would of course depend on the severity of the disease. However, Chng et al (1980) and Hall et al (1985a) found that specialist obstetricians in Aberdeen did not always identify medical problems in the *special features* area of the case record, and occasionally these women were not booked for the specialist hospital. It may be that more general practitioner involvement would be a good thing, such as the joint general practitioner–consultant booking visit practised at Sighthill (McKee 1984).

Obstetric history

Many obstetric problems have a well documented tendency to recur, for example, intrauterine growth retardation (Tejani 1982), preterm labour (Bakketeig & Hoffman 1981, Carr-Hill & Hall 1985), pre-eclampsia (Campbell et al 1985) and third-stage complications (Hall et al 1985b).

The recurrence risk is usually around three times that in women without a previous history and a careful history is therefore useful to identify women who should be booked for specialist confinement and who should be offered any preventive measures of known efficacy. However, it is very important to recognize that the attributable risk is low, and most cases of any of these problems will occur in the group of multigravidae without a previous occurrence, even though these women have a very low risk. Some will of course be identified during pregnancy but it is not possible to identify a group of women who can be sure of not having any complications. There is a wide range of recurrence risks for different congenital malformations; not all can be identified antenatally, and the method of diagnosis (chorion biopsy, amniocentesis, fetal blood sampling or ultrasonic scan) depends on the malformation being sought. Similarly, a previous perinatal death may or may not have a major recurrence risk, and a detailed analysis of previous case records is essential. Even if extra care is not medically indicated, it is usually administered for humane reasons but must be individualized. However, at least 50% of perinatal deaths occur to women with no risk factors whatever (Rooth 1979, Chng et al 1980).

There is another category of previous obstetric history which has implications for delivery — Caesarean section or previous difficult forceps delivery. Confinement under specialist care is advisable, though the appropriate mode of delivery in the next pregnancy will depend upon the indications for the first procedure and on other circumstances at the time of the next delivery. Such a history will not usually require any special arrangements for antenatal care.

The Aberdeen studies (Chng et al 1980, Hall et al 1985a) showed that obstetricians usually identified and booked women with previous intrapartum problems, but previous smallness for gestational age was apparently missed in a substantial minority of cases and specialist confinement not universally arranged.

Another way of looking at the effectiveness of first-visit screening is to assess outcomes for women identified as suitable for confinement in general practitioner or other non-specialist settings. Initial bookings seem to require to be changed quite frequently during pregnancy, varying from 24 to 30% (Lewis et al 1978, Bull 1980, Chng et al 1980) on account of antenatal complications. Of those still booked for the non-specialist setting, 8–16% are then transferred during labour (James 1977, Richmond 1977, Bull 1980, Chng et al 1980, Dixon 1982). The Aberdeen studies looked firstly at whether the transfers were really necessary (88–93% were considered so) and secondly at whether they should have been predicted by better antenatal care (only 5–9%). It seems then that there is an irreducible though small proportion of cases in which problems will arise in labour which were not predictable even by careful specialist assessment and intensive antenatal care. Where the low-risk setting is a unit integrated into a specialist unit, such transfers are not hazardous (Klein et al 1983) but in rural areas with isolated general practitioner units or with home confinements, problems may arise. Both Barron et al (1977) and Chng et al (1980) found that perinatal mortality was higher in the transfers than in those not transferred.

ROUTINE INVESTIGATIONS

The pattern of investigation in pregnancy ought to vary with the prevalence of disease (e.g. Venereal Disease Research Laboratories (VDRL) testing is clearly worthwhile if syphilis is common). In most western countries the value of most routine booking investigations (haemoglobin, blood group, rubella immunity check, hepatitis B surface antigen, VDRL) is accepted. A more critical stance was taken by Chng & Hall (1982) who showed that bacteriuria testing was much more worthwhile in women with a previous history of urinary infection. Whether serum alpha-fetoprotein screening is worthwhile must depend upon the incidence of central nervous system deformity, the attitudes of women to pregnancy termination, and on whether the high-risk women attend the antenatal clinic early enough to be included in the programme.

Routine ultrasound imaging at the booking visit is very common in Britain and in some other parts of Europe, but as with so many other obstetric procedures, this crept in without formal evaluation. The biomedical side was well documented, but the two questions — whether the good results in teaching hospitals could be generally reproduced, and whether outcomes would actually be improved — have not been satisfactorily answered. Thacker (1985) and Lilford & Chard (1985) reviewed the four controlled trials in this field and concluded that further work was necessary before routine ultrasound (either one-stage or two-stage programmes) could be recommended.

ROUTINE CARE THROUGHOUT PREGNANCY

Once antenatal care has been initiated, high-risk women may be selected for further testing or treatment using known risk factors (Fedrick & Anderson 1976, Cuckle & Wald 1982, Grant & Mohide 1982, Keirse 1984, Papiernik 1984, Newcombe 1985). A plan for subsequent care is usually suggested

Table 15.1 Recommended and actual number of antenatal visits in selected European countries (adapted from Blondel et al 1985)

Country	No. of antenatal visits Recommended	Actual
Denmark	10	8.0
Finland	14	14.0
France	7	5.9
Federal Republic of Germany	10	8.5
Luxembourg	5	5.0
Netherlands	12	12.0–14.0
Sweden	12–13	14.0
Switzerland	3–4	5.0
Scotland	12	10–12

even for healthy women without risk factors. Such care may have several aims:

1. Preparation for parturition and for parenthood is often undertaken in group classes, but may also feature in individual antenatal visits (this will sometimes be essential as not all women enjoy classes, McIntyre 1982).
2. Imparting of information to and reassurance of pregnant women are often intended by health professionals to occur, but observational studies and interviews with women often report that this rarely happens, especially in hospital clinics.
3. An important rationale for routine care is that it facilitates identification at an early stage of asymptomatic but dangerous pregnancy complications, such as pre-eclampsia, intrauterine growth retardation and malpresentation.

Other complications do of course present with symptoms (such as severe anaemia, antepartum haemorrhage, preterm labour, urinary infection) but these would normally be the subject of a patient-initiated emergency consultation. Chng et al (1980) reported that the majority of emergency antenatal admissions occurred in spite of intensive routine antenatal care and did not result directly from it.

In this chapter most attention will be paid to the identification of asymptomatic complications in low-risk women, though of course if women enjoyed routine care this would be an added benefit; if they did not, and were inconvenienced, that must be considered a cost.

Even in European countries, a very wide variation is reported in the number of routine visits recommended. Table 15.1 shows the number of antenatal visits advised and actually carried out in various European countries, all of which have perinatal mortality rates of less than 20 per 1000 (Blondel et al 1985). There is a huge variation (3–13) in the number recommended and also in the number actually performed (5–14). It seems unlikely that the large number of visits at the top of the range can be essential or justified. There is also a great deal of variation as to who is responsible for most of the care — whether obstetrician, midwife or family doctor. Obstetricians apparently undertake most care in Belgium, Luxembourg and East and West Germany; in Scandinavian countries and the Netherlands midwives play a major role. In Britain and France general practitioners tend to share care with obstetricians, though midwives conduct most deliveries. There may be historical, geographical, financial and administrative reasons for this wide variation in styles of care, but there is no clear basis for stating that any health professional is better than another or that there is an optimum number of visits which will produce the best outcomes.

In Britain there is an increasing variety of patterns of care, sometimes stimulated by dissatisfaction expressed by women, sometimes because health professionals were not enjoying what they were doing, sometimes because of overcrowding or in an effort to reach women who did not attend at all or defaulted from care, and sometimes to address neglected clinical problems.

Care by specialist obstetricians alone is rare in Britain, except for women in the private sector or those with major medical or obstetric problems, such as diabetes; even then, there is a case for continuing involvement of the general practitioner, who will normally have responsibility for the continuing care of the diabetes before and after the pregnancy. In large centres a specialist physician will also be involved.

General practitioners alone can legally take complete responsibility for antenatal care, but shared or combined care is more common, especially when the woman is to be booked for confinement under specialist care. The Royal College of Obstetricians and Gynaecologists (RCOG; 1982) and the RCOG/Royal College of General Practitioners (RCGP; 1981) have now recommended that there should be functional integration of care in this way, and therefore that all women should at least be seen by a consultant obstetrician. This may be justified by noting that the obstetric caseload of general practitioners will not usually exceed 30 per annum (Hall et al 1985a, Wilkes et al 1975); this is about 20–40 times less than that of obstetricians who may therefore be better at detecting problems. However, the hypothesis that obstetricians would be more expert has rarely been tested. Roseveare & Bull (1982) could identify no improvement in the outcome when routine referral of low-risk women was the practice. Hall et al (1985a) report direct evidence that obstetricians are more successful than general practitioners at diagnosing smallness for gestational age, and indirect evidence that they less often miss malpresentations. On the other hand general practitioner care was certainly preferred by women.

The contribution of midwives to antenatal care in Britain has frequently been an unsatisfactory one — chaperoning doctors and checking blood pressures in task-oriented clinics, with no personal responsibility. However, there has been much more interest recently in community antenatal care with midwives conducting antenatal visits independently, as in Sighthill in Edinburgh (McKee 1984), Oxford (Bull 1985) and Aberdeen (Hall et al 1985a). Midwives rarely work entirely alone in Britain, though this idea has been espoused (Wilmott 1984) as part of a programme in which teams of midwives conduct antenatal delivery and postnatal care. A recent evaluation (British Medical Journal Medical News 1986) showed excellent results.

There is also a wide variety of settings in which antenatal care takes place. Specialist care is usually provided in hospital clinics but some specialists may visit rural or urban areas outside the hospital in order to provide care which is more convenient for pregnant women. This has been done in Aberdeen, Oxford and many other centres for several decades and has recently been evaluated as an innovation in Glasgow and apparently favourably received by women. Community specialist care of this sort is sometimes provided in the general practitioner surgery or health centre (Zander et al 1978, McKee 1984, Taylor 1984). Clearly this would be possible only in a group practice in which one session at least was set aside for antenatal care. Antenatal care is sometimes offered in the woman's own home to women who are booked for home confinement under midwife care. Domiciliary visits are also used in Aberdeen for women who have defaulted from hospital visits, and for women who have been found to have raised blood pressure in hospital clinic, but where it is suspected that it may be a false positive result due to anxiety.

There is no scientific basis for a strong preference for any of the above styles of care. Women's views are of great importance but there may sometimes be a trade-off between pleasant relaxed care and safety.

How often should normal women attend? Until about 10 years ago it was apparently accepted in Britain that the 1929 pattern must be adhered to. A British Medical Journal leading article (1978) suggested that some traditional components should be left out to make way for technological innovations. Chamberlain (1978) suggested a reduction in routine care in the middle trimester of pregnancy as so little seemed to happen at that time. Edstrom (1980) deplored the fact that in developing countries midwives were still being taught that each pregnant woman must be seen at least 10 times and according to fixed schedule, rather than being trained to screen the pregnant population for at-risk women on whom they should concentrate. The first Aberdeen study (Hall et al 1980) introduced the concept of productivity which was analysed in respect of diagnosis of intrauterine growth retardation (widely recognized as a serious condition responsible for many adverse outcomes, Chiswick 1985), pre-eclampsia — an important cause of maternal and perinatal mortality — and malpresentation, a condition with implications for place and mode of delivery.

Productivity was defined as the proportion of routine visits which resulted in identification for the first time of any of these problems (for example, pre-eclampsia detection would be made by discovering a diastolic blood pressure of >90 mmHg). With a condition such as pre-eclampsia, which is known to be commoner in late pregnancy, productivity would of course increase with gestation if visits were equally frequent throughout pregnancy; but since visits increase from monthly to weekly under standard care the productivity of late visits is thereby reduced. The acceptable level of productivity must depend on the severity of the condition being sought (Redman 1982); whether any useful interventions exist; what resources are available and the costs of applying the intervention to the false positive cases. However, it is important to stress that this was the first report of what productivity actually was. The data may be used to plan for reduced visits for low-risk women, or indeed more visits for high-risk women. It seems unlikely that the best use of professional expertise could be in continuing to trawl the whole pregnant population at such frequent intervals. The Aberdeen work provided a numerical basis for rational recommendations about possible schedules which could be more productive.

Taking the example of pre-eclampsia it was found that productivity did not exceed 1% in multigravidae until after term and in primigravidae not until after 34 weeks. It was therefore recommended that normal (i.e. previously normotensive) multigravidae should be seen much less frequently (at 12, 22, 30, 36 and 40 weeks, Table 15.2) while primigravidae who have a higher risk of pre-eclampsia should in addition be seen at 26, 34, 38 and 41 weeks (Table 15.3). It was also proposed that high-risk women (the obese, those

Table 15.2 Minimum care for normal multigravidae

Gestation in weeks	Main purposes of visit*
12	History and examination, clarification of uncertain gestation, identification of risk factors for antenatal care and confinement. Advice on diet, drugs, work and exercise
16	Alpha-fetoprotein screening and/or ultrasonic scan
22	Fundal height, baseline weight
30	Fundal height, weight gain: identification of high risk for intrauterine growth retardation and pre-eclampsia
36	Fundal height, weight gain, identification of malpresentation
40	Assessment of need for induction

* Blood pressure and urinalysis at every visit.

Table 15.3 Additional visits for minimum care for normal primigravidae (to be added to the schedule for multigravidae; see Table 15.2)

Gestation in weeks	Main purpose of visit
26	Blood pressure, urinalysis, discussion of delivery and feeding
34	Blood pressure, urinalysis, discussion of delivery and feeding
38	Blood pressure, urinalysis, discussion of delivery and feeding
41	Blood pressure, urinalysis, discussion of delivery and feeding

with a high weight gain, or a strong family history of pre-eclampsia) should be seen even more frequently. This schedule was recommended by the RCOG (1982).

The evaluation of the innovation of fewer visits was complicated by the fact that there seemed to be a secular reduction in the incidence of pre-eclampsia. However, productivity did increase, at least in primigravidae, but without exposing women to any additional risk. In fact the proportion which presented for the first time during or after labour (i.e. who had not been identified by antenatal care) fell from 30 to 17%, so it appeared that the new schedules were satisfactory in this respect.

Productivity was also assessed in respect of diagnosis of smallness for gestational age which may be due to intra-uterine growth retardation. Productivity was always less than 1% and only 44% of cases were detected, with 2.5 false positives for each true positive. This was not improved by the new schedule of care, although those providing care had been alerted to the significance of previous obstetric history, smoking and poor weight gain. There are of course reports of much higher detection rates of smallness for gestational age by two-stage ultrasound examination, but since it has not been shown that such a programme results in any improvement in outcome (Neilson et al 1984, Hepburn & Rosenberg 1986) it cannot yet be recommended. What was quite clear from the Aberdeen study was that 30 weeks' gestation was not especially suitable for clinical detection of smallness for gestational age, although it might be suitable for assessment of weight gain.

Detection of malpresentation is not useful before the last 2 months of pregnancy. It was suggested by the Aberdeen workers that since fundal height assessment would be useful only with a reasonable interval between visits and since malpresentation assessment was not a priority early on, the abdomen need not be palpated at every visit. However, this was almost impossible to implement as neither the health providers nor the women thought it a good idea. The hypothesis that general practitioners would be as successful as hospital staff at detecting breeches was not confirmed (perhaps not surprising, as each general practitioner may only see a breech presentation once every 2 years or so).

The general conclusion of the Aberdeen study was that it was possible to make changes in the antenatal programme and to reduce visits for normal, i.e. low-risk, women without endangering them. Fears that there would be a major increase in the numbers of women attending their general practitioners with worries and complaints proved groundless but women did not particularly like the reduction in visits, perhaps because they suspected the change was part of the cuts in health service and also because information booklets etc. always described the standard package. However, the idea of setting out the main objectives of each antenatal visit is one that appeals greatly to the innovator and evaluator, since such specification of aims allows:

1. Rational assessment as to which health professional has the most appropriate skills to carry out the visit.
2. Subsequent analysis as to whether the objectives were fulfilled.
3. An opportunity to inform women (as suggested by Coope & Scott 1982) about the purposes of the visit so that they may take an intelligent interest in the findings.

The Aberdeen schedules (somewhat modified and expanded) have been taken up and advocated with great enthusiasm by Marsh (1985) whose approach involves full participation by midwives, and indeed the whole general practice team. Such changes should allow consultations to be more relaxed and unhurried. It was not possible to show in the Aberdeen study that this had occurred, but this was attributed to a very large increase in birth numbers with consequent pressure upon staff and facilities (Lancet 1986). Another factor may be that specialist obstetricians do not find women without problems very interesting and most of their needs may be much better met by midwives and family doctors.

Another innovation which may promote doctor–woman communication as well as interprofessional communication is to put women in charge of their own case records. This has of course recently been proposed for other fields in medicine and seems to have caused great alarm amongst physicians (Short 1986) and surgeons (Ross 1986). However, it is not such a shocking idea for obstetricians, as co-operation cards (containing at least a summary of all the relevant information) have been in use for years, and women have also been carrying their complete case record in some areas. This method has great advantages in rural areas as it ensures that the case record always accompanies the woman whenever she sees the midwife, general practitioner or specialist and when she is admitted in labour. Recent evaluations in the form of controlled trials (Draper et al 1986, Elbourne 1986, Lowitt et al 1986) have shown that fears that women would lose their notes were not borne out; mothers were on the whole positive, and anxiety was not enhanced. Access to and responsibility for notes should be given to women as this is in keeping with the modern view that women can and should have more respect for and control over their own pregnancies.

This chapter has dealt largely with outpatient antenatal care but it is interesting that recent studies have suggested that some forms of inpatient care (e.g. bedrest) are of little or no value (Lancet Leading Article 1981, Saunders et al 1985) and outpatient care is becoming more popular in pre-eclampsia (Matthews 1977, Feeney 1984). Thus the interface between outpatient and inpatient care is changing.

The trend towards scepticism and rational analysis of time-honoured practices in obstetrics should be welcomed. The possibility that social interventions may be more necessary and important than medical ones (Chalmers 1985) should engender humility in obstetricians.

REFERENCES

Abdul-Karim R N 1984 Women workers at higher risk of reproductive hazards. In: Chamberlain G (ed) Pregnant women at work. Royal Society of Medicine, London

Bakketeig L S, Hoffman H J 1981 Epidemiology of preterm birth: results from a longitudinal study of births in Norway. In: Elder M G, Hendricks C H (eds) Preterm labour. Butterworths International Medical Review, London

Barron S L, Thomson A M, Phillips P R 1977 Home and hospital confinement in Newcastle upon Tyne 1960–69. British Journal of Obstetrics and Gynaecology 84: 401–441

Blondel B, Pusch D, Schmide E 1985 Some characteristics of antenatal care in 13 European countries. British Journal of Obstetrics and Gynaecology 92: 565–568

British Medical Journal Leading Article 1978 Rethinking antenatal care. British Medical Journal 4: 1177–1178

British Medical Journal Medical News 1986 The benefits of midwife care. British Medical Journal 292: 1019

Buekens P, Delvoye P, Wallast E, Robyn C 1984 Epidemiology of pregnancies with unknown last menstrual period. Journal of Epidemiology and Community Health 38: 79–80

Bull M J V 1980 Ten years experience in a general practice obstetric unit. Journal of the Royal College of General Practitioners 30: 208–215

Bull M J V 1985 Different settings for interapartum care: the integrated general practitioner unit. In: March G N (ed) Modern obstetrics in general practice. Oxford Medical Publications, Oxford

Butler N R, Alberman E D 1969 Perinatal problems. The second report of the British perinatal mortality survey. Livingstone, Edinburgh

Butler N R, Bonham D G 1963 Perinatal mortality. The first report of British perinatal mortality survey. Livingstone, Edinburgh

Campbell D M, Gillmer M D G 1982 Nutrition in pregnancy. Proceedings of the tenth study group of the Royal College of Obstetricians and Gynaecologists. RCOG, London

Campbell D M, MacGillivray I, Carr-Hill R 1985 Pre-eclampsia in a second pregnancy. British Journal of Obstetrics and Gynaecology 92: 131–140

Carr-Hill R A, Hall M H 1985 The repetition of spontaneous preterm labour. British Journal of Obstetrics and Gynaecology 92: 921–928

Chalmers I 1985 Short, Black, Baird, Himsworth and social class differences in fetal and neonatal mortality rates. British Medical Journal 291: 231–233

Chamberlain G 1978 A re-examination of antenatal care. Journal of the Royal Society of Medicine 71: 662–668

Chamberlain G 1980a The pre-pregnancy Clinic. British Medical Journal 281: 29–30

Chamberlain G 1980b When do pregnant women attend for antenatal care? British Medical Journal 281: 515

Chamberlain R, Chamberlain G, Howlett B, Claireaux A 1975 British births 1970, vol 1. Heinemann Medical, London

Chamberlain G, Philip E, Howlett B, Masters K 1978 British births 1970, vol II. Heinemann Medical, London

Chiswick M L 1980 Antenatal care and high risk babies. British Medical Journal 280: 561

Chiswick M L 1985 Intrauterine growth retardation. British Medical Journal 291: 845–848

Chng P K, Hall M H 1982 Antenatal prediction of urinary tract infection in pregnancy. British Journal of Obstetrics and Gynaecology 89: 8–11

Chng P K, Hall M H, MacGillivray I 1980 An audit of antenatal care: the value of the first antenatal visit. British Medical Journal 281: 1184–1186

Clarke M, Clayton D G 1983 Quality of obstetric care provided for Asian immigrants in Leicestershire. British Medical Journal 286: 621–623

Coope J K, Scott A V 1982 A programme for shared maternity and child care. British Medical Journal 284: 1936–1937

Coronary Drug Project Research Group 1980 Influence of adherence to treatment and response of cholesterol on mortality in the Coronary Drug Project Group. New England Journal of Medicine 303: 1038–1041

Cuckle H S, Wald N J 1982 In: Wald N J (ed) Principles of screening in antenatal and neonatal screening. Oxford Medical Publications, Oxford

Dixon E A 1982 Review of maternity patients suitable for home delivery. British Medical Journal 284: 1753–1755

Douglas J W B 1948 Maternity services in Great Britain. Oxford University Press, Oxford

Draper J, Field S, Thomas H, Hare M J 1986 Should women carry their antenatal records? British Medical Journal 292: 603

Durnin J V G A, McKillop F M, Grant S, Fitzgerald G 1985 Is nutritional status endangered by virtually no extra intake during pregnancy? Lancet ii: 823–825

Edstrom K 1980 How can health services be made more relevant to the needs of mothers and children? In: Philpott R H (ed) Maternity services in the developing world — what the community needs. RCOG, London, pp 351–359

Elbourne D 1986 Patients' access to records. Lancet ii: 106

Fedrick J, Anderson A B M 1976 Factors associated with preterm birth. British Journal of Obstetrics and Gynaecology 83: 342–348

Feeney J G 1984 Hypertension in pregnancy managed at home by community midwives. British Medical Journal 288: 1046–1047

Garcia J 1982 Women's views of antenatal care. In: Enkin M C, Chalmers I (eds) Effectiveness and satisfaction in antenatal care. Spastics International Medical Publications/Heinemann, London

Gilligan M 1980 Perinatal enquiries at district level. In: Chalmers I, McIlwaine G (eds) Perinatal audit and surveillance. RCOG, London, pp 148–158

Graham H, McKee L 1979 The first months of motherhood, vol 4. Medical care report on a Health Education Council Project, University of York

Grant A, Mohide P 1982 Screening and diagnostic tests in antenatal care. In: Enkin M, Chalmers I (eds) Effectiveness and satisfaction in antenatal care. Spastics International Medical Publications/Heinemann, London

Hall M H, Carr-Hill R A 1985 The significance of uncertain gestation for obstetric outcome. British Journal of Obstetrics and Gynaecology 92: 452–460

Hall M H, Chng P K, MacGillivray I 1980 Is routine antenatal care worthwhile? Lancet ii: 78–80

Hall M H, McIntyre S, Porter M 1985a Antenatal care assessed. Aberdeen University Press, Aberdeen

Hall M H, Halliwell R, Carr-Hill R A 1985b Concomitant and repeated happenings in the third stage of labour. British Journal of Obstetrics and Gynaecology 92: 732–738

Hepburn M, Rosenberg K 1986 An audit of the detection and management of small-for-gestational age babies. British Journal of Obstetrics and Gynaecology 93: 212–216

James D K 1977 Patients transferred in labour from general practitioners' maternity units. Journal of the Royal College of General Practitioners 27: 414–418

Keirse M J N C 1984 Epidemiology and aetiology of the growth retarded baby. In: Howie P W, Patel N B (eds) Clinics in obstetrics and gynaecology: the small baby. Saunders, London

Kentucky Coalition for Maternal and Child Health 1983 Kentucky youth advocates inc: healthy mothers and babies: pay now or pay later. Lexington, Kentucky

Klein M, Lloyd I, Redman C, Bull M, Turnbull A C 1983 A comparison of low risk pregnant women booked for delivery in two systems of care — shared care (consultant) and integrated general practitioner unit. II Labour and delivery management and neonatal outcome. British Journal of Obstetrics and Gynaecology 90: 123–128

Kessner D M 1973 Institute of medicine: infant death. An analysis by maternal risk and health care. Contrasts in health status, vol 1. National Academy of Sciences, Washington D C

Lancet Leading Article 1981 Bed rest in obstetrics Lancet i: 1137–1138

Lancet Leading Article 1986 Antenatal care assessed. Lancet i: 1072–1074

Lewis E 1982 Attendance for antenatal care. British Medical Journal 284: 788

Lewis B V, Tipton R H, Sloper I M S 1978 Changing pattern in a general practitioner obstetric unit. British Medical Journal 1: 484–485

Lilford R J, Chard T 1985 The routine use of ultrasound. British Journal of Obstetrics and Gynaecology 92: 434–436

Lowitt A, Zander L I, James C E, Foot S, Swan A V, Reynolds A 1986 Why not give mothers their own notes? St Thomas' maternity case notes study. Northcote Trust, London

Mamelle N 1983 Travail et grossesse. Prévenir 69: 724–727

Marsh G N 1985 New programme of antenatal care in general practice. British Medical Journal 291: 646–648

Matthews D D 1977 A randomised controlled trial of bed rest and sedation or normal activity and non-sedation in the management of non-

albuminuric hypertension in late pregnancy. British Journal of Obstetrics and Gynaecology 44: 108–114
McIntyre S 1981 Expectations and experiences of pregnancy. Report of a prospective study of married primigravidae. Institute of Medical Sociology occasional paper no. 5, University of Aberdeen
McKee I 1984 Community antenatal care. In: Zander L, Chamberlain G (eds) Pregnancy care for the 1980s. Royal Society of Medicine, London
McKinlay J B 1981 From 'promising report' to 'standard procedure'. Seven stages in the career of a medical innovation. Milbank Memorial Fund Quarterly Health and Society 59: 374–411
Morehead M A, Donaldson R S, Seravalli M R 1971 Comparisons between OEO neighborhood health centers and other health care providers of ratings of the quality of health care. American Journal of Public Health 61: 1294–1306
Murphy J F, Dauncey M, Newcombe R, Garcia J, Elboume D 1984 Employment in pregnancy: prevalence, maternal characteristics, perinatal outcome. Lancet i: 1163–1166
Neilson J P, Munjauja S P, Whitfield C R 1984 Screening for small for dates fetuses: a controlled trial. British Medical Journal 289: 1179–1182
Newcombe R G 1985 A statistical view of risk factors. In: Marsh G N (ed) Modern obstetrics in general practice. Oxford Medical Publications, Oxford
Oakley A 1982 The origins and development of antenatal care. In: Enkin M, Chalmers I (eds) Effectiveness and satisfaction in antenatal care. Spastics International Medical Publications/Heinemann, London
O'Brien M, Smith C 1981 Women's visits and experiences of antenatal care. The Practitioner 225: 123–125
Papiernik E 1984 Prediction of the preterm baby. In: Howie P W, Patel N B (eds) Clinics in obstetrics and gynaecology. The small baby. Saunders, London
Pearson J 1982 Is early antenatal attendance so important? British Medical Journal 284: 1064–1065
Preventing Low Birthweight 1985 Institute of Medicine, National Academy Press, Washington D C
Redman C 1982 Screening for pre-eclampsia. In: Enkin M L, Chalmers I (eds) Effectiveness and satisfaction in antenatal care. Spastics International Medical Publications/Heinemann Medical, London
Reid M E, McIlwaine G M 1980 Consumer opinion of a hospital antenatal clinic. Social Science and Medicine 14A: 363–368
Richmond G A 1977 An analysis of 3199 patients booked for delivery in general practitioner obstetric units. Journal of the Royal College of General Practitioners 27: 406–413
Rooth G 1979 Better perinatal health in Sweden. Lancet ii: 1170–1172
Roseveare M P, Bull M J V 1982 General practitioner obstetrics; two styles of care. British Medical Journal 284: 958–960
Ross A P 1986 The case against showing patients their records. British Medical Journal 292: 578
RCOG 1982 Report of the RCOG working party on antenatal and intrapartum care. RCOG, London
RCOG/RCGP 1981 Report on training for obstetrics and gynaecology for general practitioners by a joint working party of the RCOG and RCGP. RCOG, London
Saunders M C, Dick J S, Brown I M, McPherson K, Chalmers I 1985 The effects of hospital admission for bed rest on the duration of twin pregnancy: a randomised trial Lancet ii: 793–795
Sexton M, Hebel J R 1984 A clinical trial of change in maternal smoking and its effect on birthweight. Journal of the American Medical Association 251: 911–916
Short D 1986 Some consequences of granting patients access to consultants' records. Lancet i: 1316–1318
Short report 1980 Second report from the Social Services Committee Session 1979–1980. Perinatal and neonatal mortality session, vol 1. HMSO, London
Simpson H, Walker G 1980 When do pregnant women attend for antenatal care? British Medical Journal 2: 104–106
Taylor R W 1984 Community based specialist obstetric services. In: Zander L, Chamberlain G (eds) Pregnancy care for the 1980s. Royal Society of Medicine/McMillan, London
Tejani N A 1982 Recurrence of intrauterine growth retardation. American Journal of Obstetrics and Gynaecology 59: 329–331
Thacker S B 1985 Quality of controlled trials. The case of imaging ultrasound in obstetrics: a review. British Journal of Obstetrics and Gynaecology 92: 437–444
Wilkes E, Dixon R A, Knowelden J 1975 Modern obstetrics and the general practitioner. British Medical Journal iv: 687–690
Wilmott J 1984 The community midwife and domiciliary confinements. In: Zander L, Chamberlain G (eds) Pregnancy care for the 1980s. Royal Society of Medicine, London
Zander L I, Watson M, Taylor R W, Morell D C 1978 Integration of general practitioner and specialist antenatal care. Journal of the Royal College of General Practitioners 28: 455–458

16

Alec Turnbull

Early antenatal care (up to 28 weeks)

INTRODUCTION

The object of this chapter is to describe how antenatal care is currently provided from the first visit in early pregnancy up to the 28th week. Since the arrangements for antenatal care are presently being reassessed in many UK centres, it seems best to review overall the developments and trends in antenatal care, rather than describing a single, specific regime which would give the impression of a greater uniformity than actually exists.

Chapter 15 described the development of antenatal care from its beginnings at the end of the 19th century, through a phase of increasing application to the realization in the past 20 years that for healthy, low-risk women with normal pregnancies, the benefits of hospital-based antenatal care may have been overestimated.

We have to consider how to assess the potential hazards for mother and fetus in pregnancy and how appropriate antenatal care should be provided both for low-risk women, perhaps in the community and high-risk women in specialist units. Achieving such a clearcut and apparently appropriate division of care is not so easy in practice. In low-risk women initial antenatal assessment provides a relatively poor forecast of pregnancy outcome (Chng et al 1980) and subsequent visits can fail to detect developing pathology (Hall et al 1980). Nevertheless, significant problems can be detected at the first antenatal visit. The overall standard of care during pregnancy must surely be improved by close collaboration between the primary care team and the hospital and by a continuing review of results.

The aims and objects of antenatal care are:

1. To assess the health and well-being of the mother and her fetus and make appropriate arrangements for care during pregnancy and labour.
2. To predict and, if possible, prevent or detect early and manage effectively maternal or fetal complications developing during pregnancy.
3. To help prepare the mother and her partner for the experience of childbirth and for the responsibilities of bringing up the child.
4. To provide appropriate health screening and health education.

THE PATTERNS OF ANTENATAL CARE

The usually accepted pattern of antenatal examination is of increasingly frequent assessment in late pregnancy, when the major complications such as maternal hypertensive disease or fetal intrauterine growth retardation become apparent. The pattern of monthly visits to 28 weeks, fortnightly to 36 weeks and then weekly to delivery was first recommended by the Ministry of Health in 1929 according to Hall et al (1985). In practice, this entails at least 12 to 14 visits, probably more than is required for healthy women with normal pregnancies.

Shared antenatal care

For many women, it is convenient for antenatal care to be provided partly by the family doctor and partly by the hospital. In low-risk mothers, family doctors and midwives can provide the majority of care and hospital visits are kept to a minimum. Even in high-risk cases, the patient should be cared for as much as possible by her own doctor and midwife.

Place of delivery

Nowadays in the UK, 99% of women are confined in an institution (hospital, general practitioner (GP) unit or private maternity unit). While home confinement can be a rewarding and satisfying experience for a healthy mother with a normal obstetric history when all goes well, unforeseeable major complications can only too suddenly turn it into a catastrophe. The safest place for women to be delivered must be a well equipped maternity unit with expert staff. This expertise should include not only technical and clinical skill but also an understanding of the social and psychological aspects of childbirth.

Initial assessment: the booking visit

The first antenatal visit is most important. Assessment must be comprehensive, for the findings determine the initial plan for care during pregnancy and confinement. Women should be informed before they attend that this first visit will be longer than subsequent visits and advised approximately how long it is likely to last. In some districts, all pregnant women have their first assessment at the hospital clinic. Women who wish to be cared for by their own practitioner can then be referred back to him or her. In other centres, family doctors themselves may book suitable patients for confinement in the unit, guided by a checklist of criteria for safety. These patients are a minority in most districts and most patients are referred for confinement in hospital. The second approach is satisfactory when the GP maternity unit is situated in the consultant hospital, for communication is quick and easy and transfer, if necessary, easily arranged. Isolated GP units are less satisfactory, for outcome in patients transferred from them is poor (Butler & Bonham 1963). Women booked for isolated units must therefore be healthy women with normal obstetric histories.

Ideally, the initial assessment should be conducted during the first trimester, the optimum time for establishing objectively the duration of pregnancy clinically. Since chorion villus sampling enables many fetal anomalies to be detected by 8–10 weeks' gestation (see Chapters 21–23), early referral, if necessary by telephone, is essential, while procedures such as cervical cerclage (14 weeks) or percutaneous placental biopsy (12–16 weeks) or amniocentesis (16 weeks) are less urgent.

Assessment procedure

At the initial visit, a full history is taken, clinical examination performed and appropriate investigations arranged.

History

Present pregnancy. Since the woman is usually most concerned about her present pregnancy, she should be asked how she is feeling, and if she has any symptoms such as nausea, vomiting, pain or bleeding. The obstetrician should also find out her expectations for pregnancy, labour and delivery and the baby and about any anxieties she may have in relation to previous confinements. She may be worried about induction of labour, fetal monitoring or epidural anaesthesia, for example, and having an opportunity to express her concern at this early stage of pregnancy is usually helpful.

Since women tend to see the outcome of pregnancy as successful when they achieve the experience they hope for, taking time at the first visit or at any visit to find out what she hopes for in pregnancy and childbirth helps the obstetrician to provide the type of care the woman wants and provides an opportunity to discuss potential problems realistically with women whose expectations may be unrealistic because they are in poor health or have a bad obstetric history. Much of this may have been done at a prepregnancy consultation.

In recent years, pregnant women have requested more information about their pregnancy, more discussion with their obstetrician about the options for management and the opportunity to describe their own preferences. Pregnant women therefore need to be adequately informed about pregnancy and childbirth and should be advised about suitable books, antenatal classes and discussion sessions about normal and abnormal pregnancy progress, as well as about films or videos, to ensure that they are adequately informed and able to express a preference when management decisions are discussed.

Menstrual history. In women with regular menstrual periods, a certain last menstrual period (LMP) enables the expected date of delivery (EDD) to be calculated with reasonable accuracy. Pregnancy is at full term 40 weeks or 280 days from the first day of the LMP. Although the EDD is most easily established from the LMP by use of a simple gestation calculator, in practice it is often calculated from Naegele's rule; add 7 days to the first day of the LMP and then count back 3 months or add 9 months (for example, with LMP beginning on 15 June the EDD will be 22 March of the following year).

To be sure that the calculated duration of pregnancy is correct, the details of the menstrual history must be considered, since the EDD calculated depends on the assumption that ovulation occurs 2 weeks after the LMP. The date of the LMP is uncertain in about 20% of women and even if the date is certain, the blood loss may have been scanty, implying that pregnancy could have occurred earlier and that the presumed LMP was actually a threatened abortion. In some women, the intermenstrual interval may be more or less than 28 days and since ovulation usually occurs 14 days before the next period, a prolonged intermenstrual interval implies a later EDD than calculated from Naegele's rule, while a shorter interval can mean an earlier than calculated EDD. If the LMP immediately followed stopping oral contraception, subsequent ovulation may have been considerably delayed without further menstruation so that the calculated LMP date indicates too early an EDD for the real duration of pregnancy.

Sometimes the duration of pregnancy can be calculated precisely when conception must have followed an isolated act of coitus. The date on which a pregnancy test first became positive is of little help in confirming the duration of pregnancy.

Nevertheless, the uncertainty about early pregnancy duration, allied with the need to perform certain investigations at specific times in pregnancy, encourages obstetricians to offer an ultrasound scan at booking to be sure that fetal size is in keeping with the duration of pregnancy and that the fetus is single, living and apparently normal.

Previous obstetric history. Since obstetric complications tend to recur, a knowledge of the outcome of previous pregnancies is essential for the obstetrician. While most women have normal obstetric histories, a few seem to develop recurrent complications in each pregnancy and require expert management. For each previous pregnancy, therefore, the information described below has to be obtained. (When the patient's previous confinements have been elsewhere, details of the history should be obtained by writing to the units involved.)

1. The date and place of delivery.
2. Length of gestation: Was the baby delivered at term? If preterm, at how many weeks' gestation and in what circumstances? Did the pregnancy end in abortion and if so, was curettage performed or blood transfused? If pregnancy ended in the mid-trimester, did spontaneous rupture of the membrances occur, suggesting an incompetent cervix or a uterine abnormality?
3. Birthweight: Any unduly low birthweight (<2.5 kg) in previous pregnancies indicates an increased risk in this pregnancy of prematurity, intrauterine growth retardation or fetal abnormality. An unduly heavy previous baby indicates an increased risk of abnormal carbohydrate intolerance in the mother, as well as an increased risk of difficult delivery with shoulder dystocia at delivery if there is another large baby.
4. Fetal outcome: Were previous infants normal at birth and in good condition? Have they developed normally or have handicaps become apparent? Was resuscitation required? Did any baby require transfer to a neonatal unit?
5. Onset and duration of labour: Was labour of spontaneous onset? If induced, why? Exceptionally short or very long previous labours may recur.
6. Type of delivery: Was the baby delivered spontaneously, by forceps or by Caesarean section? Was the presentation cephalic or breech? Was episiotomy performed? What analgesia was provided? How does the mother assess her previous childbirth experience?
7. Pregnancy complications: Did hypertensive disease develop during pregnancy? Was there any antepartum haemorrhage? Was any medical or surgical treatment required?
8. Labour complications: Did labour progress normally or was it augmented and if so, by what method? If Caesarean section was performed, was radiological pelvimetry performed postpartum? Were the hypertensive problems during labour or haemorrhage during or after delivery? Was blood transfusion required?
9. Postpartum complications: Was there any puerperal infection or pyrexia? Was the infection in the uterus, the breasts or elsewhere? Were there any thromboembolic complications?
10. Infant feeding: Was the baby breastfed and for how long?

Medical history. The possibility of pre-existing disease in the cardiovascular, gastrointestinal, endocrine or other systems should be established, since such diseases may be worsened by pregnancy or adversely affect the pregnancy.

Nowadays, most serious organic diseases will have been detected before pregnancy, but occasionally pregnancy may unmask previously unsuspected disorders such as latent diabetes, mitral stenosis or the lupus anticoagulant.

Surgical history. Previous gynaecological operations should be noted, especially those involving the cervix, such as cone biopsy, or late therapeutic abortion by dilatation and evacuation. Obviously, the other surgical procedures may have a bearing on pregnancy and should be noted.

Family history. A family history of diabetes may be an important pointer to the presence of a diabetic state developing during pregnancy, while a family history of hypertensive disease, tuberculosis, psychiatric disorder or inherited disease may indicate an increased risk to the patient or her baby.

A family history of inherited disease may necessitate expert genetic counselling combined with various diagnostic techniques for prenatal diagnosis, which are becoming increasingly sophisticated and effective. Amniocentesis, chorion villus sampling or percutaneous placental biopsy combined with expert ultrasound scanning may be used for the detection of fetal abnormalities such as Down's syndrome. Testing for Down's syndrome is indicated in women over 34 years and is strongly indicated in women of 40 years or more. Of course, a wide range of fetal abnormalities can be detected by such methods (see Chapters 21–23).

Physical examination. Physical examination should be thorough. The patient's height, weight and blood pressure should be measured. A mid-stream urine sample should be examined for protein and glucose and a clean-catch sample should be sent to detect significant bacteriuria (more than 10^5 organisms per ml). Physical abnormality should be looked for and the cardiovascular and respiratory systems and breasts examined. The dental state should be carefully assessed because gingivitis is common in pregnancy and further dental care is often needed. Abdominal and pelvic examination is carried out to assess the size of the uterus and exclude any other abnormality in the pelvis such as uterine fibroids or an ovarian cyst. Ideally, a speculum examination should also be performed and a cervical smear taken together with vaginal and cervical swabs to exclude infection. While pelvic examination does not cause abortion, women who have had bleeding earlier in the pregnancy or a history of first-trimester abortion in previous pregnancies seem instinctively to wish to avoid pelvic examination, at least until the risk of abortion has receded, after 16 weeks. The obstetrician should agree to this provided there are no strong reasons for an earlier examination.

The following laboratory tests should be carried out routinely at the initial assessment:

1. Full blood count.
2. ABO and rhesus grouping.
3. Rhesus antibody titre in rhesus-negative women.
4. Hepatitis antibodies.
5. Serological tests for syphilis.
6. Rubella antibodies. Women not immune to rubella are at potential risk of infection during pregnancy and should be offered vaccination after delivery of the infant and given contraceptive advice to ensure avoidance of pregnancy for at least 12 weeks after that.
7. Haemoglobin electrophoresis in patients of African or Mediterranean origin.
8. Mid-stream urine culture or slide test for bacteriuria.
9. Cervical cytology if no smear has been taken for 3 years.

Some UK obstetric units nowadays routinely offer ultrasound scanning of the pregnancy at the initial assessment visit. This provides reliable information about the size, gestational age and well-being of the fetus, detects multiple pregnancy, a blighted ovum or an anembryonic pregnancy. Normally, the fetus can be seen moving and the fetal heart beating by 8 weeks or even earlier. Occasionally fetal death, hydatidiform mole or other fetal abnormality is detected.

When the duration of pregnancy has been reliably established, arrangements can be made for the serum alpha-fetoprotein (AFP) to be measured between 16 and 18 weeks. The use of serum AFP for detecting neural tube or other fetal defects is described in Chapter 19, for detecting chromosomal abnormalities in Chapter 21 and for predicting preterm birth and intrauterine growth retardation in Chapter 24.

Risk assessment and further management options. Since initial assessment is so important it should be performed by an experienced obstetrician. A checklist may be used to ensure consistent detection of risk factors; Figure 16.1 is an example of such a checklist (Boddy et al 1982).

Healthy multiparous women with no pre-existing disease and whose previous pregnancies have progressed to normal delivery of healthy mature infants are at low risk of any serious complications in subsequent pregnancies. For such women, care should be provided as far as possible by their own general practitioner and community midwife. They are very suitable for confinement in a GP maternity unit, especially one situated within a consultant obstetric unit.

RISK CARD

NAME: .... **DOCTOR:**..............................

BOOKING HISTORY
- Age less than 18 yrs.
- Age over 38 yrs.
- Primigravid age 30 yrs. or more
- Parity =/ more than 5.

L.M.P. DETAILS
- L.M.P uncertain ± 2 weeks
- Pill stopped 1 or 2 periods before L.M.P.
- Cycle length prior to L.M.P. greater than 30 days
- IUCD in situ / on Pill after conception.
- Out of wedlock pregnancy
- Vaginal bleeding since L.M.P.

PAST OBSTETRIC HISTORY
- SB / NND
- Small for dates (< 10th Centile)
- Large for dates (> 90th Centile)
- Fetal abnormality ....
- Antibodies in previous pregnancy
- Hypertension / Eclampsia
- Termination of Pregnancy / Spon. Abortion x 2
- Premature labour (20 - 37 weeks)
- Previous Cervical Suture
- Previous Caesarean Section
- P.P.H. / M.R.O.P.
- Labour of less than 4 hours

MATERNAL HEALTH
- Chronic Illness / Drugs ....
- Hypertension / Proteinuria
- Infertility with Medical Advice
- Uterine Anomaly including Fibroids
- Smoking 10/day at Conception
- Soc. Sec. Benefits
- Isolated at Home
- Family History of Diabetes/Fetal Abnormality......................
- Completed by.. Date.........................

BOOKING EXAMINATION
- B.P. = / more than 140/90
- Maternal Weight = / more 85 kg.
- Maternal Weight = / less than 45 kg.
- Maternal Height = / less than 5 ft.
- Cardiac Murmur Detected / Referred
- Uterus large / small for dates
- Other Pelvic Mass Detected
- Blood Group Rh. Negative
- Completed by.. Date......................

Fig. 16.1 Checklist of antenatal risk factors at initial assessment. Adapted from Boddy et al (1982).

The checklist shown in Figure 16.1 shows that risk factors at initial assessment can be grouped under five headings. The level of risk can be subsequently influenced by factors arising in pregnancy, shown in Figure 16.2 (Boddy et al 1982). Thus risk factors can be classified as follows:

1. Factors relating to age and parity.
2. Factors indicating that gestational age is uncertain.
3. Factors in the previous obstetric history which relate to the main causes of fetal mortality and morbidity, including fetal malformation, preterm birth or intrauterine growth retardation.
4. Factors relating to maternal health problems with potentially adverse effects on pregnancy outcome. These would include particularly hypertension, renal or cardiovascular diseases, diabetes or rhesus disease.

FACTORS ARISING DURING PREGNANCY

Weeks of Pregnancy														
F.M. Not felt														
Hb <10 gm %														
Poor Weight Gain														
Wt. loss														
Proteinuria														
Glycosuria														
Bacilluria														
B.P. Systolic > 155														
Diastolic > 88														
Rh. Ne./Antibodies														
Uterus large for dates														
Uterus small for dates														
No increase in fundus (Zone)														
Excess liquor														
Mal presentation														
E.C.V. Successful														
Unsuccessful														
Head not engaged														
Any bleeding P.V.														
Premature labour														
Vaginal infection														
Sign when completed														
Insert Date														

Fig. 16.2 Checklist of risk factors developing during pregnancy which influence initial antenatal risk assessment. Adapted from Boddy et al (1982).

5. Factors detected at the initial assessment.
6. Factors developing during pregnancy (Fig. 16.2).

Risk assessment is an imperfect science. Complications can develop unexpectedly in a woman with a normal obstetric history, while a woman at high risk of serious complications may progress uneventfully to normal delivery. Despite such exceptions standardized methods for risk assessment should be established in each obstetric service and the method agreed by everyone involved in the service. The methods have to be agreed in district health authorities.

In practice, women at risk can be divided into those with intermediate and high risks. While there are no nationally accepted definitions for such subdivisions and all require specialist obstetric care, those at highest risk are in some units being cared for by obstetricians or physicians with special interests and expertise in fetal medicine. The Royal College of Obstetricians and Gynaecologists (1982) is promoting subspecialization and encouraging an increase in the number of fetal medicine specialists.

Women in the highest risk category include those with severe hypertensive problems, chronic renal disease, diabetes or rhesus disease of severe degree, especially with previous perinatal mortality. In such patients, sophisticated methods of investigation are required at every stage of pregnancy. In early pregnancy there is often the need for genetic counselling backed up by prenatal diagnostic techniques (see Chapters 19–23). Later in pregnancy management will involve biophysical fetal assessment techniques involving real-time and Doppler ultrasound scanning and cardiotocographic recordings of fetal heart rate in relation to fetal movements and uterine contractions (Chapter 20). These techniques can be used between 24 and 28 weeks but are more frequently used after 28 weeks. While the most seriously jeopardized fetuses have to be delivered by elective Caesarean section, fetuses at lower risk may be delivered vaginally if expert care can be provided during labour.

Further visits during pregnancy. After the initial assessment, the majority of low-risk mothers can be looked after by their own GPs during this time and the most normal and healthy women may be booked for confinement in a GP unit and have all their antenatal and intrapartum care from their own doctor and midwife. However, most women elect to be confined in hospital and their care is usually shared by the GP and the hospital obstetric team. In recent years, much thought has been given to reducing the number of potentially unnecessary hospital antenatal examinations in normal pregnancy. Hall et al (1980) suggested the format of visits shown in Table 16.1. In high-risk women, depending on the nature and severity of the risk factors, care may be shared with the GP or provided exclusively by the hospital team. In high-risk cases, antenatal visits usually have to be more frequent.

Using a checklist of the problems which could arise during pregnancy helps to ensure uniform surveillance by multiple observers. While each maternity advising committee should make its own recommendations based on local needs, Figure 16.2 illustrates the checklist for risk factors arising in pregnancy recommended by Boddy et al (1982). They also recommended the use of a symphysis–fundal height chart (Fig. 16.3). The example illustrated was developed for Oxford patients by Quaranta et al (1981). Communication between the GP and the hospital team is facilitated by a co-operation card, an example of which is shown in Figure 16.4. While the design and amount of information differs from one district to another the card should provide background information about the patient and a record of progress during pregnancy for both the GP and the hospital team.

Consumer aspects

Many women have strong views about the management of their labour and delivery and should be able to express their concerns. The obstetric team should try to ensure that any realistic expectation is achieved and that pregnant women under their care are not inhibited from discussing any concerns for fear they may be thought foolish. While it remains difficult in hospital to arrange for the patient to be seen by the same doctor at each visit, women should be informed about progress; good communication between the medical team and patient helps to reduce the extent to which apparently differing advice may be given at successive visits.

Table 16.1 Timing of antenatal examinations with shared care

Weeks' gestation	Purpose of visit	Medical staff
At 12 weeks	Initial assessment; booking for confinement; determination of gestation	Obstetrician
At 16–18 weeks	Serum alpha-fetoprotein and other blood tests	GP/midwife
At 22 weeks	Baseline weight for IUGR prediction	GP/midwife
At 26 weeks	Primigravidae only	GP/midwife
At 30 weeks	Screening for IUGR and PIH	Obstetrician
At 34 weeks	Primigravidae only	GP/midwife
At 36 weeks	Screening for malpresentation and PIH	GP/midwife
At 38 weeks	Primigravidae only	GP/midwife
At 40 weeks	Assessment for delivery	Obstetrician

IUGR = intrauterine growth retardation; PIH = pregnancy-induced hypertension.
Adapted from Hall et al (1980).

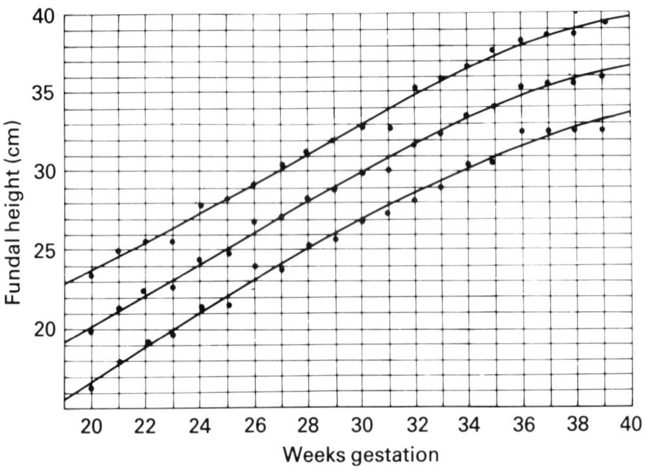

Fig. 16.3 Symphysial–fundal height chart (±1 SD). Adapted from Quaranta et al (1981).

SPECIFIC ASPECTS OF ANTENATAL CARE UP TO 28 WEEKS

Although many low-risk women need not attend hospital until after 30 weeks some abnormality may be detected before that by the GP or midwife, which will indicate referral to the specialist.

Antenatal visits

At each visit women should be asked about their general health and specifically about appetite, nausea, sickness or other gastrointestinal symptoms, abdominal pain or vaginal bleeding.

Uterine size and shape should be measured and recorded, preferably on a chart. While the variability of this measurement is well known, serial assessment of symphysis–fundal height in centimetres seems to be as sensitive as repeated ultrasonic measurement of abdominal circumference; it detects 85% of intrauterine fetal growth retardation and carries the same false positive rate, 55% (Pearce & Campbell 1983). This simple screening method is thus useful for indicating women in whom more detailed ultrasound assessment is required.

Weight gain

At each visit the women should be weighed in minimal clothing. Weight-for-height and weight gain during pregnancy are related to clinical outcome. On average, weight increases by about 0.5 kg/week between 15 and 38 weeks. The components of maternal weight gain in pregnancy are described in Chapter 10. Women within the normal range of weight-for-height who have an average weight gain tend to do best in pregnancy. Underweight women with poor weight gain during pregnancy have an increased risk of preterm birth, intrauterine fetal growth retardation or both. Excessive weight gain carries the hazards of obesity but is no longer accepted as a cause of pre-eclampsia.

Pregnant women should be encouraged to eat a good mixed diet; the ideal dietary requirements for pregnancy are considered in Chapter 10.

Blood pressure

Blood pressure should be measured at each visit. With obese patients, a large cuff may be needed to obtain accurate readings for with a normal cuff in such women the blood pressure recorded tends to be falsely high. Since blood pressure tends to fall during the middle part of pregnancy only readings before the 12th week provide a true blood pressure baseline. If, as pregnancy advances, the diastolic pressure rises by 15 mmHg above the baseline level or increases above 90 mmHg and these changes persist after a period of rest, pregnancy-induced hypertension is likely and special surveillance is required. In most cases pregnancy-induced hypertension develops after 28 weeks but in the most severe cases, it develops earlier than 28 weeks and may rapidly worsen. Ideally, blood pressure should be checked every 2 weeks in primigravidae between 24 and 30 weeks' gestation (Red-

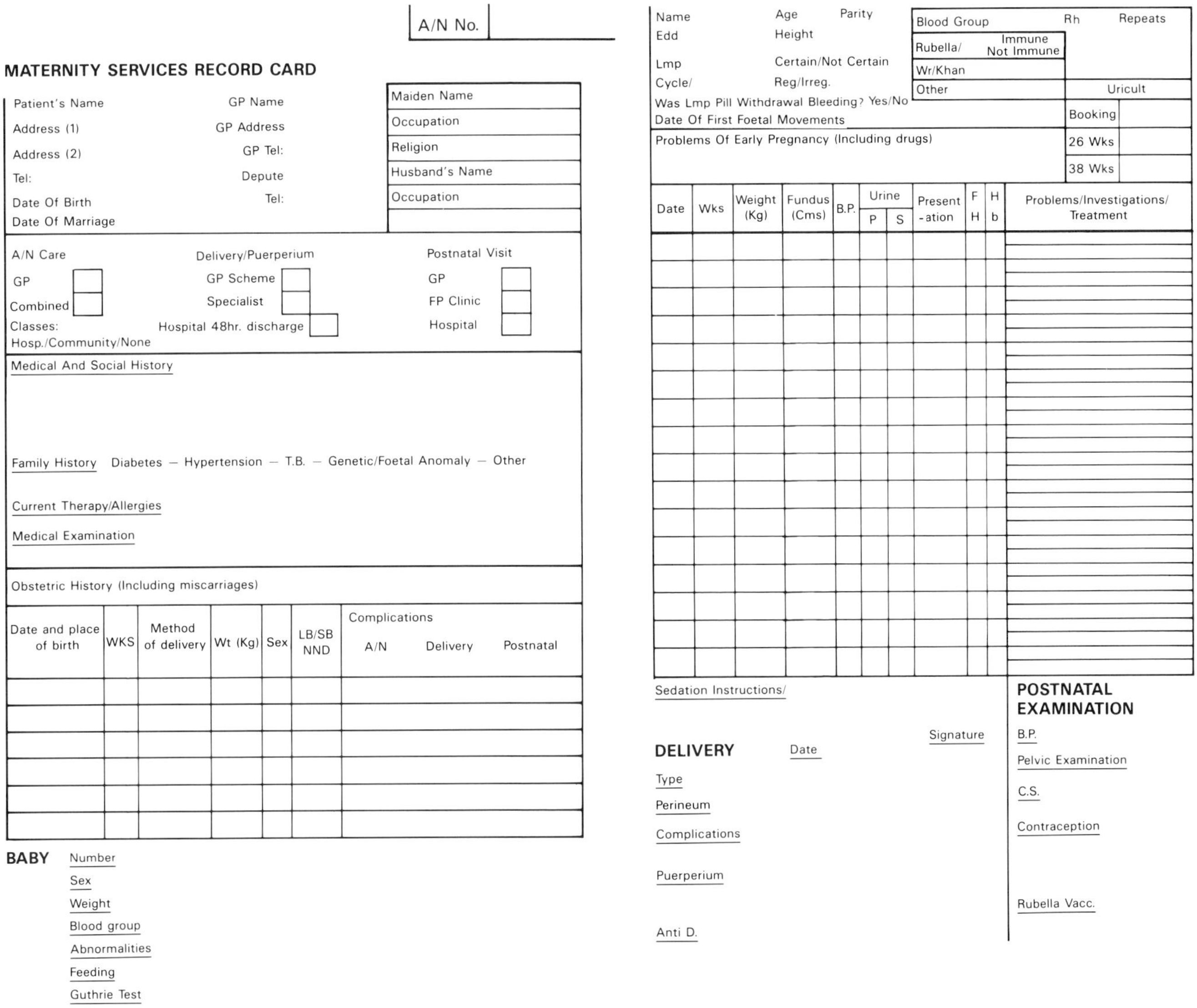
A/N No.

MATERNITY SERVICES RECORD CARD

Patient's Name — GP Name — Maiden Name
Address (1) — GP Address — Occupation
Address (2) — GP Tel: — Religion
Tel: — Depute — Husband's Name
Date Of Birth — Tel: — Occupation
Date Of Marriage

A/N Care: GP; Combined; Classes: Hosp./Community/None
Delivery/Puerperium: GP Scheme; Specialist; Hospital 48hr. discharge
Postnatal Visit: GP; FP Clinic; Hospital

Medical And Social History

Family History Diabetes — Hypertension — T.B. — Genetic/Foetal Anomaly — Other

Current Therapy/Allergies

Medical Examination

Obstetric History (Including miscarriages)

Date and place of birth	WKS	Method of delivery	Wt (Kg)	Sex	LB/SB NND	Complications A/N	Delivery	Postnatal

BABY Number; Sex; Weight; Blood group; Abnormalities; Feeding; Guthrie Test

Name — Age — Parity — Blood Group — Rh — Repeats
Edd — Height — Rubella/ Immune / Not Immune
Lmp — Certain/Not Certain — Wr/Khan
Cycle/ — Reg/Irreg. — Other — Uricult
Was Lmp Pill Withdrawal Bleeding? Yes/No
Date Of First Foetal Movements — Booking
Problems Of Early Pregnancy (Including drugs) — 26 Wks — 38 Wks

Date	Wks	Weight (Kg)	Fundus (Cms)	B.P.	Urine P	Urine S	Present -ation	FH	Hb	Problems/Investigations/ Treatment

Sedation Instructions/

DELIVERY — Date — Signature
Type; Perineum; Complications; Puerperium; Anti D.

POSTNATAL EXAMINATION
B.P.; Pelvic Examination; C.S.; Contraception; Rubella Vacc.

Fig. 16.4 First and second sides of a maternity services record card (co-operation card). From Boddy et al (1982).

man 1982). This can be conducted by the GP or midwife and does not necessitate visits to hospital.

Oedema

Since pregnant women retain water and sodium, oedema of the legs and ankles is common. Oedema may also indicate more serious disorders such as cardiac or renal disease, pre-eclampsia or anaemia and should always arouse suspicion and initiate the search for a cause. Unilateral oedema particularly associated with pain is suspicious of deep venous thrombosis.

Urine

A urine sample should be checked at every visit. Dipstick tests are generally used to detect protein or sugar. Midstream urine samples are routinely obtained for culture only at the initial assessment but should be re-examined if proteinuria or symptoms suggesting urinary infection develop.

Blood examination

After the initial assessment, standard red cell indices are usually measured at 24–26 weeks, 32–34 weeks and then close to term. Most hospitals now use electronic counters to provide accurate counts and measurements of red cells. These include the mean red cell volume, haemoglobin content and red cell haemoglobin concentration, which are calculated from the red cell count, haemoglobin concentration and packed cell volume. The earliest effect of iron deficiency is a reduction in red cell size below 80 fl and this is probably the most sensitive indicator of underlying iron deficiency during pregnancy.

Rhesus factor

Women who are rhesus(D)-positive with no abnormal antibodies usually have one further test around 36 weeks to exclude any unusual ABO or other antibodies. Women who are rhesus(D)-negative with no antibodies at the first visit are tested again at 24–26 weeks and 34–36 weeks. Some centres, recognizing that most of their remaining cases of rhesus sensitization have resulted from fetomaternal red cell transfer during pregnancy, administer 250 iu of anti-D immunoglobulin at around the 28th week and again at the 34th week of pregnancy (500 iu in all) to rhesus(D)-negative women without antibodies and with no living child.

If rhesus antibodies are found at the first visit or develop during pregnancy, more frequent antibody testing will be required and special management instituted.

Minor disorders in pregnancy

Cramps

Leg cramps are common and annoying. Without more than anecdotal evidence, these have been attributed to deficiency of diffusible serum calcium or elevation of serum phosphorus (Niswander 1982). Treatment with calcium tablets or aluminium hydroxide has been advised. Fortunately, leg cramps appear to be self-limiting and rarely persist for more than a few weeks.

Heartburn

Reduced peristalsis and relaxation of sphincteric musculature in the gastrointestinal tract in pregnancy, probably due to endocrine changes in pregnancy, predispose to heartburn with regurgitation of gastric contents into the lower oesophagus. Antacids can be helpful, as is the frequent intake of small meals and avoiding fried or fatty foods or recumbency; the pregnant woman should be encouraged to sit up as much as possible, even at night when asleep. Occasionally heartburn is associated with regurgitation of the alkaline contents of the duodenum back through the pylorus and stomach (Atlay et al 1973); it appears paradoxical but such women benefit from slightly acid therapy, and not alkaline.

Constipation

Constipation is common in pregnancy, partly because of reduced small bowel motility and partly because of increased colonic absorption (Parry et al 1970a,b). It is helpful to reassure the patient that constipation is common and physiological and can be helped by a diet containing plenty of fluid, fruit, vegetables and fibre. Regular exercise and regular bowel evacuation also help. Bulking agents such as ispaghula husk sachets or mild aperients may be required. Purgatives should be avoided.

Fainting

This is more common in late pregnancy, particularly if the pregnant woman lies flat on her back and the pressure of the uterus reduces venous return to the right heart through the inferior vena cava. Fainting may occur during the first 28 weeks, however, and is often postural, such as when sitting up from recumbency, or standing up from the sitting position. Changing posture more slowly usually avoids the problem.

Frequency of micturition

Most women develop increased frequency of micturition early in pregnancy. Although vascular engorgement in the pelvis and hormonal effects on smooth muscle have been claimed to cause this alteration in bladder function, Francis (1960) found no change in bladder tone during pregnancy and demonstrated that the urinary frequency was due partly to pressure on the bladder from the enlarging uterus and partly to polyuria associated with increased fluid intake. No treatment is indicated for urinary frequency alone but if dysuria also develops a urinary tract infection is likely.

Vaginal discharge

The physiological, white vaginal discharge normally increases during pregnancy because of increased shedding of vaginal mucosal cells and because there is increased secretion from the hypertrophied vascular cervix. If the discharge becomes yellow, offensive or associated with pruritus, vaginitis has probably developed, usually due to infection with *Monilia albicans* or *Trichomonas vaginalis*.

Vaginitis

Trichomonas vaginalis and *Monilia albicans* infections are considered in Chapter 41. Both can be detected by passing a vaginal speculum, inspecting the discharge and vaginal walls and taking vaginal swabs for culture. In women with trichomonal infections, cervical smears should also be taken as well as cervical cultures to exclude cervical gonorrhoea or chlamydia. After the 12th week of pregnancy, treating *Trichomonas vaginalis* infections with oral metronidazole has no adverse effects on the fetus (de Louvois 1983). Monilial infections should be treated with topical application of pessaries or creams containing miconazole, econazole or clotrimazole.

Varicose veins

Varicose veins tend to develop in the legs or vulva, often in women with a family history of varicosities. Signs appear early in pregnancy and women should be encouraged to use supportive elastic stockings. Surgical treatment is generally contraindicated during pregnancy since the varicosities subside after delivery, although residual varicosities of mild degree usually persist.

Haemorrhoids

These are common in pregnancy and can cause considerable discomfort. They are more likely to cause problems late in pregnancy or after delivery.

Pelvic joint pain

In the non-pregnant state, the pubic symphysis and sacroiliac joints are rigid and fixed. In pregnancy, endocrine changes can lead to relaxation of the ligaments guarding these joints; this allows a little laxity which can occasionally be considerable and very painful. The pain may be mainly in the pubic symphysis but in some women one or both sacroiliac joints become painful. It is difficult to provide completely effective treatment during pregnancy. Rest in bed and a tight girdle or orthopaedic belt around the pelvic girdle may help. Admission to hospital for rest may be necessary. Fortunately, the pain usually resolves rapidly a few days after delivery.

Backache is common in pregnancy and probably results from postural adaptation to the increasingly protuberant abdomen. Improvement in sitting or walking posture can help. Moving from the recumbent to the sitting position by rotating the trunk rather than by sitting up directly avoids stressing the back muscles and helps avoid some pain.

Paraesthesia in the hands

Numbness and tingling of the fingers is common in pregnancy and can be associated with traction on the brachial plexus due to the neck–shoulder–arm syndrome from drooping of the shoulder girdle during pregnancy. Discomfort is most common at night and early in the morning. The disorder is not serious and can be helped by physiotherapy and exercises.

Carpal tunnel syndrome

This is characterized by pain, numbness, tingling or burning in one or both hands in the area innervated by the median nerve. It is more a feature of late pregnancy than of the first 28 weeks.

NUTRITION, DRUGS, PERSONAL BEHAVIOUR AND PREGNANCY OUTCOME

Diet

The relationship between the diet of the mother and the well-being of the baby has long been a matter of interest, uncertainty and controversy. The daily recommended allowances for non-pregnant and pregnant women engaged in light work are listed in Chapter 10. The dietary requirements in pregnancy show surprisingly little increase compared with these in the non-pregnant state. For a women in good health and of normal weight-for-height, a good, well balanced, mixed diet should provide all that is required, with adequate protein (meat, fish and cheese), calcium (milk), fruit, vegetables and fibre to provide vitamins and combat the tendency to constipation.

Johnstone (1983) points out that recent nutritional guidelines have corrected an earlier tendency to over-emphasize the importance of a diet high in protein and derived from animal sources. Quoting Passmore et al (1979), he suggests a trend towards decreased consumption of fats, meat, sugar, alcohol and salt and increased consumption of potatoes, other vegetables, fruit and grain products. Protein intake should remain constant but should be derived less from animal products and more from whole-grain cereals. An increase in fibre to 30 g/day is recommended and is better obtained from whole-grain cereals than from added bran, as whole-grain products are more likely to ensure increased intake of mineral and trace elements.

The traditional dietary advice for pregnant women was to stress the need for high protein intake. This was based on the largely fallacious belief that the pregnant mother stores massive amounts of protein over and above the requirements for her baby and reproductive tissues. Johnstone et al (1981) showed that healthy pregnant women eating to appetite are not retaining nitrogen for a protein store.

Dietary supplementation

As Malhotra & Sawers (1986) point out, extremes of diet adversely affect pregnancy outcome; famine leads to low birthweight and obesity predisposes to large infants and difficult births. Marginal dietary imbalances are less well understood. In malnourished communities in developing countries the benefits of supplementation can be dramatic but in affluent western society the value of supplementation is less certain.

Preterm birth and intrauterine growth retardation are more common in women who are underweight-for-height in early pregnancy and whose weight gain between 20 and 30 weeks is significantly reduced. Dietary supplements increase the average weight of their newborn infants but do not prolong pregnancy (Campbell-Brown 1983). The increment in infant weight achieved by supplementation is usually small in comparison with the increased calorie intake and if the proportion of calories coming from protein is above approximately 20%, birthweight may actually be reduced (Rush 1982).

While prophylactic iron administration in pregnancy has been perhaps the least questioned supplement, the evidence for any benefit from it is strikingly absent (Hemminki 1982). Since Taylor & Lind (1976) have shown that increasing iron administration can lead to macrocytosis, it seems best to prescribe iron only for women with iron deficiency detected by microcytosis demonstrated by mean red cell volume (Lind 1983).

The administration of vitamin supplements and folic acid before and early in pregnancy has been reported to prevent fetal neural tube defects (Smithells et al 1980) and a similar preventive effect of folic acid alone was reported by Laurence et al (1981). Unfortunately, the double-blind trial originally proposed by Smithells et al was rejected by three hospital ethical committees and a weaker research design was used, which has left doubt about the comparability of the study and control groups, the former being volunteers and the latter including a disproportionate number from high-risk areas of Northern Ireland. The Medical Research Council decided that a randomized controlled trail was not only ethical but essential and that study is in progress, although opposed by those convinced by the work of Smithells et al (1980, Smithells 1983).

The need for supplementation with calcium and vitamin D is less controversial for population groups known to be especially vulnerable or in countries in which these deficiencies are common (Malhotra & Sawers 1986). Zinc has been of current interest, and now that more accurate measurement in blood or cells is possible, the low levels found during pregnancy have led to suggestions for routine supplementation. In a strongly worded editorial in the British Journal of Obstetrics and Gynaecology, Dr Frank Hytten (1985) explains that grossly reduced plasma nutrient levels are a normal part of pregnancy physiology and that the diagnosis of zinc deficiency is extremely difficult. Quoting three papers in the same volume of that journal, he stresses that much better evidence is required before British doctors should prescribe zinc supplements for pregnant women. Malhotra & Sawers (1986) state: 'in view of the obvious difficulties in diagnosing and treating specific dietary deficiency in pregnancy, the best approach in a relatively affluent Western society must surely be to concentrate more effort on dietary education'. Although the British public now displays a greater awareness of the importance of food for health, no national policy for healthier eating has been produced (Lancet leading article 1986). In comparison with similar countries, the British diet continues to be perhaps the least likely to promote health and longevity. The contribution of fat to total energy intake stands at record levels.

There is plenty of good advice, including the report of the National Advisory Committee on Nutrition Education in 1983. Until nutritional guidelines for pregnant women are established at national level, individual district health authorities and maternity advising committees must be responsible for publicizing the benefits of a balanced mixed diet and of avoiding food fads and excessive dependence on fast foods.

Table 16.2 Drugs very likely to be teratogenic in man

Aminopterin
Methotrexate
Vitamin D (high doses)
Tetracycline

Adapted from Lewis (1983).

Table 16.3 Drugs which may be teratogenic in man

Alcohol (in large chronic doses)	Any alkylating agent
Warfarin	Anaesthetic gases (chronic exposure)
Lithium	Penicillamine
Quinine	Sympathomimetic amines (nasal decongestants)
Any sex hormone	
Any antimetabolite	Oral contraceptives (after conception)

Adapted from Lewis (1983).

Drugs

Although the number of drugs associated with definite evidence of teratogenecity in man is quite small (see Table 16.2), there is another, larger group of drugs in which there is no conclusive evidence of teratogenecity, but which should cause an obstetrician concern if his patient had ingested one of them in the first trimester (Lewis 1983). These drugs are listed in Table 16.3.

There should be a good reason for prescribing any drug at any time in pregnancy but the indications must be particularly strong during the first 12 weeks, and even in the second half of the menstrual cycle when a woman might be unknowingly pregnant.

Smoking

Cigarette smoking has important adverse effects on pregnancy. It is particularly associated with an increased incidence of low birthweight and perinatal mortality especially from pre-eclampsia, apart from its well known ability to cause respiratory and cardiac disease. Encouraging pregnant women not to smoke is an important aspect of health education and antenatal care. Even if the pregnant woman cannot stop smoking altogether, it would be helpful if she could reduce the number of cigarettes smoked to less than five per day. While exposure to smoking by the mother reduces birthweight, Rubin et al (1986) have shown that indirect or passive exposure to smoking by the father has nearly as large an effect (66%). Birthweight was reduced by 120 g per pack of cigarettes smoked per day by the father. The effect was greatest in the more deprived socioeconomic groups.

Alcohol

Wright et al (1983), reviewing the information on alcohol ingestion in pregnancy, defined a heavy drinker as a pregnant woman who consumed more than 100 grams of alcohol per week. The authors described a Boston study in which the incidence of congenital anomalies was 32% in heavy drinkers, 14% in moderate drinkers and 9% in light drinkers or teetotallers. In contrast, a study from Colorado (Tennes & Blackard 1980) could not distinguish the effect of drinking before or during pregnancy on congenital anomalies. There seems to be no clear association between moderate drinking in pregnancy and an increased incidence of congenital abnormalities.

The congenital malformations associated with fetal alcohol syndrome were listed by Wright et al (1983) as follows:

1. Cardiac — atrial septal defect.
2. Skeletal — aberrant palmar creases; pectus excavatum.
3. Mouth — cleft lip or palate.
4. Eyes — ptosis; strabismus; prominent epicanthic folds.

Such infants, who are often small for gestational age and frequently show neurological abnormalities, tend to be delivered mainly to women who are chronic heavy alcohol drinkers.

While it is unlikely that an occasional drink taken during pregnancy has a serious effect on the fetus the safest advice for pregnant women is that alcohol should be avoided altogether.

Sexual intercourse

There has always been a suspicion that sexual intercourse may be responsible for early abortion and if abdominal cramps or vaginal bleeding follow coitus sexual intercourse should be avoided. The evidence that coitus late in pregnancy may initiate labour or premature labour is not very convincing but intercourse should certainly be avoided in women with spontaneous rupture of the membranes or antepartum haemorrhage. In healthy women with normal pregnancies, however, any prohibition is totally inappropriate (Lumley & Astbury 1982).

Bathing

Bathing or swimming is not contraindicated during normal pregnancy, but diving, snorkelling or surfing should be avoided because of possible trauma.

Dental care

In the UK, dental care is free during pregnancy and for 12 months afterwards and since gingivitis is common an important aspect of antenatal care is to encourage examination of the teeth and advise the woman if she needs dental care.

Immunization

Vaccination against smallpox was contra-indicated in pregnancy when the disease existed, as there was a risk that fetal vaccinia might develop and cause intrauterine death. By contrast, immunization against poliomyelitis is indicated if the patient is not immune. If the patient is not immune to rubella, however, she should not be immunized during pregnancy. The rubella vaccine should be administered during the early puerperium and contraceptive advice given to ensure that pregnancy does not occur for a period of 12 weeks.

Exercise

Exercise in moderation is acceptable and desirable during pregnancy, but potentially dangerous sports such as horse-riding and undue physical stress should be avoided. Advice should take into account the amount of exercise to which the women is accustomed.

Employment

Women who have sedentary jobs may continue to work throughout the pregnancy. Those whose employment requires heavy physical exertion should take leave of absence during the second trimester or seek less vigorous work. The statutory provision for maternity leave from work is 11 weeks during pregnancy and 18 weeks afterwards; the woman is entitled to a further 22 weeks of unpaid maternity leave after which she is entitled to return to her paid work.

Travel

Travel by car, train or aeroplane is not hazardous in itself but during long journeys the pregnant woman may be unable quickly to consult a doctor if an unexpected emergency arises. It is therefore inadvisable for a woman to embark on long journeys especially by air after 35 weeks of pregnancy or if she has had bleeding in pregnancy or any other complication likely to recur as an emergency.

High-risk pregnancy

The obstetrician should always be attempting to identify women antenatally whose pregnancies are at high risk for reasons which have already been described. The high risk can often be identified at the initial assessment, either because of complications of the previous obstetric history or by the detection of abnormal findings. Even women who are fit and well at initial assessment may develop complications during pregnancy such as pre-eclampsia, intrauterine growth retardation, multiple pregnancy or antepartum haemorrhage. Such women require investigation and treatment which may sometimes be provided in a day care unit, or may necessitate admission to hospital. If such a woman is then allowed home, the frequency of her subsequent antenatal clinic visits should be greater than arranged in women with uncomplicated pregnancies. Specific management arrangements therefore must be made for particular women with significant pregnancy complications. The detailed management of specific problems in pregnancy is described in detail in the appropriate chapters.

CONCLUSIONS

The potential contribution of antenatal care to health is enormous. Continuing efforts to improve the content and organization of care are needed if this potential is to be fully realized, together with continuing assessment of the effectiveness of the approach. This chapter has described the current state of antenatal care during the first 28 weeks and has indicated some of the directions in which changes may occur in the future.

REFERENCES

Atlay R, Gillison E W, Horton A L 1973 A fresh look at pregnancy heartburn. Journal of Obstetrics and Gynaecology of the British Commonwealth 80: 63–66

Boddy K, Parboosingh I J T, Shepherd N C 1982 Schematic approach to prenatal care. In: Report of the RCOG working party on antenatal and intrapartum care. Royal College of Obstetricians and Gynaecologists, London, pp 40–46

Butler N L, Bonham D G 1963 Perinatal mortality. Livingstone, Edinburgh, p 42

Campbell-Brown M 1983 Protein energy supplements in primigravid women at risk of low birthweight. In: Campbell D M, Gillmer M D G (eds) Nutrition in pregnancy. Royal College of Obstetricians and Gynaecologists, London, pp 85–98

Chng P K, Hall M H, MacGillvray I 1980 An audit of antenatal care; the value of the first antenatal visit. British Medical Journal 281: 1154–1156

de Louvois J 1983 Antimicrobial chemotherapy in pregnancy. In: Lewis P J (ed) Clinical pharmacology in obstetrics. Wright, Bristol, pp 55–71

Francis W J A 1960 Disturbances of bladder function in relation to pregnancy. Journal of Obstetrics and Gynaecology of the British Empire 67: 353–366

Hall M H, Chung P G, MacGillvray I 1980 Is routine antenatal care worthwhile? Lancet i: 78–80

Hall M H, Macintyre S, Porter M 1985 Antenatal care assessed. University Press, Aberdeen, p 6. Quote Ministry of Health 1929 memorandum

Hemminki E 1982 Effects of routine haematinic and vitamin administration during pregnancy. In: Enkin M, Chalmers I (eds) Effectiveness and satisfaction in antenatal care. Heinemann Medical, London, pp 114–121

Hytten F E 1985 Do pregnant women need zinc supplements? British Journal of Obstetrics and Gynaecology 92: 873–874

Johnstone F D 1983 Assessment of dietary intake and dietary advice in pregnancy. In: Campbell D M, Gillmer M D G (eds) Nutrition in pregnancy. Royal College of Obstetricians and Gynaecologists, London, pp 9–18

Johnstone F D, Campbell D M, MacGillvray I 1981 Nitrogen balance studies in human pregnancy. Journal of Nutrition III: 1884–1893

Lancet leading article 1986 Britian needs a food and health policy: the government must face its duty. Lancet ii: 434–436

Laurence K M, James N, Miller M H et al 1981 Double-blind randomised controlled trial of folate treatment before conception to prevent recurrence of neural tube defects. British Medical Journal 282: 1509–1511

Lewis P J 1983 Adverse effects of drugs on the fetus. In: Lewis P J (ed) Clinical pharmacology in obstetrics. Wright, Bristol, pp 17–27

Lind T 1983 Iron supplementation during pregnancy. In: Campbell D M, Gillmer M D G (eds) Nutrition in pregnancy. Royal College of Obstetricians and Gynaecologists, London, pp 181–191

Lumley J, Astbury J 1982 Advice in pregnancy: perfect remedies, imperfect science. In: Enkin M, Chalmers I (eds) Effectiveness and satisfaction in antenatal care. Heinemann Medical, London, pp 132–150

Malhotra A, Sawers R S 1986 Dietary supplementation in pregnancy. British Medical Journal 293: 465–466

Ministry of Health 1929 Memorandum on antenatal clinics: their conduct and scope. Appendix F to the Ministry of Health report 1930. HMSO, London

National Advisory Committee on Nutrition Education 1983 Proposals for nutritional guidelines for health education in Britain. Health education Council, London

Niswander K R 1982 Prenatal care. In: Benson R C (ed) Current obstetric and gynecologic diagnosis and treatment. Large, California, pp 616–629

Parry E, Shields R, Turnbull A C 1970a Colonic absorption of sodium, potassium and water in pregnancy. Journal of Obstetrics and Gynaecology of the British Commonwealth 77: 616–619

Parry E, Shields R, Turnbull A C 1970b Transit time in the small intestine in pregnancy. Journal of Obstetrics and Gynaecology of the British Commonwealth 77: 900–901

Pearce J M F, Campbell S 1983 Ultrasonic monitoring of normal and abnormal fetal growth. In: Lanvenson N H (ed) Modern management of high risk pregnancy. Plenum, New York, pp 57–101

Passmore R, Hollingsworth D F, Robertson J 1979 Prescription for a better British diet. British Medical Journal 1: 527–531

Quaranta P, Currell R, Redman C W G R et al 1981 Prediction of small for dates infants by measurement of symphysial–fundal height. British Journal of Obstetrics and Gynaecology 88: 115–119

Redman C W G R 1982 Screening for pre-eclampsia. In: Enkin M, Chalmers I (eds) Effectiveness and satisfaction in antenatal care. Heinemann Medical, London, pp 69–76

Royal College of Obstetricians and Gynaecologists 1982 Report of the RCOG working party on further specialisation within obstetrics and gynaecology. RCOG, London

Rubin D H, Krasilnikoff P A, Leventhal J M et al 1986 Effect of passive smoking on birthweight. Lancet ii: 415–417

Rush D 1982 Effects of changes in protein and calorie intake during pregnancy on the growth of the human fetus. In: Enkin M, Chalmers I (eds) Effectiveness and satisfaction in antenatal care. Heinemann Medical, London, pp 92–113

Smithells R W 1983 Diet and congenital malfunction. In: Campbell D M, Gillmer M D G (eds) Nutrition in pregnancy. Royal College of Obstetrians and Gynaecologists, London, pp 155–163

Smithells R W, Shepherd S, Schorah C J et al 1980 Possible prevention of neural tube defects by periconceptional vitamin supplementation. Lancet i: 339–340

Taylor D J, Lind T 1976 Haematological changes during normal pregnancy: iron-induced macrocytosis. British Journal of Obstetrics and Gynaecology 83: 760–769

Tennes K, Blackard C 1980 Maternal alcohol consumption, birthweight and minor physical abnormalities. American Journal of Obstetrics and Gynecology 138: 774–780

Wright J T, Topliss P J, Barrison I G 1983 Alcohol and coffee consumption during pregnancy. In: Campbell D M, Gillmer M D G (eds) Nutrition in pregnancy. Royal College of Obstetricians and Gynaecologists, London, pp 115–205

17

G. M. Stirrat

Late antenatal care (28 weeks and after)

The certain belief that antenatal care is beneficial to the pregnant woman and her unborn child is a fundamental tenet of midwifery. As such antenatal care, or rather the traditional approach to it, is often defended uncritically, such as: 'Is it not a well known fact that maternal and perinatal mortality are lower in women who have, compared with those who have not, received some antenatal care?' Although that is true, the assumption that there is a direct causal relationship rather than a mere association is not necessarily justified. Indeed, a significant proportion of the overall improvement results from environmental and social rather than medical influences (Lancet Leading Article 1986).

As Enkin & Chalmers (1982) have pointed out: 'In contrast to the convincing evidence that antenatal care is of great benefit when pregnancy is complicated or abnormal, evidence of its benefit in the absence of overt disease or complication is far less persuasive'.

The first purpose of this chapter is to assist the reader to set aside preconceived notions about the practice of late antenatal care which 'has remained unchanged and largely unchallenged for well over half a century' (Enkin & Chalmers 1982). We will then be better able to achieve our second aim of appropriate care by the appropriate person in the appropriate place.

We must begin by asking several fundamental questions:

1. What are the aims and objectives of late antenatal care?
2. How are these to be achieved?
3. By whom, when, and where is late antenatal care to be carried out?

AIMS AND OBJECTIVES

The Maternity Services Advisory Committee (1982) defined the primary aim of all antenatal care as being 'to ensure as far as possible the health and wellbeing of the woman and the unborn child'. From a different perspective, its main aim is to assess risk of harm to mother and baby, and apply the appropriate level of surveillance to minimize or eradicate its effects. Parboosingh & Kerr (1982) delineate its principal goals as:

1. The detection of previously unrecognized maternal disease.
2. The prediction, prevention, early detection and management of complications of pregnancy.
3. The amelioration of the discomforts and minor complaints of pregnancy.
4. Preparation of the couple for childbirth and child-rearing.
5. Preventive health education.

To these can be added reassurance and the alleviation of anxiety.

Screening and diagnostic function

Although frequently confused with each other, screening and diagnosis are distinct concepts. Screening is a process applied to a population to determine those at greatest risk of the specific condition being screened for. Diagnosis is the application of tests to an individual, identified because of signs and symptoms or as a result of a screening programme, to identify a particular disease. Screening procedures raise the suspicion of abnormalities in apparently normal pregnancies. Diagnostic tests confirm or refute the existence of true abnormalities in women or fetuses thought to be at high risk (Grant & Mohide 1982). The former implies a clear benefit to those examined; the latter should discriminate clearly between those who have or do not have the condition.

Given that antenatal care is predominantly a multiphasic screening programme (Enkin & Chalmers 1982), it is vital that those caring for pregnant women understand the differences between the two processes. This is therefore discussed in greater depth below.

Therapeutic aspects

One of the major benefits of antenatal care is the early detection and successful treatment of covert disease in mothers, such as diabetes, renal, cardiac or thyroid disease. Diagnosis usually occurs in the first half of pregnancy and the major tasks in late pregnancy are to assess the effectiveness of therapy, continually balancing its benefits to the mother against the hazards to the fetus and neonate, and to discern the optimum timing of delivery. Management of specific conditions is discussed in Section V of this book and the principles behind prescribing in pregnancy have been reviewed by Stirrat & Beeley (1986).

Priestly function

As Enkin & Chalmers (1982) have pointed out: 'antenatal care is a curious mixture of science and magic' and 'the reassurance that a woman may obtain from the laying on of hands and the expression of concern by a conscientious practitioner cannot be overestimated'. Nor, of course, can it be properly assessed and doctors and nurses frequently hide behind this priestly function when their uncritical practices are challenged. Even more dangerous is the irrational belief that antenatal care can act as a talisman to ward off the evil eye.

It is in this intangible area of care that mothers feel most let down by the system as can be discerned from the 1981 working party report from the National Childbirth Trust (Kitzinger 1981) and from Garcia (1982).

Educative function

There is a real and important need for encouragement, counselling and education of both mother and father, particularly in late pregnancy. The form, setting and content are discussed below, but late antenatal care must include: information on the normal changes to be expected; training for labour and delivery; discussion of a projected birth plan which will include pain relief and position for delivery, and preparation for infant-feeding.

Opportunities must be afforded to meet the midwives at the place of delivery and to see the room and facilities available there.

THE CONCEPT OF RISK AND ITS ASSESSMENT

The terms *high-risk* and *low-risk* pregnancies are used increasingly commonly, frequently without any understanding of underlying concepts. The question *at risk of what and for whom?* is seldom addressed.

The decision as to what is high risk and what is low risk is purely subjective and will vary according to the following questions:

1. *What are we trying to predict?* Although the end-point of maternal or perinatal death is easy to measure, neither is a good indicator of quality of obstetric care (Chapple 1982). Morbidity is much less easy to assess quantitatively and qualitatively. A *continuum of obstetric hazard* has been postulated frequently in which the same risk factors causing fetal death in one pregnancy lead to survival with handicap in another. No such continuum has yet been demonstrated.
2. *Who is making the assessment?* Epidemiologists and clinicians will reach very different conclusions from the same data. The former are concerned with making generalizations from individual groups of data. The latter apply the same generalizations to assess the risk of an individual developing a certain disease, and to aid diagnosis, treatment and prognosis in the patient for whom they are responsible (Chapple 1982).
3. *What is its purpose?* Conclusions reached from the same assessments will differ according to whether one wishes to evaluate the effects of intervention (including patterns of care) or discover how best to manage finite resources.
4. *How is risk being assessed?* By this is meant, how is the information gained from the tests at our disposal (alluded to later and discussed in greater detail in other chapters) to be interpreted to allow correct conclusions to be drawn and action to be taken?

This last point is undoubtedly the concept about which doctors have the least understanding and which can lead to serious errors. A potential example is given later. First we must look at basic methods of interpretation by taking a piece of paper and drawing a simple two-by-two table as shown in Figure 17.1a. Let us say we are testing for intrauterine growth retardation (IUGR). As shown in Figure 17.1b, the *true situation* is represented horizontally and the *test results* vertically. Thus, of those fetuses who are growth-retarded, i.e. (a + c), the test used has correctly predicted only a. Its ability to detect the condition is therefore the ratio of positive test results compared to the total affected, i.e. (a + c), otherwise known as the test's sensitivity. The proportion of *false negatives* is (1 − sensitivity).

The test has correctly predicted that b fetuses are not growth-retarded from the total (b + d). The test's ability to exclude the disease correctly is, therefore, the ratio of the negative test results compared to the total unaffected, i.e. b/(b + d), otherwise known as the test's *specificity*. The proportion of false positives is (1 − specificity) (Fig. 17.1c).

However, these are not the questions of most practical value to the clinician who is more interested in knowing how good the test is at predicting the true situation (Fig. 17.1d). Of those in whom the test is positive (a + b) only a are affected. Thus the *positive predictive value* of the test

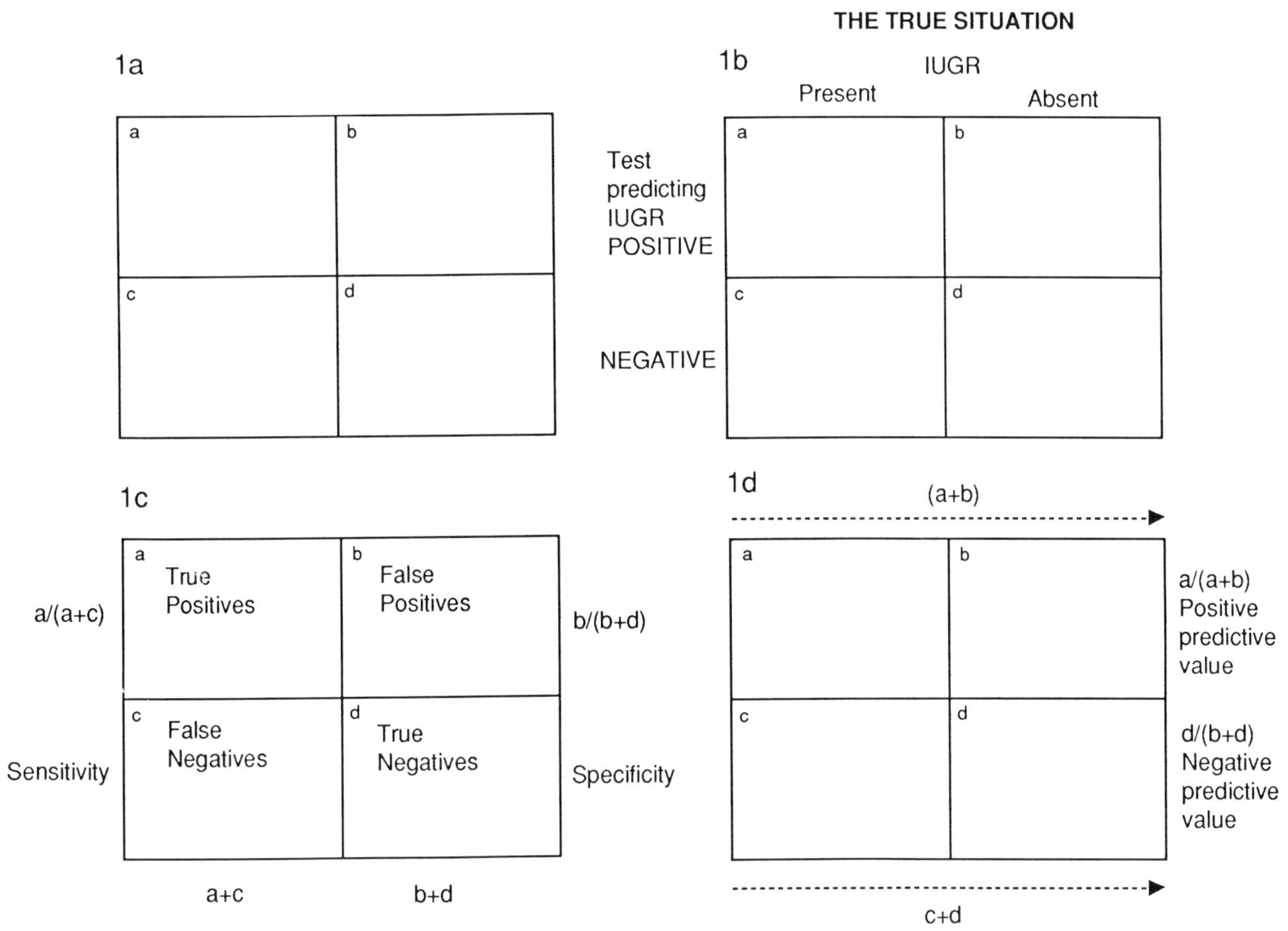

Fig. 17.1 Two-by-two table.

is a/(a + b). Of those in whom the test is negative (c + d) only d are unaffected. Thus the *negative predictive value* of the test is d/(c + d).

The overall *accuracy* of the test is found by comparing the true positives and negatives with the total tested, i.e. (a + d)/(a + b + c + d). The *prevalence* of IUGR in the population tested is expressed by the ratio of those with IUGR to the total number tested, i.e. (a + c)/(a + b + c + d). This is an extremely important concept because the positive predictive value of a test decreases dramatically as the prevalence of a condition falls. Grant & Mohide (1982) give three examples in which the same test is applied to detect a condition which has different prevalences in three populations. When the prevalence of the condition is 200/1000 (20%) the positive predictive value of their test is 53%. Reducing the prevalence to 100/1000 (10%) and 50/1000 (5%) causes the positive predictive value of the same test to fall to 33 and 19% respectively. Information from such concepts is so important and yet policies regarding intervention are seldom based on knowledge regarding the local prevalence of the condition being managed.

Working out two-by-two tables can lead to some surprising conclusions and although the example in Table 17.1 relates to early antenatal care, it is used because it makes the point very strongly. Further information on risk assessment can be found in Peters & Golding (1986).

It is, of course, important to realize that risk assessment in antenatal care can have serious problems and pitfalls. Lilford & Chard (1983), who have been in the forefront of advocating a correct approach to risk assessment, point out that the bulk of obstetric care does not consist of a single factor leading to a single decision. One of the main limitations is the inadequacy of our database, but many obstetric data are not amenable to formalized probability analysis. The former can be improved and the latter can too readily be used as an excuse for lack of rigour in making clinical decisions.

DISCRIMINATING BETWEEN NORMAL AND ABNORMAL

Pregnancy produces profound changes in the mother (see Chapter 10). One important function of antenatal care is to discriminate between what is normal and, indeed, necessary physiological adaptation and what is potentially serious

Table 17.1 Application of risk analysis to an antenatal screening programme for neural tube defect

	Alpha-fetoprotein screening	Ultrasound screening (alone)
Population to be screened and prevalence of condition	10 000 women with a 2/1000 risk of open spina bifida (OSB); therefore 20 women are carrying a fetus with OSB	
Effectiveness of screening	80% effective; therefore 16 women with affected baby will be detected	Assume 90% effective; therefore 18 women will be detected as having an affected baby
Other elements of screening programme	Assume a 2% amniocentesis rate with a 0.5% risk of miscarriage: 200 women have amniocentesis and 1 normal fetus is lost	None
False positive diagnosis rate	Approximately 1/8000 (0.01%) of women tested — therefore 1 normal pregnancy is terminated	Estimated at approximately 1/2000 (0.05%) of women tested — therefore 5 wrong diagnoses will be made
Conclusion	For every 16 OSBs detected, 2 normal babies will be lost	For every 16 OSBs correctly diagnosed, 5 wrong diagnoses will be made

N.B.: This example is not to be interpreted or used as a definitive statement comparing these two screening procedures. It is meant to illustrate how important risk analysis is when comparing suggested programmes.

Table 17.2 Continuing antenatal care

Programme for late antenatal care proposed by Royal College of Obstetricians and Gynaecologists (1982) for women at low risk of developing complications:
26 weeks — to check fetal growth
36 weeks — to check presentation
40 weeks — predelivery assessment
Additional visits must have clear objective
Care must be determined individually for higher-risk pregnancies

Programme proposed by Marsh (1985) for care by general practitioner and/or midwife for low-risk pregnancies:

Nulliparous women
Monthly from 26 to 34 weeks
Fortnightly from 34 to 40 weeks
Weekly to delivery

Multiparous women
30, 36, 40, 41 and 42 weeks

Routine examinations and investigations
Every visit: weight, urinalysis, blood pressure, check for oedema, measure fundal height
Each third-trimester visit: fetal lie and presentation, presence of fetal heart, fetal movements, relation of presenting part of pelvis (engagement)
At 36 weeks: pelvic assessment in primigravidae

pathology. Somewhere between them is a series of minor complaints which, although troublesome, are not of themselves hazardous.

As pregnancy progresses the value of the early baseline assessment (see Chapter 16) becomes apparent. Without this valid comparisons and therefore proper judgements cannot be made. Table 17.2 shows the elements of the generally accepted pattern of routine late antenatal care. As Hall & Chng (1982) have pointed out, the productivity of consultations after the booking visit is low until 32–34 weeks' gestation.

Weight gain in pregnancy

The range of weight gain in pregnancy is wide, and no single or close range of figures can be regarded as normal for any individual. It is, of course, compounded by observer bias, errors in the multiplicity of weight-scales used, and inconsistency in recorded units of measurements.

The average weight gain for European women is 12.5 kg for the whole of pregnancy and 9 kg for the second half. Mothers who gain little or no weight tend to have smaller babies than those who gain more weight. Some have static weight or even weight loss at term. The importance of weight loss as a sign of impending fetal death has been over-emphasized because it is sometimes the only adverse feature noted after sudden unexpected fetal death. Although it is neither a specific nor sensitive indicator in this context, it is part of the overall picture of maternal and fetal well-being which should be considered in the screening process.

Screening for pre-eclampsia

This enigmatic condition is discussed in detail in Chapter 36 but is highlighted here because a significant proportion of antenatal clinic routine is taken up with screening for it. Each element of the routine examination for every visit noted in Table 17.2 is, in whole or in part, designed to detect pre-eclampsia or its effects.

1. *Excessive weight gain* can occur in the terminal phase of some cases of proteinuric pre-eclampsia. On its own, however, it is a poor indicator of risk of developing pre-eclampsia.
2. Routine *urinalysis* is carried out to exclude glycosuria and proteinuria. The significance of the former in the context of abnormal carbohydrate metabolism is discussed in Chapter 39. Proteinuria of more than trace amounts is often significant and must be taken seriously. Once contamination by vaginal discharge has been excluded the major causes are urinary tract infection and pre-eclampsia. Proteinuria accompanied by even a moderate rise in blood pressure is a clear indication for immediate admission to hospital.
3. *Blood pressure* measurement in pregnancy is another area full of myths and misconceptions. It is discussed fully in Chapter 36. It is wrong to think of a critical level of blood pressure which totally discriminates between a normal and a hypertensive population of pregnant women. As Redman (1982) points out, arbitrary thresh-

old (usually around 140/90 mmHg) above which hypertension is deemed to occur is applied to the completely continuous distribution of blood pressure readings in the pregnant population. It divides the population quantitatively, not qualitatively, into those mothers and babies at higher risk of hazard and those who are not.
4. *Peripheral oedema* can be found in up to 80% of healthy pregnant women at some time, particularly during later pregnancy. Thus the same caveat about this being an adverse sign applies as to excessive weight gain. Diuretic therapy is contraindicated for peripheral oedema in pregnancy.

Pre-eclampsia occurs in its severe proteinuric form in around 6% of first pregnancies, falling to 2% of second pregnancies. Pre-eclampsia is undoubtedly overdiagnosed and up to 30% of cases present for the first time in labour or postpartum (Hall & Chng 1982). The question has therefore been asked—are all our efforts are worthwhile? In answering that, Redman (1982) emphasizes that the value of screening for pre-eclampsia is determined not by the number of diagnoses made per clinic visit but rather by the consequences if those diagnoses are not made. These can be severe for baby and mother in some cases.

Screening for fetal growth

Palpation of the pregnant abdomen is one of the rituals of antenatal care carried out as much to reassure the mother as to inform the midwife or doctor. The height of the uterine fundus is used as a rough guide to fetal size and therefore fetal growth, when measured serially. The situation is, of course, far more complex than that because of:

1. The multiplicity of observers.
2. Subjectivity of reference standards (e.g. equivalent to dates or 2 finger-breadths below xiphisternum).
3. The differing contribution to uterine size of liquor volume and fetal size.
4. The presentation, lie and position of the baby in the uterus.
5. Individuality of each mother and the baby she is carrying.

It is therefore one of the least sensitive and specific screening procedures used in medicine. Hall & Chng (1982) in a study of hospital-based and shared antenatal care in Aberdeen showed that:

1. IUGR was suspected in less than half of the cases in which it occurred.
2. Under one-third of women in whom it was suspected delivered babies weighing less than the tenth centile for gestational age and sex.
3. Diagnostic accuracy was no better for severely growth-retarded babies (less than the fifth centile) or in those who had previously delivered a growth-retarded baby.

The worrisome aspect of this is that unnecessary and possibly

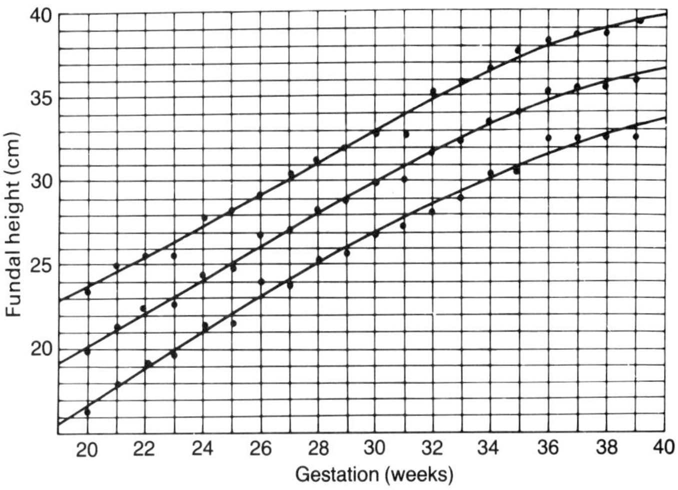

Fig. 17.2 Symphysio-fundal height.

hazardous intervention is occurring in some women while fetal problems go undetected in others.

One method for reducing subjectivity in assessing fundal height is to measure and record it in centimetres above the pubic symphysis. Figure 17.2 shows the chart derived from Quaranta et al (1981). Rosenberg and colleagues (1982) have found it to be of limited value as a screening test for IUGR with a sensitivity of only 69% and a 26% false positive rate. It is, however, superior to mere subjective assessment and is a useful part of a first-phase screening examination (see below), as long as it is recorded properly and its short-comings are appreciated. The role of ultrasonic measurement in the second phase of screening for IUGR is discussed in Chapter 27.

Other information to be gained from palpation of the uterus

1. *Fetal lie:* The relative mass of the fetus increases in the last 10 weeks of pregnancy to a far greater extent than does the volume of amniotic fluid. The freedom to move, so important for musculoskeletal development, is therefore reduced and the lie of the fetus tends to stabilize to longitudinal (with either cephalic or breech presentation). Changes in lie are uncommon in primigravidae after 32 weeks and after 36 weeks in multigravidae.

   Instability of the fetal lie in late pregnancy should not be ignored because of:
   a. potential hazard as a result of any underlying cause, e.g. placenta praevia, pelvic tumour, unsuspected multiple pregnancy.
   b. fetal hazard if labour supervenes and membranes have ruptured (e.g. shoulder presentation, obstructed labour, cord prolapse).
2. *Fetal presentation:* breech presentation occurs in 2–3% of all term deliveries, and a greater proportion of preterm deliveries.

Table 17.3 Contraindications to external cephalic version

Absolute contraindications
Multiple pregnancy
Antepartum haemorrhage (APH), whatever the cause
Ruptured membranes
Significant fetal anomaly
Caesarean section indicated for other reasons
Relative contraindications
Previous Caesarean section
Intrauterine growth retardation
Hypertension
Rhesus isoimmunization
Elderly primigravida
Grande multiparity
Anterior placenta
Obesity

Table 17.4 Physiology of fetal activity

1. Each fetus has its own rhythms and rate of daily activity. The number of perceived daily movements in a healthy fetus can vary between 10 and 1000
2. Fetal activity is greatest from 28 to 32 weeks' gestation.

Gestational age	Average number of movements/h (± 1 SD)
30 weeks	32 ± 7
40 weeks	23 ± 5

   The pattern and mean value of fetal activity do not decrease in the week preceding delivery
3. Movements differ in character. They may be strong or weak; sustained, brief or rapid; and involve the whole body, the chest wall or the limbs
4. There is no consistent change in fetal activity perceived by the mother throughout the day but ultrasonic surveillance suggests that fetal activity is greatest between 9 p.m. and 2 a.m.
5. Periods of fetal total inactivity in excess of 1 h are abnormal
6. Fetal hyperactivity does not appear to be a worrisome prognostic sign

From Rayburn (1982).

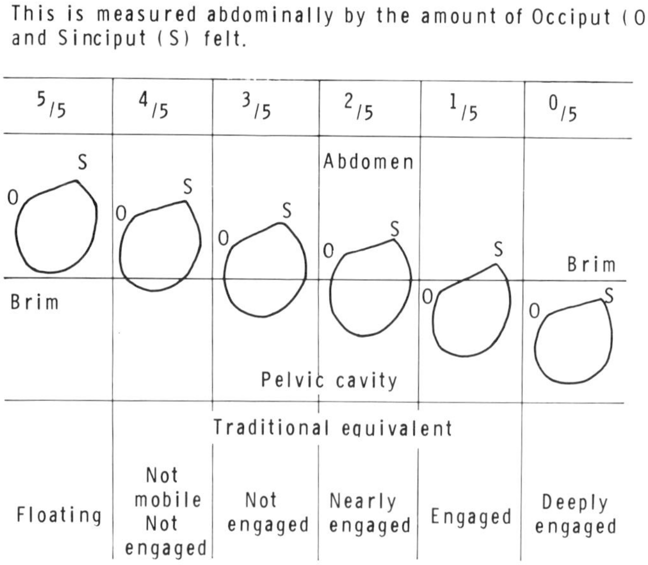

Fig. 17.3 Relationship of fetal head to pelvis assessed in fifths palpable above the brim.

External cephalic version (ECV) is safe for mother and baby in carefully selected women and reduces the need to consider elective Caesarean section. The gestational age must be known and the presentation confirmed by ultrasound before proceeding.

It is technically easier at 34 weeks (or less) but the malpresentation is more likely to recur and, if delivery is urgently necessary as a direct result of the ECV, the infant is immature. It is, therefore, becoming more common to perform ECV later, sometimes using a tocolytic agent to inhibit uterine contractions.

Table 17.3 lists the contraindications to ECV.

3. *Engagement of the presenting part:* engagement has occurred when the largest diameter of the presenting part has passed through the pelvic brim. The mechanism is described below. In a cephalic presentation it is useful to chart the extent to which the head has entered the pelvic brim, as shown in Figure 17.3.
4. *Multiplicity of fetal parts* suggests the possibility of multiple pregnancy. One would also expect the uterus to be large-for-dates. The increasing routine use of ultrasound early in pregnancy should reduce the incidence of unsuspected multiple pregnancy in late pregnancy or labour.
5. *Liquor volume:* assessment of reduced (oligohydramnios) or excessive (polyhydramnios) volumes of liquor are highly subjective. The observer should, however, still act on suspicion because of their association with fetal risk. For example, oligohydramnios may accompany IUGR; polyhydramnios may be associated with maternal diabetes and/or fetal anomaly.

Auscultation of the fetal heart is a ritual, the greatest value of which is to allow the mother to hear it with a small ultrasonic fetal heart detector. The traditional teaching that twins can be detected by the auscultation of two fetal hearts is impractical.

Fetal movement assessment

The popularization by Pearson & Weaver (1976) of a simple kick-chart on which mothers can record fetal activity has made this first-phase screening process commonplace as a rough guide to fetal welfare from 28 weeks' gestation.

Table 17.4 outlines some of the information which has been gathered on the physiology of fetal activity by Patrick et al (1982) and Rayburn (1982). The procedure for the Cardiff Count-to-Ten kick-chart of Pearson & Weaver (1976) shown in Figure 17.4 is relatively simple. Mothers are asked to count the number of discrete fetal movements beginning at 9 a.m. each day. The time at which the tenth movement is felt is marked on the chart. Instructions are given to contact the hospital if fewer than 10 movements occur in 12 hours.

In practice, however, Draper et al (1986) have shown that:

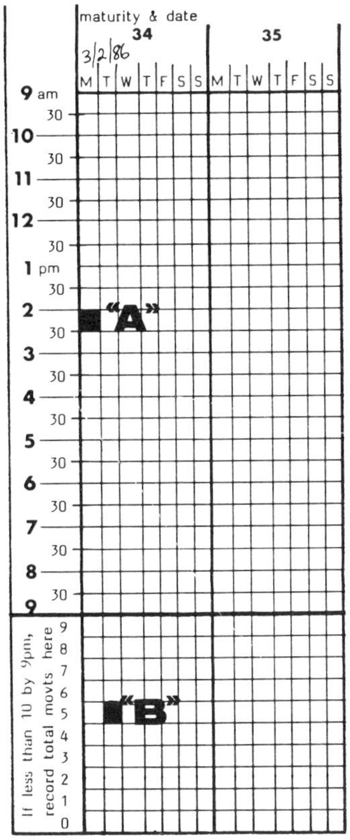

Fig. 17.4 Fetal movement chart. A = time at which tenth movement is felt; B = the number of movements felt by 9 p.m. if less than 10.

1. Many women had problems completing the chart, which reduced its value.
2. Adequate explanation on its completion was not always given.
3. The routine keeping of the chart caused anxiety in almost one-quarter of the women using it.

However, Neldam (1980) has demonstrated that maternal monitoring of fetal movements can aid the timely delivery of infants who are at increased risk of intrauterine death.

EFFECTS OF LATE-PREGNANCY PHYSIOLOGICAL CHANGES ON THE MOTHER

The endocrine milieu during pregnancy and its effect on the pregnant woman have been discussed in Section I. The predominant hormones are oestrogens (mainly oestradiol-17 beta) and progesterone and the balance between the two gradually changes towards term. They play a major role in uterine growth and activity but have other profound maternal effects.

Uterine growth is stimulated by oestrogens and mechanical stretching. Although uterine mass increases 20-fold during pregnancy, new muscle is only formed in the early weeks. Hypertrophy is the main feature up to mid-pregnancy; distension thereafter.

Uterine muscle contracts rhythmically even when isolated, but myometrial excitability is suppressed by progesterone. Oestrogen promotes prostaglandin production but the progesterone effect predominates until the late weeks of pregnancy. Thus the frequency and intensity of uterine contractions gradually increase from their low level in the first half of pregnancy. Irregular, low-frequency, high-amplitude Braxton Hicks contractions are most apparent in the last 2 months.

The balance between the effects of progesterone and oestrogens slowly swings towards the latter as labour approaches. As a result the activity of the myometrium at the fundus of the uterus increases. However, the muscle in the lower segment remains relatively inactive. Thus the unique ability of myometrium to retract (i.e. preserve the same tone but shorten) as well as contract allows the physiological lower segment to form and encourages the fetal presenting part to enter the pelvic brim (i.e. to engage).

The cervix softens early in pregnancy due to increased vascularity and gradual replacement of collagen by fluid under the influence of relaxin. As labour approaches, the cervix shortens (or effaces) and the os moves anteriorly.

One of the main functions of late antenatal care is to observe these changes and to ascertain that the fetal lie and presentation are optimal for safe labour and delivery.

Other unwanted effects

Venous pressure is greatly increased in the femoral and other leg veins due to caval compression by the uterus and fetus and pressure of blood returning from the uterus. This is one of the causes of peripheral oedema. *Varicose veins* in the leg or around the vulva may also develop or get worse during late pregnancy. Support tights and rest with legs up are advised. Mild to moderate varicose veins do not seem to predispose to deep vein thrombosis unless additional risk factors exist.

Inferior vena caval compression by the large uterus can cause hypotension and syncope on lying supine in late pregnancy. This *supine hypotensive syndrome* can be troublesome for the mother and fetus. Women should be advised to avoid this position during late pregnancy.

Pressure of the growing uterus and fetus on other organs combined with the smooth muscle-relaxing effect of progesterone produce many of the symptoms of late pregnancy, for example, regurgitation of acid stomach contents into the oesophagus and the increased incidence of hiatus hernia causing *heartburn*. Antacids should be prescribed and the woman advised to sleep propped up on several pillows. Pressure on the bladder, increasing further by engagement of the presenting part, produces *frequency of micturition* and nocturia. Once urinary infections are excluded there is no remedy for this.

In addition to its effect on the cervix, *relaxin* causes softening of the pelvic joints and supporting ligaments. This allows some flexibility in the pelvis during birth but also leads to backache, and may cause difficulty in walking. In its severest form the whole pelvis can become unstable. Pelvic girdle support from a specially designed garment (Fembrace) can give considerable relief without pressure on the uterus.

ACHIEVING AIMS

The aims of antenatal care can be summarized as appropriate care, by the appropriate person, in the appropriate place. The fetomaternal surveillance function of antenatal care is best considered in three phases:

1. First-phase antenatal screening: this is routinely applicable to all pregnant women, usually on a shared-care basis and comprises:
   a. clinical impression of uterine and fetal size.
   b. serial measurement of fundal height.
   c. daily count of perceived fetal movements from 28 weeks.
2. Second-phase antenatal screening: this is applicable to mothers in whom first-phase tests have deviated from locally accepted norms or in whom other risk factors exist (see Chapter 16). Among the second-phase tests are:
   a. serial ultrasonic assessment of fetal growth.
   b. biochemical tests of fetoplacental function.
   c. fetal heart rate monitoring — the true value of this has not yet been fully assessed. Visual assessments are liable to bias and computerized methods are not yet widely available.

   Care can continue as second-phase or return to first-phase as determined by test results.
3. Third-phase screening: this intensive surveillance is applicable to women in whom the fetus is thought to be at highest risk on the basis of second-phase screening. The available tests are:
   a. biophysical profile scoring, which reviews a variety of fetal movements, fetal heart rate and amniotic fluid volume.
   b. Doppler ultrasound measurement of fetal (umbilical or aortic) or uterine (arcuate artery) blood flow. This has not yet been validated as a reliable indicator of fetal well-being.
   c. fetoscopic sampling and analysis of umbilical cord blood may be indicated in a few instances of exceptionally high fetal risk (Nicolaides et al 1986).

Care can revert to second-phase or a decision can be made regarding timing and route of delivery if the balance of risk makes that advisable.

EDUCATIVE FUNCTION

A comprehensive programme of antenatal classes should begin around mid-pregnancy to discuss pregnancy, labour and care of the newborn infant. Classes should be co-ordinated by the midwives and the teaching should be shared among hospital and community midwives, physiotherapists, health visitors and medical staff. Table 17.5 gives an outline programme for these classes.

Table 17.5 Programme for antenatal classes

Pregnancy
Aims of antenatal care — what is done and why
Fetal growth
Remedies for troublesome symptoms such as backache and heartburn
Exercise
General advice about daily life during pregnancy; diet; smoking and alcohol (to stop former and moderate latter); sexual intercourse (no risks confirmed)
Preparation for labour
Signs and symptoms of onset of labour
Timing and procedure for admission
Basic physiology of labour
Signs of progress in labour
Induction of labour
Breathing and relaxation during labour
Analgesia — options and indications
Role of the father during labour
Deviation from normality — definitions and brief descriptions
Indications for and methods of fetal monitoring
Normal delivery — positions and policies
Instrumental delivery and Caesarean section
Third stage of labour
Indications for and repair of episiotomy
Immediate care of the newborn baby
Puerperium and care of newborn infant
The puerperium — what to expect and when
Care of the breasts
Infant-feeding and coping with a newborn baby
Routine neonatal screening tests (e.g. for phenylketonuria and thyroid function)
Contraception

Fathers should be involved as much as possible. Plenty of time should be available for discussion so that anxieties can be expressed and misunderstandings clarified. Try to make time to discuss couples' birth plans.

A tour of the hospital, including a visit to the delivery suite, should be organized to meet the midwives and see the rooms and facilities.

Enkin (1982) emphasizes that antenatal classes are as clearly interventions as any other prophylactic or therapeutic measure. They have their potential for good or harm and therefore need evaluation. The existence of classes may, in fact, be more important than what is taught. Certainly women who attend classes require less analgesia on average than those who do not attend, and they have a more positive experience of labour and delivery despite there being no difference in length of labour between the two groups.

PROGRAMME, PLACE AND PERSONNEL

Two suggested programmes for late antenatal care which are currently being tested (Royal College of Obstetricians and Gynaecologists 1982, Marsh 1985) are shown in Table 17.2.

The three quotations which follow come from a general practitioner, a group of midwives and an obstetrician respectively.

It is doubtful whether any low risk women (roughly three-quarters of all pregnancies) who are booked for delivery in a general practice or specialist unit need to be seen at hospital at all, except perhaps for a scan at 16 weeks and a consultation at 36 weeks if the specialist unit is to be responsible for the delivery (Marsh 1985).

The skills of the professionals involved in the provision of antenatal care should be more closely related to the needs of the women for whom they care. It cannot make sound economic sense to train midwives to provide antenatal care and then fail to make use of their skills. Midwives can provide the kind of care which most women need, and should be given every opportunity to do so (Robinson et al 1982).

Those providing a high level of care have no choice but to limit their patients to those specifically in need of such care. This is necessary in order to maintain both adequate experience and expertise, and to afford sufficient time to deal not only with pregnancy and its medical problems but with the pregnant woman and her family as well. The remaining pregnancies can safely be cared for by primary attendants without this being a lower level of care (Keirse 1982).

Continuing antenatal care should therefore be organized on the following basis:

1. The midwife is uniquely trained and given statutory responsibility for the care of the pregnant woman. She is therefore the key person, and not merely a handmaiden to the doctor.
2. The specialist team should concentrate their effort on those pregnancies at higher risk of fetal or maternal problems.
3. As much care as possible should take place in the community within the confines of availability of specialist staff and the willingness of general practitioners to carry out the process of risk assessment.
4. A Lancet Leading Article (1986) has emphasized that 'the actual pattern of care may be less important than the attitudes and efficiency of those providing it, particularly the degree of collaboration between specialists and generalists. Delegation of responsibility must be backed up by trust and support as well as a high standard of performance demonstrated by audit'.

Table 17.6 The elements of proper business management (from Shaw & Day 1978)

1. Define the problem
2. Locate the critical factor
3. Determine the conditions for its solution, the need to meet objectives and the balance between present and future
4. Analyse the problem
5. Find the facts necessary to a solution and capable of being obtained
6. Know where facts stop and assumptions begin
7. Develop alternative solutions, including 'do nothing'
8. Choose between solutions, using as criteria for choice: risk, economy of effort, timing, limitation of resources
9. Make the solution effective

CONCLUSIONS

Antenatal care is all about management and planning. Its most important but not sole function is risk assessment. Although different in many respects from business management, the basic principles are in fact very similar. For example, Table 17.6 shows the elements of proper business management outlined by Shaw & Day (1978). Plans must be produced and then applied. Production of a plan requires a balance between what is needed and what is possible. The way to achieve it and assess results must be decided beforehand. Application of the plan requires integrated management and good organization.

Unless these criteria can be fulfilled, the less tangible but important caring aspects of what we do amount to very little. To give an extreme and fortunately rare example, sympathy at the loss of a baby does not amount to much if properly organized care could have prevented it in the first place.

REFERENCES

Chapple J 1982 Indices of perinatal care: an epidemiologist's view. British Journal of Obstetrics and Gynaecology 89: 416–417

Draper J, Field S, Thomas H, Hare M J 1986 Women's views on keeping fetal movement charts. British Journal of Obstetrics and Gynaecology 93: 334–338

Enkin M 1982 Antenatal classes. In: Enkin M, Chalmers I (eds) Effectiveness and satisfaction in antenatal care. Spastics International, London, pp 151–162

Enkin M, Chalmers I 1982 Effectiveness and satisfaction in antenatal care. Spastics International, London, pp 266–290

Garcia J 1982 Women's views of antenatal care. In: Enkin M, Chalmers I (eds) Effectiveness and satisfaction in antenatal care. Spastics International, London, pp 81–91

Grant A, Mohide P 1982 Screening and diagnostic tests in antenatal care. In: Enkin M, Chalmers I (eds) Effectiveness and satisfaction in antenatal care. Spastics International, London, pp 22–59

Hall M, Chng P K 1982 Antenatal care in practice. In: Enkin M, Chalmers I (eds) Effectiveness and satisfaction in antenatal care. Spastics International, London, pp 60–68

Keirse M J N C 1982 Interaction between primary and secondary antenatal care, with particular reference to the Netherlands. In: Enkin M, Chalmers I (eds) Effectiveness and satisfaction in antenatal care. Spastics International, London, pp 222–233

Kitzinger S 1981 Change in antenatal care — a report of a working party set up for the National Childbirth Trust. National Childbirth Trust, London

Lancet Leading Article 1986 Antenatal care assessed. Lancet i: 1072–1074

Lilford R J, Chard T 1983 Problems and pitfalls of risk assessment in antenatal care. British Journal of Obstetrics and Gynaecology 90: 507–510

Marsh G N 1985 New programme of antenatal care in general practice. British Medical Journal 291: 646–648

Maternity Services Advisory Committee 1982 Maternity care in action I: antenatal care. HMSO, London

Neldam S 1980 Fetal movements as an indication of fetal wellbeing. Lancet i: 1222–1224

Nicolaides K H, Soothill P W, Rodeck C H, Campbell S 1986 Ultrasound-guided sampling of umbilical cord and placental blood to assess fetal wellbeing. Lancet i: 1065–1067

Parboosingh J, Kerr M 1982 Innovations in the role of obstetric hospitals in prenatal care. In: Enkin M, Chalmers I (eds) Effectiveness and satisfaction in antenatal care. Spastics International, London, pp 254–265
Patrick J, Campbell K, Carmichael L et al 1982 Patterns of gross fetal body movements over 24 hour observation periods during last 10 weeks of pregnancy. American Journal of Obstetrics and Gynecology 142: 363–371
Pearson J F, Weaver J B 1976 Fetal activity and fetal wellbeing: an evaluation. British Medical Journal i: 1305–1307
Peters T, Golding J 1985 In: Mulunsky A, Friedman E A, Gluck L (eds) Advances in Perinatal Medicine, vol. 4, pp 235–262. Plenum, New York
Quaranta P, Currell R, Redman C W G, Robinson J S 1981 Prediction of small-for-dates infants by measurement of symphysial–fundal height. British Journal of Obstetrics and Gynaecology 88: 115–119
Rayburn W F 1982 Antepartum fetal assessment: monitoring fetal activity. Clinics in Perinatalogy 9: 231–252
Redman C W G 1982 Screening for pre-eclampsia. In: Enkin M, Chalmers I (eds) Effectiveness and satisfaction in antenatal care. Spastics International, London, pp 69–80
Robinson S, Golden J, Bradley S 1982 The role of the midwife in the provision of antenatal care. In: Enkin M, Chalmers I (eds) Effectiveness and satisfaction in antenatal care. Spastics International, London, pp 234–246
Rosenberg K, Grant J M, Tweedie I, Aitchison T, Gallagher F 1982 Measurement of fundal height as a screening for FGR. British Journal of Obstetrics and Gynaecology 89: 447–450
Royal College of Obstetricians and Gynaecologists 1982 Report on antenatal and intrapartum care. Royal College of Obstetricians and Gynaecologists, London
Shaw W C, Day G J 1978 The businessman's complete check list. Business Books, London
Stirrat G M, Beeley L 1986 Prescribing in pregnancy. Clinics in Obstetrics and Gynaecology 13: 161–416

SECTION 3

Assessment of Fetal State in Early Pregnancy

J. G. Grudzinskas

The endocrinological and metabolic assessment of early pregnancy

INTRODUCTION

The detection of human chorionic gonadotrophin (hCG) in maternal blood or urine is the basis of pregnancy diagnosis by biochemical methods, since hCG is observed from the time of implantation. More recently, the systematic examination of the placenta, decidua and maternal blood has led to the identification of a new generation of proteins which may be used in the diagnosis of early pregnancy and its failure (Table 18.1). For example, measurements of Schwangerschafts protein 1 (SP1) can be used in the biochemical diagnosis of pregnancy (Grudzinskas et al 1977), and recent reports have described consistently depressed levels of pregnancy-associated plasma protein A (PAPP-A) in early pregnancy failure (Westergaard et al 1985). Furthermore, the recent detection of secretory proteins of decidual/endometrial origin holds the promise of the first non-invasive indices of function of these tissues. This chapter deals with the clinical application of measurement of hormones and proteins of fetal, maternal and placental origin in normal and abnormal early pregnancy.

Table 18.1 Placental and decidual proteins of possible diagnostic value in early pregnancy (after Bell 1986, Grudzinskas et al 1986)

Placental
Human chorionic gonadotrophin (hCG)
Schwangerschaftsprotein 1 (SP1)
Human placental lactogen (hPL)
Pregnancy-associated plasma protein A (PAPP-A)
Placental protein 5 (PP5)
Endometrial/decidual
Insulin-like growth-factor-binding protein (SBP: α_1PEG, PP12, α_1CMG, α_1PAMG)
Progestogen-dependent endometrial protein (PEP: α_2PEG, PP14, α_2CMG, α_2PAMG, AUP)

DIAGNOSIS OF PREGNANCY

The early diagnosis of pregnancy depends on the detection of hCG in maternal urine, or 1–2 days earlier in blood. The current developments in assay technology have contributed to the resolution of problems of potential non-specific results. However, it must be recognized that highly sensitive assays have shown the ubiquitous nature of hCG at low concentrations (<5 iu/l), and in clinical practice a single estimation of hCG should only be considered indicative of pregnancy if it is greater than 25 iu/l or if a lower level of hCG is seen to increase twofold at an interval of 3 days (Jones et al 1983). If hCG has been administered, estimations should be delayed until clearance of the exogenous hCG has occurred, possibly postponing the diagnosis by up to 14 days. In this circumstance, assays for other proteins of placental origin, namely SP1, may be appropriate. Other pregnancy-associated proteins, such as human placental lactogen (hPL), PAPP-A and placental protein 5 (PP5), are not serious contenders as diagnostic tests since they do not appear in the maternal blood until after 6 weeks of amenorrhoea. Finally, hCG results immediately after implantation should be interpreted with care; the earlier the diagnosis is made, the less likely is the outcome to be normal (Table 18.2) given the

Table 18.2 Pregnancy outcome in relation to time of diagnosis

Time of diagnosis	Likelihood of normal outcome (%)
Preimplantation	25–30
Postimplantation	43–60
Six weeks' amenorrhoea	85–90
Second trimester	95
Third trimester	98

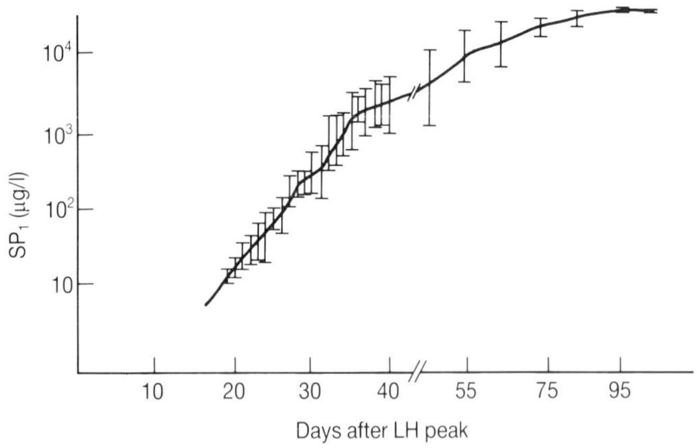

Fig. 18.1 Mean serum levels of Schwangerschaftsprotein 1 in nine women during early normal pregnancy. From Lenton et al (1981).

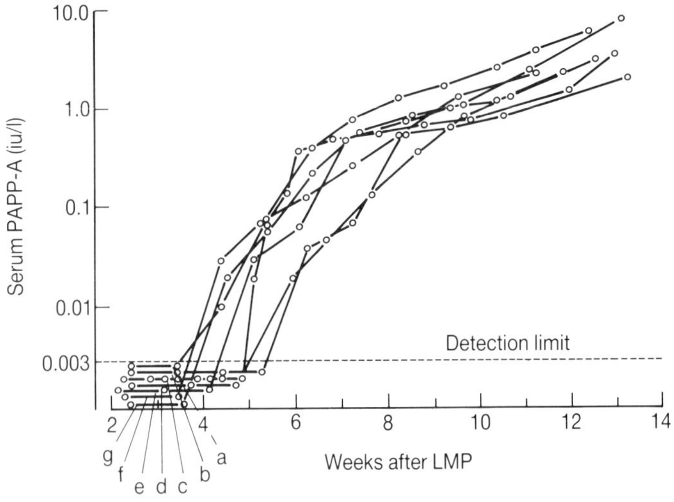

Fig. 18.2 Serum levels of pregnancy-associated plasma protein A in seven women during early normal pregnancy. From Chemnitz et al (1986).

very high rate of spontaneous pregnancy failure in the peri-implantation period (see below).

It may be desirable to restrict the use of the most sensitive hCG tests to specific clinical situations (e.g. subfertility or suspected ectopic gestation) rather than increasing the availability of diagnosis at this early stage of pregnancy in the normal population.

ENDOCRINOLOGY AND METABOLISM OF NORMAL EARLY PREGNANCY

The apparent trigger for synthesis of hCG by the conceptus is implantation. The stimulus for the production of other placental products, such as hPL, SP1 and PAPP-A, is unclear but is likely to include implantation and other as yet unrecognized events. SP1 secretion into the maternal circulation appears likely to be simultaneous with implantation and the trends in blood concentration seem to parallel the growth rate curve of functioning trophoblast (Grudzinskas et al 1977, Lenton et al 1981, Ahmed & Klopper 1985; Fig. 18.1). In normal pregnancy this pattern contrasts with that of hCG, but is similar to hPL, PAPP-A and PP5. The synthesis of SP1, at least for the initial weeks of pregnancy, seems to be independent of the presence of an embryo or fetus, and also of the site of implantation, as seen in women with ectopic gestation. In normal pregnancy the doubling times for hCG and SP1 are quite similar; concentrations of hCG and SP1 double in 2–3 days in the first 6 weeks of pregnancy (Lenton et al 1981).

The disappearance rates of these molecules after removal of the placenta are also equivalent: 40–60 hours. Curiously, there is not a large literature on hPL in early pregnancy, and this hormone is not generally considered to be useful as a pregnancy test (Letchworth 1976). Blood levels of hPL increase as pregnancy advances, and have a relationship to functioning trophoblast mass. Circulating PAPP-A can be detected in the maternal circulation consistently 28 days after conception in singleton pregnancies, but the relatively late appearance of this molecule in the peripheral blood also precludes it from use as a primary diagnostic test for pregnancy (Chemnitz et al 1986; Fig. 18.2). PAPP-A levels increase throughout gestation with a mean doubling time of 4.9 days during the first trimester; the disappearance rate after removal of the placenta is several days (Sinosich et al 1988).

The production of oestradiol and progesterone is transferred from the corpus luteum of pregnancy to the feto-placental unit in the middle of the first trimester (Klopper 1985). The synthesis of alpha-fetoprotein (AFP) by embryonal endodermal tissues is reflected by an increase in circulating levels during the first trimester; substantial amounts of AFP are detected consistently after 10 weeks' gestation (Kunz & Keller 1976). Synthesis of the secretory proteins of the endometrium may parallel the morphological changes which this tissue undergoes (Bell 1986).

Insulin-like growth-factor-binding protein of decidual origin is consistently seen in the maternal blood in the latter half of the first trimester. Peak levels are seen in mid-pregnancy. By contrast, the trends in blood levels of progestogen-dependent endometrial protein (PEP) bear a striking similarity to hCG.

CONTROL OF SYNTHESIS AND SECRETION

The mechanisms which control the synthesis of proteins of trophoblastic origin are poorly understood; uteroplacental perfusion probably plays a major role, influencing synthesis and secretion according to the law of mass action (Chard & Grudzinskas 1985). Nevertheless, it is possible to draw some conclusions on the possible effects of the ovary, the embryo and the endometrium. Firstly, following successful intrauterine pregnancy in women participating in embryo donation programmes, pregnancy seems to be independent of ovarian support as only synthetic oestrogens and progestogens were administered for the first 8–9 weeks of the pregnancies of women with ovarian failure, or after bilateral oophorectomy (Lutjen et al 1984). Secondly, whereas depressed levels of some trophoblastic proteins and hormones are seen when complications of early pregnancy become evident clinically, the initiation of synthesis and secretion appears to be unrelated to the presence of the embryo, as evidenced in blighted ovum and hydatidiform mole.

Thirdly, the site of implantation and presumably the interaction between the trophoblast and decidualized endometrium seem to be of minor relevance for the majority of the substances considered here, at least in the earliest days of pregnancy. Trophoblastic hormones and proteins have been consistently observed in ectopic gestation, but the abnormalities in synthesis have varied widely, the earliest and greatest difference being seen for PAPP-A, and the least for hCG (Sinosich et al 1985). Finally, with the possible exception of PAPP-A in association with Cornelia de Lange syndrome, fetal congenital abnormalities are not related to changes in circulating levels of trophoblastic proteins in either direction, since normal pregnancy outcome has been reported in association with the apparent absence of hPL and SP1 (Westergaard et al 1983). Gross elevations of hCG and SP1 in amniotic fluid have been reported in pregnancies complicated by Meckel's syndrome, but these changes are not reflected in the maternal circulation (Heikinheimo et al 1982). By contrast, the metabolism of progesterone and oestrogen in pregnancy is well described (see Chapter 25), and the dramatic changes in ovarian hormones observed in early pregnancy, given the work of Lutjen and his colleagues (1984), is presumably part of the maternal response to pregnancy rather than a primary phenomenon.

Currently there is little information available on endometrial and decidual proteins (Bell 1986, 1988).

COMPLICATIONS OF EARLY PREGNANCY

Early pregnancy failure

The chances of a woman desirous of pregnancy producing a viable offspring in any one ovarian cycle is approximately 25%. Detailed studies using sensitive biochemical tests confirm these conclusions; the findings are remarkably similar whether ovulation and pregnancy have occurred spontaneously, or whether they resulted from an in-vitro fertilization–embryo transfer (IVF–ET) programme (Table 18.3).

The incidence of clinically obvious miscarriage is 10–15%, whether fertilization occurred in vivo or in vitro. Estimates of the incidence of this phenomenon vary from 8 to 55%. The meticulous work of Hertig et al (1952), together with the calculations of Roberts & Lowe (1975), stimulated these studies. Differences in clinical study design, assay techniques, and populations account for the discordance in the current data; one of the major issues is the specificity of the substances is measured as an index of trophoblastic activity. In this respect, hCG measurements must still be considered as superior to those of SP1 (unless hCG has been given therapeutically). By contrast, ultrasonic findings such as uterine distension or a gestational sac cannot be considered as specific signs of pregnancy.

Table 18.3 Studies on subclinical and clinical miscarriage

Reference	Method	Pregnancy loss (%)
Hertig et al (1952)	Histology	43
Block (1976)	hLH	37.5
Braunstein et al (1977)	hCG	15
Chartier et al (1979)	hCG	30
Miller et al (1980)	hCG	43
Edmonds et al (1982)	hCG	62
Edwards & Steptoe (1983)	hCG	25–35
Jones et al (1983)	hCG	33
Whittaker et al (1983)	hCG	20
Wilcox et al (1985)	hCG	24
Seppala et al (1979a)	SP1	Not stated
Ahmed & Klopper (1983)	SP1	Not stated

hLH = human luteinizing hormone; hCG = human chorionic gonadotrophin; SP1 = Schwangerschaftsprotein 1

Threatened and spontaneous miscarriage

Circulating levels of hormones and proteins of fetal, placental and maternal origin have been used to predict the outcome in women with vaginal bleeding in early pregnancy (Niven et al 1972, Nygren et al 1973, Garoff & Seppala 1975, Kunz & Keller 1976, Braunstein et al 1978, Damber et al 1978, Jovanovic et al 1978, Schultz-Larsen & Hertz 1978, Joupilla et al 1979, Masson et al 1983a,b, Salem et al 1984). Ultrasound examination has revolutionized this practice, and some of these tests are probably obsolete if fetal life can be demonstrated by ultrasound (Joupilla et al 1980a,b, Hertz et al 1980). Nevertheless, a proportion of patients in whom fetal heart action has been demonstrated will spontaneously miscarry. We have examined serum levels of hPL, SP1, PAPP-A, progesterone, oestradiol, AFP and pregnancy-zone protein (PZP) in this situation (Westergaard et al 1985). In the 108 patients in whom the history and clinical findings were indicative of threatened miscarriage, ultrasound revealed a fetal heart action in 77, whereas examination during the first week of study gave no clearcut evidence of fetal life in the remaining 31 patients. Ultrasound scans were done at weekly intervals for 3 weeks and every 2 weeks thereafter, unless otherwise indicated by vaginal bleeding. Maternal venous blood was obtained at each ultrasound scan, and samples obtained within 24 hours of miscarriage were excluded from analysis.

Spontaneous miscarriage occurred in 42 pregnancies, 31 of which showed no sign of fetal heart action on repeated scan examination. In the remaining 11 patients, the fetal heart action was observed repeatedly until miscarriage occurred. Tables 18.4 and 18.5 summarize the sensitivity,

Table 18.4 The predictive value of abnormal (PV+) and normal (PV−) levels, sensitivity and relative risk of maternal, fetal and placental protein and hormone measurements in initial samples from patients with threatened miscarriage in the presence of fetal life. Numbers in brackets refer to the analyses if ultrasonic results are not considered

	hCG	hPL	SP1	PAPP-A	AFP	O_2	P	PZP
PV+	0	28.6	12.5	53.8	20.0	0	22.2	23.3
	(86.7)	(82.8)	(80.6)	(85.7)	(33.3)	(78.4)	(80.6)	(60.0)
PV−	84.9	87.1	85.5	93.8	86.1	84.1	86.8	88.2
	(79.5)	(77.2)	(81.9)	(90.9)	(60.8)	(81.7)	(81.9)	(64.5)
Sensitivity	0	18.2	9.1	63.6	9.1	0	18.2	27.3
	(61.9)	(57.1)	(69.0)	(85.7)	(5.0)	(67.0)	(69.0)	(21.4)
Relative risk	0	2.3	0.9	8.5	1.4	0	1.7	2.8
	(4.2)	(3.6)	(4.5)	(9.4)	(0.8)	(4.2)	4.5	(1.7)

hCG = human chorionic gonadotrophin; hPL = human placental lactogen; SP1 = Schwangerschaftsprotein 1; PAPP-A = pregnancy-associated plasma protein A; AFP = alpha-fetoprotein; E_2 = oestradiol-17β; P = progesterone; PZP = pregnancy-zone protein

Table 18.5 The predictive value of abnormal (PV+) and normal (PV−) levels, sensitivity and relative risk of maternal, fetal and placental protein and hormone measurements in all samples from patients with threatened miscarriage in the presence of fetal life. Numbers in brackets refer to the analyses if ultrasonic results are not considered

	hCG	hPL	SP1	PAPP-A	AFP	O_2	P	PZP
PV+	6.7	16.7	5.8	48.8	61.1	0	8.3	9.5
	(44.0)	(43.7)	(41.7)	(63.2)	(63.0)	(41.3)	(44.3)	(27.0)
PV−	90.8	91.8	90.6	98.8	92.9	90.1	90.9	91.1
	(89.1)	(90.0)	(90.1)	(98.4)	(86.7)	(89.7)	(90.2)	(86.5)
Sensitivity	6.5	17.4	6.5	89.1	23.9	0	8.7	8.7
	(40.7)	(38.3)	(43.2)	(91.4)	(14.8)	(40.7)	(43.2)	(17.3)
Relative risk	0.7	2.0	0.6	41.8	8.6	0	0.9	1.0
	(4.3)	(4.2)	(4.2)	(38.9)	(4.8)	(4.0)	(4.5)	(2.0)

hCG = human chorionic gonadotrophin; hPL = human placental lactogen; SP1 = Schwangerschaftsprotein 1; PAPP-A = pregnancy-associated plasma protein A; AFP = alpha-fetoprotein; O_2 = oestradiol-17β; P = progesterone; PZP = pregnancy-zone protein

predictive values and relative risk of normal and abnormal levels of the biochemical indices measured in the first sample, and in all samples in relation to the scan findings in the women who aborted. The predictive value of an abnormal level in the sample obtained at presentation was greatest for PAPP-A, particularly if there was scan evidence of fetal life (54%). When all abnormal results were considered, the predictive value was highest for AFP and PAPP-A (Table 18.5).

The differences between the indices, both in single and serial samples, were less if the ultrasound findings were not included. The sensitivity was highest for PAPP-A levels, regardless of whether the first sample (64%) or all samples were considered, in patients with ultrasound evidence of a live fetus. The predictive value of a normal test was comparable for all variables if the first sample was considered. However, when serial samples were considered and ultrasound demonstrated a live fetus, the highest value (99%) was for PAPP-A estimations.

The relative risk of miscarriage was highest for depressed levels of PAPP-A, being at least three times greater than that calculated for the other biochemical indices at clinical presentation if the fetus was alive, and 5–10 times greater if all samples were considered, regardless of the ultrasound findings. All the 11 women who had evidence of a live fetus but subsequently miscarried had depressed PAPP-A levels. In the serum obtained from these patients, PAPP-A levels were abnormal at least 4 weeks before miscarriage in four patients and in every sample obtained in the other seven (Fig. 18.3, 18.4). In contrast, the levels of the other substances measured generally remained within the normal range — the only exception was AFP.

This study examined many of the unanswered questions concerning the value of biochemical tests relative to ultrasound. Firstly, only abnormal PAPP-A levels distinguished those pregnancies which miscarried from those which did not, even when there was ultrasonic evidence of fetal heart action at the time of blood sampling. Secondly, depressed PAPP-A levels were seen several weeks before spontaneous miscarriage in some patients. Thirdly, if the heart action was not evident ultrasonically on repeated examination, depressed or abnormal levels of placental hCG, SP1, hPL, oestradiol, PAPP-A, AFP and progesterone were consistently seen. Fourthly, if miscarriage occurred after the detection of fetal heart action, the levels of these molecules were generally in the normal range, the sole exception being PAPP-A.

Finally, if the heart action was detected and the serum PAPP-A levels were normal, the chance of a normal outcome for that pregnancy was in excess of 98%. These findings (Westergaard et al 1985) do not agree with some reports on the usefulness of biochemical tests in threatened miscarriage (Huisjes 1984), but do substantiate the view that ultrasound has a useful role in the management of these disorders.

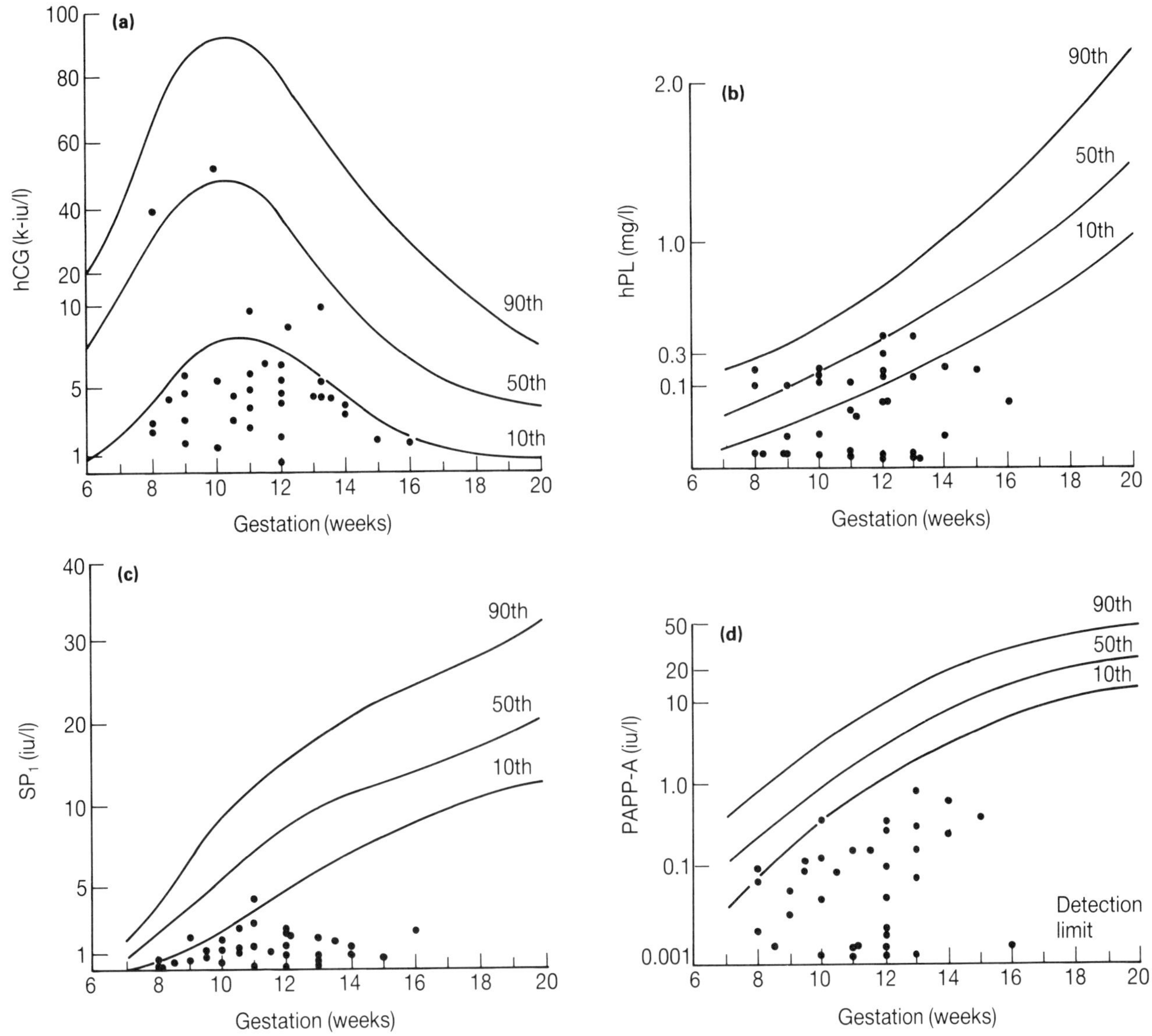

Fig. 18.3 Serum levels of (**a**) human chorionic gonadotrophin; (**b**) human placental lactogen; (**c**) Schwangerschaftsprotein 1 and (**d**) pregnancy-associated plasma protein A in 42 women with spontaneous abortion. Heavy lines represent the 10th, 50th and 90th centiles of the normal range. WHO reference material for pregnancy proteins 78/610. From Westergaard et al (1985).

ANEMBRYONIC PREGNANCY

Failure of development of the embryo makes it possible to examine the contribution of the growing conceptus to the control of protein and hormone synthesis by trophoblastic tissue. After the middle of the first trimester, ultrasonic demonstration of an empty sac is diagnostic, but prior to that time biochemical tests may be of value. Chapman and colleagues (1984) have observed depressed maternal levels of placental products in one-third of 22 women with this condition who were studied serially from 6 to 16 weeks of gestation. Furthermore, mean levels of circulating hCG were shown to be depressed at 4 weeks' gestation in a group of women studied prospectively at a subfertility clinic; mean levels of maternal PAPP-A, oestradiol and progesterone fell some 3 weeks later (Yovich et al 1986). These findings confirm that a deviation from the normal rise in blood levels of hCG is highly suggestive of failed pregnancy at a time before ultrasound can provide useful information, i.e. in the absence of fetal heart action (Grudzinskas et al 1988).

ECTOPIC PREGNANCY

The use of biochemical tests in this condition has been reviewed (Kadar 1983) and confirms the value of assays capable of detecting the very low concentrations of hCG present in this condition. These tests alert the clinician to the possibility of a pregnancy-related disorder if hCG is detected, and virtually exclude the diagnosis if a negative result (i.e. <25

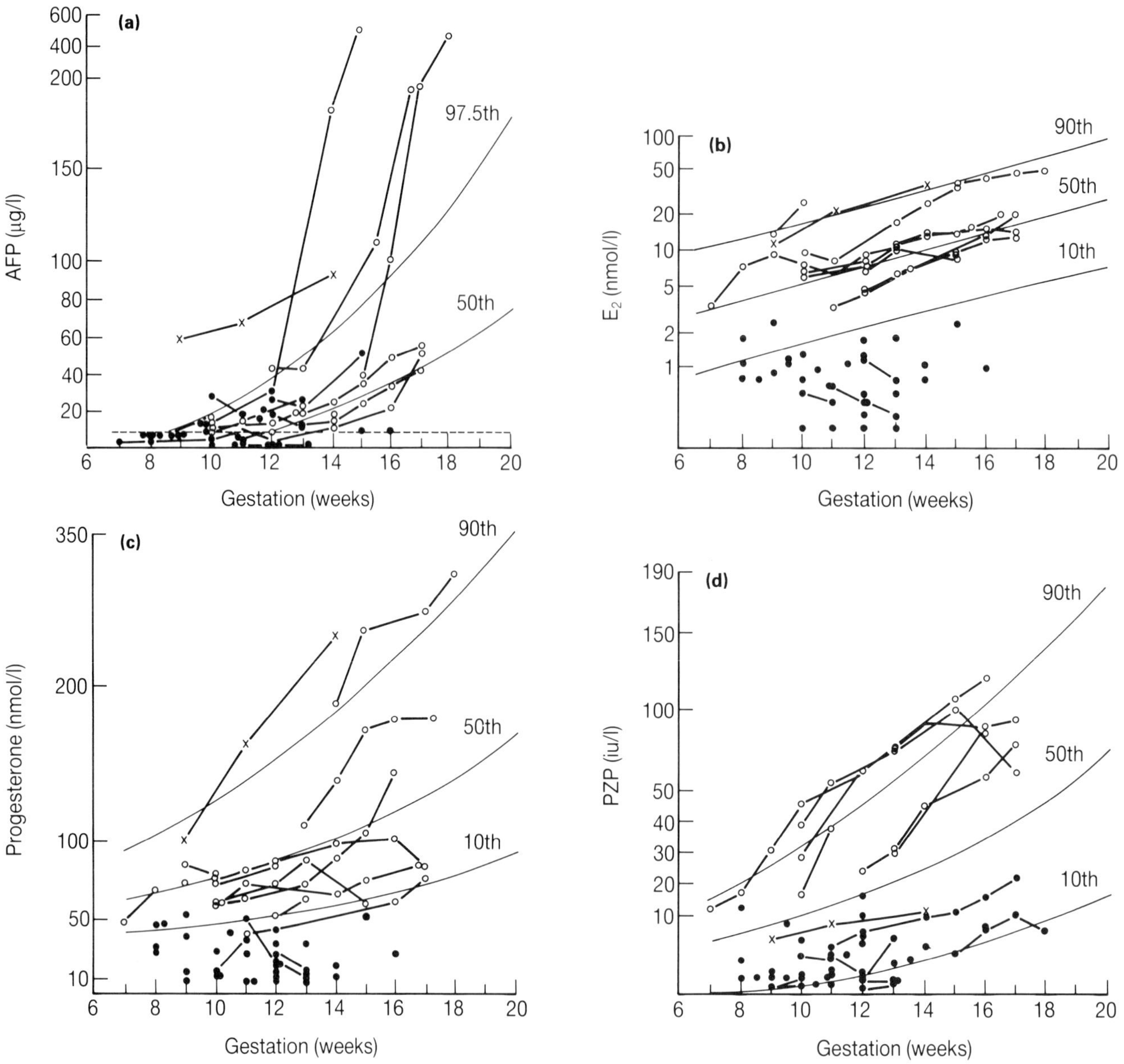

Fig. 18.4 (**a**) Alpha-fetoprotein; (**b**) prostaglandin E_2; (**c**) progesterone; (**d**) pregnancy-zone protein. ● = No ultrasonic evidence of fetal heart action; ○ = ultrasonic evidence of heart action; △ = twin pregnancy with live fetuses. Heavy lines represent the 10th, 50th and 90th centiles of the normal range. WHO reference material for pregnancy proteins 78/610. From Westergaard et al (1985).

iu/l) is obtained. Estimations of hCG used in conjunction with other tests may also facilitate the diagnosis. Quantitative estimations of hCG may also be of some value, since depressed levels are commonly seen in ectopic gestation. The combined use of hCG measurements and ultrasonic examination can often distinguish between normal or failed intrauterine pregnancy and ectopic gestation (Pittaway et al 1985). The use of a discriminatory zone for hCG in conjunction with ultrasound can also be most helpful.

If levels of hCG are greater than 6500 iu/l, ultrasound examination should reveal the presence of a live embryo in utero; if this is not the case, failed pregnancy, in particular ectopic gestation, should be suspected (Kadar 1983).

The data on SP1 are similar to that on hCG, while the findings with PAPP-A levels suggest that secretion is more severely compromised in this condition (Chemnitz et al 1984, Sinosich et al 1985). A preliminary report has shown that PAPP-A levels were depressed in all 17 women with ectopic gestation, with PAPP-A being detectable in only two women (Sinosich et al 1985). In our own study of 108 women with suspected ectopic pregnancy, the diagnosis was confirmed in 27. Low levels of hCG were found in all but four women, and of SP1 in all but three. By contrast, circulating PAPP-A was detected in only half the women with ectopic pregnancy and depressed levels were consistent (Fig. 18.5, Grudzinskas et al 1985). Thus the synthesis of PAPP-A is severely com-

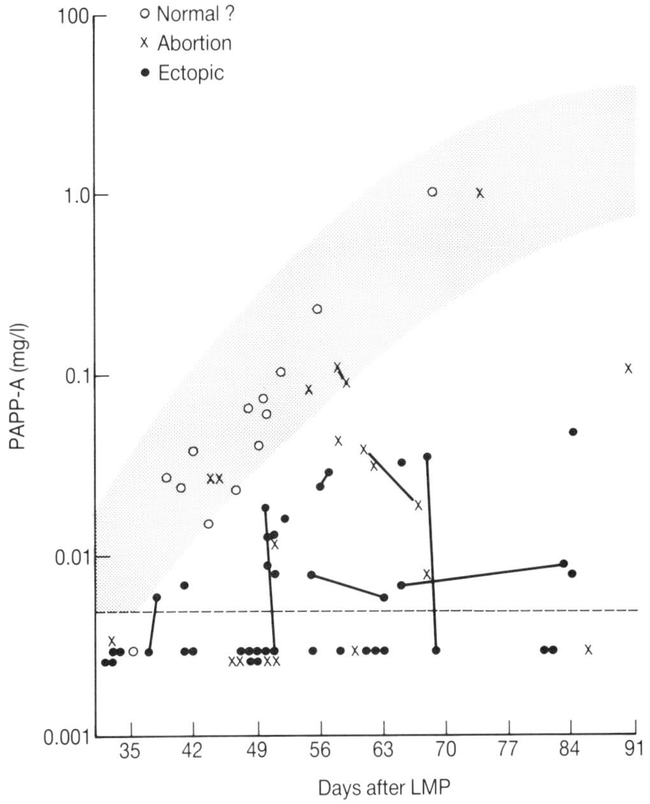

Fig. 18.5 Circulating pregnancy-associated plasma protein A in 50 women with lower abdominal pain. From Grudzinskas et al (1985).

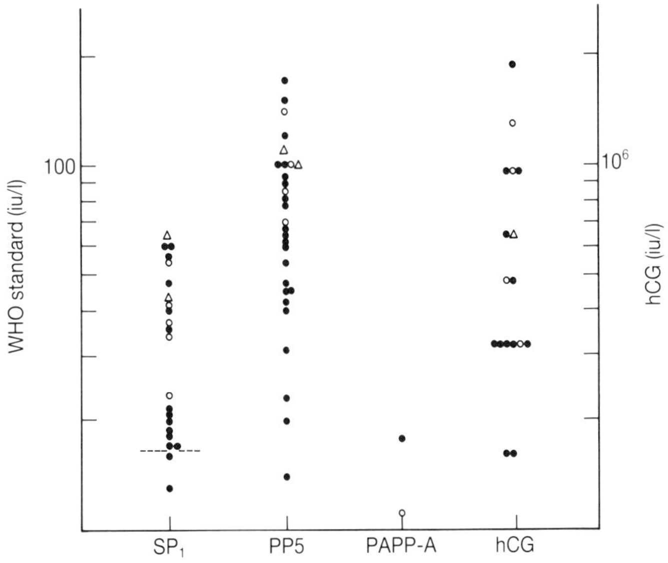

Fig. 18.6 Circulating Schwangerschaftsprotein 1 (SP1), placental protein 5 (PP5), pregnancy-associated plasma protein A (PAPP-A) and human chorionic gonadotrophin (hCG) in 31 patients with gestational trophoblastic tumours before treatment. ● = Hydatidiform mole; ○ = choriocarcinoma; △ = patient with lung metastases; dashed line = 16.5 iu/l WHO standard 78/610. Levels of proteins (SP1, PP5 and PAPP-A) < 10 iu/l or hCG < 100 000 iu/l are not shown. From Tsakok et al (1983).

promised in ectopic gestation; in conjunction with hCG, PAPP-A may form the basis of a new diagnostic test for ectopic pregnancy.

TROPHOBLASTIC DISEASE

The syncytiotrophoblast in hydatidiform mole maintains its ability to synthesize hormones and proteins, and although this capacity is reduced for hPL and steroids, it is considerably greater for hCG.

As the risk of development of choriocarcinoma and subsequent poor prognosis is higher in women in the presence of excessive hCG secretion in gestational trophoblast tumours (Newlands 1983), various centres have evaluated measurements of proteins specifically synthesized by trophoblastic tissue (e.g. SP1, PP5 and PAPP-A) in this context. In untreated hydatidiform mole reduced levels of PAPP-A have been observed in women prior to treatment, whereas elevated levels of circulating SP1 and PP5 are seen (Fig. 18.6, Tsakok et al 1983). High SP1 levels may be predictive of subsequent malignant change but these observations require confirmation. In patients with extensive choriocarcinoma, serum SP1 levels are usually lower than in benign disease and circulating PP5 cannot be detected (Seppala et al 1979b, Lee et al 1981, 1982, Soma et al 1981).

Although the place of hCG estimation in the monitoring of women with this disease is firmly established (see Chapter 31), estimations of the new trophoblastic-specific proteins may give further insight into the pathogenesis of this condition.

PLACENTAL FUNCTION TESTS AS A DIAGNOSTIC GUIDE IN PATIENTS UNDERGOING CHORIONIC VILLUS SAMPLING

Miscarriage occurring immediately and several weeks after chorionic villus sampling has been described and it is still unclear to what extent this complication is a direct result of the surgical procedure.

Ward et al (1985) examined serum levels of AFP, hCG, SP1 and PAPP-A before and 6 hours after villus sampling in 20 women. In the majority, AFP levels rose after sampling. Depressed or elevated preoperative levels of AFP, hCG and PAPP-A were associated with fetal anomalies and pregnancy loss in 7 of the 11 pregnancies which did not progress. All pregnancies but one (missed abortion) were apparently normal when assessed by ultrasound, and the two highest levels of hCG were seen in the pregnancies in which the fetus was homozygous for alpha- and beta-thalassaemia. Similar observations have been made for hPL and SP1 in pregnancies complicated by hydrops fetalis (Bellman et al 1980), suggesting that altered placental protein synthesis may be a useful early index of these conditions.

FUTURE DEVELOPMENTS

Ultrasonic examination has contributed substantially to precise assessment of early pregnancy. Nevertheless, hCG estimations are still the mainstay of the diagnosis of early pregnancy and, when used in conjunction with ultrasound, provide valuable clinical information prior to 6 weeks' gestation. After detection of the embryonic heart action at 6–7 weeks' gestation, only PAPP-A measurements seem to provide useful information. Unfortunately, they are only available on a research basis.

The diagnosis of ectopic gestation is largely dependent on awareness of a possible pregnancy-related disorder. Maternal PAPP-A measurements, used in conjunction with hCG, may increase diagnostic accuracy in this condition.

The identification of the ability of the endometrium and decidua to synthesize secretory proteins which can be measured in the uterine lumen and peripheral blood encourages their inclusion into the reproductive axis as active rather than passive participants. Since these tissues produce hormones, lipids and proteins which act locally and distally, it is possible to consider the endometrium/decidua as an endocrine organ (Healey & Hodgen 1983, Bell 1986, Grudzinskas 1987). The ability to measure these substances, in particular insulin-like growth-factor-binding protein and progestogen-dependent endometrial protein, may provide not only a non-invasive test of endometrial function in the assessment of fertility, but also an index of endometrial/decidual function in the earliest days and weeks of pregnancy.

REFERENCES

Ahmed A G, Klopper A 1983 Diagnosis of early pregnancy by assay of placental proteins. British Journal of Obstetrics and Gynaecology 90: 604–611

Ahmed A G, Klopper A 1985 Concomitant secretion of Schwangerschaftsprotein and human chorionic gonadotrophin following conception. Clinical Endocrinology 23: 677–681

Bell S C 1986 Secretory endometrial and decidual proteins: studies on clinical significance of a maternally derived group of pregnancy associated serum proteins. Human Reproduction 1: 129–143

Bell S C 1988 Synthesis and secretion of proteins by the endometrium. In: Chapman M, Grudzinskas G, Chard T (eds) Implantation. Springer, London, pp 95–118

Bellman O, Tebbe J, Lang N, Baur M P 1980 Determination of SP1 and hPL for predicting perinatal asphyxia. In: Klopper A, Genazzani A, Crosignani P G (eds) The human placenta: proteins and hormones. Academic Press, London, pp 99–108

Block S K 1976 Occult pregnancy. Obstetrics and Gynaecology 48: 365–368

Braunstein G D, Karow W G, Gentry W D, Wade M E 1977 Subclinical spontaneous abortion. Obstetrics and Gynecology 50: 415–445

Braunstein G D, Karow W G, Gentry W C, Rasor I, Wade M M 1978 First trimester chorionic gonadotrophin measurements as an aid in the diagnosis of early pregnancy disorders. American Journal of Obstetrics and Gynecology 143: 25–32

Chapman M G, Bolton A E, Mellows H, Grudzinskas J G 1984 Anembryonic pregnancy — a prospective study of placental biochemical parameters. Proceedings of the 5th International Congress of Placental Proteins, Annecy, France, p 102

Chard T, Grudzinskas J G 1985 Placental and pregnancy-associated proteins: control mechanisms and clinical application. In: Bischof P, Klopper A (eds) Proteins of the placenta. Karger, Basel, pp 104–113

Chartier M M, Roger N, Barrat J, Michelon B 1979 Measurement of plasma hCG and BhCG in the late luteal phase. Evidence of the occurrence of spontaneous menstrual abortions in infertile women. Fertility and Sterility 31: 134–137

Chemnitz J, Tornehave D, Teisner B, Poulsen H K, Westergaard J G 1984 The localisation of pregnancy proteins (hPL, SP1 and PAPP-A) in intra- and extrauterine pregnancies. Placenta 5: 489–494

Chemnitz J, Folkersen J, Teisner B et al 1986 Comparison of different antibody preparations against pregnancy-associated plasma protein A (PAPP-A) for use in localisation and immunoassay studies. British Journal of Obstetrics and Gynaecology 93: 111–118

Damber M G, von Schoultz B, Solheim F, Stigbrand T, Carlstrom K 1978 Prognostic value of the pregnancy zone protein during early pregnancy in spontaneous abortion. Obstetrics and Gynecology 51: 677–681

Edmonds D K, Lindsey K S, Miller J R, Williamson E, Wood P J 1982 Early embryonic mortality in women. Fertility and Sterility 38: 447–453

Edwards R G, Steptoe P C 1983 Current status of in vitro fertilisation and implantation of human embryos. Lancet ii: 1265–1269

Garoff L, Seppala M 1975 Prediction of fetal outcome in threatened abortion by maternal serum placental lactogen and alphafetoprotein. American Journal of Obstetrics and Gynecology 121: 257–261

Grudzinskas J G 1987 Secretory proteins of the endometrium. Tokyo Medical College Journal 45: 170–175

Grudzinskas J G, Gordon Y B, Jeffrey D, Chard T 1977 Specific and sensitive determination of pregnancy specific beta-1 glyco-protein by radioimmunoassay. Lancet i: 333–335

Grudzinskas J G, Westergaard J G, Teisner B 1985 Pregnancy-associated plasma protein A in normal and abnormal pregnancies. In: Bischof P, Klopper A (eds) Proteins of the placenta. Karger, Basel, pp 184–197

Grudzinskas J G, Westergaard J G, Teisner B 1986 Biochemical assessment of placental function: early pregnancy. Clinics in Obstetrics and Gynaecology 13: 553–569

Grudzinskas J G, Stabile I, Campbell S 1988 Early pregnancy failure: biochemical and biophysical assessment. In: Beard R W, Sharp F (eds) Early pregnancy loss: mechanisms and treatment. Peacock Press, Ashton-under-Lyme, pp 183–192

Healey D L, Hodgen G 1983 Endocrinology of the endometrium. Obstetric and Gynaecological Survey 38: 509–530

Heikinheimo M, Wahlstrom T, Aula P, Seppala M 1982 Pregnancy specific beta-1 glycoprotein in amniotic fluid. In: Grudzinskas J G, Teisner B, Seppala M (eds) Pregnancy proteins: biology, chemistry and clinical application. Academic Press, Sydney, pp 215–221

Hertig A T, Rock J, Adams E C, Menkin E C 1952 Thirty-four fertilized human ova, good, bad and indifferent recovered from 210 women of known fertility. Pediatrics 23: 202–211

Hertz J B, Mantoni M, Svenstrup B 1980 Threatened abortion studied by estradio-17-beta in serum and ultrasound. Obstetrics and Gynecology 55: 324–328

Huisjes J J 1984 Spontaneous abortion. In: Lind T (ed) Current review in obstetrics and gynaecology. Churchill Livingstone, Edinburgh, pp 132–136

Jones H W, Acosta A A, Andrews M C et al 1983 What is pregnancy? A question for in vitro fertilisation. Fertility and Sterility 40: 728–733

Joupilla P, Tapanainen J, Huhtaniemi I 1979 Plasma hCG levels in patients with bleeding in the first and second trimesters of pregnancy. British Journal of Obstetrics and Gynaecology 86: 343–349

Joupilla P, Seppala M, Chard T 1980a Pregnancy-specific beta-1 glycoprotein in complications of early pregnancy. Lancet i: 667–668

Joupilla P, Huhtaniemi I, Tapanainen J 1980b Early pregnancy failure: study by ultrasonic and hormonal methods. Obstetrics and Gynecology 55: 42–47

Jovanovic L, Dawood M Y, Landesmann R, Saxena B B 1978 Hormonal profile as a prognostic index of early threatened abortion. American Journal of Obstetrics and Gynecology 130: 274–278

Kadar N 1983 Ectopic pregnancy. In: Studd J (ed) Progress in obstetrics and gynaecology, vol 3. Churchill Livingstone, Edinburgh, pp 305–323

Klopper A 1985 Steroids in pregnancy. In: Shearman R P (ed) Clinical reproductive endocrinology. Churchill Livingstone, Edinburgh, pp 209–223

Kunz J, Keller P J 1976 hPL, oestradiol, progesterone and AFP in patients with threatened abortion. British Journal of Obstetrics and Gynaecology 83: 640–644

Lee J N, Salem H T, Al-Ani A T M et al 1981 Circulating concentrations of specific placental proteins (human chorionic gonadotrophin, pregnancy-specific beta-1 glycoprotein and placental protein 5) in untreated gestational trophoblastic tumours. American Journal of Obstetrics and Gynecology 39: 702–704

Lee J N, Salem H T, Chard T, Huang S C, Ouyang P C 1982 Circulating placental proteins (hCG, SP1 and PP5) in trophoblastic disease. British Journal of Obstetrics and Gynaecology 89: 69–72

Lenton A E, Grudzinskas J G, Gordon Y B, Chard T, Cooke I D 1981 Pregnancy specific beta-1 glycoprotein and chorionic gonadotrophin in early pregnancy. Acta Obstetricia et Gynecologica Scandinavica 60: 489–492

Letchworth A T 1976 Human placental lactogen assay as a guide to fetal wellbeing. In: Klopper A (ed) Plasma hormone assays in evaluation of fetal wellbeing. Churchill Livingstone, Edinburgh, pp 147–173

Lutjen C, Trounson A, Leeton J, Findlay J, Wood C, Renou P 1984 The establishment and maintenance of pregnancy using in-vitro fertilisation and embryo donation in a patient with primary ovarian failure. Nature 307: 174–175

Masson G M, Anthony F, Wilson M S, Lindsay K 1983a Comparison of serum and urine hCG levels with SP1 and PAPP-A levels in patients with first-trimester vaginal bleeding. Obstetrics and Gynecology 61: 223–226

Masson G M, Anthony F, Wilson M S 1983b Value of Schwangerschaftsprotein 1 (SP1) and pregnancy associated plasma protein (PAPP-A) in the clinical management of threatened abortion. British Journal of Obstetrics and Gynaecology 90: 146–149

Miller J F, Williamson E, Glue J, Gordon Y B, Grudzinskas J G, Sykes A 1980 Fetal loss after implantation. Lancet ii: 554–556

Newlands E S 1983 Treatment of trophoblastic disease. In: Studd J (ed) Progress in obstetrics and gynaecology, vol 3. Churchill Livingstone, Edinburgh, pp 158–174

Niven P A R, Landon J, Chard T 1972 Placental lactogen levels as a guide to outcome of threatened abortion. British Medical Journal iii: 799–801

Nygren K G, Johansson E D G, Wide L 1973 Evaluation of the prognosis of threatened abortion from the peripheral levels of plasma progesterone, estradiol and human chorionic gonadotrophin. American Journal of Obstetrics and Gynecology 116: 916–922

Pittaway D E, Wentz A C, Maxon W S, Herbert C, Daniell J, Fleischer A C 1985 The efficacy of early pregnancy monitoring with serial chorionic gonadotrophin determinations and realtime ultrasonography in an infertile population. Fertility and Sterility 44: 190–194

Roberts C J, Lowe C R 1975 Where have all the conceptions gone? Lancet i: 498–499

Salem H T, Ghaneimah S A, Shabaan M M, Chard T 1984 Prognostic value of biochemical tests in the assessment of fetal outcome in threatened abortion. British Journal of Obstetrics and Gynaecology 91: 382–385

Schultz-Larsen P, Hertz J B 1978 The predictive value of pregnancy specific beta-1 glycoprotein in threatened abortion. European Journal of Obstetrics, Gynecology and Reproductive Biology 8: 253–257

Seppala M, Ronnberg L, Ylostalo P, Joupilla P 1979a Early detection of implantation by pregnancy specific beta-1 glycoprotein secretion in an infertile woman treated by artificial insemination and human chorionic gonadotrophin. Fertility and Sterility 32: 608–609

Seppala M, Wahlstrom T, Bohn H 1979b Circulating levels and tissue localisation of placental protein 5 (PP5) in pregnancy and trophoblastic disease: absence of PP5 expression in the malignant trophoblast. International Journal of Cancer 24: 6–10

Sinosich M J 1988 Biological role of pregnancy-associated plasma protein A in human reproduction. In: Bischof P, Klopper A (eds) proteins of the placenta. Karger, Basel, pp 158–184

Sinosich M J, Ferrier A, Teisner B et al 1988 Pregnancy-associated plasma protein: fact, fiction, future. In: Chapman M, Grudzinskas G, Chard T (eds) Implantation. Springer, London, pp 45–82

Soma H, Kikuchi M, Takayama M et al 1981 Concentrations of SP1 and beta-hCG in serum and cerebrospinal fluid and concentrations of hCG in urine in patients with trophoblastic tumour. Archives of Gynecology 230: 321–327

Tsakok F T M, Koh M, Ratnam S S et al 1983 Pregnancy associated proteins in trophoblastic disease. British Journal of Obstetrics and Gynaecology 90: 483–486

Ward R H T, Grudzinskas J G, Bolton A E et al 1985 Fetoplacental products as a prognostic guide following chorionic villus sampling. In: Fraccaro M, Simoni G, Brambati B (eds) First trimester diagnosis. Springer-Verlag, Berlin, pp 73–76

Westergaard J G, Chemnitz J, Teisner B et al 1983 Pregnancy-associated plasma protein A — a possible marker in the classification and diagnosis of Cornelia de Lange syndrome. Placental Diagnosis 3: 225–232

Westergaard J G, Teisner B, Sinosich M J, Madsen L T, Grudzinskas J G 1985 Does ultrasound examination render biochemical tests obsolete in the prediction of early pregnancy failure? British Journal of Obstetrics and Gynaecology 92: 77–83

Whittaker P G, Taylor A, Lind T 1983 Unsuspected pregnancy loss in healthy women. Lancet i: 1126–1127

Wilcox A J, Weinberg C R, Wehmann R E, Armstrong E G, Canfield R E, Nisula B C 1985 Measuring early pregnancy loss: laboratory and field methods. Fertility and Sterility 44: 366–374

Yovich J L, McColin J C, Willcox D L, Grudzinskas J G, Bolton A E 1986 The prognostic value of beta hCG, PAPP-A, oestradiol and progesterone in early human pregnancies and the effect of medroxy progesterone acetate. Australia and New Zealand Journal of Obstetrics and Gynaecology 26: 59–64

N. J. Wald and H. S. Cuckle

Biochemical detection of neural tube defects and Down's syndrome

INTRODUCTION

Neural tube defects (NTDs) and Down's syndrome are among the most common serious congenital malformations. Their aetiology is not known so primary prevention is not yet available. Secondary prevention, through antenatal diagnosis and the selective abortion of affected pregnancies, is possible and is now an important part of antenatal care in many countries. The antenatal diagnosis of NTDs is made by performing biochemical tests on amniotic fluid collected in the second trimester of pregnancy and by ultrasound examination of the fetus after the first trimester. The diagnosis of fetal Down's syndrome is made by determining the karyotype of fetal cells collected either from the amniotic fluid in the second trimester of pregnancy or from the placenta in the first or second trimester of pregnancy. These diagnostic procedures are not carried out on all pregnant women because of the risk of harming the fetus through amniocentesis or chorion villus sampling and because of the cost, particularly that of producing a karyotype. Methods of antenatal screening are therefore needed to identify women who are at sufficiently high risk of having one or other abnormality to justify the diagnostic procedure.

NEURAL TUBE DEFECTS

Prevalence

In the UK the birth prevalence of NTDs in the absence of antenatal diagnosis and selective abortion is about 4 per 1000 births. It is approximately equal for anencephaly and spina bifida (without anencephaly), the two main types of NTD. Encephalocele is rare, accounting for only about 5% of all NTDs, and is usually included with spina bifida in tabulations of prevalence.

There is geographical variation within the UK in the prevalence of NTDs in the absence of antenatal diagnosis and selective abortion: Northern Ireland, Scotland and Wales have the highest prevalence (about 6 per 1000) and south-east England the lowest (about 2 per 1000). The rates in the rest of the world are generally lower than that in the UK but as a result of antenatal diagnosis and selective abortion the UK now has a comparatively low birth prevalence. The reason for the UK being a high-risk area is unknown but environmental factors are important. There are several observations that support this view; for example, the risk of the disorder is lower in descendants of migrants from Ireland to America than in Ireland itself.

The risk of fetal NTDs is increased about 10-fold among women who previously had one affected child, about 20-fold among those who had two affected children and about 40-fold among those who had three. These women are at sufficient risk to justify amniocentesis without first carrying out a screening test. In spite of these high risks of recurrence over 95% of infants with NTDs are born to women who have not previously had affected pregnancies, and it is primarily for such women that screening is offered.

Open lesions and closed lesions

From the point of view of screening and antenatal diagnosis an important distinction is whether the NTD is open or closed since only the former can to be detected antenatally by biochemical means. Anencephaly is an open lesion. Spina bifida lesions are classified as open if there is completely exposed neural tissue or if the lesion is covered by a thin transparent membrane. They are categorized as closed if the lesion is completely covered by skin or thick opaque membrane. Using this classification about 80% of spina bifida lesions are open.

Survival and the extent of handicap

Anencephaly is a fatal condition, either before birth or within a few hours. Infants born with open spina bifida have a poor survival and tend to be handicapped. The prognosis of infants born with closed spina bifida tends to be somewhat better. With a selective surgical policy, and in the absence of antenatal diagnosis, a study based on the ascertainment of all spina bifida births among residents of the Oxford record linkage area in 1965–1972 (Althouse & Wald 1980) showed that just over one-third of infants with open spina bifida survived for 5 years: 82% of these children were severely handicapped, 10% moderately handicapped, and only 8% had no handicap. Those who survived 5 years had spent more than 6 months in hospital by this time and undergone an average of six surgical operations. The 5-year survival rate of infants with closed spina bifida was 60% and among the survivors about one-third were severely handicapped, and a further third were moderately handicapped.

Maternal serum alpha-fetoprotein (AFP)

The only reliable screening test for open spina bifida is the measurement of AFP in maternal serum. Anencephaly can be readily detected by ultrasonography and for this reason, and because it is a fatal disorder, it will not be considered further in any detail in this chapter. Closed spina bifida is not normally detected antenatally by AFP screening and only with difficulty by ultrasonography.

AFP is an alpha-globulin of similar molecular weight to albumin. In pregnancy the main source of AFP entering the maternal circulation is AFP synthesized by the yolk sac and the fetal liver. In the second trimester of pregnancy maternal serum AFP increases from the non-pregnant level by about 17% a week, an increase which is thought to be due to fetal AFP reaching the mother across the placenta. At 17 weeks of pregnancy AFP is present in fetal serum (and cerebrospinal fluid) at a concentration of about 30 000 times greater than that in the maternal serum and 150 times greater than that in the amniotic fluid. In the presence of open spina bifida, AFP leaks into the amniotic fluid through the open defect and from there a small proportion passes into the maternal circulation. This excess AFP is the basis for the use of maternal serum AFP measurement as a screening test for open NTD.

When to screen

Table 19.1 shows the proportion of open spina bifida pregnancies with maternal serum AFP levels equal to or greater than the 95th, 97th and 99th percentiles of normal according to gestational age. This detection rate (or sensitivity) is greatest at about 19–24 weeks of gestation for anencephaly and 16–18 weeks for open spina bifida. Screening is, therefore, best done at 16–18 weeks of pregnancy when about three-quarters of open spina bifida pregnancies have maternal serum AFP levels greater than or equal to the 97th percentile of normal.

Table 19.1 Percentage of anencephalic and open spina bifida pregnancies with maternal serum AFP levels ≥ specified percentiles of normal, according to gestational age

	Anencephaly			Open spina bifida		
Gestational age (completed weeks)	Normal percentile 95th	97th	99th	Normal percentile 95th	97th	99th
10–12	20	15	15	18	18	5
13–15	72	60	49	45	37	29
16–18	88	86	84	88	76	70
19–24*	93	93	89	67	67	61

* There were too few data at 22–24 weeks to estimate seperate percentages reliably.
Adapted from the UK Collaborative AFP Study (1977).

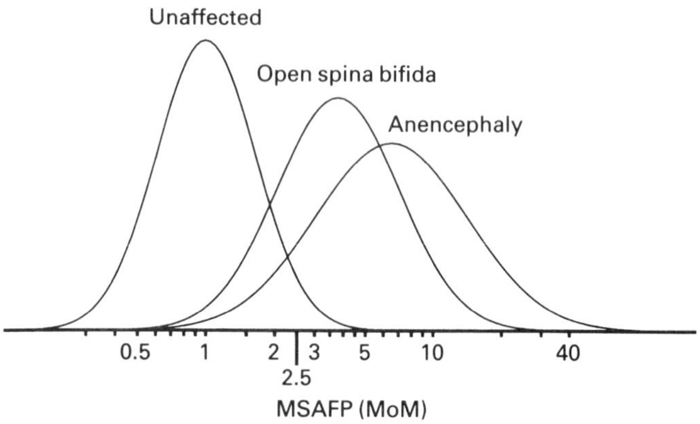

Fig. 19.1 Distribution of maternal serum alpha-fetoprotein (MSAFP) levels in unaffected, open spina bifida and anencephalic pregnancies at 16–18 weeks of gestation (based on parameters given in UK Collaborative AFP Study 1982).

Units of AFP measurement

To allow for the increase in the concentration of AFP in maternal serum during the second trimester of pregnancy it is convenient to express all AFP values as a multiple of the normal median at the relevant gestational age. This also allows for systematic differences between laboratories. The use of the median as a measure of central tendency (the middle value at a given week of pregnancy when all the values are arranged in ascending order) is preferred to the mean value since it is hardly influenced by occasional outlying values. The maternal serum AFP values are therefore usually expressed in multiples of the normal median, usually abbreviated to MoM.

Maternal serum AFP cut-off levels

Figure 19.1 shows the distribution of maternal serum AFP (in MoM) at 16–18 weeks of gestation among singleton preg-

Table 19.2 Maternal serum AFP screening at 16–18 weeks of gestation: detection rate* and false positive rate† according to AFP level

AFP (MoM)	Detection rate: Anencephaly (%)	Detection rate: Open spina bifida (%)	False positive rate (%)
⩾2.0	90	91	7.2
⩾2.5	88	79	3.3
⩾3.0	84	70	1.4
⩾3.5	82	64	0.6
⩾4.0	76	45	0.3

* The detection rate (sensitivity) is the proportion of affected pregnancies with positive results; † the false positive rate (100% specificity) is the proportion of unaffected pregnancies with positive results.
Adapted from the UK Collaborative AFP Study (1977).

nancies separately for unaffected pregnancies, open spina bifida pregnancies and anencephalic pregnancies. The distributions overlap, so there is no obvious level of serum AFP that separates affected from unaffected pregnancies. If a cut-off level was set low enough to include nearly all pregnancies with open NTD it would also include a large proportion of unaffected ones (false positives). On the other hand if the cut-off level was set so high that few unaffected pregnancies were included, then most affected pregnancies would be missed (false negatives). The selection of a particular cut-off level in antenatal screening programmes for NTDs is therefore a compromise based on various considerations such as the resources available to carry out ultrasound examinations and amniocentesis on women with positive screening results and the hazards of amniocentesis.

Table 19.2 shows the percentage of singleton pregnancies with maternal serum AFP levels equal to or greater than different cut-off levels at 16–18 weeks of gestation. Using a cut-off level of 2.5 MoM, 88% of anencephalic and 79% of open spina bifida pregnancies (69% of all spina bifidas including those with closed lesions) were detected in the UK Collaborative AFP Study (1977). At the same time 3% of unaffected singleton pregnancies had AFP levels this high or higher. Since ultrasound examination of the fetus can readily identify almost all cases of anencephaly serum AFP measurement is principally used to screen for open spina bifida.

Estimating the risk of having a fetus with open spina bifida from the maternal serum AFP level

Results shown in Table 19.2 were obtained by direct observation, whereas the distributions shown in Figure 19.1 were produced after fitting log Gaussian (normal) frequency distributions to the observed AFP values. It has been shown that the distributions fit the data well and they can be used to estimate:

1. The detection rate for spina bifida or anencephaly at any given cut-off level and the corresponding false positive rate.
2. The risk of having an affected pregnancy for women with AFP values equal to or greater than any given cut-off level.
3. The risk of having an affected pregnancy for a particular woman with a given AFP level.

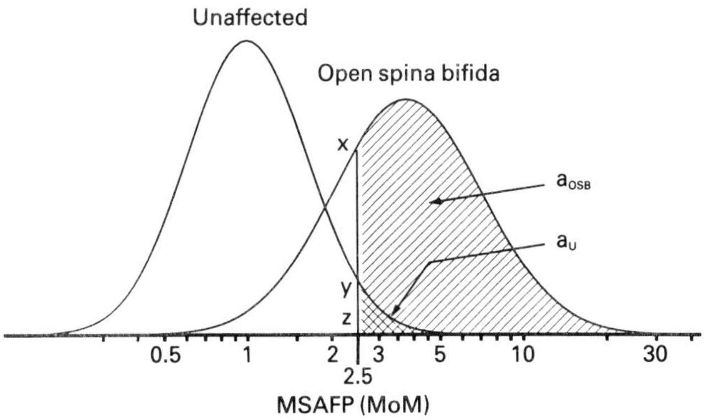

Fig. 19.2 Distribution of maternal serum alpha-fetoprotein (MSAFP) levels in unaffected and open spina bifida pregnancies showing a cut-off level at 2.5 MoM. The likelihood ratio (see text) for open spina bifida if (1) MSAFP ⩾ 2.5 MoM is a_{OSB}/a_U; (2) MSAFP = 2.5 MoM is xz/yz.

Table 19.3 Parameters of distributions of maternal serum AFP (in $\log_{10}$ MoM) in singleton unaffected and open spina bifida pregnancies at 16–18 and 19–21 weeks of gestation; gestational age based on dates (i.e. time since first day of last menstrual period)

	Open spina bifida	Unaffected pregnancy
16–18 weeks' gestation		
Mean	0.5791	0.0000
Standard deviation	0.2697	0.2163
19–21 weeks' gestation		
Mean	0.3452	0.0000
Standard deviation	0.2614	0.1844

Taken from the UK Collaborative AFP Study (1982).

The calculations involved are straightforward and can be done using tables of the Gaussian distribution. The method can be illustrated by the following example, relating to a maternal serum AFP level of 2.5 MoM. The open spina bifida detection rate and the false positive rate in a screening programme using this cut-off level can be estimated approximately by looking at the two distributions and judging what proportion of each lies to the right of 2.5 MoM, shaded in Figure 19.2. To calculate the proportions precisely it is only necessary to know the mean and standard deviation of each distribution (see Table 19.3); these define each of the distributions uniquely. The two proportions are then determined by calculating how many standard deviations 2.5 MoM is away from each of the respective means and looking up these values in tables of the Gaussian distribution. This is done in steps 1–6 in Table 19.4. The same procedure can be used for any cut-off level.

To determine the risk of having a spina bifida pregnancy

Table 19.4 Maternal serum AFP screening for open spina bifida: illustration of the calculation of (1) the detection rate (DR), false positive rate (FPR) and likelihood ratio (LR) for women with maternal serum AFP levels ≥2.5 MoM (steps 1–6) and (2) the likelihood ratio for a woman with an AFP level of exactly 2.5 MoM (steps 1–3 and 7–9)

Steps	Open spina bifida	Unaffected pregnancies
1. Convert 2.5 into $\log_{10}$	0.3979	0.3979
2. Subtract mean from Table 19.3	0.3979 − 0.5791 = −0.1812	0.3979 − 0.0 =0.3979
3. Divide by SD from Table 19.3 to determine Z	−0.1812/0.2697 = −0.67	0.3979/0.2163 =1.84
4. Look up Z in Table of normal distribution*	0.2514	0.9671
5. Subtract from 1.0 and multiply by 100% to determine DR and FPR	(1 − 0.2514) × 100% =75% (DR)	(1 − 0.9671) × 100% =3.3% (FPR)
6. Divide DR by FPR to determine LR for ≥2.5 MoM	23 (LR)	
7. Look up Z in table of heights of normal distribution†	0.3187	0.0734
8. Divide by SD from Table 19.3 to determine heights of the AFP distributions	0.3187/0.2697 =1.1817	0.0734/0.2163 =0.3393
9. Divide heights to determine LR for 2.5 MoM	3.5 (LR)	

* This table will give the area under the distribution to the left of $|Z|$, i.e. ignoring any minus sign. If Z is negative look up $|Z|$ and subtract from 1.
† This table will give the height of the standardized distribution (assuming SD = 1) at $|Z|$, i.e. ignoring any minus sign.

given a positive screening result using a cut-off level of 2.5 MoM it is only necessary to calculate how many times more likely an individual with a positive result is of having a spina bifida pregnancy compared with the risk for women in general. This factor, called the likelihood ratio, is the ratio of the shaded areas (spina bifida divided by unaffected) in Figure 19.2. It is, in fact, the detection rate divided by the false positive rate, i.e. 75%/3.3% = 23 (step 6 in Table 19.4). The likelihood ratio is used to multiply up the background birth prevalence of open spina bifida expressed as an odds. If the background prevalence is 2 per 1000 births this, expressed as an odds, would be 2:998. Multiplying 2:998 by 23 yields 46:998 which, expressed as a probability, is 46/(998 + 46), about 4%, or 1 in 25.

To determine the risk of having an affected pregnancy for a particular woman with a given AFP level the calculation is similar to the one illustrated above except that the likelihood ratio is the height of the distribution curve for affected pregnancies divided by the height of the distribution curve for unaffected individuals at the given AFP value (xz/yz in Fig. 19.2 for 2.5 MoM). The two heights are divided by each other instead of the two areas. This is calculated in Table 19.4 (steps 7–9) to be 3.5 for a woman with an AFP level of exactly 2.5 MoM. If, as before, the background prevalence of open spina bifida at birth is 2:998, her odds of having an affected pregnancy are 7:998 (3.5 × 2:998) which expressed as a probability is 7/(998 + 7), about 0.7%, or 1 in 140.

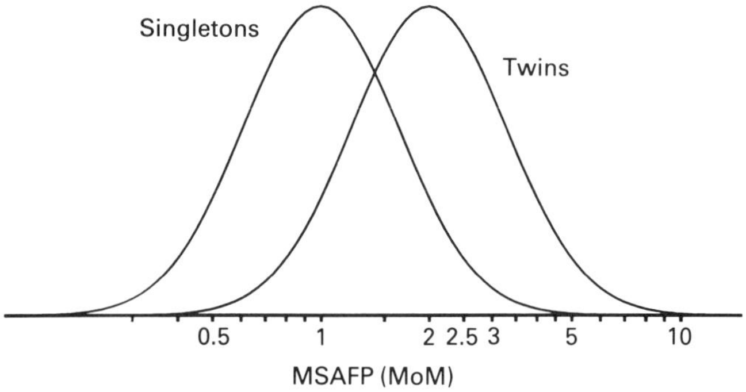

Fig. 19.3 Distribution of maternal serum alpha-fetoprotein (MSAFP) levels in unaffected singleton and twin pregnancies at 16–18 weeks of gestation.

Multiple pregnancy

Maternal serum AFP levels in twin pregnancies are on average about double those found in singleton pregnancies, monozygous twins having even higher values than dizygous twins (Wald et al 1979a), and they are about three times higher in triplet pregnancies. Values are correspondingly higher in quadruplet and quintuplet pregnancies. The distribution of unaffected singleton and twin pregnancies is shown in Figure 19.3. Insufficient data are available on AFP levels in twin pregnancies in which one fetus is affected by an open NTD.

The finding of a twin pregnancy in a woman with a raised maternal serum AFP level is often taken to be the reason for the raised level and no further action is taken. Reluctance to terminate an unaffected co-twin or to attempt a selective termination of the affected twin lends support to a policy of no action once a twin pregnancy is discovered.

If action is contemplated in such twin pregnancies, a reasonable policy would be to select a cut-off level such that the false positive rate for twin pregnancies is the same as that for singleton pregnancies. For example, a cut-off level of 5.0 MoM would identify about 3% of twins with positive AFP results, equivalent to a cut-off of 2.5 MoM in singletons. In general, the equivalent cut-off level for twin pregnancies is double the corresponding one for singleton pregnancies since the median value is double and the variances using logs are similar.

The role of ultrasonography

Women found to have a high serum AFP level should have an ultrasound examination to identify multiple pregnancy and to identify women who have high AFP levels on account

Table 19.5 Parameters of distributions of maternal serum AFP (in $\log_{10}$ MoM) in singleton unaffected and open spina bifida pregnancies at 16–18 and 19–21 weeks of gestation; calculation of MoM value using gestational age based on ultrasound biparietal diameter measurement

	Open spina bifida	Unaffected pregnancy
*16–18 weeks' gestation**		
Mean	0.7344	0.0065
Standard deviation	0.2607	0.2050
*19–21 weeks' gestation**		
Mean	0.5005	0.0065
Standard deviation	0.2521	0.1710

* Timing of test based on dates.
From Wald et al (1984a).

of the underestimation of gestational age. The latter will reduce the false positive rate by about one-third without materially affecting the detection rate.

Routine ultrasound scanning for the estimation of gestational age by the measurement of fetal biparietal diameter (BPD) during the second trimester of pregnancy will improve the performance of AFP screening by increasing the detection rate as well as by reducing the false positive rate (Wald et al 1980a, 1982). The two effects are considered separately and together.

Effect on detection rate. Spina bifida fetuses have small heads in utero, so the use of BPD measurement to estimate gestational age leads to such fetuses on average being credited with a less mature gestational age than is in fact the case (Roberts & Campbell 1980; Wald et al 1980a). A given concentration of AFP (in iu/ml) is, as a consequence, converted into a higher serum AFP level in MoMs than when gestational age is based on the time since the first day of the last menstrual period. It has been estimated that this effect will increase the detection rate for open spina bifida by about an additional 10–20% at cut-off levels above 2 MoM.

Effect on false positive rate. The use of BPD measurement to estimate gestational age influences the false positive rate in two ways (Wald et al 1982). First, the AFP values (in MoM) tend to be somewhat higher than when dates are used to estimate gestational age. This is due to the correction of the systematic overestimation of gestational age in women with uncertain gestational ages. Second, there are fewer extremely high and low values due to the increased precision of estimating gestational age by BPD measurement. The two influences exert opposite effects on the percentage of singleton unaffected pregnancies with raised serum AFP levels, the first tending to increase this proportion and the second to decrease it. The latter has a somewhat greater influence than the former, so on average the false positive rate is reduced by the routine use of BPD measurement to estimate gestational age by up to about 1% (say from 3% to 2%) at cut-off levels between 2 and 3 MoM.

Net effect on false positive rate and detection rate. The net effect is to separate the distributions of serum AFP in affected and unaffected pregnancies and also to reduce their variances so that the extent of overlap between the two distributions is reduced. The revised parameters of the maternal serum AFP distributions in open spina bifida and unaffected singleton pregnancies when gestational age based on BPD measurement is used to calculate MoM are given in Table 19.5. Separate sets of parameters are given for pregnancies at 16–18 and 19–21 weeks of pregnancy. Figure 19.4 shows the distribution of maternal serum AFP using the parameters in Table 19.5 and compares them to the parameters used in Table 19.3 where gestation is based on dates.

Table 19.6 shows the detection rates for open spina bifida and the false positive rates at 16–18 and 19–21 weeks of gestation according to the method of estimating gestational age to calculate the MoM value and the AFP cut-off level. Table 19.7 shows the corresponding odds of having a fetus with open spina bifida among women with positive AFP screening results, according to the background risk of open spina bifida at birth. The odds in Table 19.7 are relevant to the conduct of screening programmes. The equivalent odds for an individual woman with a positive result are given in Table 19.8.

Which gestational age estimate to use. When calculating maternal serum AFP MoM values, gestational age estimates based on BPD measurements should always take precedence over other estimates of gestational age even when there are only a few days difference between different estimates. Such a policy will improve the detection rate and minimize the false positive rate.

In judging when to arrange for a woman to have her AFP test, gestational age estimates based on dates should be used if no ultrasound scan has been done and the test should be scheduled for 16–18 completed weeks' gestation. If a scan has been done and a BPD is available this can be used and the test scheduled for 16 completed weeks using the BPD estimate. Though this is not optimal (since some open spina bifida pregnancies thought to be at 16 weeks based on BPD will in fact be at 19 weeks of gestation, when the test is less efficient) the loss in detection is likely to be too small to justify a change from the common practice of using BPD estimates in preference to a dates estimate when both are available.

When calculating the risk a particular woman has of a pregnancy associated with spina bifida it is important to select the AFP distribution parameters for affected and unaffected pregnancies that correspond to the correct gestational age of the pregnancy — either 16–18 weeks or 19–21 weeks. There are three factors to consider in this, namely: in unaffected pregnancies BPD estimates are more correct than menstrual date estimates; in spina bifida pregnancies this is not the case because gestational age is systematically underestimated by BPD measurement; and this underestimate rarely exceeds 1–34 days. Therefore, to select the correct gestational age, we suggest this rule: use the BPD estimate but if it is 1–34 days earlier than the dates estimate use the dates estimate. With the use of computer programs to

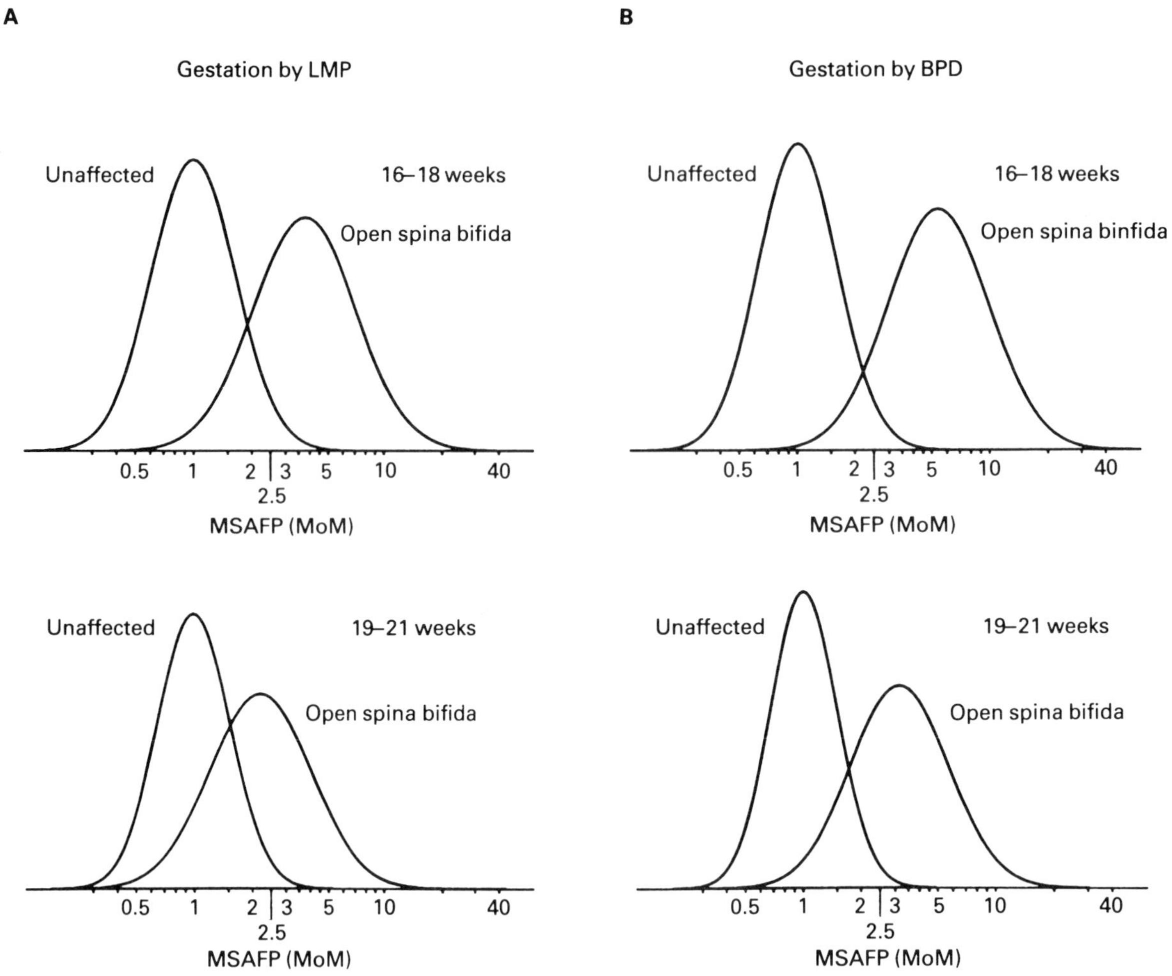

Fig. 19.4 Distribution of maternal serum alpha-fetoprotein (MSAFP) levels in unaffected and open spina bifida pregnancies at 16–18 and 19–21 weeks of gestation with gestational age estimated by (**A**) dates (LMP) and (**B**) ultrasound (BPD) to calculate the MoM value (based on parameters in Wald et al 1984a).

provide interpreted AFP reports, including the risk estimate of an affected pregnancy, the choice of which AFP parameters to use given the gestational age estimate available can be made automatically and should present no problem.

Repeat maternal serum AFP testing

About 14% of the within-week variance of serum AFP in unaffected pregnancies is due to assay error and a further 17% is due to within-person maternal serum AFP fluctuations (UK Collaborative AFP Study 1982). By collecting a fresh sample of blood from all women repeating the AFP test and taking the geometric mean of the results the assay and within-person variance will be halved. This represents only a modest change in the spread of the distributions shown in Figure 19.1 and so repeat testing can have only a relatively small effect on the performance of AFP screening. Repeating all tests is not the only option and Table 19.9 shows the effect on screening performance of three repeat testing policies (B, C and D) compared with a policy that does not involve repeat tests (A). Policy D (the retesting of women with borderline AFP results) is the most cost-effective. This is because women with values that are well above, or well below, the cut-off level are unlikely to have their results reclassified on the basis of the second test; the positives will tend to remain positive and the negatives negative and such women therefore have little to gain by having a second test. It is those with AFP levels close to the cut-off level that have most opportunity to be reclassified. Even the benefits of policy D are marginal; a 'no repeat test' policy is quite acceptable. It has the added benefits of simplicity and the avoidance of delay in making a diagnosis, at a time when the women concerned, having been told that they have a positive AFP screening test, are particularly anxious.

Table 19.6 Maternal serum AFP screening at 16–18 and 19–21 weeks of gestation: detection rate for open spina bifida and false positive rate according to method of estimating gestational age to calculate MoM value and AFP cut-off level (based on the parameters given in Tables 19.3 and 19.5)

	Method of estimating gestation age to calculate MoM value			
	Dates		Biparietal diameter	
AFP (MoM)	Detection rate (%)	False positive rate (%)	Detection rate (%)	False positive rate (%)
*16–18 weeks' gestation**				
⩾2.0	85	8.2	95	7.5
⩾2.5	75	3.3	90	2.8
⩾3.0	65	1.4	84	1.1
⩾3.5	55	0.6	77	0.4
⩾4.0	47	0.3	69	0.2
⩾4.5	39	0.1	62	0.1
⩾5.0	33	0.1	55	<0.1
*19–21 weeks' gestation**				
⩾2.0	56	5.1	79	4.2
⩾2.5	42	1.5	66	1.1
⩾3.0	31	0.5	54	0.3
⩾3.5	22	0.2	43	0.1
⩾4.0	16	0.1	34	<0.1
⩾4.5	12	<0.1	27	<0.1
⩾5.0	9	<0.1	22	<0.1

* Timing of test based on dates.

Table 19.7 Maternal serum AFP screening at 16–18 and 19–21 weeks of gestation: population odds of having a fetus with open spina bifida against having an unaffected pregnancy according to AFP cut-off level, method of estimating gestational age to calculate MoM value (dates or BPD), and the birth prevalence of open spina bifida in the absence of antenatal diagnosis and selective abortion (based on the parameters given in Tables 19.3 and 19.5)

	Birth prevalence (per 1000) of open spina bifida in the absence of selective abortion					
	0.5		1.0		2.0	
AFP (MoM)	Dates	BPD	Dates	BPD	Dates	BPD
*16–18 weeks' gestation**						
⩾2.0	1:190	1:160	1:97	1:79	1:48	1:40
⩾2.5	1:80	1:62	1:44	1:31	1:22	1:16
⩾3.0	1:42	1:26	1:21	1:13	1:11	1:6.5
⩾3.5	1:22	1:11	1:11	1:5.7	1:5.4	1:2.8
⩾4.0	1:12	1:5.3	1:5.8	1:2.6	1:2.9	1:1.3
⩾4.5	1:6.5	1:2.6	1:3.2	1:1.3	1:1.6	1.6:1
⩾5.0	1:3.7	1:1.3	1:1.9	1.5:1	1.1:1	3.0:1
*19–21 weeks' gestation**						
⩾2.0	1:180	1:110	1:90	1:54	1:45	1:27
⩾2.5	1:74	1:34	1:37	1:17	1:18	1:8.4
⩾3.0	1:31	1:11	1:16	1:5.5	1:7.9	1:2.8
⩾3.5	1:14	1:3.9	1:7.1	1:1.9	1:3.5	1.0:1
⩾4.0	1:6.7	1:1.4	1:3.4	1.4:1	1:1.7	2.8:1
⩾4.5	1:3.3	1.7:1	1:1.7	3.5:1	1.2:1	7.0:1
⩾5.0	1:1.7	4.2:1	1.2:1	8.4:1	2.3:1	17:1

BPD = biparietal diameter.
* Timing of test based on dates.

Adjustment of maternal serum AFP values for maternal weight

Maternal serum AFP levels decrease on average with increasing maternal weight (Haddow et al 1981, Wald et al 1981). This is probably due to AFP entering the maternal circulation from the fetus being diluted more in the greater plasma volume of heavier women than in that of lighter women. A simple method of adjusting AFP values to allow for mater-

Table 19.8 Maternal serum AFP screening at 16–18 and 19–21 weeks of gestation: an individual woman's odds of having a fetus with open spina bifida against having an unaffected pregnancy according to the AFP level, method of estimating gestational age to calculate MoM value (dates or BPD), and the birth prevalence of open spina bifida in the absence of antenatal diagnosis and selective abortion (based on the parameters given in Tables 19.3 and 19.5)

	Birth prevalence (per 1000) of open spina bifida in the absence of selective abortion					
	0.5		1.0		2.0	
AFP Level (MoM)	Dates	BPD	Dates	BPD	Dates	BPD
*16–18 weeks' gestation**						
1.0	1:25000	1:130000	1:12000	1:67000	1:6200	1:34000
1.5	1:5500	1:18000	1:2700	1:8900	1:1400	1:4500
2.0	1:1600	1:3600	1:800	1:1800	1:400	1:900
2.5	1:570	1:940	1:290	1:470	1:140	1:240
3.0	1:240	1:300	1:120	1:150	1:59	1:74
3.5	1:110	1:110	1:53	1:53	1:27	1:27
4.0	1:52	1:43	1:26	1:21	1:13	1:11
4.5	1:27	1:18	1:14	1:9.2	1:6.8	1:4.6
5.0	1:15	1:8.5	1:7.4	1:4.3	1:3.7	1:2.1
*19–21 weeks' gestation**						
1.0	1:6800	1:21000	1:3400	1:11000	1:1700	1:5300
1.5	1:2200	1:4100	1:1100	1:2100	1:550	1:1000
2.0	1:760	1:910	1:380	1:460	1:190	1:230
2.5	1:280	1:230	1:140	1:120	1:70	1:58
3.0	1:110	1:67	1:57	1:43	1:28	1:17
3.5	1:49	1:21	1:24	1:11	1:12	1:5.3
4.0	1:22	1:7.4	1:11	1:3.7	1:5.6	1:1.9
4.5	1:11	1:2.8	1:5.3	1:1.4	1:2.7	1.4:1
5.0	1:5.4	1:1.1	1:2.7	1.8:1	1:1.3	3.6:1

BPD = biparietal diameter.
* If gestational age estimates based on dates and BPD are both available, use the BPD estimate to select appropriate parameters but if it is 1–34 days earlier than the menstrual dates estimate, use the dates estimate (see text for justification of this rule).

Table 19.9 The effect of repeat maternal serum AFP testing (using a fresh sample) on the open spina bifida detection rate and false positive rate: singleton pregnancies at 16–18 weeks of gestation

Policy	Proportion of women rested (%)	Open spina bifida detection rate (%)	False positive rate (%)
A. No repeat test	0	75	3.3
B. Retest all women and consider positive if geometric mean of both results ⩾ 2.5 MoM	100	76	2.3
C. Retest women with levels ⩾ 2.5 MoM and consider positive if second test ⩾ 2.5 MoM	3	70	1.7
D. Retest women with levels 2.5–2.9 MoM. Those with first tests < 2.5 MoM are negative, and ⩾ 3.0 MoM are positive; consider women with second tests ⩾ 2.0 MoM as positive	2	74	2.7

Adapted from the UK Collaborative AFP Study (1982).

Table 19.10 Maternal serum AFP screening for open spina bifida at 16–18 weeks of gestation: detection rate and false positive rate according to AFP cut-off level and whether AFP values are adjusted for maternal weight

	Maternal weight adjustment No		Yes*	
AFP (MoM)	Detection rate (%)	False positive rate (%)	Detection rate (%)	False positive rate (%)
⩾2.0	85	8.2	85	7.6
⩾2.5	75	3.3	74	2.9
⩾3.0	65	1.4	64	1.2
⩾3.5	55	0.6	54	0.5
⩾4.0	47	0.3	45	0.2

* Maternal weight was adjusted by dividing the observed MoM value by 2.178×0.9874^{W}, where W is the weight in kg at the time of the AFP test.
The detection rates and false positive rates were based on the parameters given in Table 19.3, with a 0.00256 reduction in variance due to weight adjustment (Cuckle et al 1987a) and 2% decrease in the (arithmetic) mean for open spina bifida (Wald & Cuckle 1987).

nal weight is to divide the observed level (in MoM) by the expected level for the maternal weight. Adjusting AFP values for maternal weight in this way will reduce the variance of maternal serum AFP in affected and unaffected pregnancies and so tend to reduce the extent of overlap. There is a suggestion from British data (but not from US data) that women with NTD pregnancies weigh less than women with unaffected pregnancies, and maternal weight adjustment will therefore tend to reduce the mean AFP value in affected pregnancies after weight adjustment (Wald et al 1981, Haddow et al 1982). This effect, however, appears to be small and would decrease the mean AFP level for open spina bifida pregnancies by no more than 2%—too little to counteract the benefit gained by the reduction in their variances. Table 19.10 shows the spina bifida detection rate and the false positive rate at 16–18 weeks of gestation with and without maternal weight adjustment. The formula used to calculate the expected AFP level for a maternal weight is given as a footnote.

Although the benefits of weight adjustment are small the procedure is probably worthwhile, particularly since the woman is usually weighed at the time she has her AFP test, so there is no extra work involved other than to record the weight on the request card for the test.

Insulin-dependent diabetes mellitus

Women with insulin-dependent diabetes mellitus tend to have low maternal serum AFP levels—on average about two-thirds of that of unaffected pregnancies (Wald et al 1979b, Milunsky et al 1982). They also have a high risk of a pregnancy affected by an NTD. Both observations would justify adopting a serum AFP cut-off level lower than the one used in general.

Data on maternal serum AFP levels in insulin-dependent diabetic pregnancies affected by open spina bifida are not known, so an AFP cut-off level yielding a given detection rate cannot be specified. However an AFP cut-off level can be selected to yield a false positive rate for diabetic women which would be the same as for non-diabetic women. The new cut-off level is simply the usual one reduced by one-third, the extent to which serum AFP is decreased in pregnancies among insulin-dependent diabetics. For example, a cut-off level of 2.5 MoM would become 1.7 MoM. This calculation assumes that the variance of maternal serum AFP values in such women is similar to that of women in general.

Race

Blacks tend to have higher maternal serum AFP levels than whites (about 15% higher in the combined results from five studies; Wald & Cuckle 1987), though the reason for this is not known. It has been noted in the USA that the birth prevalence of NTDs is about half the rate in blacks that it is in whites (Greenberg et al 1983). The lack of data on the distribution of maternal serum AFP in blacks with NTD pregnancies precludes the definition of a cut-off level with a known detection rate. Until such data are available it is probably best to ensure that the false positive rate for blacks is the same as it is for whites and this can be done by adjusting the cut-off level—in this instance by raising it 15%—so that if a cut-off level of 2.5 MoM is used for a predominantly white community the cut-off for blacks would be 2.9 MoM.

Asian women have somewhat reduced serum AFP levels compared to white women: 6% lower in 531 Oxford women we have studied (Cuckle et al 1987b). The difference in AFP levels is probably too small to justify identifying Asians in AFP screening programmes and making appropriate adjustments to the cut-off level when interpreting a serum AFP level for Asian women.

Maternal serum AFP levels in subsequent pregnancies

Women with raised serum AFP values in one pregnancy tend to have raised levels in a second pregnancy (Wald & Cuckle 1981), but the correlation is too weak to be of practical value in screening programmes.

Fetal sex

An interesting but unexplained observation is that maternal serum AFP values are significantly associated with the sex of the fetus; higher values are more common with the male than the female fetus. In one study based on nearly 8000 singleton pregnancies at 16–18 weeks of gestation, the male:female sex ratio was 0.77 among women with serum AFP levels less than 0.5 MoM, but 1.57 among women with AFP levels ⩾ 2.5 MoM (Wald & Cuckle 1984a).

Intrauterine death, miscarriage and threatened abortion

Intrauterine death can be associated with extremely high serum AFP values — as high as 200 MoM. Serum AFP values are also high prior to a miscarriage so that the probability of a miscarriage among women with serum AFP levels ⩾ 2.8 MoM in one study was six times greater than that among women with lower AFP values (Wald et al 1977a). Vaginal bleeding early in pregnancy (i.e. threatened abortion) is associated with high serum AFP levels even if the pregnancy does not end in a miscarriage (Haddow et al 1986).

Fetomaternal haemorrhage

Women with raised maternal serum AFP levels have an increased chance of having a fetomaternal haemorrhage as evidenced by a positive Kleihauer test (Hay et al 1979, Los et al 1979). It has been shown that amniocentesis can cause a fetomaternal haemorrhage and elevate the serum AFP level, possibly for weeks after the procedure. For this reason collecting serum for AFP measurement should be done before an amniocentesis is performed.

Low birthweight

High maternal serum AFP levels in the second trimester of pregnancy are associated with the delivery of low birthweight infants. Women with maternal serum AFP levels above 2.5 MoM have 4–5-fold increased risk of having a low birthweight infant. Unfortunately only about 15% of all low birthweight infants can be identified in this way (Brock et al 1977, Wald et al 1977b) and so serum AFP screening is not an effective method of identifying pregnancies at risk of low birthweight, even if there were an effective method of preventing low birthweight delivery.

The mechanism for the inverse association between AFP and birthweight is not known but it may be due to abnormalities in the placenta which have been shown to be associated with both raised serum AFP and low birthweight (Boyd & Keeling 1986).

Other conditions associated with raised serum AFP

About three-quarters of pregnancies affected by fetal anterior abdominal wall defects in the absence of a fetal NTD have AFP levels above 2.5 MoM (Wald et al 1980b). Congenital nephrosis is associated with high serum AFP values, and the detection rate may be greater than for open NTD (Ryynänen et al 1983) although this autosomal recessive condition is very rare in most countries other than Finland where in certain regions the frequency of heterozygotes can be as high as 1 in 10. High serum AFP levels can also occur in the presence of oligohydramnios arising for no obvious reason, a condition which suggests a very poor fetal prognosis (Stirrat et al 1981).

Table 19.11 Outcome of pregnancies with maternal serum AFP levels equal to or greater than specified cut-off levels in Oxford from 1975 to 1980. Each specified outcome excludes those listed above it (based on a total of 24 660 women tested at 16–22 weeks of gestation)

	Maternal serum AFP level (MoM)			
	⩾3.0	⩾3.5	⩾4.0	⩾4.5
Number of pregnancies	402 (100%)	246 (100%)	164 (100%)	119 (100%)
Outcome	(%)	(%)	(%)	(%)
Miscarriage	16.4	21.1	19.5	19.3
Multiple pregnancy*	12.2	11.4	9.1	10.1
Anencephaly	5.2	8.1	9.1	11.8
Open spina bifida	5.0	7.7	9.1	8.4
AAWD	1.2	2.0	3.0	4.2
Non-NTD, non-AAWD termination	3.7	5.3	6.7	6.7
Stillbirth ⩽ 2.5 kg	0.7	0.8	1.2	1.7
Stillbirth > 2.5 kg	0.2	0.0	0.0	0.0
Neonatal death				
1st week†	1.5	2.4	3.7	3.4
2nd–4th week	0.5	0.8	0.6	0.8
Birthweight ⩽ 2.5 kg	7.7	4.9	4.9	5.9
Healthy singleton	45.5	35.4	32.9	27.7

* The proportion of multiple pregnancies among women with raised serum AFP levels has decreased in recent years since they are more often recognized by ultrasound scan before 16 weeks of gestation and as a result an AFP test is not performed.
† All ⩽ 2.5 kg.
AAWD = anterior abdominal wall defect.
From Wald & Cuckle (1984a).

Outcome of pregnancy in women with high serum AFP levels

Table 19.11 shows the outcome of pregnancies in women with high serum AFP values among 24 660 women who underwent AFP screening at 16–22 weeks of pregnancy in Oxford between 1975 and 1980 (Wald & Cuckle 1984a). Prognosis in these women was substantially poorer than for women in general. The outcomes, other than the NTD and anterior abdominal wall defects, represent a mixed group for which, in general, no effective intervention is available.

Amniotic fluid AFP

The main biochemical diagnostic test for open NTD is amniotic fluid AFP measurement. Amniotic fluid AFP levels decline on average by about 13% per week in the second trimester, and as with maternal serum AFP, are usually expressed in MoM (UK Collaborative AFP Study 1979). The best time for the test is at 16–18 weeks of pregnancy. Figure 19.5 shows the distribution of amniotic fluid AFP in singleton unaffected and open spina bifida pregnancies at 16–18 and 19–21 weeks. Unaffected pregnancies associated with serious abnormalities other than an NTD or ending in a miscarriage have been excluded since such conditions produce positive results and many would not regard them as genuine false positives. The false positive rate determined in this way has been termed the practical false positive rate. Table 19.12, derived from the distributions shown in Figure 19.5, shows the detection rate and practical false positive rate using different cut-off levels. For example, using a cut-

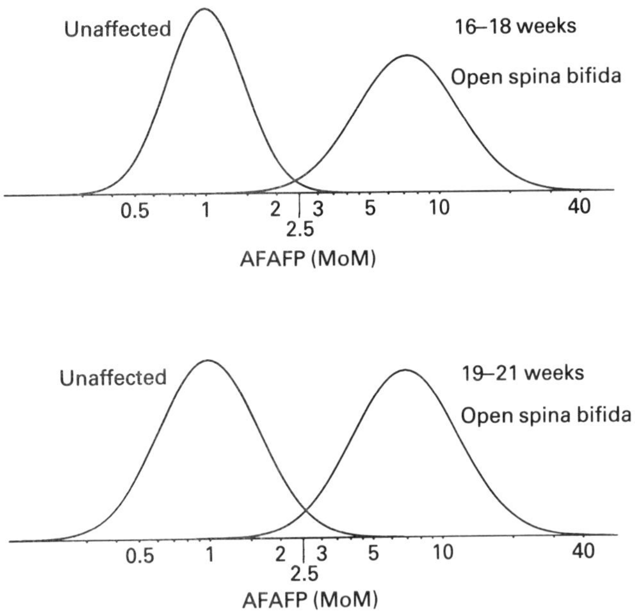

Fig. 19.5 Distribution of amniotic fluid alpha-fetoprotein (AFAFP) levels in unaffected and open spina bifida pregnancies at 16–18 and 19–21 weeks of gestation (based on parameters given in the UK Collaborative AFP Study 1982).

Table 19.12 Amniotic fluid AFP at 16–18 and 19–21 weeks of gestation in women with a positive maternal serum AFP test*: detection rate for open spina bifida, practical false positive rate† and population odds of having an affected fetus given a positive result according to AFP cut-off level calculated using gestational age based on dates. The odds are based on a birth prevalence of open spina bifida in the absence of antenatal diagnosis and selective abortion of 2 per 1000

AFP (MoM)	Detection rate (%)	Practical false positive rate (%)	Odds of being affected given a positive result
16–18 weeks' gestation			
⩾2.5	98	0.76	10:1
⩾3.0	96	0.18	41:1
⩾3.5	93	0.06	160:1
⩾4.0	88	0.01	680:1
⩾4.5	83	<0.01	2100:1
⩾5.0	77	<0.01	59000:1
19–21 weeks' gestation			
⩾2.5	97	3.07	2.4:1
⩾3.0	95	1.22	5.9:1
⩾3.5	90	0.52	13:1
⩾4.0	85	0.23	28:1
⩾4.5	80	0.11	57:1
⩾5.0	74	0.05	110:1

* ⩾2.5 MoM at 16–18 weeks' gestation and AFP MoM value calculated using gestational age based on biparietal diameter measurement.
† Percentage of non-NTD pregnancies with positive results excluding miscarriages and serious fetal malformations.
Calculated using parameters given in UK Collaborative AFP Study (1982).

off level of 3.0 MoM at 16–18 weeks of gestation, the detection for open spina bifida is 96% and the practical false positive rate is 0.2%.

Table 19.13 Amniotic fluid AFP at 16–18 and 19–21 weeks of gestation in women with a positive maternal serum AFP test*: individual woman's odds of having a singleton fetus with open spina bifida† according to actual AFP level. The odds are based on a birth prevalence of open spina bifida in the absence of antenatal diagnosis and selective abortion of 2 per 1000

Actual AfP level (MoM)‡	Odds of being affected at 16–18 weeks' gestation‡	Odds of being affected at 19–21 weeks' gestation‡
2.0	1:84	1:86
2.2	1:32	1:42
2.4	1:13	1:22
2.6	1:5.6	1:12
2.8	1:2.5	1:6.8
3.0	1:1.2	1:4.0
3.2	1.8:1	1:2.5
3.4	3.6:1	1:1.5
3.6	7.0:1	1:1.0
3.8	13:1	1.5:1
4.0	24:1	2.3:1

* ⩾2.5 MoM at 16–18 weeks' gestation; maternal serum AFP MoM value was calculated using gestational age based on biparietal diameter measurement.
† Excluding miscarriages and serious fetal malformations other than open spina bifida.
‡ Using gestational age based on the BPD estimate but if it is 1–34 days earlier than the dates estimate use the dates estimate.
Calculated using parameters given in UK Collaborative AFP Study (1982).

Table 19.12 shows how the performance of the test is better at 16–18 than at 19–21 weeks of gestation. Table 19.12 also shows the odds of open spina bifida for women with raised maternal serum AFP levels (after the use of ultrasound to exclude multiple pregnancy and the effect of underestimated gestational age) who also have amniotic fluid AFP levels equal to or greater than the specified cut-off levels. The table assumes a birth prevalence of 2 per 1000. The odds should be halved for a birth prevalence of 1 per 1000 and reduced to a quarter for a birth prevalence of 0.5 per 1000. Table 19.13 shows the corresponding odds for individual women with particular amniotic AFP levels.

Amniotic fluid blood staining

At 17 weeks of pregnancy the concentration of AFP in fetal serum is about 150 times that in amniotic fluid. The introduction of small amounts of fetal blood into amniotic fluid can therefore lead to raised amniotic fluid AFP levels. Such a mixture may arise as a result of amniocentesis, especially if the needle enters the placenta; it can also occur naturally with spina bifida pregnancies, presumably from the blood vessels close to the lesion. Amniotic fluid blood staining may therefore complicate the interpretation of a raised AFP level. Amniotic fluid acetylcholinesterase determination may resolve the uncertainty but sometimes it may be necessary to do a repeat amniocentesis or rely more on the results of the detailed ultrasound examination of the fetus.

Table 19.14 Fetal abnormalities associated with raised second trimester amniotic fluid AFP levels according to the probable or possible mechanism for the elevation

Probable or possible mechanism	Abnormality
Leakage through lesion or skin	Open NTD
	Anterior abdominal wall defect
	Turner's syndrome (cystic hygroma)
	Trisomy 13 (scalp defect)
	Nuchal bleb
	Pilonidal sinus
	Amniotic band syndrome
	Epidermolysis bullosa
	Prune belly syndrome
Leakage through kidneys	Congenital nephrosis
	Polycystic kidneys
Reduced clearance in gut	Oesophageal atresia
	Duodenal atresia
AFP loss from fetal autolysis	Intrauterine death and miscarriage
	Rhesus haemolytic disease
Decreased volume of amniotic fluid	Renal agenesis
	Urethral obstruction
Not known	Hydrocephaly
	Hydrocele
	Median palatoschisis

The use of ultrasound in the interpretation of amniotic fluid AFP results

The use of gestational age estimates based on ultrasound BPD measurements to calculate MoM values will decrease the detection of open spina bifida through amniotic fluid AFP measurement for the same reason that it increases detection through maternal serum AFP measurement. The opposite effect will occur because amniotic fluid levels decrease, whereas maternal serum levels increase in the second trimester. The simplest way of using ultrasound most effectively to estimate gestational age is, for the reasons given on page 273, to use the BPD estimate, but if this is 1–34 days earlier than the dates estimate, the latter should be used.

Other fetal abnormalities

Various fetal abnormalities other than NTD and certain adverse outcomes of pregnancy may be associated with raised amniotic AFP values in the second trimester. Table 19.14 gives a list of such abnormalities classified according to the probable or possible explanation for the raised AFP level. Apart from open NTDs, anterior abdominal wall defects and intrauterine death or miscarriage, the conditions are either rare, or only rarely have raised amniotic fluid AFP levels.

Acetylcholinesterase

The second main biochemical diagnostic test for open NTDs is acetylcholinesterase (AChE) determined by polyacrylamide gel electrophoresis. The cerebrospinal fluid is rich in AChE and it is therefore not surprising that a fetal lesion in which cerebrospinal fluid is exposed to amniotic fluid is associated with high amniotic fluid AChE levels. Table 19.15 shows results from the Collaborative AChE Study (1981) which investigated the value of performing a gel AChE test on amniotic fluid samples collected from women with positive amniotic fluid AFP tests. A result was regarded as positive if there was an AChE band in the gel which migrated to the same position as AChE from cerebrospinal fluid. The detection rate in this group of women was 99.6% for anencephaly and 99.4% for open spina bifida. The practical false positive rate was 6%, two-thirds of which were associated with fetal blood staining. The odds of having a fetus with open spina bifida given a positive gel AChE test in women with a single positive amniotic fluid AFP ($\geqslant$3.0 MoM) at 16–18 weeks of gestation in relation to the background prevalence of open spina bifida, the reasons for the amniocentesis and the presence of amniotic fluid blood staining are given in Table 19.16. If the amniotic fluid sample is not visibly contaminated with fetal blood the odds of being affected are high, regardless of the birth prevalence or the reasons for the amniocentesis. However, in amniotic fluids that are contaminated with substantial amounts of fetal blood the error rate can be quite high.

Table 19.15 Gel AChE results in pregnancies with positive amniotic fluid AFP results (from about 34 000 tests for AFP)

Outcome	Number of pregnancies	AChE-positive number (%)
Anencephaly	478	476 (99.6)
Open spina bifida	335	333 (99.4)
Anterior abdominal wall defect	63	47 (75)
Congenital nephrosis	11	0 (0)
Other serious malformations	14	7 (50)
Miscarriage	73	34 (47)
No serious malformation or miscarriage	125	8 (6)
Total	1099	905

Adapted from the Collaborative AChE Study Report (1981).

Three prospective studies have examined the use of the gel AChE test in women with negative amniotic fluid AFP tests (Read et al 1982, Aitken et al 1984, Wyvill et al 1984). Combining their results, out of 5021 unaffected pregnancies without serious malformations, nine had positive AChE tests — a false positive rate of 0.2%. There were only two open spina bifida pregnancies with negative amniotic fluid AFP tests; both had positive AChE tests. The results are promising, but until larger series are published the value of the gel AChE test in such women is uncertain.

Blood-stained amniotic fluid

Amniotic fluid containing *maternal* blood is not a source of AChE false positives provided the test is performed correctly. Maternal blood does yield a band in the gel at the position where AChE from NTD pregnancies is found, but this is not due to AChE and as a result the band is not inhibited by the specific AChE inhibitor (BW284C51) which should be used on all apparently positive gels.

Table 19.16 AChE test in women with a positive amniotic fluid AFP test*; population odds of having a fetus with open spina bifida given a positive AChE test† according to prevalence of open spina bifida; reason for amniocentesis and aminiotic fluid blood staining

Birth prevalence of open spina bifida‡	Reason for amniocentesis	Before AChE test	After AChE found to be positive		
			Amniotic fluid blood staining Not known	Mainly fetal	None or mainly maternal
1 per 1000	Raised serum AFP (≥2.5 MoM)	9:1	140:1	18:1	480:1
	Previous infant with an NTD	2:1	32:1	4:1	106:1
	Other	1:4	4:1	1:2	13:1
2 per 1000	Raised serum AFP (≥2.5 MoM)	18:1	290:1	36:1	950:1
	Previous infant with an NTD	5:1	80:1	10:1	260:1
	Other	1:2	8:1	1:1	26:1

* ≥3.0 MoM at 16–18 weeks of gestation.
† Excluding miscarriages and serious fetal malformations other than open spina bifida.
‡ In the absence of antenatal diagnosis and selective abortion.
Adapted from the Collaborative AChE Study Report (1981).

Table 19.17 Gel-AChE density ratio in gel-AChE positive samples: positive rate* according to fetal defect in four studies

Centre	Criteria for sample selection	Open spina bifida (%)	Anterior abdominal wall defect (%)
Maine[1]	Positive AF-AFP	100 (20/20)	0 (0/10)
Oxford[2]	Positive AF-AFP not visibly blood-stained†	100 (24/24)	0 (0/8)
Edinburgh[3]	None	100 (14/14)	0 (0/10)
N. Carolina[4]	Positive AF-AFP	100 (21/21)	0 (0/12)
Combined	—	100 (79/79)	0 (0/40)

*Proportion of pregnancies with AChE/PChE density ratio ≥0.15 (numbers in parentheses).
†Visible blood contamination can produce ratios typical of either defect.[1,3]
[1]Goldfine et al (1983)
[2]Wald et al (1984b)
[3]Peat and Brock (1984)
[4]Burton (1986)

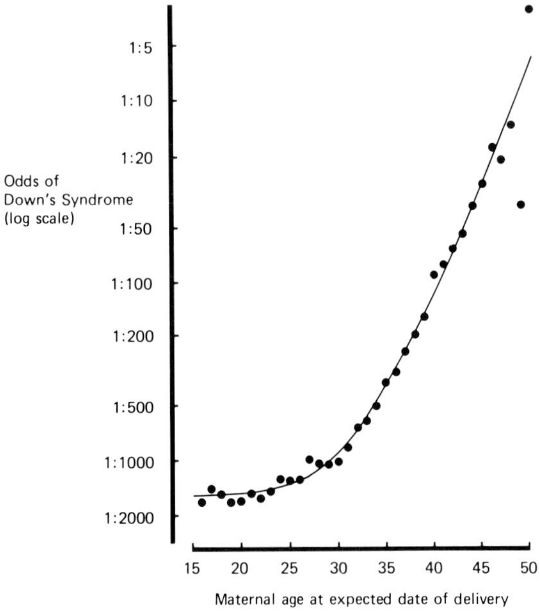

Fig. 19.7 Risk of a Down's syndrome birth according to maternal age at expected date of delivery, derived from the pooled results of eight series. The observed odds are shown together with a fitted regression line (from Cuckle et al 1987).

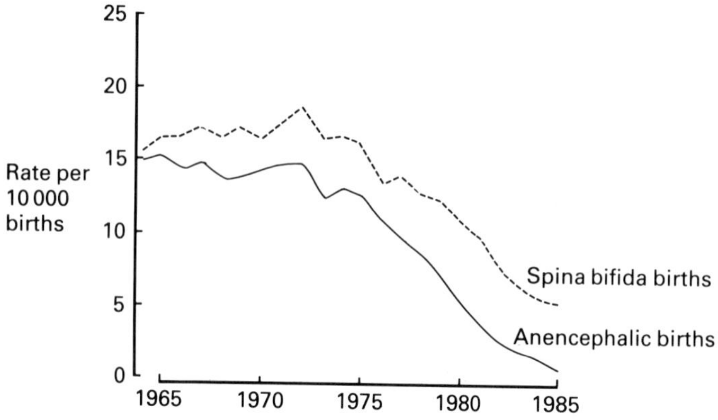

Fig. 19.6 Birth prevalence of anencephaly and spina bifida in England and Wales from 1964 to 1985 (from Cuckle & Wald 1987a).

Amniotic fluid containing *fetal* blood can be a source of AChE false positives. Fetal serum contains AChE and false positives begin to occur when the concentration of fetal blood in amniotic fluid reaches about 60 million cells per ml, a level of contamination which is easily seen by the naked eye (Barlow et al 1982a). In clinical practice if a gel AChE test turns out to be positive in the presence of more than 60 million fetal red cells per ml it is sensible to repeat the amniocentesis 1–2 weeks later.

Fetal calf serum contamination of amniotic fluid and AChE

Fetal calf serum contains AChE which in the gel AChE test yields a band in the gel at a similar position to that where

AChE from NTD pregnancies is found, and like the NTD band it is inhibited by BW284C51. Often samples for amniotic fluid AFP and AChE determination are first processed in the laboratory for cytogenetic studies and at this stage it is occasionally possible, through technical error, to contaminate the amniotic fluid supernatant with fetal calf serum which is used in the culture medium to grow amniotic fluid cells for chromosome studies. Fetal calf serum is such a rich source of AChE that very small traces of fetal calf serum in the amniotic fluid at dilutions as low as 1:20 000 can cause false positives. It is possible that as many as half of AChE false positives in clear samples are due to fetal calf serum contamination.

If an AChE result is positive in a clear sample, paticularly one with a negative amniotic AFP result, amniotic fluid fetal calf serum contamination may be the explanation. The presence of contamination can be demonstrated by performing a sensitive immunological test for bovine serum albumin (Brock et al 1982). If this is positive, fetal calf serum contamination is the probable cause for the AChE positive result (Barlow et al 1984).

Anterior abdominal wall defects and AChE

Gel AChE tests can distinguish between open spina bifida and anterior abdominal wall defects (Goldfine et al 1983, Peat & Brock 1984, Wald et al 1984b, Burton 1986). Both defects yield two bands in the gel, one due to AChE and the other due to pseudocholinesterase (PChE). With anterior abdominal wall defects the AChE band is faint and the PChE band relatively dense, whilst with open spina bifida the AChE band is relatively denser and the PChE band less dense. The densities of the two bands can be quantified by scanning densitometry. Table 19.17 shows the striking separation and the distribution of AChE/PChE density ratios according to the type of defect. Anterior abdominal wall defects are associated with ratios less than 0.15; open spina bifida is associated with ratios greater than this. Ultrasound examination of the fetus is probably the most effective way of distinguishing open spina bifida from abdominal wall defects; the band pattern of the AChE test however, provides a powerful complementary diagnostic test. The importance of distinguishing the diagnosis of these two defects lies in the fact that the prognosis of infants with abdominal wall defects is often good with appropriate early surgery soon after birth, so that a termination of pregnancy may be contraindicated. This is particularly the case with gastroschisis but less so with exomphalos, which is often associated with other severe abnormalities.

Alternative methods of AChE determination

Various modifications to the original gel AChE test have been suggested. The most useful is the use of the slab gel technique rather than the disc gel to enable as many as 20 samples to be assayed simultaneously and to permit adequate quality control (Barlow et al 1982b). Assays based on the use of antibodies to AChE have been introduced (Nørgaard-Pedersen et al 1983, Brock et al 1985). While they are effective and have the advantage of being quantitative, none have been sufficiently evaluated to show whether they have a better diagnostic accuracy than the qualitative test, but one (R431) looks very promising (Rasmussen et al 1987).

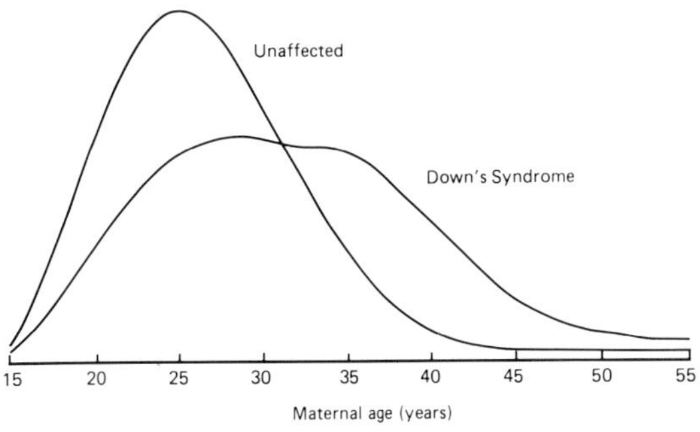

Fig. 19.8 Distribution of maternal age in unaffected and Down's syndrome births in England and Wales in 1981–1985 derived by applying the regression line in Figure 19.7 to the age distribution of maternities in that period.

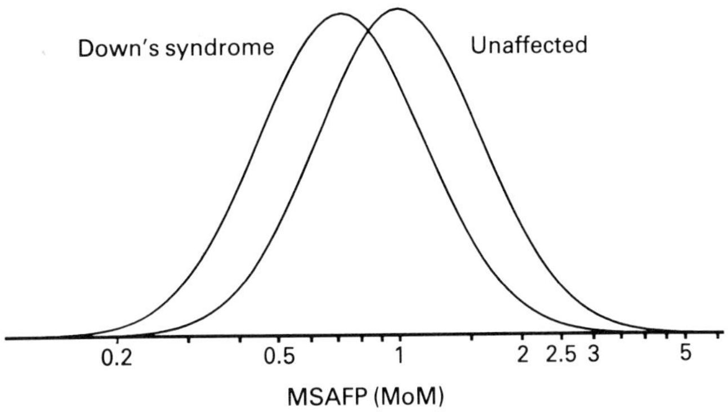

Fig. 19.9 Distribution of maternal serum alpha-fetoprotein (MSAFP) levels in unaffected and Down's syndrome pregnancies at 14–20 weeks of gestation (based on parameters given in Cuckle et al 1987).

Combining information on maternal serum AFP, amniotic fluid AFP and AChE on women with borderline amniotic fluid AFP levels

Women with borderline amniotic fluid AFP levels are occasionally seen; these cases can pose diagnostic problems. A nomogram has been devised for use in such cases (Wald & Cuckle 1982). The nomogram can be used for tests done at 16–18 and or 19–21 weeks of gestation and it permits information on maternal serum AFP, amniotic fluid AFP and gel AChE results to be used in combination to determine an individual woman's risk of having spina bifida. Since amniocentesis can itself elevate the maternal serum AFP

Table 19.18 An individual woman's odds of a Down's syndrome birth according to maternal age and maternal serum AFP level at 14–20 weeks of gestation; gestational age based on dates

Maternal age at EDD (years)	Maternal serum AFP level (MoM)															
	0.40	0.45	0.50	0.55	0.60	0.65	0.70	0.75	0.80	0.85	0.90	0.95	1.00	1.50	2.00	2.50
25	1:430	1:520	1:610	1:710	1:810	1:910	1:1000	1:1100	1:1300	1:1400	1:1500	1:1600	1:1700	1:3100	1:4700	1:6400
26	1:410	1:490	1:580	1:670	1:770	1:870	1:970	1:1100	1:1200	1:1300	1:1400	1:1500	1:1700	1:3000	1:4500	1:6100
27	1:380	1:460	1:550	1:630	1:720	1:820	1:920	1:1000	1:1100	1:1200	1:1300	1:1400	1:1600	1:2800	1:4200	1:5700
28	1:360	1:430	1:510	1:590	1:670	1:760	1:850	1:940	1:1000	1:1100	1:1200	1:1300	1:1400	1:2600	1:3900	1:5300
29	1:320	1:390	1:460	1:530	1:610	1:690	1:770	1:860	1:940	1:1000	1:1100	1:1200	1:1300	1:2400	1:3500	1:4800
30	1:290	1:350	1:410	1:480	1:540	1:620	1:690	1:760	1:840	1:920	1:1000	1:1100	1:1200	1:2100	1:3200	1:4300
31	1:250	1:300	1:360	1:420	1:480	1:540	1:600	1:670	1:740	1:810	1:880	1:950	1:1000	1:1800	1:2800	1:3800
32	1:220	1:260	1:310	1:360	1:410	1:460	1:520	1:570	1:630	1:690	1:750	1:820	1:880	1:1600	1:2400	1:3200
33	1:180	1:220	1:260	1:300	1:340	1:390	1:430	1:480	1:530	1:580	1:630	1:690	1:740	1:1300	1:2000	1:2700
34	1:150	1:180	1:210	1:250	1:280	1:320	1:360	1:400	1:440	1:480	1:520	1:570	1:610	1:1100	1:1600	1:2200
35	1:120	1:150	1:170	1:200	1:230	1:260	1:290	1:320	1:360	1:390	1:420	1:460	1:500	1:890	1:1300	1:1800
36	1:98	1:120	1:140	1:160	1:180	1:210	1:230	1:260	1:280	1:310	1:340	1:370	1:400	1:710	1:1100	1:1400
37	1:77	1:93	1:110	1:130	1:140	1:160	1:180	1:200	1:220	1:250	1:270	1:290	1:310	1:560	1:840	1:1100
38	1:60	1:72	1:85	1:99	1:110	1:130	1:140	1:160	1:170	1:190	1:210	1:230	1:240	1:440	1:660	1:890
39	1:46	1:56	1:66	1:76	1:87	1:99	1:110	1:120	1:140	1:150	1:160	1:170	1:190	1:340	1:510	1:690
40	1:36	1:43	1:51	1:59	1:67	1:76	1:85	1:94	1:100	1:110	1:120	1:130	1:140	1:260	1:390	1:530
41	1:27	1:33	1:39	1:45	1:51	1:58	1:65	1:72	1:79	1:87	1:94	1:100	1:110	1:200	1:300	1:400
42	1:21	1:25	1:29	1:34	1:39	1:44	1:49	1:54	1:60	1:66	1:72	1:77	1:84	1:150	1:220	1:310
43	1:16	1:19	1:22	1:26	1:29	1:33	1:37	1:41	1:45	1:50	1:54	1:59	1:63	1:110	1:170	1:230
44	1:12	1:14	1:17	1:19	1:22	1:25	1:28	1:31	1:34	1:37	1:41	1:44	1:47	1:85	1:130	1:170
45	1:9	1:11	1:12	1:14	1:16	1:19	1:21	1:23	1:26	1:28	1:30	1:33	1:36	1:64	1:96	1:130
46	1:7	1:8	1:9	1:11	1:12	1:14	1:16	1:17	1:19	1:21	1:23	1:25	1:27	1:48	1:71	1:97
47	1:5	1:6	1:7	1:8	1:9	1:10	1:12	1:13	1:14	1:15	1:17	1:18	1:20	1:35	1:53	1:72
48	1:4	1:4	1:5	1:6	1:7	1:8	1:9	1:9	1:10	1:11	1:12	1:13	1:14	1:26	1:39	1:53
49	1:3	1:3	1:4	1:4	1:5	1:6	1:6	1:7	1:8	1:8	1:9	1:10	1:11	1:19	1:29	1:39

EDD = expected date of delivery; MoM = multiple of normal median.
From Cuckle et al (1987a).

level, only values from serum samples collected before the amniocentesis should be used.

Other diagnostic tests on amniotic fluid

Other biochemical diagnostic tests for open NTD have been suggested but none offer the sensitivity and specificity of amniotic fluid AFP and AChE determination. Two such tests have been suggested for the measurement of two molecular variants of amniotic fluid AFP, distinguished on the basis of their reactivity to concanavalin A (Smith et al 1979), and the identification of morphologically characteristic amniotic fluid cells which rapidly adhere to glass in culture (Gosden & Brock 1977).

Risks of amniocentesis

There is no doubt that there is a risk of fetal damage associated with amniocentesis. The main risk appears to be miscarriage and the best estimate of the excess risk is 0.8% (2.1%; 48/2302 versus 1.3%; 30/2304) based on the results of a randomized trial of amniocentesis (Tabor et al 1986). During the first few months of the study, an 18 gauge needle was used and thereafter a finer needle (20 gauge) was used (Tabor et al 1988). The National Institute for Child Health and Development study of amniocentesis (1976) and that carried out by the Canadian Medical Research Council (1977) both demonstrated that the risk of miscarriage was related to the needle size: for ⩽19, 20–21 and ⩾22 gauge needles the risks were 6.1, 3.1 and 2.4% respectively in the former study and 10, 2.8 and 1.7% in the latter. 21 and 22 gauge needles are satisfactory and probably generate an excess risk of miscarriage considerably less than that observed in the study of Tabor and colleagues.

The Medical Research Council Working Party on Amniocentesis (1978) suggested that amniocentesis was also associated with two non-fatal adverse outcomes of pregnancy, namely compression abnormalities (specifically congenital dislocation of the hip and talipes) and neonatal respiratory difficulties. The suggestion of an association with compression abnormalities was reinvestigated and excluded as a hazard by a large-scale case-control study (Wald et al 1983). The link between amniocentesis and neonatal respiratory difficulties has not been further investigated and remains a possible complication. It is one, however, that can be satisfactorily treated by appropriate neonatal intensive care.

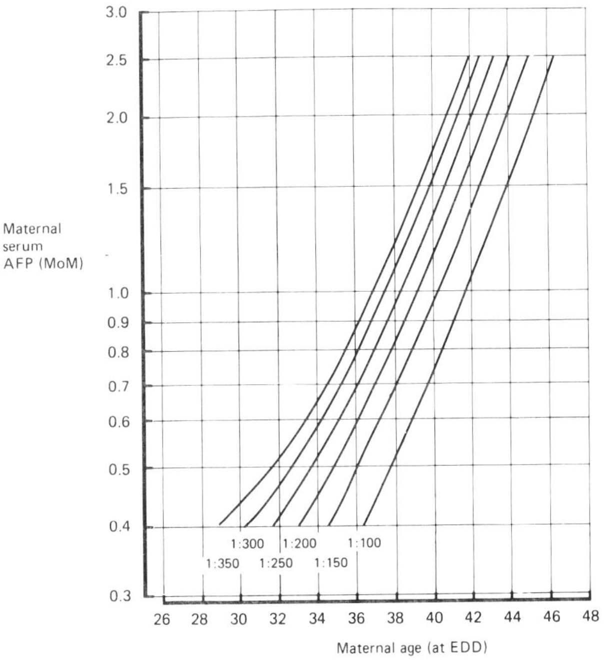

Fig. 19.10 Six maternal serum AFP and maternal age Down's syndrome iso-risks (14–20 weeks of gestation, restricted to 0.40–2.50 MoM). The iso-risks specified in the figure are the risks of a Down's syndrome birth (based on the risk equations in Cuckle et al 1987).

Table 19.19 Combined maternal serum AFP and maternal age screening for Down's syndrome at 14–20 weeks of gestation: detection rate, false positive rate and odds of a Down's syndrome birth according to iso-risk cut-off*

Iso-risk cut-off†	Detection rate (%)	False positive rate (%)	Average Down's syndrome risk in positives
1:100	17	0.9	1:41
1:150	23	1.7	1:61
1:200	27	2.7	1:79
1:250	31	3.8	1:97
1:300	35	5.2	1:117
1:350	39	6.7	1:137

* The rates are derived as in Cuckle et al (1987a) except that the proportions of affected and unaffected pregnancies less than or equal to a given AFP level were estimated from the log Gaussian AFP distributions rather than directly, and distribution of births in 1981–1985 are used.
† A woman has a positive result if the risk of a Down's syndrome birth based on her serum AFP level and age is equal to or greater than the specified iso-risk.
Adapted from Wald & Cuckle 1987.

Diagnostic ultrasound

The increasing use of ultrasound as a method of antenatal diagnosis sometimes leads to a positive diagnosis being made on the basis of the ultrasound findings alone without first performing an amniocentesis and an amniotic fluid AFP and gel AChE determination. With anencephaly the accuracy of ultrasound is sufficiently great for amniocentesis to be avoided. However, as far as the diagnosis of spina bifida is concerned there is no study that has shown that an ultrasound diagnosis is more accurate. The desire to avoid the trauma and hazards of amniocentesis is understandable but is not a sufficient reason for adopting alternative inadequately evaluated procedures. It is therefore best at present to offer women who are known to be at risk of having a fetus with spina bifida both a detailed diagnostic ultrasound examination and an amniocentesis, and only avoid one or other of these investigations in exceptional circumstances.

Outcome of screening in England and Wales

The birth prevalence of anencephaly and spina bifida has declined by 80% from 31.5 to 6.2 per 10 000 total births between 1964–1972 and 1985 (see Fig. 19.6). Over the same period notified terminations of pregnancy with a suspected fetal central nervous system abnormality increased from less than 1 to 56% of NTD births and central nervous system terminations combined. The under-reporting of the suspected abnormality on the termination of pregnancy notification form makes it difficult to assess the contribution that screening for NTD has made on the decline of the birth prevalence but it probably accounts for one-half or more of the decline. This decline in one of the most common causes of serious childhood handicap represents a major public health achievement. It has also had the effect of focusing research into primary prevention instead of simply early detection and selective abortion.

DOWN'S SYNDROME

Prevalence

The maternal age-specific birth prevalence of Down's syndrome is remarkably similar in different parts of the world. It is about 0.7, 1, 9, 140 per 1000 births for women aged 20, 30, 40 and 50 respectively (see Fig. 19.7 which is derived from the pooling of data from eight surveys). Paternal age exerts a separate but small influence on the risk when maternal age has been taken into account. In England and Wales the overall prevalence is about 1.3 per 1000 births.

Most births associated with Down's syndrome are unexpected, over 99% being born to couples who have not previously had infants with Down's syndrome and do not themselves have a balanced translocation of chromosome 21. The recurrence risk in women who have had one infant with Down's syndrome in the absence of a parental balanced translocation can be approximately estimated by adding a risk of 5 per 1000 to the background age-specific risk. It is not known why such women have an increased risk. In the rare event of one of the parents having a balanced reciprocal translocation (about 1 in 5000 couples are affected) the risk of Down's syndrome is about 10%.

Survival and extent of handicap

About two-thirds of pregnancies associated with fetal Down's syndrome end in a miscarriage (Creasey & Crolla

Table 19.20 An individual woman's odds of a Down's syndrome birth according to maternal age and maternal serum AFP level at 14–20 weeks of gestation; gestational age based on BPD

Maternal age at EDD (years)	Maternal serum AFP level (MoM)															
	0.40	0.45	0.50	0.55	0.60	0.65	0.70	0.75	0.80	0.85	0.90	0.95	1.00	1.50	2.00	2.50
25	1:360	1:440	1:530	1:630	1:740	1:850	1:960	1:1100	1:1200	1:1300	1:1500	1:1600	1:1800	1:3400	1:5300	1:7500
26	1:340	1:420	1:510	1:600	1:700	1:810	1:920	1:1000	1:1200	1:1300	1:1400	1:1500	1:1700	1:3200	1:5100	1:7200
27	1:320	1:400	1:480	1:570	1:660	1:760	1:860	1:970	1:1100	1:1200	1:1300	1:1400	1:1600	1:3000	1:4800	1:6700
28	1:300	1:370	1:440	1:520	1:610	1:700	1:800	1:900	1:1000	1:1100	1:1200	1:1300	1:1500	1:2800	1:4400	1:6200
29	1:270	1:330	1:400	1:480	1:560	1:640	1:730	1:820	1:910	1:1000	1:1100	1:1200	1:1300	1:2600	1:4000	1:5700
30	1:240	1:300	1:360	1:430	1:500	1:570	1:650	1:730	1:810	1:900	1:990	1:1100	1:1200	1:2300	1:3600	1:5100
31	1:210	1:260	1:320	1:370	1:430	1:500	1:570	1:640	1:710	1:790	1:870	1:950	1:1000	1:2000	1:3200	1:4400
32	1:180	1:220	1:270	1:320	1:370	1:430	1:490	1:550	1:610	1:680	1:750	1:820	1:890	1:1700	1:2700	1:3800
33	1:150	1:190	1:230	1:270	1:310	1:360	1:410	1:460	1:510	1:570	1:630	1:690	1:750	1:1400	1:2300	1:3200
34	1:130	1:160	1:190	1:220	1:260	1:300	1:340	1:380	1:420	1:470	1:520	1:570	1:620	1:1200	1:1900	1:2600
35	1:100	1:130	1:150	1:180	1:210	1:240	1:270	1:310	1:340	1:380	1:420	1:460	1:500	1:970	1:1500	1:2100
36	1:81	1:100	1:120	1:140	1:170	1:190	1:220	1:250	1:270	1:300	1:330	1:370	1:400	1:770	1:1200	1:1700
37	1:64	1:79	1:96	1:110	1:130	1:150	1:170	1:190	1:220	1:240	1:260	1:290	1:310	1:610	1:960	1:1300
38	1:50	1:62	1:75	1:88	1:100	1:120	1:130	1:150	1:170	1:190	1:210	1:230	1:250	1:470	1:750	1:1100
39	1:39	1:48	1:58	1:68	1:80	1:91	1:100	1:120	1:130	1:140	1:160	1:170	1:190	1:370	1:580	1:810
40	1:30	1:37	1:44	1:52	1:61	1:70	1:80	1:90	1:100	1:110	1:120	1:130	1:150	1:280	1:440	1:620
41	1:23	1:28	1:34	1:40	1:47	1:53	1:61	1:68	1:76	1:85	1:93	1:100	1:110	1:210	1:340	1:480
42	1:17	1:21	1:26	1:30	1:35	1:41	1:46	1:52	1:58	1:64	1:71	1:77	1:84	1:160	1:260	1:360
43	1:13	1:16	1:19	1:23	1:27	1:31	1:35	1:39	1:44	1:48	1:53	1:58	1:64	1:120	1:190	1:270
44	1:10	1:12	1:15	1:17	1:20	1:23	1:26	1:29	1:33	1:36	1:40	1:44	1:48	1:93	1:150	1:200
45	1:7	1:9	1:11	1:13	1:15	1:17	1:20	1:22	1:25	1:27	1:30	1:33	1:36	1:69	1:110	1:150
46	1:5	1:7	1:8	1:10	1:11	1:13	1:15	1:16	1:18	1:20	1:22	1:25	1:27	1:52	1:81	1:110
47	1:4	1:5	1:6	1:7	1:8	1:10	1:11	1:12	1:14	1:15	1:17	1:18	1:20	1:38	1:60	1:85
48	1:3	1:4	1:4	1:5	1:6	1:7	1:8	1:9	1:10	1:11	1:12	1:13	1:15	1:28	1:44	1:63
49	1:2	1:3	1:3	1:4	1:4	1:5	1:6	1:7	1:7	1:8	1:9	1:10	1:11	1:21	1:32	1:46

BPD = biparietal diameter; EDD = expected date of delivery; MoM = multiple of normal median.
From Cuckle et al (1987a).

1974). Most of the fetal loss occurs in the first trimester of pregnancy but there is also a selective loss in the second and third trimesters, the prevalence at about 18 weeks of pregnancy being about 25% higher than it is at birth.

Infants with Down's syndrome are invariably mentally handicapped and also may have associated physical congenital abnormalities affecting the heart (about 30%), gastrointestinal tract, eye and ear. Life expectancy is now about 50 years (Øster et al 1975, Masaki et al 1981, Baird & Sadovnick 1987). In the first years of life the use of health services is about double that of unaffected infants (Gill et al 1987). The main burden of care, however, arises from the fact that individuals with Down's syndrome are completely dependent on others and require considerable personal supervision throughout their lives. Recently Alzheimer's disease has been recognized as a common complication in adults with Down's syndrome. Virtually all Down's syndrome adults aged over 30 years get neuritic plaques and neurofibrillary tangles in their brains typical of Alzheimer's disease, and a large proportion of them become clinically demented (Dalton 1982, Kolata 1985). The amyloid polypeptide of Alzheimer's disease is coded by a gene on chromosome 21 (Goldgaber et al 1987). It is found in adults with Down's syndrome as well as in the brains of patients with Alzheimer's disease (Glenner & Wong 1984, Masters et al 1985).

Maternal age screening

Figure 19.8 shows the distribution of pregnancies with and without Down's syndrome according to maternal age. There is considerable overlap in the two distributions so that at the outset it is clear that the use of maternal age as a screening method cannot be very effective. Using an age cut-off level of 40 years, about 1% of women will be offered an amniocentesis and this would lead to the detection of about 16% of Down's syndrome. Even if the oldest 10% of women were offered an amniocentesis (age cut-off level of 34) this would lead to the detection of only 40% of Down's syndrome. In practice the detection of Down's syndrome by maternal age screening is much less than would be expected from the distributions shown in Fig. 19.8 because many women are not explicitly identified to be at risk on account of their age and offered an amniocentesis, and others decline the test (Knott et al 1986). As a result few screening programmes have achieved a reduction in the birth prevalence of Down's syndrome of more than 15%.

Table 19.21 An individual woman's odds of a Down's syndrome birth according to maternal age and maternal serum AFP level at 14–20 weeks of gestation; AFP adjusted for maternal weight, gestational age based on dates

Maternal age at EDD (years)	Maternal serum AFP level (MoM)															
	0.40	0.45	0.50	0.55	0.60	0.65	0.70	0.75	0.80	0.85	0.90	0.95	1.00	1.50	2.00	2.50
25	1:400	1:490	1:580	1:680	1:780	1:890	1:1000	1:1100	1:1200	1:1400	1:1500	1:1600	1:1800	1:3300	1:5100	1:7000
26	1:380	1:460	1:550	1:640	1:740	1:850	1:960	1:1100	1:1200	1:1300	1:1400	1:1600	1:1700	1:3100	1:4800	1:6700
27	1:360	1:430	1:520	1:610	1:700	1:800	1:900	1:1000	1:1100	1:1200	1:1300	1:1500	1:1600	1:3000	1:4500	1:6300
28	1:330	1:400	1:480	1:560	1:650	1:740	1:830	1:930	1:1000	1:1100	1:1200	1:1400	1:1500	1:2700	1:4200	1:5800
29	1:300	1:370	1:440	1:510	1:590	1:670	1:760	1:850	1:940	1:1000	1:1100	1:1200	1:1300	1:2500	1:3800	1:5300
30	1:270	1:330	1:390	1:460	1:530	1:600	1:680	1:760	1:840	1:920	1:1000	1:1100	1:1200	1:2200	1:3400	1:4700
31	1:230	1:290	1:340	1:400	1:460	1:530	1:590	1:660	1:730	1:810	1:890	1:960	1:1000	1:1900	1:3000	1:4100
32	1:200	1:250	1:290	1:340	1:400	1:450	1:510	1:570	1:630	1:690	1:760	1:830	1:900	1:1700	1:2600	1:3500
33	1:170	1:210	1:250	1:290	1:330	1:380	1:430	1:480	1:530	1:580	1:640	1:700	1:750	1:1400	1:2200	1:3000
34	1:140	1:170	1:200	1:240	1:270	1:310	1:350	1:390	1:440	1:480	1:530	1:570	1:620	1:1200	1:1800	1:2500
35	1:110	1:140	1:160	1:190	1:220	1:250	1:290	1:320	1:350	1:390	1:430	1:470	1:500	1:940	1:1400	1:2000
36	1:90	1:110	1:130	1:150	1:180	1:200	1:230	1:60	1:280	1:310	1:340	1:370	1:400	1:750	1:1200	1:1600
37	1:71	1:87	1:100	1:120	1:140	1:160	1:180	1:200	1:220	1:250	1:270	1:290	1:320	1:590	1:910	1:1300
38	1:56	1:68	1:81	1:95	1:110	1:120	1:140	1:160	1:170	1:190	1:210	1:230	1:250	1:460	1:710	1:980
39	1:43	1:52	1:62	1:73	1:84	1:96	1:110	1:120	1:130	1:150	1:160	1:180	1:190	1:360	1:550	1:760
40	1:33	1:40	1:48	1:56	1:65	1:74	1:83	1:93	1:100	1:110	1:120	1:140	1:150	1:270	1:420	1:580
41	1:25	1:31	1:37	1:43	1:49	1:56	1:63	1:71	1:79	1:87	1:95	1:100	1:110	1:210	1:320	1:440
42	1:19	1:23	1:28	1:32	1:37	1:43	1:48	1:54	1:60	1:66	1:72	1:78	1:85	1:160	1:240	1:340
43	1:14	1:18	1:21	1:25	1:28	1:32	1:36	1:41	1:45	1:50	1:54	1:59	1:64	1:120	1:180	1:250
44	1:11	1:13	1:16	1:18	1:21	1:24	1:27	1:31	1:34	1:37	1:41	1:45	1:48	1:90	1:140	1:190
45	1:8	1:10	1:12	1:14	1:16	1:18	1:20	1:23	1:25	1:28	1:31	1:33	1:36	1:67	1:100	1:140
46	1:6	1:7	1:9	1:10	1:12	1:14	1:15	1:17	1:19	1:21	1:23	1:25	1:27	1:50	1:77	1:110
47	1:4	1:5	1:7	1:8	1:9	1:10	1:11	1:13	1:14	1:15	1:17	1:18	1:20	1:37	1:57	1:79
48	1:3	1:4	1:5	1:6	1:6	1:7	1:8	1:9	1:10	1:11	1:12	1:14	1:15	1:27	1:42	1:58
49	1:2	1:3	1:4	1:4	1:5	1:5	1:6	1:7	1:8	1:8	1:9	1:10	1:11	1:20	1:31	1:43

EDD = expected date of delivery; MoM = multiple of normal median.
From Cuckle et al (1987a).

Combined maternal serum AFP and maternal age screening

Maternal serum AFP levels are, on average, 76% of those found in unaffected pregnancies in the second trimester (based on the weighted geometric mean value of 0.76 MoM from the 13 series included in Table 6 of Wald & Cuckle 1987). The reason for the low levels in Down's syndrome pregnancies is probably due to reduced fetal production, as evidenced by the low levels in fetal umbilical cord serum (0.45 MoM, Cuckle et al 1986) and the low levels in amniotic fluid (0.68 MoM based on the weighted geometric mean value from 11 series published in Table 6 of Wald & Cuckle 1987). The extent of reduction in maternal serum AFP levels seems to be similar between 14 and 20 weeks of gestation and data from 22 cases suggest that levels may also be low in the first trimester (Cuckle et al 1988).

Figure 19.9 shows the distribution of maternal serum AFP levels in Down's syndrome and unaffected pregnancies at 14–20 weeks of gestation. The overlap between the distributions is great but there is still sufficient discrimination for AFP to be of value as a screening test, particularly since maternal serum AFP and maternal age are independent determinates of the risk of Down's syndrome. Table 19.18 shows the risk of a Down's syndrome birth according to an individual pregnant woman's age and serum AFP level based on the age-specific risks given in Figure 19.7 and the log Gaussian AFP distributions shown in Figure 19.9.

For a given false positive rate the maximum Down's syndrome detection rate can be achieved by choosing maternal age-specific maternal serum AFP cut-off levels such that the risk of Down's syndrome for women with AFP levels exactly at the cut-off level is the same at each age. A curved line on the graph of maternal serum AFP against maternal age joining these points of identical risk can be termed an iso-risk. Figure 19.10 shows six such iso-risks. The detection rate and false positive rate associated with each iso-risk are shown in Table 19.19.

The risk estimates given in Table 19.18 relate to AFP results interpreted using gestational age based on dates, and not adjusted for maternal weight. The fetal BPD in Down's syndrome pregnancies is similar to that in unaffected pregnancies (Cuckle & Wald 1987b) as is the maternal weight (see Figure 6 in Wald & Cuckle 1987). The only effect of using BPD and weight adjustment is therefore to reduce the variance in the distributions of serum AFP in affected and unaffected pregnancies. Tables 19.20–19.22 show the

Table 19.22 An individual woman's odds of a Down's syndrome birth according to maternal age and maternal serum AFP level at 14–20 weeks of gestation; AFP adjusted for maternal weight, gestational age based on BPD

Maternal age at EDD (years)	Maternal serum AFP level (MoM) 0.40	0.45	0.50	0.55	0.60	0.65	0.70	0.75	0.80	0.85	0.90	0.95	1.00	1.50	2.00	2.50
25	1:320	1:410	1:500	1:600	1:700	1:820	1:940	1:1100	1:1200	1:1300	1:1500	1:1600	1:1800	1:3600	1:5900	1:8500
26	1:310	1:390	1:470	1:570	1:670	1:780	1:890	1:1000	1:1100	1:1300	1:1400	1:1600	1:1700	1:3500	1:5600	1:8100
27	1:290	1:360	1:450	1:530	1:630	1:730	1:840	1:950	1:1100	1:1200	1:1300	1:1500	1:1600	1:3300	1:5300	1:7600
28	1:270	1:340	1:410	1:490	1:580	1:680	1:780	1:880	1:990	1:1100	1:1200	1:1400	1:1500	1:3000	1:4900	1:7100
29	1:240	1:310	1:380	1:450	1:530	1:620	1:710	1:800	1:900	1:1000	1:1100	1:1200	1:1400	1:2700	1:4500	1:6400
30	1:220	1:270	1:340	1:400	1:470	1:550	1:630	1:720	1:810	1:900	1:1000	1:1100	1:1200	1:2400	1:4000	1:5700
31	1:190	1:240	1:290	1:350	1:410	1:480	1:550	1:630	1:710	1:790	1:870	1:960	1:1100	1:2100	1:3500	1:5000
32	1:160	1:210	1:250	1:300	1:360	1:410	1:470	1:540	1:610	1:680	1:750	1:830	1:910	1:1800	1:3000	1:4300
33	1:140	1:170	1:210	1:250	1:300	1:350	1:400	1:450	1:510	1:570	1:630	1:690	1:760	1:1500	1:2500	1:3600
34	1:110	1:140	1:170	1:210	1:250	1:290	1:330	1:370	1:420	1:470	1:520	1:570	1:630	1:1300	1:2100	1:3000
35	1:92	1:120	1:140	1:170	1:200	1:230	1:270	1:300	1:340	1:380	1:420	1:460	1:510	1:1000	1:1700	1:2400
36	1:74	1:92	1:110	1:140	1:160	1:190	1:210	1:240	1:270	1:300	1:340	1:370	1:410	1:830	1:1300	1:1900
37	1:58	1:73	1:89	1:110	1:130	1:150	1:170	1:190	1:210	1:240	1:270	1:290	1:320	1:650	1:1100	1:1500
38	1:45	1:57	1:70	1:83	1:98	1:110	1:130	1:150	1:170	1:190	1:210	1:230	1:250	1:510	1:830	1:1200
39	1:35	1:44	1:54	1:64	1:76	1:88	1:100	1:110	1:130	1:140	1:160	1:180	1:190	1:390	1:640	1:920
40	1:27	1:34	1:41	1:49	1:58	1:68	1:78	1:88	1:99	1:110	1:120	1:140	1:150	1:300	1:490	1:710
41	1:20	1:26	1:31	1:38	1:44	1:52	1:59	1:67	1:76	1:84	1:94	1:100	1:110	1:230	1:370	1:540
42	1:16	1:20	1:24	1:29	1:34	1:39	1:45	1:51	1:57	1:64	1:71	1:78	1:86	1:170	1:280	1:410
43	1:12	1:15	1:18	1:22	1:25	1:30	1:34	1:39	1:43	1:48	1:54	1:59	1:65	1:130	1:210	1:310
44	1:9	1:11	1:14	1:16	1:19	1:22	1:26	1:29	1:33	1:36	1:40	1:44	1:49	1:99	1:160	1:230
45	1:7	1:8	1:10	1:12	1:14	1:17	1:19	1:22	1:24	1:27	1:30	1:33	1:37	1:74	1:120	1:170
46	1:5	1:6	1:8	1:9	1:11	1:12	1:14	1:16	1:18	1:20	1:23	1:25	1:27	1:55	1:90	1:130
47	1:4	1:5	1:6	1:7	1:8	1:9	1:11	1:12	1:14	1:15	1:17	1:18	1:20	1:41	1:67	1:96
48	1:3	1:3	1:4	1:5	1:6	1:7	1:8	1:9	1:10	1:11	1:12	1:14	1:15	1:30	1:49	1:71
49	1:2	1:2	1:3	1:4	1:4	1:5	1:6	1:6	1:7	1:8	1:9	1:10	1:11	1:22	1:36	1:52

BPD = Biparietal diameter; EDD = expected date of delivery; MoM = multiple of normal median.
From Cuckle et al (1987a).

Table 19.23 Risk of a 35-year-old woman having a Down's syndrome term pregnancy according to selected maternal serum AFP, unconjugated oestriol (uE_3) and human chorionic gonadotrophin (hCG) levels

uE_3 (MoM)	hCG (MoM)	AFP (MoM) 0.4	1.0	2.5
0.4	0.5	1:370	1:2800	1:22000
	1.0	1:84	1:480	1:2800
	2.0	1:16	1:69	1:310
1.0	0.5	1:820	1:4800	1:28000
	1.0	1:330	1:1400	1:6400
	2.0	1:110	1:360	1:1200
1.4	0.5	1:2200	1:11000	1:52000
	1.0	1:1300	1:4600	1:17000
	2.0	1:630	1:1700	1:4700

MoM = multiple of normal median.
Derived from formulae in Wald et al (1988b).

Table 19.24 Combined maternal age and serum AFP, unconjugated oestriol and human chorionic gonadotrophin screening for Down's syndrome at 14–20 weeks' gestation; detection rate, false positive rate and odds of a Down's syndrome birth according to risk cut-off level*

Risk cut-off level	Detection rate (%)	False positive rate (%)	Average Down's syndrome risk in positives
1:100	44	1.7	1:29
1:150	52	2.8	1:42
1:200	57	3.9	1:54
1:250	61	5.0	1:65
1:300	64	6.1	1:75
1:350	67	7.2	1.85

*A woman has a positive result if the risk of Down's syndrome is equal to or greater than the risk cut-off.
Adapted from Wald et al (1988b).

risk of Down's syndrome applicable to women for whom these adjustments have been made.

When a maternal serum AFP test is repeated on a fresh sample of blood because the first result was positive (i.e. below some iso-risk) Tables 19.18 and 19.20–19.22 cannot be used to estimate the risk of Down's syndrome. If the repeat MoM value is higher than the original this would not necessarily imply that the risk is reduced. For AFP levels below about 0.7 MoM, regression to the mean ensures that most repeat tests on Down's syndrome pregnancies will be higher than the original. It is not, in general, useful to carry out repeat AFP tests when screening for Down's syndrome but if two tests are done both need to be used to estimate the woman's risk of having an affected pregnancy. A table has been produced for this purpose (Cuckle et al 1989).

Table 19.25 A basic serum screening programme for open NTD and Down's syndrome

1. A maternal serum AFP, unconjugated oestriol and hCG test is carried out at 16–18 weeks of gestation based on dates and an ultrasound BPD measurement is made. (Anencephaly should be identified at this stage.) The values are expressed in MoM, using the gestational age estimate based on BPD. If a scan has already been done the AFP tests should be carried out at 16 weeks based on BPD.
2. The result is regarded as positive if (a) the AFP level is raised, say ≥2.5 MoM*, or (b) the risk of Down's syndrome calculated from the serum levels and age is high, say ≥1:250.
3. If the result is positive an amniocentesis is performed; an amniotic fluid AFP test is carried out on women with raised serum AFP levels; a karyotype is carried out on women with a high risk of Down's syndrome.
4. An amniotic fluid AFP result is regarded as positive if it is equal to or greater than a cut-off level of 3.0 MoM, using gestational age based on the BPD estimate, but if it is 1–34 days earlier than the dates estimate use the dates estimate.
5. If the amniotic fluid AFP result is positive a gel AChE test is done.
6. An offer of a termination of pregnancy is made if the AChE result is also positive, or if the karyotype is positive.

BPD = biparietal diameter; MoM = multiple of normal median.
* It has become common practice to carry out a detailed ultrasound examination to visualize the lesion in women with raised maternal serum AFP levels. There are insufficient data to estimate the diagnostic accuracy of this compared to the use of amniotic fluid AFP and AChE tests.

Table 19.26 Expected outcome of screening for open NTD and Down's syndrome at 16–18 weeks of gestation in all pregnancies in England and Wales (say 600 000 births per year) using the scheme given in Table 19.25

	Anencephaly	Open spina bifida	Anterior abdominal wall defect	Down's syndrome	Unaffected*
Total	1080	960	150	780	597 030
Positive screening test	1080	864	110	476	46 568
Positive amniotic fluid AFP test	ND	829	74	ND	30
Positive AChE test	ND	824	56	ND	2
Positive karyotype	ND	ND	ND	476	0
Termination of pregnancy	1080	824	56	476	2

ND = Not done.
* Excludes miscarriages and closed spina bifida.
Notes
1. Birth prevalences per 1000 births are as follows: 1.8 anencephaly, 1.6 open spina bifida, 0.25 anterior abdominal wall defects and 1.3 Down's syndrome.
2. The screening tests involve maternal serum AFP and biparietal diameter measurement; the latter can be expected to detect all cases of anencephaly.
3. Open spina bifida screening detection rate is 90% and the false positive rate is 2.8% (see Table 19.6).
4. Down's syndrome screening detection rate is 61% and the false positive rate is 5.0% (see Table 19.24). Nearly all the false positives will be additional to those for open spina bifida screening.
5. Anterior abdominal wall defect screening detection rate is 73% (Wald et al 1980b).
6. Open spina bifida amniotic fluid AFP detection and false positive rates are 96% and 0.18% (see Table 19.12) and the anterior abdominal wall defect detection rate is 67% (Wald et al 1980b).
7. In women with positive amniotic fluid AFP tests the gel AChE open spina bifida detection rate is 99.4% and the false positive rate is 6% (see Table 19.15).

As with AFP screening for NTDs, it may be necessary to use different cut-off levels for twins, insulin-dependent diabetics and blacks. Since the distribution of AFP in pregnancies such as those which are affected by fetal Down's syndrome is unknown, iso-risk cut-offs cannot be calculated. However to ensure that the false positive rate is similar to that in the general population the maternal age-specific AFP cut-off level equivalent to an iso-risk in a singleton pregnancy in a white non-diabetic should be doubled for twins, reduced by one-third for insulin-dependent diabetics and increased by 15% for blacks.

RECENT DEVELOPMENTS

Maternal serum unconjugated oestriol (uE_3) (Canick et al 1988, Wald et al 1988a) and human chorionic gonadotrophin (hCG) (Bogart et al 1987, Wald et al 1988b), as well as AFP, are effective markers of Down's syndrome. As with AFP, uE_3 and hCG levels can be expressed in MoMs to take account of changes in their concentrations with gestational age; uE_3 increases and hCG decreases with gestational age in the second trimester. On average, uE_3 levels are about 25% lower in affected pregnancies than in unaffected pregnancies and hCG levels are about double. The best way to screen for Down's syndrome using maternal age and the three serum markers is, as with age and AFP alone, to estimate an individual's risk of having an affected pregnancy from all four variables, taking appropriate account of the correlations that exist between them (Wald et al 1988b). Table 19.23 shows how the risk for a 35-year-old woman varies according to the serum levels. Table 19.24 shows the detection rate and false positive rate associated with different risk cut-off levels. For example, using a 1:250 cut-off, the detection rate is 61% and false positive rate 5.0%; both compare favourably with the rates of 35% and 5.2% respectively using a 1:300 cut-off for age and AFP alone (Table 19.19).

With the introduction of serum screening some women formerly thought to be at high risk on account of their age will, because their serum AFP or uE_3 level is relatively high or their serum hCG level relatively low, now be classified as being at low risk and may therefore choose not to have amniocentesis. Other women previously thought to be at low risk on account of their youth will now be classified as being at high risk on account of their low AFP or uE_3 levels or high hCG level. This reassignment of women and the improved effectiveness of screening that it confers will need to be supported by adequate education.

The serum screening results may in future be improved further by the addition of information derived from ultrasound fetal biometry. One measure is likely to be of value, namely femur length, which is shorter in Down's syndrome fetuses than in unaffected fetuses (Benacerraf 1987, Lockwood et al 1987) as may be expected in view of the fact that infants with Down's syndrome are short.

CONCLUSIONS

A simplified summary of a basic maternal serum and maternal age screening programme for open NTD and Down's syndrome is summarized in Table 19.25. Although there are acceptable deviations, the basic scheme is common to all satisfactory AFP screening programmes for NTD and the recent extension to Down's syndrome screening is being adopted in several centres. Table 19.26 indicates the expected results of screening all pregnancies in England and Wales using this scheme. If every woman was offered and accepted screening, an estimated total of 2436 affected and 2 unaffected pregnancies would be terminated—all 1080 anencephalic pregnancies, 86% of pregnancies with open spina bifida (824), more than one-third of pregnancies with anterior abdominal wall defects (56) and more than half of thosewith Down's syndrome (476). No other single method of antenatal screening can avoid as much severe physical and mental handicap.

Acknowledgements

We thank Glenn Palomaki for help in producing the figures showing the distributions of AFP and Kiran Nanchahal for her computer programming assistance.

REFERENCES

Aitken D A, Morrison N M, Ferguson-Smith M A 1984 Predictive value of amniotic acetylcholinesterase analysis in the diagnosis of fetal abnormality in 3700 pregnancies. Prenatal Diagnosis 4: 329–340
Althouse R, Wald N J 1980 Survival and handicap in infants with spina bifida. Archives of Disease in Childhood 55: 845–850
Baird P A, Sadovnick A D 1987 Life expectancy in Down syndrome. Journal of Pediatrics 110: 849–854
Barlow R D, Cuckle H S, Wald N J, Rodeck C H 1982a False positive gel-acetylcholinesterase results in blood-stained amniotic fluids. British Journal of Obstetrics and Gynaecology 89: 821–826
Barlow R D, Wald N J, Cuckle H S 1982b A simple method for amniotic fluid acetylcholinesterase determination suitable for routine use in the antenatal diagnosis of open neural-tube defects. Clinica Chimica Acta 119: 137–142
Barlow R D, Cuckle H S, Wald N J 1984 The identification of false-positive amniotic fluid acetylcholinesterase results due to fetal calf serum contamination. British Journal of Obstetrics and Gynaecology 91: 986–988
Benacerraf B R, Gelman R, Frigoletto F D 1987 Sonographic identification of second-trimester fetuses with Down's syndrome. New England Journal of Medicine 317: 1371–1376
Bogart M H, Pandian M R, Jones C W 1987 Abnormal maternal serum chorionic gonadotropin levels in pregnancies with fetal chromosome abnormalities. Prenatal Diagnosis 7: 623–630
Boyd P A, Keeling J W 1986 Raised maternal serum alpha-fetoprotein in the absence of fetal abnormality—placental findings. A quantitative morphometric study. Prenatal Diagnosis 6: 369–373
Brock D J H, Barron L, Jelen P, Watt M, Scrimgeour J B 1977 Maternal serum alpha-fetoprotein measurements as an early indicator of low birthweight. Lancet ii: 267–268
Brock D J H, Barlow R D, Wald N J et al 1982 Fetal calf serum as cause of false positive amniotic fluid acetylcholinesterase gel tests. Lancet ii: 1044
Brock D J H, Barron L, van Heyningen V 1985 Prenatal diagnosis of neural-tube defects with a monoclonal antibody specific for acetylcholinesterase. Lancet i: 5–7
Burton B K 1986 Positive amniotic fluid acetylcholinesterase: distinguishing between open spina bifida and ventral wall defects. American Journal of Obstetrics and Gynecology 155: 984–986
Canadian Medical Research Council 1977 Diagnosis of genetic disease by amniocentesis during the second trimester of pregnancy. A Canadian study. Report no 5. Supply Services, Ottawa
Canick J A, Knight G J, Palomaki G E, Haddow J E, Cuckle H S, Wald N J 1988 Low second trimester maternal serum unconjugated oestriol in pregnancies with Down's syndrome. British Journal of Obstetrics and Gynaecology 95: 330–333
Collaborative Acetylcholinesterase Study Report 1981 Amniotic fluid acetylcholinesterase electrophoresis as a secondary test in the diagnosis of anencephaly and open spina bifida in early pregnancy. Lancet ii: 321–324
Creasy M R, Crolla J A 1974 Prenatal mortality of trisomy 21 (Down's syndrome) Lancet i: 473–474
Cuckle H S, Wald N J 1987a The impact of screening for open neural tube defects in England and Wales. Prenatal Diagnosis 7: 91–99
Cuckle H S, Wald N J 1987b The effect of estimating gestational age by ultrasound cephalometry on the sensitivity of alpha-fetoprotein screening for Down's syndrome. British Journal of Obstetrics and Gynaecology 94: 274–276
Cuckle H S, Wald N J, Lindenbaum R H 1986 Cord serum alpha-fetoprotein and Down's syndrome. British Journal of Obstetrics and Gynaecology 93: 408–410
Cuckle H, Wald N J, Thompson S G 1987a Estimating a woman's risk of having a pregnancy associated with Down's syndrome using her age and maternal serum alpha-fetroprotein level. British Journal of Obstetrics and Gynaecology 94: 387–402
Cuckle H S, Nanchahal K, Wald N J 1987b Maternal serum alpha-fetoprotein and ethnic origin. British Journal of Obstetrics and Gynaecology 94: 1111–1112
Cuckle H S, Wald N J, Barkai G et al 1988 First trimester biochemical screening for Down's syndrome. Lancet ii: 851–852
Cuckle H S, Wald N J, Nanchahal K, Densem J W 1989 Repeat maternal serum testing in antenatal screening programmes for Down syndrome. British Journal of Obstetrics and Gynaecology 96: 52–60
Dalton A J 1982 A prospective study of Alzheimer's disease in Down's syndrome. Cited in: Pueschel S M 1982 Health concerns in persons with Down syndrome. In: Pueschel S M, Tingey C, Rynders J E, Crocker A C, Crutcher D M (eds) New perspectives on Down syndrome. Brookes, Baltimore, pp 113–133
Gill M, Murday V, Slack J 1987 An economic appraisal of screening for Down's syndrome in pregnancy using maternal age and serum alpha fetoprotein concentration. Society of Science and Medicine 24: 725–731
Glenner G G, Wong W C 1984 Alzheimer's disease and Down's syndrome: sharing of a unique cerebrovascular amyloid fibril protein. Biochemical Biophysical Research Communication 122: 1131–1135
Goldfine C, Miller W A, Haddow J E 1983 Amniotic fluid gel cholinesterase density ratios in fetal open defects of the neural tube and ventral wall. British Journal of Obstetrics and Gynaecology 90: 238–240
Goldgaber D, Lerman M I, McBride O W, Saffiotti U, Gajdusek D C 1987 Characterisation and chromosomal localisation of a cDNA encoding brain amyloid of Alzheimer's diseases. Science 235: 877–880
Gosden C M, Brock D J H 1977 Morphology of rapidly adhering amniotic-fluid cells as an aid to the diagnosis of neural-tube defects. Lancet i: 919–922
Greenberg F, James L J, Oakley G P 1983 Estimates of birth prevalence rates of spina bifida in the United States from computer-generated maps. American Journal of Obstetrics and Gynaecology 145: 570–573
Haddow J E, Kloza E M, Knight G J, Smith D E 1981 Relationship between maternal weight and serum alpha-fetoprotein concentration during the second trimester. Clinical Chemistry 27: 133–134
Haddow J E, Smith D E, Sever J 1982 Effect of maternal weight on maternal serum alpha-fetoprotein. British Journal of Obstetrics and Gynaecology 89: 93
Haddow J E, Knight G J, Kloza E M, Palomaki G E 1986 Alpha-

fetoprotein, vaginal bleeding and pregnancy risk. British Journal of Obstetrics and Gynaecology 93: 589–593
Hay D L, Barrie J V, Davison G B et al 1979 The relationship between maternal serum alpha-fetoprotein levels and fetomaternal haemorrhage. British Journal of Obstetrics and Gynaecology 86: 516–520
Knott P D, Penketh R J A, Lucas M K 1986 Uptake of amniocentesis in women aged 38 years or more by the time of the expected date of delivery: a two-year retrospective study. British Journal of Obstetrics and Gynaecology 93: 1246–1250
Kolata G 1985 Down syndrome — Alzheimer's linked. Science 230: 1152–1153
Lockwood C, Benacerraf B R E, Krinsky A et al 1987 A sonographic screening method for Down syndrome. American Journal of Obstetrics and Gynecology 157: 803–808
Los F J, de Wolf B T H M, Huisjes H J 1979 Raised maternal serum-alpha-fetoprotein levels and spontaneous fetomaternal transfusion. Lancet ii: 1210–1212
Masaki M, Higurashi M, Iijim K et al 1981 Mortality and survival for Down syndrome in Japan. American Journal of Human Genetics 33: 629–639
Masters C L, Simms G, Weinman N A, Multhaup G, McDonald B L, Beyreuther K 1985 Amyloid plaque core protein in Alzheimer's disease. Proceedings of the National Academy of Science USA 82: 4245–4249
Medical Research Council Working Party on Amniocentesis Report 1978 An assessment of the hazards of amniocentesis. British Journal of Obstetrics and Gynaecology 85 (suppl 2)
Milunsky A, Alpert E, Kitzmiller J L, Younger M D, Neff R K 1982 Prenatal diagnosis of neural tube defects. VIII The importance of serum alpha-fetoprotein screening in diabetic pregnant women. American Journal of Obstetrics and Gynaecology 142: 1030–1032
National Institute for Child Health and Development 1976 National registry for amniocentesis study group. Mid-trimester amniocentesis for prenatal diagnosis. Safety and accuracy. Journal of the American Medical Association 236: 1471–1476
Nørgaard-Pedersen B, Hangaard J, Bjerrum O J 1983 Quantitative enzyme antigen immunoassay of acetylcholinesterase in amniotic fluid. Clinical Chemistry 29: 1061–1064
Øster J, Mikkelsen M, Nielsen A 1975. Mortality and life-table in Down's syndrome. Acta Paediatrica Scandinavica 64: 322–326
Peat D, Brock D J H 1984 Quantitative estimation of the density ratios of cholinesterase bands in human amniotic fluids. Clinica Chimica Acta 138: 319–324
Rasmussen A G, Sorensen K, Selmer J et al 1987 Immunochemical determination of acetylcholinesterase in amniotic fluid — an evaluation of 11 monoclonal antibodies. Clinica Chimica Acta 166: 17–25
Read A P, Fennell S J, Donnai D 1982 Amniotic fluid acetylcholinesterase: a retrospective and prospective study of the qualitative method. British Journal of Obstetrics and Gynaecology 89: 111–116
Roberts A, Campbell S 1980 Small biparietal diameter of fetus with spina bifida. British Journal of Obstetrics and Gynaecology 87: 927–928
Ryynänen M, Seppälä M, Kuusela P et al 1983 Antenatal screening for congenital nephrosis in Finland by maternal serum alpha-fetoprotein. British Journal of Obstetrics and Gynaecology 90: 437–442
Smith C J, Kelleher P C, Belanger L, Dallaire L 1979 Reactivity of amniotic fluid alpha-fetoprotein with concanavalin A in diagnosis of neural tube defects. British Medical Journal i: 920–921
Stirrat G M, Gough J D, Bullock S, Wald N, Cuckle H 1981 Raised maternal serum AFP, oligohydramnios and poor fetal outcome. British Journal of Obstetrics and Gynaecology 88: 231–235
Tabor A, Medsen M, Obel E B et al 1986 Randomised controlled trial of genetic amniocentesis in 4606 low-risk women. Lancet i: 1287–1293
Tabor A, Philip J, Bang J, Madsen M, Obel E B, Norgaard-Pedersen B 1988 Needle size and risk of miscarriage after amniocentesis. Lancet i: 183–184
UK Collaborative Study on Alpha-Fetoprotein in Relation to Neural Tube Defects 1977 Report Maternal serum alpha-fetoprotein measurement in antenatal screening for anencephaly and spina bifida in early pregnancy. Lancet i: 1323–1332
UK Collaborative Study on Alpha-Fetoprotein in Relation to Neural Tube Defects Second Report 1979 Amniotic-fluid alpha-fetoprotein measurement in antenatal diagnosis of anencephaly and open spina bifida in early pregnancy. Lancet ii: 651–662
UK Collaborative Study on Alpha-Fetoprotein in Relation to Neural Tube Defects 1982 Fourth Report Estimating an individual's risk of having a fetus with open spina bifida and the value of repeat alphafetoprotein testing. Journal of Epidemiology and Community Health 36: 87–95
Wald N J, Cuckle H S 1981 Raised maternal serum alpha-fetoprotein levels in subsequent pregnancies. Lancet i: 1103
Wald N J, Cuckle H S 1982 Nomogram for estimating an individual's risk of having a fetus with open spina bifida. British Journal of Obstetrics and Gynaecology 89: 598–602
Wald N J, Cuckle H S, 1984a Open neural tube defects. In: Wald N J (ed) Antenatal and neonatal screening for disease. Oxford University Press, Oxford, pp 25–73
Wald N J, Cuckle H S 1984b Neural-tube defects: screening for biochemical diagnosis. In: Rodeck C H, Nicolaides K H (eds) Prenatal diagnosis. Proceedings of the 11th Study Group of the Royal College of Obstetrics and Gynaecology. RCOG, London, pp 214–219
Wald N J, Cuckle H S 1987 Recent advances in screening for neural tube defects and Down syndrome. In: Rodeck C (ed) Prenatal diagnosis. Baillière Tindall, London, pp 649–676
Wald N J, Barker S, Cuckle H, Brock D J H, Stirrat G M 1977a Maternal serum AFP and spontaneous abortion. British Journal of Obstetrics and Gynaecology 84: 357–362
Wald N J, Cuckle H S, Stirrat G M, Bennett M J, Turnbull A C 1977b Maternal serum alpha-fetoprotein and low birth-weight. Lancet ii: 268–270
Wald N J, Cuckle H S, Peck S, Stirrat G M, Turnbull A C 1979a Maternal serum alpha-fetoprotein in relation to zygosity. British Medical Journal 1: 455
Wald N J, Cuckle H, Boreham J, Stirrat G M, Turnbull A C 1979b Maternal serum alpha-fetoprotein and diabetes mellitus. British Journal of Obstetrics and Gynaecology 86: 101–105
Wald N, Cuckle H S, Boreham J, Stirrat G 1980a Small biparietal diameter of fetuses with spina bifida: implications for antenatal diagnosis. British Journal of Obstetrics and Gynaecology 87: 219–221
Wald N, Cuckle H, Barlow R et al 1980b Early antenatal diagnosis of exomphalos. Lancet i: 1368–1369
Wald N, Cuckle H, Boreham J, Terzian E, Redman C 1981 The effect of maternal weight on maternal serum alpha-fetoprotein levels. British Journal of Obstetrics and Gynaecology 88: 1094–1096
Wald N J, Cuckle H S, Boreham J, Turnbull A C 1982 Effect of estimating gestational age by ultrasound cephalometry on the specificity of alpha-fetoprotein screening for open neural tube defects. British Journal of Obstetrics and Gynaecology 89: 1050–1053
Wald N J, Terzian E, Vickers P A, Weatherall J A C 1983 Congenital talipes and hip malformation in relation to amniocentesis: a case control study. Lancet ii: 246–249
Wald N J, Cuckle H S, Boreham J 1984a Alpha-fetoprotein screening for open spina bifida: effect of routine biparietal diameter measurement to estimate gestational age. Revue d'Epidemiologie et de Santé Publique 32: 62–69
Wald N J, Barlow R D, Cuckle H, Turnbull A C, Goldfind C, Haddow J E 1984b Ratio of amniotic fluid acetylcholinesterase to pseudocholinesterase as an antenatal diagnostic test for exomphalos and gastroschisis. British Journal of Obstetrics and Gynaecology 91: 882–884
Wald N J, Cuckle H S, Densem J W et al 1988a Maternal serum unconjugated oestriol as an antenatal screening test for Down's syndrome. British Journal of Obstetrics and Gynaecology 95: 334–341
Wald N J, Cuckle H S, Densem J W et al 1988b Maternal serum screening for Down syndrome in early pregnancy. British Medical Journal 297: 883–887
Wyvill P C, Hullin D A, Elder G H, Laurence K M 1984 A prospective study of amniotic fluid cholinesterases: comparison of quantitative and qualitative methods for the detection of open neural tube defects. Prenatal Diagnosis 4: 319–327

20

J. Malcolm Pearce

The biophysical diagnosis of fetal abnormalities

INTRODUCTION

Since Professor Ian Donald introduced ultrasound into obstetrics in the late 1950s vast improvements have been made in electronics so that equipment is now cheaper and easy to use. This together with the fact that examinations may be repeated and are apparently without hazard (Royal College of Obstetricians and Gynaecologists 1984) has revolutionized obstetrics. Confirmation or determination of gestational age, monitoring of fetal growth (see Chapter 9) and the assessment of the biophysical aspects of fetal well-being (see Chapter 26) are well known examples of the use of ultrasound antenatally.

Antenatal diagnosis of many fetal structural abnormalities is possible only by ultrasound and its availability in the last decade has allowed many women to continue through pregnancy knowing that their fetus would not be handicapped by the same abnormality as a previous baby. The use of ultrasound to complement amniocentesis, chorion villus sampling, fetoscopy and direct umbilical cord needling is discussed in Chapter 23. This chapter will consider ultrasound in its unique role as both a screening and a diagnostic test for fetal abnormalities.

GENERAL PRINCIPLES OF DIAGNOSIS AND MANAGEMENT

The images displayed on the television monitor of an ultrasound machine are essentially computer reconstructions based on echoes reflected from tissue junctions and discontinuities within tissues. They are two-dimensional pictures and the skill of the ultrasound operator comes from interpreting these in a three-dimensional fashion and from avoiding incorrect interpretations due to artefacts. Unlike conventional X-rays or computer tomography, ultrasound produces many artefactual appearances to trap the novice operator.

The diagnosis of fetal abnormalities is made in one of three ways (Campbell & Pearce 1984):

1. By direct visualization of a structural defect, for example the absence of the fetal skull vault in anencephaly.
2. By demonstrating disproportionate size or growth of a particular fetal part, for example, the short limbs in cases of dwarfism.
3. By recognition of the effect of an anomaly on an adjacent structure, for example the presence of posterior urethral valves which may be diagnosed by the consequent dilatation of the renal tract.

The widespread use of ultrasound to confirm gestational age and for the early diagnosis of multiple pregnancy has led to the diagnoses of many abnormalities being made in the first half of pregnancy. In this respect ultrasound examination performed in the routine setting by ultrasonographers, doctors or midwives is best seen as a screening test. If an abnormality is suspected at this examination facilities should be available for an early referral to an operator who is able to make a definitive diagnosis. As fetal abnormalities are often multiple the entire fetus should be examined carefully by ultrasound and if the diagnosed abnormality is known to be associated with chromosome anomalies then karyotyping either by amniocentesis or directly from leukocytes in the fetal blood (see Chapter 23) should also be offered. It therefore behoves the doctor carrying out diagnostic ultrasound examinations to be fully aware of the associations of individual abnormalities and to keep abreast of the management of such conditions.

Having arrived at a definitive diagnosis there are then three options open to the parents:

1. The pregnancy may be terminated. At the present time the law in England, Wales and Scotland allows termination of pregnancy up to 28 weeks' gestation although

this may be reduced to 24 weeks in the near future. If, following discussion of the prognosis the parents opt for termination, facilities must be available to allow this to be carried out right up to 28 weeks' gestation. Diagnosis of fetal abnormalities made late in pregnancy often creates a much more emotionally charged situation. If the abnormality will lead to death in utero or shortly after delivery, most obstetricians will opt to let nature take its course. This, however, seems to be unacceptable to many patients who, having been told the situation, will often request that the pregnancy is ended as soon as possible. A sympathetic approach to early induction of labour should be adopted but this must be balanced against the risk to the mother and to future pregnancies.

2. The pregnancy may be allowed to continue with continuing ultrasound surveillance. Many abnormalities do not carry a threat to the life of the fetus and usually do not deteriorate in utero. An example of this is pelviureteric junction obstruction. In such cases continued monitoring with appropriate measurements will determine if the condition is worsening. If deterioration does occur then the options are usually premature delivery or possibly in utero surgery. Again a balanced judgement should be made, assisted by the free use of amniocentesis to determine the lecithin : sphingomyelin ratio and to assay for phosphatidylglycerol to help in management. In general the obstetrician and his paediatric colleagues should lean towards early delivery with subsequent appropriate management rather than attempting intervention in utero.
3. Prenatal therapy or surgery. This is only available at present for a few conditions and should only be carried out by people who are expert at intrauterine manipulation. Where such manoeuvres are available, they are discussed under the specific diagnosis.

The decision as to which line of management to adopt is difficult and should be made by a multidisciplinary team. The parents should obviously be involved to the extent of their understanding but the timing of delivery and discussion of the long-term treatment and prognosis should be done in conjunction with a neonatologist and a paediatric surgeon, if appropriate. Furthermore although most obstetricians involved in prenatal diagnosis by ultrasound become amateur geneticists by necessity, it is important to refer the patient after the pregnancy for formal genetic counselling.

Terminating pregnancies complicated by fetal abnormalities is best performed by extra-amniotic prostaglandin infusion as dilatation and evacuation or intra-amniotic instillations renders the tissue unsuitable for diagnosis. Consent should be sought for a post-mortem examination; although consent is only legally required if the fetus is more than 28 weeks' gestation, it must be remembered that the parents will still consider this fetus as a baby. The parents should also be given a chance to see and hold the baby after it has been suitably clothed. A consent form of the type shown in Figure 20.1 should also be provided for parents who wish to bury or cremate their baby. In addition, whether consent is given for post-mortem or not the following investigations should be carried out before the fetus is put in formalin:

St George's Hospital
Medical School

UNIVERSITY OF LONDON

Patron: Her Majesty the Queen

DEPARTMENT OF OBSTETRICS
AND GYNAECOLOGY

CRANMER TERRACE
LONDON SW17 0RE

Tel: 01-672 1255 Ext. 4175
Telex: 945291 SAGEMS G

Professor G. V. P. Chamberlain
Mr. J. M. Pearce
Dr. T. R. Varma
Dr. C. Wilson
Mr. A. G. Amias
Mr. S. L. Stanton
Mrs. U. Lloyd

To: A local undertaker

Dear Sir

Re: The baby of Mr & Mrs Smith

This is to confirm that I was present at the birth of baby Smith who was born before 28 weeks gestation without signs of life. I should be grateful if you would give the parents your assistance in burying/cremating their baby.

Yours faithfully

Fig. 20.1 A specimen consent form to allow burial or cremation of a fetus born before 28 weeks' gestation without signs of life.

1. Blood should be obtained by direct cardiac puncture for karyotyping.
2. The fetus should be X-rayed.
3. The baby should be photographed. This should be done by the hospital photographer and should include a full facial view, a view of the whole body and of any obvious abnormalities. A copy of a photograph of the whole baby should be offered to the parents and if refused should be carefully filed in case they later change their minds. These photographs should be available for the geneticist. If a Polaroid camera is used do not stand closer than the 1 m minimum focusing distance.
4. The placenta should be sent in formalin for histology.

Ideally the post-mortem should be carried out by a trained perinatal pathologist and if intracranial abnormalities are suspected the brain should be fixed by perfusion before it is cut.

ULTRASOUND AS A SCREENING TEST

Ultrasound in the first half of pregnancy has been shown to be superior to bimanual pelvic examination in early pregnancy (Campbell 1974) and to X-rays for maturity in later pregnancy (Robinson et al 1979) in the assessment of gestational age in patients with unknown dates. Controversy still exists as to whether ultrasound examination in the first half

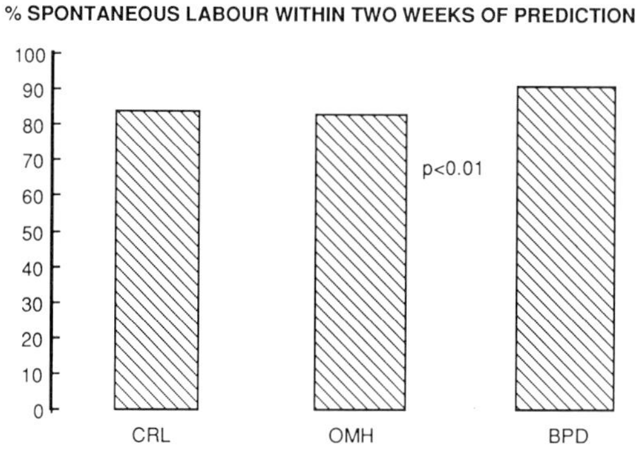

Fig. 20.2 A comparison of ultrasound parameters with optimal menstrual history in predicting the date of delivery of a mature fetus. CRL = Crown–rump length; OMH = optimal menstrual history; BPD = biparietal diameter.

Table 20.1 Prenatal diagnosis made at the time of routine early ultrasound (from Campbell & Pearce 1984)

Detected	Missed
6 Anencephaly	
6 Spina bifida	
5 Hydrocephaly	
1 Microcephaly	1 Microcephaly
1 Encephalocele	
1 Holoprosencephaly	
2 Omphaloceles	
1 Duodenal atresia	
1 Obstructive uropathy	
1 Renal agenesis	1 Renal agenesis
4 Fetal tumour	1 Single atrium
	1 Pulmonary atresia
	1 Hypertrophic cardiomyopathy

$n = 11\,664$.

of pregnancy should be reserved for those patients in whom there is doubt about the validity of their last menstrual period or whether it should be a matter of routine. Evidence from a study based on historical controls (Grennert et al 1978) and from a prospective non-randomized study (Warsof et al 1983) is in favour of routine ultrasound. The three prospective randomized studies reported in the literature (Bennett et al 1982, Bakketeig et al 1984, Eik-Nes et al 1984) tend to support the concept that ultrasound measurements are more accurate at predicting the date of delivery and hence reduce the number of patients who exceed 42 weeks' gestation. Only one study, however (Eik-Nes et al 1984), shows a benefit from this. This is to be expected, as it would need a very large study to demonstrate the significance of reducing the number of people who exceed 42 weeks' gestation from 12 to 6%. What is certain, however, is that the use of ultrasound reduces the number of babies who are born unexpectedly premature after induction of labour (Chapman et al 1979). Apart from establishing gestational age, routine ultrasound examination in early pregnancy is very accurate at diagnosing multiple gestations (Grennert et al 1978, Persson et al 1978, Warsof et al 1983) and in localizing the placenta. Placental localization is worthwhile at this time as over 95% of the population will have a fundal placenta which will not become a placenta praevia.

With the widespread use of ultrasound, pregnant women and their attendants are coming to expect to deliver babies free from any structural abnormalities. With increasing litigation against health care practitioners it is important to realize what can reasonably be expected from the average ultrasonographer in the exclusion of abnormalities.

Timing of the first ultrasound examination

Many ultrasound departments have now recognized the value of scanning the patient at 16–18 weeks' gestation (Warsof et al 1983). Practitioners of ultrasound know that examining the anatomy of the fetus is a great deal easier at 18 weeks' than at 16 weeks' gestation. Figure 20.2 demonstrates that in predicting the date of delivery routine ultrasound is superior to optimal menstrual dates up to about 22 weeks' gestation. Since most obstetricians will not be more than 4 weeks out in estimating gestation age in the first half of pregnancy, ultrasound planned at 18 weeks' gestation is unlikely to be performed at more than 22 weeks.

If ultrasound examinations are performed in the first trimester and crown–rump length is measured, there is little hope of diagnosing major structural abnormalities with the possible exception of anencephaly.

What abnormalities may be diagnosed at the time of routine ultrasound?

Table 20.1 illustrates the diagnosis made at King's College Hospital from routine early ultrasound (Campbell & Pearce 1984). It is important to realize that although the majority of the examinations were carried out by ultrasonographers, they worked in a department where referral for the diganosis of fetal abnormalities was common and so were exposed to ultrasonically diagnosed anomalies much more frequently than the average ultrasonographer. If the ultrasound examinations for 3000 patients are carried out by two or three ultrasonographers, each can only expect to see three or four abnormalities a year. Since many of the abnormalities are subtle they may be overlooked.

Despite this it is reasonable to expect all ultrasonographers to diagnose such gross conditions as anencephaly and not to miss masses attached to the fetus such as cystic hydromata or omphaloceles. Cystic dilatation or masses within the fetal abdomen or chest are usually easily detectable and after a few months of training all ultrasonographers should be able to spot reduced amniotic fluid volume in the first half of pregnancy. Oligohydramnios at this stage has an extremely poor outcome and should encourage the ultrasonographer to look in detail for associated abnormalities or to refer the patient to an appropriate centre.

Table 20.2 A specimen checklist for use at routine ultrasound examination in early pregnancy

Anatomy	Measurement
Number of fetuses	
Beating fetal heart	
Fetal head	Biparietal diameter
Intact cerebral vault	
Normal shape	
Normal ventricles	VH ratio
Normal cerebellum	
Normal spine	
Longitudinal view	
Transverse view of each vertebra	
Normal chest, appearance	
Four-chamber view of heart	
Intact abdominal wall	
Single stomach bubble	
Normal kidneys	
Normal bladder	
Limbs	Femur length
Amniotic fluid volume (subjective impression)	
Placental site	
Three vessels in cord	

VH = ventricular hemisphere

In order to achieve such diagnosis a mental checklist is necessary for every ultrasound examination. Even a routine examination to confirm gestational age which lasts for only 10–15 minutes should involve the ultrasonographer following a checklist similar to that given in Table 20.2.

The question of what measurements should be made at routine examination is debatable. Most would believe that the minimum should be measurement of the biparietal diameter and of the fetal femur length. If both of these agree with the postmenstrual age derived from the first day of the last menstrual period no further measurements are necessary. If the measurements differ from the menstrual dates and more particularly, if the measurements differ from each other then it is necessary to measure the fetal head circumference and abdominal circumference (or area). A value judgement should be made on these measurements and the fetal gestational age confirmed or altered as appropriate. If there is a discrepancy between the measurements of the femur and the fetal head then the possibility of microcephaly, spina bifida or dwarfism should be considered. Despite the fact that 80% of babies with spina bifida have large cerebral ventricles at 18 weeks' gestation, the fetal head is often reduced in size (Roberts & Campbell 1980, Wald et al 1980) and therefore a small fetal head compared with other measurements should lead to a detailed examination of the fetal spine.

Should screening for neural tube defects (NTD) be by serum alpha-fetoprotein or ultrasound?

This is a question which at present cannot clearly be answered. It depends largely upon the following factors:

The prevalence of NTD

If the upper confidence limit on maternal serum alpha-fetoprotein (MSAFP) is set at 2.5 times the multiple of the median (2.5 MoM) as recommended by the UK Collaborative Study (1977) then approximately 2% of all pregnant women screened will be positive. If the prevalence of NTD is 5 per 1000 then for every 5000 deliveries 100 women will require further investigations in order to detect 25 NTD. This is obviously an extremely good balance particularly if the further investigation is detailed ultrasound, rather than amniocentesis. If, however, the incidence of NTD is only 1 per 1000, then only 5 of the 100 positive-screened women will have an abnormality and the test becomes less acceptable.

It is not surprising therefore that many areas where there is a low prevalence of NTD have stopped screening by MSAFP (Standing et al 1981). The arguments for not screening by MSAFP are further strengthened if the diagnostic test is amniocentesis, which probably carries at least 1 in 200 risk of miscarrying a normal pregnancy (see Chapter 23).

The incidence of NTD is falling (Owens et al 1981) and in future screening for all by means of ultrasound will probably be routine.

The quality of the local ultrasound

Many hospitals have now opted to spend valuable resources on ultrasound machinery and technicians rather than on screening by MSAFP. If routine ultrasound for establishing gestational age is delayed until 18 weeks' gestation then it is not unreasonable to expect to diagnose all anencephaly and at least 80% of cases of spina bifida at that time. Although the diagnosis of spina bifida by ultrasound requires a degree of skill, at least 80% of all such babies will have enlarged cerebral ventricles at the 18 weeks' ultrasound and this is much more readily recognizable and diagnosed by direct measurements. This compares favourably with the direct diagnosis of spina bifida by ultrasound (UK Collaborative Report 1977).

Ideally all patients should be screened by means of a routine ultrasound at approximately 18 weeks' gestation and also by MSAFP. The interpretation of MSAFP should be made on the gestational age estimated from the ultrasound examination (Fig. 20.3). A combination of the two tests should be expected to detect more than 90% of all NTD with no concomitant increase in the false positive rate.

What to tell the patient thought to be carrying an abnormal fetus at the time of routine ultrasound

As a general rule ultrasound scanning is a joyous occasion for the parents and if the operator takes time to point out the baby on the screen it can improve the woman's compliance with antenatal advice (Cambell et al 1982). Thought-

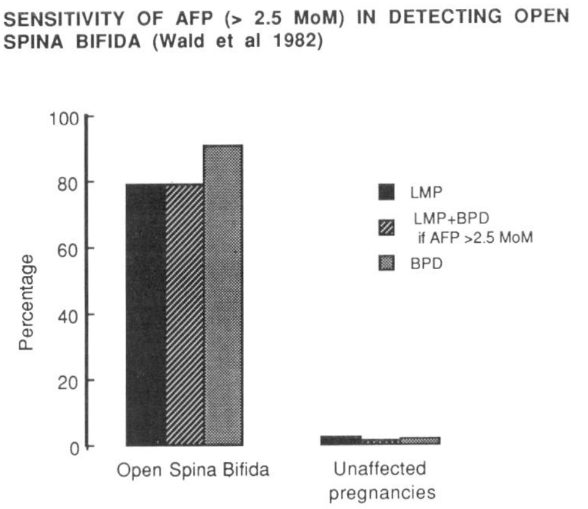

Fig. 20.3 The effect of ultrasound estimation of gestation on the specificity of alpha-fetoprotein screening. AFP = alpha-fetoprotein; BPD = biparietal diameter; LMP = last menstrual period.

less comments or reports, or unnecessary recall for further examination may however create anxiety and stress. This is more so when an anomaly is suspected.

If the operator is confident of the diagnosis then the parents should probably be told but without embarking on management discussions (Lind 1986). Early referral to the obstetrician is essential. The situation is more complex when an abnormality is only suspected. Patients are extremely sensitive to a variation in routine (Furness 1987) and will commonly ask: 'Is my baby normal?' The choice of approach lies between the following:

1. Telling the truth. This involves telling the patient what is suspected and arranging a definitive scan, preferably immediately or certainly within 48 hours. This approach is extremely helpful to the person performing the second scan as the patient will have recovered from the initial shock of a possible abnormality and be more capable of comprehending the options offered once the diagnosis is established.
2. Telling the patient that a particular measurement cannot be obtained because of fetal position or that the placenta cannot be accurately localized. This approach may provoke less anxiety.

The referring obstetrician must retain the prerogative of deciding which lines of management to discuss with the patient, and each hospital should have its own policy on what to tell patients. Probably the best situation occurs when one obstetrician performs the definitive scan and, with the prior agreement of all the other referring obstetricians, performs the necessary counselling.

DIAGNOSTIC ULTRASOUND EXAMINATION FOR FETAL ABNORMALITIES

Table 20.3 indicates patients who should be offered detailed untrasound examination. Although this examination has

Table 20.3 Reasons for referral for detailed ultrasound examination (from Chudleigh & Pearce 1986)

Raised maternal serum alpha-fetoprotein
Patients undergoing amniocentesis
Patients with a personal or family history of a structural anomaly
Patients with a personal or family history of a chromosome anomaly that has a structural marker
Oligohydramnios
Polyhydramnios
Maternal diabetes mellitus
Patients in preterm labour, especially with a breech presentation
Multiple gestation
Patients exposed to teratogens in early pregnancy
Patients with suspicious findings on ultrasound
Patients with symmetrically small fetuses

often been called high-resolution ultrasound, most modern ultrasound equipment is capable of producing the images necessary to make the diagnosis. The diagnosis is extremely operator-dependent and in good centres accurate diagnosis can be made in 99% of cases with a false negative rate of under 1% (Campbell & Pearce 1984).

Diagnosis of structural fetal abnormalities comes from a sound knowledge of normal fetal anatomy which can only be gained with experience. As the fetus has a limited way in which it can express abnormalities, once it is recognized that the anatomy is abnormal the differential diagnosis is not too difficult. Well over 50% of fetal abnormalities are craniospinal.

THE DIAGNOSIS OF SPECIFIC ABNORMALITIES

Craniospinal abnormalities

Figure 20.4 is an ultrasound picture of a transverse section of a fetal head on which the biparietal diameter is usually measured. Figure 20.5 is a pathological section taken at the same level and demonstrates how well the ultrasound image echoes the intracranial anatomy. The main reasons for referral for detailed examination to exclude craniospinal abnormalities are a raised maternal alpha-fetoprotein, previous history of an affected infant or, more recently, because of abnormality suspected at the time of routine ultrasound examination.

Figure 20.6 illustrates an anencephalic fetus; this is an easy diagnosis to make with ultrasound if due care is taken. The main reason for overlooking the diagnosis is because inability to measure the biparietal diameter is wrongly attributed to fetal position. In order to measure correctly the biparietal diameter, the fetal head needs to be in occipito-transverse position, that is with the midline echo from the fetal brain at right angles to the ultrasound beam. Failure to achieve such a measurement should lead to the patient being re-scanned 1 week later. Patients should never have gestation estimated on the basis of femur length measurement alone because unless the fetal head is seen in the correct position all chance of examining the intracranial anatomy

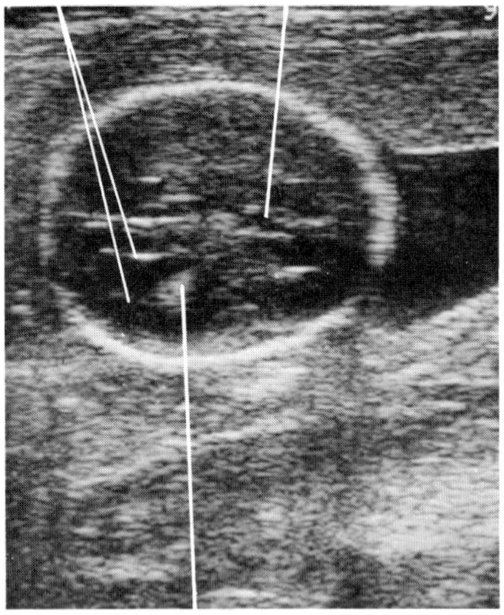

Fig. 20.4 Transverse section of a fetal head on which the biparietal diameter is measured. From Chudleigh & Pearce (1986).

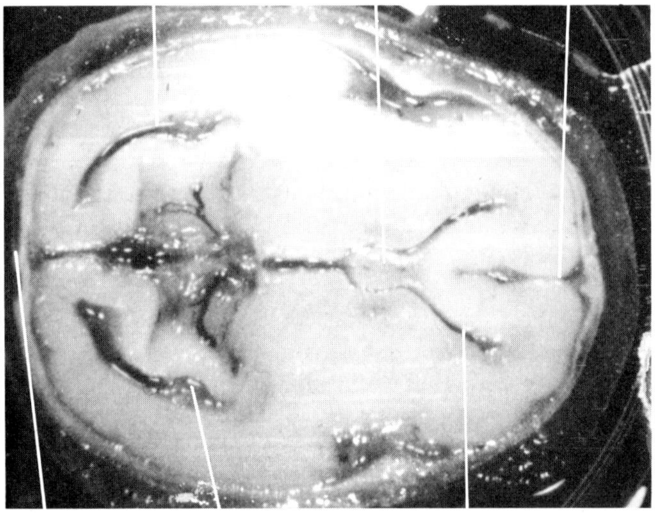

Fig. 20.5 Pathological specimen of a fetal head taken at the same level as Figure 20.4. From Chudleigh & Pearce (1986).

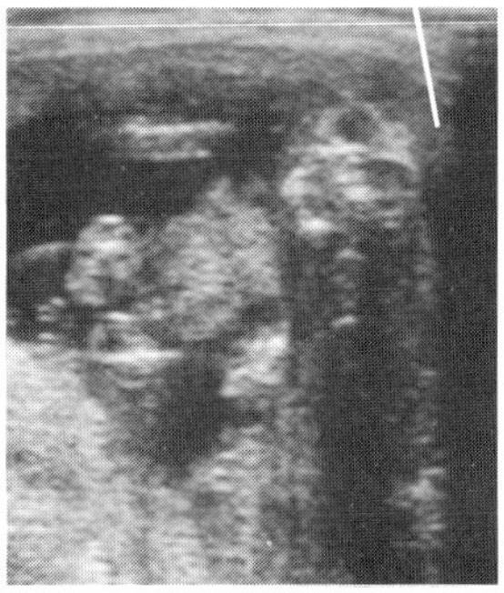

Fig. 20.6 Anencephalic fetus. The absence of the fetal cranial vault is readily appreciated. From Chudleigh & Pearce (1986).

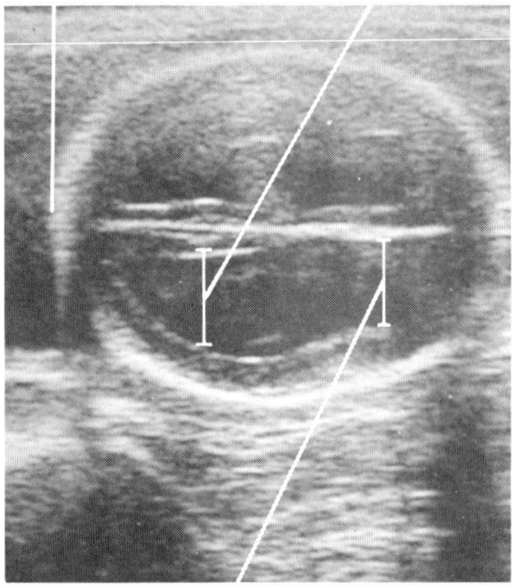

Fig. 20.7 Hydrocephaly. The section is the same as Figure 20.4 but the massive dilatation of the ventricles can be readily appreciated. From Chudleigh & Pearce (1986).

is lost. As long as these patients are recalled (this only refers to about 10%) such abnormalities should not be overlooked.

Figure 20.4 also illustrates the lateral cerebral ventricles. These should be easily visible on the same transverse section as is used to measure the biparietal diameter. With experience it is easy to recognize hydrocephaly or, more strictly, ventriculomegaly, as at this stage the head circumference is not usually large while the lateral ventricles are. Normality can be confirmed by measuring ventricular hemisphere ratio. This is usually done for both the anterior and posterior horns and plotted on an appropriate chart. Figure 20.7 illustrates a case of hydrocephaly; Figure 20.8 is a nomogram of the anterior horn ventricular hemisphere ratio together with cases of proven hydrocephaly. As can be seen, all cases of hydrocephaly had measurements well outside the confidence intervals.

Ventricular dilatation does not usually increase the bipar-

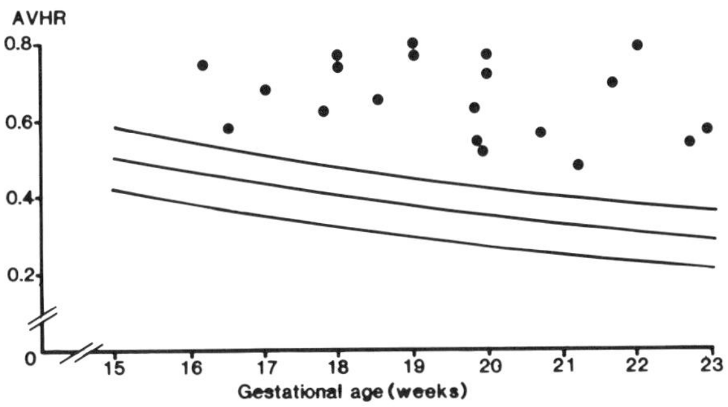

Fig. 20.8 Nomogram of the anterior ventricular hemisphere ratio (AVHR) together with proven cases of hydrocephaly.

Table 20.4 Outcome of intrauterine therapy for hydrocephaly (from Report of International Fetal Surgery Registry 1986)

7 Deaths
4 procedure-related
3 from coexisting anomalies
12 Normal infants
All had aqueduct stenosis as the cause of the hydrocephaly
These were 43% of all cases of aqueduct stenosis
4 Mild/moderate handicap
Developmental delay
Developmental quotients <80
18 Severe handicap
Developmental quotients <60
5 cortical blindness
3 fits
2 spastic displegia

$n = 11\,664$.

ietal diameter or head circumference measurement before 24 weeks' gestation and in cases of spina bifida associated with hydrocephaly these measurements may even be small for gestational age (Roberts & Campbell 1980, Wald et al 1980). In the UK the most common cause of ventriculomegaly in early pregnancy is spina bifida. A careful examination should therefore be made of the fetal spine.

Isolated hydrocephaly is uncommon. In early pregnancy the condition may be due to aqueduct stenosis, occasionally inherited as a sex-linked condition, but more commonly of unknown aetiology; it carries a recurrence risk of about 1 in 30. In general, isolated hydrocephaly tends to be more severe than hydrocephaly associated with spina bifida. In the USA this condition is more common than NTD and intrauterine drainage by means of ventrioculo-amniotic shunting has been attempted (Birnholz & Frigoletto 1981). Initially this was by means of ultrasonically guided puncture of the cerebral ventricles but this failed to stop fluid re-accumulating and later a rubber shunt with a one-way valve was introduced which could be inserted under ultrasound guidance. The results in 41 fetuses were reported in 1986 (Report of the International Fetal Surgery Registry) and are summarized in Table 20.4. It is apparent from this table

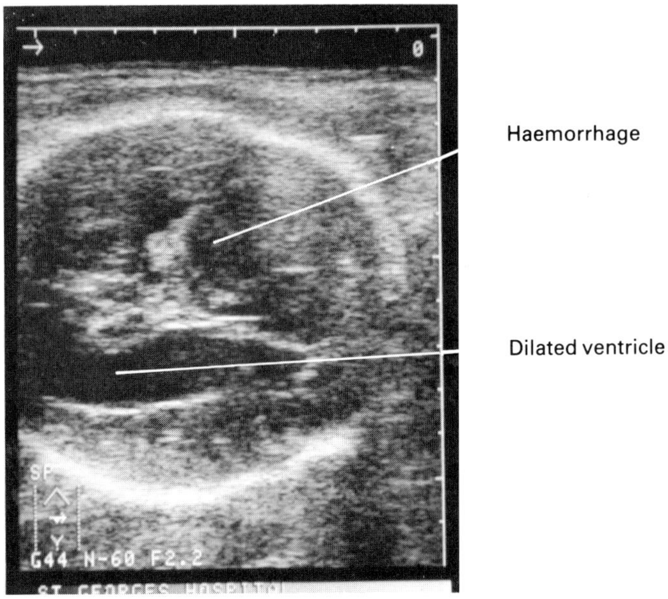

Fig. 20.9 Oblique section of a fetal head at 34 weeks' gestation illustrating mild dilatation of the ventricles due to a periventricular haemorrhage.

that the outcome in all these babies was extremely poor and the procedure has now largely been abandoned.

Hydrocephaly in the first half of pregnancy may also be associated with abnormal kidneys (Meckel's syndrome). This condition is usually fatal and is inherited in an autosomal recessive fashion.

Mild dilatation of the cerebral ventricles causes serious concern. Having carefully excluded a coexisting abnormality serious consideration should be given to obtaining a fetal karyotype. If karyotyping is normal and there is no evidence of a recent TORCH virus infection, then patients can be given a favourable prognosis. Ultrasound examination should be carried out fortnightly to assess the growth of the fetal head and to determine if the degree of ventricular dilatation is worsening. Very occasionally a cause will be found for this, as in Figure 20.9 which illustrates a prenatal periventricular haemorrhage of unknown aetiology. Figure 20.10 illustrates the postnatal scan of this baby, who demonstrates no neurological abnormality.

Having determined that the ventricles are of normal size, the skull vault should be carefully examined looking for the defect of an encephalocele (Fig. 20.11). These are rare lesions and constitute less than 1% of all NTD. They range in size from a small bony defect without brain tissue in the herniated meninges to a major vault defect in which there are large amounts of brain in the herniated sac, usually called exencephaly. The prognosis depends on how much brain tissue there is within the lesion (Lorber 1967); the more extruded the brain, the worse the prognosis. In severe lesions the fetal head measurements usually indicate microcephaly. Encephaloceles may be occipital, parietal or frontal in origin although occipital encephaloceles are by far the most com-

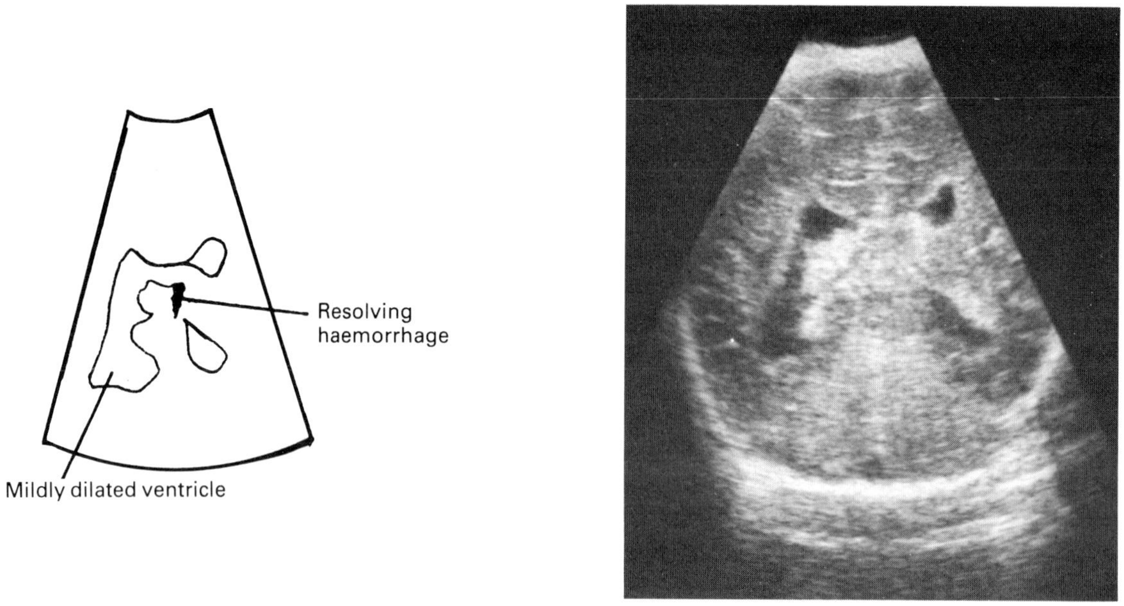

Fig. 20.10 Postnatal scan of the fetus illustrated in Figure 20.9 demonstrating the resolving haemorrhage together with mild dilatation of the ventricles. Courtesy of Professor Neil McIntosh.

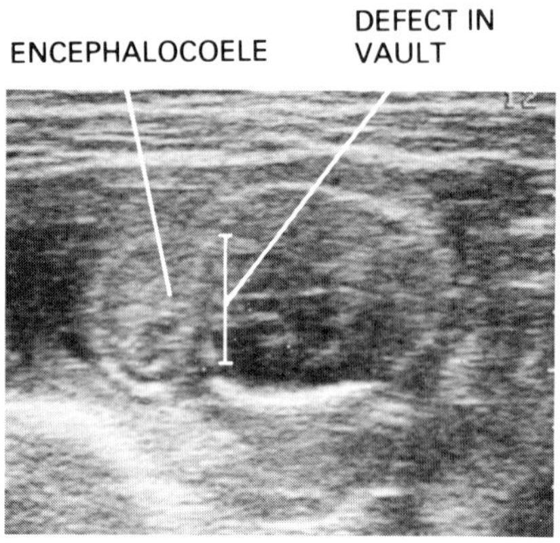

Fig. 20.11 Encephalocele.

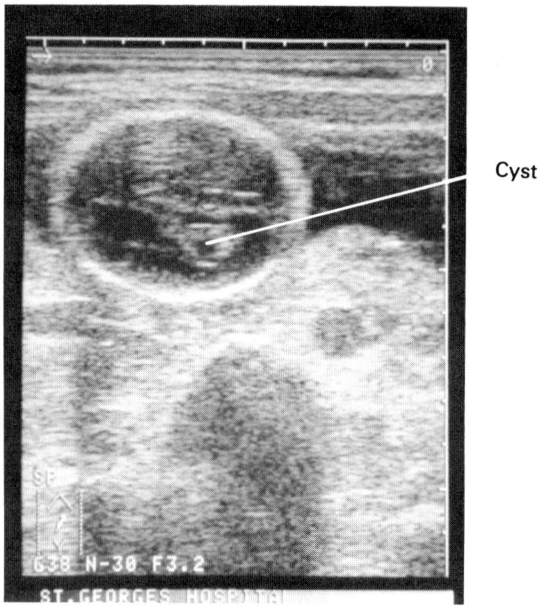

Fig. 20.12 Choroid plexus cyst. This cyst was small and disappeared by 24 weeks' gestation.

mon. The lesion is easy to diagnose but has been confused with cystic hygroma. Clear guidelines on the differential diagnosis have been given by Pearce et al (1985); essentially there is always a vault defect in the presence of an encephalocele. Encephaloceles are rarely associated with elevated MSAFP levels as the lesions are skin-covered.

Whilst examining the fetal head, the cerebral ventricles should be further examined for the presence of cysts. Figure 20.12 illustrates a choroid plexus cyst. Most are thought to be developmental and will usually disappear by 24 weeks' gestation (Chudleigh et al 1984). Large choroid plexus cysts that fill the cerebral ventricle have been associated with chromosome abnormalities and therefore karyotyping is essential before the patients are given a favourable prognosis. Other brain cysts are rare; that seen in Figure 20.13 is a porencephalic cyst which resulted from maternal asphyxia due to her status epilepticus. Prognosis in these cases is difficult as world experience is limited but such an extensive cyst was felt to have a poor outcome.

Finally before leaving the fetal head the posterior fossa should be examined for abnormalities which, although uncommon, generally have a poor prognosis. Figure 20.14 illustrates normal cerebellar hemispheres which are dumb-

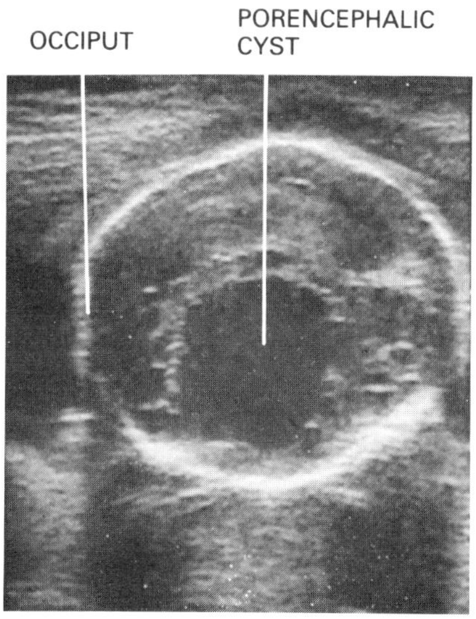

Fig. 20.13 Porencephalic cyst; end-result of a periventricular haemorrhage which burst out into the fetal brain. In this case the asphyxial insult to the fetus was maternal status epilepticus. From Chudleigh & Pearce (1986).

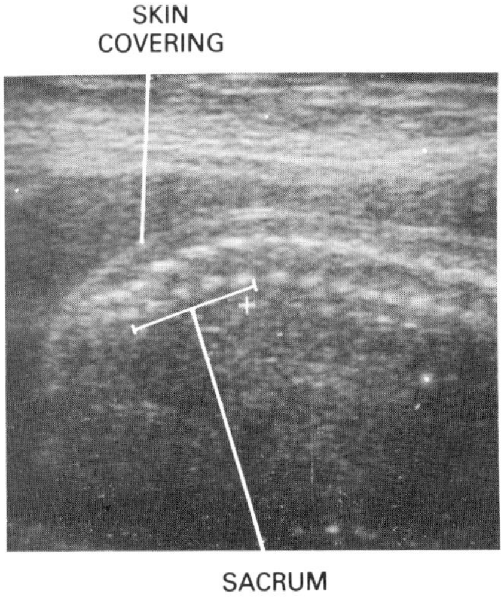

Fig. 20.15 Longitudinal section of a normal fetal spine. The skin covering can be seen along the entire length of the spine. From Chudleigh & Pearce (1986).

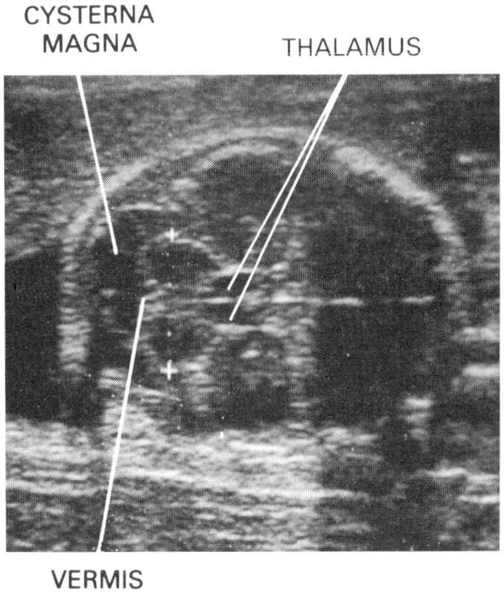

Fig. 20.14 Normal appearance of the fetal cerebellum. From Chudleigh & Pearce (1986).

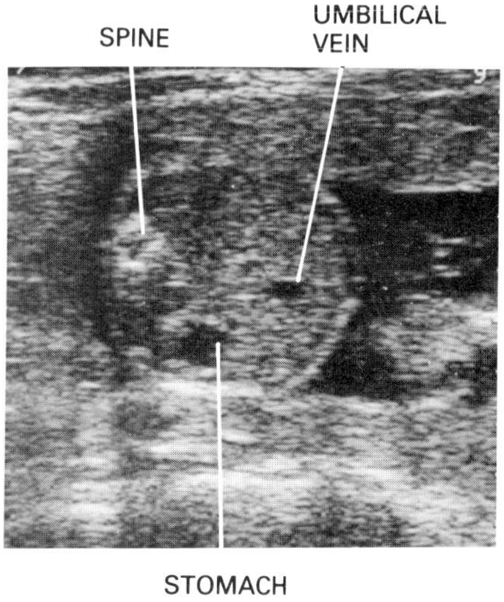

Fig. 20.16 The appearance of a normal vertebra viewed in transverse section. From Chudleigh & Pearce (1986).

bell-shaped. Absence of the cerebellum is usually associated with trisomies but may also be associated with spina bifida, microcephaly or hydrocephaly. The Arnold–Chiari malformation may lead to a change in the shape of the fetal head which looks more like a lemon than a rugby ball. Enlargement of the fourth ventricle constitutes the Dandy–Walker malformation which may readily be diagnosed by ultrasound (Dempsey & Hobbs 1981). Absence of all or part of the cerebellum is also easily diagnosed by ultrasound.

Examination of the fetal spine requires some care and must never be done in one single view. Figure 20.15 shows a normal spine seen in longitudinal section; the skin covering the whole length of the spine can clearly be seen. This view alone, however, can lead to grave errors and each vertebra should be examined in transverse section. The typical normal vertebra is illustrated in Figure 20.16; Figure 20.17 illustrates the abnormality seen in cases of spina bifida. The term *spina bifida* refers to the bony abnormality and Figure 20.18 illustrates the correct terminology for other abnormalities.

Ultrasound diagnosis of spina bifida has advantages over the diagnosis made by means of amniotic fluid alpha-fetoprotein levels. Ultrasound will confirm that the cause of the raised maternal serum or amniotic fluid alpha-fetoprotein is a spina bifida. In addition the type of lesion can be determined; the separate strands of neural tissue that exist in

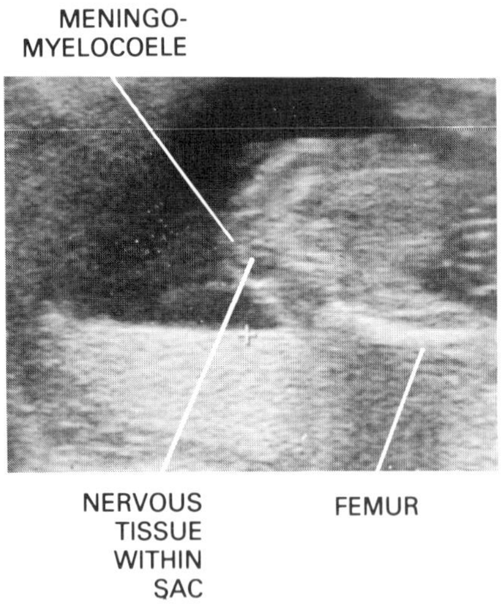

Fig. 20.17 Transverse section of the spine in cases of spina bifida. Compare with Figure 20.16. From Chudleigh & Pearce (1986).

Table 20.5 Predicting outcome of spina bifida diagnosed before 26 weeks' gestation

Feature	Favourable	Unfavourable
Hydrocephaly	Absent or mild	Severe
Spine	Not deformed	Deformed
Lesion	Closed Meningocele	Open Meningomyelocele
Number of vertebrae involved*	Less than 2	More than 2
Associated anomalies (rare — 5%)	No	Yes

* If more than 2 lumbosacral vertebrae are involved there will be bowel and bladder sphincter problems.

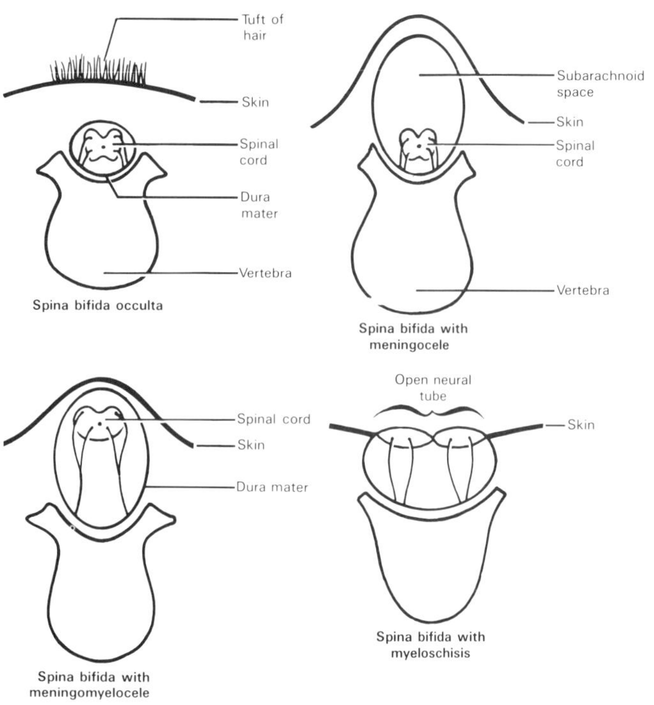

Fig. 20.18 Terminology of spina bifida.

the meningomyelocele are visible with careful scanning. The association of hydrocephaly with the lesion can be readily determined and the parents can be given a sensible prognosis based on that proposed by Lorber (1972). Table 20.5 lists the criteria used in determining the prognosis.

Patients with a normal fetus but a raised MSAFP can be strongly reassured at the end of the detailed ultrasound examination and should be shown their baby on the screen as this significantly reduces anxiety levels (Tsoi et al 1987). This is preferable to the wait necessitated by laboratory analysis of amniotic fluid alpha-fetoprotein. Many patients who have a raised MSAFP and undergo amniocentesis are told: 'If you do not hear in 2 weeks, everything is normal'. They have high anxiety levels throughout their pregnancy (Fearn et al 1982) even after hearing the subsequent normal result.

Patients with a normal fetus and a raised MSAFP have a higher incidence of intrauterine growth retardation and preterm delivery. They should therefore be subsequently managed by serial measurements to estimate growth.

Diagnosis of microcephaly by ultrasound may be extremely difficult and is one of the abnormalities that will almost always be over-looked at the time of routine ultrasound in the first half of pregnancy. The primary defect in microcephaly is in brain growth, but since brain growth determines head growth (Warkany 1975) the skull is also small. Microcephalic infants are nearly always severely abnormal intellectually and, as brain growth appears to affect stature, the infants are often underweight. Amongst the better known causes for microcephaly are rubella infections in the first trimester, cytomegalovirus and toxoplasmosis infections, severe irradiation, maternal addiction to heroin and other drugs, for example the hydantoin syndrome. A few cases are associated with an autosomal mode of inheritance. In the absence of an obvious cause the recurrence rate appears to be about 1 in 30.

A reduced rate of head growth may be due to intrauterine growth retardation or microcephaly. Growth rates must therefore be related to the size of the abdominal circumference and the femur length. The diagnosis by ultrasound is not easy and nearly always relies on serial measurements (Fig. 20.19). It is not possible to make the diagnosis of microcephaly on an isolated measurement unless the head measurements are at least three standard deviations below those expected for gestational age whilst the abdominal circumference and femur are appropriate. The diagnosis of microcephaly in women who have had a previously affected infant may be delayed as late as 24 weeks' gestation. Late termination of pregnancy is usually strongly requested by all patients with this diagnosis following a previously abnormal child.

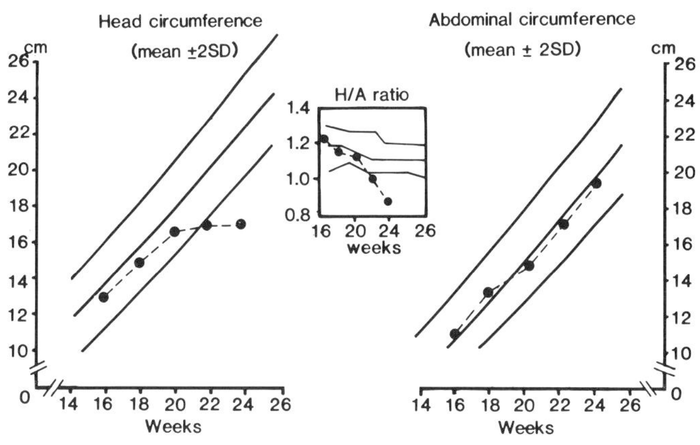

Fig. 20.19 Biparietal diameter and head/abdominal (H/A) ratio measurements in the case of microcephaly. Note that diagnosis was not made until almost 24 weeks' gestation.

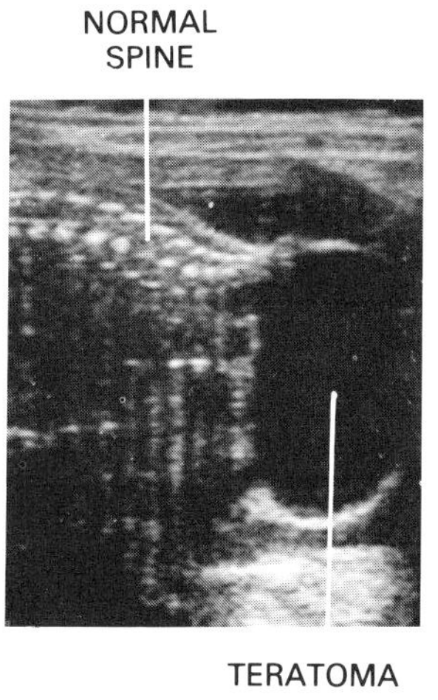

Fig. 20.20 Longitudinal view of the fetal spine demonstrating a sacrococcygeal teratoma.

Rare abnormalities of the fetal head are usually easy to recognize. Holoprosencephaly is the presence of a single centrally placed cerebral ventricle and may be associated with midline abnormalities of the fetal face. Hydranencephaly is complete absence of the cerebral hemispheres thought to be due to failure of carotid arteries to cannulate. It is easily recognized on ultrasound as the cerebral vault contains only fluid. Abnormalities of the fetal head shape are rare, apart from the well recognized dolichocephalic shape of the head of the breech presentation.

Fetal tumours

The commonest reason for referral in this category is because of a suspicious finding on routine ultrasound. The two most common fetal tumours are cystic hygroma and sacrococcygeal teratoma. The latter is easy to diagnose in that the fetal spine is obviously normal and the tumour is apparent (Fig. 20.20). These teratomas are benign in two-thirds of patients (Donnelan & Swenson 1968) but there are no antenatal characteristics which allow the prediction of the nature so all such patients should be delivered by Caesarean section as these teratomas are associated with dystocia.

Fetal cystic hygroma is almost always associated with Turner's syndrome. The outcome of pregnancies associated with Turner's syndrome has been reviewed (Connor 1986). This review also dealt with the question of what to tell parents who have an incidental diagnosis of Turner's syndrome based on amniocentesis. The natural history of Turner's syndrome based on ultrasound findings in the mid-trimester is poor (Chervenak et al 1983, Pearce et al 1985). This is because most coexist with chylothorax and ascites and these findings carry a grave prognosis (Chervenak et al 1983). The finding of a cystic hygroma should therefore warrant karyotyping and detailed fetal echocardiography. In many of these pregnancies intrauterine death occurs but in the absence of a chromosome abnormality or ascites the outlook is favourable and the cystic hygroma may be dealt with surgically after delivery.

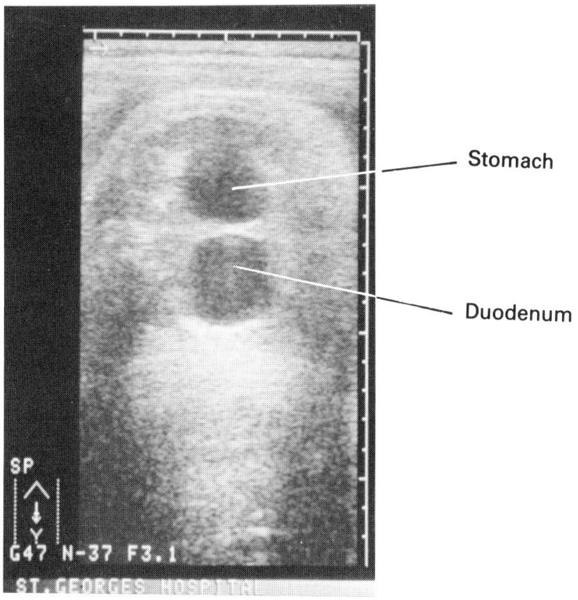

Fig. 20.21 Transverse section of the fetal abdomen illustrating a double bubble sign associated with duodenal atresia.

Gastrointestinal anomalies

Bowel obstruction above the ileum in the fetus usually results in polyhydramnios due to failure of absorption of swallowed amniotic fluid. Excess of amniotic fluid is the usual reason for referral for detailed ultrasound. Bowel obstruction such as duodenal atresia is easy to recognize as it presents a classical appearance known as the double bubble sign (Fig. 20.21). These lesions are readily amenable to surgery but as up to one-third are associated with Down's syndrome, karyotyping should be considered before a prognosis is given. Oeso-

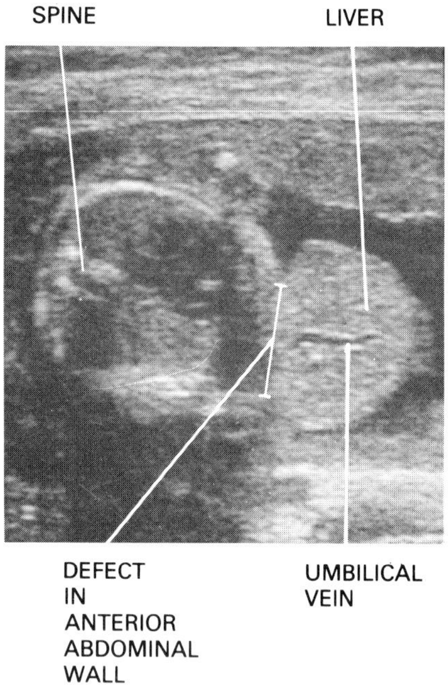

Fig. 20.22 Omphalocele. The defect in the abdominal wall is clearly seen and the liver bulges through this defect. From Chudleigh & Pearce (1986).

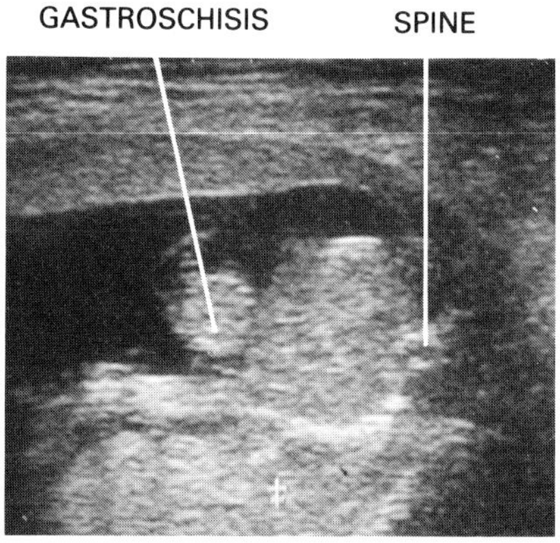

Fig. 20.23 Gastroschisis. This can be differentiated from an omphalocele by the presence of a normal umbilical vein within the fetal abdomen. From Chudleigh & Pearce (1986).

phageal atresia may be suspected because of the presence of polyhydramnios and the absence of a stomach bubble on repeated examinations. Colonic obstruction in Hirschsprung's disease or anal atresia may be detected by ultrasound because of distended loops of descending colon. Such diagnoses, however, are not usually made until the third trimester. Meconium peritonitis is usually recognizable prenatally because of the intense intra-abdominal calcification that it excites and although it is nearly always associated with cystic fibrosis, it may result from maternal antidepressant therapy (such as lithium and tricyclic antidepressants).

One of the more unusual causes of raised MSAFP is an omphalocele or a gastroschisis. These conditions are easy to diagnose on ultrasound and can usually be differentiated. Omphaloceles are due to a midline defect in the abdominal wall, through which the peritoneal sac containing the liver and varying amounts of small bowel bulges (Fig. 20.22). The most common variety is due to failure of the physiological hernia to return at 9 weeks' gestation.

More severe abnormalities may also occur and may be associated with midline defects involving the bladder (ectopia vesicae) or the thorax and heart (ectopia cordis). Approximately half of all fetuses with an omphalocele will have associated cardiac or chromosome abnormalities. Karyotyping and detailed cardiac ultrasound are therefore important before providing a prognosis. As a general guideline the outlook for a fetus that has both an omphalocele and a cardiac abnormality (usually the tetralogy of Fallot) is poor, whereas if the omphalocele is an isolated defect surgical repair after birth has an excellent prognosis. There is conflicting evidence in the literature as to the best mode of delivery but the problem often solves itself as the condition is often associated with polyhydramnios and an unstable lie. If, however, the pregnancy does continue to term there seems to be no overwhelming reason to deliver by Caesarean section as the peritoneal sac is often toughened by exposure to amniotic fluid.

Gastroschisis is a much less common condition than omphalocele; the insertion of the umbilical cord into the abdominal wall is intact, but usually to the right and somewhat lower than the umbilicus, and the small bowel can be seen to be extruded (Fig. 20.23). Counselling of patients is best done in conjunction with the paediatric surgeon but in general an encouraging prognosis can be given. The abdominal wall defect is usually small and the bowel can be readily replaced. The only caveat, however, is that the extruded small bowel does not have a peritoneal covering and may therefore become oedematous, matted and stenosed at the site of the extrusion. This may necessitate extensive resection of bowel with concomitant long-term intravenous feeding and malabsorption syndromes.

Diaphragmatic hernias may be diagnosed prenatally as cystic spaces seen within the chest. The literature on the outcome of such lesions is poor but up to one-third of such babies die antenatally. The outcome for the baby appears to be determined by the amount of bowel within the chest cavity. If the lesion is extensive and there is stomach, colon and small bowel in the chest then the baby commonly dies from pulmonary hypoplasia. Smaller lesions carry a good prognosis. The condition deteriorates after birth due to the child swallowing air, distending the bowel in the chest which leads to increased displacement of the neonatal heart. This is perhaps one of the conditions which may in future be treated with fetal surgery. Experimental work in monkeys (Harrison 1983) has demonstrated that if the diaphragmatic hernia is reduced by mid-pregnancy the fetal lungs continue to grow. In the next few years, it may become possible to consider opening the uterus, temporarily removing the fetus, correcting the hernia and replacing the fetus. Diaphragmatic

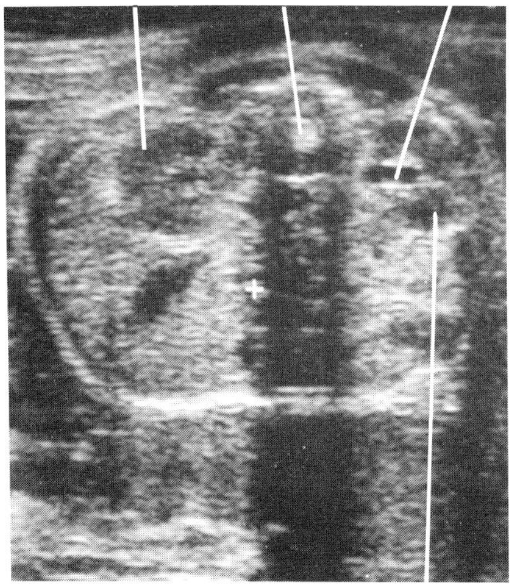

Fig. 20.24 Transverse section of the fetal abdomen demonstrating both kidneys. From Chudleigh & Pearce (1986).

hernias are usually isolated defects, and do not tend to recur in future pregnancies.

Renal tract abnormalities

Normal fetal kidneys are clearly seen from 18 weeks' gestation (Fig. 20.24). The fetal bladder is also easily visible at this time and this, together with a normal amount of amniotic fluid, is an added reassurance of good renal function. The diagnosis of renal agenesis, however, is extremely difficult. This is because it is based on the absence of renal echoes, the absence of bladder-filling and severe oligohydramnios. Visualization of kidneys is difficult due to lack of amniotic fluid and the inability to see one kidney which usually lies in the shadow produced by the spine. Furthermore perirenal fat or large adrenal glands may mimic the renal shadow. The difficulty in making the diagnosis of renal agenesis is widely recognized (Kierse & Meeran 1978, Hobbins et al 1979, Pearce & Campbell 1983) and the diagnosis should only be made by an experienced ultrasonographer. If there is doubt it is perhaps best to err on the side of caution but extreme oligohydramnios in the first half of pregnancy carries a very poor prognosis (Table 20.6).

Polycystic disease of the kidneys is divided into infantile and adult types. The infantile variety shows an autosomal recessive pattern of inheritance and is almost always associated with death from renal failure in early childhood. Patients referred for detailed ultrasound to exclude infantile polycystic disease usually have a past history of an affected child. Since the disease process tends to recur if bilateral cystic disease of the kidneys is seen in the current fetus it is safe to assume the diagnosis and offer a poor prognosis. Infantile polycystic kidneys may well be missed at the time

Table 20.6 Outcome of oligohydramnios before 26 weeks' gestation

Finding	Percentage
Urinary tract anomalies	39
Renal agenesis	
Urethral valves	
Urethral atresia	
Infantile polycystic kidneys	
Multicystic kidneys	
Other structural anomalies	7
Cardiac	
Neural tube	
Chromosomal anomalies	7
Structurally normal fetus	7
Spontaneous abortion	
Intrauterine death	13
Neonatal death	14
Alive and well	13

$n = 11\,664$.

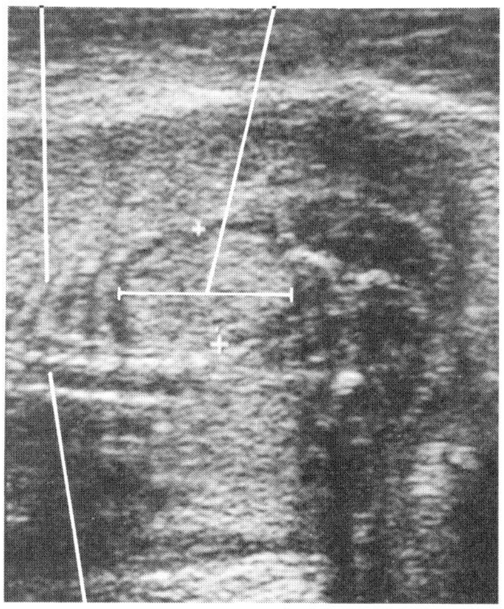

Fig. 20.25 Infantile polycystic kidneys. The kidneys take on an unusually bright appearance because of microcysts within them. From Chudleigh & Pearce (1986).

of routine ultrasound, however, as the cysts are usually microscopic and interpretation of the pattern requires skill (Fig. 20.25).

Obstructive uropathy is the term applied to anatomical or physiological obstruction in any part of the urinary tract. In the fetus such conditions show a wide spectrum of pathological, clinical and ultrasonical features. Those with the most favourable prognosis present as the pelviureteric junction obstruction. The diagnosis is readily made by demonstrating an enlarged renal pelvis (Fig. 20.26). The condition may be bilateral although it is not uncommon for it to be expressed unilaterally in utero.

The large majority of these fetuses need only frequent

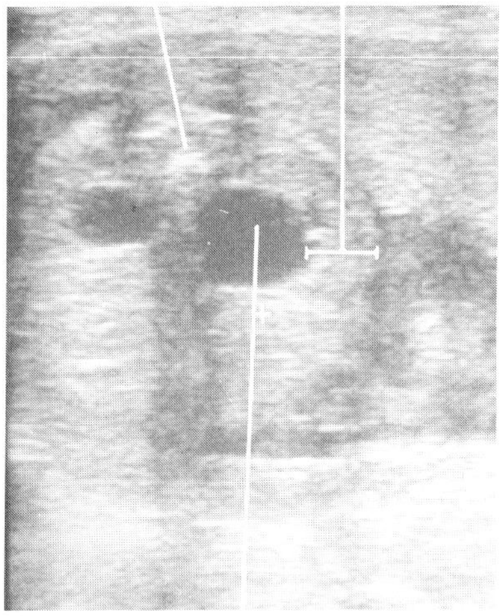

Fig. 20.26 Pelviureteric junction obstruction. From Chudleigh & Pearce (1986).

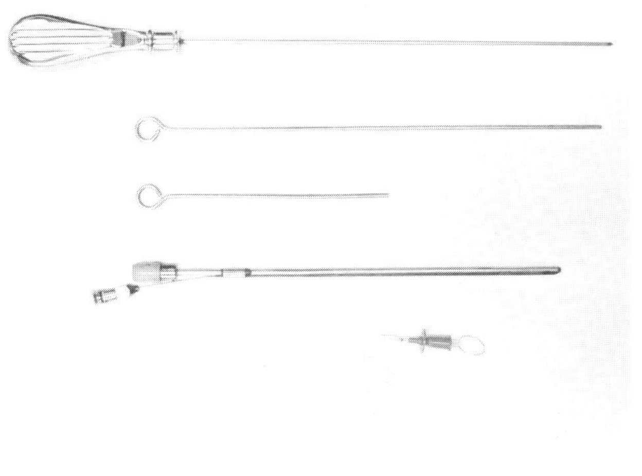

Fig. 20.27 Vesicoamniotic shunt set (Rocket Ltd, UK). The catheter is a double pigtail catheter. One end is inserted into the fetal bladder and the other remains in the amniotic fluid cavity.

monitoring and as the condition is usually an isolated defect, a good prognosis can be given to the parents. If deterioration occurs the renal pelvis gets bigger and the cortical thickness decreases; this is usually late in the third trimester when delivery is the most appropriate means of treatment. Although the insertion of nephrostomy tubes in utero has been described the author has never found it necessary. Pelviureteric junction obstruction is now considered as a series of acute obstructions, rather than a chronic obstruction. The management of these children has changed over the last few years and in the absence of grade IV reflux (reflux of urine into the renal pelvis at the time of micturition) or of hypertension, long-term monitoring seems to be all that is necessary.

The other end of the spectrum of obstructive uropathy is of complete urethral stenosis. This condition presents ultrasonically as a complete absence of amniotic fluid together with gross dilatation of the renal tract. In addition the kidneys are often small and of increased echogenecity, suggesting severe dysplasia. The outcome is inevitably fetal demise and no therapy can be offered.

Posterior urethral valves occur almost exclusively in male infants and cause varying degrees of dilatation of the renal tract. It is in this group of babies that in utero surgery by means of suprapubic catheterization (the vesicoamniotic shunt; Fig. 20.27) may perhaps alter the outcome. The condition is diagnosed by dilated bladder and renal pelves in a male fetus. Before considering vesicoamniotic shunting, detailed ultrasound should be carried out to exclude other abnormalities. Approximately 25% of these babies will have a chromosome abnormality so at the time of insertion of the shunt, blood should be taken from the umbilical cord for karyotyping. Inserting the shunt should be regarded as

Table 20.7 Outcome of vesicoamniotic shunt (73 fetuses) (from Report of the International Fetal Surgery Registry 1986)

Outcome	Number (percentage)
Elective termination	11 (15)
Abnormal chromosomes	6
Renal dysplasia	5
Other abnormalities	5
Deaths	32 (44)
Pulmonary hypoplasia	27
Chronic renal failure	1
Associated anomalies	1
Procedure-related	3
Survivors	30 (41)
Chronic renal failure	2
Cloacal syndrome	1

a diagnostic test. The following lines of management are suggested depending upon initial results:

1. If the karyotype is abnormal, termination of pregnancy should be offered.
2. If the urinary sodium is more than 80 mmol/l or the vesicoamniotic shunt is not working, termination should be offered. Severely dysplastic kidneys seem unable to conserve sodium. It is easy to determine if the shunt is working because the amount of amniotic fluid should rapidly increase. If this does not occur then most babies die from pulmonary hypoplasia.
3. If the fetus is chromosomally normal and the amniotic shunt is working, weekly ultrasound examination should be performed to determine fetal growth, bladder volume and size, and amniotic fluid volume. The shunts are relatively small and have a tendency to become blocked but may be replaced. If the shunt blocks after 32 weeks' gestation fetal lung maturity should be assessed by measurement of amniotic fluid lecithin : sphingomyelin ratio and

Table 20.8 Ultrasonic features of lethal limb reduction deformities

Syndrome	Limbs	Other features
Achondrogenesis	Severe micromelia	Polyhydramnios Hydrops
Thanatophoric dwarfism	Severe micromelia	Megalocaphaly Small chest Polyhydramnios Absent corpus
Jeune's syndrome	Severe micromelia	Polydactyly Dysplastic kidneys
Camptomelic dwarfism	Severe micromelia Bowed tibia	Polyhydramnios Macrocephaly Cardiac defects Cleft palate

Table 20.9 Ultrasonic features of less than lethal limb reduction deformities

Syndrome	Limbs	Other features
Achondrogenesis	Micromelia — onset after mid-pregnancy	Mild hydrocephaly
Hypochondroplasia	Micromelia — onset after mid-pregnancy	
Acromesomelic dwarfism	Micromelia with more distal than proximal limb reduction	
Ellis-van Creveld syndrome	Micromelia — onset after mid-pregnancy	Polydactyl ASD
Diastrophic dwarfism	Late-onset micromelia Flexion deformities	
Cleidocranial dysostosis	Late-onset micromelia	Absent clavicles Hypomineralized skull

phosphatidyl glycerol. If the fetus is mature, delivery is preferable to inserting a further shunt. Table 20.7 illustrates the outcome for these fetuses.

Limb reduction deformities

All fetal long bones can easily be measured on ultrasound but measurement may be time-consuming due to fetal movements. Nomograms are available for all the long bones (Queenan et al 1980). Tables 20.8 and 20.9 illustrate the ultrasound findings in cases of dwarfism together with its common associations. All lethal forms of dwarfism are associated with early shortening of the limb bones, readily recognizable before 22 weeks' gestation. Less than lethal conditions commonly result in slow growth which may not be apparent until later in pregnancy. This is best seen in achondroplastic fetuses. Homozygous achondroplasia leads to severe early limb reduction and usually results in death after birth because of reduced size of the fetal chest, whereas heterozygous achondroplasia tends not to show deviation in fetal growth until well after 24 weeks' gestation (Filly & Golbus 1983).

In addition to dwarfism, hypomineralization due to conditions such as achondrogenesis, hypophosphatasia and osteogenesis imperfecta can be recognized on ultrasound. The genetics of osteogenesis imperfecta is difficult and at least four types are described. In the most severe degree, intrauterine fractures can be diagnosed. Isolated limb deformities are easily missed at the time of routine ultrasound but with care amelia, phocomelia and amputation deformities can be detected. Likewise, abnormalities of fetal fingers and toes can be determined in the second trimester but examination is extremely time-consuming. If the structural abnormalities being sought of the hands or fingers are not clearly seen and are markers for a more severe syndrome, fetoscopy should be considered.

Rocker bottom feet can be recognized on ultrasound with experience and postural deformities such as talipes can also be detected.

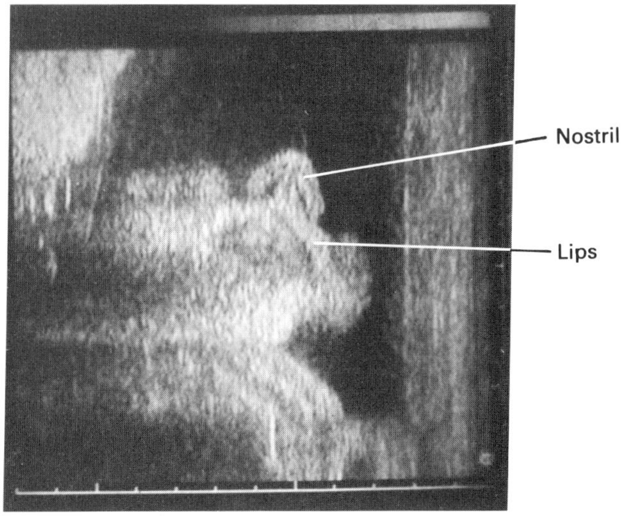

Fig. 20.28 Frontal view of a normal fetal face. The fetal lips and nostrils are clearly visible.

Facial abnormalities

Full frontal views of the face, and views of the face in profile, are possible with ultrasound. Abnormalities of the face are therefore recognizable and may be associated with various syndromes. For example, the arrhinencephaly cyclops syndrome is usually detected by the presence of a single, abnormal orbit. Soft tissues of the face are more difficult to visualize (Fig. 20.28) but with care, harelip and cleft palate may also be diagnosed.

Cardiac abnormalities

These constitute the second most common group of abnormalities and occur in approximately 8 per 1000 live births. Half of these defects however are small, self-correcting or easily correctable defects but one-quarter of all children born with congenital heart disease die of their defect; in over half of this group, death occurs in the first year of life.

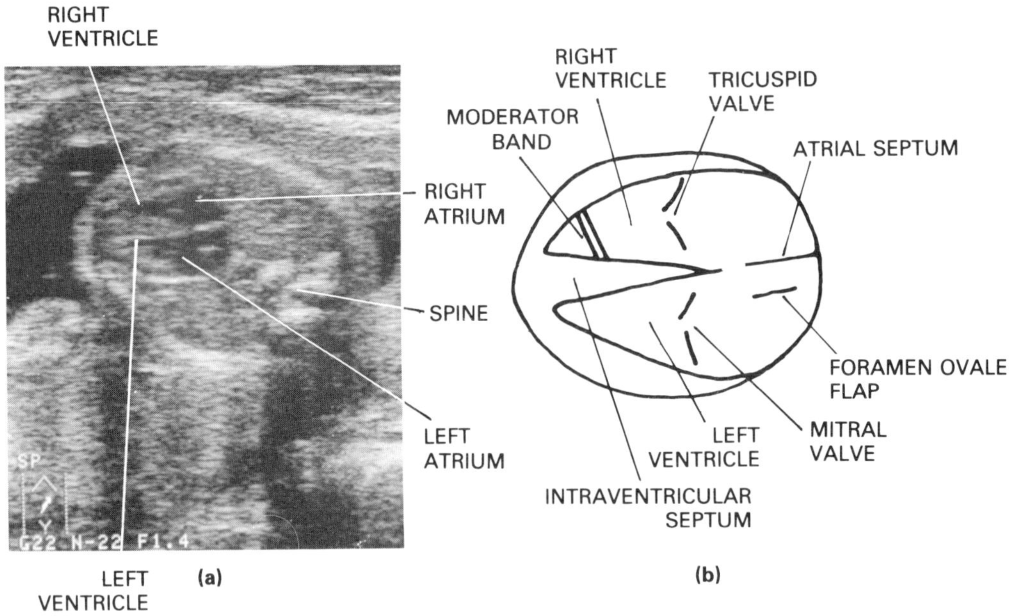

Fig. 20.29 (**a**) Four-chamber view of the fetal heart; (**b**) diagram to illustrate the normal anatomy. From Chudleigh & Pearce (1986).

The prenatal diagnosis of cardiac lesions may therefore lead to termination of pregnancy for lesions which carry a high mortality. More optimistically, recognizing the defect during pregnancy leads to the baby being transferred in utero to be born in a hospital with the appropriate cardiac facilities to offer early surgery.

Although detailed diagnosis is time-consuming and demands clear understanding of cardiac anatomy, many major structural abnormalities can be diagnosed from the simple four-chamber view (Fig. 20.29). If this view is extended to show the origin of the aorta from the left ventricle to the pulmonary outflow tract from the right ventricle, most major abnormalities can be excluded by 24 weeks' gestation. Interested readers should consult Allan (1986).

CONCLUSIONS

Ultrasound examination is now routine in most pregnancies. Its primary aim in early pregnancy is to confirm or establish gestational age and to diagnose multiple pregnancies. Its use at this time should be regarded as a screening procedure for fetal anomalies, and with care, most major anomalies can be detected. In this role it may replace MSAFP in screening for NTD.

As a diagnostic instrument for women at high risk of fetal anomalies it is extremely accurate. The subsequent management of fetal anomalies diagnosed necessitates sensitive communication between the parents, the perinatal obstetrician, neonatologist and paediatric surgeon. Final counselling also requires the expertise of the geneticist and the perinatal pathologist.

Acknowledgement

I am grateful to Mrs Jill Edwards for typing the manuscript.

REFERENCES

Allan L D 1986 Manual of fetal echocardioagraphy. MTP Press, New York
Bakketieg L S, Eik-Nes S H, Jacobsen G et al 1984 Randomised controlled trial of ultrasonographic screening in pregnancy. Lancet ii: 207–211
Bennett N Y, Little G, Dewhurst J, Chamberlain G V P 1982 Predictive value of ultrasound measurement in early pregnancy: a randomised controlled trial. British Journal of Obstetrics and Gynaecology 89: 338–341
Birnholz J C, Frigoletto A 1981 In utero decompression of obstructive hydrocephalus. New England Journal of Medicine 304: 1021–1023
Campbell S 1974 Fetal growth. In: Beard R W, Nathanielsz P W (eds) Fetal physiology and medicine, 1st edn. Saunders, London, pp 271–301
Campbell S, Pearce J M F 1984 The prenatal diagnosis of fetal structural anomalies by ultrasound. Clinics in Obstetrics and Gynaecology 10: 475–506
Campbell S, Reading A E, Cox D N et al 1982 Ultrasound scanning in pregnancy; the short term effects of early real time scans. Journal of Psychosomatic Obstetrics and Gynaecology 1: 57–61
Chapman M, Sheat J H, Furness E T, Jones W R 1979 Routine ultrasound screening in early pregnancy. Medical Journal of Australia 2: 62–63
Chervenak F A, Isaacson G, Blakemore K J 1983 Fetal cystic hygroma. Cause and natural history. New England Journal of Medicine 309: 822–825
Chudleigh P, Pearce J M F 1986 Obstetric ultrasound: how, why and when. Churchill Livingstone, Edinburgh, p 85
Chudleigh P, Pearce J M F, Campbell S 1984 The prenatal diagnosis of transient cysts of the fetal choroid plexus. Prenatal Diagnosis 4: 135–137
Connor J M 1986 Prenatal diagnosis of the Turner syndrome; what to tell the parents. British Medical Journal 293: 711–712
Dempsey P J, Hobbs H J 1981 The in utero diagnosis of the Dandy–Walker syndrome. Journal of Clinical Ultrasound 9: 403–405
Donnelan W A, Swenson O I 1968 Benign and malignant sacrococcygeal teratomas. Surgery 64: 834–836
Eik-Nes S H, Okland O, Aure J C, Ulstein M 1984 Ultrasound screening in pregnancy: a randomised controlled trial. Lancet i: 1347

Fearn J, Hibbard B M, Laurence K M, Roberts A 1982 Screening for neural tube defects and maternal anxiety. British Journal of Obstetrics and Gynaecology 89: 218–221
Filly R A, Golbus M S 1983 Ultrasonography of the normal and abnormal fetal skeleton. In: Callan P W (ed) Ultrasonography in obstetrics and gynaecology. Saunders, Philadelphia, pp 81–96
Furness M E 1987 Reporting obstetric ultrasound. Lancet i: 675–676
Grennert L, Persson P-H, Gennser G 1978 Benefits of ultrasound screening of a pregnant population. Acta Obstetricia et Gynecologica Scandinavica (suppl) 78: 5–14
Harrison M R 1983 Prenatal management of the fetus with a correctable defect. In: Callan P W (ed) Ultrasonography in obstetrics and gynaecology. Saunders, Philadelphia, pp 177–192
Hobbins J C, Grannum P A T, Berkowitz R L 1979 Ultrasound in the diagnosis of congenital abnormalities. American Journal of Obstetrics and Gynecology 134: 331–338
Kierse M J N C, Meeran R H 1978 Antenatal diagnosis of Potter's syndrome. Obstetrics and Gynecology (suppl) 52: 64–67
Lind T 1986 Obstetric ultrasound: getting good vibrations. British Medical Journal 299: 576–577
Lorber J 1967 The prognosis of occipital encephalocoeles. Developmental Medicine and Child Neurology (suppl) 13: 75–79
Lorber J 1972 Spina bifida cystica. Archives of Disease in Childhood 47: 854–873
Owens J R, McAllister E, Harris F, West L 1981 19 Year incidence of neural tube defects in area under constant surveillance. Lancet ii: 1032–1034
Pearce J M F, Campbell S 1983 The prenatal diagnosis of fetal urinary tract anomalies. In: Rodeck C H, Nicolaides K H (eds) Prenatal diagnosis. Proceedings of the 11th Study Group of the Royal College of Obstetricians and Gynaecologists, London, pp 313–324
Pearce J M F, Griffin D, Campbell S 1985 The differential prenatal diagnosis of cystic hygromata and encephalocoele by ultrasound examination. Journal of Clinical Ultrasound 13: 317–320
Persson P-H, Grennert L, Gennser G, Kullander S 1978 On improved outcome of twin pregnancies. Acta Obstetricia et Gynecologica Scandinavica 58: 3–7
Queenan J T, O'Brien G B, Campbell S 1980 Ultrasound measurements of fetal limb bones. American Journal of Obstetrics and Gynecology 138: 297–301
Report of the International Fetal Surgery Registry 1986 New England Journal of Medicine 315: 336–340
Roberts A B, Campbell S 1980 Fetal head measurements of spina bifida. British Journal of Obstetrics and Gynaecology 87: 927–931
Robinson H P, Sweet E M, Adam A H 1979 The accuracy of radiological estimates of gestation age using fetal crown rump length measurements by ultrasound as a basis for comparison. British Journal of Obstetrics and Gynaecology 82: 702–710
Royal College of Obstetricians and Gynaecologists 1984 Report of the RCOG working party on routine ultrasound examination in pregnancy. RCOG, London
Standing S J, Brindle M J, MacDonald A P, Lacey R W 1981 Maternal alpha-fetoprotein screening: two years' experience in a low risk district. British Medical Journal 283: 705
Tsoi M M, Hunter M, Pearce J M F, Chudleigh P, Campbell S 1987 Ultrasound scanning in women with raised serum alphafetoprotein: short term psychological effect. Journal of Psychosomatic Research 31: 35–39
UK Collaborative Study 1977 Alphafetoprotein in relation to neural tube defects. Lancet i: 1323–1332
Wald N, Cuckle H, Boreham J 1980 Biparietal diameter measurements in fetuses with spina bifida. British Journal of Obstetrics and Gynaecology 87: 219–221
Wald N, Cuckle H, Boreham J 1982 Effect of estimating gestational age by ultrasound cephalometry on the specificity of alphafetoprotein screening for open neural tube defects. British Journal of Obstetrics and Gynaecology 89: 1050–1053
Warkany J 1975 Cogenital malformations. Year Book Medical Publishers, New York, p 237
Warsof S L, Pearce J M F, Campbell S 1983 The present place of routine ultrasound screening. Clinics in Obstetrics and Gynaecology 10: 445–458

21

M. d'A. Crawfurd

Diagnosis of chromosomal abnormalities

HISTORICAL INTRODUCTION TO CYTOGENETIC METHODOLOGY

Following the early works of Painter (1923) it was for many years accepted that the normal diploid chromosome number of man was 48. In 1956 Tjio & Levan, studying human fetal lung fibroblasts, found only 46 chromosomes and gave the first clear description of the individual chromosome pairs. It shows the strength of the erroneous belief in a diploid number of 48 that Tjio & Levan comment that they gained the courage to publish from the knowledge that other workers had abandoned a research project because those workers could only find 46 chromosomes in human somatic cells. Tjio & Levan's findings were rapidly confirmed by Ford & Hamerton (1956) on meiotic preparations from testicular biopsies. The clear analysable karyotypes first obtained by these workers depended on three advances in cytogenetic technique that had just become available: the use of colchicine as a spindle inhibitor which led to an accumulation of cells in metaphase in cell cultures; the use of hypotonic solution to swell cells and thereby disperse the chromosomes during the harvesting procedure; and the technique, borrowed from the botanical cytogeneticists, of squashing the preparation between slide and coverslip to disperse the cells further.

These techniques are still fundamental in human cytogenetics except that nowadays we use less disruptive methods of final chromosomal dispersal than squashing. An important early advance was the development of a technique for culturing peripheral blood lymphocytes (Nowell & Hungerford 1960). This depended on the chance discovery that phytohaemagglutinin is a mitogen for the T-lymphocytes of peripheral blood and permitted chromosome analysis from blood samples. The major new technical advance in chromosomal analysis since these early studies has been the introduction of a variety of methods of differential staining or banding. These started with the introduction of quinacrine banding by Caspersson et al (1970); this required the use of a fluorescence microscope. Giemsa banding, needing only the usual high quality optical microscope used by cytogeneticists, was introduced by Sumner et al (1971) and the simplified trypsin Giemsa method by Marina Seabright in 1971. Variants of this last technique are now standard in most cytogenetic laboratories. In addition to quinacrine (Q) and Giemsa (G) banding several further methods of differential staining are used to clarify the findings in individual cases. These include reverse (R) banding in which the dark bands of G banding stain light and vice versa, facilitating visualization of telomeres; C-banding for centromeric regions; silver staining to reveal the nucleolar organizer regions (NOR) of the satellited chromosomes; DAPI staining for the heterochromatic regions of several chromosomes including the short arm of number 15, as well as other methods.

Even with this broad armamentarium of staining techniques there are cases in which small deletions, inversions that do not substantially alter the position of the centromere or the banding pattern, or reciprocal translocations involving short equal-length segments may be suspected by the cytogeneticist but be impossible to prove or even pass wholly undetected. Such cases are potentially resolvable using recombinant DNA techniques. If a deleted chromosome segment or one involved in a rearrangement is known to carry a DNA sequence for which there is a probe available then the presence or absence or position within the chromosomes of that sequence may be detected. The presence or absence of a DNA sequence may be demonstrated by the presence or absence of a specific band on Southern blotting (see Chapter 22). Its precise chromosomal localization may be determined by in situ hybridization of the probe to metaphase spreads. Recent examples of the application of this approach include the demonstration that the supernumerary chromosome in cat eye syndrome is either a dicentric chro-

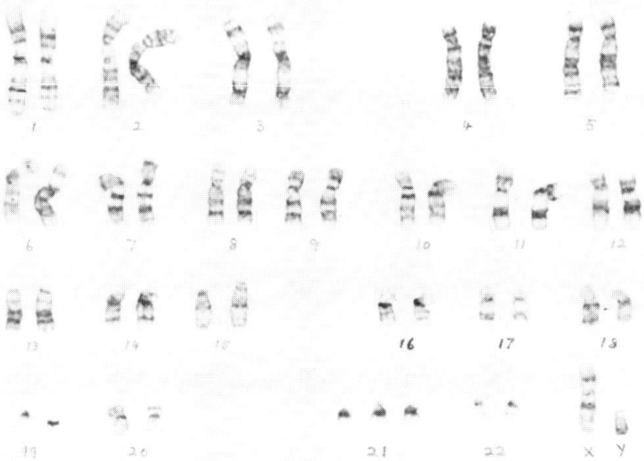

Fig. 21.1 G-banded karyotype of a male Down's syndrome patient with standard trisomy 21.

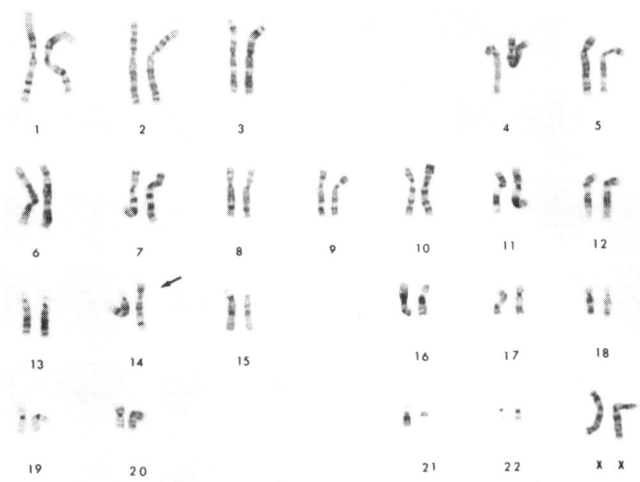

Fig. 21.2 G-banded karyotype of a Down's syndrome patient with a Robertsonian translocation between chromosomes 14 and 21, resulting in effective trisomy for chromosome 21.

mosome 22 incorporating the q 11 region or an interstitial duplication of the 22q 11 region (McDermid et al 1986) and an analysis of chromosome 15 proximal long arm abnormalities in Prader–Willi syndrome (Donlon et al 1986). This approach is likely to become increasingly important over the next few years.

HUMAN CONSTITUTIONAL CHROMOSOMAL ABNORMALITIES

The first human chromosome abnormality to be discovered was that in Down's syndrome. In 1959 Lejeune et al reported the observation of an extra small acrocentric chromosome in fibroblast cultures of patients with Down's syndrome. At that time the two pairs of small acrocentrics, 21 and 22, were not readily distinguished and it was decided that the extra chromosome was probably one of the second smallest pairs, number 21. Subsequent studies with meiotic preparations and with banding techniques have shown this conclusion to be wrong and that it is after all the smallest chromosome which is affected. However the term trisomy 21 for the chromosome abnormality in Down's syndrome (Fig. 21.1) had become so well established that we now define the smallest chromosome pair as being number 21 and the second smallest pair as number 22.

Although trisomy 21 was confirmed as the abnormality in the great bulk of cases it was found that in about 3% of Down's syndrome children there were 46 chromosomes but that one of these was an abnormal chromosome arising from the centric fusion of a chromosome 21 with another acrocentric chromosome, 13–15 or 21–22, in a Robertsonian translocation (Fig. 21.2; Polani et al 1960). These children are effectively trisomic for 21, having two independent chromosomes 21 and a third 21 fused to another acrocentric chromosome. No differences have been detected between patients with trisomic or translocation Down's syndrome. In about half of these translocation cases, when involving fusion of a 21 with one of the pairs 13–15, usually 14, it is found that one or other parent carries the translocation in a symptomless balanced form (Fig. 21.3; Penrose et al 1960, Penrose & Delhanty 1961, Sergovich et al 1962, Carter et al 1986). It is important to recognize such cases, both because a parent with a balanced translocation is at increased risk of further Down's children, and because further relatives may also carry the balanced translocation and should be identified. It should be noted that an individual who carries a 21;21 translocation cannot have a normal child; all will be either trisomic or monosomic for chromosome 21 (Bavin et al 1963).

The well known association of Down's syndrome births with maternal age is specifically arising with trisomic Down's syndrome through maternal meiotic errors in the formation of the ovum. There has been speculation for many years as to the likely mechanism for the maternal age effect. Only recently has evidence been produced leading to the hypothesis that the older the mother the less likely she is to abort a trisomic fetus spontaneously (Stein et al 1986). The results of studies on a possible paternal age effect have been conflicting but the consensus of the more recent research fails to demonstrate any such effect (Roth et al 1983).

Following Lejeune's discovery of trisomy 21 in Down's syndrome there was in 1959 and the early 1960s a spate of discoveries of human syndromes of chromosomal abnormality. These included D trisomy (trisomy 13; Patau et al 1960); E trisomy (trisomy 18; Edwards et al 1960); XXY and variants in Klinefelter's syndrome (Jacobs & Strong 1959) and complete or mosaic 45, X karyotype in Turner's syndrome (Ford et al 1969). Subsequent studies have revealed further sex chromosomal anomalies, including the XXX and XYY syndromes and their variants, structural sex chromosome anomalies, the XY sex constitution in testicular feminization and XX males who carry Y chromosomal material translocated to their X (Affara et al 1986). There have also been many new autosomal anomaly syndromes described, including further trisomies, such as that for chromosome 8; and many structural deletions or rearrangements such as cri du chat syndrome in which there is a deletion of the short arm of chromosome 5, and deletions in several syndromes that are not always chromosomal, at least at a microscopic level, such as bilateral retinoblastoma, Wilms' tumour and Prader–Willi syndrome.

In recent years an important new sex chromosomal syndrome has been defined which accounts for a high proportion of the excess of males among the mentally subnormal. This is the Martin–Bell syndrome of X-linked mental subnormality associated with macro-orchidism and minor dysmorphic facial features (Martin & Bell 1943). In 1969 Lubs described a family in which a marker X chromosome with a constriction near the tip of the long arm was segregating in an X-linked manner. It was subsequently shown that the marker X chromosome described by Lubs, now known as the fragile X or fra(X) characterizes the Martin–Bell syndrome (Giraud et al 1976). Cytogenetic laboratories now spend an appreciable proportion of their time screening patients for the presence of the fragile X chromosome.

Apart from these well known syndromes of chromosome abnormality there are many patients with less common trisomies, partial trisomies and monosomies, triploidies and inversions arising from chromosomal breakage giving rise to simple deletions, inversions, translocations and more complex rearrangements. When these result in an aneuploid or unbalanced chromosomal constitution they are nearly always associated with phenotypic abnormality ranging from early loss of the embryo to minor dysmorphic changes in a baby born at term. Nevertheless the finding of an unexpected deletion or other aneuploid rearrangement at prenatal diagnosis should always be checked against the parental karyotypes before any prediction of fetal abnormality is made. The author has recently been involved in a case in which amniocentesis revealed a deletion of the whole of band 11p12. This was found to be segregating in the family without phenotypic effect.

The significance of balanced chromosomal rearrangements for offspring depends on the mode of ascertainment. When detected in the parent or other relative of an abnormal child with aneuploidy, risks for further children are high. They may also be high when ascertained through investigation of a couple for recurrent miscarriage. When discovered as a chance finding, risks for children are relatively low.

Studies in which tissue from spontaneous abortuses have been karyotyped, especially early abortuses, show a high incidence of chromosomal abnormality—up to 50% or more. Many of the trisomies and other abnormalities found are never seen in term or near term births, indicating that they are inevitably lethal. Yet other abnormalities, especially most monosomies, which must occur, are not seen even in the earliest abortuses, indicating an even earlier lethality.

PRENATAL DIAGNOSIS OF CHROMOSOMAL ABNORMALITY

Amniocentesis

Technique of cell culture and analysis

The discovery of mammalian sex chromatin soon led to its demonstration in human amniotic cells and to the suggestion that such cells might be cultured to reveal the fetal karyotype (Fuchs & Riis 1956, Sachs et al 1956, Riis & Fuchs 1960, Austin 1962). In 1966 Steele & Breg demonstrated that human amniotic fluid does contain viable cells, and that they can be cultured and used for the demonstration of sex chromatin or for chromosomal analysis. Their observations were confirmed by Jacobson & Barter (1967) who evaluated 91 amniotic fluid samples taken at varying times from 5 weeks' gestation to term. Their highest success rates were from 12 weeks on and the successful cultures included one in which they demonstrated the transmission of a maternal Robertsonian translocation in balanced form to the fetus. Nadler (1968) made similar observations and was one of the first to make a prenatal diagnosis of an abnormal fetus, with an inherited D;G translocation Down's syndrome. Valenti and colleagues (1968) also made a prenatal diagnosis of an inherited D;G translocation Down's syndrome fetus at about the same time as Nadler. In their case, following termination of pregnancy, the fetus showed features of Down's syndrome but was too macerated for successful cell culture.

Following these early observations several groups of workers published studies on small series of amniocenteses establishing the optimum period of gestation for amniocentesis for chromosomal analysis at about 16 weeks and the best methods of cell culture, harvesting and chromosomal preparation and analysis (Lisgar et al 1970, Nadler & Gerbie 1970, Wahlstrom et al 1970, Fuchs 1971, Nadler 1971, Timson et al 1971, Milunsky et al 1972, Warburton & Miller 1972). The chromosomal banding techniques discussed earlier have greatly increased the precision of prenatal as well as postnatal diagnosis of chromosomal disorder. It is now possible to detect many small deletions, inversions, reciprocal translocations and other rearrangements that could not have been detected hitherto, as well as whole chromosomal aneuploid states. The only other major subsequent technical advance in amniocentesis for chromosomal or other prenatal diagnostic indications has been the increasing use of ultrasound control at the time of amniocentesis (Lachman 1977). This has reduced the frequency of placental puncture with consequent bloody taps and is now sufficiently widely available that amniocentesis should not be undertaken without

Table 21.1 Rates per 1000 of chromosomal abnormality at amniocentesis (amnio) and livebirths (LB) by maternal age

	47, +21		47, +18		47, +13		47, XXX		47, XXY		Other clinically significant abnormalities‡		All abnormalities§	
Maternal age (years)	Amnio*	LB**	Amnio	LB	Amnio†	LB††	Amnio	LB	Amnio	LB	Amnio	LB	Amnio	LB
33	2.4	1.6	0.6	0.2	0.4	0.2	0.4	0.4	0.4	0.4	1.1	0.8	4.6–5.4	2.9–3.5
34	3.1	2.0	0.8	0.2	0.4	0.2	0.5	0.5	0.5	0.4	1.2	0.8	5.8–6.5	3.7–4.2
35	4.0	2.6	1.0	0.3	0.5	0.3	0.6	0.5	0.6	0.6	1.3	0.9	7.4–8.0	4.7–5.2
36	5.2	3.4	1.3	0.4	0.6	0.3	0.7	0.6	0.8	0.7	1.3	0.9	9.5–9.9	5.9–6.4
37	6.7	4.4	1.6	0.5	0.6	0.4	0.8	0.8	1.0	0.9	1.4	1.0	12.1–12.2	7.6–7.9
38	8.7	5.7	2.1	0.6	0.7	0.4	1.0	0.9	1.2	1.1	1.5	1.0	15.4–15.2	9.7–9.8
39	11.2	7.3	2.6	0.8	0.9	0.5	1.2	1.1	1.5	1.4	1.6	1.1	19.6–19.0	12.3–12.1
40	14.5	9.4	3.3	1.0	1.0	0.5	1.4	1.3	1.9	1.7	1.7	1.2	25.0–23.8	15.7–15.2
41	18.7	12.2	4.2	1.2	1.1	0.6	1.7	1.6	2.4	2.2	1.8	1.2	31.9–29.9	20.1–19.0
42	24.1	15.7	5.2	1.6	1.3	0.7	2.0	1.9	3.0	2.7	1.9	1.3	40.7–37.6	25.6–23.9
43	31.1	20.2	6.6	2.0	1.5	0.8	2.4	2.2	3.8	3.4	2.0	1.4	51.9–47.5	32.6–30.2
44	40.1	26.1	8.4	2.5	1.8	1.0	2.9	2.7	4.7	4.3	2.2	1.5	66.1–60.1	41.6–38.1
45	51.8	33.7	10.6	3.2	2.0	1.1	3.4	3.2	5.9	5.4	2.3	1.6	84.3–76.0	53.0–48.2
46	66.8	43.4	13.3	4.0	2.4	1.3	4.1	3.8	7.4	6.8	2.4	1.7	107.5–96.5	67.6–61.0
47	86.2	56.0	16.9	5.1	2.7	1.5	4.9	4.6	9.3	8.5	2.6	1.8	137.1–122.6	86.2–77.5
48	111.2	72.3	21.3	6.4	3.1	1.8	5.9	5.5	11.7	10.7	2.7	1.9	174.8–155.9	109.9–98.5
49	143.5	93.3	26.9	8.1	3.6	2.0	7.0	6.5	14.6	13.4	2.9	2.0	222.9–198.6	140.1–125.3

*, ** Values of 0.08 and 0.06 respectively should be added to these values to allow for structural rearrangements associated with Down's syndrome.
†, †† Values of 0.06 and 0.03 respectively should be added to these values to allow for structural rearrangements associated with trisomy 13.
‡ Include structural rearrangements associated with trisomies 13 and 21.
§ First value of range given is derived from the regression analysis on all abnormalities; the second by adding the values for all abnormalities.
Reproduced from Tables 1–4 from Hook et al (1983), with permission.

it, not just immediately prior to the procedure but throughout the amniocentesis (Miskin et al 1974).

Abnormalities detected

Several studies on large series of amniocenteses have reported on the frequency of chromosomal abnormality. These have reported the experience of either a single or multiple centres (Littlefield et al 1974, Galjaard 1976, Boue et al 1979, Golbus et al 1979, Polani et al 1979, Crandall et al 1980, Daniel et al 1982, Diernaes et al 1982, Simoni et al 1982, Squire et al 1982). Comparing data from these studies, mothers aged 35 years or over consistently yield chromosomal abnormality on amniocentesis at a frequency of between 1.9 and 2.8%, with an overall frequency of 2.3%. Similarly, mothers with a previous child or other relatives with Down's syndrome or other chromosomal abnormality have given consistently lower frequencies of fetal chromosomal abnormality of 0.7–1.3% or have failed to detect any abnormalities with an overall frequency of 0.99%. In contrast the presence of a parental translocation carries a higher risk, ranging between 5.7 and 18.3% in different series (Galjaard 1976, Polani et al 1979, Daniel et al 1982, Simoni et al 1982, Squire et al 1982), or 9.4% overall.

Hook et al (1983), using several sources of data on the rates of cytogenetic abnormality at amniocentesis in women aged 35 years and over, have calculated maternal age-specific estimates for ages 33–49 years of the rates that would apply at livebirth. They used regression methods to remove the scatter that arises from sampling variation and estimated the rates separately for trisomies 13, 18 and 21, triple X and XXY syndromes, and other abnormalities. The figures they give for both frequencies at amniocentesis and at livebirth, which are valuable for genetic counselling, are quoted in Table 21.1.

Hazards

The hazards — real and potential — of amniocentesis are sufficiently rare as to make their true frequency difficult to assess. They may involve either the mother or the fetus. There have been individual reports of maternal complications, including infection, most commonly amnionitis, but this seems to be exceedingly rare (NICHD 1976). Other maternal complications include vaginal bleeding, usually minor, and leakage of amniotic fluid. The potentially most serious maternal complication is fetomaternal blood transfusion, especially when the placenta is penetrated (Wang 1967, Curtis et al 1972) but rhesus sensitization of Rh-negative mothers can be avoided if all such mothers are given anti-D immunoglobulin at amniocentesis. The Kleihauer test cannot be relied on to detect all of those at risk (Lawrence 1977). Nevertheless, the risk of Rh immunization following uncomplicated amniocentesis is low, probably around 11% (Tabor et al 1986).

Similarly, there have been reports of fetal complications including injury and abortion (Fairweather & Walker 1964, Broome et al 1975). Fetal injury is more common in association with amniocentesis done late in pregnancy than in mid-trimester amniocentesis and in association with amniography (Greasman et al 1968). Serious injury to the fetus in mid-trimester amniocentesis, especially when done under ultrasound control, is rare. About 2% of infants whose mothers had mid-trimester amniocentesis showed needle scars (Raimer & Raimer 1984). The frequency of abortion resulting from amniocentesis has proved especially difficult to determine because of the relatively high frequency of spontaneous abortion. Early studies suggested a relatively small, if any, increase in the frequency of abortion after amniocentesis (Gerbie et al 1971, Kalbac & Newman 1974).

Five major studies published between 1976 and 1978 attempted to assess the frequency of fetal loss and other complications of amniocentesis. A Canadian study of over 1000 pregnancies found an incidence of fetal loss similar to that in pregnant women aged 35 years or more in the general population (Simpson et al 1976). Galjaard (1976) collated results from nearly 3500 amniocenteses performed at 20 European centres and found an absolute abortion rate of only 1.4%. A later Danish study of over 1000 pregnancies with amniocenteses found an absolute abortion rate of 2.4% and the authors suggested an increased frequency of abortion of 0.3–0.7% (Philip & Bang 1978). An American study carried out by the National Institute of Child Health and Human Development (NICHD 1976) examined the outcome of 1000 pregnancies with amniocentesis and just under 1000 controls, not all of whom were matched. No significant difference in fetal loss rates between the subjects and controls was found.

In none of these studies were all the subjects matched against satisfactory controls. The Medical Research Council (MRC) therefore set up a UK survey to attempt a proper assessment of the hazards of amniocentesis which reported in 1978. The survey looked at the course and outcome of pregnancy and delivery and the progress of any consequent child in a group of 2424 pregnant women who had an amniocentesis within the first 20 weeks of pregnancy, and in a similar group of matched controls who did not have an amniocentesis. The difficulties of obtaining matched controls in such studies are highlighted by the fact that the working party were unable to find suitable controls for a further 505 patients. They found an increased fetal loss among the subjects of 1.0–1.5% and an increased frequency among the infants born to these women of respiratory distress, including hyaline membrane disease, congenital dislocation or subluxation of the hip and talipes, as well as maternal antepartum haemorrhage, also of a similar order of 1.0–1.5%. Subsequent evidence suggests that the infantile morbidity may be due to postural defects due to maternal leakage of amniotic fluid following amniocentesis. Even the MRC study faced difficulties in finding matching controls and has been accused of bias in this respect. However any bias was allowed for by the working party in calculating the frequencies of abnormality.

However, as with the other studies of that time, not all the amniocenteses were done under ultrasound control, or even with prior ultrasound examination, as would be the case now. A Swedish study with ultrasound control found a fetal loss rate of 2.3% in subjects, a value similar to that in controls in previous studies (Bartsch et al 1980), and a more recent Dutch follow-up of 3000 pregnancies with mid-trimester amniocentesis found a fetal loss rate of 1.53% for the first 1500 cases and 0.47% for the second 1500 cases (Leschot et al 1985). The authors conclude that mid-trimester amniocentesis performed by an experienced obstetrician under ultrasound control carries a risk of fetal death of about 0.5%.

A long-term 5–7-year follow-up of 62 children born after mid-trimester amniocentesis of the mother and compared with 60 matched control children showed no difference between the two groups for paediatric or neurodevelopmental disorder, orthopaedic or respiratory problems (Gillberg et al 1982). The authors have observed needle scars in two cases in a previous uncontrolled series. The lack of evidence of any increased risk of orthopaedic problems, especially talipes or hip problems, was confirmed in a study by Wald et al (1983).

A recent controlled randomized study of 4606 women at low genetic risk, of whom half were assigned to amniocentesis and half were not, found an increased spontaneous abortion rate in the study group of 1%. The study group also showed more frequent leakage of amniotic fluid and respiratory problems after birth, but not postural problems (Tabor et al 1986). These hazard rates are higher than those of other recent studies.

Fetoscopy and ultrasound

Fetoscopy and fetal blood sampling are discussed more fully in Chapter 23. Fetoscopy using an endoamnioscope with aspiration of blood from placental blood vessels was introduced in 1973 (Valenti 1973). This method, which requires a laparotomy and a rigid fetoscope, is applicable when there is posterior placenta and has been used by Kan et al (1974) and by Hobbins & Mahoney (1978). This technique was introduced for diagnosis of haemoglobin disorders and, because it could not be safely used when the placenta was anterior, it was replaced by placental aspiration. Subsequently Rodeck & Campbell (1978) showed that fetoscopy could be used to obtain pure fetal blood even when the placenta is anterior, thereby widening the scope for the application of this technique. It is now mainly used for the diagnosis of haemoglobin and metabolic disorders, severe dysmorphic syndromes, the confirmation of neural tube defect and the diagnosis of fetal rubella (Daffos et al 1984) or toxoplasmosis (Desmonts et al 1985).

Fetoscopy is clearly not a method of choice for the routine diagnosis of chromosomal fetal abnormality, as even in skilled hands the consequent abortion rate is about 4%

(Rodeck & Campbell 1978). However, occasionally in high-risk situations, such as a parental balanced translocation, amniocentesis cultures may fail to grow. Alternatively amniotic fluid cell cultures may yield an ambiguous result. Common examples of the latter situation are the detection of mosaicism for a significant chromosomal anomaly, or of an unidentified marker chromosome in more than one culture flask that may or may not reflect the constitution of the fetal tissues. In such circumstances fetoscopy may be justified to resolve the uncertainty. Direct vision of the fetus may reveal external dysmorphology consistent with a suspected or possible chromosomal abnormality, and fetal blood sampling will permit chromosomal analysis of cells that are definitely fetal. This approach may also be adopted when a mother at high risk presents at a late stage of the second trimester (Cordesius et al 1980), for selective prenatal diagnosis of twins, and for confirmation of fetal abnormality detected by ultrasound (Gosden et al 1985). Fetoscopy is also the method of choice for the prenatal diagnosis of the X-linked Martin–Bell syndrome of mental retardation (fragile X syndrome), which cannot be readily demonstrated in amniotic fluid cells, or rare syndromes with increased chromosome breakage such as Fanconi's anaemia (Gosden et al 1985).

Ultrasound is of course used as an adjunct to all of these techniques and to chorionic villus biopsy, discussed below. High-resolution fetal ultrasound scanning is being increasingly used by itself for the diagnosis of dysmorphic syndromes. Unlike fetoscopy it can detect internal as well as external malformations, is non-invasive and harmless to both fetus and mother. Its use for the detection of neural tube defect and many other malformation syndromes is discussed in Chapters 20, 25 and 26. Ultrasonic examination may give rise to a suspicion of chromosomal abnormality, as for example detection of the cystic hygroma of a fetus with Turner's syndrome or of exomphalos in a fetus with trisomy 18, especially when the latter is associated with a heart defect (Crawford et al 1985). The cephalic index of children with Down's syndrome is reduced. This is so even at birth (author's personal observation). The hope that this might also be a consistent observation at mid-trimester fetal ultrasonography was raised by a single observation of brachycephaly in a fetus subsequently shown to have Down's syndrome (Buttery 1979). Unfortunately, this has not subsequently proved to be a consistent finding in Down's fetuses (P. Farrant, personal communication).

Chorionic villus sampling

Development of the technique

Amniocentesis, fetoscopy and fetal ultrasound scanning all suffer from the disadvantage that they cannot be done until at least the start of the second trimester. Furthermore culture of cells and their chromosomal analysis involves further delay so that mothers have an appreciable period of anxious waiting for results, and in those who proceed to termination this is perforce relatively late with increased risk of complications.

This major disadvantage led several groups of workers to explore the possibility of obtaining tissues of fetal origin for diagnosis in the first trimester. Probably the earliest reported attempts were those of Kullander & Sandahl who in 1973 reported fetal chromosomal analysis from transcervical placental biopsy in early pregnancy, and Hahnemann who in 1974 reported a similar study which had been carried out earlier. Both groups undertook their studies immediately prior to termination of pregnancy. The first report of successful prenatal diagnosis — of fetal sex — in the first trimester was from China (Department of Obstetrics and Gynaecology, Tietung Hospital 1975). Rhine and colleagues (1977) aspirated exfoliated trophoblastic tissue from the endocervical canal. A team from the USSR have also reported fetal sexing and enzyme assay on chorion biopsies taken at 6–12 weeks' gestation (Kazy et al 1982). Niazi and colleagues (1981) at St Mary's Hospital, London, reported a successful method of culture of fibroblasts from trophoblast villi.

Application to diagnosis of chromosomal abnormality and sex determination

The earliest application of this technique was in the prenatal diagnosis of haemoglobinopathies utilizing DNA methods (Williamson et al 1981, Old et al 1982) and this has continued as a major application (see also Chapter 22). Reliable fetal sex determination, using fetal karyotype analysis of chorion tissue combined with use of a Y chromosome-specific DNA probe, was also reported relatively early in the development of the clinical application of chorionic villus sampling (Gosden et al 1982).

The earliest report of prenatal diagnosis of a chromosome abnormality by this technique was that of Brambati & Simoni from Milan (1983). The authors diagnosed trisomy 21 in the fetus of a 37-year-old woman at 11 weeks' gestation by direct analysis of mitoses in the biopsy material.

The St Mary's group published the first survey of a series of biopsies performed on women about to undergo termination, and obtained chorionic villi in 40% of cases (Horwell et al 1983). Subsequent improvements in techniques, especially the use of real-time ultrasound to guide the aspirating cannula or direct vision, have led to a marked improvement in the success rate — to 90% or more (Ward et al 1983, Gustavii 1983, 1984a, Rodeck et al 1983a,b, Gustavii et al 1984, Maxwell et al 1985, Perry et al 1985b, Czepulkowski et al 1986). Further improvements in methods of processing the biopsy material have led to minimization of maternal cell contamination and rapid cell growth (Simoni et al 1983, Czepulkowski et al 1986, Heaton et al 1984). The latter has been achieved by culture with Chang medium.

Further reports of chromosome abnormalities detected in

chorion villus samples, either by direct analysis (Gregson et al 1983, MacKenzie et al 1983, Sachs et al 1983, Simoni et al 1983, Szabo et al 1984, Brambati et al 1985, Perry et al 1985) or following initial cultures (Heim et al 1985, Hogge et al 1985, 1986, Simoni et al 1986) have followed Brambati & Simoni's initial report. Most of the larger series of cases have used cultured cells for analysis rather than direct chromosomal analysis; either long-term culture (Heim et al 1985, Hogge et al 1985, 1986) or short-term (12–48 h) incubation (Simoni et al 1986). Although direct analysis provides an immediate result and avoids the risk of overgrowth of fetal by maternal cells it provides, in the hands of most cytogeneticists, fewer metaphase spreads of poorer quality than those obtained from cultured cells (Brambati et al 1983, Maxwell et al 1985, Czepulkowski et al 1986); this has resulted in chromosomal rearrangements being undetected on direct analysis, and in a few instances in detection of chromosomal aberrations not present in fetal tissue (Kalousek & Dill 1983, Liu et al 1983). Moreover maternal metaphases may even be present in direct preparations (Simoni et al 1986). There have even been reports of chromosomal abnormality, detected in long-term villus culture and confirmed in the fetus, not detectable in direct or short-term cultured preparations (Eichenbaum et al 1986, Martin et al 1986). In only one of two such cases was the fetal abnormality mosaic (Eichenbaum et al 1986).

There have also been further reports on fetal sexing for X-linked disorders in chorionic villus material. The methods used include the use of Y-specific DNA probes for rapid sexing by the dot hybridization technique (Gosden et al 1984a, b) by standard Southern blotting (Gosden et al 1984b, Lau et al 1984) and by direct chromosome analysis for fetal sexing (Lilford et al 1983, Gibbs et al 1984, Gosden et al 1984b, Simoni et al 1984); several groups have used both methods. Karyotyping has the advantage of also revealing any chromosomal abnormality that may be coincidentally present (Simoni et al 1984). The fragile X associated with mental retardation, especially in males, can be detected in cells cultured from chorionic villi, but not by direct analysis and not wholly reliably (Tommerup et al 1985).

Transabdominal chorionic villus biopsy

Some workers have preferred the transabdominal approach, with aspiration of villus tissue from the placenta, to the more widely adopted transcervical approach. Lilford's group in particular has pioneered the transabdominal approach, arguing that this reduces the risk of maternal infection or endotoxic shock (Maxwell et al 1986a). Others have reported on their experience of this approach (Bovicelli et al 1986, Gustavii et al 1986a), which seems to be gradually gaining wider acceptance. The only disadvantage of transabdominal sampling found by Bovicelli and colleagues in a comparison of the two routes was a smaller sample size. One advantage of transabdominal biopsy is that it need not be confined to the first trimester and can therefore be used to bridge the 12–16 weeks gap between transcervical biopsy and amniocentesis, or as an alternative to the latter for later diagnosis (Gustavii et al 1986b, Maxwell et al 1986b, Nicolaides et al 1986). However Szabo and colleagues (1986) claim that in certain circumstances the transcervical route can also be used in the second trimester.

Hazards

A major concern in the development of chorionic villus sampling for prenatal diagnosis has been the fear that the frequency of complications would be higher than with amniocentesis, despite the lack of such complications in the early Russian series (Kazy et al 1982), and in a more recent small Canadian series (Perry et al 1985). The main anxieties have been of induced fetal death or abortion — whether associated with fetal infection or sac rupture or not — fetomaternal haemorrhage and maternal infection. Two cases of fatal fetal Neisserial infection were reported by Kullander & Sandahl (1973). One such case was recorded in an early series of seven transcervical biopsies, done for diagnosis of a haemoglobin disorder, in which there was intrauterine death associated with infection (Petrou et al 1983); and a further isolated case of septic abortion was reported by Blakemore et al (1985). Brambati & Varotto (1985) recorded two probable cases among 700 samplings. The frequency of complications is certainly higher when blind transcervical aspiration is undertaken compared to direct vision or aspiration under ultrasound control, and there is also a lower success rate (Liu et al 1983). Mild to moderate, or even severe, maternal bleeding is fairly common following transcervical chorionic biopsy (Maxwell et al 1985).

The King's College Hospital group have assessed fetomaternal haemorrhage after chorionic villus sampling and obtained negative Kleihauer tests on all of 161 patients, but a rise in maternal serum alpha-fetoprotein in half of them, with the level of increase correlated with the number of attempts at biopsy (Warren et al 1985). As with amniocentesis all rhesus-negative women undergoing chorionic villus sampling should be given anti-D immunoglobulin.

The major problem in assessing the frequency of abortion as a result of chorionic villus sampling in the first trimester is the relatively high rate of spontaneous abortion in early pregnancy and the lack of precise data on frequency in relation to length of gestation and maternal age. Gustavii (1984b) has provided figures, which although based on relatively small numbers at the older maternal ages, do provisionally give some guidance. It is clear that the spontaneous abortion rate for older mothers (40 years and over) is appreciably increased up to the 14th week. For example, at 8 weeks' gestation a mother of 40 years or more has a 1 in 3 risk of fetal loss, compared to a 1 in 14 risk under 30 years. From 14 weeks on there appears to be no maternal age difference.

Several groups have published series in which spontaneous abortions after sampling are recorded but most do not give sufficient information for a direct comparison with Gustavii's figures (Heim et al 1985, Hogge et al 1985, Jahoda et al 1985, Jackson et al 1986, Simoni et al 1986). Taken overall they indicate a spontaneous abortion rate of about 4% following chorionic villus sampling. However there is a suggestion that the fetal loss rate has declined in the more recent studies; the figures from Philadelphia (Jackson et al 1986) are no more than those for recent amniocentesis series, as demonstrated by the authors, and probably only marginally worse than those to be expected without prenatal diagnosis. Hogge and colleagues' (1986) figures suggest higher fetal loss rates following sampling before 9 weeks and after 11 weeks than between 9 and 11 weeks' gestation, but these numbers are too small for confidence. No such dip appears in Gustavii's figures for naturally occurring spontaneous abortion.

A more informed verdict on the rate of spontaneous abortion after chorionic villus sampling compared with amniocentesis will have to await the outcome of a current controlled trial by the MRC in Britain.

QUALITY CONTROL AND INTERPRETATION OF FINDINGS

An essential element of the work of cytogenetic laboratories undertaking prenatal diagnosis is the monitoring of the outcome of pregnancies in which they have performed analyses on chorionic villus or amniotic fluid samples. In order to confirm normal findings and to confirm that fetal and not maternal cells have been analysed, they need to know the outcome of every pregnancy in which they have been involved. The required information includes whether the pregnancy ended in a termination, spontaneous abortion, live or stillbirth; the sex of the fetus or infant; and the presence or absence of clinical abnormality. Laboratories depend on maternity units to provide this information, without which they cannot ensure the continuing reliability of their reports.

Laboratories will of course need to undertake cytogenetic confirmation of any abnormality detected prenatally, either in the aborted fetus or the newborn infant. This is important in all cases, but especially in those in which mosaicism has been detected in villus tissue or only in one flask of cultured amniotic fluid cells. In such cases the mosaicism is likely to have arisen in trophoblast, or artefactually in cultures and would not be expected to be present in the fetus. However this should always be confirmed. Abortuses, stillborn infants and those dying in the neonatal period should have an autopsy by a paediatric pathologist, especially where the more uncommon chromosomal abnormalities are concerned. Where a female karyotype is detected antenatally there may be some doubt as to whether the cells are of fetal rather than maternal origin. A laboratory may wish to check this by looking for chromosomal polymorphisms of paternal origin in the putative fetal cells. Alternative methods are human leukocyte antigen determination of the parental and fetal cells or the use of DNA polymorphisms, especially those associated with minisatellite DNA or other hypervariable loci. The DNA approach has not yet been reported in this context but would be more convenient to use if the new non-radioactive biotin-labelled probes were adapted to this purpose.

Parental karyotypes may also need to be determined when a chromosomal abnormality is detected prenatally. This is important when a translocation, balanced or unbalanced, an inversion, small deletion or other complex rearrangement is found. If a balanced translocation is found in a normal parent then a similar translocation in the fetus is unlikely to be a cause of clinical abnormality. Balanced Robertsonian translocations (fusion of acrocentric chromosomes with loss of inessential short arm DNA) are invariably without direct phenotypic effect. However, balanced reciprocal translocations, although usually harmless, are not always so. Similarly inversions are usually harmless but cannot be assumed to be so. The commonest inversion, that of the pericentric region of chromosome 9, is virtually a normal variant but if it extends beyond the pericentric heterochromatin could have clinical significance. Unbalanced fetal chromosomal rearrangements do of course nearly always carry grave implications. From time to time small marker chromosomes, with or without satellites, are detected on prenatal diagnosis. Sometimes special stains indicate an origin from chromosome 15 but otherwise the precise origin is uncertain. When these prove to be familial they are harmless and a good prognosis can be given for the child. However when parental karyotyping indicates that a marker chromosome has developed de novo there is a high risk of clinical abnormality, of the order of 10–30% (Warburton 1982).

When a balanced rearrangement is found in a parent, other relatives as well as the parents themselves may need investigation and counselling because of the risk of transmission of the rearrangement in an unbalanced form.

INDICATIONS FOR CYTOGENETIC PRENATAL DIAGNOSIS

Maternal age

By far the most common indication for prenatal cytogenetic diagnosis, either chorionic villus sampling or amniocentesis, is high maternal age. The decision as to the cut-off age to use in offering prenatal diagnosis to mothers is by its nature arbitrary and different centres use different ages, mostly between 35 and 40 years. The precise risks differ slightly among the published studies but for women of 33 years and over the risk figures given in Table 21.2, based on the estimates of E. B. Hook (Hook et al 1983), are as reliable as any for the findings at amniocentesis or livebirth. Compar-

Table 21.2 Outcome of first-trimester chorionic villus sampling in published series

Authors	No. of diagnostic cases analysed	No. abnormal: Chromosomal	No. abnormal: Biochemical	No. abnormal: Male sex in X-linked disorders	No. of pregnancies terminated	Fetal losses (% of those not terminated): Spontaneous abortions	Fetal losses: Late losses	Fetal losses: Total
Heim et al (1985)	80	6	0	2	8	6(8.3)		
Jahoda et al (1985)	294	11		11	22	9(5.3)*		
Hogge et al (1985, 1986)	983	50	3	8	43	51(5.4)	15(1.6)	66(7.0)
Simoni et al (1986)	986	70	Not stated	22	56	39(5.8)†	7(1.0)	46(6.8)
Jackson et al (1986)	846				75	17(2.2)	5(0.7)	22(2.9)

* In a control amniocentesis series there were 9/134 spontaneous abortions (6.7%). In both the chorion villus and the amniocentesis series the spontaneous abortions reported relate only up to 16 weeks' gestation.

† Fetal losses are for 677 concluded pregnancies that were not terminated. This study was based on two centres: Milan and Genoa. The spontaneous abortion rate for Milan was appreciably lower than in Genoa—4% compared to 9.3%. This difference may have been related to a higher number of sampling attempts in Genoa.

able figures for the findings in the first trimester are not yet available but would be expected to be somewhat higher, especially for trisomies 13 and 18. One factor, at least within public health services such as the UK National Health Service, influencing the choice of cut-off age is unfortunately the resources available for laboratory cultures and analysis. The growth of demand for cytogenetic analysis in recent years is such that few hospital laboratories have all the staff and equipment to meet the full potential demand for their services and they find themselves obliged to place restrictions on the indications for which they will accept samples, unlike a commercial laboratory that can expand to meet demand. This difficulty necessitates close liaison between the laboratory and its client clinicians. However this does have the counter advantage that the clinician gets sound advice on when to undertake prenatal diagnosis and on the interpretation of results.

When resources permit, an increased uptake of facilities for prenatal diagnosis on higher maternal age groups can be achieved by professional education and early pregnancy counselling (Knott et al 1986).

The observation by Merkatz and colleagues (1984) of a correlation between low maternal serum alpha-fetoprotein levels and fetal trisomy raised the possibility of an alternative, or preferably complementary, method of selecting mothers for chromosomal prenatal diagnosis. This observation was rapidly confirmed (Chard et al 1984, Cuckle et al 1984, Fuhrmann et al 1984, Tabor et al 1984, Baumgarten et al 1985) by several centres and there is a relatively low maternal serum alpha-fetoprotein even in the additional presence of a neural tube defect or ventral wall defect (Macri et al 1986). Cuckle and colleagues (1984) have proposed the use of a scale of cut-off values for maternal serum alpha-fetoprotein related to maternal age for selection of patients for amniocentesis. The only study failing to find a low mean maternal serum alpha-fetoprotein in Down's syndrome pregnancies assayed the alpha-fetoprotein on samples stored for up to 3 years (Cowchock & Ruch 1984). Amniotic fluid alpha-fetoprotein also tends to be low in the presence of a Down's fetus, but is curiously not related to other trisomies (Tabor et al 1984, Cuckle et al 1985a, Davis et al 1985, Hullin et al 1985, Nelson & Petersen 1985, Doran et al 1986, Jones et al 1986, Trigg et al 1986).

Several workers have expressed reservations about using maternal serum alpha-fetoprotein to select women for amniocentesis on the grounds of a too high false positive rate (7–12%) necessitating too many amniocenteses on women with an unaffected fetus (Houlsby 1984, Seller 1984, Spencer & Carpenter 1985, Wyatt 1985), with consequent maternal anxiety and some increase in miscarriages. In response to these criticisms Cuckle and colleagues (1985) point out that pooling the results of published studies and applying their age-related cut-offs, a 30% detection rate could be expected for Down's syndrome with an $11\frac{1}{2}$% false positive rate. The authors believe this justifies at least a pilot study. Murday & Slack (1985) tested Cuckle and colleagues' (1985b) proposed strategy against their own experience in the north-east Thames region of the National Health Service. They concluded that the measurement of maternal serum alpha-fetoprotein is only useful in women aged 32 years and over as risks below this age are too low, even with a very low serum alpha-fetoprotein. Since some previous studies have included women below that age this limitation reduces the number of unnecessary amniocenteses. In Murday & Slack's study if 50% of women of 32 years and over with a combined risk of 1 in 200 or greater for Down's syndrome had amniocenteses this would have generated 800–900 additional amniocenteses over a 1-year period. Ultrasound confirmation of gestational age along with exclusion of all cases with maternal serum alpha-fetoprotein greater than 2.5 multiples of the median would further reduce the number of amniocenteses. Hershey and colleagues (1986) have also calculated birth risks combining maternal age and serum alpha-fetoprotein; their results gave appreciably higher risks. Similar but less complete calculations have been presented by Martin & Liu (1986), using different assumptions regarding the sensitivity and specificity of maternal serum alpha-fetoprotein assay. These authors suggest—rather unconvincingly — that when prospective studies provide better estimates of sensitivity and specificity, age criteria may become obsolete. Martin & Liu are certainly correct that wholly reliable risk figures will only comes from prospective studies.

Maternal serum alpha-fetoprotein is also lower in trisomic pregnancies at the time of chorionic villus sampling in the first trimester (Brambati et al 1986). This gives hope that it could be used for screening at this earlier stage of pregnancy with the prospect of early termination of detected trisomic fetuses for those mothers requesting this.

A further marked improvement in the antenatal detection of Down's syndrome comes with the additional assay of human chorionic gonadotrophin (Bogart et al 1987) and unconjugated oestriol (Wald et al 1988a) in maternal serum. When these two assays are combined with that for maternal serum alpha-fetoprotein and with maternal age, Wald and colleagues (1988b) estimate that 60% of affected pregnancies would be detected at a similar amniocentesis rate to that in existing programmes. Even better detection might be achieved with the addition of fetal femur length:biparietal diameter ratio ultrasonic measurement (Lockwood et al 1987, Benacerraf et al 1987).

Previous child with chromosomal abnormality

Apart from maternal age there are several further indications for prenatal diagnosis of chromosomal abnormality. One of the relatively common indications is a previous child with a chromosomal abnormality. Following the birth of a child with trisomic Down's syndrome the risk to the parents of having a further Down's child is about 1 in 200 up to a maternal age of 35 years and about twice the population age risk from 35 years on (Mikkelsen 1979). There is some evidence that there may be a rather higher recurrence risk at very young maternal ages and that the risk of Down's syndrome and other trisomies is also increased after the birth of a trisomy other than Down's syndrome. The risk for all chromosomal abnormalities, following the birth of a Down's child, is about double that for Down's syndrome itself, at either birth or amniocentesis.

Where one or other parent has mosaic trisomy 21 the risk for children should be regarded as high, although it is not possible to measure this risk. Only about 30 cases of Down's syndrome women having a child have been reported. One-third of the children born to these women had Down's syndrome and this proportion holds good where both mother and child have had a chromosomal analysis (Bovicelli et al 1982). There are no reports of proven paternity by a non-mosaic Down's syndrome man. In one case studied by the author (in preparation) red cell blood groups and white cell human leukocyte antigen phenotypes were compatible with a Down's husband being the father of his wife's normal daughter. However minisatellite DNA analysis excluded paternity, which may have been by an untested male relative.

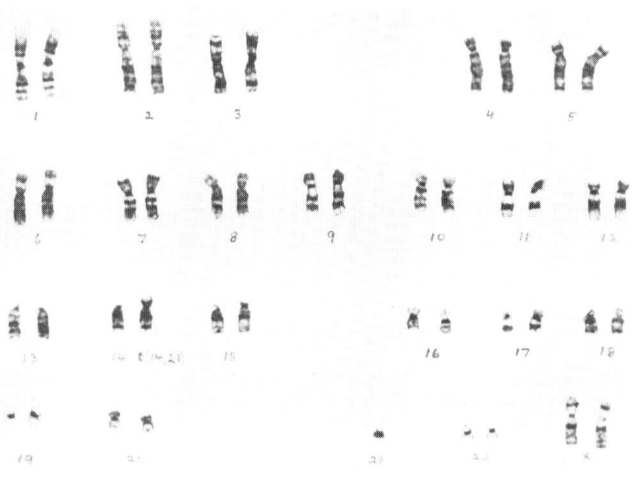

Fig. 21.3 G-banded karyotype of clinically normal female patient with a balanced Robertsonian translocation between chromosomes 14 and 21.

Apart from a previous child with aneuploidy there are several inherited disorders with increased frequency of chromosome instability. In Fanconi's anaemia there are increased numbers of non-specific chromosomal breaks and chromatid rearrangements involving non-homologous chromosomes (Schroeder & German 1974). Bloom's syndrome also has frequent non-specific chromatid breaks but exchanges tend to involve homologous chromosomes and are most readily demonstrated in the form of increased sister–chromatid exchanges (Chaganti et al 1974, Schroeder & German 1974). A third syndrome of chromosomal instability is ataxia-telangiectasia but here breaks at 14q 12 are specifically involved, and also pericentric inversions of chromosome 7 (Oxford et al 1975). A distinct chromosomal abnormality, centromeric puffing, is seen in Robert's syndrome (Tomkins et al 1979). All of these syndromes are inherited in an autosomal recessive manner and therefore carry a 1 in 4 recurrence risk in siblings. They should be detectable at prenatal diagnosis by appropriate techniques of chromosomal analysis.

Parental chromosomal rearrangement

Apart from parental Down's syndrome or other aneuploidy a parental balanced chromosomal rearrangement, or marker chromosome, carries the highest risk for a clinically abnormal unbalanced rearrangement in a child. Balanced translocations are of two types: centric fusions, or Robertsonian translocations, in which two acrocentric chromosomes (pairs 13, 14, 15, 21 and 22) fuse together; and reciprocal translocations in which breaks occur in any two chromosomes and fragments are exchanged. Balanced Robertsonian translocations themselves produce no phenotypic abnormality (Fig. 21.3) but may be transmitted in an unbalanced form (see Fig. 21.2). In the most common example, a 14;21 translocation, the effectively 14 trisomic unbalanced offspring is lethal, as would be any monosomic offspring and is not seen either at amniocentesis or birth. The surviving offspring are chromosomally normal, have a balanced 14;21 translocation like the parent, or have an unbalanced translocation with effective trisomy 21 and Down's syndrome. The frequency of the different products of this translocation and other rearrangements was assessed in a collaborative European study (Boue 1979). Frequency depends on whether the carrier parent is male or female. Where the father carries the 14;21 translocation less than 1% of children will have Down's syndrome due to the unbalanced form of the translocation, with 40% being normal and 60% having the balanced translocation. Where the mother carries the translocation the risk is higher, the comparable percentages being 13, 35 and 52% respectively. The available data for other Robertsonian translocations involve smaller numbers and are less reliable but indicate similar proportions for 21;22 and a lower unbalanced frequency (0.7%) for 13;14 translocations. Robertsonian translocations between homologous chromosomes, as for example 21;21, are devastating obstetrically as all offspring will be either trisomic or lethally monosomic. The carrier of such a translocation cannot have a normal child.

Reciprocal translocations are more varied and their consequences less predictable. Balanced reciprocal translocations, like Robertsonian ones, usually produce no clinical abnormality. However in the case of reciprocals this is not invariable as the breakpoint may disrupt a gene or produce a position effect and it is difficult always to be sure that reciprocal translocations are truly balanced. If an apparently balanced reciprocal translocation is present in several healthy members of a family then it can be accepted as being without clinical effect. A de novo reciprocal translocation in a neonate, if balanced, can be accepted as indicative of a low risk (about 10%) for siblings; but of a high risk if unbalanced. The risk of clinical abnormality in the children of carriers of balanced reciprocal translocations varies with the chromosomes involved and the method of ascertainment. When detected through a previous fetus or child or other close relative with an unbalanced translocation recurrence risks are likely to be high; when ascertained as a chance finding of the balanced translocation, risks for the unbalanced state will be lower.

Similar arguments apply to inversions. A pericentric inversion segregating in a family with no history of abnormal children will carry a low risk, whereas an inversion detected through a child with an unbalanced duplication–deletion product of the parental inversion implies a relatively high risk for siblings.

When a balanced rearrangement is found the carrier should be offered prenatal diagnosis. This is clearly important when the risks are high, but even with relatively low risks (1% or less) it should still be offered as this is still substantially higher than the population risk of a chromosomally abnormal child. When the risks for children are considered to be appreciable it may also be necessary to investigate all relatives who are at risk of carrying the balanced rearrangement; this frequently involves a substantial family study.

Occasionally a fetus is found at amniocentesis or chorion villus sampling to carry a supernumerary small marker chromosome. The origin of such chromosomes is often obscure. Many carry satellites and they can be assumed to derive from acrocentric chromosomes. In a few, DAPI staining may indicate derivation from chromosome 15. When these chromosomes prove to be familial they are usually harmless but, as discussed earlier, when de novo they carry a high risk of fetal abnormality (Warburton 1982).

Recurrent miscarriage is not of itself an indication for prenatal diagnosis. As discussed earlier, if a mother presents in early pregnancy with such a history she and her husband should have a chromosomal analysis if this has not already been done. Only if an abnormality is found should prenatal diagnosis be considered.

Sex determination

Sex determination may be requested in the first or second trimester when there is known to be a risk of the fetus having an X-linked recessive disorder. Chromosomal analysis is the preferred method. Sex chromatin examination is not sufficiently reliable. Ultrasound visualization of the external genitalia can also be misleading since male genitalia may be missed or a short length of cord misinterpreted as a penis. Probes for Y chromosomal repetitive DNA performed on DNA extracted directly from a chorionic villus sample is a quick and reliable method and may be used to provide an immediate answer. However full chromosomal analysis provides information on any chromosomal abnormality that might be coincidentally present, as well as on chromosomal sex.

Fetal sex determination alone may be used when there is a high risk of a severely handicapping X-linked recessive disorder for which prenatal diagnosis is not feasible. For example, if the mother is known on pedigree evidence to be a carrier then a male fetus will have a 1 in 2 risk of being affected — a risk high enough to justify termination if the mother so wishes. A female fetus will at worst only be a carrier. Even when specific prenatal diagnosis is available sex determination is a necessary adjunct as the finding of a female fetus will take the urgency out of the situation, whereas that of a male fetus will indicate that it is necessary to establish as soon as possible whether or not he is affected.

FUTURE DEVELOPMENTS IN PRENATAL DIAGNOSIS FOR CHROMOSOMAL DISORDER

Screening methods

At present we lack reliable simple screening methods for the early detection of fetal chromosomal disorders. The value of a low maternal serum alpha-fetoprotein as an indicator of possible fetal trisomy has already been discussed. Although a potentially useful approach, especially when combined with maternal age, it is not sensitive or specific enough to be the ideal screening method. As also already discussed, prenatal high-resolution fetal ultrasound may alert the operator to the possibility of chromosomal disorder but is not sensitive enough to be a general screening method. Unfortunately in the near future there is no other technique likely to provide a screening method superior to these, except possibly the isolation of fetal cells from maternal circulation.

Isolation of fetal cells from the maternal circulation

It is known from studies of rhesus isoimmunization that small numbers of fetal cells, including white blood cells (Freese & Titel 1963) and trophoblast cells (Covone et al 1984), cross the placental barrier to enter the maternal circulation throughout pregnancy. Theoretically if these could be isolated from the mother's blood they could be used for chromosomal analysis as well as for biochemical or DNA analysis. Several groups of workers have attempted to do this. The general approach of most such studies has been to incubate cells from the mother's blood with fluorochromatic dyes bound to antibodies specific for paternal HLA or fetal antigens. The fetal cells are then sorted from the maternal cells on a fluorescence-activated cell sorter. This method at present only yields a cell mixture enriched in fetal cells rather than a pure fetal cell population. Furthermore, too few fetal cells are isolated from any reasonably sized maternal blood sample to be of practical value. Whether or not the efficiency of this or any other method could be improved sufficiently to yield enough pure fetal cells for diagnosis remains to be seen.

Flow cytometry of fetal chromosomes from cell cultures

A theoretical alternative to microscopic analysis of cultured fetal cells would be chromosomal analysis on a fluorescence-activated cell sorter, using DNA-binding fluorochromes. The sorter generates a series of peaks, each one representative of those chromosomes giving the same amount of fluorescence. This in turn reflects the amount of DNA in the chromosomes, which is roughly related to chromosome length. The height of each peak is indicative of the number of chromosomes of the specified relative fluorescence (Fig. 21.4). The procedure thus generates a series of peaks with a characteristic normal profile which is subject to minor normal variation. Aneuploid cells or cells in which a chromosomal rearrangement alters the length of one or more chromosomes will give an abnormal profile.

At present this technique is a valuable research tool. However the equipment is expensive and the analysis requires a substantial yield of cultured cells and the constant attention of the operator while the profile is being generated. It is possible that future developments in the equipment will permit a more automated procedure than at present and will increase the sensitivity of the machine in measuring fluorescence of chromosomes, but currently it does not offer any advantage over current methods of chromosomal analysis, except for occasional selected cases.

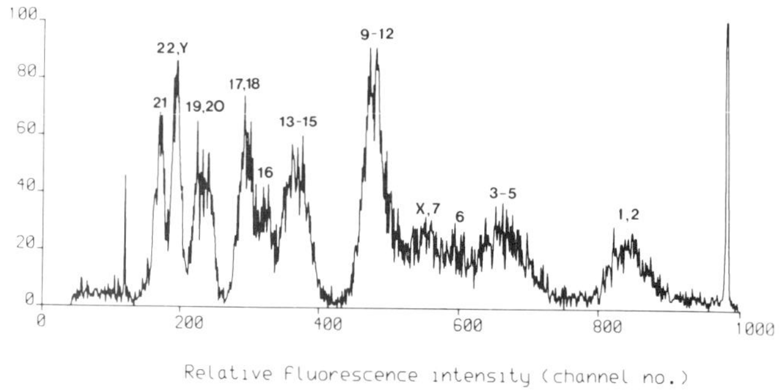

Fig. 21.4 Flow profile of the chromosomes of a normal male subject generated by a fluoresence activated cell sorter.

Automation and standardization of cultures and microscopical techniques

Considerable effort has gone into the development of automated methods of chromosomal analysis using a 'flying spot' microscope slide scanner linked to a computer programmed to analyse the images constructed by the scanner. These programmes can be designed to recognize metaphase spreads for analysis by the operator or to display a karyotype on a visual display unit; an editing facility can be built in. In theory such an assembly should be able to eliminate many hours of direct visual microscopic analysis by highly paid scientific staff in cytogenetic laboratories. Nevertheless such systems have not come into widespread use. This is partly due to the high capital cost of such systems and partly to the fact that most were developed before chromosome banding became routine. It is much more difficult to achieve successful scanning of bands than of whole chromosomes, as the quality of differential staining varies enormously from cell to cell and even from chromosome to chromosome, in a way that the experienced cytogeneticist can evaluate. It is virtually impossible to write a computer program that could cope effectively with the degree of variation routinely seen.

The development of practical routine automated analysis will probably have to await improvements in the techniques of chromosome preparation, including culture, harvesting and staining, that will give results of consistently much higher quality than at present.

Cell culture and harvesting are also procedures that give variable end-results. Again the achievement of consistently high mitotic rates and well spread metaphases awaits better techniques, one of which is a fully defined culture medium including appropriate growth factors or mitogens. When this has been achieved it will be possible both to automate these procedures and to provide standardized material for analysis.

DNA probes

Reference has been made at the beginning of this chapter to the use of DNA probes for chromosomal analysis. A panel of probes, each specific for a particular chromosome arm or region, could be used in place of microscopic analysis, either by Southern blotting techniques, or by in situ hybridization in interphase cells (Pinkel et al 1986). This approach has already been used with probes for Y chromosomal heterochromatin in sex determination, but for other chromosomes would have to be analysed on a gene dosage basis. Its more general use, as for example for the detection of the common trisomies, has still to be evaluated. Probes that have been regionally localized within a short chromosome segment can be used for in situ hybridization as discussed earlier, to detect small deletions or other arrangements that may not be detectable microscopically. The author, working in collaboration with Dr Mattei, has used this approach to decide whether a small terminal deletion of the short arm of chromosome 18 segregating in a family is balanced or not.

The recent improvement in sensitivity of non-autoradiographic methods of probe labelling and their likely continuing improvement may lead to a wide application of these techniques in cytogenetics.

ETHICAL ISSUES

The ethical issues involved in prenatal diagnosis have been discussed elsewhere (Crawfurd 1983, 1988, Crawford et al 1988). Termination of pregnancy for an inevitably lethal fetal abnormality is relatively uncontroversial, as in for example the detection of a lethal chromosomal anomaly such as trisomy 13. Termination for a severely handicapping abnormality, or especially for a high risk of such an abnormality, is highly controversial. Probably the majority of women in the UK would wish to have a pregnancy terminated where the fetus could be shown to be severely handicapped and many feel that they should have the right to termination entirely at their own discretion. Others, on religious grounds or from a general conscientious objection, feel that such termination is only permissible if there is a threat to the mother's life.

A doctor who has such conscientious objections is not obliged to collaborate in prenatal diagnosis or termination. However if he sees a patient who wishes, or might wish to have this done he should refer her to a colleague willing to undertake such work. The touchstone in all such situations is the wishes of the patient within the law and failure to give appropriate advice or to refer to a colleague who will do so could be negligent.

Increasingly the medical profession is having to recognize that it is not sufficient to listen to a patient's request and then give positive advice, for that is directive counselling. Patients should be advised on the risks of abnormality in the fetus and on the advantages and disadvantages of possible options so that they can make informed decisions for themselves. This implies adequate counselling before prenatal diagnosis, including the opportunity to opt out of any screening test. It also implies that if the woman opts for prenatal diagnosis proper procedures are followed with the right equipment and a skilled experienced operator, or at least a trainee under skilled supervision, a competent laboratory and prompt efficient follow-up of results. When abnormality is detected further counselling may be necessary before the patient decides whether or not to proceed to termination. This is especially so where a chromosomal abnormality other than Down's syndrome is detected, when the parents will have no prior understanding of the implications.

The concept of informed consent is vital where a mother is being invited to participate in a trial as, for example, of a new method of prenatal diagnosis. Great care must always be exercised by the research worker not to allow his enthusiasm to abuse the patient's willingness to help.

At the laboratory level there are differing views on what to report to the clinician. There are two problems. The first is whether or not to report a full karyotype with a detailed description of all the normal variations present or only an abbreviated karyotype distinguishing between normal and abnormal. This is best resolved by discussion between the laboratory and the clinicians it serves. The second problem is more difficult. Many laboratories report the karyotype of the fetus, full or abbreviated, including a statement of the sex chromosomal constitution. Others do this if any abnormality has been found but otherwise merely report that no abnormality has been detected. The reason for this practice is that some patients when given the full result will seek an abortion, contrary to the intention of the 1967 Abortion Act, if the sex is not that wished. This is likely to become a more prevalent practice with the increasing availability of early chorionic villus sampling. Certainly the laboratory has no right to withhold the full result from the clinician if he requests it, or in the case of a private laboratory from a patient with direct access. Again the procedure needs to be agreed between the laboratory and its clinical colleagues.

REFERENCES

Affara N A, Ferguson-Smith M A, Tolmie J et al 1986 Variable transfer of Y-specific sequences in XX males. Nucleic Acids Research 14: 5375–5387

Austin C R 1962 Sex chromatin in embryonic and fetal tissue. Acta Cytologica 6: 61–68

Bartsch F K, Lundberg J, Wahlstrom J 1980 One thousand consecutive midtrimester amniocenteses. Obstetrics and Gynecology 55: 305–308

Baumgarten A, Schoenfeld M, Mahoney M J, Greenstein R M, Saal H M 1985 Prospective screening for Down syndrome using maternal serum AFP. Lancet i: 1280–1281

Bavin J T R, Marshall R, Delhanty J D A 1963 A mongol with a 21:22 type chromosomal translocation. Journal of Mental Deficiency Research 7: 84–89
Benacerraf B R, Gelman R, Frigoletto F D 1987 Sonographic identification of second-trimester fetuses with Down's syndrome. New England Journal of Medicine 317: 1371–1376
Blakemore K J, Mahoney M J, Hobbins J C 1985 Infection and chorionic villus sampling. Lancet ii: 339
Bogart M H, Pandian M R, Jones O W 1987 Abnormal maternal serum chorionic gonadotrophin levels in pregnancies with fetal chromosome abnormalities. Prenatal Diagnosis 7: 623–630
Boue A 1979 European collaborative study on structural chromosome anomalies in prenatal diagnosis. In: Murken J D, Stengel-Rutkowski S, Schwinger E (eds) Proceedings of the third European conference on prenatal diagnosis of genetic disorders. Enke, Stuttgart, pp 34–54
Boue J, Morer I, Laisney V, Boue A 1979 Diagnostic prénatals. Résultats de 1532 ponctions amniotiques et étude prospective de 1023 cas. Nouvelle Presse Médicale 8: 2949–2953
Bovicelli L, Orsini L F, Rizzo N, Montacuti V, Bacchetta M 1982 Reproduction in Down syndrome. Obstetrics and Gynecology (suppl) 59: 13S–17S
Bovicelli L, Rizzo N, Montacuti V, Morandi R 1986 Transabdominal versus transcervical routes for chorionic villus sampling. Lancet ii: 290
Brambati B, Simoni G 1983 Diagnosis of fetal trisomy 21 in first trimester. Lancet i: 586
Brambati B, Varotto F 1985 Infection and chorionic villus sampling. Lancet ii: 609
Brambati B, Oldrini A, Simoni G et al 1983 First trimester fetal karyotyping in twin pregnancy. Journal of Medical Genetics 20: 58–60
Brambati B, Simoni G, Danesino C et al 1985 First trimester fetal diagnosis of genetic disorders: clinical evaluation of 250 cases. Journal of Medical Genetics 22: 92–99
Brambati B, Simoni G, Bonacci I, Piceni L 1986 Fetal chromosomal aneuploidies and maternal serum alpha-fetoprotein levels in first trimester. Lancet ii: 165–166
Broome D L, Kellogg B, Weiss B A, Wilson M G 1975 Needle puncture of the fetus during amniocentesis. Lancet ii: 604
Buttery B 1979 Occipitofrontal-biparietal diameter ratio: an ultrasonic parameter for the antenatal evaluation of Down's syndrome. Medical Journal of Australia 2: 1662–1664
Carter C O, Hamerton J L, Polani P E, Gunalp A, Weller S D V 1986 Chromosome translocation as a cause of familial mongolism. Lancet ii: 678–680
Caspersson T, Zech L, Johansson C 1970 Analysis of human metaphase chromosome set by aid of DNA-binding fluorescent agents. Experimental Cell Research 62: 490–492
Chaganti R S K, Schonberg S, German J 1974 A many-fold increase in sister chromatid exchanges in Bloom's syndrome lymphocytes. Proceedings of the National Academy of Sciences (USA) 71: 4508–4512
Chard T, Lowings C, Kitau M J 1984 Alphafetoprotein and chorionic gonadotrophin levels in relation to Down's syndrome. Lancet ii: 750
Cordesius E, Gustavii B, Mitelman F 1980 Prenatal chromosomal analysis of fetal blood obtained at fetoscopy. British Medical Journal 1: 1107
Covone A E, Muton D, Johnson P M, Adinolfi M 1984 Trophoblast cells in peripheral blood from pregnant women. Lancet ii: 841–843
Cowchock F S, Ruch D A 1984 Low maternal serum AFP and Down syndrome. Lancet ii: 161–162
Crandall B F, Lebherz T B, Rubinstein L et al 1980 Chromosome findings in 2500 second-trimester amniocenteses. American Journal of Medical Genetics 5: 345–356
Crawford D C, Chapman M G, Allan L D 1985 Echocardiography in the investigation of anterior abdominal wall defects in the fetus. British Journal of Obstetrics and Gynaecology 92: 1034–1036
Crawfurd M d'A 1983 Prenatal diagnosis: ethical and legal aspects. British Medical Bulletin 39: 310–314
Crawfurd M d'A 1988 Ethical guidelines in fetal medicine. Fetal Therapy (in press)
Crawfurd M d'A, Cooke P, Harper P S 1988 Guideline on medico-legal aspects of medical genetics: a discussion document prepared by a working party of the Clinical Genetics Society. Clinical Genetics Society, London
Cuckle H S, Wald N J, Lindenbaum R H 1984 Maternal serum alpha-fetoprotein measurement: a screening test for Down's syndrome. Lancet i: 926–929
Cuckle H S, Wald N S, Lindenbaum R H, Jonasson J 1985 Amniotic fluid AFP levels and Down syndrome. Lancet i: 290–291
Cuckle H S, Wald N J, Lindenbaum R H 1985 Screening for Down's syndrome using serum alpha-fetoprotein. British Medical Journal 291: 349
Curtis J D, Cohen W N, Richerson H B, White C A 1972 The importance of placental localization preceding amniocentesis. Obstetrics and Gynecology 40: 194–198
Czepulkowski B H, Heaton D E, Kearney L U, Rodeck C H, Coleman D V 1986 Chorionic villus culture for first trimester diagnosis of chromosome defects: evaluation by two London centres. Prenatal Diagnosis 6: 271–282
Daffos F, Forestier F, Grangeot-Keros L et al 1984 Prenatal diagnosis of congenital rubella. Lancet ii: 1–3
Daniel A, Stewart L, Saville T et al 1982 Prenatal diagnosis in 3000 women for chromosome, X-linked and metabolic disorders. American Journal of Medical Genetics 11: 61–75
Davis R O, Cosper P, Huddleston J F et al 1985 Decreased levels of amniotic fluid alpha-fetoprotein associated with Down syndrome. American Journal of Obstetrics and Gynecology 153: 541–544
Department of Obstetrics and Gynaecology, Tietung Hospital Anshan 1975 Fetal sex prediction by sex chromatin of chorionic villi cells during early pregnancy. Chinese Medical Journal 1: 117–126
Desmonts G, Daffos F, Forestier F, Capella-Pavlovsky M, Thulliez Ph, Chartier M 1985 Prenatal diagnosis of congenital toxoplasmosis. Lancet i: 500–503
Diernaes E, Filtenborg J A, Hasch E 1982 Three years' experience with prenatal diagnosis in a Danish county. Lancet ii: 1044–1045
Donlon T A, Lalande M, Wyman A, Bruns G, Latt S A 1986 Isolation of molecular probes associated with the chromosome 15 instability in the Prader–Willi syndrome. Proceedings of the National Academy of Sciences (USA) 83: 4408–4412
Doran T A, Cadesky K, Wong P Y, Mastrogiacomo C, Capello T 1986 Maternal serum alpha-fetoprotein and fetal autosomal trisomies. American Journal of Obstetrics and Gynecology 154: 277–281
Edwards J M, Harnden D G, Cameron A H, Crosse V M, Wolff O H 1960 A new trisomic syndrome. Lancet i: 787–790
Eichenbaum S Z, Krumins E J, Fortune D W, Duke J 1986 False-negative finding on chorionic villus sampling. Lancet ii: 391
Fairweather D V I, Walker W J 1964 Obstetrical considerations in the routine use of amniocentesis in immunized Rh negative women. Journal of Obstetrics and Gynaecology of the British Commonwealth 71: 48–53
Ford C E, Hamerton J L 1956 The chromosomes of man. Nature 178: 1020–1023
Ford C E, Jones K W, Polani P E, de Almeida J C, Briggs J H 1969 A sex chromosome anomaly in a case of gonadal dysgenesis (Turner's syndrome). Lancet i: 711–713
Freese U E, Titel J H 1963 Demonstration of fetal erythrocytes in the maternal circulation. Obstetrics and Gynecology 22: 527–532
Fuchs F 1971 Amniocentesis and abortion: methods and risks. Birth Defects Original Article Series 7: 18–19
Fuchs F, Riis P 1956 Antenatal sex determination. Nature 177: 330
Fuhrmann W, Wendt P, Weitzel H K 1984 Maternal serum-AFP as screening test for Down syndrome. Lancet ii: 413
Galjaard H 1976 European experience with prenatal diagnosis of congenital disease: a survey of 6121 cases. Cytogenetics Cell Genetics 16: 453–467
Gerbie A B, Nadler H L, Gerbie M V 1971 Amniocentesis in genetic counselling: safety and reliability in early pregnancy. American Journal of Obstetrics and Gynecology 109: 765–770
Gibbs D A, McFadyen I R, Crawfurd M d'A et al 1984 First-trimester diagnosis of Lesch-Nyhan syndrome. Lancet ii: 1180–1183
Gillberg C, Ramussen P, Wahlstrom J 1982 Long-term follow-up of children born after amniocentesis. Clinical Genetics 21: 69–73
Giraud F, Ayme S, Mattei J F, Mattei G M 1976 Constitutional chromosome breakage. Human Genetics 34: 125–136
Golbus N S, Loughman W D, Epstein C J, Halbasch G, Stephens J D, Hall B D 1979 Prenatal genetic diagnosis in 3000 amniocenteses. New England Journal of Medicine 300: 157–163
Gosden J R, Gosden C M, Christie S, Morsman J M, Rodeck C H 1984a Rapid fetal sex determination in first trimester prenatal diagnosis by dot hybridisation of DNA probes. Lancet i: 540–541

Gosden J R, Gosden C M, Christie S, Cooke H J, Mosman J M, Rodeck C H 1984b The use of cloned Y chromosome-specific DNA probes for fetal sex determination in first trimester prenatal diagnosis. Human Genetics 66: 347–351
Gosden C, Rodeck C H, Nicolaides K H, Campbell S, Eason P, Sharp J C 1985 Fetal blood chromosome analysis: some new indications for prenatal karyotyping. British Journal of Obstetrics and Gynaecology 92: 915–920
Gosden J R, Mitchell A R, Gosden C M, Rodeck C H, Morsman J M 1982 Direct vision chorion biopsy and chromosome-specific DNA probes for determination of fetal sex in first-trimester prenatal diagnosis. Lancet ii: 1416–1419
Gregson N M, Seabright M 1983 Handling chorionic villi for direct chromosome studies. Lancet ii: 1491
Greasman W T, Lawrence R A, Thiede H A 1968 Fetal complications of amniocentesis. Journal of the American Medical Association 204: 91–94
Gustavii B 1983 First-trimester chromosomal analysis of chorionic villi obtained by direct vision technique. Lancet ii: 507–508
Gustavii B 1984a Chorionic villi sampling under direct vision. Clinical Genetics 26: 297–300
Gustavii B 1984b Chorionic biopsy and miscarriage in the first trimester. Lancet i: 562
Gustavii B, Chester M A, Edvall H et al 1984 First-trimester diagnosis on chorionic villi obtained by direct vision technique. Human Genetics 65: 373–376
Gustavii B, Edvall H, Dahlander K, Jonsson N, Carlen B 1986a Transabdominal chorionic villus sampling. Lancet i: 440–441
Gustavii B, Edvall H, Szalenius E, Dahlander K, Jorgensen C 1986b Second trimester chorionic villus (placental) biopsy. Lancet i: 969
Hahnemann N 1974 Early prenatal diagnosis: a study of biopsy techniques and cell culturing from extra-embryonic membrane. Clinical Genetics 6: 294–306
Heaton D E, Czepulkowski B H, Horwell D H, Coleman D V 1984 Chromosome analysis of first trimester chorionic villus biopsies prepared by a maceration technique. Prenatal Diagnosis 4: 279–287
Heim S, Kristoffersson U, Mandahl N et al 1985 Chromosome analysis in 100 cases of first trimester trophoblast sampling. Clinical Genetics 27: 451–457
Hershey D W, Crandall B F, Perdue S 1986 Combining maternal age and serum alpha-fetoprotein to predict the risk of Down syndrome. Obstetrics and Gynecology 68: 177–180
Hobbins J C, Mahoney M J 1978 Fetal blood drawing. Lancet ii: 107–109
Hogge W A, Schonberg S A, Golbus M S 1985 Prenatal diagnosis by chorionic villus sampling: lessons of the first 600 cases. Prenatal Diagnosis 5: 393–400
Hogge W A, Schonberg S A, Golbus M S 1986 Chorionic villus sampling: experience of the first 1000 cases. American Journal of Obstetrics and Gynecology 154: 1249–1252
Hook E B, Cross P K, Schreinemachers D M 1983 Chromosomal abnormality rates at amniocentesis and in live-born infants. Journal of the American Medical Association 249: 2034–2038
Horwell D H, Loeffler F E, Coleman D V 1983 Assessment of transcervical aspiration technique for chorionic villus biopsy in the first trimester of pregnancy. British Journal of Obstetrics and Gynaecology 90: 196–198
Houlsby W T 1984 Maternal serum AFP as screening test for Down syndrome. Lancet i: 1127
Hullin D A, Gregory P J, Dyer C L, Dew J O 1985 Place of amniotic fluid AFP in prenatal diagnosis of trisomies. Lancet ii: 662
Jackson L G, Wapner R A, Barr M A 1986 Safety of chorionic villus biopsy. Lancet i: 674–675
Jacobs P A, Strong J A 1959 A case of human inter-sexuality having a possible XXY sex-determining mechanism. Nature 183: 302–303
Jacobson C B, Barter R H 1967 Intrauterine diagnosis and management of genetic defects. American Journal of Obstetrics and Gynecology 99: 796–807
Jahoda M G S, Voster R P L, Sachs E S, Galjaard H 1985 Safety of chorionic villus sampling. Lancet ii: 941–942
Jones S R, Evans S E, Bowser-Riley S M, Hulten M A, Leedham P, McMahon G 1986 Amniotic fluid alpha-fetoprotein levels and trisomy 21. Lancet i: 1506–1507
Kalbac R W, Newman R L 1974 Amniotic fluid analysis in complicated pregnancies. Obstetrics and Gynecology 44: 814–818
Kalousek D K, Dill F J 1983 Chromosomal mosaicism confined to the placenta in human conceptions. Science 221: 665–667
Kan Y W, Valenti C, Carmazza V, Guidotti R, Rieder R F 1974 Fetal blood sampling in utero. Lancet i: 79–80
Kazy Z, Rozousky I S, Bakharev V A 1982 Chorion biopsy in early pregnancy: a method of early prenatal diagnosis for inherited disorders. Prenatal Diagnosis 2: 39–45
Knott P D, Ward R H T, Lucas M K 1986 Effect of chorionic villus sampling and early pregnancy counselling on uptake of prenatal diagnosis. British Medical Journal 293: 479–480
Kullander S, Sandahl B 1973 Fetal chromosome analysis after transcervical placental biopsies during early pregnancy. Acta Obstetricia et Gynecologica Scandinavica 52: 355–359
Lachman K 1977 Ultrasound during amniocentesis. Lancet ii: 832
Lau Y-F, Huang J C, Dozy A M, Kan Y W 1984 A rapid screening test for antenatal sex determination. Lancet i: 14–16
Lawrence M 1977 Diagnostic amniocentesis in early pregnancy. British Medical Journal 2: 191–192
Lejeune J, Gautier M, Turpin R 1959 Les chromosomes humains en culture de tissus. Compte Rendus de l'Académie de Science (Paris) 248: 602–603
Leschot N J, Verjaal M, Treffers P E 1985 Risks of midtrimester amniocentesis; assessment in 3000 pregnancies. British Journal of Obstetrics and Gynaecology 92: 804–807
Lilford R, Maxwell D, Coleman D, Czepulkowski B, Heaton D 1983 Diagnosis, 4 hours after chorion biopsy, of female fetus in pregnancy at risk of Duchenne muscular dystrophy. Lancet ii: 1491
Lisgar F, Gertner M, Cherry S, Hau L Y, Hirschhorn K 1970 Prenatal chromosome analysis. Nature 225: 280–281
Littlefield J W, Milunsky A, Atkins L 1974 An overview of prenatal genetic diagnosis. In: Motulsky A G, Lenz W (eds) Proceedings of the International Conference of Birth Defects. Excerpta Medica, Amsterdam, pp 221–225
Liu D T Y, Mitchell J, Johnson J, Wass D M 1983 Trophoblast sampling by blind transcervical aspiration. British Journal of Obstetrics and Gynaecology 90: 1119–1123
Lockwood C, Benacerraf B, Krinsky A et al 1987 A sonographic screening method for Down's syndrome. American Journal of Obstetrics and Gynecology 157: 803–808
Lubs H A 1969 A marker X chromosome. American Journal of Human Genetics 21: 231–244
MacKenzie I Z, Lindenbaum R H, Patel C, Clarke G, Crocken M, Jonasson J A 1983 Prenatal diagnosis of an unbalanced chromosome translocation identified by direct karyotyping of chorionic biopsy. Lancet ii: 1426–1427
Macri J N, Buchanan P D, Gold M P 1986 Low alpha-fetoprotein and trisomy. Lancet ii: 405
Martin J P, Bell J 1943 A pedigree of mental defect showing sex-linkage. Journal of Neurology and Psychiatry 6: 154–157
Martin A O, Liu K 1986 Implications of 'low' maternal serum alpha-fetoprotein levels: are maternal age risk criteria obsolete? Prenatal Diagnosis 6: 243–247
Martin A O, Elias S, Rosinsky B, Bombard A T, Simpson J L 1986 False-negative finding on chorionic villus sampling. Lancet ii: 391
Maxwell D, Czepulkowski B H, Heaton D E, Coleman D V, Lilford R 1985 A practical assessment of ultrasound-guided transcervical aspiration of chorionic villi and subsequent chromosomal analysis. British Journal of Obstetrics and Gynaecology 92: 660–665
Maxwell D, Lilford R, Czepulkowski B, Heaton D, Coleman D 1986a Transabdominal chorionic villus sampling. Lancet i: 123–126
Maxwell D, Modell B, Petrou M, Ward R H T 1986 Second trimester chorionic villus (placental) biopsy. Lancet i: 969
McDermid H E, Duncan A M V, Brasch K R et al 1986 Characterization of the supernumerary chromosome in cat eye syndrome. Science 232: 646–648
Medical Research Council Working Party on Amniocentesis 1978 An assessment of the hazards of amniocentesis. British Journal of Obstetrics and Gynaecology 85 (suppl 2)
Merkatz I R, Nitowsky H M, Macri J N, Johnson W E 1984 An association between low maternal serum alpha-fetoprotein and fetal chromosomal abnormalities. American Journal of Obstetrics and Gynecology 148: 886–894
Mikkelsen M 1979 Previous child with Down syndrome and other

chromosome aberration. In: Murken J D, Stengel-Rutkowski S, Schwinger E (eds) Prenatal diagnosis. Enke, Stuttgart, pp 22–29
Milunsky A, Atkins L, Littlefield J W 1972 Amniocentesis for prenatal genetic studies. Obstetrics and Gynecology 40: 104–108
Miskin M, Doran T A, Rudd N, Gardner H A, Liedgren S, Benzie R 1974 Use of ultrasound for placental localization in genetic amniocentesis. Obstetrics and Gynecology 43: 872–877
Murday V, Slack J 1985 Screening for Down's syndrome in the north east Thames region. British Medical Journal 291: 1315–1318
Nadler H L 1968 Antenatal detection of hereditary disorders. Pediatrics 42: 912–918
Nadler H L 1971 Indications for amniocentesis in the early prenatal detection of genetic disorders. Birth Defects Original Article Series 7: 5–9
Nadler H L, Gerbie A B 1970 Role of amniocentesis in intrauterine detection of genetic disorders. New England Journal of Medicine 282: 596–599
Nelson M M, Petersen E M 1985 Prospective screening for Down syndrome using maternal serum AFP. Lancet i: 1281
Niazi M, Coleman D V, Loeffler F E 1981 Trophoblast sampling in early pregnancy. Culture of rapidly dividing cells from immature placental villi. British Journal of Obstetrics and Gynaecology 88: 1081–1085
NICHD National Registry for Amniocentesis Study Group 1976 Midtrimester amniocentesis for prenatal diagnosis: safety and accuracy. Journal of the American Medical Association 236: 1471–1476
Nicolaides K H, Soothill P W, Rodeck C H, Warren R C, Gosden C M 1986 Why confine chorionic villus (placental) biopsy to the first trimester? Lancet i: 543–544
Nowell P C, Hungerford D A 1960 Chromosome studies on normal and leukemic human leucocytes. Journal of the National Cancer Institute 25: 85–109
Old J M, Ward R H T, Petrou M, Karagozlu F, Modell B, Weatherall D J 1982 First-trimester fetal diagnosis for haemoglobinopathies: three cases. Lancet ii: 1413–1416
Oxford J M, Harnden D G, Parington J M, Delhanty J D A 1975 Specific chromosome aberrations in ataxia-telangiectasia. Journal of Medical Genetics 12: 251–262
Painter T S 1923 Studies in mammalian spermatogenesis. II. The spermatogenesis of man. Journal of Experimental Zoology 37: 291–321
Patau K, Smith D W, Therman E, Inhorn S L, Wagner H P 1960 Multiple congenital anomaly caused by an extra autosome. Lancet i: 790–793
Penrose L S, Delhanty J D A 1961 Familial Langdon Down anomaly with chromosomal fusion. Annals of Human Genetics 25: 243–252
Penrose L S, Ellis J R, Delhanty J D A 1960 Chromosomal translocations in mongolism and in normal relatives. Lancet ii: 409–410
Perry T B, Vekemans M J J, Lippman A, Hamilton E F, Fournier P J R 1985 Chorionic villi sampling: clinical experience, immediate complications, and patient attitudes. American Journal of Obstetrics and Gynecology 151: 161–166
Petrou M, Ward R H T, Modell B et al 1983 Obstetric outcome in first trimester fetal diagnosis for the haemoglobinopathies. Lancet ii: 1251
Philip J, Bang J 1978 Outcome of pregnancy after amniocentesis for chromosome analysis. British Medical Journal 2: 1183–1184
Pinkel D, Straume T, Gray J W 1986 Cytogenetic analysis using quantitative, high-sensitivity fluorescent hybridization. Proceedings of the National Academy of Sciences (USA) 83: 2934–2938
Polani P E, Briggs J H, Ford C E, Clarke C M, Berg J M 1960 A mongol girl with 46 chromosomes. Lancet i: 721–723
Polani P E, Alberman E, Alexander B J et al 1979 Sixteen years experience of counselling, diagnosis and prenatal detection in one genetic centre, progress, results and problems. Journal of Medical Genetics 16: 166–175
Raimer S S, Raimer B G 1984 Needle puncture scars from midtrimester amniocentesis. Archives of Dermatology 120: 1360–1362
Rhine S A, Palmer C G, Thompson J F 1977 A simple alternative to amniocentesis for first trimester prenatal diagnosis. Birth Defects 13: 231–247
Riis P, Fuchs F 1960 Antenatal determination of foetal sex in prevention of hereditary diseases. Lancet ii: 180–182
Rodeck C H, Campbell S 1978 Sampling pure fetal blood by fetoscopy in second trimester of pregnancy. British Medical Journal 2: 728–730
Rodeck C H, Morsman J M, Nicolaides K H, McKenzie C, Gosden C M, Gosden J R 1983a A single-operator technique for first-trimester chorion biopsy. Lancet ii: 1340–1341
Rodeck C H, Morsman J M, Gosden C M, Gosden J R 1983b Development of an improved technique for first-trimester microsampling of chorion. British Journal of Obstetrics and Gynaecology 90: 1113–1118
Roth M-P, Feingold J, Baumgarten A, Bigel P, Stoll C 1983 Re-examination of paternal age effect in Down's syndrome. Human Genetics 63: 149–152
Sachs L, Serr D M, Danon M 1956 Analysis of amniotic fluid cells for diagnosis of fetal sex. British Medical Journal 2: 795–798
Sachs E S, Van Hemel J O, Galjaard H, Niermeijer M F, Johoda M G J 1983 First-trimester chromosomal analysis of complex structural rearrangements with RHA banding on chorionic villi. Lancet ii: 1426
Schroeder T M, German J 1974 Bloom's syndrome and Fanconi's anaemia: demonstration of two distinctive patterns of chromosome disruption and rearrangement. Humangenetik 25: 299–306
Seabright M 1971 A rapid banding technique for human chromosomes. Lancet ii: 971–972
Seller M J 1984 Prenatal screening for Down syndrome. Lancet i: 1359
Sergovich F R, Soltan H C, Carr D H 1962 A 13–15/21 translocation chromosome in carrier father and mongol son. Canadian Medical Association Journal 87: 852–858
Simoni G, Fraccaro M, Arslanion A et al 1982 Cytogenetic findings in 4952 prenatal diagnoses. An Italian collaborative study. Human Genetics 60: 63–68
Simoni G, Brambati B, Danesino C et al 1983 Efficient direct chromosome analysis and enzyme determinations from chorionic villi samples in the first trimester of pregnancy. Human Genetics 63: 349–357
Simoni G, Brambati B, Danesino C, Fraccaro M 1984 Antenatal sex determination. Lancet i: 397
Simoni G, Gimelli G, Cuoco C et al 1986 First trimester fetus karyotyping: 1000 diagnoses. Human Genetics 72: 203–209
Simoni G, Rossella F, Lalatta F, Fraccaro M 1986 Maternal metaphases on direct preparation from chorionic villi and in cultures of villi cells. Human genetics 72: 104
Simpson E, Dallaire L, Miller J R et al 1976 Prenatal diagnosis of genetic disease in Canada: report of a collaborative study. Canadian Medical Association Journal 115: 739–746
Spencer K, Carpenter P 1985 Screening for Down's syndrome using serum alpha-fetoprotein: a retrospective study indicating caution. British Medical Journal 290: 1940–1943
Squire J A, Nauth L, Ridler M A C, Sutton S, Timberlake C 1982 Prenatal diagnosis and outcome of pregnancy in 2036 women investigated by amniocentesis. Human Genetics 61: 215–222
Steele M W, Breg W R 1966 Chromosome analysis of human amniotic fluid cells. Lancet i: 383–385
Stein Z, Stein W, Susser M 1986 Hypothesis: attrition of trisomies as a maternal screening device, an explanation of the association of trisomy 21 with maternal age. Lancet i: 944–947
Sumner A T, Evans H J, Buckland R A 1971 New technique for distinguishing between human chromosomes. Nature New Biology 232: 31–32
Szabo J, Herczeg J, Thurzo L, Szemere G 1984 Karyotyping from uncultured human trophoblast in first trimester of pregnancy. Obstetrics and Gynecology 64: 807–810
Szabo J, Gellen J, Szemere G 1986 Why confine chorionic villus (placental) biopsy to the first trimester? Lancet i: 1030
Tabor A, Philip J, Madsen M, Bang J, Obel B, Norgaard-Pedersen B 1946 Randomised controlled trial of genetic amniocentesis in 4606 low-risk women. Lancet i: 1287–1293
Tabor A, Nørgaard-Pedersen B, Jacobsen J C 1984 Low maternal serum AFP and Down syndrome. Lancet ii: 16
Tabor A, Jerne D, Bock J E 1986 Incidence of rhesus immunization after genetic amniocentesis. British Medical Journal 293: 533–536
Timson J, Harris R, Gadd R L, Ferguson-Smith M E, Ferguson-Smith M A 1971 Down's syndrome due to maternal mosaicism, and the value of antenatal diagnosis. Lancet i: 549–550
Tjio J H, Levan A 1956 The chromosome number of man. Hereditas 42: 1–6
Tomkins D, Hunter A, Roberts M 1979 Cytogenetic findings in Roberts-SC phocomelia syndrome(s). American Journal of Medical Genetics 4: 17–26
Tommerup N, Sondergaard F, Tonneson T, Kristensen M, Aveiler B, Schinzel A 1985 First trimester prenatal diagnosis of a male fetus with fragile X. Lancet i: 870

Trigg M E, Hitchens J, Geier M R, Hutchinson G 1986 Low maternal serum AFP and Down syndrome. Lancet ii: 161

Valenti C 1973 Antenatal detection of hemoglobinopathies: a preliminary report. American Journal of Obstetrics and Gynecology 115: 851–853

Valenti C, Schutta E J, Kehaty T 1968 Prenatal diagnosis of Down's syndrome. Lancet ii: 220

Wahlstrom T, Brosset A, Bartsch F 1970 Viability of amniotic cells at different stages of gestation. Lancet ii: 1037

Wald N J, Terzian E, Vickers P A, Weatherall J A C 1983 Congenital talipes and hip malformation in relation to amniocentesis: a case-control study. Lancet ii: 246–249

Wald N J, Cuckle H S, Densem J W et al 1988a Maternal serum unconjugated oestriol as an antenatal screening test for Down's syndrome. British Journal of Obstetrics and Gynaecology 95: 334–341

Wald N J, Cuckle H S, Densem J W et al 1988b Maternal serum screening for Down's syndrome in early pregnancy. British Medical Journal 297: 883–887

Wang M Y F W, McCutcheon E, Desforges J C F 1967 Fetomaternal hemorrhage from diagnostic transabdominal amniocentesis. American Journal of Obstetrics and Gynecology 97: 1123–1128

Warburton D 1982 De novo structural rearrangements: implications for prenatal diagnosis. In: Willey A M, Carter T P, Kelly S, Porter I H (eds) Problems in diagnosis and counselling. Academic Press, Paris, pp 63–75

Warburton D, Miller O J 1972 Present status and future trends in prenatal diagnosis of chromosomal disorders. Clinics in Obstetrics and Gynaecology 15: 272–282

Ward R H T, Modell B, Petrou M, Karagozlu F, Douratsos E 1983 Method of sampling chorionic villi in first trimester of pregnancy under guidance of real time ultrasound. British Medical Journal 286: 1542–1544

Warren R C, Butler J, Morsman J M, McKenzie C, Rodeck C H 1985 Does chorionic villus sampling cause fetomaternal haemorrhage? Lancet i: 691

Williamson R, Eskdale J, Coleman D V, Niazi M, Loeffler F E, Modell B M 1981 Direct gene analysis of chorionic villi: a possible technique for first trimester antenatal diagnosis of haemoglobinopathies. Lancet ii: 1125–1127

Wyatt P R 1985 Screening for Down's syndrome using serum alpha-fetoprotein. British Medical Journal 291: 740

22

M. d'A. Crawfurd

Diagnosis of inborn errors of metabolism

INTRODUCTION

The inborn errors of metabolism are single gene defects inherited in a recessive manner. They may be either autosomal or X-linked. With the autosomal recessive disorders the realization that a pregnancy is at risk will usually come from the recognition that a previous child of the parents was affected. Occasionally such realization will come from a carrier screening test indicating that both parents are carriers, as in the screening of an Ashkenazi couple for Tay–Sachs disease. The haemoglobin disorders present further examples but these are discussed elsewhere (Chapter 23). Apart from the haemoglobin disorders in populations with a high incidence, it is most unusual for a carrier couple to be detected because one partner has been found to be a carrier in a family in which an autosomal recessive inborn error of metabolism has been diagnosed and the other partner is found by chance to also be a carrier. This would only have an appreciable likelihood when the frequency of carriers in the general population is high, as for example the 1 in 22 frequency for the cystic fibrosis carrier state in the white population.

A fetal risk of X-linked recessive disorder may also arise from a previous affected child. However if that was a sporadic case it may have been due to fresh mutation with the mother being a non-carrier. When a woman has a family history of a brother or maternal uncle with an X-linked disease she is also at risk herself of being a carrier of the gene for it. Her percise initial risk will depend on the specific pedigree findings, including the results of carrier detection studies on female relatives. The estimation of such risks is one of the few clinical situations requiring fairly sophisticated probability calculations with which clinical geneticists are familiar. When such calculations indicate an appreciable risk further tests are necessary to establish whether the pregnant woman is herself a carrier. Clearly it is preferable for diagnostic investigations on the affected child and carrier tests on parents to be completed before the mother becomes pregnant again. When the obstetrician sees a family in which there is a risk of a child with an inborn error of metabolism, before the mother becomes pregnant he should ensure that the necessary preliminary investigations are completed. Since the inborn errors of metabolism are by definition inherited diseases in which the gene product, usually an enzyme, is known, prenatal diagnosis should be relatively easy. In autosomal recessive diseases the affected fetus will be homozygous for the abnormal gene and in X-linked recessive diseases hemizygous, with little or no enzyme activity. Often prenatal diagnosis is indeed straightforward with well separated distributions of the levels of enzyme activity in cells readily obtainable at prenatal diagnosis between the affected homozygote or hemizygote on the one hand and the normal or carrier fetus on the other.

However, several factors may complicate this hopeful expectation. There may be some overlap of residual minimal activity in cells from an affected fetus and the lower end of the range for a carrier fetus. Fortunately this is a rare problem. More often the enzyme involved is not expressed in cultured amniotic fluid or trophoblast cells, as in phenylketonuria where the enzyme, phenylalanine hydroxylase, is expressed only in liver (Crawfurd et al 1981).

Carrier detection by enzyme assay may be unreliable in X-linked recessive diseases owing to the very wide range of enzyme activity in carrier females due to the random variation arising from X inactivation. In such carrier females the X chromosome bearing the normal allele will be expressed in some cells, and that bearing the mutant allele in others. The randomly varying proportions of the normal and mutant cells can result in overall enzyme levels ranging from little more than those in affected males to levels well within the normal range. This problem can sometimes be overcome by using an autoradiographic method to score uptake and metabolic conversion of a radiolabelled substrate by individual cells, as from a fibroblast culture. The carrier female should show a dual cell population: labelled and unlabelled. However, even this method is not always reliable.

In general a larger number of cells is needed for biochemical analysis than for karyotyping. For this reason close liaison among obstetricians, cytogeneticists and biochemists is vital. The laboratories will require a good quality specimen of adequate quantity for both chromosomal and biochemical analysis. It often takes longer to grow up a sufficient quantity of cells for enzyme assay than for chromosomal analysis. For this reason chorionic villus sampling may be the method of choice and where an amniocentesis has to be done it may be worth doing this at 15 rather than 16 weeks' gestation. Each laboratory should check with colleagues before discarding any cultures, as these may be useful if the cells cultured for one or other purpose have grown slowly, or even failed. The expression of specific enzymes in chorionic villus tissue varies and may be best determined directly on uncultured tissue if sensitive micromethods are available or after culture. Usually it is best to do both. As with cytogenetic analysis special care needs to be taken in analyses from chorionic villus tissue to exclude maternal cell contamination.

BIOCHEMICAL DIAGNOSIS

The methods available for prenatal diagnosis of inborn errors of metabolism vary. Since many of these diseases are very rare the diagnostic methods for many are performed only in a few specialist laboratories. Furthermore new methods for specific diseases are being continuously reported. For these reasons it is advisable when a family presents requiring prenatal diagnosis for such a disease to check with a genetic centre or appropriate laboratory on the current availability of suitable methods.

Probably the ideal method is a reliable enzyme assay that can be performed on uncultured and cultured chorionic villus tissue and on cultured amniotic fluid cells. Fujimoto and colleagues (1968) used an autoradiographic method for the detection of hypoxanthine-guanosine ribosyl transferase activity in cultured and uncultured amniotic fluid cells of a female fetus heterozygous for Lesch–Nyhan disease. Quantitative enzyme assay is used in the prenatal diagnosis of Hurler's disease (Stirling et al 1979) and Tay–Sachs disease (Milunsky 1973), using assay of alpha-L-iduronidase and hexosaminidase A, respectively. When such an assay gives an unequivocal result from chorion villus sampling it is not necessary to confirm the result from an amniocentesis but this may be necessary if there is any doubt.

For inborn errors for which an enzyme assay method is not available it may be possible to measure a specific metabolite in amniotic fluid, or even maternal urine. One of the earliest reports of metabolic prenatal diagnosis for Hunter's disease utilized the assay of mucopolysaccharides in the amniotic fluid (Crawfurd et al 1973), but this is not always reliable (Matalon et al 1972). Where enzyme assay is performed the measurement of a metabolite in the amniotic fluid may provide a valuable check against, for example, contamination of the cell culture by maternal cells. A good illustration of this approach is the measurement of organic acids in amniotic fluid by gas chromatography and mass spectrometry. This method has been used to demonstrate raised methylcitrate in the amniotic fluid in pregnancies with a fetus with proprionic acidaemia (Sweetman et al 1979a, Buchanan et al 1980). Similarly, raised amniotic fluid methylmalonic acid has been found in pregnancies with a fetus with methylmalonic aciduria (Morrow et al 1970, Gompertz et al 1974). Increased excretion of 3-hydroxy-3-methylglutaric and 3-methylglutaconic acids in maternal urine has been reported in a pregnancy in which the fetus was shown after birth to have 3-hydroxy-3-methylglutaryl-CoA lyase deficiency (Duran et al 1979).

RECOMBINANT DNA DIAGNOSIS

An alternative approach to prenatal diagnosis of inborn errors of metabolism is the application of the new techniques of molecular biology which have already been so successfully exploited in the haemoglobin disorders. DNA methods of prenatal diagnosis may be used to confirm the results of biochemical methods. More importantly they may be used when the limitations of biochemical methods, already discussed, might result in no or equivocal results. These methods depend on the extraction of DNA from cultured cells or directly from biopsy tissue, as obtained at chorionic villus sampling for example and its cleavage at specific sites by restriction endonucleases, the separation of the fragments formed by gel electrophoresis and the detection of specific fragments of interest by the hybridization of a radioisotope-labelled DNA probe of known constitution to the fragments following their transfer to a filter (Southern blotting). The final detection of probe bound to its complementary DNA fragment is made by autoradiography. This technique has the advantage that it can be applied to any tissue containing nucleated cells, such as amniotic fluid cells, trophoblast cells, fibroblasts or white blood cells. Whether the relevant DNA in the nuclei is 'switched on' with synthesis of its gene product is irrelevant. Nor is it essential that the gene product be known. Hence the method can also be applied to inherited diseases where the gene product is unknown, such as cystic fibrosis or Huntington's chorea, as well as to the true inborn errors of metabolism where it is known.

There are two possible ways in which DNA methods may be applied to such prenatal diagnoses. The preferred method uses a probe which directly recognizes the mutant site in the DNA fragments formed by restriction cleavage, either by the use of a short oligonucleotide probe complementary to the mutant sequence or by recognition of a restriction site either created or lost at the site of the mutation. Thus it recognizes a specific mutation in an individual and is not dependent on establishing the status of relatives. Such probes may be isolated from cloned DNA from affected individuals or may be synthesized as short oligonucleotides when the nucleic acid base sequence around the mutation is known. This method is used in the diagnosis of sickle cell disease but unfortunately has severe limitations when applied to inborn errors of metabolism. The first limitation is that for most such diseases a restriction enzyme cleaving exactly at the mutant site is so far unknown. This may be overcome with time.

A second limitation is more fundamental. Most inborn errors of metabolism are rare and unlike sickle cell disease are not maintained by selection. In consequence many different mutations may result in the same enzyme deficiency, in the rarer diseases possibly an almost unique mutation for each affected family. The exceptions will probably turn out to be those diseases with a high frequency in a particular population, such as cystic fibrosis in whites and Tay–Sachs disease in Ashkenazi Jews.

In general, therefore, for the inborn errors of metabolism we have to fall back on an alternative approach. This depends on the fact that restriction enzyme cleavage sites occur with high frequency in DNA and that many such sites may be either present or absent in normal individuals. When DNA from a number of normal subjects is cleaved with an appropriate restriction enzyme, and a specific DNA probe is hybridized to the fragments generated, differing patterns of fragments are seen. Furthermore these patterns of fragments are inherited, often with two or more patterns occurring with high frequency. These normal variations in DNA fragments, which genetically are analogous to normal blood groups or to enzyme or serum protein polymorphisms, have been rather clumsily termed restriction fragment length polymorphisms (RFLP), or more simply just DNA polymorphisms. They are sufficiently frequent that several such polymorphisms are likely to be found within and on either side of any given gene. They may thus be used, in a particular family, as markers of the disease gene whose presence can be deduced from the presence of such a linked variant. The principal limitation of this approach is that it is necessary to determine the RFLP phenotypes within a family as a whole in order to establish which of the variants is coupled to the disease allele rather than its normal counterpart. If a key member of the family proves to be homozygous for the DNA polymorphism being used then it will not be possible to determine whether the allele transmitted to a child is the one coupled to the disease allele or not — this is termed a non-informative or only partially informative situation. Some examples of this and other non-informative situations are shown in Figures 22.1 and 22.2. This problem of non-informative findings can be reduced if more than one polymorphism is used, especially if polymorphisms with gene frequencies of about 0.5 are chosen.

A further limitation arises from the fact that linked genes may be separated by crossing over at meiosis. The closer

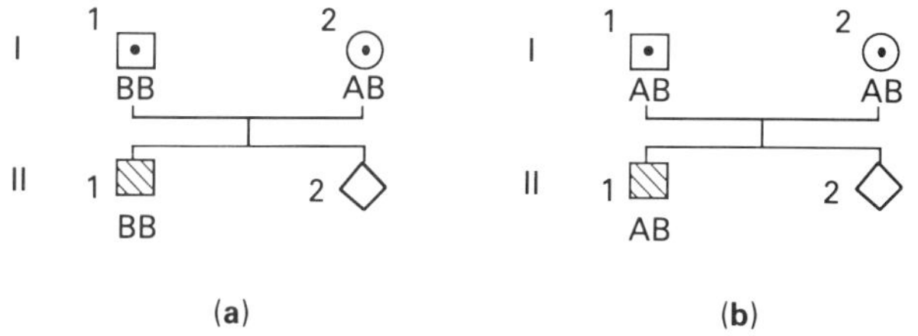

Fig. 22.1(a) II1 is an affected son of carrier parents I1 and 2. He is of phenotype BB for an RFLP, indicating that it is a B allele which is coupled to the disease gene in each parent. If the fetus II2 is AB it will be either normal or a carrier but if it is BB it will be either a carrier or affected; **(b)** Here it is not possible to say which of the parents contributed which disease allele. If II2 is AA or BB the fetus must be a carrier, but it AB it may be normal or affected.

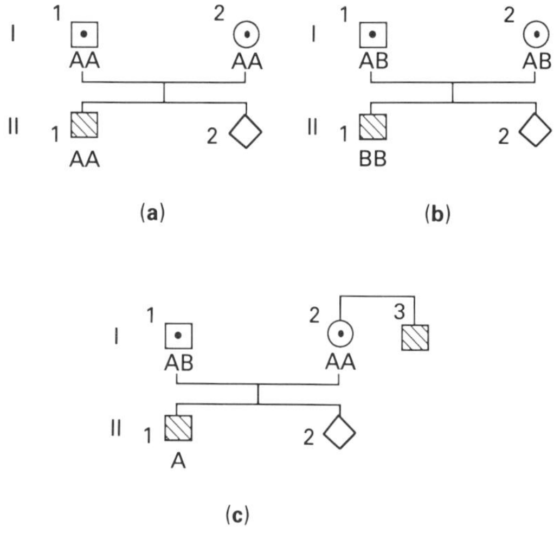

Fig. 22.2(a) This situation is of course totally non-informative. **(b)** This situation is fully informative. **(c)** This X-linked situation is totally uniformative as there is no way of telling which of I2's A alleles is linked to the disease gene. If she had been heterozygous, AB, the situation would have been informative.

they are the less the chance of crossing over, or recombination. Provided adequate linkage studies have been done the recombination frequency can be calculated and, therefore, so can the risk of a misleading result. This enables the risk of an affected child to be given as a mathematical probability. Again the use of multiple polymorphisms, especially polymorphisms that are closely linked to the disease gene and lie either side of it, minimizes the risk of recombination giving a misleading result.

DNA methods are especially valuable in diseases where the enzyme defect is not expressed in tissues available for prenatal diagnosis, such as phenylketonuria. It can also be of great value in the preliminary determination of carrier status of mothers for X-linked disorders such as Lesch–Nyhan disease and Anderson–Fabry's disease.

See Table 22.1 for inborn errors of metabolism for which prenatal diagnosis has been reported.

Table 22.1 Inborn errors of metabolism for which prenatal diagnosis has been reported

Disease	Inheritance	Prenatal diagnostic methods	References
Carbohydrate disorders			
Galactosaemia, classical	AR	1. Transferase assay in AF cells 2. Galactitol assay in AF	Fensom et al 1974, 1975; Benson et al 1979 Allen et al 1980
Glycogen storage disease, type II or Pompe's disease	AR	α-glucosidase assay in AF cells	Fensom et al 1976
Pyruvate carboxylase deficiency (Leigh's disease)	AR	Pyruvate carboxylase assay in AF cells	Marsac et al 1982
Mucopolysaccharidoses			
Hurler's disease (MPS IH)	AR	1. Iduronidase assay in AF cells 2. AF glycosaminoglycan assay	Pedersen et al 1979; Stirling et al 1979 Whiteman & Henderson 1977
Hunter's disease (MPS II)	XR	1. Sulphoiduronate sulphatase assay in AF cells 2. AF glycosaminoglycan assay	Liehbaers et al 1977; Lykkelund et al 1983 Whiteman & Henderson 1977
Sanfilippo A disease (MPS IIIA)	AR	1. Sulphamidase assay in AF cells 2. AF glycosaminoglycan assay	Hopwood & Elliot 1981 Mossman & Patrick 1982
Sanfilippo B disease (MPS IIIB)	AR	α-N-acetylglucosaminidase in AF cells and AF heparan sulphate assay	Mossman et al 1983
Morquio A disease (MPS IVA)	AR	N-acetylgalactosamine-6-sulphate deficiency in AF cells	von Figura et al 1982
Maroteaux–Lamy disease (MPS VI)	AR	Arylsulphatase B assay in AF cells	van Dyke et al 1981
Sly disease (MPS VII)	AR	β-Glucuronidase assay in AF cells	Poenaru et al 1982
Aminoacidopathies			
Homocystinuria	AR	Cystathionine-β-synthase assay on AF cells or cultured chorionic villus cells	Fowler et al 1982; Benson et al 1983
Methylene tetrahydrofolate reductase deficiency	AR	MTHFR enzyme assay in AF	Wendel et al 1983
Cystinosis	AR	^{35}S-cystine cellular uptake and conversion	Willcox & Patrick 1974
Classical phenylketonuria	AR	RFLP detection with a phenylalanine gene probe	Lidsky et al 1985a,b; Daiger et al 1986
Ornithine carbamyl transferase deficiency	XR	Enzyme assay in fetal liver biopsy	Rodeck et al 1982
Citrullinaemia	AR	Radioisotopic enzyme assay of argininosuccinate synthetase deficiency in AF cells	Fleischer et al 1983
Argininosuccinic aciduria	AR	Argininosuccinase assay in AF cells	Goodman et al 1973; Fleischer et al 1983
Maple syrup urine disease	AR	Assay of branched chain 2-ketoacid decarboxylase	Wendel & Claussen 1979
Organicacidurias			
Glutaric aciduria type I	AR	Glutaryl-CoA dehydrogenase assay in AF cells	Goodman et al 1980
Glutaric aciduria type II	AR	GC/MS of glutaric acid and 2-hydroxyglutaric acid in AF	Mitchell et al 1983; Bone et al 1984
Proprionic acidaemia	AR	1. GC/MS of methylcitrate in AF 2. Assay of proprionyl-Co A carboxylase in cultured AF cells	Sweetman et al 1979b Fensom et al 1984
Methylmalonic aciduria	AR	GC/MS of methylmalonic acid in AF and assay of adenosylcobalamin synthesis in AF cells	Fensom et al 1984

REFERENCES

Allen J T, Gillet M, Holton J B, King G S, Pettit B R 1980 Evidence of glactosaemia in utero. Lancet i: 603

Aula P, Rapalo J, von Kuskull H, Ammälä P 1984 Prenatal diagnosis and fetal pathology of aspartylglucosaminuria. American Journal of Medical Genetics 19: 359–367

Benson P F, Brandt N J, Christensen E, Fensom A H 1979 Prenatal diagnosis of galactosaemia in six pregnancies — possible complications with rare alleles of the galactose-1-phosphate uridyl transferase locus. Clinical Genetics 16: 311–316

Benson P F, Fensom A H, Cress M J et al 1983 Recent advances in prenatal diagnosis of inborn errors of metabolism. Symposium on progress in perinatal medicine. Excerpta Medica, Amsterdam, p 165

Booth C W, Gerbie A B, Nadler H L 1973 Intrauterine detection of GM_1-gangliosidosis type 2. Pediatrics 52: 521–524

Boue J, Chalmers R A, Tracey B M 1984 Prenatal diagnosis of dysmorphic neonatal-lethal type II glutaricaciduria. Lancet i: 846–847

Boyle J A, Raivio K O, Astrin K H 1970 Lesch–Nyhan syndrome: preventive control by prenatal diagnosis. Science 169: 688–689

Buchanan P D, Kahler S G, Sweetman L, Nyhan W L 1980 Pitfalls in the prenatal diagnosis of proprionic acidaemia. Clinical Genetics 18: 177–183

Coates P M, Cortner J A, Mennuti M T, Wheeler J E 1978 Prenatal diagnosis of Wolman disease. American Journal of Medical Genetics 2: 397–407

Crawfurd M d'A, Dean M F, Hunt D M et al 1973 Early prenatal diagnosis of Hurler's syndrome with termination of pregnancy and confirmatory findings of the fetus. Journal of Medical Genetics 10: 144–153

Crawfurd M d'A, Gibbs D A, Shepherd D M 1981 Studies on human phenylalanine mono-oxygenase. I. Restricted expression. Journal of Inherited Metabolic Diseases 4: 191–195

Daiger S P, Lidsky A S, Chakraborty R, Koch R, Güttler F, Woo S L C 1986 Polymorphic DNA haplotypes at the phenylalanine hydroxylase locus in prenatal diagnosis of phenylketonuria. Lancet i: 229–232

Duran M, Schutgens R B H, Ketel A et al 1979 3-Hydroxy-3-methylglutaryl coenzyme A lyase deficiency: postnatal management following prenatal diagnosis by analysis of maternal urine. Journal of Pediatrics 95: 1004–1007

Durand P, Gatti R, Borrone C et al 1979 Detection of carriers and prenatal diagnosis for fucosidosis in Calabria. Human Genetics 51: 195–201

Ellis R B, Ikonne J U, Patrick A D, Stephens R, Willcox P 1973 Prenatal diagnosis of Tay-Sachs disease. Lancet ii: 1144–1145

Fensom A H, Benson P F, Blunt S 1974 Prenatal diagnosis of galactosaemia. British Medical Journal 4: 386–387

Fensom A H, Benson P F, Blunt S 1974 Assay of galactose-1-phosphate uridyl transferase in cultured amniotic cells for prenatal diagnosis of galactosaemia. Clinica Chimica Acta 62: 189–194

Table 22.1 Inborn errors of metabolism for which prenatal diagnosis has been reported (*contd.*)

Disease	Inheritance	Prenatal diagnostic methods	References
Sphingolipidoses			
Classic Tay–Sachs disease	AR	Hexosaminidase assay on AF and cells cultured from it	Ellis et al 1973
Heat-labile hexosaminidase B variant of Tay–Sachs disease	AR	Hexosaminidase B assay on AF cells	Momoi et al 1983
Sandhoff disease	AR	Hexosaminidase A and B assay on AF cells	Norby & Schwartz 1979
Generalized gangliosidosis	AR	Assay of GM_1-β-galactosidase on AF cells	Kleijer et al 1976
Juvenile GM_1 gangliosidosis	AR	Assay of GM_1-β-galactosidase on AF cells	Booth et al 1973
Metachromatic leukodystrophy	AR	Assay of arysulphatase A in AF cells	Wiesemann et al 1975
Gaucher's disease, infantile type	AR	Assay of β-glucocerebrosidase in AF cells	Svennerholm et al 1981
Gaucher's disease, adult and juvenile types	AR	Assay of β-glucocerebrosidase in AF cells	Kitigaura et al 1978
Niemann–Pick disease, type A	AR	Assay of sphingomyelinase in AF cells	Patrick et al 1977
Niemann–Pick disease, type B	AR	Assay of sphingomyelinase in AF cells	Wenger et al 1981
Krabbe's disease (globoid leukodystrophy)	AR	Assay of galactocerebroside β-galactosidase in AF cells	Tsutsumi et al 1982
X-linked ichthyosis	XR	Assay of steroid sulphatase in AF cells and of dehydroepiandrosterone in AF	Hähnel et al 1982
Anderson-Fabry disease	XR	1. Assay of α-galactosidase A in AF or CVS cells	Galjaard et al 1974; Morgan et al 1987
		2. RFLP detection with a probe linked to the Fabry locus	Morgan et al 1987
Farber's disease	AR	Assay of ceramidase on AF cells	Fensom et al 1979
Other lipidoses			
Mucolipidosis I (sialidosis)	AR	Assay of neuraminidase on AF cells	Mueller & Wenger 1981
Mucolipidosis II (I-cell disease)	AR	Demonstration of multiple lysosomal enzyme deficiencies on AF cells, and elevated activities in AF	Gehler & Cantz 1976
Mucolipidosis IV	AR	By transmission electron microscopy	Kohn et al 1982
Wolman's disease	AR	Assay of acid lipase on AF cells	Coates et al 1978
Mannosidosis	AR	Assay of α-mannosidase on AF cells	Poenaru et al 1979
Fucosidosis	AR	Assay of α-fucosidase on AF cells	Durand et al 1979
Aspartylglycosaminuria	AR	Assay of 1-aspartamido-β-N-acetylglucosamine amidohydrolase in AF cells	Aula et al 1984
Purine and pyrimidine disorders			
Lesch–Nyhan disease	XR	1. Assay of hypoxanthine guanine phosphoribosyl transferase (HGPRT) in AF cells	Boyle et al 1970
		2. Assay of HGPRT in CVS cells	Gibbs et al 1984
		3. Linked RFLP analysis in CVS cells	Gibbs et al 1986

AR = autosomal recessive; XR = X-linked recessive; AF = amniotic fluid; CVS = chorionic villus sample; RFLP = restriction fragment length polymorphism.

Fensom A H, Benson P F, Blunt S, Brown S P, Coltart T M 1976 Amniotic cell 4-methylumbelliferyl-alpha-glucosidase for prenatal diagnosis of Pompe's disease. Journal of Medical Genetics 13: 148–149

Fensom A H, Benson P F, Neville B R G, Moser H W, Moser A E, Dulaney J T 1979 Prenatal diagnosis of Farber's disease. Lancet ii: 990–992

Fensom A H, Benson P F, Chalmers R A et al 1984 Experience with prenatal diagnosis of proprionic acidaemia and methylmalonic aciduria. Journal of Inherited Metabolic Diseases 7 (suppl 2): 127–128

Fleischer L D, Harris C J, Mitchell D A, Nadler H L 1983 Citrullinemia: prenatal diagnosis of an affected fetus. American Journal of Human Genetics 35: 85–90

Fowler B, Børresen A L, Boman N 1982 Prenatal diagnosis of homocystinuria. Lancet ii: 875

Fujimoto W Y, Seegmiller J E, Uhlendorf B W, Jacobson C B 1968 Biochemical diagnosis of an X-linked disease in utero. Lancet ii: 511–512

Galjaard H, Niermeijer M F, Hahnemann N, Mohr J, Sorensen S A 1974 An example of rapid prenatal diagnosis of Fabry's disease using microtechniques. Clinical Genetics 5: 368–377

Gehler J, Cantz M, Stoeckenius M, Spranger J 1976 Prenatal diagnosis of mucolipidoses II (I-cell disease). European Journal of Pediatrics 122: 201–206

Gibbs D A, McFadyen I R, Crawfurd M d'A et al 1984 First-trimester diagnosis of Lesch–Nyhan syndrome. Lancet ii: 1180–1183

Gibbs D A, Headhouse-Benson C M, Watts R W E 1986 Family studies of the Lesch–Nyhan syndrome: the use of a restriction fragment length polymorphism (RFLP) closely linked to the disease gene for carrier state and prenatal diagnosis. Journal of Inherited Metabolic Disease 9: 45–88

Gompertz D, Goodey P A, Saudubray J M, Charpentier C, Chignolle A 1974 Prenatal diagnosis of methylmalonic acidemia. Pediatrics 54: 511–513

Goodman S I, Mace J W, Turner B, Garrett W J 1973 Antenatal diagnosis of argininosuccinic aciduria. Clinical Genetics 4: 236–240

Goodman S I, Gallegos D A, Pullin C J 1980 Antenatal diagnosis of glutaric acidemia. American Journal of Human Genetics 32: 695–699

Hähnel R, Hähnel E, Wysocki S J, Wilkinson S P, Hockey A 1982 Prenatal diagnosis of X-linked ichthyosis. Clinica Chimica Acta 120: 143–152

Hopwood J J, Elliot H 1981 Sulphamidase activity in leukocytes, cultured skin fibroblasts and amniotic cells: diagnosis of Sanfilippo A syndrome with the use of a radiolabelled disaccharide substrate. Clinical Science 61: 729–735

Kitigaura T, Owada N, Sakiyama T et al 1978 In utero diagnosis of Gaucher disease. American Journal of Human Genetics 30: 322–327

Kleijer W J, Van de Veer E, Niermeijer M F 1976 Rapid prenatal diagnosis of GM_1-gangliosidoses using microchemical methods. Human Genetics 33: 299–305

Kohn G, Sekeles E, Arnon J, Ornoy A 1982 Mucolipidosis IV: prenatal diagnosis by electron microscopy. Prenatal Diagnosis 2: 301–307

Lidsky A S, Guttler F, Woo S L C 1985a Prenatal diagnosis of classic phenylketonuria by DNA analysis. Lancet i: 549–551

Lidsky A S, Ledley F D, DiLella A G et al 1985b Extensive restriction site polymorphism of the human phenylalanine hydroxylase locus and its application in prenatal diagnosis of phenylketonuria. American Journal of Human Genetics 37: 619–634

Liehbaers I, DiNatale P, Neufeld E F 1977 Iduronate sulfatase in amniotic fluid: an aid in the prenatal diagnosis of the Hunter syndrome. Journal of Pediatrics 90: 423–425

Lykkelund C, Søndergaard F, Therkelsen A J et al 1983 Feasibility of first trimester prenatal diagnosis of Hunter syndrome. Lancet ii: 1147

Marsac C, Augereau Ch, Feldman G, Wolf B, Hansen T L, Berger R 1982 Prenatal diagnosis of pyruvate carboxylase deficiency. Clinica Chimica Acta 119: 121–127

Matalon R, Dorfman A, Nadler H L 1972 A chemical method for the antenatal diagnosis of mucopolysaccharidoses. Lancet i: 798–799

Milunsky A 1973 The prenatal diagnosis of hereditary disorders. Thomas, Springfield, Illinois

Mitchell G, Saudubray J M, Benoit Y et al 1983 Antenatal diagnosis of glutaricaciduria type II. Lancet i: 1099

Momoi T, Kikuchi I, Shigematsu Y, Sudo M, Tanioka K 1983 Prenatal diagnosis of Tay–Sachs disease with heat-labile beta-hexosaminidase B. Clinica Chimica Acta 133: 331–334

Morgan S H, Cheshire J K, Wilson T M, MacDermot K, Crawfurd M d'A 1987 Anderson-Fabry disease—family linkage studies using two polymorphic X-linked DNA probes. Pediatric Nephrology 1: 536–539

Morrow G III, Schwarz R H, Hallock J A, Barness L A 1970 Prenatal detection of methylmalonic acidemia. Journal of Pediatrics 77: 120–123

Mossman J, Patrick A D 1982 Prenatal diagnosis of mucopolysaccaridosis by two-dimensional electrophoresis of amniotic fluid glycosaminoglycans. Prenatal Diagnosis 2: 169–176

Mossman J, Young E P, Patrick A D et al 1983 Prenatal tests for Sanfilippo disease type B in four pregnancies. Prenatal Diagnosis 3: 347–350

Mueller O T, Wenger D A 1981 Mucolipidosis I: studies of sialidase activity and a prenatal diagnosis. Clinica Chimica Acta 109: 313–324

Norby S, Schwartz M 1979 Prenatal diagnosis of Sandhoff disease (GM_2 gangliosidosis type 2). Danish Medical Bulletin 26: 353–356

Patrick A D, Young E, Kleijer W J, Niermeijer M F 1977 Prenatal diagnosis of Niemann–Pick disease type A using a chromogenic substrate. Lancet ii: 144

Pedersen C, Schwartz M, Guttler F, Hobolth N 1979 Prenatal diagnosis of the Hurler syndrome. Danish Medical Bulletin 26: 357–359

Poenaru L, Girard S, Thepot F et al 1979 Antenatal diagnosis in three pregnancies at risk for mannosidosis. Clinical Genetics 16: 428–432

Poenaru L, Castelnau L, Mossman J, Boue J, Dreyfus J C 1982 Prenatal diagnosis of heterozygote for mucopolysaccaridosis type VII (beta-glucuronidase deficiency). Prenatal Diagnosis 2: 251–256

Rodeck C H, Patrick A D, Pembrey M E, Tzannatos C, Whitfield A E 1982 Fetal liver biopsy for prenatal diagnosis of ornithine carbamyl transferase deficiency. Lancet ii: 297–300

Speer A, Bollman R, Michel A et al 1986 Prenatal diagnosis of classical phenylketonuria by linked restriction fragment length polymorphism analysis. Prenatal Diagnosis 6: 447–450

Stirling J L, Robinson D, Fensom A H, Benson P F, Baker J E, Button L R 1979 Prenatal diagnosis of two Hurler fetuses using an improved assay for methylumbelliferyl-alpha-L-iduronidase. Lancet ii: 37

Svennerholm L, Hakansson G, Lindsten J, Wahlström J, Dreborg S 1981 Prenatal diagnosis of Gaucher disease. Assay of beta-glucosidase activity in amniotic cells cultivated in two laboratories with different cultivation conditions. Clinical Genetics 19: 16–22

Sweetman L, Weyler W, Shafai T, Young P E, Nyhan W L 1979 Prenatal diagnosis of proprionic acidemia. Journal of the American Medical Association 242: 1048–1052

Sweetman L, Weyler W, Shafai T, Young P E, Nyhan W L 1979 Prenatal diagnosis of proprionic acidemia. Journal of the American Medical Association 242: 1048–1052

Tsutsumi O, Satoh K, Sakamoto S, Suzuki Y, Kato T 1982 Application of a galactosylceramidase microassay to early prenatal diagnosis of Krabbe's disease. Clinica Chimica Acta 125: 265–273

Van Dyke D L, Fluharty A L, Schafer I A, Shapiro L J, Kihara H, Weiss L 1981 Prenatal diagnosis of Maroteaux–Lamy syndrome. American Journal of Medical Genetics 8: 235–242

Von Figura K, van de Kamp J J, Niermeijer M F 1982 Prenatal diagnosis of Morquio's disease type A (N-acetylgalactosamine-6-sulphate sulphatase deficiency). Prenatal Diagnosis 2: 67–69

Wendel U, Claussen U 1979 Antenatal diagnosis of maple syrup urine disease. Lancet i: 161–162

Wendel U, Claussen U, Diekmann E 1983 Prenatal diagnosis for methylene-tetrahydrofolate reductase dificiency. Journal of Pediatrics 102: 938–940

Wenger D A, Kudoh T, Sattler M, Palmieri M, Yudkoff M 1981 Niemann–Pick disease type B: prenatal diagnosis and enzymatic studies on fetal brain and liver. American Journal of Human Genetics 33: 337–344

Whiteman P, Henderson H 1977 A method for the determination of amniotic fluid glycosaminoglycans and its application to the prenatal diagnosis of Hurler and Sanfilippo diseases. Clinica Chimica Acta 79: 99–105

Wiesemann U N, Meier C, Spycher M A et al 1975 Prenatal metachromatic leukodystrophy. Helvetica Paediatrica Acta 30: 31–42

Willcox P, Patrick A D 1974 Biochemical diagnosis of cystinosis using cultured cells. Archives of Disease in Childhood 49: 209–212

23

Elizabeth A. Letsky

Prenatal diagnosis of haemoglobinopathies

Inherited haemoglobin defects are responsible for significant morbidity and mortality worldwide and present a vast public health problem, which is concentrated in the populations of the eastern Mediterranean, Middle East, parts of India, South-east Asia, Africa and the West Indies. Following the influx of immigrants from these parts of the world, obstetricians in the United Kingdom are encountering women with genetic defects of haemoglobin seldom seen in the indigenous populations.

Prenatal diagnosis of a fetus at risk of a serious haemoglobin defect is now possible and such a fetus has to be identified early enough for the relevant procedures to be planned in advance.

It is obvious that population screening in communities at risk is a prerequisite for identification of those who carry and can transmit genes for abnormal haemoglobin production. When this screening should take place and who should be responsible for it are the subject of active debate. This is a very sensitive area and beyond the scope of this chapter, but suffice to say that education within communities which have a high incidence of these genetic defects ideally leads to early and voluntary screening for the carrier state. Couples can then plan their families without fear of producing a child with a serious haemoglobin defect or, if indicated, make their own decision about prenatal diagnosis before pregnancy is embarked upon.

In some countries, e.g. Greece and Cyprus, where beta-thalassaemia is a sizeable public health problem, premarital blood-testing for identification of beta-thalassaemia is obligatory, but most workers in these communities agree that this is rather late in the emotional life of a couple who are already committed to each other. It creates many problems for those unfortunate enough to find that they are both carriers. Some of them, but by no means all, will have the oppportunity of prenatal diagnosis if they decide to go ahead with their marriage.

Unfortunately, the techniques for prenatal diagnosis are limited to a few centres around the world, mainly in countries where the defects in haemoglobin occur in a comparatively small number of immigrants. It is hoped that eventually it will be possible to set up units of adequate size to deal with the numbers in the countries where these haemoglobinopathies are a major health problem.

A brief outline of haemoglobinopathies and the associated problems arising during pregnancy with a fuller account of the techniques currently available for prenatal diagnosis of these conditions follows, to enable those involved in obstetric practice to appreciate the desirability of prepregnancy identification of the woman and fetus who are at risk. This is of particular relevance now that antenatal diagnosis for an increasing number of these defects is possible by DNA analysis of fetal tissue obtained as early as 8 weeks' gestation.

NATURE OF THE DISORDERS

The genetic disorders of haemoglobin structure and synthesis are probably the commonest single gene disorders in the world population. They consist of two main groups:

1. The structural haemoglobin variants.
2. Inherited abnormalities of the synthesis of the globin chains of haemoglobin, the thalassaemias.

The genetic disorders of haemoglobin can only be appreciated against the background of an understanding of the structure, genetic control, and developmental genetics of normal haemoglobin. A brief simplified description follows; those who require further detail will find it in Weatherall & Clegg's (1981) masterly monograph.

All normal human haemoglobins have a similar basic structure. They consist of two different pairs of peptide chains (Fig. 23.1), each of which has a haem molecule

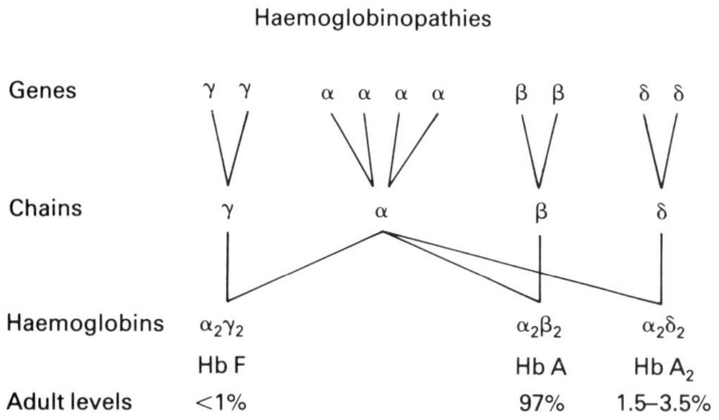

Fig. 23.1 Genetic control of globin chain synthesis. Adult levels achieved by 6 months of age.

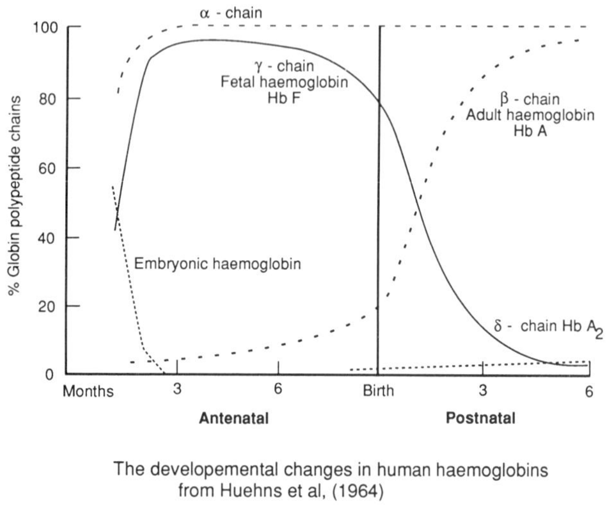

Fig. 23.2 The developmental changes in human haemoglobins. After Huehns et al (1964).

attached to it. Normal adults have a major and a minor haemoglobin component called haemoglobins A and A_2; these have a molecular formula $\alpha_2\beta_2$ and $\alpha_2\delta_2$ respectively. In fetal life the major haemoglobin is haemoglobin F ($\alpha_2\gamma_2$), although small amounts of haemoglobin A are being synthesized from as early as 6 weeks' gestation. The major change from fetal to adult haemoglobin production, i.e. gamma to beta chain synthesis, occurs from about 32 weeks postconception (Fig. 23.2). At birth there is approximately 70–90% haemoglobin F in the cord blood, although at this time of development gamma and beta chains are being produced in approximately equal amounts. Gamma chain synthesis declines rapidly after birth and by the end of the first year normal infants have only 1–2% haemoglobin F in their red cells. In addition to fetal and adult haemoglobin there are several different embryonic haemoglobins which disappear from the fetal blood by about the sixth week of development (Fig. 23.2).

The synthesis and structure of the four globin chains (alpha, beta, gamma and delta) are under separate control (Fig. 23.1). The adult levels shown in Figure 23.1 are those achieved by 6 months of age. It is obvious that only those conditions which affect the synthesis or structure of haemoglobin A ($\alpha_2\beta_2$), which should comprise over 95% of the total circulating haemoglobin in the adult, will be of significance for the mother during pregnancy. Alpha chain production is under the control of four genes, two inherited from each parent, located on chromosome 16 and, as can be seen, the alpha chains are common to all three haemoglobins. Beta chain production, on the other hand, is under the control of only two genes — one inherited from each parent; the beta together with gamma and delta genes are located on chromosome 11.

Although there are many different structural haemoglobin variants and disorders of alpha and beta chain synthesis, the most important ones from the public health point of view are the thalassaemias and the sickling disorders. Under normal circumstances the states for beta-thalassaemia and sickle cell haemoglobin are symptomless, with no direct effect on the quality of life or life expectancy. However, with the increased stress on haemopoiesis during the antenatal period, the clinical effects of these haemoglobin defects, even in the heterozygous or carrier state, may complicate obstetric management.

It will be obvious that any child born with homozygous defects of beta chain synthesis or structure will be perfectly healthy at birth and will not develop symptoms and signs of sickle cell disease or thalassaemia until 3–6 months of age, when beta chain production normally becomes predominant.

THE THALASSAEMIAS

The thalassaemias are an extremely heterogeneous group of genetic disorders of haemoglobin synthesis, all of which are characterized by a reduced rate of production of one or more of the globin chains of haemoglobin (Weatherall & Clegg 1981). They are classified according to the chain which is inefficiently produced. Although there are many different forms of thalassaemia they fall into two broad groups: the alpha-thalassaemias and the beta-thalassaemias. In the account of the different forms of alpha- and beta-thalassaemia which follows, the beta-thalassaemias will be dealt with first because they are the most important from a clinical point of view.

Beta-thalassaemias

The beta-thalassaemias are characterized by an inability to synthesize adult beta chains. Hence these disorders do not present in intrauterine life but only after birth when the effect of the switch from gamma to beta chain synthesis becomes significant. The heterozygous states for these conditions are symptomless. However, in the homozygous state for beta-thalassaemia there is a marked deficiency of beta chain production and although gamma chain synthesis persists it is usually insufficient to compensate for the deficiency of beta chains and hence there is a severe anaemia. For as yet obscure reasons, the homozygous states for delta–beta thalassaemia are much less severe because compensation by gamma chain synthesis is much more efficient in this disorder.

There are two main forms of beta-thalassaemia, the beta^0-thalassaemia in which no beta chains are produced, and the beta$^+$-thalassaemias in which there is a reduction in the amount of beta chains.

Prevalence

The beta-thalassaemias occur particularly commonly in the Mediterranean island populations, parts of Italy and Greece, throughout the Middle East, in parts of the Indian subcontinent, and throughout South-east Asia. The carrier rates in these populations range from 5 to 20%. The beta^0-thalassaemias are particularly common in Sardinia, the Po Valley region of Italy, and throughout South-east Asia. The beta$^+$-thalassaemia gene is particularly common in Cyprus, parts of southern Italy, and in the Middle East. In many populations both varieties of beta-thalassaemia are encountered.

Thalassaemia major, homozygous thalassaemia resulting from the inheritance of a defective beta globin gene from each parent, was the first identified form of the thalassaemia syndromes. It was described in the 1920s by Cooley, a physician practising in the United States. The first few cases were found in the children of Greek and Italian immigrants. The name *thalassaemia* was derived from the Greek *thalassa* meaning sea, or in the classical sense, the Mediterranean, because it was thought to be confined to individuals of Mediterranean origin.

Thalassaemia is a rare inherited abnormality among the indigenous British population. The heterozygote state is found in roughly 1 in 1000 individuals (compared with 1 in 7 in Cyprus) and the birth rate of homozygotes is of the order of 1 in 4 million. Some of the genes involved may be new mutations and some may have been imported from the Mediterranean from as far back as Phoenician times. However, thalassaemia has been brought to the United Kingdom in recent years by movements of populations and the arrival of immigrant groups of various ethnic origins.

In the 1950s and 1960s the main source of thalassaemia major cases was from the immigrant Cypriot populations who settled in the Greater London Area. From the 1960s onwards there has been a steady increase in the proportion of Asian cases.

Although the majority of the 360 or so cases currently living in the UK are still to be found in and around the Greater London Area there are increasing numbers of cases in the Midlands, Manchester, Bradford and Leeds. This is not only due to the fact that there has been an influx of Asian immigrants to these areas but that the Cypriot population of Greater London is a homogenous group which has taken advantage of the availability of prenatal diagnosis and consequently there has been a dramatic reduction in the number of homozygotes born to Cypriot couples at risk.

The Asian immigrant population, unlike the Cypriot, is very heterogenous, with incidences of thalassaemia varying markedly from group to group. They continue to have a high incidence of first-cousin marriages. A large group of rural Indians and Pakistanis has settled in the industrial towns of the Midlands and north-west. Few of this group make use of genetic counselling or fetal diagnosis and the incidence of thalassaemic children in this group continues to rise.

Before the days of regular transfusion, a child born with homozygous beta-thalassaemia would die in the first few years of life from anaemia, congestive cardiac failure, and intercurrent infection. Now that regular transfusion is routine where blood is freely available, survival is prolonged into the teens and early 20s. The management problem becomes one of iron overload derived from the transfused red cells. This results in hepatic and endocrine dysfunction and, most important of all, myocardial damage — the cause of death being cardiac failure in the vast majority of cases. Puberty is delayed or incomplete.

Modern management of thalassaemia consists of regular blood transfusions, timely splenectomy and iron chelation therapy. There has been no fundamental change since 1964 but we have learnt how to use these tools to their best advantage.

Bone marrow transplanation has been successfully performed in homozygous beta-thalassaemia and is a therapeutic option in younger patients who have human leukocyte antigen-compatible siblings. It should be offered to those patients for whom regular blood transfusion and iron chelation therapy are not available. In centres with adequate facilities children can be offered at least 15–20 years of reasonable life with conventional therapy, during which time an oral chelating agent should become available and genuine advances in gene therapy will be made. The fact that bone marrow transplantation can be successful in thalassaemia suggests that the disease will be amenable to gene therapy in the future (Lancet Editorial 1987). Prenatal diagnosis programmes have already led to a remarkable fall in the number of cases of severe forms of thalassaemia.

It is too early yet to know whether children started in the first 2 years of life on the more recently introduced intensive subcutaneous iron chelation programmes will achieve normal puberty and have a normal expectation of life. Successful pregnancy in a truly transfusion-dependent thalassaemic woman is very rare (Goldfarb et al 1982). It remains to be seen how effective recently instituted intensive iron chelation programmes will be.

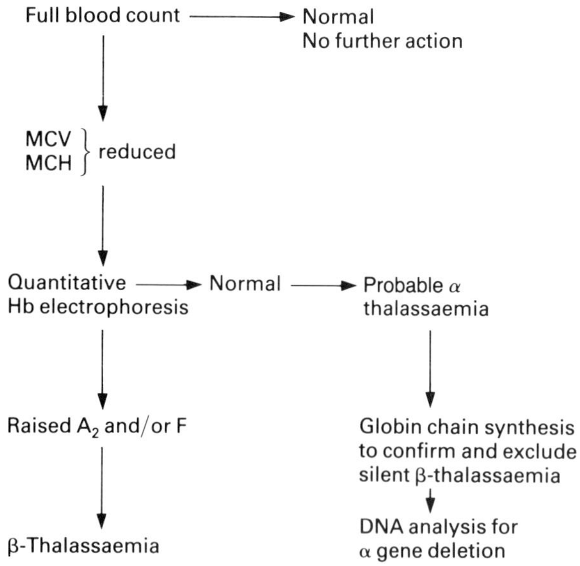

Fig. 23.3 Scheme for identifying individuals who are thalassaemia carriers. MCV = mean cell volume; MCH = mean corpuscular haemoglobin; Hb = haemoglobin.

Table 23.1 Red cell indices in thalassaemia and iron deficiency

		Normal range	Iron deficiency	Thalassaemia
PCV/RBC	MCV	75–99 fl	↓	↓
Hb/RBC	MCH	27–31 pg	↓	↓
Hb/PVC	MCHC	32–36 g/dl	↓	→

PCV = packed cell volume; RBC = red blood count; Hb = haemoglobin; MCV = mean corpuscular volume; MCH = mean corpuscular haemoglobin; MCHC = mean corpuscular haemoglobin concentration.

Management of beta-thalassaemia in pregnancy

Sometimes survival is possible without regular transfusion in homozygous beta-thalassaemia, a condition named thalassaemia intermedia, but this usually results in severe bone deformities due to massive expansion of marrow tissue, the site of largely ineffective erythropoiesis.

Although iron loading still occurs from excessive gastrointestinal absorption, stimulated by the accelerated marrow turnover, it is much slower than in those who are transfused and pregnancy may occur in this situation. Extra daily folate supplements should be given but iron in any form is contraindicated. The anaemia should be treated by transfusion during the antenatal period.

Perhaps the commonest problem associated with haemoglobinopathies and pregnancy in developed countries today is the anaemia in the antenatal period in women who have thalassaemia minor, heterozygous beta-thalassaemia. They can be identified for further examination of the blood by simple screening tests (Fig. 23.3). The red cells produced are very small with inadequate haemoglobin content, resulting in low mean cell volume (MCV) and mean cell haemoglobin (MCH), together with a normal or near normal mean corpuscular haemoglobin concentration (MCHC) (Table 23.1). The level of haemoglobin may be normal or slightly below the normal range. The diagnosis will be confirmed by finding a raised concentration of HbA_2 ($\alpha_2\delta_2$), with or without a raised HbF ($\alpha_2\gamma_2$). This is caused by excess alpha chains combining with delta and gamma chains because of the relative lack of beta chains (Fig. 23.1). Rare cases of heterozygous beta-thalassaemia with normal A_2 can only be identified by globin chain synthesis studies.

Women with beta-thalassaemia minor require the usual oral iron and folate supplements in the antenatal period. Oral iron for a limited period will not result in significant iron loading, even in the presence of replete iron stores, but *parenteral* iron should never be given (Letsky 1987). Iron deficiency has been shown in women in the UK with thalassaemia minor in a study of serum ferritin levels (Hussein et al 1975) and is regularly observed on investigation of anaemia, particularly in women of Asian origin who attend the antenatal clinic at Queen Charlotte's Maternity Hospital (Letsky, personal observation). If the anaemia does not respond to oral iron, and intramuscular folic acid has been tried, transfusion is indicated to achieve an adequate haemoglobin for delivery at term.

Alpha-thalassaemia

The alpha-thalassaemias are characterized by an inability to produce the alpha chains which are common to haemoglobins A ($\alpha_2\beta_2$), A_2 ($\alpha_2\delta_2$), and F ($\alpha_2\gamma_2$). In fetal life a deficiency of alpha chains results in the production of excess gamma chains which form γ_4 molecules or haemoglobin Barts. In adult life a deficiency of alpha chains leads to excess of beta chains which form β_4 tetramers of haemoglobin (Hb,H). Haemoglobin Barts and H are unstable and also useless as oxygen carriers. There are many different alpha-thalassaemia determinants which are associated with either a reduced or total absence of alpha chain production. In their heterozygous states these disorders are symptomless but in the homozygous or compound heterozygous states they give rise to a spectrum of disorders ranging from intrauterine death to a haemolytic anaemia of variable severity in adult life.

Normal individuals have four functional alpha genes. Alpha-thalassaemia, unlike beta-thalassaemia, is often but not always a gene deletion defect. There are two forms of alpha-thalassaemia trait which are the result of inheriting two or three normal alpha genes instead of the usual four. These are called $alpha^0$- and $alpha^+$-thalassaemia (Fig. 23.4), sometimes known as $alpha^1$- and $alpha^2$-thalassaemia, respectively. HbH disease is an intermediate form of alpha-thalassaemia in which there is only one functional alpha gene; HbH is the name given to the unstable haemoglobin formed

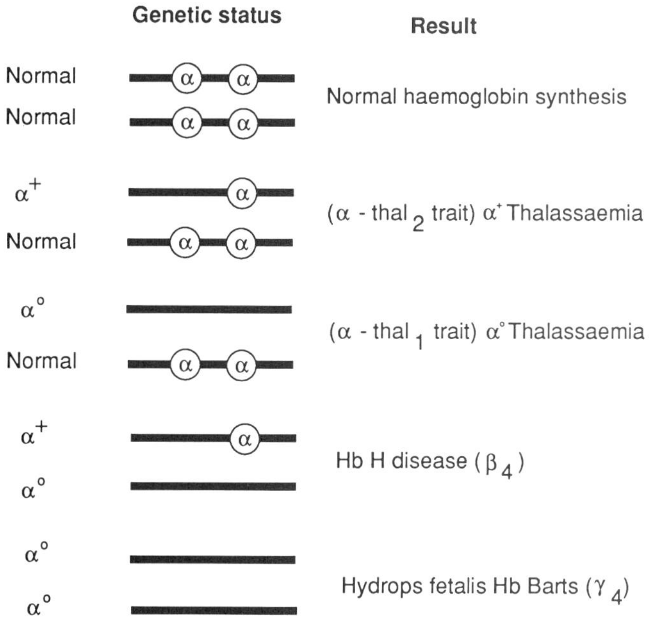

Fig. 23.4 Alpha genes and the various thalassaemias resulting from alpha gene deletion.

Table 23.2 Some of the therapeutic agents, chemicals and foodstuffs known to trigger haemolysis in glucose-6-phosphate dehydrogenase-deficient subjects. These can also augment haemolysis in HbH disease

Antimalarials	*Sulfones*
Primaquine	Sulfoxone (Diazone)
Pamaquine	Thiazolsulfone (Promizole)
Mepacrine	Diaminodiphenyl sulphone (DDS)
Quinine	
Chloroquine	*Others*
	Dimercaprol (BAL)
Sulphonamides	Methylene blue
Sulphanilamide	Naphthalene (moth balls)
Sulphacetamide	Aminosalicylic acid (PAS)
Sulphamethoxypyridazine (Lederkyn)	Phenylhydrazine
Sulphisoxazole (Gantrisin)	Acetylphenylhydrazine
Sulphafurazole	Probenecid (Benemid)
	Vitamin K (water-soluble analogues)
	Chloramphenicol
Nitrofurans	Quinidine
Nitrofurantoin (Furadantin)	Trinitrotoluene
Furazolidone (Furazone)	Mesantoin
Nitrofurazone (Furacin)	Broad beans
Antipyretics and analgesics	
Acetylsalicylic acid (aspirin)	
Acetanilide	
Acetophenetidin (Phenacetin)	
Aminopyrine (Pyramidon)	
Antipyrine	

by tetramers of the beta chain (β_4) when there is a relative lack of alpha chains. Alpha-thalassaemia major, in which there are no functional alpha genes (both parents having transmitted alpha^0-thalassaemia), is incompatible with life and pregnancy usually ends prematurely in a hydrops which will only survive a matter of hours if born alive. This is a common condition in South-east Asia. The name Hb Barts was given to tetramers of the gamma chain of fetal haemoglobin (γ_4) because it was first identified in a Chinese baby born at St Bartholomew's Hospital, London.

Management

During pregnancy, with its stress on the haemopoietic system, carriers of alpha-thalassaemia, particularly those with alpha^0-thalassaemia (two deleted genes on the same chromosome) may become very anaemic. They can be identified for further tests at booking, by finding abnormal red cell indices (Table 23.1), as in beta-thalassaemia trait. They have smaller red cells (MCV) and a reduced individual cell content of haemoglobin (MCH), although the mean cell haemoglobin concentration (MCHC) is usually within or just below the normal range. These changes are often minimal in alpha$^+$-thalassaemia (one deleted gene; Fig. 23.4), but this condition is not as important as alpha^0-thalassaemia in terms of genetic counselling and prenatal diagnosis. The diagnosis can only be confirmed by globin chain synthesis studies or, in the case of gene deletion, by DNA analysis of nucleated cells (Fig. 23.3).

There is no easily identifiable haemoglobin made or excess or lack of one or other of the normal haemoglobins. These individuals need iron and folate oral supplements throughout the antenatal period. Sometimes intramuscular folic acid is helpful but parenteral iron should *never* be given (as in beta-thalassaemia). If the haemoglobin is not thought to be adequate for delivery at term, transfusion is indicated.

Patients with HbH disease have a chronic haemolytic anaemia; they have 5–30% HbH in their peripheral blood, which can be identified on haemoglobin electrophoresis of freshly taken specimens as a fast-moving band. Sufferers have a normal life expectancy but require daily oral folate supplements to cover the demands of increased marrow turnover. During pregnancy it is recommended to give 5.0 mg folate daily to women with HbH disease. These women will transmit either alpha^0- or alpha$^+$-thalassaemia to their offspring.

It is perhaps not widely appreciated that because HbH is an unstable haemoglobin, it is susceptible to the oxidant effects of the same drugs and toxins as listed for glucose-6-phosphate dehydrogenase deficiency. Individuals with HbH disease should be given a list of compounds to be avoided, some of which are shown in Table 23.2. Exposure to them may trigger acute on chronic haemolysis.

Pregnancy with an alpha-thalassaemia hydrops is associated with severe, sometimes life-threatening pre-eclampsia (as in severe rhesus haemolytic disease). Vaginal deliveries are associated with obstetric complications due to the large fetus and very bulky placenta. If routine screening of the parents indicates that the mother is at risk of carrying such a child because both parents have alpha^0-thalassaemia, she should be referred for prenatal diagnosis.

The recent massive movement of refugees from Indo-

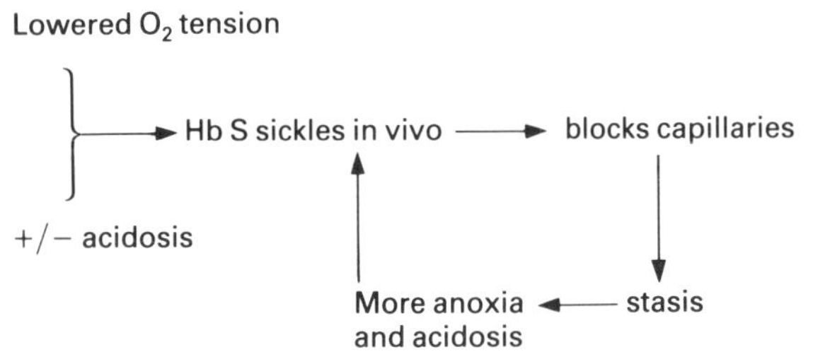

Fig. 23.5 Sequence of events in intravascular sickling.

China has produced populations in Europe, America and Australia, but perhaps not to the same extent in the UK, in which there is a high incidence of thalassaemia, particularly alpha^0-thalassaemia; these women obviously require prepregnancy screening if the mothers are to be best managed in pregnancy. Because the alpha^0 determinant is rare in Africans, alpha-thalassaemia does not pose a serious clinical problem in African populations and fetuses are not at risk of either alpha-thalassaemia hydrops or HbH disease (see Fig. 23.4).

HAEMOGLOBIN VARIANTS

Over 250 structural variants of the globin chains of normal human haemoglobins have been described but the most important by far, both numerically and clinically, is sickle cell haemoglobin (HbS). This is a variant of the beta globin chain where there is one amino acid substitution at the sixth position, a glutamine replacing a valine residue. HbS has the unique physical property that, despite being a soluble protein in its oxygenated form, in its reduced state the molecules become stacked on one another, forming tactoids, which distort the red cells to the characteristic shape which gives the haemoglobin its name. These sickled cells, because of their rigid structure, tend to block small blood vessels. The sickling phenomenon occurs particularly in conditions of lowered oxygen tension but may also be favoured by acidosis, dehydration or cooling, causing stasis in small blood vessels (Fig. 23.5).

Sickle cell syndromes

The sickling disorders include the heterozygous state for sickle cell haemoglobin, sickle cell trait (HbAS); homozygous sickle cell disease (HbSS); compound heterozygotes for Hb variants, the most important of which is sickle cell/HbC disease (HbSC), and sickle cell thalassaemia. Although these disorders are more commonly seen in black people of African origin, they can be seen in Saudi Arabians, Indians and Mediterraneans.

The characteristic feature of homogygous sickle cell anaemia (HbSS) is the occurrence of periods of health punctuated by periods of crisis. Between 3 and 6 months of age, when normal HbA production usually becomes predominant, a chronic haemolytic anaemia develops—haemoglobin level is between 6 and 9 g/dl. Even if the haemoglobin is in the lower range, symptoms due to anaemia are surprisingly few. This is because of the low affinity of HbS for oxygen; oxygen delivery to the tissues is facilitated, and there is little or no cellular anoxia even on exertion.

The acute episodes due to intravascular sickling are of far greater practical importance since they cause vascular occlusion resulting in tissue infarction (Fig. 23.5). The affected part is painful and the clinical manifestations are extremely variable, depending on the site at which sickling takes place. Sickling crises are often precipitated by infection and may be exacerbated by an accompanying dehydration. The majority of deaths are due to massive sickling following an acute infection.

Renal complications are a constant finding; there is a progressive inability to concentrate the urine and haematuria is common. Both these defects result from sickling in the renal medullary circulation. Inability to concentrate the urine adequately makes pregnant women unduly prone to dehydration during labour.

Prognosis depends greatly on environment; in Africa, a large proportion of children with this disorder die within the first 5 years and probably less than 10% reach adulthood. In contrast, in the West Indies, where prompt treatment and prophylaxis of infection are more easily available, many women with sickle cell disease need management during pregnancy (Serjeant 1983). Thomas et al (1982), reviewing 241 mortalities from homozygous sickle cell disease in the West Indies, found that 10 were associated with pregnancy and often due to pulmonary embolus which has been reported with hyterozygotes (Van Dinh et al 1982).

Sickle cell haemoglobin C disease (HbSC) is a milder variant of HbSS with normal or near normal levels of haemoglobin. One of the dangers of this condition is that, owing to its mildness, neither the woman nor her obstetrician may be aware of its presence. These women are at risk of massive, sometimes fatal, sickling crises during pregnancy and particularly in the puerperium. It is therefore vital that the abnormality is detected, preferably before pregnancy, so that the appropriate precautions can be taken.

Clinical manifestations of the doubly heterozygous condition, sickle cell thalassaemia, are usually indistinguishable from HbSS although those who make detectable amounts of HbA are usually less severely affected but still at risk from sickling crises during pregnancy.

Sickle cell trait (HbAS) results in no detectable abnormality under normal circumstances although it is easily diagnosed by specific investigations including haemoglobin electrophoresis. Affected subjects are not anaemic even under the additional stress of pregnancy, unless there are additional complications. Sickling crises occur only in situations of extreme anoxia, dehydration and acidosis.

Management of sickle cell syndromes

At present there is no effective long-term method of reducing the liability of red cells to sickle in vivo. Once a crisis is established, there is no evidence that alkalis, hyperbaric oxygen, vasodilators, plasma expanders, urea or anticoagulants are of any value. Where beneficial effects have been reported they can usually be attributed to the meticulous care and supportive therapy received by the patient, rather than to the specific measures themselves. Adequate fluid administration alone probably accounts for the benefit.

Contraception and sickle cell syndromes

There is much more longitudinal experience in the USA than there is as yet in the UK. Methods of contraception vary (Samuels-Rein et al 1984), but problems arise from the assumption that sicklers are at increased risk of thromboembolism if they use oral contraception. The patient's risk of thromboembolism is less than that of pregnancy and there are almost no data to suggest that patients with sickle cell disease run a greater risk than any other patients using low-oestrogen preparations (Charache & Niebyl 1985). The usual contraindications hold true, of course, and patients should be monitored meticulously for alterations in blood pressure and liver function.

Recommendations for tubal ligation should be made only after difficult pregnancies and sterilization should not be advised routinely for patients with sickle cell disease.

Sickle cell disease and pregnancy

Women with sickle cell disease present special problems in pregnancy (Charache et al 1980, Tuck et al 1983). Fetal loss is high, presumably due to sickling infarcts in the placental circulation. Abortion, preterm labour and other complications are more common than in women with normal haemoglobin. Although many women with sickle cell disease have no complications, the outcome in any individual case is always in doubt. The only consistently successful way of reducing the incidence of complications due to sickling is by regular blood transfusion at approximately 6-week intervals, to maintain the proportion of HbA at 60–70% of the total (Huehns 1982). Between 3 and 4 units of blood should be given at each transfusion. This regime has two effects; it dilutes the circulating sickle haemoglobin and, by raising the haemoglobin, reduces the stimulus to the bone marrow and therefore the amount of sickle haemoglobin produced.

Sickle cells have a shorter life than normal red cells and so the effect of each successive transfusion is more beneficial. If this regime has been instituted a general anaesthetic may be given with safety and sickling crises in the course of normal labour are much less likely. The management of sickle cell syndromes in pregnancy in the UK is a relatively recent problem but it is clear on review of the American literature that modern obstetric care alone, without transfusion, has reduced the maternal morbidity and mortality dramatically and also improved fetal outcome, although risk rates still remain higher for pregnancy complicated by sickle cell disease (Charache et al 1980, Serjeant 1983). Increasing numbers of obstetric centres have adopted prophylactic transfusion regimens but the real benefit of such regimens remains to be proved by a large trial with proper controls (Tuck et al 1987). At the time of writing one such trial is in progress in Britain.

These regular transfusion protocols are not without complications. Of course there is a risk of transmitting infection, particularly non A non B hepatitis and the pregnant woman with her altered immunity is particularly susceptible.

Now that all blood donors are screened for exposure and response to the acquired immune deficiency syndrome (AIDS) virus, the much publicized and feared hazard of human immunodeficiency virus (HIV) infection resulting from 1-unit blood donations (non-pooled blood products) is extremely small. The risk of infected blood being undetected has been calculated to be 0.7 per million donations and that is if high-risk donors (homosexuals and drug addicts) are giving blood, which they are asked not to do in the UK (Acheson 1987).

The most worrying complication has been the development of atypical red cell antibodies (Tuck et al 1987), resulting from the fact that the donor populations differ in ethnic origin from the recipients and carry different minor red cell antigens. This has resulted in extreme difficulties in finding compatible blood (Miller et al 1981, Tuck et al 1983), and even in haemolytic disease of the newborn (Tuck et al 1983). There is a real danger that regular top-up transfusions or partial exchange transfusion regimes may become accepted therapy in pregnancy complicated by sickle cell disease, before their true benefits and hazards have been properly evaluated (Tuck et al 1987). The general consensus from the USA is that until results of properly planned trials with correctly chosen controls are available it would seem wise to give close obstetric supervision, and deliver women where there are special care baby units available. Transfusion should only be given in preparation for general anaesthetic or where there is evidence of maternal distress (Charache et al 1980, Charache & Niebyl 1985). If the disorder presents late in pregnancy and there is more urgency because, for instance, the woman is profoundly anaemic or suffering a crisis, exchange transfusion can be used.

Clinical supervision and awareness of early signs of possible complications are probably more important in improved outcome than regular transfusion.

It is obvious that it would be far better to prevent the emergency situation during pregnancy by identification of women before pregnancy and early booking for antenatal care. However, even after preparation with regular transfusion, tissue hypoxia, acidosis and dehydration should be avoided because they make the patient's own remaining red cells more likely to sickle. Tourniquets should not be used. To minimize pulmonary infection, prophylactic antibiotics are desirable to cover all anaesthetics.

The worry concerning aspiration pneumonitis, hypoxia and other perioperative pulmonary problems may be avoided by using regional anaesthesia, but this substitutes the risk of hypotension and venous pooling in vessels of the lower extremities. Wrapping the legs in elastic bandages and elevating them will reduce venous pooling and subsequent hypotension. Epidural is preferred to spinal anaesthesia because there is less risk of hypotension if proper preoperative hydration regimes with left uterine displacement are adopted. Although a number of sicklers in the obstetric literature have been reported to have suffered pulmonary emboli there is no good evidence to incriminate regional anaesthesia as a significant additional risk factor and indeed there are good physiological data to support the concept that it has a protective role. In an emergency both regional and general anaesthesia may have to be given without ideal preparation. Good communication and co-operation between anaesthetist, obstetrician and haematologist together with meticulous postoperative care help most such emergencies result in a happy outcome. Again, as with the controversy over blood transfusion, it is simple lack of awareness of potential problems and relaxation of vigilance which change the story (Charache & Niebyl 1985) rather than the details of the measures adopted to deal with the many and varied hazards of sickle haemoglobin in pregnancy.

No special preparation with blood transfusion is required in pregnancy for women with sickle cell trait (HbAS). However, as in patients with HbSS, it is essential that hypoxia and dehydration are avoided during anaesthesia and labour, particularly in the immediate post-delivery period. In fact the majority of unexpected deaths associated with HbS have occurred in patients with sickle cell trait in the immediate postoperative or postpartum period (Pastorek & Seiler 1985).

The single most important pregnancy precaution is for the woman's partner to be screened, so that the couple can be advised of the risk of a serious haemoglobin defect in their offspring.

Detection of HbS

Any test designed to screen for the presence of HbS should detect not only sickle cell disease but also distinguish HbSC, HbS thalassaemia and sickle cell trait. The classic sickling test in which the red cell is suspended in a reducing agent is difficult to interpret and may occasionally give false negative results. Furthermore it is time-consuming and its usefulness is limited when diagnosis is urgent. A proprietary product, Sickledex, overcomes these drawbacks; it detects HbS by precipitation of deoxygenated HbS. It is rapid, reliable, and does not give false negatives. Definitive diagnosis of the particular sickle cell syndrome involved requires haemoglobin electrophoresis and sometimes, in the case of sickle cell states and thalassaemia, family studies. Screening early in pregnancy where there is no absolute urgency is probably better carried out by performing Hb electrophoresis. The sickling test will then only have to be carried out on blood from those women with an abnormal band in the S region on conventional electrophoresis (on cellulose acetate in tris buffer at pH 8.9) to distinguish it from HbD, which has similar electrophoretic mobility.

SCREENING FOR HAEMOGLOBINOPATHY

Unfortunately, screening procedures are currently often not carried out until the woman is pregnant. In most cases this means that early prenatal diagnosis by DNA analysis of a chorion biopsy is not possible. Selection for screening in a busy antenatal clinic may be more time-consuming than it is worth and, to be efficient, should involve detailed documentation of a woman's heritage before excluding her from testing. For this reason, and because of the remote possibility of missing such a defect in the non-immigrant population, general screening for haemoglobinopathies is carried out routinely on every pregnant woman's blood at Queen Charlotte's Maternity Hospital, which serves a cosmopolitan population. This involves examination of red cell indices (Table 23.1), haemoglobin electrophoresis, and, where indicated, quantitation of HbA_2 and HbF on every sample of blood taken at booking (Fig. 23.3). If a haemoglobin variant or thalassaemia is found, the partner is requested to attend so that his blood can also be examined. By this means medical staff are able to assess the chances of a serious haemoglobin defect in the fetus early in pregnancy, to advise the parents of the potential hazard and to offer them prenatal diagnosis by fetal blood sampling, if they so desire.

Inevitably this results in late prenatal diagnosis and a painful, demoralizing second-trimester termination if indicated, but unless couples at risk are identified before pregnancy is embarked upon there is no other alternative, with few exceptions. These include all couples with sickle haemoglobin and some rare but easily identified forms of thalassaemia for which DNA probes are readily available. In addition these couples have to be identified within the first 8–10 weeks of fetal development, which is unusual with standard booking procedures.

PRENATAL DIAGNOSIS OF HAEMOGLOBINOPATHIES

Fetal blood sampling: globin chain synthesis

Until the mid 1970s the prenatal diagnosis of thalassaemia major and of sickle cell disease (also a beta globin chain defect) was thought to be a relatively unrealistic goal for two reasons. Firstly, because information concerning beta chain synthesis in the first and second trimesters of human pregnancy was lacking and secondly, because it was believed that any techniques necessary for acquisition of fetal blood would prove to be prohibitively dangerous with respect to the maintenance of the pregnancy.

Huehns and his colleagues at University College Hospital showed that adult haemoglobin (HbA $\alpha_2\beta_2$) could be detected in the red cells of the fetus at as early as 8–10 weeks of gestation (Huehns et al 1964; Fig. 23.2). If the haemoglobin is labelled with a radioactive amino acid and then globin chain separation is effected by use of carboxymethyl cellulose urea chromatography (Clegg et al 1966), the amount of beta chain synthesis can be quantitated and compared to gamma chain derived from fetal haemoglobin (HbF $\alpha_2\gamma_2$) (Wood & Weatherall 1973). The beta : gamma ratio was determined in fetuses with normal haemoglobins at various gestations on abortion material when termination was being carried out for non-haematological reasons. The next stage was to find the beta : gamma ratios in fetuses of Cypriot women in London, where offspring were at risk for thalassaemia and the women had already opted for a termination. The normal beta : gamma ratio at 18 weeks' gestation is about 0.11. It was found that those fetuses who had thalassaemia minor had beta : gamma ratios at or above 0.045, and those with thalassaemia major had ratios of 0.025 or below (Chang et al 1975).

The diagnosis of sickle cell disease using fetal blood samples is much simpler, and does not require quantitation of beta globin chain synthesis because structural differences give the haemoglobin different electrophoretic properties.

Various methods for obtaining fetal blood have been tried. The first and simplest approach is that of placental aspiration, pioneered in the UK by Fairweather at University College Hospital. The placenta is located by ultrasound, a 20 gauge needle is placed in the fetal surface of the placenta and a small sample (less than 0.1 ml) is aspirated with or without ultrasound guidance. There is bleeding into the amniotic fluid immediately following withdrawal of the needle and a sample of the blood-stained amniotic fluid often contains a high percentage of fetal cells.

The second approach, developed at Yale (Hobbins & Mahoney 1974), involves the modification of fetoscopy to equip a small fibreoptic fetoscope with an aspirating needle such that a fetal vein on the surface of the placenta can be identified. The fetal blood sampling is performed at 18–20 weeks' gestation when the placenta is sufficiently thick and the vessels large enough to provide a specimen of fetal blood. By both these methods of placental aspiration a mixture of fetal and maternal blood may be obtained, since the end of the needle might not be precisely and completely within the lumen of a vessel containing fetal blood. It may therefore extract a small amount of maternal blood from the comparatively close pool accumulating around the villae. A Coulter particle size analyser can be used in the operating room to determine rapidly the relative proportion of the large fetal erythrocytes and small maternal red cells. The obstetrician can stop as soon as an adequate sample is taken.

In the absence of maternal reticulocytosis, as little as 10 μl of fetal cells would suffice, even in the presence of as much as 80% maternal cell contamination. The reason for this is that fetal red cells synthesize globin chains at a much higher rate than do mature adult red cells. It is also possible to concentrate fetal red cells in a mixture of maternal and fetal cells because of the antigenic and biochemical difference between the two (Kan et al 1974, Boyer et al 1976, Alter et al 1979). Pure fetal blood samples, therefore, are not required for the diagnosis of haemoglobinopathies, but Rodeck & Nicolaides (1983) perfected a technique for sampling pure fetal blood from the umbilical cord. Samples uncontaminated by maternal blood or amniotic fluid are obtained. This facilitates the direct examination of fetal red cells for globin chain content without prior manipulation and also provides samples of pure fetal plasma for prenatal diagnosis of genetic coagulation defects (Nicolaides et al 1985). However, this technique has the same disadvantages that the others share, for the sampling is carried out at approximately 18 weeks' gestation and will result in second-trimester termination of pregnancy if indicated.

The procedure has some risks. The most important by far is fetal loss which may be due to fetal exsanguination (associated more commonly with placental aspiration) or may be secondary to premature labour (more frequent when the fetoscope is used). Sometimes amniotic fluid leak follows the investigations, usually when the fetoscope is used, but does not necessarily herald preterm labour and the pregnancy may continue to term with no ill effect (Alter 1979).

It is now possible to obtain pure fetal blood from the umbilical cord by means of an ultrasound-guided needle (Nicolaides et al 1986). The risks to the pregnancy of this procedure are considerably less than when the fetoscope is used. Many obstetricians are adopting the use of ultrasound guidance for sampling amniotic fluid, chorionic villus sampling and for oocyte recovery, so that blood sampling by ultrasound-guided needling in high-risk pregnancies need not be restricted to a few specialized centres. The safety of the method needs further investigation, but it would appear to compare very favourably with other methods. Daffos (cited in Nicolaides et al 1986) sampled 1050 pregnancies with only two fetal losses related to the procedure and no significant maternal morbidity.

Studies of fetal blood from cases at risk for haemoglobinopathies began in 1974 in collaborative work between Boston Children's Hospital and University College Hospital in London (Alter et al 1975) and in San Francisco (Kan et al 1977). Almost 4000 cases had been studied by the early 1980s in 21 centres around the world (Alter 1983). In all, 90% were at risk for thalassaemia and the others for sickle cell disorders. It is of interest that most of the prenatal tests have been performed for thalassaemia, although sickle cell disease is more common in the USA where prenatal diagnosis using fetal blood analysis started. However, sickle cell disease has variable severity, while thalassaemia is more often fatal in children. Current treatment for thalassaemia is cumbersome, expensive and difficult. Thus the decision regarding abortion of the affected fetuses is perhaps easier.

The overall fetal loss rate is now 5%—under 2% in centres in London—which is much less than the 12–15% loss rate of earlier reported studies (Alter 1979). A total of 1% of diagnoses have been incorrect. These were primarily due to overlap in beta : gamma ratio between the heterozygote and beta$^+$ homozygote, resulting either in termination of pregnancies in which the fetus proved to have thalassaemia minor or allowing pregnancies with thalassaemia major to go to term. It is obvious that if fetal blood sampling could be avoided the risks of prenatal diagnosis would be considerably less.

Globin gene analysis

In the last few years there have been remarkable advances in molecular biology and in particular the development of techniques for isolating and analysing DNA (Weatherall 1985a). Normal globin genes have been examined using molecular hybridization and restriction endonuclease mapping techniques (Old & Higgs 1983). For the study of human genetic diseases DNA is usually obtained from the nuclei of white blood cells in a peripheral blood sample. However, in the prenatal diagnosis of haemoglobinopathies there are two possible alternative sources of DNA for diagnosis of fetal disease—amniotic fluid fibroblasts and trophoblast tissue obtained by a transcervical chorion biopsy technique (Rodeck & Morsman 1983, Nicolaides et al 1985). The use of these techniques depends on being able to identify an abnormality of DNA of the globin gene involved in the haemoglobinopathy or a closely linked polymorphism which is inherited with the relevant gene.

The application of recombinant DNA technology for the detection of human genetic disorders involves a few basic steps (Fig. 23.6). The limiting factor is to be able to make a gene probe which will recognize and combine with the targeted genomic DNA. Fetal DNA is prepared from chorionic biopsy tissue or from amniotic fluid fibroblasts. This DNA is then cleaved into fragments with restriction endonuclease enzymes derived from bacteria. Each enzyme recognizes a specific sequence of bases and cuts at a prescribed point. These DNA fragments are then separated on the basis of size by agarose gel electrophoresis and transferred to nitrocellulose papers by a blotting technique. The DNA material is then submitted to a search by the appropriate radiolabelled probe. If an area of DNA complementary to the probe is present in one of the fragments then hybridization will occur between the probe and fragment, and this can be visualized with autoradiography (Fig. 23.6). In conditions resulting from gene deletion the expected fragments may be absent in homozygote individuals or less intense in heterozygotes.

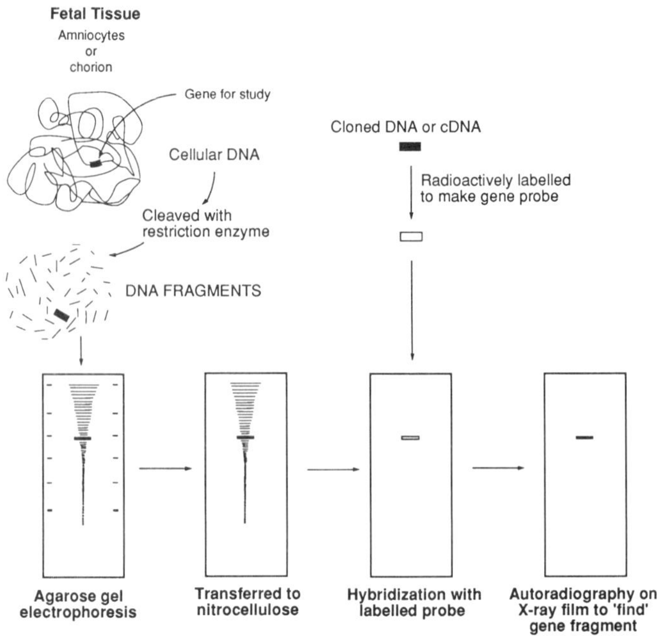

Fig. 23.6 Simplified representation of the basic steps involved in DNA analysis for prenatal diagnosis of haemoglobinopathies. From Weatherall (1985b).

Alternatively a probe may be used to identify a linked polymorphism. Polymorphisms close to the gene represent stable inheritable non-functional variants—unlikely to be separated from the gene in question during meiosis—and can be used to identify mutated genes because the polymorphisms alter the DNA fragment lengths which hybridize with the selected probes.

All cases of sickle cell disease can now be diagnosed prenatally by DNA analysis because of an identifiable base change in the beta gene structure which synthesizes sickle haemoglobin. Most fetuses at risk for serious alpha-thalassaemia syndromes can be identified because the abnormalities result from alpha gene deletion (Kan et al 1976). Delta-beta thalassaemias are also diagnosable because they result from gene deletions (Orkin et al 1978). The majority of beta-thalassaemias are still prenatally diagnosed by fetal blood sampling but a rapidly increasing number are becoming identifiable by DNA analysis because of linked polymorphisms or partial gene deletions (Kan et al 1980). Unfortunately in these cases however, unless the couple has been identified and there is a large family available for study and plenty of time to perform the laboratory investigations required, the technique has not usually been used until an affected child has been brought into the world.

A recent study of the Mediterranean populations including UK Cypriot immigrants suggests that in 70% of first pregnancies at risk for beta-thalassaemia an affected fetus could be identified with oligonucleotide probes (see Weatherall 1985a). These are small, synthetic DNA fragments which are specifically constructed to detect single base changes in DNA. Although oligonucleotide probe technology is still being developed, it has already been possible to construct probes which identify the single base changes causing human single gene disorders (Weatherall 1985b).

A new rapid method of DNA analysis for prenatal diagnosis of sickle cell anaemia using a radiolabelled oligonucleotide probe has recently been described (Embury et al 1987). In vitro enzymatic amplification of the genomic beta globin gene sequences to be analysed provides sufficient DNA for analysis and prenatal identification of sickle cell haemoglobin on the same day that the fetal tissue is made available. Even if direct analysis without culturing the tissue provided is possible, standard procedures in the molecular genetics laboratory can take up to 2 weeeks.

Amniotic fluid fibroblasts

Although amniocentesis is safer than fetal blood sampling, sufficiently large samples of cells for analysis are not obtained any earlier with this procedure. This means that termination of an affected pregnancy may be delayed until late in the second trimester. However, in Hong Kong Chan et al (1984) have shown that they can diagnose alpha-thalassaemia by direct analysis of the globin genes in fetal DNA obtained from amniotic fluid fibroblasts without culture (usually 3–4 weeks' culture is required to get sufficient DNA). An earlier termination is therefore facilitated using a technique with very little associated risk.

It may be asked why prenatal diagnosis for alpha-thalassaemia should be attempted when the major form of the disease is incompatible with life, and HbH disease probably does not adversely affect life expectancy. One reason is that pregnancy with an alpha-thalassaemia hydrops is associated with severe, sometimes life-threatening pre-eclampsia in the mother. Also, vaginal deliveries are associated with obstetric complications due to the large fetus and very bulky placenta; the mothers are usually of Oriental origin and so are small in stature (Liang et al 1985).

Chorion biopsy

Details of a new technique were initially published by Williamson and colleagues (1981); these authors demonstrated that prenatal diagnosis was possible in the first trimester. They showed that samples of trophoblast could be obtained by transcervical aspiration before elective abortion in 8–14-week pregnancies. DNA is extracted from chorionic villi and sufficient is obtained to perform restriction endonuclease mapping (Old et al 1982). The potential advantages of DNA analysis may be utilized in this way in the future for prenatal diagnosis not only of haemoglobinopathies but other conditions such as cystic fibrosis, where there is no means, as yet, of detecting the carrier state (Lancet Editorial 1984, Weatherall 1984, 1985a). However, the realization of this technique depends not only on the ability to analyse DNA variations in the laboratory; the method of obtaining chorionic villi must be proved to be safe, with risks of fetal loss and morbidity no greater than with current procedures. Family DNA studies are required as soon as it is recognized that a couple are at risk and before pregnancy is embarked upon, so that their suitability for this type of prenatal diagnosis can be assessed. This facilitates practical arrangements for early chorion biopsy if the couple has identifiable DNA abnormalities associated with the haemoglobinopathy.

Old et al (1986) reported on 200 cases of first-trimester fetal diagnosis for haemoglobinopathies carried out in the UK using chorionic villus sampling and DNA analysis. The results suggest that, provided that chorionic villus sampling is proven to be associated with an acceptably low fetal loss rate and has no significant long-term effects on fetal development, it will become the method of choice for fetal diagnosis of haemoglobinopathies and of other single gene disorders. The current chorionic villus sampling fetal loss rate is little more than 2% which compares favourably with other methods used in prenatal diagnosis.

Initially transcervical villus sampling was carried out using an endoscope but this technique has been largely abandoned and biopsy specimens are obtained using a fine-bore needle and cannula under ultrasound guidance. Even so the procedure still probably carries a risk of abortion at least two to three times greater than that of amniocentesis, plus a maternal risk of endotoxic shock ascribed to penetration of a contaminated cervix. For these reasons some workers in the field have adopted the transabdominal approach (Maxwell et al 1986). They claim that this avoids the potentially infected endocervical canal and also that needle-guided transabdominal chorionic villus sampling is more easily learned than transcervical techniques. High abortion rates seemed to be associated with transcervical biopsy until the operator becomes skilled. In addition the transabdominal method may be used over a wider gestational age range — 9–14 weeks as opposed to 9–12 weeks using the transcervical route. Maxwell and colleagues (1986) suggest that the technique should be widely evaluated in clinical practice, possibly as part of a controlled trial comparing transabdominal with transcervical routes.

Meanwhile the procedure of fetal blood sampling remains the method used in many cases of beta-thalassaemia. However, recent indications are that an increasing number of thalassaemia syndromes will become susceptible to diagnosis by examination of chorion biopsy and, of course, all cases of sickle cell disease can now be diagnosed by DNA analysis of either chorion, or, later in pregnancy, amniotic fluid fibroblasts.

COST IMPLICATIONS

The major limitation of DNA technology is that it requires specialist laboratories and uses expensive materials.

On the basis of current figures in the UK it has been

calculated (Old et al 1986) that the cost of a family DNA study followed by a separate fetal diagnosis for thalassaemia is £480, including materials and labour. The diagnosis of sickle cell disease does not require a family study and therefore costs half this amount.

Chorion villus sampling costs about £250; therefore the cost for a first-trimester diagnosis of beta-thalassaemia is £730 and for sickle cell anaemia is £490. Diagnosis by prenatal fetal blood sampling is much less costly. The current cost of managing a patient with thalassaemia major is around £5000 per annum, and about £2000 for sickle cell disease.

It is obvious that in time even a prenatal diagnosis programme based entirely on expensive DNA technology will prove to be highly cost-effective.

Rationale for screening

The main reason why prepregnancy screening programmes for haemoglobinopathies should be set up is the handicap associated with homozygous beta-thalassaemia. The management of homozygous beta-thalassaemia by regular blood transfusion and chelating agents is extremely expensive and places a major burden on the health services, particularly in those developing countries where the disease is so common. Undoubtedly, the most cost-effective approach to the problem of thalassaemia is the development of programmes for the prepregnancy screening of potential mothers and, in cases where they are found to be carriers, of their partners (Weatherall & Letsky 1984). Where both parents are affected they should be offered the possibility of antenatal diagnosis by fetal blood or trophoblast sampling and of abortion of homozygous fetuses. This type of programme is now well established in many parts of the world, but screening usually takes place in the antenatal period when conception has already occurred. Even if the couple is known to be at risk, having already had an affected child, there may not be time for proper investigation. Advantage cannot then be taken of the more acceptable trophoblast sampling technique for DNA analysis of the fetus.

IMPLICATIONS FOR THE FUTURE

Now that first-trimester fetal diagnosis is becoming possible for an increasing number of serious haemoglobinopathies and the technique becomes available in more centres over the world, screening procedures should be extended beyond the antenatal clinic. It has been suggested (Modell 1983) that education and counselling should be directed at three points in people's lives — at school, at marriage, and at family planning clinics. The information given should include details of where blood testing can be carried out and when this should be done, although it should probably be left to the informed individual to request the test. This involves education of the communities at risk and also — a component which is often forgotten — education of the medical practitioners caring for these communities.

REFERENCES

Acheson D 1987 Press Release 87/5. Department of Health and Social Security, London

Alter B P 1979 Prenatal diagnosis of haemoglobinopathies and other haematological diseases. Journal of Pediatrics 95: 501–513

Alter B P 1983 Antenatal diagnosis using fetal blood. In: Weatherall D J (ed) The thalassaemias. Churchill Livingstone, Edinburgh, pp 114–133

Alter B P, Modell C B, Fairweather D, et al 1976 Prenatal diagnosis of haemoglobinopathy: a review of 165 cases. New England Journal of Medicine 295: 1437–1443

Alter B P, Metzger J B, Yock P G, Rothchild S B, Cover G J 1979 Selective hemolysis of adult red blood cells: an aid to prenatal diagnosis of haemoglobinopathies. Blood 53: 279–287

Boyer S H, Noyes A N, Boyer M L 1976 Enrichment of erythrocytes of fetal origin from adult–fetal blood mixtures via selective haemolysis of adult blood cells: an aid to antenatal diagnosis of haemoglobinopathies. Blood 47: 883–897

Chan V, Ghosh A, Chan T K, Wong V, Todd D 1984 Prenatal diagnosis of homozygous α thalassaemia by direct DNA analysis of uncultured amniotic fluid cells. British Medical Journal 288: 1327–1329

Chang H, Modell C B, Alter B P et al 1975 Expression of the β thalassaemia gene in the first trimester fetus. Proceedings of the National Academy of Sciences (USA) 72: 3633–3637

Charache S, Niebyl J R 1985 Pregnancy in sickle cell disease. In: Letsky E A (ed) Haematological disorders in pregnancy. Clinics in haematology. Saunders, London, pp 729–746

Charache S, Scott J, Niebyl J, Bonds D 1980 Management of sickle cell disease in pregnant patients. Obstetrics and Gynecology 55: 407–410

Clegg J B, Naughton M A, Weatherall D J 1966 Abnormal human haemoglobins; separation and characterisation of the γ and β chains by chromatography and the determination of two new variants Hb Chesapeake and Hb J (Bangkok). Journal of Molecular Biology 19: 91–108

Embury S H, Scharf S J, Saiki R K et al 1987 Rapid prenatal diagnosis of sickle cell anaemia by a new method of DNA analysis. New England Journal of Medicine 316: 656–661

Goldfarb A E, Hochner-Celnikier D, Beller U, Menashe M, Dargan I, Palti Z 1982 A successful pregnancy in transfusion dependent homozygous β-thalassaemia: a case report. International Journal of Gynaecology and Obstetrics 20: 319–322

Hobbins J C, Mahoney J M 1974 In utero diagnosis of haemoglobinopathies: techniques for obtaining fetal blood. New England Journal of Medicine 290: 1065–1067

Huehns E R 1982 The structure and function of haemoglobin: clinical disorders due to abnormal haemoglobin structure. In: Hardisty R M, Weatherall D J (eds) Blood and its disorders, 2nd edn. Blackwell Scientific, Oxford, p 364

Huehns E R, Dance N, Beavan G H, Hect F, Motulsky A G 1964 Human embryonic haemoglobin. Cold Spring Harbor Symposium on Quantitative Biology 29: 327–331

Hussein S S, Hoffbrand A V, Laulicht M, Attock B, Letsky E A 1975 Serum ferritin levels in beta thalassaemia trait. British Medical Journal 2: 920

Kan Y W, Nathan D G, Cividalli E, Crookston M C 1974 Concentration of fetal red blood cells from a mixture of maternal and fetal blood anti-i serum; an aid to prenatal diagnosis of haemoglobinopathy. Blood 43: 411–415

Kan Y W, Golbus M S, Dozy A M 1976 Prenatal diagnosis of α thalassaemia: clinical application of molecular hybridization. New England Journal of Medicine 295: 1165–1167

Kan Y W, Trecartin R F, Golbus M S, Filly R A 1977 Prenatal diagnosis of β thalassaemia and sickle cell anaemia. Experience with 24 cases. Lancet i: 269–271

Kan Y W, Lee K Y, Forbetta M, Angua A, Cao A 1980 Polymorphism of DNA sequence in β globin gene region. Application to prenatal

diagnosis of β thalassaemia in Sardinia. New England Journal of Medicine 302: 185–188
Lancet Editorial 1984 Molecular genetics for the clinician. Lancet i: 257–259
Lancet Editorial 1987 Marrow transplantation for thalassaemia. Lancet i: 1246
Letsky E A 1987 Anaemia in obstetrics. In: Studd J (ed) Progress in obstetrics and gynaecology, vol 6. Churchill Livingstone, Edinburgh, pp 23–59
Liang S T, Wong V C W, So W W K, Ma H K, Chan V, Todd D 1985 Homozygous α-thalassaemia; clinical presentation, diagnosis and management. A review of 46 cases. British Journal of Obstetrics and Gynaecology 92: 680–684
Maxwell D, Czepulkowski B, Lilford R, Heaton D, Coleman D 1986 Transabdominal chorionic villus sampling. Lancet i: 123–126
Miller J M, Horger E O, Key T C, Walker E M 1981 Management of sickle haemoglobinopathies in pregnant patients. American Journal of Obstetrics and Gynecology 141: 237–241
Modell B 1983 Prevention of haemoglobinopathies. British Medical Bulletin 39: 386–391
Nicolaides K H, Rodeck C H, Mibashan R S 1985 Obstetric management and diagnosis of haematological disease in the fetus. In: Letsky E A (ed) Haematological disorders in pregnancy. Clinics in haematology. Saunders, London, pp 775–805
Nicolaides K H, Soothill P W, Rodeck C H, Campbell S 1986 Ultrasound-guided sampling of umbilical cord and placental blood to assess fetal wellbeing. Lancet i: 1065–1067
Old J M, Higgs D R 1983 Gene analysis. In: Weatherall D J (ed) The thalassaemias. Churchill Livingstone, Edinburgh, pp 74–102
Old J M, Ward R H T, Petrou M, Karagozlu F, Modell B, Weatherall D J 1982 First trimester fetal diagnosis for haemoglobinopathies: three cases. Lancet ii: 1413–1416
Old J M, Warren R, Modell B et al 1986 First-trimester fetal diagnosis for haemoglobinopathies: report on 200 cases. Lancet ii: 763–767
Orkin S H, Alter B P, Altay C et al 1978 Application of endonuclease mapping to the analysis and prenatal diagnosis of thalassaemias caused by globin gene deletion. New England Journal of Medicine 229: 166
Pastorek J G II, Seiler B 1985 Maternal death associated with sickle cell trait. American Journal of Obstetrics and Gynecology 151: 295–297
Rodeck C H, Morsman J M 1983 First trimester chorion biopsy. British Medical Bullein 39: 338–342
Rodeck C H, Nicolaides K H 1983 Fetoscopy and fetal tissue sampling. British Medical Bulletin 39: 332–337
Samuels-Rein J H, Scott R B, Brown W E 1984 Contraceptive practices and reproductive patterns in sickle cell disease. Journal of the National Medical Association 76: 879–883
Serjeant G R 1983 Sickle haemoglobin and pregnancy. British Medical Journal 287K: 628–630
Thomas A N, Pattison C, Serjeant G R 1982 Causes of death in sickle-cell disease in Jamaica. British Medical Journal 285: 633–635
Tuck S M, Studd J W W, White J M 1983 Pregnancy in sickle cell disease in the United Kingdom. British Journal of Obstetrics and Gynaecology 90: 112–117
Tuck S M, James C E, Brewster E M, Pearson T C, Studd J W W 1987 Prophylactic blood transfusion in maternal sickle cell syndromes. British Journal of Obstetrics and Gynaecology 94: 121–125
Van Dinh T, Boor P J, Garza J R 1982 Massive pulmonary embolism following delivery of a patient with sickle cell trait. American Journal of Obstetrics and Gynecology 143: 722–724
Weatherall D J 1984 Prenatal diagnosis of thalassaemia. British Medical Journal 288: 1321–1322
Weatherall D J 1985a The new genetics and clinical practice, 2nd edn. Oxford University Press, Oxford
Weatherall D J 1985b Prenatal diagnosis of inherited blood disorders. In: Letsky E A (ed) Haematological disorders in pregnancy. Clinics in haematology 14. Saunders, London, pp 747–774
Weatherall D J, Clegg J B 1981 The thalassaemia syndromes, 3rd edn. Blackwell Scientific, Oxford
Weatherall D J, Letsky E A 1984 Genetic haematological disorders. In: Wald N J (ed) Antenatal and neonatal screening. Oxford University Press, London
Williamson R, Eskdale J, Coleman D V, Niazi M, Loeffler F E, Modell B M 1981 Direct gene analysis of chorionic villi: a possible technique for first trimester antenatal diagnosis of haemoglobinopathies. Lancet ii: 1125–1127
Wood W G, Weatherall D J 1973 Haemoglobin synthesis during human fetal development. Nature 244: 162–165

24

C. H. Rodeck

Invasive intrauterine procedures

INTRODUCTION

The uterus is no longer an iron curtain and the fetus has become a patient because of the increased accessibility provided by modern technology. Palpation, auscultation and radiology are no longer the only tools available. Of the non-invasive methods, ultrasound is the most useful, although other modalities such as magnetic resonance imaging show promise.

Imaging is only one part of the diagnostic and therapeutic armamentarium. A large variety of samples can now be acquired for analysis by an impressive array of techniques. They will be briefly reviewed in this chapter. All should be regarded as ultrasound-guided procedures, as maximal safety and success can only be achieved with the combined use of ultrasound. A good way to start, therefore, is to consider the contribution that ultrasound makes to the performance of invasive procedures.

ULTRASOUND AND INVASIVE PROCEDURES

Information obtained

1. Fetal viability should be confirmed before carrying out the procedure.
2. Menstrual age should be checked by sonographic fetal measurements. This is best done before the procedure so that it can be planned for the optimal gestational age.
3. Multiple pregnancy must be diagnosed. If present, it considerably complicates the procedure and its implications, e.g. if twins are discordant for an abnormality.
4. As detailed an anomaly scan as possible should always be done, and lack or excess of amniotic fluid noted.
5. Other uterine or adnexal abnormalities can be excluded.
6. The placenta is localized and its margins defined. The latter may not be possible in the first trimester, but for chorion villus biopsy (CVB), the instrument clearly needs to be guided into the centre of the placenta. For ultrasound-guided cord blood sampling with an anterior placenta, the needle usually passes through the placenta into the base of the cord. In most other invasive procedures, the placenta is avoided as far as possible.
7. The objective of the procedure is identified, e.g. placenta for CVB, pool of amniotic fluid for amniocentesis, placental insertion of cord for fetal blood sampling (FBS), or part of the fetus for skin biopsy or fetoscopic examination.
8. Selection of site and direction of entry of trocar or needle.
9. Identification of the needle tip if position is uncertain.
10. Simultaneous guidance of needle for FBS, amniocentesis, CVB or shunting procedure.
11. Simultaneous monitoring of fetal heart rate and direction of blood flow during intravascular transfusions.
12. Early warning of complications, e.g. intra-amniotic bleeding or fetal bradycardia.
13. Immediate postoperative scan, e.g. fetal heart rate.
14. Follow-up scan, usually the next day for procedures more major than CVB or amniocentesis. The presence of the fetal heart beat and amniotic fluid are noted.

Methods of using ultrasound

Most of the above items of information are relevant to all invasive procedures. How ultrasound is used, however, can differ considerably; there has been a trend towards increasingly close involvement.

At first, lip service was paid to placental localization, some hours or even the day before the procedure. It is no surprise that this failed to show any benefit (Levine et al 1978) but it was not appreciated how much intrauterine and intra-abdominal topography could change in a few minutes. The fault lay not with ultrasound but the way it was used.

It became clear that amniocentesis should be performed in the ultrasound department and as quickly as possible after the entry point had been selected sonographically (Kerenyi & Walker 1977, Harrison et al 1975). This technique is extremely successful and widely used.

For more complex procedures, e.g. fetoscopy, fetal catheterization, a similar technique can be used, but with the ultrasound probe wrapped in a sterile polythene bag and using a sterile medium such as liquid paraffin, for acoustic coupling (Rodeck 1980). This enables scanning at any time before, during and after the procedure.

The unsterile ultrasound probe can be held on the patient's abdominal wall during the passage of the needle through the layers, thus providing simultaneous guidance. Many prefer this method for amniocentesis (Jonatha 1974), although it can be slower and a little more painful than the speedier performance already outlined. However, it is mandatory for cord sampling and CVB, usually with a sterile probe.

Special sterilized ultrasound biopsy transducers can be used (Bang & Northeved 1972) but a cheaper alternative is to attach a needle guide to the ultrasound probe. Freedom of movement is limited by this approach, but it has been widely used for amniocentesis, cord sampling and transabdominal CVB.

Type of probe

Many find orientation easier with linear array probes but they may be bulky and cumbersome. Sector probes are smaller and better for first-trimester work. An excellent compromise between the two is a curvilinear probe.

The ultrasonographer

In many centres, invasive procedures are done very successfully by a team consisting of operator, assistant and ultrasonographer. This requires extremely close team work and a change in sonographer can be disturbing. The information derived from the scanning is so vital to the decision-making that it is more straightforward and in principle better if this is done by the operator. There is then no doubt where the responsibility lies.

COUNSELLING

No patient should have an invasive procedure without detailed counselling and in many instances a consent form is necessary. Counselling may require a geneticist, and may already have been done, but this does not absolve the obstetrician from responsibility for ensuring that the patient is informed. She (and her partner) should have knowledge of:

Table 24.1 Techniques of amniocentesis

Without ultrasound
Ultrasound immediately before procedure
Simultaneous ultrasound
Ultrasound biopsy transducer

Table 24.2 Indications for amniocentesis

Before 20 weeks
1. Chromosome abnormalities (maternal age, translocation carrier, previous affected child)
2. Fetal sexing in X-linked disorders
3. Neural tube defects — raised alpha-fetoprotein or acetylcholinesterase levels
4. Inborn errors of metabolism
5. DNA analysis
After 20 weeks
1. Bilirubin (Δ OD at 450 nm)
2. Phospholipids (for fetal pulmonary maturity)
3. Fetal maturity
4. Amniography or fetography

1. The disease or abnormality that is being investigated.
2. The prognosis.
3. The risk of occurrence and recurrence.
4. The nature of the procedure, its risks and success rate.
5. The possibility of other tests or options, or of having none.
6. The diagnostic accuracy and when the result will be available.
7. Termination of pregnancy, methods and risks.
8. What to do in the event of complications.

In an ideal world, most of these points will have been covered before the pregnancy. All too often this is not possible, or the problem may have arisen during the pregnancy. More than one session may be required and women should have the opportunity to go away to think and discuss. It is quite unacceptable hastily to burden the patient with new information in a darkened ultrasound room immediately before a procedure.

DIAGNOSTIC PROCEDURES

Amniocentesis

Technique

Regular use of amniocentesis was first advocated by Bevis (1952) in the management of rhesus disease. Many practitioners achieved a high degree of success before ultrasound was available, but few would now wish to do without it. Table 24.1 shows various techniques for performing amniocentesis, aspects of which have been discussed above.

The needle most commonly used is a 21 gauge spinal one with stylet. Full scrub, gowning and draping are not necessary provided a meticulous no-touch technique is used. Neither is local anaesthesia necessary, although some prefer to use it.

A transvaginal approach has been tried (Scrimgeour 1973a) but the procedure is now exclusively transabdominal.

Indications

The indications for amniocentesis are shown in Table 24.2. For fetal chromosome analysis and the diagnosis of inborn errors of metabolism, the procedure is performed at 15–16 weeks' gestation. By this time the uterus is readily accessible transabdominally; it contains 150–200 ml of amniotic fluid, so that 15–20 ml can be removed with impunity, and the extraembryonic coelom is obliterated by the amnion and chorion coming into contact. The result is usually available in 3–4 weeks, i.e. by 18–20 weeks. Amniocentesis is more commonly performed at 18–20 weeks for the diagnosis of neural tube defects after suspicion has been raised by an elevated maternal serum alpha-fetoprotein level. However, high-resolution ultrasound is increasingly being used to diagnose neural tube defects, particularly anencephaly, for which amniocentesis should rarely be necessary now. DNA analysis is possible using the appropriate gene probe, but amniocytes are not as good a source of DNA as chorionic villi and the latter have the advantage of being obtainable in the first trimester.

The main diagnostic uses of amniocentesis after 20 weeks' gestation are in the management of haemolytic disease and for fetal pulmonary maturity. The assessment of fetal maturity (gestational age) by amniotic fluid studies is inaccurate and rarely used: neither is amniography or fetography. All these procedures have been supplanted by ultrasound.

Chorion villus biopsy (CVB)

Techniques

CVB is an example of a technique arriving at the wrong time. The pioneering work in the late 1960s using endoscopes (Hahnemann & Mohr 1968, Kullander & Sandahl 1973) was not taken up, partly because there appeared to be a high complication and failure rate, and partly because it was becoming clear that amniocentesis was safe and reliable for fetal chromosome analysis. Even earlier studies had already been performed on placental biopsy (Alvarez 1964), but within another context.

The report from China (Tietung Hospital 1975) of the successful use of an aspiration cannula, passed blindly with continuing pregnancies, re-awakened interest in the West, although work with ultrasound-guided forceps was also being done in the USSR (Kazy et al 1982). The demonstration that villi could be used for gene analysis (Williamson et al 1981) led to the development of further methods. Blind aspiration was shown to be unreliable (Horwell et al 1983) and endoscopy too complicated (Gosden et al 1982). Ultrasound-guided transcervical catheters have become the most widely used techniques (Rodeck et al 1983, Ward et al 1983; Fig. 24.1); application increased greatly when it was shown that chromosome analysis could be done on direct preparations of villi (Simoni et al 1983). The similar use of a biopsy forceps is also very successful (Goossens et al 1983). Sector or curvilinear ultrasound probes are preferable to lin-

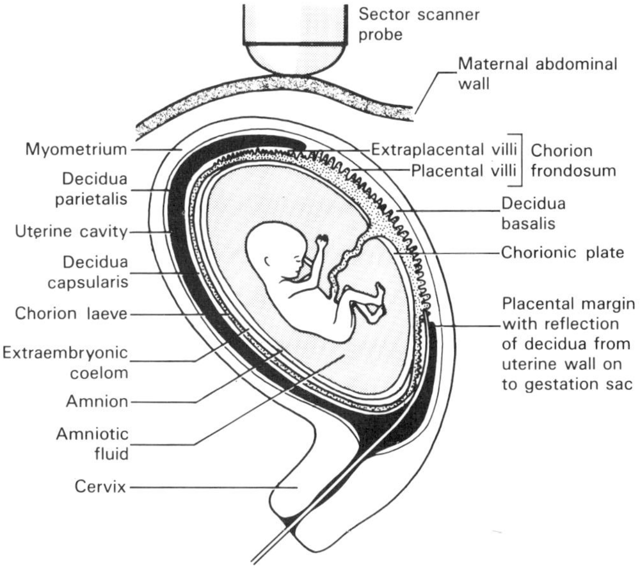

Fig. 24.1 Transcervical passage of an aspiration cannula into the placental site under ultrasound guidance.

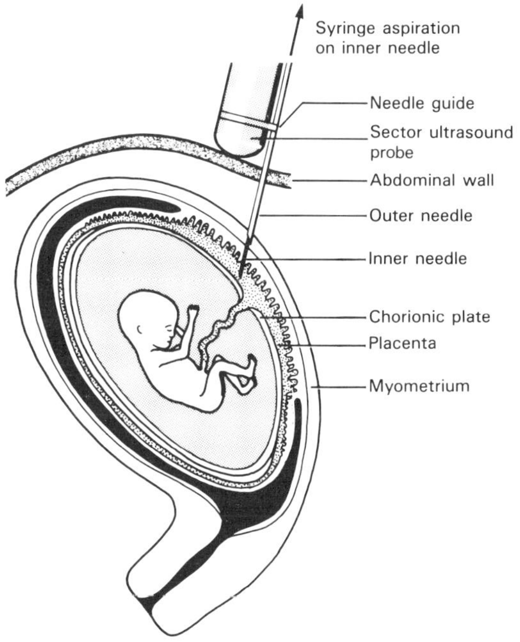

Fig. 24.2 Transabdominal needle aspiration of chorionic villi under ultrasound guidance.

Table 24.3 Techniques of chorion villus biopsy

Transcervical
Blind aspiration
Endoscopic
Ultrasound-guided
Cannula (plastic or metal)
Biopsy forceps
Transabdominal
Ultrasound-guided needle aspiration

ear array. All the above methods are transcervical, but a transabdominal approach has also been devised which is increasingly being used (Smidt-Jensen & Hahnemann 1984; Fig. 24.2). Table 24.3 summarizes the various techniques. They have recently been reviewed in detail (Rodeck 1987, Ward 1987).

It is not clear at present whether one method is better than the others. All are performed without analgesia or anaesthesia and sufficient material for diagnosis should be obtainable in over 98% of cases. Transabdominal CVB may have a lower risk of introducing infection into the uterus than transcervical, but the fetal loss rate seems similar for both. Undoubtedly, operator preference and experience are the most important factors.

The advantages of CVB are summarized in Table 24.4. Clearly the most important, particularly from the patient's point of view, is the possibility of first-trimester diagnosis. Most authors state the optimal time for CVB is 9–10 weeks' gestation, with a possible range from 8 to 12 weeks. However, one advantage of transabdominal over transcervical CVB is that the former can be performed at any stage of pregnancy, while the latter can only be carried out in the first trimester.

Table 24.4 Advantages of chorion villus biopsy

1. Enables first-trimester fetal diagnosis, i.e. early reassurance or early termination; avoidance of long delay and late termination
2. Villi are a good source of DNA
3. Villi are (nearly always) genetically, chromosomally and biochemically identical to the fetus
4. Villi can be sampled without perforating the membranes or fetus

Indications

The indications for CVB are given in Table 24.5.

The advances in molecular genetics have been particularly rapid in the last decade and as more genes are cloned and probes developed, more diseases can be diagnosed by this technology: only the main ones are listed here.

The enzyme deficiency underlying most of the inborn errors of metabolism is expressed in villi, and in many cases the villi can be assayed directly, giving a result by the next day; in some, culture is required.

Table 24.5 Indications for chorion villus biopsy

DNA analysis
Haemoglobinopathies — sickle cell disease, alpha-thalassaemia, most beta-thalassaemias
Most haemophilias — A and B
Duchenne muscular dystrophy (not all families)
Cystic fibrosis (not all families)
Alpha$_1$-antitrypsin deficiency
Chromosome abnormalities
Inborn errors of metabolism

Chromosome analysis on villi can be by direct preparation or after culture: most laboratories use both methods. The indications are similar to those for amniocentesis.

More information is required on the diagnostic accuracy of tests on chorionic villi. For example, false positive chromosomal diagnoses may occur due to abnormalities such as mosaicism being present in the villi but not in the fetus. The precise incidence of such problems has yet to be determined.

The questions of who should have CVB and whether it will replace amniocentesis are being asked. CVB is most clearly beneficial to patients with genetic histories and a 1:2 or 1:4 recurrence risk of having an affected fetus: in such patients it is already replacing amniocentesis and FBS. Most patients eligible for fetal chromosome analysis (i.e. on grounds of maternal age) have a much lower risk of an affected child and although increasing numbers are now having CVB, it is not wise to offer this routinely yet until more is known of the diagnostic accuracy and its risk. The outcome of several randomized controlled trials is awaited. In practical terms, neither the obstetric nor the laboratory facilities exist for a major switch from amniocentesis to CVB. In order to achieve this, equipment, staff and training would have to be provided on a large scale.

Table 24.6 Techniques for fetal blood sampling

Placentacentesis (blind needling)
Fetoscopy
Chorionic plate vessels
Cord insertion
Ultrasound-guided needling
Cord insertion
Fetal heart
Intrahepatic umbilical vein

Fetal blood sampling (FBS)

Techniques

Techniques of FBS are listed in Table 24.6.

Placentacentesis

This was the first technique (sometimes called blind needling) to be used clinically to obtain fetal blood (Kan

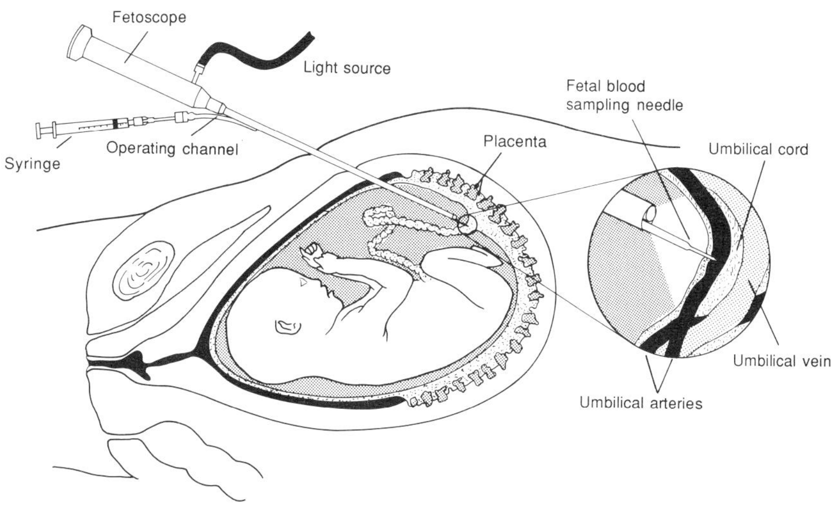

Fig. 24.3 Fetoscope in utero with puncture of umbilical artery (inset) at base of cord, under direct vision. By courtesy of General Practitioner.

et al 1974). Multiple punctures were made in the chorionic plate with a 19 or 20 gauge needle in the hope that a fetal vessel would bleed into the amniotic fluid, which was then aspirated. Samples often contained a very low proportion of fetal cells and 10–15% of patients required a repeat procedure. The fetal mortality was about 10% (Fairweather et al 1980) and this technique is now obsolete.

Fetoscopy

Early attempts concentrated on visualization and required a laparotomy (Valenti 1972, Scrimgeour 1973b). Fetoscopy is now rarely required for fetal examination, and only when small or subtle lesions of diagnostic importance cannot be adequately assessed by ultrasound scanning. Diagnostic application of FBS awaited the development of a percutaneous technique (Hobbins & Mahoney 1974). Fetal blood was obtained by puncture of chorionic plate vessels although these samples were also contaminated by amniotic fluid and/or maternal blood. Since then fetoscopy has become a precise ultrasound-guided technique and pure fetal blood samples can be aspirated from the umbilical cord vessels at the placental insertion with 100% reliability (Rodeck & Campbell 1978, Rodeck & Nicolaides 1986). A 1.7 mm diameter Olympus Selfoscope is used with a special cannula (RM Surgical Developments) that will also accept needles or biopsy forceps (Fig. 24.3). The procedure can be performed from 15 weeks' gestation onwards into the third trimester and is a versatile means of access to the fetus, permitting a variety of diagnostic and therapeutic manoeuvres (Rodeck & Nicolaides 1986). It is not easy to learn and recent improvements in ultrasound technology have led to a wider adoption of sonographically guided needling for fetal blood sampling.

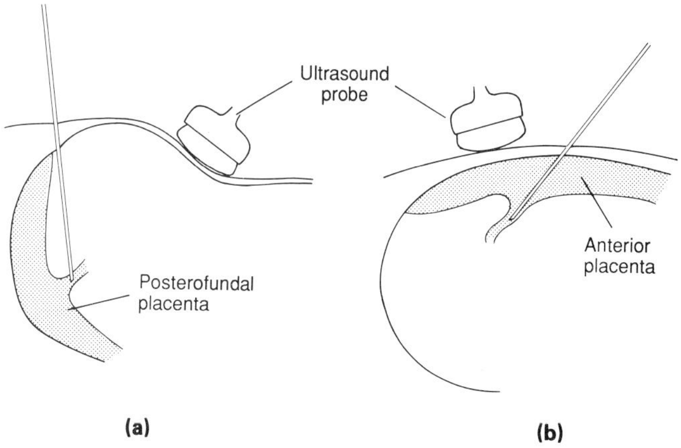

Fig. 24.4 Ultrasound-guided needling in (**a**) posterofundal placenta; (**b**) anterior placenta. A curvilinear ultrasound probe is shown.

Ultrasound-guided cord needling

A sector probe (Daffos et al 1983) or a curvilinear probe (Nicolaides et al 1986a) can be used to guide a 20 or 21 gauge needle into an umbilical cord vessel; the base of the cord at the placental insertion is again the optimal site. For anterior placentae the route is transplacental and for posterior it is transamniotic (Fig. 24.4). In the latter circumstance, difficulties may occur due to the fetus or loops of cord obscuring the cord insertion. Most centres performing FBS are now using a variant of this technique.

Other methods

Fetal blood may also be obtained by sonographically guiding a needle into the fetal heart or the intrahepatic umbilical vein (Bang 1983). Neither method is widely used.

Table 24.7 Indications for fetal blood sampling

1.	Haemoglobinopathies
2.	Bleeding disorders
3.	Chromosome disorders
4.	Immunodeficiencies
5.	Viral and other infections
6.	Metabolic disorders
7.	Unexplained (non-haemolytic) hydrops
8.	Fetal blood grouping
9.	Assessment of fetal anaemia
10.	Assessment of fetal blood gas and acid–base status

Indications

The groups of disorders that can be investigated with fetal blood are shown in Table 24.7.

The *haemoglobinopathies* were the classical indication for which the early blood sampling techniques were evolved (Hobbins & Mahoney 1974, Kan et al 1974). The diagnosis is made by studying the biosynthesis of globin chains. As this is far more active in fetal than in maternal reticulocytes, mixed samples are tolerable, although pure fetal samples have greatly simplified laboratory work. More recently, most of these patients have first-trimester CVB and DNA analysis, provided the latter is feasible and the pregnancy is sufficiently early.

Pure fetal blood samples, in which clotting has not been initiated, can be used for bioassay of factor VIIIC and factor IX for diagnosis of fetal *haemophilia A* and *B* respectively (Mibashan & Rodeck 1984). Many other coagulopathies and platelet disorders can be diagnosed as the relevant normal ranges are available (Mibashan & Rodeck 1984). First trimester diagnosis is also now the primary method, provided the family is informative for a DNA marker.

A *karyotype* can be obtained from cultured fetal lymphocytes within 3 days—far more rapidly than from amniocytes. This is particularly useful in the further investigation of fetal malformations discovered by ultrasonography, such as omphalocele, hydrops, obstructive uropathy, as these have a much higher incidence of chromosome aberrations in the second trimester than at term (Nicolaides et al 1986b). This is now the largest group of patients having FBS. Other indications include fragile X-linked mental retardation and amniotic fluid culture failure and mosaicism.

Many of the severe combined *immunodeficiences* can be diagnosed by monoclonal anti-T cell lymphocyte antibodies and a fluorescence-activated cell sorter.

Fetal *rubella*, *cytomegalovirus* and *toxoplasmosis* infection can be diagnosed by sensitive radioimmunoassays for specific IgM.

Fetal blood enables the rapid diagnosis of many *inborn errors of metabolism*, although this is usually done on amniotic fluid, and increasingly now by CVB.

When detailed ultrasonography has failed to make a diagnosis in a *hydropic fetus*, FBS may reveal a chromosome disorder or viral infection.

Fetal blood grouping may be useful in cases of blood group incompatibility.

In *erythroblastosis fetalis*, the severity of anaemia and the adequacy of a fetal transfusion can be directly monitored.

Fetal blood gas and acid–base measurements are valuable in high-risk fetuses (Rodeck & Nicolaides 1986). This will become an expanding indication, particularly when used in combination with cardiotocography and Doppler studies of blood flow velocities.

Fetal skin biopsy

Techniques

These can also be fetoscopic or ultrasound-guided. Small biopsies (2 mm) can be taken under direct vision by passing 21 gauge cupped biopsy forceps down the side arm of the fetoscope cannula (Rodeck et al 1980). Larger specimens can be obtained, albeit with less precision, by introducing 18 gauge forceps into the cannula after withdrawal of the fetoscope, the biopsy site having been first selected by inspection. Several variants of ultrasound-guided techniques have been developed.

Indications

These include many of the severe genodermatoses such as epidermolysis bullosa fetalis and dystrophica, epidermolytic hyperkeratosis, harlequin ichthyosis and oculocutaneous albinism. Light and electron microscopy can be performed on the biopsies.

Fetal liver biopsy

Techniques

A fetoscopic method was developed so that an aspiration needle was introduced into the fetal hypochondrium (Rodeck et al 1982a). Fetal liver can also be biopsied by ultrasound guidance (Holzgreve & Golbus 1984).

Indications

The fragments of liver are very small but suitable for biochemical analysis. Obviously, this tissue is only required when more accessible ones cannot be used such as in the genetic enzyme deficiences of the urea cycle, ornithine carbamyl transferase and carbamyl phosphate synthetase.

Fetal tumour biopsy

Needle biopsies can be taken under ultrasound guidance for histological examination. This may confirm the diagnosis of fetal masses such as teratomas or congenital adenomatoid malformation of the lung.

Aspiration of fluid

Diagnostic information can be obtained by ultrasound-guided needle puncture and aspiration of the fetal bladder or cysts. If the bladder is enlarged due to obstructive uropathy, biochemical analysis of fetal urine and in particular its sodium content may help in the assessment of fetal renal function. Emptying of the bladder will allow the rate of refilling to be studied. Aspirated cyst fluid can be subjected to cytological and biochemical analysis. Pleural fluid with a high white cell count is suggestive of chylothorax.

Other fetal endoscopic procedures

Rarely, if a fetus has massive ascites or megacystis in the presence of anhydramnios, a fetoscope may be introduced directly into the fetal peritoneal cavity or bladder. Inspection and biopsy may then be performed.

Contrast radiography

Radio-opaque contrast media are no longer used intra-amniotically for amniography or fetography, or intraperitoneally during intraperitoneal transfusions. However, their use may still occasionally be helpful, e.g. when considering the differential diagnosis of a cystic lesion in the fetal chest, which includes diaphragmatic hernia and cystic adenomatoid malformation of the lung. Ultrasound-guided injection of contrast medium into the fetal chest in one such case showed dispersal of opacity throughout the peritoneal cavity (Fig. 24.5), proving that the lesion was a diaphragmatic hernia.

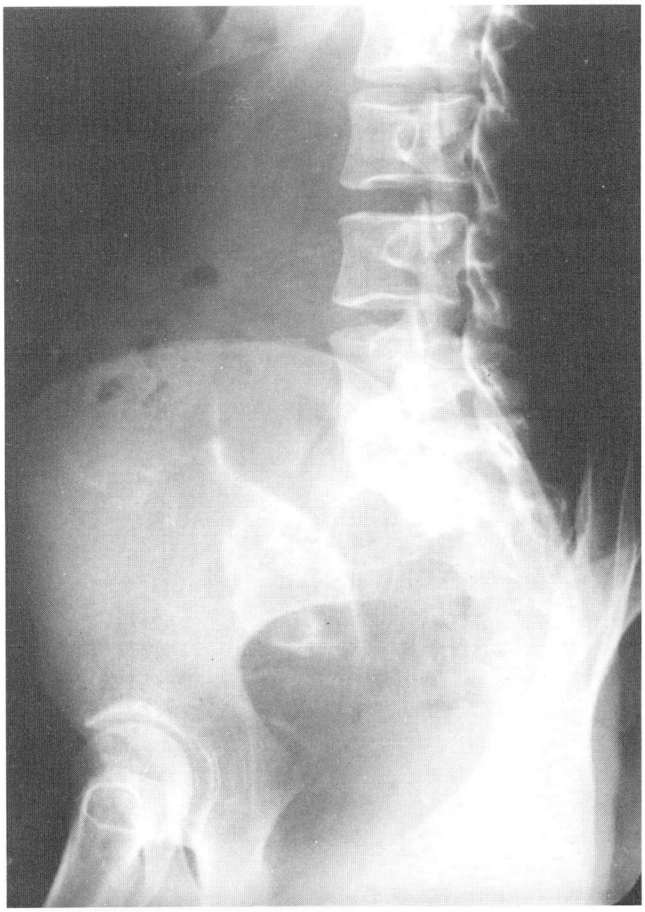

Fig. 24.5 X-ray of 18-week fetus with congenital diaphragmatic hernia showing dispersal of injected contrast throughout pleural and peritoneal cavities.

THERAPEUTIC PROCEDURES

Amniocentesis

Amniocentesis can be used therapeutically:

1. To instil prostaglandins, hypertonic saline or urea into the amniotic cavity to initiate a second-trimester abortion.
2. To drain amniotic fluid in polyhydramnios. There is a risk of stimulating labour or causing abruptio placentae if too much is removed too quickly. It is best to take off small quantities (e.g. 0.5–1 litres) fairly frequently and before the uterus becomes too distended.
3. To instil nutrients or drugs: a beneficial effect has never been proven.

Fetal transfusion

Hysterotomy

Open intrauterine exchange transfusions have been performed using the fetal femoral artery (Freda & Adamsons 1964) or saphenous vein (Ascensio et al 1966). These methods did not become widely used because of their extreme invasiveness and the high postoperative morbidity and fetal mortality.

Intraperitoneal transfusion

The original technique described by Liley in 1963 used X-ray guidance. This was the first direct therapeutic fetal intervention and the technique was widely adopted. The fetal mortality was at least 10% because the relatively imprecise method of guidance could lead to trauma in a fetus that was already severely compromised.

Improved results were obtained when ultrasound was used to guide the needle into the fetal peritoneal cavity (Frigoletto et al 1981, Harman et al 1983) and sonography has now replaced X-ray image intensification.

Intraperitoneal transfusion can also be performed fetoscopically using a fine 21 gauge Tuohy needle which can be passed down the side arm of the cannula and placed under direct vision into the fetal abdomen. However, this would only be required as an adjunct to some other fetoscopic procedure, e.g. blood sampling or intravascular transfusion.

Table 24.8 Types of fetal transfusion

Hysterotomy
Intraperitoneal
X-ray-guided
Ultrasound-guided
Fetoscopic
Intravascular
Fetoscopic
umbilical vessel
Ultrasound-guided
umbilical cord (vein)
intrahepatic (umbilical vein)
intracardiac

Intravascular transfusion

The first percutaneous intravascular transfusions were reported in 1981 by Rodeck et al and this technique has led to an improved fetal survival rate of 80–90% even in severely affected fetuses (Rodeck et al 1984). An umbilical vessel at the base of the cord is punctured and a fetal blood sample is taken for immediate haematocrit estimation. The severity of anaemia thus having been established, packed O-negative donor cells are transfused to achieve a haematocrit of 35–45%. A final blood sample is taken after the transfusion to confirm this. Straight transfusions are given and exchanges are not necessary. The interval between transfusions is 2–3 weeks and five or six may be required from 18–20 weeks' gestation onwards, until planned delivery at about 34 weeks.

As with FBS, most centres now use ultrasound-guided needle puncture of the umbilical vein at the cord insertion, although the intrahepatic umbilical vein is also satisfactory (Bang et al 1982) and occasionally the heart has been used. With a combination of ultrasound-guided transfusions into the umbilical vein and the peritoneal cavity, the interval between transfusions can be lengthened to 4 weeks, thus leading to a reduction in the number of procedures required (author's unpublished observations). The various types of ltransfusion that can be given are summarized in Table 24.8.

Fetal immobilization is beneficial for the performance of these procedures and can be achieved by heavy maternal sedation. However, this is not always successful, and if it is desired to avoid heavy sedation, the fetus can be effectively paralysed by intramuscular or intravenous curare or pancuronium (De Crespigny et al 1985).

Intrauterine shunting procedures

Obstructive uropathy

The most common cause of obstructive uropathy is a posterior urethral valve leading to megacystis, megaureter, varying degrees of renal damage, oligohydramnios, and pulmonary hypoplasia. It may be difficult to distinguish this from the low-pressure functional dilatation of the urinary tract associated with the prune belly syndrome. Work in experimental animals suggested that the reversal of a blockage led to improvement in renal function and on this basis, treatment of the human fetus was attempted. A few surgical procedures at hysterotomy have been performed (Harrison et al 1982) but the great majority have been percutaneous (Golbus et al 1982, Rodeck & Nicolaides 1984).

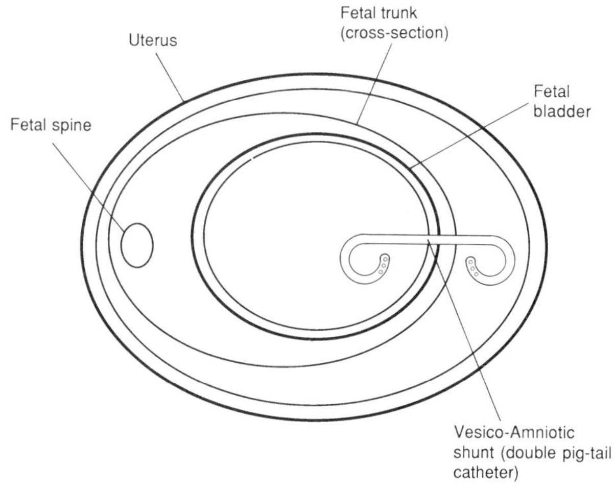

Fig. 24.6 Cross-section of uterus and fetal trunk showing double pigtail catheter (vesico-amniotic shunt) in position.

A trocar and cannula are introduced into the fetal bladder with ultrasound guidance and a plastic, double pigtailed catheter or shunt is inserted so that one end coils in the bladder and the other in the amniotic cavity (Fig. 24.6). Technically this is not difficult, but the major problem lies in selection of cases. At one extreme, the fetus may have irreparably damaged kidneys while at the other its prognosis may be good without intervention. An attempt must therefore be made to assess renal function, albeit crudely, by a combination of sonographic observations, biochemical analysis of a sample of fetal urine, rate of refilling of bladder if this has been emptied by needling, or appearance of amniotic fluid after a shunt has been placed for initially diagnostic purposes (i.e. observing urine production). Where renal function exists there is the hope that this may be preserved. From data collected by the International Fetal Surgery Registry (Manning et al 1986), this appears to be so but follow-up is limited and there is as yet no proof that intrauterine intervention has benefited these fetuses.

It is also of vital importance to exclude other fetal abnormalities, particularly chromosome defects, before embarking on fetal therapy.

Hydrocephalus

Similar reasoning to that applied to obstructive uropathy was also used for obstructive hydrocephalus, provided that infections, chromosome defects and other abnormalities had been excluded.

The first such fetus to be treated had repeated encephalocentesis under ultrasound-guidance, but the cerebrospinal fluid reaccumulated rapidly and the outcome was poor (Birnholz & Frigoletto 1981). Chronic drainage with a ventriculo-amniotic shunt was attempted in a number of centres (Clewell et al 1981). However, there were considerable problems in keeping the shunts in position and in maintaining patency; repeat procedures were frequently required. Follow-up of the survivors revealed a high incidence of severe retardation (Manning et al 1986) and enthusiasm for this form of therapy has vanished. It may become re-established in the future if improvements are made in shunt design and in the prognostic assessment of fetal hydrocephalus.

Hydrothorax

Long-standing fetal pleural effusions are likely to cause pulmonary hypoplasia and, by pressure on the heart and decrease in venous return, may lead to generalized secondary hydrops.

Needle aspiration has been performed successfully (Schmidt et al 1985), but in the author's experience, the effusions rapidly re-accumulate. Therefore, in this situation also, there is a place for chronic drainage. Pleuro-amniotic shunts, similar to the double pigtail vesico-amniotic catheter, have been inserted in eight fetuses with good neonatal outcome in six (Rodeck et al 1988).

Careful selection of cases and exclusion of additional fetal abnormalities are important principles, as in other forms of fetal therapy.

Aspiration of fluid

Large fetal cysts may exert damaging pressure and occasionally ultrasound-guided aspiration may be a simple remedy. Such cysts or massive ascites can also cause dystocia and aspiration of fluid may lead to safer delivery.

Selective fetocide

With increasing use of prenatal diagnosis in twin pregnancies, one fetus may be found to have a severe abnormality and the other to be normal. This places the parents in a serious dilemma, and given the option, most prefer to keep the healthy twin but not the affected one.

To date, most cases have arisen in the second trimester, and a number of different solutions have been employed, e.g. hysterotomy and removal of the affected fetus (Beck et al 1980), cardiac puncture and fetal exsanguination (Aberg et al 1978) and fetoscopic air embolization (Rodeck et al 1982b).

The advent of first-trimester diagnosis has stimulated new techniques for dealing with the problem of discordancy. The most effective appears to be the transabdominal injection of a small quantity of potassium chloride (0.5–1 ml) into the fetal chest or heart, which causes immediate asystole (author's unpublished observations). This method could be used for an ectopic pregnancy provided the diagnosis was made before the patient was symptomatic.

Table 24.9 Possible adverse effects of invasive intrauterine procedures

Delay in receiving result
Failure to obtain a sample
Incorrect sample obtained
Failure in diagnosis
False positives and negatives — wrong diagnosis
Trauma and haemorrhage
Maternal abdominal wall, bowel or bladder
Uterus
Placenta
intra-amniotic bleeding
retroplacental haematoma
fetomaternal haemorrhage
Membranes
amniotic fluid leakage
Cord
haematoma
Fetus
perforation, necrosis, death
Infection
Maternal abdominal wall, septicaemia, chorioamnionitis, fetal aspiration pneumonia
Spontaneous abortion
Intrauterine death
Malformations
Rhesus isoimmunization
Intrauterine growth retardation
Spontaneous premature rupture of membranes
Preterm labour
Abruptio placentae
Neonate
Preterm delivery
Small-for-dates
Infection
Talipes
Respiratory difficulties

The operator must ascertain by ultrasound that the pregnancy is dichorionic to be assured that there are no vascular connections between the fetal circulations, and must be certain which of the fetuses is affected.

RISKS OF INVASIVE INTRAUTERINE PROCEDURES

The hazards of penetrating the uterus depend not so much on the procedure itself but rather on how it is done and the experience of the operator. The large number of possible adverse effects, many of which are theoretical, are listed in Table 24.9. Many occur spontaneously and one of the ever-present problems of assessing the risks of a procedure is the need for knowledge — rarely available — of the background incidence of those complications in the population being studied.

Amniocentesis

The vast majority of amniocenteses are simple and straightforward; diagnostic success and accuracy are high. An important and under-rated problem is the anxiety associated with the long wait (3–4 weeks) for a result.

Much debate has focused on the extent to which sponta-

Table 24.10 Spontaneous abortion rate (%) in amniocentesis subjects and controls in four studies

	Subjects	Controls
Canadian MRC (1977)	0.9	1.6–1.9
NICHD (1978)	2.8	2.4
MRC (UK; 1978)	2.7	1.3
Tabor et al (1986)	1.7	0.7

neous abortion is increased after amniocentesis. This has been examined in four studies: the Canadian Medical Research Council (MRC; 1977), the US National Institute of Child Health and Development (NICHD) Amniocentesis Register (1978), the UK MRC (1978) and more recently one from Denmark (Tabor et al 1986). The results are summarized in Table 24.10. In the first three studies there were problems in selecting controls: only in the Danish study were the two groups comparable because of randomization. It would appear, therefore, that amniocentesis causes a 1% increase in abortion rate. However, a larger needle (18 gauge) was used in the Danish study than in most centres, and increasing size of needle is associated with a higher abortion rate, as is repeated insertion of the needle (Canadian MRC 1977, NICHD 1978).

An increase in perinatal mortality has not been demonstrated. However, the UK study suggested that there was a higher incidence of postural deformities (talipes) and respiratory difficulties in the neonates. The former has not been confirmed but the Danes also found an increase in respiratory distress syndrome in the subjects as compared with the controls. Work in non-human primates supports the view that amniocentesis may sometimes interfere with normal lung development, although it has not been established whether this is a consequence of chronic leakage of amniotic fluid or of some other mechanism (Hislop & Fairweather 1982).

Amnionitis occurs in about 1 in 1000 amniocenteses and fetal trauma is very rare. In the UK study, more skin marks and dimples were found in the control neonates than in the subjects.

Chorion villus biopsy

Less scientific information is available for this relatively new procedure, although some 21 000 have been performed worldwide. The average rate of fetal loss before 28 weeks' gestation for all centres is 3–4% (Rodeck 1987) but in some with the largest experience, it is as low as 2%. It appears to be the same for transcervical and transabdominal procedures although it is likely that the former carries a higher risk of intrauterine infection.

Spontaneous fetal losses vary more in the first trimester with gestational age and maternal age than in the second trimester, making comparison between centres more difficult. It is to be hoped that the outcome of randomized trials will clarify the position. Similar data on the medium-term complications of later pregnancy and long-term effects on the neonates are also urgently needed. There are as yet no suggestions of any specific adverse consequences of CVB.

The diagnostic accuracy of CVB has not yet been firmly established. Results from villi, fetal and neonatal tissues must be collected and compared.

Fetal blood sampling

In the most experienced centres, fetal losses associated with fetoscopy are about 2% (Rodeck & Nicolaides 1986). Some 4% of patients leak amniotic fluid after the procedure, although this often stops and most pregnancies continue normally. There may be a slight increase in preterm delivery (8–10%) although the mechanism is unclear. The risk of amnionitis after fetoscopy is probably somewhat higher than after amniocentesis.

Ultrasound-guided needling, again in experienced hands, appears to have a fetal loss rate of 1.5% and no obvious increase in preterm delivery or amniotic fluid leakage (Daffos et al 1983). The diameter of the needle is of course less than that of fetoscope. It may also be relevant that most needling procedures have been done later in gestation than have fetoscopies, and therefore in a population with a slightly lower background abortion rate. While it seems reasonable to conclude that needling is less invasive than fetoscopy, there are unfortunately no controls available for any of the published series. It should be re-emphasized that such excellent results can only be achieved after a considerable amount of experience and training.

Therapeutic procedures

It is still more difficult to quote accurate risk figures for procedures such as transfusions or shunting. The immediate fetal mortality and subsequent abortion rates do not seem to be significantly different from those associated with needling or fetoscopy. The picture is compounded by the fact that these fetuses are not normal — there may be concomitant polyhydramnios, etc. It is clear, however, that ventriculo-amniotic shunting for hydrocephalus has a high procedure-related fetal mortality of some 10%.

CONCLUSIONS

Advances in ultrasound technology have in some instances largely removed the need for invasive procedures, e.g. most neural tube defects are diagnosable sonographically and amniocentesis for alpha-fetoprotein and acetylcholinesterase estimation is usually not necessary. Paradoxically, ultrasound has also made possible a wide range of invasive procedures which can be performed with great precision and a remarkable degree of safety. The combined approach will lead to further opportunities to study and treat fetal physiology and pathology.

REFERENCES

Aberg A, Metelman F, Cantz M, Gehler J 1978 Cardiac puncture of fetus with Hurler's disease avoiding abortion of unaffected co-twin. Lancet ii: 990–991

Alvarez H 1964 Morphology, pathophysiology of the human placenta. I. Studies of morphology and development of the chorionic villi by phase-contrast microscopy. Obstetrics and Gynecology 23: 813

Ascensio S H, Figueroa-Longo J G, Pelegrina I A 1966 Intrauterine exchange transfusion. American Journal of Obstetrics and Gynecology 95: 1129–1133

Bang J 1983 Ultrasound-guided fetal blood sampling. In: Albertini A, Crosignani P F (eds) Progress in perinatal medicine. Excerpta Medica, Amsterdam, p 223

Bang J, Northeved A 1972 A new ultrasonic method for transabdominal amniocentesis. American Journal of Obstetrics and Gynecology 114: 599–601

Bang J, Bock J E, Trolle D 1982 Ultrasound-guided transfusion for severe rhesus haemolytic disease. British Medical Journal i: 373–374

Beck L, Terinde R, Dolff M 1980 Zwillingschwangerschaft mit freier Trisomie 21 eines Kindes; Sectio parva mit Entfernung des kranken und spatere gebust des gesunden Kindes. Geburtshilfe und Frauenheilkunde 40: 397–400

Bevis D C A 1952 The antenatal prediction of haemolytic disease of the newborn. Lancet i: 395–398

Birnholz J C, Frigoletto F D 1981 Antenatal treatment of hydrocephalus. New England Journal of Medicine 303: 1021–1023

Canadian Medical Research Council 1977 Diagnosis of genetic disease by amniocentesis during the second trimester of pregnancy. A Canadian study. Report no. 5. Supply Services, Ottowa, Canada

Clewell W H, Johnson M L, Meier P R et al 1981 Placement of ventriculoamniotic shunt for hydrocephalus in a fetus. New England Journal of Medicine 305: 955

Daffos F, Capella-Pavlovksy M, Forestier F 1983 Fetal blood sampling via the umbilical cord using a needle guided by ultrasound. Prenatal Diagnosis 3: 271–274

De Crespigny L Ch, Robinson H P, Ross A W, Quinn M 1985 Curarisation of fetus for intrauterine procedures. Lancet i: 1164

Fairweather D V I, Ward R H T, Modell B 1980 Obstetric aspects of mid-trimester fetal blood sampling by needling or fetoscopy. British Journal of Obstetrics and Gynaecology 87: 87–91

Freda V F, Adamsons K J 1964 Exchange transfusion in utero. American Journal of Obstetrics and Gynecology 89: 817–821

Frigoletto F D, Umansky I, Birnholz J et al 1981 Intrauterine fetal transfusion in 365 fetuses during 15 years. American Journal of Obstetrics and Gynecology 139: 781–790

Golbus M S, Harrison M R, Filly R A, Callen P W, Katz M 1982 In utero treatment of urinary tract obstruction. American Journal of Obstetrics and Gynecology 143: 383–388

Goossens M N, Dumez Y, Kaplan L, Lupker M, Chabret C, Henrion R, Rosa J 1983 Prenatal diagnosis of sickle cell anaemia in the first trimester of pregnancy. New England Journal of Medicine 309: 831–833

Gosden J R, Mitchell A R, Gosden C M, Rodeck C H, Morsman J M 1982 Direct vision chorion biopsy and chromosome specific DNA probes for determination of fetal sex in first trimester prenatal diagnosis. Lancet ii: 1418–1420

Hahnemann N, Mohr J 1968 Genetic diagnosis in the embryo by means of biopsy from extra-embryonic membranes. Bulletin of European Society of Human Genetics 2: 23–29

Harman C R, Manning F A, Bowman J M, Lange I R 1983 Severe rhesus disease — poor outcome is not inevitable. American Journal of Obstetrics and Gynecology 145: 823–829

Harrison M R, Golbus M S, Filly R A et al 1982 Fetal surgery for congenital hydronephrosis. New England Journal of Medicine 326: 591–593

Harrison R, Campbell S, Craft I 1975 Risks of fetomaternal haemorrhage resulting from amniocentesis with and without ultrasound placental localisation. Obstetrics and Gynecology 46: 389–391

Hislop A, Fairweather D V I 1982 Amniocentesis and lung growth: an animal experiment with clinical implications. Lancet ii: 1271–1272

Hobbins J C, Mahoney M J 1974 In utero diagnosis of hemoglobinopathies. Technic for obtaining fetal blood. New England Journal of Medicine 290: 1065–1067

Holzgreve W, Golbus M S 1984 Prenatal diagnosis of ornithine transcarbamylase deficiency utilising fetal liver biopsy. American Journal of Human Genetics 36: 320–324

Horwell D H, Loeffler F E, Coleman D V 1983 Assessment of transcervical aspiration technique for chorionic villus biopsy in the first trimester of pregnancy. British Journal of Obstetrics and Gynaecology 90: 196–198

Jonatha W D 1974 Amniozentese in der Fruhschwangerschaft unter Sichtkontrolle mit Ultraschall. Elektromedica 3: 94–96

Kan Y W, Valenti C, Guidotti R, Carnazza V, Rieder R F 1974 Fetal blood sampling in utero. Lancet i: 79–80

Kazy Z, Rozovsky I S, Bakharev V A 1982 Chorion biopsy in early pregnancy: a method of early prenatal diagnosis for inherited disorders. Prenatal Diagnosis 2: 39–45

Kerenyi T D, Walker B 1977 The preventability of 'bloody taps' in second trimester amniocentesis by ultrasound scanning. Obstetrics and Gynecology 50: 61–64

Kullander S, Sandahl B 1973 Fetal chromosome analysis after transcervical placental biopsies during early pregnancy. Acta Obstetricia et Gynecologica Scandinavica 52: 355–359

Levine S C, Filly R A, Golbus M A 1978 Ultrasonography for guidance of amniocentesis in genetic counselling. Clinical Genetics 14: 133

Liley A W 1963 Intrauterine transfusion of fetus in haemolytic disease. British Medical Journal ii: 1107–1108

Manning F A, Harrison M R, Rodeck C H 1986 Catheter shunts for fetal hydronephrosis and hydrocephalus. Report of the International Fetal Surgery Registry. New England Journal of Medicine 315: 336–340

Medical Research Council 1978 An assessment of the hazards of amniocentesis. British Journal of Obstetrics and Gynaecology 85 (suppl 2)

Mibashan R S, Rodeck C H 1984 Haemophilia and other genetic defects of haemostasis. In: Rodeck C H, Nicolaides K H (eds) Prenatal diagnosis. Wiley, Chichester, pp 179–194

National Institute of Child Health and Development Amniocentesis Register 1978 The safety and accuracy of mid-trimester amniocentesis. US Department of Health, Education and Welfare, No. 78–190

Nicolaides K H, Soothill P W, Rodeck C H, Campbell S 1986a Ultrasound-guided sampling of umbilical cord and placental blood to assess fetal well being. Lancet i: 1065–1967

Nicolaides K H, Rodeck C H, Gosden C M 1986b Rapid karyotyping in non-lethal malformations. Lancet i: 283–286

Rodeck C 1980 Fetoscopy guided by real-time ultrasound for pure fetal blood samples, fetal skin samples and examination of the fetus in utero. British Journal of Obstetrics and Gynaecology 87: 449–456

Rodeck C H 1987 Chorion villus biopsy. Oxford Reviews in Reproductive Biology 9: 137–160

Rodeck C H, Campbell S 1978 Sampling pure fetal blood by fetoscopy in second trimester of pregnancy. British Medical Journal ii: 728–730

Rodeck C H, Nicolaides K H 1984 Ultrasound guided invasive procedures in obstetrics. Clinics in Obstetrics and Gynaecology 10: 529–539

Rodeck C H, Nicolaides K H 1986 Fetoscopy. British Medical Bulletin 42: 296–300

Rodeck C H, Eady R A J, Gosden C M 1980 Prenatal diagnosis of epidermolysis bullosa letalis. Lancet i: 949–952

Rodeck C H, Kemp J R, Holman C A, Whitmore D N, Karnicki J, Austin M A 1981 Direct intravascular fetal blood transfusion by fetoscopy in severe rhesus isoimmunisation. Lancet i: 625–628

Rodeck C H, Patrick A D, Pembrey M E, Tzannatos C, Whitfield A E 1982a Fetal liver biopsy for prenatal diagnosis of ornithine carbamyl transferase deficiency. Lancet ii: 297–299

Rodeck C H, Mibashan R S, Abramovicz J, Campbell S 1982b Selective fetocide of the affected twin by fetoscopic air embolism. Prenatal Diagnosis 3: 83–89

Rodeck C H, Morsman J M, Nicolaides K H, McKenzie C, Gosden C M, Gosden J R 1983 A single operator technique for first trimester chorion biopsy. Lancet ii: 1340–1341

Rodeck C H, Nicolaides K H, Warsof S L, Fysh W J, Gamsu H R, Kemp J R 1984 The management of severe rhesus isoimmunisation by fetoscopic intravascular transfusion. American Journal of Obstetrics and Gynecology 150: 769–774

Rodeck C H, Fisk N M, Fraser D I, Nicolini U 1988 Long-term in utero

drainage of fetal hydrothorax. New England Journal of Medicine 319: 1135–1138
Schmidt W, Harms E, Wolf D 1985 Successful prenatal treatment of non-immune hydrops fetalis due to congenital chylothorax. British Journal of Obstetrics and Gynaecology 92: 685–687
Scrimgeour J B 1973a Amniocentesis: technique and complications. In: Emery A C H (ed) Antenatal diagnosis of genetic diseases. Churchill Livingstone, Edinburgh, pp 11–39
Scrimgeour J B 1973b Other techniques for antenatal diagnosis. In: Emery A E H (ed) Antenatal diagnosis of genetics disease. Churchill Livingstone, Edinburgh pp 40–57
Simoni G, Brambati B, Danesino C, Rosella F, Terzoli G L, Ferrari M, Fraccaro M 1983 Efficient direct chromosome analysis and enzyme determination from chorionic villi samples in the first trimester of pregnancy. Human Genetics 63: 349
Smidt-Jensen S, Hahnemann N 1984 Transabdominal fine needle biopsy from chorionic villi in the first trimester. Prenatal Diagnosis 4: 163–169
Tabor A, Philip J, Marsen M, Bang J, Obel F B, Norgaard-Pedersen B 1986 Randomised controlled trial of genetic amniocentesis in 4606 low-risk women. Lancet i: 1287–1293
Tietung Hospital of Anshan Steelworks, Department of Obstetrics and Gynaecology 1975 Fetal sex prediction by sex chromatin of chorion villi cells during early pregnancy. Chinese Medical Journal 1: 117–126
Valenti C 1972 Endoamnioscopy and fetal biopsy; a new technique. American Journal of Obstetrics and Gynecology 114: 561–564
Ward R H T 1987 Techniques of chorion villus sampling. In: Rodeck C H (ed) Fetal diagnosis of genetic defects. Baillière's Clinical Obstetrics and Gynaecology 1: 489–511
Ward R H T, Modell B, Petrou M, Karagozlou F, Douratsos E 1983 Method of sampling chorionic villi in first trimester of pregnancy under guidance of real-time ultrasound. British Medical Journal 286: 1542–1544
Williamson R, Eskdale J, Coleman D V, Niazi M, Loeffler F E, Modell B 1981 Direct gene analysis of chorionic villi; a possible technique for the first trimester diagnosis of haemoglobinopathies. Lancet ii: 1125–1127

SECTION 4

Assessment of Fetal State in Late Pregnancy

25

Arnold Klopper

Biochemical methods of fetal assessment

INTRODUCTION

In so far as such things have a beginning, the biochemical measurement of fetal metabolism began in 1930 when Guy Marrian, evaporating great pans of urine from pregnant women on a flat roof at University College, London, isolated a trihydroxy phenol, later called oestriol. He deserved a Nobel Prize but got instead the Chair of Biochemistry in Edinburgh whence flowed a stream of discoveries about oestrogens — how to measure them and how they changed in the menstrual cycle and pregnancy. Pregnancy urine proved to be the source of all manner of exciting new things. A few years earlier, Aschheim & Zondek (1927) had found in it a protein peculiar to pregnancy. So specific to pregnancy was chorionic gonadotrophin, as it came to be called, that its demonstration was ipso facto a proof of pregnancy. These authors did not get the Nobel Prize either, although Zondek was made Professor of Obstetrics and Gynaecology at the Hadassah Medical School in Jerusalem after the Nazis drove him out of Germany. Marrian's work laid the foundation for steroid assay as a means of fetal assessment: chorionic gonadotrophin did not prove so useful and protein assays did not come into their own until the discovery of quite a different protein, placental lactogen, by Ito & Higashi some 30 years later in 1961.

For quarter of a century after Aschheim & Zondek and Marrian, we remained shackled by methodology. There was no chemical method for estimating chorionic gonadotrophin or oestriol. All one could do was look at the effects of these substances on the ovaries or uteri of a variety of laboratory animals. These biological tests were laborious, slow, nonspecific and expensive. As a means of assessing the well-being of the fetus they never got off the ground in spite of being backed by statistics so complex that a sound mathematical education was essential for a bioassayist. All this before computers, too. When chemical methods were evolved everyone turned from bioassay with relief.

Biochemical assays for a variety of steroids were introduced in the mid 1950s. It was nearly a decade later that the first useful protein assay — for human placental lactogen — was introduced. The early history of fetal assessment was dominated by steroid assay methodology. At first it was always urine. Steroids are a great deal more concentrated in urine than in blood and you could start with much more urine than blood. The turning point in oestrogen measurement was the work of James Brown, a pupil of Marrian's in Edinburgh. Brown's method for the assay of oestrone, oestradiol and oestriol in urine, published in 1955, dominated the scene for many years and scientists from all over the world made the pilgrimage to Edinburgh. As often in science, Brown was standing on the shoulders of another man. This was Kober, who devised the colour reaction of oestrogens in sulphuric acid which bears his name and which made the spectrophotometric measurement, the centrepiece of the Brown method, possible. Kober published his work in 1931, only a year after Marrian discovered oestriol, and vanished in a concentration camp a few years later. Brown made fetal assessment by oestriol assay his life's work and in 1985 retired from his Chair in Melbourne, full of honour.

After a few years urinary assays became tedious and unpleasant and everybody dreamt of speedy clean assays done on blood. But that had to wait for another technological innovation — radioimmunoassay. Now that radioimmunoassay has been with us for 30 years, we begin to see its shortcomings. For the measurement of proteins, radioimmunoassay is fast being replaced by enzyme-linked methods and soon it will be yesterday's method, even for steroids. With the coming of radioimmunoassay went urinary assays; with the going of radioimmunoassay may come assays in saliva or sweat. Looking back now it is clear that we lost much when we gave up urine. We shall have to re-examine what we stand to gain by passing from blood to saliva.

Progesterone was isolated at about the same time as oestriol but its escape from bioassay was indirect. Another of Marrian's pupils designed a method for measuring the inert metabolite of progesterone, pregnanediol, in urine (Klopper et al 1955). For the author's sake I shall treat it kindly but the truth of the matter is progesterone is not a useful indicator of fetal well-being and pregnanediol assays have been consigned to the slagheap of history.

We are now more or less free from the shackles of methodology. We can measure any protein or steroid in any fluid we like. We cannot measure it quickly enough to be of use to a woman in labour, but that is only a matter of time. More to the point however we cannot measure the concentration where it matters — at the site of action. That is not always because the site of action cannot be reached without causing damage. It is sometimes because we neither know what the test substance does nor where.

Why does the pregnant woman produced large amounts of oestriol? What can this molecule do that other oestrogens cannot? Pregnant women with a deficiency of placental suphatase produce very little oestrogen and pregnancies with no measurable placental lactogen have been recorded. Yet these pregnancies are to all intents and purposes normal. The implication is that the fetoplacental unit pours into the mother an increasing stream of steroids and proteins for no purpose at all. The hypothesis, that the concentration of placental products in the mother's circulation is determined solely by the placental mass and the uterine blood flow, has been seriously advanced (Gordon & Chard 1979). Certainly there is no good evidence of any feedback control; of any system that stimulates or reduces the production of placental proteins in response to greater or lesser need for them. We would be in a much better case with our measurements if the changes in the substance we measure were the cause of the disease we study rather than a secondary consequence.

In 1980 Goebelsmann wrote 'daily oestriol assays are mandatory for fetal surveillance in diabetic pregnancy'. Four years later, Chamberlain (1984) said that oestrogen assays for fetal monitoring had been abandoned in his hospital without any consequent rise in perinatal mortality. Why the change in opinion? Who is right? Of course the rise of physical methods of fetal assessment, such as ultrasound, have contributed to the decline in biochemical methods, but that is not the whole story. Either biochemical methods are no use or we are using them wrongly. In order to assess the proper place of biochemical methods in obstetric practice we shall have to examine what expectations of them we have entertained and why they were not fulfilled.

THE USE OF BIOCHEMICAL TESTING

At first the expectations based on biochemical assays were simple, although hidden behind Greek letters signifying statistical evaluations of significance. In essence what was expected of a biochemical measurement was that it should tell you what to do. You measured the oestriol level or the placental lactogen concentration and the result was supposed to indicate whether to do a Caesarean section next day, induce labour or wait a little longer. It took a long time to discover that biochemical assays do not provide that sort of answer, at least not very clearly, and not by themselves. A lot of that time was accounted for by the time it took to explore the blind passageways such as substituting blood for urine or Schwangerschaftsprotein 1 for placental lactogen.

The reason why biochemical tests did not give definitive answers about management lay in their variability from subject to subject and from time to time. The difference between one healthy woman and another at the same stage of gestation was often as great as the difference between a normal pregnancy and one that was failing. There is no doubt that if you compared the mean plasma oestriol in a group of normal women with that of a group of women carrying a growth-retarded fetus, the latter would have a significantly lower value. But clinicians do not treat groups: they need to decide about Mrs Jones.

The variation from time to time is even greater. From day to day urinary oestriol excretion has a coefficient of variation of 21.3% (Klopper et al 1974). If instead of 24-hour collections you compare 48-hour urines, the variation is less. The longer the period of collection, the less the variation, but a test which took several days before you could even begin the assay had little practical application. The pendulum swung the other way and many studies using overnight urine collections were published. But these were so variable that only those who had staked their reputation on them persisted for any length of time. In the end, 48-hour urines were probably the best compromise. Better things were hoped for from plasma assays but when these came along, the variability (30.9%) was worse. Nor did going from steroids to proteins improve matters notably.

All manner of tricks were tried to reduce variability for plasma assays. Buster (1981) suggested taking multiple samples at 5 minute intervals and assaying the pooled plasma. Not surprisingly this was not greeted with any enthusiasm. Using the cumulative mean of daily serial assays was a more reliable device (Chard & Klopper 1982), but this once again introduced the problem that the better answers took a lot longer to obtain.

Failure to allow for variability was not all that went wrong. There are three main ways in which biochemical tests can be applied: as a means of diagnosis, as a device to decide management, or as a screen to categorize an obstetric population. Biochemical tests have to be judged in terms of these objectives. Unless the purpose is clearly defined the results cannot be properly evaluated. There is nothing characteristic about plasma oestriol concentration in retarded fetal growth and placental lactogen assay will not enable you to distinguish between antepartum haemorrhage due to abruptio placenta or to placenta praevia.

Fortunately the range of obstetric diagnosis is not large and making the diagnosis is seldom taxing. The problem is knowing what to do. In this respect biochemical tests may have more of a role to play. Assays of placental lactogen may not tell you the cause of a threatened abortion but they may help to decide whether the fetus is still viable or whether you should evacuate the uterus directly. If the clinical situation is such that you can wait long enough to establish a trend, biochemical assays may have much to say. Of course, setting them out in this way restricts their role but makes them more valuable in the smaller area assigned. Much of antenatal care is screening for specific conditions — for anaemia, syphilis, rhesus incompatibility, spina bifida. Few would deny the value of such biochemical tests. Much of the future application of biochemical tests lies in an extension of the screening function. One such extension is only just taking shape. Many diseases of late pregnancy have their genesis in early pregnancy. If biochemical tests can detect early the changes which later will give rise to premature labour, haemorrhage or pre-eclampsia, they would be more valuable. There are some hints that some of the early discovered placental products, such as placental protein 5 or pregnancy-associated plasma protein A, can sort high from low risks in these diseases, albeit uncertainly.

Much depends on how close a biochemical test is to the cause rather than the consequence of the disease being studied. If some event in early pregnancy results in a woman developing pre-eclampsia in late pregnancy; if the pre-eclampsia causes a reduction in uterine blood flow; if the reduced blood flow causes damage to the placenta and if that damage reduces the production of pregnancy-associated plasma protein A by the placenta, there is not much percentage in measuring the last event in the series. But suppose pre-eclampsia is really an immunological disease which starts in early pregnancy long before the overt manifestations of hypertension and proteinuria. Suppose also that pregnancy-associated plasma protein A is a factor in the immunological response to pregnancy and is affected by the early events that result in pre-eclampsia. Then measurements of pregnancy-associated plasma protein A could have quite a different use, particularly if the object is to identify a group at high risk of subsequently developing pre-eclampsia.

We have concentrated too much on the sick women in the antenatal ward and too little on healthy women in the antenatal clinic in early pregnancy or even in the prepregnancy clinic. Certainly by the time most obstetricians first see their antenatal patients at 12 or 14 weeks' gestation, all the important definitive events of the pregnancy and most of the wastage of pregnancy is over. All that happens after 12 weeks is that the fetus grows bigger. We have just began to explore what tests at 4–8 weeks' can tell us.

STEROIDS

The steroids are a large family of substances distributed throughout the plant and animal kingdom. Although they consist of carbon, hydrogen and oxygen, they are not used as energy sources or as structural raw material. A great variety of substituents can be attached at various points in the basic molecule, altering its shape. It is as though steroids were keys, differently shaped to fit different locks. This is a helpful simile for it explains how steroids act as universal signals. They fit into protein molecules, shaped to fit them as a lock receives a key. Although different steroids may be isomers, having the same formula, any substituents with a different space orientation in relation to the rest of the molecule will fit the lock badly or not at all. This accounts for their specificity as biological signals and is a property used in many ways, both by nature and by man. When the body needs the signal only for a short while, nature switches it off by changing the substituents. When man requires a synthetic steroid to act for a long while, he synthesizes one with substituents which can only be changed slowly and with difficulty.

The nucleus to which substituents are attached in the formation of different steroids consists of four carbon rings fused together — the cyclophenanthrene nucleus. Even with all their characteristic substituents added, steroids are small molecules compared to other biological entities. Common mammalian steroids range from 18 carbon atoms in oestrogens to 28 carbon atoms in cholesterol. Their molecular weight is in the 300–400 range, as compared to proteins which can go over a million daltons. They are for the most part highly lipid-soluble, and penetrate cell membranes freely. They are thus universally distributed but only convey a message to a small population of target cells which alone possess proteins with the configuration which will bind a particular steroid during the short period in its biological life when it possesses the particular array of substituents which fit the lock. In some ways this is central to the problem of using steroids as biochemical test substances. The prime object is to read the strength of the signal. But we have to measure the steroid in blood or urine, remote from its site of action and often in a biologically inactive form.

The rapid metabolism of steroids influences their usefulness as biochemical indicators of the state of the fetoplacental unit. They are synthesized by an array of enzymes which trim precursor molecules step by step to the desired shape. This takes place in the adrenal, the testis, the ovary and the placenta — the site which most concerns us in this chapter. Their rate of production is determined by the amount of enzyme and of substrate, as with all enzyme-controlled processes. The amount of enzyme is largely dependent on the bulk of functional enzyme-containing tissue.

Indirectly many steroid measurements in pregnancy are simply measures of the bulk of functional placental tissue, which can be a very useful measure if areas of trophoblast are being put out of action by obstetric disease. The substrates on which the placental enzymes act come from either the mother or the fetus. In the case of many steroids, e.g. oestradiol, the substrate supply from the mother is an important rate-limiting factor. The substrate supply is determined by the concentration of the substrate and the uterine blood flow. Many obstetric diseases are associated with a reduction in uterine blood flow and it is likely that this is the factor which plays a part in the reduction of steroid synthesis in obstetric disease.

The relationship between steroid production in the placenta and the effects of obstetric disease is blunted by two further factors: firstly, there appears to be no feedback control between placental synthesis and the sites of steroid action. Nothing that we can determine tells the placenta that more or less oestradiol or progesterone is needed, wherever these steroids may act. Secondly, there is no single step in steroid synthesis which is clearly rate-limiting, more so than any other step in the process. In the case of fetal substrate supply, the matter might be somewhat different. The main fetal precursor for placental oestrogen synthesis is a 19-carbon androgen, dehydroepiandrosterone, from the fetal adrenal. The placenta is able to utilize maternal dehydroepiandrosterone for synthesis of oestrogens such as oestradiol and oestrone, but it cannot do so for oestriol. The reason is that oestriol has a substituent (a hydroxyl at C_{16}) which is added to the molecule of dehydroepiandrosterone by a C_{16}-hydroxylating system which is for the most part limited to the fetal adrenal and liver. The state and size of these fetal organs have a discernible effect on the ability of the trophoblast to produce oestriol.

Steroids are carried in the maternal blood stream strongly bound to specific carrier proteins or more weakly bound to non-specific proteins, such as albumin. Only a tiny fraction, around 2%, is present in free solution. The 98% of steroid which is protein-bound cannot enter cells and is biologically inactive. Normal steroid measurements take in this protein-bound fraction and attempts to separate bound and free steroid before measurement have proved cumbersome and difficult. Steroids are present in the free form in saliva and high hopes were entertained of steroid measurements made on this fluid. It appears, however, that the ratio of free to bound steroid is fixed and measurements of free steroid in saliva are closely related to those of total steroid in serum at perhaps 1/50th of the serum concentration.

Of course the concentration of a substance in blood is controlled as much by the rate at which it runs out as by the rate at which it runs in. Indeed in the case of some placental proteins, this is comparatively slow so that there is a tendency for the substance to accumulate. The high plasma concentration gives a falsely high impression of the production rate in the placenta. Worse still, if something goes wrong with the placenta and the production falls off, it takes some time for this event to evidence itself by a fall in serum concentration.

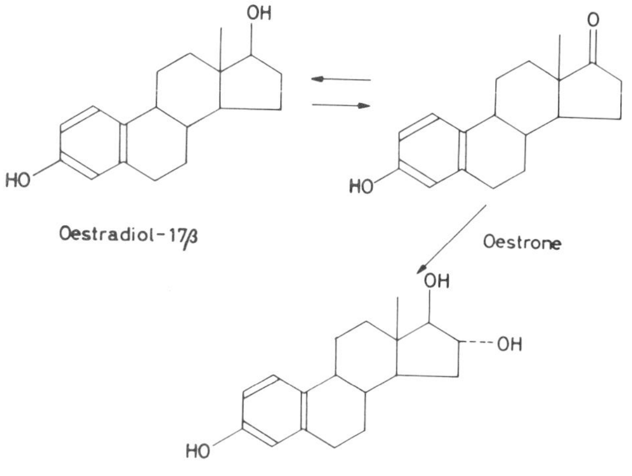

Fig. 25.1 The structure and metabolic relationships of the three classical oestrogens.

None of this applies to placental steroids. They have short half-lives in the circulation (approximately 5–10 minutes) and the plasma concentration bears a close relationship to the rate of secretion from the placenta. This is due to the nature of their catabolism. They are either converted to the next compound in the metabolic chain, e.g. progesterone to pregnanediol, or the free steroid or metabolite is conjugated to a sulphate or a glucosiduronate moiety and rapidly excreted in urine. Either way the steroid is excluded from the fraction measured in blood.

THE OESTROGENS

The oestrogens are 18 carbon steroids at the end of a metabolic chain, starting with cholesterol which has 28 carbon atoms. Their common feature is that ring A of the cyclophenanthrene nucleus is aromatic, i.e. has double bonds between alternate pairs of carbon atoms and there is a hydroxyl group attached to carbon 3. Such a configuration puts oestrogens into the class of phenols and gives them some chemical properties useful for their measurement when such measurements had to be preceded by laborious purification. All oestrogens have at least one hydroxyl (the one attached to C_3) but may have up to three more attached to other carbon atoms. The structure of the three classical oestrogens is shown in Fig. 25.1. It can be seen that, although oestradiol and oestrone are interconvertible and can act as precursors for oestriol, the latter cannot be metabolized to oestradiol or oestrone.

The number, position and orientation in space of the hydroxyl groups is the basis for the classification of oestrogens, although there are other structural differences between different oestrogens. Although 27 different molecular configurations have been identified, in terms of biochemical tests, we are concerned with only four: oestrone (one hydroxyl), oestradiol (two hydroxyls), oestriol (three hydroxyls) and oestetrol (four hydroxyls).

Oestrone–oestradiol

These two oestrogens are interconvertible by enzyme systems which are widely distributed in the body. They exist in the circulation as an equilibrium mixture and as biochemical test substances there is little to choose between them. In this role oestradiol has been overshadowed by oestriol. This may be a mistake as far as assays in serum are concerned. Oestriol is by far the major oestrogen in urine, but the serum concentration of oestradiol is higher. It is likely, therefore, that some urinary oestriol is derived from plasma oestradiol. There is, however, no good evidence that oestradiol assays will tell anything about fetal well-being which cannot be learnt from measuring oestriol.

The raw material for the synthesis of oestradiol is a C_{19} androgen, dehydroepiandrosterone, which is produced by the maternal and fetal adrenals. Under normal circumstances about 40% of the oestradiol produced by the placenta comes from maternal precursor. When dehydroepiandrosterone in the form of its sulphate is injected into the maternal circulation the rate-limiting step of precursor supply to the placenta is upset, and within 45 minutes plasma oestradiol rises to 4–5 times the pre-injection level. This constitutes a searching test of the capacity of the enzyme systems in the placenta involved in the conversion of dehydroepiandrosterone sulphate to oestradiol. At one time high hopes were entertained of the procedure as a dynamic test of placental function—plotting over a 3-hour period the change produced in plasma oestradiol by a bolus injection of 50 mg dehydroepiandrosterone sulphate. Unfortunately, the response was highly variable from one individual to another and the tests have fallen into disuse (Klopper et al 1976). This is a pity for although not useful as a test of placental function it could have been a powerful tool for the study of the role of oestradiol in pregnancy.

Oestriol

Oestriol is synthesized from the 16-hydroxy derivative of dehydroepiandrosterone sulphate. This 16-α hydroxyl group is retained throughout the further metabolism of the steroid. It is the characteristic feature of oestriol and has direct bearing on oestriol assays to assess fetal well-being. The main part of the dehydroepiandrosterone which goes into the making of all steroids is supplied by the fetal adrenal. The 16-hydroxylation of oestriol takes place to some extent in the fetal adrenal but for the most part in the fetal liver. The adult adrenal and liver are deficient in the 16-hydroxylating enzyme and virtually all the 16-hydroxydehydroepiandrosterone used by the placenta to make oestriol comes from the fetus. Herein lies the importance of oestriol: it is a fetal as well as placental product.

The supply of dehydroepiandrosterone by the fetal adrenal as well as its 16-hydroxylation by the fetal liver are rate-limiting steps with direct bearing on the rate of oestriol production by the placenta.

Another enzyme system at the very end of the oestriol pathway is also of fetal origin. This is the sulphuryl transferase system which converts free oestriol into biologically inert oestriol sulphate. Sulphurylation is a common way of protection against biologically active compounds and it is likely that this is a mechanism for protecting the fetus against the high concentration of oestriol in its circulation. The fetus has no way of getting rid of the oestriol sulphate and this form of the steroid cannot cross the placental barrier into the maternal circulation. It has first to be desulphurylated by sulphatase in the placenta. These two steroid sulphate metabolizing enzymes, one fetal and one placental, control the inflow of oestriol into the maternal circulation. The fetal liver has large reserves of sulphuryl transferase and it is unlikely that this system is ever rate-limiting. Placental damage is more common and extensive than fetal liver damage and it is possible that sulphatase depletion plays a part in the fall of maternal serum oestriol or the urinary excretion seen in extensive infarction or retroplacental haemorrhage.

One finding concerning sulphatase has contributed to the disillusion about the usefulness of oestriol assay. The production of sulphatase is genetically controlled and through genetic defect the placenta may be severely deficient in sulphatase. In such cases the plasma oestriol or its urinary excretion may be very low. On this account patients have been subjected to unnecessary Caesarean section as the low levels are not indicative of fetal hazard.

There is no accumulation of oestriol sulphate on the fetal side. The sulphatase deficiency also affects earlier steps in oestriol metabolism as 16-hydroxydehydroepiandrosterone sulphate also has to be converted to the free steroid before it can be metabolized to oestriol. Not only does this indicate that oestriol is not essential to fetal well-being, it also suggests that substrate supply rather than its subsequent metabolism is the link between oestriol level and fetal well-being.

The fetal adrenals are very large in relation to other organs and their steroidogenetic pattern is different from that of the baby after the first few weeks of life. The large fetal adrenals produce mainly dehydroepiandrosterone, a minor product of the adult adrenal. Presumably this is to supply substrate for the synthesis of oestriol—a strange procedure if oestriol is unnecessary. The size of the fetal adrenals, and therefore their capacity to generate oestriol substrate, is related to the overall fetal weight. Not surprisingly there is a correlation between plasma or urinary oestriol and the weight of the fetus. This leads to the most useful application of oestriol assay in clinical obstetrics: the diagnosis and management of retarded intrauterine growth. It is wise not to oversimplify this situation. There are many ifs and buts. Small babies with small adrenals and a low oestriol production are not necessarily sick babies. True growth-retarded babies, functioning poorly in many respects including adrenal growth, may die suddenly without dramatic prior change in adrenal function. The progressive deviation of oestriol levels from normal with a slow rise or none at all, is the significant feature. It is this which contributes to management rather than the expectation of a dramatic fall indicating imminent fetal death.

The fact that fetal adrenal substrate supply is such an important factor in determining oestriol explains why oestriol assays are sometimes less than helpful. In the USA oestriol assays were at one time *de rigueur* for the management of diabetic pregnancy, but now their use has declined. It is true that when a diabetic has a small infarcted placenta and growth-retarded fetus the oestriol levels will give warning of the hazardous state of the fetus. But few diabetic pregnancies produce such a baby; many result in a large fetus with large adrenals and a hypertrophic placenta. These are more than enough to keep oestriol production normal in spite of the deleterious effect of the disease on the fetus.

The role of the fetal liver is less obtrusive. One would have thought that fetal diseases which damage liver function, such as rhesus incompatibility, would result in lowered oestriol production. There is in fact no correlation between the fetal state and oestriol level in this disease and moribund fetuses may have normal oestriol just before delivery. Perhaps in this situation the hypertrophic placenta compensates for the ailing fetus.

The placental enzyme system most likely to have an effect on oestriol levels in obstetric disease is placental aromatase; the enzyme system which causes the unsaturation of ring A of all the oestrogens. This enzyme is very oxygen-sensitive and reduction in placental blood flow will quickly affect its activity. This is one situation in which the reduction of oestriol output may be sudden and severe. This is probably the basis for the usefulness of oestriol assays in pre-eclampsia, a disease associated with reduced uterine blood flow and given to sudden deterioration.

The theoretical basis for the use of oestriol assays as a measure of fetal well-being arises from the concept of the fetoplacental unit as enunciated by Diczfalusy in 1962. In essence this states that with regard to oestriol, neither the fetus or the placenta is a complete endocrine unit. The molecules are shuttled back and forth between the two so that together they form a complete unit. Oestriol assays measure not placental function or the fetal state alone but the two together.

Oestetrol

Oestetrol has four hydroxyl groups. It is synthesized in the fetal liver from oestradiol of fetal origin (Gurpide et al 1966). Being entirely of fetal origin, high hopes were entertained of its assay as a measure of placental function. These hopes were disappointed and the test is now falling into disuse. Fetal liver enzyme systems appear to be immune from the problems which beset intrauterine life.

PROGESTERONE

In the early days of steroid assays it was not possible to measure plasma progesterone so its main urinary metabolite, pregnanediol, was determined instead. This gave sufficient promise as a placental function test that attempts to measure the active hormone in blood were energetically pursued. When this became possible, investigators were disappointed to find that progesterone assays were a good deal less informative than oestrogen measurements. The link between progesterone and the fetal state, even in the obvious case of threatened abortion, was vague and uncertain. Progesterone levels are very variable; the changes are often without rhyme or reason.

PROTEIN HORMONES OF THE PLACENTA

In the beginning it was easy. When in 1927 Aschheim & Zondek discovered a pregnancy-specific protein in urine it was soon found that chorionic gonadotrophin was of placental origin and had effects on the ovary. This fitted the classical concept of a hormone — a substance secreted into the circulation to act catalytically at a distance on another tissue — and the endocrine career of the placenta began. It continued smoothly some 34 years later when Ito & Higashi (1961) isolated a second protein from the placenta and Josimovich & MacLaren (1962) demonstrated its endocrine nature. But we were already running into difficulties with definitions. Is adrenalin a hormone when secreted by adrenal glands, but not when it comes from a nerve ending? The turmoil grew worse when Hans Bohn (1971) started isolating more and more different proteins from the placenta. Others joined in and by now the total is well into the twenties. Are they all hormones? Some we can exclude because they are structural proteins of the placenta not secreted into the circulation; others because they are not peculiar to the placenta, being produced and secreted by other tissues. For example, chorionic gonadotrophin has been isolated from the male pituitary. We are left with a small but probably growing list of secreted proteins, undoubtedly of placental origin and as specific to the placenta as chorionic gonadotrophin. We do not know their target tissue, or what they do, but think they are chemical messengers and as such classify them with chorionic gonadotrophin and placental lactogen.

Although all the proteins which I shall designate as placental hormones can be found in the maternal circulation, we are running into trouble with the concept that hormones require to be carried from the cell of origin to a distant site in the general circulation. It is clear that sometimes messages are passed from one cell to an adjacent one of a different nature, without requiring the signal substance to be conveyed in the endovascular space. This has come to be called a paracrine activity and it is likely that some of the proteins discussed below are acting in a paracrine manner. From our point of view all that matters is that we can measure the strength of the signal and from that make deductions about the state of the placenta.

The placental proteins are a world apart from the placental steroids. For one thing they are very much larger. The steroids range from 300 to 400 in molecular weight, while the proteins range from 20 000 to 800 000. The size difference alone has many consequences. The proteins cannot enter cells, except occasionally by a complex process of *internalization*, and have to exert their effects on cells after binding to the limiting membrane. The steroids move freely in and out and are distributed through every nook and cranny of the body. They diffuse out from the placenta in either direction, toward the fetus and toward the mother. The proteins are secreted unidirectionally toward the mother. Only traces of the placental proteins can be found in the fetal circulation.

Another difference lies in their metabolism. Steroids drain away as fast as they are produced. Oestrogens have a half-life of 5–10 minutes in the biologically active form. Their plasma concentration is determined by their rate of synthesis in the placenta, not by their outflow in urine or transformation into other molecules. With the exception of human placental lactogen, which has a half-life of 15 minutes, the placental proteins have half-lives measured in days rather than minutes. They tend to accumulate and their plasma concentration may give a falsely high impression of their rate of production. Because of their slow turnover the concentration of the proteins is more steady from time to time than that of the steroids. On the other hand, the placental protein concentrations are slow to respond when rapid changes take place in placental production.

We have failed thus far to identify the factors which control the production of any of the placental proteins. There appears to be no feedback mechanism which throttles back placental production when less is needed or stimulates it when more is required. The only factors which appear to determine the plasma concentration of a placental protein are the functioning mass of the placenta and the uterine blood flow. It is difficult to ascribe a function to any of the placental proteins when there appears to be no means of modulating their production. Perhaps they have all-or-none effects and operate constantly at well above threshold level. It has even been suggested that they have no particular function at all; the placenta is simply programmed to produce them for no good reason (Gordon & Chard 1979). If this is true, it detracts from their value as placental function tests. We would be in a better position to use the assays if we knew which function they represented. Of course if their activity is paracrine, limited to their immediate vicinity, the distant plasma concentration may have no physiological significance. It is smoke, drifting away from the conflagration and gives no indication of the temperature of the fire.

Human chorionic gonadotrophin

Human chorionic gonadotrophin (hCG) can first be detected in the circulation of the mother about 7 days after fertilization, i.e. at implantation and a week before a period has been missed. At this stage the conceptus is only a speck of tissue and it is astonishing that it can produce enough protein to be measurable, when diluted throughout the whole maternal intravascular volume. It must take a few days for the concentration to build up to the point where hCG can be detected. It is likely, therefore, that the secretion begins a few days earlier, while the fertilized ovum is lying free in the uterine cavity or still in the Fallopian tube, which makes one wonder whether the stimulation of the corpus luteum is the whole story of the function of hCG. Perhaps it has a paracrine role in relation to the tissues with which it comes into contact before implantation.

Once hCG is present in the maternal blood it increases very rapidly, doubling in concentration every 2–3 days. It is presumed that this steep rise reflects the rapid proliferation of the trophoblast. If, therefore, hCG assays hold up a mirror to the early growth of the embryo they should be valuable in the first few weeks of pregnancy. This is a stage of pregnancy which does not usually impinge upon the obstetrician; yet it is likely that much of the wastage of pregnancy takes place at that time, perhaps without the mother being aware of her pregnancy. Induction of ovulation, in vitro fertilization and artificial insemination are all giving us access to this area. The borderland between unexplained infertility and early pregnancy loss is now being explored. The results are promising and the next few years are likely to see an upsurge in hCG assays in infertility clinics.

Until now the main application for hCG assays has been somewhat later in pregnancy, for the management of threatened abortion at 8–12 weeks. The results have been disappointing and no refinement of technique or improvement of study design is likely to change that. This is for two reasons: firstly at this stage any change in hCG is the consequence of irrevocable trophoblast damage rather than the reversible cause of impending abortion. Secondly, hCG concentration peaks at 10 weeks and then declines to a lower level for the rest of the pregnancy. Are you looking at trophoblast deterioration or a normal physiological event? Why hCG peaks so early and what turns it off is one of the fascinating mysteries of reproductive physiology. The placenta continues to grow and if, in spite of that, hCG does not keep pace there must be something that turns it off. If we can find the answer to that question we may be a long way toward understanding the control of hCG production. It surely cannot be just trophoblast mass and uterine blood flow.

Two technical advances will greatly affect the assay of hCG and indeed all other proteins. One is the substitution of enzyme or other labels for radioactive atoms. This enables the assay end-points to be read by less sophisticated apparatus than a gamma counter. It gives the reagents a much longer shelf-life and puts placental protein assays within the reach of clinical services with a limited access to laboratory technology.

The other advance is the development of monoclonal antisera. However pure the antigen which is used to raise an antiserum in a whole animal, such an antiserum consists of a large population of antibodies directed at different binding sites on the antigenic molecule. Monoclonal antibodies consist of a single antibody species directed at a single binding site constituted by a particular amino acid sequence in the antigen. Thus there is now available a monoclonal antibody against hCG which recognizes only the 15 amino acid sequence at the carboxy terminal of the beta chain of the molecule. This confers absolute specificity on the assay, as this sequence is unique to hCG.

Human placental lactogen

There is a strange relationship between pituitary and trophoblastic hormones. Luteinizing hormone and hCG are so close that one can be used therapeutically in the place of the other. Of the 190 amino acids in the chain of human placental lactogen (hPL), 163 have the same sequence as pituitary growth hormone and hPL has growth-promoting properties. It might be supposed that hPL is a hormone operative in the field of carbohydrate metabolism but there is no good evidence of interaction between hPL and plasma glucose or insulin. Nor have hPL assays been found to be notably useful in the management of diabetic pregnancy.

Of all the placental proteins, hPL comes closest to the picture of the placenta running free, without restraint or stimulus. Indeed the mean curve of plasma hPL closely resembles the growth curve of the placenta, even flattening off between 37 and 40 weeks, as does the placental weight. But to regard hPL measurements as an indirect way of weighing the placenta in utero is an over-simplification. Few have found a significant correlation between hPL and placental weight. It appears in the circulation later than hCG, although much of the difference between the two may be a matter of assay sensitivity. It rises less steeply and is not as useful an indicator of the viability of the conceptus in very early pregnancy as is hCG.

A little later, say 8–9 weeks, hPL is a more reliable indicator. As most overt abortions take place at a stage of gestation when hCG is already starting to fall in normal pregnancy, hPL has a better record than hCG in the management of threatened abortion. It has been claimed that a single assay on admission can do much to reduce time spent in hospital. The pregnancy may not continue even if the hPL is normal but if it is low the outlook is so poor that curettage should be considered.

Like other placental proteins hPL assay may be deceptive when the threatened abortion is due to an anembryonic gestation sac. In such cases the trophoblast development may be normal and the hPL equally so, although the pregnancy is doomed to failure.

The relationship between hPL levels and fetal weight is indirect, presumably through the relationship with placental weight. Nevertheless the most useful application of hPL assays in late pregnancy is the diagnosis and management of retarded fetal growth particularly when it occurs in association with hypertension. In this context an experiment by Spellacy and colleagues (1975) has captured the clinical imagination. The authors did hPL assays on a group of patients at risk. The results were available to the clinicians in half the patients and were used in management of these patients. In the other half, where the hPL value was not revealed, the perinatal mortality was 15% whereas in those patients where it was known the perinatal mortality was 3.4%.

Apart from fetal growth, hPL assays have no strong specific application in late pregnancy. Indeed, in conditions such as rhesus incompatibility and diabetes which may be associated with a large placenta, the general rule that hPL levels fall when there is fetal hazard may be reversed. With these exceptions hPL assays are as good a predictor of poor fetal outcome as oestriol assays and better than clinical observations such as severe pre-eclampsia, low maternal weight gain and heavy smoking.

Schwangerschaftsprotein 1

This protein, much to the comfort of English speakers, was formerly known as pregnancy-specific $beta_1$ glycoprotein. Unfortunately, it is not pregnancy-specific and there are other placental glycoproteins with $beta_1$ electrophoretic mobility. It has, therefore, had to revert to the specificity of the number given to it by one of its discoverers, Hans Bohn (1971). It is likely to remain Schwangerschaftsprotein 1 (SP_1) until we securely assign a unique function to it and so admit it to the company of hCG and hPL.

SP_1, like hCG, can be detected very early in pregnancy—around the time of implantation, 7–10 days after ovulation. Like hCG, SP_1 rises very steeply in early pregnancy. Indeed there is a good deal of physiological resemblance between SP_1 and hCG, the most notable difference being that hCG falls after 10 weeks' gestation while SP_1 continues to rise steadily. The clinical applications in early pregnancy are very much the same as those of hCG and hPL, with the addition that it combines the particular virtues of both. Because it appears so early in pregnancy and rises so steeply it can be used, like hCG, to detect pregnancy and subclinical abortion. Because it reflects faithfully trophoblast vitality it is about as useful as hPL in the management of threatened abortion.

An interesting new application for the assay of these pregnancy proteins has appeared in recent years. They all rise so steeply in early pregnancy that the large difference between one week and the next tends to cancel out the difference between one individual and another at the same stage of pregnancy. Consequently the value at any time will be in a range characteristic of that stage of pregnancy. In other words hCG, hPL or SP_1 assays can be used to determine the stage of gestation. hCG assays have a limited use because the downturn after 10 weeks makes it impossible to use them after that time, but SP_1 or hPL concentration up to 14 weeks is at least as reliable as ultrasound in determining the stage of pregnancy. This opens possibilities for routine screening of obstetric populations.

The uses for, and the reliability of, SP_1 assays in late pregnancy are much as those of hPL. There is, however, one important difference between the two proteins: SP_1 has a much longer half-life — 22 hours as opposed to 15 minutes. SP_1 tends to accumulate in the circulation and its high concentration does not indicate a high rate of synthesis. Small, non-significant variations in production do not affect the plasma levels. It keeps remarkably steady; the coefficient of variation from day to day (5%) is barely higher than the experimental error of replicate determinations. But this absence of day-to-day variability is bought at the cost of a speedy response to large important changes in production. SP_1 will persist in the circulation for weeks after the placenta is delivered. The patient-to-patient variation is no smaller than that of hPL.

Consequently the application of SP_1 assays to the problems of the management of obstetric disease in late pregnancy are as much obfuscated by a large normal range as is the application of hPL assays. As there is little to choose between them, obstetricians tend to lean toward the test they know. The literature on hPL is much more extensive.

Pregnancy-associated plasma protein A

Pregnancy-associated plasma protein A (PAPP-A) does not fit the picture of a typical placental protein. Indeed there have been doubts whether it is purely a placental protein or whether the endometrium might be contributing to the synthesis of this large molecule of 800 000 daltons. An endometrial element in PAPP-A would fit neatly with one hypothesis about the function of the protein. If the trophoblast presents to the maternal immune recognition system a protein which is at least partly maternal in origin, the possibility of it provoking an immune response is diminished. It has also been suggested that PAPP-A is an inhibitor of fibrinolysis. It could, therefore, be involved in the maintenance of a protective fibrin screen over the placenta, a suggestion supported by the finding that immunohistochemical techniques show a high concentration in the fibrin on the surface of the trophoblast.

The evidence that PAPP-A concentration is determined by placental size and therefore by uterine blood flow is weak. PAPP-A continues to rise until term, while placental weight flattens off in the last 2–3 weeks. PAPP-A levels are, if anything, raised in pre-eclampsia while uterine blood flow is reduced. The fact that PAPP-A is so much of a maverick among placental proteins makes it difficult to assign it a place in the hierarchy of placental function tests. On rather empirical grounds there appears to be one clinical application for its application. This is in respect of the prognosis of anembryonic pregnancy. Such pregnancies are doomed to abortion but, as the trophoblast may function normally, this fact is not evident when SP_1 or hPL assays are done for threatened abortion. It appears that PAPP-A might give a more reliable prognosis in this situation. So would an ultrasonic scan. Surprisingly PAPP-A assays also give a better assessment of the prognosis when threatened abortion occurs in the presence of a live fetus.

Placental protein 5

Placental protein 5 (PP_5) has had little exposure as a placental test, but has potential value in coagulation disorders as it has been classified as the antithrombin III of pregnancy. The suggestion that its concentration may be indicative of the risk of abruptio placentae and even premature labour is worth exploring further.

PLACENTAL ENZYMES

The distinction between placental proteins with presumed hormonal activity such as SP_1 and other proteins of placental origin is unreal and has been operated here only as an arbitrary basis of classification. Even so it is by no means certain that the protein hormones do not have enzymatic activity or that the enzymes do not also act as chemical messengers. A review of placental enzymes published nearly 20 years ago (Hagerman 1969) listed 85 known enzymes in the human placenta. Many more have been added since then. Very few are germane to the present discussion. The steroid metabolizing enzymes have already been mentioned. A casual count shows nine of these for which claims as rate-limiting catalysts in steroid metabolism have been entered. All of them could, therefore, have a direct bearing on biochemical tests of placental function. They may in future play a larger role in chemical evaluation, but as they are not presently directly accessible for evaluation they will not be pursued further.

Two enzymes, not related to steroid metabolism, are released into the maternal circulation and have been proposed as biochemical indices of placental function. Alkaline phosphatase is mainly a liver enzyme but a group of isoenzymes, distinguished by the fact that they are not inactivated by being heated to 60–70°C, are produced by the placenta and secreted into the maternal circulation in increasing measure as pregnancy advances. Cystine aminopeptidase (CAP) is an N-terminal endopeptidase which, among other substrates, will hydrolyse oxytocin (and hence the name oxytocinase). It may be, therefore, that in pregnancy it acts as a control on oxytocin levels. Both enzymes owe their brief career as placental function tests to the fact that they are enzymes acting on known substrates which can be linked to spectrophotometric readouts. It was, therefore, possible to measure the small amounts of enzyme protein in blood long before radioimmunoassay made measurements of oestrogens or placental proteins possible. They are not closely linked to the fetal state and their claims to attention rest more on their history than on any evidence of clinical usefulness.

Enzymes (gamma glutamyl transpeptidase, alkaline phosphatase and amino peptidase) play a role in the diagnosis and management of cystic fibrosis. Genetic probes can pinpoint the carriers of the disease. Their relatives should, therefore, be examined by genetic probes to establish whether they are liable to transmit the disease. When such women get pregnant, the state of the fetus as regards cystic fibrosis may be determined by measuring the named enzymes in amniotic fluid. Not surprisingly the enzymes can only be measured in a few university laboratories.

TESTS ON THE AMNIOTIC FLUID

It is difficult to know where to stop for the list has no end. Any biochemical test can be performed in pregnancy, while some can only be done during pregnancy. That is the first criterion in limiting our list. This still leaves as candidates all the substances which can be measured in amniotic fluid. The fluid, if not the substances, is peculiar to pregnancy.

Amniocentesis is an invasive procedure, only to be ventured upon if the information to be gained is essential and reliable. For the most part it is not. Even when the fluid is available without risk from the vagina in premature rupture of the membranes, the answers are seldom reliable and it is not worthwhile keeping an assay method set up for such occasional use. Three tests, two of them applicable only to amniotic fluid, need to be briefly considered. They are lecithin: sphingomyelin ratio, liquor bilirubin and alpha-fetoprotein.

Lecithin: sphingomyelin ratio

This test enjoyed a brief but considerable vogue. At a time when respiratory distress syndrome caused the death of many more babies than it does now, it was worth an amniocentesis to lessen the risk of delivering a premature baby with deficient pulmonary function. The use of the lecithin: sphingomyelin ratio declined *pari passu* with the declining risk from prematurity, but nobody noticed until it was firmly pointed out (James et al 1983). That article spelt the near extinction of the test.

Liquor bilirubin

The bilirubin concentration of the amniotic fluid can be determined by direct spectrophotometry without preliminary chemical work-up. It is a simple test and was much used to assess the amount of fetal damage in rhesus isoimmunization. Like the lecithin: sphingomyelin ratio, it has declined in keeping with the decline in the disease for which it was used.

Alpha-fetoprotein

Although the measurement of alpha-fetoprotein (AFP) in liquor is a reliable indication of spina bifida or anencephaly, this test is ancillary to the measurement of the protein in blood. There is a good deal of controversy about whether whole obstetric populations should be screened at 16 weeks' gestation to identify the small number of women who have raised AFP and are therefore at risk of carrying a fetus with a central nervous system defect. The incidence of the disease is less in England than in Scotland and many hospitals south of the border have abandoned routine screening. The positive findings, even in Scotland, are rare and can sometimes be anticipated by a history of previous babies with a central nervous system defect, or its existence in other members of the family. In addition it is very difficult to define a cut-off point which would identify reliably all pregnancies with a central nervous defect without including some fetuses in which the high AFP was without sinister significance.

AFP is produced by the fetal liver and it has been claimed that a raised AFP indicates a significant risk of subsequent fetal growth retardation. This is surprising as one would expect a small liver to produce less AFP. The explanation offered is that the high level of AFP indicates extra permeability of placenta and membranes. This somewhat devious argument is not convincing and the evidence that has been put forward in support of the original claim is less so.

THE WAY FORWARD

There is a substantial basis to the disillusionment about biochemical tests of placental function. If we merely repeat the present tests in the same manner as hitherto, their credibility will continue to decline. We need either to develop new tests or to apply old tests in new ways. The case for whole population screening such as gestation determination by hPL or SP_1 assay and for measurements in very early pregnancy has already been made. Other possibilities are just over the horizon. Until now our attention has been focused on the products of the fetoplacental unit. But the fetoplacental unit receives many signals from the mother, some of which determine its growth and vitality. We are increasingly aware that the communication between fetus and mother is a dialogue, not a monologue. We are learning to read these maternal signals, some of which come from the decidua. At the last count 17 different proteins, synthesized by the endometrium of pregnant women, have been detected (Bell et al 1986). Some must pass through the chorion and amnion, for they have been found in the liquor. They can be measured in maternal blood. If any are directed at the fetoplacental unit, the maternal blood concentration may be some indication of the strength of the signal going to the fetus.

Perhaps we are looking in the wrong place by examining what the fetoplacental unit sends to the mother. Perhaps we should look more at what goes to the fetus, not only maternal products such as endometrial proteins; some trophoblastic products are as likely to be directed at the fetus as at the mother. There is no doubt that the trophoblastic proteins are secreted only into the maternal circulation but the case is quite otherwise with placental steroids. For the most part they are present in higher concentration in the fetal circulation than in the maternal. The concentration of both progesterone and of oestradiol is higher in the umbilical vein than in the umbilical artery (Farquharson & Klopper 1984). There is little doubt that there is active uptake of these steroids by the fetus. Is this only a catabolic exercise? There seems little point in sending steroids to the fetus if they do nothing. If they have some function to fulfil, the degree to which they do so may be important.

In the past, we have not been able to sample the fetal circulation without undue risk but each passing year concentrates the attention of the obstetrician more upon the second patient — the fetus. Already intrauterine fetal blood sampling can be done and soon we will be able to probe the biochemistry of the fetus as well as we can today see its morphology with ultrasound.

REFERENCES

Aschheim S, Zondek B 1927 Hypophysen Vorderlappenhormon und Ovarialhormon im Harn von Schwangeren. Klinische Wochenschrift 6: 1322

Bell S C, Patel S R, Kirwan P H, Drife J O 1986 Protein synthesis and secretion by the human endometrium during the menstrual cycle and the effect of progesterone in vitro. Journal of Reproduction and Fertility 77: 221

Bohn H 1971 Nachweis und Charakterisierung von Schwangerschaftsproteinen in der menschlichen Plazenta sowie ihre quantitative Bestimmung im Serum schwangerer Frauen. Archiv für Gynäkologie 21: 440

Brown J B 1955 A chemical method for the determination of oestriol, oestrone and oestradiol in urine. Biochemical Journal 60: 185

Buster J 1981 Clinical applications of steroid assay tests of fetal–placental function. In: Abraham G E (ed) Radioimmunoassay systems in clinical endocrinology. Marcel Dekker, New York, p 349

Chamberlain G V 1984 An end to antenatal oestrogen monitoring. Lancet i: 1171

Chard T, Klopper A 1982 Placental function tests. Springer Verlag, Heidelberg

Diczfalusy E 1962 The endocrinology of the fetus. Acta Obstetricia et Gynecologica Scandinavica 41: 45

Farquharson R G, Klopper A I 1984 Progesterone concentrations in maternal and fetal blood. British Journal of Obstetrics and Gynaecology 91: 133

Goebelsmann U 1980 Hormonal assessment of fetoplacental function. In: Givens J R (ed) Endocrinology of pregnancy. Year Book Medical, Chicago, p 364

Gordon Y B, Chard T 1979 The specific proteins of the human placenta: some new hypotheses. In: Klopper A, Chard T (eds) Placental proteins. Springer Verlag, Heidelberg, pp 1–21

Gurpide E, Schwers J, Weich M T, Van de Wiele R, Lieberman S 1966 Fetal and maternal metabolism of oestradiol during pregnancy. Journal of Clinical Endocrinology 26: 1355

Hagerman D 1969 The enzymology of the placenta. In: Klopper A, Diczfalusy E (eds) Foetus and placenta. Blackwell, Oxford, p 413

Ito Y, Higashi K 1961 Studies on the prolactin-like substance in the human placenta. Endocrinologica Japanica (Tokyo) 8: 269

James D K, Tindall V R, Richardson T 1983 Is the lecithin/sphinogomyelin ratio outdated? British Journal of Obstetrics and Gynaecology 90: 995

Josimovich J, MacLaren J 1962 Presence in the human placenta and term serum of a highly lactogenic substance immunologically related to pituitary growth hormone. Endocrinology 71: 209

Klopper A, Michie E, Brown J B 1955 A method for the determination of urinary pregnendiol. Journal of Endocrinology 12: 209

Klopper A, Wilson G, Masson G 1974 The variability of plasma hormone levels in late pregnancy. In: Scholler R (ed) Hormonal investigations in human pregnancy. Editions Sepe, Paris, p 77

Klopper A, Varela-Torres R, Jandial V 1976 Placental metabolism of dehydroepiandrosterone sulphate in normal pregnancy. British Journal of Obstetrics and Gynaecology 83: 478

Kober S 1931 Ein kolorimetrische Bestimmung des Brunshormons. Biochemische Zeitung 239: 209

Marrian G F 1930 The chemistry of oestrin. Biochemical Journal 24: 1021

Spellacy W N, Buhi W C, Birk S A 1975 The effectiveness of human placental lactogen as an adjunct in decreasing perinatal deaths. American Journal of Obstetrics and Gynecology 121: 835

26

Naren Patel

Fetal assessment by biophysical methods: cardiotocography

INTRODUCTION

Obstetricians have for a long time looked for antenatal tests that would identify the fetus at risk of intrauterine hypoxia and death. Ideally such a test should not only be reliable, but performed easily and repeatedly. The result should be available immediately and the cost should be minimal. Whilst many biochemical tests, such as estimations of oestriol and placental lactogens, have been carried out in the past, these correlate poorly in predicting fetal outcome (Varma 1981).

The test for fetal well-being most commonly used currently is antenatal cardiotocography — either the stress test which is popular in the USA or the non-stress test used widely in Europe. The sophisticated equipment needed for fetal heart rate recording and the significance of the various changes that occur in heart rate are the results of many years of observations and research.

Marsac, a French obstetrician, was probably the first to observe the fetal heart sounds (Pinkerton 1976). On 22 December 1822, Jean Alexandre Le Jumeau, Vicomte de Kergaradec, read his monograph 'Mémoir sur l'auscultation appliquée à l'étude de la grossesse' in the Royal Academy of Medicine in Paris. He recognized the distinct fetal tones and sounds which he thought were from the umbilical cord and the placenta. In 1833, Kennedy, an obstetrician in Dublin, published his monograph on obstetrical auscultation. Von Hoefft in 1836 described the normal range of fetal heart rate and the fact that the rate decreased with gestational age. Hohl (1833) and Huter (1862) thought that tachycardia was associated with fetal compromise and maternal fever. Kennedy (1833) thought that the most ominous fetal heart signs were 'slowness of its return following a contraction'. With further evaluation of the fetal heart the importance of auscultation throughout labour was stressed by Schwartz (1858) and Von Winckel (1893).

The introduction of continuous fetal heart rate recording using the averaging technique developed by Hon & Lee (1963) in the 1960s and 1970s changed the pattern of monitoring in labour (Hon 1972). However, it was Hammacher (1962, 1966) who not only developed the first antenatal cardiotocograph equipment with the phonocardiograph but also reported on the fetal heart rate characteristics associated with fetal compromise in the antepartum period. Kubli et al (1969) noted the association of late decelerations, baseline tachycardia and loss of variability with fetal compromise associated with pathological pregnancies. For monitoring the fetus antenatally the contraction stress test (CST) began to be evaluated in the USA while the non-stress test (cardiotocography; CTG) was being used in Europe.

METHODOLOGY

Antenatal cardiotocography employs external (indirect) methods of monitoring the fetal heart rate. The signals obtained are often small, sometimes discontinuous and constantly shifting, and therefore the qualities of tracing are often not as good as those obtained by direct methods, e.g. fetal scalp electrode as used during labour. Three techniques have been evaluated to obtain fetal heart recordings antenatally — phonocardiography, fetal electrocardiography and ultrasound Doppler cardiography.

Phonocardiography

In phonocardiography the signal is obtained by pressing a microphone on the maternal abdomen and the natural fetal heart sounds are amplified and converted into electrical signals. However, although theoretically this should allow the fetal heart signal to be identified clearly, in practice sound generated by the placenta, umbilical vessels and maternal intra-abdominal blood vessels as well as other extraneous noises are also picked up by the abdominal microphone and may mask the sounds from the fetal heart.

Due to the presence of additional unwanted sound, a system of signal filtration is required to produce a fetal heart rate signal free of artefacts. The clinical usefulness of this method in recording the fetal heart sounds has been looked at both antenatally and during the intrapartum period. The results indicate that there is a high incidence of poor tracings obtained using this method.

Saling (1969), examining 282 fetal heart rate tracings, found that only 22% could be considered of good quality; 15% were of very poor quality and the rest were of intermediate quality. Ruttgers & Kubli (1969) found that 51% of the 408 antepartum phonocardiograms they obtained were of good quality and 11% were considered useless. However Jauer et al (1976) found in their study of 95 antenatal patients between 27 and 41 weeks' gestation that as many as 77% of tracings were of good quality.

Clearly, although satisfactory recordings of the fetal heart rate may be obtained using this method, the recording is affected by many factors, is found to be difficult in practice and has a high incidence of poor-quality tracings. Currently work is in progress attempting to improve on the lead signal and recognition of patterns using microprocessors.

Fetal electrocardiography

By pressing electrodes on the maternal abdominal wall it is possible to record the fetal ECG. However the maternal ECG is also recorded; the elimination of this maternal ECG complex requires electronic filtration of the signals and amplification of the fetal component before a clear fetal heart rate recording is obtained.

In abdominal fetal ECG, the fetal R waves of the fetal ECG complex are used as trigger signals. The potential of this part of the ECG signal varies throughout pregnancy.

From the 18th week of gestation until the 27th, the R wave potential is high. Following this, there is a decline to a minimum potential at 30 weeks' gestation. Between 27 and 34 weeks of gestation it is impossible to obtain continuous fetal heart rate tracings in 70% of cases (Steer 1986). Thereafter the fetal R wave potential increases until delivery. This variation is thought to be due to the effect of vernix caseosa altering the electrical resistance of the fetal skin (Wheeler et al 1978).

A number of studies have been performed during the antenatal period to determine the frequency with which satisfactory recordings of the fetal heart can be made. Obviously direct comparisons between different studies are difficult because of the imprecise assessment of tracings, which in most cases are simply divided into good, intermediate and poor quality. However, many groups have reported successful use of abdominal ECG to record the fetal heart, particularly when used in the last 4 weeks of pregnancy (Wheeler et al 1978, Keegan & Paul 1980). The newer equipment using noise reduction techniques may be more satisfactory (Greene 1987, Jenkins 1984, Jenkins et al 1986).

Ultrasound fetal cardiotocography

This is now the most commonly used method for recording fetal heart rate antenatally. It utilizes the physical principle of the Doppler effect in which sound waves hitting a moving object are reflected back at an altered frequency. Using this principle, the fast opening and closing of the fetal heart valves can be detected. Since they cause a definite ultrasound frequency shift, this physical movement can be used to generate well defined trigger pulses.

Initially the ultrasound transducers used consisted of a single transmitter and a single piezoelectric crystal receiver. This combination of narrow beam transducers had the disadvantage that the ultrasound beam required precise positioning to produce a good signal. Due to this difficulty, broad beam array transducers were devised, consisting of several pairs of transmitter and receiver crystals, which detected the movement of a large area of the fetal heart wall and produced smaller, slower frequency shifts compared with those produced by the fetal heart valves themselves. Using this method, most studies have indicated that a reliable recording of the fetal heart can be obtained (Bishop 1968, Solum 1980). However using ultrasound fetal cardiotocography with a broad beam transducer, true beat-to-beat variability of the fetal heart or short-term variability cannot be recorded accurately. Assessment of baseline variability is possible in clinical practice with good-quality recordings (Solum et al 1981).

In spite of the difficulties in obtaining recordings of suitable quality for analysis with Doppler ultrasound monitors, this method has become the most useful in clinical practice with good recordings being obtained relatively easily, independent of gestational age.

Some more recent machines incorporate the technique of autocorrelation, which uses the techniques of signal processing of ultrasound signal with microprocessors. Two types of correlation are possible — the cross-correlation and autocorrelation. The advantage of the latter is that more precise calculation of the periodicity of the wave forms can be achieved (Steer 1986). The disadvantages however are halving or doubling of true fetal heart rate and detection of maternal instead of fetal heart rate.

PHYSIOLOGY

Details of fetal cardiovascular physiology are fully dealt with in Chapter 8. A brief discussion follows with particular reference to the clinical relevance of the fetal heart rate changes.

The parasympathetic and sympathetic components of the autonomic nervous system control fetal cardiac behaviour. The regulation of fetal heart rate is also influenced by vasomotor centres, chemo- and baroreceptors and cardiac antoregulation. Pathological events such as fetal hypoxia modify these influences and fetal cardiac responsors. Minor changes in fetal blood gases do not produce a change in fetal heart rate (Wood et al 1979).

Baseline fetal heart rate

Fetal heart rate falls with increasing gestational age (Schifferle & Caldeyro-Barcia 1973) and also becomes more variable (Ruttgers et al 1972). The decrease in fetal heart rate is due to development of vagal tone (Hon & Yeh 1969). Therefore the mean baseline fetal heart rate is a reflection of a balance of sympathetic and parasympathetic autonomic influences. The mean normal baseline fetal heart rate in late pregnancy is between 120 and 150 beats/min.

Rates between 100 and 120 beats/min are regarded as fetal bradycardia. If the variability is abnormal, it is usually a reflection of increased vagal tone. If observed spasmodically it may suggest cord compression. Persistent marked bradycardia is associated with congenital heart defect (Garite et al 1979). Baseline bradycardia is rarely associated with antepartum hypoxia (Young et al 1979) unless placental abruption is present.

Baseline tachycardia of over 160 beats/min is associated with maternal fever or chorioamnionitis; in the latter there may also be loss of variability. Kubli et al (1972) showed that with chronic fetal hypoxia the fetal heart rate is within normal range, in contrast to the situation in acute or subacute fetal hypoxia where there is baseline tachycardia present. This may be due to an increase in the levels of catecholamines. Administration of beta-mimetic drugs to the mother leads to mild fetal tachycardia. A persistent high fetal tachycardia over 200 beats/min is associated with cardiac arrhythmia (Kline et al 1979).

Fetal heart rate variability

Under normal physiological conditions the interval between each heart beat (beat-to-beat) is different and this is referred to as short-term variability; it increases with increasing gestational age (Goodlin 1977, Wheeler et al 1979). Long-term variability is due to the periodic changes in the direction and size of the changes from hypoxia resulting in oscillations around the mean baseline fetal heart rate. These oscillations occur approximately two to six times per minute. Short-term variability, normally of the order of 1–3 beats/min, cannot be identified visually (Wheeler et al 1979).

The factors that influence fetal heart rate variability are fetal sleep states, accelerations and decelerations, as well as gestational age (deHaan et al 1971, Romer et al 1979). Fetal heart rate variability increases with gestational age. Under normal physiological situations the fetal heart rate variability is the product of opposing sympathetic and parasympathetic influence on the heart. Several investigators have shown the relationship between reduced variability and chronic fetal hypoxia (Hammacher 1966, Kubli et al 1972) and severe fetal hypoxia resulting in loss of variability (Dalton et al 1977). Mild and early stages of hypoxia on the other hand may be associated with a reduction in fetal heart rate variability (Flynn et al 1979). Fetal infection is associated with tachycardia and loss of variability. Drugs that cause depression of the central nervous system, such as hypnotics and opiate alkaloids, are also associated with reduced fetal heart rate variability (Petrie et al 1978, Keegan et al 1979).

The fetus is known to undergo sleep–wake cycles of 60–70 min (Sterman 1967, Junge 1979). The quiet phase can average from 20–30 min. True wakefulness is associated with acceleration and increased fetal heart rate variability, while sleep cycles are associated with reduced variability. Motor and respiratory movements are similarly affected (Dalton et al 1977). Fetal breathing movements are also associated with short-term variability (Dawes et al 1981b). Millar et al (1979) showed that a maternal glucose injection had an influence on the fetal cardiovascular system by altering fetal metabolism. Diurnal variation in fetal heart rate variability may also be present, as it is in motor and respiratory functions.

Sinusoidal pattern

This pattern is commonly associated with an anaemic fetus, as a result of either rhesus sensitization or cardiac failure (Manseau et al 1972, Modanlouh et al 1977). Sinusoidal fetal heart rate pattern resembles a sine wave of fixed periodicity of 2–5 cycles/min (Young et al 1980). Original publications describing this pattern of fetal heart rate all reported a very high perinatal loss (Kubli et al 1972, Manseau et al 1972, Rochard et al 1976). However, apart from cases of rhesus sensitization, its usefulness in clinical management antenatally requires further evaluation. Transient or irregular sinusoidal patterns and those with higher frequency than 2 cycles/min are not an indication for intervention.

FETAL HEART RATE ACCELERATIONS

Accelerations are usually transient, of about 15–20 beats/min, and are commonly associated with fetal movement, external stimuli or uterine contractions. They are rarely seen in association with fetal hypoxia (Wood et al 1979). The presence of accelerations suggests intact fetal sympathetic activity and is therefore a major component in the evaluation of antenatal cardiotocography or non-stress tests (Fischer 1976, Paul & Millar 1978).

FETAL HEART RATE DECELERATIONS

Decelerations of a transient nature are a frequent occurrence. The non-recurring early or mildly variable type, in association with uterine activity or fetal movement, are normally associated with normal fetal outcome (Kidd et al 1985a). Late and recurrent decelerations are of hypoxic origin (Perar et al 1980, Kidd et al 1985a). Decelerations in the presence of loss of baseline variability are associated with fetal hypoxia (Kubli et al 1972). Occasional late decelerations without any other fetal heart rate characteristics, such as loss of variability, are not an indication for intervention (Kidd et al 1985b). Decelerations associated with marked or atypical contractions may be associated with fetal hypoxia (Kubli et al 1978, Visser et al 1980). Marked decelerations may also be associated with maternal supine hypotensive syndrome. Several publications have reported the association of repeated late decelerations and fetal death, particularly in the high-risk cases (Kubli et al 1978, Lenstrup & Falck-Larsen 1979, Visser & Huisjes 1977, Solum & Sjoberg 1980). Recurrent late decelerations, particularly when present in association with loss of variability, are a poor prognostic sign.

Based on the physiology and pathophysiology of fetal heart rate the following criteria could be used in the diagnosis of fetal hypoxia in the intrapartum period.

Normal and abnormal antepartum fetal heart rate

A normal trace is one with a baseline of 120–160 beats/min with a variability of 5–25 beats/min, with at least two accelerations of an amplitude of 10–15 beats/min over a 15–20-minute interval. There should be no decelerations, except for an occasional sporadic mild variety. An abnormal fetal heart rate pattern is characterized by marked baseline tachycardia (over 180 beats/min) or bradycardia (less than 100 beats/min) and a marked increase in the amplitude of the baseline variability (over 25–30 beats/min). Further, loss of variability and recurrent late or atypical decelerations are associated with fetal compromise; these are the most important features in the prognostic index of the test.

PERFORMING OF NON-STRESS CARDIOTOCOGRAPHY

The pregnant woman should be comfortable either in a left lateral position or semi-recumbent to avoid supine hypotension. Blood pressure and maternal pulse rate should be recorded prior to performing the test. An external ultrasound transducer for the recording of fetal heart rate and tocodynamometer for recording of uterine activity are attached to the maternal abdomen. The ultrasound transducer is located to obtain the best fetal heart signal. The tocodynamometer is usually placed on the fundus of the uterus.

The recording is carried out over a period of 30 minutes.

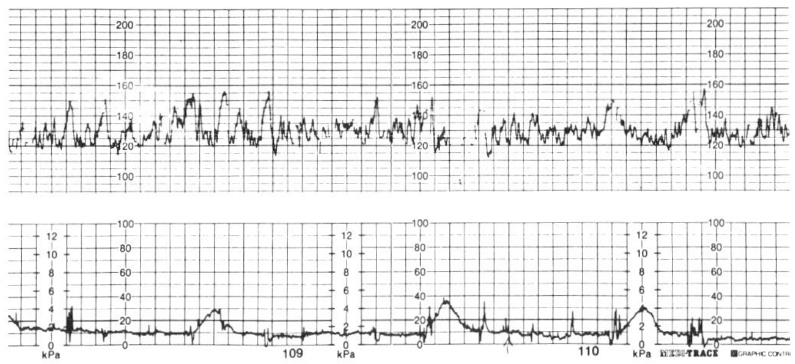

Fig. 26.1 Normal non-stress test showing fetal movement and uterine activity, normal fetal heart rate with normal long-term variability and accelerations.

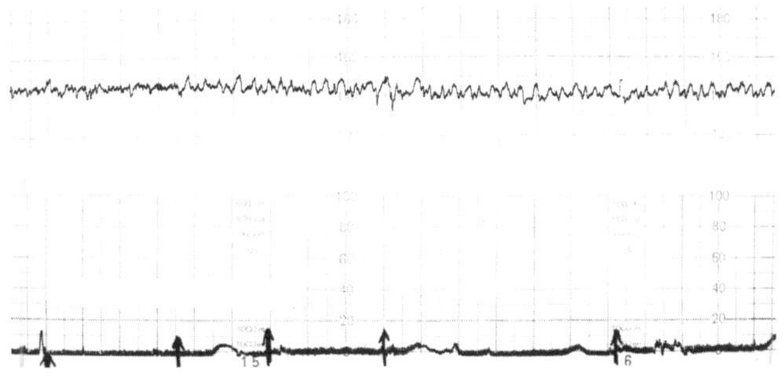

Fig. 26.2 Antenatal non-stressed fetal heart rate recording showing reduced long-term variability with no accelerations. Arrows are event markers during fetal movements. Tracing is an effect of sedative drugs.

External stimulus in the nature of palpation or gentle movement of the fetus is perfomed if the non-stress test is non-reactive after 20 minutes. Alternatively, other stimulatory tests such as an acoustic test as described by Luz (1979) are sufficient to wake the fetus. Maternal blood pressure and pulse are recorded at the end of a 30-minute period.

For clinical purposes the antenatal fetal heart rate patterns can be divided into:

1. Normal.
2. Showing transient abnormality.
3. Suspicious.
4. Abnormal, requiring intervention.

The tracing is regarded as normal when the baseline is within normal range, has normal variability and when accelerations are present with fetal activity or uterine contractions (Fig. 26.1). Shallow spiked occasional decelerations are not an ominous sign.

Transient reduction in variability and lack of accelerations may be related to fetal sleep states or medication (Fig. 26.2). Maternal blood pressure may also be responsible. Tests of fetal stimulation should be carried out in these situations.

Suspicious tests are associated with reduced fetal activity and reactivity. There may be reduced variability and accele-

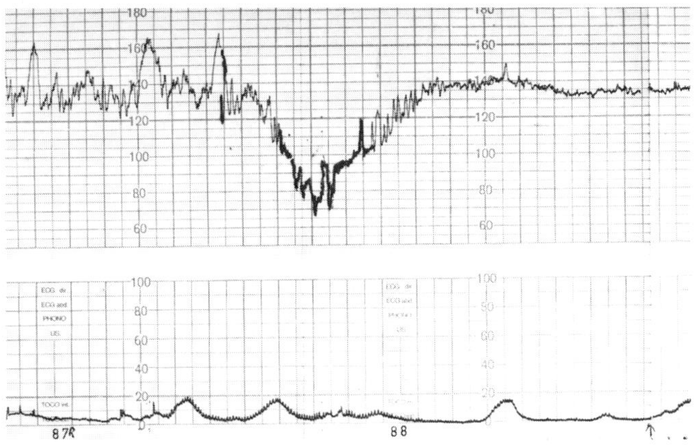

Fig. 26.3 Isolated marked late deceleration of fetal heart rate which had previously followed a normal reactive pattern. Tracing is of suspicious but doubtful significance and should be repeated.

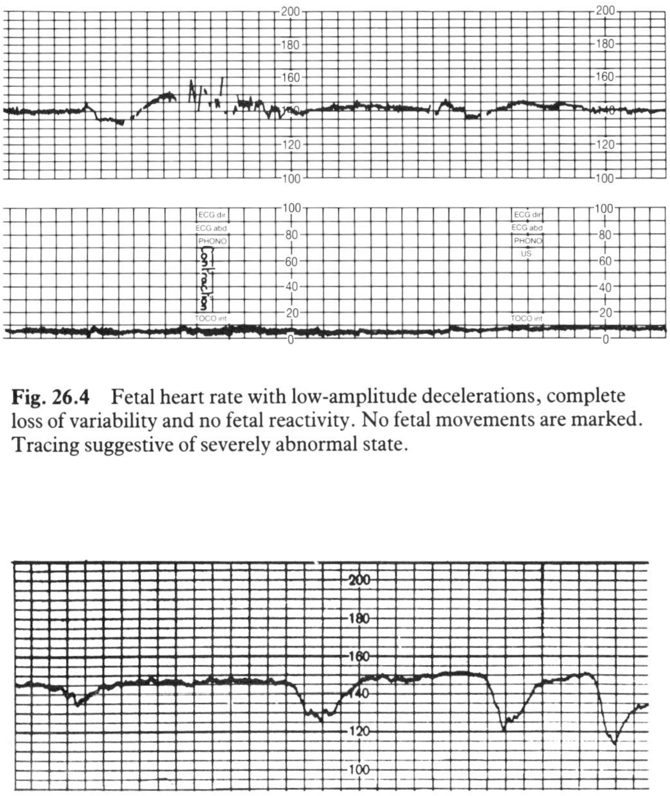

Fig. 26.4 Fetal heart rate with low-amplitude decelerations, complete loss of variability and no fetal reactivity. No fetal movements are marked. Tracing suggestive of severely abnormal state.

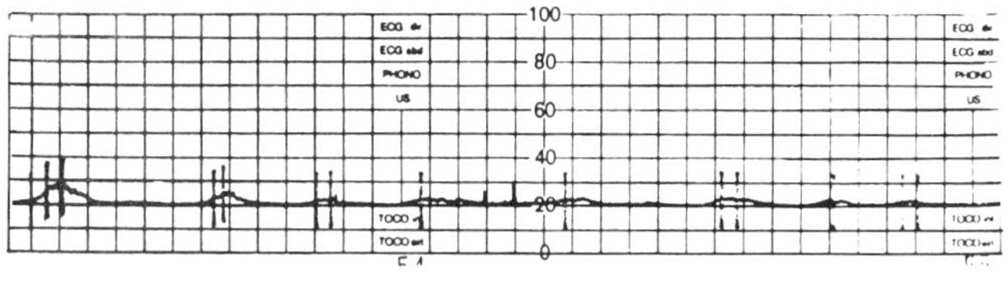

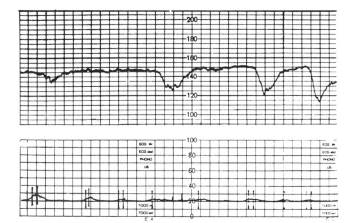

Fig. 26.5 Antenatal heart rate tracing showing loss of variability with recurrent decelerations following fetal movements. Tracing suggests fetal hypoxic state.

rations may be absent. Sporadically occurring, non-repeating late decelerations may be present in the presence of fetal activity and reactivity (Fig. 26.3). Similarly, mild repeating decelerations in the presence of accelerations are suspicious signs requiring repeat tests to be performed. Minor deviations of baseline fetal heart rate and sinusoidal patterns require further evaluation to assess the worth of these patterns in diagnosing pathological fetal states.

Fetal heart rate tracings showing marked reduction in variability and accelerations with isolated or recurrent decelerations should be regarded as abnormal (Fig. 26.4, 26.5).

The need for a uniform method of interpretation of antenatal cardiotocography trace is obvious. It will make the results more comparable and the task of teaching staff in training easier. Various attempts have been made in the form of devising scoring systems. Kubli & Ruttgers (1972) described the first of these. Others followed and all are based on the changes in the fetal heart rate as described by Schifferle & Caldeyro-Barcia (1973) and others. Each system tried to modify or add to the original system (Hammacher et al 1974, Fischer et al 1976, Krebs & Petres 1978, Pearson & Weaver 1978, Lyons et al 1979, Breart et al 1981). Some of these scoring systems did not include accelerations and the more recent quantitative methods which include accelerations and decelerations have a better prognostic index in diagnosing fetal compromise (Garoff et al 1978, Wilken et al 1980).

The two commonly used scoring systems in Europe are those devised by Fischer et al (1976) and Meyer-Menk et al (1976). They are similar and are based on a 10-point scoring system (Table 26.1). The simplified system by Pearson & Weaver does not take into account the variability of the fetal heart rate and is based on a 6-point scoring system. Trimbose & Keirse (1978) showed that the assessment of cardiotocographs using scoring systems improved the inter- and intraobserver reliability compared to subjective assessment. Keirse & Trimbose (1980) found that using the Meyer-Menk scoring system there were no false positive scores, in contrast to other systems in which the false positive rate could be as high as 20%. Adis et al (1978) showed a strong correlation between cardiotocograph scores and umbilical artery pH (Fig. 26.6). Flynn et al (1982) compared the Meyer-Menk/Fischer, the Cardiff and the Birmingham scoring systems with a subjective assessment of the cardiotocographs as either reactive or non-reactive and found the scoring systems to have a poor correlation with fetal outcome compared to the subjective assessment of experienced observers.

Some of the American scoring systems have tried to simplify the interpretation further by only looking at acceleration patterns (Paul & Millar 1978, Schifrin et al 1979, Mandenhall et al 1980). As periods of non-reactive tracings in relation to fetal sleep–wake periods are common, further evaluation of tracings without accelerations becomes necessary.

The efforts at developing computer-assisted analyis and

Table 26.1 Scoring system for interpretation of antenatal cardiotocography trace

	Score		
Parameter	0	1	2
Baseline level (beats/min)	<100, >180	⩾100, <120; >160; ⩽180	⩾120, ⩽160
Amplitude of fluctuation (4 beats/min)	⩽5, sinusoidal	>5, ⩽10 (⩾25)	>10, <25
Frequency of fluctuation (cpm)	<2, sinusoidal	⩾2, ⩽4	>4
Deceleration pattern with uterine contractions	Late deceleration pattern frequency ⩾25%, marked variable pattern, severe supine syndrome	Late deceleration pattern frequency <25%, moderate or mild variable deceleration pattern, early deceleration pattern	Lack of deceleration, single mild variable, deceleration, dip 0
Acceleration with arousal test or fetal movements	Absolute lack of acceleration (negative response)	Atypical shape, no spontaneous acceleration	Acceleration with fetal movements (positive response)

A total of 10 points is optimal; 0 is the worst result: 8–10 points, normal; 5–7 points, prepathological or suspicious record; 0–4 points, pathological. From Meyer-Menk et al (1976).

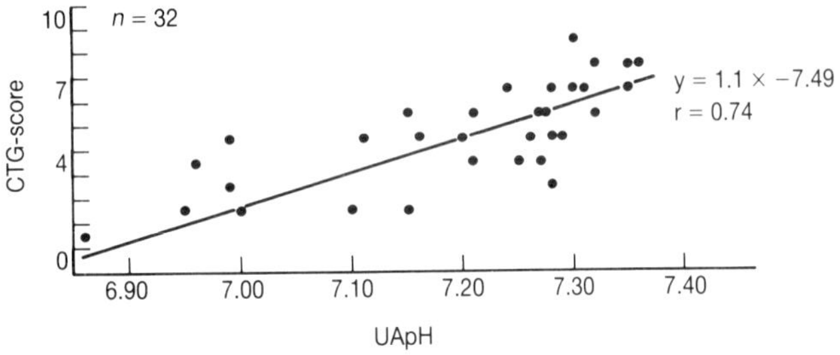

Fig. 26.6 Correlation between the cardiotocograph (CTG) score of the last antepartum record and the umbilical artery pH in 32 high-risk pregnancies with prelabour Caesarean section. From Adis et al (1978).

quantitation have not been successful (Escarcena et al 1979). The problem in computerization of antenatal fetal heart signals is related to the poor quality of the signals obtained and the signal-to-noise ratio (Wheeler et al 1979, Ammala 1983). Dawes et al (1981a, 1982) described a system of computerized numerical analysis of fetal heart periods. Although when using Doppler ultrasound failure time averaged 40%, the system may be useful in the analysis of antenatal fetal heart records and has potential in clinical use.

CLINICAL APPLICATION

According to the Scottish stillbirth and neonatal death report (Cole 1985), 275 normally formed infants died before labour started; the majority of them weighed less than 2500 g. In an attempt to prevent these deaths, obstetricians have always looked for a reliable, quick test to identify fetuses who are at risk. Antepartum fetal heart rate monitoring has become widely accepted over the last few years but the stillbirth rate still remains high. The overall incidence of antepartum death is approximately 3–4/1000. In an unselected population the risk of antenatal fetal death rate is 1/1000 within 1 week of a negative cardiotocograph (Kubli et al 1978, Schifrin et al 1979). The incidence of normal and pathological

Table 26.2 Incidence of normal and pathological cardiotocography in low- and high-risk pregnancies (from Solum 1980)

Cardiotocograph	Low risk ($n = 411$)	High risk ($n = 401$)
Normal	384 (93.5%)	311 (77.6%)
Suspect	22 (5.4%)	29 (7.2%)
Pathological	5 (1.1%)	61 (15.2%)

cardiotocographs in low- and high-risk obstetric population varies, as shown in Table 26.2. In the management of 250 pregnancies with intrauterine growth retardation, Varma (1984) found that non-reactive cardiotocographs were significantly associated with adverse intrapartum factors and neonatal outcome. Similar findings have been reported by Lenstrup & Haase (1985) in 454 high-risk pregnancies.

Several other reports of a randomized trial in high-risk pregnancies do not support these findings (Brown et al 1982, Flynn et al 1982, Lumley et al 1983, Kidd et al 1985b). Most of these series however were not reporting on frequent fetal heart testing in high-risk pregnancies. In most cases the results were related to one or two isolated cardiotocographs prior to delivery or death of the fetus. Kubli would have quite rightly argued that the concept of antenatal fetal heart testing demands frequent testing, particularly in the compromised fetus, as the fetal heart rate changes occur in a progressive fashion. There is an increasing duration of low fetal activity periods (Halberstadt 1981). However, in situations of acute hypoxia, fetal death may occur shortly after a normal reactive tracing is obtained. Freeman (1981) has shown that with frequent proper antenatal monitoring, the rate of fetal death can be reduced to 3.2/1000 in high-risk pregnancies. In terms of adverse intrapartum neonatal events the false negative rate varies from 2 to 20% (Rochard et al 1976, Keirse & Trimbose 1980, Weingold et al 1980). A normal tracing is therefore not reassuring in all cases but a pathological tracing relates closely to poor fetal outcome (Solum 1980).

Table 26.3 Neonatal neurological outcome in relation to antepartum fetal heart rate (FHR) patterns in small-for-dates (SFD) term and preterm fetuses (from Visser et al (1980)

	n	CS	pH_{ua} (mean)	Neonatal neurological diagnostic category: Normal	Suspect	Abnormal	NNOS (median)
SFD term							
Normal FHR	9	9	7.25	8	1	–	56
Decelerations	14	14	7.14	3	7	4	51.6
Total	23						
SFD preterm							
Normal FHR	12	—	7.18	7	5	–	53
Decelerative FHR	14	11	7.16	4	6	4	50.5
Terminal FHR	7	7	6.99	–	3	4	48.5
Total	33						

CS = Caesarean section, NNOS = neonatal neurological optimality score; pH_{ua} = pH in umbilical artery blood.

As the natural course of chronic fetal hypoxia is slow, antenatal fetal heart monitoring if carried out once a week in low-risk (as opposed to no-risk) pregnancies, may be sufficient. However in high-risk pregnancies, with uteroplacental insufficiency or maternal disease such as hypertension or diabetes, the test will need to be repeated more frequently, even daily. The mode of delivery will be determined by the severity of the pathological tracing and other clinical features. With very non-reactive tracings and late decelerations, the incidence of subsequent brain damage is nearly 10% (Visser et al 1980), particularly so in small-for-dates and preterm babies (Table 26.3).

ANTENATAL STRESS TESTS

Oxytocin challenge tests

The commonest of these tests is the contraction stress test or oxytocin challenge test. It was developed in the USA by Kubli et al (1968) and is still more popular there than in Europe. The test is carried out in the same way as a non-stress test, recording fetal heart rate and uterine contractions using external ultrasound transducers and tocodynamometer. If spontaneous uterine activity is not recorded after 20 minutes, oxytocin infusion is started intravenously with 0.5 ml/min to produce three uterine contractions in a 10-minute period. A positive test is where fetal heart rate decelerations occur with uterine activity. A vast literature has now accumulated on the oxytocin challenge test (Freeman 1975, Schifrin et al 1975, Huddleston et al 1979, Staisch et al 1980, Lin et al 1981, Devoe 1984) in the management of high-risk pregnancies. The incidence of false positive is between 5 and 10%; the incidence of hyperstimulation is in the same range. Correlation of positive tests with intrapartum events is poor (Paul & Millar 1978); the test is invasive and time-consuming. It is currently being recommended as a second-line test following unsatisfactory non-stress cardiotocograph tests (Keegan & Paul 1980).

Nipple stimulation tests

To overcome the problems with oxytocin challenge test, nipple stimulation tests are currently being investigated. Nipple stimulation during human lactation institutes a neurohypophyseal reflex resulting in the release of oxytocin from the posterior pituitary (Cobo 1974). Stimulation of one or both nipples in late pregnancy produces a uterine contraction, presumably due to the release of endogenous oxytocin. Nipple stimulation is used instead of oxytocin infusion to produce uterine contractions if a non-reactive trace is obtained after a 20-minute recording of fetal heart rate (Huddleston et al 1984, Lanke & Nemes 1984, Chayen et al 1985, Copel et al 1985). The hyperstimulation rate is about 4%, with a failure rate of 4 to 15%. The correlation with intrapartum events and neonatal outcome is poor. The test, however, is easier to perform and is non-invasive and needs to be evaluated further.

Other tests

Other stimulatory tests studied include acoustic stimulation (Reid & Millar 1977); light stimulation (Peleg & Goldman 1980) and exercise tolerance (Brotanek & Sureau 1985). When the non-stress test is non-reactive an auditory stimulus of 105–120 dB is applied and repeated at a few seconds' interval. The test is regarded as negative if a fetal heart rate acceleration of 15 beats/min or more is evoked. Fetuses who failed to respond to the auditory stimulus subsequently had a significantly high positive oxytocin challenge test. It is suggested from this study that the auditory stimulus may eliminate the need for many oxytocin challenge tests.

In the light stimulation test the fetus is exposed to a cold light source for 30 seconds through an amnioscope following a vaginal examination. Again the idea is to replace the oxytocin challenge test if there is an unsatisfactory non-stress test. The procedure is invasive in that it requires the woman to be put in the lithotomy position and a vaginal examination is necessary. A reported series is too small to make further comment.

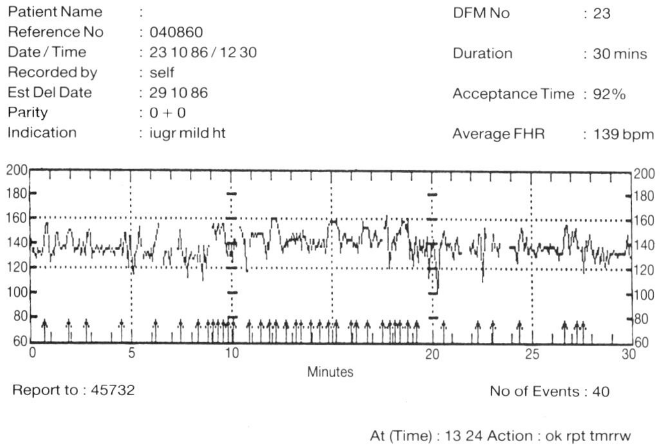

Patient Name :
Reference No : 040860
Date / Time : 23 10 86 / 12 30
Recorded by : self
Est Del Date : 29 10 86
Parity : 0 + 0
Indication : iugr mild ht
DFM No : 23
Duration : 30 mins
Acceptance Time : 92%
Average FHR : 139 bpm
200
180
160
140
120
100
80
60
0
5
10
20
25
30
Minutes
Report to : 45732
No of Events : 40
At (Time) : 13 24 Action : ok rpt tmrrw

Fig. 26.7 Antenatal fetal heart rate tracing obtained using Huntley technology. Distant fetal monitor with home monitoring equipment. Compressed signal transmitted via telephone line.

The exercise test is employed in patients where the non-stress test is unsatisfactory, rather than carrying out an oxytocin challenge test. The principle is to challenge the placental reserve by application of hypoxic stimulus in the form of maternal exercise. The patient is asked to carry out a mild form of exercise by stepping up and down three steps for 3 minutes. The fetal heart rate is recorded prior to and following this procedure. Fetal heart rate deceleration patterns are classed as ominous. The authors carried out the test in 375 pregnant women and felt that the test helped working practices of pregnant women at home and at work in high-risk pregnancies.

CONCLUSIONS

Antepartum fetal heart rate monitoring is the most widely accepted diagnostic test for assessment of the fetus at risk of hypoxia. The non-stress test or the antenatal cardiotocography is most commonly employed and the various stress tests, particularly the oxytocin challenge test, are used now rather as second-line tests. For monitoring a normal pregnancy the non-stress test has been found to be lacking and is probably not cost-effective. For monitoring high-risk pregnancies, the test is used serially and identifies fetuses at risk of hypoxia with a high degree of reliability. A normal test predicted a normal outcome in 90% of cases, whilst a pathological test, particularly one in which there was repeatedly loss of variability with decelerative patterns, was associated with fetal compromise in nearly all cases. The test needs to be done frequently to identify the changing fetal heart rate pattern associated with hypoxia, and whilst this can be carried out on an outpatient basis, it does involve the pregnant women attending the hospital or antenatal clinic. With the development of a digital system for distant heart rate recording and subsequent rapid transmission by telephone to the hospital, this problem could be overcome (Gough et al 1986). The complete recording of fetal heart rate carried out by the mother at home is transmitted to hospital in less than 30 seconds and stored on computer for analysis. Preliminary reports are promising and the tracings obtained appear to be satisfactory (Fig. 26.7). While stress tests, particularly oxytocin challenge tests, are still used in certain countries, they are rarely used in Europe now.

REFERENCES

Adis B, Wurth G, Stuke P 1978 Grundlagen und Ergebnisse fur die Beurtelung der Kardiotokographie mit einem neuren CTG-score. Inaugural dissertation, Heidelberg

Ammala P 1983 Antepartum non-stress cardiotography and quantified short term variability of fetal heart rate in high risk pregnancies. Annales Chirurgiae et Gynaecologiae 72: 347–352

Bishop E H 1968 Ultrasonic fetal monitoring. Clinical Obstetrics and Gynecology 11: 1154

Breart G, Coupil F, Legrand H et al 1981 Antepartum fetal heart rate monitoring. A semi-quantitative evaluation of the 'non-stress' fetal heart rate. European Journal of Obstetrics, Gynecology and Reproductive Biology 11: 227–237

Brotanek V, Sureau C 1985 Exercise test as a physiological form of antepartum stress test. International Journal of Gynaecology and Obstetrics 23: 327–333

Brown V A, Sawers R S, Parsons F J, Duncan S L B, Cooke I D 1982 The value of antenatal cardiotocography in the management of high risk pregnancy: a randomised control trial. British Journal of Obstetrics and Gynaecology 98: 716–722

Chayen B, Scott E, Cheng C, Perera C, Schiffer M A 1985 Contraction stress test by breast stimulation as part of antepartum monitoring. Acta Obstetricia et Gynecologica Scandinivica 64: 3–6

Cobo E 1974 Neuroendocrine control of milk ejection in women. In: Josimovich J F, Renaulds M, Cobo E (eds) Lactogenic hormones, fetal nutrition and lactation. Wiley, New York, p 433

Cole S 1985 Perinatal mortality survey. Information Services Division, Edinburgh

Copel J A, Otis C S, Stewart I, Rosetti C, Weiner S 1985 Contraction stress testing with nipple stimulation. Journal of Reproductive Medicine 30: 465–471

Dalton K J, Dawes G C, Partick J E 1977 Diurnal, respiratory and other rhythms of fetal heart rate in lambs. American Journal of Obstetrics and Gynecology 127: 414

Dawes G S, Visser G H A, Goodman J D S, Vevene D H 1981a Numerical analysis of the human fetal heart rate; the quality of ultrasound records. American Journal of Obstetrics and Gynecology 141: 43

Dawes G S, Visser G H A, Goodman J D S, Levene D H 1981b Numerical analysis of the human fetal heart rate; modulation by breathing and movement. American Journal of Obstetrics and Gynecology 140: 535

Dawes G S, Houghton R S, Redman C W G 1982 Base line in human fetal heart records. British Journal of Obstetrics and Gynaecology 89: 270–275

deHaan J, Bemmel J H, von Veth A F L et al 1971 Quantitative evaluation of FHR patterns. European Journal of Obstetrics and Gynaecology 3: 95

Devoe L D 1984 Clinical features of the reactive positive contraction stress test. Obstetrics and Gynecology 63: 523

Escarcena L, McKinney R D, Depp R 1979 Fetal base line heart rate variability estimation. I. Comparison of clinical stochastic quantification techniques. American Journal of Obstetrics and Gynecology 135: 615

Fischer W M (ed) 1976 Kardiotokography, Geburtshilfe. Thieme, Stuttgart

Fischer W M, Stude J, Brandl H 1976 Ein Vorschlag zur Beurteilung des antepartalen Kardiotokogramms. Zeitschrift für Perinatologie 180: 117

Flynn A M, Kelly J, O'Connor M 1979 Unstressed antepartum cardiotocography in the management of the fetus suspected of growth retardation. British Journal of Obstetrics and Gynaecology 86. 106

Flynn A M, Kelly J, Matthews K, O'Connor M, Viegas O 1982 Predictive

value of an observer variability. British Journal of Obstetrics and Gynaecology 89: 434–440
Freeman R K 1975 The use of the OST for antepartum clinical evaluation of utero-placental function. American Journal of Obstetrics and Gynecology 121: 481
Freeman R 1981 Antepartum fetal heart rate. Rate monitoring lecture: the world symposium of perinatal medicine. San Francisco
Garite T J, Linzee M E, Freeman R K, Dorchester W 1979 FHR patterns and fetal distress in fetuses with congenital anomalies. Obstetrics and Gynecology 53: 716
Garoff L, Vansellow H, von Hagen C, Grothe W, Ruttgers H, Kubli F 1978 Evaluation of 6000 antepartum CTG according to the previously published CTG code. Lecture presented to the 6th European Congress of Perinatal Medicine, Vienna
Goodlin R C 1977 Fetal cardiovascular responses to distress. A review. Obstetrics and Gynecology 49: 371
Gough N A G, Dawson A A J, Tomkins T J 1986 Antepartum fetal heart rate recording and subsequent fast transmission by a distributed microprocessor based dedicated system. International Journal of Biomedical Computing 18: 61–65
Greene K R 1987 The ECG waveform. Baillière's Clinical Obstetrics and Gynaecology 1: 131
Halberstadt E 1981 Zeitdauer und Assagekraft des antepartelen CTG. Perinatal Magazine 8
Hammacher K 1962 Neue Metode zur selecktiven Registrierung der fetalen Herzschlagfrequenz. Geburtshilfe und Frauenheilkunde 22: 1542
Hammacher K 1966 Fruherkennung intrauteriner Gefahrenzustand durch Elektophonokardiographie und Tokographie. In: Elert R, Huter K (eds) Die Parophylaxe fruhkindlicher Hirnschaden. Thieme, Stuttgart
Hammacher K, Brundell R E, Gaudenzp R, Grandi D E P, Richter R 1974 Kardiotocographischer Nachweis einer fetalen Gefahrdung mit einen CTG-score. Gynaekologische Rundschau 14: 61
Hohl A F 1833 Die geburtschilfliche Exploration. Theil I. Halle, p 34
Hon E H 1972 The present status of electronic monitoring of the human fetal heart. International Journal of Gynaecology and Obstetrics 10: 191
Hon E H, Lee S T 1963 Noise reduction in fetal electrocardiography. 2. Averaging techniques. American Journal of Obstetrics and Gynecology 87: 1086
Hon E H, Yeh S Y 1969 Electronic evaluation of fetal heart rate. X. The fetal arrhythmia index. Medical Research Engineering 8: 14
Huddleston J F, Sutcliffe G, Kerry F E, Flowers C E 1979 Oxytocin challenge test for antepartum fetal assessment. American Journal of Obstetrics and Gynecology 135: 609
Huddleston J F, Sutcliffe G, Robinson D 1984 Contraction stress test by intermittent nipple stimulation. Obstetrics and Gynecology 63: 669
Huter V 1862 Uber dem Fotalpuls Monatz. Geburtskunde Frauenkrankheiten XVIII supplement, Berlin
Jauer P C, Heinrich J, Koepck E, Hopp H, Seidenschnur G 1976 Vergleichende Untersuchungen zur Frage der Wertigkeit der Impulsaufnahmeverfahren der vorgeburtlichen Kardiotokographie. Zentralblatt für Gynaekologie 98: 990
Jenkins H 1984 A study of the intrapartum fetal electrocardiogram using a real-time computer. Thesis submitted for the Degree of Doctor of Medicine, Nottingham University
Jenkins H M L, Symonds E M, Kirk D L, Smith P R 1986 Can fetal electrocardiography improve the prediction of intrapartum fetal acidosis? British Journal of Obstetrics and Gynaecology 93: 6–12
Junge H D 1979 Behavioural state related heart rate and motor activity patterns in the newborn infant and the fetus antepartum. I. Technique, illustration of recordings and general results. Journal of Perinatal Medicine 7: 85
Keegan K A, Paul R H 1980 Antepartum fetal heart rate testing, IV. The non-stress test as a primary approach. American Journal of Obstetrics and Gynecology 136: 75
Keegan K A, Paul R H, Brouissard P M, McCart T, Smith M A 1979 Antepartum fetal heart rate testing. III. The effect of phenobarbital on the non-stress test. American Journal of Obstetrics and Gynecology 133: 579
Keirse M C, Trimbose J M 1980 Assessment of antepartum cardiotocograms in high risk pregnancy. British Journal of Obstetrics and Gynaecology 87: 261
Kennedy E 1833 Observations of obstetrical auscultation on obstetrical auscultation. Dublin
Kidd L C, Patel N B, Smith R 1985a Non-stress antenatal cardiotocography — a prospective blind study. British Journal of Obstetrics and Gynaecology 92: 1152
Kidd L C, Patel N B, Smith R 1985b Non-stress antenatal cardiotocography — a prospective randomised clinical trial. British Journal of Obstetrics and Gynaecology 92: 1156
Kline M A, Holsman J R, Austen E M 1979 Fetal tachycardia prior to the development of hydrox attempted pharmacologic cardio version. Case report. American Journal of Obstetrics and Gynecology 134: 346
Krebs H B, Petres R E 1978 Clinical application of a scoring system for evaluation of antepartum fetal heart rate monitoring. American Journal of Obstetrics and Gynecology 130: 765
Kubli F 1986 Development of fetal heart rate pattern. Workshop of cerebral handicap, Heidelberg
Kubli F, Ruttgers H 1972 Semi-quantitative evaluation of antepartum fetal heart rate. International Journal of Gynaecology and Obstetrics 10: 182
Kubli F W, Kaeser O, Hinselmann M 1968 Diagnostic management of chronic placental insufficiency. In: The fetal placental unit. Excerpta Medica, Amsterdam
Kubli F W, Hon E H, Khazin A F, Takemura H 1969 Observations on heart rate and pH in the human fetus during labour. American Journal of Obstetrics and Gynecology 104: 1190
Kubli F, Ruttgers H, Heller U, Bogdan C, Ramzin M 1972 Die antepartal fetal Herzfrequnz 2. Zeitschrift für Geburtshilfe und Perinatologie 176: 309
Kubli F, Boos R, Ruttgers H, von Hagens C, Vansclow H 1978 Antepartum FHR monitoring. In: Beard R W, Campbell S (eds) Current status of FHR monitoring and ultrasound in obstetrics. Royal College of Obstetricians and Gynaecologists, London
Lanke R R, Nemes J M 1984 Use of nipple stimulation to obtain contraction stress test. Obstetrics and Gynecology 623: 345
Lenstrup C, Falck-Larson J 1979 Cardiotocogram in fetuses at risk. Ugeskrift for Laeger 1141: 1485
Lenstrup C, Haase N 1985 Predictive value of antepartum fetal heart rate non-stress test in high risk pregnancy. Acta Obstetricia et Gynecologica Scandinavica 64: 133
Lin C, Devoe L, River P, Moawa D, Moawa A 1981 Oxytocin challenge test in intrauterine growth retardation. American Journal of Obstetrics and Gynecology 140: 282
Lumley J, Lester A, Anderson I, Renou P, Wood C 1983 A randomised trial of weekly cardiotocography in high risk obstetric patients. British Journal of Obstetrics and Gynaecology 90: 1018
Luz N P 1979 Audiotory evoked response. In: Scientific exhibition monograph. VIIII World Congress of Gynaecology and Obstetrics, Tokyo
Lyons E R, Blysma-Howel L M, Shamshee S, Toll M E 1979 Scoring system for non-stress antepartum FHR monitoring. American Journal of Obstetrics and Gynecology 133: 242
Mandenhall H W, O'Leary J A, Phillips K O 1980 The non-stress test: the value of a single acceleration in evaluating the fetus at risk. American Journal of Obstetrics and Gynecology 136: 87
Manseau P, Vaquier J, Chavinine J, Sureau C 1972 Le rythme cardiaque foetal 'sinocoidal'. Aspect evocatur de souffrance foetal au cours de la grosse. Journal of Gynecology, Obstetrics and Reproductive Biology 1: 343
Meyer-Menk W, Ruttgers H, Boos R, Wurth G, Eddis B, Kubli F 1976 A proposal for a new matter of CTG evaluation. In: Abstracts of the 5th European congress of perinatal medicine in Uppsala. Armquist and Wiksel, Stockholm, p 138
Millar F C, Skiba H, Klapholz H 1979 The effects of maternal blood sugar levels on fetal activity. Obstetrics and Gynecology 52: 662
Modanlouh D, Freeman R K, Braly P, Rasmussen S B 1977 A simple matter of fetal and neonatal heart rate beat to beat variability quantitation; preliminary report. American Journal of Obstetrics and Gynecology 127: 861
Paul R H, Millar F C 1978 Antepartum FHR monitoring. Klinische Obstetrische und Gynaekologie 21: 375
Pearson J F, Weaver J B 1978 A six point scoring system for antenatal cardiotocographs. British Journal of Obstetrics and Gynaecology 85: 321
Peleg T, Goldman J 1980 Fetal heart rate acceleration and response to light stimulation as a clinical measure of fetal well being. A preliminary report. Journal of Perinatal Medicine 8: 38
Perar J T, Kuueger T R, Harris J L 1980 Fetal oxygen cosumption and

mechanisms of heart rate response during artificially produced late decelerations of fetal heart rate in sleep. American Journal of Obstetrics and Gynecology 136: 478
Petrie R H, Yeh S Y, Manata Y et al 1978 The effect of drugs on fetal FHR variability. American Journal of Obstetrics and Gynecology 130: 294
Pinkerton J H M 1976 Fetal auscultation — some aspects of its history and evolution. Journal of the Irish Medical Association 69: 363
Reid J, Millar F 1977 Fetal heart rate acceleration in response to acoustic stimulation as a measure of fetal wellbeing. American Journal of Obstetrics and Gynecology 129: 512
Rochard F, Chiforene B, Gone-Pogonpil F, Legrand H, Blottiere J, Sureau C 1976 Non-stress fetal heart rate monitoring in the antepartum period. American Journal of Obstetrics and Gynecology 126: 699
Romer V M, Heinzl S, Peters F E, Mietzner S, Bruhl G, Heening P 1979 Auscultation frequency in baseline FHR in the last 30 minutes of labour. British Journal of Obstetrics and Gynaecology 86: 472
Ruttgers H, Kubli F 1969 Kontinuierliche Registrierung von fetaler Herzfrequenz bie gleichzeitiger Wehenschreibung. II Probleme der Instrumentierung. Gynäkologie 2: 82
Ruttgers H, Kubli F, Haler U, Bachmann M, Grunder E 1972 Die antepartale fetal Herzfrequnz. Zeitschrift für Geburtshilfe und Perinatology 176: 294
Saling E 1969 Verbesserung der apparativen Herzschlagregisdrierung beim Feten unter der Geburt. Fortschritte der Medizin 87: 777
Schifrin B, Lapidus M, Geetis De, Leviton N A 1975 Contraction stress test for antepartum evaluation. Obstetrics and Gynecology 45: 433
Schifrin B S, Foy G, Amato J, Kates R, McKenna J 1979 Routine FHR monitoring in the antepartum period. Obstetrics and Gynecology 54: 21
Schifferle P, Caldeyro-Barcia R 1973 Effects of atropine and beta adrenergic drugs on the heart rate of the human fetus. In: Boreus L (ed) Fetal pharmacology. Raven Press, New York, pp 259–279
Schwartz H 1858 Die vorzeitigen Atembewgungen. Leipzig
Solum T 1980 Antenatal cardiotocography methods, interpretation and clinical application. Acta Obstetricia et Gynecologica Scandinavica (suppl 96)
Solum T, Sjoberg N O 1980 Antenatal cardiotocography and intrauterine death. Acta Obstetricia et Gynecologica Scandinavica 59: 481
Solum T, Ingemarsson I, Nygren A 1981 The accuracy of ultrasonic fetal cardiotocography. Journal of Perinatal Medicine 9: supplement
Staisch K J, Wesleg J R, Barshore L A 1980 Blind oxytocin challenge test and perinatal outcome. American Journal of Obstetrics and Gynecology 138: 399
Steer P J 1986 Evaluation of cardiotocographs. DHSS scientific and technical branch. British Medical Journal 292: 827
Sterman M B 1967 The relationship of intrauterine fetal activity to maternal sleep state. Experiments in Neurology (suppl) 19: 98
Trimbose J M, Keirse M 1978 Significance of antepartum cardiotocography in normal pregnancy. British Journal of Obstetrics and Gynaecology 85: 907
Varma T R 1981 Clinical experience in non-stressed antepartum cardiotocography in high risk pregnancies. International Journal of Gynaecology and Obsteterics 19: 433
Varma T R 1984 Unstressed antepartum cardiotocography in the management of pregnancy complicated by intrauterine growth retardation. Acta Obstetricia et Gynecologica Scandinavica 63: 129–134
Visser G H A, Huisjes H J 1977 Diagnostic value of the unstressed antepartum cardiotocogram. British Journal of Obstetrics and Gynaecology 84: 321
Visser G H A, Redman C W G, Huisjess J, Turnbull A C 1980 Non-stress antepartum heart rate monitoring; implication of decelerations after spontaneous contraction. American Journal of Obstetrics and Gynecology 138: 429
Von Hoefft H 1836 Beobachtungen uber Auskultation der Schwengeren. Zeitschrift fur Geburtskunde VI: 1
Von Winckel F 1893 Lehrbuch der Geburtshilf. Leipzig
Weingold A B, Yonekura M L, O'Kieffe J 1980 Non-stress testing. American Journal of Obstetrics and Gynecology 138: 195
Wheeler T, Murrills A, Shelley T 1978 Measurements of the fetal heart rate during pregnancy by a new electrocardiographic technique. British Journal of Obstetrics and Gynaecology 85: 12
Wheeler T, Cooke E, Murrills A 1979 Computer analysis of fetal heart rate variation during normal pregnancy. British Journal of Obstetrics and Gynaecology 86: 186
Wilken H P, Hackel B, Wilken H 1980 Klinische Erfahrungn mit den antepartalen CTG-auswerterverfahren nach Fischer, Hammacher, Huch und Kubli. IV Score nach Kubli. Zentralblatt für Gynaekologie 102: 909
Wood C, Walker A, Yardley R 1979 Acceleration of the fetal heart rate. American Journal of Obstetrics and Gynecology 86: 186
Young B K, Katz M, Klein S A 1979 The relationship between heart rate patterns and tissue pH in the human fetus. American Journal Obstetrics and Gynecology 134: 685
Young B K, Katz M, Wilson S J 1980 Sinusoidal fetal heart rate. I. Clinical significance. American Journal of Obstetrics and Gynecology 136: 587

27

Frank A. Manning, Savas Menticoglou and Chris Harman

Fetal assessment by biophysical methods: ultrasound

INTRODUCTION

The concept of target imaging by analysis of reflectance characteristics of biophysical energies has its origins in the military, being developed and quickly advanced in World War II: target recognition by detecting reflected electromagnetic energy (radar) and particle compression energy (sonar) are the principal examples. With wonderful irony these have been adapted to image a more important target, the human fetus, and the information has been transformed from the intent of destruction to the intent of preservation. The almost unfathomable wealth of new information about the human fetus derived from ultrasound imaging has created and will continue to create major changes in the practical and psychological basis for the practice of perinatal medicine.

Beginning with the pioneer work of Professor Ian Donald in Glasgow, where crude sonar devices were used to create the first human fetal images (Donald & Brown 1961), obstetrical ultrasound has advanced so that highly sophisticated computer-assisted ultrasound imaging methods are now available to produce two-dimensional dynamic (real-time) fetal images of remarkable clarity and detail (Fig. 27.1). Technological developments continue and in the near future three-dimensional (holographic) ultrasound fetal images will become available.

This chapter will review some of the contemporary practical applications of this new technology in modern perinatal medicine with some reference to probable future uses. The primary intent is to describe the clinical applications of ultrasound in perinatal medicine. However, the new practical uses of ultrasound may describe only part of the clinical significance of this new technology. Traditional obstetrics involves care of a patient — the fetus — who cannot be seen or easily examined and this physical impediment has slowed the development of rational and reliable methods for detection and treatment of fetal diseases. Ultrasound imaging overcomes much of this handicap and in so doing creates the concept of the fetus as a patient. This subtle and sustained shift in psychological basis of prenatal care, wrought in part by ultrasound fetal imaging, may be expected to produce as great an advance in the quality of prenatal care as will the practical applications. It is now becoming possible to begin to apply the time-honoured extrauterine methods of physical examination such as monitoring of biophysical

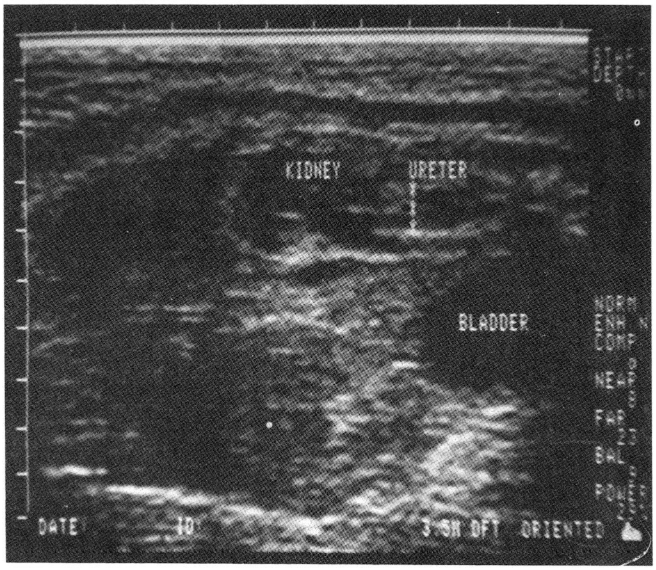

Fig. 27.1 Ultrasound scan of a fetus in the longitudinal coronal plane demonstrating the left urogenital tract. Note the kidney is well visualized, including the renal pelvis and ureter. The renal vessels are visualized and in dynamic mode visualized to pulsate. The echolucent structure on the upper pole of the kidney is the fetal adrenal gland.

markers, such as vital signs, to the intrauterine patient. Further, as the diagnosis of pathophysiology in the individual fetus improves in accuracy through application of these methods, the concept of disease-specific testing and therapy methods will also evolve. These concepts form an integral part of the application and clinical interpretation of ultrasound fetal imaging.

ULTRASOUND METHODS

Ultrasound is a form of particle compression energy of a frequency beyond the upper range of human hearing: diagnostic instruments used in obstetrics most commonly operate at a frequency of 3.5 million cycles per second (MHz). All ultrasound transducers use a synthetic crystal, usually zirconium, to produce the sound waves. Generation of the signal is based upon a piezoelectric phenomenon by which infusion of electrical energy (electrons) causes realignment in an atomic lattice structure of the crystal with resultant physical deformation of the crystal surface. Conversely physical compression of the crystal, produced by returning echoes, releases electrons within the lattice, producing a minute electrical signal. Therefore the crystal serves as both the transmitter and receiver. The crystal, when coupled to the skin surface, emits a repetitive high-frequency low-energy signal that penetrates tissues. Some of the signal energy is reflected at each tissue density interface, the portion being a direct function of the magnitude of the tissue density variation. The reflected echoes are detected in time and intensity by the transducer and displayed as two-dimensional co-ordinates on a cathode ray tube. A detailed description of signal processing falls beyond the scope of this chapter and is well described elsewhere (Manning 1984).

For practical purposes the clinician should know that these signals are displayed by intensity or brightness (B-mode) in up to 132 shades of grey (grey scale). A dynamic or real-time ultrasound image is produced by repeating the frequency of ultrasound image rapidly enough to capture the movement of the target. This is achieved in one of two ways:

1. Electronic interrogation of several crystals aligned longitudinally (linear array) or concentrically (annular array).
2. Moving a single transducer through a prescribed arc (sector scanning).

Dynamic B-mode ultrasound imaging has been a great advance since the method permits assessment of both structural and functional characteristics of the fetus. More detailed spectral analysis of echoes may be useful in the future to assess tissue density and structure. Thus, for example, spectral analysis of fetal lung echoes holds promise as a method for determination of lung maturity and detection of conditions such as pulmonary hypoplasia (Harman, personal communication). Spectral analysis of the Doppler shift of ultrasound signals produced by blood flow and fetal and maternal vessels has already been shown to be a useful marker of perinatal disease (Eik-Nes et al 1980, Gill et al 1981, Kurjak & Rajhvajn 1982).

SAFETY

The safety of ultrasound has been and will continue to be a subject of intense research efforts in obstetrics. Ultrasound transducers cause the application of physical energy to the mother and fetus. The energy is maximal at the signal source and decreases as a function of the distance squared. This diagnostic method has been used in obstetrics since as early as 1961 (Donald & Brown 1961). In 25 years of experience, there has never been a single reproducible deleterious fetal effect reported as a consequence of this energy exposure. During this time, signal strength has continued to be reduced as detection sophistication improves: most diagnostic systems now operate at a mean intensity of less than 10 mW/cm^2. At the University of Manitoba where diagnostic ultrasound has been used in obstetrics since 1967, more than 10 000 children exposed to ultrasound in utero have been followed without recognition of any adverse effect (Lyons E. A., personal communication). Detailed examination of subsets of matched sibling cohorts (exposed and non-exposed) has failed to detect any biologically significant effect in the exposed groups (Lyons E. A., personal communication). Further, data of second-generation effects of ultrasound exposure are now becoming available, again showing no recognizable adverse effect of ultrasound on exposed individuals' progeny. Thus, although by definition the definitive answer concerning the safety of ultrasound may never be reached, the results to date imply remarkable safety.

The human error of misuse of ultrasound and misinterpretation of ultrasound data is no doubt real. The equipment is complex and requires training for proper use, and the information obtained must always be considered within the entire clinical context. In our centre in earlier days, iatrogenic perinatal death has resulted from elective intervention for presumed fetal maturity based on ultrasound data. It is likely that this tragedy has been repeated elsewhere and illustrates the need for rational clinical consideration of ultrasound-derived data. It would seem that the potential for human error is the major safety concern regarding in ultrasound in modern obstetrics.

DETERMINATION OF FETAL AGE AND GROWTH

An accurate estimate of gestational age (fetal age) is of fundamental importance in obstetrical practice. To the mother the information regarding her expected date of confinement is essential for the anticipation and planning of the arrival of her child. To the physician the information is critical since disease recognition and subsequent management decisions are to a large extent dependent upon knowing the fetal age; for example, recognition of abnormal variations in fetal growth and abnormal durations of pregnancy depend extensively upon accurate dates. Similarly most critical perinatal management decisions are based on this information. In the compromised fetus with progressive disease, management decisions are usually based on balancing the risks of continued in utero existence against potential neonatal risks incurred by delivery: the estimate of gestational age invaribly forms a pivotal point in these deliberations. In the immature fetus with progressive acquired or congenital disease, planning the appropriate method of in utero therapy depends on knowing fetal age precisely. Thus for example calculation of intraperitoneal blood transfusion volumes in the severely affected rhesus-immunized fetus is dependent upon an accurate estimate of gestational age (Bowman & Manning 1983).

Traditionally, physicians have used the maternal menstrual history as the basis for calculation of gestational age (Naegele's rule); as the seasoned clinician knows, this method is subject to considerable error and all too frequently lacks the precision necessary for critical diagnostic and management decisions. Ultrasound-based fetal age estimation, derived from direct evaluation of fetal morphometric and functional data, is an attractive alternative, particularly in the patient with uncertain menstrual data or in the patient in whom subsequent perinatal management decisions may be made at particular gestational ages (for example in insulin-dependent diabetics).

Ultrasound assessment of fetal age is a complex subject, being the product of history and change and a volatile mixture of art and science. The earliest ultrasound indices selected to determine fetal age, for example biparietal diameter measurements, were selected not by rational choice, but by being one of the few reproducible fetal landmarks that could be identified by early-generation ultrasound equipment. To this day the biparietal diameter measurement remains exclusively an obstetrical phenomenon and is not used in assessment of neonatal age.

The tremendous improvement in the resolution quality of ultrasound fetal images has created major changes in the determination of fetal age. The criteria for biparietal diameter determination has become increasingly precise, now bearing only a passing resemblance to the original images. A wide assortment of new variables to assess fetal age have been introduced, ranging from long bone measurement (O'Brien & Queenan 1981), to renal volume determination (Grannum et al 1980) and intraorbital diameter measurement (Mayden et al 1982).

The introduction to dynamic ultrasound imaging has also altered the concept of fetal age determination. Fetal functional activities, while clearly in the research area at present, may ultimately be used to refine the accuracy of age estimates (Prechtl 1985). In the nursery, neonatal age determination is usually based on both morphometric and functional data (Dubowitz et al 1970). Functional variables will probably also be of considerable importance in the assessment of the fetus of later but uncertain gestation, for example, the presumed third-trimester fetus. Knowing the striking inaccuracy of morphometric estimates in late gestation and the quite remarkable accuracy of well-being predicted by functional variable assessment, it seems reasonable to question the use of dating parameters at all in late gestation. Separating the art from the science of ultrasound dating remains a very important clinical challenge. The science of fetal morphometric study is relatively precise, in good hands yielding negligible error. The art remains as the clinical ability to weave the myriad of ultrasound data into the clinical context of the individual case. Despite the reliability of the measurements, the variability of biological expression between healthy and sick fetuses requires constant consideration to arrive at appropriate management decisions.

Using contemporary high-resolution ultrasound instruments it has now become possible to begin to determine fetal age from as early as a few days after completion of implantation, by determination of gestational sac volume (Robinson 1975). As ultrasound has developed, it is now possible to measure growth of virtually any fetal organ system and to correlate these measurements with gestational age. It is unlikely that any specific organ measurement would yield clearly superior accuracy. Despite a bewildering range of new nomogram tables for specific organ systems and gestational age that have become available, it is still best to use accepted morphometric variables, including head size measurements (biparietal diameter, head circumference), long bone (femur length), abdominal circumference and crown–rump length.

Growth begins at conception and continues to delivery and beyond; the rate is exponential from conception, progressively flattening out with advancing gestation. At any given point in time, biological variation in morphometric indices of fetal growth are inversely proportional to the rate of growth. This relationship forms the basis of an important clinical rule, namely that the accuracy of ultrasound for estimating gestational age is inversely related to the duration of gestation.

The sources of error in ultrasound estimates of gestational age are diverse but in general can influence all the morphometric indices used. True measurement error in experienced hands makes only a minor contribution to estimate error: the inter- and intraobserver error of biparietal diameter measurement in our clinical laboratory consistently runs at less than 5%. Other published studies have shown similar accuracies (Hughey & Sabbagha 1978). Measurement error is more likely to occur when marginal quality images are used, emphasizing the need for strictly regulated criteria within the clinical laboratory setting. Variations in population demographics contribute to estimate error. Genetic influences on growth rate, for example in fetuses of oriental

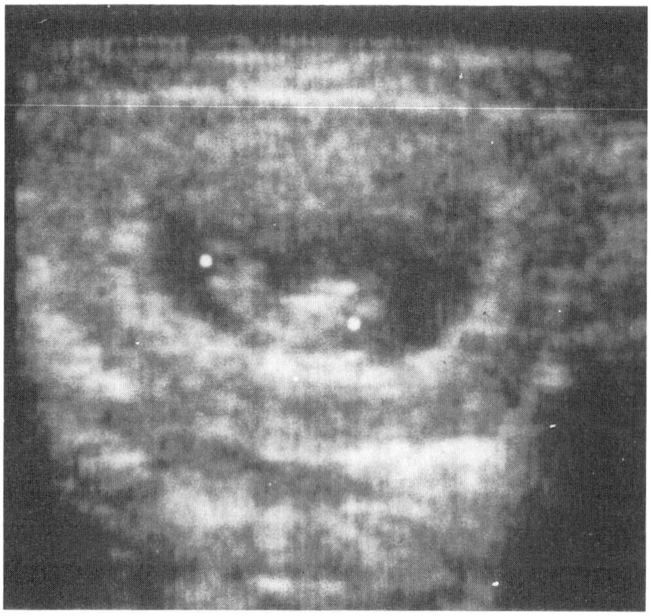

Fig. 27.2 Crown–rump measurement in utero. The cephalic pole with the developing fetal eye is well visualized.

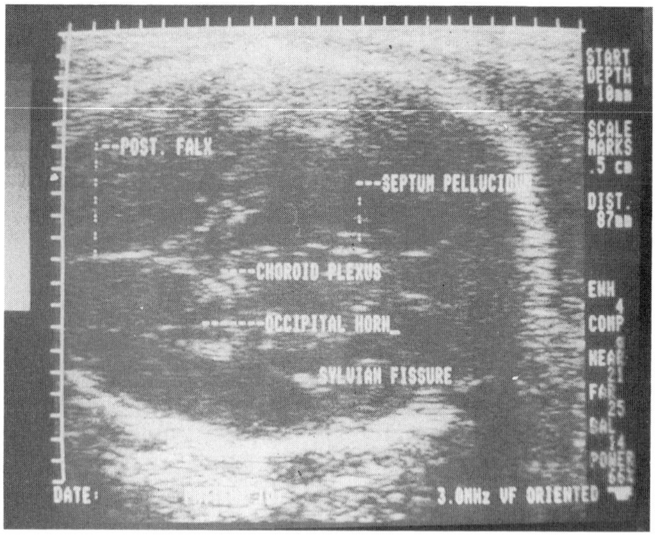

Fig. 27.3 Ultrasound scan of the fetal head in the plane of the biparietal diameter, demonstrating the basic landmarks. In dynamic mode the vascular pulsation of the posterior and middle cerebral arteries may be visualized.

and Caucasian parentage, the socioeconomic status of the parents, and the altitude, are all known to affect fetal growth rate (Lubchenco et al 1963, Greunwald 1966, Ounsted & Ounstead 1966). These variables no doubt influence the growth rate of the ultrasound indices used to measure fetal age. Most nomograms used for calculation of fetal age by ultrasound do not compensate for these factors and probably represent the local blend of the diversities (Weiner et al 1977). Fetal growth rates in multiple pregnancy are clearly different from those in single pregnancies and require specific and separate nomograms (Crane et al 1980). The greatest source of error of estimate, however, results from the interaction between the genetically determined growth potential of the fetus and its intrauterine environment, yielding individual biological variation. This variation may be quite striking, especially in late gestation. For example, whereas a biparietal diameter of 9.0 cm is the average for 36 weeks in our laboratory, similar measurements may, on occasion, be observed in a 32-week fetus with accelerated growth and in a 40-week fetus with a lesser but normal growth potential.

From a practical standpoint ultrasound indices of fetal age determination depend on the gestational age at the time of assessment. *Crown–rump measurement* can be obtained between 6 and 12 weeks of gestation and is the single most accurate method of fixing fetal age. It is obtained from an image of the embryo in its maximal longitudinal plane, by recording the distance between the crown of the head and the caudal end of the torso (Fig. 27.2). This method yields an estimate error of ±3.5 days (Robinson 1973), rivalling, if not exceeding, the predictive accuracy of reliable, normal menstrual history

The *biparietal diameter* can be measured from as early as 12 weeks and reliably from 14 weeks onward. The plane of the biparietal diameter, a purely obstetrical concept, describes an oval shape that passes through the fetal head in a very slightly depressed occipitofrontal tilt so that in the midline of the plane, the septum pellucidum cavernosum, is visualized anteriorly and the thalamic nuclei are seen slightly posteriorly to the midpoint. Moving laterally from the midline, a portion of the circle of Willis vessels, the choroid plexus, portions of the mid-component of the lateral ventricle and the middle cerebral artery sylvian gyrus are seen (Fig. 27.3).

The biparietal diameter is measured from the outer calvarium to the far wall inner calvarium bone at or just anterior to the thalamic nuclei. Most of the clinical research data relating biparietal diameter to gestational age was collected by Campbell (1962). The method yields an accuracy of estimate that varies with gestational age, ranging from an average error of estimate of 1 week in a pregnancy of less than 20 weeks, to an average error of estimate of up to 3 weeks when performed after 34 weeks of gestation.

The biparietal diameter measurement may occasionally be rendered inaccurate by variations in head shape, most commonly in the fetus in a persistent breech presentation with the apparent elongation of the occipitofrontal length (dolichocephaly). Comparison of the biparietal diameter to the occipitofrontal diameter, the cephalic index described by Hohler (1982), is a simple means of recognizing this and other potential measurement errors. Intrinsic fetal cranial abnormalities, such as microcephaly or hydrocephaly, invalidate the use of biparietal diameter in determining gestational age.

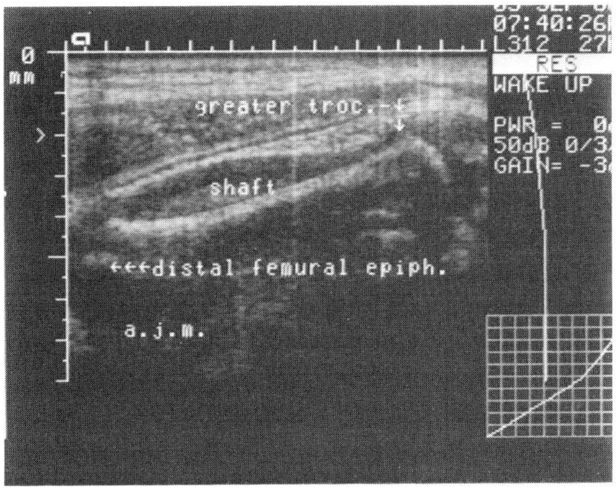

Fig. 27.4 Ultrasound scan of the fetal thigh demonstrating the femur. The distal femoral epiphysis is also visible.

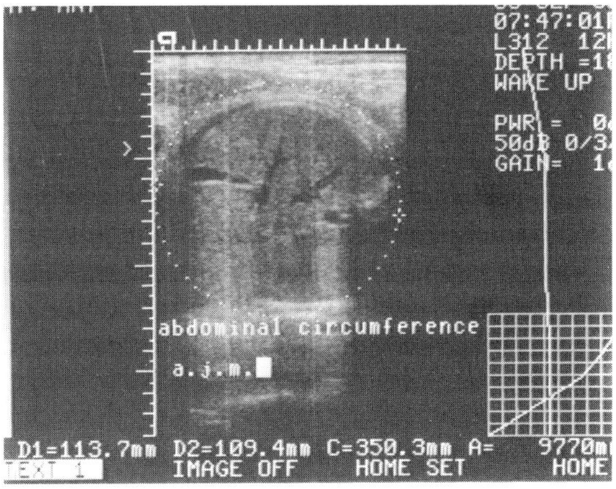

Fig. 27.5 Ultrasound scan of the fetal abdomen in the transverse plane at a level slightly superior (cranial) to the insertion of the umbilical vein into liver substance. Note that a portion of the umbilical vein and branch of the hepatic vein are visualized. The abdominal circumference, measured by light pencil, is 35.0 cm.

Calculation of *head circumference*, now achieved with considerable ease using computer-assisted light pencils, is an alternative method to biparietal diameter determination. To date however this method has not been shown to be superior in estimate accuracy to conventional biparietal diameter measurement (Hadlock et al 1982a).

The use of *femur measurements* is a relatively new method of fetal age determination, first described by O'Brien & Queenan (1981) and subsequently investigated in detail by Hadlock et al (1982b). The measurement requires imaging the fetal thigh in the longitudinal axis and recording the distance from the greater trochanter along the shaft of the femur to the distal end (Fig. 27.4). The measurement can reliably be obtained from as early as 14 weeks' gestation. As with biparietal diameter measurements the error of estimate varies with gestational age, ranging from an average estimate error of 1 week before 20 weeks and an error of up to 3 weeks after 34 weeks' gestation (Hadlock et al 1982b). Interestingly, femur length in late gestation is closely related to body length: in 123 fetuses studied within 3 days of delivery (36–43 weeks), body length calculated from femur length by the formula body length (cm) = ((femur length × 6.44) + 4.51) yielded an average percentage error of less than 1% (Manning et al 1986b) The relationship of other long bone measurement (for example humerus) to fetal age has been studied and catalogued (Hobbins et al 1982), but, in general, these measurements are used primarily for the assessment of the fetus at risk of short-limbed dystrophies.

Fetal abdominal circumference has been described as a method to estimate fetal age (Hadlock & Deter 1982). This measurement is obtained by recording the skin surface circumference at a plane passing perpendicular to the long axis of the fetus at or near the level of the intrahepatic portion of the umbilical vein (Fig. 27.5). In contemporary obstetrics the measurement is rarely used for fetal age determination but is of critical importance in estimation of fetal weight and weight gain. The use of derived values, such as abdominal circumference area, have not been shown to enhance predictive accuracy of fetal abdominal biometry, but may introduce further measurement error. Accordingly, these measures are rarely used and are not recommended.

Recently several innovative approaches have improved estimation of fetal age. Sabbagha et al (1978) have described the concept of growth-adjusted sonographic age, by which serial measurements of biparietal diameter fetal growth can be assigned according to fixed percentile ranking. Making serial measurements of the common ultrasound indices, either alone or in combination, improves the accuracy of predicted gestational age (Deter & Hadlock 1981, Hadlock et al 1983).

Ultrasound assessment of fetal growth

The rate of fetal growth is the net expression of a complex interaction between the inherent genetic growth potential and the ability of the fetal–maternal interface to supply the required metabolic needs. The rate of fetal growth is intimately related to fetal age. In both intra- and extrauterine life, growth is measured by incremental increase in body mass, length and linear and volumetric organ parameters. Abnormal variation from the expected rate of growth, either excessive or reduced, is associated with a sharp increase in the risk of perinatal death or damage (Jones & Battaglic 1977). In the Manitoba experience, more than 60% of all stillbirths in the untested population exhibited unequivocal signs of growth failure (Morrison & Olsen 1985). Ultrasound now plays a key role in the prenatal recognition of abnormalities of fetal growth, morphometric stigmata of abnormal growth, and evaluation of the immediate and future risk of the affected fetus.

Intrauterine growth retardation is a general term describing infants whose birthweight is likely to fall below the 10th percentile for gestational age and sex. The widespread use of this term with its broad pathological overtones is unfortunate because fetuses at the lower end of the distribution curve are clearly heterogeneous. The majority (approximately 70%) of intrauterine growth-retarded fetuses are, in fact, normal small fetuses. Fetuses with serious potentially lethal extremity growth impairment (approximately 20%) and those with inherent genetic or structural abnormalities (approximately 10%) make up the remainder of the population. The ratio of normal small to pathological small fetuses shifts progressively towards an increase in probability of abnormal fetuses as the birthweight percentile falls (Streeter et al 1984). In contrast, serious and potential lethal growth failure can exist without the fetal weight falling below the arbitrary lower linear cut-off.

The appropriate perinatal management for the fetus with suspected growth failure is critically dependent upon accurate differentiation of the underlying aetiology. The scope of management decisions is wide, ranging from conservative observation in the normal small fetus, through avoidance of intervention for fetal indications when growth failure is due to lethal chromosome abnormalities (i.e. chromosomal trisomy) or structural abnormalities (i.e. renal agenesis), to early and aggressive intervention for the fetus with non-correctable extrinsic growth impairment (i.e. uteroplacental failure). Fetal assessment by ultrasound now plays an essential and critical role in evaluating the fetus with suspected growth failure, in determining the presence and extent of disease, the extent of functional compromise and risk of death or damaging the fetus in utero, and, when combined with invasive procedures, in determining the presence of associated lethal anomalies.

Clinical recognition of growth failure, except in extremis, is notoriously difficult. Over- and under-reporting are common, even in the hands of the most experienced clinician. Campbell (1974) reported an English experience in which less than 40% of growth-retarded fetuses were detected by clinical examination alone. In our own experience of more than 2200 fetuses referred because of clinical suspicion of growth failure, less than 10% were confirmed as intrauterine growth-retarded at delivery. The not infrequent difficulty in estimating gestational age from menstrual history is an obvious compounding factor.

The diverse range of ultrasound data now available has proved extremely useful in solving this common dilemma. The ultrasound data are derived from three sets of observation and should always be used in combination.

1. The biparietal diameter and femur length are used to define fetal age and to assess linear growth.
2. Fetal mass (weight), the second critical component, is derived from selected fetal volume determinations. In the newborn, detailed measurements of limb, trunk, and head volume correlate closely with actual weight (average error 4.1%); most of the error is due to a normal variation of neonatal density (Thompson & Manning 1983). In the fetus, volume : mass may be determined either by extrapolation from the neonatal method (Thompson & Manning 1983) or, more simply, by determining abdominal circumference alone (Campbell & Wilkin 1975), or in combination with the biparietal diameter (Shepard et al 1983) and/or the femur length (Hadlock et al 1985). These methods all yield approximately the same error of estimate — about 16% (± 2 SD). The error of the estimate, both absolute and percentage, is not constant across weight ranges but rather varies inversely with actual weight. Thus the error of estimate is least in the small fetus.
3. Examination of fetal well-being and the functional signs of extrinsic growth impairment is the third critical ultrasound component. Dynamic ultrasound monitoring of central nervous system-regulated fetal functional parameters (breathing, movement, tone, heart rate activity) offers an accurate insight into the immediate fetal condition. Amniotic fluid volume plays a critical role in detection and assessment of severity of extrinsic fetal growth failure. The volume of amniotic fluid is the result of an equilibration between fluid production, primarily by the fetal lung and kidney, and fluid removal, primarily by fetal swallowing (Seeds 1980). Fetal renal and pulmonary perfusion fall dramatically when the fetus becomes hypoxaemic or acidaemic; the decrease is a result of the fetal aortic arch chemoreceptor stimulation and selected redistribution of cardiac output away from renal and pulmonary tissue (Cohn et al 1974). Amniotic fluid is easily visualized by ultrasound methods and the relative volume of the fluid can be categorized according to a semi-quantitative method (Chamberlain et al 1984c). By this method oligohydramnios is defined as when general scanning of the uterus fails to detect any pocket of fluid that measures at least 1 cm in two perpendicular axes: this definition is severe and describes the extremes of fluid distribution (Fig. 27.6). Most centres, including our own, are now beginning to use a 2-cm maximal pocket to define oligohydramnios. This more liberal definition of oligohydramnios results in minimal loss of specificity while causing a substantial increase in sensitivity. In the fetus with suspected growth failure, provided the membranes are intact and functional renal tissue is known to be present, the presence of oligohydramnios is a virtual hallmark of severe extrinsic growth failure (Manning et al 1981b, Philipson et al 1983). While the absence of oligohydramnios does not exclude the diagnosis of growth failure (Hoddick et al 1984, Bastide et al 1986, Bottoms et al 1986), it tends to imply disease of lesser severity (Chamberlain et al 1984c).

To date we have used this composite ultrasound method to guide management of more than 5000 patients referred for suspected growth failure and among more than 1400

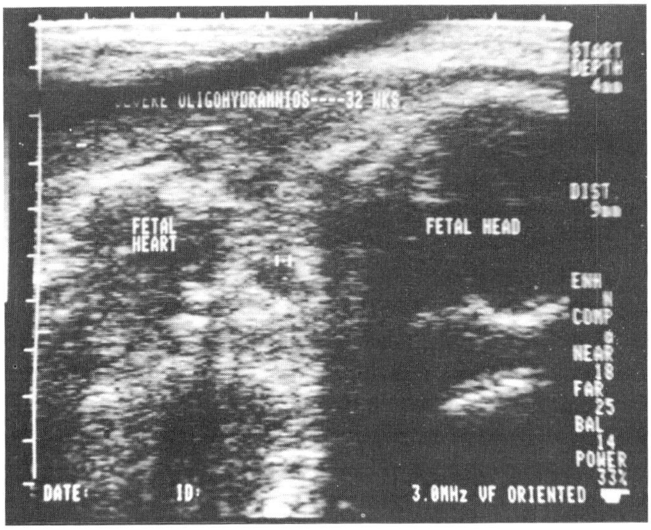

Fig. 27.6 Ultrasound scan of a 32-week fetus with severe oligohydramnios. The largest pocket of fluid, located between the chin and thorax, measures 0.9 cm. Note that the fetus is compacted in the uterus with the head and chest applied to the uterine wall. This finding in the presence of intact membranes and normal functioning renal tissue is usually a sign of chronic fetal compromise.

newborn infants with proven growth failure (less than the 10th percentile for age and sex). The ultrasound data are used to guide clinical decisions in the following sequential arrangement. At the initial referral the patient's records are reviewed to assess certainty of gestational age estimate: the patient is defined as having certain dates if the last normal menstrual period is recorded reliably and validated by an early urine pregnancy test (less than 8 weeks of gestation) and if ultrasound dating parameters have been obtained before 20 weeks' gestation. Patients who fail to meet these criteria are assumed to have uncertain dates.

The initial ultrasound step is a detailed anatomical screening for detection of lethal anomalies: when positive, subsequent management is based solely upon maternal risk factors. In our experience renal anomalies, particularly renal agenesis, are the most common anomaly seen with suspect growth failure. Since fetuses with either renal agenesis or severe extrinsic growth failure may both present with extreme oligohydramnios, differentiation can on occasion be difficult. The presence of functioning renal tissue can be established by noting bladder-filling during an extended observation period (up to 6 hours). Failure to detect bladder-filling over short intervals may be misleading since in the normal fetus urine production varies in a diurnal way (Chamberlain et al 1984a). The validity of maternal frusemide (Lasix) injection to induce fetal diuresis is unproven in man but is known to be ineffective in animal models (Chamberlain et al 1985).

In the structurally normal fetus the next ultrasound step is to determine fetal well-being. We use the fetal biophysical profile scoring method which includes estimation of amniotic fluid volume. An alternate approach may be to combine stress or non-stress antenatal cardiotocography with amniotic fluid volume estimation. If the fetal biophysical profile score is persistently abnormal (equal to or less than 4) or oligohydramnios is present, or both are observed, delivery is instituted provided the gestational age is estimated to be at least 26 weeks. This lower age limit at which intervention is contemplated is determined by survival rates in the neonatal nursery and is moving steadily downwards.

In the structurally normal fetus with normal functional assessment, management is based on serial linear growth and mass estimates and on the certainty of gestational age. In the fetus with certain gestational age, fetal mass is plotted against a weight : age nomogram specific for our population. Fetuses with estimated weight above the 10th percentile are considered not to exhibit growth failure and are discharged from the protocol. Management of fetuses with weight estimates below the 10th percentile depend upon fetal age and cervical favourability: when gestational age is at least 37 weeks and the cervix is favourable, delivery is recommended. If gestational age is 37 weeks or greater and the cervix is unfavourable or if gestational age is less than 37 weeks, conservative management is recommended with serial (once-weekly) ultrasound assessment. Conservative management is continued until either the cervix becomes favourable or functional assessment of fetal well-being becomes abnormal.

We do not recommend delivery solely upon failure to demonstrate continued growth in either linear or mass estimate, or based on the inter-relationship between these variables (head : abdominal circumference). We use a similar management plan in women with uncertain dates whose fetuses have suspected growth failure, withholding any intervention until the cervix becomes favourable for induction and fetal maturity has been ascertained, usually by amniocentesis and phospholipid profile, or functional assessment of the fetus becomes abnormal.

We have used this composite ultrasound method for the diagnosis and management of the fetus with suspected growth failure since 1979: more than 1400 babies whose birthweight fell below the 10th percentile for gestational age and sex have been studied and the results have been encouraging. In this selected at risk population, we have recorded 10 perinatal deaths among structurally normal fetuses (corrected perinatal mortality rate 7.1/1000, eight stillbirths and two neonatal deaths. Three of these 10 deaths were unpreventable, being associated with extreme prematurity of less than 27 weeks and stillbirth in two cases, and severe neonatal asphyxia with death despite immediate intervention in the remaining case. The corrected perinatal mortality (7.1/1000) in this group contrasts favourably with the observed rate in the comparable untested high-risk population of 65/1000 (Baskett 1979).

Fetal macrosomia, defined as birthweight in excess of the 90th percentile for gestational age and sex, is also associated with increased perinatal risk, including mortality and morbidities such as shoulder dystocia, brachial plexis injury, traumatic delivery and a neonatal metabolic disorder such as hypoglycaemia). As with intrauterine growth retardation, macrosomic fetuses are also the result of diverse aetiologies, including normal but increased genetic growth potential and disease states such as maternal diabetes mellitus. Some recent studies have suggested that fetal macrosomia may by itself be a more reliable predictor of maternal glucose imbalance than the formal glucose tolerance test (Helewa et al 1986).

The ultrasound diagnosis of macrosomia is based both on estimate of the fetal mass: age relationships and on the recognition of specific physical stigmata. The confidence limits of fetal weight estimation deteriorate sharply beyond about 4000 g; the primary error is an underestimation of actual weight. At present the detection of macrosomia by fetal weight estimation is not a totally reliable clinical method. In the fetus with suspect macrosomia, ultrasound detection of subcutaneous fat deposits, especially in the malar regions, may be useful; marked exaggeration of cheek-pad fat strongly suggests underlying maternal diabetes.

ASSESSMENT OF THE PLACENTA AND FETAL ENVIRONMENT

The placenta, a unique fetal mammalian organ, is now visualized easily in considerable detail using contemporary high-resolution ultrasound instruments. The valuable information garnered by placental ultrasonography can be categorized into two general areas: the accurate localization of the placenta and the assessment of placental architecture, in both normal and abnormal states.

Placental localization

Placental ultrasonography is now the firstline method of placental localization, having virtually replaced the older and less accurate methods such as isotope scans and its specialized radiographic techniques (of soft tissue placentography, contrast amniography and arteriography). In the clinical medium, ultrasound placental localization is used for three major purposes: to evaluate the patient with antepartum haemorrhage, to guide needle placement for amniocentesis and other invasive intrauterine procedures, and to identify the placental insertion of the umbilical vein for ultrasound-guided percutaneous fetal blood sampling (cordocentesis).

The ultrasound evaluation of the patient with suspected *placenta praevia*, usually initiated by an episode of painless antepartum haemorrhage, is perhaps the most graphic example of how ultrasound and clinical data must be considered together to improve diagnostic accuracy. The term placenta praevia describes the spectrum of degrees of abnormal placental implantation, ranging from minor encroachment into the lower uterine segment to complete coverage of the internal cervical os (see Chapter 32). Whereas the placental margin can always be identified by ultrasound, the relationship of the placental edge to the internal os is much more difficult to determine. Therefore, with the exception of complete placenta praevia, the ultrasound diagnosis of placenta praevia is always a relative diagnosis.

Several changing clinical factors influence the accuracy of the ultrasound diagnosis of praevia. Firstly, the position of the cervix and its internal os may vary widely in the anteroposterior position. The variability of the position of the cervix noted at vaginal examination in the normal patient is well known to the experienced clinician. Exact determination of the position of the internal os by ultrasound methods is extremely difficult and generally unreliable. Secondly, the lower uterine segment, which arises primarily from the internal cervical canal, develops at different rates and at different gestational ages in different patients. The extent of development of the lower uterine segment cannot be determined accurately by ultrasound methods. Thus, what may appear to be a complete placenta praevia in early gestation may resolve entirely by late pregnancy. The change is a result of the development of the lower uterine segment below the lower margin of the placenta — the term *migrating placenta* was used in the old radiographic literature to describe this normal physiological process.

These anatomical and dynamic events dictate the clinical interpretation of the ultrasound diagnosis of placenta praevia and from these associations, several useful clinical rules may be developed. Firstly, the clinical significance of the ultrasound diagnosis of placenta praevia varies directly with gestational age at diagnosis. This clinical rule is illustrated by the reported incidence of ultrasound-diagnosed placenta praevia in the second trimester of up to 30% (Mittelstadt et al 1979), whereas the overall true incidence of the disease is known to be about 0.5% (Goplerud 1977). For practical purposes the ultrasound diagnosis before about 26 weeks of gestation may be considered to be of little clinical significance. Secondly, the clinical significance of the ultrasound diagnosis varies with an anterior or posterior placental location. In most patients the cervix and internal os are displaced towards the posterior aspect of the vaginal vault. Therefore, the probability of true placenta praevia is increased when a posterior praevia is suspected using ultrasound.

The probability of persistence of the ultrasound diagnosis of praevia is increased by about threefold when the placenta is posterior as compared with an anterior implantation (Gillieson et al 1982). Thirdly, overfilling of the maternal bladder, by exaggerating the posterior rotation of the cervix, may contribute to the incorrect diagnosis of placenta praevia (Williamson et al 1978). This potential diagnostic error is easily overcome by studying placental position at varying maternal bladder volumes. In our experience, using dynamic ultrasound methods, we have found studies after maternal voiding to be the most accurate. Fourthly, the ultrasound diagnosis of placenta praevia may change dramatically with development of the lower uterine segment, especially in early labour.

Therefore it follows that repeated ultrasound examination, including even examination in labour, is a key step in ensuring diagnostic accuracy. Examination under anaesthesia with all arrangements for immediate Caesarean section is required in all patients with suspected praevia, except in those with an ultrasound diagnosis of complete praevia. There are few, if any, indications for elective Caesarean section for the ultrasound diagnosis of placenta praevia, the exception being complete praevia where the placenta is seen to extend from both the anterior and posterior walls of the lower uterine cavity, covering the lowermost portion. Finally, determination of the relationship between the presenting fetal part and the lowermost placental margin can be clinically very useful. When the leading edge of the presenting part is below the lowermost portion of the placental margin, the probability of vaginal delivery is high.

Ultrasound localization of the placenta and fetus immediately prior to intrauterine invasive procedures has a significant and positive impact on success rates and on the rate of complications. Localization of the placental site and the amniotic fluid pockets has sharply improved the success rate of amniocentesis while reducing the risks of fetomaternal bleeding (Platt et al 1978). In selected circumstances, continuous dynamic ultrasound imaging during amniocentesis may be indicated (Crane & Kopla 1984). Similarly, the success rate of fetal invasive procedures, such as intrauterine transfusion, is improved by dynamic ultrasound guidance while at the same time reducing the risk of fetal death (Harman et al 1983). More recently, the converse, i.e. deliberate ultrasound-guided puncture of fetal vessels for either diagnostic (e.g. rapid karyotype determination) or therapeutic (e.g. fetal intravascular transfusion) procedures, has become a practical reality (Crespigny et al 1985, Daffos et al 1985, Copel et al 1986, Menticoglou et al 1986). The significance of these new procedures remains to be fully explored but the potential is likely to be enormous.

Placental architecture

The clinical significance of ultrasound evaluation of placental architecture remains uncertain at present. Grannum et al (1975), from Yale, described a method of grading placental maturity based upon ultrasound recognition of cotyledon architectural characteristics, including the extent and distribution of echogenic (calcium) deposits; in a retrospective study they reported the presence of a grade III placenta (most mature) to be associated with a mature L:S ratio in 23 cases. Harman et al (1982) studied the relationship of placental grade by the Grannum criteria to pulmonary maturity (by L:S ratio) in 563 pregnancies in which amniocentesis was done; an immature L:S ratio ($<2:1$) was observed in 7% of patients with a grade III placenta, and no significant difference in predictive accuracy of pulmonary maturity was noted between the grade III and grade II placenta classification. The authors noted that while the placenta did undergo a series of changes, identifiable by ultrasound and related to gestational age in a progressive fashion, the method of placental grading was of little value in estimating gestational age and maturity. They concluded that placental grading by ultrasound was not accurate enough to eliminate the need for amniocentesis.

A relationship between placental grade and intrauterine growth retardation has been postulated (Hills et al 1984). Again, however, prospective studies have not sustained this hypothesis. Harman (1984) made serial observations of placental grade in 200 small-for-dates fetuses, noting that neither the frequency of grade III placenta nor the average gestational age from transition between grades was related to birthweight percentile. Therefore, it seems that the clinical value of placental grading remains undetermined at present.

The ultrasound diagnosis of *abruptio placentae* by ultrasound monitoring architectural change remains a largely unexplored clinical area but with a major abruption, ultrasound signs include detachment of the placenta from the uterine wall, retroplacental haematoma formation, free-flowing blood or clot extending from the placental edge, and acute functional signs of fetal compromise. In practice, however, ultrasound is of little value in assessing the patient with major abruption, since the diagnosis is clinically obvious.

The pathogenesis of abruption is not well documented, but a growing body of ultrasound evidence suggests that the pathological process, at least in some cases, may evolve over considerable time. Either isolated intracotyledonary bleeding or subchorionic haematoma may be the initial event preceding a major abruption; both can be recognized by ultrasound (Fig. 27.7). The concept of an abruption in evolution, a process that may be recognized by ultrasound, might ultimately permit timed early intervention, thereby reducing both the maternal and fetal risks.

Specific placental architectural changes may be observed in other pathological conditions. Placental oedema, characterized by placental thickening, a loss of cotyledon structure and a diffuse ground-glass appearance, may be seen in the severely rhesus-immunized hydropic fetus, and occasionally in the twin-to-twin transfusion syndrome. Primary placental disorders such as chorioangioma and neoplastic degeneration (hydatidiform mole, choriocarcinoma) are easily recognized by ultrasound (see Chapter 31).

Recognition of umbilical cord position by ultrasound may be a useful method of antepartum recognition of the fetus at risk for intrapartum cord prolapse. Lange et al (1985) studied cord position in 1471 high-risk singleton pregnancies; in nine patients (0.61%) the umbilical cord was noted to lie within the region of the lower uterine segment, below the presenting fetal parts. The ultrasound diagnosis of a

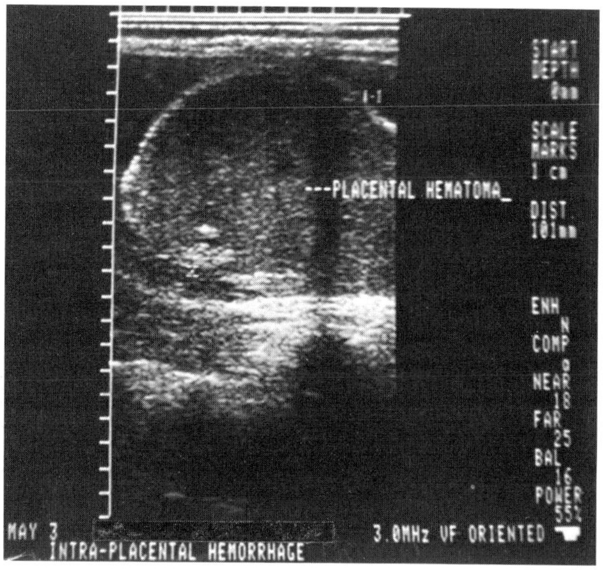

Fig. 27.7(a) Ultrasound scan demonstrating isolated intracotyledonary haematoma measuring 10.1 cm maximal diameter. Note the loss of normal placental architecture. This patient developed massive clinical abruption 2 days later.

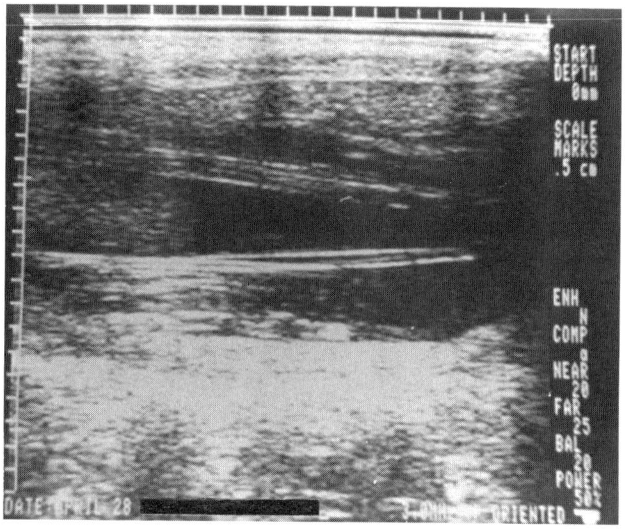

Fig. 27.7(b) Ultrasound scan demonstrating fetal membranes stripped off the placenta due to subchorionic bleeding. The patient developed clinical abruption within 1 week.

cord presentation was persistent in most patients and was confirmed at delivery in eight of the nine cases. One of the nine infants died as a result of the spontaneous rupture of membranes and cord prolapse. It is important to note that there were no instances of cord prolapse among the remaining 1452 patients in whom cord position by ultrasound was normal. These data strongly suggest that the antenatal diagnosis of impending cord prolapse is now a practical reality.

Clinicians have long known that abnormal amniotic fluid volumes, both excessive and diminished, are often associated with perinatal problems. The accurate estimation of amniotic fluid volume by clinical methods is difficult but it is now possible with ultrasound. Chamberlain et al (1984b,c) described an ultrasound-based, semi-quantitative method for fluid volume determination, in which the largest pocket is identified and then measured. In serial observations in 7562 patients the distribution of fluid pocket size was documented; fluid was defined as normal when the largest pocket measured >2 cm and <8 cm in its maximal vertical diameter; it was increased when the measurements exceeded 8.0 cm; it was defined as marginally decreased when the measurements were between 1 and 2 cm, and decreased when the measurements were <1.0 cm (Chamberlain et al 1984b). Perinatal outcome was strongly related to amniotic fluid volume measurements (Table 27.1). The incidence of major lethal anomalies was lowest in patients with normal fluid and was increased 17-fold with increased fluid and 32-fold with decreased fluid. Perinatal mortality, both gross and corrected, was least in patients with normal fluid and increased seven-fold with increased fluid and 40-fold with decreased fluid. Intervention for oligohydramnios has been shown to improve perinatal survival rates (Bastide et al 1986). The incidence of intrauterine growth retardation was increased almost eightfold in patients with decreased fluid, and the incidence of macrosomia was 3.8-fold greater in patients with increased fluid.

FETAL BIOPHYSICAL PROFILE SCORING

Ultrasound assessment of fetal health

The purpose of any form of antenatal fetal surveillance must be to recognize accurately fetal and environmental conditions which adversely influence perinatal mortality and morbidity, at an early enough stage to use whatever corrective measures may be available. Whereas perinatal morbidity is of equal clinical importance to mortality, the latter outcome determination is sharp, well defined and not subject to observer bias. Therefore, perinatal mortality forms the most reproducible measure of the impact of any fetal assessment programme. The demographic stability and homogeneity of our population in Manitoba and the fact that the perinatal mortality statistics have been recorded annually for some years prior to the institution of the fetal assessment programme, makes this a unique study population in which to determine the effects of any new surveillance and testing methods. In our population, in the absence of antepartum testing, the most commonly recognized causes of perinatal death were asphyxia (60%) and congenital anomalies (25%), while the remaining 15% of deaths were primarily due to prematurity complications (Baskett 1979). Clearly, an effective antepartum assessment programme must detect both fetal asphyxia and congenital anomalies. These two aspects of fetal assessment may be achieved either by separate testing for asphyxia, using antepartum fetal heart rate testing methods and diag-

Table 27.1 Qualitative amniotic fluid volume by ultrasound and perinatal outcome (from Chamberlain et al 1984c)

Qualitative amniotic fluid volume*	No. of patients	Lethal anomaly(%)	Gross PNM per 1000	Corrected PNM per 1000	IUGR (%)	Macrosomia (%)
Normal (>2.0 <8.0 cm)	7096	0.24	4.65	1.97	4.9	8.7
Marginal decreased (>1.0 <2.0 cm)	159	1.9	56.6	37.7	20	0
Decreased (<1.0 cm)	64	7.8	185.5	109.4	38.6	0
Increased (>8.0 cm)	243	4.12	32.9	4.12	0	33.3
Total	7562	0.42	8.2	3.7	5.49	9.5

* Defined by measurement of the largest pocket of amniotic fluid.
PNM = perinatal mortality; IUGR = intrauterine growth retardation.

nostic imaging, or by a combined method based on dynamic ultrasound imaging. In our opinion the latter method is superior.

Fetal asphyxia is manifest by central nervous system depression and resultant loss or alteration of the fetal biophysical activities under direct central nervous system regulation. In this regard fetal responses to asphyxia mirror neonatal effects, i.e. asphyxia induces a coma-like state in the fetus. The characterization of fetal biophysical responses to asphyxia is complex, since responses may be expected to vary with the pre-asphyxial fetal condition, the magnitude and duration of the asphyxial insult and whether it is repeated.

In experimental fetal animals, fetal asphyxia is usually produced by administering a hypoxic gas mixture to the mother, creating maternal hypoxaemia with subsequent fetal hypoxaemia. Under these conditions fetal biophysical variables such as fetal breathing movements and forelimb movements are abolished, and their absence persists for some time after the restoration of normal fetal gases (Boddy & Dawes 1975, Natale et al 1981). In the human fetus, asphyxia is rarely the result of maternal hypoxaemia, although this cause is occasionally seen in pathological conditions (Manning & Platt 1979), or as a consequence of cigarette smoking in pregnancy (Manning & Feyerabend 1976, Socol et al 1982). However, the most common cause of fetal asphyxia is uteroplacental dysfunction, aggravated by repetitive flow interruption due to uterine contractions during late pregnancy. Chronic repetitive episodes of fetal hypoxaemia produce both acute and chronic fetal biophysical variable changes. During and for some time after fetal hypoxaemia, acute or active biophysical variables regulated by central nervous system outflow are lost; these include fetal breathing; gross body movement; fetal flexor tone, and heart rate acceleration with fetal movement (non-stress test). Chronic responses to hypoxaemia (oligohydramnios, extrinsic growth failure) are the result of hypoxia-induced aortic body chemoreceptor stimulation with subsequent redistribution of fetal cardiac output, often to a profound degree (Cohn et al 1974). Blood flow during hypoxaemia is directed towards fetal brain, heart, adrenals, placenta and away from other organ systems. The effect of this reflex change is readily identified in asphyxiated newborns: the peripheral cyanosis, oliguria, thrombocytopenia, hyperbilirubinaemia, respiratory distress syndrome and necrotizing enterocolitis may all be attributed to this fetal protective reflex.

Fetal biophysical profile scoring encompasses simultaneous measurement of both acute (breathing, movement, tone and heart rate) and chronic (amniotic fluid) indices of fetal asphyxia. Unlike amniotic fluid volume, the acute variables are profoundly influenced by fetal central nervous system state changes or rhythm. For reasons and mechanisms which are poorly understood, central nervous system activity and energy outflow are not constant but vary in discrete temporal patterns. The time base for these patterns or rhythms is complex and inter-related. At least two major rhythms may be identified: short-term rhythm of appropriately 20–40-minutes' duration and long-term (24–26 hours) diurnal or circadian rhythms. The short-term rhythms, often called sleep–wake cycles, can cause marked changes in acute fetal biophysical activities. During active or rapid eye movements (REM) sleep, a state in which the fetus spends about 70–80% of its time, cortical electrical activity is characterized by low-voltage high-frequency discharge and fetal movements are vigorous, sustained and frequent; fetal breathing movements are present for most of the time; flexor tone is normal or even exaggerated and there are heart rate accelerations with fetal movements. In contrast, in quiet fetal sleep states, occupying about 20–30% of the time, cortical electrical activity is characterized by high-voltage low-frequency discharge; fetal movements are infrequent isolated events; episodes of fetal breathing activity occur less often; flexor tone may be normal or diminished and heart rate accelerations with fetal movements are uncommon. Quiet sleep state in the fetus and particularly phases of deep sleep produce much the same reduction in biophysical activities as does asphyxia. Indeed the mechanism which affects biophysical events in normal and abnormal conditions may be similar: there is a general reduction in central nervous system activity. The two states may be differentiated by observing some biophysical activities, even though the frequency of these activities may be reduced, or by extending the observation time until, in normal cases, transition to an active sleep state is observed. In applying the concept of fetal biophysical profile scoring, it is essential to extend the observations either until normal biophysical activities are recognized or until there has been at least 30 minutes' continuous observation. Fortunately in clinical practice the need

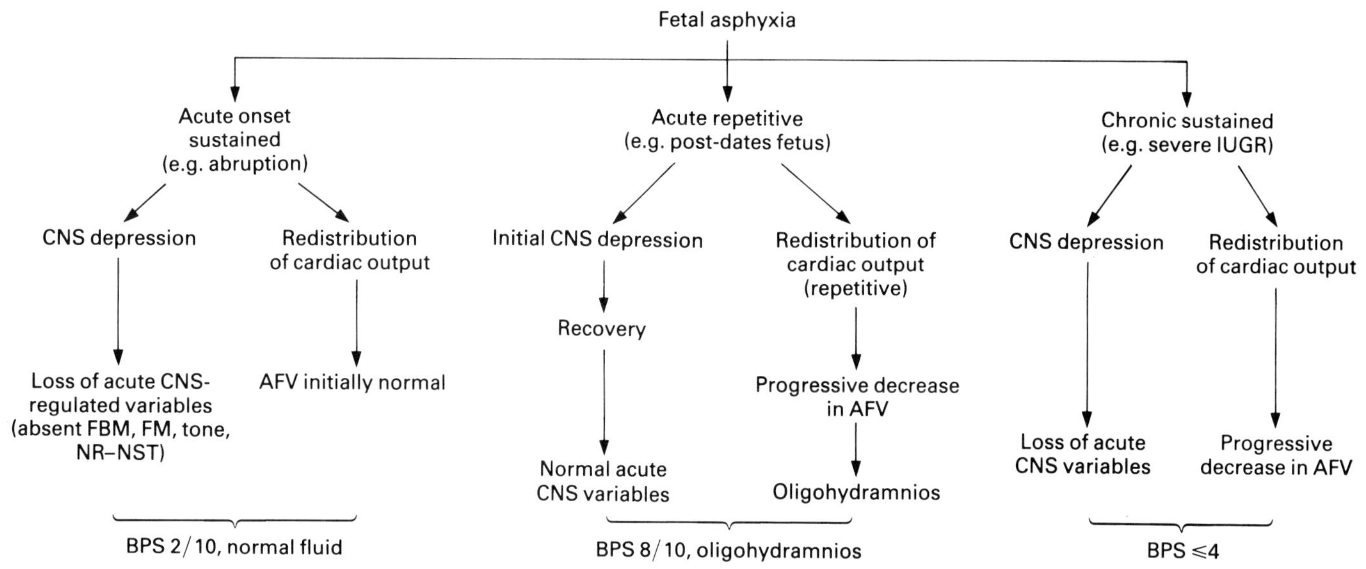

Fig. 27.8 Schematic representation of the mechanisms by which fetal asphyxia may affect the fetal biophysical profile score. The fetal adaptive responses may be expected to vary with the rate of onset, severity, duration and repetitive frequency of the asphyxial insult. Consideration of both acute (central nervous system-regulated) and chronic fetal responses (oligohydramnios) to fetal asphyxia are necessary to achieve maximal detection of disease. CNS = central nervous system; IUGR = intrauterine growth retarded; FBM = fetal breathing movements; FM = fetal body movements; NR–NST = non-reactive non-stress test; AFV = amniotic fluid volume; BPS = biophysical profile score.

to maintain observation for 30 minutes to complete the test is rare — average testing time is 8 minutes. In our experience of more than 40 000 tests, we have encountered abnormal scores in less than 2% of all tests (Manning et al 1985, 1986a).

The effect of fetal asphyxia on the fetal biophysical profile score will vary with the duration, magnitude and repetitive frequency of hypoxic insults, producing a spectrum of test results (Fig. 27.8). In the previously normal fetus subjected to acute sustained asphyxia, the acute variables will be abnormal but amniotic fluid volume may be normal. In contrast, repetitive episodes of intermittent hypoxaemia will cause the absence of acute variables during the period of fetal hypoxaemia with recovery during normoxaemic period, but will produce a net decrease in amniotic fluid production, leading to oligohydramnios. Finally, chronic progressive hypoxaemia will result in both a loss of acute biophysical variables and in the development of oligohydramnios.

Table 27.2 Biophysical profile scoring: technique and interpretation

Biophysical variable	Normal	Abnormal
Fetal breathing movements	>1 episode of >30 s in 30 min	Absent or no episode of >30 s in 30 min
Gross body movements	>3 discrete body/limb movements in 30 min (episodes of active continuous movement considered as single movement)	<2 episodes of body/limb movements in 30 min
Fetal tone	>1 episode of active extension with return to flexion of fetal limb(s) or trunk. Opening and closing of hand considered normal tone	Slow extension with return to partial flexion or movement of limb in full extension or absent fetal movement
Reactive fetal heart rate	>2 episodes of acceleration of >15 beats/min and of >15 s associated with fetal movement in 10 min	<2 episodes of acceleration of fetal heart rate or acceleration of >15 beats/min in 20 min
Qualitative amniotic fluid	>1 pocket of fluid measuring >1 cm in two perpendicular planes	Either no pockets or a pocket <1 cm in two perpendicular planes

The method

In our centre, fetal biophysical profile scoring is the primary method of fetal risk assessment. The gestational age at which testing begins is set to the minimum at which intervention would be considered should an abnormal result be encountered. Over the years since the inception of the programme the lower limit of age for testing has fallen as the possibility of safe transition from fetal to neonatal life at lower gestational ages has improved, and is currently 26 weeks. At each testing episode, in addition to scoring the fetal biophysical profile, fetal morphometric data are obtained (biparietal diameter, femur length, abdominal circumference); the fetus is examined for structural and functional anomaly and the placenta and umbilical cord are assessed. The fetal biophysical profile score is obtained by components.

Firstly, variables recorded by dynamic ultrasound methods are assessed and coded numerically using a binary approach to variable recognition. These variables are coded as normal or abnormal according to fixed criteria and then assigned an arbitrary score of 2 if normal and 0 if abnormal (Table 27.2). In original design the variables were considered

Table 27.3 Biophysical profile scoring: management protocol

Score	Interpretation	Recommended management
10	Normal infant, low risk for chronic asphyxia	Repeat testing at weekly intervals. Repeat twice weekly in diabetic patients and patients >42 weeks' gestation
8	Normal infant, low risk for chronic asphyxia	Repeat testing at weekly intervals. Repeat twice weekly in diabetic patients and patients >42 weeks' gestation. Indication for delivery = oligohydramnios
6	Suspected chronic asphyxia	Repeat testing within 24 h. Indication for delivery = oligohydramnios or remaining <6
4	Suspected chronic asphyxia	>36 score and favourable cervix. If <36 weeks and lecithin: sphingomyelin ratio <2.0, repeat test in 24 h. Indication for delivery = repeat score >6 or oligohydramnios
0–2	Strong suspicion of chronic asphyxia	Extend testing time to 120 min. Indication for delivery = persistent score <4, regardless of gestational age

to be of equal significance and accordingly assigned the same binary numerical value. A recent in-depth review of some 342 abnormal score results supports this original premise (Manning et al 1989). Composite variable analysis of abnormal test results reveals that the distribution of score variables is not skewed, but rather almost equally distributed among possible combinations. Amniotic fluid volume is assessed using a semi-quantitative method, as described previously (Chamberlain et al 1984c). In our original description of the method the presence or absence of fetal heart rate acceleration with fetal movements was performed regardless of the results obtained by dynamic ultrasound monitoring (Manning et al 1980). However, in a more recent review of 26 257 tests among 12 620 referred high-risk patients we noted that the predictive accuracy of the four ultrasound-monitored variables, when normal, was equal to that achieved by the addition of the non-stress test (Manning et al 1985). This observation prompted a prospective study in which the non-stress test was only used when one or more of the ultrasound variables was abnormal (Manning et al 1987). Since these results confirmed our hypothesis, we have modified the profile scoring method so that the non-stress test is now used only when one or more of the ultrasound-monitored variables are abnormal.

The frequency of testing is modified in accordance with the nature of the condition prompting referral (Table 27.3) and more recently, with the gravity and progression of the condition. Thus, for example, in most patients with hypertension, testing is done on a weekly basis, but in some patients with rapidly progressive or very severe disease, testing may occur more frequently and in some extreme cases on a daily basis. Arbitrary and fixed regimens for the frequency of testing are no longer in order.

Clinical results

Clinical testing of the concept of fetal biophysical profile scoring began with a prospective blind clinical study in 216 referred high-risk patients (Manning et al 1980). Each of the five variables was recorded serially in these patients and the relationship between the result of the last test and perinatal outcome was determined. Each variable considered independently was related to outcome. The overall perinatal mortality for the study group was 50.9 per 1000 (11 deaths), the corrected mortality (excluding deaths due to anomaly) was 32.4 per 1000 (seven deaths). The false negative rate, that is stillbirth within 1 week of a last normal test result, was least for normal fetal tone (rate 6.9 per 1000) and greatest with a normal (reactive) non-stress test (12.8 per 1000). The positive predictive accuracy, that is stillbirth within 1 week of the last abnormal test result, was greatest with the absence of fetal breathing movements (115.5 per 1000) and least with an abnormal (non-reactive) non-stress test (58.5 per 1000). When variables were considered in various combinations, all measures of predictive accuracy improved as more variables were considered.

When all five variables were considered collectively the perinatal mortality rate ranged from 600 per 1000 when all variables were abnormal to 0 per 1000 when all variables were normal. Intermediate combinations of normal and abnormal variables yielded intermediate perinatal mortality values. This initial study, while confirming the predictive accuracy of the testing method could not, by the blind design, offer insight into the value of any of the testing methods in reducing perinatal mortality.

A second study, prospective in design and in which fetal biophysical profile scores were used to guide clinical management, was performed (Manning et al 1981a). Serial fetal biophysical profile scoring was done in 1184 consecutive referred high-risk pregnancies (2238 tests) and management was based upon fixed criteria (Table 27.3). The frequency of abnormal test results (fetal biophysical profile scoring <6) was surprisingly and unexpectedly low, occurring in only 47 instances among 2238 tests (2.1%).

In the entire study group, perinatal mortality was reduced to 5.06 per 1000 (six deaths); this perinatal mortality rate was significantly less than that observed in a comparable but untested high-risk population (65 per 1000) and the rate observed in the general population (14.3 per 1000, Baskett 1979). The false negative rate in this study, that is stillbirth within 1 week of a normal test result, was 0.8 per 1000 (one death). These data strongly suggest that intervention, based upon recognition of fetal asphyxia by biophysical profile scoring, was responsible for this fall in perinatal mortality.

This preliminary study has been expanded and the result in 12 620 referred high-risk pregnancies (26 257 tests) has been reported (Manning et al 1985). The results of this study are very similar to the pilot study in 1184 patients but the large patient experience garnered now permits interpretation of data in a more assured manner. Firstly, the very high proportion of normal test results was again confirmed (25 606 of 26 257 tests; 97.52%). Since despite recognizable maternal risk factors, the majority of fetuses in any population may be expected to be normal, it is encouraging that the frequency of normal test results was so high. Furthermore, these data again confirm a very low false negative rate with this method (0.634 per 1000), indicating that normal test results accurately reflect a normal fetus and do not underestimate the incidence of fetal disease.

The clinical significance of this point becomes apparent when comparing the results with single variable testing such as the non-stress test. With the latter method the frequency of normal test results is lower (85–90%) and the false negative rate is higher (3 per 1000; Lavery 1982). Secondly the positive predicted accuracy of the abnormal fetal biophysical profile score (<4) is again confirmed. Despite clinical intervention, the corrected perinatal mortality rate rose progressively as the score fell, ranging from 22 per 1000 with a score of 4, to 187 per 1000 with a score of 0. Thirdly, overall perinatal mortality was again demonstrably reduced by this method. The gross perinatal mortality among these 12 620 patients was 7.37 per 1000 (93 deaths); corrected perinatal mortality was 1.90 per 1000 (24 deaths). These mortality rates are significantly less than observed in the general population (14.3 per 1000) or the untested high-risk population (65 per 1000). Further, the distribution of death by primary aetiology varied between the tested and untested population. In the tested population 66.7% of deaths (62 deaths) were due to major lethal anomaly; the comparable figure in the general population was 25%. This shift in distribution is interpreted as being the result of a reduction of deaths in structurally normal fetuses in the tested population and is viewed as additional evidence of the validity of the testing method. Finally, as with all clinical testing methods, independent confirmation of results by other centres is essential, since in any given centre factors other than the testing scheme described may influence the overall reported results. Some other institutions have reported similar or even better results than those reported here (Baskett et al 1983, Platt et al 1983, Vintzileos et al 1983, Manning et al 1989).

CONCLUSIONS

The now widespread use of dynamic ultrasound imaging methods in the specialty of obstetrics and gynaecology will continue to create remarkable positive changes in the scientific and clinical endeavours. We may anticipate that as we continue to add the information garnered from visual assessment of the patient and her fetus to our time-honoured methods of clinical assessment, we will continue to improve the outcome for our patients. The visionary work of the pioneer Ian Donald, outlined most clearly in his treatise 'Sonar — the story of an experiment' (1974), has now been visited upon our specialty. It seems likely that as we further explore this modality and its many applications, including assessment of fetal biometry, structural and functional integrity and newer invasive therapies, we will move even closer to the elusive goal of elimination of perinatal death and disease.

REFERENCES

Baskett T F 1979 Review of perinatal mortality and morbidity at the Health Sciences Center: a 10 year review. University of Manitoba, Manitoba

Baskett T F, Grag J H, Pewett S T et al 1983 Antepartum fetal assessment using a fetal biophysical profile score. Obstetrics and Gynecology 61: 480

Bastide A, Manning F A, Harrison C R et al 1986 Ultrasound evaluation of amniotic fluid: outcome of pregnancies with severe oligohydramnios. American Journal of Obstetrics and Gynecology 154: 895

Boddy K, Dawes G S 1975 Fetal breathing. British Medical Bulletin 31:1

Bottoms S F, Welch R A, Zador R A et al 1986 Limitation of using maximal vertical pocket and other sonographic evaluations of amniotic fluid volume to predict fetal growth: technical or physiologic? American Journal of Obstetrics and Gynecology 1555: 154

Bowman J M, Manning F A 1983 Intrauterine transfusion: Winnipeg 1982. Obstetrics and Gynecology 61: 203

Campbell S 1969 The prediction of fetal maturity by ultrasound measurement of the biparietal diameter. Journal of Obstetrics and Gynaecology of the British Commonwealth 76: 603

Campbell S 1974 The assessment of fetal development by diagnostic ultrasound. Clinics in Perinatology 1: 507

Campbell S, Wilkin D 1975 Ultrasonic measurement of the fetal abdominal circumference in the estimation of fetal weight. British Journal of Obstetrics and Gynaecology 83: 689

Chamberlain P F, Manning F A, Morrison I et al 1984a Circadian rhythm in bladder volumes in the term human fetus. Obstetrics and Gynecology 64: 657

Chamberlain P F, Manning F A, Morrison I et al 1984b Ultrasound valuation of amniotic fluid volume. II The relationship of increased amniotic fluid volume to perinatal outcome. American Journal of Obstetrics and Gynecology 150: 250

Chamberlain P F, Manning F A, Morrison I et al 1984c Ultrasound evaluation of amniotic fluid volume. I. The relationship of marginal and decreased amniotic fluid volumes to perinatal outcome. American Journal of Obstetrics and Gynecology 150: 245

Chamberlain P F, Cumming M, Forchia M G et al 1985 Ovine fetal urine production following maternal intravenous furosemide administration. American Journal of Obstetrics and Gynecology 151: 815

Cohn H E, Sacks E T, Heyman M A et al 1984b Cardiovascular responses to hypoxemia and acidemia in fetal lambs. American Journal of Obstetrics and Gynecology 120: 817

Copel J A, Scioscia A, Grannum P A et al 1986 Percutaneous umbilical blood sampling in the management of Kell isoimmunization. Obstetrics and Gynecology 67: 288

Crane J P, Kopla M M 1984 Genetic amniocentesis: impact of placental position upon the risk of pregnancy loss. American Journal of Obstetrics and Gynecology 150: 813

Crane J P, Tokmich P G, Kopta M 1980 Ultrasound growth patterns in normal and discordant twins. Obstetrics and Gynecology 55: 678

de Crespigny L C, Robinson H P, Quin M et al 1985 Ultrasound guided fetal transfusion for severe Rh isoimmunization. Obstetrics and Gynecology 66: 529

Deter R L, Hadlock F P 1981 Evaluation of three methods for obtaining fetal weight estimates using dynamic image ultrasound. Journal of Clinical Ultrasound 9: 421

Donald I 1974 Sonar — the story of an experiment. Ultrasound in Medicine and Biology 1: 109

Daffos F, Capella-Pavlovsky M, Forestier F 1985 Fetal blood sampling

during pregnancy with use of a needle guided by ultrasound: a study of 606 consecutive cases. American Journal of Obstetrics and Gynecology 153: 655
Donald I, Brown T G 1961 Demonstration of tissue interfaces within the body by ultrasonic echo sounding. British Journal of Radiology 34: 539
Dubowitz L M S, Dubowitz V, Goldberg C P 1970 Clinical assessment of gestation age in the newborn. Journal of Pediatrics 77: 1
Eik-Nes S H, Brubakk O, Ulsteir M K 1980 Measurement of human fetal blood flow. British Medical Journal 280: 283
Gill R W, Trudinger B J, Garrett W T et al 1981 Fetal umbilical venous flow measured in utero by pulsed Doppler and B-mode ultrasound. I. Normal pregnancies. American Journal of Obstetrics and Gynecology 139: 720
Gillieson M S, Winer-Mural H T, Muram D 1982 Lowlying placenta. Radiology 144: 577
Goplerud C P 1977 Bleeding in late pregnancy. In: Danforth D N (ed) Obstetrics and gynecology. Harper & Row, Hagerstown, Maryland, p 378
Grannum P A T, Berkowitz R L, Hobbins J C et al 1975 The ultrasonic changes in the maturing placenta and the relationship to fetal pulmonic maturity. American Journal of Obstetrics and Gynecology 133: 915
Grannum P, Brachen M, Silverman R et al 1980 Assessment of fetal kidney size in normal gestation by comparison of ratio of kidney circumference to abdominal circumference. American Journal of Obstetrics and Gynecology 136: 249
Greunwald P 1966 Growth of the human fetus. I. Normal growth and its variation. American Journal of Obstetrics and Gynecology 94: 1112
Hadlock F P, Feter R L 1982 Fetal abdominal circumference as a predictor of menstrual age. American Journal of Roentgenology 139: 367
Hadlock F P, Deter R L et al 1982 Fetal biparietal diameter: a critical re-evaluation of the relation to menstrual age by means of real time ultrasound. Journal of Ultrasound Medicine 1: 197
Hadlock F P, Deter R L, Marrest R B et al 1982a Fetal head circumference: relation to menstrual age. American Journal of Radiology 138: 649
Hadlock F P, Harrist R B, Deter R L et al 1982b Ultrasonically measured fetal femur length as a predictor of menstrual age. American Journal of Roentgentology 138: 875
Hadlock F P, Deter R L, Harrist R B et al 1983 Computer assisted analysis of fetal age in the third trimester using multiple fetal growth parameters. Journal of Clinical Ultrasound 11: 313
Hadlock F, Harrist R B, Deter R L et al 1985 Estimation of fetal weight by head, body and femur measurements: a prospective study. American Journal of Obstetrics and Gynecology 151: 333
Harman C R 1984 Ultrasound placental grading: relationship to fetal age, birth weight and birth weight percentile. Proceedings of the Society of Obstetricians and Gynecologists of Canada, Toronto
Harman C R, Manning F A, Sterns E et al 1982 The correlation of ultrasonic placental grading and fetal pulmonary maturity in 563 pregnancies. American Journal of Obstetrics and Gynecology 143: 941
Harman C R, Manning F A, Bowman J M et al 1983 Severe Rh disease: poor outcome is not inevitable. American Journal of Obstetrics and Gynecology 145: 823
Helewa M E, Lange I R, Davi M et al 1986 The neonatal outcome of macrosomic fetuses born to mothers with a normal glucose tolerance test. Proceedings of the Society of Obstetricians and Gynecologists of Canada, Toronto
Hills D, Irwin G A L, Tuck S et al 1984 Distribution of placental grade in high risk gravidas. American Journal of Roentgenology 143: 1101
Hobbins J C, Bracken M B, Mahoney K J 1982 Diagnosis of fetal skeletal dysplasias by ultrasound. American Journal of Obstetrics and Gynecology 142: 306
Hoddick W K, Callen P W, Filly R A et al 1984 Ultrasonographic determination of qualitative amniotic fluid volume in intrauterine growth retardation: reassessment of the 1 cm rule. American Journal of Obstetrics and Gynecology 149: 758
Hohler C W 1982 Cross checking pregnancy landmarks by ultrasound. Contemporary Obstetrics and Gynecology 20: 169
Hughey M, Sabbagha R E 1978 Cephalometry of real time imaging: a critical appraisal. American Journal of Obstetrics and Gynecology 131: 825
Jones M D, Battaglic F C 1977 Intrauterine growth retardation. American Journal of Obstetrics and Gynecology 127: 540
Kurjak A, Rajhvahn B 1982 Ultrasound measurement of umbilical blood flow in normal and complicated pregnancies. Journal of Perinatal Medicine 10: 3
Lange I R, Manning F A, Morrison I et al 1985 Cord prolapse: is antenatal diagnosis possible? American Journal of Obstetrics and Gynecology 151: 1083
Lavery J P 1982 Non stress fetal heart rate testing. Clinical Obstetrics and Gynecology 25: 689
Lubchenco L V, Harsman C, Dressler M et al 1963 Intrauterine growth as estimated from liveborn birth weight data at 24–42 weeks of gestation. Pediatrics 32: 793
Manning F A 1984 Ultrasound in perinatal medicine. In: Creasy R K, Resnick R (eds) Maternal–fetal medicine: principles and practice. W B Saunders, Philadelphia, p 203
Manning F A, Feyerabend C 1976 Cigarette smoking and fetal breathing movements. British Journal of Obstetrics and Gynaecology 83: 2612
Manning F A, Platt L D 1979 Maternal hypoxemia and fetal breathing movements. Obstetrics and Gynecology 53: 758
Manning F A, Platt L D, Sipos L 1980 Antepartum fetal evaluation: development of a fetal biophysical profile score. American Journal of Obstetrics and Gynecology 136: 787
Manning F A, Baskett T F, Morrison I et al 1981a Fetal biophysical profile scoring: a prospective study in 1184 high risk patients. American Journal of Obstetrics and Gynecology 140: 289
Manning F A, Hill L M, Platt L D 1981b Qualitative amniotic fluid volume determination by ultrasound: antepartum detection of IUGR. American Journal of Ostetrics and Gynecology 139: 254
Manning F A, Morrison I, Lange I R et al 1985 Fetal assessment based on fetal biophysical profile scoring: experience in 12 620 referred high risk pregnancies. I. Perinatal mortality by frequency and etiology. American Journal of Obstetrics and Gynecology 151: 343
Manning F A, Harman C R, Lange I R et al 1986a Fetal assessment by biophysical profile scoring: 1985 update. European Journal of Obstetrics, Gynecology and Reproductive Biology 21: 331
Manning F A, Morrison I, Lange I R et al 1986b Fetal length determination in utero: an ultrasound method. Obstetrics and Gynecology Proceedings of the Society of Obstetricians and Gynecologists of Canada, (abstract)
Manning F A, Harman C R, Morrison I et al 1987 Modified fetal biophysical profile scoring by selective use of the NST: a prospective study. American Journal of Obstetrics and Gynecology 156: 709
Manning F A, Morrison I, Harman C R et al 1989 The abnormal BPS: analysis of distribution of abnormal variables. American Journal of Obstetrics and Gynecology (in press)
Mayden K L, Tortora M, Berkowitz R et al 1982 Orbital diameters: a new parameter for prenatal diagnosis and dating. American Journal of Obstetrics and Gynecology 144: 298
Menticoglou S M, Manning F A, Harman C R 1986 Ultrasound guided percutaneous aspiration of fetal blood for prenatal diagnosis. Proceedings of the Society of Gynecologists and Obstetricians of Canada, Toronto
Mittelstadt C A, Partain C L, Boyce I L 1979 Placenta previa: significance in the second trimester. Radiology 131: 465
Morrison I, Olsen J 1985 Weight specific stillbirths and associated causes of death: an analysis of 675 stillbirths. American Journal of Obstetrics and Gynecology 152: 975
Natale R, Clewlow F, Dawes G S 1981 Measurement of forelimb movement in the fetal lamb. American Journal of Obstetrics and Gynecology 140: 548
O'Brien G D, Queenan J T 1981 Growth of the ultrasound femur length during normal pregnancy. American Journal of Obstetrics and Gynecology 141: 833
Ounsted M, Ounstead C 1966 Maternal regulation of intrauterine growth. Nature 187: 777
Philipson E H, Sokol R J, Williams T 1983 Oligohydramnios: clinical association and predictive value for intrauterine growth retardation. American Journal of Obstetrics and Gynecology 146: 271
Platt L D, Manning F A, LeMay M 1978 Real time B-scan directed amniocentesis. American Journal of Obstetrics and Gynecology 240: 700
Platt L D, Eglington G S, Sipos L 1983 Further experience with the fetal biophysical profile score. Obstetrics and Gynecology 672: 271
Prechtl H F R 1985 Ultrasound studies of human fetal behaviour. Early Human Development 12: 91
Robinson H 1973 Sonar measurements of fetal crown–rump lengths as

a means of assessing fetal maturity in early pregnancy. British Medical Journal 4: 28
Robinson H P 1975 Gestational sac volumes as determined by sonar in the first trimester of pregnancy. British Journal of Obstetrics and Gynaecology 82: 100
Sabbagha R E, Hughey M, Depp R 1978 Growth adjusted sonographic age: a simplified method. Obstetrics and Gynecology 51: 383
Seeds A E 1980 Current concepts of amniotic fluid dynamics. American Journal of Obstetrics and Gynecology 138: 575
Shepard M J, Richards V A, Benkowitz R L et al 1983 An evaluation of two equations for predicting fetal weight by ultrasound. American Journal of Obstetrics and Gynecology 1432: 47
Socol M L, Manning F A, Murata Y et al 1982 Maternal smoking causes fetal hypoxemia: experimental evidence. American Journal of Obstetrics and Gynecology 142: 214
Streeter H, Manning F A, Lange I R 1984 Perinatal mortality and morbidity in IUGR fetuses by birth weight percentile. Proceedings of the Society of Obstetricians and Gynecologists of Canada, Toronto
Thompson T, Manning F A 1983 Estimation of volume and weight of the perinate: relationship to morphometric measures by ultrasonography. Journal of Ultrasound Medicine 2: 113
Vintzileos A M, Campbell W A, Ingardia P T et al 1983 The fetal biophysical profile score and its predictive value. Obstetrics and Gynecology 672: 271
Weiner S N, Flynn M J, Kennedy A W et al 1977 A composite curve of ultrasonic biparietal diameters for estimating gestational age. Radiology 122: 781
Williamson D, Bjorgen J, Baier B et al 1978 Ultrasound diagnosis of placenta previa: value of the postvoid scan. Journal of Clinical Ultrasound 6: 58

SECTION 5

Abnormal Pregnancy

28

Alec Turnbull

Spontaneous abortion

In the United Kingdom, abortion is defined as the expulsion of a fetus showing no signs of life before the completed 28th week of pregnancy. Spontaneous abortion is often termed miscarriage by non-medical persons because abortion tends to be regarded as induced, either therapeutic or criminal. Although Beard (1985) has argued in favour of the term miscarriage being used more officially to describe spontaneous abortion, it has not as yet been generally accepted and the term abortion is still generally used in medical practice to describe both spontaneous and induced types.

Spontaneous abortion is common and carries physical and psychological risks for women. Abortion can be early, in the first trimester or late, in the second trimester. Early abortions have been considered to be particularly associated with fetal anomalies while the late abortions are more often associated with maternal factors. Abortion may occur as a single isolated event, or may be recurrent; a woman is said to suffer from recurrent spontaneous abortion (RSA) if she has had three or more abortions.

VIABILITY

The concept of a duration of pregnancy after which the fetus is 'capable of being born alive' is the product of the Infant Life (Preservation) Act 1929; this and other subsequent Acts of Parliament have used 28 completed weeks (196 days from the first day of the last menstrual period) as an acceptable limit between likely survival or death of an infant after birth. The complexity of the legal situation arising from these Acts is worsened by the lack of any adequate definition of the terms 'capable of being born alive' or, for that matter, 'viability'.

All this legislation is of importance because it defines the gestational age up to which legal abortion may be performed.

In 1974 the Lane Committee recommended that the Abortion Act should be amended to authorize abortion only up to the 24th week of pregnancy instead of up to the 28th week, as at present (Report of the Committee of the Working of the Abortion Act 1974). Certainly the 28th week limit has become unrealistic because of the great improvement in the management of very small babies which means that many infants born well before the 28th week of gestation now survive. In 1985, a committee comprising representatives of the Royal College of Obstetricians and Gynaecologists, the British Paediatric Association, the Royal College of General Practitioners, the Royal College of Midwives, the British Medical Association and the Department of Health and Social Security, published their Report on Fetal Viability and Clinical Practice and made the following recommendations:

1. The gestational age after which a fetus is considered as viable should be changed from the present limit of 28 weeks (196 days) to 24 weeks (168 days) of gestation.
2. In accordance with the World Health Organization (WHO) recommendation, a record should be kept of all babies born alive or dead of 22 weeks' (154 days') gestational age, or weighing 500 g or more, if born earlier.
3. Confirmation of the gestational age of the fetus by all reasonable available methods including ultrasound, in addition to a careful clinical assessment, should be carried out before a decision is taken to terminate a pregnancy thought to be of a gestational age of 20 weeks or more.

The appendix to this report helps clarify the confusion about what current Acts of Parliament have to say about the question of viability and lists the Acts which have a bearing on the protection of the fetus. These aspects are also considered in Chapter 29.

The legal position relating to fetal viability has recently been under review, with several bills relating to the latest

Table 28.1 Indication for sonar and subsequent pregnancy outcome

Indication	All	Continuing >28 weeks	Blighted ovum	Missed abortion	Live abortion	Hydatidiform mole	Miscellaneous	Total pregnancy failure	Percentage failure
Threatened abortion	182	56	47	56	12	9	2	126	69
Recurrent abortion	90	64	10	7	9	–	–	26	29
Other	153	119	12	6	3	1	2	24	15.6
Total	425	249	69	69	24	10	4	176	

From Robinson (1975).

gestation permissible at therapeutic abortion being presented to Parliament. These attempts to change the law were unsuccessful.

GENERAL FEATURES OF SPONTANEOUS ABORTION

Of all clinically diagnosed pregnancies, between 15 and 20% end in a spontaneous abortion (WHO 1970) and of all these abortions, approximately 80% take place before 13 weeks (Jeffcoate 1975). These figures refer to clinically diagnosed pregnancies but it is likely that conception loss is much greater. Roberts & Lowe (1975) provided statistical arguments for the hypothesis that at least 75% of very early pregnancies were aborted spontaneously. Even earlier, Hertig (1968) showed in a histological study of preimplantation blastocysts that 50% were abnormal. In a prospective study, Miller et al (1980) reported a total postimplantation conception loss of 43%. Of these, 33% were diagnosed only on the evidence of raised beta-human chorionic gonadotrophin while 11% were clinically evident pregnancies.

Aetiology

Abortion in early pregnancy is almost always preceded by death of the embryo or fetus, unlike later abortions in which the fetus is born alive and some other explanation must be invoked. In first-trimester abortions, fetal death may be associated with abnormalities of the ovum itself, immunological factors, abnormalities in the reproductive tract or systemic disease in the mother. In early spontaneous abortion, abnormality of development of the embryo, fetus or placenta is often reported. In 1943, Hertig & Sheldon observed abnormal blighted ova in which embryos were degenerate or absent in 49%, showed visible localized anomalies in 3%, and placental abnormalities in 10%. In spontaneous abortions of increasing gestational age the incidence of abnormal development decreased considerably. Boué & Boué (1978) estimated that 50–60% of early spontaneous abortions were associated with a chromosomal abnormality in the conceptus. As Underwood & Mowbray (1985) point out, however, such studies do not make it clear that the 50% of abnormality is achieved in the minority of cases (less than 20%) in which chromosome culture is possible.

A very careful study by Robinson (1975) clarified the types of pregnancy failure associated with spontaneous abortion. The author reported the details of subsequent pregnancy outcome in 425 patients referred for sonar evaluation — 182 because of threatened abortion, 90 because of recurrent abortion and 153 for other reasons, including pregnancy considered large- or small-for-dates, pregnancy associated with an irregular menstrual cycle, uncertain date of last menstrual period, excessive sickness, or simply to confirm normal pregnancy. Of these pregnancies, 249 progressed beyond the 28th week and Robinson described the sonar findings in the 176 cases who subsequently aborted. The findings are summarized in Table 28.1. Abortion occurred in 69% of threatened abortions, 29% of RSA and 15.6% of the others — a figure in keeping with the spontaneous abortion rate previously quoted.

Robinson classified the categories of pregnancy failure as follows:

1. *Blighted ovum or anembryonic pregnancy*. These terms were used synonymously and their diagnosis was restricted to pregnancies in which a gestation sac could be defined by sonar but in which neither sonar nor subsequent examination of the products of conception demonstrated a fetus.
2. *Missed abortion*. This diagnosis was made when a fetus could clearly be demonstrated within the gestation sac but no fetal heart could be detected. Pathological confirmation was usually obtained by finding a very macerated fetus within the products of conception although this was not considered to be essential when the scan clearly demonstrated a fetus with no heartbeat.
3. *Live abortion*. Abortion was considered to be live if the fetal heart had been clearly demonstrated by sonar a few days prior to the spontaneous abortion or if the fetus at the time of abortion showed no maceration and had a crown–rump length compatible with the period of amenorrhoea. Pregnancy duration was designated early or late depending on whether abortion occurred before or after the 12th week.
4. *Hydatidiform mole*. This was diagnosed when the uterus

Table 28.2 Fetal disorder detected by sonar in 176 cases in which early pregnancy failure later recurred

Disorder	No.	%
Blighted ovum	69	39.2
Missed abortion	69	39.2
Live abortion		
Early	6	3.4
Late	18	10.2
Hydatidiform mole	10	5.7
Miscellaneous	4	2.3
Total	176	100

Adapted from Robinson (1975).

was seen to be filled with echoes of similar size and amplitude and no gestational sac or fetus could be seen.

5. *Miscellaneous*. The four patients in this group were either lost to follow-up or aborted at home. In each case, a provisional diagnosis of blighted ovum had already been made.

Table 28.2 shows that of the 176 cases of early pregnancy failure, almost 80% were associated with either a blighted ovum (39%) or a missed abortion (39%). A further 8% also showed absence of a fetus, with hydatidiform mole in 5.7% and probable blighted ovum in 2.3%.

CAUSES OF SPONTANEOUS FIRST-TRIMESTER ABORTION

It is clear that first-trimester abortion is overwhelmingly associated with a process which leads to the death and absorption of the fetus but knowledge of the proportion of abortuses associated with lethal chromosomal abnormalities is limited by the difficulty of culturing fetal material once the fetus is dead.

Chromosomal abnormalities are clearly very common amongst fetuses aborted alive or soon enough after death to allow culture of cells but cases may represent only a small minority of all first-trimester abortuses.

Immunological factors

Immunological factors may be responsible for the missed abortions and blighted ova described earlier. Couples with RSA are more likely than control couples to share common human leukocyte antigens (Beer et al 1981, Taylor & Faulk 1981, Underwood & Mowbray 1985). The first two research groups demonstrated sharing of class I antigens, while Underwood & Mowbray (1985) demonstrated only sharing of class II antigens.

An incomplete maternal immunological response to pregnancy seems to be of particular importance in RSA rather than in single isolated abortions, but it may prove relevant in both types. Immunological aspects are considered in more detail below, in the section on RSA.

Maternal disease

Many maternal disorders have been implicated in abortion although the evidence for such an association is not very convincing. These conditions are generally implicated more in RSA than in single isolated abortions and they are considered at greater length below.

The diseases implicated, however, include chronic infections such as toxoplasmosis, cytomegalovirus, chlamydia or herpes. Brucella abortus seems a more important cause of abortion in cattle than in the human.

Endocrine disorders

Abortion has often been attributed, sometimes without adequate reason, to deficient secretion of progesterone. The incidence of abortion also seems to be increased in women with diabetes (Sutherland & Pritchard 1987), or with thyroid disease, especially hypothyroidism (Stray-Pedersen & Stray-Pedersen 1984).

Laparotomy

Laparotomy may occasionally be followed by abortion, particularly during the first 12 weeks of pregnancy. It is therefore customary to delay removal of an ovarian cyst until after the 16th week of pregnancy when the risk of abortion has fallen. Peritonitis increases the likelihood of abortion so that early laparotomy for, say, suspected appendicitis, is likely to be safer for both fetus and mother than delay.

Abnormalities of the uterus

Abnormalities of the shape of the uterine cavity associated with abnormal Müllerian fusion predispose to recurring abortion, as does cervical incompetence. Both are discussed in the section on RSA, as well as in Chapter 33. Submucous fibromyomata may also increase the risk of spontaneous abortion.

Physical and psychological trauma

Patients and their relatives tend to attribute abortion to a recent fall, accident, blow or psychological shock. It is unlikely that these factors are of much importance in causing abortion, since the fetus probably died some time before the abortion occurred, particularly with those in the first trimester.

On the other hand, the psychological effects of spontaneous abortion on the mother should not be underestimated. Recent studies (Friedman & Gath 1988) have shown that the bereavement response following abortion may be intense; it is greater in women who have no living child or who have only had previous abortions and is greater with increasing gestation at abortion.

Predisposing factors

Several factors influence the incidence of abortion without being specifically causal in themselves. Kline et al (1978) showed that the risk of abortion increased with increasing maternal age, while Naylor & Warburton (1979) showed that the rate of abortion also increased with high gravidity.

Kline et al (1977) showed that smoking was a risk factor for spontaneous abortion and Roberts & Lloyd (1973) showed that abortion was commoner in low socioeconomic groups.

The pathology of spontaneous abortion in the first trimester

Histological examination of the products of conception after spontaneous abortion reveals haemorrhage into the decidua basalis and necrotic changes in the tissues adjacent to the bleeding. The ovum becomes detached in part or whole and the concentration of prostaglandin E in the decidua increases markedly (Jaschevatsky et al 1983), presumably playing a part in the expulsion of the ovum. If there is an intact sac, it usually contains a small macerated fetus with a little fluid but commonly there is no visible fetus in the sac. In other cases, hydatidiform degeneration of the placental villi is seen (see Chapter 37). A carneous mole is an ovum surrounded by layers of blood clot of varying thickness depending on the duration of the process. In such cases bleeding has been occurring at intervals over a considerable period with layers of blood forming at different times, before the mole is finally extruded.

CAUSES OF SPONTANEOUS SECOND-TRIMESTER ABORTION

While most of the factors which cause abortion in the first trimester also do so in the second trimester, later abortions are said to be less often associated with chromosomally abnormal fetuses (Mikamo 1970). By contrast, the proportion of couples with abnormalities predisposing to abortion is higher in the second- than in the first-trimester abortions, stressing the greater importance of parental factors in late abortions.

Cervical incompetence is the maternal disorder most commonly associated with second-trimester abortion. Stray-Pedersen & Stray-Pedersen (1984) detected it in 30% of second-trimester abortions. While it is often regarded as the result of previous cervical trauma such as cervical dilatation for primary dysmenorrhoea or legal abortion (especially more than one), cervical conization or partial amputation, these investigators noted that in 13 of 25 women in whom they detected cervical incompetence during pregnancy, no previous cervical dilatation had ever taken place, implying a congenital origin in more than half the cases.

Abnormalities of the uterine body, such as bicornuate or septate uterus, are classically regarded as causing late abortion, but while they may do so (see Chapter 33), Stray-Pedersen & Stray-Pedersen (1984) found they were associated with primary RSA (20%) or with first-trimester abortion (12%) as often as with second-trimester abortion (12%).

Endometrial infection was commoner in first-trimester abortion (16%) but still relatively common in second-trimester abortion (12.7%).

Listeria monocytogenes can cause late abortion, usually associated with high fever. A rare but dangerous cause of late abortion is infection of the pregnant human with sheep *Chlamydia psittaci*. High fever, intrauterine death and disseminated intravascular coagulation can develop (Johnson 1985). Since the pregnant woman is infected as a result of caring for an infected sheep during its parturition, the infection almost always occurs in the wife of a sheep farmer.

Overall, a reproductive abnormality was found in 69% of second-trimester abortions, compared with only 49% of first-trimester abortions (Stray-Pedersen & Stray-Pedersen 1984).

Pathology of spontaneous second-trimester abortion

In many late abortions, the fetus has been growing normally until close to the event when abortion is due to maternal causes. When intrauterine death occurs, the fetus becomes macerated. The skull bones collapse, the abdomen becomes distended and the fetus takes on a dull, reddish-brown colour; the skin peels readily and the internal organs degenerate, becoming friable, soft and necrotic. If the amniotic fluid is absorbed, the fetus may become compressed to form a *fetus compressus*. Occasionally this process continues to such an extent that a *fetus papyraceus* develops. This is particularly liable to occur in twin pregnancy if one fetus dies early in pregnancy and the other continues to develop.

CLINICAL FEATURES OF SPONTANEOUS ABORTION

In the *first trimester* abortion, the clinical progression is threatened, inevitable, incomplete or missed abortion and the clinical features of these problems are described below. Septic abortion is another important clinical complication and is also described later.

Threatened abortion

Vaginal bleeding in the first half of pregnancy is first diagnosed as threatened abortion. Approximately 15% of all pregnancies are complicated by threatened abortion and of these, 16–18% progress to abortion depending on the amount of bleeding (Evans & Beischer 1970). A useful clinical rule is that if vaginal bleeding in the first 12 weeks of pregnancy is as heavy as the patient's normal menstrual blood loss, pregnancy is rarely successful (Peckham 1970). When bleeding is slight and resolves, pregnancy may continue satisfactorily, but the threatened abortion tends to affect subsequent perinatal outcome adversely (Thompson & Lein 1961).

Hertig (1968) showed that bleeding in early pregnancy may be physiological. Bleeding can occur from necrotic decidua parietalis over the implanting ovum between 12 and 28 days after fertilization or from the decidua vera as the developing gestation sac obliterates the uterine cavity between 2 and 8 weeks after fertilization. In neither of these situations would the bleeding compromise the developing embryo. In contrast, where a threatened abortion progresses to abortion, bleeding usually starts only after the embryo is dead.

Ultrasound assessment of the condition of the fetus is therefore of vital importance in the management of such cases.

Inevitable abortion

When abortion is inevitable, pain increases, the cervix dilates and the membranes may rupture with a leak of fluid from the vagina.

Incomplete abortion

In first-trimester abortions, the fetus and placenta are usually expelled together. If the placenta, either in whole or in part, is retained in the uterus, bleeding ultimately occurs — the commonest feature of incomplete abortion. This can be profuse and lead to hypovolaemia.

Missed abortion

In the first trimester, missed abortion is usually diagnosed on ultrasound examination, which reveals a fetus but no fetal heartbeat. Sometimes a further examination 1 or 2 weeks later to review the situation reveals simply that the pregnancy was less far advanced than had been calculated from the date of the last menstrual period, and is now actually progressing normally.

If the dead products of conception are retained for more than approximately 30 days, a coagulation defect may develop, with the risk of severe uterine haemorrhage when the uterus is emptied.

It is not known why early intrauterine fetal death in some cases is quickly followed by spontaneous abortion while in others there is prolonged retention of the dead conceptus. In some cases, treatment with long-acting progestogens predisposes to this situation (Smith et al 1978).

In the *second-trimester abortion* the clinical features may be similar to those in the first trimester, especially in those occurring early in the second trimester. Later abortions may present clinical features like the onset of labour at term or pre-term, with increasing uterine contractions leading to expulsion of the fetus and placenta. There is often persistent intermittent bleeding, however, which may have begun earlier in pregnancy, even in the first trimester. Pregnancy continuing after bleeding in the second trimester is also associated with increased risks of subsequent prematurity, low birthweight and increased perinatal mortality (Turnbull & Walker 1956, Chamberlain et al 1978, Federick & Adelstein 1978, South & Naldrett 1973). Such a presentation may be associated with uterine abnormalities, submucous fibroids or endometrial infections.

Cervical incompetence typically presents with unexpected spontaneous rupture of the membranes not associated with abdominal pain. In women with suspected cervical incompetence, repeated vaginal examination or ultrasound scanning in pregnancy may reveal progressive silent dilatation of the cervix commencing at the internal os, unlike labour at term in which cervical dilation commences at the external os and only later involves the internal os (Varma et al 1986). Abortion of the fetus results when the rupture of the membranes induces labour. This may occur quickly, especially if intrauterine infection develops, or may be delayed for days or even weeks.

Spontaneous rupture of the membranes may occur in the second trimester without an incompetent cervix, sometimes after amniocentesis.

If the pregnancy continues with little or no amniotic fluid in the uterus, the fetus may appear to grow and develop satisfactorily but lung development is often retarded and when born preterm, the infant is liable to die of pulmonary hypoplasia with pneumothorax and pneumomediastinum (Thibeault et al 1985). However, the outcome is not uniformly bad (Thomas & Smith 1974). It has not been possible before delivery to detect which fetuses will have normal or abnormal lung development. Recent work on this subject is considered in the section on treatment.

TREATMENT OF SPONTANEOUS ABORTION

In the first trimester the management of abortion has been revolutionized by the development of ultrasound. Robinson (1972a) showed that threatened abortion could be differentiated from an incomplete or complete abortion at a single examination, thereby avoiding unnecessary treatment by evacuation of the uterus. Robinson (1972b, 1978) also showed that the fetal heartbeat could normally be demonstrated by 7 weeks' gestation and Jouppila et al (1980) showed that it could always be demonstrated by 9 weeks. Approximately 50% of pregnancies complicated by threatened abortion have a successful outcome, but if the fetal heartbeat is identified, outcome is successful in 89–92% of cases (Bennett & Kerr-Wilson 1980, Jouppila et al 1980).

Threatened abortion in the first trimester with only slight bleeding, a uterus enlarged in keeping with the calculated gestational age and a closed cervix, is most likely associated with a continuing pregnancy. Even without real-time ultrasound, a simple ultrasound fetal heart monitor will detect a fetal heartbeat, although not usually before the 13th week.

Inevitable abortion

If there is increased bleeding, rhythmical uterine contractions and a loss of clear fluid suggesting rupture of the membranes, abortion is almost certainly inevitable. Ultrasound assessment can exclude the unlikely possibility that the fetal heartbeat is present. If not, and unless complete expulsion of the uterine contents quickly follows, the uterus should be emptied surgically under general anaesthesia.

Incomplete abortion

In this situation, the cervix is dilated and placental debris may be lying free in the lower uterus, or partly adherent there or in the dilated cervical canal and protruding through the external os. The uterine size is smaller than would be expected from the calculated gestation. Bleeding may be free and the vagina full of blood clot.

If bleeding causes hypovolaemia the patient will have a rapid, thready pulse, pallor and hypotension and surgical evacuation of the uterus should be delayed until normovolaemia has been restored. Bleeding can usually be controlled by intravenous injection of 0.25 mg ergometrine and an intravenous infusion should be set up. The patient's blood group and rhesus factor should be determined and crystalloid fluids and plasma-expanding preparations administered as soon as possible until blood is available.

When the cervix is dilated with placental debris protruding it may be possible to remove these products of conception with suitable forceps without general anaesthesia. Alternatively, the uterine cavity can be evacuated without anaesthesia by means of a suction curette. In most gynaecological emergency units, however, patients requiring evacuation of an incomplete abortion are dealt with under general anaesthesia to ensure that the uterine cavity is properly explored and emptied. Examination under general anaesthesia is also essential if there is any doubt about the diagnosis. Ectopic pregnancy may already be suspect, since very little material may have been found in the uterus on curettage or because pain has been a particular feature as well as bleeding. In such circumstances, laparoscopy would clearly be indicated to exclude ectopic pregnancy and could be performed immediately in the anaesthetized patient.

Missed abortion

When intrauterine fetal death is detected early in pregnancy — before 12 weeks — by ultrasound, the uterus should be emptied by curettage under general anaesthesia. Pretreatment with a vaginal pessary containing 1 mg of 16,16-dimethyl-prostaglandin E_1 generally ensures easy dilatation of the cervix and facilitates the procedure. If missed abortion is diagnosed later in pregnancy, after 14–16 weeks or later, it is safer to induce spontaneous abortion by vaginal or extra-amniotic administration of prostaglandins. Potent analogues such as 16,16-dimethyl-prostaglandin E_1 can be given vaginally at 3-hourly intervals in a dose of 1 mg (Cameron & Baird 1984) or prostaglandin E_2 1.5–2 mg administered extra-amniotically in a slow-release gel (MacKenzie & Embrey 1976).

If a missed abortion is retained within the uterus for more than about 4 weeks, a coagulation defect may develop with hypofibrinogenaemia. If a missed abortion is not detected until it has been present for several weeks' duration, coagulation failure must be detected and corrected before the uterus is evacuated.

Differential diagnosis of first-trimester abortion

Several conditions can mimic spontaneous abortion by causing delayed menstruation, bleeding or pelvic pain. In older women, metropathia haemorrhagica may present as spontaneous abortion. Unopposed oestrogen stimulation causes endometrial hyperplasia and uterine enlargement initially associated with amenorrhoea. Subsequently, the hyperplastic endometrium begins to degenerate with prolonged and sometimes profuse bleeding. A degree of cervical dilatation occurs and white, gelatinous endometrium may be expelled spontaneously or evacuated by curettage. These symptoms and signs simulate spontaneous abortion and demonstrate the need for histological examination of material obtained at curettage to establish the diagnosis. Such histological examination is essential to detect the cases in which abortion is associated with the hydatidiform degeneration of the trophoblast, which usually presents as abortion but requires subsequent surveillance (see Chapter 31).

Another condition which can simulate abortion is a pedunculated submucous fibroid being expelled spontaneously through the cervix. A large cervical polyp or a cervical carcinoma may mimic spontaneous abortion although they would usually present a previous history of persistent bleeding or offensive vaginal discharge.

Nowadays, ectopic pregnancy is probably the most important differential diagnosis of abortion. Its incidence is increasing, its presentation is frequently atypical and it often simulates spontaneous abortion. Classically, ectopic pregnancy presents with severe episodic pelvic pain, exquisite tenderness on pelvic examination and a unilateral mass in the pelvis. There may be severe intra-abdominal bleeding with hypovolaemia. This syndrome is instantly recognizable and is usually resolved by rapid resuscitation, laparotomy and removal of the ectopic pregnancy. The diagnostic difficulties which arise are related to the often atypical presentations of ectopic pregnancy. If there is amenorrhoea and bleeding, but no pain or pelvic tenderness, the condition may not be suspected. Unruptured tubal pregnancy may present with such symptoms and the gynaecologist must always be alert to the possibility—and to the very rare coexistence of tubal and intrauterine pregnancy, the latter proceeding to spontaneous abortion.

Bimanual pelvic examination should always be performed very gently in cases of spontaneous abortion lest an intact tubal pregnancy is inadvertently ruptured. A high degree of suspicion is essential. If ectopic pregnancy is suspected, rapid sensitive assay of beta-human chorionic gonadotrophin in urine will be positive, despite the apparent absence of intrauterine pregnancy on clinical examination or on transabdominal ultrasound scanning. This combination is suspicious of ectopic pregnancy. Transvaginal ultrasound scanning produces a clearer picture and can demonstrate the ectopic pregnancy without the patient having a full bladder (Urquhart & Fisk 1988).

A large corpus luteum can delay the onset of menstruation until it ruptures spontaneously, leading to a delayed period and acute pelvic pain and tenderness, due to intrapelvic bleeding from the rupture. Thus, a ruptured corpus luteum cyst can simulate either a spontaneous abortion or an ectopic pregnancy.

Similar clinical pictures may be associated with an exacerbation of chronic pelvic inflammatory disease or with spontaneous rupture of endometriotic cysts in the ovaries.

If there is any suspicion of ectopic pregnancy or other serious pelvic pathology, laparoscopy will rapidly establish the diagnosis. It is an essential investigation for patients in good condition and with doubt about diagnosis. In patients who have an obvious acute abdominal emergency with probable intra-abdominal bleeding, however, laparotomy should be performed at once and no time should be lost in performing laparoscopy.

Treatment of second-trimester abortion

Abortion occurring early in the second trimester is managed in the same way as in the first trimester. When bleeding or pain develops later in the second trimester, at say 18–24 weeks, however, treatment is usually aimed at maintaining the pregnancy, provided the fetus is alive and normal. Ultrasound examination is therefore of vital importance for assessing the condition of the intrauterine fetus.

Serum alpha-fetoprotein (AFP)

The level of serum AFP measured before bleeding began may serve as a pointer to later outcome. Very high levels (>2.5 multiples of the median; MOM), in the absence of detectable neural tube defects or exomphalos are associated with early delivery, intrauterine growth retardation and a generally jeopardized pregnancy (Chapter 19). Very low levels (<0.4 MOM) are associated with an increased risk of Down's syndrome (Chapter 19) and, especially if scanning reveals the cardiac or intestinal abnormalities which are often associated with this syndrome, placental biopsy or cordocentesis should be performed to karyotype the fetus quickly as the information could be of vital importance in deciding about maintaining the pregnancy (see Chapter 24).

Tocolysis

If the fetus is normal it may be possible to suppress uterine contractions with beta-mimetics or other drugs described in Chapter 51. Maintaining the fetus in utero for even a few days may be very important for the future outcome for the fetus if abortion threatens at 23 or 24 weeks. Tocolysis is useful if the problem is of excessive uterine contractions, but if there is profuse bleeding or intrauterine infection, pregnancy may have to be terminated for the sake of the mother. More often, however, bleeding is intermittent and infection controllable and the patient's condition can be maintained by blood transfusion and appropriate antibiotics if pregnancy is continuing satisfactorily for the fetus. Serious intrauterine infection usually causes abortion with early delivery of the fetus and placenta.

Cervical incompetence

Cervical incompetence may present as silent cervical dilatation without painful uterine contractions. There may be some mucoid vaginal discharge following a feeling of fullness in the lower abdomen and sometimes frequency or urgency of micturition. The membranes bulge through the dilating cervical canal and ultimately rupture spontaneously. This condition may be detected by chance on speculum examination, or may have been looked for because of a previous history suggesting cervical incompetence. Cervical dilatation usually commences after 14 weeks, usually between 16 and 24 weeks. Treatment is to close the cervical canal surgically by inserting a non-absorbable suture of nylon or mersilene at the level of the internal cervical os and tying it firmly with a 4 Heger dilator in the cervical canal. If performed before 20 weeks and without rupturing the membranes, there is a good chance of a successful outcome (between 40 and 90% according to Beischer & Mackay (1986) and 70% according to Stray-Pedersen & Stray-Pedersen (1984)). Beta-mimetic drugs are often given intravenously for a day or two after the operation and then orally until pregnancy is clearly seen to be progressing satisfactorily (see Chapter 24).

The simplest and most widely used form of cervical cerclage was described by MacDonald (1957) and is illustrated in Fig. 28.1. The other is the more complicated operation described by Shirodkar (1960). Prophylactic cerclage is best performed around 12–14 weeks in women with known cervical incompetence before cervical dilatation begins and after the main risk of first-trimester abortion has passed. Emergency cerclage can be performed after the cervix has dilated and the membranes are bulging but failure is more common,

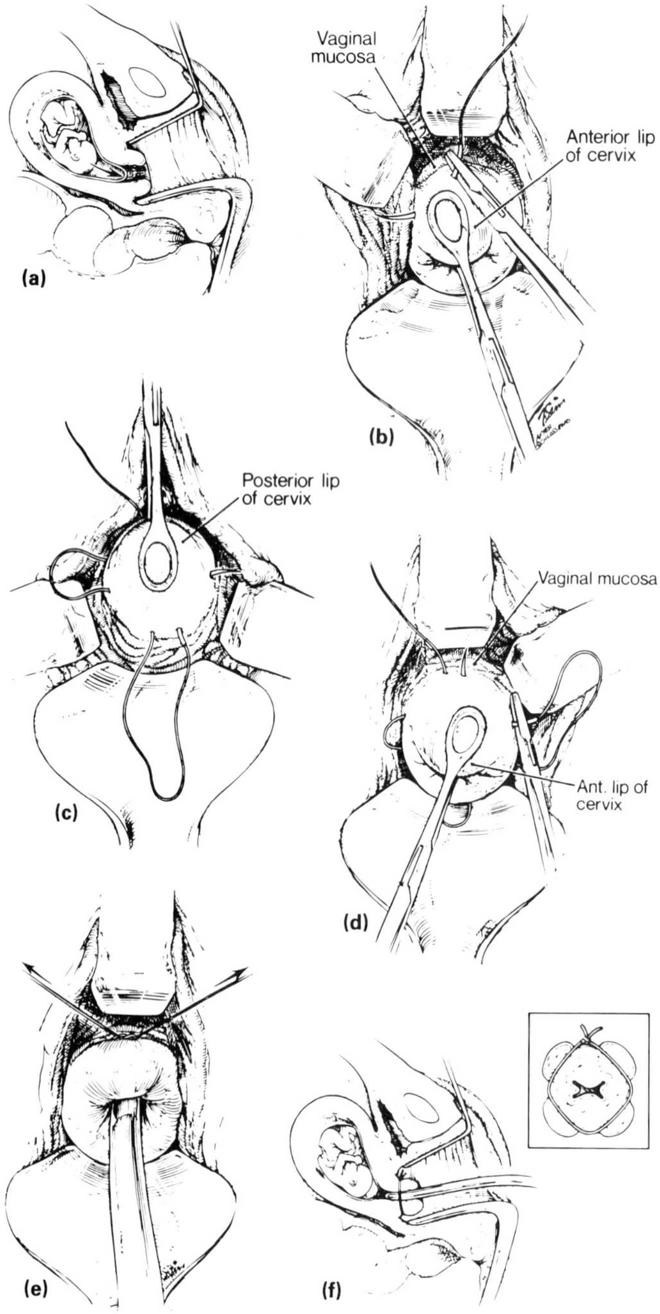

Fig. 28.1 Incompetent cervix treated by the McDonald procedure. (**a**) Somewhat dilated cervical canal and beginning prolapse of membranes (arrow). (**b**) Start of the cerclage procedure with a suture of number 2 Prolene being replaced superiorly in the body of the cervix very near the level of the internal os. (**c**) Continuation of the replacement of the suture in the body of the os. (**d**) Completion of the encirclement. (**e**) The suture is tightened around the cervical canal sufficiently to reduce the diameter of the canal to a few millimetres and is then securely tied. In the illustration a *small* dilator has been placed just through the level of ligation to maintain patency of the canal when the suture is tied. (**f**) The effect of the suture placement on the cervical canal is apparent. From Pritchard & MacDonald (1980), with permission.

since the membranes may be inadvertently ruptured during insertion of the suture, the suture may cut through the thin wall of the dilated cervix or intrauterine infection may develop.

If pregnancy continues satisfactorily with the cervical cerclage suture in position, it is generally removed around the 37th week of pregnancy and the subsequent spontaneous onset of labour is awaited — it does not generally begin when the suture is removed, but usually a week or two later.

Spontaneous rupture of membranes with oligohydramnios

Spontaneous rupture of the membranes without cervical incompetence can lead to second-trimester abortion especially if intrauterine infection develops. If there is no infection, however, pregnancy may continue despite oligohydramnios. As described earlier, the fetus may appear to be growing satisfactorily but pulmonary hypoplasia is common and when present causes early neonatal death. It has not been possible to know which fetuses are affected by pulmonary hypoplasia until delivery. Recently, Blott et al (1987) reported that if fetal breathing movements could be detected in such cases, pulmonary development was most likely to be normal, but if fetal breathing movements were not present, pulmonary hypoplasia was usually present. Soon after this report, however, Moessinger et al (1987) reported that fetal breathing movements were not a reliable predictor of continued lung development in pregnancies complicated by oligohydramnios. Their observations were confirmed by Kilbride et al (1988), whose experience was that measurement of amniotic fluid volume was the most reliable predictor of fetal pulmonary hypoplasia. At present, management of these cases must continue to be expectant (Chapter 51).

Differential diagnosis of second-trimester abortion

The patient with second-trimester abortion presents with an abdominal mass associated with lower abdominal pain, vaginal bleeding or vaginal leakage of fluid. If a fetal heart is detectable with a stethoscope or an ultrasound fetal heart detector, abdominal pain may be associated with complications such as uterine fibroids undergoing necrobiosis (red cell degeneration), torsion of an ovarian cyst or an acute abdominal emergency such as appendicitis, cholecystitis or intestinal obstruction. If there has been previous uterine surgery, rupture of the uterus might explain both pain and vaginal bleeding, although the fetal heart would probably not be present. Advanced extrauterine pregnancy is rare in the UK, but does occur and may present considerable diagnostic difficulty, as does pregnancy in the rudimentary horn of a double uterus, again a rare differential diagnosis of second-trimester abortion (see Chapter 33).

Nowadays, expert ultrasound imaging helps to resolve most of the problems of differential diagnosis but if an acute surgical emergency is a possibility, laparotomy is better performed too early than too late.

Septic abortion

Serious infective complications of abortion are often, but not always, associated with criminal interference. Septic abortion used to be one of the commonest causes of maternal death before the 1967 Abortion Act, death being due to complications such as haemorrhage, septicaemia, endotoxic shock, disseminated intravascular coagulation and renal failure. Since the 1967 Abortion Act in this country began to operate in 1968 and more liberal legislation for therapeutic abortion was enacted in other developed countries, there has been a dramatic reduction in maternal mortality and morbidity from septic abortion and a great fall in the number of emergency admissions to hospital for septic abortion. The Confidential Enquiries into Maternal Mortality in England and Wales for 1982–1984 for the first time report no deaths from criminal abortion. Avoiding the need for women to seek criminal abortion has therefore reduced maternal deaths from this cause far more effectively than did treating the consequences of criminal interference in the past. Septic abortions still occur, however, for even nowadays criminal interference is not unknown. Other factors can also predispose. For example, sepsis can readily develop when an intrauterine contraceptive device has been retained within the uterus during pregnancy (Williams et al 1975).

Microbiology

Septic abortion is most often associated with pathogenic organisms of the bowel and vaginal flora; anaerobic organisms are more common, including anaerobic streptococci, *Bacteroides* and clostridia. Aerobic organisms include *Escherichia coli* and group B beta-haemolytic streptococci (Smith et al 1970).

Clinical features

In addition to signs of threatened or incomplete abortion, the patient is febrile and usually has significant tenderness over the uterus and lower abdomen. There may be offensive as well as blood-stained vaginal discharge. Initially, infection is confined to the uterus but it tends to spread through the uterine wall into the connective tissues of the broad ligament and lateral pelvic wall, leading to pelvic cellulitis and possibly septicaemia. In severe cases, endotoxic shock can develop, sometimes with disseminated intravascular coagulation. Such patients are at risk of acute renal failure.

Investigation should include general and pelvic examination; blood samples should be obtained for full blood count, blood grouping and cross-matching; urine analysis; swabs taken for culture from the endocervix and lower uterine cavity and peripheral blood also sent for culture. Ultrasound scan of the pelvis should be performed and if there is peritonitis, an abdominal X-ray should be obtained to detect any intra-abdominal or intrauterine gas (suggesting clostridial infection or uterine perforation). An X-ray or ultrasound should also demonstrate an intrauterine foreign body.

Treatment

The treatment of septic abortion is to evacuate the infected products of conception as soon as possible. Although mild infection can be treated successfully with broad-spectrum antibiotics given by mouth in the usual dosage, serious infections have to be treated vigorously from the outset. Large doses of penicillin should be given intravenously together with an antibiotic such as cephradine to deal with aerobic organisms and metronidazole to deal with anaerobic organisms. The management of haemorrhage, shock and endotoxic shock is considered in detail in Chapters 60, 61 and 64. In clinical practice consultation with the clinical microbiologist is essential in the management of severe septic complications of abortion.

RECURRENT SPONTANEOUS ABORTION (RSA)

RSA is generally defined as a history of three or more consecutive spontaneous abortions. It is classified as primary if the patient has never had a successful pregnancy and secondary if she has delivered one or more infants before the series of abortions.

Some authorities consider RSA in most cases to be a chance phenomenon (Pritchard & MacDonald 1980), pointing out that whichever of a great variety of treatments is used, pregnancy outcome is ultimately successful in 70–90% of cases. As early as 1962, Javert stressed that psychotherapy was the most important factor in treatment and that whether or not drugs were included in treatment, most series reported a salvage rate of 74–82%. On the other hand, Stray-Pedersen & Stray-Pedersen (1984) calculated that the expected probability of a woman having three consecutive abortions was between 0.3 and 0.4%, but that the actual frequency of habitual abortion was significantly higher, between 0.4 and 0.8%, according to reports by Javert (1967) and by Glass & Golbus (1978). They suggested that the difference between the actual and expected rates indicated that recurrent abortion was not just a random occurrence but the result of specific disorders which needed to be identified in this type of reproductive failure.

Stray-Pedersen & Stray-Pedersen (1984) found that reproductive abnormalities were significantly more frequent in the primary than in the secondary RSA group and also more frequent in couples with second- than first-trimester abortions. The frequency of positive findings also correlated with the number of previous abortions, for in those who had had three repetitive abortions, fewer abnormalities were detected than in women who had had a larger number. In the primary RSA group and in women with first-trimester abortions, the

Table 28.3 Causes of recurrent spontaneous abortion (RSA)

As generally listed		Investigated by Stray-Pedersen & Stray-Pedersen (1984)		
Category	Subdivision	110 couples with cause (56%) in 190 couples with RSA		
Maternal				
Infective	*Brucella* (antibody)	29 positive endometrial cultures (15%)		
	Toxoplasma (culture)			
	Cytomegalovirus (culture)			
	Chlamydia (culture)	(*Ureaplasma urealyticum* 22)		
	Herpes simplex (culture)	(*Toxoplasma gondii* 7)		
Genetic	Chromosomal anomaly	5 — Translocations 2 (probably not significant 1)		
Systemic	Debilitating disease	2 — Ulcerative colitis		
Metabolic	Diabetes			
	Thyroid disease	4 — Hyperthyroid 1 Hypothyroid 3		
Reproductive, endocrinological	Progesterone deficiency	6 — Luteal deficiency		
Anatomical	Uterus	30 — Fixed retroversion	5	(15%)
		Submucous fibroids	4	
		Synechiae	2	
		Abnormal Müllerian fusion	19	
	Cervix	25 — Cervical incompetence (13%)		
Paternal				
Genetic	Chromosomal anomaly	2 — Translocation 1 Probably not significant 1		
Reproductive system	Sperm abnormalities	8 — Polyspermia 1 Oligospermia 7		
No cause found 85 (of 195 couples) = 44%				

Adapted from Stray-Pedersen & Stray-Pederson (1984).

commonest abnormalities they found were malformations of the uterine body and endometrial infections. In women with secondary RSA and second-trimester abortions, cervical incompetence was the most common abnormality.

Reviews, such as the one by Glass & Golbus (1978), list groups of causal factors, but different studies use different classifications of RSA. Some include only primary RSA while others include both primary and secondary types. Some include only women with three or more abortions while others include women with two or more abortions.

Causes of RSA

Women with a history of RSA should be assessed by a diagnostic screening programme which should identify potential reproductive abnormalities. No positive finding should be regarded as the absolute cause of RSA but its detection may indicate necessary treatment. Stray-Pedersen & Stray-Pedersen (1984) investigated 195 couples with three or more previous consecutive spontaneous abortions. They carried out a comprehensive screening programme, kept the couples under observation for 1–9 years afterwards, and were involved in the management of subsequent pregnancies. Table 28.3 lists the maternal and paternal abnormalities found in the 195 couples and illustrates how the findings in this exceptionally careful long-term study compare with causes usually listed. A potential cause for RSA was found in 110 or 56% of the couples they investigated, as follows:

Maternal causes

Endometrial infection was present in 29 of 110 (15%) of women; 22 were positive for *Ureaplasma urealyticum* and seven for *Toxoplasma gondii*. Subsequent pregnancy outcome was significantly improved following treatment of the *U. urealyticum* with doxycycline (200 mg followed by 100 mg daily for 2 weeks). The seven patients with *T. gondii* were treated for 4 weeks with pyrimethamine/sulphadiazine/folinic acid, as described by Stray-Pedersen et al (1978). Four subsequently conceived and three continued to full term. One aborted at 26 weeks; she was found also to have an incompetent cervix.

Genetic causes. Chromosomal abnormalities were found in five of the 390 individuals examined. These included balanced reciprocal translocations in two women, Robertsonian translocation in one man, large satellites on one G-chromosome in one woman and a tendency to breakage close to the centromere of chromosome number 1 in one man. The latter two anomalies were considered to be probably without significance for reproduction.

Although chromosomal abnormalities were clearly not more than occasionally associated with RSA in this investigation, it is important to karyotype both the woman and her partner, for those with abnormal chromosomes, particularly translocation, should be advised to have amniocentesis in subsequent pregnancy to exclude the possibility of fetal chromosomal abnormality since they are at much increased risk (see Chapter 21). Many women disregard this advice however, fearing an increased risk of abortion from amniocentesis.

Systemic disorders. In two women, previously unrecognized ulcerative colitis was detected. Following colectomy and ileostomy, both patients achieved uneventful term pregnancies.

Metabolic causes. Although diabetes and thyroid disease are thought to be associated with RSA, Stray-Pedersen & Stray-Pedersen (1984) found no case of diabetes in their series nor any abnormality of glucose tolerance, although Sutherland & Pritchard (1987) have confirmed the increased risk of abortion in diabetic women. Four cases of thyroid disease were detected, however—one with hyperthyroidism and three with hypothyroidism. Two of the latter achieved normal pregnancies after replacement therapy with thyroxine.

Progesterone deficiency has long been regarded as a potentially important cause of abortion and of RSA. In fact, there is little evidence that abortion results from de novo progesterone deficiency, although progesterone levels may fall when placental function has been disrupted by haemorrhage (Mellows 1983). Radwanska et al (1978) showed that there was no significant difference in plasma progesterone levels between the sixth and the 12th week in pregnancy with successful outcome in women with or without threatened abortion. At least one-third of patients who presented with threatened abortion and proceeded to abort had normal plasma progesterone levels when first sampled (Radwanska et al 1978, Hertz et al 1980). Such findings have not discouraged innumerable obstetricians from treating threatened or recurrent abortion with progesterone or synthetic progestogens or with human chorionic gonadotrophin (hCG) to stimulate progesterone production by the corpus luteum.

Luteal phase deficiency and RSA. Stray-Pedersen & Stray-Pedersen (1984) identified six women with luteal deficiency before pregnancy, diagnosed because the luteal phase lasted less than 10 days in three successive cycles, was combined with low progesterone levels (<15 nmol/l) and histological immaturity of the secretory endometrium as described by Jones (1975).

In the subsequent pregnancies, Stray-Pedersen & Stray-Pedersen treated these patients with hCG in a dose of 3000 iu twice weekly from the fifth to the 14th weeks of gestation. All continued successfully to term. No large randomized control trial of this therapy has yet been published.

A meticulous small study of hCG treatment was conducted in four groups of patients by Sandler & Baillie (1979). Their four groups were: 15 normal primigravidae; 13 pregnant women with three or more abortions treated weekly with 10 000 iu hCG; 10 pregnant women with a history of three or more abortions treated monthly with 40 000 iu hCG, and 18 patients with a history of three or more abortions, given no hCG. There was no difference in the abortion rate in the four groups but a much larger series would have been required to achieve statistical significance. In the group receiving the largest doses of hCG there was actually a fall in plasma progesterone, implying a potentially adverse effect. While treatment with hCG may have a place in the management of RSA its widespread use should meantime be discouraged until larger trials have been reported.

There is certainly some evidence that a defective luteal phase before pregnancy predisposes to subsequent early RSA, the implication being that the deficient corpus luteum cannot maintain early pregnancy. If this deficiency *is* important in human pregnancy failure it can only influence very early pregnancy. Csapo et al (1972) showed that removal of the corpus luteum at 49 ± 2 days after the last period caused abortion in human pregnancy but lutectomy at 61 ± 4 days did not affect pregnancy maintenance. It is therefore unlikely that corpus luteum deficiency causes abortion after 8 weeks' gestation.

Horta et al (1977) found lower progesterone levels in the luteal phase in 10 women with a history of RSA than in 15 control women with normal obstetric histories. When pregnancy subsequently occurred in RSA patients, plasma progesterone levels remained low and abortion occurred. Recently, Daya et al (1988) reported that 40% of women investigated because of a history of RSA suffered from luteal phase deficiency in the non-pregnant state, judged by the histological appearances of luteal phase endometrium and repeated measurements of plasma progesterone. They claimed that daily vaginal administration of 50 mg micronized progesterone in the luteal phase, reinforced by weekly injections of 250 mg 17α-hydroxyprogesterone caproate during pregnancy up to the 12th week, led to successful pregnancy outcome in 81% of patients so far treated. Improvement in the quality of the luteal phase has been claimed for treatment with clomiphene (Garcia et al 1977), hCG and progesterone. There is, however, an urgent need to identify a more reliable method of establishing the diagnosis of luteal phase deficiency than is presently available, and to conduct large and well planned randomized controlled trials.

Progestogens. Progestogens have continued to be prescribed generally for RSA despite the evidence that treatment with them does not improve the outcome of pregnancy. There are at least potential maternal and fetal consequences, apart from the possibility that presently unrecognized long-term effects could later be discovered, similar to those resulting from the administration of diethylstilbestrol (Herbst et al 1971, 1975, 1980, Bibbo et al 1977, Beral & Colwell 1981).

In the mother, progestogen treatment may result in the retention of a dead fetus for 8 weeks or more (Piver et al 1967) and may also lead to prolonged menstrual disturbances after the pregnancy (Turner et al 1966). In the fetus, the effects of progestogens depend on the type of preparation used. Jacobson (1962) recommended that Norethindrone (norethisterone) should not be used in pregnancy after finding that 15 of 80 female infants had been masculinized (and that some of the mothers also showed masculinization effects) after administration of this compound in pregnancy. Wilkins

Table 28.4 Results of four double-blind controlled trials of the treatment of recurrent abortion

Author and drug	Control group			Treatment group		
	Patients	Abortions	Success (%)	Patients	Abortions	Success (%)
Shearman & Garrett (1963)						
17-Hydroxy-progesterone caproate	27	5	82	23	5	78
Goldzicher (1964)						
Metroxyprogesterone acetate	31	5	84	23	5	78
Levine (1964)						
17-Hydroxy-progesterone caproate	12	4	67	12	3	75
Klopper & Macnaughton (1965)						
Quingesterone	15	5	67	18	8	56

(1960) reported masculinization of 70 female infants following maternal ingestion of 17α-ethinyl testosterone or 17α-ethinyl-19-noretestosterone during pregnancy. The effects were worst when the drug had been taken before 12 weeks of pregnancy.

Nowadays, progestogens with such masculinizing potential are no longer used. Although compounds such as 17-hydroxyprogesterone caproate seem unlikely to masculinize the female fetus, they do not appear to provide better pregnancy outcome than controls. Table 28.4 summarizes the findings of four double-blind control studies of progestogens in RSA in which the incidence of successful pregnancy outcome was approximately 70–80% whether treatment was given or not. Those who favour the concept of luteal phase deficiency as a factor in RSA would argue that treatment was begun too late in those studies, usually not being commenced until at least 8 weeks' gestation.

Anatomical causes. Table 28.3 shows that abnormalities of the uterus and cervix were extremely common. Stray-Pedersen & Stray-Pedersen (1984) found that 30 women (15%) had abnormality of the uterus, including fixed retroversion in five and submucous fibroids distorting the uterine cavity in four, intrauterine adhesions (synechiae) in two and disorders associated with abnormal Müllerian fusion in 19. Correcting the retroversion surgically was uniformly successful, they reported, but removing fibroids was apparently successful in only one woman. Treatment of intrauterine adhesions produced only one successful pregnancy. Of eight women with a bicornuate uterus and eight with a major subseptate uterus, all were operated on and eight subsequently carried pregnancies to term. In the others, it was subsequently demonstrated that the reconstruction had been unsuccessful, leaving abnormality of the uterine cavity still present. Cervical incompetence was found in 25 patients and in those with a history of late second-trimester abortion, a Macdonald type of cerclage was performed in the 14th week of subsequent pregnancy. Of the 18 patients who conceived, 13 had successful pregnancies and five aborted. Surprisingly, the majority (13) of the 25 women with cervical incompetence suffered from primary RSA, suggesting that in them the condition was of congenital origin. None had earlier undergone any cervical operation such as amputation or conization. Overall, the pregnancy success rate for cervical incompetence treated by cerclage was 71%.

Paternal causes

Male genetic factors were found in two — one a Robertsonian translocation and one a tendency to breakage close to the centromere of chromosome number 1. This latter finding was considered to be insignificant for reproduction.

Sperm abnormalities were found in eight, with polyspermia (more than 300 million per ml) in one and oligospermia (8–15 million sperms per ml) in seven.

Fetal causes

These are not listed in Table 28.3 but it should be noted from Table 28.1 (Robinson 1975) that of the 90 women with a history of RSA, 26 aborted, 10 in association with a blighted ovum.

Fetal and maternal chromosome anomalies in RSA

Tharapel et al (1985) published a major review of the results from 79 surveys of couples with two or more pregnancy losses (8208 women and 7834 men) and also of the chromosomal anomalies found in 6261 successfully karyotyped abortuses.

In the parents, there was an overall prevalence of major chromosomal abnormalities of 2.9%. This is five to six times higher than that of the general adult population. Approximately 50% of all chromosome abnormalities detected were balanced reciprocal translocations, 24% were Robertsonian translocations, 12% were sex chromosomal mosaicisms in females and the rest consisted of inversions and other sporadic abnormalities. Tharapel et al (1985) advise that parents with two or more idiopathic pregnancy losses should be karyotyped to aid in management and counselling. When a chromosomal abnormality is identified, prenatal diagnosis is indicated in future pregnancies.

In the abortuses, chromosomal abnormalities were frequent. In data from 14 studies, Tharapel et al (1985) noted abnormalities in 2698 of 6261 abortuses which were successfully karyotyped. Table 28.5 lists the findings and shows

Table 28.5 Pooled cytogenetic data on successfully karyotyped abortuses from 14 surveys

Total abortuses	6261
Normal karyotype	3563
Abnormal karyotype	2698
X monosomy	528
XXX and XXY	10
Sex chromosome mosaic	12
Triploidy	428
Tetraploidy	152
Autosomal trisomies (A–G)	1339
Double trisomy	36
Autosomal monosomy	6
Autosomal mosaicism	56
Structural abnormality of autosomes	98
Others	33

Adapted from Tharapel et al (1985).

that the numerical abnormality most often seen was aneuploidy (monosomy and trisomy) followed by polyploidy (triploidy and tetraploidy). Unbalanced structural abnormalities, including duplication and deletion, accounted for a considerable number of abortions.

These findings are in general agreement with the idea that a high proportion of early first-trimester abortuses are grossly abnormal. However, Underwood & Mowbray (1985) point out that these conclusions are based on successfully karyotyped abortuses which probably represent less than 20% of all abortuses since the great majority are anembryonic or associated with a dead fetus whose cells cannot be successfully cultured. Underwood & Mowbray argue that the majority of spontaneous abortions result from immunological causes, discussed below.

Implications of investigating the clinical causes of RSA

While the study by Stray-Pedersen & Stray-Pedersen (1984) was conducted most carefully, it shares with many other clinical studies lack of information about investigations in control women with a normal obstetric history. It is therfore impossible to know how relevant the abnormal findings reported are to the history of RSA.

Nevertheless, the incidence of Müllerian anomalies they observed was 20–60 times higher than that reported in the normal population by Green & Harris (1976). The fact that metroplasty led to a marked improvement in the pregnancy success rate accords with the importance of fundal malformation in RSA (see Chapter 33). While hysterography may be required to establish the diagnosis, the value of a puerperal ultrasound scan in detecting uterine abnormalities after preterm delivery (Bennett 1976) suggests that a post-abortal scan might indicate the cases of RSA with a likely uterine abnormality and the work of Fedele et al (1988) seems to confirm this.

More work on the clinical significance of chronic endometrial infection is required. Stray-Pedersen & Stray-Pedersen noted that the incidence of *Ureaplasma urealyticum* infection in the endocervix was similar to that found in the fertile female population, while the incidence of *Toxoplasma* antibodies among those with habitual abortion did not differ from the overall Norwegian population. Nevertheless, the finding of positive endometrial cultures at least draws attention to a disorder which could be unfavourable for normal pregnancy development. The improved outcomes of pregnancies following eradication of these infections supports the value of the investigation and of the treatment of positive findings.

Pregnancy outcomes

In the 110 couples investigated by Stray-Pedersen & Stray-Pedersen in whom an abnormality was found, 70 subsequently became pregnant and 56 had a successful outcome — a success rate of 80%. In the 85 couples in whom no abnormality was found, 61 became pregnant and 37 were treated by 'tender loving care', with weekly attendance at the hospital and advice about rest and the avoidance of coitus. No hormone therapy was given. Of these, 32 had successful pregnancies — a success rate of 86%. Of the 24 who had no specific treatment and were simply referred back to their own clinic, only eight had a successful outcome — a success rate of 33%. However, the allocation to the two groups was not random, although many agree with Javert (1962) that psychotherapy is of real value in the management of women with a history of RSA.

Immunological causes and treatment of RSA

In recent years there has been much interest in the possibility that RSA is associated with an immunological cause. The basis for this was considered to be the sharing of class 1 major histocompatibility complex (MHC) antigens by mother and father (MacIntyre & Faulk 1979, Beer et al 1981), or sharing of class II MHC antigens (Underwood & Mowbray 1985). As a result, pregnancy fails to induce the antipaternal antibody usually found in successful pregnancies. The absence of this lymphocytotoxic antipaternal antibody is thought to indicate the absence of an immunological blocking factor which normally prevents rejection of the fetus (see Chapter 11).

While controversy remains about the exact immunological mechanism which may predispose to RSA, a review by Underwood & Mowbray (1985) makes clear their belief, and that of other workers in the immunological field, that the great majority of recurrent abortions are associated with an immunological rejection process. They suggest that the incidence of genetic abnormality in these abortuses may have been greatly exaggerated. As they point out, figures of 50% abnormality are frequently reported in such studies without it being made clear that the 50% abnormality comes from the fewer than 20% of abortuses which can successfully be cultured and karyotyped. They suggest that the genetically abnormal fetuses may be aborted without first dying, as do the majority of immunological abortions. In support of this idea, they report that hCG levels in most RSA patients fall days or even weeks before abortion. Only a minority do not do so and may represent those associated with fetal chromosomal abnormalities.

In the experience of Underwood & Mowbray in investigating a large number of RSA couples, the commonest association with RSA after the absence of antipaternal immunity was the presence of triploidy and partial molar pregnancies. They say it is normally assumed that recurrent triploidy is impossible because it would be due to random double fertilization, a highly unlikely event not expected to occur twice in the same woman. Fetal triploidy is found in about 5% of RSA couples having abortions, however, and in one woman, three proven triploid or partial molar pregnancies were seen, followed by normal pregnancy. It may be that diploid spermatozoa were the explanation of the recurrence of the triploid pregnancies. The authors now recommend screening husbands for this possibility since separating haploid from diploid spermatozoa is now a practical procedure which can be used for treatment.

Immunological treatment

An understanding of the immunological basis for RSA has lagged behind attempts to treat it. Treatment has been based on the assumption that some fault in maternal immunization is responsible for the abortion. Taylor & Faulk (1981) considered that because of shared antigens in the parents, maternal immunization against placental polymorphic determinants could not occur. They therefore attempted to produce cross-reacting antibodies by immunization with buffy coat leukocytes from many unrelated donors. Several donors were used on each of several occasions, both before and during the next pregnancy. Obviously the donors had to be carefully matched for red cell antigens but rhesus-incompatible donors were not used. Of the four RSA patients treated, three had normal pregnancies and the fourth was in the 28th week of pregnancy at the time the report was published.

Beer et al (1983) immunized 38 women with leukocytes taken only from their husbands. At the time of their report, 20 had not achieved pregnancy but in the remaining 18, four (22%) had delivered a living child, 10 (56%) were more than 16 weeks' pregnant, two (11%) had aborted and two (11%) had had ectopic pregnancies. There were no controls.

Mowbray et al (1985) reported a very important control trial of treatment of women with RSA by immunizing once with either paternal or maternal cells. In this paired sequential double-blind trial, women were admitted with a history of either primary or secondary RSA. Criteria for inclusion to the trial were:

1. No detectable antibody demonstrable against paternal lymphocytes;

Table 28.6 Outcome of pregnancies in trial

	Outcome			
Source of cells	Live	Abortion	Total	Live (%)
Husband	17	5	22	77
Wife	10	17	27	37
Total	27	22	49	55

After Mowbray et al (1985).

Table 28.7 Outcome of pregnancies in trial by previous number of live births

		Outcome		
Previous live births	Source of cells	Success	Abortion	Success (%)
0	Husband	12	4	75
	Wife	8	15	35
1	Husband	5	1	32
	Wife	2	2	50

After Mowbray et al (1985).

2. No cause found for the abortions;
3. Women were rhesus-positive;
4. Women were seen before pregnancy had occurred;
5. Participants were resident in the UK.

Women admitted to the trial subsequently received a preparation of lymphocytes, either from their husband or from themselves, given intravenously together with additional intradermal and subcutaneous injections of the same lymphocyte preparations. Allocation was random. Results are shown in Table 28.6. At the completion of the trial, results were available in 47 patients. Of the 22 treated with their husband's lymphocytes, 17 achieved live pregnancies (77%) and only five aborted. Of the 27 women who received their own cells, however, only 10 delivered live infants and 17 aborted — a success rate of 37%.

Table 28.7 shows that the results were influenced by whether the woman had a history of primary or secondary RSA. With primary RSA, immunization with the husband's cells gave a success rate of 75%, compared with 35% for women who received their own cells. With secondary RSA, the success rate following injection of paternal lymphocytes was 82% compared with 50% following injection of the woman's own cells.

Subsequently, Mowbray (1986) reported having immunized 414 women with paternal lymphocytes with a continuing success rate just below 80%. Some of the failures of treatment had been shown to have non-recurrent genetic causes for abortion, predominantly trisomy.

Underwood et al (1986) also reported that approximately 50% of women produced detectable cytotoxic antipaternal antibody following a single immunization with paternal lymphocytes. Of the cytotoxic antibody-positive women, 80%

had successful pregnancies if they fell pregnant within 50 days of immunization. Subsequently, however, the success rate declined, mainly in antibody-negative women. A single immunization therefore seems to be effective in some women only for a short time and booster immunization may be useful in women who do not rapidly become pregnant.

A randomized double-blind control trial is a powerful research tool and the large difference found by Mowbray et al (1985) between women immunized with their husband's lymphocytes and those immunized with their own cells is very impressive and convincing. However, the results of the trial were significant not so much because the results in the women immunized by paternal lymphocytes were so good, but because the results in those receiving their own lymphocytes were so bad. The success rate of 77% in the women immunized with paternal lymphocytes is on a par with the treated and control cases in Table 28.4 illustrating randomized controlled trials of progestogens in RSA. They are also similar to the 86% success rate obtained with counselling and psychological support achieved by Stray-Pedersen & Stray-Pedersen (1984), although that was not a randomized allocation. However, the success rate of 33% observed in women who were given no specific antenatal care by Stray-Pedersen & Stray-Pedersen was similar to the women immunized with their own cells in the study by Mowbray et al (1985). The poor results in controls in the study by Mowbray et al may reflect recruitment of women with an exceptionally large number of previous abortions.

While there seem to be more optimists than pessimists about immunotherapy by RSA in the UK, current American opinion seems cautious. Simpson (1986) writes: 'especially controversial are treatment programs that include sensitisation of women with lymphocytes from either their husband or from a typed specific donor'. However, he continues: 'physicians desiring couples to be evaluated for an immunological basis for fetal wastage should refer these patients to a center actively investigating this subject'. Perhaps he was mainly concerned to ensure that couples received expert immunological care. Much work is in progress and the true value of immunotherapy for RSA should be established before long.

Lupus anticoagulant

The lupus anticoagulant is an immunoglobulin which is sometimes but not always associated with systemic lupus erythematosus. It prolongs phospholipid-dependent coagulation times and is paradoxically associated with an increased risk of thrombotic episodes (Lubbe et al 1984). Table 28.8 shows the indications on which Lubbe and colleagues proceed to investigate for the possible presence of lupus anticoagulant in pregnancy. Repeated first-trimester spontaneous abortions are common as are unexpected intrauterine deaths in the second or third trimester. The major feature in the placentas examined in such pregnancies is infarction, usually in the form of multiple scattered infarcts at different stages of evolution. Thrombotic episodes are common and should always raise suspicion of the lupus anticoagulant especially when other features in Table 28.8 are present.

Table 28.8 Indications for investigating for lupus anticoagulant in pregnancy

Fetal losses
Repetitive in first trimester
Unexpected in second or third trimester
Clinical suspicion or activity of systemic lupus erythematosus
Deep venous or arterial thrombosis
Positive antinuclear antibody test
Platelet count reduced to $<175\times 10^9/l$
Biologically false positive Venereal Disease Research Laboratories test
Positive anti-smooth muscle antibody test

From Lubbe et al (1984).

Table 28.9 Outcome of pregnancies in 10 women with lupus anticoagulant with and without treatment with prednisone and aspirin

				Fetal losses		
Treatment	No. of patients	Pregnancies	Live births	0–20 weeks	21–28 weeks	29–40 weeks
Without	10	28	3	9	8	8
With	10	7	6	1	–	–

After Lubbe et al (1984).

Diagnosis. Lubbe et al (1984) describe extensive serological and haematological investigations. The most useful indicators of the presence of the lupus anticoagulant are prolongation of the activated partial thromboplastin time (APTT) and of the kaolin clotting time (KCT; see Chapter 38).

Treatment. The importance of detecting the lupus anticoagulant in women with RSA or repeated fetal losses in later pregnancy is that the disturbed clotting can be returned to normal by administration of prednisone in immunosuppressive doses (40–60 mg/day) together with aspirin (75 mg/day) to counteract platelet adhesiveness. Table 28.9 shows that in the 10 women with lupus anticoagulant studied by Lubbe et al (1984) there had been 28 pregnancies before the diagnosis was established. Of these, livebirth occurred in only three and fetal loss occurred before 20 weeks in nine, between 21 and 28 weeks in eight and after 29 weeks in eight. Subsequently, seven of the 10 women again became pregnant and on treatment with prednisone and aspirin, six had livebirths and only one had an early pregnancy loss.

Complications of treatment. A Cushingoid facies developed in most of the women treated with prednisone over a mean period of 17 weeks. Complete resolution of the facies occurred on reduction or discontinuation of prednisone. No complications were ascribable to the aspirin therapy; the dose was equivalent only to one paediatric tablet per day.

Implications for clinical obstetrics. The incidence of this disorder remains unknown but in the near future the incidence is likely to be resolved because an antibody to cardiolipin, measured by an enzyme-linked immunosorbent assay, identifies specifically and early in pregnancy women at risk of fetal deterioration or death during apparently normal pregnancy as the result of developing the lupus anticoagulant.

BEREAVEMENT REACTION FOLLOWING SPONTANEOUS ABORTION

It is generally suggested that emotional symptoms are frequent after spontaneous abortion (Corney & Horton 1974, Siebel & Graves 1980, Leppert & Pahlika 1984, Oakley et al 1984). The findings have been difficult to evaluate because none of the studies used standardized measures to assess psychiatric symptoms and some enquiries were made years after the abortion. Friedman & Gath (1988) have conducted a study using standardized psychiatric measures to examine a representative sample of women. They found that 4 weeks after spontaneous abortion, women were four times as likely to be suffering from significant depression as women in the general population. The psychological response to abortion was uniformly one of depression. The intensity of the reaction was greater in women with no living child, in those who had had one or more abortions previously and in those whose abortion was in the second, rather than in the first trimester of pregnancy.

Following spontaneous abortion, many women require support and reassurance before making an adequate recovery from the pregnancy loss. When counselling, it is essential for the obstetrician to have as much factual information as possible about the abortion. In particular, it is helpful to have available the pathology report on the fetus and placenta, as well as various relevant pathology and microbiology reports. Counselling in such cases needs to be conducted in much the same way as that following stillbirth or neonatal death (see Chapter 67).

REFERENCES

Beard R W 1985 Miscarriage or abortion. Lancet ii: 122–123

Beer A E, Quebbeman J F, Ayers J W T, Haines R F 1981 Major histocompatibility complex antigens, maternal and paternal immune response and chronic habitual abortions in humans. American Journal of Obstetrics and Gynecology 141: 987–998

Beer A E, Quebbeman J F, Semprini A E, Smouse P E, Haines R F 1983 Recurrent abortion: analysis of the roles of parental sharing of histocompatibility antigens and maternal immunological responses to paternal antigens. In: Isogima S, Billington N D (eds) Reproductive immunology. Elsevier Science Publishers, Amsterdam, pp 185–195

Beischer N A, Mackay E V 1986 Bleeding in early pregnancy. In: Beischer N A, Mackay E V (eds) Obstetrics and the newborn. Baillière Tindall, London, p 140

Bennett M J 1976 Puerperal ultrasonic hysterography in the diagnosis of congenital uterine malformation. British Journal of Obstetrics and Gynaecology 83: 389

Bennett M J, Kerr-Wilson R H J 1980 Evaluation of threatened abortion by ultrasound. International Journal of Gynaecology and Obstetrics 17: 382–384

Beral V, Colwell L 1981 Randomised trial of high doses of stilboestrol and ethisterone in pregnancy: long term follow up of the children. Journal of Epidemiology and Community Health 35: 155–160

Bibbo M, Gill W B, Azizi F et al 1977 Follow up study of male and female offspring of DES-exposed mothers. Obstetrics and Gynecology 49: 1–8

Blott M, Greenough A, Nicolaides K H, Moserso G, Gibb D, Campbell S 1987 Fetal breathing movements as predictor of favourable pregnancy outcome after oligohydramnios due to membrane rupture in second trimester. Lancet ii: 129–131

Boué A, Boué J 1978 Chromosomal anomalies associated with fetal malformation. In: Scrimgeour J B (ed) Towards the prevention of fetal malformation. Edinburgh University Press, Edinburgh

Cameron I I, Baird D T 1984 The use of 16,16-dimethyl trans Δ2 prostaglandin E methyl ester (gemeprost) vaginal pessary for termination of pregnancy in early second trimester. A comparison with extra-amniotic prostaglandin E_2. British Journal of Obstetrics and Gynaecology 91: 1136–1140

Chamberlain G V P, Phillips E. Howlett B et al 1978 British births, 1970, vol 2. Obstetric care. Heinemann Medical, London, p 56

Confidential Enquiries into Maternal Deaths in England & Wales. (1982–1984). HMSO, London

Corney R T, Horton F T 1974 Pathological grief following spontaneous abortion. American Journal of Psychiatry 131: 825–827

Csapo A I, Pulkkinen M O, Ruttner B et al 1972 The significance of human corpus luteum in pregnancy maintenance. American Journal of Obstetrics and Gynecology 112: 1061–1067

Daya S, Ward S, Burrows E 1988 Progesterone profiles in luteal phase defect cycles and outcome of progesterone treatment in patients with recurrent spontaneous abortion. American Journal of Obstetrics and Gynecology 158: 225–232

Evans J H, Beischer N A 1970 The prognosis of threatened abortion. Medical Journal of Australia 2: 165–168

Fedele L, Dorta M, Vercellini P, Brioschi D, Candiane G B 1988 Ultrasound in the diagnosis of unicornuate uterus. Obstetrics and Gynecology 71: 274–277

Federick J, Adelstein P 1978 Factors associated with low birthweight of infants delivered at term. British Journal of Obstetrics and Gynaecology 85: 1–7

Friedman T, Gath D 1988 The psychiatric consequences of spontaneous abortion (submitted for publication)

Garcia J, Jones G S, Wentz A C 1977 The use of clomiphene citrate. Fertility and Sterility 28: 707

Glass R H, Golbus M S 1978 Habitual abortion. Fertility and Sterility 29: 257–265

Goldzicher J W 1964 Double blind trial of a progesterone in habitual abortion. Journal of the American Medical Association 188: 651–654

Green L K, Harris 1976 Uterine anomalies. Frequency of diagnosis and associated obstetric complications. Obstetrics and Gynecology 47: 427–429

Herbst A L, Ulfelder H, Poskanzer D C 1971 Adenocarcinoma of the vagina; association of maternal stilbestrol therapy with tumor appearance in young women. New England Journal of Medicine 284: 878–881

Herbst A L, Poskanzer D C, Roberg J J, Friedlander L, Scully R E 1975 Prenatal exposure to stilbestrol; a prospective comparison of exposed female offspring with unexposed controls. New England Journal of Medicine 292: 334–339

Herbst A L, Hubby M M, Blough R R, Azizi F 1980 A comparison of pregnancy experience in DES-exposed and DES-unexposed daughters. Journal of Reproductive Medicine 24: 62–69

Hertig A T, Sheldon W H 1943 Minimal criteria required to prove prima facie case of traumatic abortion or miscarriage. An analysis of 1,000 spontaneous abortions. Annals of Surgery 117: 596–606

Hertz J B, Larsen J F, Arends J et al 1980 Progesterone and human chorionic gonadotrophin in serum and pregnenediol in urine in threatened abortion. Acta Obstetricia et Gynecologica Scandinavica 59: 23–27

Horta J L H, Fernandez J G, Soto de Leon B et al 1977 Direct evidence of luteal insufficiency in women with habitual abortion. Obstetrics and Gynecology 49: 705–708

Jacobson B D 1962 Hazards of norethisterone during pregnancy. American Journal of Obstetrics and Gynecology 84: 962–968
Jaschevatsky O E, Shalit A, Grunstein S, Kaplanski J, Danon A 1983 Increased decidual prostaglandin E concentration in human abortion. British Journal of Obstetrics and Gynaecology 90: 958
Javert C T 1962 Further follow up on habitual abortion. American Journal of Obstetrics and Gynecology 84: 962–968
Javert C T 1967 Spontaneous and habitual abortion. McGraw-Hill, New York
Jeffcoate N 1975 Principles of gynaecology, 3rd edn. Butterworths, London
Johnson F W 1985 Abortion due to infection with *Chlamydia psittaci* in a sheep farmer's wife. British Medical Journal [Clinical Research] 290: 592–594
Jones G E S 1975 Luteal phase defects. In: Behrman S J, Kestner R W (eds) Progress in infertility. Little, Brown, Boston
Jouppila P, Huhtaniemi I, Tapaneinen J 1980 Early pregnancy failure: a study by ultrasonic and hormonal methods. Obstetrics and Gynecology 55: 42–47
Kilbride H W, Thibeault D N, Yast J, Manlik D, Grundy H O 1988 Fetal breathing is not a predictor of pulmonary hypoplasia in pregnancies complicated by oligohydramnios. Lancet i: 305–306
Kline J, Stein Z A, Susser M et al 1977 Smoking: a risk factor for spontaneous abortion. New England Journal of Medicine 297: 793–796
Kline J, Shrout P E, Stein Z A et al 1978 An epidemiological study of the role of gravidity in spontaneous abortion. Early Human Development 1: 345–356
Klopper A, Macnaughton M 1965 Hormones in recurrent abortion. Journal of Obstetrics and Gynaecology of the British Commonwealth 72: 1022–1028
Leppert P C, Pahlika B S 1984 Grieving characteristics after spontaneous abortions: a management approach. Obstetrics and Gynecology 64: 119–122
Levine L 1964 Habitual abortion: a controlled study of progestational therapy. Western Journal of Surgery Obstetrics and Gynecology 72: 30–36
Lubbe W F, Butter W S, Palmer S J, Liggins G C 1984 Lupus anticoagulant in pregnancy. British Journal of Obstetrics and Gynaecology 91: 357–363
MacDonald I A 1957 Suture of the cervix for inevitable miscarriage. Journal of Obstetrics and Gynaecology of the British Commonwealth 64: 346–350
MacKenzie I Z, Embrey M P 1976 Single extra-amniotic injection of prostaglandins to induce abortion. British Journal of Obstetrics and Gynaecology 83: 505
McIntyre J A, Faulk W P 1979 Maternal blocking factors in human pregnancy are found in plasma not in serum. Lancet ii: 821–823
Mellows H J 1983 Treatment of threatened and recurrent abortion. In: Lewis P J (ed) Clinical pharmacology in obstetrics. Wright P S G, Bristol, pp 166–181
Mikamo K 1970 Anatomic and chromosomal anomalies in spontaneous abortion. American Journal of Obstetrics and Gynecology 106: 243–254
Miller J F, Williamson E, Glue J et al 1980 Fetal loss after implantation. A prospective study. Lancet ii: 554–556
Moessinger A C, Fox H E, Higgins A, Rey H R, Al Haideri M 1987 Fetal breathing movements are not a reliable predictor of continued lung development in pregnancies complicated by oligohydramnios. Lancet ii: 1297–1300
Mowbray J F 1986 Effect of immunisation with paternal cells in recurrent spontaneous abortion. Journal of Reproduction and Immunology (suppl): 1–178
Mowbray J F, Gibbings C, Liddell H, Regnald P W, Underwood J L, Beard R W 1985 Controlled trial of treatment of recurrent spontaneous abortion by immunisation with paternal cells. Lancet i: 941–943
Naylor A F, Warburton D 1979 Sequential analysis of spontaneous abortion. II. Collaborative study data show that gravidity determines a very substantial rise in risk. Fertility and Sterility 31: 282–286
Oakley A, McPherson A, Roberts H 1984 Miscarriage. Fontana, London
Peckham C H 1970 Uterine bleeding during pregnancy. Obstetrics and Gynecology 35: 937–941
Piver M S, Bolognese R J, Feldman J D 1967 Long acting progesterone as a cause of missed abortion. American Journal of Obstetrics and Gynecology 97: 579–581
Pritchard J A, MacDonald P C 1980 In: Pritchard J A, MacDonald P C (eds) Abortion. Williams obstetrics, 16th edn. Appleton-Century-Crofts, New York, pp 587–621
Radwanska E, Frankenberg J, Allen E 1978 Plasma progesterone levels in normal and abnormal early human pregnancy. Fertility and Sterility 30: 398–402
Report of the Committee of the Working of the Aborton Act 1974 Chairman the Hon Mrs Justice Lane, Vol. 1, HMSO, London
Report of Fetal Viability and Clinical Practice 1985 Royal College of Obstetricians and Gynaecologists, London
Roberts C J, Lloyd S 1973 Area differences in spontaneous abortion rates in South Wales and their relation to neural tube defect incidence. British Medical Journal 4: 20–22
Roberts C J, Lowe C R 1975 Where have all the conceptions gone? Lancet i: 498
Robinson H P 1972a Sonar in the management of abortion. Journal of Obstetrics and Gynaecology of the British Commonwealth 79: 90–94
Robinson H P 1972b Detection of fetal heart movement in the first trimester of pregnancy using pulsed ultrasound. British Medical Journal 4: 466–468
Robinson H P 1975 The diagnosis of early pregnancy failure by sonar. British Journal of Obstetrics and Gynacology 82: 849–857
Robinson H P 1978 Normal development in early pregnancy. In: de Vlieger M, Kazner E, Kossot G et al (eds) Handbook of clinical ultrasound. Wiley, New York, pp 121–134
Sandler S W, Baillie P 1979 The use of human chorionic gonadotropins in recurrent abortion. South African Medical Journal 55: 832–835
Shearman R P, Garrett W J 1963 Double blind study of effect of 17-hydroxyprogesterone caproate on abortion rate. British Medical Journal 1: 292–295
Shirodkar V N 1960 Habitual abortion in the second trimester. In: Shirodkar V N (ed) Contributions to obstetrics and gynaecology. Livingstone, Edinburgh
Siebel M, Graves W 1980 The psychological implications of spontaneous abortions. Journal of Reproductive Medicine 25: 161–165
Simpson J L 1986 Fetal wastage. In: Gabbe S G, Niebyl J R, Simpson J L (eds) Obstetrics. Churchill Livingstone, New York, pp 651–673
Smith C, Southern H, Lehmann L 1970 Bacteraemia in septic abortion. Obstetrics and Gynecology 35: 704
Smith C, Gregori C A, Breen J L 1978 Ultrasonography in threatened abortion. Obstetrics and Gynecology 51: 173
South J, Naldrett J 1973 The effect of vaginal bleeding in early pregnancy on the infant born after the 28th week of pregnancy. Journal of Obstetrics and Gynaecology of the British Commonwealth 80: 236–241
Stray-Pedersen B, Stray-Pedersen S 1984 Etiologic factors and subsequent reproductive performance in 195 couples with a prior history of habitual abortion. American Journal of Obstetrics and Gynecology 148: 140–146
Stray-Pedersen B, Eng J, Reikvam T M 1978 Uterine *T. mycoplasma* colonization in reproductive failure. American Journal of Obstetrics and Gynecology 130: 307
Sutherland H W, Pritchard C W 1987 Increased incidence of spontaneous abortion in pregnancies complicated by maternal diabetes mellitus. American Journal of Obstetrics and Gynecology 156: 135–138
Taylor C, Faulk W P 1981 Prevention of recurrent abortion with leucocyte transfusions. Lancet ii: 68–69
Tharapel A T, Tharapel S A, Bannerman R M 1985 Recurrent pregnancy losses and parental chromosome abnormalities: a review. British Journal of Obstetrics and Gynaecology 92: 899–914
Thibeault D N, Beatty E C, Hall R T, Bowen S K, O'Neill D H 1985 Neonatal pulmonary hypoplasia with premature rupture of the fetal membranes and oligohydramnios. Journal of Pediatrics 107: 273–277
Thomas I T, Smith D W 1974 Oligohydramnios, cause of the non-renal features of Potters' syndrome, including pulmonary hypoplasia. Journal of Pediatrics 84: 811–814
Thompson J F, Lein J N 1961 Fetal survival following threatened abortion. Obstetrics and Gynecology 18: 40–43
Turnbull E P N, Walker J 1956 The outcome of pregnancy complicated by threatened abortion. Journal of Obstetrics and Gynaecology of the British Empire 63: 553–559
Turner S J, Mizrek G B, Feldman G L 1966 Prolonged gynecologic and endocrine manifestations subsequent on medroxyprogesterone acetate during pregnancy. American Journal of Obstetrics and Gynecology 95: 222–227

Underwood J L, Mowbray J F 1985 Treatment of recurrent spontaneous abortion. Clinics in Immunology and Allergy 5: 33–42
Underwood J L, Day J D J, Mowbray J F 1986 Correlations of antibodies with success rate following immunisation with paternal cells for recurrent spontaneous abortion. Journal of Reproduction and Immunology (suppl): 1–178
Urquhart D R, Fisk N M 1988 Transvaginal ultrasound in suspected ectopic pregnancy. British Medical Journal 296: 465–466
Varma T, Patel R, Pillai U 1986 Ultrasound assessment of the cervix. Acta Obstetricia et Gynecologica Scandinavica 65: 229–233
WHO 1970 Spontaneous and induced abortion. WHO Technical Report Series no 41, Geneva
Wilkins L 1960 Masculinization of female fetus due to use of orally given progestogens. Journal of the American Medical Association 10: 118–122
Williams P, Johnson B, Vessey M 1975 Septic abortion in women using intrauterine devices. British Medical Journal 4: 263

29

Wendy Savage

Therapeutic abortion

INTRODUCTION

It is estimated that every year in the world, 40–60 million abortions are induced, that is between one-quarter to one-third of all known conceptions, irrespective of the legal status of this procedure (Tietze & Henshaw 1986). In countries where the law does not permit abortion, mostly in the Third World, a heavy toll is paid by women resorting to this method of controlling their unwanted fertility (Measham et al 1983). Septic abortion is still a major cause of maternal mortality in these countries (Liskin 1980, Kahn et al 1986) and leads to much ill health and subsequent infertility due to chronic pelvic inflammatory disease. The effect on maternal mortality following a change in the previously liberal law in Romania is shown clearly in Figure 29.1. The birth rate climbed initially then fell slowly as the death rate from illegal abortion rose — an important natural experiment. This needs to be kept in mind as obstetricians who witnessed such deaths in their early professional lives retire. The majority of consultants in the UK have been trained since the 1967 Abortion Act became law and will have no personal experience of these tragedies.

In the 20 years since the law was changed in the UK, liberalization of abortion legislation has occurred throughout the world, and now about two-thirds of the global population live in countries in which there is at least a possibility of obtaining a legal abortion (Fig. 29.2). In the UK the changes in the law in other countries have been reflected by the nationalities of those women who travel to the UK to obtain abortions. The number rose from 5000 in 1969 to a peak of 56 000 in 1973 and has remained around 30 000 a year

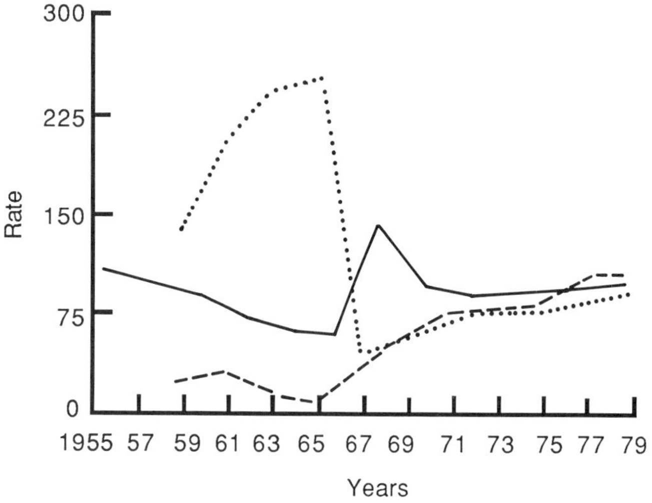

Fig. 29.1 Number of known abortions (. . .) and livebirths (—) per 1000 women aged 15–44 years and number of deaths attributed to abortion per million women aged 15–44 years (— — —) in Romania from 1955 to 1979.

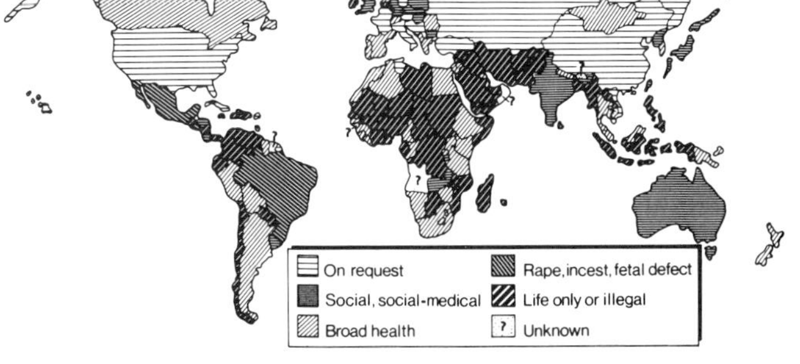

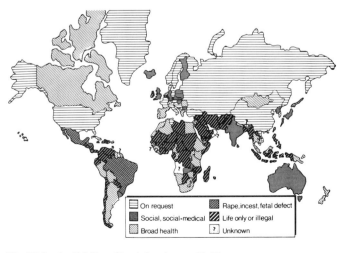

Fig. 29.2 Availability of legal abortion worldwide.

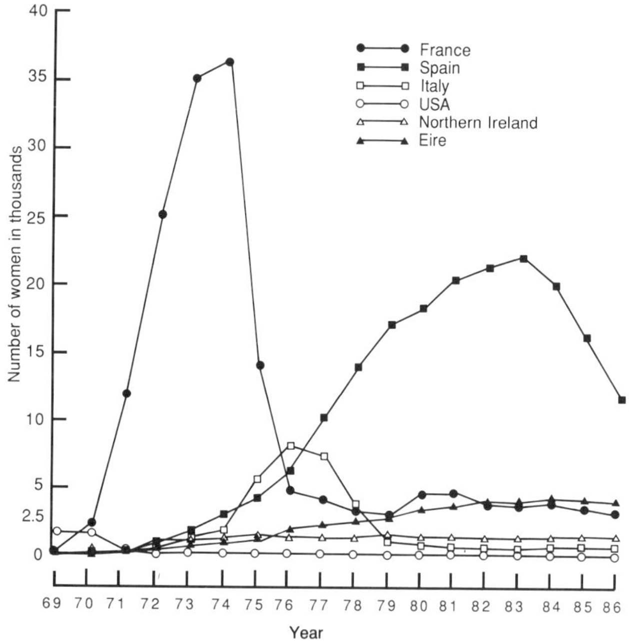

Fig. 29.3 Number of foreign women and those from Northern Ireland having abortions in England and Wales between 1969 and 1986. From Office of Population Censuses and Surveys figures.

since 1975 (Fig. 29.3). The injustice that those who had money to travel were able to terminate their pregnancies whilst poor women could not has been used by well-known women in Italy, France and Spain to further the public debate, which led to the law being changed in these predominantly Catholic countries.

This change in the medical and legal climate has aroused strong resistance from the antiabortion lobby, many of whom have religious objections to abortion in almost any circumstance. The bombing of clinics and demonstrations outside them aimed at persuading women to change their minds have not been seen in the UK, unlike in the USA or New Zealand; pressure through Parliament or the law has been the main thrust of the campaign in the UK.

In Eire a referendum in 1983 led to the unborn child being protected by law; an unsuccessful attempt to do this in the UK was made by Enoch Powell in 1985.

Abortion is unique amongst medical operations in that the interests of the woman are best served by the destruction of the developing fetus—a potential human being. Some doctors hold that this position can rarely be right, and the debate about the ethics of abortion will continue as long as there is need for the operation. The pragmatic view—that if a woman is going to terminate a pregnancy then it is better done quickly and safely by a doctor rather than allowing her to risk her life and future health in unqualified hands—is held by an increasing proportion of physicians and nurses. This reflects the experience since the law was changed (BMJ Leader 1981) and the climate in society in general; polls have shown that 70–80% of those sampled believe that the decision to abort a pregnancy should be taken by the woman in consultation with her doctor—a position a long way from the law as it stands at present (Francome 1984).

As the world population has now reached 5 billion and the rate of increase is approximately 1 billion every 10 years, abortion is likely to be used increasingly to limit the growth of population in the Third World (Cook & Dickens 1982).

HISTORY AND INCIDENCE OF LEGAL ABORTION

Induced abortion has been described in every preliterate culture studied, and seems to have existed in some form or another in all those with written records. In England from 1307 to 1803, abortion 'at the woman's will' before quickening was not a crime, and even after this stage was only a misdemeanour; the same was true in the USA from 1607 to 1928 (David 1981).

Several laws were passed in the 19th century, culminating in the 1861 Offences Against the Person Act which made surgical abortion a crime punishable by life imprisonment in England and Wales. This law did not apply to Scotland, which allowed Professor Dugald Baird to embark on a cautiously liberal policy of abortion in Aberdeen from the 1940s.

In 1929 the Infant Life Preservation Act was passed in order to close a gap in the legislation between abortion and infanticide, i.e. a child being killed at the moment of birth. This has rarely been invoked but is of importance in that it mentions that 28 weeks' gestation is prima-facie evidence of viability; this is referred to in the 1967 Abortion Act (House of Lords Select Committee 1987).

In the 1930s, the high rate of maternal mortality, which reached a peak of 6 per 1000 women in 1933, and to which illegal abortion made an increasing contribution, prompted the British Medical Association (BMA) to set up a committee to look into this tragic loss of life. Despite internal efforts to prevent the publication of their report, the committee recommended in 1936 that abortion should be legalized on grounds of the physical and mental health of the woman, and on social grounds, which they said was a 'matter for consideration by the community as a whole, and not by the medical profession alone' (British Medical Association 1936). The Government then set up the Birkett Committee to examine the question of abortion in 1937. The gynaecologist Aleck Bourne performed an abortion on a 14-year-old girl raped by two soldiers in 1938 and reported his action to the police. His subsequent trial and acquittal provided a precedent that allowed doctors to do an abortion if they considered that continuing the pregnancy 'was likely to render a woman a mental or physical wreck' (Hindell & Simms 1971).

After World War II legal cases and private members' bills were discussed each decade, until the thalidomide disaster raised public consciousness. Increasing parliamentary lobbying by the Abortion Law Reform Association changed the political climate. In 1966, 30 years after the BMA recommendation, David Steel introduced the Medical Termination of Pregnancy Bill which became law in October 1967 and came into force in April 1968. The lack of financial and administrative planning has shaped the services which are available for women in Britain today, excluding those in Northern Ireland where the Act does not apply.

THE PRESENT LAW AND ITS EFFECTS

The 1967 Act allowed women to have a legal abortion if two doctors agreed that continuance of the pregnancy was a threat to her life (clause 1), or to her mental or physical health (clause 2), greater than if the pregnancy was terminated. The importance of social circumstances was acknowledged and the effect on the mental or physical health of an existing child or children (clause 3) was included. Eugenic grounds were recognized in clause 4 which allows abortion if there is a substantial risk of fetal abnormality. The clauses or statutory grounds relate to the form which must be completed before or within 24 hours of an abortion being carried out by doctors who have seen and examined the woman. In an emergency there is another form which only requires the signature of one doctor to certify that the woman's life is in immediate danger, but this is rarely used—only six times out of 147 619 operations performed in 1986 (Office of Population Censuses and Survey).

Some 89% of forms in 1986 gave clause 2, while only 9.5% used clause 3 as the indication for abortion. In all, 1.2% were solely on clause 4, of which the majority were done in the NHS, making up 2.3% of NHS abortions compared with 0.3% of those in the non-NHS. In addition only 1.5% of all abortions were done at 20 weeks' gestation and later; almost 18% of all abortions done because of a risk of fetal abnormality were done as late as this.

The rate of abortion in England and Wales rose rapidly in the first few years after the Act was passed and by 1972 had reached 11.3 per 1000 women aged 15 to 44 years. By the 1980s the rate was relatively stable at just over 12 per 1000 women (Fig. 29.4), which is low by international standards. The provisional figure for 1986 is 13.42 per 1000. Countries in parts of Eastern Europe and Russia where abortion is used as a method of fertility regulation have rates which are 3–5 times as high. The USA and Singapore have rates twice that of the UK, while Scandinavian countries' rates are about 1.5 times times greater (Fig. 29.5). The abortion ratio (the number of abortions per 100 known pregnancies) ranges from about 1 in India to 100 in Poland, while in England and Wales it was 21 and in Scotland 15.2 in 1984.

In the UK the collection of these statistics is facilitated by the statutory duty laid upon doctors to complete yet another form after performing an abortion; these can be

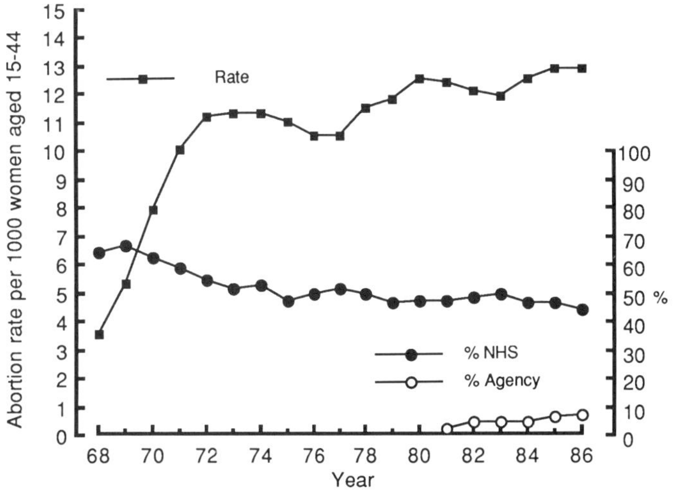

Fig. 29.4 Legal abortions carried out on residents of England and Wales between 1968 and 1986. Abortion rate is given per thousand women aged 15–44. From Office of Population Censuses and Surveys figures and Registrar General abortion statistics.

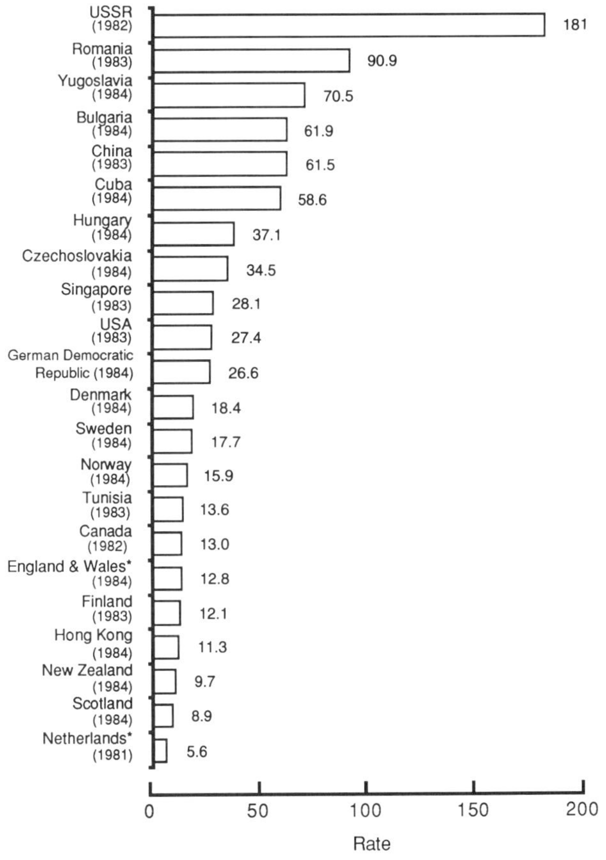

* Residents only

Fig. 29.5 Legal abortion rate per 1000 women aged 15–44: selected areas. Data are from latest available year.

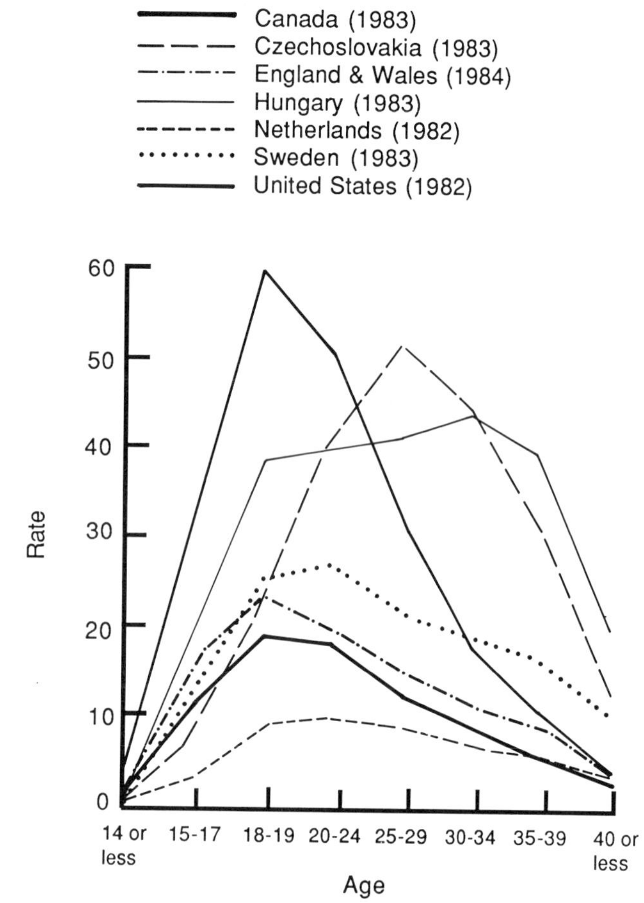

Fig. 29.6a Legal abortion rate per 1000 women by age: selected areas. Data are from latest available year.

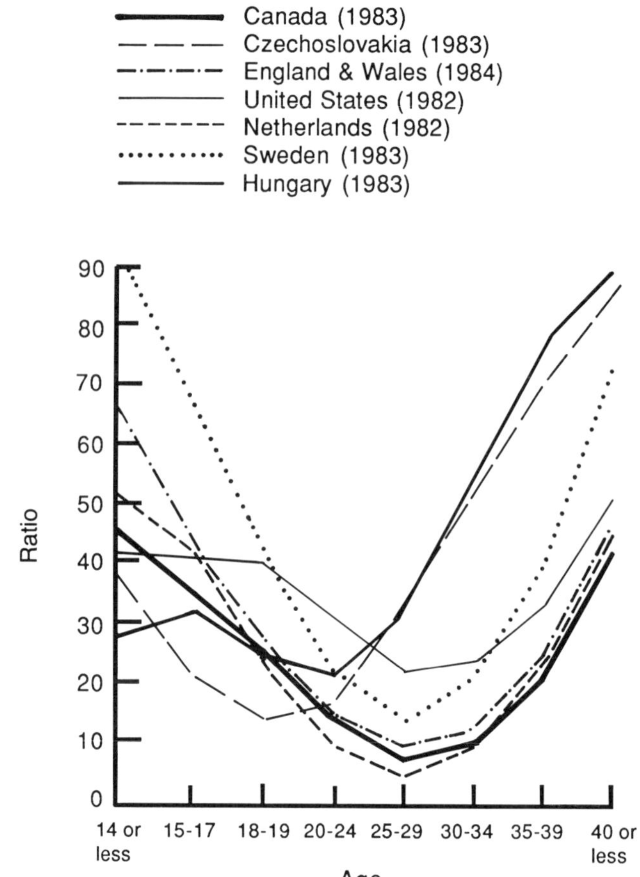

Fig. 29.6b Legal abortion ratio per 100 known pregnancies (legal abortions plus livebirths 6 months later) by age of woman: selected areas. Data are from latest available year.

compared with the long-established system of birth and death registration. In many countries the same reliance cannot be placed upon official statistics, which probably underestimate considerably the number of operations performed legally. The rate of abortion is lowest in women at the extremes of reproductive life, whereas the abortion ratio is highest (Fig. 29.6). In western countries single women have higher abortion rates than married women of the same age. In Singapore and China extramarital pregnancy is socially unacceptable and, as in Japan, the majority of abortions are carried out on married women in their 20s. In the UK about half of all operations are performed on NHS premises; the persistence of the inequalities in provision led to some districts entering into agency agreements with the non-profit-making sector, notably in the West Midlands Region. Since this solution was introduced in 1981, about 4% of women have had their pregnancies terminated outside the NHS but paid for by the NHS (see Fig. 29.4).

MORBIDITY AND MORTALITY

Abortion has been a leading cause of maternal mortality in the UK until the last decade and sepsis was a major cause of abortion deaths (Fig. 29.7). Legally induced abortion is a very safe operation and the operation most frequently performed outside the NHS. Over 2 million abortions have now been done since the law was changed, and the proportion of women operated on in the first trimester has risen from 65% to over 85%. Between 1980 and 1985 the mortality rate for England and Wales was 1.4 per 100 000 procedures (Office of Population Censuses and Surveys 1985).

In the first trimester the mortality should be less than 1 per 100 000 operations—approximately the same risk as dying in an air crash or from an injection of penicillin. The rate in the NHS has always been higher than in the non-NHS sector (Table 29.1), and vigorous debate followed Diggory's comments (1984) restating this fact. Initially, difference in methods used in the two sectors probably explained many of the excess deaths, as more late abortions by hysterotomy and hysterectomy were done in the NHS and the use of concurrent sterilization was greater as was the death rate from pulmonary embolism (Savage 1981a). In the 1976–1978 enquiry, in five of seven legal-abortion deaths, care was considered to be substandard but by the 1979–1981 report the assessors found no avoidable factors in the abortion deaths

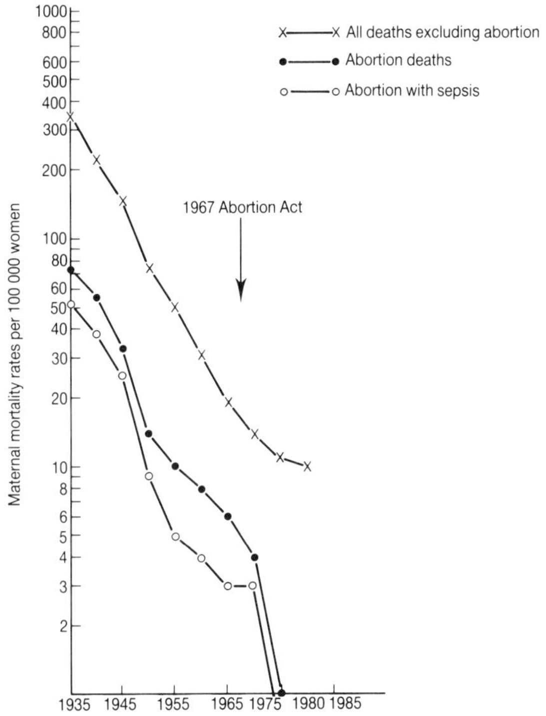

Fig. 29.7 Maternal mortality between 1935 and 1985 in England and Wales. Calculated from data in Macfarlane & Mugford 1984.

Table 29.1 Number of deaths from abortion in resident and non-resident women operated on in NHS and non-NHS premises between 1968 and 1985 in England and Wales

	NHS	non-NHS	% of abortions in NHS
1968–1971	42	6	61.3
1972–1975	24	7	50.4
1976–1979	17	0	48.9
Total	83	13	52.2
Rate per 100 000 operations	14.2	1.45	
1980–1982	5	2	47.7
1983–1985	4	2	47.6
Total	9	4	
Rate per 100 000 operations	2.4	0.65	47.6
Total 1968–1985	92	17	
Rate per 100 000 operations	9.6	1.13	

Data from Registrar General's Reports 1968–1974; Office of Population Censuses and Surveys 1975–1985.

(Confidential Enquiries into Maternal Deaths 1982, 1986).

The most likely explanation is that the non-NHS sector has a few highly experienced doctors working in a small number of clinics with a high volume of patients. In contrast there are a large number of NHS gynaecological units throughout the country where each consultant trains junior staff on a relatively small number of patients. In the study of late abortion carried out in 1982, 502 doctors notified abortions after 20 weeks' gestation — 466 between 1 and 4 cases during the 6-month period but 11 doctors notified over 100 cases each (Alberman & Dennis 1984).

Since the liberalization of abortion law the morbidity of legal abortion has been less than was initially feared (British Medical Journal 1981). Morbidity is related to age, parity, social class and pre-existing health of the woman, gestation at operation and the skill, experience and fatigue of the operator. Apart from the characteristics of the operator all these variables have been subjected to epidemiological analysis (Grimes & Cates 1979) and the most important factor is the length of gestation at operation. These authors calculated that delaying the operation from 8 until 10 weeks increased the risk of a major complication by 60%, whilst delaying from 8 until 16 weeks increased the risk by 300–1300%, depending on the method used. The study of late abortions by the Royal College of Obstetricians and Gynaecologists and the Department of Health and Social Services (RCOG/DHSS) led by Professor Alberman found that 39% of women operated on at 15–16 weeks had been medically referred before the 12th week of pregnancy, and that delays after this were much greater in the NHS than in the non-NHS sector (Alberman & Dennis 1984). Delay due to irregular menstruation or over-confidence in the method of contraception used were thought by the doctors who completed the questionnaires to be responsible for delay in 30% of the women operated on in the second trimester. Human factors such as indecision, fear and changed relationships were found in 50% of the women. In those operated upon from 20 weeks, financial barriers were quoted in 20% and in 1 in 200 there had been a previous attempt at a legal abortion.

METHODS OF ABORTION

Abortion before 8 weeks

Interception

There is debate as to when pregnancy begins; some workers consider that it is not until implantation. However before this time a potential pregnancy can be interrupted. This method is known as interception: 100 μg ethinyloestradiol plus 500 mg norgestrel given within 48 hours of unprotected mid-cycle intercourse is effective in preventing pregnancy in over 95% of women (Yuzpe et al 1974). It is important to inform the woman about the possibility of failure, and of our lack of knowledge about the effect of hormones given at this stage of embryogenesis, as well as the side-effects such as nausea and vomiting which may interfere with absorption; menstrual cycle disturbance; the possibility of ectopic pregnancy and the need for a follow-up examination and future contraception.

The insertion of a postcoital intrauterine contraceptive device has been remarkably effective with one reported failure (Kubba & Guilleband 1984), but it is not suitable in rape cases or if there is a risk of sexually transmitted disease (Lippes et al 1976).

Menstrual regulation or aspiration

Despite the simplicity of this method and its acceptability to women (Stringer et al 1975), it has never become widely available in the UK. Karman developed the flexible plastic cannula with which the uterine contents can be aspirated using a syringe for suction and without anaesthaesia, before the law was changed in California (Karman & Potts 1972). Edelman et al (1974) confirmed the low rate of complications and Goldthorpe (1977) described its use in a district general hospital in the NHS. The availability of the newer more sensitive pregnancy tests should reduce the proportion of women (up to 10%) operated on who are not pregnant, but gynaecologists need to inform general practitioners and women that this service is available.

Aspiration has a major role in countries in which the law, unlike British law, does not require the intention to terminate a pregnancy to be sanctioned, but where the fact of having terminated a proven pregnancy is illegal (Laufe 1979, Paxman & Barberis 1980). In Bangladesh paramedics have been trained in the technique and have as low complication rates as doctors (Akhtar, personal communication, quoted in Tietze & Henshaw 1986).

Unfortunately, when the new abortion notification form was introduced (Savage 1981b), the opportunity of introducing a category for this method was missed, so information about its exact use in the UK is lacking. In our experience in Tower Hamlets, London, less than 1% of women present early enough for this method to be used, and these women have been without exception nurses, doctors or medical students.

In the non-NHS sector it has been difficult to find a clinic or individual doctor doing this simple operation, although the unit run by University College Hospital at the National Temperance Hospital was oversubscribed by Camden residents (Grahame, personal communication).

Prostaglandins and RU486: contragestational agents

In 1973 Segal & Atkinson suggested the term contragestational agents for a variety of methods which could interrupt an early pregnancy without using surgical techniques. Prostaglandins were first used by Karim & Filshie in 1970 to cause early abortion, but natural prostaglandins caused too many gastrointestinal side-effects and had a high incidence of retained products. Complete abortion rates of 60–80% have been achieved using synthetic prostaglandin analogues as pessaries to induce uterine contractions (Bygdeman et al 1983); gastrointestinal side-effects are still common whether administered by intramuscular injection or per vaginam. Antiprogesterone agents such as RU486, which blocks progesterone receptors in the uterus, or Epostane, which reduces progesterone production by inhibiting the steroid dehydrogenase enzyme which converts pregnenolene to progesterone, are still undergoing trials (Healy & Fraser 1985, Elia 1985).

Abortion from 8 to 15 weeks' gestation

Evidence from large-scale studies in the USA suggests that the traditional division of abortion methods into first and second trimester is artificial; vaginal methods by vacuum alone up to about 12 weeks, supplemented by evacuation with sponge forceps up to 15+ weeks, is the method of choice (Stubblefield 1981, Beekhuizen et al 1982, Castadot 1986). It was British authors who in the early 1970s, pioneered the vaginal methods (Bierer & Steiner 1971, Davis 1972, Slome 1972, Finks 1973) but the Americans have extended the use of this method, which became standard in some states by 1978.

Cates & Grimes (1981) analysed all abortion deaths from 1972 to 1978 and concluded that, while dilatation and evacuation (D&E) between 13 and 16 weeks was more dangerous than suction alone performed up to 12 weeks, it was three times safer than abortion performed after 16 weeks. On epidemiological grounds there is no justification for delaying until 16 weeks to perform an instillation method, as is still done in some units in the UK. One-third of women in the non-NHS sector and one-quarter of those in the NHS operated on between 15 and 19 weeks in a late abortion study had been delayed waiting for a prostaglandin abortion (Alberman & Dennis 1984). Grimes et al (1980) randomized 200 women to D&E as outpatients compared with prostaglandin $F_{2\alpha}$ given as inpatients and found fewer complications, better patient compliance and thus less delay in performing the operation. They further assessed in 1982 3711 D&E procedures done by four physicians in ambulatory settings and showed that the complication rates were significantly less than for either prostaglandin or saline instillations (Cates et al 1982). They concluded that laws requiring these operations to be done in a hospital setting should be repealed.

Cadesky et al (1985) compared 100 women who underwent D&E at 13–16 weeks' gestation with 100 women matched for age and parity who had undergone prostaglandin $F_{2\alpha}$ instillation and found a small but significantly smaller complication rate and much shorter hospital stay.

Grimes & Schultz (1985) again reviewed the literature of D&E compared with other methods in the 13–16-week period; they showed that between 1972 and 1981 in the USA amniotic fluid embolism, a rare but lethal complication, caused no deaths under 12 weeks; only one death followed D&E whereas 18 followed instillation procedures.

In the USA laminaria tents are often used to soften the cervix (Newton 1972) but only one study of their use has been reported in the UK (Nicolaides et al 1983). In the UK prostaglandin pessaries in various dose regimens, as described by MacKenzie & Fry (1981) and Fisher & Taylor (1984) have shown in a controlled study to be effective, are more commonly used.

In England and Wales in 1986 over 87% of abortions were done by 12 weeks, 5.6% at 13–14 weeks and 3% at 15–16 weeks. Table 29.2 shows how the methods used in

Table 29.2 Percentage of second-trimester abortions performed by different methods in the NHS and non-NHS sectors in England and Wales in 1973, 1979 and 1985. Totals may be <100% as some were unrecorded

	1973	1979		1985	
	All	NHS	non-NHS	NHS	non-NHS
Vaginal					
VA/D&C	53.9	32.7	49.1	31.1	50.6
D&E	0.0	3.2	11.2	2.9	9.9
Medical					
Prostaglandin	0.0	54.1	10.3	57.0	33.6
Other	0.0	0.2*	21.7*	5.2	4.8
Surgical					
Hysterectomy	0.8	0.5	0.03	0.34	0.009
Hysterotomy	10.0	4.3	1.3	1.9	0.009
Other	26.7	4.3	5.7	0.7	0.7

VA = vacuum aspiration; D&C = dilatation and curettage; D&E = dilatation and evacuation.
*Saline instillation.
From Registrar General's Report 1974; Office of Population Censuses and Surveys 1985.

the second trimester have changed over the last decade. There are still differences between the NHS and non-NHS sectors.

Technique of abortion at 8–15 weeks

In the UK almost all operations in this gestational range are done under general anaesthaesia, whereas in the USA the majority are done using local anaesthaesia. Peterson et al (1981) showed that between 1972 and 1978 the use of general anaesthesia increased the risk of death two- to fourfold in women undergoing first-trimester procedures. The lower death rate between 1980 and 1985 in the USA (0.4 per 100 000 in 1981) compared with the UK (1.1 per 100 000) may be partly explained by this difference in anaesthesia as well as the lower use of sterilization in the USA — 1.4% in the USA in 1980 compared with 7.3% in England and Wales in 1980 and 5.0% in 1985.

Operative technique

The vulva and vagina are cleansed with antiseptic solution and, using a sterile technique with gloves and drapes but dispensing with operating gowns and leggings, a bimanual examination is performed to assess the size and position of the uterus and check the adnexae. It is usually not necessary to catheterize the bladder.

Some operators use a paracervical or intracervical block of not more than 20 ml of 0.5% lignocaine possibly to facilitate dilatation of the cervix and to reduce blood loss. The anterior lip of the cervix is grasped by a volsellum. Two will distribute the load but in the conscious patient use one fine single-toothed tenaculum. The uterus is sounded to confirm the size and direction of the canal, and then dilated using tapered dilators; 10 mm should rarely be exceeded in a nulliparous woman, but if resistance is encountered this should not be forcibly overcome even if the uterus is 15 weeks in size, as evacuation can proceed through 8–9 mm, although it is slower. In a multiparous woman 12 mm is permissible if there is no resistance.

Before attempting to aspirate the uterus, most surgeons give Syntocinon 10 u intravenously to make the uterus contract. A sponge forceps is introduced to rupture the membranes at the same time. The curette is attached to an electric pump by suction tubing using a metal handle with an air inlet. The uterus is aspirated with a plastic curette of approximately the same diameter as the number of weeks' gestation of the pregnancy, up to 10–12 mm as described above.

From 12 to 15 weeks, after the liquor has been removed the suction curette is removed and a sponge forceps are used to remove placental and fetal tissue; the left hand is placed over the fundus to check how the uterus is contracting down. Once the uterus feels almost empty, the cavity is checked with a sharp curette which is stroked over the walls rather than used to scrape off the endometrium, to show where the cavity still seems rough. The suction curette can then be directed to the appropriate place until it is felt to be gripped by the contracted uterus and only frothy blood is obtained. The fetal tissue should be examined by the operator or a trained assistant to reduce the possibility of fetal products having been retained, and subsequent haemorrhage, infection and the need for re-evacuation.

Kiel (1986) from Texas, in a report of 13 477 cases examined by a pathologist, found that pregnancy was confirmed in 98.68%, decidua alone was found in 0.79%, 0.52% of the specimens were not diagnostic of pregnancy and 0.01% had a hydatidiform mole. There were two ectopic pregnancies in the 31 women followed up, one with decidua and one with no evidence of pregnancy — about 1% of each group. If there are no obvious fetal parts, the tissue needs to be examined either in the theatre by floating in saline or water or under the low power of a microscope. If this is not feasible a specimen should be sent for histological examination and arrangements made for a follow-up examination so that the complications mentioned above, or a continuing pregnancy, are not missed.

Hysterectomy and hysterotomy are rarely indicated on medical grounds at this gestation. Morbidity and mortality are higher and sterilization at the time of hysterotomy is associated with an increased risk of pulmonary embolism (Table 29.3). Fibroids rarely prevent access to the uterine cavity and carcinoma is probably the only true medical indication for using hysterectomy. These methods are rarely used in the non-NHS sector or the USA but continue to be used significantly more often in the NHS and in some regions (Fig. 29.7), although the rates have fallen since these variations were first reported (Savage 1979).

Abortion from 16 to 24 weeks

The methods available at this stage of gestation are listed in Table 29.4.

Table 29.3 Deaths by procedure in England and Wales 1970–1981

	Method of operation				
	Hysterotomy hysterectomy	Utus paste	D&C	VA	Other methods, incl. combination
Number of deaths	16	8	13	9	13
Operations	55 765	3977	465 137	963 462	61 201
Rate/100 000	2.87	20.1	0.28	0.13	2.45
PE deaths	8	0	2	4	1
PE rate/10^6	14.3	0	0.43	0.42	1.63

Calculated from Office of Population Censuses and Surveys data and Confidential Enquiry data.
PE = Pulmonary embolism.

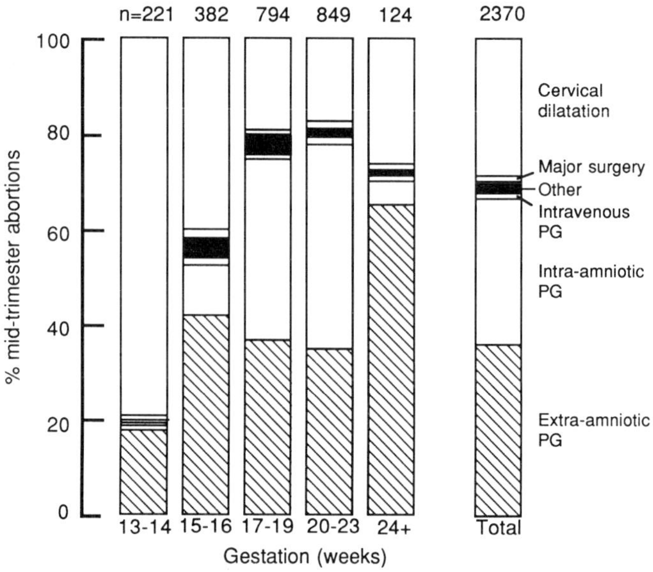

Fig. 29.8 Methods of second-trimester abortion used in England and Wales during the period January–June 1982, obtained by a survey conducted by the RCOG (1984) of 2370 terminations.
PG = prostaglandins.

Table 29.4 Methods of late abortion for 16 weeks' gestation and over

Method	Range (weeks)	Use in UK	Advisability
Intra-amniotic methods			
Hypertonic saline	16–26	Minimal since 1981	Safety = $PGF_{2\alpha}$
Hypertonic glucose	16–26	? nil since 1960s	No, infection
Hypertonic urea	16–26	Not used alone	With PGs useful
$PGE_2/F_{2\alpha}$	16–26	PGE_2 used in UK	D&V unpleasant
PGs + urea	16–26	Exact use unknown	Safe & effective
These methods may be combined with i.v. Syntocinon or PGs, and/or tents, PGs to ripen cervix			
Extra-amniotic methods			
Saline	16–26	Not used in UK	Not recommended Safety
Ethacridine	16–26	Not used in UK	Not recommended Slow
Utus paste	16–26	Not used since 1980	Not recommended/ High risk of infection
$PGE_2/F_{2\alpha}$	16–26	PGE_2 in UK	Slow live fetus
PGs i.m. or p.v.	16–26	Experimental	High incidence of D&V
Surgical			
D&E	16–18/20	Mainly non-NHS	Recommended method
D&E—two stage method	18/20–26	Mainly private	Safe in skilled hands
D&E—two stage with PG	16–26	Not yet used	Dutch experience safe
Anti-progesterones may be added in future to assist with IA/EA and surgery			
Hysterectomy	16–26	Use declining	Risk of PE/rarely need
Hysterotomy	16–26	Use declining	PE, scar/rarely need
Vaginal hysterectomy or hysterotomy not used since sixties in UK			

PG = prostaglandin; D&V = diarrhoea and vomiting; PE = pulmorary embolism; D&E = dilatation and evacuation.

D&E can be used safely up to 18 weeks in the nulliparous woman and up to 20 weeks in those who have had children, if the operator has been trained in this technique. Preoperative preparation of the cervix with prostaglandin pessaries or insertion of a Foley catheter or of laminaria tents reduces the risk of cervical damage.

The cervix may need to be dilated to 14 or 15 mm to insert the heavier bone-crushing forceps designed by Bierer. Blood loss is likely to be greater and an intravenous line is often inserted by the anaesthetist in the UK, although in the USA the procedure is done under local anaesthetic as a day-case procedure in some states. For fuller descriptions of the technique see Diggory (1977), Savage (1979) and Hodgson (1981).

Two-stage methods

Davis (1972) and Finks (1981) described dilating the cervix, rupturing the membranes and pulling down a loop of cord which was then cut. Antibiotics were then given and then next day evacuation of the softened fetus was performed. Finks reported that in 1008 cases there were no infections, 15 cervical lacerations of minor degree and two women required blood transfusion. In the late abortion study (Alberman & Dennis 1984) it was recorded that some operators dilated the cervix to 22 mm, with apparent safety in the hands of experienced practitioners. A variant of this is where prostaglandin or Epostane is injected intra-amniotically and 2–4 hours later D&E is performed under local anaesthaesia. Several hundred of these procedures have been done without problems in Netherlands.

Table 29.5 Selected trials of prostaglandins for abortion — intramuscular and vaginal routes

Reference	Method	Number of women	Mean induction–abortion time	% aborting in 24 h	% D&V
Cameron & Baird 1984*	Vaginal PGE_1	57	13 h 59 min	77	19 + 12
	cf. $EAPGE_2$	58	14 h 57 min	79	14 + 2
WHO PG Task Force 1977	Vaginal $PGF_{2\alpha}$	310	14 h 12 min	88 in 48 h	67 + 70
WHO PG Task Force 1982	i.m. sulprostone	145	14 h 48 min	88	50 + 26

Adapted from MacKenzie 1987
*Randomized open trial.
PGE_1 = 16, 16-dimethyl-trans-Δ_2-prostaglandin E_1 methyl ester vaginal pessaries = gemeprost
$PGF_{2\alpha}$ = 15-methyl-$PGF_{2\alpha}$
D&V = diarrhoea and vomiting
For further information see Toppozada 1986

Instillation techniques

Injections of saline, prostaglandin with or without urea, rivanol and hypertonic glucose have all been and are still being used in some parts of the world (MacKenzie 1985). In the UK, intra-amniotic urea and prostaglandin E_2 tend to be the method most often chosen, as the induction abortion interval is shortened compared with prostaglandin alone, and the chance of the fetus being born alive is very low. Selinger et al (1986) have reported a reduced induction–abortion interval by using Epostane, a 3-beta-hydroxy steroid inhibitor, prior to prostaglandin. In the USA, prostaglandin $F_{2\alpha}$ has been used in most of the trials and urea is less commonly added.

Intra-amniotic prostaglandin and urea technique

Ultrasound is used to confirm the gestation and localize the placenta. Timing of the admission with sensitivity towards staff and other patients in the gynaecology ward is important. Amniocentesis is performed in a sterile manner and as much liquor as possible is drained before instilling 40 g urea in 200 ml of normal saline and 5 mg Prostin E_2. With this dose, vomiting and diarrhoea are less of a problem. Occasional reactions with shivering, vomiting, diarrhoea or hypotension should be treated rapidly with intravenous hydrocortisone, antihistamines and intravenous fluids.

A cannula (epidural type) is left in place in the amniotic cavity to give another dose of prostaglandin if necessary. Abortion usually takes place within 12 hours and if incomplete is followed by ERPC under general anaesthesia. Anti-D should be given if the woman is rhesus-negative. Recent work suggests that 75 μg may be needed (Gravenhorst et al 1986).

Extra-amniotic prostaglandin

Little has been written about this method since Embrey et al described its use in 1972; the data collected by the DHSS do not allow a distinction to be made between the various routes of administration of prostaglandins. The DHSS/RCOG study (Alberman & Dennis 1984) which asked gynaecologists to give supplementary information showed that abortions in the second trimester were approximately evenly divided between vaginal, intra-amniotic and extra-amniotic methods; Figure 29.8 shows which method is used at the various gestational ages.

The disadvantages of the method are the likelihood of delivery of a live fetus, long induction delivery interval unless Syntocinon is used, risk of infection if there is cervicitis and restriction of the woman's mobility. Prostaglandins given by intramuscular injection or vaginally have been tried in recent years; Table 29.5 gives some information about the success rate in these trials. Although extra-amniotic prostaglandins are widely used in the UK, they are rarely used in the USA and consequently little has been written about this method since its introduction.

Technique. At preoperative assessment, any woman with cervicitis should be referred for investigation by a sexually transmitted diseases clinic and adequate therapy given before embarking on the abortion.

A Foley catheter is passed through the cervix, which may have been softened using a 3 mg prostaglandin E_2 pessary, and connected to a syringe pump. It is important to measure the dead space before injecting the prostaglandin solution as a total of 1.5–2.0 mg is usually sufficient; 100–200 μg/h is given, i.e. 1–2 ml/h. The induction–abortion interval is about 18 hours but may be as long as 32 hours. Intravenous Syntocinon may be used after some hours, but attention must be paid to the prevention of water intoxication as 10–20 u/l may be needed before the uterus contracts. Feeney (1982) noted that 3 litres is the point at which problems begin to occur. Observations, analgesia and incomplete abortion are treated as described above.

Hysterotomy and hysterectomy are described in standard texts and again are rarely the methods of choice, although in the hands of those who rarely do a second-trimester termination, this operation may be safer than embarking on an instillation technique with which none of the staff are familiar. The risk of an unanticipated hysterectomy is not easy to ascertain from the statistics prepared by the Office of Population Censuses and Surveys but if one assumes that the category 'other surgical' replaces 'hysterectomy with other methods', the differences between the NHS and non-

Table 29.6 Presumed unplanned surgery in NHS and non-NHS abortions

Year	NHS		non-NHS	
*Hysterectomy with other methods**				
1977	12	2.3	6	1.2
1978	9	1.6	3	0.5
1979	9	1.6	2	0.3
1980	9	1.5	3	0.4
Total	39	1.7	14	0.6
Unexpected hysterectomy risk:	1 : 3333		1 : 12 500	
'Other surgical' not hysterectomy or hysterotomy only				
1981	14	2.3	3	0.4
1982	11	1.8	2	0.3
1981–1982 Other surgical risk	1 : 5000		1 : 26 724	
1983	15	2.4	42*	6.5
1984	42†	6.4	38	5.3
1985	46	7.1	9	1.2
1983–1985 Other surgical risk	1 : 1800		1:2378	

*Number and rate per 10 000 operations
†The discontinuity in these data suggests that a different interpretation has been used after 1983.

Table 29.7 The number of abortions performed after 20 weeks and percentage of total abortions (in parentheses) on women resident in England and Wales, 1977–1985

Year	20–23 weeks	≥24 weeks		Total ≥20 weeks
1977	912 (0.9)	183 (0.18)		1095 (1.1)
1978	1249 (1.1)	261 (0.23)		1510 (1.3)
1979	1486 (1.2)	281 (0.23)		1767 (1.5)
1980	1853 (1.4)	381 (0.29)		2232 (1.7)
	21–22 weeks	23–24 weeks	≥ 25 weeks	Total >20 weeks
1981	585 (0.45)	296 (0.23)	104 (0.08)	985 (0.8)
1982	610 (0.47)	290 (0.22)	78 (0.06)	978 (0.8)
1983	697 (0.55)	311 (0.24)	57 (0.07)	1065 (0.8)
1984	722 (0.53)	447 (0.33)	57 (0.04)	1226 (0.9)
1985	836 (0.59)	440 (0.31)	31 (0.02)	1309 (0.9)

Abortions performed after 23 weeks by place of operation 1981–1985 as a percentage of total abortions on women resident in England and Wales

Year	NHS (including agency)		non-NHS (excluding agency)	
	23–24 weeks	≥25 weeks	23–24 weeks	≥25 weeks
1981	79 (0.1)	45 (0.07)	217 (0.3)	59 (0.09)
1982	61 (0.09)	42 (0.06)	229 (0.3)	36 (0.05)
1983	80 (0.1)	50 (0.07)	231 (0.4)	37 (0.06)
1984	67 (0.1)	34 (0.05)	380 (0.6)	23 (0.03)
1985	66 (0.09)	27 (0.04)	374 (0.5)	4 (0.006)

NHS sectors persist (Table 29.6). In Canada between 1976 and 1980, there were 28 unanticipated hysterectomies in 305 000 abortions — a rate of 0.9 per 10 000 cases (Tietze & Henshaw 1986).

Very late abortion: 25–26 weeks

The 1967 Abortion Act refers back to the 1929 Infant Life Preservation Act which states that 28 weeks' gestation is taken as prima-facie evidence of viability. This means that below 28 weeks' gestation the onus is on the prosecution to show that the fetus could have lived, whereas at 28 weeks the onus is on the operator to show that the fetus could not have survived. In anencephaly, for example, most doctors would terminate the pregnancy at 32 weeks or later if the diagnosis was made late and would be acting within the law.

With the advances in neonatal intensive care many gynaecologists have felt uneasy about both the moral and legal position if a pregnancy is terminated at 24 weeks or above (Bromwich 1987) and in 1985 the DHSS gained a voluntary agreement from the non-NHS clinics that they would not perform abortions after 24 weeks — a position that the charitable sector had adopted 2 years earlier. Table 29.7 shows the effect that this has had on the number of very late abortions, which have always made up a very small proportion of the total number of abortions performed. Although most of these very late abortions are done for fetal abnormality (Alberman et al 1984), some are done for complex social problems, frequently in teenagers or for mental disorders (Savage 1985).

The problem of teenage pregnancy has been well reviewed by Bury (1984) and Barron (1986). In a national study Simms & Smith (1982) found that 5% of their sample of teenage mothers had seriously considered an abortion but 10 of these were told that they were too late, despite the fact that six saw their general practitioner between 5 and 9 weeks of gestation.

The methods used are similar to those described. Labour usually ensues quickly after instillation of prostaglandin E_2 and urea; abortion is more likely to be complete than in earlier pregnancy. With the increasing use of ultrasound after 20 weeks to detect cardiac, central nervous system and renal abnormalities which may be compatible with life, albeit with a severely handicapped existence, and the likelihood that young teenagers and depressed women will continue to present on an occasional basis requesting late termination, the author is against a change in the law, which works well in practice, although future challenges to the 1967 Act similar to David Alton's 1987/88 attempt are to be expected.

Counselling and preoperative examination

The provision of lay counsellors in the charitable sector has been essential to their approach to dealing with requests for abortion (Simms 1977, Rowe 1988), but provision of this service has taken longer in the NHS. Allen (1981) showed that some women were counselled by all those they saw whereas others, who were often isolated single parents, did not get the support they needed.

Lilford et al (1985) reported satisfactory acceptance by women of a computerized program of history-taking administered by a nurse. The authors showed that more important

Table 29.8 Women not suitable for day-care operation

Social	No adult in home overnight
Psychological	Severe depression requiring observation
Medical	History of pulmonary embolism asthma/cardiac disease sickle cell trait previous adverse anaesthetic reactions weight >90 kg (1977 >70 kg) serious neurological disease blood disorders interfering with haemostasis
Gynaecological	Gestation 13 weeks or over Previous cone biopsy or Manchester repair Large fibroid uterus Request for co-incident tubal ligation

In 1977, previous uterine scar was considered an indication for admission but this policy has been revised in the light of experience.

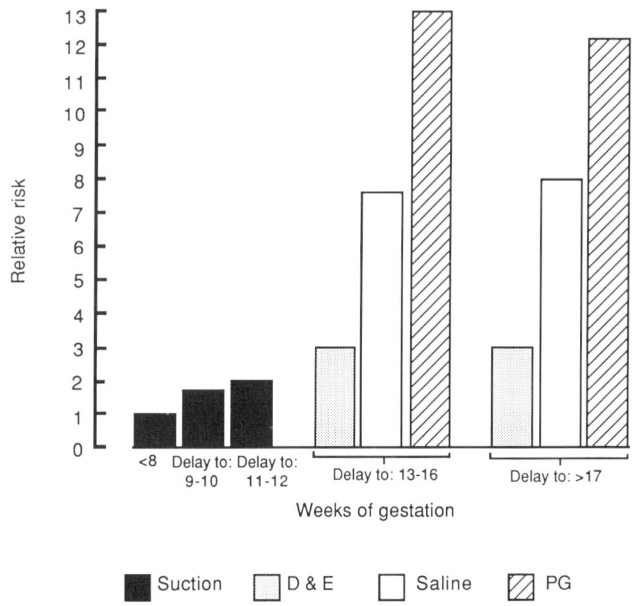

Fig. 29.9 Relative risk of major abortion-related morbidity due to length of gestation and choice of method, compared with risk associated with suction at 8 weeks' gestation. Data from JPSA/CDC study, USA 1971–1975. D&E = dilatation and evacuation; PG = prostaglandin.

Table 29.9 Routine tests done at Tower Hamlets DCAS

Blood
- Haemoglobin
- Blood group and antibody screen
- Rhesus factor
- Serological tests for syphilis
- Rubella status
- To at-risk groups only:
  - Haemoglobin electrophoresis in Asian, Afro-Caribbean and Mediterranean women
  - Hepatitis antigen in Asian women, recent jaundice, i.v. drug abusers
  - HIV—Partner of haemophiliac, bisexual, i.v. drug abusers, prostitutes or, on request, rape victim

Other tests
- Cervical swab for culture and sensitivity
- Cervical smear for cytology if not done, or abnormal, in last 3 years
- Urine tested for sugar and protein

features of the history were elicited than by the standard medical model and that a psychosocial profile could be prepared to alert staff.

A full general examination of the woman should be made, with particular note of cardiorespiratory or genital abnormalities which might influence the operation. Complications are higher in obese women and a list of criteria for day-case procedures should be agreed by the gynaecologist and anaesthetist in charge of this. Table 29.8 shows the current exclusion criteria in Tower Hamlets, which have become fewer as experience has been gained in the 10 years since Peter Huntingford started this service.

The routine investigations suggested are listed in Table 28.9. Screening for human immunodeficiency virus (HIV) is not recommended as a routine but would be offered after suitable counselling (Millar 1987) to women who are in high-risk groups, such as intravenous drug abusers, partners of haemophiliacs whose HIV status is not known, or partners of bisexual men. The woman who is found to be HIV-positive should be placed at the end of the operating list, as should those who are hepatitis-positive, to facilitate cleaning of the theatre. Visors should be worn and all specimens clearly labelled; careful technique to avoid needlestick injuries or contamination of non-intact skin by blood should be followed.

IMMEDIATE AND EARLY COMPLICATIONS

Operative and immediate complications are well documented in numerous studies (Diggory 1969, Beric & Kupresanin 1971, Lewis et al 1971, Tietze & Lewit 1972, Kerslake 1973, Hull et al 1974, Grimes & Cates 1979) but long-term sequelae are difficult to follow in a prospective manner and much of the evidence is indirect. The on-going joint study conducted by the RCOG and Royal College of General Practitioners (RCGP) has already confirmed in a prospective study of 6105 women undergoing abortion that the incidence of morbidity was 10% and that of more major problems 0.7% (Joint study of the RCGP and RCOG—Frank et al 1985a).

Haemorrhage, infection, uterine trauma, retained products and anaesthetic complications are the main complications and 5–10% of women having abortions experience one of these. Some 3–5/1000 experience a major complication, such as haemorrhage requiring transfusion, laparotomy for perforation of the uterus, or salpingitis. Figure 29.9 shows how the relative risk of a major complication rises with increasing gestation (Cates & Grimes 1981). Edelman & Berger (1981), reviewing the literature on menstrual aspiration or very early abortion, give rates of 1–10% for total

Table 29.10 Operative and early complication rates reported in selected studies

Reference	Number of women	Complication rate per 100 women: Haemorrhage	Infection	Trauma to: Cervix	Uterus
First trimester operations					
Tietze & Lewit 1972	47 618	1.0	0.6	0.9	0.3
Edelman et al 1974 VA	2498	2.4	2.5	1.0	0.4
VEA	613	0.0	0.5	0.0	0.0
Hodgson et al 1975 (based on 65% follow-up)	20 248	0.05	0.7	0.01	0.1
Kerslake 1973	4511	0.7	1.0	0.01	0.12
(followed)	3005				
Grimes & Cates 1979	54 155	0.4	0.7	1.0	0.2
RCGP/RCOG Study 1985					
<9 weeks	1497	0.2	3.5	0.53	
9–12 weeks	3719	1.4	3.4	0.56	
>12 weeks	889	2.7	4.2	0.89	
The operations were carried out between 1976 and 1979. Follow-up by the woman's GP prospective study from time of request					
RCOG/DHSS Study 1984					
<12 weeks	370	0.3	0.8	0.5	1.1
13–14	221	0.5	0.5	0.9	0.5
15–16	382	0.5	1.8	0.6	0.8
17–19	794	0.9	0.6	1.6	0.5
20–23	849	0.8	0.7	2.2	0.5
24–27	124	0.8	0.8	4.8	0.5
The operations were performed Jan–June 1982. Reports by operator using case notes in retrospect, 4/52 follow-up					

complications with this method and point out that the rate of uterine perforation is only 0.03% in the 10 000 cases reported.

Table 29.10 shows the incidences of the various complications for selected studies; the low rates are notable in contrast to early studies in this country (Stallworthy et al 1971).

Anaesthaesia

General anaesthesia has been used for the majority of operations in this country, in contrast to the widespread use of local anaesthesia in the USA, especially in free-standing clinics such as *Pre-term.* Grimes & Cates (1979) compared 36 430 first-trimester procedures under local anaesthesia with 17 725 under general anaesthesia. Major complications were similar in incidence, 0.3 and 0.35% respectively, but the rates of haemorrhage, perforation, and cervical trauma were lower in the local anaesthesia group. Convulsions were not seen in any of the general anaesthesia group but were present in 0.3% of the local anaesthesia group. One death in the general anaesthesia group was reported.

Of the 51 deaths following legal abortion between 1973 and 1978 in the UK, eight were caused by, and one was associated with, general anaesthesia but in the latest Confidential Enquiry into Maternal Death (1986) there was only one anaesthesic death among the six abortion deaths analysed between 1979 and 1981. From 1970 to 1975 17.6% of deaths in England and Wales and 15.5% of those in the USA were associated with anaesthesia (12 using general anaesthesia, 6 local anaesthesia, and 2 narcotic analgesic techniques).

Haemorrhage

This is rarely a problem in early abortions done by vacuum extraction. Haemorrhage of more than 500 ml occurred in 79 (1.3%) of the 6105 women in the RCGP/RCOG study (Frank et al 1985a). NHS operations were four times as likely to have this amount of loss as non-NHS procedures and operations over 12 weeks' gestation were seven times as likely to be complicated in this way as those under 12 weeks.

Retained products

If the products of conception are routinely inspected, the incidence of retained products requiring evacuation of the uterus should be less than 1%. When using intra-amniotic methods between one-half and one-third of placentas are retained. The uterus should be evacuated under general anaesthesia if the placenta is retained for more than 30 minutes since haemorrhage becomes more likely if the placenta is retained for over 2 hours (Berger & Kerenyi 1974).

Infection

Infection may be associated with retained products, so measures that reduce the incidence of incomplete termination will also reduce the rates of infection. Collection of the aspirated products in a gauze or mesh bag is recommended by Hodgson (1981) to facilitate examination; Hodgson mentions that weighing is advocated by Burnhill & Armstead (1978).

Hodgson et al (1975) and Brewer (1980), in sequential trials using tetracyclines, demonstrated a reduction in complications due to infection during the period when antibiotics were given. Burkman et al (1976) found that endometritis was three times higher in women with untreated gonorrhoea than in women who did not have a positive culture. Sonne-Holm et al (1981) in a controlled trial found a reduction in pelvic inflammatory disease from 10.9% in the placebo group to 5.5% in women given penicillin G followed by pivampicillin. Further analysis showed that of 105 women who had previously had pelvic inflammatory disease, 22.4% of those receiving placebo but only 2.1% of those having antibiotics had infections. The numbers in the study are small (493) and the rates of infection and previous pelvic inflammatory disease higher than one would expect in this country, but the finding of such a high rate of infection with a history of pelvic inflammatory disease has very important implications for management.

Mills (1984) reported 12 (2.4%) cases of pelvic infection

in 500 women screened by plating endocervical swabs directly on to Thayer-Martin medium and treating the nine women who were found to have gonorrhoea. Ridgeway et al (1983) isolated chlamydia from 5.2%, compared with Mills (1983) who found an incidence of 1.75% of 347 women attending the Tower Hamlets Day Care Abortion Service (DCAS), none of whom developed pelvic inflammatory disease. MacKenzie & Fry (1981) reported a rate of 1.75% whereas the RCGP/RCOG study (Frank et al 1985a) found 3.8% of women to have pelvic infection. Duthie et al (1987) screened 167 women in Liverpool; 19 (11%) had *Chlamydia trachomatis* isolated. Seven women (4%) had pelvic inflammatory disease post-operatively; five of the seven had had positive cultures for *Chlamydia*. Another 8% of the women had minor morbidity, and high count cultures of *Mycoplasma* or *Chlamydia* were more likely to have been found in these women beforehand.

Making a diagnosis and treating the woman prior to the operation is preferable to giving all women prophylactic antibiotics. This is done by either screening all women with the appropriate swabs or selectively, by taking a careful sexual history and referring all women who have become pregnant as a result of a casual encounter, who are found to have *Trichomonas* infection or clinical evidence of cervicitis, to the sexually transmitted disease clinic.

If treatment is not prompt, 5–10% of these women may have tubal damage and without adequate therapy, 1–2/1000 women may develop tubal infertility.

Uterine trauma

In the USA predilatation of the cervix with laminaria tents has been used commonly since the mid 1970s (Golditch & Glasser 1974, Newton 1975, Harlap et al 1979). On both sides of the Atlantic the use of tapered Pratt dilators, rather than straight Hegar dilators, has increased and the realization that forcible dilatation of the cervix is harmful has led to greater care being taken (Hulka et al 1974, Johnstone et al 1976). The introduction of flexible and firm plastic curettes, in place of the glass Kerslake or metal Bierer curettes, has also helped to reduce the diameter to which the cervix is dilated. Prostaglandin pessaries to soften the cervix, especially in the young adolescent, have been advocated by some workers (Brenner et al 1973). In large-scale studies it is not easy to distinguish between cervical lacerations caused by external tears from the volsella, which can easily be repaired, and serious lacerations of the internal os, which may be damaged permanently or the damage may extend into the broad ligament. These are rare but important complications. In the RCGP/RCOG study (Frank et al 1985a) 37 women (0.6%) had uterine trauma, 11 cervical lacerations and 22 perforations which required laparotomy for repair; one woman had a hysterectomy. These rates are comparable with many studies but the authors comment that women having non-NHS abortions only had one-third of the risk of trauma compared with those in the NHS.

Uterine perforation with a sound is probably commoner than reported (Hodgson 1981); usually it only requires observation (Frieman & Wulff 1977). Perforations with the curette or sponge forceps may occur before evacuation is complete and damage to bowel, omentum and, less commonly, Fallopian tube and ureter has occurred. Immediate laparoscopy allows the abortion to be completed and damage to be assessed (Lauerson & Birnbaum 1973); it also reduces the incidence of laparotomy. King et al (1980) found an incidence of 1/1000 laparotomies for abortion complications in 11 885 consecutive operations.

With later abortions, perforation of the uterus is more likely with D&E than with intra-amniotic methods, but bucket-handle tears of the cervix or cervicouterine fistulas have been reported in 1.0% of cases by Lowensohn & Ballard (1974). Augmentation of prostaglandin or saline abortions with oxytocin before the cervix has dilated appears to be the precipitating factor (Horwitz 1974) and uterine rupture has been reported following the use of intravenous, intra-amniotic and extra-amniotic prostaglandins combined with oxytocin (Propping et al 1977, Emery et al 1979, Traub & Ritchie 1979).

Water intoxication

The combination of high doses of oxytocin with electrolyte-free solutions may lead to fluid overload (Lauerson & Birnbaum 1973) and one death from this cause has been reported in England and Wales. Monitoring urine output, and discontinuing the infusion if this falls or if signs of mental confusion or restlessness occur, prevents this complication. Awareness of the dangers among medical and nursing staff and instructions to discontinue the infusion after every 6 hours for 30 minutes is a worthwhile precaution.

Disseminated intravascular coagulation

This was originally thought to be a complication of saline abortions alone but Cohen & Ballard (1974) found an incidence of only 0.2% in a series of 5000 cases. Disseminated intravascular coagulation has now been described in association with urea abortions (Grundy & Craven 1976) and late D&E procedures (Davis 1972) as well as with prostaglandin and oxytocin methods. Oxytocin increased the risk of disseminated intravascular coagulation five times in women having saline abortions in Cohen & Ballard's (1974) study, whereas Burkman et al (1976) found that the risk of disseminated intravascular coagulation in women given urea plus oxytocin or prostaglandin was only one-quarter of that for women having saline alone.

Thromboembolic disease

Pulmonary embolism is most likely to follow abdominal surgical procedures; however, in Confidential Enquiries into

Maternal Deaths (1986), three of the four deaths due to pulmonary embolism followed abortions performed by suction curettage at 9–10 weeks and only one of these was combined with sterilization. The fourth woman, who was only 21, had an abnormal fetus aborted by extra-amniotic prostaglandin at 18 weeks' gestation. In the RCOG/RCGP study (Frank et al 1985a) 29 women (0.5%) had a thrombosis but only three had pulmonary infarction and two had deep vein thromboses of the legs. There were no deaths.

Air embolism

This complication may occur following incorrect connection of suction apparatus and is a rare but totally preventable complication (Munsick 1972). Two of the 51 deaths in England and Wales between 1970 and 1975 were due to air embolism but none were reported between 1976 and 1981 (Office of Population Censuses and Surveys and Confidential Enquiries).

The uterine distension syndrome

A complication originally reported by Nathanson (1973) and which occurred 42 times in 26 560 abortions reviewed by Hodgson (1981)—a rate of 1.5 per 1000 cases—is that of uterine distension by blood, leading to hypotension and severe pain. Vacuum aspiration gives rapid relief. Uterine distension seems to occur if the uterus is evacuated through a small-calibre curette and the placental site is low-lying. The author has now seen three cases, two performed under 9 weeks' gestation and one at 14 weeks.

Livebirths

Movement of a non-viable fetus may cause distress both to the woman and her attendants, and it is most likely to occur if either extra-amniotic prostaglandin or intra-amniotic prostaglandin alone is used. Hypertonic solutions are fetocidal in the majority of cases. In 1988, a 21 week fetus aborted because of a risk of Ehlers-Danlos syndrome received much media and parliamentary attention, and the case was reported to the DPP who ruled that there was no case to answer. Four other cases of livebirths have been reported in the popular press in this country. In one an error of dates had occurred and in two the fetus was only at 18 weeks' gestation—this was confirmed by ultrasound scan. The last baby was delivered by Caesarean section for antepartum haemorrhage at 29 weeks, although claimed to be an abortion at 26 weeks initially (Daily Mirror, 21 January 1978, Evening Star Ipswich, 27 April 1979, Liverpool Daily Post, 20 April 1979, Sunday People, 25 March 1979). Pakter & Nelson (1972) reported 62 live fetuses with two long-term survivors in 36 000 saline abortions; Stroh & Hinman (1976) reported 27 live fetuses in 16 000 urea or saline abortions and 9 in 1000 born by hysterotomy. The change in climate of opinion about very late abortion and the use of ultrasound to date the pregnancy in cases of uncertain dates should reduce the incidence of this problem, which poses considerable ethical dilemmas.

LONG-TERM SEQUELAE

Rhesus isoimmunization

This is an entirely preventable complication provided that blood is taken for rhesus typing prior to operation and anti-D gamma globulin is administered to those women at risk. Freda et al (1970) estimated the risk of sensitization to be 2% at 2 months and about 9% at 3 months' gestation. Studies in the USA show rates of administration of anti-D globulin from 44 to 99% of women at risk (Grimes & Cates 1979). About 5–10% of new cases of rhesus isoimmunization in the UK result from failure to give anti-D at the time of an abortion (Tovey 1986, 1987, Contreras et al 1986, Hussey 1987).

Evidence available to quantify long-term sequelae

Although literally hundreds of papers on this important topic have been published, almost none of them satisfy the criteria of a good study for the reasons listed below:

1. Few are prospective from the time of abortion.
2. There is inadequate documentation of the abortion history in either the study group or the group used for comparison.
3. There is insufficient information about the previous abortion procedure being studied as a potential risk factor, for example the abortion technique, gestational age, skill of the operator, or even whether or not the abortion was legal.
4. There is failure to control for a variety of confounding variables common to both the risk factor being studied, that is induced abortion, and the late complication being investigated. For example, if considering the effect of previous abortion on birthweight, birthweight is also affected by age, parity, marital status, social class, income, smoking, alcohol and drug abuse, as well as relevant medical factors. All these factors must be controlled for if one is to conclude that the difference found is due to abortion.
5. When selecting the control group, some have used women who have had a prior spontaneous abortion, a group whose increased risk was documented in the Perinatal Mortality Survey of 1958 (Butler & Bonham 1963). Is comparison with women having their first pregnancy valid, or is it better to compare with women having their second child? Some workers have used two or more comparison groups in order to solve this dilemma, resulting in very complex statistical analyses of the various groups.

Menstrual irregularities, ectopic pregnancy, secondary infertility, increased rates of spontaneous abortion and preterm delivery have all been said to follow induced abortion, but other studies have failed to find any effects.

Menstrual irregularities

Beric et al (1973) found myometrium in 54.3% of cases after sharp curettage but in only 7.8% after vacuum aspiration, thus providing an explanation of the increased incidence of intrauterine synechiae (Asherman's syndrome) reported by Prudan (1964). Andolesk (1974) did not find any difference in menstrual patterns in 4664 women seen before and after abortion. Beric (1981) stated that young women are more likely to suffer from menstrual problems following abortion but admitted that he had no control group to confirm this impression. British and American workers have not reported this complication.

Ectopic pregnancy

After Shinagawa & Nayagama (1969) reported that 18 of 19 women with cervical pregnancies had previously had abortions, several authors looked at the relationship between induced abortion and ectopic pregnancy with conflicting results (Panayotou et al 1972, Roht & Aoyama 1974, Beric 1981). Three studies — by Daling & Emanuel (1977) in Seattle, Dalaker et al (1979) in Norway, and Chung et al (1980) in Hawaii — did not find any significant relationship. Beral (1975) examined the rate of ectopic pregnancy during the transition period from legal to illegal abortion in England and Wales; she found an increase up to 1970 and stable rates after this date. In Confidential Enquiries into Maternal Deaths (1986) the death rate per million pregnancies had declined from 12.4 in 1970–1972 to 8.2 in 1979–1981; infection and tubal surgery were reported to be the most common predisposing causes.

Secondary infertility

Most of the studies show no significant effect (Daling et al 1981); Hogue et al (1979) even found a higher rate of conception after induced abortion than in the control group. Obel (1979a), in a prospective study, noted a higher incidence of infertility in women who had pelvic infection following abortion. Table 29.11 lists selected studies; there does not seem to be a British one addressing the topic (Hogue et al 1982).

Spontaneous abortion

The majority of the studies follow women booking for antenatal care and are therefore subject to bias in several ways. MacKenzie & Hillier (1977) have reported a truly prospective study of women followed from the time of prostaglandin abortion through to the next pregnancy. The majority of this group of women, of whom 168 became pregnant, had had second-trimester abortions but not all had elective terminations — some had missed abortions. Compared with a control group matched reasonably well for age and parity (although those in the study group were more likely to be unmarried and have unplanned pregnancies) there was no significant increase in first-trimester abortions and a possibly significant increase in second-trimester abortion. The histories of these women did not suggest cervical incompetence.

The RCGP/RCOG (Frank et al 1985b) study has reported on the post-index pregnancy in 745 women in a prospective study compared with 1339 pregnancies in the control group. A small increase was found in the relative risk of first-trimester abortion × 1.24 (confidence limits: 0.81–1.90) while a smaller decrease was found in the relative risk of a second-trimester miscarriage × 0.97 (confidence limits: 0.51–1.83), both of which could have arisen by chance. The study recruited over 7000 women to each arm of the trial (Frank et al 1985b).

Table 29.12 summarizes the major studies and supports personal experience, which includes a follow-up study of 200 women in New Zealand (75% of whom were seen 3–6 years later) and over 5000 women seen at the Tower Hamlets DCAS. The conclusions are that:

1. First-trimester abortion done by vacuum aspiration without excessive dilatation of the cervix does not increase the risk of first-trimester abortion in a subsequent pregnancy. There may be a risk of an increase in second-trimester abortion but if so this is low — 1.5–2 times the normal risk.
2. Second-trimester abortion, whether by intra-amniotic or D&E techniques, has been insufficiently studied, but if there is a risk it is low. The small amount of evidence about extra-amniotic prostaglandins from Oxford is reassuring (MacKenzie & Hillier 1977).
3. First-trimester abortion by dilatation and curettage has been associated with higher rates of subsequent abortion — 1.5–2.5 times the normal risk in studies mainly from Eastern Europe.
4. The increased risk demonstrated in some studies of women who have had repeated abortions has not been adequately confirmed, since the controls differ in important respects (Table 29.13). These women may be an inherently high-risk group in countries with adequate contraceptive services.

Delivery of preterm or low birthweight infants

The majority of studies which have looked at this problem have not found an increase in preterm delivery compared with controls, even when the controls have not been matched. Reports from Hungary (Czeizal et al 1970, Klinget 1970) suggested that the incidence of both prematurity and low birthweight was increased in the population, where

Table 29.11 Selected studies of infertility after induced abortion

Reference	Study location and date	Design	Abortion procedure*	Controlled variables	Results
Roht & Aoyama 1973	Japan 1971	Cross-sectional	Mostly D&C	Age, duration of marriage	Gravidity was similar for those reporting and not reporting previous induced abortions
Hogue et al 1978	Yugoslavia 1966–1972	Abortion cohort	Mostly VA	Contraceptive use	Pregnancy-to-conception intervals were significantly shorter after induced abortion
Trichopoulous et al 1976	Greece 1974	Case-control	Illegal D&C	Age, parity, education	For secondary infertility >18 months, relative risk (RR) = 1.1 (0.59, 1.9)
			Illegal D&C	Age, parity, education, spontaneous abortion history	RR = 12.5 (2.3, 66.9)
Obel 1979a	Denmark 1967–1975	Pregnancy cohort	Mostly VA	Age, parity, socioeconomic status, regular menstrual cycle, contraceptive use	For pregnant women, the preceding interpregnancy interval did not significantly differ according to outcome of the preceding pregnancy
Daling et al 1981	Washington 1976–1978	Case-control	Mostly VA	Age, gravidity, race or ethnic status, marital status, socioeconomic status	For secondary infertility >12 months, RR = 1.3 (0.071, 2.4)
			Mostly VA	Age, gravidity, race or ethnic status, marital status, socioeconomic status, spontaneous abortion history	RR = 1.2 (0.41, 3.8)
Chung et al 1980	Hawaii 1970–1979	Abortion cohort	Mostly VA	Age, gravidity, menstrual regularity, contraceptive use	Several analytic techniques resulted in conclusion that induced abortion had not impaired ability to conceive
Stubblefield et al 1984	Boston 1976–1979	Abortion cohort/ controls:pregnancy/ contraceptive	Mixed	Groups reasonably comparable	Pregnancy rates for all three groups influenced by age, parity, race, marital status, etc. Induced abortion did not affect rates except those with history of 3 abortions, who had higher rate

Adapted from Hogue et al 1982
*VA = vacuum aspiration, D&C = dilatation and curettage.

women might experience several induced abortions. Later reports from Eastern Europe (Hogue 1975, Beric 1981) did not show an increase in preterm delivery; Roht & Aoyama (1974) in Japan, MacKenzie & Hillier (1977) in Oxford, Van der Slikke & Treffers (1978) in the Netherlands, Obel (1979b) in Denmark, and Schoenbaum et al (1980) in Boston confirmed these findings. Table 29.14 summarizes some of the most recent studies.

Hogue et al (1979) in Singapore and the World Health Organization (1979) multicentre trial showed no difference in outcome when first-trimester abortion was performed by vacuum aspiration. However, these studies did show an increase in the number of low birthweight infants born to women in whom dilatation and curettage had been used to terminate the previous pregnancy.

Russell's (1974) follow-up of teenagers undergoing abortion in the 1960s is a reminder that damage to the small teenage cervix may have serious effects on the woman's future reproductive performance.

Psychological sequelae

A considerable amount has been written on this subject; Simon & Senturia (1966) reviewed the literature from 1935 to 1964, while Gibbons (1984) assessed the more recent publications. The results from the on-going RCOG/RCGP study are awaited with interest, as few studies are prospective. In the earlier literature the bias of the author or of those quoting the work of others is often striking. The majority of the studies have found that mental health is better after abortion than before. Transient feelings of guilt or regret are found in most women; however, providing that the abortion is carried out in a supportive atmosphere, adjustment is rapid. Between 0.5 and 2% of women regret the decision (Greer et al 1976). If abortion is combined with sterilization—especially if sterilization was made a condition for

Table 29.12 Risk of spontaneous abortion following induced abortion

Reference	Place and date of study	Method of abortion	Number of subjects	Type of study	Results
Hogue 1978*	Yugoslavia 1968–1972	First trimester VA and D&C	144 A 352 C	Prospective cohort	Increased risk of an adverse outcome
Van der Slikke & Treffers 1978	Netherlands 1972–1976	VA 95% in country	504 A 13 991 C	Retrospective cohort	First-trimester abortion not studied; no significant difference in rate of second-trimester abortion, although the rate of 2.6% is double that of controls
WHO 1979	European multicentre 1973–1976	VA and D&C	1643 A 5585 C	Prospective cohort	Second-trimester abortion studied, no significant difference with VA but 3–4 times risk with D&C
Hogue et al 1979*	Singapore 1970–1974	VA and D&C	1617 A 1915 C	Prospective cohort	Midtrimester abortion studied; no significant difference with VA but 3 times risk with D&C
Harlap et al 1979	California 1974–1976	First and second trimesters VA and D&C	4512 A 28 401 C	Prospective cohort	No increase in rate of first-trimester abortion; 1.8 times risk of second-trimester abortion with one abortion, 3 times risk with two; most of risk related to pre-1973 period
Obel 1979b	Denmark 1975–1977	First and second trimesters	431 A 2611 C	Prospective cohort	No significant difference
Levin et al 1980	Boston 1976–1978	VA 73%	240 A 1072 C	Retrospective cohort	No significant risk of midtrimester abortion with one prior abortion, 2–3 times risk with two or more
Ratten & Beischer 1979	Melbourne 1977–1978	First and second trimesters	520 A 520 C	Prospective cohort	No difference with first-trimester abortion, but 3 times risk of second-trimester abortion; controls prior spontaneous abortion; 4% of aborters clinically had cervical incompetence
Madore et al 1981	California 1976–1978	First and second trimesters	2081 A 4098 C	Prospective cohort	Midtrimester abortion times 2 in subjects; if controlled for marital status, smoking, and socioeconomic class differences disappeared
Frank et al 1985b	UK 1976–1979	First and second trimester Mixed ops	745 A 1339 C	Prospective cohort GP FU	First trimester abortion RR 1.24 ns Second trimester abortion RR 0.97 ns

*From Cates 1980
(A = abortion; C = controls; VA = vacuum aspiration; D&C = dilatation and curettage)

performing the abortion—much higher rates of regret may be found (Ottoson 1971). Psychosis is more common after full-term delivery than abortion (Brewer 1977).

The changing attitudes of feminists towards abortion are exemplified by Petchesky (1986):

> Thus Adrienne Rich wrote in the mid-1970s: 'No free woman, with 100% effective non-harmful birth control readily available, would "choose" abortion' and 'Abortion is violence: a deep, desperate violence, inflicted by a woman, upon, first of all, herself'. The basis of this victim-blaming position is a perspective that reduces a woman's condition universally to 'male violence'. It is a strain of feminist tradition which idealizes motherhood, implying that the termination of every unwanted pregnancy is somehow a tragedy. Whatever its intention, this view does not accord with the facts. Many, perhaps most, abortions performed today (and as far as we can tell through much of history) are not the product of 'grim driven desperation', as Rich calls it, but of women's sober determination to take hold of their lives and, sometimes, of a sense of enlarged power for being able to do so.

This viewpoint seems to me to lack an understanding of the desperation of women before modern methods of contraception and legal abortion were available, when repeated childbearing was the lot of most working-class women (Hall 1976), although it is a stand taken by some activists in the pro-choice movement. In the author's experience, the decision to terminate a pregnancy is not taken lightly although regret is rare if the woman has been allowed to make her own decision.

ADMINISTRATIVE AND PREVENTIVE MEASURES

More than 20 years after the Abortion Act was passed, the NHS has not been able to provide a comprehensive service for all the women who request legal abortions. Figure 29.10 shows how the rates of NHS abortions still vary regionally, so that many women have to travel some distance to a private or charitable service to obtain this operation. Although the simplicity and safety of day-care abortion are clear from well documented work in the USA and in the UK, the proportion of day-case operations has risen only slowly from 25 to 35% in the non-NHS and from 13 to 38% in the NHS between 1977 and 1985. Day care was planned for 44% of women in the NHS in 1986 (Office of Population Censuses and Surveys 1987), although 75–80% of women are suitable for this type of care, which is cheaper and preferred by women with young children.

Delay in the abortion referral process leads to a higher

Table 29.13 Selected studies of the effect of multiple induced abortion

Reference	Place and date of study	Type of study	Method	Matched variables	Effect studied	Results
Lerner & Varma 1981	New York City 1976–1980	Pregnancy cohort	VA and D&C	Age, race or ethnic status, gestation at booking, height of mother, smoker, sex of infant	Low birthweight	Compared with G2P1, RR = 2.6 (1.2, 6.0); compared with G1, RR = 1.9 (0.73, 4.9)
			VA and D&C	Age, race or ethnic status, gestation at booking, height of mother, smoking, sex of infant	Shortened gestation	Compared with G2P1, RR = 1.5 (0.36, 6.2); compared with G1, RR = 1.4 (0.31, 5.9)
			VA and D&C	Age, race or ethnic status, gestation at booking, height of mother, smoking, sex of infant	Toxaemia	Compared with G2P1, RR = 4.2 (1.5, 11.4); compared with G1, RR = 1.5 (0.19, 2.3)
			VA and D&C	Age, race or ethnic status, gestation at booking, height of mother, smoking, sex of infant	Premature rupture of the membranes	Compared with G2P1, RR = 1.7 (0.81, 3.6); compared with G1, RR = 1.0 (0.88, 1.2)
Harlap et al 1979	California 1974–1976	Pregnancy cohort	Mostly VA (after 1973)	Age, gestation at booking	Spontaneous abortion	For second-trimester spontaneous abortion compared with G1, RR = 3.1 (1.6, 6.2)
Chung et al 1980	Hawaii 1970–1978	Abortion cohort	Mostly VA	None	Ectopic pregnancy	Compared with 1 prior abortion, RR = 0.94
			Mostly VA	Multivariate confounder score including parity	Spontaneous abortion	Compared with no prior abortion, RR = 1.01 for first-trimester spontaneous abortion; RR = 0.80 for second-trimester spontaneous abortion
			Mostly VA	Multivariate confounder score including parity	Low birthweight	Compared with no prior abortion, RR = 0.86
			Mostly VA	Multivariate confounder score including parity	Shortened gestation	Compared with no prior abortion, RR = 1.00
			Mostly VA	Multivariate confounder score including parity	Pregnancy complications	Compared with no prior abortion, RR = 0.91
			Mostly VA	Multivariate confounder score including parity	Labour complications	Compared with no prior abortion, RR = 0.94
			Mostly VA	Multivariate confounder score including parity	Congenital malformations	Compared with no prior abortion, RR = 1.44
			Mostly VA	Multivariate confounder score including parity	Postneonatal death	Compared with no prior abortion, RR = 1.03
Pickering & Forbes 1985	Scotland 1980–1981	Pregnancy cohort	Mostly VA	Age, height, parity, sex of infant, marital status, social class	SGA infant	Compared with P1 + 0, RR = 1.13 P2 + 0 0.68, IA × 10.9
					Preterm delivery	Compared with P1 + 0, RR = 1.27 P2 0.79 1IA 1.35

Adapted from Table 7 in Hogue et al (1982) Refs 1–3 from this paper.
RR = relative risk; VA = vacuum aspiration; D&C = dilatation and curettage.

proportion of late operations (Alberman & Dennis 1984) and morbidity rises with each week of gestation. Sterilization is still used more often in the NHS than in any comparable country; Figure 29.11 shows these variations.

The greater efficiency, lesser mortality and morbidity of the non-NHS sector has been documented by the RCGP/RCOG study (Frank et al 1985b), in addition to the RCOG late abortion study (Alberman & Dennis 1984). Lawson et al (1976) and Ashton (1980, Ashton et al 1983) have shown how to reduce waiting time; Chalmers & Anderson (1972) looked in detail at referral practices. The Camden study (Clarke et al 1983) suggested that some younger more affluent women bypassed the NHS and found the attitudes preferable in the non-NHS sector.

The suggestion of regional NHS abortion units has not yet been taken up but may commend itself to regional general managers (Savage & Paterson 1982). The later abortions would be centralized for teaching and research, supported by satellite day-care units. It should not be difficult to find nurses and doctors who have no conscientious objection to abortion, and such a unit would relieve many hospital staff of a task they dislike. Kaltreider et al (1979) have looked

Table 29.14 Risk of preterm delivery or low birthweight, taken from selected studies since 1978

Reference	Place and date of study	Method of abortion	Number of subjects	Type of study	Results
Van der Slikke & Treffers 1978	Netherlands 1972–1976	Mainly VA	504 A 13 991 C	Retrospective cohort	No significant relationship primiparae, age-matched preterm delivery
WHO 1979	European multicentre 1973–1976	VA and D&C	1643 A 5585 C	Prospective cohort	No significant differences in babies weighing under 2500 g when VA used; 2.5 times increase in preterm delivery in Scandinavian cities
Hogue et al 1979*	Singapore 1970–1974	VA and D&C	2975 A 3130 C	Prospective cohort	Increased risk of low birthweight infant after D&C but not after VA
Ratten & Beischer 1979	Australia 1977–78	First trimester	520 A 520 C	Prospective cohort	Preterm delivery rate times 2 in aborted patients: controls not matched for important variables
Obel 1979b	Denmark 1974–1975	All methods	576 A 6684 C	Prospective cohort	No significant relationship
Logrillo et al 1980	USA 1970–1976	All methods	20 306 A 20 306 C	Record linkage, prospective cohort	1.3–1.7 times risk of low birthweight infant or preterm delivery in aborted group compared with women having second baby but not if compared with primigravidae
Schoenbaum et al 1980	1975–1976	VA 73%	205 A 3041 C	Retrospective cohort	No significant relationship
Madore et al 1981	USA 1976–1978	All methods	2081 A 4098 C	Retrospective cohort interviewed	No difference in preterm deliveries or low birthweight infants
Frank et al 1985b	UK 1976–1978	All methods	745 A 1339 C	Prospective GPFU	RR low birthweight 1.39 NS RR delivery less than 37 weeks, 1.13 NS

*from Cates 1980
RR = relative risk; NS = not significant; A = abortion; C = controls; VA = vacuum aspiration; D&C = dilatation and curettage; GPFU = general practitioner follow-up.

at the attitudes of staff to abortion by different methods; an anonymous article in the British Medical Journal (1984) described how one young doctor felt about her work in the abortion field, arguing that the surgical technique did not require the skills of a consultant gynaecologist. Freedman et al (1986) reported no difference in the complication rates of physicians and physician assistants in 2458 first-trimester abortions. Women doctors with family planning training could easily be taught the necessary skills and would provide a better service than a shifting population of often poorly supervised trainee gynaecologists.

Morbidity and mortality rise with increasing gestation. The aim should be to set up sympathetic, accessible services which have the minimum of delay. In the Tower Hamlets' experience in an inner city area, less than 10% of women present in the second trimester. Prompt referral by the general practitioner, avoidance of delay in waiting for pregnancy testing and the provision of pregnancy testing at the general practitioner surgery or family planning clinic help. Open access to a well publicized abortion facility can also do much to reduce delay. Doctors with a conscientious objection to abortion could be identified as such in the list of general practitioners published by the Family Practitioner Committee; doctors' own moral beliefs do sometimes lead to long delays.

The establishment in each district of a director of well women's services should be facilitated. This person could have responsibility for services for abortion, contraception, sterilization, cervical cytology and perhaps mammography screening. Prepregnancy clinics and healthy living clinics for both sexes would be a positive first step to improve the health of women.

THE FUTURE

We need an acceptance politically that women should be able to control their own fertility and have a right to enjoy their sexuality, as men have usually done throughout history.

Ory (1983) updated the work started by Tietze in 1969 and showed that logically the safest way for a woman in the 15–34-year age group to prevent pregnancy is to rely on the condom, with abortion as a back-up. Sterilization is increasingly used by women over this age and carries a small risk of death — 1 in 250 000 operations in American hospitals according to Peterson et al (1981). Vasectomy carries no risk to the woman and only a 1 in 1 000 000 chance of death to the man. Wider contraceptive provision has made a significant impact on conception rates, which have fallen from 89.1 in 1969 to 71.4 per 1000 women aged 15–44 years in 1983 (Office of Population Censuses and Surveys 1985) — a reduction of 20%. The addition of abortion to the analysis increases this to a fall of 30% in the birth rate, with the result that the UK is approaching zero population growth.

Condoms should be widely advertised and easy to obtain in places where young people meet. Sex education should stress the need for responsibility in sexual relationships to counteract the influence of the advertising industry and the

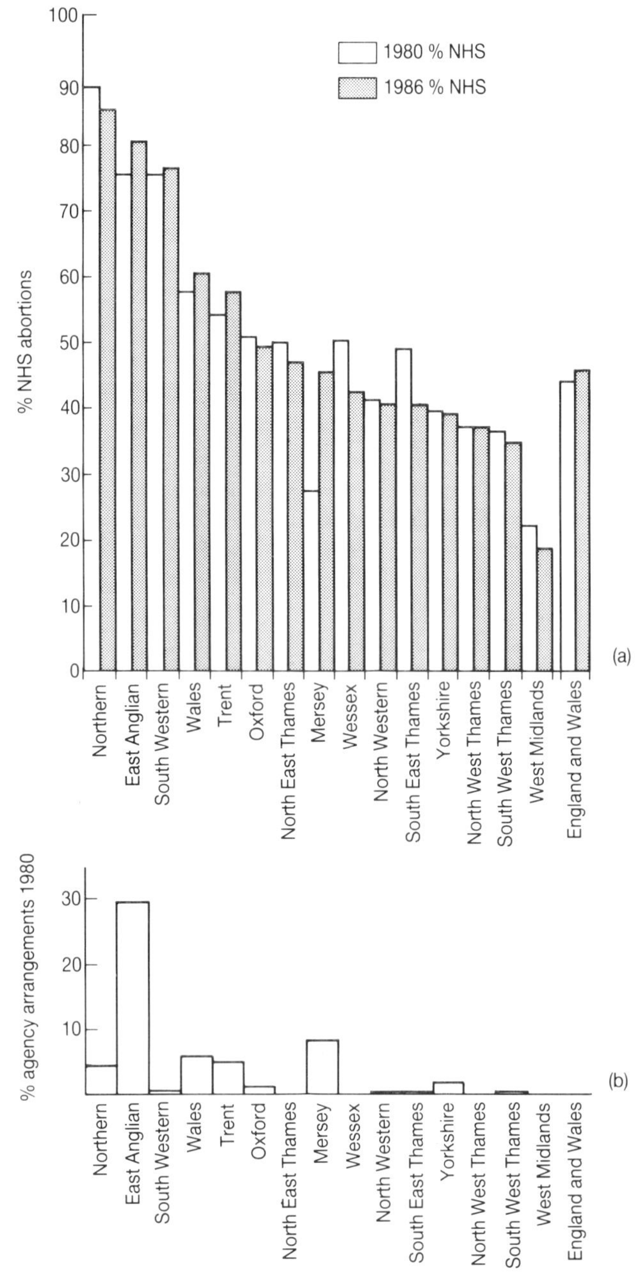

Fig. 29.10 Proportion of operations done in NHS or on an agency basis for England and Wales by region.

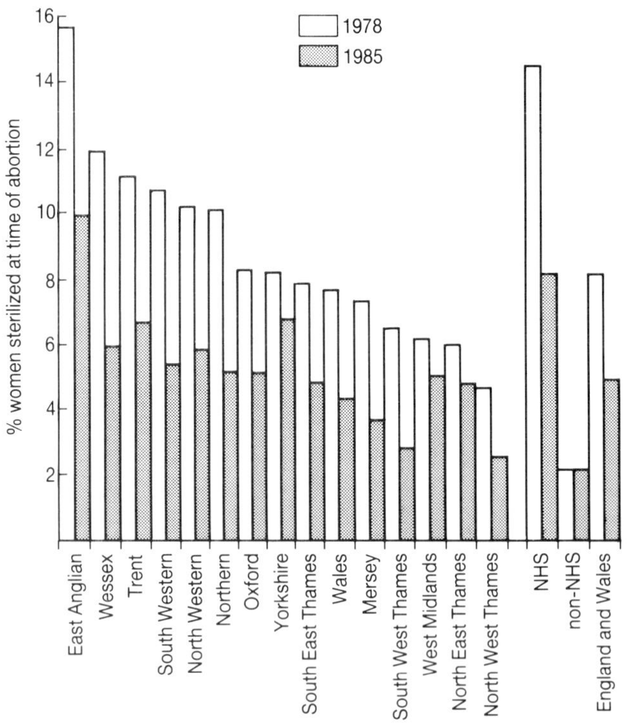

Fig. 29.11 Sterilization at time of abortion by region in 1978 and 1985. OPCS figures for England and Wales.

media where sex is never followed by pregnancy, abortion or venereal disease but used to sell everything.

Doctors should support legislation to give women the right to choose an abortion, at least in the first trimester, and take the necessary steps to provide a more efficient service. This would be cheaper, more humane and medically safer than the present system. The experience in Sweden should be noted; there a change in the law in 1975 allowing the woman to choose to have an abortion up to the 18th week of pregnancy led to a fall in the number of second-trimester procedures from 20% in 1973 to 5% in 1983. The rate of abortion also fell because of a well planned sex education and contraceptive programme. In teenagers, the fall in conception rates was 30% over the 10 years (Rolen 1984).

Regional NHS abortion units should be set up, possibly on an agency basis. The RCOG should consider a subspecialty of fertility control to encourage centres of excellence such as the Margaret Pyke Centre, where teaching and research thrive.

Educating young people about health and increasing awareness of their bodies should help to reduce the number of women presenting late in pregnancy; the fall in the rate of unplanned teenage pregnancies in Sweden after the passage of the 1975 law relating to contraception, abortion and sex education does suggest that adequate knowledge can prevent unplanned pregnancy (Rolen 1984).

Research into ways of terminating very early pregnancies, so that the self-administered abortion pill becomes a reality, will continue. The replacement of amniocentesis for prenatal diagnosis by chorion villus sampling (Brambati 1987) should help to reduce the number of late abortions required on these grounds. Prospective studies comparing the effects of different methods of second-trimester pregnancy termination on future reproductive performance are still needed, while research into new drugs to improve the medical methods available will continue.

Perhaps by the end of the century the abortion rate will have fallen below 5 per 1000 and every child will be a wanted child.

REFERENCES

Alberman E, Dennis K J 1984 Late abortions in England and Wales. Royal College of Obstetricians and Gynaecologists, London

Alberman E, Kani W, Stanwell-Smith R 1984 Congenital abnormalities in legal abortions at 20 weeks' gestation or longer. Lancet i: 1226–1228

Allen I 1981 Family planning — sterilisation and abortion services. Policy Studies Institute, London

Andolesk L 1974 The Ljublana abortion study 1971. Center for Population Research, Bethesda, USA, p 32

Ashton J R 1980 Components of delay amongst women obtaining termination of pregnancy. Journal of Biosocial Science 12: 261–273

Ashton J R, Machin D, Osmond C, Balajaran R, Adam S A, Donnan S P B 1983 Trends in induced abortion in England and Wales. Journal of Epidemiology and Community Health 37: 105–110

Barron S L 1986 Sexual activity in girls under 16 years of age. British Journal of Obstetrics and Gynaecology 93: 787–793

Beekhuizen W, van Schie K J, van Lith D A F, du Plessis M, Keirse M J N C 1982 Aspirotomy for outpatient termination of pregnancy in the second trimester. In: Keirse M J N C, Bennebroek Gravenhorst J, van Lith D A F, Embrey M P (eds) Second trimester pregnancy termination. Leiden University Press, The Hague

Beral V 1975 An epidemiologic study of recent trends in ectopic pregnancy. British Journal of Obstetrics and Gynaecology 82: 775–782

Berger G S, Kerenyi T D 1974 Analysis of retained placenta associated with saline abortion: methodologic considerations. American Journal of Obstetrics and Gynecology 120: 479–483

Beric B 1981 Late somatic sequelae/delayed complications of induced abortion. In: Hodgson J (ed) Abortion and sterilization. Academic Press, London, pp 379–393

Beric B M, Kupresanin M 1971 Vacuum aspiration, using para-cervical block for legal abortion as an outpatient procedure up to the 12th week of pregnancy. Lancet ii: 619–621

Beric B, Kupresanin M, Kapor-Stanulovic N 1973 Accidents and sequelae of medical abortions. American Journal of Obstetrics and Gynecology 116: 813–821

Bierer I & Steiner V 1971 Termination of pregnancy in the second trimester with the aid of laminaria tents. Medical Gynaecology and Sociology 6: 9–10

Brambati B 1987 Chorionic villus sampling: a safe and reliable alternative in fetal diagnosis? Research in Reproduction 19: 1–4

Brenner W E 1975 Second trimester interruption of pregnancy. In: Taymour M L, Green T H (eds) Progress in gynaecology, vol 6. Grune & Stratton, New York, pp 421–444

Brenner W E, Dingfelder J R, Staurovsky L G, Hendricks C H 1973 Vaginally administered $PGF_{2\alpha}$ for cervical dilatation in multiparas prior to suction curettage. Prostaglandins 4: 819

Brewer C 1977 Incidence of postabortion psychosis: a prospective study. British Medical Journal 1: 476–477

Brewer C 1980 Prevention of infection after abortion with a supervised single dose of doxycycline. British Medical Journal 281: 780–781

British Medical Association 1936 Report of the committee on medical aspects of abortion. British Medical Association, London

British Medical Journal Leader 1981 Late consequence of abortion. British Medical Journal i: 1564

British Medical Journal 1984 Personal view. British Medical Journal 289: 1377

Bromwich P 1987 Late abortion. British Medical Journal 294: 526–528

Burkman R T, Tonascia J H, Atienza M F, King T M 1976 Untreated endocervical gonorrhoea and endometritis following elective abortion. American Journal of Obstetrics and Gynecology 126: 648–651

Burnhill M, Armstead J W 1978 Reducing the morbidity of vacuum aspiration abortion. International Journal of Gynaecology and Obstetrics 16: 204–209

Bury J 1984 Teenage pregnancy in Britain. Birth Control Trust, London

Butler N R, Bonham D G 1963 Perinatal mortality. The first report of the 1958 British Perinatal Mortality Survey. Livingstone, Edinburgh

Bygdeman M, Bergstrom S 1976 Clinical use of prostaglandins for pregnancy termination. Population Reports, series G, No. 7

Bygdeman M, Christensen N, Green K et al 1983 Menses induction and second-trimester pregnancy termination using a polymeric controlled release vaginal delivery system containing 15(s) 15-methyl $PGF_{2\alpha}$ methyl ester. Contraception 27: 141–151

Cadesky K I, Ravinsky E, Lyons E R 1985 Dilation and evacuation: a preferred method of mid-trimester abortion. American Journal of Obstetrics and Gynecology 153: 329–332

Castadot R G 1986 Pregnancy termination: techniques, risks, and complications and their management. Fertility and Sterility 45: 5–17

Cates W 1980 A Bibliography: studies of long-term effects of induced abortion. Center for Diseases Control, Atlanta

Cates W, Grimes D A 1981 Deaths from second trimester abortion by dilatation and evacuation: causes, prevention, facilities. Obstetrics and Gynecology 58: 401–408

Cates W, Schultz K F, Grimes D A et al 1982 Dilatation and evacuation procedures and second trimester abortions: the role of physician skill and hospital setting. Journal of the American Medical Association 248: 559–563

Chalmers I, Anderson A 1972 Factors affecting gestational age at therapeutic abortion. Lancet i: 1324–1326

Chung C S, Steinhoff P G, Mi M P, Smith R G 1980 Long term effects of induced abortion. Presented at the 105th Annual meeting of the American Public Health Association, Washington DC, October 1980

Clarke L, Farrell C, Beaumont B 1983 The Camden Abortion Study: the view and experiences of having NHS and private treatment. British Pregnancy Advisory Service, Solihull

Cohen E, Ballard C A 1974 Consumptive coagulopathy associated with intra amniotic saline instillation and the effect of intravenous oxytocin. Obstetrics and Gynecology 43: 300–303

Confidential Enquiries into Maternal Deaths 1975 (1970–1972). HMSO, London

Confidential Enquiries into Maternal Deaths 1979 (1973–1975). HMSO, London

Confidential Enquiries into Maternal Deaths 1982 (1976–1978). HMSO, London

Confidential Enquiries into Maternal Deaths 1986 (1979–1981). HMSO, London

Contreras M, de Silva M, Hewitt P E 1986 Why women are not receiving anti-Rh prophylaxis. British Medical Journal 293: 1373

Cook R J, Dickens B M 1982 Emerging issues in Commonwealth abortion laws. Commonwealth Secretariat, London

Czeizal A, Bognar A, Tusnady A, Revesz P 1970 Changes in mean birth weight and proportion of low-weight births in Hungary. British Journal of Preventive and Social Medicine 24: 146–153

Dalaker K, Lichtenberg S M, Okland G 1979 Delayed reproductive complications after induced abortion. Acta Obstetricia et Gynecologica Scandinavica 58: 491–494

Daling J R, Emanuel I 1977. Induced abortion and subsequent outcome of pregnancy in a series of American women. New England Journal of Medicine 297: 1241–1245

Daling J R, Spadoni L R, Emanuel I 1981 Role of induced abortion in secondary infertility. Obstetrics and Gynecology 57: 59–61

David H 1981 Abortion policies. In: Hodgson E (ed) Abortion and sterilization: medical and social aspects. Academic Press, London, pp 1–38

Davis G 1972 Mid trimester abortion. Lancet ii: 1026

Diggory P L C 1969 Some experiences of therapeutic abortion. Lancet i: 873–874

Diggory P L C 1977 Techniques of abortion. In: Potts M, Diggory P, Peel J (eds) Abortion. Cambridge University Press, Cambridge, p 212

Diggory P 1984 Safety of termination of pregnancy: NHS vs private. Lancet ii: 920

Duthie S J, Hobson D, Tait I A et al 1987 Morbidity after termination of pregnancy in the first trimester. Genito-urinary Medicine 63: 182–187

Edelman D A, Berger G S 1981 Menstrual regulation. In: Hodgson J (ed) Abortion and sterilization. Academic Press, London, p 216

Edelman D A, Brenner W E, Davis G L R, Child P 1974 An evaluation of the Pregnosticon-Dri-Dot test in early pregnancy. American Journal of Obstetrics and Gynecology 119: 521–524

Elia D 1985 Uses of RU 486: a clinical update. IPPF Medical Bulletin 20(5): 1–2

Embrey M P, Hillier K, Mahendran P 1972 Induction of abortion by extra-amniotic administration of prostaglandin E_2 and $F_{2\alpha}$. British Medical Journal ii: 146–149

Emery S, Jarvis G J, Johnson D A N 1979 Uterine rupture after intra-amniotic injection of prostaglandin E_2. British Medical Journal ii: 51

Feeney J G 1982 Water intoxication and oxytocin. British Medical Journal 285: 243–285
Finks A A 1973 Mid trimester abortion. Lancet i: 263–264
Finks A A 1980 Presented at the 2nd Trimester Pregnancy Termination Course, University of Leiden, The Netherlands
Francome C 1984 Abortion freedom. George Allen & Unwin, London
Frank P I, Kay C R, Wingrave S J, Lewis T L T, Osborne J, Newell C 1985a Induced abortion operations and their early sequelae: joint study of the Royal College of General Practitioners and the Royal College of Obstetricians and Gynaecologists. Journal of the Royal College of General Practitioners 35: 175–180
Frank P I, Kay C R, Lewis T L T, Parish S 1985b Outcome of pregnancy following induced abortion. Report from the joint study of the Royal College of General Practitioners and the Royal College of Obstetricians and Gynaecologists. British Journal of Obstetrics and Gynaecology 92: 308–316
Freda V J, Gorman J G, Galen R S, Treacy N 1970 The threat of rhesus immunization from abortion. Lancet ii: 147–148
Freedman M A, Jillson D A, Coffin R R, Novick L F 1986 Comparison of complication rates in first trimester abortions performed by physician assistants and physicians. American Journal of Public Health 76: 550–555
Frieman S M, Wulff G J L 1977 Management of uterine perforation following elective abortion. Obstetrics and Gynecology 50: 647–650
Gibbons M 1984 Psychiatric sequelae of induced abortion. Journal of the Royal College of General Practitioners 34: 146–150
Golditch I M, Glasser M H 1974 The use of laminaria tents for cervical dilatation prior to vacuum aspiration abortion. American Journal of Obstetrics and Gynecology 119: 481–484
Goldthorpe W O 1977 Ten-minute abortions. British Medical Journal ii: 562–564
Gravenhorst Bennebroek J, Beinteman-Dubbeldam A, van Lith D A F, Beekhuizen W 1986 Elevation of maternal alpha-fetoprotein serum levels in relation to fetomaternal haemorrhage after second trimester pregnancy termination by aspirotomy. British Journal of Obstetrics and Gynaecology 93: 1302–1304
Greer H S, Lal S, Lewis S C, Belsey E M, Beard R W 1976 Psychosocial consequences of therapeutic abortion, King's termination study III. British Journal of Psychiatry 128: 74–79
Grimes D A, Cates W 1979 Complications from legally-induced abortion: a review. Obstetrical and Gynecological Survey 34: 177–191
Grimes D A, Schulz K F 1985 Morbidity and mortality from second-trimester abortions. Journal of Reproductive Medicine. 20: 505–514
Grimes D A, Hulka J F, McCutchen M E 1980 Midtrimester abortion by dilatation and evacuation versus intra-amniotic instillation of prostaglandin $F_{2\alpha}$. A randomized clinical trial. American Journal of Obstetrics and Gynecology 137: 785–790
Grundy M F B, Craven E R 1976 Consumption coagulopathy after intra-amniotic urea. British Medical Journal ii: 677–678
Hall R (ed) 1976 Dear Dr Stopes: sex in the 1920s. Letters to Marie Stopes. Andre Deutsch, London
Harlap S, Shiono P, Ramcharan S, Berendes H, Pellegrin F 1979 A prospective study of spontaneous fetal losses after induced abortions. New England Journal of Medicine 301: 677–681
Healy D L, Fraser H M 1985 The antiprogesterones are coming: menses induction, abortion, and labour? British Medical Journal 290: 580–581
Hindell K, Simms M 1971 Abortion law reformed. Peter Owen, London
Hodgson J 1981 Late midtrimester abortion. In: Hodgson J (ed) Abortion and sterilization. Academic Press, London
Hodgson J, Major B, Portman K, Quattlebaum F W 1975 Prophylactic use of tetracycline for first trimester abortions. Obstetrics and Gynecology 45: 574–578
Hogue C 1975 Low birth weight subsequent to induced abortion. A historical prospective study of 948 in Skopje, Yugoslavia. American Journal of Obstetrics and Gynecology 123: 675–681
Hogue C, Schoenfelder J R, Gesta W M 1978 The interactive effects of induced abortion, inter-pregnancy interval and contraceptive use on subsequent pregnancy outcome. American Journal of Epidemiology 107: 15–26
Hogue C, Wood J L, Lean T H 1979 Long-term sequelae in dilatation and curettage versus vacuum aspiration: report of an epidemiologic study in Singapore. In: Satuchni G I, Sciarra J J, Speidel J J (eds) Pregnancy termination; procedures, safety and new developments. Harper & Row, London, p 149
Hogue C J R, Cates W Jr, Tietze C 1982 The effects of induced abortion on subsequent reproduction. Epidemiologic Reviews 4: 66–94
Horwitz D A 1974 Uterine rupture following attempted saline abortions with oxytocin in a grand multiparous patient. Obstetrics and Gynecology 43: 921–922
House of Lords Select Committee on the Infant Life (Preservation) Bill 1987 Special report with evidence. HMSO, London
Hulka J F, Lefler H T, Anglone A, Lachenbruch P A 1974 A new electronic force monitor to measure factors influencing cervical dilation for vacuum curettage. American Journal of Obstetrics and Gynecology 120: 166–173
Hull M G R, Gordon C, Beard R W 1974 The organisation and results of a pregnancy termination service in an NHS hospital. Journal of Obstetrics and Gynaecology of the British Commonwealth 81: 577–587
Hussey R M 1987 Why women are not receiving anti-Rh prophylaxis. British Medical Journal 294: 119
Johnstone F D, Beard R J, Boyd I E, McCarthy T G 1976 Cervical diameter after suction termination of pregnancy. British Medical Journal i: 68–69
Kahn A R, Rochat R W, Jahan F A, Begum S F 1986 Induced abortion in a rural area of Bangladesh. Studies in Family Planning 17: 95–99
Kaltreider N B, Goldsmith S, Margolis A J 1979 The impact of midtrimester abortion techniques on patients and staff. American Journal of Obstetrics and Gynecology 135: 235–238
Karim S M M, Filshie G M 1970 Therapeutic abortion using prostaglandin $F_{2\alpha}$. Lancet i: 157–159
Karman H, Potts M 1972 Very early abortion using syringe as vacuum source. Lancet i: 1051–1052
Kerslake D 1973 Abortion in the private sector — Fairfield Nursing Home. Medical Gynaecology, Andrology and Sociology 8: 10–16
Kiel F W 1986 The medical value of examining tissue from therapeutic abortions: an analysis of 13 477 cases. British Journal of Obstetrics and Gynaecology 93: 594–596
King T M, Atienza M F, Burkman R T 1980 The incidence of abdominal surgical procedures in a population undergoing abortion. American Journal of Obstetrics and Gynecology 137: 530–533
Klinget A 1970 Demographic consequences of the legalization of induced abortion in Europe. International Journal of Obstetrics and Gynecology 8: 680–691
Kubba A A, Guillebaud J 1984 Failure of post-coital contraception after insertion of an intra-uterine device. Case report. British Journal of Obstetrics and Gynaecology 91: 596–597
Lauerson N H, Birnbaum S 1973 Laparoscopy as a diagnostic and therapeutic technique in uterine perforations during first trimester abortions. American Journal of Obstetrics and Gynecology 117: 522–529
Laufe L E 1979 Menstrual regulation: international perspective. In: Zatuchni G I, Sciarra J J, Speidel J J (eds) Pregnancy termination: procedures, safety, and new developments. Harper & Row, London pp 78–81
Lawson J, Barron S L, Yave D, Quierdo A M E, Phillip P R 1976 Management of the abortion problem in an English city. Lancet ii: 1288–1291
Lerner R C, Varma A O 1981 Prospective study of the outcome of pregnancy subsequent to previous induced abortion. Final report. New York Downstate Medical Center, State University of New York
Levin A A, Schoenbaum S C, Monson R, Stubblefield P, Ryan K D 1980 Association of induced abortion with subsequent pregnancy loss. Journal of the American Medical Association 243: 2495–2499
Lewis S C, Lal S, Branch B, Beard R W 1971 Outpatient termination of pregnancy. British Medical Journal 4: 606–610
Lilford R J, Bingham P, Bourne G L, Chard T 1985 Computerized histories facilitate patient care in a termination of pregnancy clinic: the use of a small computer to obtain and reproduce patient information. British Journal of Obstetrics and Gynaecology 92: 333–340
Lippes J, Malik T, Tatum H J 1976 The post-coital copper-T. Advances in Planned Parenthood 11: 1
Liskin L 1980 Complications of abortion in developing countries. Population Reports, series F, no. 7, Johns Hopkins University, Maryland
Logrillo V 1981 Family Planning Perspectives 13: 80
Logrillo V, Quickenton P, Therriault G D et al 1980 Effect of induced

abortion on subsequent reproductive function. Final report to NICHD. New York State Health Department, Albany, New York
Lowensohn R, Ballard C A 1974 Cervicovaginal fistula; an apparent increased incidence with $PGF_{2\alpha}$. American Journal of Obstetrics and Gynecology 119: 1057–1061
Macfarlane A, Mugford M 1984 Birth counts: statistics of pregnancy and childbirth. HMSO, London
MacKenzie I Z 1987 Methods of second trimester pregnancy termination. Prostaglandin Perspectives 3: 18–21
MacKenzie, I Z, Fry A 1981 Prostaglandin E_2 pessaries to facilitate first trimester aspiration termination. British Journal of Obstetrics and Gynaecology 88: 1033–1037
MacKenzie I Z, Hillier K 1977 Prostaglandin induced abortion and outcome of subsequent pregnancies: a prospective controlled study. British Medical Journal ii: 1114–1117
Madore C, Hawes W E, Many F, Hexter A G 1981 A study on the effects of induced abortion on subsequent pregnancy outcome. American Journal of Obstetrics and Gynecology 139: 516–521
Measham A R, Obaidullah M, Rosenberg M J, Rochat R W, Khan A R, Jabeen S 1981 Complications from induced abortion in Bangladesh related to types of practitioner and methods and impact on mortality. Lancet ii: 199–202
Millar D 1987 ABC of AIDS: counselling. British Medical Journal 294: 1671–1674
Mills A 1983 Therapeutic abortion and chlamydial infection. British Medical Journal 286: 1649
Mills A M 1984 An assessment of pre-operative microbial screening on the prevention of post-abortion pelvic inflammatory disease. British Journal of Obstetrics and Gynaecology 91: 182–186
Munsick R A 1972 Air embolism and maternal death from therapeutic abortion. Obstetrics and Gynecology 36: 688–690
Nathanson B N 1973 The postabortal pain syndrome; a new entity. Obstetrics and Gynecology 41: 739–742
Newton B 1972 Laminaria tents: relics of the past or modern medical devices? American Journal of Obstetrics and Gynecology 113: 442–448
Newton B 1975 A practitioner's report on laminaria tents. Contemporary Obstetrics and Gynecology 5: 29–42
Nicolaides K H, Welch C C, MacPherson M B A, Johnson I R, Filshie G M 1983 Lamicel — a new technique for cervical dilatation before first trimester abortion. British Journal of Obstetrics and Gynaecology 90: 475–479
Obel E B 1979a Fertility following legally induced abortion. Acta Obstetricia et Gynecologica Scandinavica 58: 539–542
Obel E B 1979b Pregnancy complications following legally induced abortion. Acta Obstetricia et Gynecologica Scandinavica 58: 485–490
Office of Population Censuses and Surveys 1975–1985 Abortion statistics. HMSO, London
Ory H W 1983 Mortality associated with fertility and fertility control: 1983. Family Planning Perspectives 15: 57–63
Ottoson J O 1971 Legal abortion in Sweden: 30 years experience. Journal of Biosocial Science 3: 173–192
Pakter J, Nelson F G 1972 Effect of a liberalised abortion law in New York City. Mount Sinai Journal of Medicine 39: 535
Panayotou P P, Kaskerelis D B, Miettinen O S, Trichopoulos D B, Kalamdidi A K 1972 Induced abortion and ectopic pregnancy. American Journal of Obstetrics and Gynecology 114: 507
Paxman J M, Barberis M 1980 Menstrual regulation and the law. International Journal of Gynecology and Obstetrics 6: 823–829
Petchesky R P 1986 Abortion and woman's choice. Verso, London
Peterson H B, Grimes D A, Cates W, Rubin G L 1981 Comparative risk of death from induced abortion at <12 weeks' gestation performed with local versus general anesthesia. American Journal of Obstetrics and Gynecology 141: 763–768
Pickering R M, Forbes J F 1985 Risks of preterm delivery and small-for-gestational-age infants following abortion: a population study. British Journal of Obstetrics and Gynaecology 92: 1106–112
Population Reports 1976 Post-coital contraception, series J, no. 9. Johns Hopkins University, Baltimore, p 142
Potts M, Diggory P, Peel D 1977 Abortion. Cambridge University Press, Cambridge
Propping D, Stubblefield P G, Golub J, Zucherman J 1977 Uterine rupture following mid-trimester abortion by laminaria, prostaglandin $F_{2\alpha}$ and oxytocin. Report of two cases. American Journal of Obstetrics and Gynecology 128: 689–690
Prudan D 1964 Neki menstruacioni poreme ćaji zbeg endouterinih sinehija posle poloačaja. Quoted in Abortion and sterilization (edited by Hodgson J) Academic Press, London p 381
Ratten G J, Beischer N A 1979 The effect of termination of pregnancy on maturity of subsequent pregnancy. Medical Journal of Australia i: 479–480
Registrar General's statistical tables: supplement on abortion 1968–1974. HMSO, London
Ridgeway G L, Mumtax G, Stephens R A, Oriel J D 1983 Therapeutic abortion and chlamydial infection. British Medical Journal 286: 1478–1479
Roht L H, Aoyama H 1973 Induced abortion and its sequelae: prematurity and spontaneous abortion. American Journal of Obstetrics and Gynecology 120: 868–874
Rolen M 1984 Free means fewer. An evaluation of the Swedish Abortion Act and family planning programme of 1984. Regeringskansliets Offsetcentral, Stockholm
Rowe J (ed) 1988 Reducing late abortions: access to NHS services in early pregnancy. Proceedings of a conference held in September 1987. Birth Control Trust, London
Russell J K 1974 Sexual activity and its consequences in the teenager. Clinics in Obstetrics and Gynaecology 1: 683–698
Savage W D 1979 Methods of midtrimester abortion. Fertility and Contraception 3: 53
Savage W D 1981a Abortion and sterilisation — should the operations be combined? British Journal of Family Planning 7: 8–12
Savage W D 1981b New form for termination of pregnancy. British Medical Journal 282: 478–479
Savage W D 1985 Requests for late termination of pregnancy: Tower Hamlets 1983. British Medical Journal 299: 621–623
Savage W D, Paterson I 1982 Abortion methods and sequelae. British Journal of Hospital Medicine 28: 364–384
Schoenbaum S C, Monson R R, Stubblefield P G, Darney P D, Ryan K J 1980 Outcome of the delivery following an induced or spontaneous abortion. American Journal of Obstetrics and Gynecology 136: 19–24
Segal S J, Atkinson L E 1973 Systemic contragestational agents. In: Osofsky H J, Osofsky Y D (eds) The abortion experience. Psychological and medical impact. Harper & Row, Hagerstown, p 400
Selinger M, Gillmer M D, MacKenzie I Z, Phipps S 1986 Midtrimester myometrial sensitisation following anti-progesterone therapy. Abstracts. 24th British Congress of Obstetrics and Gynaecology, RCOG, London, p 273
Shinagawa S, Nayagama M 1969 Cervical pregnancy as a positive sequela of induced abortion. Report of 19 cases. American Journal of Obstetrics and Gynecology 105: 282–284
Simms M 1977 Report on non-medical abortion counselling. Birth Control Trust, London
Simms M, Smith C 1982 Teenage mothers and abortion. British Journal of Sexual Medicine 9 (89): 45–47
Simon N M, Senturia A 1966 Psychiatric sequelae of abortion. Review of the literature 1935–1964. Archives of General Psychiatry 15: 378–389
Slome J 1972 Termination of pregnancy. Lancet ii: 881–882
Sonne-Holm S, Heisterberg L, Hebjørn S et al 1981 Prophylactic antibiotics in first trimester abortions; a clinical controlled trial. American Journal of Obstetrics and Gynecology 139: 693–696
Stallworthy J A, Moolgaoker A S, Walsh J J 1971 Legal abortion: a critical assessment of its risks. Lancet ii: 1245–1249
Stringer J, Anderson M, Beard R W, Fairweather D V I, Steele S J 1975 Very early termination of pregnancy (menstrual extraction). British Medical Journal iii: 7–9
Stroh G, Hinman A R 1976 Reported live births following induced abortion: $2\frac{1}{2}$ years experience in upstate New York. American Journal of Obstetrics and Gynecology 126: 83–91
Stubblefield P G 1981 Midtrimester abortion by curettage procedures: an overview. In: Hodgson J E (ed) Abortion and sterilization: medical and social aspects. Academic Press, London
Stubblefield P G, Schoenbaum S C, Wolfson C E, Cookson D J, Ryan K J 1984 Fertility after induced abortion: a prospective follow-up study. Obstetrics and Gynecology 62: 186–193

Tietze C 1969 Mortality with contraception and induced abortion. Studies in Family Planning 1: 1
Tietze C, Henshaw S K 1986 Induced abortion: a world review. Alan Guttmacher, London
Tietze C, Lewit S 1972 Joint programme for the study of abortion (JPSA): early medical complications of legal abortion. Studies in Family Planning 3: 97
Toppozada M K 1986 Prostaglandins in mid-trimester abortion. Prostaglandin Perspectives 2: 1–3
Tovey L A D 1986 Haemolytic disease of the newborn — the changing scene. British Journal of Obstetrics and Gynaecology 93: 960–966
Tovey L A D 1987 Why women are not receiving anti-Rh prophylaxis. British Medical Journal 294: 508
Traub A I, Ritchie J W K 1979 Rupture of the uterus during prostaglandin-induced abortion. British Medical Journal ii: 496
Trichopoulos D, Handanos N, Danezis J, Kalandidi A, Kalapothaki V I 1976 Induced abortion and secondary infertility. British Journal of Obstetrics and Gynaecology 83: 645–650
Van der Slikke J W, Treffers P E 1978 Influence of induced abortion on gestational duration in subsequent pregnancies. British Medical Journal i: 270–272
World Health Organization task force on sequelae of abortion 1979 Gestation, birthweight and spontaneous abortion in pregnancy after induced abortion. Lancet i: 142–145
Yuzpe A A, Thurlow H J, Ramzey I, Leyshon J I 1974 Post-coital contraception — a pilot study. Journal of Reproductive Medicine 13: 53–58

30

Gillian Turner

Ectopic pregnancy

Ectopic pregnancy is of increasing concern to gynaecologists. It is a major cause of maternal mortality since deaths from other causes have fallen so much, and accounts for about 10% of maternal deaths (Confidential Enquiries into Maternal Deaths 1986). Ory (1981) found ectopic pregnancy to be the main cause of maternal death in the black female population in the USA in 1977. The aetiology remains obscure and rarely is a precise anatomical or histological cause found in any specific case. Reduced fertility, sterility and recurrent ectopic pregnancy are sequelae with distressing psychological effects. New techniques have meant that the diagnosis is being made more frequently before rupture has occurred and management of the condition is currently under review with many centres adopting a more conservative surgical approach than heretofore.

An ectopic pregnancy is one sited outside the normal nidation site within the uterine cavity (see Fig. 30.1). Implantation occurs in the absence of decidualized endometrium and endometrial glands. The commonest site for ectopic gestation is in the ampulla of the Fallopian tube (Breen 1970; Fig. 30.2) but other sites within the tube are recognized, the interstitial portion being the least common while implantation in the abdominal cavity, ovary, cervix, on the broad ligament and elsewhere has been recorded. Ectopic pregnancy may be bilateral, and may be concurrent with an intrauterine pregnancy. However, these circumstances are rare.

HISTORY

There is little in the writings of the ancients and the Middle Ages regarding ectopic pregnancy, perhaps because of the natural history of the condition. It may resolve spontaneously even before the diagnosis is confirmed, or it may cause death, the source and nature of the catastrophic intraperitoneal haemorrhage only determined by careful postmortem examination. In Lund's study (1955) 33% of 387 ectopic pregnancies resolved without surgery.

Ectopic pregnancy seems peculiar to the human species (Woodruff & Pauerstein 1969), although it is uncertain why, since anatomically the genital tract is similar to that of higher primates. If it does occur in animals it does so only rarely. Pelvic inflammatory disease, so often a precursor to ectopic gestation, seems to be a condition confined to humans (Vasquez et al 1983) and a further factor may be the particularly invasive property of human trophoblast (Ramsey et al 1976).

INCIDENCE

The incidence of ectopic pregnancy varies geographically and in many countries appears to be rising. However, the oft-quoted figure of one ectopic for every 28 births at the University Hospital in Jamaica (Douglas 1963) has only changed marginally by 1985 in the same unit. In that year there were 108 ectopic pregnancies and 2863 births — one ectopic for 26.5 births (Palmer & Matadial 1986). There is as much variation and controversy about how the figures should be expressed as there is in the figures themselves (Table 30.1).

Texts requoting figures from standard reviews fail to emphasize the increasing incidence of the condition. Rubin et al (1983) reviewing two data sets from the National Center for Health and Statistics covering ectopic pregnancy in the USA for the years 1970–1978 found the rate per 1000 reported pregnancies more than doubled in that time — the final rate was 9.4 ectopics per 1000 reported pregnancies.

The death rate from ectopic pregnancy varies geographi-

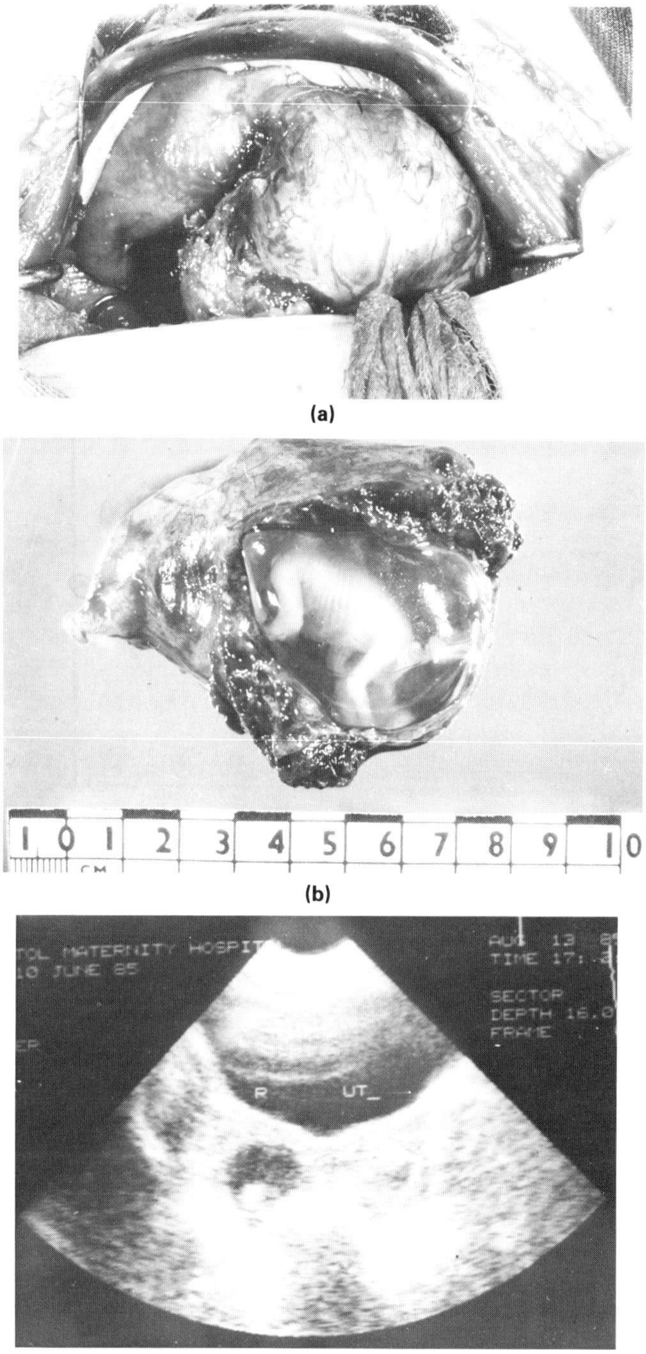

Fig. 30.1 (**a**) Unruptured tubal ectopic pregnancy at laparotomy; (**b**) salpingectomy specimen; unruptured tubal ectopic pregnancy dissected to show intact ectopic gestational sack; (**c**) ultrasound scan of ectopic pregnancy shown in (**b**). Right tubal ectopic with gestation sac seen entirely separate from uterus, which shows decidual change.

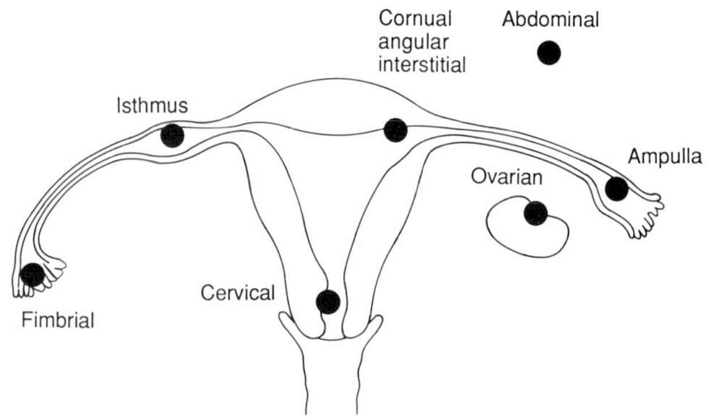

Fig. 30.2 Diagram showing different sites of ectopic pregnancy.

cally, as would be expected, and is assuming a more prominent position as a cause of maternal death as other causes decrease. The death rate from ectopic pregnancy in England and Wales from 1979 to 1981 was 8.2 per million pregnancies (Confidential Enquiries into Maternal Deaths 1986), while Walker (1985), reviewing maternal deaths in Jamaica for the triennium 1981–1983, found the death rate from ectopic pregnancy to be 118 per million births. It now appears in England and Wales that 1 in about 500 ectopic pregnancies ends in maternal death (Confidential Enquiries into Maternal Deaths 1986).

PATHOPHYSIOLOGY

Robertson et al (1985) reviewed placentation in ectopic and abdominal pregnancy. They describe how the blastocyst embeds in the tubal stroma having penetrated the surface epithelium; attempted placentation is towards the nearest major blood supply on the mesosalpingeal aspect of the tube. Woodruff & Pauerstein (1969) point out that in the absence of endometrium there are no endometrial glandular secretions available to the developing blastocyst. Perhaps tubular secretions are a substitute. Rewell (1971), discussing extra-uterine decidua, observes that there is little or no stromal decidual response in the tubal mucosa. Since the tubal wall is thin and has no protective decidual layer, the migrating trophoblast is able to penetrate through to the subserosa rapidly (Robertson et al 1985). The bulk of the non-villous trophoblast is cytotrophoblast, as in early intrauterine pregnancy. Placental bed giant cells are seen from the second trimester on in normal pregnancy (Pijnenborg et al 1981), but as most ectopic pregnancies end by 8–10 weeks, non-villous syncytial giant cells are a rare finding in ectopic nidation. The physiological vascular changes that occur in the uteroplacental spiral arteries in normal pregnancy (Brosens et al 1967) are mimicked in tubal ectopic pregnancy by the interaction between the endovascular trophoblast and the tubal vessels.

The blood supply to the Fallopian tube is from the anastomosis between branches of the uterine and ovarian vessels which lie in the mesosalpinx. Penetrating vessels from the anastomosis divide into smaller branches which supply the tubal muscularis and mucosa. It is these smaller vessels that are first breached and colonized by endovascular trophoblast which then continues to invade against the blood flow; it reaches the penetrating vessels in the subserosa and con-

Table 30.1 Incidence of ectopic pregnancy — geographical variation

Author	Year	Location	Years studied	Incidence
Douglas	1963	Jamaica	1954–1961	1:28 births
Benson	1980	USA	1980	1:150–200 conceptions
Scott	1981	UK	1981	1:300 mature intrauterine pregnancies
Rubin et al	1983	USA	1970–1978	1:108 reported pregnancies
Macafee	1982	Leicestershire	1980	1:175 live and stillbirths
Pillai	1984	Bristol*	1980–1984	1:99 deliveries
Palmer & Matadial	1986	Jamaica	1985	1:26.5 births

* Approximation as the unit services a larger population for gynaecology than for obstetrics.

tinues invading further into the mesosalpinx and the anastomosis. There is usually only one wave of endovascular trophoblastic migration as tubal ectopic pregnancy frequently ends before the second wave which in normal pregnancy occurs at about 16 weeks (Pijnenborg et al 1980). The tuboplacental vasculature is thus fragile and unsupported, and with the conceptus growing within the wall of the tube is extremely vulnerable. The view that the conceptus grows not within the lumen but within and outside the wall of the tube is held by Budowick et al (1980) and supported by Robertson et al (1985). At operation the tube is distended by blood, caused by tubal placental abruption as the invading trophoblast breaches the vessel walls, which, being thin and unsupported, disrupt and bleed.

Placentation in advanced extrauterine pregnancy is according to Robertson et al (1985): 'an exceedingly complex matter which has never been fully elucidated'. Trophoblast appears to penetrate superficially when implantation occurs in the peritoneal cavity and rare cases establish a blood supply and functioning placenta that carry the fetus to term. There is much discussion among those few persons with experience of this condition as to how or whether to deliver the placenta at laparotomy. When implantation has involved a major organ like the liver, consensus seems to be to leave the placenta in situ. However, it may start to separate and bleed, in which case it has to be removed. In other less vascular implantation sites such as the broad ligament the placenta can be peeled off in a relatively haemostatic manner (Lawson 1988, personal communication).

Macroscopic examination of the Fallopian tube at operation and even gross histological examination often reveal no obvious abnormalities (Novak & Woodruff 1969, Westrom et al 1981, Pillai 1984), yet tubal disease is responsible for much female infertility — 30% according to Case & Zuspan (1969); 16% in Westrom's (1975) study involving 3956 couples and 14% in Hull's population study (1985); salpingitis is an acknowledged precursor of ectopic pregnancy. Brosens & Vasquez (1976) using scanning electron microscopy have shown loss of ciliated cells in the fimbriae to be a feature of pelvic inflammatory disease; Vasquez et al (1983) using the same techniques have demonstrated that there are changes in the tubal anatomy with marked lack of cilia in cases of ectopic pregnancy, particularly close to the implantation site. They suggest that this may be because the pregnancy implants at the site of maximal damage, and support the hypothesis that previously unrecognized pelvic inflammatory disease is an antecedent for at least some cases of ectopic pregnancy.

AETIOLOGY

The aetiology continues to pose a puzzle, although certain high-risk factors have been identified. A history of pelvic inflammatory disease, a previous ectopic pregnancy or past tubal surgery, particularly for tubes damaged by pelvic inflammatory disease, is paramount. Contraceptive practice may also influence the likelihood of ectopic pregnancy — intrauterine devices and progestogen usage in various forms have been specifically questioned. Age, parity, socioeconomic factors and race are additional factors that influence ectopic pregnancy. In several large American studies those women at greatest risk of ectopic pregnancy were identified as non-whites of 35 years or more (Kohl 1976, Glebatis & Javeerich 1983, Rubin et al 1983).

Although tubal damage resulting from inflammatory processes causing macroscopic or microscopic damage is the main cause of ectopic pregnancy, other anatomical abnormalities such as congenital diverticula, accessory ostia or atresia have been implicated. These specific identifiable features are rarely found in any particular case of ectopic pregnancy and perhaps they are more theoretical than proven aetiological factors, although listed as such in most traditional texts. Excessive length of the tube, tortuosity, and distortion by fibroids or ovarian cysts are further features which possibly come into the same category. Distortion of the tube by peritubular adhesions consequent upon pelvic inflammation is more truly an aetiological factor. Transperitoneal migration of the zygote has been implicated and may on occasion be a factor.

The incidence of sexually transmitted diseases and pelvic inflammatory disease has risen over the last 25 years in an alarming fashion in most of the western world. It must be remembered that the true incidence of pelvic inflammatory disease in any population is difficult, if not impossible, to obtain since the criteria for diagnosis vary widely. The diagnosis is frequently unconfirmed, the disease is not notifiable and not all cases are treated in hospital. These variables

Table 30.2 Conservative treatment of ectopic pregnancy: risk of recurrent ectopic pregnancy (Brosens, 1987, personal communication)

	Subsequent pregnancy			
	Number	Intrauterine	Ectopic	Ratio of ectopic: intrauterine
No infertility problem	41	28 (68%)	4 (9%)	1 : 7
Previous infertility problem	29	6 (20%)	4 (13%)	1 : 1.5

Table 30.3 Ectopic pregnancy after tubal surgery (Brosens, 1987, personal communication)

	Number of conceptions	Ectopic pregnancy
Salpingostomy	166	51 (31%)
Tubocornual anastomosis	37	5 (13%)
Reversal of sterilization	210	10 (5%)

must not be forgotten in any discussion of pelvic inflammatory disease.

Adler (1980) found in England and Wales that between 1966 and 1977 the rate of gonorrhoea in women rose by 130%, and that the number of cases of acute salpingitis increased by 50% over a similar period, but evidence of a direct association between this increase and the concurrent increase in the incidence of ectopic pregnancy is lacking. A study of returns made nationally in England and Wales of information about hospitalized patients found that between 1966 and 1972 there was an increase in the incidence of pelvic inflammatory disease and ectopic pregnancy, but failed to find an association between the two (Beral 1975). There was a steady rise in the incidence of pelvic inflammatory disease from 1964 but the sudden increase in ectopic pregnancies dated from 1970. Moreover the incidence of pelvic inflammatory disease was increased most markedly in the 15–24-year-olds but the incidence of ectopic pregnancy was not. Beral (1975) suggested that if there is a delay between the time of infection and the development of the tubal changes predisposing to ectopic pregnancy then an association between the two could not be excluded. Since salpingitis affects the young typically, these women still have many potentially fertile years ahead of them and the proportion of women at risk of ectopic pregnancy will increase.

There is a generally recognized recurrence rate of ectopic pregnancies of 10–12% (Hallatt 1975, Schoen & Nowak 1975). Schoen & Nowak in their 16-year study found that the majority of recurrences (80%) occurred within 4 years. The recurrence may occur because the causal factor of the initial ectopic is still present, for example tubal damage from pelvic inflammatory disease, or because a new factor subsequent upon the treatment of the initial ectopic pregnancy, for example adhesions, has occurred. Brosens (personal communication) has related the risk of recurrent ectopic pregnancy to a history of infertility (Table 30.2), indicating that recurrent ectopic pregnancy is more likely in those with a previous infertility problem. These results support the deciliation findings described earlier.

Any patient who has had tubal surgery for whatever reason and becomes pregnant must be regarded as having an ectopic pregnancy until it is proved otherwise, even if the tubal surgery was for sterilization. Brosens (personal communication 1987) reported the collective results of ectopic pregnancies following tubal surgery of various sorts; surgery on damaged rubes resulted in the highest number of ectopic pregnancies (Table 30.3).

Hughes (1979) reported that between 12 and 33% of pregnancies occurring in women previously sterilized will be ectopic, and Tatum & Schmidt (1979) also report a rate of up to 42.9% depending on the method used for sterilization.

Other contraceptive practices have been implicated in the aetiology of ectopic pregnancy. Kadar (1983) addressed the question: 'Does intrauterine contraceptive device (IUCD) use increase the risk for ectopic pregnancy?' and reviewing the literature in detail, quoted the summary of the current position from Ory (1981) as follows:

1. Permanent users of IUCDs have the same risk of ectopic pregnancy as those who have never used them.
2. Use of any form of contraception (including IUCDs) reduces the risk of ectopic pregnancy.
3. Pill users are at least risk. Those using all other forms of contraceptives have a three times greater risk.
4. For IUCD users the risk increases threefold after 2 years, but even then is only equal to the rate of ectopics in those who have never used them.
5. The type of device — copper or plain plastic — makes no difference to the ectopic rate.

Progestogens in various forms have been said to increase the likelihood of ectopic pregnancy. There seems little doubt that this is true for progestogen-loaded intrauterine devices (Snowden 1977; Diaz et al 1980) but the evidence that the progestogen-only mini contraceptive pill causes ectopic pregnancy is weak. It is more likely that the minipill protects against any pregnancy, and in particular intrauterine pregnancies. However if a pregnancy occurs, taking the minipill increases the likelihood of its being ectopic in just the same way as intrauterine devices and sterilization do.

Other risk factors may be considered iatrogenic, such as ectopic pregnancy occurring as a complication of embryo transfer following in vitro fertilization (IVF). The first human pregnancy following IVF and embryo transfer was a tubal pregnancy (Steptoe & Edwards 1976) and ectopic pregnancies continue to be reported (Table 30.4).

Other combinations of intra- and extrauterine gestations are likely to be reported unless the recommendation that cornual tubal occlusion should be performed on all patients

Table 30.4 Ectopic gestation following in vitro fertilization

Type	Reference
Unilateral single tubal ectopic	Smith et al (1982)
Unilateral tubal twin ectopic	Dor et al (1984)
Bilateral tubal ectopic	Hewitt et al (1985)
Unilateral tubal ectopic and intrauterine twin gestation	Sondheimer et al (1985)

with hopelessly damaged tubes before undertaking IVF is followed (Hewitt et al 1985). It appears that there will always be a small risk of ectopic pregnancy following multiple embryo replacement if the cornua are patent and the tubes damaged; this risk is estimated as approximately 22% by Hewitt et al (1985).

DIAGNOSIS

The problems of diagnosis are legion, although there is seldom doubt when the patient presents with a short history of acute abdominal pain, amenorrhoea followed by vaginal bleeding, and on examination is shocked, has abdominal tenderness and cervical excitation pain. These classic signs and symptoms are the exception rather than the rule, however. The most important criterion for the clinician is to *think ectopic*, as urged by Zlatnik (1986) and have a high index of suspicion if there is a history of pelvic inflammatory disease, a previous ectopic pregnancy, tubal surgery or an intrauterine device.

Kadar (1983) suggests that at surgery only 5–15% of ectopic pregnancies are unruptured, but Sherman et al (1982) reported that 58% of their ectopics were unruptured at surgery, and Pillai (1984) found a similarly high incidence of 57% in her study. With increasing use of conservative surgery, prompt treatment before rupture occurs offers the best chance for a fertile future.

The most significant symptoms are amenorrhoea, unilateral lower abdominal pain and vaginal bleeding, although not all symptoms are always present. Amenorrhoea is not invariable, as rupture may occur before the missed period. Cycles may be irrregular and dates unknown or uncertain, but generally amenorrhoea is present in about 75% of cases. Douglas (1963) found 14% of cases had no amenorrhoea and Lucas & Hassim (1970), reporting a series of 144 cases from Zambia, found 15% gave a normal menstrual history.

The most significant signs are lower abdominal tenderness, marked tenderness to one side of the cervix, and pain on moving the cervix. A mass may be palpable. The symptoms and signs will vary depending on the stage of development of the ectopic pregnancy, and the amount of intraperitoneal bleeding that has occurred. Abdominal pain is more common in the acute presentation, whereas vaginal bleeding occurs frequently in the chronic case. Only nine patients in Douglas' series (1963) of 438 ectopic pregnancies were noted to have the 'classical' prune juice vaginal loss.

Delay in making the diagnosis and diagnostic errors are common. Kadar (1983), reviewing the literature, reports that an incorrect diagnosis is made initially in 20–25% of cases; the presentation-to-surgery interval exceeded 48 hours in 40–50% of cases and was longer than a week in 20–25%. An initial error in diagnosis occurred in 14% (Douglas 1963); 13% (Pillai 1984) and in 10% (Aikin 1982).

Twice as many ectopic pregnancies are suspected as actually occur. The index of suspicion for ectopic pregnancy is rising as the incidence increases and early diagnosis should be made in increasing numbers of cases, but casting the net wider means that fewer of the patients under suspicion actually have ectopic pregnancies. The differential diagnosis includes salpingitis and pelvic inflammatory disease, acute appendicitis, intrauterine pregnancy problems such as threatened abortion, and ovarian problems such as torsion of a cyst or rupture of a corpus luteum cyst.

INVESTIGATIONS

Generally it is considered that routine pregnancy tests using standard immunological methods demonstrating the presence of human chorionic gonadotrophin (hCG) in urine are not helpful as an ectopic pregnancy may not produce enough to give a positive result, although Robinson et al (1985) suggest that they do have a place (see later). Estimation of the concentration of the beta subunit of hCG (beta hCG) in maternal serum has been shown to be a much more useful test in the diagnosis of ectopic pregnancy (Schwartz & di Pietro 1980; Khoo & Molloy 1983). Serial measurement of beta hCG may improve the diagnostic rate (Holman et al 1984). Kadar et al (1981) measured two samples of maternal serum for beta hCG 48 hours apart, and showed that in normal pregnancy the increase in beta hCG as a percentage of the original value was more than 66%. The increase was less than this in 87% of ectopic pregnancies.

Ultrasound is of more value in showing an intrauterine pregnancy than in demonstrating extrauterine pregnancy (Kelly et al 1979a) (Fig. 30.3, 30.4a,b) but ultrasound used in conjunction with beta hCG assay has improved diagnostic accuracy. Kadar et al (1981) described a beta hCG range of 6000–6500 miu/ml, below which gestation is not normally present, and above which the intrauterine gestation sac should be seen on ultrasound scanning. They called this the discriminatory zone. Although agreeing that this concept was valid, Holman et al (1984) felt that it was not often useful clinically as most patients with ectopic pregnancy in their study had beta hCG levels below this zone.

Robinson et al (1985), reporting a study of 260 consecutive patients with a clinical suspicion of ectopic pregnancy from the Royal Women's Hospital in Melbourne, concluded that the combined use of diagnostic ultrasound and serum assays of beta hCG was valuable in discriminating between those patients with and without ectopic pregnancy. They felt sim-

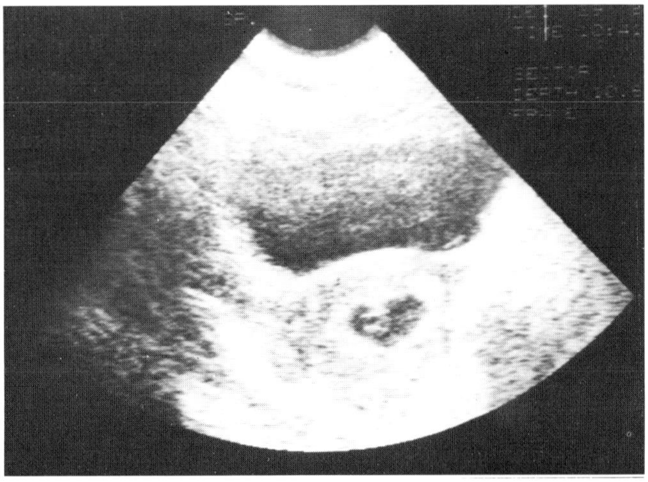

Fig. 30.3 Transverse ultrasound scan of intrauterine pregnancy at 6½ weeks' gestation.

ple urine pregnancy tests were also of value, reducing the use of the more costly beta subunit assays as the initial screening test. Of practical clinical importance was the finding that a negative serum beta hCG test virtually excluded an ectopic pregnancy. Conversely, an ectopic pregnancy was highly likely if there was an empty uterus and adnexal mass or free fluid in the pouch of Douglas, together with a positive urine test. In only 8% of their cases was an absolute diagnosis of ectopic pregnancy made with ultrasound with the demonstration of a living fetus outside the uterus. The use of a vaginal ultrasound probe should improve the diagnostic accuracy of ultrasound.

Weckstein et al (1985), reporting 60 consecutive women presenting to the University of California Irvine Medical Center with acute lower abdominal pain, found that clinical examination and urine pregnancy testing were poor predictors of either the absence or the presence of an early ectopic pregnancy. However, the combination of positive serum hCG analysis and ultrasound examination predicted accurately 93% of proven cases of ectopic pregnancy. This study also looked at the predicted accuracy of culdocentesis alone and in combination with ultrasound or qualitative serum pregnancy testing, and found that the combination of ultrasound and serum pregnancy testing was superior. Culdocentesis (Lucas & Hassim 1970), culdoscopy and colpotomy are rarely used in the UK at present because of the availability and acceptance of laparoscopy, although Holman et al (1984) concluded that culdocentesis was still an important diagnostic procedure in suspected ectopic pregnancy.

Laparoscopy should be carried out in all cases where there is a suspicion of ectopic pregnancy, but at all times it must be remembered that laparotomy should be carried out regardless of all other findings if the patient's condition dictates. Detailed and serial ultrasound examinations, pregnancy tests, whether urine or serum, and observation are only to be advocated when the patient's condition is stable

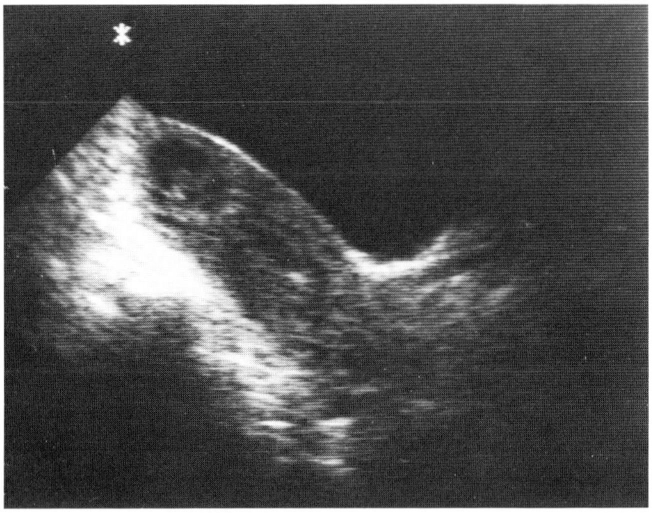

(a)

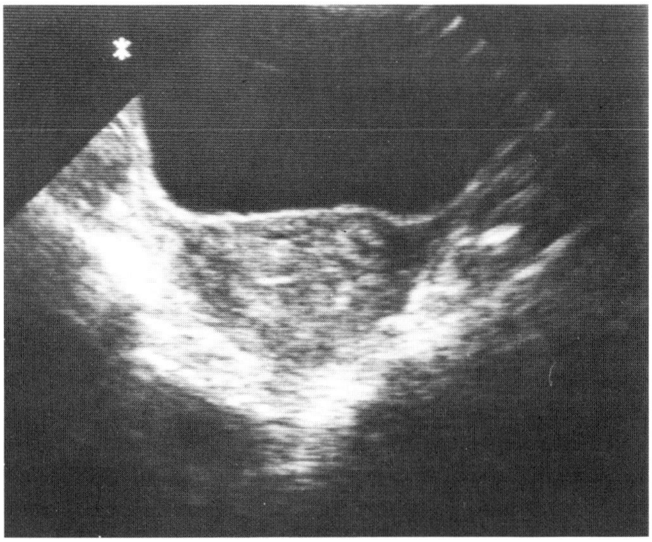

(b)

Fig. 30.4 (**a**) Longitudinal scan and (**b**) transverse scan. Uterine cavity shadow is entirely separate from left cornual ectopic pregnancy, but within the outline of the myometrium, at 6½ weeks' gestation.

and the diagnosis has yet to be made. For such patients in whom an early ectopic pregnancy is suspected and the patient's condition is stable, various management flow charts have been devised (Fig. 30.5; Kadar 1983, Robinson & de Crespigny 1983).

When the diagnosis of ectopic pregnancy is uncertain and the patient's condition stable, the first step is a pregnancy test (a negative urinary test should be reinforced by a serum test), followed by ultrasound if positive. If ultrasound examination reveals an empty uterus with an adnexal mass or free fluid in the peritoneal cavity, laparoscopy follows. The

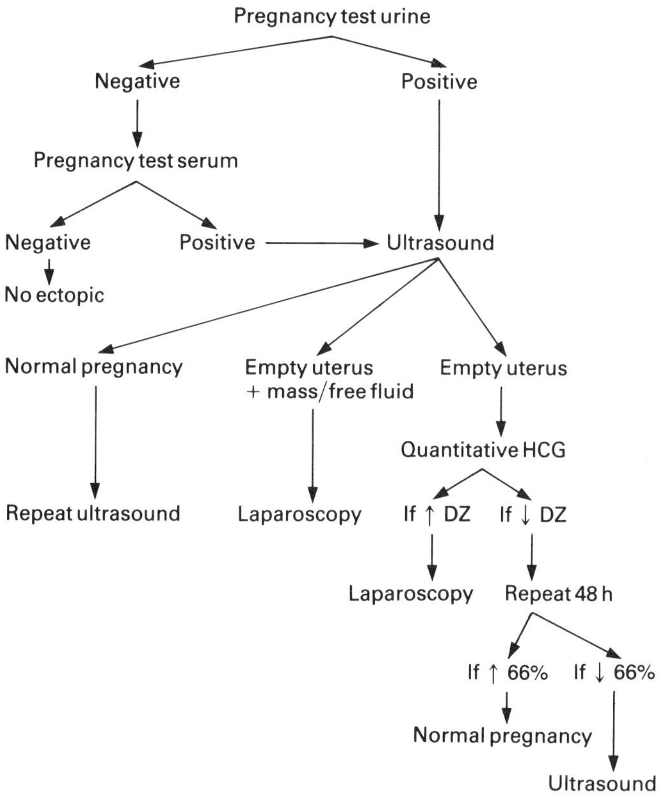

Fig. 30.5 Management flow chart of ectopic pregnancy. DZ = discriminatory zone. After Kadar 1983, Robinson & de Crespigny 1983.

finding of an empty uterus per se requires that detailed consideration be given to the quantitative hCG report and if the level is above the discriminatory zone then laparoscopy should be carried out. If a low hCG level is found an expectant course can be followed, repeating the hCG level in 48 hours. The percentage increase in hCG dictates the next step: if more than 66% increase, then a normal intrauterine pregnancy is likely; if less, then repeated ultrasound examination is advised. Even if on initial ultrasound the finding is of an intrauterine pregnancy, further careful observation should be maintained as a cause for the presenting symptoms is sought.

Only patients whose condition is stable should be investigated and observed as suggested by the above (Fig. 30.5). Delay can mean death for the patient with a ruptured ectopic pregnancy.

TREATMENT

Traditionally the treatment for ectopic pregnancy has been salpingectomy and the majority of cases are still treated in this way. Salpingo-oophorectomy with the ipsilateral ovary being removed was advocated by Jeffcoate (1955) in the belief that this would reduce the likelihood of transperitoneal migration of the zygote and reduce the incidence of recurrent ectopic pregnancy. Data supporting this contention, however, are lacking, and removing a healthy-looking ovary is to be deprecated.

Allan C. Barnes has been quoted as instructing his junior staff over a quarter of a century ago: 'You should work as hard as possible to conserve a lady's tube in her first ectopic, just as you would if this were her second ectopic in her only remaining tube' (Israel 1982). Reluctance to attempt to conserve the tube containing an ectopic pregnancy probably arises from the belief that such a tube may increase the likelihood of recurrence of ectopic pregnancy. However Stromme (1973), reviewing conservative surgery for ectopic pregnancy over a 20-year period, reported that in those patients with two tubes with recurrent ectopic pregnancy, the ectopic occurred as often in the previously uninvolved tube as in the tube that had been operated on for the first ectopic. Bender (1956), comparing the outcome in patients who conceived after salpingectomy and after salpingo-oophorectomy, found the recurrent ectopic rate to be 7.8 and 7% respectively, but more patients had intrauterine conceptions after salpingo-oophorectomy (49%) than after salpingectomy (36%).

A further reason for the apparent lack of enthusiasm for a conservative approach to surgery for ectopic pregnancy may be that it is felt that it would entail a lengthier operation, predispose to increased blood loss, and require the attentions of a surgeon of greater seniority than is usually on first call for emergency gynaecology. Schenker & Evron (1983) demonstrated that conservation of the tube at the time of surgery for ectopic pregnancy is both safe and feasible; Langer et al (1982) agreed that unless the tube was ruptured conservative surgery should be considered in all women who want to retain fertility. It is very important to be aware of the woman's wishes regarding her fertility, since this knowledge before undertaking laparoscopy or laparotomy can and should influence the surgical approach. In the acute situation where perhaps there is little or no opportunity to learn the woman's wishes regarding her fertility, Barnes' advice should be borne in mind and the tube conserved if this can be done without hazard to the woman's life. In the more common situation where the diagnosis is initially in doubt and investigations are proceeding, discussion with the woman should include learning her wishes regarding her fertility. The woman who conceives an ectopic pregnancy after sterilization is likely to have different views from the woman who conceives an ectopic after tubal surgery for infertility, and the surgical procedure should be tailored according to the woman's wishes.

In the acute case, the priority is to stop haemorrhage and to prevent further bleeding. The woman's survival is of paramount importance. Salpingectomy is the traditional operation to achieve this, but over 50% of women who have had an ectopic pregnancy will want to conceive again. Only one-third of them will achieve a live infant, and around 15%

will have another ectopic (Rubin 1934). According to Pouly et al (1986) the risk of ectopic pregnancy following conservative surgery is comparable to that after salpingectomy and in their study is about 20%. Attention is now therefore directed towards improving the outlook for fertility by improving the number of subsequent live births, and reducing the recurrent ectopic rate. Conservation of the damaged tube with conservative treatment of the ectopic does not significantly increase the likelihood of a subsequent ectopic. Pouly et al (1986) reporting on conservative management found that of 122 subsequent pregnancies, 24 were repeat ectopics and 12 were in the involved tube.

Approximately 10% of tubal pregnancies occur in the outer third of the tube (Stromme 1973, Hallatt 1975, Pillai 1984) and this area is most amenable to a conservative surgical approach. The principle is to conserve the maximum amount of tube possible. It may be possible to milk the ectopic pregnancy from the end of the tube without excessive bleeding and achieve haemostasis, although trophoblastic tissue may be left behind and cause bleeding later (Bruhat et al 1980). Linear salpingostomy over the site of the ectopic pregnancy on the antimesenteric border of the tube using needle cautery may be necessary if the 'milking' method is not applicable. The pregnancy products can be shelled out if they do not extrude spontaneously. Manual compression is the best way of controlling bleeding at the implantation site (Kadar 1983). If haemostasis is a problem, fine atraumatic haemostatic sutures placed in the mesentery adjacent to the implantation site have been advocated (Rosenblum et al 1960); this has been recommended as a routine procedure by others (Kelly et al 1979b) to prevent delayed haemorrhage due to remaining trophoblastic tissue. The salpingostomy incision can be left open to close by secondary intention, with any bleeding controlled by diathermy or oversewing the cut edge with fine, absorbable material, or closed in one or two layers to heal by primary intention using 6–0 synthetic absorbable or non-absorbable sutures (De Cherney & Kase 1979). All such procedures should be carried out using the principles of atraumatic surgery — gentle tissue handling, continuous irrigation and appropriate instruments.

Laparoscopic aspiration of the ectopic pregnancy has been carried out, and high patency and pregnancy rates have been reported by Bruhat et al (1980) and Gordts et al (1983). The tube is incised, aspirated and left open, but the technique requires considerable experience with laparoscopic techniques and the risks and complications remain to be evaluated. Adjunctive procedures, such as reconstructive procedures on the non-pregnant tube, are contraindicated in acute cases with haemoperitoneum, but reconstructive procedures may be considered in cases where the ectopic pregnancy has not ruptured, and where the procedure is planned (Brosens et al 1984). The value of ventrosuspension, hydrotubation and hydrocortisone is highly debatable but after conservative surgery it may be important to monitor hCG levels for 2 or 3 weeks to detect active remnants of trophoblastic tissue (Johnson et al 1980).

Conservative management of ectopic pregnancy with methotrexate has been reported. Ory et al (1986) treated six patients with tubal ectopic pregnancy diagnosed at laparoscopy. All six desired future pregnancies and five had had previous ectopics. In five complete resolution occurred; the sixth patient had an acute haemoperitoneum requiring surgery.

Feichtinger (1987) reported the use of methotrexate in a woman with an ectopic pregnancy following IVF 34 days previously. The ectopic gestational sac was located by ultrasound, punctured transvaginally and after aspiration 10 mg methotrexate was injected into the sac. There were no side-effects and menstruation occurred 13 days later.

NON-TUBAL ECTOPIC PREGNANCY

Other sites, though much rarer, are to be remembered; Beischer (1980) draws attention to the cervix as a particularly dangerous site. The cervical ectopic pregnancy is particularly hazardous because of the excessive bleeding that frequently occurs. The cervix has no decidua and trophoblast invades deeply; the cervix is a very vascular structure with little muscle and does not retract as myometrium does. Prompt attention to resuscitation by an experienced team of senior staff, including adequate blood replacement and monitoring with central venous pressure line while urgent surgery is carried out by an equally experienced team, is mandatory. Removal of the products of conception from the ballooned-out cervix may seem like dealing with an ordinary abortion except that the bleeding becomes much worse afterwards. The endocervix should be packed, and the question of hysterectomy may arise (Stewart 1967). Suturing the cervix with a pursestring suture to compress it against a large Foley catheter held in its canal may be life-saving. Fortunately it is a rare site.

Acosta (1984) states that ovarian pregnancy is not as infrequent as was previously thought and that the differential diagnosis is from a bleeding ruptured corpus luteum. Excision of the bleeding area rather than oversewing to achieve haemostasis is advocated if pregnancy is suspected.

In cases of interstitial ectopic pregnancy cornual resection may be necessary but this is not advised as a routine procedure as it predisposes to rupture in a subsequent intrauterine pregnancy.

Pregnancy in a rudimentary horn, although not strictly ectopic, presents the same problems and can lead to much low abdominal pain and later to catastrophic haemorrhage.

Advanced extrauterine pregnancy is a rarity, the likelihood of which should be considered whenever induction of labour is attempted and fails or when midtrimester termination of pregnancy is attempted and fails. The diagnosis is often missed because it is not considered (King 1954). Dixon & Stewart (1960) discussed the difficulties in diagnosis, offering no absolute reliable clinical signs apart from the overlapping of the maternal spine by fetal parts on a lateral abdominal X-ray, which they considered to be conclusive proof of extrauterine pregnancy. Careful ultrasound examination should provide the same proof but if the diagnosis is not even considered, it may be missed in less than experienced hands. Of the 10 cases presented, all the mothers and four of the babies survived (Dixon & Stewart 1960). There continues to be debate regarding whether the placenta should be removed in cases of advanced extrauterine pregnancy. If there is an obvious vascular pedicle which can be divided, or if the placenta is attached to the uterus or broad ligament, it can be removed together with those organs. If it is attached to bowel or mesentery, it can be left in situ after trimming the membranes and cutting the cord. If the placenta tries to separate, alarming haemorrhage will occur and it will have to be removed. The decision is made at laparotomy depending on the findings (Stewart 1967).

Autotransfusion is a procedure rarely resorted to in areas where there is plenty of donor blood available. Serious reaction can occur during autotransfusion if the blood is contaminated during transfer from abdomen to bottle, if it haemolyses even partially, and if it is somewhat defibrinated and contaminated by peritoneal fluid. But if donor blood is unavailable, as happens in many remote parts of the world, autotransfusion can be life-saving. It is also acceptable to some Jehovah's Witnesses who will not permit donor transfusion. Stewart (1967) describes in detail the simple equipment and procedure needed. The fluid blood is scooped from the open abdomen with a gallipot or ladle. It is filtered through sterile gauze into a sterile bowl or jug containing sodium citrate solution, and when 500 ml has been collected it can be decanted into a sterile transfusion bottle and used immediately. Since Stewart's detailed description, transfusion fluids in many parts of the world are now packed in plastic bags but this should not deter one from considering autotransfusion if the need arises.

CONCLUSIONS

Ectopic pregnancy is a cause of death and severe morbidity. The aetiology, which may be multifactorial, is poorly understood but, remembering that the majority of women afflicted are in their 20s and want children, attention should be directed to early diagnosis before rupture and conservative surgical care designed to maintain fertility should be attempted. A very early ultrasound scan demonstrating an intrauterine pregnancy in patients at risk of ectopic gestation is reassuring to both parent and doctor.

Acknowledgements

I am grateful to Dr Peter Wardle for supplying illustrations and ultrasound pictures.

REFERENCES

Acosta A A 1984 Discussion. American Journal of Obstetrics and Gynecology 150: 155
Adler M W 1980 Trends for gonorrhea and pelvic inflammatory disease in England and Wales and for gonorrhea in a defined population. American Journal of Obstetrics and Gynecology 138: 901–904
Aikin D R 1982 Personal communication reported in Macafee C A J (1982) Ectopic pregnancy. British Journal of Hospital Medicine 9: 246–247
Beischer N 1980 Unanswered questions on ectopic pregnancy. British Medical Journal i: 1127–1128
Bender S 1956 Fertility after tubal pregnancy. British Journal of Obstetrics and Gynaecology of the British Empire 68: 400–403
Benson R C 1980 Ectopic pregnancy. In Handbook of obstetrics and gynecology. Lange, California, p 248
Beral V 1975 An epidemiological study of recent trends in ectopic pregnancy. British Journal of Obstetrics and Gynaecology 82: 775–782
Breen J L 1970 A 21-year survey of 654 ectopic pregnancies. American Journal of Obstetrics and Gynecology 106: 1004–1019
Brosens I, Vasquez G 1976 Fimbrial microbiopsy. Journal of Reproductive Medicine 16: 171
Brosens I, Robertson W B, Dixon H G 1967 The physiological response of the vessels of the placental bed to normal pregnancy. Journal of Pathology and Bacteriology 93: 569–579
Brosens I, Gordts S, Vasquez G, Boeckx W 1984 Function-retaining surgical management of ectopic pregnancy. European Journal of Obstetrics, Gynecology and Reproductive Biology 18: 395–402
Bruhat M A, Manhes H, Mage G, Pouly J L 1980 Treatment of ectopic pregnancy by means of the laparoscope. Fertility and Sterility 33: 411–414
Budowick M, Johnson T R B, Genadry R, Parmley T H, Woodruff J D 1980 The histopathology of the developing tubal ectopic pregnancy. Fertility and Sterility 34: 169–171
Case A L, Zuspan F P 1969 Infertility. Surgical Clinics of North America 49: 121–135
Confidential Enquiries into Maternal Deaths in England and Wales 1979–1981. 1986 HMSO, London
De Cherney A, Kase N 1979 The conservative surgical management of unruptured ectopic pregnancy. Obstetrics and Gynecology 54: 451–455
Diaz S, Croxatto H B, Pavez M et al 1980 Ectopic pregnancies associated with low dose progestagen-releasing IUD's. Contraception 22: 259–269
Dixon H G, Stewart D B 1960 Advanced extrauterine pregnancy. British Medical Journal ii: 1103–1111
Dor J, Rudak E, Mashiach S, Goldman B, Nebell L 1984 Unilateral tubal twin pregnancy following in-vitro fertilisation and embryo transfer. Fertility and Sterility 42: 297–299
Douglas C P 1963 Tubal ectopic pregnancy. British Medical Journal ii: 838–841
Feichtinger W 1987 Proceedings of the 3rd ESHRE Meeting, Cambridge
Glebatis D M, Javoerich D T 1983 Ectopic pregnancies in upstate New York. Journal of the American Medical Association 249: 1730–1735
Gordts S, Boeckx W, Brosens I 1983 Results of conservative surgery of the unruptured tubal pregnancy. XI World Congress of Fertility and Sterility, Dublin, abstract no. 559
Hallatt J G 1975 Repeat ectopic pregnancy: a study of 123 consecutive cases. American Journal of Obstetrics and Gynecology 122: 520–523
Hewitt J, Martin R, Steptoe P C, Rowland G F, Webster J 1985 Bilateral tubal ectopic pregnancy following in-vitro fertilisation and embryo replacement. Case report. British Journal of Obstetrics and Gynaecology 92: 850–852
Holman J F, Tyrey E L, Hammond C B 1984 A contemporary approach to suspected ectopic pregnancy with list of quantitative and qualitative assays for the beta subunit of human chorionic gonadotrophin and sonography. American Journal of Obstetrics and Gynecology 150: 151–155
Hughes G J 1979 The early diagnosis of ectopic pregnancy. British Journal of Surgery 66: 789–792

Hull M G R, Glazener C M A, Kelly N J et al 1985 Population study of causes, treatment and outcome of infertility. British Medical Journal 291: 1693–1697

Israel R 1982 Footfalls echo in the memory. Fertility and Sterility 38: 403–405

Jeffcoate T N A 1955 Salpingectomy or salpingo-oophorectomy? Journal of Obstetrics and Gynaecology of the British Empire 62: 214–215

Johnson T R B, Stanborn J R, Wagner K S, Compton A A 1980 Gonadotrophin surveillance following conservative surgery for ectopic pregnancy. Fertility and Sterility 33: 207–208

Kadar N 1983 Ectopic pregnancy: a reappraisal of aetiology, diagnosis and treatment. In Studd J (ed) Progress in obstetrics and gynaecology, vol 3. Churchill Livingstone, Edinburgh, p 310

Kadar N, Caldwell B V, Romero R 1981 A method for screening ectopic pregnancy and its indications. Obstetrics and Gynecology 58: 162–165

Kelly M T, Santos-Ramos R, Duenhoelter J H 1979a The value of sonography in suspected ectopic pregnancy. Obstetrics and Gynecology 53: 703–708

Kelly R W, Martin S A, Strickler R C 1979b Delayed haemorrhage in conservative surgery for ectopic pregnancy. American Journal of Obstetrics and Gynecology 133: 225–226

Khoo S K, Molloy D 1983 A prospective study of pHCG RIA of serum and urine in the diagnosis of ectopic and other complicated early pregnancies. Australian and New Zealand Journal of Obstetrics and Gynaecology 23: 155–160

King G 1954 Advanced extrauterine pregnancy. American Journal of Obstetrics and Gynecology 67: 712–740

Kohl S, 1976 Contraceptive and sterilisation practices and extrauterine pregnancy: a realistic perspective. In Tatum H J, Schmidt F H (eds) Modern trends in infertility and conception control, Williams & Wilkins, Baltimore, p 825

Langer M D, Bukovsky I, Herman A 1982 Conservative surgery for tubal pregnancy. Fertility and Sterility 38: 427–430

Lucas C, Hassim A M 1970 Place of culdocentesis in the diagnosis of ectopic pregnancy. British Medical Journal i: 200–202

Lund J J 1955 Early ectopic pregnancy. Comments on conservative treatment. Journal of Obstetrics and Gynaecology of the British Empire 62: 70–76

Macafee C A J 1982 Diagnoses not to be missed: ectopic pregnancy. British Journal of Hospital Medicine 9: 246–248

Novak E R, Woodruff J D 1969 Ectopic pregnancy. In Novak E R, Woodruff J D (eds) Novak's gynecological and obstetric pathology, 6th edn. W B Saunders, Philadelphia, p 432

Ory H W 1981 Ectopic pregnancy and intrauterine contraceptive devices: new perspectives. Obstetrics and Gynecology 57: 137–144

Ory S J, Villanueva A L, Sand P K, Tamura R K 1986 Conservative treatment of ectopic pregnancy with methotrexate. American Journal of Obstetrics and Gynecology 154: 1299–1306

Palmer O, Matadial L 1986 Personal communication

Pijnenborg R, Dixon G, Robertson W B, Brosens I 1980 Trophoblastic invasion of human decidua from 8 to 18 weeks of pregnancy. Placenta 1: 3–19

Pijnenborg R, Bland J M, Robertson W B, Dixon G, Brosens I 1981 The pattern of interstitial trophoblastic invasion of the myometrium in early human pregnancy. Placenta 2: 303–315

Pillai M 1984 Current trends in ectopic pregnancy. Unpublished

Pouly J L, Mahnes H, Mage G, Canis M, Bruhat M A 1986 Conservative laparoscopic treatment of 321 ectopic pregnancies. Fertility and Sterility 46: 1093–1097

Ramsey E M, Houston M L, Harris J W S 1976 Interactions of the trophoblast and maternal tissues in three closely related primate species. American Journal of Obstetrics and Gynecology 124: 647–652

Rewell R E 1971 Extrauterine decidua. Journal of Pathology 105: 219–229

Robertson W B, Brosens I, Landells W N 1985 Abnormal placentation. In Wynn R M (ed) Obstetrics and gynecology annual, vol 14. Appleton-Century-Crofts, Connecticut, pp 421–424

Robinson H P, de Crespigny L J Ch 1983 Ectopic pregnancy. Clinics in Obstetrics and Gynaecology 10(3): 418

Robinson H P, de Crespigny L J Ch, Harvey J, Hay D L, 1985 Ectopic pregnancy — potentials for diagnosis using ultrasound and urine and serum pregnancy tests. Australian and New Zealand Journal of Obstetrics and Gynaecology 25: 49–53

Rosenblum J M, Dowling R W, Barnes A C 1960 Treatment of tubal pregnancy. American Journal of Obstetrics and Gynecology 80: 274–277

Rubin I C 1934 The stauts of the residual tube following ectopic pregnancy in relation to sterility and further pregnancy. American Journal of Obstetrics and Gynecology 28: 698–706

Rubin G L, Peterson H B, Dorfman S F et al 1983 Ectopic pregnancy in the United States: 1970 through 1978. Journal of the American Medical Association 249: 1725–1729

Schenker J G, Evron S 1983 New concepts in the surgical management of tubal pregnancy and the consequent post-operative results. Fertility and Sterility 40: 709–723

Schoen J A, Nowak R J 1975 Repeat ectopic pregnancy. A 16-year clinical survey. Obstetrics and Gynecology 45: 542–545

Schwartz R O, Di Pietro D L 1980 B-HCG as a diagnostic aid for suspected ectopic pregnancy. Obstetrics and Gynecology 56: 197–203

Scott J S 1981 Ectopic pregnancy. In Dewhurst J (ed) Integrated Obstetrics and Gynaecology for postgraduates. Blackwell, London, p 222

Sherman D, Langer R, Sadovsky G 1982 Improved fertility following ectopic pregnancy. Fertility and Sterility 37: 497–502

Snowden R 1977 The progestasert and ectopic pregnancy. British Medical Journal 4: 1600–1601

Sondheimer S J, Turek R W, Blasco L, Strauss J, Arger P, Mennuti M 1985 Simultaneous ectopic pregnancy with intrauterine twin gestations after in vitro fertilisation and embryo transfer. Fertility and Sterility 43: 313–316

Steptoe P C, Edwards R G 1976 Reimplantation of a human embryo with subsequent tubal pregnancy. Lancet i: 880–882

Stewart D B 1967 Extrauterine pregnancy. In Lawson J B, Stewart D B (eds) Obstetrics and gynaecology in the tropics and developing countries. Arnold, London, p 375

Stromme W B 1973 Conservative surgery for ectopic pregnancy. A 20-year review. Obstetrics and Gynecology 41: 215–223

Tatum H, Schmidt F H 1979 Contraceptive and sterilisation practices and extrauterine pregnancy: a realistic perspective. In Wallach E H, Kempers R D (eds) Modern trends in infertility and conception control. Williams & Wilkins, Baltimore, p 583

Vasquez G, Winston R M L, Brosens I A 1983 Tubal mucosa and ectopic pregnancy. British Journal of Obstetrics and Gynaecology 90: 468–474

Walker G J A 1985 Maternal mortality review: Jamaica 1981–1983. Ministry of Health, Jamaica

Weckstein L N, Boucher A R, Tucker I, Gibson D, Rettenmaier M A 1985 Accurate diagnosis of early ectopic pregnancy. Obstetrics and Gynecology 63: 393–398

Westrom L 1975 Effects of acute pelvic inflammatory disease on fertility. American Journal of Obstetrics & Gynecology 121: 707–713

Westrom L, Bengtsson L D M, Mardh P-H 1981 Incidence, trends, and risks of ectopic pregnancy in a population of women. British Medical Journal 1: 15–18

Woodruff J D, Pauerstein C J 1969 The Fallopian tube. Williams & Wilkins, Baltimore, p 182

Zlatnik F J 1986 Abortion and ectopic pregnancy. In Pitkin R M, Zlatnik F J (eds) 1986 Year book of obstetrics and gynecology. Year Book Medical Publisher, Chicago, p 477

K. D. Bagshawe and Sylvia D. Lawler

Hydatidiform mole and choriocarcinoma

INTRODUCTION

Gestational trophoblastic diseases include hydatidiform mole, a conceptus which in most patients has no serious sequelae, and choriocarcinoma, a cancer which, without specific treatment, progresses rapidly to a fatal outcome. Since the trophoblast forms the fetal side of the interface with maternal tissue, these diseases present a series of unique problems in biology and clinical practice. We now have the knowledge and resources to eliminate morbidity and mortality and the challenge which remains is how to use these assets to full effect in the widely differing circumstances of clinical practice around the world.

Definition of terms

In 1983 a World Health Organization (WHO) scientific group made recommendations for the histopathological and clinical terminology for gestational trophoblastic disease. They are quoted in the Appendix at the end of this chapter, with the comments of the present authors in italics in brackets.

EPIDEMIOLOGY

For many years it has been generally accepted that the incidence of gestational trophoblastic disease (GTD) is greater in some Asian than in most European populations. There is now reason to ask whether this difference may have been exaggerated.

Incidence of hydatidiform mole (HM)

The accuracy of data on the incidence of HM depends partly on the diagnosis; errors can arise because a macroscopic diagnosis cannot always be precise. At the microscopic level pathological entities of complete hydatidiform mole (CHM) and partial hydatidiform mole (PHM) recognized in 1977 (Vassilakos et al) could not be defined in earlier studies and still present difficulties. Another factor is whether hospital-based statistics or population data are used to provide the estimate of incidence.

In Table 31.1 the data on the geographical incidence of HM are summarized. The source of information up to 1980 was the WHO report (WHO 1983). Recently published population-based figures for England and Wales (Bagshawe et al 1986) have also been included. It can be seen that the data based on hospital statistics generally gave a higher incidence than those based on population data for the same geographical region. The range of incidence throughout the world is 0.2–1.96/1000 pregnancies for population-based studies and 0.7–11.6/1000 births for hospital-based statis-

Table 31.1 Summary of reported incidence of hydatidiform mole

	Rate per 1000		
Territory	Pregnancies	Deliveries	Livebirths
Latin America			
Population-based studies	0.2	—	—
Hospital-based studies	0.9–4.6	1.1–1.9	1.1–2.0
North America			
Population-based studies	1.1	1.2	0.7
Hospital-based studies	0.7–0.8	0.5–3.9*	1.0–4.6†
Asia			
Population-based studies	1.96	1.2	3.02
Hospital-based studies	1.1–10.0	1.5–11.6‡	0.8–3.7
Europe			
Population-based studies	0.6	0.8	1.5§
Hospital-based studies	—	0.8	—
Africa			
Hospital-based studies	—	1.0–5.8‖	—
Oceania			
Hospital-based studies	0.9	1.0	—

*Alaska; †Hawaii; ‡Indonesia; §England and Wales; ‖Nigeria.

Table 31.2 Morphology of complete and partial hydatidiform moles

Partial mole	Complete mole (triploid)	(diploid)
Embryo/fetus	Present (direct or indirect evidence): tends to die early	Absent
General features	Pronounced scalloping, increasing with villous fibrosis. No mesenchymal cell necrosis	Round to ovoid outline. Delayed maturation. Random mesenchymal cell necrosis during cistern formation
Hydropic swelling Oedema to cistern formation	Distinctly focal, less pronounced and slow in evolution. Slow maturation of unaffected villi. Maze-like cisterns after mid-gestation in some cases	Pronounced. All villi affected early in molar evolution
Vascularity	Persistent and functioning capillaries that tend to disappear late from cistern walls. Often fetal (nucleated) erythroblasts. Avascularity and fibrosis of villous mesenchyme after fetal death	Capillaries formed in situ, empty of blood, disappear with cistern formation
Trophoblast	Immaturity and focal, mild to moderate hyperplasia, mostly syncytial. Trophoblastic inclusions in villous stroma in most cases	Gross cyto- and syncytial hyperplasia of haphazard distribution unrelated to mesenchymal changes

Modified from WHO (1983).

tics. The higher incidences reported from Asia and Africa have been based on hospital statistics and, when population-based figures are available, the difference between Asian and European populations is reduced.

Temporal trends

Data on temporal trends on the incidence of HM are limited. In two hospitals in the USA, the incidence of HM declined during World War II but subsequently rose above pre-war levels (Yen & McMahon 1968). An increase in incidence was reported from Israel between 1950 and 1965 (Matalon & Modan 1972); during the period 1950–1970 the incidence among indigenous women in Greenland increased after 1965 (Nielson & Hansen 1979).

Between 1973 and 1983, 6842 women resident in England and Wales were registered as having had HM. During this 11-year period, 6 853 224 livebirths were recorded in England and Wales, giving an overall incidence of 1.00 HM per 1000 livebirths. The number of HM registrations increased progressively over the years and the incidence for 1983 was 1.54 per 1000 livebirths (Bagshawe et al 1986). This progressive increase may reflect an increasing incidence but it could also be due to a greater use of the registration scheme or a broadening of the criteria for the diagnosis of HM. Histopathological analysis was restricted to 317 patients from whom tissue was available in 1983 and on this basis the ratio of complete hydatidiform mole to livebirths was 1.01/1000. These data may be compared with the data of Cohen et al (1979) from Baltimore, USA where there were 8 HM in 4829 elective abortions — 1.67/1000.

Incidence of choriocarcinoma

The data available for regional differences in the incidence of choriocarcinoma are scanty. In population-based studies in Latin America and Europe similar incidences per 10 000 pregnancies have been reported, but figures from Japan based on the rate per 10 000 pregnancies or livebirths are higher (WHO 1983).

HYDATIDIFORM MOLE

On the basis of histopathological and genetic studies HM can now be defined in two major entities: complete hydatidiform mole (CHM) and partial hydatidiform mole (PHM). The morphological criteria for the differential diagnosis are summarized in Table 31.2.

Partial hydatidiform mole

PHM are associated with the presence of a fetus (Szulman & Surti 1978a, b) and are triploid (Szulman & Surti 1978a). Triploidy occurs in 1–3% of all recognized conceptions and in about 20% of spontaneous abortions with an abnormal karyotype (Boue et al 1975). Not all of these become PHM. Genetic studies have demonstrated that triploid PHM have one maternal and two paternal sets of chromosomes, whereas triploid conceptuses that are not PHM can arise by digyny, having two maternal and one paternal set of chromosomes (Jacobs et al 1982a, Lawler et al 1982a). In PHM the triploid fetus usually dies at about 8–9 weeks of gestational age, the vessels collapse, the endothelium degenerates and the erythroblasts disappear (Table 31.2).

Tetraploids with an excess of paternal chromosomes have also been described (Sheppard et al 1982; Surti et al 1986), and in the two recently described cases these were classified as PHM.

The most important clinical aspect of PHM is whether or not they can give rise to choriocarcinoma. In a prospective study of well characterized HM in the UK, all 38 PHM resolved spontaneously (Lawler & Fisher 1987) but a requirement for chemotherapeutic intervention has been reported in cases of histologically diagnosed PHM (Stone & Bagshawe 1976; Szulman & Surti 1982). Choriocarcinoma has occurred in patients who have had PHM (Looi & Sivanesaratnam 1981, and personal observation), but a causal relationship between the PHM and the choriocarcinoma has not yet been established in any case. Particularly where the obstetrical history is complicated, the pregnancy immediately antecedent to the choriocarcinoma need not necessarily be the causative one (Lawler et al 1976).

Complete hydatidiform mole

Macroscopically, CHM usually resemble the form described classically as a bunch of grapes. CHM lack evidence of the presence of an embryo — it dies before the placental circulation is established. Swelling of the villi results in compression of the peripheral mesenchyme of the villus and the formation of cisterns. Trophoblastic hyperplasia occurs, which is more marked in some villi than in others; the degree of trophoblastic hyperplasia varies between different CHM (Table 31.2). CHM have a diploid nuclear genome that is derived androgenetically (Kajii & Ohama 1977, Wake et al 1978). The majority of CHM are homozygous with a 46,XX karyotype, the most likely mode of origin being fertilization of an egg by a duplicated haploid sperm (Lawler et al 1979, 1982b, Jacobs et al 1980). A minority (about 10%) of the CHM are heterozygous, usually 46,XY, but they can be 46,XX (Fisher & Lawler 1984). The most likely mode of origin is fertilization of an enucleated egg by two sperms (Ohama et al 1981).

The egg therefore does not contribute to the nuclear genome of homozygous or heterozygous CHM but it does supply the cytoplasm. In a normal conceptus the mitochondrial DNA is maternal in origin (Giles et al 1980) and it has been shown that the mitochondrial DNA of CHM is also maternally derived (Wallace et al 1982, Edwards et al 1984). Thus CHM represent a unique cell type because they combine a paternal nuclear genome with a maternal mitochondrial genome.

Occasionally CHM can present with a fetus. This occurs in a twin pregnancy if one develops normally and the other forms a CHM. Genetic studies can be used to show that such twins have a dizygotic origin, giving rise to an androgenetically derived CHM and a normal conceptus (Fisher et al 1982). Where a fetus is present every effort should be made to distinguish between CHM with twin fetus and PHM (see below), since the potential for progression to gestational trophoblastic tumour (GTT) is much less with the latter.

Relative frequency of partial and complete HM

The relative frequency of PHM and CHM in a series of HM depends on how the cases are ascertained. Among a series of 1602 spontaneous abortions examined histologically and by cytogenetic methods in Hawaii, 88 PHM (69%) and 40 CHM (31%) were diagnosed (Jacobs et al 1982b). On the other hand in cases diagnosed clinically as HM the majority are found to be CHM; the frequency of PHM varies between 16% (Bagshawe et al 1986) and 23% in the UK (Lawler & Fisher 1987).

Risk factors for hydatidiform mole

In order to account for differences in incidence of HM in different populations in future it will be necessary to analyse the data regarding PHM and CHM as separate entities. Various factors have been suggested as playing a causative role in HM and these will now be considered.

Age

The age when the pregnancy occurs has an important influence on the risk of HM. The UK data of Bagshawe et al (1986) showed that there is a progressive increase in risk with increasing age over 30, and that for women aged over 50 years the risk of a pregnancy resulting in HM was 400 times greater than for women aged between 25 and 29 years. Evidence of increase in HM for younger age groups has also been suggested (Bagshawe 1969, Slocumb & Lund 1969, Teoh et al 1971, Matsuura et al 1984) and a high risk for girls aged under 15 was found in the most recent data (Bagshawe et al 1986). Thus since the majority of HM are CHM, the chance of the egg becoming enucleated is increased at the extremes of reproductive life. The risk of PHM appears not to be increased at late maternal age (Parazzini et al 1986, Lawler & Fisher 1987).

Ethnic group

Differences have been observed in the incidence of HM in different ethnic groups living in the same country. In the USA between 1970 and 1977 HM was found to be only half as frequent among black women as among women of other racial groups (Hayashi et al 1982). From 1963 to 1965 in Singapore, women of Eurasian descent had twice the frequency of HM as did those of Chinese, Indian or Malaysian origin (Teoh et al 1971).

In a case control study in Hawaii of patients with CHM no difference was seen in the prevalence of moles between oriental women born in the Orient and those born and raised in Hawaii (Matsuura et al 1984). These findings suggest that environmental factors did not affect the risk of CHM among the immigrant groups.

Obstetric history

It is difficult to study the independent effects of the number of preceding pregnancies on the risk of HM. Since gravidity and age are correlated, gravidity-specific rates of HM would be expected to increase with increasing gravidity. It has been reported that gravidity has no significant effect on the incidence of HM (Matalon et al 1972).

It has been known for many years that women who have had one previous HM appear to have an increased risk of HM in a subsequent pregnancy (Chesley et al 1946). In the UK series (Bagshawe et al 1986) the risk that a subsequent pregnancy was molar was 1:76. Thus although the risk of a second HM is probably 10–20 times higher than for a first HM, most patients who want a further pregnancy have a successful livebirth.

Even if a patient has had two HM there is a good chance of her having a subsequent livebirth; 76% of such patients succeed. The risk of a third HM in patients at risk is 1:6.5.

The risk of choriocarcinoma may be increased for term deliveries if they follow HM, but the data are scanty and in such cases it may be impossible to determine which pregnancy was causal.

Women who have given birth to twins may also be at increased risk of having HM (De George 1970). Twinning and HM may be different expressions of an underlying problem with fertilization or gametogenesis.

Other risk factors

There are no reliable data on the influence of consanguinity or family history on the incidence of HM. The ABO blood group distribution of the patients and their husbands does not differ from those in the normal control population (WHO 1983). The same applies to the human leukocyte antigen (HLA) system (Lawler 1978).

The published data for an effect of diet on the aetiology of HM are contradictory. There is evidence from Italy of an increased risk of HM in smokers and in women married to men over 40 years of age (La Vecchia et al 1985).

Diagnosis

Diagnosis of HM depends heavily on clinical suspicion and on ultrasound examination. Well known warning signs include excessive nausea, vomiting, malaise, uterus large for gestational age, pre-eclampsia early in pregnancy, vaginal passage of vesicles and uterine haemorrhage. Many cases of PHM present as missed or incomplete abortions. Although human chorionic gonadotrophin (hCG) values may be >100 000 iu/l in serum and higher in urine, particularly with CHM, most patients have values within the normal pregnancy range. The fall in values that occurs after the 10th–12th week in normal pregnancy may not occur in HM. Very high values of hCG may be accompanied by signs of thyrotoxicosis (Kock et al 1966, Kenimer et al 1975).

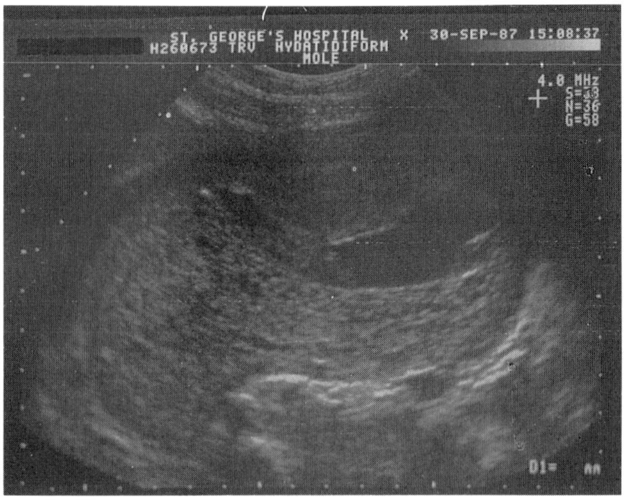

Fig. 31.1 Longitudinal ultrasound scan showing transonic areas in hydatidiform mole.

Ultrasound

The sonographic diagnosis of HM was first described by MacVicar & Donald in 1963 and its usefulness in differentiating between molar and viable pregnancies is well established (Baird et al 1977). The classic appearances of hydatidiform mole were based on images using B-mode bistable scanners which showed a speckled pattern of multiple mixed echoes, giving a snowstorm effect (MacVicar & Donald 1963, Donald 1965, Baird et al 1977). This resulted from the reflection of the ultrasound waves from the walls of the hydropic villi. Additionally, single or multiple transonic areas of variable size were occasionally seen due to haemorrhage or blood clot. In CHM there is an absence of fetal parts (Fig. 31.1, 31.2).

Although the ultrasonic features of HM are characteristic, they are not pathognomonic and in some cases the appearances are identical with those of retained products of conception, missed abortion with fetal maceration, blood clots within the uterine cavity and degenerating fibroids (Sauvage et al 1974). Grey-scale and real-time techniques have added little to this description, except that it is now realized that the snowstorm effect of the bistable scanners is made of

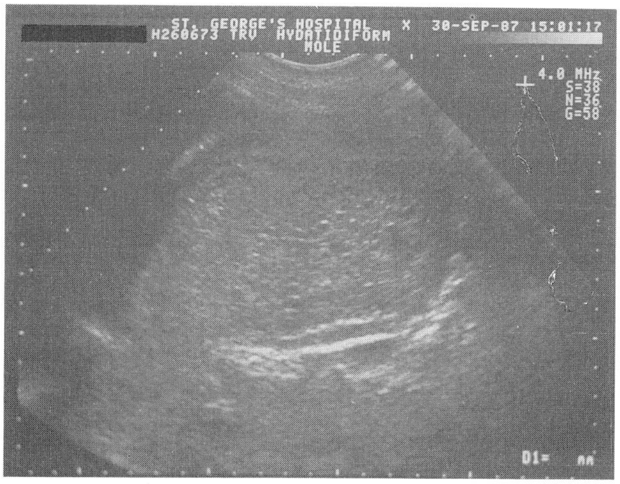

Fig. 31.2 Transverse ultrasound scan showing transonic area in theca lutein cyst.

complex heterogeneous echoes. These techniques also facilitate the detection of fetal parts.

Uterine size with HM may be larger or smaller than expected for gestational age. Baird et al (1977) reported 78% of patients with a larger and 17% with a smaller than expected uterus, whilst Santos-Ramos et al (1980) reported 64 and 22% respectively.

There are few ultrasound reports of an HM and a coexistent fetus; the problem is to distinguish PHM with a surviving fetus from a twin pregnancy in which one conceptus is CHM (see above). Suzuki et al (1980) reported a patient with a threatened miscarriage at 20 weeks' gestation in whom ultrasound showed a viable fetus and placenta with a separate snowstorm-like mass within the uterus; a normal fetus and a CHM were delivered spontaneously at 32 weeks.

Theca lutein cysts may be present; these appear as transonic areas of variable size in the pelvis adjacent to the uterus in approximately 40–50% of patients (Baird et al 1977, Requard & Mettler 1980, Santos-Ramos et al 1980). Fleischer et al (1978) described the appearances of myometrial invasion using ultrasound but Requard & Mettler (1980) failed to confirm this. Woo et al (1985) found a correlation between serum beta-hCG in patients with GTD and uterine size, but Requard & Mettler (1980) did not find this relationship in patients with HM.

Before evacuation HM may be associated with severe nausea, vomiting and pre-eclampsia. Disseminated intravascular coagulation has been described (Henderson & Lund 1971, Egley et al 1975) and trophoblastic cells or villi or both may embolize to the pulmonary arteries and cause acute right heart failure (Lipp et al 1962, French et al 1977). At Charing Cross we have seen three patients in severe cardiorespiratory failure with HM in situ; oxygen, diuretics and methotrexate with folinic acid were required but all survived.

Evacuation

In recent years vacuum aspiration has become the preferred method for evacuating HM. There is some evidence that the method of evacuation may influence the likelihood of sequelae (Curry et al 1975, Baja-Panlilio & Sanchez 1976). Hysterotomy or induction of evacuation with oxytocin or prostaglandins was unfavourable compared with spontaneous evacuation, curettage or suction evacuation (Bagshawe et al 1986).

Risks following HM

Although HM often has no more immediate consequences than any other failed pregnancy, for some patients it constitutes a more serious event. There may be malaise, coagulopathies, blood loss and increased anxiety from awareness of an abnormal pregnancy, fear of sequelae and fear for subsequent pregnancies. There are risks of uterine perforation before and after evacuation, trophoblastic embolism, persisting or sporadic haemorrhage, as well as the risk of malignant sequelae. Malnutrition rarely seems to be a complicating factor in western countries but may be so in developing countries.

Much depends on how the problem is handled by the obstetrician. Patients want to know the facts about risks and time is well spent explaining the need for follow-up.

The Charing Cross data indicate that risk of choriocarcinoma after CHM is probably not more than 3%. The risk of invasive mole (IM) after CHM is difficult to define because many moles are more invasive than normal placental tissue. However, many regress spontaneously and only 5–10% of CHM patients require specific treatment for choriocarcinoma or IM (Bagshawe 1976). The risk of choriocarcinoma after PHM may be no higher than after a normal pregnancy. The risk of IM is much lower after PHM than after CHM, although a precise figure cannot yet be given.

Uterine perforation in the first 6–10 weeks following evacuation of HM is a risk that needs better recognition. It may occur with either choriocarcinoma or IM. A high persisting hCG level (>20 000 iu/l) and uterine pain or tenderness on palpation are important warnings of this serious complication.

The risks of a second mole have been discussed. There are reports of women having multiple consecutive HM and it is sometimes asserted that these patients do not get sequelae (Bagshawe 1969, Sand et al 1984).

The criteria adopted for therapeutic intervention for sequelae to HM differ according to national and local conditions, so that the frequency of intervention also differs. In addition to the mode of evacuation of HM several other factors may influence the risk of sequelae. A high hCG value at the time of evacuating the uterus is often accompanied by a large-for-dates uterus and these patients have a higher risk of requiring chemotherapy (Chun et al 1964, Curry et al 1975, Morrow et al 1977, Requard & Mettler 1980, Santos-Ramos et al 1980, Bagshawe et al 1986). Theca lutein cysts have been claimed to carry a high risk of sequelae but this is controversial and may simply reflect the amount of trophoblastic tissue and hCG levels.

A report that oral contraceptives, taken whilst hCG values were still elevated (Stone & Bagshawe 1979) following evacuation of HM, increased the risk of requiring chemotherapy also proved controversial and contrary evidence has come from the USA (Eddy et al 1983). However, a recent case control analysis of UK data supports the earlier UK evidence of a twofold increase in the risk when applying the criteria for therapeutic intervention used in the UK (Bagshawe, personal observation). The UK data do not allow analysis of the type of oral contraceptive taken and it may be that the amount of oestrogen is critical (Yuen & Burch 1983).

Age over 45 years is associated with a slight increase in the risk of sequelae but parity has not been identified as a risk (Shiina & Ichinoe 1979). Ethnic group is not a significant risk factor for sequelae in the UK (Bagshawe et al 1986); there are no comparable data from other countries.

Follow-up after HM

The purpose of follow-up is to provide a basis for knowing when therapeutic intervention is required and avoiding it if not. Depending on the criteria used for defining HM and for intervention, between 7 and 30% of patients receive chemotherapy for sequelae after HM compared with 1 in 50 000 or less after normal term pregnancies. Follow-up for CHM should still be regarded as essential and limited follow-up for PHM is appropriate at least until there are more solid data. Patients with products of conception showing hydropic change do not require follow-up but it is better to follow up if the diagnosis is in doubt. A standard 2-year follow-up for all patients from the time of evacuation of HM is no longer necessary but greater flexibility requires an understanding of what is at stake.

For many years follow-up has been based on hCG assays; when properly performed, this has proved reliable. The renal clearance rate of hCG is close to 1 ml/min and values fall to <5 iu/ml serum within about 25 days of the end of a non-molar pregnancy. Continued detection of hCG after this time indicates that viable trophoblast has persisted in the uterus or at other sites. Urine values tend to be about 1.5 times higher than serum values but, close to the lower limit of detection, serum values are more reliable.

Patients with high hCG values (>20 000 iu/l) more than 4 weeks post-evacuation have a high risk of uterine perforation and generally require chemotherapy.

In some patients hCG values fall quickly after HM; in a recent UK study (Bagshawe et al 1986) 42% of a series of 5124 cases attained normal serum or urine values by 56 days post-evacuation and none of these developed sequelae. It was therefore suggested that such patients need to be followed up only for 4–6 months and can then proceed to a new pregnancy without delay. This 42% of patients probably includes many with PHM and those with hydropic change wrongly categorized as HM.

Some patients whose hCG became normal after more than 56 days post-evacuation subsequently had rising hCG values and required treatment for choriocarcinoma, so it should not be assumed that a normal hCG first obtained more than 56 days post-evacuation excludes risk.

In many patients hCG elevation persists beyond 56 days but still falls to the detection limit by 4–6 months and does not increase again. Once hCG values have been normal for 6 months it seems reasonable to inform women keen to start a new pregnancy of the level of residual risk to help them decide whether to wait for 2 years before becoming pregnant again. Patients whose hCG has fallen to normal after more than 56 days post-evacuation and who are known to have had normal hCG values for 6 months subsequently still have a risk of 1:286 for GTT. So far no case of GTT has been identified after completing a 2-year follow-up, but some instances of GTT have been detected as late as 22 months post-evacuation. Where a histological diagnosis has been made in a case of GTT arising more than 9 months following HM in the present series, it has always been of choriocarcinoma.

Serum tests for hCG should be performed every 2 weeks until the limit of detection is reached, then monthly till 1 year post-evacuation and then 3-monthly for the second year. For patients in whom short follow-up is appropriate, follow-up arrangements remain similar up to the point of discontinuation.

Prophylactic chemotherapy for HM

The essential issue here is whether the amount of chemotherapy acceptable as a prophylactic eradicates all or most of the early trophoblastic proliferations that would, if untreated, go on to kill. There is no doubt that prophylactic chemotherapy can accelerate the elimination of lesions that would die out anyway but an overall reduction in mortality and morbidity in a substantial series of mole patients has not been demonstrated. A recent paper by Kashimura et al (1986) provides a valuable review. Also, is it justifiable to give many women of reproductive age potentially mutagenic cytotoxic agents for the unproven benefit of a few?

The answer to this in western countries is generally negative even though no excess fetal abnormalities have been shown to result from methotrexate/folinic acid treatment (Walden & Bagshawe 1976, Rustin et al 1984). In developing countries where follow-up is not possible, there may be a case for prophylactic chemotherapy which may reduce overall morbidity.

Invasive mole (IM)

When HM is found deeply invading the uterine wall or producing metastases, it is described as IM. There may be extensive sheets of trophoblast while villi may be scarce or plentiful. It is probable that many moles penetrate the uterine wall but they are rarely identified since hysterectomy is usually inappropriate. Curettage frequently fails to produce a prompt fall in hCG values although the uterine cavity is often clear. IM usually dies out spontaneously, as indicated by falling hCG values in the weeks following evacuation, but uterine perforation and haemorrhage from vaginal metastases are important potential complications. There have been reports of fatal brain metastases from IM; on the other hand small opacities on chest X-ray may resolve spontaneously. If hCG values are falling, therapeutic intervention for one or two pulmonary opacities of <2 cm diameter may be unnecessary.

If hCG values have not reached the limit of detection by 4–6 months post-evacuation, intervention with chemotherapy is usually indicated.

PLACENTAL SITE TROPHOBLASTIC TUMOUR (PSTT)

This is a rare form of trophoblastic tumour with distinctive features. Most cases have followed term pregnancies or non-mole abortions, usually within 1–3 years. PSTT appears to rise from placental bed trophoblast, in contrast to villous trophoblast associated with choriocarcinoma. Morphologically it consists of relative uniform cytotrophoblast with few syncytial cells. Some of the syncytial cells stain for hCG but more markedly for human placental lactogen (hPL). Serum levels of hCG are usually in the low hundreds but may reach 1–2000 iu/l. PSTT may also be associated with nephrotic syndrome and hypertension (Kurman et al 1976, Scully & Young 1981, Eckstein et al 1982).

The response to chemotherapy is relatively poor and hysterectomy should always be performed promptly unless there is already evidence of unresectable metastases. Chemotherapy in patients with nephrotic syndrome presents great difficulties but renal function has returned to normal after hysterectomy. PSTT may represent the most malignant end of a spectrum of lesions characterized at the benign level by placental site reaction.

CHORIOCARCINOMA

Choriocarcinoma is distinguished from IM mainly by the absence of villi. Characteristically there are cores of cytotrophoblastic cells, often showing marked pleomorphism; these cells are surrounded by syncytial elements with extensive areas of haemorrhage. The cytotrophoblastic cells are the stem cells. Syncytial cells are often multinucleate and are differentiated end cells. The bluish hue of the lesions on mucous membranes and skin indicates the presence of both blood vessels and blood clot. Choriocarcinoma may follow any antecedent pregnancy and is generally evident within 2 years of the causal pregnancy, but there are many exceptions; one patient in the Charing Cross series presented with choriocarcinoma 17 years after hysterectomy for HM.

Risk factors for choriocarcinoma

Obstetric history

The median age of women with choriocarcinoma is somewhat higher than that for normal pregnancy. This may be an effect of the association of CHM with age. Bad obstetric histories with increased fetal wastage have been found in association with GTT (Baltazar 1976, Walden & Bagshawe 1976). In European populations, term deliveries, non-molar abortions and HM contribute approximately equal numbers of cases of choriocarcinoma although in reports published since 1960 the percentage of cases of choriocarcinoma preceded by HM ranges from 29% (Kolstad & Hognestad 1965, Baltazar 1976) to 83% (Teoh et al 1972). This higher percentage of cases of choriocarcinoma following HM, an uncommon outcome of pregnancy, indicates that HM is a powerful risk factor for choriocarcinoma. In reviewing the data Matalon et al (1972) concluded that the risk of a patient with HM developing choriocarcinoma ranged from 2 to 19%. Overall the risk of choriocarcinoma after HM is about 1000 times higher than after a normal term delivery.

Genetics of choriocarcinoma

When gestational choriocarcinoma occurs after a term birth, the conceptus would be diploid, XX or XY, with one maternal and one paternal chromosome set. In the UK, where the sex of the relevant child was studied there were equal numbers of male and female children in pregnancies preceding the one complicated by choriocarcinoma (WHO 1983).

When gestational choriocarcinoma arises from CHM the expectation is that the majority of the conceptuses would be homzygous, 46, XX. A minority arising by dispermy would be heterozygous either 46, XY or, rarely, 46, XX.

Although the karyotypes of only a few choriocarcinomas have been described, sex has been determined by Y-body staining of tissue sections. Davis et al (1984) found 14 out of 19 histologically proven choriocarcinoma to be Y-body-positive, indicating an excess of XY. The small number of tumours studied cytogenetically have yielded an approximately equal number of tumours with and without a Y chromosome. These cytogenetic studies in choriocarcinoma have also shown that whether the causal pregnancy was a term birth, non-molar abortion or CHM, the tumours have all been heterozygous for some genetic loci demonstrated, either by the presence of the Y chromosome, or by heteromorphism of the autosomes (non-sex chromosomes). Thus genetic studies of choriocarcinoma are consistent with the suggestion that heterozygous CHM have more malignant potential than the homozygous ones which have a doubled haploid genome (Lawler & Fisher 1986). Trophoblastic tumours that follow molar pregnancies have been shown to have a high incidence of heterozygosity. This applies to invasive mole (Wake et al 1984) and to choriocarcinoma cell lines (Wake et al 1981, Sasaki et al 1982, Sheppard et al 1985).

In a prospective study in the UK Lawler & Fisher (1987) found that 13 out of 73 (17.8%) of patients with homozygous CHM and 2 out of 8 (25%) patients with heterozygous CHM required chemotherapy for the development of GTT. The difference is not statistically significant.

It is possible that requirement for treatment in cases of heterozygous CHM is higher in the Japanese population; Wake et al (1984) found that 60% of the patients with heterozygous CHM were treated.

ABO blood groups

In 1971 Bagshawe et al reported that spontaneous regression of trophoblast after evacuation of HM was most likely in cases where the patient and male partner had the same ABO group. Recently a similar observation has been made in a prospective study of 88 cases of CHM (Lawler & Fisher 1987). A highly significant correlation was found between ABO mating type and fate of CHM. All patients in this series who required chemotherapy after the evacuation of CHM were partners of a male of dissimilar ABO group.

Data from the USA (Scott 1962), the UK (Bagshawe et al 1971, Bagshawe 1976) and Singapore (Dawood et al 1971) on patients with choriocarcinoma showed a slight excess of blood group A and a deficit of blood group O. The UK data also suggested that the risk of a woman developing choriocarcinoma is influenced by the blood group of her male partner. This effect was most marked in cases where GTT was preceded by a term delivery. In a population in which the phenotype frequency of blood groups O and A are approximately equal, the expectation is that the ratio of matings:

$$\frac{(A \times O) + (O \times A)}{(A \times A) + (O \times O)}$$

would be 1.0. In a series of 115 cases of choriocarcinoma following a term birth, treated at Charing Cross Hospital, London, this ratio was 2.19, showing that the risk of choriocarcinoma was increased when the patient had a different ABO group from her partner.

As far as prognosis following treatment is concerned, the mortality rate for unlike matings (A × O, O × A) was less favourable than for like matings (A × A, O × O, Bagshawe 1982). These data on CHM and choriocarcinoma suggest that, as far as groups A and O are concerned, an ABO-incompatible environment favours trophoblastic proliferation.

When considering the B or AB types, which are the rarer types in Europeans, group B or AB patients had a relatively poor prognosis, whereas patients with group B or AB spouses tended to have a good prognosis.

The HLA system

In general it has been found that patients in the clinical high-risk category (Bagshawe 1976) are as a group more compatible with the spouses at the HLA-B locus than patients in the low-risk group (Lawler 1978). Although in the majority of cases when choriocarcinoma follows a term birth the child from the pregnancy antecedent to the tumour is HLA-incompatible, as compared with normal controls there is a small excess of compatible fetuses (Lewis & Terasaki 1971, Lawler 1978). Thus an increased risk of GTT is associated with a trend towards HLA compatibility.

TREATMENT

Selection for chemotherapy

Following HM

Some centres report giving chemotherapy to any patient who still has detectable hCG 6–8 weeks after evacuation of HM (Hammond et al 1967, Lurain et al 1983). This results in 15–30% of all HM patients receiving chemotherapy, compared with the 3–5% who are known to develop choriocarcinoma. This policy is sometimes justified in the USA by litigation risks if treatment is deferred longer; unnecessary use of cytotoxic agents has so far been assumed to be a lesser risk. More cogent arguments for this policy are the difficulty in sustaining follow-up, a shorter period of waiting for possible treatment and possibly shorter duration of treatment. In the UK and other countries where systematic follow-up of HM patients has been established, the objective has been to give chemotherapy to as few patients as is consistent with achieving eradication. Using appropriate criteria, about 5–10% of HM patients require chemotherapy depending on the definition of HM.

The following criteria for intervention with chemotherapy have been used in the UK since the early 1970s (Bagshawe et al 1973) and more recently were recommended by the WHO study group (WHO 1983) on trophoblastic diseases:

1. High levels of hCG more than 4 weeks after evacuation; serum value >20 000 iu/l; urine >30 000 iu/l. These patients are at risk of uterine perforation.
2. Progressively increasing hCG values at any time after evacuation (minimum of three rising values).
3. Persistent uterine blood loss.
4. Evidence of metastases in central nervous system, kidney,

liver or gastrointestinal tract; or pulmonary metastases >2 cm diameter or three in number.
5. Any level of hCG persisting 4–6 months after evacuation.

Within the group of patients requiring chemotherapy after HM some have IM and others choriocarcinoma. A histological diagnosis is not often obtained and both forms are treated with the same protocols. Those whose tumours prove difficult to eradicate are presumed to have choriocarcinoma and whenever surgical intervention has proved necessary in the Charing Cross series this histological diagnosis has been made. The fact that the opportunity to distinguish IM and choriocarcinoma histologically is exceptional does not mean that they are equivalent lesions. GTT present a broad spectrum, with curability readily attained at one end and high potential to kill at the other.

No history of HM

Trophoblastic tumours are a unique exception to the rule that histological diagnosis of a neoplasm is essential. This arises from the desirability and feasibility of retaining reproductive function in young women but there are several supporting considerations. Hysterectomy may cause dissemination, particularly since the remarkable vascularity of the tumour can prevent effective clamping of all the relevant vessels early in the operation and haemorrhage from large friable vessels is a hazard. Biopsy of vaginal metastases may cause torrential haemorrhage. Hepatic needle biopsy has proved fatal and should not be attempted when choriocarcinoma is suspected. Attempted resection of intestinal and cerebral metastases as a diagnostic or first therapeutic procedure has also proved fatal.

These potentially fatal interventions are unnecessary. No premenopausal woman with a tumour presenting in the vulva, vagina, cervix, corpus uteri, ovary, kidney, spleen, liver, lungs, spinal cord or brain should be subjected to biopsy or other surgical procedure without a sensitive test for hCG being done and if this is positive, the procedure is rarely necessary or desirable. It is, of course, necessary to consider the possibility of an intercurrent pregnancy, a germ cell tumour of the ovary, ectopic production of hCG by a non-trophoblastic tumour and PSTT.

Prognostic factors

It is somewhat ironic that as management methods and chemotherapy have improved during the past 30 years so drug resistance has emerged as the cause of two-thirds of deaths. It has become an essential first step to assess each tumour for its potential to become resistant. Patients whose tumours have low potential for resistance do not need to be subjected to the toxic regimens which are essential to get the best results in those with high potential. Prognostic factors are used to assess this potential for drug resistance.

A prognostic scoring system has been presented in several publications and is not discussed in detail here (Bagshawe 1976, WHO 1983). It is summarized in Table 31.3. The two most powerful factors are hCG values reflecting tumour burden and the interval between the last known pregnancy and time of instituting chemotherapy. It is however important to distinguish high hCG values associated with HM in utero or immediately following evacuation of HM from those associated with trophoblastic tumour, and also to identify PSTT as a separate entity.

Table 31.3 Scoring system, based on prognostic factors

	Score			
Prognostic factors	0	1	2	6*
Age (years)	<39	>39		
Antecedent pregnancy	HM	abortion	term	
Interval (months)†	4	4–6	7–12	12
hCG (iu/l)	10^3	10^3–10^4	10^4–10^5	10^5
ABO groups (female × male)		O × A A × O	B × – AB × –	
Largest tumour, including uterine tumour		3–5 cm	5 cm	
Site of metastases		spleen kidney	GI tract liver	brain
Number of metastases identified		1–4	4–8	8
Prior chemotherapy			single drug	two or more drugs

*The weighting has been increased from 4 in the original WHO scoring table.
†Interval between end of antecedent pregnancy and start of chemotherapy.
The total score for a patient is obtained by adding the individual scores for each prognostic factor.
hCG = human chorionic gonadotrophin; HM = hydatidiform mole; GI = gastrointestinal.

Clinical staging

Clinical staging of trophoblastic tumours has been proposed (Sung et al 1983). This has the considerable virtue of conformity with gynaecological practice for other tumours. Staging systems do not however incorporate all the information about a patient and the tumour which may be valuable in clinical management. Clinical staging is also highly dependent on the sensitivity of the imaging techniques used. It is therefore not a substitute for prognostic scoring but may provide a useful shorthand system for comparisons between different series of patients.

Stage 1 Lesion confined to uterus.
Stage 2 Extends outside uterus but still confined to pelvis.
Stage 3 Lung metastases.
Stage 4 Metastases at non-pelvic, non-pulmonary sites.

Monitoring chemotherapy with hCG

hCG was the first tumour marker to be identified and used to monitor trophoblastic tumours. It remains the best marker available for any tumour. In addition to its diagnostic role discussed elsewhere, it is valuable in monitoring the viable mass of residual tumour. A quantitative assay sensitive to 5 iu/l or less is required for this purpose. One cell produces about 10^4–10^5 iu hCG/day and at the limit of sensitivity a good assay will detect about 10^4–10^6 viable tumour cells, something less than 1 mm^3 of viable tumour. Thus if treatment is discontinued as soon as a negative result is obtained the tumour will not have been eliminated.

Management and treatment of trophoblastic tumours

Surgical intervention in early stages of management

Constraints on biopsy and other surgical intervention have already been discussed but surgery still has a place. Vaginal metastases which break down and bleed spontaneously can usually be controlled by carefully placed mattress sutures (Bower et al 1965). Biopsy or attempted excision can result in serious haemorrhage because the vascular bed may be extensive and continuous with grossly dilated pelvic vessels.

In the event of uterine or tubal perforation hysterectomy or salpingectomy may be unavoidable although local resection and repair of the uterine wall are sometimes possible with IM (Wilson et al 1965, Takeuchi 1982). Oophorectomy is not usually necessary and even large theca lutein cysts only require aspiration.

Elective hysterectomy may be judged appropriate for the near-menopausal patient with HM but it must be emphasized that this does not eliminate the risk of sequelae and therefore does not obviate the need for hCG follow-up. Up to 10% of patients were found not to have a uterine tumour; it had either died out or it must be presumed that malignant transformation had occurred in deported trophoblast. For the patient with an established uterine choriocarcinoma the hazards of early hysterectomy have been emphasized. However, prompt hysterectomy is at present probably essential if PSTT is likely on clinical or histological evidence.

Uterine haemorrhage due to a trophoblastic tumour usually subsides in a few days with appropriate chemotherapy, as does bleeding from gastrointestinal metastases. The influence of chemotherapy on wound healing and postoperative infection is complex. Modest single-dose therapy at the time of surgery may reduce the risk of dissemination with no significant impairment of wound healing. If methotrexate is used there is danger of temporary postoperative renal dysfunction leading to drug retention and potentially fatal toxicity. Methotrexate (50 mg i.m.) may be used and followed after 24 hours and again after 36 hours by folinic acid (15 mg i.m.).

Radiotherapy

Although there is no substantial evidence that choriocarcinoma is radioresistant, radiotherapy has not played a major part in the development of effective therapy for choriocarcinoma, with the possible exception of brain metastases. Choriocarcinoma spreads largely by the haematogeneous route and this may limit the effectiveness of radiotherapy.

Chemotherapy

Introduction

During the 1950s and 1960s it became clear that whereas some trophoblastic tumours remitted readily with methotrexate or actinomycin D, others remitted only with difficulty or remission was not achieved. As new drugs became available the question arose whether the available effective drugs should be introduced sequentially as single agents and in simple combinations or whether they should all be given from the start of treatment in expectation of reducing therapeutic failures due to drug resistance. It was observed that resistance to one drug appeared to increase the probability of resistance to others (Bagshawe 1975). However, using all the drugs in effective concentration would have incurred greater toxicity than was necessary for many patients.

Analysis of the Charing Cross series up to 1973 suggested that the prognostic scoring system (Table 31.3) could be used to indicate the probability that a tumour would become resistant to the therapeutic protocols used up to that time. Using the prognostic score, subsequent policy has been to stratify patients according to their risk of resistance into low-, middle- and high-risk groups. Those with low risk have been treated with a low-toxicity protocol avoiding alopecia.

Those with medium risk received a cycle of protocols consisting of single agents or simple combinations so that most of the useful drugs were introduced during a 3–4-week cycle of treatment. This incurred moderate toxicity and usually partial alopecia but comparatively quick recovery has allowed intervals between treatments to be limited to about 7 days.

For the high-risk patients all the known effective agents were combined in a single complex protocol. The first of these, decribed originally as CHAMOMA, received various modifications and is sometimes described as the Bagshawe protocol in the USA. Although in our hands and many others it appeared more effective than earlier treatments it soon underwent modification at Charing Cross. Cyclophosphamide was substituted for melphalan (CHAMOCA) and, following identification of etoposide as an effective agent, CHAMOCA was used alternately with etoposide. These protocols were toxic and it was emphasized that CHAMOMA and CHAMOCA were frequently truncated to CHAMO and individual dosages reduced to minimize the recovery interval between courses. Such protocols were not intended or suitable for multicentre trials.

As experience with these drugs advanced it became possible to combine features from the middle- and high-risk protocols in the present protocol of EMA/CO which is better

Table 31.4 Low-risk regimen: methotrexate (MTX)/folinic acid (FA)

Day 1	MTX 50 mg i.m. at 12.00 noon
Day 2	FA 6 mg i.m. at 6.00 p.m. at 30 h later
Day 3	MTX 50 mg i.m. at 12.00 noon
Day 4	FA 6 mg i.m. at 6.00 p.m.
Day 5	MTX 50 mg i.m. at 12.00 noon
Day 6	FA 6 mg i.m. at 6.00 p.m.
Day 7	MTX 50 mg i.m. at 12.00 noon
Day 8	FA 6 mg i.m. at 6.00 p.m.

Courses are repeated after an interval of 6 days. Start each course on the same day of the week, unless toxicity contraindicates.

tolerated and makes it possible for most patients to have weekly treatment with a minimal stay in hospital.

Disease at certain sites requires special consideration. Patients with respiratory insufficiency or confluent radiological shadowing may experience respiratory failure in the early stages of treatment. There is loss of pulmonary compliance and enlargement of the radiological opacities. The effects are minimized by dose reduction and administration of dexamethasone. Assisted respiration has not proved advantageous. Liver metastases may necrose rapidly, resulting in intrahepatic or intra-abdominal haemorrhage. Impaired renal function, even of quite minor degree, results in prolonged retention of methotrexate as does a pleural effusion or haemothorax, so that methotrexate may need to be omitted from the initial therapy. Retention of methotrexate requires prompt treatment with leucovorin (folinic acid) for it can be fatal, even with modest amounts of methotrexate.

Preliminary investigations include careful assessment of renal and hepatic function. Patients must be instructed to maintain a high fluid intake throughout each course of treatment, particularly with protocols that include methotrexate and cyclophosphamide. Renal and hepatic function should be assessed weekly during treatment and full blood counts performed twice weekly.

Low-risk patients

Patients with scores of 5 or less according to the prognostic scoring system (Table 31.3) include most of those with postmolar trophoblastic tumours and some of those following other pregnancies. The most widely used therapeutic protocol for this purpose is shown in Table 31.4. It consists of methotrexate and folinic acid on alternating days for 8 days followed by 6 days' rest before the next course; this is known as the MTX/FA protocol.

With normal renal function and high fluid intake, toxicity is often negligible and rarely causes more than a moderate mucositis. A few patients require more folinic acid. Some patients get pleuritic or peritoneal pain and blepharitis may occur. Mild erythema of exposed skin may be seen but photosensitivity can be marked and sunbathing is inadvisable for the duration of treatment. Alopecia does not occur. Marked elevation of liver enzymes occurs in a few patients and may

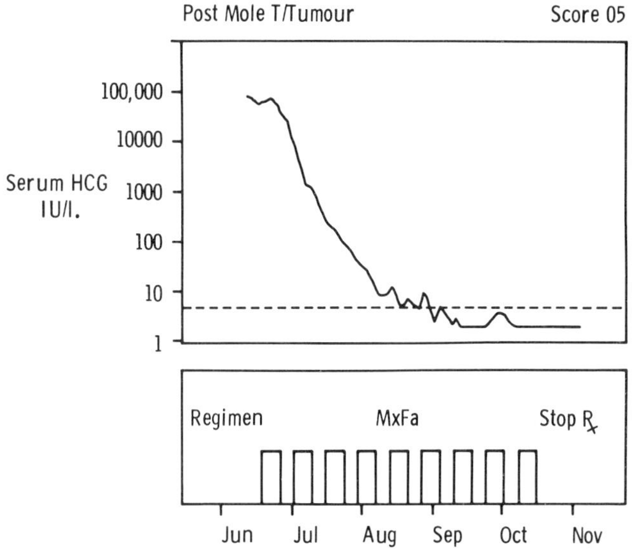

Fig. 31.3 Following evacuation of hydatidiform mole on 20 May hCG values persisted at a high level and chemotherapy was instituted promptly because of the risk of uterine perforation. WHO score 5. A total of nine courses of methotrexate (Mx) and folinic acid (Fa) was given.

require a change of therapy. Haemorrhage may result as uterine tumours undergo lysis during the first two or three courses of treatment.

Patients with hepatotoxicity or severe pleuritic pain may be treated with actinomycin D 0.5 mg daily i.v. for 4–5 days, repeated after an interval of 7–9 drug-free days. Extravasated actinomycin D causes pain and tissue necrosis. It is usually well tolerated but causes mucositis, nausea, vomiting, diarrhoea, myelosuppression and some alopecia. Pigmentation may occur and some patients become intolerant after several courses.

hCG values may increase during the first 10 days after starting treatment. Subsequently values should fall at least 10-fold with each 2-week cycle (Fig. 31.3). The interval between treatments should be as short as is consistent with safety. Courses should be continued until hCG has been undetectable (<5 iu/l) in serum for at least 6 weeks and longer if hCG has taken more than 8 weeks to reach normal levels.

About 15–20% of patients in the low-risk category do not attain normal hCG levels on the MTX/FA protocol alone. Patients scoring 5 are more likely to need additional drugs. If hCG values level off in the 10–500 iu/l range, switching to actinomycin D may suffice and the patient may still be spared the toxicity of multidrug therapy. However, if normal values are not attained after two courses of actinomycin a change to the high-risk protocol may be necessary.

Some workers have advocated use of higher doses of MTX/FA given on a once-a-week schedule. A small trial with such a protocol at Charing Cross proved less satisfactory than the standard one, now widely used in trophoblastic disease centres around the world. No doubt this regimen

Table 31.5 EMA/CO regimen

This regimen consists of two courses. Course 1 is given on days 1 and 2. Course 2 is given on day 8. Course 1 may require overnight admission; course 2 does not.	
Course 1 EMA	
Day 1	Etoposide 100 mg/m^2 by i.v. infusion in 200 ml saline
	Actinomycin D 0.5 mg i.v. stat
	Methotrexate 100 mg/m^2 i.v. stat
	Methotrexate 200 mg/m^2 by i.v. infusion over 12 h
Day 2	Etoposide 100 mg/m^2 by i.v. infusion in 200 ml saline over 30 min
	Actinomycin D 0.5 mg i.v. stat
	Folinic acid 15 mg i.m. or orally every 12 h for 4 doses beginning 24 h after starting methotrexate
Course 2 CO	
Day 8	Vincristine (Oncovin) 1.0 mg/m^2 i.v. stat
	Cyclophosphamide 600 mg/m^2 i.v. in saline
The courses can usually be given on days 1 and 2, 8, 15 and 16, 22 etc. The intervals should not be extended without cause.	

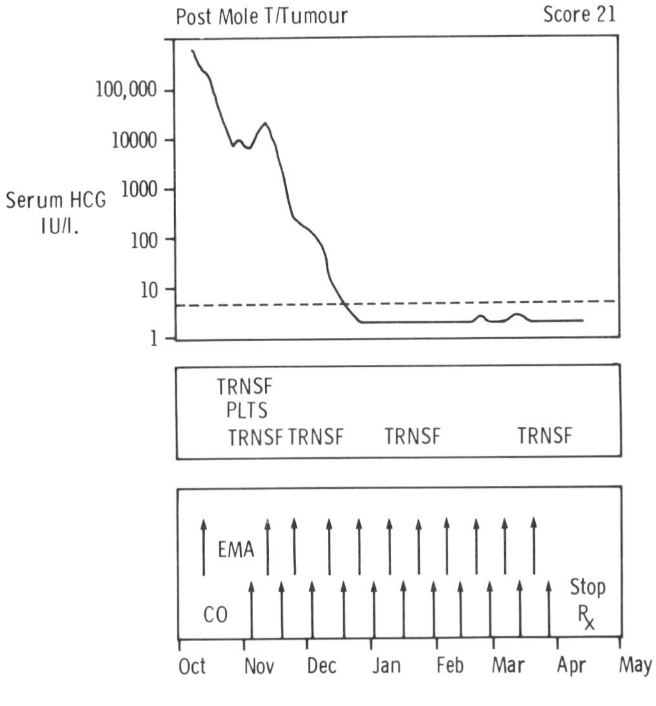

Fig. 31.4 This patient was referred from abroad 2 years after evacuation of hydatidiform mole with a large uterine mass, extensive pulmonary metastases and paraparesis from spinal cord compression at level L2–3. Her WHO score was 21. Treatment was with the EMA/CO regimen. Dosages were reduced with the first course because of respiratory failure and this delayed giving the second course. Note the increase in hCG which followed the initial fall. Subsequently the EMA/CO schedule included methotrexate at 1 g/m^2 because of spinal cord involvement.

will be replaced in time but improvement is unlikely to come by random experimentation which puts lives at risk.

Medium- and high-risk patients

Patients with WHO scores of 6 or more have a risk of becoming drug-resistant to MTX/FA; the higher the score the greater the risk. Several protocols have evolved for the treatment of patients who fall into the group where the risk of drug resistance is a major consideration (Rustin & Bagshawe 1985). There has also been a steady evolution in the development of these protocols. The EMA/CO protocol described here (Table 31.5) has been found the most acceptable regimen so far used at Charing Cross. It is as effective as any previously used and is better tolerated than the earlier alternatives. It is essesntial to keep the courses as close together as possible (Fig. 31.4). The protocol also requires hospital admission for one night only every 2 weeks, although treatment is given weekly. The amount of chemotherapy delivered is greater than in many earlier high-risk protocols and incorporates the five most potent drugs.

Table 31.6 POMB regimen

Day 1	Vincristine (Oncovin) 1.0 mg/m^2 (max 2 mg) i.v.
	Methotrexate 300 mg/m^2 i.v. infusion over 12 h
Day 2	Bleomycin 15.0 mg i.v. as a 24 h infusion
	Folinic acid 15 mg twice a day for 4 doses, begun 24 h after the start of methotrexate
Day 3	Bleomycin 15.0 mg i.v. as a 24 h infusion
Day 4	Cis-platinum 120 mg/m^2 i.v. with forced diuresis and magnesium sulphate supplement

Our experience with EMA/CO has been gained in patients with WHO scores of 8–26. Patients who have not had prior therapy have a better than 90% survival rate and about 80% of those who have relapsed or become resistant to prior therapy have also achieved sustained remission.

Although most patients in the high-risk category achieve remission on EMA/CO alone, there are exceptions. Some of these achieve remission on a cis-platinum-containing protocol. Cis-platinum has become the pivot of therapy for germ cell tumours but its place in gestational choriocarcinoma is less well established. It has helped to achieve remission in about 30–40% of patients showing resistance to EMA/CO. Cis-platinum plus etoposide has been used as a substitute for the CO part of the EMA/CO protocol. Cis-platinum administration requires full hydration, weighing bed facilities and magnesium supplements. Bleomycin has a transient effect on choriocarcinoma and it may be used with cis-platinum in the POMB regimen (Table 31.6). Although vinblastine is often used with cis-platinum and bleomycin in the treatment of germ cell tumours, it is more myelosuppressive than the POMB regimen, which includes vincristine. When patients have become multidrug-resistant the more myelosuppressive drugs are best avoided.

All the high-risk protocols cause alopecia. Mucositis is usually avoided with EMA/CO provided a high fluid intake is taken and dose adjustments are made for any impairment of renal function. With all high-risk protocols there is a tendency for toxicity to be cumulative and whilst myelosuppression is not usual in the early stages it is rarely absent where treatment lasts several months. Treatment should however be sustained on a weekly basis as long as the total white

Table 31.7 Summary of risks associated with trophoblastic tumour

1. Uterine perforation and haemorrhage
2. Haemorrhage from biopsy etc.
3. Death from massive pulmonary, hepatic, intestinal or brain metastases or from haemorrhage into metastases
4. Death from complications of chemotherapy
5. Drug resistance
6. Loss of function in central nervous system, lungs or reproductive system

blood cell count >2000 mm³ and platelets >100 000 mm³. Sometimes it is necessary to give treatment when counts are lower than these values.

Patients with prognostic scores of 6–7 should continue therapy until hCG has been undetectable for 8–10 weeks. Those with scores of 8 or more should continue treatment for 12–14 weeks after hCG has become undetectable.

Central nervous system metastases

All patients should be examined for occult brain metastases at the start of chemotherapy. Computerized tomography scan is convenient but not infallible: early results with magnetic resonance imaging suggest that this is superior. Serum: cerebrospinal fluid ratios of hCG below 60:1 are a valuable means of detection and may be positive when computerized tomography is negative (Bagshawe & Harland 1976, Athanassiou et al 1983). Low-risk patients with lung metastases and all high-risk patients should have lumbar punctures both to obtain serum:cerebrospinal fluid ratios and to give intrathecal methotrexate (10 mg) every 2 weeks, at least until hCG is in the normal range.

Brain metastases can become established at any time before or during chemotherapy so long as there are viable tumour cells able to enter the vascular system. Sometimes tumour emboli are presumed to have caused vascular occlusions with infarction without the development of true metastases. Cerebral haemorrhage may be the presenting feature but headaches, visual disturbance due to retinal deposits or damage to any part of the visual tracts and cortex, hemiparesis, cerebellar dysfunction or spinal cord compression with root pain and bladder symptoms may all occur.

Management of central nervous system metastases

Treatment is a medical emergency but must be carefully considered. If the patient has not had prior chemotherapy, drugs are the main component of treatment but surgery may have a place, particularly if the metastasis is on, or close to, the cortex. If the patient has already received multidrug chemotherapy then the objective should be elective surgical removal provided the location of the metastasis or metastases is not a contraindication. Although there have been a few reports of remissions from brain metastases being achieved with radiation therapy, data for prolonged survival are limited and experience at Charing Cross Hospital leads us to believe it is not contributory to survival.

Chemotherapy for established brain metastases has incorporated high-dose methotrexate (1 g/m³) in the EMA/CO regimen with increased folinic acid rescue. Intrathecal methotrexate 10 mg is given with the CO regimen provided there is no evidence of raised intracranial pressure. If lesions are large or multiple, or if there is raised intracranial pressure, it is essential to try to minimize cerebral oedema during the initial chemotherapy. This requires use of corticosteroids (dexamethasone 4 mg 6-hourly) and may require osmotic diuretics and reduction in the dosage of chemotherapeutic agents in the early phase of treatment.

Surgery for drug-resistant choriocarcinoma

Surgery plays an important part in drug-resistant disease. Chemotherapy over several months may succeed in eliminating disease at most sites but residual disease is indicated by persistence of hCG. Identification of focal sites of residual disease by ultrasound, computerized tomography and magnetic resonance imaging is then undertaken. Immunoscintigraphy may help locate small foci of tumour and distinguish viable from non-viable tumour (Begent & Bagshawe 1983). Resistant tumour is most commonly located in the lungs and brain and at this stage removal of residual foci can be life-saving. As chemotherapy has improved residual uterine disease has become a rarity but if there is doubt about residual tumour in the uterus at this stage hysterectomy should be undertaken.

APPENDIX

Diagnostic note (after WHO 1983) (*Authors' comments in italics in brackets*)

HISTOPATHOLOGICAL ENTITIES

Hydatidiform mole (*HM*). A general term that includes two distinct entities — complete hydatidiform mole and partial hydatidiform mole. The features common to both forms are a hydropic state of some or all villi and trophoblastic hyperplasia.

Partial hydatidiform mole (*PHM*). An abnormal conceptus with an embryo or fetus that tends to die early, with a placenta subject to focal swelling of the villi leading to cistern formation, and with focal trophoblastic hyperplasia, usually involving the syncytiotrophoblast only. The unaffected villi appear normal and vascularity of the villi disappears following fetal death.

Complete hydatidiform mole (*CHM*). An abnormal conceptus without an embryo or fetus, with gross hydropic swelling of the placental villi and usually pronounced trophoblastic hyperplasia of both layers (cyto- and syncytiotrophoblast). The swelling of the villi leads to central cistern formation with a concomitant compression of the maturing connective tissue that has lost its vascularity.

Invasive mole (*IM*). A tumour or tumour-like process invading the myometrium and characterized by trophoblastic hyperplasia and persistence of placental villi. It commonly results from complete hydatidiform mole and may do so from partial hydatidiform mole. It may metastasize but it does not exhibit the progression of a true cancer and it may regress spontaneously. The following terms are synonyms which the WHO scientific group considered should no longer be used: malignant mole, molar destruens, chorioadenoma destruens.

(Invasive mole, though not a cancer, can be lethal)

Gestational choriocarcinoma. A carcinoma arising from the trophoblastic epithelium that shows both cytotrophoblastic and syncytiotrophoblastic elements. It may arise from conceptions that give rise to a livebirth, an abortion at any stage, an ectopic pregnancy, or a hydatidiform mole and it may possibly arise *ab initio*. Chorionepithelioma is a synonym which the WHO scientific group considered should no longer be used.

Placental site trophoblastic tumour. A tumour that arises from the trophoblast of the placental bed and is composed mainly of cytotrophoblastic cells. It encompasses lesions of low- and high-grade malignancy. Trophoblastic pseudotumour is a synonym which the WHO scientific group considered should no longer be used.

The following conditions may be involved in the differential diagnosis of trophoblastic disease, but do not themselves constitute trophoblastic disease.

Placental site reaction. A term that refers to the physiological finding of trophoblastic and inflammatory cells in the placental bed. The term syncitial endometritis has sometimes been applied to this process but it is inappropriate and confusing, and the WHO scientific group recommended that it should no longer be used.

Hydropic degeneration. A condition of placental villi characterized by dilatation and increased fluid content or liquefaction of the stroma, but without trophoblastic hyperplasia. It must be distinguished from hydatidiform mole and is not associated with increased risk of neoplastic sequelae. Molar degeneration, hydatidiform degeneration and hydropic change are synonyms which the WHO scientific group considered should no longer be used.

The following terms were considered by the WHO scientific group to have no further use.

Transitional mole. A term that has been applied in the past to conceptions with a recognizable embryo or gestational sac and hydatidiform villi.

Villous choriocarcinoma. A term that was suggested as a name for lesions that show villi but metastasize. These lesions are in fact invasive moles and therefore the term villous choriocarcinoma is superfluous.

CLINICAL TERMS

Although it is recognized that invasive mole and choriocarcinoma show important biological and prognostic differences, clinical management of these conditions often has to proceed without a histopathological diagnosis and this has resulted in the use of terms intended to embrace both conditions. It is important, however, that these terms should closely reflect the histopathological entities and their natural histories wherever possible.

Gestational trophoblastic disease (GTD). A general term that covers hydatidiform mole, invasive mole, placental site tumour and choriocarcinoma. It therefore includes both benign and malignant conditions in variable proportions.

Gestational trophoblastic tumour (GTT). A disease state in which there is clinical evidence of invasive mole or choriocarcinoma. This category is further subdivided according to antecedent pregnancy as postmole, postabortion, postdelivery or unknown pregnancy. The WHO scientific group considered that the term gestational trophoblastic tumour should replace gestational trophoblastic neoplasia since invasive mole is not regarded as a true neoplasm.

Metastatic trophoblastic tumour (MTT). A disease state in which there is clinical evidence of invasive mole or choriocarcinoma that has extended beyond the body of the uterus.

(Although clinical intervention in trophoblastic disease may sometimes be appropriate in the absence of relevant histological evidence, histological criteria continue to have a central place in our understanding.)

Acknowledgements

We thank Dr Matthew Long for contributing the section on ultrasound of hydatidiform mole. We thank the Cancer Research Campaign and Medical Research Council for support.

REFERENCES

Athanassiou A, Begent R H J, Newlands E S, Parker D, Rustin G J S, Bagshawe K D 1983 Central nervous system metastases in choriocarcinoma. Twenty-three years experience at Charing Cross Hospital. Cancer 52: 1728–1735

Bagshawe K D 1969 Choriocarcinoma. Edward Arnold, London

Bagshawe K D 1975 Medical oncology. Medical aspects of malignant disease. Blackwell, London, p 305

Bagshawe K D 1976 Risk and prognostic factors in trophoblastic neoplasia. Cancer 38: 1373–1385

Bagshawe K D 1982 Some facets of trophoblastic neoplasia in man. Journal of Reproduction and Fertility 31 (suppl): 175–179

Bagshawe K D, Harland S 1976 Immunodiagnosis and monitoring of gonadotrophin producing metastases in the central nervous system. Cancer 38: 112–118

Bagshawe K D, Rawlins G, Pike M C, Lawler S D 1971 The ABO blood groups in trophoblastic neoplasia. Lancet i: 553–557

Bagshawe K D, Wilson H, Dublon P, Smith A, Baldwin M, Kardana A 1973 Follow-up after hydatidiform mole. Journal of Obstetrics and Gynaecology of the British Commonwealth 80: 461–468

Bagshawe K D, Dent J, Webb J 1986 Hydatidiform mole in England and Wales 1973–83. Lancet ii: 673–677

Baird A M, Beckly D E, Ross F G M 1977 The ultrasound diagnosis of hydatidiform mole. Clinical Radiology 28: 637–645

Baja-Panlilio H, Sanchez F S 1976 A better incidence of chorionic malignancy following hydatidiform mole. A longitudinal study of 868 cases admitted in a maternity hospital in Manila. Proceedings of the First Inter-Congress of the Asian Federation of Obstetrics and Gynaecology 2: 89

Baltazar J C 1976 Epidemiological features of choriocarcinoma. Bulletin of World Health Organization 54: 523–532

Begent R H J, Bagshawe K D 1983 Radioimmunolocalisation of cancer. In: Fishman W H (ed) Oncodevelopmental markers. Academic Press, New York, pp 167–188

Boue J G, Boue A, Lazar P 1975 Retrospective and prospective epidemiological studies of 1500 karyotyped spontaneous human abortions. Teratology 12: 11–26

Bower D B, Bagshawe K D, Brewis R A L 1965 Vaginal bleeding from chorionepithelioma. British Medical Journal 1: 249

Chesley L C, Cosgrove S A, Preece J 1946 Hydatidiform mole with special reference to recurrence and associated eclampsia. American Journal of Obstetrics and Gynecology 52: 311–320

Chun D, Braga C, Chow C et al 1964 Clinical observations on some aspects of hydatidiform moles. Journal of Obstetrics and Gynaecology of the British Commonwealth 71: 180–184

Cohen B A, Burkmam R J, Rosenshein N B, Atienza M F, King J M, Parmley T H 1979 Gestational trophoblastic disease within an elective abortion population. American Journal of Obstetrics and Gynecology 135: 452–454

Curry S L, Hammond C B, Tyrey L et al 1975. Hydatidiform mole, diagnosis, management and long term follow up. Obstetrics and Gynecology 45: 1–8

Davis J R, Surwit E A, Garay J P, Foriter K J 1984 Sex assignment in gestational trophoblastic neoplasia. American Journal of Obstetrics and Gynecology 148: 722–725

Dawood M Y, Teoh E S, Ratnam S S 1971 ABO blood group in trophoblastic disease. Journal of Obstetrics and Gynaecology of the British Commonwealth 78: 918–923

De George F V 1970 Hydatidiform mole in other pregnancies of mothers of twins. American Journal of Obstetrics and Gynecology 108: 369–371

Donald I 1965 Diagnostic uses of sonar in obstetrics and gynaecology. Journal of Obstetrics and Gynaecology of the British Commonwealth 72: 907

Eckstein R P, Paradinas F J, Bagshawe K D 1982 Placental site trophoblastic tumour (trophoblastic pseudotumour): a study of four cases requiring hysterectomy including one fatal case. Histopathology 6: 211–226

Eddy G L, Schlaerth J B, Nalick R H, Gaddis O, Nakamura R M, Morrow C P 1983 Postmolar trophoblastic disease in women using hormonal contraception with and without oestrogen. Obstetrics and Gynecology 62: 736–740

Edwards Y H, Jeremiah S J, McMillan S L, Povey S, Fisher R A, Lawler S D 1984 Complete hydatidiform mole combines maternal mitochondria with a paternal molecular genome. Annals of Human Genetics 48: 119–127

Egley C C, Simon L R, Haddox T 1975 Hydatidiform mole and disseminated intravascular coagulation. American Journal of Obstetrics and Gynecology 121: 1122

Fisher R A, Lawler S D 1984 Heterozygous complete hydatidiform moles: do they have a worse prognosis than homozygous complete moles? Lancet ii: 51

Fisher R A, Sheppard D M, Lawler S D 1982 Twin pregnancy with complete hydatidiform mole (46, XX) and fetus (46, XY): genetic origin proved by analysis of chromosome polymorphisms. British Medical Journal 284: 1218–1220

Fleischer A C, James A E, Krause D A, Millis J B 1978 Sonographic patterns in trophoblastic diseases. Radiology 126: 215–220

French W, Freund U, Carlson R W, Weil M H 1977 High output heart failure associated with pulmonary edema complicating hydatidiform mole. Archives of Internal Medicine 137: 367–369

Giles R E, Blanc H, Cann H M, Wallace D C 1980 Maternal inheritance of human mitochondrial DNA. Proceedings of the National Academy of Sciences of the United States of America 77: 6715–6719

Hammond C B, Hertz R, Ross G T, Lipsett M B, Odell W D 1967 Primary chemotherapy for non-metastatic gestational trophoblastic neoplasms. American Journal of Obstetrics and Gynecology 98: 71–78

Hayashi K, Bracken M B, Freeman D H Jr, Hellenbrand K 1982 Hydatidiform mole in the United States (1970–1977): a statistical and theoretical analysis. American Journal of Epidemiology 115: 67–77

Henderson S R, Lund C J 1971 Severe pre-eclampsia, disseminated intravascular coagulopathy and hydatidiform mole complicating a 20-week pregnancy with a fetus. Obstetrics and Gynecology 37: 722–729

Jacobs P A, Wilson C M, Sprenkle J A, Rosensheim N B, Migeon B E 1980 Mechanisms of origin of complete hydatidiform mole. Nature 286: 714

Jacobs P A, Szulman A E, Funkhouser J, Matsuura J S, Wilson C C 1982a Human triploidy: relationship between parental origin of the additional haploid complement and development of partial hydatidiform mole. Annals of Human Genetics 46: 223–231

Jacobs P A, Hunt P A, Matsuura J S, Wilson C C, Szulman A E 1982b Complete and partial hydatidiform mole in Hawaii: cytogenetics, morphology and epidemiology. British Journal of Obstetrics and Gynaecology 89: 256–266

Kajii T, Ohama K 1977 Androgenetic origin of hydatidiform mole. Nature 268: 633–634

Kashimura Y, Kashimura M, Sugimori H et al 1986 Prophylactic chemotherapy for hydatidiform mole. Cancer 58: 624–629

Kenimer J G, Hershman J M, Higgins H P 1975 The thyrotropin in hydatidiform moles is human chorionic gonadotrophin. Journal of Clinical Endocrinology and Metabolism 40: 482–491

Kock H, Kessel H, Van Stolte L et al 1966 Thyroid function in molar pregnancy. Journal of Clinical Endocrinology 26: 1128–1134

Kolstad P, Hognestad J 1965 Trophoblastic tumours in Norway. Acta Obstetricia et Gynecologica Scandinavica 44: 80–88

Kurman R J, Scully R E, Norris H J 1976 Trophoblastic psuedotumour of the uterus. Cancer 38: 1214–1246

La Vecchia C, Franceschi S, Parazzini F et al 1985 Risk factors for gestational trophoblastic disease in Italy. American Journal of Epidemiology 121: 457–464

Lawler S D 1978 HLA and trophoblastic tumours. British Medical Bulletin 34: 305–308

Lawler S D, Fisher R A 1986 Genetic aspects of gestational trophoblastic tumours. In: Inchinoe K (ed) Trophoblastic diseases. Igaku-Shoin, Tokyo

Lawler S D, Fisher R A 1987 Genetic studies in hydatidiform mole with clinical correlations. Placenta 8(1): 77–88

Lawler S D, Klouda P T, Bagshawe K D 1976 The relationship between HLA antibodies and the causal pregnancy in choriocarcinoma. British Journal of Obstetrics and Gynaecology 83: 651–655

Lawler S D, Pickthall V J, Fisher R A, Povey S, Wyn Evans M, Szulman A E 1979 Genetic studies of complete and partial hydatidiform moles. Lancet ii: 580

Lawler S D, Fisher R A, Pickthall V J, Povey S, Wyn Evans M 1982a Genetic studies on hydatidiform moles. 1. The origin of partial moles. Cancer Genetics and Cytogenetics 5: 309–320

Lawler S D, Povey S, Fisher R A, Pickthall V J 1982b Genetic studies on hydatidiform moles. II The origin of complete moles. Annals of Human Genetics 46: 209–222

Lewis J L, Terasaki P I 1971 HLA leukocyte antigen studies in women with trophoblastic tumours. American Journal of Obstetrics and Gynecology 111: 547–554

Lipp R G, Kindschi J D, Schmitz R 1962 Death from pulmonary embolism associated with hydatidiform mole. American Journal of Obstetrics and Gynecology 83: 1644–1647

Looi L M, Sivanesaratnam V 1981 Malignant evolution with fatal outcome in a patient with partial hydatidiform mole. Australian and New Zealand Journal of Obstetrics and Gynaecology 21: 51–52

Lurain J R, Brewer J I, Torok E E 1983 Natural history of hydatidiform mole after primary evacuation. American Journal of Obstetrics and Gynecology 145: 591

MacVicar J, Donald I 1963 Sonar in the diagnosis of early pregnancy and its complications. Journal of Obstetrics and Gynaecology of the British Commonwealth 70: 387–395

Matalon M, Modan B 1972 Epidemiological aspects of hydatidiform mole in Israel. American Journal of Obstetrics and Gynecology 101: 126–132

Matalon M, Paz B, Modan M, Modan B 1972 Malignant trophoblastic disorders. American Journal of Obstetrics and Gynecology 112: 101–106

Matsuura J, Chiu D, Jacobs P A, Szulman A E 1984 Complete hydatidiform mole in Hawaii: an epidemiological study. Genetic Epidemiology 1: 271

Morrow C P, Kletzky O A, DiSaia P J et al 1977 Clinical and laboratory correlates of molar pregnancy and trophoblastic disease. American Journal of Obstetrics and Gynecology 128: 424

Nielson N H, Hansen J P H 1979 Trophoblastic tumours in Greenland. Journal of Cancer Research and Clinical Oncology 95: 177–186

Ohama K, Kajii T, Okamoto E 1981 Dispermic origin of XY hydatidiform moles. Nature 292: 551–552

Parazzini F, La Vecchia C, Pampallona S 1986 Parental age and risk of complete and partial hydatidiform mole. British Journal of Obstetrics and Gynaecology 93: 582–584

Requard C K, Mettler F A 1980 The use of ultrasound in the evaluation of trophoblastic disease and its response to therapy. Radiology 135: 415–422

Rustin G J S, Bagshawe K D 1985 Gestational trophoblastic tumors. Critical Reviews in Oncology/Haematology 3: 103–142

Rustin G J S, Booth M, Dent J, Salt S, Rustin F, Bagshawe K D 1984 Pregnancy after cytotoxic chemotherapy for gestational trophoblastic tumours. British Medical Journal 288: 103–106

Sand P K, Lurain J R, Brewer J I 1984 Repeat gestational trophoblastic disease. Obstetrics and Gynecology 63: 140–144

Santos-Ramos R, Forney J P, Schwarz B E 1980 Sonographic findings and clinical correlations in molar pregnancy. Obstetrics and Gynecology 56: 186–192

Sasaki S, Katayama P K, Roesler M, Pattillo R A, Mattingly R F, Onkawa K 1982 Cytogenetic analysis of choriocarcinoma cell lines. Acta Obstetricia et Gynecologica Japan 34: 2253–2256

Sauvage J P, Crane J P, Kopta M M 1974 Difficulties in the ultrasonic diagnosis of hydatidiform mole. Obstetrics and Gynecology 44: 546

Scott J S 1962 Choriocarcinoma: observations on the etiology. American Journal of Obstetrics and Gynecology 83: 285–293

Scully R E, Young R H 1981 Trophoblastic psuedotumour: a reappraisal. American Journal of Surgical Pathology 5: 76
Sheppard D M, Fisher R A, Lawler S D, Povey S 1982 Tetraploid conceptus with three paternal contributions. Human Genetics 62: 371–374
Sheppard D M, Fisher R A, Lawler S D 1985 Karyotypic analysis and chromosome polymorphisms in four choriocarcinoma cell lines. Cancer Genetics and Cytogenetics 16: 251–259
Shiina Y, Ichinoe K 1979 The age incidence of hydatidiform mole and the secondary occurrence rate of invasive mole. Acta Obstetricia et Gynecologica Japan 31: 82–86
Slocumb J C, Lund C J 1969 Incidence of trophoblastic disease. Increased rate in younger age group. American Journal of Obstetrics and Gynecology 104: 421–423
Stone M, Bagshawe K D 1976 Hydatidiform mole: two entities. Lancet i: 535
Stone M, Bagshawe K D 1979 An analysis of the influences of maternal age, gestational age, contraceptive method and the primary mode of treatment of patients with hydatidiform moles on the incidence of subsequent chemotherapy. British Journal of Obstetrics and Gynaecology 86: 782–792
Sung H Z, Wu P C, Wang Y E, Tang M Y, Yang H Y 1983 A proposal of clinical staging of malignant trophoblastic diseases based on a study of the development of the diseases. In: Pattillo R A, Hussa R O (eds) Human trophoblast neoplasms. Plenum Press, New York, p 327
Surti U, Szulman A E, Wagner K, Leppert M, O'Brien S J 1986 Tetraploid partial hydatidiform moles: two cases with a triple paternal contribution and a 92, XXXY karyotype. Human Genetics 72: 15–21
Suzuki M, Matsunobu A, Wakita K et al 1980 Hydatidiform mole with a surviving co-existing fetus. Obstetrics and Gynecology 56: 384–388
Szulman A E, Surti U 1978a The syndromes of hydatidiform mole. I. Cytogenetic and morphological correlations. American Journal of Obstetrics and Gynecology 131: 665–671
Szulman A E, Surti U 1978b The syndromes of hydatidiform mole. II. Morphological evolution of the complete and partial mole. American Journal of Obstetrics and Gynecology 132: 20–27
Szulman A E, Surti U 1982 The clinicopathologic profile of the partial hydatidiform mole. Obstetrics and Gynecology 59: 597–602
Takeuchi S 1982 The nature of invasive mole and its rational management. Seminars in Oncology 9: 181–186
Teoh E S, Dawood M Y, Ratnam S S 1971 Epidemiology of hydatidiform mole in Singapore. American Journal of Obstetrics and Gynecology 110: 415–420
Teoh E S, Dawood M Y, Ratnam S S 1972 Observations on choriocarcinoma in Singapore. Obstetrics and Gynecology 40: 519–524
Vassilakos P, Riotten G, Kajii T 1977 Hydatidiform mole: two entities. A morphologic and cytogenetic study with some clinical considerations. American Journal of Obstetrics and Gynecology 127: 167–170
Wake N, Takiyi N, Sasaki M 1978 Androgenesis as a cause of hydatidiform mole. Journal of the National Cancer Institutute 60: 51–57
Wake N, Tanaka K, Chapman V, Matsui S, Sandberg A A 1981 Chromosomes and cellular origin of choriocarcinoma. Cancer Research 41: 3137–3143
Wake N, Seki T, Fujita H et al 1984 Malignant potential of homozygous and heterozygous complete moles. Cancer Research 44: 1226–1230
Walden P A M, Bagshawe K D 1976 Reproductive performance of women successfully treated for gestational trophoblastic tumours. American Journal of Obstetrics and Gynecology 125: 1108–1114
Wallace D C, Surti U, Adams C W, Szulman A E 1982 Complete moles have paternal chromosomes but maternal mitochondrial DNA. Human Genetics 61: 145–147
Wilson R B, Beecham C T, Symmonds R E 1965 Conservative surgical management of chorioadenoma destruens. Obstetrics and Gynecology 26: 814–820
Woo J S K, Wong L C, Ma H-K 1985 Sonographic patterns of pelvic and hepatic lesions in persistent trophoblastic disease. Journal of Ultrasound Medicine 4: 189–198
World Health Organization 1983 Gestational trophoblastic diseases. Technical report series 692. World Health Organization, Geneva
Yen S, McMahon B 1968 Epidemiologic features of trophoblastic disease. American Journal of Obstetrics and Gynecology 101: 126–132
Yuen B H, Burch P 1983 Relationship of oral contraceptives and the intrauterine contraceptive devices to the regression of concentrations of the beta sub-unit of human chorionic gonadotrophin and invasive complications after molar pregnancy. American Journal of Obstetrics and Gynecology 145: 214–217

32

S. L. Barron

Antepartum haemorrhage

INTRODUCTION

A survey of all births in Britain in 1970 found that there was a history of bleeding in one in 10 of all pregnancies (Chamberlain et al 1978). The bleeding varied from a small episode before 28 weeks (4.2%) to placenta praevia (0.5%; Table 32.1). In practice, it is often difficult to allocate cases to simple diagnostic categories, such as premature separation of placenta or placenta praevia, and there is little doubt that small episodes of bleeding often go unreported.

The placenta contains, within the intervillous space, about 700 ml of maternal blood which reaches it via the uterine and ovarian arteries. The open arterioles discharge into the choriodecidual space, which depends for its integrity only on the adherence of the placenta to the maternal decidua. This normally remains intact until after delivery of the fetus, so long as the placenta is inserted into the upper segment of the uterus. Effacement and dilatation of the cervix cause separation from the chorion, from its attachment to the myometrium, sometimes producing a small amount of bleeding (a show). If, however, the placenta is inserted either wholly or partly into the lower segment (placenta praevia) bleeding not only becomes inevitable but may be very heavy.

When bleeding occurs from a normally sited placenta, separation from the decidual bed may lead to a cycle of massive haemorrhage and further separation (placental abruption). The fetus is deprived of placental function and the uterine muscle is suffused with extravasated blood — the Couvelaire uterus (Speert 1957). Such separation is not always catastrophic and the bleeding may be trivial. Nevertheless, the perinatal mortality following even minor episodes of antepartum haemorrhage (APH) is about double that in women without a history of such bleeding (Table 32.1).

Fetal blood in the placenta circulates within the capillaries of the villi and is separated from maternal blood in the intervillous space by the capillary wall and trophoblast. In vasa praevia a placental blood vessel lies in front of the presenting part of the fetus, usually because of anatomical variation such as velamentous insertion of the cord. Rupture of the vessel causes not only vaginal bleeding but also exsanguination of the fetus.

Finally, there are causes of bleeding which are best described as incidental APH because they are unrelated to the placenta. Polyps or carcinoma of the cervix may cause bleeding, especially following coitus; or bleeding can occur from varicosities of the vulva.

Table 32.1 Bleeding in pregnancy: frequency and perinatal mortality

Type of bleeding	Incidence (%)	Perinatal mortality rate (per 1000 births)
None	88.7	16.8
Placenta praevia	0.5	81.4
Accidental APH	1.2	143.6
Bleeding <28 weeks	4.2	61.0
Other specified cause	2.2	39.7
Unspecified	2.4	32.6
No information	0.8	30.3
Total in survey	17005 (100%)	21.4

From Chamberlain et al (1978).
APH = antepartum haemorrhage.

Nomenclature

Students of all ages are understandably confused by the term accidental APH, which is sometimes used as a synonym for abruption. The expression dates from the 19th century when obstetricians distinguished unavoidable bleeding due to placental presentation from inadvertent or accidental bleeding (Kerr et al 1954); this had nothing to do with the present-day association of the word accidental with trauma. Abruptio placentae, also called ablatio placentae, indicates that the placenta has separated from its implantation in the uterine wall before delivery of the fetus. In the UK it is usual to use the anglicised version placental abruption.

Timing

Until about 10 years ago, APH was defined simply as bleeding from the genital tract after the 28th week of pregnancy and before labour; however, two major advances have changed our understanding and management of bleeding in late pregnancy. The first is the contribution of diagnostic ultrasound which has enabled the placental site to be identified in early pregnancy before the appearance of symptoms. The second advance has been in the paediatric care of very low birthweight infants so that even infants born as early as 24 weeks' gestation now have a good chance of survival. This means that intervention in pregnancy for the sake of the infant can now be undertaken before the arbitrary 28 weeks boundary.

The 28 weeks rule was convenient because in the UK it is the legal limit of viability and the registration of stillbirth. Changing that concept would mean a change in the law, but meanwhile the International Federation of Gynaecology and Obstetrics (FIGO) has recommended that perinatal death statistics should include any fetus born after 22 weeks or weighing 500 g or more. It therefore seems reasonable that 22 weeks should also form the new boundary between the definition of APH and bleeding of early pregnancy.

World Health Organization (WHO) rubrics

The International Classification of Diseases (ICD, ninth revision, WHO 1977) recognizes premature separation of placenta (641.2), other APH (641.8) and unspecified APH (641.9). The term accidental haemorrhage is so well established that it is unlikely to disappear, but it is tolerable only if its meaning is defined. The following nomenclature (with the appropriate ICD code) is therefore suggested as a way of resolving the confusion:

Incidental APH (ICD 641.8)
Placenta praevia
  with haemorrhage (ICD 641.1)
  without haemorrhage (ICD 641.0)
  vasa praevia (ICD 663.5)
Accidental APH
  abruption (ICD 641.2)
unspecified APH (ICD 641.9)

PLACENTA PRAEVIA

Definitions

The placenta is partly or wholly inserted in the lower uterine segment and its condition is usually divided into four grades (Fig. 32.1):

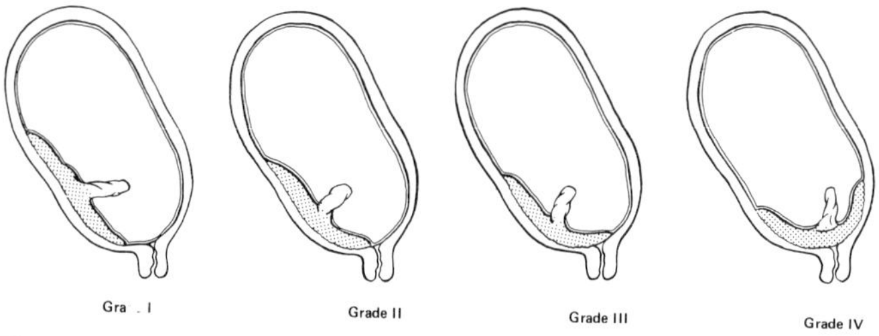

Fig. 32.1 The four grades of placenta praevia (see text for explanations).

Grade I (lateral placenta praevia):
  the placenta just encroaches on the lower uterine segment.
Grade II (marginal placenta praevia):
  the placenta reaches the margin of the cervical os.
Grade III (partial placenta praevia):
  the placenta covers part of the os.
Grade IV (complete placenta praevia):
  the placenta is centrally placed in the lower uterine segment.

The routine use of ultrasound has revealed that the relationship between the placental site and the lower segment can change as pregnancy progresses, so that the placenta appears to migrate up the uterus. For this reason there is a tendency to over-diagnose grade I placenta praevia. The use of ultrasound also increases the likelihood of diagnosing placenta praevia before there has been any bleeding (ICD 641.0).

Incidence

Estimates of incidence based on a defined population are hard to find. One source of error is the practice of many American authors of using 20 weeks as the lower limit of APH and rejecting as irrelevant cases of placenta praevia delivered vaginally. Nevertheless, there is reasonable agreement that placenta praevia occurs in between 0.4 and 0.8% of pregnancies. The incidence of placenta praevia by maternal age and parity is summarized in Table 32.2.

Aetiology

The placenta develops as a discoid condensation of trophoblast on the surface of the chorion at about 8–10 weeks' gestation; the position is determined by the site of implantation (Hamilton & Mossman 1972). Routine ultrasound examination in pregnancy has provided interesting information on the changing anatomical relationship of placental site to the cervix as the uterus enlarges. Low implantation has been observed in 5–28% of pregnancies during the second trimester, but as the uterus grows, the placental site appears to migrate upwards and by term only 3% are praevia. It is possible that the observed migration is due in part to differential development of the placenta, possibly affected

Table 32.2 The incidence of placenta praevia in relation to maternal age and parity (rates are per 100 pregnancies)

	Maternal age				
Reference	<20	20–24	25–29	30–34	35+
Chamberlain et al (1978)	0.1	0.3	0.5	0.6	1.5
Paintin (1962)	0.1	0.2	0.4	├ 0.7 ┤	
Clark et al (1985)	0.1	0.2	0.3	0.4	0.9
Naeye (1980)					
Non-smokers	0.2	├ 0.4 ┤		├ 0.8 ┤	
Smokers	0.3	├ 0.7 ┤		├ 1.8 ┤	

	Pregnancy number			
	1	2	3–4	5+
Naeye (1980)				
Non-smokers	1.5	1.8	1.7	1.8
Smokers	1.8	1.9	2.2	2.9
Paintin (1962)	0.3	0.3	├ 0.7 ┤	
Clark et al (1985)	0.1	0.2	0.4	0.6
Chamberlain et al (1978)	1.1	├ 1.4 ┤		1.7

by previous scarring or changes in vascularization. There is evidence for this from the observation that the umbilical cord in placenta praevia frequently has a marginal insertion (Hibbard 1986). Adherence to a lower segment scar may also explain the increased incidence of placenta praevia following a previous Caesarean section.

Increased surface area

It is generally accepted that conditions in which the area of the placenta is increased, such as twins, succenturiate lobe and placenta membranacea, have an increased incidence of placenta praevia, but there is little published evidence on the subject apart from the association with placenta extrachorialis (Scott 1960).

Age, parity and previous Caesarean section

The increased incidence of placenta praevia with age and parity is shown in Table 32.2. The relationship between parity and placenta praevia was also found to be true in cases of low implantation diagnosed in the second trimester but which did not prove to be praevia at term (Newton et al 1984). In a study of 147 cases of major placenta praevia, McShane et al (1985) found that 22 (15%) had had a previous Caesarean section. In their study of 97 799 deliveries, Clark et al (1985) found that the incidence of placenta praevia in those who had not had previous Caesarean section was 0.26%; in those with one scar it was 0.65% and with three or more Caesarean section scars it was 2.2% (Table 32.3).

Other gynaecological surgery

It has been suggested that an induced abortion increases the risk of placenta praevia in a subsequent pregnancy, but

Table 32.3 Placenta praevia, placenta accreta and previous Casearean section

No. of Caesarean sections	Patients (no.)	Placenta praevia (no.)	Placenta praevia %	Placenta accreta (no.)	Placenta accreta %
0	92 917	238	0.26	12	5
1	3 820	25	0.65	6	24
2	850	15	1.8	7	47
3	183	5	3.0	2	40

From Clark et al (1985).

the studies of Grimes & Techman (1984) and of Newton et al (1984) showed no evidence of such an association. Rose & Chapman (1986) compared the gynaecological history of 80 women with placenta praevia with controls who were matched for age and parity. As well as confirming the association with parity and a history of previous Caesarean section, they also found a significant relation to a history of dilatation and curettage, a less significant relationship to evacuation of retained products of conception, but no relation to a previous induced abortion. They concluded that endometrial damage was a factor in the aetiology of placenta praevia.

Cigarette smoking

In a paper based on the large US collaborative study, Naeye (1980) showed that placenta praevia was more frequent in mothers who smoked during pregnancy than those who did not, or who had already stopped smoking. The relationship was not as strong as with placental abruption (Table 32.2) but the finding is difficult to explain.

Association with placenta accreta

Not only does the risk of placenta praevia increase with the number of previous Caesarean sections, but so does the likelihood of placenta accreta (Table 32.3). McShane et al (1985) also reported that of the 22 women in their series with a previous Caesarean section scar, 6 (27%) of them had placenta accreta.

Clinical aspects

Signs and symptoms

The characteristic feature of placenta praevia is painless bleeding, usually in the third trimester. As pregnancy advances, Braxton Hicks contractions cause the lower segment to thin and in multiparae there is often some dilatation of the cervix. As a result, the abnormally inserted placenta separates from the decidua and bleeding results from the exposed uterine blood vessels. The bleeding is usually unprovoked, although there is sometimes a history of coitus just before. Commonly, the woman wakes because she feels wet and is then alarmed to discover that she has been bleeding. Sometimes there is a history of episodes of bleeding in the second trimester, but fortunately, the first episode of bleeding is often minor. Since the lower uterine segment has poor contractility, the bleeding from placenta praevia can be very severe and although it is unusual for the bleeding to be severe before the 34th week of pregnancy, the exceptions that do occur amply justify hospital admission even for apparently trivial episodes of bleeding. The most catastrophic cases of haemorrhage from placenta praevia occur from ill-advised attempts at vaginal examination.

With routine ultrasound scanning in early pregnancy, most cases of placenta praevia are suspected before there has been any bleeding; there may be a problem of overdiagnosis and the unnecessary anxiety that it provokes.

Diagnosis

In placenta praevia, the abdomen is soft with no tenderness. The presenting part should be easily felt and the fetal heart unaffected. The low placenta acts as a pelvic tumour, and displaces the presenting part, with a high incidence of malpresentation (Hibbard 1986). In some cases, the condition is suspected because of an unstable lie even before there has been any bleeding. A deeply engaged presenting part is strong evidence that the praevia is of minor degree.

Vaginal examination in a case of placenta praevia may provoke serious bleeding and should therefore only be undertaken in an operating theatre with everything ready for an immediate Caesarean section.

The diagnosis can be particularly difficult when the episode of bleeding occurs with the onset of labour, and there is a grade I praevia. In these circumstances, the presenting part is engaged and the presence of labour contractions obscures the abdominal palpation.

There is some justification for passing a vaginal speculum where there is a suspicion that the bleeding is coming from a local lesion of the vagina or cervix, but this can usually wait until more serious causes have been eliminated. The other reason for inserting a speculum is in order to collect a blood sample to test for fetal haemoglobin. Bleeding from vasa praevia is a rare cause of APH but unless it is recognized and the baby delivered by immediate Caesarean section, fetal exsanguination will occur.

Placental localization

Ultrasonography has overtaken other methods of placental localization because of its convenience, safety and accuracy. It is the practice in many British and European obstetric units to offer routine ultrasound scanning at about 16 weeks' gestation. Doubts have been expressed about the wisdom of routine scanning, partly on the grounds that ultrasound has not been proven to be absolutely safe to the fetus, but also (and perhaps more cogently) on the grounds that routine scanning raises false fears which may lead to unnecessary obstetric intervention. This criticism applies particularly to the diagnosis of placenta praevia and the condition should not be diagnosed on the basis of a single observation in the second trimester.

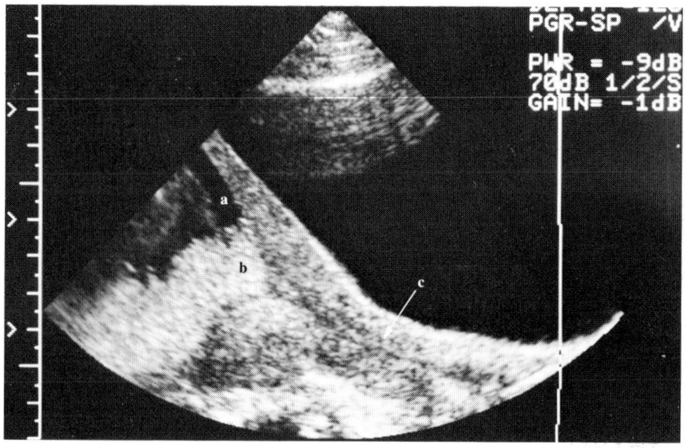

Fig. 32.2 Real-time ultrasonograph showing the edge of placenta overlying the cervical canal. a = liquor; b = edge of placenta; c = cervical canal. Reproduced by kind permission of Dr P. G. Rose.

Table 32.4 Prediction of placenta praevia from early ultrasound scans: results of 632 scans in 503 women

Gestation (weeks)	Praevia at first scan	Significant bleeding or praevia at term (no.)	%
10–14	65	2	3.1
15–19	157	3	1.9
20–24	125	4	3.2
25–29	97	5	5.2
30–34	46	11	23.9
35–term	13	3	23.1
Total	503	28	5.6

From Comeau et al (1983).

Chapman et al (1979) found a low-lying placenta in 28% of women who were scanned routinely before 24 weeks' gestation; by 24 weeks the incidence had fallen to 18% and by term it was 3%. The apparent change in position is due to formation of the lower segment and the enlargement upwards of the upper uterine segment. There may also be technical errors when the lower margin of the placenta is difficult to define because the bladder is not adequately filled.

Real-time scanners can produce high-quality images (Fig. 32.2) and it is now possible, because of the reduction in size of the equipment, to carry out ultrasound scanning within the delivery room. In early pregnancy, although the placenta can be visualized without difficulty, the diagnosis of placenta praevia cannot be made with confidence, for the reasons given above. The later in pregnancy the scan is performed, the more accurate the prediction (Table 32.4). Of 222 cases of placenta praevia predicted by scan before 20 weeks, only 5 (2.2%) had significant bleeding or placenta praevia at term (Comeau et al 1983).

Once bleeding has occurred, diagnosis by ultrasound is difficult because of the resemblance of placenta to blood clot and the indistinct appearance of the cervical os. This is particularly true close to term and in such circumstances clinical examination may be necessary (Table 32.4).

Radioisotope placentography is an acceptable alternative when sonar is not available or unsatisfactory. The method uses an intravenous injection of ^{99m}Tc bound to red blood cells or radioactive albumin bound to ^{132}I. These substances remain within the vascular compartment and the very vascular placental bed shows up as an area of high radioactivity. By means of a Picker scanner, the area can be pictured as a coloured print-out which delineates the placenta, but of course it does not show the site of the fetus or the lower uterine segment (Robertson et al 1968). The isotopes used are considered safe for use in pregnancy because of their short half-life; the procedure itself involves only minimal discomfort to the mother.

Soft-tissue radiography

Although largely eclipsed by ultrasound, X-rays are still used when ultrasound is not available. A lateral film of the lower abdomen is taken with low voltage X-rays. This shows up the lower margin of the placenta by distinguishing it from uterine muscle. If the head presents, then the internal limit of the placenta may also be seen. When the placenta is on the posterior wall, it is more difficult to define because of the overlying bony pelvis, but it may be demonstrated by its ability to displace the presenting part forwards when the patient is X-rayed in a sitting position.

Pelvic angiography involves the injection of a radiopaque medium into the femoral artery after retrograde catheterization with the catheter tip at the bifurcation of the aorta. It gives a good and reliable picture of the placental site but the procedure is uncomfortable, especially the intra-arterial injection, and carries some risk; it is therefore rarely used where easier and less invasive methods are available.

Magnetic resonance imaging (MRI)

This is a new but expensive method of tissue imaging available at present in only a few centres. If a very powerful magnetic field is passed through the body, the hydrogen atoms are polarized so that the H^+ ions are aligned. The protons (the hydrogen atom nuclei) are displaced by radio pulses and in returning to their basal state, give out a small radio signal. A series of images can be built up from the proton density maps of a section of the body. The sections may be at any plane of the body and no ionizing radiation is used.

Unfortunately, at the present time the tissues need to be still for some seconds while the imaging is performed, hence clear fetal images are difficult but localization of the placenta is excellent since both the placental edge and the cervical canal can be readily identified (Powell et al 1986). This may be the most precise method of diagnosing placenta praevia in the future, but at present MRI equipment is available in very few centres in the UK.

Clinical management

Most patients with placenta praevia appear with a history of painless APH, sometimes precipitated by coitus. There may have been more than one warning show of blood but insufficient to have alarmed the patient. The priority is to assess and deal with the blood loss and arrange for an adequate supply of blood should transfusion become necessary.

Where routine ultrasound is done in early pregnancy, the diagnosis should be easy and further localization of the placenta is not necessary. Only in cases of serious haemorrhage is it necessary to make an immediate diagnosis; the important point is to distinguish placenta praevia from vasa praevia and placental abruption. In such circumstances, ultrasound, if available, may be very helpful.

Examination under anaesthesia and amniotomy

The procedure should only be carried out under anaesthesia in an operating theatre, with everything prepared for an immediate transfusion and Caesarean section, should the examination provoke heavy bleeding. The stage of gestation for delivery should be right; there is no point in carrying out an examination when conservative management would be more appropriate. It is a mistake to hurry the examination and it should be performed with the patient in the lithotomy position and using sterile drapes. After catheterizing the bladder, two fingers are introduced into the vagina, avoiding the cervical os. Each vaginal fornix is palpated in turn, the object being to feel whether there is a placenta between the presenting head and the finger. If the four fornices are empty, then a finger can be introduced into the cervical os. If the cervical os is tightly closed and there is significant bleeding it is unwise to use force to dilate the cervix and Caesarean section should be performed.

The presence of clot often makes it difficult to define the edge of the placenta, but if the membranes can be identified then a forewater amniotomy is carried out. Heavily blood-stained liquor is suspicious of an abruption, but if the bleeding is separate from the liquor and it does not stop within a few minutes, it is best to proceed to Caesarean section.

Examination under anaesthesia is also justified where clinical or ultrasound evidence suggests an anterior grade I placenta praevia. Vaginal delivery is therefore possible and amniotomy may be all that is necessary. Once the membranes are ruptured and the uterus is contracting, the presenting part compresses the lateral edge of the placenta and arrests the bleeding.

Expectant management

Unless the bleeding is severe there is much to be gained by expectant management, with the aim of making a correct diagnosis and postponing delivery until about 37 weeks. The benefits of conservative management and the history of its introduction have been well reviewed by Myerscough (1982). The advantage of adequate transfusion is self-evident, but the advantages of avoiding premature delivery to the baby are perhaps less than they used to be, thanks to the improvements in neonatal paediatrics.

Use of tocolytics

When bleeding is complicated by premature labour, it is logical to inhibit uterine activity by means of tocolytic agents. Sampson et al (1984) reported the benefits from an intravenous infusion of terbutaline sulphate, starting with a bolus of 0.25 mg and continuing with 10 μg/min. Silver et al (1984) also advocated aggressive conservatism, which include the use of blood transfusion and tocolytics (type unstated) in all cases of placenta praevia after 21 weeks' gestation. They claimed that by postponing delivery in most cases they achieved a low perinatal mortality rate of 42/1000. The danger of using tocolytic agents is that they produce tachycardia and palpitations, neither of which are desirable in someone already suffering from hypovolaemia. Furthermore, since they are contraindicated in placental abruption, the diagnosis of placenta praevia must be secure.

Vasa praevia is difficult to diagnose, but must always be borne in mind, particularly where the clinical picture is unusual. The diagnosis is made by testing the vaginal blood for fetal haemoglobin using the alkaline denaturation test or by examining the blood microscopically for the presence of nucleated red cells.

Vaginal delivery

There is no point in postponing delivery beyond 37 weeks' gestation except in women with minor degrees of placenta praevia in whom the placenta is anterior and the head engaged. Such a situation may not be apparent until labour starts or an attempt is made to rupture the membranes. In such circumstances, the bleeding is usually controlled by amniotomy augmented by Syntocinon infusion.

Caesarean section

With the exception mentioned above, delivery by Caesarean section is the method of choice but the operation can be hazardous. When the placenta is anterior the lower segment can be very vascular with huge veins coursing across the potential site of the incision. Once the lower segment has been opened, the placenta must either be incised or separated in order to reach the baby.

Each method has its problems. Incising the placenta may be speedy, but dividing fetal vessels can cause fetal exsanguination. On the other hand, separating the placenta may be difficult especially if it is adherent. Once placental separation has been started, the fetus is deprived of maternal oxygen and delivery becomes urgent. Further difficulty can arise if there is a transverse lie and this is one of the few occasions in which it may be prudent to resort to an upper segment incision. An alternative to the classical incision is to convert the transverse lower segment incision into an inverted T, an approach which many obstetricians consider does not heal well, although there is no published evidence on the matter.

Much will depend on the exact circumstances, but the author's preference is for a lower segment approach, underrunning the large vessels with a catgut suture before dividing them. The anterior placenta is then separated with the finger until the edge is reached and the amniotic sac can be opened. If necessary the incision is extended into an inverted T.

Placenta accreta is a serious complication of placenta praevia, leading to uncontrollable bleeding. Hysterectomy may be necessary. It is one of the reasons why Caesarean section for placenta praevia should always be carried out under the supervision of an experienced obstetrician. It is not an operation for the tyro (DHSS 1986). It is particularly liable to be present in association with anterior placenta praevia in a woman who has had one or more previous Caesarean sections (Clark et al 1985).

Table 32.5 Maternal and fetal mortality in placenta praevia before and after introduction of conservative management in Belfast

Year	No. of cases	Maternal mortality (%)	Caesarean section (%)	Fetal mortality (%)
1932–1936	76	2.6	—	51
1937–1944	174	0.6	31	24
1945–1952	206	0.0	68	15

From Macafee (1945) and Macafee et al (1962).

Maternal mortality

The dramatic fall in maternal mortality from APH since the beginning of the century is partly due to the availability of blood transfusion and improved understanding of coagulation failure, but there have also been important changes in management. In placenta praevia the outlook for mother and child were greatly improved by the introduction of conservative management, pioneered in Belfast and rapidly adopted elsewhere. An expectant regime was used, with bedrest, blood transfusion and more liberal use of Caesarean section (Macafee et al 1962). The effects of this change in policy on maternal and fetal mortality are shown in Table 32.5.

Perinatal mortality

The fetal outlook following placenta praevia is more favourable than in placental abruption and has continued to

Table 32.6 The incidence of placental abruption in relation to maternal age and partity (rates per 100 pregnancies)

<table>
<tr><th></th><th colspan="5">Maternal age</th></tr>
<tr><th>Reference</th><th><20</th><th>20–24</th><th>25–29</th><th>30–34</th><th>35+</th></tr>
<tr><td>Hibbard & Hibbard (1963)</td><td>0.85</td><td>0.9</td><td>1.1</td><td>1.2</td><td>1.7</td></tr>
<tr><td>Chamberlain et al (1978)</td><td>1.4</td><td>1.2</td><td>1.0</td><td>1.2</td><td>1.8</td></tr>
<tr><td>Paintin (1962)</td><td>0.9</td><td>0.7</td><td>0.7</td><td colspan="2">0.8</td></tr>
<tr><td>Naeye (1980)</td><td></td><td></td><td></td><td></td><td></td></tr>
<tr><td>Non-smokers</td><td>1.3</td><td colspan="2">1.7</td><td colspan="2">2.3</td></tr>
<tr><td>Smokers</td><td>1.6</td><td colspan="2">2.1</td><td colspan="2">3.3</td></tr>
<tr><th></th><th colspan="4">Pregnancy number</th><th></th></tr>
<tr><th></th><th>1</th><th>2</th><th>3–4</th><th>5+</th><th></th></tr>
<tr><td>Naeye (1980)</td><td></td><td></td><td></td><td></td><td></td></tr>
<tr><td>Non-smokers</td><td>1.5</td><td>1.8</td><td>1.7</td><td>1.8</td><td></td></tr>
<tr><td>Smokers</td><td>1.8</td><td>1.9</td><td>2.2</td><td>2.9</td><td></td></tr>
<tr><td>Paintin (1962)</td><td>0.7</td><td>0.6</td><td>0.9</td><td>0.9</td><td></td></tr>
<tr><td>Hibbard & Hibbard (1963)</td><td>0.8</td><td colspan="2">1.0</td><td>2.3</td><td></td></tr>
<tr><td>Chamberlain et al (1978)</td><td>1.1</td><td colspan="2">1.4</td><td>1.7</td><td></td></tr>
</table>

Description of samples

Hibbard & Hibbard (1963)	23 043 consecutive deliveries, Mill Road Hospital, Liverpool, UK
Naeye (1980)	53 518 pregnancies in 12 university hospitals, USA, 1959–1966 (collaborative perinatal project)
Chamberlain et al (1978)	17 005 pregnancies born in UK during April 1970 (British births 1970 survey)
Paintin (1962)	30 383 singleton pregnancies to married women resident in Aberdeen, UK, 1949–1958

improve over the past 50 years (Macafee et al 1962, Crenshaw et al 1973). In 1980, Cotton et al reported a perinatal mortality rate of 126/1000 total births, which is little different from that of Paintin (1962). There have, however, been two reports from the USA that the perinatal mortality rate has been reduced by a more active approach, with perinatal mortality rates of 81/1000 (McShane et al 1985) and 42/1000 (Silver et al 1984). Scotland, with its system for detailed recording of every pregnancy in the country, provides excellent epidemiological data. During the two years 1984 and 1985 there were 800 cases of placenta praevia with 19 perinatal deaths — a mortality of only 24/1000 (Scottish Health Service, personal communication). Unlike placental abruption, placenta praevia does not cause intrauterine hypoxia and premature delivery is the greatest cause of morbidity and mortality.

PLACENTAL ABRUPTION

Incidence

In the British Births study (Chamberlain et al 1978), placental abruption occurred in about 1% of pregnancies, in close agreement with other reports from the UK. Table 32.6 shows a good deal of variation in the recorded incidence, probably due to differences in definition and accuracy of diagnosis.

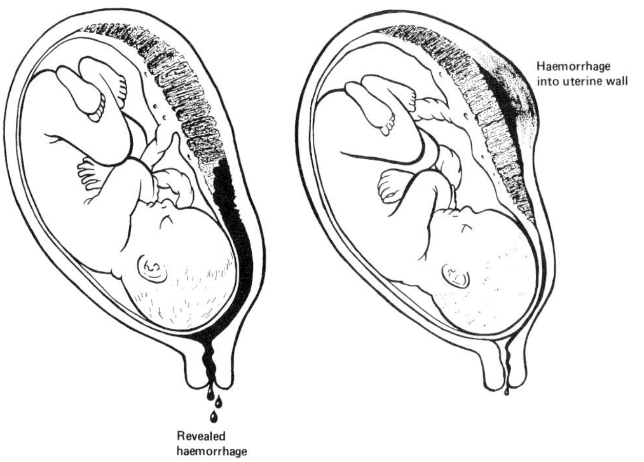

Fig. 32.3 Placental abruption (see text for explanation).

There is no agreement as to whether the condition is more common with increasing age and parity. Although Naeye (1980) believes that it is, a comparison of the data in Table 32.6 shows that although the rise with these parameters is consistent, it is not impressive.

Mechanism

The term abruption (Latin: breaking away from a mass) describes the process by which the placental attachment to the uterus is disrupted by haemorrhage. According to Egley & Cefalo (1985), the process of abruption begins with uterine vasospasm, followed by relaxation and subsequent venous engorgement and arteriolar rupture into the decidua. The blood then attempts to escape by dissecting under the membranes, sometimes getting into the amniotic sac and producing blood-stained liquor — a common finding in cases of placental abruption. The alternative path is for the blood to dissect under the placenta, causing it to separate from its maternal attachment and often extending into the uterine muscle itself (Fig. 32.3). The effect on the myometrium is to cause a tonic contraction, which makes the uterus feel woody and hard. The increase of intrauterine pressure embarrasses the placental circulation, adding to the hypoxia already caused by the separation of the placenta.

Examination of the placenta after birth typically shows an area of organizing blood clot with an underlying compression of the maternal surface. Fox (1978) found evidence of retroplacental clot in 4.5% of placentas which he examined routinely. This suggests that small episodes are more common than is realized.

Aetiology

The aetiology remains an enigma. Although the cause is sometimes obvious, as in cases of direct trauma to the uterus, such cases are uncommon and in the majority the cause is obscure. A woman who has suffered from the condition once has a recurrence rate with subsequent pregnancy of about 6%; this suggests that there may be an underlying abnormality in the uterus or its vasculature.

Egley & Cefalo (1985) found that women who had an unexplained high level of serum alpha-fetoprotein on routine screening had an increased risk of placental abruption. They suggested that this was evidence of faulty implantation, but it could equally well be due to repeated small episodes of fetomaternal bleeding resulting from decidual necrosis.

Maternal hypertension

There is a wealth of evidence to link maternal hypertension to the occurrence of placental abruption, but there is no agreement on whether the hypertension precedes the abruption or vice versa. Paintin (1962) and Hibbard & Hibbard (1963) looked at the epidemiology of APH in Aberdeen and Liverpool respectively. They concluded that there was no evidence of pre-existing hypertension in most cases of placental abruption and that the hypertension and proteinuria happened as a consequence of the abruption. Naeye et al (1977) came to a similar conclusion from their study of 212 perinatal deaths following placental abruption in the US collaborative study. More recently, Abdella et al (1984) came to the opposite conclusion. They examined 265 consecutive cases of placental abruption in Memphis, USA. The overall incidence in the 24 258 deliveries was 1.2%, but it was 2.3% in those with pre-eclamptic toxaemia, 10% in those with chronic hypertension and 23.6% in those with eclampsia.

Abdominal trauma

A direct blow to the abdomen is a dramatic but infrequent cause of abruption. It can occur from assault or more commonly as a result of injury in a car collision. Crosby & Costiloe (1971), using data from the state of California, found an incidence of 4% of placental abruption in women who survived a car crash whilst wearing a seat belt. Their findings suggest that seat belts, whilst reducing fatal accidents, can also traumatize the pregnant uterus: however, this is not an argument against the use of seat belts.

Abruption was a well recognized complication of external cephalic version when it was a common practice, especially when performed under anaesthesia. According to Savona-Ventura (1986), who quotes four series of cases, the incidence of abruption following version was between 2 and 9%. The practice of external version is now being revived, with the addition of tocolytic drugs, and the complication rates are reported to be low (Lancet Leader 1984).

Toxins, drugs and nutritional deficiencies

Epidemiological evidence suggests that the incidence of placental abruption is related to social factors. Perinatal mortality rates from APH increase with maternal age and with decreasing social class, suggesting that environmental factors play an important part (Baird & Thomson 1969). Placental abruption was found to be the commonest cause of fetal loss in an African village and was strongly associated with maternal poverty and malnutrition (Naeye et al 1979).

The theory that placental abruption was due to folate or vitamin deficiency was suggested by Hibbard & Hibbard (1963) from their study of APH in Liverpool, but it was not confirmed by others, notably Pritchard (1970). For a time it was fashionable to give folate supplements to reduce the risk of recurrent placental abruption, but the results were disappointing.

Abruption has been reported following snake bite (Zugaib et al 1985) but is not reported as a complication of anticoagulant therapy (Howell et al 1983). It has also been reported in relation to cocaine abuse, possibly related to transient hypertension (Acker et al 1983). One drug, however, is repeatedly implicated — nicotine.

Cigarette smoking

Evidence is accumulating that cigarette smoking increases the risk of placental abruption. Using data from the US collaborative study, Naeye (1980) reported that the incidence of abruption was 1.69% in non-smokers, 2.46% in smokers and 1.87% in smokers who had given up in early pregnancy. These rates were independent of age and parity and the fact that its effect was also found to be dose-related suggests that the effect was pharmacological. Naeye found evidence of decidual necrosis at the edge of the placenta and thought that this was ischaemic in origin. Cigarette smoking is known to affect uteroplacental blood flow and to induce uterine contractions (Lehtovirta & Forss 1978).

Uterine decompression

Sudden decompression of the uterus occurs when the membranes rupture in the presence of polyhydramnios. The reduction of uterine volume causes a corresponding loss of surface area and as a result the placenta sheers off. Nevertheless, according to Pritchard (1970), it is an uncommon cause of abruption.

Abnormalities of the placenta and uterus

In a comprehensive study, Scott (1960) identified a strong association between placenta extrachorialis and all forms of APH, including abruption. This is supported by Wilson & Paalman (1967) who believed that the commonest specific abnormality associated with placental abruption was a circumvallate placenta, in which there is a rim of placental tissue outside the chorial plate. On the other hand, Fox (1978) stated that the commonest findings in placental abruption are necrosis of the decidua and infarcts of the villi, but made no mention of anatomical anomalies.

Vena caval compression syndrome

Although experimental occlusion of the vena cava in animals can produce placental abruption, Pritchard (1970) found no evidence that compression of the inferior vena cava by the uterus (supine hypotension syndrome) was a cause of abruption. In fact, two patients in their series underwent ligation of the inferior vena cava during pregnancy without harm to the fetus.

Lupus anticoagulant

There has been considerable interest in the role of the lupus anticoagulant as a cause of fetal death in the second trimester (Carreras et al 1981, Lubbe et al 1984, Lubbe & Liggins 1985). The factor causes thrombosis of the vessels in the placental bed with severe fetal growth retardation and fetal death. The prognosis can sometimes be improved by the administration of low-dose aspirin and corticosteroids. No evidence has yet been adduced for its role in the genesis of abruption.

Signs and symptoms

The presenting symptoms are bleeding, pain and the onset of premature labour. Hurd et al (1983) reported that 35% of women admitted with abruption were already in labour. About 10% give a history of previous small episodes of vaginal bleeding (Egley & Cefalo 1985). If the separation starts near the placental margin, then vaginal bleeding occurs early and, because there is little concealed haemorrhage, pain is minimal. Here, the diagnosis may be less obvious. Tenderness over the placental site may not be apparent for several hours and since the event may stimulate uterine contractions, the clinical presentation may resemble premature onset of labour with a heavy show.

When bleeding occurs into the uterine muscle there is pain, increased uterine tone and a deceptive absence of vaginal bleeding. When seen at Caesarean section, the Couvelaire uterus is deeply suffused with haematoma, looking like a huge bruise (Speert 1957). The patient looks distressed and unwell, the abdomen is tender and the uterus has a woody consistency. If placental separation is extensive, fetal parts are difficult to identify and the fetal heart beat may be very slow or absent. If the placenta is posterior, tenderness is less marked and the patient complains of backache. The blood pressure is a poor guide to the extent of bleeding. The coexistence of hypertension (whether it is cause or effect) confuses the usual association of haemorrhage with hypotension. Some cases are unsuspected (the silent abruption) and only diagnosed in retrospect (Notelovitz et al 1979).

With such a variation in clinical presentation, the division of placental abruption into three grades (Sher & Statland 1985) has much to commend it as a guide to management.

Grade I—not recognized clinically before delivery and usually diagnosed by the presence of a retroplacental clot.

Grade II—intermediate. The classical signs of abruption are present but the fetus is still alive.

Grade III—severe. The fetus is dead, IIIa without coagulopathy or IIIb with coagulopathy.

Differential diagnosis

When vaginal bleeding, a tonically contracted tender uterus and fetal hypoxia occur together, there is little doubt about the diagnosis of placental abruption, but a very similar picture is produced by a ruptured uterus. If the rupture is through a previous Caesarean section scar, the tenderness tends to be localized to the suprapubic area, but real confusion can occur if the scar is from some other operation, such as a myomectomy, or is spontaneous.

In the absence of vaginal bleeding, other conditions causing acute abdominal pain and uterine tenderness in pregnancy which will have to be considered include:

1. Haematoma of the rectus sheath;
2. Retroperitoneal haemorrhage;
3. Rupture of an appendix abscess;
4. Acute degeneration or torsion in a uterine fibroid.

A more common problem occurs when there is a small amount of bleeding associated with uterine contractions and a slightly tender uterus. The difficulty is to distinguish a grade I placental abruption from spontaneous preterm labour with a heavy show, especially since a small abruption can itself provoke labour.

Bleeding without pain can also be confusing; it is important to make the distinction from placenta praevia. An ultrasound scan can be very helpful; with a good-quality machine and an experienced operator it is possible to visualize the retroplacental clot or intraperitoneal bleeding. Previous knowledge of the placental site from routine examination in early pregnancy is, of course, very helpful in these circumstances.

Coagulopathy

The first description of a haemophilia-like syndrome associated with a Couvelaire uterus is credited to De Lee in 1901, but it was not until 1936 that Dieckman described the presence of hypofibrinogenaemia (see Myerscough 1982). The condition is thought to originate from disseminated intravascular clotting stimulated by the release of thromboplastin from damaged muscle or a dead fetus. The condition is discussed in more detail in Chapter 38.

In a woman already shocked by an abruption, coagulopathy adds considerably to the dangers to the mother and to the problems of management. Successful treatment requires the resources of a competent haematology laboratory and blood transfusion service.

Hypovolaemic shock

The blood loss in cases of placental abruption is nearly always under-estimated. This is partly because of the invisible bleeding behind the placenta and into the myometrium, but also because of the association with hypertension which tends to mask the signs of hypovolaemia. Renal necrosis, a serious complication, is the result of under-transfusion rather than anything to do with the hypertension and should be preventable (Pritchard & Brekken 1967).

Management

Initial assessment

Once placental abruption has been suspected, action should be swift and decisive since the prognosis for mother and fetus is worsened by delay. The first step is to set up an intravenous line and to correct blood loss as soon as possible. In severe cases two lines should be set up in different veins (DHSS 1986). A central venous catheter is invaluable because it helps to prevent under-transfusion before delivery and over-infusion during the vital hours following delivery. In pre-eclampsia, the circulating blood volume is reduced and there is a risk of pulmonary oedema if too much fluid is infused. The temptation to over-infuse occurs during recovery when there is anxiety about the return of renal function and the central venous pressure should be maintained at about +10 cmH_2O. Blood is taken for cross-matching and to screen for clotting factors including a platelet count. Urinary output should be monitored by a self-retaining catheter in the bladder, using one of the calibrated collecting systems now available. Secretion of at least 30 ml/h indicates adequate renal perfusion; less raises the possibility of under-transfusion.

There are three practical options for management:

1. Expectant — in the hope that pregnancy will continue.
2. Immediate Caesarean section.
3. Rupture the membranes and aim at vaginal delivery.

Expectant treatment. There is a place for conservative treatment when the diagnosis is in doubt or the abruption very minor. Such cases usually present with a small painless vaginal bleed and a localized area of uterine tenderness appears only after several hours; or an ultrasound shows a suspicious area of placental separation. In such circumstances, there is something to be gained from allowing the pregnancy to continue, but the decision will depend on the length of gestation, whether or not there has been a previous episode, the state of the fetus and the extent of the placental separation. Abruption occurring in a posteriorly sited placenta can be treacherous because the only symptom may be backache and the site of tenderness is out of reach.

However innocuous the incident of abruption seems to have been, some damage has likely been done to the integrity and function of the placenta and the fetus should be carefully monitored. It is a good principle to induce labour in all such patients at or before term.

Caesarean section. If the baby is still alive (grade II abruption), electronic fetal monitoring should be started and immediate preparations made for Caesarean section, although the decision to proceed is not always easy. In the first place, the outlook for the fetus is poor, not only in terms of immediate survival but also because 15.4% of liveborn infants did not survive the neonatal period (Abdella et al 1984). Secondly, the presence of coagulopathy adds considerably to the risks of the operation; it can be difficult to achieve haemostasis when the myometrium is engorged by haematoma without the added problem of hypofibrinogenaemia. If the uterus is already contracting well and delivery appears to be imminent within a few hours, then the membranes should be ruptured and the decision to operate postponed, so long as the fetal heart is satisfactory. In a series reported by Hurd et al (1983), the perinatal mortality following Caesarean section was 3/20 (15%), compared with 6/30 (20%) for those delivered vaginally.

Rupturing the membranes and hastening delivery. The main purpose of forewater amniotomy is to hasten the onset of labour and, by encouraging uterine contractions, to reduce uterine bleeding. In most cases it is effective, but also has dangers. If the uterus has become atonic, as happens rarely, the reduction of intrauterine pressure encourages further bleeding which fills the space. Simple observation of the uterine outline gives warning of such continued bleeding. An intravenous infusion of Syntocinon should always be running before starting. The other disadvantage is that a small premature breech baby may slip through a partially dilated cervical os. Rupture of the membranes should therefore be reserved for cases in which the fetus is already dead or labour is already well advanced.

Management of grade III placental abruption

When the baby is dead the only indication for Caesarean section is uncontrollable bleeding or failure of conservative management. If labour has not already started, the membranes should be ruptured and an infusion of Syntocinon started. The outline of the uterus should be marked with a pen and the girth around the umbilicus measured at hourly intervals to detect bleeding which is not being expelled because the uterus has lost its ability to contract. This is fortunately rare but if there is no response to Syntocinon and amniotomy, and bleeding, visible or concealed, continues, Caesarean section may become necessary. Although such an operation is hazardous it may be life-saving.

The management of coagulopathy

The sequence of events which lead to coagulopathy involves a cascade of changes affecting both thrombus formation and fibrinolysis and is considered in detail in Chapter 38. The consequences go beyond the loss of fibrinogen from the circulation because the peripheral deposition of fibrin may also affect the blood vessels in other organs such as kidney and liver. In addition there is sometimes a consumptive thrombocytopenia. With the delivery of the placenta and the extrusion of old clot, the whole process reverts to normal and there is a dramatic improvement within a few hours. Rapid delivery is therefore the key to the treatment of coagulopathy.

Adequate blood transfusion is essential, not only to maintain the circulating haemoglobin, but also to replace platelets. If possible the blood should be fresh and supplemented by fresh platelet concentrate if the platelet count falls below 50 000 ml. Although whole blood is preferable, alternatives will usually be necessary initially. Packed red cells, with fresh or frozen plasma can be used together with plasma-expanding agents such as degraded gelatin products. Dextrans are nowadays better avoided because they may inhibit blood clotting as well as interfering with cross-matching (see Chapter 38).

Replacement of fibrinogen is of doubtful value, since it is immediately deposited in peripheral veins, but it may be of value in desperate circumstances such as Caesarean section. An alternative is to use cryoprecipitate. The use of fibrinolytic inhibitors (such as aminocaproic acid or aprotinin) is controversial because it is said that they consolidate the intravascular clot, with serious consequences in the lungs or liver (Sher & Statland 1985). Heparin has also been advocated because of its effect in augmenting antithrombin III, but Sher & Statland do not advocate it and to most obstetricians it seems illogical (see Chapter 38) and dangerous.

Postpartum haemorrhage

The delivery of the placenta often indicates the end of the acute phase of anxiety, but the battle is not yet over. By this time there are high circulating levels of fibrin degradation products which can have an inhibiting effect on the myometrium (Basu 1969). Postpartum haemorrhage occurs in about 25% of cases and, coupled with the continuing coagulopathy and the heavy blood loss already sustained, severe postpartum haemorrhage can be a *coup de grâce*. This is one of the occasions on which the use of aprotinin is justified.

Renal failure

Ischaemic necrosis of the kidney is a serious complication of placental abruption and the most likely cause is inadequate perfusion during the phase of acute blood loss but it can also occur from fibrin deposits resulting from disseminated intravascular clotting.

Oliguria during the first 12 hours following an abruption is common and does not necessarily imply permanent renal damage. Even when urinary output falls below the optimum of 30 ml/h, diuretics should be used only with the greatest caution, if at all. They cannot improve renal perfusion and may do harm (Sher & Statland 1985). If the oliguria persists after 12 hours and the central venous pressure indicates a normal circulating blood volume, the most important step is to prevent fluid and electrolyte overload by reducing the volume of the infusion to that of the urinary output. If the serum potassium, blood urea and creatinine start to rise then help is needed from a nephrologist; such experts prefer to be consulted too early rather than too late.

Rhesus prophylaxis

Transplacental haemorrhage is likely to occur with any bleeding in pregnancy and can be quite extensive following placental abruption (Pritchard et al 1985). Anti-D immunoglobulin should therefore be given to every rhesus (D)-negative woman within 48 hours of placental abruption. The usual dose in the UK is 100 μg, but this is inadequate if the volume of transplacental haemorrhage exceeds 5 ml fetal blood. A Kleihauer test will give an estimate of the amount of transplacental haemorrhage, but the assessment is complicated by the effect of blood loss and replacement.

Management of a subsequent pregnancy

Abruption is a serious condition, with a high perinatal mortality and a risk of recurrence, estimated as about 7% (Pritchard et al 1985). Although the causes are not known, there is an understandable desire to do something positive in the following pregnancy.

The value of folate supplements during pregnancy has not been proven, but there is little to be lost from their use, preferably before conception. In spite of the uncertainty of the role of hypertension in the causation of abruption, hypertension discovered in such patients should be investigated after the pregnancy is over and then treated accordingly, with antihypertensive treatment maintained during the next pregnancy. The harmful effects of cigarette smoking are well documented and Naeye (1980) has shown that to stop smoking even during pregnancy reduced the risk of abruption by 23%.

It is important to motivate the patient to take prevention seriously and, above all, to give up smoking. Admission to hospital around the time when the previous episode occurred has no proven value, but it is reassuring to both patient and doctor. It also provides an opportunity to measure fetal well-being, to treat any existing hypertension, to reinforce the non-smoking advice and to encourage early reporting of pregnancy bleeding.

Maternal mortality

Maternal mortality from placental abruption has fallen from 8% in 1917 to under 1% (Egley & Cefalo 1985) and the

Table 32.7 Maternal deaths from antepartum haemorrhage in England and Wales (DHSS 1986)

	1970–72	1973–75	1976–78	1979–81
Placental abruption	6	6	6	2
Placenta praevia	6	2	2	3
Maternal mortality per million	5.2	4.1	4.7	2.7

Table 32.8 Perinatal mortality from placental abruption

Author	Period of study	Perinatal mortality (%)
Paintin (1962)	1949–1958	51
Hibbard & Hibbard (1963)	1952–1958	25.2
Lunan (1973)	1966–1970	38 (58, 1966; 27.8, 1970)
Chamberlain et al (1978)	1970	14.4
Paterson (1979)	1968–1975	34.8
Hurd et al (1983)	1979–1981	30.0
Abdella et al (1984)	1970–1980	33.5

most recent Report on Confidential Enquiries into Maternal Deaths for 1978–1981 (DHSS 1986) registered only three deaths from placenta praevia and two from placental abruption. Since these reports only contain information about deaths, there are no denominators from which mortality rates can be derived. Nevertheless, haemorrhage is now making a smaller contribution to maternal mortality and ranks sixth in the causes of maternal deaths (Table 32.7).

Perinatal mortality

Perinatal mortality is increased by any kind of bleeding in pregnancy, but is highest following placental abruption. The perinatal mortality of 14.4%, reported in the British births study (Chamberlain et al 1978; see Table 32.1) is rather low. Although Lunan (1973) reported that perinatal mortality from placental abruption declined during the 5 years of his study, a comparison with six other reports does not show much evidence of an improvement over the years (Table 32.8).

More than half of the perinatal deaths are stillborn. In a series of 274 admissions with abruption reported by Abdella et al (1984), 57 (23%) babies were stillborn, and of these, 44 (16%) were dead before arrival in hospital. Of the remaining 217 live births, 35 (16%) died within 28 days, most of them weighing under 2500 g. As would be expected, the chances of survival depended on the gestation and increased from 23% at 28–32 weeks to 87.6% at 37–40 weeks (Paterson 1979). For liveborn babies weighing 2500 g or more the survival rate is reported as 98% (Lunan 1973). According to Abdella et al (1984), the presence of chronic hypertension trebles the fetal mortality from abruption.

There is also concern about the quality of life for the survivors. The Apgar score and the incidence of respiratory distress syndrome are both worse in babies following abruption than would be expected in infants of equivalent birthweight (Niswander et al 1966). The incidence of congenital anomalies was 4.4%, which is about twice that of the population as a whole, and anomalies of the central nervous system are said to be as much as five times as high (Egley & Cefalo 1985).

Placental abruption still makes a significant contribution to perinatal mortality. In the US collaborative study it was the second most frequent cause and accounted for 15% of all perinatal deaths (Naeye et al 1977). More recent population-based statistics from Scotland (Scottish Health Service 1986) reported 72 deaths from placental abruption (12.3% of the total); 81% of these weighed less than 2500 g. There were another 10 deaths among late abortions between 20 and 28 weeks' gestation. Under current British law these were not registered as stillbirths.

UNEXPLAINED ACCIDENTAL HAEMORRHAGE

In the British births study of 1970 (Chamberlain et al 1978), of 1079 cases of APH, 406 (38%) had bleeding of unspecified cause. The fact that perinatal mortality was twice that of those with no history of bleeding (Table 32.1) suggests that something is compromising placental function. Placental anomalies such as circumvallate placenta (Scott 1960) have been implicated and the idea of a ruptured marginal sinus was a popular explanation, but has never been supported by placental anatomists.

Management

Once other causes of APH have been excluded, the possibility of a silent abruption must be constantly reviewed. Even when no uterine tenderness develops and there is no ultrasound evidence of retroplacental clot, fetal monitoring with cardiotocography should be performed and the pregnancy should not be allowed to go beyond term.

It is not clear why perinatal mortality is increased in cases of unexplained APH. In some there will have been minor episodes of silent abruption (Notelovitz et al 1979) or there may be anatomical anomalies of the placenta (Scott 1960).

CONCLUSIONS

Antepartum haemorrhage remains an important cause of fetal loss. Ultrasound has made the diagnosis of placenta praevia possible in early pregnancy and has contributed to the improvement in the outcome of pregnancy for both mother and child. One cause for concern remains: the rising Caesarean section rate, which is happening all over the world, will probably lead to an increase in the incidence of placenta praevia and of placenta accreta.

The causes and prevention of placental abruption are still not understood and further research is needed. Such evidence as there is suggests that environmental factors play an important part in aetiology and the same factors may be important in the cause of unexplained hypoxic stillbirths. The seed of abruption is probably sown soon after implantation and future improvements in management will depend on a better understanding of the pathology of the placental bed in early pregnancy.

REFERENCES

Abdella T N, Sibai B M, Hays J M, Anderson G D 1984 Relationship of hypertensive disease to abruptio placentae. Obstetrics and Gynecology 63: 365–370

Acker D, Sachs B J, Tracey K J, Wise W E 1983 Abruptio placentae associated with cocaine use. American Journal of Obstetrics and Gynecology 146: 220–221

Baird D, Thomson A M 1969 The effects of obstetric and environmental factors on perinatal mortality. In: Butler N R, Alberman E D (eds) Perinatal problems. Livingstone, Edinburgh, p 223

Basu H K 1969 Fibrinolysis and abruptio placentae. Journal of Obstetrics and Gynaecology of the British Commonwealth 76: 481–495

Carreras L O, Defreyn G, Machin S J et al 1981 Arterial thrombosis, intrauterine death and lupus anticoagulant: detection of immunoglobulin interfering with prostacyclin formation. Lancet i: 244–246

Chamberlain G V P, Philipp E, Howlett B, Masters K 1978 British births, 1970. Heinemann, London, pp 54–79

Chapman M G, Furness E T, Jones W R, Sheat J H 1979 Significance of the ultrasound location of the placental site in early pregnancy. British Journal of Obstetrics and Gynaecology 86: 846–848

Clark S L, Koonings P P, Phelan J P 1985 Placenta previa/accreta and prior cesarean section. Obstetrics and Gynecology 66: 89–92

Comeau J, Shaw L, Marcell C C, Lavery J P 1983 Early placenta previa and delivery outcome. Obstetrics and Gynecology 61: 577–580

Cotton D B, Read J A, Paul R H, Quilligan E J 1980 The conservative aggressive management of placenta previa. American Journal of Obstetrics and Gynecology 137: 687–695

Crenshaw C, Jones D E D, Parker R T 1973 Placenta previa: a survey of 20 years experience with improved perinatal survival by expectant therapy and caesarian delivery. Obstetrical and Gynecological Survey 28: 461–470

Crosby W M, Costiloe J P 1971 Safety of lap-belt restraint for pregnant victims of automobile collisions. New England Journal of Medicine 284: 632–635

DHSS 1986 Report on confidential enquiries into maternal deaths in England and Wales. Report on health and social subjects no 29. HMSO, London

Egley C, Cefalo R C 1985 Abruptio placenta. In: Studd J (ed) Progress in obstetrics and gynaecology 5. Churchill Livingstone, London

Fox H 1978 Pathology of the placenta. Saunders, London, pp 108–112

Grimes D A, Techman T 1984 Legal abortion and placenta previa. American Journal of Obstetrics and Gynecology 149: 501–504

Hamilton W J, Mossman H W 1972 Human embryology, 4th edn. Macmillan, London, p 130

Hibbard L T 1986 Placenta previa. In Sciarra J J (ed) Gynecology and obstetrics. Harper & Row, Philadelphia

Hibbard B M, Hibbard E D 1963 Aetiological factors in abruptio placentae. British Medical Journal 2: 1430–1436

Howell R, Fidler J, Letsky E, de Swiet M 1983 The risks of antenatal subcutaneous heparin prophylaxis in a controlled trial. British Journal of Obstetrics and Gynaecology 90: 1124–1128

Hurd W W, Miodovnik M, Hertzberg V, Lavin J P 1983 Selective management of abruptio placentae: a prospective study. Obstetrics and Gynecology 61: 467–473

Kerr J M M, Johnstone R W, Phillips M H 1954 Historical review of British obstetrics and gynaecology, Livingstone, Edinburgh, pp 1800–1950

Lancet Leader 1984 External cephalic version. Lancet i: 385

Lehtovirta P, Forss M 1978 The acute effect of smoking on intervillous blood flow of the placenta. British Journal of Obstetrics and Gynaecology 85: 729

Lubbe W F, Liggins C G 1985 Lupus anticoagulant and pregnancy. American Journal of Obstetrics and Gynecology 153: 322–327

Lubbe W F, Butler W S, Palmer S J, Liggins C G 1984 Lupus anticoagulant in pregnancy. British Journal of Obstetrics and Gynaecology 91: 357–363

Lunan C B 1973 The management of abruptio placentae. Journal of Obstetrics and Gynaecology of the British Commonwealth 80: 120–124

Macafee C H G, Millar W G, Harley G 1962 Maternal and foetal mortality in placenta praevia. Journal of Obstetrics and Gynaecology of the British Commonwealth 69: 203–212

McShane P M, Heyl P S, Epstein M F 1985 Maternal and fetal morbidity resulting from placenta previa. Obstetrics and Gynecology 65: 176–182

Myerscough P 1982 Munro Kerr's operative obstetrics, 10th edn. Baillière Tindall, London, p 417

Naeye R 1980 Abruptio placentae and placenta previa: frequency, perinatal mortality, and cigarette smoking. Obstetrics and Gynecology 55: 701–704

Naeye R L, Harkness W L, Utts J 1977 Abruptio placentae and perinatal death: a prospective study. American Journal of Obstetrics and Gynecology 128: 740–746

Naeye R L, Tafari N, Marboe C C 1979 Perinatal death due to abruptio placentae in an African city. Acta Obstetricia et Gynecologica Scandinavica 58: 37–40

Newton E R, Barss V, Cetrulo C L 1984 The epidemiology and clinical history of asymptomatic midtrimester placenta previa. American Journal of Obstetrics and Gynecology 148: 743–748

Niswander K R, Friedman E A, Hoover D B, Petrowski H, Westphal M C 1966 Fetal morbidity following potentially anoxigenic obstetric conditions. 1 Abruptio placentae. American Journal of Obstetrics and Gynecology 95: 838–845

Notelovitz M, Bottoms S F, Dase D F, Leichter P J 1979 Painless abruptio placentae. Obstetrics and Gynecology 53: 270–272

Paintin D 1962 The epidemiology of ante-partum haemorrhage. Journal of Obstetrics and Gynaecology of the British Commonwealth 69: 614–624

Paterson M E L 1979 The aetiology and outcome of abruptio placentae. Acta Obstetricia et Gynecologica Scandinavica 58: 31–35

Powell M C, Buckley J, Price H, Worthington B S, Symonds E M 1986 Magnetic resonance imaging and placenta previa. American Journal of Obstetrics and Gynecology 154: 565–569

Pritchard J A 1970 Genesis of severe placental abruption. American Journal of Obstetrics and Gynecology 108: 22–27

Pritchard J A, Brekken A L 1967 Clinical and laboratory studies on severe abruptio placentae. American Journal of Obstetrics and Gynecology 97: 681–700

Pritchard J, MacDonald P C, Gant N F 1985 Williams obstetrics, 17th edn. Appleton-Century-Croft, Norwalk, p 399

Robertson E G, Millar D G, Day M J 1968 Placental localization by colorscan using iodine 132 labelled human serum albumin. Journal of Obstetrics and Gynaecology of the British Commonwealth 75: 636–641

Rose G L, Chapman M G 1986 Aetiological factors in placenta praevia. British Journal of Obstetrics and Gynaecology 93: 586–589

Sampson M B, Lastres O, Thomasi A M, Thomason J L, Work B A 1984 Tocolysis with terbutaline sulfate in patients with placenta previa complicated by premature labor. Journal of Reproductive Medicine 29: 248–250

Savona-Ventura C 1986 The role of external cephalic version in modern obstetrics. Obstetrical and Gynecological Survey 41: 393–400

Scott J S 1960 Placenta extrachorialis (placenta marginata and placenta circumvallata). Journal of Obstetrics and Gynaecology of the British Empire 67: 904–918

Scottish Health Service Information Services Division 1986 Perinatal mortality survey, Scotland 1985. Common Services Agency, Edinburgh

Sher G, Statland B E 1985 Abruptio placentae with coagulopathy: a

rational basis for management. Clinical Obstetrics and Gynecology 28: 15–23
Silver R, Depp R, Sabbagha R E, Dooley S L, Socol M L, Tamura R K 1984 Placenta previa: aggressive expectant management. American Journal of Obstetrics and Gynecology 150: 15–22
Speert H 1957 Alexandre Couvelaire and uteroplacental apoplexy. Obstetrics and Gynecology 9: 740–743
Wilson D, Paalman R J 1967 Clinical significance of circumvallate placenta. Obstetrics and Gynecology 29: 774–778
World Health Organization 1977 International classification of diseases, 9th revision. World Health Organization, Geneva
Zugaib M, de Barros A C D, Bittar R E, Burdmann E de A, Neme B 1985 Abruptio placentae following snake bite. American Journal of Obstetrics and Gynecology 151: 754–755

33

C. J. T. Craig

Genital tract abnormalities

EMBRYOLOGY

Although given in detail in Chapter 6, the elements of applied embryology are given here for the reader's convenience.

The paramesonephric (Müllerian) ducts form the Fallopian tubes, uterus and the upper two-thirds of the vagina. The lower third of the vagina is a development from the urogenital sinus. The paramesonephric ducts develop from an invagination of the coelomic epithelium lateral and parallel to the mesonephric ducts about day 38 (England 1983). They progress caudally and cross ventrally to the mesonephric ducts and fuse to form a Y-shaped uterovaginal primordian at week 8 (40 mm crown–rump length). This lower uterovaginal primordian projects into the urogenital sinus. Canalization of the paramesonephric ducts commences before fusion of the ducts and proceeds craniocaudally (Hamilton & Mossman 1972). The breakdown of the epithelium between the canals of the paramesonephric ducts and the urogenital sinus occurs late in fetal life (Hamilton & Mossman 1972).

Complete fusion of the paramesonephric ducts occurs by mid-pregnancy (Thomas 1968). The exact time for the loss of the median septum between the two duct systems is not apparently known (Thomas 1968, Hamilton & Mossman 1972, Arey 1975, Corliss 1976, England 1983). The fusion progresses both cranially and caudally, with the vaginal septum disappearing before the uterine septum. The stimulus for and the mechanism by which the median septum is lost is unknown. The mechanism is believed to depend either on loss of vascularity or as a result of the septum being retracted into the myometrium at the uterine fundus. In adult patients with a partial or complete septum, the septum is relatively avascular. The fetal uterus shows a preponderance of muscle tissue in the fundus compared with other areas.

In the final embryological development of the uterus the fundus bulges cranially so that its concave appearance turns into a convex dome. This is said to occur after a time (Arey 1975).

The embryological development is summarized in Table 33.1.

CLASSIFICATION: DEVELOPMENTAL ANOMALIES OF THE GENITAL TRACT

Every anomaly should be accurately described so that it can be correctly classified. Only in this way will reliable data about fetal wastage be correctly assigned to each type of genital tract abnormality (Buttram 1983). For example, a bicornuate uterus causes minimal fetal wastage whereas a septate uterus almost invariably leads to poor reproductive outcome (Jones 1981). Accurate classification also permits a true comparison of the efficacy of different treatments.

Many classifications exist (Hamilton & Mossman 1972, Jones 1981, Buttram 1983) but they have the disadvantage of being in Latin and unrelated to the actual times of embryo-

Table 33.1 Summary of embryological development

Paramesonephros
1. Paramesonephric duct system development (day 38)
2. Canalization of the duct systems (commences weeks 7–8)
3. Fusion of the two duct systems (week 8)
4. Median septum loss between the two canalized systems (date unknown)
5. Fundal dome formation (date unknown)
Urogenital sinus
1. Urogenital sinus development (weeks 6–7)
2. Junction of paramesonephric duct system and urogenital sinus (week 8)
3. Transverse septum loss between paramesonephric duct system and urogenital sinus (late in fetal life)

logical development. The following classification eliminates these disadvantages.

1. *Failure of development.*
   No paramesonephric duct development*.
   Unilateral paramesonephric duct development.
2. *Failure of paramesonephric duct canalization**.
   a. Total (Rokitansky-Küster–Hauser syndrome).
   b. Partial.
      (i) Fallopian tubes canalized.
      (ii) Fallopian tubes and uterus canalized.
      (iii) Fallopian tubes, uterus and cervix canalized.
3. *Failure of fusion of paramesonephric ducts.*
   a. Total.
      (i) Complete duplication of uterus, cervix and vagina. One Fallopian tube to each uterus.
   b. Partial.
      (i) Duplication of uterus and cervix. Single vagina.
      (ii) Cornual duplication of uterus. Single uterine lower segment, cervix and vagina.
   Total and partial variants may be associated with a normal contour to the uterus or with major or minor fundal indentations on the serosal surface. Partial fusion abnormalities may be associated with an incompetent cervix.
4. *Failure of median septum loss.*
   a. Total.
      (i) Septum present in uterus, cervix and upper two-thirds of vagina.
   b. Partial.
      (i) Septum present in uterus and cervix.
      (ii) Septum present in uterus.
      (iii) Septum present in fundal portion of uterus.
   Partial septum loss abnormalities are often associated with an incompetent cervix.
5. *Failure of fundal dome development.*
6. *Failure of fusion of paramesonephric ducts with urogenital sinus**.
7. *Failure of transverse septum loss between paramesonephric system and urogenital sinus.*
   a. In isolation.
   b. In combination.

INCIDENCE

The incidence of genital tract abnormalities in obstetrics reported in the literature varies greatly due to many factors, the most important being the interest and awareness of the observers.

Where there is a high index of suspicion the correct diagnosis can be made in most cases by the diligent use of readily available diagnostic methods (Craig 1973, Bennett 1976, Green & Harris 1976). It is not necessary to wait for a specific number of pregnancy losses before initiating diagnostic procedures (Craig 1973, Gibbs 1973).

*These abnormalities are associated with primary amenorrhoea, haematometra or haematocolpos and are not relevant to the subject of genital tract abnormalities in obstetrics.

Table 33.2 Presentation of congenital abnormalities of the uterus

Method of diagnosis	Incidence (%)	Source
1. Retrospective	0.1	Elias et al 1984
2. Retrospective	1:10 to 1:1500	Greiss & Mauzy 1961
3. Retrospective	1:200 to 1:600	Heinonen et al 1982
4. Retrospective	0.25	Green & Harris 1976
5. Premature labour	1–3	Gibbs 1973
6. Hysterosalpingograms in infertility cases	3	Craig 1973
7. Uterine pocketing postpartum	12	Hay 1961
8. Uterine pocketing postpartum	1:30	Greiss & Mauzy 1961
9. Immediately postpartum	2–3	Elias et al 1984
10. Preterm labour	5	Landesman & Wilson 1983
11. Retrospective	3–4	Scott 1976
12. 155 women with recurrent pregnancy losses	27	Harger et al 1983
13. 110 of 195 women with three or more consecutive abortions		Stray-Pedersen & Stray-Pedersen 1984

The reported incidence of uterine anomalies has also been influenced by whether or not fundal dome abnormalities (Tompkins 1962) or congenital cervical incompetence (Stray-Pedersen & Stray-Pedersen 1984) are included. As both are true congenital anomalies they should be included in calculations of incidence. They can be associated with clinical problems. Since asymptomatic women have never been studied, however, the overall incidence is unknown.

Women with congenital abnormalities of the uterus often have renal tract anomalies as well. For example, abnormalities of the renal tract were found in 9% of patients with a double uterus (Rock & Zacur 1983).

It is unlikely that there is a single genetic cause for these anomalies. Elias et al (1984) studied 24 women with an abnormality of the uterus and 156 close female relatives; in only one of the relatives was there a congenital uterine abnormality. They conclude that there is a polygenic multifactorial aetiology.

PRESENTATION IN PREGNANCY AND CHILDBIRTH (Table 33.2)

First-trimester abortions

The decreased vascularity of any intrauterine septum can be a cause of first-trimester abortions. In one study 12% of patients with three previous first-trimester abortions were found to have a uterine abnormality (Stray-Pedersen & Stray-Pedersen 1984). Other factors, such as increased fundal myometrium development, may also play a role. Buttram & Gibbons (1979) found that, of 19 patients with a unicornuate uterus, who had had 14 pregnancies, 12 aborted in the first trimester.

Second-trimester abortions

Once the fetus has grown beyond 12 weeks two factors are essential for continued maintenance of intrauterine pregnancy: the competence of the cervix and the ability of the fundus to undergo continuing distension. If one or both of these is deficient the risk of second-trimester abortion or preterm labour must be increased.

Craig (1973) found congenital fundal abnormalities to be present in 15 (31%) of 48 cases of congenital cervical incompetence. Heinonen et al (1982) found a similar association in 10% of patients with congenital cervical incompetence. Most reports on cervical incompetence have not investigated a possible association with fundal abnormalities. The author's experience since 1973 continues to be that cervical incompetence coexists with fundal anomalies in 30% of cases.

Stray-Pedersen & Stray-Pedersen (1984) found that 7% of patients with recurrent second-trimester abortions had a uterine abnormality. Daly et al (1983) reported on 40 pregnancies in 25 patients who had either a partial or total uterine septum. In these women there had been only one term delivery, five preterm third-trimester deliveries and 34 abortions, mainly in the second trimester. McShane et al (1983) state that abnormal uteri can be detected in 10–15% of habitual aborters.

Because of varying classifications of uterine abnormalities and definitions of preterm labour, it is difficult to quantitate reproductive outcome in women with congenital uterine abnormalities. Jones (1981) claims that the bicornuate uterus causes only minimal problems with pregnancy, while the septate uterus is almost always involved with pregnancy failure. Buttram (1983) writes that the abortion rate for septate uteri is twice as high as with bicornuate uteri. On the other hand, Heinonen et al (1982) and Craig (1973) have not observed such a difference.

Thus considerable confusion exists about the exact incidence of second-trimester abortion in women with uterine fundal abnormalities and whether particular types of fundal abnormality predispose to abortion. In women who have had a mid-trimester abortion, however, it is essential to investigate both for fundal abnormalities and for cervical incompetence (Craig 1973, Gibbs 1973).

Third trimester

Preterm labour

Gibbs (1973) states that 1–3% of preterm labours are associated with uterine abnormalities, not dissimilar to the 5% quoted by Landesman & Wilson (1983), but significantly less than the 12.5% found by Daly et al (1983) in patients with septate or subseptate uteri. Carr-Hill & Hall (1985), in an analysis to determine the incidence of uterine abnormality in preterm birth, noted that the incidence was tripled in women with one previous preterm birth with or without a preceding abortion, but increased sixfold in women who had had two previous preterm births. The authors emphasized however that the risk was relatively low, i.e. 15.4% after one preterm birth and 32.0% after two preterm births.

Abnormal fetal presentation

There are many causes for an abnormal fetal lie, of which a duration of pregnancy of less than 32 weeks is the most common. For practical purposes therefore a congenital uterine anomaly should only be considered as a potential cause in the last 8 weeks of pregnancy. None the less, a persistent abnormal presentation earlier in pregnancy should arouse suspicion.

Most publications on abnormal presentation fail to list anomalies of the uterus as a cause. Green & Harris (1976), however, found a 24% incidence of uterine anomalies with breech presentation—six times higher than the 4% incidence generally quoted for all patients.

Semmens (1962) found the incidence of transverse lie to be 14.5% in women with uterine anomalies.

Unexpected failure of external cephalic version to correct a breech presentation or transverse lie should lead to the suspicion of fundal abnormality.

Intrauterine growth retardation

It seems possible that nidation on a poorly vascular uterine septum or partial septum could hinder placental development, leading to placental insufficiency and intrauterine growth retardation (IUGR). This hypothesis is supported by the studies of Bennett (1976) who found that the placenta was to some extent implanted on a uterine septum in three cases of severe IUGR associated with fundal abnormality.

Multiple pregnancy

Tompkins (1962) suggested an association between uterine anomaly and multiple pregnancy, but other authors only mentioned occasional twin pregnancies without suggesting any causal relationship.

Craig (1973) found that in 57 patients with uterine anomalies there were only two twin pregnancies in the 113 previous pregnancies although 30 of the 57 women had a family history of multiple pregnancy.

Early engagement of the presenting part

Engagement of the head before the 34th week suggests preterm labour.

First stage of labour

Abnormal presentation

With the onset of labour and rupture of the membranes prolapse of the cord is possible if the presentation is abnormal.

Incoordinate uterine action

Greiss & Mauzy (1961) found only two cases of uterine inertia in 77 patients, while Craig (1973) found only one instance of incoordinate uterine action in 57 patients. Green & Harris (1976) reported an increased incidence of abnormal presentation with dystocia and Caesarean section delivery. These reports, and that of Semmens (1962) suggest that the incidence of abnormal uterine action itself is not increased by uterine anomalies. Hay (1958) found that the incidence of 4% for incoordinate uterine action with uterine abnormalities was the same as the overall hospital rate.

Second stage of labour

Outlet obstruction from a vertical vaginal septum has been seen by the author on only two occasions and must be very rare. In 77 cases of genital anomalies in pregnant women reported by Greiss & Mauzy (1961) only one required division of a vaginal septum in labour.

Third stage of labour

Retained placenta

The association between abnormalities of the uterine fundus and retained placenta is relatively common and most obstetricians have personal knowledge of one or more cases. Hay (1958) found that in women with retained placenta the incidence of uterine abnormality was 18%, while Green & Harris (1976) found a 17% incidence.

Postpartum haemorrhage

Although uterine abnormalities predispose to retained placenta, they do not seem to increase the incidence of postpartum haemorrhage.

DIAGNOSIS

The diagnosis of congenital abnormality of the uterus rests mainly on a strong index of suspicion. Suspicion may be aroused by any of the presentations described, occurring on even a single occasion. Particularly with second-trimester abortion or preterm labour, the old textbook teaching is incorrect that two of these presentations must occur in succession before any diagnostic procedure is undertaken. This dogma was based on the false assumption that the prognosis for a successful outcome improved with subsequent pregnancies and that the first incident could be fortuitous. Carr-Hill & Hall (1985), Craig (1973) and Gibbs (1973) have all published evidence that there is no justification for delaying appropriate diagnostic investigation. Glass & Globus (1978), however, still advocate investigation only after two successive abortions.

Different diagnostic methods are used depending on whether the investigation is undertaken during pregnancy and childbirth, immediately postpartum or postabortal or in the interval phase between pregnancies.

Diagnostic methods

Probing the fundus of the uterus with an intrauterine sound is a simple, office procedure which can readily detect subseptate or arcuate uteri.

Testing for *competence of the cervix* with Hegar's dilators is another readily performed office procedure. If a number 7 dilator passes easily through the internal os in a patient at least 6 weeks postpartum, cervical incompetence is almost certainly present.

Dilatation and curettage: when this procedure is performed, and especially in postabortal evacuations of the uterus, an instrument should be passed from cornu to cornu, seeking a partial septum.

Craig (1973) reported a series of 18 patients in whom dilatation and currettage had been performed specifically as part of the investigation of previous fetal loss, in whom the diagnosis of fundal abnormality was missed presumably because careful assessment of the fundus was not made.

Manual removal of the placenta: Hay (1961) suggested that cornual pocketing, detected during manual removal of the placenta, was diagnostic of a congenital uterine anomaly. Greiss & Mauzy (1961) agree.

Hysterography: this is an invaluable investigation for establishing uterine abnormality, but it is essential that the axis of the uterus is parallel to the X-ray plate. This can only be achieved with certainty if the procedure is performed with an image intensifier and the patient is lightly enough sedated to be able to co-operate in changing position. Manipulation of the uterus into the ideal position is neither difficult nor painful and with a good hysterograph gives an accurate picture of the internal cervical os, the shape of the cavity of the uterus and the appearance of the fundus. Major abnormalities of the cavity of the uterus are easy to interpret and cervical incompetence is usually self-evident (Fig. 33.1, 33.2).

Minor fundal abnormalities of the arcuate type or the broad, bicornuate uterus have to be specially sought and the author believes that all hysterographs should be measured according to the *criteria of Tompkins* (1962; Fig. 33.3, 33.4). Arey (1975) has shown that the development of a fundal dome is a late but definite embryological occurrence. Heinonen et al (1982) do not consider the arcuate uterus

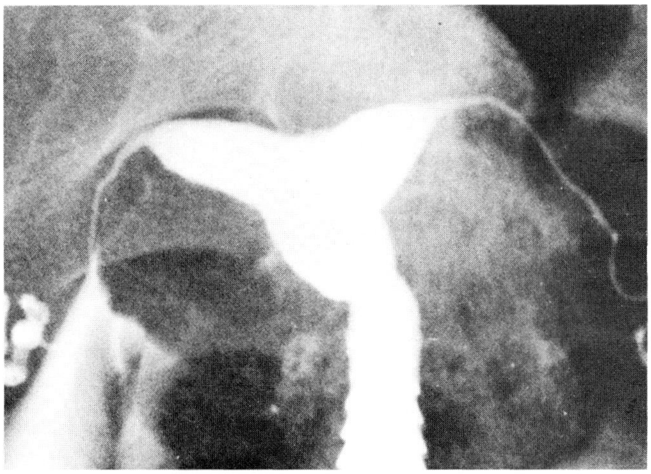

Fig. 33.1 Failure of fusion of paramesonephric ducts. Cornual duplication of uterus with breast forms.

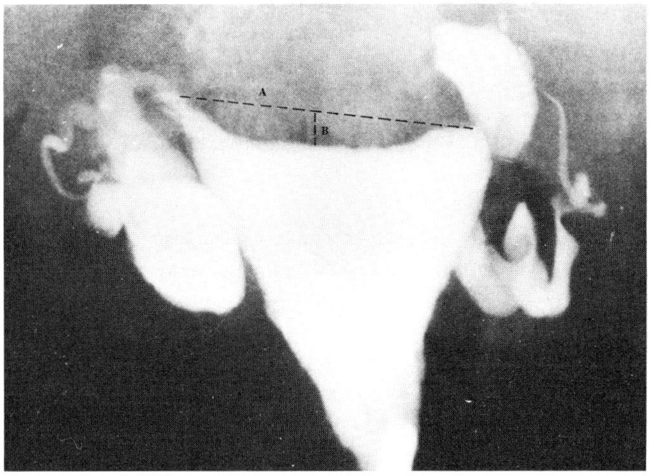

Fig. 33.3 Failure of fundal dome development. Tompkins type II uterus. Length of B is greater than 10% of length of A.

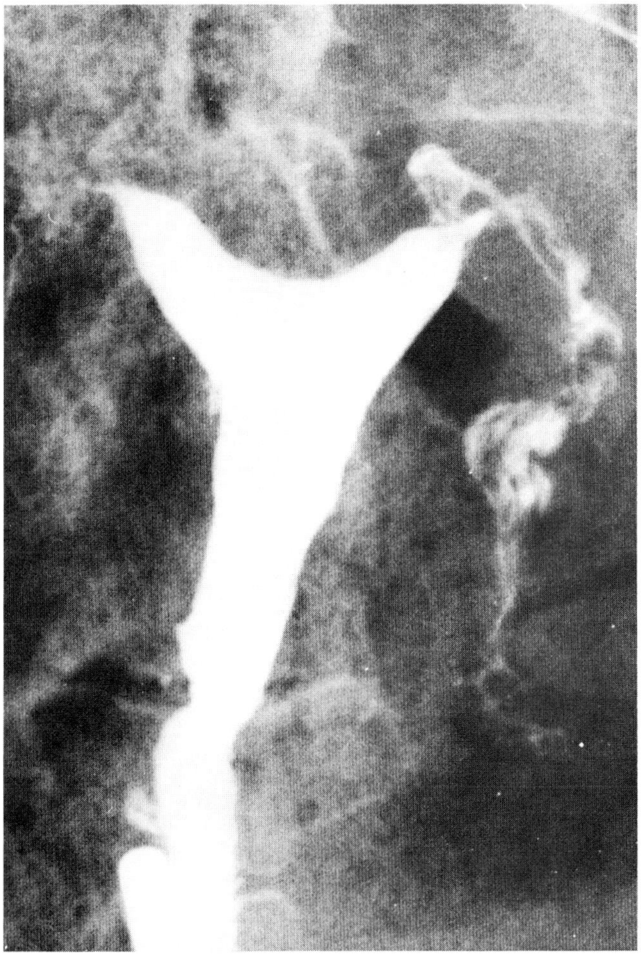

Fig. 33.2 Failure of fusion of paramesonephric ducts. Cornual duplication of uterus. Incompetent cervix.

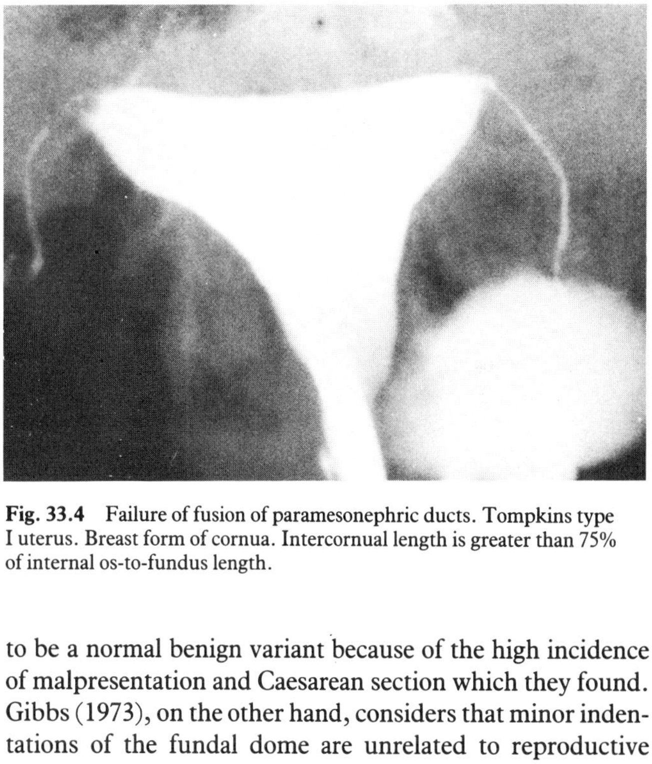

Fig. 33.4 Failure of fusion of paramesonephric ducts. Tompkins type I uterus. Breast form of cornua. Intercornual length is greater than 75% of internal os-to-fundus length.

to be a normal benign variant because of the high incidence of malpresentation and Caesarean section which they found. Gibbs (1973), on the other hand, considers that minor indentations of the fundal dome are unrelated to reproductive function and may be ignored. While this particular aspect still needs clarification, present evidence suggests that minor abnormalities should not be discounted.

Another abnormal finding is the uterine cornu with a rounded 'breast and nipple' appearance. The normal uterus has relatively sharp cornua.

Hysteroscopy: hysteroscopy enables the presence and length of uterine septum to be determined and the breadth of the base.

Ultrasound: postpartum ultrasound examinations can give a useful indication as to which uteri are probably abnormal and identify patients who need a hysterograph for accurate anatomical diagnosis (Bennett 1976).

Ultrasound examinations done during the second and third trimester may reveal cervical incompetence with membranes bulging into the internal os (Jackson et al 1984). Sonar may also confirm a suspected abnormal uterus in cases of persistently abnormal presentation.

Laparoscopy. Laparoscopic examination is an ancillary tool used to differentiate between a bicornuate uterus with a two-horned or notched fundus and a septate uterus with an externally normal uterine appearance. This differentiation is essential if hysteroscopic resection of a septum is contemplated. The procedure can only be performed in septate uteri.

MANAGEMENT

The management of genital abnormalities, particularly of the uterus, depends on a number of factors including:

1. the time of diagnosis;
2. the previous obstetric history;
3. the exact nature of the lesion;
4. the mode of presentation.

Each case must be individually assessed and all other possible causes that could account for a similar presentation must be excluded. Only then may the uterine abnormality be assumed to be the cause and treated.

DIAGNOSIS DURING PREGNANCY

Cervical cerclage

Cervical cerclage is indicated if a clinical and/or ultrasound diagnosis of incompetence of the internal os is made before the 27th completed week of pregnancy. The later in pregnancy the procedure is performed, the less satisfactory is the outcome for the fetus, because the procedure is technically more difficult and the risk of amnionitis increases. It should not be performed if the cervix is 3 cm or more dilated or more than 80% effaced.

Tocolytic drugs

In some patients who have undergone cervical cerclage and in those not selected for cerclage because of advanced duration or pregnancy (27–32 weeks), tocolytic drugs may be used in the hope of postponing or arresting labour. Steroid therapy is given if labour does not ensue (5 mg dexamethasone 6-hourly for four doses). There is a reduced incidence of respiratory distress syndrome (Curet et al 1984). Tocolytic drugs are not used if the membranes are ruptured or if the pregnancy has passed 32 weeks' duration.

Bell (1983), studying intrauterine pressure changes with an external guard ring tocodynamometer, was able to select those patients who would most benefit from tocolytic and steroid therapy.

Bedrest

Clinical experience suggests that bedrest with the foot of the bed elevated can allow the presenting part to fall away from the cervix for short periods (24–36 hours). This may delay the onset of labour in high-risk cases diagnosed during pregnancy (Manabe & Sagawa 1983).

Intrauterine growth assessment

As previously noted, placentation on a septum could lead to IUGR. Serial ultrasound is necessary to confirm whether this is so, and if present, further follow-up with cardiotocography is essential (see Chapter 26).

DIAGNOSIS DURING LABOUR

Epidural anaesthesia

This together with intravenous oxytocin infusion to augment uterine contractility may enable labour to progress satisfactorily in women whose slow cervical dilatation is associated with congenital uterine anomaly.

Caesarean section

This may be necessary if there is an abnormal presentation or if there are signs of fetal hypoxia associated with IUGR.

Vaginal septum

Division or excision of this may be required if the septum is delaying progress in the second stage of labour.

Prevention of postpartum haemorrhage

The reports of Hay (1958, 1961) and Greiss & Mauzy (1961), implying that the incidence of retained placenta is increased in the presence of uterine abnormalities, were published before active management of the third stage was generally accepted. Since 1961 only Green & Harris (1976) have noted an increased frequency of retained placenta.

Apart from ensuring that an intravenous infusion is established, third-stage management should therefore be conducted in line with modern custom, an oxytocin preparation such as Syntocinon being administered intramuscularly with the birth of the anterior shoulder and the placenta delivered by controlled cord traction. Since there have been so few reports of retained placenta with uterine anomaly since 1961, active management of the third stage seems likely to have reduced this risk.

DIAGNOSIS POSTPARTUM OR IN THE INTERVAL PHASE BETWEEN PREGNANCIES

It is at this time that the diagnosis is made and treatment provided in the majority of patients. Treatment may or may not include surgery.

Non-surgical treatment

Pregnant patients with only one previous first-trimester abortion and in whom no other abnormality has been found may be treated expectantly. Patients with a previous obstetric history of preterm delivery where the infant survived without respiratory complications require no special treatment.

Danezis et al (1978) have reported on cases of primary and secondary infertility associated with uterine abnormalities. Conservative treatment with a variety of intrauterine devices for 2–3 months was said to provide satisfactory correction in 78%. Hysterograph appearances after treatment show little difference compared with those before treatment, however, and this approach does not seem justified in women with a previous history of fetal wastage.

Surgical treatment

Surgical treatment is indicated for women in whom uterine anomaly appears to be the only ascertainable cause of previous second-trimester abortion, previous preterm delay of less than 32 weeks or preterm delivery later in pregnancy resulting in stillbirth, neonatal death or the development of severe respiratory distress.

Cervical cerclage

This may be performed in women in whom the only abnormality is cervical incompetence or in women with a fundal abnormality in whom previous pregnancy has not progressed beyond the 32nd week of pregnancy. Cerclage in these cases may enable fundal expansion to accommodate the growing fetus for between 4 and 8 weeks, so that a more mature fetus with a reduced risk of respiratory distress syndrome may be delivered.

The suture can be inserted prior to pregnancy but unfortunately in many cases causes an unpleasant discharge and in others, secondary infertility. The optimum time to perform cervical cerclage is 14–16 weeks of pregnancy. Bennett (1984) advocates early cerclage once sonar confirmation of a viable pregnancy has been made. Postoperatively, patients should be seen every 2 weeks until 3 weeks before the duration of pregnancy when the previous abortion or preterm labour occurred, and then weekly. At each visit a vaginal examination is made to check that the cervix is not effacing with the suture either cutting into the substance of the cervix or rolling down towards the external os. If this occurs before the 28th week of pregnancy a second suture is indicated. If the membranes rupture, the suture should usually be removed, otherwise amnionitis and infection of the fetus may soon ensue.

There is no advantage in prescribing oral tocolytics for patients who have undergone cervical cerclage.

Uteroplasty

Three forms of uteroplasty are commonly used: those of Strassman (1966; Fig. 33.5), Jones & Jones (1953; Fig. 33.6) and Tompkins (1962; Fig. 33.7). The former two operations excise the septum transversely and longitudinally respectively and thus reduce the size of the uterine cavity. The Tompkins operation excises no material, heals with a better scar and recreates a normal fundal dome. Craig (1973), Gibbs (1973), Heinonen et al (1982) and McShane et al (1983) have all emphasized the simplicity of and good results from the Tompkins operation. Scott (1976) advocates the Strassman operation but acknowledges that some patients may end up with a worse result.

The major drawback of uteroplasty is that all subsequent deliveries must be by Caesarean section.

In a series of more than 60 pregnancies following uteroplasty, the author has not encountered a case of uterine rupture.

The operation is performed in cases with a fundal abnormality but no evidence of an incompetent cervix and where no previous pregnancy has reached 32 weeks.

Uteroplasty combined with cervical cerclage

This procedure is carried out in all patients with defects at both fundal and cervical levels and where no previous pregnancy has reached 32 weeks.

Hysteroscopic incision of a uterine septum

Chervenak & Neuwirth (1981), Daly et al (1983) and Israel & March (1984) have all reported successful incision of uterine septa with direct visualization through a hysteroscope. The procedure is indicated in septate and subseptate uteri and simultaneous laparoscopic control is required to exclude uterine perforation. The publications report a total of 42 patients, not all of whom have subsequently become pregnant. Initial results indicate an impressive improvement in outcome closely approaching the improvement achieved by transabdominal uteroplasty.

Treatment with Nd:YAG laser has been used in the removal of uterine septa (Goldrath & Fuller 1985).

An important advantage of this form of treatment is that in subsequent pregnancy the patient does not need Caesarean section.

The postoperative hysterograph appearance in these cases demonstrates the uterus is left arcuate. This failure to re-

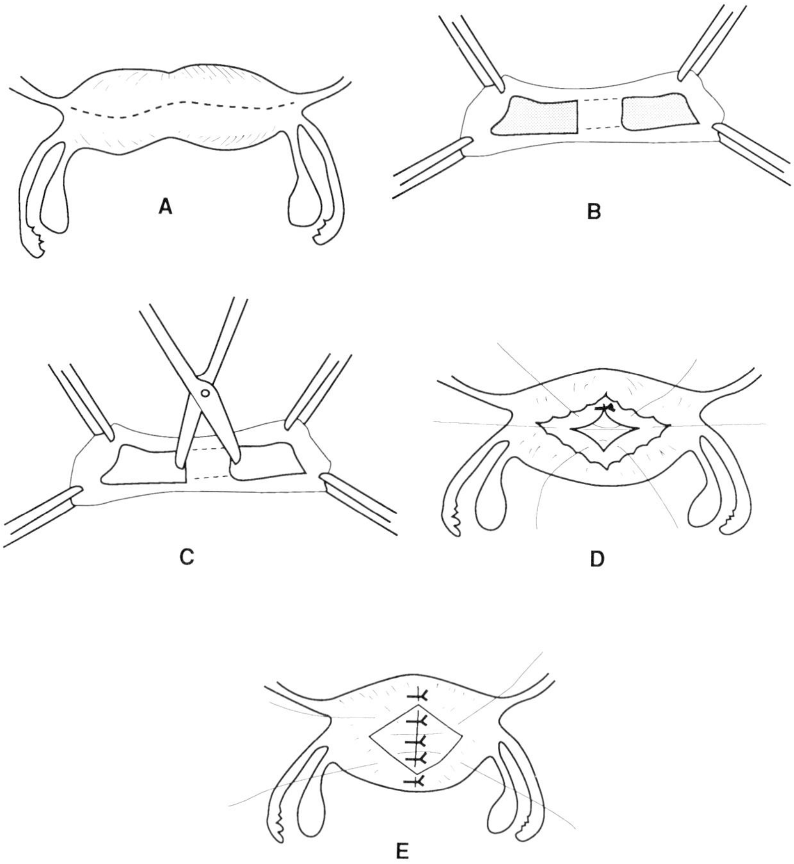

Fig. 33.5 Strassman uteroplasty (after Strassman 1966). Dashed lines indicate lines of incision.

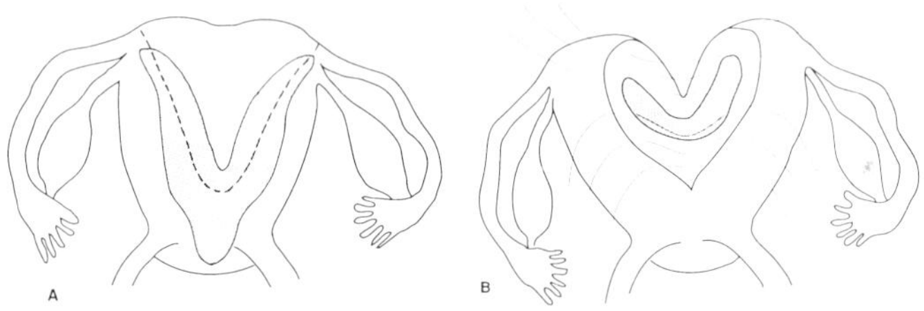

Fig. 33.6 Jones uteroplasty (after Jones & Jones 1953). Dashed lines indicate lines of incision.

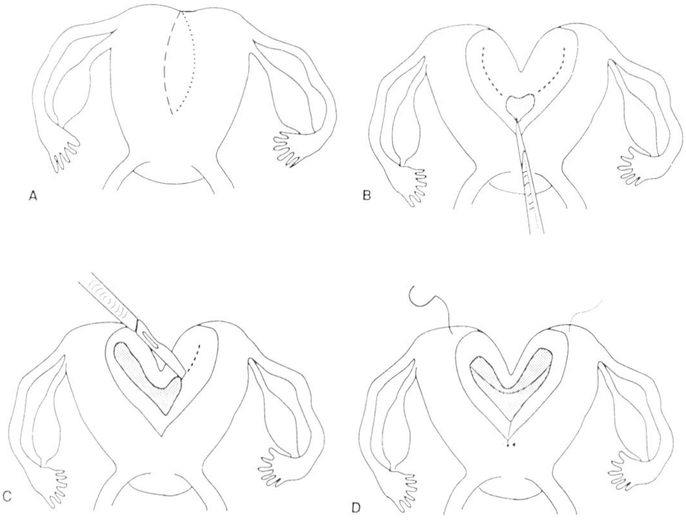

Fig. 33.7 Tompkins uteroplasty (after Tompkins 1962). Dashed lines indicate lines of incision.

create a fundal dome may explain why 2 of 8 pregnancies ended spontaneously at 21 and 33 weeks respectively (Daly et al 1983).

Final assessment of the place for hysteroscopic incision of uterine septa will depend on the results from larger series, with many more subsequent pregnancies and deliveries (Goldrath & Fuller 1985).

PROGNOSIS

It is not possible to assess accurately the place of treatment for individual uterine abnormalities as most authors have reported the outcome of series of cases which include a variety of uterine abnormalities. None the less, before treatment, only 10–20% of infants survive. With correct diagnosis and appropriate treatment of the anomaly, fetal survival increases to between 80 and 95% (Strassman 1966,

Capraro et al 1968, Craig 1973, Jones & Wheeless 1968, Rock & Jones 1977, Rock & Zacur 1983, Stray-Pedersen & Stray-Pedersen 1984, Narita et al 1985).

However, many patients with uterine abnormalities have good obstetric histories and are never diagnosed. The overall prognosis may not be as poor as indicated. Nevertheless, once mid-trimester abortions or preterm labour has occurred, investigation and diagnosis, followed by the correct treatment, are essential to prevent further fetal wastage.

While the alert obstetrician can often establish the presence of a uterine anomaly after only a single late abortion or preterm labour, it is not usually appropriate to advise immediate recourse to major surgical treatment. While cervical incompetence can effectively be treated by the relatively minor cerclage procedure, uteroplasty usually necessitates not only laparotomy, but also delivery by Caesarean section in any subsequent pregnancy.

It is therefore generally advisable for the patient to attempt another pregnancy, or even two, before she and the obstetrician can be reasonably certain that uterine anomaly is the *only* ascertainable cause of pregnancy loss. Even in a woman with a normal uterus a first pregnancy may end in spontaneous abortion or preterm labour and subsequent pregnancies may be uneventful. When the obstetrician detects a uterine anomaly, therefore, the patient must be fully informed of the diagnosis and its implications, and subsequent management arranged with her understanding and agreement.

REFERENCES

Arey L B 1975 Developmental anatomy. Saunders, Philadelphia, pp 318, 326

Bell R 1983 The prediction of preterm labour by recording spontaneous antenatal uterine activity. British Journal of Obstetrics and Gynaecology 90: 884–887

Bennett M J 1976 Puerperal ultrasonic hysterography in the diagnosis of congenital uterine malformations. British Journal of Obstetrics and Gynaecology 83: 389–392

Buttram V C Jnr 1983 Müllerian anomalies and their management. Fertility and Sterility 40: 159–163

Buttram V C, Gibbons W E 1979 Müllerian anomalies: a proposed classification (an analysis of 144 cases). Fertility and Sterility 32: 40–46

Capraro V J, Chuang J T, Randall L L 1968 Improved fetal salvage after metroplasty. Obstetrics and Gynecology 31: 97–103

Carr-Hill R A, Hall M H 1985 The repetition of spontaneous preterm labour. British Journal of Obstetrics and Gynaecology 92: 921–928

Chervenak F A, Neuwirth R S 1981 Hysteroscopic resection of the uterine septum. American Journal of Obstetrics and Gynecology 141: 351–353

Corliss C E 1976 Patten's human embryology. Elements of clinical development. McGraw-Hill, New York, pp 361–369

Craig C J T 1973 Congenital abnormalities of the uterus and foetal wastage. South African Medical Journal 47: 2000–2003

Curet L B, Rao A V, Zachman R D et al and the collaborative group on antenatal steroid therapy 1984 Association between ruptured membranes, tocolytic therapy and respiratory distress syndrome. American Journal of Obstetrics and Gynecology 148: 263–268

Daly D C, Walters C A, Soto-Albors C E, Riddick D H 1983 Hysteroscopic metroplasty. Surgical techniques and obstetrical outcome. Fertility and Sterility 39: 623–628

Danezis J, Soumpus A, Papathanassiou Z 1978 Conservative correction of uterine anomalies in cases of congenital and posttraumatic infertility. International Journal of Fertility 23: 118–122

Elias S, Simpson J L, Carson S A, Malinak L R, Buttram V C 1984 Genetic studies in incomplete Müllerian fusion. Obstetrics and Gynecology 63: 276–279

England M A 1983 A colour atlas of life before birth. Normal fetal development. Wolfe Medical Publications, London, pp 157–163

Gibbs C E 1973 Diagnosis and treatment of uterine conditions that may cause prematurity. Clinics in Obstetrics and Gynaecology 16: 159–170

Glass R H, Golbus M A 1978 Habitual abortion. Fertility and Sterility 29: 257–265

Goldrath M H, Fuller J A 1985 Intrauterine laser therapy. In: Keye W R (ed) Laser surgery in gynaecology and obstetrics. Castle House, Tunbridge Wells, pp 105–106

Green L K, Harris R E 1976 Uterine anomalies. Frequency of diagnosis and associated obstetric complications. Obstetrics and Gynecology 47: 427–429

Greiss F C Jnr, Mauzy C H 1961 Genital anomalies in women. An evaluation of diagnosis, incidence and obstetric performance. American Journal of Obstetrics and Gynecology 82: 330–339

Hamilton W J, Mossman H W 1972 Human embryology. Williams & Wilkins, Baltimore, pp 407–411

Harger J H, Archer D F, Marchese S G, Muracca-Clemens M, Garver K L 1983 Etiology of recurrent pregnancy losses and outcome of subsequent pregnancies. Obstetrics and Gynecology 62: 574–581

Hay D J 1958 The diagnosis and significance of minor degrees of uterine abnormality in relation to pregnancy. Journal of Obstetrics and Gynaecology of the British Empire 65: 557–582

Hay D J 1961 Uterus umcollis and its relationship to pregnancy. Journal of Obstetrics and Gynaecology of the British Empire 68: 361–377

Heinonen P K, Saarikoski S, Pystynen P 1982 Reproductive performance of women with uterine anomalies. Acta Obstetricia et Gynecologica Scandinavica 61: 157–162

Israel R, March C M 1984 Hysteroscopic incision of the septate uterus. American Journal of Obstetrics and Gynecology 149: 66–73

Jackson G, Pendelton H J, Nichol B 1984 Diagnostic ultrasound in the assessment of patients with incompetent cervix. British Journal of Obstetrics and Gynaecology 91: 232–236

Jones H W Jnr 1981 Reproductive impairment and the malformed uterus. Fertility and Sterility 36: 137–148

Jones H W, Jones G E S 1953 Double uterus as an etiological factor of repeated abortion; indication for surgical repair. American Journal of Obstetrics and Gynecology 65: 323

Jones H W Jnr, Wheeless C R 1969 Salvage of the reproductive potential of women with anomalous development of the Müllerian ducts. American Journal of Obstetrics and Gynecology 104: 348–364

Landesman R, Wilson K H 1983 Management of preterm labour. In: Zuspan F P, Christian C D (eds) Reid's controversy in obstetrics and gynecology III. Saunders, Philadelphia, p 44

McShane P M, Reilly R J, Schiff I 1983 Pregnancy outcome following Tompkins metroplasty. Fertility and Sterility 40: 190–194

Manabe Y, Sagawa N 1983 Changes in the mechanical forces of cervical distention before and after rupture of the membranes. American Journal of Obstetrics and Gynecology 147: 667–671

Narita O, Asai M, Masahashi T, Suganuma N, Mizutani S, Tomoda Y 1985 Plastic unification of a double uterus and the outcome of pregnancy. Surgical Gynecology and Obstetrics 161: 152–156

Rock J A, Jones H W Jnr 1977 The clinical management of the double uterus. Fertility and Sterility 28: 798–806

Rock J A, Zacur H A 1983 The clinical management of repeated early pregnancy. Fertility and Sterility 39: 123–137

Scott J S 1976 Abortion, ectopic pregnancies and trophoblastic growths. In: Dewhurst C J (ed) Integrated obstetrics and gynaecology for post graduates. Blackwell Scientific Publications, Oxford, pp 229–232

Semmens J P 1962 Congenital anomalies of female genital tract. Obstetrics and Gynecology 19: 328

Strassman E O 1966 Fertility and unification of double uterus. Fertility and Sterility 17: 165–176

Stray-Pedersen B, Stray-Pedersen S 1984 Etiologic factors and subsequent reproductive performance in 195 couples with a prior history of habitual abortion. American Journal of Obstetrics and Gynecology 148: 140–146

Thomas J B 1968 Introduction to human embryology. Lea & Febiger, Philadelphia, p 269

Tompkins P 1962 Comments on the bicornuate uterus and twinning. Surgical Clinics of North America 42: 1049–1062

I. MacGillivray

Multiple pregnancy

Since ancient times there has been a fascination with multiple human births. In smaller mammals large litters are common but in large mammals, including man, multiple births are relatively uncommon. It has even been suggested that multiple human births are evidence of atavistic reversion.

In some primitive societies twins were welcomed and indeed idolized, but in others both mothers and twins were ostracized and in some cases one or both twins were killed. In more recent times, interest has centred around the greater risk to the mothers and the babies compared with singleton pregnancies. In 1865, the Scottish obstetrician James Matthews Duncan wrote: 'The rarity of plural births in women and increased danger to mother and offspring in these circumstances render such an event in a certain limited sense a disease or an abnormality.'

TYPES OF TWINNING

It has been suggested that there are three types of twin pregnancy but the third type, due to fertilization of one ovum by two sperms, apparently does not occur in humans. The two other types are:

1. *monozygotic*; one ovum may divide early, giving rise to the dichorionic diamniotic (separate or fused) type, or it may divide later, giving rise to the monochorionic diamniotic or the rare monochorionic monoamniotic types;
2. *dizygotic* twins arise from two separate ova and give rise to dichorionic diamniotic placentation which may be separate or fused (Fig. 34.1).

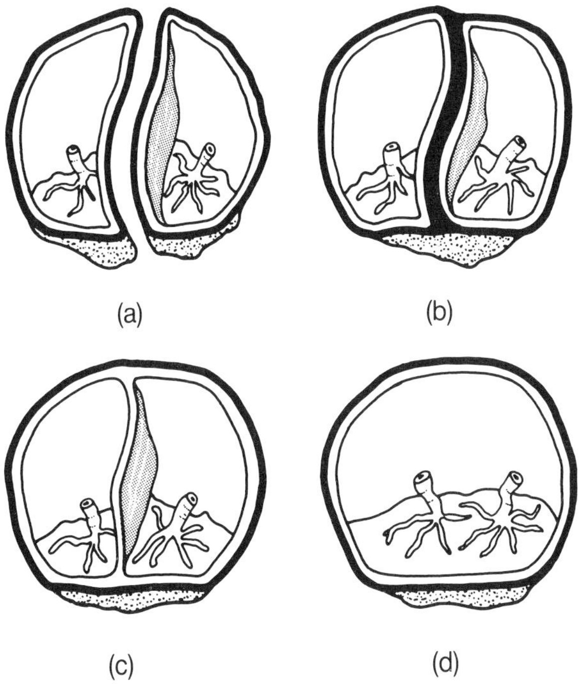

Fig. 34.1 Zygosity and placentation in twin pregnancies. Monozygotic or dizygotic: (a) separate diamniotic; (b) fused diamniotic. Monozygotic: (c) monochorionic diamniotic; (d) monochorionic monoamniotic.

Differentiation of the two types of twin

When the sexes are different, the twins are always dizygotic. On examination of the membranes, those which have only one chorionic membrane must be monozygotic. If the sexes are the same and the placentation is dichorionic then the twins may be either monozygotic or dizygotic. In such cases the zygosity is determined by examination of genetic markers (Corney & Robson 1975) based on blood groups and various placental and blood enzymes or by recombinant fragment

Table 34.1 Twinning rates per 1000 pregnancies in various countries

Country	Monozygotic	Dizygotic	Total
Nigeria	5.0	49.0	54.0
USA			
Black	4.7	11.1	15.8
White	4.2	7.1	11.3
England and Wales	3.5	8.8	12.3
Japan	3.0	1.3	4.3

Adapted from Nylander (1975).

Table 34.2 Multiple births per 1000 pregnancies in various countries

Country	Twins	Triplets	Quadruplets
Nigeria*	66.5	1.78	0.06
USA†			
Black	13.4	0.14	0.0018
White	10.0	0.09	0.001
England and Wales‡	9.6	0.12	0.009
Japan§	6.4	0.056	0.001

*Nylander (1975); †Statistical Bulletin of Metropolitan Life Insurance Company (1960); ‡Registrar General (1979); § Imaizumi & Inouye (1984).

length polymorphism using DNA probes. Alternatively, the zyogosity may be determined by finger- or palm-printing the babies. In monozygotic twins the prints are very similar but never exactly the same. The latest method using mini-satellite DNA probes is extremely sensitive and specific (Hill & Jeffreys 1985).

INCIDENCE OF TWINNING

The highest recorded incidence of twinning is in Nigeria and possibly this accounts for the varying attitudes to twinning found there. In some areas of Nigeria twins are welcomed; in others they are disliked and in yet others they are taboo.

The lowest recorded incidence of twinning is in Japan (Table 34.1). The difference in incidence is only found in dizygotic twins arising from two ova; there is a remarkably constant rate of monozygotic twinning throughout the world.

The incidence of higher multiples was until recently very uncommon. The reported frequencies in various countries differ (Table 34.2) and surprisingly, the incidence of triplets and quadruplets is as high in Japanese as it is in whites. It is usually calculated by Hellin's law (1895) which states that twins occur in every 89 births, triplets in 89^2 and quadruplets in 89^3. The widespread use of ovulation stimulators, and more recently in vitro fertilization, has caused a great increase in the number of twins and higher multiples.

It appears that monozygotic twinning is a chance phenomenon and women who have monozygotic twins have no particular features, although there is a rare tendency for monozygotic twinning in some families and a tendency for the incidence to increase with increasing maternal age and ovulation induction (MacGillivray et al 1988). In contrast, dizygotic twinning is influenced by many factors. As long ago as 1865 Matthews Duncan reported a higher incidence of twinning in older women who had a large number of children. This was shown by Campbell and co-workers in 1975 to apply only to dizygotic twinning. Similarly, mothers of dizygotic twins tend to be taller and heavier than mothers of singletons. There is a well known but ill defined familial tendency to dizygotic twinning, possibly through both maternal and rather more weakly the paternal line (Parisi et al 1983). The maturation of more than one oocyte in a menstrual cycle might be an inherited characteristic, possibly from mother to daughter; on the male side it has been suggested that the sperms of fathers of dizygotic twins are more active and motile. There is evidence that the levels of follicle-stimulating hormone and luteinizing hormone are higher in women who have had twin pregnancies than those who have had singleton pregnancies (Nylander 1973, Martin et al 1984). It is not certain, however, whether taller, heavier women are more likely to produce more of these hormones than smaller women, nor is it known whether there is a familial tendency to higher follicle-stimulating hormone and luteinizing hormone levels.

Famine and war are known to reduce the incidence of twinning (Bulmer 1959). There is some evidence to suggest that mothers of twins are more fertile, but it is difficult to obtain accurate information about this because of widespread contraceptive practice. There have been conflicting reports on the effects of oral contraceptives on twinning rates. It was shown by Macourt and co-workers (1982) that oral contraception increased a woman's chances of having monozygotic twins if she became pregnant within 6 months of coming off the pill. However, Hemon et al (1981) in a matched control study of a sample of twins and singletons showed use of the pill had a significant negative association with unlike sex twinning, and that the relationship remained after adjustment for age, parity and maternal weight. They also found no relation between twinning and the cessation of oral contraceptives and last menstrual period. Recent Aberdeen data show that oral contraception does not influence the incidence of either monozygotic or dizygotic twinning (MacGillivray et al 1988).

There is some suggestion of a seasonal variation in twinning in some parts of the world (Miura et al 1984, Richter et al 1984), and there are also definite secular trends. There has been a widespread world fall in the twinning rate, but this appears to have stabilized (British Medical Journal Editorial 1976) or even risen slightly in countries with widespread fertility programmes that make use of ovarian stimulation.

Table 34.3 Weight gain (kg/week) in primigravidae with singleton and twin pregnancies

Weeks	Singleton	Twin
13–20	0.42	0.60
20–30	0.47	0.54
30–36	0.40	0.64

MATERNAL ADAPTATION DURING PREGNANCY

Maternal response during a twin pregnancy is much greater than in a singleton and even greater with higher multiples. If this is not recognized then the pregnancy may be considered pathological; for example, there is a very marked increase in plasma volume, with a relatively low increase in red cell volume. This causes the haemoglobin concentration to fall and thus levels of 10% g/dl haemoglobin are quite common in twin pregnancies by 30 weeks' gestation. There is a greater increase in haemoglobin mass than in singleton pregnancies and the mean corpuscular volume remains around 85.

Similarly, the increase in erythrocyte sedimentation rate and leukocyte count is also greater in twin pregnancies than in singletons. Cardiac output and stroke volume do not differ in twin pregnancies compared with singletons (Campbell et al 1985), although the fall in blood pressure is slightly greater in mid-trimester in twin pregnancies than in singletons (Campbell & MacGillivray 1977).

Just as the birthweight of singletons correlates with the amount of plasma volume, so too does the combined birthweights of the twins. The greater the plasma volume, the greater the combined birthweight. Similarly, total body water, measured by deuterium oxide (Campbell & MacGillivray 1977), relates to the combined birthweight of twins in primigravidae, but not so much in parous women as happens with singleton pregnancies.

In view of the marked increase in total body water in twin pregnancies, weight gain is also greater, even in the first trimester (Table 34.3). The total intravascular mass of protein is greater in twin than in singleton pregnancies, although total protein concentration rises to 6 g per 100 ml in singletons compared with only 5.5 g per 100 ml in twin pregnancies. There is a greater increase in glomerular filtration rate (Swapp 1975) and in respiratory tidal volume in twin compared with singleton pregnancies (Templeton & Kelman 1974). Serum osmolarity is the same in twin pregnancies as it is in singletons, as are serum concentrations of sodium, potassium and chloride.

With the larger amount of placental tissue in twin pregnancies, the levels of placental hormones are about 50% above singleton values for oestrogens and progesterone in the plasma and urine. The placental protein hormones SP1, PAPPA, PP5 and human placental lactogen are also increased in twin pregnancies, as is the fetal product, alphafetoprotein. Unfortunately, it is not possible to differentiate the contribution of hormones from each twin and only a combined value can be obtained. Thus, interpretation of hormone results in twin pregnancies can be difficult.

Carbohydrate metabolism is altered in twin pregnancies. Campbell (1979) found that the response to an intravenous glucose tolerance test was decreased during twin pregnancies. It is not clear, however, whether this signifies a greater tendency to diabetes or greater resistance to insulin.

Many minor disturbances, particularly of the alimentary system, are more troublesome in twin than in singleton pregnancies. These include reduced gastric motility, hypochlorhydria, oesophageal reflux and constipation.

DIAGNOSIS IN PREGNANCY

Early diagnosis is highly desirable so that gestational length can be determined accurately and the woman can be warned of possible complications. The diagnosis may be suspected from increased weight gain, fundal height, fetal parts and movements. The high values found in tests such as alfafetoprotein may alert the clinician; ultrasonic scanning, which is commonly done routinely nowadays, is usually the first indication of twin pregnancy. Examination may reveal that the uterus is larger than would be expected from calculated gestation, and that multiple fetal parts are palpable. More than two fetal poles may be palpable, e.g. two heads and one breech. When a fetal head is smaller than would be expected from the size of the baby, multiple pregnancy should be suspected. Fetal cardiac auscultation is only of value if two observers are listening simultaneously at two different areas and recording fetal heart rates differing by at least 10 beats/min. An ultrasonic fetal heart monitor gives a better indication because it detects the flow of blood in the baby's heart. In the differential diagnosis, factors such as wrong dates, uterine fibroids, ovarian cysts, hydatidiform moles and polyhydramnios must be taken into account.

COMPLICATIONS OF TWIN PREGNANCIES

In the first half of pregnancy there is little difference between a twin and singleton pregnancy. In the second half however, as the uterus becomes larger, the mechanical discomforts from the over-distended uterus become noticeable and more trying for the patient. Lower abdominal pain and backache are common, as are varicose veins, increased frequency of micturition, constipation and oedema of the abdominal wall, vulva and lower limbs. During the later weeks of pregnancy, it is difficult for the women with twins to be comfortable and walking is difficult, partly because of locomotor difficulties and partly because of breathlessness.

Table 34.4 Percentage of women developing pre-eclampsia in monozygotic (MZ) and dizygotic (DZ) twin pregnancies by parity (from MacGillivray 1984)

	Primigravidae (%)		Multigravidae (%)	
	MZ	DZ	MZ	DZ
Proteinuric pre-eclampsia	17.65	18.64	7.18	8.28
Gestational hypertension	26.89	24.15	13.45	17.20
Normotensive	55.46	57.21	79.37	74.52
Total	100 $n = 119$	100 $n = 236$	100 $n = 223$	100 $n = 628$

Pre-eclampsia

There are many reports of the danger of pre-eclampsia in twin pregnancies compared with singletons. This was shown in a large series of 1206 twin births in Aberdeen in which the zygosity was accurately determined by examination of cord blood and placental tissue for blood groups and enzymes (MacGillivray 1984). There is no difference between the incidence of proteinuric pre-eclampsia in monozygotic, compared with dizygotic, twins. This incidence was high in both types, particularly in primigravidae (Table 34.4). This is contrary to the report of Stevenson and co-workers in 1971 that there was a higher incidence in dizygotic twinning. These authors' study, however, was based on the determination of zygosity by the sex of the twins. However, MacFarlane & Scott (1976) found no variation in the incidence of pre-eclampsia between monozygotic and dizygotic twin pregnancies differentiated on the sex of the twins.

Polyhydramnios

This is more common in twin than singleton pregnancies; the incidence of chronic polyhydramnios is about the same in both types of twin pregnancies. However the incidence of acute hydramnios is much higher in monozygotic than in dizygotic twin pregnancies.

Antepartum haemorrhage

This is usually considered to be more common in twin pregnancies than in singletons, probably because of the greater incidence of pre-eclampsia and because of the larger bulk of placental tissue leading to a greater likelihood of placental praevia. However, a careful study of a large number of twin pregnancies by Nylander (1975) showed that there was no greater incidence of antepartum haemorrhage in twin than in singleton pregnancies. This was confirmed in a study of twins in Scotland (Scottish Twin Study 1983).

Abortion

It is difficult to determine the frequency of abortions in twin pregnancies because in any large series of cases some of the twin pregnancies are not recognized. In a study of an unselected series of spontaneous abortions, the twinning rate was 1/44, compared with 1/103 live and stillbirths (Uchida et al 1983). The frequency of the phenomenon of the vanishing twin is also difficult to determine, but by frequent ultrasound scanning it is possible to detect a number of these cases.

Anaemia

A greater expansion of plasma volume than red cell volume, causing a lowering of haemoglobin concentration, is found in twin pregnancies; this has suggested that anaemia is more common. However, the total haemoglobin mass is greater in twin pregnancies. The haemoglobin concentration is therefore an unreliable indicator and the packed cell volume should be less than 27% before anaemia is diagnosed (Nylander 1975). On this basis Nylander found that the incidence of anaemia was 10.4% for twin pregnancies compared with 10.6% for singleton pregnancies. However, Chanarin et al (1968) found megaloblastic haemopoiesis on sternal narrow aspiration in 30% of 27 twin pregnancies compared with 13% of singletons. Hall et al (1979) in 123 twin pregnancies found that 2.4% had macrocytosis and nuclear hypersegmentation in the peripheral blood, which is about the same as in singleton pregnancies not treated with folic acid.

Anaemia (haemoglobin < 9.5 g) was no more common in twin pregnancies (6%) than in single pregnancies (5.1%) in the Scottish Twin Study (1983).

Hall et al (1979) concluded that there was a reduction in both iron and folic acid stores in twin pregnancy but that the incidence of clinically significant anaemia was low. They suggested that prophylactic iron and folic acid should not be recommended but that specific treatment should be given where there was evidence of significant anaemia, as the authors considered that any deficiency would be transient and self-limiting in nature.

Preterm labour

The incidence of preterm labour in twin pregnancies is about 30% compared with about 10% in singleton pregnancies, and in large measure accounts for the perinatal mortality being higher in twin than in singleton pregnancies. In most cases, the cause of this increased incidence of preterm delivery is unknown, but is influenced both by the zygosity and the sex of the twins. In a study of 879 twin pregnancies in the Aberdeen area between 1968 and 1983 (MacGillivray et al 1988), the commonest cause of preterm delivery in twins was difference in the two zygosity types, but not influenced by placentation.

In monozygotic twinning there may be a higher incidence of preterm delivery than in dizygotic twins (Table 34.5). This higher incidence was partly due to more frequent rupture of the membrane in the monozygotic preterm delivery than in the dizygotic (Table 34.6). In monozygotic twinning

Table 34.5 Preterm (< 37 weeks) delivery by zygosity and placentation in the Aberdeen area from 1968 to 1983

	Preterm (%) ($n = 310$)	Term (%) ($n = 569$)	All (%) ($n = 879$)
Monozygotic monochorionic ($n = 155$)	51.0	49.0	100
Monozygotic dichorionic ($n = 142$)	42.3	59.7	100
Monozygotic dichorionic ($n = 441$)	34.2	65.8	100
Not known ($n = 141$)	14.2	85.8	100
Total ($n = 879$)	35.3	64.7	100

From MacGillivray 1983.

Table 34.6 Type of preterm delivery of twins by zygosity and placentation

	Elective (%)	Spontaneous rupture of membranes (%)	Contraction and retraction (%)
Monozygotic monochorionic ($n = 79$)	22.8	43.0	34.2
Monozygotic dichorionic ($n = 60$)	8.3	56.7	35.0
Dizygotic dichorionic ($n = 151$)	13.3	39.7	47.0
Not known ($n = 20$)	15.0	30.0	55.0
Total ($n = 310$)	14.8	43.2	41.9

From MacGillivray 1983.

Table 34.7 Sex ratio and preterm delivery in twin pregnancies by zygosity and placentation

	Elective	Spontaneous rupture of membranes	Contraction and retraction
Monozygotic monochorionic ($n = 79$)			
BB	9	19	18
GG	9	15	9
BB:GG	100:100	127:100	200:100
Monozygotic dichorionic ($n = 60$)			
BB	3	23	13
GG	2	11	8
BB:GG	150:100	209:100	163:100
Dizygotic dichorionic ($n = 151$)			
BB	8	16	20
GG	5	16	17
BG	7	28	34
BB:GG	160:100	100:100	118:100
B:G	135:100	100:100	109:100

From MacGillivray 1983.

there was a very high boy:girl sex ratio in cases of preterm labour (Table 34.7), in agreement with the findings in preterm singletons (Hall & Carr-Hill 1982). However, in dizygotic twinning there was no great difference in sex ratio. While it is easy to postulate about the causes of preterm labour being more common in monozygotic twin pregnancies, there is no obvious reason why the dizygotic preterm labour rate should also be high in this series, and for different reasons.

MANAGEMENT OF TWIN PREGNANCIES

Antenatal care

As some complications are so much more likely to arise in twin pregnancies, it is desirable that these women should be seen more frequently for antenatal care. They also require more support and advice and probably have more questions than women with singleton pregnancies. Although these mothers should be seen more often, they probably do not need to be examined any more frequently than women with singleton pregnancies, provided that they are feeling adequate fetal movements. Blood pressure and weight should be measured and urine tested more frequently than would be done in singletons because of the greater incidence and earlier onset of pre-eclampsia. Two other major complications to be dealt with are fetal growth retardation and preterm labour.

Weekes et al (1977) found that low maternal age, low parity and monozygosity were significantly related to preterm labour in twin pregnancies.

Preterm delivery is even more common in triplet pregnancies. Syrop & Varner (1985) reported a 75% incidence of preterm delivery in triplet pregnancies and Itzkowic (1979), a rate of 78%.

Uterine height and waist measurements can be valuable in assessing the growth of twins (Schneider et al 1978, Leroy et al 1982). Recording fetal movements can also be useful but the movements are greater in twin than single pregnancies if recorded by maternal daily fetal movement recordings; mothers of triplets record even more movements than those of twins (Samueloff et al 1983).

Antepartum fetal heart rate monitoring is difficult in multiple pregnancy but non-stress cardiotocography was of value in 50 cases of multiple pregnancy reported by Bailey et al (1980). In five cases there was a non-reactive pattern and in four of these a baby died (two antepartum and two neonatal deaths). All were growth-retarded at birth. They found non-stress cardiotocography was better than serial oestrogens or serial biparietal diameter measurements in multiple pregnancy and this was confirmed in 27 twin pregnancies by Lenstrup (1984).

Bedrest

There has been considerable debate regarding the value or desirability of rest in twin pregnancies. This has been advocated to avoid or delay the development of pre-eclampsia, to encourage fetal growth and to prevent the onset of preterm delivery. Whether rest in bed should be carried out at home or in hospital is not clear and this has bedevilled most of the studies attempting to evaluate bedrest. It was suggested by Russell (1952) that larger twins were born to middle-class women because they were rested more than working-class women. Since this difference also accounted for the lower perinatal mortality rate, he advocated admitting all women with twin pregnancy at the 30th week for rest and diet.

Subsequently, several authors recommended bedrest for patients in the third trimester of twin pregnancy (Bender 1952, Anderson 1956, Guttmacher & Kohl 1958). A comparison by Dunn (1961) of two groups of women with twin pregnancy showed that there were no differences in birthweight or gestational length in the groups who were rested or not rested. In contrast, Jeffrey et al (1974), in a study of 114 twin pregnancies in which 41 patients had bedrest, 31 had no bedrest and 42 women in whom twin pregnancy was not diagnosed until labour, it was found that bedrest promoted intrauterine growth. There was a significant difference ($P < 0.05$) in small-for-dates babies: 23.4% in the bedrest group, 41.4% in the group not diagnosed until labour and 34.6% in the group which had no bedrest.

In a series of 491 twin pregnancies, Komorony & Lampé (1977) found that the perinatal mortality rate was 5.4% in 242 women who were hospitalized from 24–26 weeks onwards, compared with 21.7% in 249 women who did not have bedrest. There was also a higher preterm delivery rate of 75% compared with 41%, and 77.2% of babies were below 2500 g compared with 42.9% in the rested, hospitalized group.

There is still controversy about the results of studies, even in this decade. Thus, van der Pol et al (1982) found no effect of clinical bedrest on gestational age. In rested primigravidae there was a small significant increase in birthweight compared with non-rested women. On the other hand, a shorter duration of pregnancy was found in hospitalized cases by Weekes et al (1977), Hartikainen-Sorri & Jouppila (1984) and Saunders et al (1985). However, Kappel et al (1985) demonstrated a reduced frequency of preterm delivery after bedrest in hospital, compared with bedrest at home or no bedrest at all, and an increase in gestational age and birthweight with rest, but the difference in weight disappeared after correction for gestation. There were no significant differences in the perinatal mortality rates between the two groups.

On balance there appears to be no obstetrical advantage from admitting women with twin pregnancies routinely for bedrest in hospital, and there is a considerable disadvantage in the disruption this causes the family and, as has been pointed out by Powers & Miller (1979) and Tresmontant et al (1983), the cost of hospitalization is considerable.

On the other hand, it is essential that women with twin pregnancies should be admitted to hospital if there are specific indications, such as pre-eclampsia, antepartum haemorrhage or threatened preterm labour. In fact it may be necessary to admit some women with twin pregnancies to hospital from about 30 weeks, because of the distance they live from the central hospital, to ensure that the babies are delivered under the best circumstances and receive immediate urgent neonatal care. The detection of threatened preterm labour is difficult, but there is much to be said for routine examination of the cervix weekly from about 28 weeks onwards, as advocated by Houlton et al (1982), who found a significant association between the cervical score and the impending onset of labour ($P < 0.0001$). Sixty per cent of preterm labours would have been predicted, with a false positive rate of 20%. When multiparae were excluded, the predictive value was 80% and the false positive rate was less than 5%. Cervical screening has been found valuable in the Aberdeen Twins Clinic. Nevertheless, O'Connor et al (1981) did not find that cervical assessment and uterine activity were helpful in predicting preterm labour.

The other suggestion, made by Russell (1952), was that diet could be improved if women with twin pregnancies were admitted to hospital. Women liable to have twin pregnancies tend to be heavier but do not have a higher dietary intake than women with singletons. From a 7-day weighed dietary intake and a 24-hour urinary nitrogen test, energy and protein intake proved to be the same in twin as in singleton pregnancies. In both, on average, it was 300–400 kcal less than that recommended by the Department of Health and Social Security — 2400 kcal (Campbell et al 1982). These authors also found that there were no significant differences in the levels of dietary intake of zinc, copper and iron between twin and singleton pregnancies. The diet recommended in women with twin pregnancy should not therefore differ from women with singleton pregnancy.

Other specific measures

Cervical suture has been recommended for the prevention of preterm labour in multiple pregnancies, but was not found to be of value by Sinha et al (1979), Dor et al (1982) or Weekes et al (1977) in twin pregnancies, or by Itzkowic (1979) in triplet pregnancies.

Beta-adrenergic stimulants have also been shown to be ineffective in the prevention (or treatment) of preterm labour, or in increasing intrauterine fetal growth in twin pregnancies (Cetrulo & Freeman 1976, Marivate et al 1977, O'Connor et al 1979).

There is therefore no means of preventing preterm labour or of increasing intrauterine growth in twin pregnancies. Hospitalization is thus only to be advocated if complications develop such as pre-eclampsia, or impending preterm labour. Wherever possible, preterm labour with twin pregnancy should be conducted in a specialized hospital. It may be necessary in certain geographic circumstances to admit women with twin pregnancies to hospital in late pregnancy to avoid preterm delivery at home or in transit. The timing of admission is difficult, but in general should be from about 34 weeks or earlier, depending on circumstances.

ELECTIVE CAESAREAN SECTION

Elective Caesarean section may be carried out at or after 38 weeks' gestation to avoid trauma at delivery, or at any gestation when there are complications such as pre-eclampsia or haemorrhage. The decision to deliver by Caesarean section in cases of malpresentation is a matter of individual preference and depends on the obstetrician's attitude towards breech presentation. Some extremists would suggest Caesarean section for all twins even in the multiparous mother, but there are risks from the operation itself, such as respiratory distress syndrome. The second twin can also suffer at Caesarean section, particularly if born by a difficult breech extraction through the lower segment incision. In early preterm deliveries some advocate the upper segment classical incision for the delivery of twin breeches; the vertical incision may also be useful in transverse lie.

It is the author's preference to aim for a vaginal delivery if the baby or babies are presenting by the breech near to term and if the pelvis is adequate and the babies are well grown; this applies even in primigravidae, provided the mother is young. Elective Caesarean section, however, is indicated if the first twin or more particularly if both babies are lying transversely. Most obstetricians would prefer to do an elective Caesarean section if the first baby is presenting by the brow or the face, but some may allow a short trial of labour to see whether conversion occurs in labour.

Although the great majority of twin pregnancies will end before 40 weeks, some twin pregnancies may be prolonged beyond 40 completed weeks. Most obstetricians agree that twin pregnancies should be delivered by the end of the 40th week. Since it is difficult by cardiotocography or examination of the amniotic fluid to determine whether or not the pregnancy should be allowed to continue beyond 40 weeks, an arbitrary decision is usually made to deliver.

MANAGEMENT OF LABOUR

An anaesthetist should always be available for twin deliveries, and preferably an epidural anaesthesic is administered during the first stage of labour. This allows any manipulation required for the delivery of first and second twins to be carried out, including Caesarean section if required. Pudendal nerve block may be used to deliver the first baby, but it may be necessary to use general anaesthesia for delivery of the second. This is much less satisfactory than epidural anaesthesia as it may be necessary to induce general anaesthesia very rapidly.

The condition of the baby during the first stage of labour is monitored, when possible, by cardiotocography. The fetal heart can be located by real-time B-scan, even in a triplet pregnancy, or for antepartum monitoring (Powell-Phillips et al 1979).

Should fetal distress develop in either twin during the first stage of labour, Caesarean section must be performed, but if the cervix is fully dilated when fetal distress has developed, the first baby should be delivered expeditiously by the means employed by the obstetrician for singleton deliveries. If the breech is presenting, however, and it is not possible to carry out an assisted breech delivery, breech extraction should be avoided and Caesarean section performed. If the cervix is fully dilated and the cord prolapses, the baby should be delivered vaginally as quickly as possible. If not, Caesarean section should be considered.

Obstructed labour is dealt with in much the same way as for a singleton pregnancy. This is liable to occur in many parts of Africa where facilities are poor and the twinning rate is high. Shock and infection are the greatest risks in these cases; active and rapid resuscitation is necessary before delivery. Extraperitoneal Caesarean section was recommended by Crichton (1973) for cases of established or potential intrauterine infection. On the other hand, Philpott (1980) recommended destructive operations as an alternative to an unnecessary and hazardous Caesarean section when the babies are dead.

When the first stage of labour is not progressing sufficiently rapidly, oxytocic stimulation is frequently used and is of great value. An infusion of not more than 5 iu oxytocin in 150 ml 5% dextrose should be set up during the first stage of labour. This can be alternated with 5% dextrose as required, depending on the strength of contractions. Oxytocin can also be given to stimulate the second and third stages of labour as required.

Once the first twin is delivered by whatever means, the lie of the second twin is checked and corrected, if necessary, by external version to a longitudinal lie. The fetal heart is checked and the membranes of the second sac are ruptured; an oxytocin drip is started if contractions are not present.

In general, the longer the second baby is retained, the higher the perinatal mortality risk. Malpresentation and uterine inertia were the main causative factors in the retention of the second twin in a series of 160 cases reviewed by Adeleye (1972) in Nigeria. Active intervention reduced the length of retention and consequently the perinatal mortality rate.

In some circumstances in which the first twin has been delivered at a very early gestation, it is possible to continue the pregnancy for several weeks and deliver a live, second twin.

In exceptional circumstances it may be necessary to perform Caesarean section for the second twin after the first has been delivered vaginally. This may be indicated when the cervix has closed down and there is fetal distress or in cases of incorrectable transverse lie in which a fetal shoulder has become impacted.

A rare cause of obstruction is the locking or entanglement of the twins; it occurs in about 1 in 1000 twin deliveries (Nissen 1958). The condition should be suspected when part of the first baby has been born but the delivery cannot be completed. It may be necessary to give a general anaesthetic to decide the degree of locking and whether it is possible to disengage the head. Disengagement will be difficult because the amniotic fluid will have largely drained away. In the technique of Kimball & Rand (1950), forceps are applied to the head of the second twin and traction and hyperextension are applied to the first twin in the classic type of chin-to-chin locking when the first twin presents as a breech and the second cephalic. The head of the first twin is delivered by flexion. When the first twin is dead, decapitation is carried out and the second twin delivered as quickly as possible. The Kimball & Rand technique is likely to succeed only where the babies are small; it is dangerous for both mother and babies.

Another rare complication is conjoined twins. This was reported only once in 546 twin deliveries by Tan et al (1971). When possible, the conjoined twins should be delivered by Caesarean section. The condition can be suspected either on ultrasonic scanning or on radiological examination.

Delivery of higher multiples has a higher rate of abnormal presentation which is likely to occur in at least one-half of these fetuses. Subsequent babies are at greater risk than the first. However, with triplets, provided that the presentations are not abnormal, vaginal delivery can be attempted if there are no other contraindications. In higher multiples the usual practice is to deliver by Caesarean section unless labour starts at a very early gestation. The optimum timing for delivery depends on the degree of intrauterine growth retardation and presence of complications, but generally, delivery should be performed by 37 weeks.

PERINATAL MORTALITY AND MORBIDITY

The perinatal death rate in twins is usually five or six times greater than in singletons. In Scotland in 1983, for example, the perinatal mortality rate in twins was 55.9 per 1000, compared with 9.7 per 1000 in singletons (Scottish Twin Study 1983). Perinatal mortality is said to be higher in monozygotic than in dizygotic twin pregnancies, but the difference is not as great as was previously thought. Thompson et al (1983) showed that the highest perinatal mortality was in the group in which zygosity had not been determined (Table 34.8).

Table 34.8 Perinatal mortality rates by zygosity in Aberdeen

	Alike	Dizygotic	Not stated	All twins
Perinatal deaths	26	38	32	96
Total babies	550	958	170	1678
Perinatal mortality rate (per 1000 total births)	47.3	39.7	188.2	57.2

From MacGillivray 1983.

Table 34.9 Cause and gestation length in 54 twin deaths in Aberdeen

		Gestation		
Cause	Uncertain (745–2000 g)	30 weeks	30–34 weeks	35+ weeks
Pre-eclampsia Antepartum haemorrhage Infection deformity	0	0	1	7
Immaturity	4	21	17	4

Immaturity: no cause other than small size (2500 g or less).
From MacGillivray 1983.

Even if all those of unknown zygosity were included in the alike or monozygotic group, the difference between monozygotic and dizygotic would only just reach statistical significance.

Low birthweight infants (birthweight less than 2500 g) account for over 50% of multiple births compared to less than 10% of singleton births. In a study of 54 twin pregnancy deaths in Aberdeen in 1976–1981 (MacGillivray, unpublished data) (Table 34.9), 52% of the perinatal deaths were due to small babies, compared with 25% in singletons. Four times as many low birthweight twins die compared with twins weighing 2500 g or more. Infants of shorter pregnancy duration are usually of average weight for dates. Those born later are usually smaller. If infant birthweight is over 2500 g perinatal mortality is similar to that in singletons. The weight of twins deviates from normal singleton standards early in the third trimester, to a mean, peak birthweight of 2900 g for twins reached at 39 weeks' gestation.

Fetal abnormalities are more common in twin pregnancies than singletons and the incidence of malformations in monozygotic twin pregnancies is higher than in dizygotic twins (Myrianthopoulos 1978, Corney et al 1983). In both the Aberdeen study by Corney et al (1983) and the American study of Myrianthopoulos (1978), the incidence of malformations was twice as high in monozygotic as in dizygotic twins, but the much higher incidence of malformations in the American study than in Aberdeen was because babies were followed up for 7 years in America, while in Aberdeen only malformations occurring in the first week of life were reported. The incidence of fetal malformations in twins was not influenced by the type of placentation.

The many studies which have been carried out to follow up twins are all in agreement that there are more physiological and psychological differences, lower intelligence quotients and more language and verbal reasoning difficulties in twins than in singletons.

When a major malformation is detected early in pregnancy in one twin and the other appears normal, selective feticide can be carried out on the affected twin by injecting air into a large fetal vessel through a fetoscope (Rodeck 1984).

More first than second twins die; Sherman & Lowe (1970) showed that there were 50% more perinatal deaths in second than first born twins. Trauma accounts for twice as many deaths in first born twins compared with singletons and four times as many in second born twins. The neonatal mortality rate is twice as high for second as for first born twins, but the stillbirth rate is about the same as for first born (Little & Friedman 1958, Sherman & Lowe 1970).

Growth retardation is a common feature of twins. There is greater discordance of weight with monozygotic twins while the risks to the babies is greater than with dizygotic twins. Growth retardation is best confirmed by ultrasound scanning to measure crown–rump length or cross-sectional scanning of the trunk.

The size of the two babies is of great importance in determining the date of the delivery, particularly if the second baby appears to be smaller than the first. The risks to the two babies differ somewhat, in that the first baby is more likely to be at risk from prolapse of the cord, while the second is more likely to have problems because of malpresentations and placental insufficiency.

Non-stress cardiotocography, when expertly carried out, can be of great value in assessing the condition of the twins and should be carried out particularly in women with complications or suspected growth retardation.

The incidence of cerebral palsy in twins is three times that of singletons (Dunn 1965); the risk of cerebral palsy is greater in second twins, especially those delivered by the breech. Apgar scores in second were poor compared with those in first twins, especially those delivered by breech extraction or version and extraction (Ware 1971). The second twin was more severely asphyxiated than the first, especially when both babies were delivered by the vertex (MacDonald 1962) and there were twice as many second than first born babies with low Apgar scores in the Aberdeen series (MacGillivray 1980). There are more second twins with low Apgar scores than first twins and assisted breech delivery resulted in lower Apgar scores than any other type of delivery. However, breech deliveries in multigravidae were at greater risk than those in primigravidae, possibly suggesting that it was early gestation as much as presentation that predisposed to low Apgar scores. It is interesting that Calvert (1980) showed that on the basis of Apgar scores delivery by lower segment Caesarean section is more dangerous when the baby presents by the breech than cephalic, even in the best circumstances. The author believed that this was due to an inherent abnormality which had itself caused the breech presentation.

REFERENCES

Adeleye J A 1972 Retained second twin in Ibadan: its fate and management. American Journal of Obstetrics and Gynecology 114: 204–207

Anderson W J R 1956 Stillbirth and neonatal mortality in twin pregnancy. Journal of Obstetrics and Gynaecology of the British Empire 63: 205–215

Bailey D, Flynn A M, Kelly J, O'Connor M 1980 Antepartum fetal heart monitoring in multiple pregnancy. British Journal of Obstetrics and Gynaecology 87: 561–564

Bender S 1952 Twin pregnancy. A review of 472 cases. Journal of Obstetrics and Gynaecology of the British Empire 59: 510–517

British Medical Journal Editorial 1976 Worldwide decline in dizygotic twinning. British Medical Journal i: 1553

Bulmer M G 1959 Twinning rate in Europe during the war. British Medical Journal i: 29–30

Calvert J P 1980 Intrinsic hazard of breech presentation. British Medical Journal 281: 1319–1320

Campbell D M 1979 Glucose tolerance in complicated pregnancies. In: Sutherland H W, Stowers J M (eds) Carbohydrate metabolism in pregnancy and the newborn. Springer, Berlin, p 509

Campbell D M, MacGillivray I 1977 Maternal physiological responses and birthweight in singleton and twin pregnancies. European Journal of Obstetrics, Gynecology and Reproductive Biology 7: 7–12

Campbell D M, Campbell A, MacGillivray I 1975 Maternal characteristics of women having twin pregnancies. Journal of Biosocial Science 6: 463–470

Campbell D M, MacGillivray C, Tuttle S 1982 Maternal nutrition in twin pregnancy. Acta Geneticae Medicae et Gemellologiae 31: 221–227

Campbell D M, Haites N, MacLennan F, Rawles J 1985 Cardiac output in twin pregnancy. Acta Geneticae Medicae et Gemellologiae 34: 225–228

Cetrulo C L, Freeman R K 1976 Ritodrine HC1 for the prevention of premature labor in twin pregnancies. Acta Geneticae Medicae et Gemellologiae 25: 321–324

Chanarin I, Rothman D, Ward A, Peng J 1968 Folate studies and requirements in pregnancy. British Medical Journal 2: 390–394

Corney G, Robson E B 1975 Types of twinning and determination of zygosity. In: MacGillivray I, Corney G, Nylander P P S (eds) Multiple human reproduction. Saunders, London, pp 16–39

Corney G, MacGillivray I, Campbell D M, Thompson B, Little J 1983 Congenital anomalies in twins in Aberdeen and NE Scotland. Acta Geneticae Medicae et Gemellologiae 32: 31–35

Crichton D 1973 A simple technique of extraperitoneal lower segment caesarean section. South African Medical Journal 47: 2011–2012

Dor J, Shaler J, Mashiach S, Blankenstein J, Serr D M 1982 Elective cervical suture of twin pregnancies diagnosed ultrasonically in the first trimester following induced ovulation. Gynecologic and Obstetric Investigation 13: 55–60

Dunn B 1961 Bed rest in twin pregnancy. Journal of Obstetrics and Gynaecology of the British Commonwealth 68: 685–687

Dunn P M 1965 Some observations on twins. Developmental Medicine and Child Neurology 7: 121–134

Guttmacher A F, Kohl S G 1958 The fetus of multiple gestations. Obstetrics and Gynecology 12: 528–541

Hall M H, Carr-Hill R 1982 The weaker sex? Impact of sex ratio on onset and management of labour. British Medical Journal 285: 401–403

Hall M H, Campbell D M, Davidson R J L 1979 Anaemia in twin pregnancy. Acta Geneticae Medicae et Gemellologiae 28: 279–284

Hartikainen-Sorri A L, Jouppila P 1984 Is routine hospitalisation needed in antenatal care of twin pregnancy? Journal of Perinatal Medicine 12: 31–34

Hellin D 1895 Die ursache der multiparitat der unipaeten. Tiere Uberhaupt und der Zwillingsschwangerschaft beim Menschen Insbesondere. Seltz und Schanet, Munich

Hemon D, Berger C, Lazar P 1981 Twinning following oral contraception discontinuation. International Journal of Epidemiology 10: 319–328

Hill A V, Jeffreys A J 1985 Use of minisatellite DNA probes for determination of twin zygosity at birth. Lancet ii: 1394–1395

Houlton M C, Marivate M, Philpott R H 1982 Factors associated with pre-term labour and changes in the cervix before labour in twin pregnancy. British Journal of Obstetrics and Gynaecology 89: 190–194

Imaizumi Y, Inouye E 1984 Multiple birth rates in Japan. Further analysis. Acta Geneticae Medicae et Gemellologiae 33: 107–114

Itzkowic D 1979 A survey of 59 triplet pregnancies. British Journal of Obstetrics and Gynaecology 89: 23–28

Jeffrey R L, Bowes W A, Delaney J J 1974 Role of bed rest in twin gestation. Obstetrics and Gynecology 43: 822–826

Kappel B, Hansen K B, Moller J, Faaberg-Andersen J 1985 Bed rest in twin pregnancy. Acta Geneticae Medicae et Gemellologiae 34: 67–71

Kimball A P, Rand P R 1950 A maneouver for the simultaneous delivery of chin-to-chin locked twins. American Journal of Obstetrics and Gynecology 59: 1167–1172

Komorony B, Lampé L 1977 The value of bed rest in twin pregnancies. International Journal of Gynecology and Obstetrics 15: 262–266
Lenstrup C 1984 Predictive value of antepartum non-stress test in multiple pregnancies. Acta Obstetricia et Gynecologica Scandinavica 63: 597–601
Leroy B, Lefort F, Jeny R 1982 Uterine height and umbilical perimeter curves in twin pregnancies. Acta Geneticae Medicae de Gemellologiae 31: 195–198
Little W A, Friedman E A 1958 The twin delivery — factors influencing second twin survival. Obstetrics and Gynecology Survey 13: 611–623
MacDonald R R 1962 Management of second twin. British Medical Journal i: 518–522
MacFarlane A, Scott J S 1976 Pre-eclampsia/eclampsia in twin pregnancies. Journal of Medical Genetics 13: 208–211
MacGillivray I 1980 Twins and other multiple deliveries. Clinics in Obstetrics and Gynaecology 7: 588
MacGillivray I 1984 The Aberdeen contribution to twinning. Acta Geneticae Medicae et Gemellologiae 33: 5–12
MacGillivray I, Thompson B, Campbell D M 1988 Twinning and twins. John Wiley, Chichester
Macourt D C, Stewart P, Zaki M 1982 Multiple pregnancy and fetal abnormalities in association with oral contraceptive usage. Australia and New Zealand Journal of Obstetrics and Gynaecology 22: 25–28
Marivate M, de Villiers K Q, Fairbrother P 1977 The effect of prophylactic outpatient administration of feneterol on the time of onset of spontaneous labour and fetal growth in twin pregnancy. American Journal of Obstetrics and Gynecology 128: 707–708
Martin N G, El Beaimi J L, Olsen M C, Bhatnagar A S, Macourt D 1984 Gonadotrophin levels in mothers who have had two sets of DZ twins. Acta Geneticae Medicae et Gemellologiae 33: 131–139
Matthews Duncan J 1865 On the comparative frequency of twin-bearing in different pregnancies. Edinburgh Medical Journal 10: 928–929
Miura T, Nakamura I, Shimura M, Nonaka K, Aman Y 1984 Twinning rates by month of mothers' birth in Japan. Acta Geneticae Medicae et Gemellologiae 33: 125–130
Myrianthopoulos N C 1978 Congenital malformations: the contribution of twin studies. Birth Defects: Original Articles Series XIV: 151
Nissen E D 1958 Twins: collision impaction, compaction and interlocking. Obstetrics and Gynecology 11: 154–159
Nylander P P S 1973 Serum levels of gonadotrophins in relation to multiple pregnancy in Nigeria. Journal of Obstetrics and Gynaecology of the British Commonwealth 80: 651–653
Nylander P P S 1975 In: MacGillivray I, Corney G, Nylander P P S (eds) Human multiple reproduction. Saunders, London, p 142
O'Connor M C, Murphy H, Dalrymple I J 1979 Double blind trial of ritodrine and placebo in twin pregnancy. British Journal of Obstetrics and Gynaecology 86: 706–709
O'Connor M C, Arias E, Royston J P, Dalrymple I J 1981 The merits of special antenatal care for twin pregnancies. British Journal of Obstetrics and Gynaecology 88: 222–230
Parisi P, Gatti M, Prinzi G, Caperna G 1983 Familial incidence of twinning. Nature 304: 626–627
Philpott R H 1980 Obstructed labour. Clinics in Obstetrics and Gynaecology 7: 601–602
Powell-Phillips W D, Wittmann A, Davison B M 1979 Fetal monitoring of a triplet pregnancy. British Journal of Obstetrics and Gynaecology 86: 666–667
Powers W F, Miller T C 1979 Bed rest in twin pregnancy: identification of a critical period and its cost implications. American Journal of Obstetrics and Gynecology 134: 23–29
Registrar General 1979 Multiple pregnancies. OPCS series FM1 no. 6. HMSO, London
Richter J, Miura T, Nakamura I, Nonaka K 1984 Twinning rates and seasonal changes in Görlitz, Germany from 1611–1860. Acta Geneticae Medicae et Gemellologiae 33: 121–124
Rodeck C H 1984 Fetoscopy in the management of twin pregnancies discordant for a severe abnormality. Acta Geneticae Medicae et Gemellologiae 33: 57–60
Russell J K 1952 Maternal and fetal hazards associated with twin pregnancies. Journal of Obstetrics and Gynaecology of the British Empire 59: 208–213
Samueloff A, Eurow S, Sadovsky E 1983 Fetal movements in multiple pregnancy. American Journal of Obstetrics and Gynecology 146: 789–792
Saunders M C, Dick J S, Brown I McL, McPherson K, Chalmers I 1985 The effects of hospital admission for bed rest on the duration of twin pregnancy. Lancet ii: 793–795
Schneider L, Bessis R, Hajeri H, Papiernik E 1978 On twin care: early detection of twin pregnancies with the use of charts of normal uterine height and waist measurements. Progress in Clinical and Biological Research 24: 143–146
Scottish Twin Study 1983 Preliminary report. Social Paediatric and Obstetric Research Unit, University of Glasgow and Greater Glasgow Health Board, Glasgow
Sherman G H, Lowe E W 1970 Do twins carry a high risk for mother and baby? Journal of the American Medical Association 62: 217–220
Sinha D P, Nandakumar V C, Brough A K, Beebejaun M S 1979 Relative cervical incompetence in twin pregnancy. Acta Geneticae Medicae et Gemellologiae 28: 327–331
Statistical Bulletin of Metropolitan Life Insurance Company 1960
Stevenson A C, Davison B C C, Say B et al 1971 Contribution of fetal/maternal incompatibility to aetiology of pre-eclamptic toxaemia. Lancet ii: 1286–1289
Swapp G H 1975 In: MacGillivray I, Corney G, Nylander P P S (eds) Multiple human reproduction. Saunders, London, p 11
Syrop C H, Varner M W 1985 Triple gestation: maternal and neonatal implications. Acta Geneticae Medicae et Gemellologiae 34: 81–88
Tan T K, Goon S M, Salmon Y, Wee J H 1971 Conjoined twins. Acta Obstetricia et Gynecologica Scandinavica 50: 373–380
Templeton A, Kelman R 1974 Tidal volume in twin pregnancy. In MacGillivray I, Corney G, Nylander P P S (eds) Human multiple reproduction. Saunders, London, p 110
Thompson B, Samphier M, MacGillivray I, Campbell D M, Corney G 1983 Outcome of twin pregnancies in relation to birthweight and zygosity. Fourth Congress of International Society for Twin Studies, London
Tresmontant R, Helvin G, Papiernik E 1983 Cost of care and prevention of preterm births in twin pregnancies. Acta Geneticae Medicae et Gemellologiae 32: 99–103
Uchida I A, Freeman V C P, Gedeon M, Goldmaker J 1983 Twinning rate in spontaneous abortions. American Journal of Human Genetics 35: 987–993
van der Pol J G, Bleker O P, Treffers P E 1982 Clinical bed rest in twin pregnancy. European Journal of Obstetrics and Gynecology 14: 75–80
Ware H D 1971 The second twin. American Journal of Obstetrics and Gynecology 110: 855–873
Weekes A R L, Menzies D N, de Boer C H 1977 The relative efficiency of bed rest, cervical suture and no treatment in the management of twin pregnancy. British Journal of Obstetrics and Gynaecology 84: 161–164

35

D. V. I. Fairweather

Rhesus affect

INTRODUCTION

Rhesus haemolytic disease, like tuberculosis, can now be listed among the diseases which used to be common, indeed lethal, but have now reduced in incidence and in importance as causes of mortality. In less than 30 years after its aetiology was first discovered, remarkable progress has been made not only in its treatment but also in its prevention. By the mid 1970s rhesus isoimmunization was considered as a disappearing phenomenon but the rate of progress in finally eliminating it has been much slower in the last 10 years. Most major obstetric centres in the UK still have referrals of cases of severe rhesus affection requiring specialized management techniques and facilities.

HISTORY TO DISCOVERY OF RHESUS FACTOR

According to Ballantyne (1892), Hippocrates in the year 400 BC described a syndrome which appears to be the first report of hydrops fetalis (massive oedematous swelling of the fetus found at delivery), though Pickles (1949) credits Plater, a famed Renaissance physician, with the first clear-cut account of hydrops fetalis in 1641. Jaundice in newborn infants was certainly described as early as the 17th century. Ballantyne (1892) first brought the disease into prominence by describing the clinical and pathological criteria for the diagnosis of hydrops — oedema, anaemia and enlargement of the liver, spleen and placenta. In addition he noted bilirubin staining of the amniotic fluid. Buchan & Comrie (1909) first noted the relationship between congenital anaemia and jaundice in the newborn. Diamond et al (1932) reported that hydrops fetalis, icterus gravis neonatorum and anicteric anaemia of the newborn were manifestations of the same disease process — erythroblastosis fetalis (although that term recognizing the haemolytic process was first introduced in 1912). Interestingly, they also noted that there were no cases of fetal–maternal incompatibility in the ABO blood group in their patients.

A major breakthrough occurred when Ruth Darrow (1938) concluded that the pathogenesis of erythroblastosis fetalis was based on the formation of a maternal antibody against a component of fetal blood, and in the same year Hellman & Hertig reported the peculiar familial occurrence of erythroblastosis and noted its rarity among first born infants. The stage was now set for the observations revealing the aetiology of this disorder, of which aspects had been so well recognized and documented for so many years.

Levine & Stetson (1939) described an atypical agglutinin in the blood of a woman who had just given birth to a stillborn macerated fetus and who subsequently suffered a transfusion reaction when transfused with apparently compatible blood. They postulated that the maternal immunization was the result of a fetal antigen inherited from the father and lacking in the mother. Then Landsteiner & Wiener (1940) discovered the antigen — which they called the Rh antigen (Rh because the same antigen had been noted in the rhesus monkey) — on red blood cells, revealing the rhesus system. In the following year Levine et al (1941) confirmed that Rh sensitization did cause erythroblastosis and Landsteiner & Wiener (1941) rounded off the story by working out the Mendelian dominant inheritance of the Rh factor.

Table 35.1 Frequency of Rh genes in the population of western Europe and North America

Gene terminology		Approximate frequency	
Fisher–Race	Wiener	(%)	
CDe	R^1	42	95 (CDe + cde + cDE)
cde	r	39	
cDE	R^2	14	
cDe	R^0	2.5	
Cde	r^1	1	
cdE	r^{11}	1	

Table 35.2 Frequency of the commoner genetic constitutions in the white population of western Europe and North America

CDe/cde	33%	(Rh-positive; heterozygous)
CDe/CDe	18%	(Rh-positive; homozygous)
cde/cde	15%	(Rh-negative)
CDe/cDE	12%	(Rh-positive; homozygous
cDE/ced	11%	(Rh-positive; heterozygous)

GENETICS AND MECHANISM OF RHESUS ISOIMMUNIZATION

Although the genetic locus for Rh antigen has been located on the short arm of chromosome 1, there is no consensus as to the number of antigens in the Rh system or to the number of genes controlling their synthesis (Rote 1982). Two possible systems are usually quoted; the first is that of *Fisher–Race* (1946), which assumed that three genes are responsible for the production of Rh antigens: each gene has two major alleles designated c or C; d or D; e or E, located close together on the chromosome and enabling transmission in inheritance as a block of three closely linked genes, e.g. CDe or cde, the antigens being represented by the single letters.

The second model, *Wiener* (1944), assumes that a single gene locus is responsible for the synthesis of Rh antigen and that antigenic variations are controlled by several alleles which may be present at the single locus in a similar fashion to the human leukocyte antigen (HLA) system in man. This model uses an alternative nomenclature (r or R).

Table 35.1 shows (using both terminologies) the approximate frequencies of the genes in the population of western Europe and the USA. It is obvious that three of the complexes are much commoner than the others, accounting for about 95% of all chromosomes in that population. In other populations the frequencies vary greatly, e.g. in Africa cDe has a prevalence of 60%.

Each individual possesses two of these complexes and Table 35.2 shows the approximate frequencies of the commoner genetic constitutions (again for western Europe and the USA—white population).

The D antigen is the most potent and d the weakest (anti-d has never appeared) in stimulating antibody formation; persons possessing the D gene are termed rhesus-positive (DD = homozygous+ or Dd = heterozygous+). When the D is absent from both chromosomes in any individual and its place is occupied by the d allele, the individual is rhesus-negative (dd).

In practice, problems from rhesus isoimmunization arise only where a rhesus-negative mother carries a rhesus-positive fetus. Early understanding of the basic mechanism leading to rhesus affection had indicated that when rhesus-positive fetal red cells enter the maternal circulation, being foreign to the mother (i.e. the rhesus gene was not present in the mother's chromosomes), the first exposure caused sensitization, but that it was not until a further exposure to rhesus-positive cells, giving another antigenic stimulus, that the production of antibodies began. These maternal antibodies to the rhesus-positive cells of the baby then passed back into the fetal circulation, causing destruction of the baby's erythrocytes (erythroblastosis). More than 95% of cases of rhesus incompatibility are due to the D antigen. If, however, both mother and fetus are rhesus-negative there is no problem, even if fetal cells leak into the maternal circulation.

The rhesus status of the fetus depends on the combination of one of the two complexes from the mother (ovum) with one of the two complexes from the father (sperm) at reduction, division and fertilization. Thus for example, shown diagrammatically:

If *father* is Rh-positive heterozygous and *mother* is Rh-negative genotype

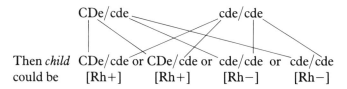

CDe/cde   cde/cde

Then *child* could be: CDe/cde [Rh+] or CDe/cde [Rh+] or cde/cde [Rh−] or cde/cde [Rh−]

i.e. there is a 50–50 chance of a Rh-positive child when the father is heterozygous (Dd).

It can be appreciated similarly that if the father is homozygous (e.g. CDe/CDe) then all the infants produced would be rhesus-positive. The genetic make-up of the father is therefore important in terms of the risk of immunization. Although it is estimated that the chance is 1 in 8 that a rhesus-negative woman will have a partner who is rhesus-positive, it was noted in the past that the number of rhesus-affected births was only about 1/20 of that expected. This can be explained by the effect of various naturally occurring protective factors.

One such factor which determines whether or not the process of immunization is initiated in the mother is the ABO blood group of the mother and of the fetus. Although, as mentioned earlier, Diamond et al (1932) had noted the absence of erythroblastosis if there was incompatibility of fetal–maternal ABO blood groups and Levine (1943) had also noted a negative relationship between ABO incompatibility and Rh sensitization, it was not until much later that Levine (1958) described the protective mechanism invoked against Rh sensitization by nature's destruction of the fetal red cells in the maternal circulation if they were of an incompatible ABO group to that of the mother. As indicated above, immunization of the mother is set in train by the escape of fetal red cells into the maternal circulation. Wiener (1948) first postulated that the starting point for the haemolytic process in the newborn was the occurrence of occult placental haemorrhage, although with another worker (Wiener & Silverman 1940) he had earlier shown the placenta to be permeable to antibodies. Fetal bleeding into the maternal circulation was first shown by Chown (1954) and the first clinically useful laboratory test to demonstrate the presence of fetal red cells which had escaped into the maternal circulation was devised by Kleihauer et al (1957), using the knowledge that fetal haemoglobin, unlike adult haemoglobin, was resistant to elution by acid or alkali. Recently, because it has been realized that some patients may have raised concentrations of haemoglobin F in their own red cells and that these cells may be confused with fetal cells on elution, McWilliams & Davies (1985) described an immunofluorescence technique for the detection of feto-maternal haemorrhage whereby Rh D positive cells in maternal blood fluoresce intensively while Rh D negative cells do not fluoresce. This method is clearly more specific and should be used when the results of the acid elution method are in doubt.

Reference has already been made to variation in the distribution of rhesus gene frequencies between different countries and populations. There are of course also variations in the distribution of ABO blood groups and taken together these factors account for the finding that in some parts of the world, such as the Far East, rhesus disease is relatively uncommon.

Despite continuing study of the human Rh blood group system, it remains a genetic enigma. Its antigen system is second only in complexity to the HLA system. Rh antigen synthesis is probably controlled by 1–3 structural genes and an undetermined number of regulatory genes. The antigen, a protein mosaic, apparently has multiple variable antigenic determinants. The immunological response against Rh antigenic sites is also variable and one-third of the rhesus-negative population are non-responders, failing to elicit a measurable anti-D antibody response. In those sensitized individuals who carry a rhesus-positive fetus, the rhesus disease may vary in severity from mild anaemia or jaundice in the neonatal period (associated with little or no ill effect) to severe hydrops fetalis with death in utero before the 28th week of pregnancy. For certain families, therefore, rhesus diseases was in the past a great tragedy as in the natural course of events 15% of those babies affected were stillborn and 20% of those who were born alive died.

DEVELOPMENTS IN THE ASSESSMENT AND MANAGEMENT OF RHESUS AFFECTION

Perhaps the first step which was to aid the practical management of rhesus disease came when Coombs et al (1945) described a new test (subsequently referred to as the Coombs test) for the detection of weak and incomplete rhesus agglutinins in maternal serum. In the test the strength of immunization was determined by antibody titre level measured by a serial dilution technique. Values were indicated by dilutions (e.g. 1/2: mild; 1/4–1/8 . . . 1/256–1/512: severe) and the level of antibody titre was thought to reflect reasonably accurately the severity of disease in the fetus. Much use was to be made of this approach over the next 20 years; however, the following year, another breakthrough occurred when Wallerstein (1946) described the treatment of severe erythroblastosis by simultaneous removal and replacement of blood of the newborn infant—one of the first reports of the technique which is now known as exchange transfusion. Historically speaking, however, Diamond (1947) deserves credit for the principle of treatment by transfusion of newborn infants suffering from jaundice and anaemia (then called simple transfusion) which he had begun in his unit as early as 1927.

Exchange transfusion, by reducing the blood volume and simultaneously raising the haemoglobin level, overcame heart failure, which was one of the causes of death. By replacing rhesus-positive erythrocytes coated with antibody with rhesus-negative cells unaffected by antibody, haemolysis was reduced to almost normal levels, which meant that anaemia and severe hyperbilirubinaemia—which could lead to kernicterus, another cause of damage or death—rarely developed, as confirmed by Mollison & Walker (1952), reporting the first British controlled trials. Exchange transfusion—repeated if necessary, and sometimes supplemented by further simple transfusion in the weeks after delivery—together with the introduction of routine blood group and antibody testing of the mothers, which allowed antenatal prediction of haemolytic diseases of the newborn (HDN) in about 95% of cases, meant that by the 1950s the neonatal death rate from the affects of Rh disease was reduced to less than one-fifth of the earlier level.

Having reached this point the main effort was directed towards preventing stillbirth. This was a complex problem and when more became known about the significance of high or rising titres of maternal antibody, premature induction of labour became the treatment of choice. Because of the dangers of prematurity it had to be restricted to patients where stillbirth was almost inevitable and delayed as late in pregnancy as was compatible with livebirth. In practice, at that time, this meant not earlier than 35 weeks of gestation, because earlier delivery led to deaths not from rhesus disease but from the effects of prematurity, particularly on the fetal lungs.

Of course it had also been recognized that in selecting

Table 35.3 Relationship between previous obstetric history of HDN and risk of stillbirth if fetus is Rh-positive (Northumberland and Durham 1952–61)

Previous history	Risk of stillbirth (%)	Number of cases studied
No infant previously affected	8	1644
Previously affected infant		
mild	2	205
moderate	18	459
very severe	46	43
1 previous stillbirth	58	132
>1 previous stillbirth	76	59
Total		2542

From Walker et al 1966.

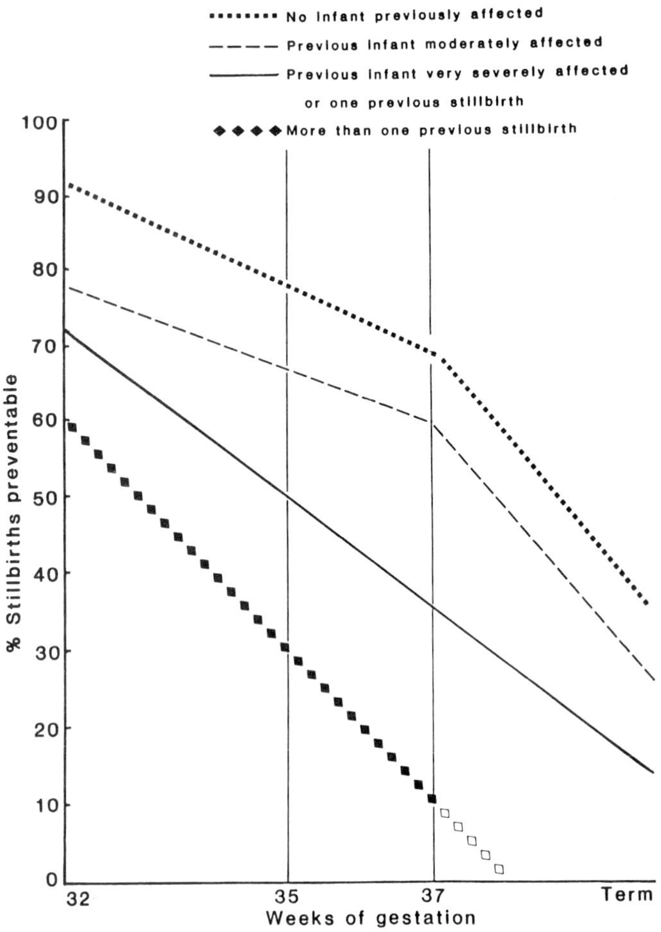

Fig. 35.1 Percentage of stillbirths preventable by induction of labour at varying intervals before term. From Walker et al 1966.

patients who might be at risk of stillbirth for premature induction of labour, the history relative to the severity of disease in previous infants was a helpful guide. Walker et al (1966) quantified this (Table 35.3), indicating that the risk of stillbirth was small (2%) if the previous affected infant was only mildly affected by HDN, but rose to over 50% if previous stillbirth had occurred. Unfortunately, before the previous obstetric history could be usefully applied, a family had to lose or almost lose an infant and once this had occurred the prospect of successful prevention of stillbirth by premature induction in a subsequent pregnancy was significantly reduced (Fig. 35.1).

In patients with a previous history of stillbirth premature induction could prevent at most 50% of stillbirths. While it might have been expected that within a family the stage of gestation when stillbirth occurred in one pregnancy would indicate the probable time of stillbirths in subsequent pregnancies and therefore be useful in deciding the optimal time for premature induction, it was found (Walker et al 1966) that in consecutive pairs of stillbirths the later one occurred at an earlier stage of gestation in 46%; at the same time in 23%, but in a later stage in 31%. In cases where livebirth succeeded stillbirth, 35% were delivered earlier, 24% at the same time and 41% at a later stage of gestation. The time of stillbirth in one pregnancy was therefore not a reliable guide to the optimal time for induction in a later one.

The maternal serum antibody titre was statistically related to the severity of the disease, as demonstrated in Table 35.4, so that with an antibody titre of 1 in 4 or less, the risk of stillbirth was only 2% but it was as high as 45% when the titre was 1 in 512 or higher. However, as shown, all grades of severity occurred at all titres so that the practical application of this relationship to individual cases was not reliable, although it was noted that there was a somewhat better correlation in patients developing antibodies for the first time.

Table 35.4 Antibody titre in relation to severity of HDN (1952–1961) (indirect Coombs technique at 30–36 weeks' gestation)

	Severity of HDN (%)		
Antibody titre	Liveborn	Stillborn	Number (%) of cases
1/1–1/4	98	2	190 (23)
1/8–1/32	94	6	397 (48)
1/64	87	13	92 (11)
1/128	74	26	78 (9)
1/256	66	34	47 (6)
1/512	55	45	31 (3)
Total	89	11	835 (100)

From Walker et al 1966.

A third factor of importance in the identification of patients whose infants were at risk emerged as a result of the observation of Bevis (1952) that in samples of amniotic fluid taken from affected pregnancies at various stages of gestation, the concentration of certain yellow pigments (of iron and bile) offered a reliable guide to the outcome for the fetus in terms of predicting the degree of severity of affection. Soon examination of the amniotic fluid for the presence of bilirubin became an established procedure. However three main concerns limited its usefulness: firstly, that amniocentesis was necessary to obtain the samples and

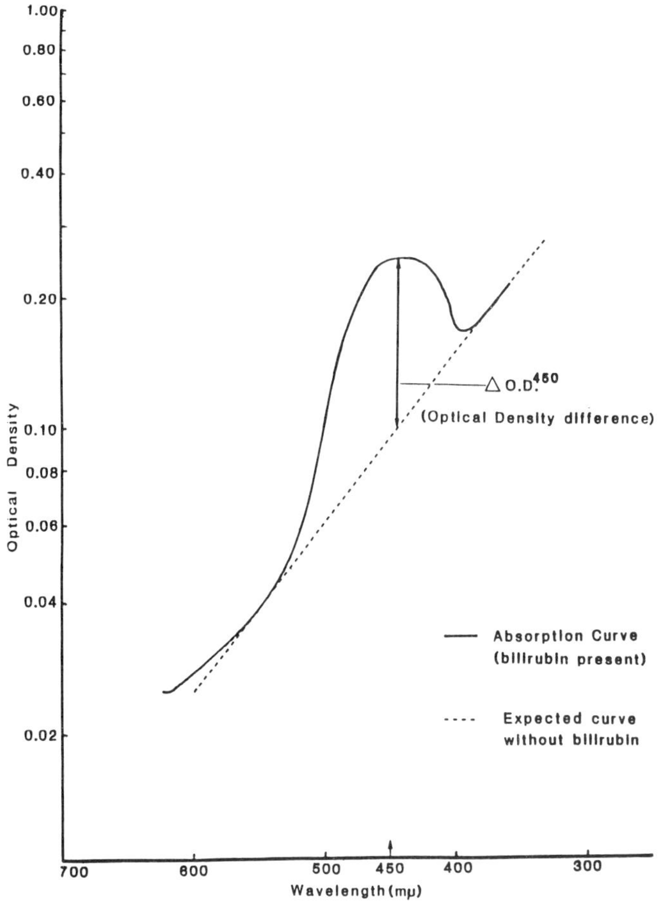

Fig. 35.2 Measurement of optical density difference.

this was potentially dangerous, though Fairweather & Walker (1964) showed the risk of failure or injury to the fetus, including fetal or fetomaternal bleeding, or premature onset of labour etc. was very small. These risks were practically eliminated once ultrasound techniques became available. Secondly, the amount of bile pigment/bilirubin in the amniotic fluid depended not only on severity of the disease but also the stage of gestation, tending to fall in parallel with the protein level as term approached (Walker & Jennison 1962). Thirdly, the quantitative measurement of bilirubin presented difficulties.

Chemical methods had proved unsatisfactory, so most workers elected to be guided by measuring the absorption band at 450 μm, using spectrophotometry to calculate the difference between the absorption measured in the sample and an arbitary line omitting absorption due to pigmentation, expressed as optical density difference (ΔOD450, Liley 1961, 1963b, Fig. 35.2).

By a combination of the three methods of prediction (history, antibody titre and liquor pigmentation), in the early 1960s we were able to reduce the number of stillbirths and neonatal deaths due to rhesus disease with a combination of premature induction and exchange transfusion. Even given a perfect method of selecting patients so that the optimal time for interference could be determined, it proved only a partial solution to the problem because 50% of stillbirths occurred before 35 weeks and 30% before 32 weeks' gestation; when some workers tried induction of labour before 32 weeks in very bad history cases, although preventing stillbirth they often provoked neonatal deaths not from the treatable rhesus problem but from the effects of prematurity.

It was another milestone when Liley (1963a) described the technique of intrauterine transfusion whereby rhesus-negative donor cells were injected into the fetal peritoneal cavity early in pregnancy and absorbed into the fetal circulation, countering the anaemia which is a constant feature of severe HDN and offering the possibility that intrauterine life could be prolonged to a stage where premature induction could be more safely and successfully employed. This technique was clearly reserved for those patients whose babies were severely affected very early in the pregnancy and, because of the technical difficulties, it was and still is performed only in a limited number of centres throughout the country by teams of doctors specially trained and interested in the problem.

INTRAUTERINE TRANSFUSION AND ITS FURTHER DEVELOPMENT

When Liley (1963a) first described his technique at 32 and 33 weeks' gestation, the placenta was localized by injection of radiopaque dye into the amniotic cavity (amniography). The fetus swallowed some of the dye with the amniotic fluid and so outlined some of the fetal bowel, enabling the target area (the fetal peritoneal cavity) to be visualized so that under local anaesthesia an 8 cm 16 gauge Touhy needle could be passed into the amniotic cavity and thence through the fetal abdominal wall. When the needle was thought to be in the fetal peritoneal cavity — free injection of saline was used to check the position — a fine polythene catheter was then fed through the Touhy needle and the needle was withdrawn. Group O Rh-negative blood (100 ml) was then injected over a 20-minute period. Ten days later a second transfusion was given and then a further week later the infant was delivered by Caesarean section. Obviously the transfusion needle had to avoid vital fetal structures (e.g. heart, liver) but radiography could not provide a detailed cross-sectional image of the fetal abdomen and so needle placement was difficult and sometimes failed or injuries were caused. In addition radiation exposure to the fetus could be significant, particularly as many fetuses required more than one transfusion. Because of those concerns Hobbins et al (1976) suggested the use of ultrasound; in subsequent years the techniques have been further improved and refined as more sophisticated ultrasound machines (real-time sector scanners) allowed accurate visualization of the needle tip during fetal intraperitoneal placement.

Shortly after Liley (1963a) suggested intraperitoneal fetal transfusion, Freda & Adamsons (1964) reported the technique of intrauterine intravascular fetal blood transfusion using hysterotomy to gain access to the fetal femoral artery. Others also tried similar approaches but soon abandoned this route because of high fetal mortality, mainly due to preterm delivery. More recently, it has been possible to locate the umbilical cord of the fetus accurately using ultrasound and to place needles or catheters into the fetal abdomen under ultrasound (Berkowitz & Hobbins 1981) or into umbilical vessels by fetoscopy (Rodeck et al 1981) control. Intravascular (as oppposed to intraperitoneal) transfusion of the fetus was again advocated (Rodeck et al 1984), the claim being that it allowed earlier transfusion if necessary in severely affected cases.

Nicolaides et al (1986a), reporting their results of 96 intravascular fetal blood transfusions, confirmed the successful use of repeated rapid transfusions of large volumes of blood by percutaneous cordocentesis under ultrasound control in the management of fetal anaemia from 18 to 36 weeks' gestation. Mackenzie et al (1987) also suggested that the results of these in utero intravascular transfusions were better if ultrasound rather than fetoscopic guidance is used for the percutaneous needle placement.

These intravascular procedures can undoubtedly be associated with technical problems and Berkowitz et al (1987) have advised that unless severe hydrops is present, an intraperitoneal transfusion should always be strongly considered as an alternative to performing an intravascular transfusion which seems as if it will be unusually difficult. At present therefore both intraperitoneal and intravascular transfusion techniques should still be available in the specialized centres dealing with reducing numbers of these problem cases.

Over the years many schemes (the majority based on that described by Liley in 1963) have been developed for plotting ΔOD450 values of the liquor bilirubin against the weeks of gestation in order to determine the need for intrauterine transfusion or premature delivery. Each centre or laboratory nowadays tends to have its own version of a prediction chart based on local experience. As shown in Figure 35.3, three zones are usually delineated and the cases where intrauterine transfusion should be considered are those with values in or approaching the upper zone before 32 weeks of gestation.

The decision on when to perform the first intrauterine transfusion depends primarily on the liquor bilirubin levels, though again the advent of ultrasound has enabled visualization of the fetus so that other factors may be assessed, such as fetal or placental oedema, presence of fetal ascites and more recently fetal liver enlargement (Vintzileos et al 1986), which may also indicate increasing severity of affection. Once an intrauterine transfusion has been performed, repeat transfusions should be carried out until preterm delivery is reasonable. Various schedules have been devised: most advocate the second tranfusion 7–14 days after the first and subsequent transfusions at intervals of around 2 weeks.

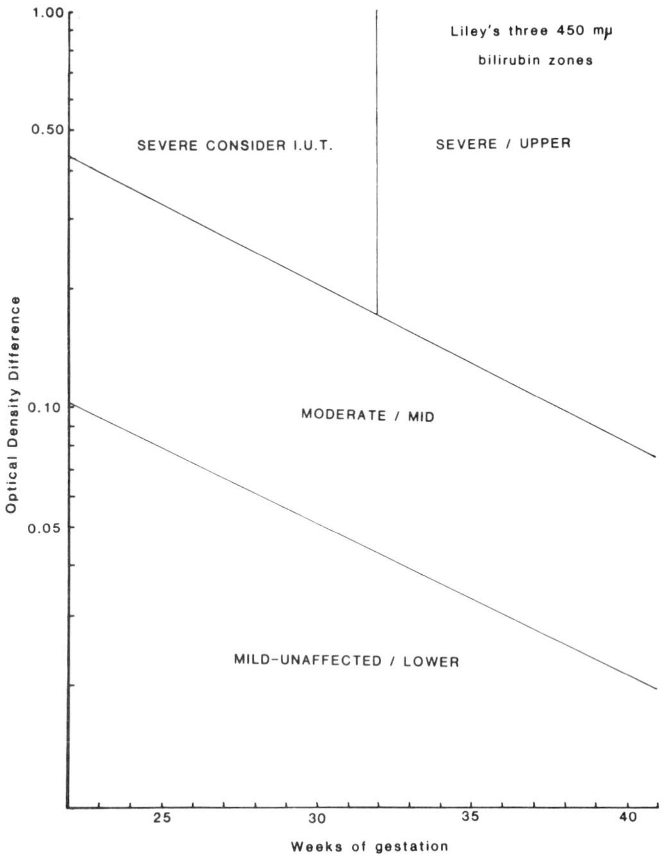

Fig. 35.3 Specimen prediction chart indicating Liley's zones and expected severity of disease based on liquor analysis.

The amount of blood transfused varies depending on the stage of gestation, roughly following a formula: (number of weeks of gestation) $-$ 20 $\times$ 10 ml (Bowman 1975). Most authors advise removing ascitic fluid if it is present before commencing intraperitoneal transfusion, in order to avoid excessive intra-abdominal pressure which could cause fetal death. Transfusion is done at a rate of around 5 ml/min and monitoring fetal heart rate throughout is advisable. Fresh group O Rh negative, leukocyte-poor red cells, packed to a haematocrit of about 80% and maternally cross-matched, are used. The decision when to deliver the infant depends on the intensive neonatal support care available and the survival rates achieved by the particular centre. Many elect to deliver (rather than continue intrauterine transfusions) after 32 weeks' gestation when a greater than 95% neonatal survival rate might be expected.

Survival rates in initial published series (Fairweather et al 1967) averaged 50%, though they were dependent upon the time at which initial transfusion was instituted (before 30 weeks, survival averaged only 25%) and accordingly the number of repeat transfusions required. Recent survival rates quoted, however, range from 70 to 75% (Larkin et al 1982) for specialized referral centres and obviously also depend on the severity of fetal involvement and the experience of the operators, together with the use of small gauge needles and more accurate placement techniques.

Intrauterine transfusion poses little risk to the mother. Infection can be avoided by aseptic technique and some also advocate prophylactic antibiotics. Other problems reported include premature labour, premature rupture of the membranes and abruptio placentae. The fetal risks are usually secondary to trauma and malplacement of the transfusion needle.

Follow-up studies on the quality of life of surviving infants have continued to be encouraging and in controlled studies the only significant difference in intrauterine transfusion survivors was an increased risk of inguinal and umbilical hernias. Intellectual and behavioural development was normal (Stewart et al 1978).

PREVENTION: DEVELOPMENT OF ANTI-D IMMUNOGLOBULIN PROPHYLAXIS PROGRAMMES

As already noted, Levine (1958) first suggested that ABO incompatibility was protective against erythroblastosis but Finn (1960) made the first reference, suggesting that it might be possible to destroy any fetal red cells found in the maternal circulation following delivery by means of a suitable antibody. With his Liverpool colleagues (Finn et al 1961) he and other workers in the USA went on to elaborate experimental studies in male and postmenopausal female volunteers which laid the foundation for the first multicentre controlled clinical trial (British Medical Journal 1966) of prevention of Rh haemolytic disease in primigravidae using high-titre anti-D gamma globulin administered by intramuscular injection within 36 hours of delivery. By 1967 it was clear that suppression of Rh immunization by the post-delivery administration of anti-D was successful; throughout the world prophylaxis programmes were introduced, resulting in a marked reduction in the incidence of Rh immunization as a pregnancy complication. However, new cases still occurred, either because the need for prophylaxis was overlooked after delivery, or because the prophylaxis failed to prevent sensitization. In those latter cases, however, subsequent Rh D positive infants are seldom severely affected.

Postpartum prophylaxis was instituted because larger numbers of fetal cells were found in the maternal circulation immediately following delivery as a result of transplacental haemorrhage during the third stage. However, earlier studies by Zipursky et al (1963) showed that fetal erythrocytes are often found in the blood of pregnant women and on this basis Zipursky & Israels (1967) argued that in order to make prophylaxis programmes more efficient antepartum administration of anti-D should be instituted. In Canada and other countries antenatal prophylaxis programmes were introduced; anti-D was administered once or twice during the third trimester to avoid antenatal sensitization. It was also recognized that sensitization caused by feto-maternal bleeding precipitated by other obstetric occurrences, such as termination of pregnancy, amniocentesis, mid-trimester fetal blood sampling etc., could be prevented by antenatal administration of anti-D at the time of such occurrences.

The preferred dose of anti-D has varied in different countries and different situations (100–300 μg postpartum, 50–100 μg antenatally), depending on the estimated volume of the feto-maternal bleed.

RATIONALE FOR CURRENT PROPHYLAXIS PROGRAMMES IN THE UK

Postnatal prophylaxis

As indicated above, the value of postnatal prophylaxis has been accepted for many years. If the mother has no anti-D antibody at booking she is usually re-tested at 28 weeks and 32–36 weeks, and again at delivery. After delivery the blood group of the baby is tested and if Rh D positive, the mother is given anti-D immunoglobulin. The number of fetal cells in the maternal circulation is also ascertained by the Kleihauer test to indicate the severity of any feto-maternal transfusion, so that the appropriate dose of anti-D may be given (20 μg anti-D neutralizes 1 ml fetal red blood cells; Urbaniak 1985). In fact, fetal transplacental haemorrhage exceeding 15 ml of fetal cells is rare — less than 0.3% — (Bowman 1985) and although routine American practice has been to use 300 μg doses of anti-D, UK practice of using 100 μg doses for postnatal prophylaxis has provided comparable protection rates. It is, however, always advisable to check the Kleihauer result so that if there is evidence of a greater than average fetomaternal bleed (e.g. as in obstetric complications such as placental abruption, manual removal of placenta or fulminating pre-eclampsia) the dose can be increased. Although the prophylactic injection should be given as soon as possible after delivery, administration up to 72 hours or even longer after delivery is worthwhile.

Prophylaxis following abortion or antenatal procedures

Significant fetomaternal transfusion may occur antenatally during procedures such as amniocentesis or external cephalic version and after threatened or other types of abortion, or termination of pregnancy. It is also recognized in association with antepartum haemorrhage. Prophylaxis (50 μg standard dose — 100 μg or more if indicated by Kleihauer test) should be given at the time and repeated at 6-weekly intervals in the case of antepartum haemorrhage if intermittent bleeding continues. Some authorities also advise anti-D administration following ectopic pregnancy.

Antenatal prophylaxis

Some Rh D negative women develop anti-D antibodies during their first Rh D positive pregnancy well before delivery and the possibility of routine postnatal prophylaxis. Clarke et al (1985) found in England and Wales that the current prophylaxis programme still failed to prevent some 600–700 Rh D negative women being immunized. They identified three main reasons for failure:

1. failure to give anti-D when indicated;
2. failure of protection by the passive anti-D immunoglobulin;
3. intrapartum immunization.

Failures because of point 1 above can be reduced by increasing general awareness to the problem. Those due to point 2 may be lessened by better assessment of the necessary anti-D dose in relation to the size of bleed, but those due to point 3 result from occult transplacental haemorrhage, particularly in the third trimester, and it is for this group that antenatal prophylaxis is relevant.

Although in the UK there had previously been resistance to the introduction of routine antenatal prophylaxis programmes because they were thought not to be cost-effective, the statement by Clarke et al (1985) that: 'clearly the virtual elimination of rhesus haemolytic disease can be achieved only by giving anti Rh immunoglobulin antenatally as well as postnatally' has led to the new advice as stated in Drug and Therapeutics Bulletin (1985) being adopted for a limited progamme of antenatal prophylaxis.

It has now been recognized that those Rh D negative women who develop antibodies during their first Rh positive pregnancy are particularly liable to have subsequent babies with severe Rh disease. Such antenatal sensitization can be avoided by giving anti-D at 28 and 34 or 36 weeks. Trials have shown that this is more effective — approaching 100% in preventing sensitization than post-partum prophylaxis alone (Drug and Therapeutics Bulletin 1985).

Accordingly in the UK it is now advised that this regime, using 100 μg doses, is offered to all Rh D negative mothers except those who already have antibodies who have no living children. This antenatal prophylaxis has also been shown to be more than twice as cost-effective in treating primiparae than multiparae. The need for postnatal (within 72 hours) prophylactic administration of anti-D still exists in those patients who receive antenatal anti-D injections. Unwanted side-effects with anti-D immunoglobulin are rare and mild, usually confined to redness around the injection site and mild allergic reactions.

Finally it must be remembered that anti-D protection is temporary and must be repeated with every pregnancy.

Footnote on the mechanism of anti-D protection

It is of interest to note that although prophylaxis programmes have reduced the numbers of women with anti-D in their sera (Tovey 1986), there has been no effect on the incidence of other blood group antibodies (those most likely to cause clinical problems are anti-c, anti-E and anti-Kell). If, as alleged, anti-D immunoglobulin acts in a non-specific way simply by removing fetal cells (Woodrow et al 1975), the introduction of anti-D should have caused reduction in the incidence of other antibodies as well as anti-D in Rh negative women. In Tovey's series this was not the case, suggesting that the protection may occur in the more specific way suggested by Pollack et al (1982) of antibody-mediated immune suppression.

Plasmapheresis in pregnancy for the management of rhesus isoimmunization

Attempts were made (Carter 1959) to absorb antibodies already in the maternal circulation using *Rh hapten* but proved unsuccessful. Thereafter attempts at the removal of maternal antibodies by plasmapheresis were instituted, as reported by Powell (1968). Over the last decade intense maternal plasmapheresis has been utilized by several investigators in an attempt to decrease the severity of erythroblastosis fetalis (Fraser et al 1976, Rock 1981, Robinson 1984, Knott 1987). Although there is often a transient decrease in the amount of circulating anti-Rh D after treatment, this is often followed by a rebound increase in antibody production. There is controversy about whether fetal survival or transfusion rate is improved with this technique and the outcome of pregnancy does not appear to be significantly affected.

The cost of treatment is high and plasmapheresis is very time-consuming, involving either small-volume (500 ml) or large-volume (2000 ml) exchanges at least weekly or sometimes twice weekly, depending upon initial titre. Usually anti-D levels of 4 iu/l are used as the critical level to commence plasmapheresis. It appears that this form of treatment even in combination with other methods of therapy is of doubtful value.

SUGGESTED ROUTINE INVESTIGATION FOR RHESUS-NEGATIVE MOTHER AT BOOKING

Where the mother is known to be rhesus-negative or has a previous history of rhesus-affected infants, reference to a consultant obstetrician by 12 weeks is advised.

1. Ascertain previous history in relation to rhesus-affected infants. Cross-check patient's history from relevant hospital maternity and neonatal records to clarify management adopted in previous pregnancy, investigations, treatment, complications, method of and gestation at delivery, outcome for infant — including cord Hb and bilirubin levels at birth, rhesus and blood group status, treatment given and current health
2. Check rhesus and blood group of mother.

3. Check for presence of/titre of antibodies in maternal serum.
4. If antibodies are present request blood check on partner to determine his ABO and Rh status. If rhesus-positive, determine genotype and zygosity.
5. Enquire whether mother is given anti-D injection antenatally and/or postnatally in previous pregnancies.

MANAGEMENT ROUTINE DEPENDING UPON PREVIOUS RHESUS HISTORY

This is determined by category of worst affected previous infant fathered by current partner.

1. *Where the previous infant is only mildly affected* (Rh+ Coombs+ — no treatment required). No special investigative measures are required as risk of the infant being severely affected before term is unusual (2%). Await spontaneous delivery at term. Facilities should be available for exchange transfusion of the neonate if necessary.
2. *Where there is no previously affected infant*, i.e. antibodies are detected for first time in current pregnancy. Antibody titre testing should be performed on rhesus-negative mothers at the time of booking and again at 28–32 weeks' gestation.
   2.1. *If antibody titre is less than 1/16* at 32 weeks, no other investigative measures are required. Manage as for (1) above.
   2.2. *If repeat antibody titre is 1/16 or higher* (this will identify the 8% at risk of stillbirth), recommend amniocentesis at 32 weeks, then depending upon ΔOD450 (bilirubin level):
      a. If no or minimal pigmentation, i.e. lower zone, await spontaneous delivery at term. Facilities should be available for exchange transfusion of the neonate if necessary.
      b. If mid-zone pigmentation level repeat amniocentesis in 10–14 days.
         i. If repeat amniocentesis shows pigmentation level has risen to upper zone advise induction of labour forthwith.
         ii. If pigmentation level remains in mid zone consider induction of labour around 37–38 weeks. Decide time for induction by cross-reference with other methods for determining intrauterine fetal status—fetal movements, ultrasound appearances, cardiotocography, etc.
      c. If upper zone pigmentation level, repeat amniocentesis in 7–10 days. If still in upper zone advise induction of labour forthwith.

      If repeat amniocentesis shows level has fallen to mid zone proceed as in (b) above.

   Patients in categories (b) and (c) above should be managed in regional centres where specialized obstetric and neonatal facilities are available.
3. *Where previous stillbirth was due to rhesus disease or previous infant was very severely affected* (cord haemoglobin <9 g/100 ml or cord bilirubin >7 mg/100 ml): in this category of patient amniocentesis should be commenced around 20 weeks' gestation and management will depend upon the changes in bilirubin level of the liquor samples.

   Amniocentesis should be repeated within 7–10 days if the level is in the upper zone, otherwise in 14 days. If consecutive samples show worsening of the haemolytic process (increased bilirubin levels) with levels in the upper zone before 32 weeks' gestation, intrauterine transfusion should be advised. If severe affection is predicted from 18–24 weeks, consideration might be given to use of intravascular transfusion (via fetoscopy or directly under ultrasound control), otherwise the intraperitoneal route should be chosen. If expertise is available, fetal intravascular transfusion can be done by cordocentesis under ultrasound control. Careful ultrasound assessment of the fetus to detect the presence of ascites and oedema is also necessary in order to monitor the progress of treatment. If ascites is present, the fluid should be removed before the intraperitoneal transfusion is given.

   It is likely that repeat transfusions will be required about every 2 weeks until delivery can be contemplated. Interpretation of liquor bilirubin levels post intrauterine transfusion is difficult, due to contamination with leakage of blood from the transfusion. The timing of delivery will depend upon the response to treatment, the stage of gestation and the neonatal intensive care facilities available. A balance will have to be struck between the risks of further intrauterine transfusion and those of prematurity. The decision should be made jointly by obstetrician and neonatologist and of course delivery should take place in the regional centre where the experienced team is based.

   The method of delivery chosen will reflect other obstetric considerations, such as the presentation, the state of cervix, the maternal condition and the previous obstetric history as well as the severity of the fetal disease and the stage of gestation. If straightforward labour and delivery are thought unlikely to follow induction of labour, preference for elective Caesarean section will be understandable, particularly if delivery is to be undertaken before 34 weeks or if the presentation is other than cephalic.
4. *Where previous infant was moderately affected:* amniocentesis need not be commenced before 28 weeks' gestation. Repeat amniocentesis will again be required every 10–14 days depending on the liquor bilirubin level and the prediction chart zone. Where levels are or remain in the mid or lower zones, management should be as considered in 2.2 above. If levels enter or remain in the upper zone before 32 weeks' gestation, intrauterine transfusion

should be advised and further management organized as in 3.

NEWER METHODS OF RECOGNITION AND ASSESSMENT OF SEVERITY OF RHESUS DISEASE

Whilst measurement of amniotic fluid ΔOD450 has been and still is the common method used for the assessment of severity of rhesus disease in the fetus, Liley's (1963b) approach was designed for application after 28 weeks. The advent in recent years of safer techniques for fetal intraperitoneal or intravascular transfusion has encouraged obstetric intervention much earlier in pregnancy and the validity of extrapolating the Liley graph backwards to the middle of the second trimester of pregnancy has led to re-examination of the predictive value of the ΔOD450. Nicolaides et al (1986b) found that the severity of fetal anaemia could not be predicted accurately in second-trimester pregnancies by the trend in ΔOD450 and suggested that the only reliable method was by direct measurement of fetal haemoglobin.

Mackenzie et al (1987), also noting that amniotic fluid ΔOD450 values do not always correlate with the severity of disease and that there have been doubts about the critical level of maternal anti-D which should be taken as a threshold for advising intrauterine transfusions, drew attention to the importance of using the fetal haematocrit as the main indicator of erythropoietic compensation so that premature initiation of intrauterine transfusion therapy may be avoided. Nicolaides et al (1987) have also drawn attention to the value of measurement of fetoplacental blood volume to enable better calculation of the volume of donor blood for fetal transfusion and prediction of the post-transfusion haematocrit value.

The increasing availability of chorionic villus sampling now widely used for the diagnosis of genetic disorders in the first trimester has led to this technique being applied in the first trimester for fetal blood group determination and the management of severe immunization (Kanhai et al 1987). This work so far has demonstrated the feasibility of this approach but there are clearly many problems still to be addressed (Fuhrman et al 1987). At present chorionic villus sampling for fetal blood group typing must be reserved for a highly selected group of patients, who will require detailed follow-up.

CONCLUSIONS

The prevention and virtual elimination of Rh haemolytic disease will only be achieved by giving anti-Rh immunoglobulin antenatally as well as postnatally.

It has still not proved possible to eliminate antibodies successfully from the maternal circulation once Rh isoimmunization has occurred, though efforts using this approach still continue (plasmapheresis, drug therapies etc.) and it is hoped that when this has been achieved Rh haemolytic disease can be eradicated.

In the meantime, better surveillance of the immunized mother during pregnancy should allow early prediction of the severity of disease in at-risk pregnancies. Thereafter, premature induction of labour, if necessary combined with intrauterine fetal transfusion to combat fetal anaemia and enable pregnancy to be maintained until the fetus is mature enough to survive, followed by exchange transfusion if indicated, have significantly improved the outcome for affected pregnancies and reduced fetal and neonatal mortality to minimal levels. Improved management of very low birthweight infants in neonatal intensive care units has also enhanced survival figures.

REFERENCES

Ballantyne J W 1892 General dropsy of the foetus. In: The diseases and deformities of the foetus, vol. I. Oliver and Boyd, Edinburgh
Berkowitz R L, Hobbins J C 1981 Intrauterine transfusion using ultrasound. Obstetrics and Gynecology 57: 33
Berkowitz R L, Chitkara U, Wilkins I, Lynch L, Mehalek M 1987 Technical aspects of intravascular intrauterine transfusions: lessons learned from 33 procedures. American Journal of Obstetrics and Gynecology 157: 4–9
Bevis D C A 1952 The antenatal prediction of haemolytic disease of the newborn. Lancet i: 395
Bowman J M 1975 Rh erythroblastosis. Seminars in Hematology 12: 189
Bowman J M 1985 Controversies in Rh prophylaxis. Who needs Rh immune globulin and when should it be given? American Journal of Obstetrics and Gynecology 151: 289–294
British Medical Journal 1966 Prevention of Rh haemolytic disease: results of the clinical trial. A combined study from centres in England and Baltimore. British Medical Journal 2: 907
Buchan A H, Comrie J D 1909 Four cases of congenital anaemia with jaundice and enlargement of the spleen. Journal of Pathology and Bacteriology 13: 398
Carter B B 1959 A survey of the Rh hapten. Texas Report on Biology and Medicine 17: 175
Chown B 1954 Anaemia from bleeding of the fetus into mother's circulation. Lancet i: 1213
Clarke C A, Mollison P L, Whitfield A G W 1985 Deaths from rhesus haemolytic disease in England and Wales in 1982 and 1983. British Medical Journal 291: 17–19
Coombs R R A, Mourant A E, Race R R 1945 Rh factor: detection of weak 'incomplete' Rh agglutinins: new test. Lancet ii: 15
Darrow R R 1938 Icterus gravis (erythroblastosis) neonatorum: examination of aetiologic considerations. Archives of Pathology 25: 378
Diamond L K 1947 Erythroblastosis foetalis or haemolytic disease of the newborn. Proceedings of the Royal Society of Medicine 40: 546
Diamond L K, Blackfan K D, Baty J M 1932 Erythroblastosis fetalis and its association with universal oedema of fetus, icterus gravis neonatorum and anaemia of the newborn. Journal of Pediatrics 1: 269
Drug and Therapeutics Bulletin 1985 Anti D immunoglobulin prophylaxis—are we doing enough? 23: 93
Fairweather D V I, Walker W 1964 Obstetrical considerations in the routine use of amniocentesis in immunised Rh negative women. Journal of Obstetrics and Gynaecology of the British Commonwealth 71: 48
Fairweather D V I, Tacchi D, Coxon A, Hughes M I, Murray S, Walker W 1967 Intrauterine transfusion in Rh-isoimmunization. British Medical Journal 4: 189
Finn R 1960 Erythroblastosis. Lancet i: 536
Finn R, Clarke C A, Donohoe W T A et al 1961 Experimental studies on the prevention of Rh haemolytic disease. British Medical Journal 1: 1486

Fisher R A, Race R R 1946 Rh gene frequencies in Britain. Nature 157: 48–49
Fraser I D, Bennett M O, Bothamley J E et al 1976 Intensive antenatal plasmapheresis in severe rhesus isoimmunisation. Lancet i: 6
Freda V J, Adamsons K 1964 Exchange transfusion in utero. American Journal of Obstetrics and Gynecology 89: 817–821
Furhman H C, Klink F, Grzejszczyk G et al 1987 First trimester diagnosis of $Rh_O(D)$ with an immunofluorescence technique after chorionic villus sampling. Prenatal Diagnosis 7: 17–21
Hellman L M, Hertig A T 1938 Pathological changes in the placenta associated with erythroblastosis of the fetus. American Journal of Pathology 14: 111
Hobbins J C, Davis C D, Webster J 1976 A new technique utilising ultrasound to aid intrauterine transfusion. Journal of Clinical Ultrasound 4: 135
Kanhai H H, Gravenhorst J B, Gemke R J, Overbeeke M A, Bernini L F, Beverstock G C 1987 Fetal blood group determination in first-trimester pregnancy for the management of severe immunization. American Journal of Obstetrics and Gynecology 156: 120–123
Kleihauer E, Braun H, Betke K 1957 Demonstration von fetaleim Haemoglobin in den Erythrocyten eines Blutansstrichs. Klinische Wisschenschaft 35: 637
Knott P D 1987 Plasmapheresis in pregnancy for the management of rhesus isoimmunisation. Journal of Obstetrics and Gynaecology 8: 6–8
Landsteiner K, Wiener A S 1940 An agglutinable factor in human blood recognised by immune sera for rhesus blood. Proceedings of the Society for Experimental Biology and Medicine 43: 223
Landsteiner K, Wiener A S 1941 Studies on an agglutinogen (Rh) in human blood reacting with anti-rhesus sera and with human iso-antibodies. Journal of Experimental Medicine 74: 309
Larkin R M, Knochel J Q, Lee T G 1982 Intrauterine transfusions: new techniques and results. Clinical Obstetrics and Gynecology 25: 303
Levine P 1943 The pathogenesis of erythroblastosis fetalis. Journal of Pediatrics 23: 656
Levine P 1958 The influence of the ABO system on Rh haemolytic disease. Human Biology 30: 14
Levine P, Stetson R E 1939 Unusual cases of intra group agglutination. Journal of the American Medical Association 113: 126
Levine P, Katzin E M, Burnham L 1941 Isoimmunisation in pregnancy: its bearing on the aetiology of erythroblastosis fetalis. Journal of the American Medical Association 116: 825
Liley A W 1961 Liquor amnii analysis in the management of the pregnancy complicated by rhesus sensitisation. American Journal of Obstetrics and Gynecology 82: 1359
Liley A W 1963a Intrauterine transfusion of foetus in haemolytic disease. British Medical Journal 2: 1107
Liley A W 1963b Errors in the assessment of hemolytic disease from amniotic fluid. American Journal of Obstetrics and Gynecology 86: 485
Mackenzie I Z, Bowell P J, Ferguson J, Castle B M, Entwistle C C 1987 In utero intravascular transfusion of the fetus for the management of severe rhesus isoimmunisation — a reappraisal. British Journal of Obstetrics and Gynaecology 94: 1068–1073
McWilliam A C, Davies S C 1985 Detection of fetomaternal haemorrhage by an immunofluorescence technique. Journal of Clinical Pathology 38: 919–921
Mollison P, Walker W 1952 Controlled trials of the treatment of haemolytic disease of the newborn. Lancet i: 429
Nicolaides K H, Soothill P W, Clewell W, Rodeck C H 1986a Rh disease: intravascular fetal blood transfusion by cordocentesis. Fetal Therapy 1: 185–192
Nicolaides K H, Rodeck C H, Mibashan R S, Kemp J R 1986b Have Liley charts outlived their usefulness? American Journal of Obstetrics and Gynecology 155: 90–94
Nicolaides K H, Clewell W H, Rodeck C H 1987 Measurement of human fetoplacental blood volume in erythroblastosis fetalis. American Journal of Obstetrics and Gynecology 157: 50–53
Pickles M M 1949 In: Haemolytic disease of the newborn. Blackwell, Oxford
Pollack W, Gorman J G, Freda V J 1982 Rh immune suppression, past present and future. In: Frigoletto F D Jr, Jewett J F, Konugres A A (eds) Rh hemolytic disease, new strategy for eradication. G K Hall Medical Publishers, Boston, pp 9–70
Powell L C 1968 Intensive plasmapheresis in the pregnant Rh-sensitised woman. American Journal of Obstetrics and Gynecology 101: 153
Robinson E A E 1984 Principles and practice of plasma exchange in the management of Rh haemolytic disease of the newborn. Plasma Therapy and Transfusion Technology 5: 7–14
Rock G A 1981 Plasma exchange in the treatment of rhesus haemolytic disease: review. Plasma Therapy 2: 211
Rodeck C H, Holman C A, Karnicki J, Kemp J R, Whitmore D N, Austin M A 1981 Direct intravascular fetal blood transfusion by fetoscopy in severe rhesus isoimmunisation. Lancet i: 625
Rodeck C H, Nicolaides K H, Warsof S L, Fysh W J, Gamsu H R, Kemp J R 1984 The management of severe rhesus isoimmunisation by fetoscopic intravascular transfusion. American Journal of Obstetrics and Gynecology 150: 769–774
Rote N S 1982 Pathophysiology of Rh isoimmunisation. Clinical Obstetrics and Gynecology 25: 245
Stewart A, Turcan D, Rawlings G, Hart S, Gregory S 1978 Outcome for infants at high risk of major handicap. In: Elliot K, O'Connor M (eds) Major mental handicap — methods and costs of prevention. Elsevier, Amsterdam, pp 151–164
Tovey L A D 1986 Haemolytic disease of the newborn — the changing scene. British Journal of Obstetrics and Gynaecology 93: 960–966
Urbaniak S J 1985 Rh (D) haematolytic disease of the newborn: the changing scene. British Medical Journal 291: 4–6
Vintzileos A M, Campbell W A, Storlazzi E, Mirochnick M H, Escoto D T, Nochimson D J 1986 Fetal liver ultrasound measurements in isoimmunized pregnancies. Obstetrics and Gynecology 68: 162–167
Walker W 1960 Factors influencing the role of premature induction in the prevention of hydrops foetalis. Proceedings of the 7th Congress of the European Society for Haematology, London, part II: 1189
Walker A H C, Jennison R F 1962 Antenatal prediction of haemolytic disease of newborn. Comparison of liquor amnii and serological studies. British Medical Journal 2: 1152
Walker W, Murray S, Fairweather D V I 1966 Haemolytic disease of the newborn at the crossroads. Newcastle Medical Journal 29: 142
Wallerstein H 1946 Treatment of severe erythroblastosis by simultaneous removal and replacement of blood of newborn infant. Science 103: 583
Wiener A S 1944 The Rh series of allelic genes. Science 100: 595
Wiener A S 1948 Diagnosis and treatment of anaemia of the newborn caused by occult placental haemorrhage. American Journal of Obstetrics and Gynecology 56: 717
Wiener A S, Silverman I J 1940 Permeability of the human placenta antibodies. Journal of Experimental Medicine 71: 21
Woodrow J C, Clarke C A, Donohue W T A 1975 Mechanism of Rh prophylaxis: an expanded study on specificity of immunosuppression. British Medical Journal 2: 57–59
Zipursky A, Israels L G 1967 The pathogenesis and prevention of Rh immunisation. Canadian Medical Association Journal 97: 1245
Zipursky A, Polock J. Neelands P, Chown B, Israels L G 1963 The transplacental passage of fetal red blood cells and the pathogenesis of Rh immunisation during pregnancy. Lancet ii: 489

36

C. W. G. Redman

Hypertension in pregnancy

The arterial pressure of pregnant women would be of little or no interest to obstetricians were it not for the conditions of pre-eclampsia and eclampsia. These specific disorders of pregnancy are common, dangerous and poorly understood. Hypertension is one of the signs by which they are recognized and for that reason has become a focus of obstetric interest and research. In this chapter, pre-eclampsia and its sequelae will be described. Other hypertensive conditions will also be mentioned. They can predispose to, or mimic, pre-eclampsia but otherwise, conceptually, should be considered a completely separate topic.

TERMINOLOGY

Hypertension

The concept of hypertension is convenient, but imprecise and usually invested with a spurious significance. An arbitrary threshold is used to divide normotensive from hypertensive individuals, although there is no intrinsic difference between people whose pressures are just below or just above a cut-off reading. To label some as hypertensive is to say no more than that their blood pressures are in an upper centile range; they may be unusual but they are not necessarily abnormal.

Even if there is evidence that a particularly high blood pressure is abnormal, hypertension is a sign not a disease (Pickering 1968). In clinical terms, a discussion of hypertension is as useful as a discussion of pyrexia. The sign may reveal the disease, but not its origin, significance or all of its dangers. After all, individuals with pulmonary tuberculosis may die, but not of the pyrexia by which their condition may be first recognized. In this chapter the term hypertension is used loosely to mean a blood pressure that is higher than average.

Pre-eclampsia and pregnancy-induced hypertension

A multiplicity of terms is often used to hide a lack of knowledge or understanding. This is true of the condition of pre-eclampsia. Pre-eclampsia, pre-eclamptic toxaemia (PET), pregnancy-induced hypertension (PIH), pregnancy-associated hypertension (PAH), hypertensive disease of pregnancy (HDP) or gestosis are roughly synonymous terms describing various aspects of transient hypertension in late gestation. Many will argue forcefully about the refined distinctions inherent in their favoured term but these are not firmly based and make a difficult subject unnecessarily more difficult.

In this chapter, the single term pre-eclampsia is used to label a pregnancy-specific syndrome which may terminate in eclampsia (convulsions) and is characterized by a group of signs of which hypertension is one. The use of one word to describe the syndrome does not exclude the possibility that it may have several causes. Toxaemia is an obsolete expression previously used to describe any hypertension or proteinuria in pregnancy, whether pregnancy-induced or not.

THE THREE LEVELS OF PRE-ECLAMPTIC PATHOLOGY

There are three levels of the pathology of pre-eclampsia. The primary pathology is not known for certain but is local-

Table 36.1 Secondary pathology of pre-eclampsia

System	Symptoms or signs
Cardiovascular system	Increased arterial sensitivity to angiotensin II
	Increased peripheral resistance
	Raised blood pressure
	Reduced circulating blood volume
Renal system	Reduced uric acid clearance
	Reduced glomerular function
	Reduced renal blood flow
	Proteinuria
	Glomerular endotheliosis
Coagulation system	Increased fibrinogen–fibrin turnover
	Reduced platelet count
Hepatic system	Raised liver enzymes
	Jaundice
Miscellaneous	Abnormal fluid retention

ized within the gravid uterus; the condition always resolves after delivery. Although the presence of trophoblast is necessary, the fetus is not, because pre-eclampsia can develop with hydatidiform mole (Chun et al 1964). The abnormality of pre-eclampsia must therefore be either an abnormality of the trophoblast itself or of the maternal adaptation to the presence of trophoblast. The latter is more likely because there are several maternal-specific factors for pre-eclampsia such as primigravidity (MacGillivray 1958), family history (Chesley et al 1968), and underlying medical disorders (Felding 1969).

The secondary pathology of pre-eclampsia includes the maternal adaptation to the abnormal relationship between the uterus and trophoblast. Normal pregnancy imposes changes on maternal physiology resulting from factors which enter the maternal circulation from the placenta and amniochorion. It is likely that the abnormal uteroplacental relationship of pre-eclampsia is mediated by a disturbed balance of the same factors, leading to the secondary pathology which includes the defining signs of pre-eclampsia (hypertension and proteinuria) and other comparable changes (Table 36.1).

Under certain circumstances the secondary disturbances of pre-eclampsia can become so severe that they initiate new or tertiary pathology—when the regulation of the affected maternal systems is pushed beyond its limits. The tertiary pathology of pre-eclampsia is what makes it so dangerous for the mother.

THE PRIMARY PLACENTAL PATHOLOGY

In pre-eclampsia the uteroplacental circulation is compromised by two lesions involving the spiral arteries which are the end-arteries supplying the intervillous space. The first is a relative lack of the trophoblast infiltration of the arterial walls during placentation (Brosens et al 1972). This occurs between weeks 8 and 18, and is thought to be essential to dilate the arteries for the expanded uteroplacental blood flow of the second half of the pregnancy (Fig. 36.1). The second is acute atherosis—aggregates of fibrin, platelets and lipid-loaded macrophages (lipophages) which partially or completely block the arteries (Robertson et al 1967). Neither change is specific to pre-eclampsia but can also occur with intrauterine growth retardation without a maternal syndrome (Brosens et al 1977, De Wolf et al 1980)—an observation of which the implications are not yet fully understood. It could mean that the spiral artery changes are an associated but not primary feature of pre-eclampsia or that pre-eclampsia is a broader disorder than previously considered, not necessarily including hypertension. Once pre-eclampsia is established uteroplacental blood flow is reduced (Johnson & Clayton 1957, Dixon et al 1963). Earlier, at 18–24 weeks, before the disorder is overt, abnormalities in the flow velocity wave forms of the uterine arcuate arteries have been detected by ultrasound Doppler techniques (Campbell et al 1986). This is consistent with the view that the uteroplacental circulation is never normally developed in pre-eclampsia.

It is believed that these circulatory problems cause placental ischaemia which in turn causes the maternal signs (Page 1972). There is no direct evidence that this is so, but in various animal models a pre-eclamptic-like illness can be induced by placental ischaemia (Wardle & Wright 1973, Abitbol 1977, Cavanagh et al 1977). Hypoxia is thought to stimulate trophoblast both to proliferate and to form syncytial knots (Tominaga & Page 1966) and these changes are prominent in pre-eclamptic placentas (Burstein et al 1957, Wentworth 1967). In addition, placental infarcts occur more commonly (Little 1960), although they are not specific to pre-eclampsia. The ischaemia may extend to the decidua, in which haemorrhages are a feature (Brosens 1964).

THE SECONDARY AND TERTIARY PATHOLOGY

Involvement of the cardiovascular system

The hypertension of pre-eclampsia is caused by an increased peripheral resistance (Assali et al 1964, Groenindijk et al 1984). Measurements or estimates of the cardiac output have been variable, ranging from normal (Assali et al 1964) to increased (Benedetti et al 1980) or decreased (Kuzniar et al 1982, Groenindijk et al 1984). Some of the differences between studies may reflect drug use rather than the characteristics of the disease itself. For example, treatment with vasodilators stimulates cardiac output in pre-eclamptic women by reducing afterload (Groenindijk et al 1984).

Many have looked for a circulating vasoactive substance in pre-eclamptic women, so far without success. Increased circulating concentrations of serotonin, catecholamines or angiotensin II have not been consistently found. However, arterial reactivity to exogenous vasopressor substances such as vasopressin (Dieckmann & Michel 1937), catecholamines (Raab et al 1956, Talledo et al 1968, Zuspan et al 1964) and angiotensin II is increased, the last having been demon-

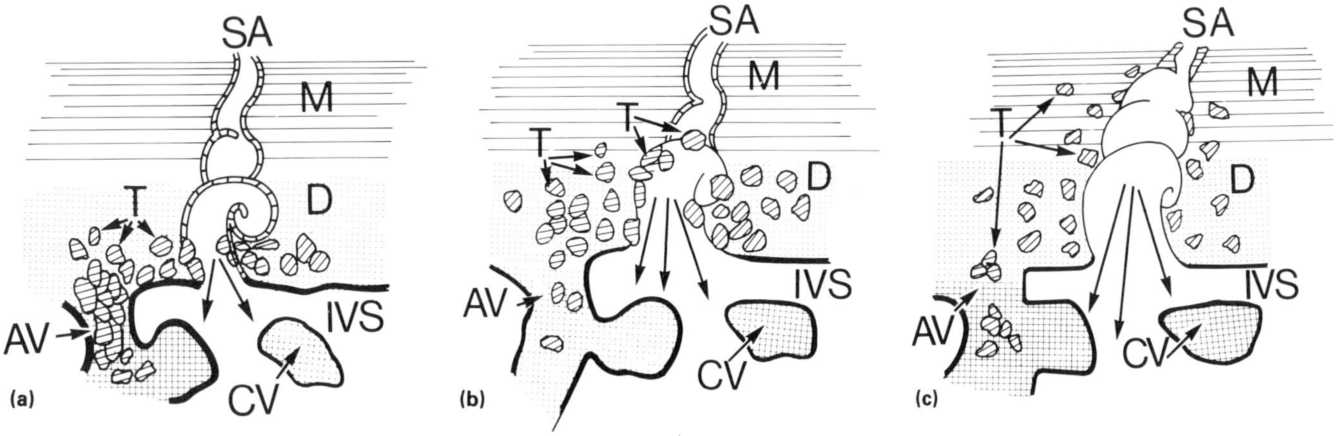

Fig. 36.1 Placentation and pre-eclampsia at (**a**) 6 weeks; (**b**) 12 weeks; (**c**) 18 weeks. Trophoblast (T) from an anchoring villus (AV) invades the decidua (D) and the distal end of a spiral artery (SA)—a process well established by 6 weeks after the last menstrual period (see Fig. 36.1a). At this stage the spiral artery is thick-walled but the action of the trophoblast breaks down the arterial structure so that the vessel becomes thin-walled and dilated, at first in its decidual segment (Fig. 36.1b), extending by 18 weeks into the myometrial (M) segment (Fig. 36.1c). The effect is to allow the blood flow into the intervillous space (IVS) to increase. A chorionic villus (CV) is also shown.

In pre-eclampsia this process fails to extend beyond the normal stage for 12 weeks so that the ability of the spiral artery to deliver an adequate flow of blood is impaired.

strated both in vivo (Talledo et al 1968, Gant et al 1973, Kaulhausen et al 1982) and ex vivo using omental vessels taken at Caesarean section (Aalkjaer et al 1985). In normal pregnancy, arterial reactivity to exogenous angiotensin II is reduced relative to the non-pregnant state (Abdul-Karim & Assali 1961, Lumbers 1970) whereas the responses to catecholamines are unchanged (Raab et al 1956). Vascular responses to angiotensin II are affected by prostaglandins. For example, the pressor response is attenuated by infusing prostaglandin E_2 (Broughton Pipkin et al 1982) but enhanced by giving prostaglandin synthetase inhibitors (Everett et al 1978). These observations have led to various theories that pre-eclampsia may result from a disturbed balance of prostaglandins.

Plasma volume, colloid osmotic pressure and oedema

Maternal plasma volume increases during the second and third trimesters of pregnancy (Hytten & Paintin 1963, Pirani et al 1973). The extent of the increase depends on the size of the conceptus, being higher in women with multiple pregnancy (Fullerton et al 1965, Rovinsky & Jaffin 1965) and least in those with fetuses which are small-for-gestational-age (Hytten & Paintin 1963, Duffus et al 1971, Pirani et al 1973). Maternal plasma volume is reduced in pre-eclampsia compared with normal pregnancy (Freis & Kenny 1948, MacGillivray 1967, Gallery et al 1979). Pre-eclampsia is frequently associated with intrauterine growth retardation (see p. 521), which accounts for some of the observed change in plasma volume. But whether the plasma volume is further decreased, given fetal size, has not been determined. Hypertension itself may be a factor because it is associated with reduced plasma volumes in non-pregnant subjects (Bing & Smith 1981). More important may be the hypoalbuminaemia characteristic of the disorder (Horne et al 1970, Studd et al 1970) which causes a lower colloid osmotic pressure (Benedetti & Carlson 1979, Zinaman et al 1985). This alters the Starling forces governing fluid transport across the capillaries, so that the vascular system in pre-eclampsia becomes leaky, with a maldistribution of fluid—too much in the interstitial spaces (oedema) and too little in the vascular compartment (hypovolaemia).

Involvement of the renal system

The involvement of the kidneys in pre-eclampsia has long been recognized and is one of its more consistent features. Proteinuria reflects advanced disease, associated with a poorer prognosis (Naeye & Friedman 1979) than if it is absent. Pre-eclampsia is characteristically variable in its presentation—certainly more than is commonly recognized. Thus, cases of eclampsia have been documented without proteinuria (Chesley 1978a); that is, neurological complications can be severe without apparent renal involvement. When there is proteinuria it is not preceded by a phase of microalbuminuria undetected by the crude techniques of clinical screening (Lopez-Espinoza et al 1986). Once present it has no specific features. It is moderately selective (Simanowitz et al 1973), increases until delivery and not uncommonly exceeds 10 g/24 h; pre-eclampsia is the commonest cause of heavy proteinuria in pregnancy (Fisher et al 1977). A nephrotic syndrome may ensue: apart from generalized oedema, there is hypoproteinaemia (Horne et al 1970), a reduced plasma oncotic pressure (Zinaman et al 1985), and hypovolaemia (Liley 1970). Serous effusions, particularly ascites, are not uncommon. The oedema may cause tertiary pathology such as respiratory difficulties resulting from laryngeal oedema (Jouppila et al 1980) and pulmonary oedema (Benedetti & Carlson 1979). Cerebral oedema (Kirby

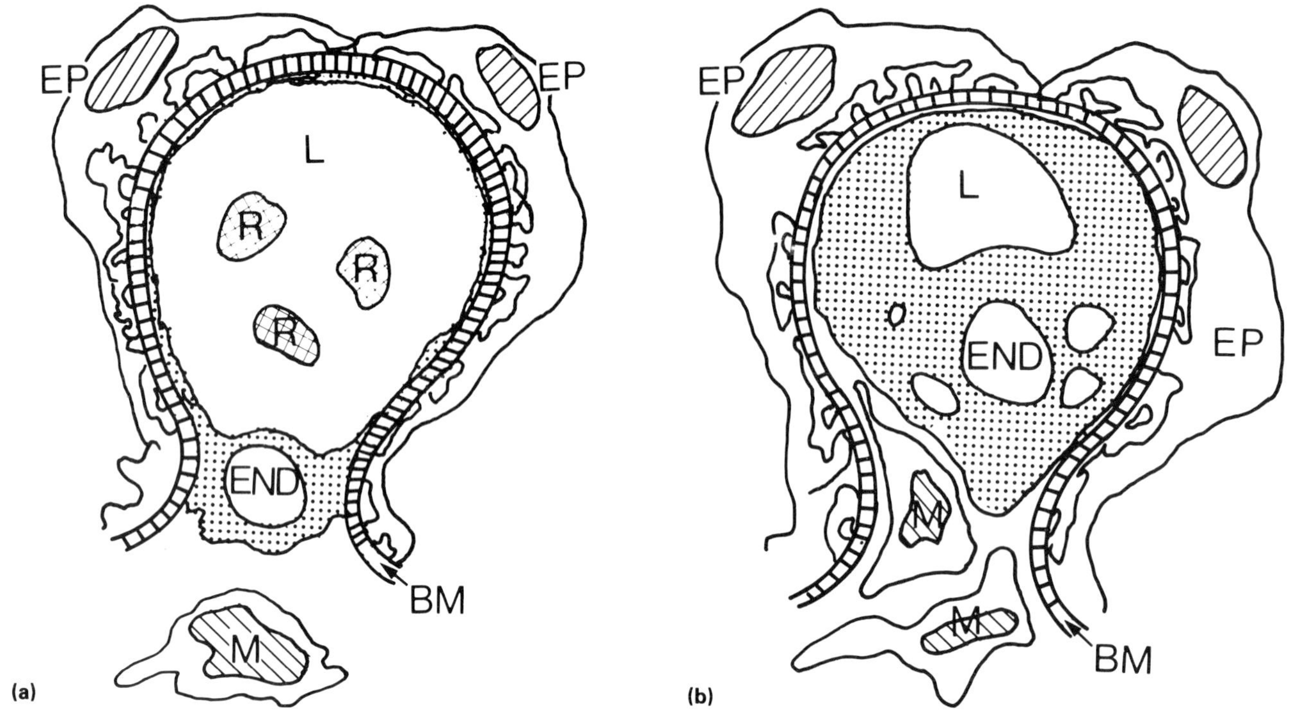

Fig. 36.2 Two diagrams of one capillary loop in a normal (**a**) and pre-eclamptic (**b**) glomerulus. The main change is gross swelling of the endothelial (END) cell's cytoplasm with partial obliteration of the capillary lumen (L). The basement membrane (BM) is intact, as are the foot processes of the epithelial (EP) cells. There is a slight increase in the numbers of the mesangial (M) cells. Red blood cells (R) are squeezed out of the glomerulus, which on light microscopy appears swollen and bloodless.

& Jaindl 1984) is a feature and is possibly the cause of at least some cases of eclampsia.

Renal involvement in pre-eclampsia has other well documented features, including characteristic glomerular histology and changes in function. The typical renal glomerular lesion of pre-eclampsia is glomerular endotheliosis (Fig. 36.2); the endothelial cells of the glomeruli swell and block the capillary lumina so that the glomeruli appear enlarged and bloodless (Spargo et al 1959).

Renal biopsy is never indicated to resolve the differential diagnosis of pre-eclampsia, however atypical or difficult the presentation. The investigation is reserved for those who continue to have significant proteinuria and renal impairment at a remote time after delivery. It has been claimed (Spargo et al 1959) and denied (Fisher et al 1969) that the glomerular lesions are pathognomonic. The former view makes pre-eclampsia a primary renal disease, whereas renal involvement must always be secondary to the uteroplacental problem. Normal renal histology has been found in some cases of eclampsia (Dennis et al 1963). Since it does not exclude the diagnosis, renal biopsy does not provide a completely specific or sensitive diagnosis for pre-eclampsia.

The glomerular pathology correlates with the degree of hyperuricaemia (Pollak & Nettles 1960), the latter being a well documented component of the condition. It is usually an early feature (Redman et al 1976a), preceding the onset of proteinuria and useful for diagnosis at that stage. The hyperuricaemia results from a reduced renal urate clearance (Chesley & Williams 1945), also observed in pre-eclampsia superimposed on chronic hypertension (Hayashi 1956). It may be exacerbated by eclamptic fits (Crawford 1941), probably depending on the degree of hypoxia and ensuing metabolic acidosis. The reduction in the renal clearance of urate is proportionally more than that of inulin (Chesley & Williams 1945). As the plasma urate rises, the plasma concentrations of urea and creatinine at first remain steady, tending to increase slowly after proteinuria has become established. The mechanisms underlying these changes are not understood.

The tertiary pathology of renal involvement in pre-eclampsia is acute renal failure arising from either tubular or cortical necrosis.

Involvement of the clotting system

The blood in normal pregnancy is said to be hypercoagulable; the response to clotting stimuli is brisker and the spontaneous intravascular conversion of fibrinogen to fibrin is increased three- to fivefold (Fletcher et al 1979). This is probably the result of local activity in the uteroplacental circulation rather than systemic changes. The concentrations of several circulating clotting factors increase (fibrinogen, factors VII, VIII, X and XI; Bonnar 1975). The activity of the fibrinolytic system measured by the euglobulin lysis time appears to be inhibited (Bonnar et al 1969).

In normal pregnancy the platelet counts are unchanged (Tygart et al 1986) or slightly reduced (Bonnar et al 1969, Sejeny et al 1975). Platelet turnover may be moderately increased (Rakoczi et al 1979), although this is disputed by some (Wallenburg & van Kessel 1978). There is greater platelet reactivity (Lewis et al 1980, Morrison et al 1985), with higher concentrations of the platelet-specific protein beta-thromboglobulin in peripheral plasma (Douglas et al 1982). These trends are exaggerated in some, but not all, cases of pre-eclampsia with a progressive fall in the platelet count (Redman et al 1978), a reduced platelet lifespan (Rakoczi et al 1979, Boneu et al 1980) and circulating plasma concentrations of beta-thromboglobulin which are increased (Redman et al 1977a, Douglas et al 1982, Oian et al 1986). The platelets tend to be larger (that is, probably younger, Giles & Inglis 1981), even in the absence of thrombocytopenia (Stubbs et al 1986).

It is hard to interpret these results and impossible at present to identify the trigger to the platelet abnormalities. One hypothesis is that pre-eclampsia results from a primary disturbance of prostanoid metabolism particularly affecting the balance between the opposing actions of prostacyclin and thromboxane on platelet aggregation and vascular tone. The attraction of this hypothesis is that it unifies the potential causes of pre-eclamptic hypertension and of platelet dysfunction. The disadvantage is that it cannot explain why platelet abnormalities are an inconsistent part of the syndrome; for example, only 29% of one series of eclamptic women showed thrombocytopenia, that is, platelets less than $150\,000 \times 10^9/l$ (Pritchard et al 1976).

Nevertheless the fall in the platelet count may be an early sign of the start of pre-eclampsia (Redman et al 1978). This may progress to decompensation to give the tertiary pathology of overt disseminated intravascular coagulation (DIC). Before then, other signs of coagulation disturbances are hard to elicit but may include an increased ratio of factor VIII-related antigen to pro-coagulant activity (Redman et al 1977c), thought to reflect factor VIII consumption (Denson 1977). DIC, an example of tertiary pathology, is a rare end-stage to this process for which the original evidence was obtained post-mortem (McKay et al 1953). When it develops, clotting factors such as fibrinogen, factors VII and VIII, are consumed and serum fibrin and fibrinogen degradation products are increased.

A further complication is microangiopathic haemolysis (Vardi & Fields 1974) which may cause a sudden drop in haemoglobin, associated with haemoglobinuria and fragmented or distorted red cells (schistocytes) on the peripheral blood film. The red blood cells are thought to be disrupted in their passage through damaged small arteries and arterioles (Brain et al 1962). The severe clotting abnormalities of pre-eclampsia are particularly associated with liver pathology, now recognized as an important and dangerous component of the disorder (see Chapter 37).

Involvement of the liver

About two-thirds of women dying from eclampsia have specific lesions in the liver (Sheehan & Lynch 1973a) which are periportal lake haemorrhages and various grades of ischaemic damage, including complete infarction (Sheehan & Lynch 1973b). The haemorrhages arise from the arteries and arterioles of the portal tract, which show the same diffuse mural damage as occurs elsewhere in severe pre-eclampsia and eclampsia, namely, insudation of the media by fibrin — so-called fibrinomedia or plasmatic vasculosis (Sheehan & Lynch 1973c). In addition there are thromboses in the portal tract vessels which may extend into the tributaries of the portal vein.

Most of this pathology has been defined post mortem although it has also been confirmed in biopsy studies. The earliest abnormality that has been detected in mild cases of pre-eclampsia, without thrombocytopenia or disturbances of the plasma liver enzymes, is fibrin–fibrinogen deposition in the hepatic sinusoids (Arias & Mancilla-Jimenez 1976). This may merely be a sign of clearance of an increased burden of intravascular fibrin by the reticuloendothelial system of the liver. The cause of the portal arterial lesions which precede periportal haemorrhages may be extreme hypertension or some other unidentified insult to the arterial tree.

The tertiary pathology of the liver disease includes jaundice and hepatic encephalopathy (Long et al 1977, Davies et al 1980) as well as the bleeding problems of the associated severe DIC. The liver disturbances may be out of proportion to the severity of the pre-eclampsia as judged by the conventional signs of hypertension and proteinuria. Epigastric pain and vomiting are the typical symptoms associated with liver involvement but are not always present (Sheehan & Lynch 1973d). Unless evidence for hepatic derangement is sought in all cases of proteinuric pre-eclampsia, dangerous presentations will be missed.

In certain severe cases, typically of multiparae rather than primiparae, there may be bleeding under the liver capsule (Sheehan & Lynch 1973e). Subsequently this may rupture to cause massive haemoperitoneum, shock and usually maternal death (Bis & Waxman 1976).

Liver damage is particularly associated with DIC in pre-eclampsia. When there is also the associated complication of microangiopathic haemolysis the acronym HELLP syndrome has been used to label the concurrence of haemolysis, elevated liver enzymes and low platelet counts (Weinstein 1982). This is merely a convenient way of bringing the presentation — which has been documented, albeit incompletely, for many years (Pritchard et al 1954, Killam et al 1975) — into focus. It is a dangerous presentation that is often not associated with marked hypertension or other conventional indices of severe pre-eclampsia (Weinstein 1982). Indeed liver damage and low platelet counts have been documented in primigravidae without hypertension or proteinuria, but with the typical hepatic histology of pre-eclampsia, including fibrin deposition in the sinusoids (Aarnoudse et al 1986).

Involvement of the nervous system

The reported incidence of eclampsia in hospital populations has varied from 2 per 10 000 in Sweden (Svensson et al 1984) to 80 per 10 000 in Calcutta (Bhose 1964). In New Zealand, where the condition was notifiable, its incidence dropped from 32 to 8 per 10 000 maternities between 1928 and 1958 (Corkill 1961). In more recent years, the incidences have been 6–9 per 10 000 in the Grampian region (Templeton & Campbell 1979), 4–10 per 10 000 in South Wales (Wightman et al 1978), and 8.8 per 10 000 in the National Birthday Trust Survey of 1958 (Butler & Bonham 1963). In Oxford, where the numerator is increased by transferred cases, but the denominator comprises all the maternities in and around the city, there were 18 cases of eclampsia between 1978 and 1986, a rate of 3.6 per 10 000.

Eclampsia, malignant hypertension and hypertensive encephalopathy

Malignant hypertension is a syndrome of severe hypertension with papilloedema or retinal haemorrhages associated with characteristic intimal cellular hyperplasia of the renal interlobular arteries at autopsy (malignant nephrosclerosis; Kincaid-Smith et al 1958). Typically, there is proteinuria, renal impairment and DIC (Linton et al 1969), which are also features of severe pre-eclampsia. However, in pre-eclampsia or eclampsia, papilloedema or retinal haemorrhages are usually absent and malignant nephroscelerosis is not found at autopsy. Therefore, according to the usual terminology, most cases of severe pre-eclampsia or eclampsia cannot be classified as malignant hypertension.

Hypertensive encephalopathy is a separate, acute or subacute syndrome of diffuse rather than focal cerebral dysfunction, not ascribable to uraemia, which is reversed by treatment of the raised arterial pressure. Headaches, nausea, vomiting and convulsions are typical symptoms (Chester et al 1978). It is a rare complication of malignant hypertension (Clarke & Murphy 1956), frequently occurs in the context of acute nephritis, and, like eclampsia, is not normally associated with gross papilloedema or retinopathy (Jellinek et al 1964). Eclampsia is certainly an encephalopathy. Average blood pressures are high (170–195/110–120 mmHg; Sibai et al 1981) but cases with much lower blood pressures are not rare, although some may result from errors in sphygmomanometry.

Hypertensive encephalopathy can also occur at relatively low blood pressure levels. One of the complications of hypertensive encephalopathy is cortical blindness (Jellinek et al 1964), also a feature of severe pre-eclampsia and eclampsia (Grimes et al 1980, Liebowtiz 1984). The medical condition can be reversed by control of the blood pressure, although it is not clear from the anecdotal reports how much of the recovery may arise from spontaneous resolution, for example, of an underlying acute nephritis. The obstetric condition is resolved by delivery so it would not be sensible or ethical to test stringently the effect of antihypertensive medication on the encephalopathy. Therefore, it cannot be formally proved that eclampsia is a form of hypertensive encephalopathy, although it probably is.

The cerebrovascular pathology of hypertensive encephalopathy and eclampsia

The cerebral pathology of eclampsia resembles that of hypertensive encephalopathy and comprises thrombosis, fibrinoid necrosis of the cerebral arterioles, diffuse microinfarcts and petechial haemorrhages (Sheehan & Lynch 1973f, Chester et al 1978). These changes are not found in malignant hypertension. In women with eclampsia, computerized tomography has shown diffuse (Kirby & Jaindl 1984) and focal oedema (Beeson & Duda 1982) as well as haemorrhages (Beck & Menezes 1981) and infarcts (Gaitz & Bamford 1982).

The cause of cerebral dysfunction of hypertensive encephalopathy

The traditional view is that the problem is of ischaemia secondary to intense vasoconstriction (Sheehan & Lynch 1973f). But some argue that vasoconstriction, far from being abnormal, is an appropriate, indeed essential protective response to extremes of arterial pressure (Johansson et al 1974). Otherwise a rise in the blood pressure would cause an uncontrolled increase in tissue perfusion and rupture the microcirculation distal to the arterioles. Protective vasospasm is the result of a local smooth muscle reflex dependent on stretch receptors (Vinall & Simeone 1981). In normal individuals arterial constriction maintains constant cerebral perfusion when the mean arterial pressure varies from 60 to 150 mmHg (Strandgaard et al 1973).

As the arterial pressure increases, the arterial smooth muscle must maintain a greater opposing constriction to regulate distal perfusing pressure. But beyond the limit of its strength the smooth muscle begins to yield, at first in short segments which progressively extend until the whole length of the small artery or arteriole is blown-out. This sequence can be demonstrated experimentally on cerebral or mesenteric vessels when extreme hypertension is induced (Byrom 1954, Giese 1964, Rodda & Denny-Brown 1966). Ultimately, the vessels become distended more than they would be with complete relaxation under normal pressure. As forced dilatation begins, so cerebral blood flow increases. The high pressure perfusion begins to rupture the more delicate distal microcirculation. Dilatation is associated with damage to the vessel wall, allowing insudation of plasma; abnormal permeability is confined to the dilated segments (Giese 1964, Goldby & Beilin 1972). Thus hypertensive encephalopathy is not caused by vasoconstriction but by pressure-forced loss of tone in the small arteries and arterioles.

The upper limit of cerebral autoregulation in elderly normotensive individuals is at a mean arterial pressure of 130–150 mmHg (Strandgaard et al 1973). In middle-aged chronically hypertensive individuals this limit is shifted to 170–200 mmHg. In previously normotensive pregnant women it is probably no higher than 150 mmHg (an actual reading of about 200/130 mmHg) but has never been measured directly. Various factors may increase the susceptibility of the cerebral arteries and arterioles of pregnant women to hypertensive damage. The most important is vascular permeability. If this were increased, plasmatic vasculosis and the sequelae of vessel wall leakage and damage could both occur at a lower threshold. In particular, cerebral oedema would be an expected feature during pregnancy. Vascular permeability is increased in other circulations (Oian et al 1985), although permeability of cerebral vessels has not been directly measured.

Thus the extreme hypertension of pre-eclampsia can damage the cerebral circulation and is a key factor underlying maternal convulsions and death.

Involvement of the fetus

Impairment of the uteroplacental circulation affects the functions which sustain the fetus. Pre-eclampsia is conventionally considered to be a maternal disorder in which the fetus is an incidental participant. From the fetal viewpoint, however, pre-eclampsia could be seen as a fetal syndrome, with maternal involvement being incidental. In fact pre-eclampsia is a placental disorder causing both maternal and fetal features. Whether or not pre-eclampsia is truly a *sick placenta syndrome* remains to be proved, but it is a concept which fits well with clinical experience.

Perinatal mortality increases once proteinuria is established. About three-quarters of the excess mortality can be explained by overt placental pathology (Naeye & Friedman 1979), consistent with the view that pre-eclampsia is a primary placental disease. Intrauterine deaths were previously the most significant (Nelson 1955a, Claireaux 1961), sometimes comprising as many as 85% of all perinatal deaths from pre-eclampsia (Fitzgerald & Clift 1958). It is one of the achievements of modern antenatal care that this is no longer the case. However, perinatal mortality remains high in eclampsia, ranging from 13% in Memphis (1977–1980, Sibai et al 1981) to 64% in Cardiff (1965–1974, Wightman et al 1978). Not surprisingly, it is also very high if the mother dies (Department of Health and Social Security 1986). As a certified cause of perinatal death pre-eclampsia ranks seventh in importance (Edouard & Alberman 1980). This may not be an accurate estimate because complications caused by the pre-eclampsia (prematurity, abruption, placental insufficiency) may be given precedence on the death certificate. A well timed elective delivery should pre-empt the fetal and maternal complications, but may expose the neonate to the hazards of prematurity — pre-eclampsia is the commonest reason for elective preterm delivery (Rush et al 1976).

Pre-eclampsia is the most important cause of intrauterine growth retardation in singletons with no malformations (Gruenwald 1966). The studies where fetal growth has been found to be normal (Beaudry & Sutherland 1960, De Souza et al 1976) have depended on inappropriate definitions which include a large but undefined number of cases of chronic hypertension without superimposed pre-eclampsia. Fetal growth failure is more a feature of early-onset disease (Baird et al 1957, Long et al 1980). A total of 90% of a series presenting with proteinuria before 34 weeks delivered infants weighing less than the 25th centile (Moore & Redman 1983).

Table 36.2 Tertiary pathology of pre-eclampsia

Convulsions
Cerebral haemorrhage
Cerebral oedema
Retinal detachment
Pulmonary oedema
Laryngeal oedema
Disseminated intravascular coagulation
Renal cortical necrosis
Hepatic rupture

TERTIARY PATHOLOGY AND MATERNAL MORTALITY

It is the tertiary pathology (summarized in Table 36.2) that kills women suffering from pre-eclampsia. Pre-eclampsia and eclampsia are the most important causes of maternal death in the USA (Kaunitz et al 1985), in the Nordic countries comprising Scandinavia, Iceland and Finland (Augensen & Bergsjo 1984) and England and Wales (Department of Health and Social Security 1986). The pattern of pathology varies but in England and Wales cerebral pathology is the most significant, particularly cerebral haemorrhage (Table 36.3).

In that cerebral haemorrhage is a known complication of severe hypertension in other contexts, it must be assumed, although it has not been proved, that it is a major predisposing factor in this situation. For this reason, pre-eclamptic hypertension is extremely important, as well as being an early defining sign of the disorder.

The other causes of maternal death include hepatic pathology, to the extent that liver involvement must be regarded

Table 36.3 Maternal deaths from hypertensive disease (England and Wales)

Cause of death	1973–75	1976–78	1979–81
Cerebral haemorrhage	17 (44%)	17 (59%)	9 (25%)
Other cerebral pathology	6 (15%)	4 (14%)	8 (22%)
Anoxic cardiac arrest	1	3	2
Hepatic pathology	4	1	8
Other	11	4	9

From Department of Health and Social Security 1986.

Table 36.4 Progression of pre-eclampsia

	Stage 1	Stage 2	Stage 3
Hypertension	+	+	+
Proteinuria	–	+	+
Symptoms	–	–	+
Eclampsia	–	–	–
Duration	2 weeks–3 months	2–3 weeks	2 h–3 days
Timing of admission	Elective	Today	Flying squad
Anticonvulsants	No	No	Yes
Delivery	After 38 weeks	After 34–36 weeks	After stabilization

as the second most dangerous presentation of the disorder after eclampsia itself.

MANAGEMENT OF PRE-ECLAMPSIA

The principles of management are early diagnosis, early admission to hospital, well timed delivery to pre-empt complications and postpartum follow-up to define underlying medical problems and the outlook for another pregnancy. Although this sounds simple in theory, it is difficult in practice. Only if the clinician can keep one step ahead of events at all stages will dangerous situations be avoided. For convenience, the progression of pre-eclampsia can be divided into three stages leading to eclampsia (Table 36.4). This grossly over-simplifies the problem: every clinician will regularly see cases that do not conform to this pattern. However, the staging dovetails with the requirements of management and provides a convenient framework for dealing with the problem in everyday practice. Cases should be diagnosed in stage 1, admitted to hospital as soon as stage 2 is detected, and delivered before the onset of stage 3. Stage 3 is an obstetric emergency which in an ideal world should never occur. This sequence requires delivery to be expedited before the patient herself begins to feel unwell. Thus diagnosis and management depend on the results of screening asymptomatic women. This is one of the central features and requirements of antenatal care.

Screening for pre-eclampsia

The screening interval

Screening for pre-eclampsia begins at 20 weeks although in rare cases pre-eclampsia has presented earlier. One of the most critical features of the screening procedure is the interval between examinations. The speed of progression of pre-eclampsia is variable, although it is only rarely that the exact evolution of a case is fully documented. Certainly some cases evolve into stage 3 in less than 2 weeks. This means that an interval of more than 2 weeks between examinations is dangerous if fulminating pre-eclampsia is going to develop. Even an interval of 2 weeks may be too long in these instances. The standard pattern of antenatal care in this country is of monthly visits at 20, 24 and 28 weeks. This leaves two dangerous gaps where early-onset pre-eclampsia can evolve undetected, that is in the months before and after 24 weeks, which are sometimes the lacunae of antenatal care. This is why, for example, nearly half the cases of antenatal eclampsia seen in Oxford and an undue proportion of maternal deaths in England and Wales from eclampsia occur at this time.

To identify all cases of pre-eclampsia under all circumstances, women would need to be screened at weekly intervals from 20 weeks. Clearly this is impossible and some compromise needs to be sought. This can be achieved by reviewing expectant women at the end of the first trimester and estimating their individual risks of pre-eclampsia as low, medium or high. Low-risk women need to be screened for pre-eclampsia every 4 weeks to 32 weeks and then every 2 weeks to delivery. Medium-risk women need to be screened at 20 and 24 weeks then every 2 weeks to 36 weeks, then every week to delivery. This closes the gap between 24 and 28 weeks. High-risk women need to be seen more often, on a schedule tailored to their needs, but particularly closing the gap between 20 and 24 weeks. This determines the basic programme of observations, assuming that the woman is completely free of all signs of pre-eclampsia. Once these signs begin to appear the risks increase and the intervals between observations need to be shortened, ultimately requiring inpatient rather than outpatient observations. Until this time is reached, screening is usually best done in the community rather than in a hospital clinic.

Estimating the risks of pre-eclampsia

Some of the risk factors are listed in Table 36.5 and include fetal-specific as well as maternal-specific components. It is universally agreed that primigravidae are several times more prone to the condition. Some investigators even claim that it is a disorder restricted to first pregnancies. However, the proportion of primigravidae amongst eclamptic women varies in different series from 44% (Maqueo et al 1964) to 85% (McLane & Kuder 1943), and most report incidences around 65–75% (e.g. Templeton & Campbell 1979). Because there

Table 36.5 Risk factors for pre-eclampsia

Maternal	
First pregnancy	
Previous severe pre-eclampsia	
Age under 20 or over 35	
Family history of pre-eclampsia or eclampsia	
Underweight and short	
Migraines	
Chronic hypertension	
Chronic renal disease	
Fetal	
Multiple pregnancy	
Hydatidiform mole	
Placental hydrops	

can be less doubt about the diagnosis of eclampsia compared with pre-eclampsia it must be accepted that multiparous women have some susceptibility to the disorder. However, all primigravid women are at least in a medium-risk group. The preponderance of primigravidae amongst pre-eclamptic women has led to the concept of a protective effect of a first pregnancy. However, the protection is not always complete so that the parous women who are particularly at risk are those who have had the problem before. Thus the incidence of proteinuric pre-eclampsia in a second pregnancy is 10–15 times more in those in whom it is recurrent than in those in whom the first pregnancy was normal (Davies et al 1970, Campbell & MacGillivray 1985). One of the few factors that can help to identify women at risk of early-onset pre-eclampsia is a history of previous pre-eclampsia (Moore & Redman 1983). If the only previous pregnancy is nonviable the likelihood of pre-eclampsia is slightly reduced—but only if the pregnancy progressed into the second trimester (Campbell & MacGillivray 1985).

The predisposition to pre-eclampsia is inherited. The daughters of eclamptic women are eight times more likely to suffer pre-eclampsia than expected (Chesley et al 1968). The pattern of inheritance can be explained on the basis of a single recessive gene for which the mother must be homozygous (Cooper & Liston 1979, Chesley & Cooper 1986). It is easy but not usual to take a family history of pre-eclampsia. If, for example, a primigravida is the daughter of a woman who suffered eclampsia, she should be categorized as high- rather than medium-risk, and screened accordingly.

Maternal age is closely linked to parity. In most series the incidence of pre-eclampsia with age is J-shaped with higher incidences in teenage women and those more than 30 years old. The increased incidence in teenage women is mostly the result of the high proportion of primigravidae in this group, although amongst primigravidae the risk may be increased in the very young (Hauch & Lehmann 1934). Otherwise, increasing age is the key risk factor (summarized by Davies 1971). Hence if primigravidae are in a medium-risk group, older primigravidae (35 years or more) are in a high-risk group. Age is the most influential risk factor for death from pre-eclampsia or eclampsia (Lopez-Llera et al 1976).

It has been believed for many years that overweight women are more prone to pre-eclampsia (Stewart & Hewitt 1960, MacGillivray 1961). However, the more stringent the diagnostic criteria the more this association disappears (Lowe 1961) and is replaced by the opposite effect. Eclampsia affects women of all body builds, but particularly underweight women (Chesley 1984). Short stature is also important (Baird 1977). Thus the short, underweight primipara is in a high-risk category for pre-eclampsia and her antenatal care should be adjusted accordingly.

Certain medical problems seem to predispose to pre-eclampsia. The problem is complicated because they include those (chronic hypertension, renal disease) that can mimic the disorder. In the absence of a specific diagnostic test for pre-eclampsia it is sometimes difficult or impossible to disentangle those elements of proteinuric hypertension caused by a chronic medical problem from those arising from superimposed pre-eclampsia. The conventional definitions of pre-eclampsia cease to be applicable. If a women is permanently proteinuric there are no accepted criteria for diagnosing proteinuric pre-eclampsia.

Nevertheless it is generally agreed that chronically hypertensive women are three to seven times more likely to develop high blood pressures and proteinuria (superimposed pre-eclampsia) than normotensive women (Chesley et al 1947, Butler & Bonham 1963, Harley 1966, Walters 1966). Women with hypertension associated with chronic renal disease have a particular susceptibility to superimposed pre-eclampsia (Felding 1969).

A history of migraine predisposes to early-onset pre-eclampsia (Moore & Redman 1983) and eclampsia (Rotton et al 1959), although this association was not noted in one other series (Wainscott et al 1978).

Social class does not appear to have a marked effect on the incidence of pre-eclampsia (Nelson 1955b, Baird 1977). Indeed those classified in the upper social classes (non-manual occupations) have a higher incidence of severe pre-eclampsia than the wives of manual workers (skilled and unskilled; Baird 1977). Lower social class is associated with shortness and a poorer diet, the former definitely and the latter possibly predisposing to the problem. Another key factor is cigarette smoking—which increases in the lower social classes but is associated with a reduced incidence of pre-eclampsia (Zabriskie 1963, Underwood et al 1965, Duffus & MacGillivray 1968). Because the perinatal mortality in smokers is high it would seem likely that the effect of smoking is to diminish the maternal responses to the placental problems of pre-eclampsia. Certainly smoking cannot be prescribed to prevent pre-eclampsia.

The maternal-specific risk factors for pre-eclampsia are simple to elicit. The fetal-specific factors only become apparent as pregnancy evolves and have in common an enlarged trophoblast mass. They include multiple pregnancy (Mac-

Gillivray 1958), hydatidiform mole (Chun et al 1964—a cause of atypical pre-eclampsia at mid-gestation), and hydrops fetalis (Jeffcoate & Scott 1959) from all causes, including rhesus isoimmunization.

The baseline assessment

In the first half of pregnancy the risk factors can be assessed to decide how often a woman needs to be screened for pre-eclampsia after 20 weeks of pregnancy. In addition, this is the time to determine the baseline for diagnosing pre-eclampsia should it occur. This should obviously include a careful and accurate measurement of the arterial pressure. If proteinuria is detected, its amount and significance must be evaluated without delay; the problem cannot be avoided until the third trimester. In women who are classified as high-risk, for example elderly primigravidae, or primigravidae with underlying medical problems, the baseline should include laboratory measurements which will be used later if pre-eclampsia supervenes—platelet count, plasma creatinine and uric acid, and liver function tests. It is important to screen for asymptomatic bacteriuria and treat any confirmed infection.

Naturally, other baseline aspects of the pregnancy, for example, reliable assessment of gestational age, are equally important.

PRINCIPLES OF DIAGNOSIS

None of the known features of pre-eclampsia is specific. Even grand mal convulsions in pregnancy can have causes other than eclampsia. Nor is there an absolute criterion for judging the accuracy of a diagnosis retrospectively or assessing the correctness of the various definitions of the syndrome. This is an unsatisfactory situation which will not be resolved until the pathophysiology of the disorder is fully defined. If it is accepted that the clinical condition of pre-eclampsia is a secondary maternal adaptation to a primary uteroplacental problem, it will present in many forms, reflecting individual differences in the susceptibility of maternal target-organ systems. So, pre-eclampsia cannot be stereotyped and the balance of its different components will vary from case to case. One woman may have severe hypertension but little renal involvement; another, severe renal involvement but little hypertension, and a third, predominantly hepatic involvement. It may even be possible to have pre-eclampsia without hypertension (Redman et al 1977a). For diagnostic purposes all the secondary features of the disorder should be considered as possible components. The presence of only one component is never diagnostic. The absence of any one component never excludes the diagnosis with certainty. There is no simple formula which allows the clinician to stop thinking and make the diagnosis by rote.

One consequence of these considerations is that it is impossible to diagnose stage 1 pre-eclampsia without resorting to additional investigations. It cannot be detected by observing changes in the blood pressure alone.

Diagnosis of pre-eclamptic hypertension

Measurement of arterial pressure

Sphygmomanometry is a non-invasive way of estimating the true intra-arterial pressure. Phase I of the Korotkoff sounds defines the systolic pressure. In non-pregnant subjects phase V (extinction of the Korotkoff sounds) is preferred to phase IV (muffling) for the diastolic end-point (Kirkendall et al 1981). However, in some pregnant women, the Korotkoff sounds can be heard at zero cuff pressure—that is, phase V does not exist. For this reason phase IV has to be used (Davey & MacGillivray 1986) even though phase V, when present, is slightly better correlated with direct measurements (Raftery & Ward 1968). The differences between phase IV and V end-points are usually trivial—2 mmHg or less in 75% of middle-aged men, for example (Lichtenstein et al 1986). The Korotkoff sounds are produced by vibrations in the arterial wall (Wiggers 1956). They are less distinct if the arterial wall is rigid, for example in shock (Cohn 1967) or eclampsia (Seligman 1971), when the indirect readings may grossly underestimate the arterial pressure.

When the blood pressure is measured in the third trimester the lateral position is often used to avoid the supine hypotension syndrome. If the blood pressure is taken in the uppermost arm it will seem to be reduced because the cuff is above the heart (Van Dongen et al 1980). If the patient sits or stands, diastolic pressure is increased (Redman 1984) because of vasoconstriction in the lower extremities and increased peripheral resistance. There is therefore no ideal position for measuring blood pressure in pregnancy. The semi-recumbent position is to be preferred and if lateral tilt is needed to avoid supine hypotension, the cuff must be kept level with the heart.

Hypertension is over-diagnosed in obese individuals if too small a cuff is used. The standard cuff (12 × 23 cm) is adequate for arms with circumferences of less than 35 cm (Maxwell et al 1982). Since less than 5% of chronically hypertensive pregnant women exceed this measurement the problem is not common and can be resolved by using a larger arm cuff (15 × 33 cm) or a thigh cuff (18 × 36 cm).

The definition and grading of hypertension

The conventional dividing line is 140/90 mmHg (Hughes 1972) but some use only the diastolic pressure limit of 90 mmHg or higher (Nelson 1955b, Butler & Bonham 1963). In the second half of pregnancy more than 20% of pregnant women have a blood pressure of 140/90 mmHg or higher at least once. However, only 1% of women reach or exceed 170/110 mmHg. In the first half of pregnancy 2% of women have a blood pressure at or above 140/90 mmHg (Redman 1984).

Hypertension can therefore be graded as mild to moderate for readings in the range 140–165/90–105 mmHg, and severe for readings of 170/110 mmHg and higher. The relevance of this grading is that the purpose of using antihypertensive treatment is to prevent severe hypertension, however transient.

The differential diagnosis of hypertension in pregnancy

In the first half of pregnancy a raised blood pressure tends to reflect a permanent state — chronic hypertension. In the second half, it identifies in addition those who have an acquired pregnancy-induced hypertension including cases with pre-eclampsia. An abnormal increase in blood pressure from an early baseline is important in these cases; for example, one definition specifies systolic and diastolic changes of +30 and +15 mmHg respectively (Hughes 1972). Since the average diastolic increment for all women in the third trimester is nearly 15 mmHg (10–12 mmHg; MacGillivray et al 1969, Chesley 1976), a higher threshold is more appropriate for diagnosing pre-eclampsia, such as 20 mmHg, or even 25–30 mmHg (Redman & Jefferies 1988). Many definitions of pre-eclamptic hypertension have no requirement for a diastolic increment; instead an absolute level above 90 mmHg after 26 (Nelson 1955b) or 20 weeks (Butler & Bonham 1963) is considered to be diagnostic provided that no previous reading reached this limit. Individuals whose pressures rise from a diastolic pressure of 85 mmHg (mild chronic hypertension) may be grouped with those whose pressures have risen from baseline levels of 70 mmHg or less (normotension). Many women with normal pregnancies, but chronic hypertension, are therefore wrongly considered to have pre-eclampsia.

Even a pronounced rise in the arterial pressure from normal to abnormal levels does not distinguish pre-eclamptic from chronic hypertension. The fall in arterial pressure which occurs mainly during the second half of the first trimester may in some cases of chronic hypertension be exaggerated. An extreme case has been reported of a woman whose pre-pregnancy readings were 224–280/140–180 mmHg; during pregnancy the pressure fell, without hypotensive treatment which was not available at the time, to levels of 110–130/60–80 mmHg (Chesley & Annitto 1947), that were apparently normal. In the third trimester blood pressure normally rises to pre-pregnant levels; the increase is exaggerated in these cases.

A rise in the arterial pressure by more than a defined amount above a hypertensive threshold is therefore not pathognomonic of pre-eclampsia. Other signs are needed to confirm the diagnosis. These may include new proteinuria, hyperuricaemia or thrombocytopenia. Whereas oedema is, in general, not helpful, accelerated weight gain (≥2.0 kg/week) is. Evidence of placental disease supports the diagnosis. For example, if the fetus is well grown, pre-eclampsia is less likely, although not impossible. Hydatidiform mole should be sought if the problem presents at mid-gestation. Hydramnios increases the likelihood of fetal and placental hydrops which can be diagnosed by ultrasonography. In many circumstances the diagnosis is beset by doubt that can be dispelled only if the disorder worsens. Often induced or spontaneous delivery curtails the sequence of events before the diagnosis can be established with certainty (Redman 1987). The diagnosis of mild or moderate pre-eclampsia at the end of pregnancy is therefore almost always suspect.

In women with pre-existing hypertension, renal disease or both, there may be acute exacerbations of the hypertension and proteinuria in the second half of pregnancy. Sometimes these episodes are labelled superimposed pre-eclampsia and sometimes they are perceived only as an underlying medical problem coinciding with pregnancy. Often the disorders affect second or later pregnancies and on this basis alone a pre-eclamptic process is discounted. However, the alternative should also be considered, that some such women may be unusually susceptible to pre-eclampsia and constitutionally unable to benefit from the protective effect of a first pregnancy. Without a specific test for pre-eclampsia these opinions cannot be tested. For the present, if the episode is transient, confined to the second half of pregnancy and associated with evidence of placental disease, it may be reasonably called pre-eclampsia superimposed on whatever chronic disorder has been identified.

These considerations relate to phaeochromocytoma coinciding with pregnancy. This rare but dangerous complication of pregnancy causes a maternal mortality which was previously as high as 50% (Blair 1963). The presentation frequently simulates severe pre-eclampsia with extreme but unstable hypertension, proteinuria and pre-eclamptic-like symptoms such as headaches (Schenker & Chowers 1971). All patients with proteinuric hypertension in pregnancy should therefore be screened for phaeochromocytoma, although the diagnosis can still be missed by false negative results (Coden 1972). If the condition is identified and treated before delivery, the maternal mortality is reduced (to zero in cases where alpha-adrenergic blockade has been used). Methods of diagnosis are the same as in non-pregnant individuals except that radiological localization is precluded.

Diagnosis of pre-eclamptic renal disease

Early involvement of the renal system (usually before or during stage 1) leads to reduced uric acid clearance despite a normal glomerular filtration rate. Plasma uric acid will rise, a useful change to indicate stage 1 pre-eclampsia and to distinguish pre-eclamptic from chronic hypertension. Pregnant women with chronic hypertension alone have normal plasma urate concentrations. Hyperuricaemic hypertension in the second half of pregnancy therefore is more likely

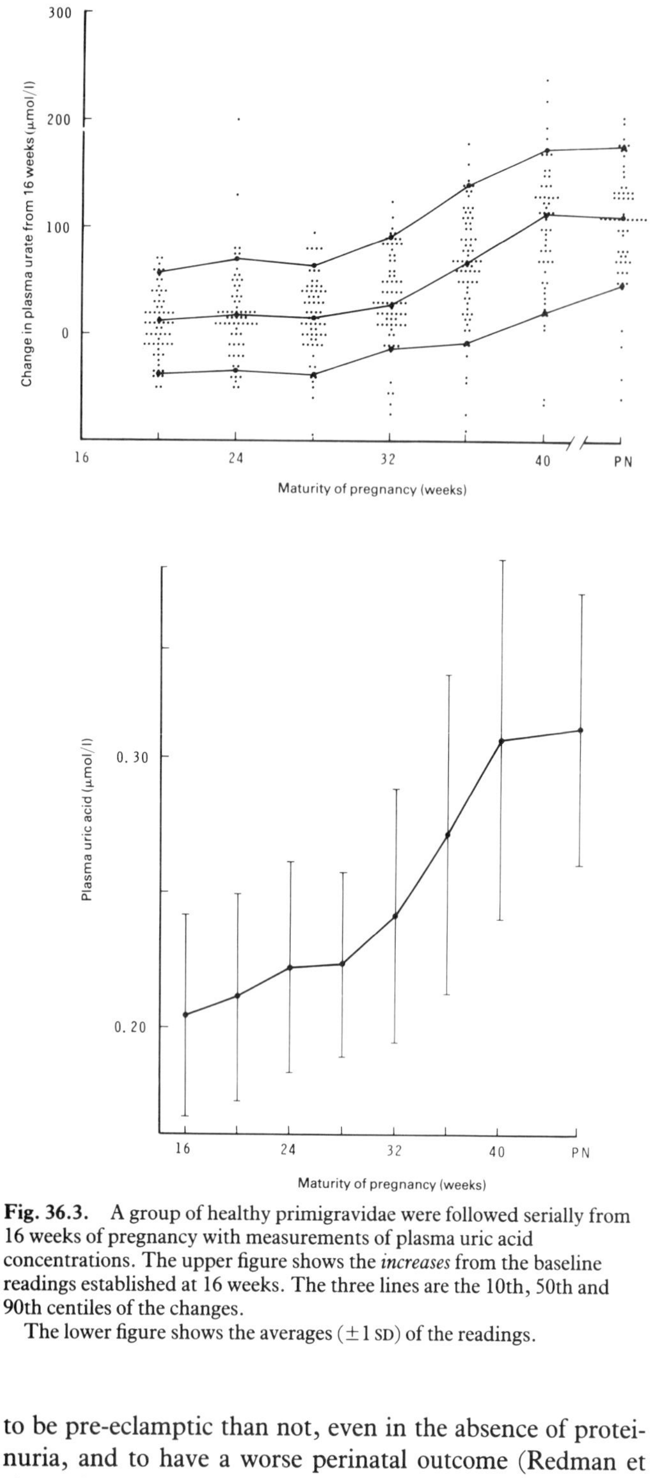

Fig. 36.3. A group of healthy primigravidae were followed serially from 16 weeks of pregnancy with measurements of plasma uric acid concentrations. The upper figure shows the *increases* from the baseline readings established at 16 weeks. The three lines are the 10th, 50th and 90th centiles of the changes.

The lower figure shows the averages (±1 SD) of the readings.

to be pre-eclamptic than not, even in the absence of proteinuria, and to have a worse perinatal outcome (Redman et al 1976b). The normal range of plasma urate concentrations rises in the third trimester (Fig. 36.3). As a rough guide, values above 0.30, 0.35, 0.40 and 0.45 mmol/l at 28, 32, 36 and 40 weeks, respectively, are likely to reflect abnormality. But just as pre-existing hypertension can muddle the presentation of pre-eclamptic hypertension, so can pre-existing or constitutional hyperuricaemia. Transient hyperuricaemia may have other causes including treatment with diuretics or acidosis (Goldfinger et al 1965, Fadel et al 1976). Like other signs of pre-eclampsia, hyperuricaemia is a variable component of the condition and may not be observed even in cases of eclampsia (Dennis et al 1963).

Proteinuria is what distinguishes the second stage of the disease. Screening depends on the use of dipsticks which may give false positive results if the urine is alkaline, and false negative results if it is highly dilute or contains proteins other than albumin. Any positive result (1+ or more) must be immediately evaluated in a mid-stream sample of urine taken whilst a vaginal tampon excludes contamination. If urinary infection can be ruled out, the amount of proteinuria should be measured—ideally over 24 hours. With a single sample an albumin:creatinine ratio can help to correct for the degree of concentration of the urine. A 24-hour excretion of 0.5 g represents about 0.1 g albumin/mmol/l creatinine. Even with this correction the amount of proteinuria typically fluctuates on an hour-by-hour basis (Chesley 1939). It is still not universally appreciated that dipstick assessment of proteinuria does not allow the progression of pre-eclampsia to be charted. However, in clinical practice, new proteinuria of 1+ or more in all urine samples tested, combined with new hypertension, can be used to identify the onset of stage 2. Proteinuria is usually associated with glomerular dysfunction, which is most simply estimated by measuring the plasma concentrations of creatinine and urea. In the absence of pre-existing renal disease a plasma creatinine above 80 mmol/l is rarely normal and above 100 mmol/l is always abnormal. The plasma urea is more variable but values above 6.0 and 7.0 mmol/l correspond to possible and probable renal impairment. Measurement of creatinine clearance is in theory a better approach; in practice it is so difficult to guarantee complete collection that it is less helpful than it should be.

Once proteinuria is established, hypoalbuminaemia and other features of a nephrotic syndrome may appear, including oedema.

The diagnostic significance of oedema

A total of 85% of women with proteinuric pre-eclampsia have oedema (Thomson et al 1967). This pathological oedema is easily confused with the physiological oedema found in 80% of normal pregnant women (Robertson 1971). Physiological oedema has not been shown to be the precursor of pathological oedema, but will appear to be so if definitions of pre-eclampsia are used which emphasize oedema, even in the absence of hypertension (such as those of the American Committee on Maternal Welfare; Chesley 1978b). In the best prospective study of pregnant women with no oedema, or early- or late-onset oedema, all had a similar incidence of hypertension (Robertson 1971). For all these reasons the detection of oedema is not clinically useful, nor should oedema be included in the definition of pre-eclampsia (Vosburgh 1976). Development of oedema is associated with a higher rate of weight gain, hence the numerous reports associating excessive weight gain with the development of pre-eclampsia (Abitbol 1969). A sudden acceleration in the rate of weight gain is a useful diagnostic feature. More than 1.0 kg per week is unusual, more than 2.0 kg per week is always abnormal. In 15% of cases of pre-eclampsia and eclampsia there is no oedema — dry pre-eclampsia — a particularly dangerous variant for both mother (Eden 1922) and baby (Chesley 1978c).

Diagnosis of clotting and hepatic abnormalities

The early disturbances of the clotting system are relatively inaccessible to clinical monitoring. Only the platelet count, among routinely available tests, is likely to be informative. Serial readings from a baseline early in pregnancy are more helpful than later single measurements. Counts of less than $100 \times 10^9/l$ are not normal, but must always be confirmed by examination of the blood film to exclude clumping, a cause of spurious thrombocytopenia (Solanki & Blackburn 1985). A consistent decline by more than $100 \times 10^9/l$ from the baseline to less than $200 \times 10^9/l$ is unusual and can confirm the diagnosis if other signs are present. The platelet count should be checked at least every week once stage 2 disease is established. If the count is less than $100 \times 10^9/l$ or if the disease has progressed beyond stage 2, evidence for DIC should be sought. A prolonged thrombin time, reduced fibrinogen concentration and evidence for haemolysis on the blood film are the simplest screening tests. Fibrin–fibrinogen degradation products can also be measured, although usually the results are available only to confirm the diagnosis retrospectively.

Evidence for liver dysfunction should be sought once proteinuria is established or if there is thrombocytopenia. It is our practice to measure plasma aspartate transaminase activity as a screening test, repeated at least every week until delivery.

MISTAKES COMMONLY MADE IN DIAGNOSIS

The commonest mistake is to discount a raised blood pressure and ascribe it to nervousness. Systolic readings should not be ignored: a pressure of 160/80 mmHg needs to be viewed with the same caution as one of 140/90 mmHg. Antenatal screening not infrequently fails to include urine testing or at least a record of the result if the test is done: this is an unacceptable omission. The importance of proteinuria is often underestimated if it is associated with moderate hypertension. Such presentations are frequently labelled mild pre-eclampsia, whereas all proteinuric pre-eclampsia is severe. The significance of abdominal pain and vomiting may be missed, particularly by general practitioners who encounter such symptoms every day in their non-pregnant patients with trivial problems. All too often the complaints by the patient of prodromal symptoms are not heeded, even by specialist staff; as elsewhere in clinical practice, the patient tells you the diagnosis. Jaundice is a rare and regularly misunderstood presentation. Finally, clinicians still fail to appreciate that the unseen complications of the disorder may be worse than those that are 'visible' (hypertension and proteinuria). This is particularly true of the fetal, coagulation and hepatic complications.

WHEN TO ADMIT TO HOSPITAL

Stage 3 pre-eclampsia and eclampsia itself are both obstetric emergencies which justify admission by flying squad if the patient presents first at home, or in an outlying clinic.

If new proteinuria (1+ or more) is detected in association with hypertension (diastolic pressure of 90 mmHg or more) then the gravida should be admitted on the same day. Failure in this practice is one of the commonest causes of preventable obstetric disasters. The fact that the hypertension may be only mild does not alter this requirement. The reason for admission is that if stage 2 pre-eclampsia has begun the disease has entered a short-lived and unstable phase. No obstetrician can guarantee the safety of a woman with proteinuric pre-eclampsia for as long as 24 hours if she remains out of hospital.

The reason for admission is not that bedrest is therapeutic, but to achieve the aim of keeping one step ahead of events. To do this, the interval between screening observations must be shortened to at least 6 hours, with the option of immediate intervention if necessary. Thus admission to an isolated general practitioner unit is not adequate.

Some women admitted with apparent stage 2 pre-eclampsia will not have the diagnosis confirmed and can be allowed home. However, if the diagnosis is confirmed, even if the woman's condition appears stable, it is dangerous to allow the patient home — she is now committed to staying in hospital until delivery.

Mild to moderate hypertension alone is not a reason for hospital admission, even if it is a new development in the third trimester. However, because it is commonly the earliest indication of pre-eclampsia it demands more frequent monitoring. If stage 1 pre-eclampsia is diagnosed it may be necessary to admit to hospital non-urgently to sort out the extent of the problems, but a well organized day-care unit where the patient can be seen as often as required is all that is needed for continuing supervision thereafter.

THE TREATMENT OF PRE-ECLAMPTIC HYPERTENSION

Although the hypertension of pre-eclampsia is a secondary feature it causes tertiary pathology and must be considered the major cause of maternal death from cerebral haemorrhages. The threshold at which pressure-induced arterial injury occurs is high, and varies from individual to individual, but once exceeded dangerous situations develop rapidly. In these circumstances good control of the blood pressure is mandatory although it is always no more than a temporary expedient pending delivery. The level at which treatment is started is a compromise between the needs for safety and the desire to avoid unnecessary medication. Our practice is to prevent readings at or above 170 mmHg systolic or 110 mmHg diastolic, which gives a generous safety margin. If in any 24-hour period two measurements reach this threshold then treatment is started. Systolic hypertension is as dangerous as diastolic hypertension. There are two requirements: to gain control in the short term, and to maintain control long enough after delivery until the risk of extreme hypertension has receded.

The acute control of pre-eclamptic hypertension

If the women presents in stage 2 or 3 pre-eclampsia, the evolution of the pre-eclampsia may be so fast and severe as to create a situation where control of the blood pressure has to be achieved within 1–3 hours. A smooth and sustained reduction is to be preferred. A number of vasodilating agents given parenterally can be used.

Hydralazine

Hydralazine has been the preferred antihypertensive agent for the treatment of acute severe pre-eclampsia (Pritchard & Pritchard 1975, Chamberlain et al 1978a, Lindberg & Sandstrom 1981). It may be given intravenously by continuous infusion (Joyce & Kenyon 1972) or intermittent boluses (Pritchard & Pritchard 1975), or by intramuscular or subcutaneous injections (Redman 1980). After intravenous administration there is a significant delay of 20–30 minutes in the onset of action.

Hydralazine is a vasodilator, directly inhibiting the contractile activity of smooth muscle (Jacobs 1984). In the cerebral circulation it first dilates the capacitance vessels, causing a rapid and marked increase in intracranial pressure (Overgaard & Skinhoj 1975), which probably accounts for the common side-effect of severe headaches. This is an undesirable action of the drug, particularly in the context of actual or impending eclampsia where intracranial pressure may already be increased because of oedema. Subsequently the resistance vessels dilate and cerebrovascular flow increases (McCall 1953, Overgaard & Skinhoj 1975). Cardiac output increases (Assali et al 1953, Freis et al 1953) because of the increased venous return (Tarazi et al 1976). A marked tachycardia nearly always occurs. Originally this was thought to result from stimulation of baroceptor reflexes. But hydralazine also causes a prolonged activation of noradrenaline release (Lin et al 1983) which correlates closely with the tachycardia, and could also explain the anxiety, restlessness and hyper-reflexia commonly encountered. These symptoms and signs, together with headaches, may affect 50% of women (Assali et al 1953) and simulate the features of impending eclampsia. Then the symptoms of the disease cannot be disentangled from those caused by the treatment.

It is relevant that hydralazine stimulates the release of noradrenaline, which is a potent vasoconstrictor of the uteroplacental circulation in sheep (Ladner et al 1970), guinea pigs (Girard et al 1971) and rhesus monkeys (Wallenburg & Hutchinson 1979), and therefore probably in humans. Thus although it increases cardiac output, hydralazine fails to improve indices of uteroplacental perfusion in pre-eclamptic women (Lunell et al 1983, Jouppila et al 1985, Suonio et al 1986). Signs of fetal distress (heart rate decelerations) have been noted after its use (Vink et al 1980, Vink & Moodley 1982).

Thus hydralazine is not an ideal drug. It is easier to use if the sympathetic nervous system is already inhibited by methyldopa or beta-adrenergic blocking agents. A continuous infusion is not a rational way to achieve control of the blood pressure for more than 4–6 hours, for which either methyldopa or labetalol should be given orally. Our own practice has been to give intermittent intramuscular hydralazine (10 mg) combined with an oral loading dose of methyldopa (500–1000 mg). The hydralazine can be repeated every 2 or 3 hours until the action of methyldopa begins 6–8 hours later. Monitoring of the fetus is essential but in our experience fetal distress is rare, and more related to the severity of the pre-eclampsia than the administration of hydralazine.

Other drugs for the acute control of hypertension

Labetalol is a combined alpha- and beta-adrenergic blocking agent which can be given intravenously. It lowers the blood pressure smoothly and rapidly without the tachycardia characteristic of treatment with hydralazine. A typical regimen starts with 20 mg/h, which is doubled every 30 minutes until control has been gained (Garden et al 1982). Since alpha-adrenergic stimulation is thought to constrict the uteroplacental circulation, labetalol would be expected to enhance flow; in fact no effect, good or bad, has been observed (Lunell et al 1982). There are no adequate trials of its parenteral use in pregnancy to show how it might affect perinatal outcome.

Diazoxide is a powerful and rapid vasodilator; an intravenous bolus dose may cause severe hypotension, cerebral ischaemia or death from cerebral infarction (Ledingham & Rajagopalan 1979). A maternal death in this setting has been reported (Henrich et al 1977). It must therefore be given with extreme care, either as a series of mini-boluses (Ram & Kaplan 1979) or by slow intravenous infusion (Thien et al 1980). It probably should not be given by obstetric staff who are unlikely to have enough experience of its use or enough time to monitor its administration properly.

Sodium nitroprusside has been used during human pregnancy for the treatment of severe pre-eclampsia (Strauss et al 1980) and other medical complications (Donchin et al 1978, Lipson et al 1978), but it must be used only by specialists in intensive care with a high level of cardiovascular monitoring not available in obstetric units. Sodium nitroprusside is potentially toxic to the fetus but normal fetal survival has been associated with its use (Stempel et al 1982, Goodlin 1983).

The calcium channel blocking agent, nifedipine, is an effective vasodilator which acts rapidly when given by mouth. Two oral preparations are available: nifedipine capsules act within 10–15 minutes; nifedipine in slow-release tablets has a slower onset of action (about 60 minutes) but a more prolonged effect. The experience of nifedipine in pregnancy is limited, but so far it appears to be at least as safe as hydralazine (Redman unpublished observations; Walters & Redman 1984). Tachycardia occurs but is less of a problem than with hydralazine. Nifedipine is used for the treatment of heart failure because it reduces after-load. Nevertheless it has a negative inotropic action on the myocardium and, in combination with beta-adrenergic blockade, can precipitate heart failure (Robson & Vishwanath 1982). If magnesium sulphate is used as an anticonvulsant agent, possible but as yet undocumented interactions with calcium channel blockers may be a problem. The advantage of nifedipine over hydralazine is its ease of oral administration; like hydralazine it can cause severe headaches.

Longer-term control of pre-eclamptic hypertension

The control of pre-eclamptic hypertension must always be extended for a few days at least, and frequently for longer. Therefore, once the blood pressure has been controlled acutely the effects should be prolonged by medication which will lower the blood pressure in a more sustained way. The requirements are for a drug that is safe in pregnancy, has an onset of action in 6–12 hours, allows some titration of effect and can be safely combined with a second drug if needed. The choice lies between methyldopa and various beta-adrenergic blocking agents (beta-blockers).

Methyldopa, in adequate doses, can control blood pressure within 6–12 hours. A loading dose of 500–1000 mg is followed by 250–750 mg four times a day. If necessary, it can be given by slow intravenous infusion, but not by intramuscular injection. Sedation is the rule for the first 48 hours and tiredness thereafter is common. Postural hypotension is rarely a problem in the antenatal patient.

The safety of methyldopa in pregnancy has been established by case control studies (Leather et al 1968, Redman et al 1976c, Redman et al 1977b). No serious adverse fetal effects have yet been documented. Methyldopa crosses the placenta and accumulates in relatively high concentrations in amniotic fluid (Jones & Cummings 1978). Fetal heart rate variability is unaffected but there is a slight but discernible slowing of the fetal heart rate, and neonatal blood pressure is transiently reduced for a short period after delivery (Whitelaw 1981), yet none of these effects is clinically important. The infants in one case control study were followed up and assessed at the age of 7 years. The group exposed to methyldopa in utero were as well as their controls (Cockburn et al 1982); this establishes the longer-term safety of methyldopa in pregnancy.

The beta-blockers have the advantage of causing fewer subjective side-effects but their safety in pregnancy has not been so exhaustively investigated. A preparation such as atenolol has a slow onset of action and flat dose–response curve, which make the day-to-day titration of blood pressure control almost impossible. However, its short-term safety for the fetus and neonate has been adequately demonstrated (Rubin et al 1983). Oxprenolol and labetalol are faster-acting alternatives. Claims that oxprenolol promotes fetal growth (Gallery et al 1985) have not been substantiated (Fidler et al 1983). The agent preferred probably matters less than the clinician's familiarity with its use in achieving good control of blood pressure.

Postpartum hypertension

Arterial pressure progressively rises during the first 5 days after normal delivery (Walters et al 1986). This trend may be exaggerated in hypertensive women, so that the highest readings of all may be recorded during this period. Concurrently, the signs and symptoms of severe pre-eclampsia can appear for the first time postpartum, with the onset of epigastric pain (McKay 1972) and eclampsia. A maternal death has been reported following an eclamptic convulsion on the sixth day after delivery (Chapman & Karimi 1973). It is relatively unusual for these potential problems to be sought after delivery and inappropriately early postpartum discharge is one preventable factor associated with maternal death from pre-eclampsia or eclampsia (Hibbard 1973).

Postpartum hypertension needs to be managed, like antepartum hypertension, with treatment titrated so that severe hypertension is avoided. It is better not to use methyldopa because of the tiredness and depression that it causes. Labetalol is to be preferred to other beta-blocking agents because of its quick onset of action, but postural hypotension may be a problem. The patient can usually be discharged 6–8 days after delivery. Within 2–3 weeks of discharge antihypertensive treatment can normally be reduced or stopped, a decision which can be delegated to the general practitioner.

MANAGEMENT OF FLUID BALANCE AND PLASMA VOLUME

Salt restriction and diuretics

Pre-eclamptic oedema used to be treated both by salt restriction and the use of diuretics. Salt restriction can be an important part of the management of hypertension in non-pregnant patients but its use in pregnancy has been tested in only one controlled trial (Robinson 1958). Perinatal mortality in the salt-restricted group was significantly increased nearly twofold and was associated with more toxaemia in both nulliparous and parous patients. Other studies suggest that at least a high-salt diet is not detrimental (Chesley & Annitto 1943, Mengert & Tacchi 1961). Salt restriction is not without hazards, however, for it may aggravate renal impairment (Mule et al 1957) to the point of iatrogenic acute renal failure (Palomaki & Lindheimer 1970), or it may contribute to the puerperal shock syndrome once seen in severely pre-eclamptic patients (Tatum & Mule 1956). The evidence available provides no case for salt restriction in the prophylaxis or management of pre-eclampsia.

After their introduction, thiazide diuretics were widely prescribed for the prevention and treatment of pre-eclampsia. Nearly 7000 women were randomized in 11 controlled trials of varying size and quality. In the pooled data, the incidence of stillbirth was reduced by one-third, a difference which was not statistically significant (Collins et al 1985). Otherwise there was no evidence of benefit.

A number of serious side-effects have been associated with the use of thiazide diuretics. The fetal consequences of their diabetogenic action have not been defined. Diuretics have caused maternal death from pancreatitis, can cause hypokalaemia and, by causing hyperuricaemia, obscure one of the more useful signs of early pre-eclampsia. There is indirect evidence for reduced placental perfusion following diuretic therapy (Gant et al 1975). Diuretics should therefore not now be used in the management of pre-eclampsia, except for specific indications such as the rare complication of left ventricular failure.

Plasma volume expansion

Diuretics aggravate the hypovolaemia of severe pre-eclampsia and may precipitate renal failure. Some believe that the reduced circulating volume of pre-eclampsia induces a latent or actual state of shock (Cloeren & Lippert 1972) and that it is beneficial to expand the plasma volume to correct poor renal and placental function (Goodlin et al 1978, Morris & O'Grady 1979). No one questions that pre-eclamptic women are more vulnerable to blood loss and that this should be corrected promptly. But the evidence that there is a primary underfilling of the intact circulation is not good. Available data point to an abnormal leakiness with loss of fluid and plasma proteins from the vascular compartment. This may be temporarily corrected (over 30–60 minutes, for example) by infusing colloid solutions, but in the longer term such management may simply predispose to oedema formation in the lungs, brain or other tissues. Plasma volume expansion cannot therefore be considered part of the routine management of the pre-eclamptic patient.

Oliguria associated with pre-eclampsia or eclampsia

It is rare for a woman with stage 2 pre-eclampsia to require an indwelling urinary catheter, except during and for about 6 hours after Caesarean section. Oliguria (consistently less than 30 ml of urine per hour) is not necessarily abnormal. If it occurs, the most important priority is to define the reason why, before any treatment is given. The clinical reflex of giving more fluid and a diuretic without further thought is always incorrect. Oliguria may be a normal response to a poor fluid intake or to the stress of surgery. A reduction in urine output is to be expected after the arterial pressure has been effectively reduced by antihypertensive drugs. In two situations oliguria can be a cause for concern: pre-renal failure associated with blood loss at delivery and renal failure associated with DIC. The two problems may be combined with antepartum haemorrhage.

To assess blood volume depletion and its correction, it may be necessary to insert a central venous pressure (CVP) line in those who have had a massive blood loss or whose pre-eclampsia has progressed beyond the second stage. If the CVP is low it is better to infuse whole blood than colloid solutions, which in turn are preferable to electrolyte solutions. Overloading with the electrolyte solutions carries the risk of inducing pulmonary oedema. Some advocate pulmonary artery catheterization so that the pulmonary capillary wedge pressure can be measured and the results used to monitor the circulation whilst blood volume is being corrected (Clark et al 1986). This may be justified in rare cases, but only after the patient's supervision has been transferred to an intensive care team.

Renal failure associated with renal intravascular thrombosis as a result of DIC may be prevented but will not be reversed by expanding the blood volume. DIC can develop extremely rapidly so that the situation may need to be re-assessed every 4 hours. The platelet count, fibrinogen titre and thrombin time are simple screening tests, the last being prolonged when there are increased circulating fibrin and fibrinogen degradation products.

Diuretics should be reserved to control the complications of fluid overload. A single large intravenous dose of frusemide may be given as a diagnostic test in patients whose oliguria has not responded to volume replacement. If the urine output fails to increase then renal necrosis (tubular or cortical) may have already occurred.

MANAGEMENT OF THE COAGULATION DISTURBANCES

In general the only remedy for DIC is to correct the underlying problem. In pre-eclampsia this means ending pregnancy by delivery. With the knowledge that abnormal coagulation probably mediates at least some of the terminal complications of the disorder, various regimens of anticoagulation have been tried. Heparinization failed to modify the course of severe pre-eclampsia (Howie et al 1975). Prostacyclin infusion corrected the hypertension in one case, but not the underlying fetal problems which necessitated premature delivery (Fidler et al 1980). Successful prophylactic anticoagulation with warfarin has been reported twice (Valentine & Baker 1977, Schramm 1979). The dangers of anticoagulation in patients at risk of cerebral haemorrhage must be emphasized.

In routine clinical practice, anticoagulation should not be used either prophylactically or therapeutically. More recently, a prophylactic antiplatelet regimen (aspirin and dipyridamole) was associated with a significantly better perinatal outcome in a randomized controlled trial in high-risk subjects (Beaufils et al 1985). A further controlled trial of low-dose aspirin on its own successfully ameliorated the progression of pre-eclampsia in selected high-risk primigravidae (Wallenburg et al 1986). Thus there may be a place for antiplatelet therapy using low-dose aspirin if further trials give equally favourable results.

The poor haemostasis of individuals recovering from severe DIC postpartum can rarely cause intractable haemorrhage. Transfusions of platelets and fresh frozen plasma may be needed in addition to the replacement of whole blood as supportive treatment.

MANAGEMENT OF ECLAMPSIA

Time of occurrence

Eclampsia has been documented as early as 16 weeks of pregnancy (Lindheimer et al 1974), but is usually confined to the second half of pregnancy, occurring more commonly towards term (Templeton & Campbell 1979). In about half the cases convulsions begin before labour (Eden 1922, Bhose 1964, Porapakkham 1979). Most postpartum fits happen within 24 hours of delivery (Porapakkham 1979). Previously, it was disputed whether or not convulsions later than 48 hours after delivery could result from eclampsia (Jeffcoate & Scott 1959), but definite examples have now been described up to 23 days postpartum (Samuels 1960). Perhaps as many as half the cases of postpartum eclampsia occur more than 48 hours after delivery (Watson et al 1983).

Impending eclampsia — who to treat

The commonest difficulty is to identify accurately which patients are likely to have fits. Hyper-reflexia is an unreliable sign observed in most anxious individuals. The presence of ankle clonus is probably more informative: one or two beats is not uncommonly found and has little significance, but three or four beats is unusual and sustained clonus is definitely abnormal. More important is the subjective well-being of the patient. If she feels entirely well she is most unlikely to be about to have an eclamptic fit. Headaches, vomiting, or epigastric pain are all ominous complaints. The symptoms are, however, non-specific and all too easily discounted as the consequence of viral gastroenteritis or simply influenza. This should not happen in the hospitalized patient but the symptoms represent a diagnostic trap in the community when they are the first indication of the problem. A sudden cessation of urine output may be a premonitory sign in the catheterized patient. The level of the blood pressure, the degree of proteinuria and the presence or absence of oedema cannot be used to forecast whether fits are likely in the next few hours.

In some units the problem is side-stepped by treating all women with stage 2 pre-eclampsia with anticonvulsants. This is undesirable because it greatly increases the number of women treated, and therefore the risks of major side-effects.

Prevention and treatment of eclamptic fits

Because eclampsia is rare few have substantial experience of its management, so that individual investigators are unable to compare different regimens systematically. Different protocols of management have been recommended on the basis of uncontrolled case series but no controlled trials have been reported.

Given that the aim of good care is to prevent fits, it is disappointing that in the majority of cases the first eclamptic convulsion occurs after admission to hospital (Templeton & Campbell 1979, Gedekoh et al 1981, Sibai et al 1981). This indicates that either the women who are likely to have convulsions are not identified accurately or that the treatment given is ineffective.

It is not the grand mal convulsions themselves that are the dangerous feature of eclampsia so much as the severity of the underlying disturbances, which may include cerebral microinfarcts, oedema or haemorrhages. The priorities are to maintain the airway, stop the convulsions, control the blood pressure, then expedite delivery.

The use of anticonvulsants

The purpose of medical treatment is to prevent or control fitting, not to sedate the patient. Not all sedatives are anticonvulsants, nor all anticonvulsants sedatives. If a patient is deemed to need anticonvulsants she also needs urgent delivery. Treatment is a short-term holding measure whilst the underlying cause of the problem, the pregnancy, is ended. In the UK intravenous benzodiazepines or chlormethiazole have been preferred. Although these are the agents of choice for stopping convulsions, they are inappropriate for longer-term prevention of fits. In the USA parenteral magnesium sulphate is used. This is not a good agent for stopping seizures, but it appears to be effective for preventing them. Although not a routine in obstetric practice, it is better to consider the problems of stopping and preventing convulsions as separate. Thus diazepam is the treatment of choice to stop fits and magnesium sulphate or phenytoin to prevent recurrences.

Diazepam and chlordiazepoxide

The anticonvulsant action of these drugs is achieved only by intravenous administration. Diazepam is the treatment of choice to stop fits but its action is short-lived. A dose of 10 mg intravenously can be repeated intermittently as necessary with each new convulsion to a total of 50 mg. The continuous infusion of 10 mg/h (Lean et al 1968) should not be necessary except in the most intractable cases. Diazepam impairs consciousness and in high doses may depress respiration. It crosses the placenta rapidly, causing loss of fetal heart rate variation within 2 minutes of administration (Scher et al 1972). When maternal doses exceed 30 mg neonatal side-effects become prominent, including low Apgar scores, respiratory depression, poor feeding and hypothermia (Cree et al 1973). For these reasons diazepam should be used only to stop fits, not to maintain anticonvulsant treatment thereafter.

It has been claimed that the use of intravenous chlormethiazole avoids these neonatal problems. It is given as a 0.8% solution, with a loading dose of 40–100 ml to stop convulsions and then 60 ml/h to keep the patient drowsy but easily aroused. Neonatal depression is more likely if the total dose exceeds 12 g (1500 ml infusion; Duffus et al 1969). Respiratory depression is the main maternal risk.

Since it is preferable to avoid sedative preparations once fits have stopped, the choice lies between intravenous phenytoin or parenteral magnesium sulphate.

Phenytoin

There is little experience of the use of phenytoin in obstetrics (Slater et al 1987), although it is routinely prescribed in medical practice. It has a long half-life so that once an adequate loading dose has been given phenytoin should be given only once a day. It is absorbed slowly, variably and sometimes incompletely from the gut. To prevent recurrent fits acutely, 18 mg/kg is given intravenously at the rate of not more than 50 mg/min, with an onset of action after 20 minutes. If given too quickly cardiovascular collapse or central nervous system depression may occur. Electrocardiogram monitoring is desirable. The intravenous preparation is very alkaline and irritant to veins but should not be diluted to avoid precipitation.

Magnesium sulphate

This is administered intramuscularly or intravenously, achieving therapeutic plasma concentrations of 4–7 mmol/l. Its advantage is that it does not cause depression of the cerebral nervous system of either mother or neonate (Mordes & Wacker 1978). The mode of action is not known. A high extracellular magnesium concentration reduces the excitability of smooth muscle (Altura & Altura 1981), possibly by inhibiting entry of calcium ions into the cell. Responses of vascular smooth muscle to vasoconstrictor agents are diminished in vitro in this circumstance. In vivo, the effect of magnesium administration on pre-eclamptic hypertension is transient and slight (Pritchard 1955). However, extreme hypermagnesaemia has been associated with refractory hypotension in a non-gravid patient (Mordes et al 1975). Cardiac and uterine muscle contractility are also impaired. The side-effect of an overdose is cardiac arrest (McCubbin et al 1981). At high concentrations it also causes a relative blockade of the neuromuscular junction, which can lead to a loss of deep tendon reflexes or respiratory depression (Pritchard & Stone 1967).

Although in skilled hands it is clearly a safe and effective preparation, its side-effects include failure to control fits (Pritchard & Stone 1967, Sibai et al 1981), maternal death from overdosage (Hibbard 1973), hypocalcaemic tetany (Eisenbud & LoBue 1976) and neonatal hypermagnesaemia associated with hyporeflexia and respiratory depression (Lipsitz 1971). Its major disadvantages are the risk of toxicity and the lack of an understanding of its mode of action.

CARE OF THE FETUS

Pre-eclampsia is a placental disorder. The extent to which the associated maternal and fetal syndromes predominate varies from case to case. A severe maternal problem can coincide with relatively minor fetal problems or vice versa. Monitoring of the fetal state is therefore an essential part of management. It is vital to keep ahead of events, perhaps more so than in the care of the mother, because the fetus is inaccessible to direct examination and so assessment is harder and more time-consuming. In stage 1 pre-eclampsia it is necessary to estimate fetal size and monitor fetal growth. A baseline ultrasound assessment at 16–18 weeks is helpful as a reference point. Serial abdominal circumference measurements should be done every 2 weeks. In stage 2 pre-eclampsia it is important to monitor the fetus daily. Methods include fetal heart rate analysis (Smith et al 1988), ultrasound biophysical profiles (Manning et al 1980) and Doppler wave form analyses of the fetal circulation (Trudinger et al 1987).

WHEN TO DELIVER

The best timing of delivery is a matter of opinion and judgement, with few facts or absolute guidelines to help the inexperienced clinician. However, all women who have either stage 3 pre-eclampsia or eclampsia should be delivered without delay once their condition has been stabilized. This must be done regardless of gestational maturity. In the rare instances where these problems present at 26 weeks or earlier the decision is, in effect, one of late termination of pregnancy.

There must be compelling special reasons to leave women with proteinuric pre-eclampsia undelivered beyond 36 weeks. Indeed, after 34 weeks it becomes increasingly more difficult to justify conservative management. The same arguments can be transposed to women with definite non-proteinuric pre-eclampsia at 38–40 weeks. However, the practice of inducing *all* women with hypertension indiscriminately before term has little or no justification.

The most difficult problems arise with stage 2 pre-eclampsia presenting between 26 and 34 weeks of pregnancy. Although delivery is desirable it is not essential. If it can be deferred for 2 weeks or longer, significant maturation of the fetus may be achieved to reduce the problems of immaturity after birth. Conservative management of proteinuric pre-eclampsia can only be undertaken by an experienced team offering continuous monitoring and care. It is not easy, and sometimes impossible, for this to be achieved in understaffed busy units with heavy routine commitments. It is thus desirable for such patients to be moved at an early stage to specialized regional centres.

The conservative approach needs to be used with discretion and in the knowledge that in some patients it will achieve little or no gain in time. To defer delivery safely it is essential to know how all the maternal systems are affected by the disorder. The fetal state must also be reviewed continually. Delivery is necessary if the maternal blood pressure cannot be controlled, if the platelet count is less than $50 \times 10^9/l$, if the plasma creatinine has risen from normal levels to more than 120 mol, if there is evidence for liver damage or if the pre-eclampsia progresses to stage 3. Alternatively, increasing fetal problems may make extrauterine life safer. Any of these developments can happen unpredictably and suddenly, and will be missed unless the monitoring and care are maintained at a high level.

Of 122 cases of stage 2 pre-eclampsia presenting before 32 weeks in Oxford in 1980–1985, conservative management extended the life of the pregnancy beyond the onset of proteinuria by an average time of 15 days. A total of 31% were delivered because of maternal problems, 48% because of fetal problems and 7% because of both. The remainder were delivered non-urgently because adequate maturation had been achieved, or because they went into spontaneous labour. Five infants, all weighing less than 1000 g and all but one at less than 28 weeks, died in utero.

If premature delivery is necessary then the question arises as to whether corticosteroids should be given to accelerate fetal pulmonary maturation. There is no convincing evidence that there is benefit and there must be concern about the high doses of steroids which need to be given to women who are already suffering major systemic disturbances as a result of their pre-eclampsia. Possible side-effects of steroids given for this indication include gastrointestinal haemorrhage (Semchyshyn 1981), pulmonary oedema (Elliott et al 1979) and cardiopulmonary arrest (Iams et al 1980). Unless better evidence is forthcoming, steroids should not be given to pre-eclamptic women for this indication.

The mode of delivery is determined, amongst other variables, by the speed with which it must be expedited, the ability of the fetus to withstand labour and the chances of successful induction of labour at early gestational ages. As in other circumstances, vaginal delivery is always to be preferred if it is safe.

Even low doses of oxytocin (2–5 mu/min) are antidiuretic within 10–15 minutes of the start of the infusion (Abdul-Karim & Rizk 1970). If given intravenously with large volumes of 5% dextrose and water, this can cause hyponatraemia and convulsions (McKenna & Shaw 1979). The drug causes peripheral vasodilatation with a reflex tachycardia which may stimulate significant increases in cardiac output. If cardiac function is already compromised, as happens in rare cases of severe pre-eclampsia, myocardial failure may occur (Tepperman et al 1977).

In the management of the third stage, ergometrine should be avoided because it causes hypertension (Forman & Sullivan 1952) and Syntocinon should be used instead. The pre-eclamptic patient is particularly prone to hypertension following ergometrine (Baillie 1963) and headaches, convulsions and death have been reported as major sequelae (Tepperman et al 1977).

A woman with a shrunken intravascular compartment is less tolerant of blood loss than is the normal pregnant woman. Blood replacement must therefore be initiated sooner, but very carefully, to guard against the dangers of underfilling and overfilling.

Analgesia and anaesthesia for labour and delivery

Epidural analgesia has (Hibbard & Rosen 1977, Moore et al 1985) and has not (Pritchard & Pritchard 1975, Lindheimer & Katz 1985) been recommended for the management of pre-eclamptic women in labour. Those in favour point out that maternal cardiac output is unaffected (Newsome et al 1986), placental intervillous blood flow appears to be enhanced (Jouppila et al 1982) and that control of maternal blood pressure is improved (Willocks & Moir 1968, Graham & Goldstein 1980, Newsome et al 1986), although there is no effect on the maximum recorded pressures (Greenwood & Lilford 1986). No controlled trials have been reported, but if it is done with care, the procedure seems to be safe for the baby (Graham & Goldstein 1980, Moore et al 1985). The risk is of precipitating hypovolaemia through vasodilatation and pooling of the blood in the veins of the lower extremities. These problems can be anticipated and avoided, so that the benefits seem to outweigh the disadvantages. However, epidural analgesia is contraindicated if there is evidence of actual or incipient DIC. A knowledge of at least the platelet count is essential and, if less than $100\,000 \times 10^9/l$, the procedure should be avoided.

In many cases a Caesarean section has to be done too quickly to consider using epidural anaesthesia. Although general anaesthesia allows more precise control of the speed and timing of surgery, there are particular risks for pre-eclamptic women as well as those risks inherent in the procedure. Intubation may be difficult (Jouppila et al 1980) or impossible (Heller et al 1983) because of laryngeal oedema, which may also cause postoperative respiratory obstruction and cardiac arrest (Tillman Hein 1984). Laryngoscopy is a well known cause of extreme transient reflex hypertension in all individuals. The problem is aggravated in pre-eclamptic women (Hodgkinson et al 1980) and may be so extreme as to cause acute pulmonary oedema (Fox et al 1977).

Anticipating these problems is the key to their management. Laryngeal oedema is one of the few indications for the use of diuretics in pre-eclampsia; if it is anticipated an experienced and well briefed anaesthetist should do the intubation. The blood pressure swings at laryngoscopy are ameliorated if adequate control has been gained before the anaesthetic is given.

CHRONIC HYPERTENSION IN PREGNANCY

This group comprises women with essential and renal hypertension, and hypertension caused by miscellaneous but rare conditions. The first problem is most commonly encountered. Women with essential hypertension tend to be older and parous, heavier and to have a family history of hypertension. As already mentioned, an individual with chronic hypertension may appear normotensive when she starts antenatal care early in the second trimester and then show a rise in blood pressure in the third trimester of a degree which resembles pre-eclampsia. This has led to considerable diagnostic confusion but explains why third-trimester hypertension segregates into two groups: non-recurrent, affecting primigravidae and with a raised perinatal mortality, and recurrent, affecting multiparae with a good perinatal outcome (Adams & MacGillivray 1961, MacGillivray 1982). The former group would have pre-eclampsia as defined in this chapter, while the latter probably have chronic hypertension. The only sure way to detect chronic hypertension in pregnancy is to refer to pre-pregnancy readings, or if as is usual these are not available, to reassess the blood pressure at a remote time after delivery. If blood pressures are consistently at or above 140/90 mmHg in the first half of pregnancy, then chronic hypertension can be inferred. Not uncommonly the presentation is of mild hypertension alone in the second half of pregnancy without any antecedent readings. It is not possible in these circumstances to distinguish chronic hypertension from pre-eclampsia with absolute certainty.

Chronic hypertension is one of the major predisposing factors to pre-eclampsia; the two conditions, which in their pure forms are easily separable, may commonly occur together. Pre-eclampsia superimposed on chronic hypertension tends to be recurrent in later pregnancies, whereas it is not in normotensive individuals. It used to be thought that chronic hypertension was extremely dangerous when combined with pregnancy (Browne & Dodds 1942). It is now clear that the particular risks of chronic hypertension in pregnancy are entirely attributable to the increased chance of developing superimposed pre-eclampsia, and that the majority of chronically hypertensive women who do not develop pre-eclampsia can expect a normal perinatal outcome (Chamberlain et al 1978b).

The signs of pre-eclampsia in chronically hypertensive women are the same as in other women, except that the blood pressure levels start from a higher baseline. Thus a rise in the blood pressure, progressive hyperuricaemia or abnormal activation of the clotting system herald the appearance of superimposed pre-eclampsia which will progress to proteinuria unless pre-empted by delivery. When proteinuria develops, intrauterine growth retardation is almost the rule.

It is not uncommon for a woman with chronic hypertension to be on antihypertensive treatment before conception. None of the commonly used antihypertensive drugs is known to be teratogenic. However, some women treated for mild or moderate chronic hypertension can safely stop their treatment before conception to keep fetal drug exposure to a minimum. Amongst those who must continue are some whose blood pressures will fall enough by 3 months of pregnancy to be able to stop treatment at that time. Diuretics and angiotensin-converting enzyme inhibitors are the two preparations to avoid if possible. Although angiotensin-converting enzyme inhibitors have been given to women who have had successful pregnancies, there are anxieties about their safety for the fetus, based on animal experiments. In the last 3 months of pregnancy it can be anticipated that more medication will be needed to maintain blood pressure control.

In general medical practice, the purpose of treating blood pressures in the range of 140–170/90–110 mmHg is to prevent the long-term complications of hypertension. On this timescale, whether or not treatment is used during the brief period of gestation is irrelevant. For this reason, the indication for treatment in women with this degree of chronic hypertension would be to prevent the superimposition of pre-eclampsia, the only major short-term problem. In fact, there is clear evidence, based on a large randomized controlled trial, that the early control of moderate chronic hypertension does not confer this benefit (Redman 1980). Thus there is no fetal indication for the control of moderate hypertension in pregnancy — medical management should be decided solely on considerations of maternal safety.

POSTPARTUM FOLLOW-UP

Severe pre-eclampsia and eclampsia can cause irreversible maternal damage, particularly acute renal and cortical necrosis or cerebral haemorrhage. In the absence of these complications there is no evidence that long-term health is impaired by a pre-eclamptic illness. In terms of life expectancy pre-eclamptic women fall into two groups: those who have an episode only in their first pregnancy and become normotensive soon after delivery have a normal life expectancy. The second group have recurrent pre-eclampsia in several pregnancies, or blood pressures which remain elevated in the puerperium. They have a higher incidence of later cardiovascular disorders and a reduced life expectancy, compatible with the diagnosis that the initial episode of pre-eclampsia was superimposed on pre-existing hypertension (Chesley et al 1976).

The postpartum follow-up of a woman who has had severe pre-eclampsia should include assessment of blood pressure and renal status not earlier than 6 weeks after delivery. Pre-eclampsia may be the event which reveals chronic renal disease or pre-existing hypertension, indicating the need for further investigation and management. Women with persisting renal impairment with or without proteinuria need an intravenous pyelogram; occasionally renal biopsy is required to define the cause of their problem. Women with persisting hypertension need to have the nature of their problem fully explained. For most, all that is required is to organize a regular review of the blood pressure once or twice a year. For some, it is necessary to continue treatment indefinitely. The reasons need to be fully explained and other measures which can mitigate the problem should be emphasized: weight loss, avoidance of excessive salt intake, stopping smoking. Very rarely an individual with severe hypertension is identified who may need further investigation, for example, angiography to exclude renal artery stenosis. Advice about family planning needs to be given. Oral contraceptives are a cause of hypertension which may be severe and rarely malignant. For this reason chronic hypertension is a relative contraindication to their use. The advice given to postpartum women should be guided by whether or not hypertension persists as a chronic problem. If a pre-eclamptic woman's blood pressure returns to normal, then she need not be denied the benefits of oral contraceptives provided adequate and continuing medical supervision is available.

Women who have suffered severe pre-eclampsia want to know the outlook for another pregnancy, an issue which is made more difficult if the recent pregnancy resulted in a perinatal death. In general, the outlook is better than the patients think, but not as good as they would like. The risk of recurrence in a second pregnancy is about 1 in 20. The odds should be increased if there are underlying medical problems to about 1 in 10. Every obstetrician will encounter rare individuals who have repeated episodes of severe pre-eclampsia, often without a surviving child. Each further episode increases the risk of recurrence in another pregnancy.

CONCLUSIONS

Pre-eclampsia and eclampsia are the commonest causes of curable hypertension in medical practice. They are primarily disorders of the placenta and placental bed which cause both maternal and fetal syndromes; they constitute a major cause of maternal death as well as of perinatal death, prematurity and fetal growth retardation.

The disorder is unpredictable and variable in its onset and evolution, but is always reversed by delivery. Pre-eclampsia is detected by screening the asymptomatic patient; its complications are pre-empted by well timed delivery.

The onset of proteinuria indicates advanced disease requiring admission to hospital on the day of detection, even if the blood pressure is only mildly elevated. The onset of symptoms is a terminal development which precedes eclamptic convulsions. Ideally all women should be delivered before this stage is reached. Control of the maternal blood pressure is an essential part of management to protect the mother from the risk of cerebral haemorrhage and generalized arteriolar injury.

REFERENCES

Aalkjaer C, Danielsen H, Johannesen P, Pedersen E B, Rasmussen A, Mulvany M J 1985 Abnormal vascular function and morphology in pre-eclampsia: a study of isolated resistance vessels. Clinical Science 69: 477–482

Aarnoudse J G, Houthoff H J, Weits J, Vellenga E, Huisjes H 1986 A syndrome of liver damage and intravascular coagulation in the last trimester of normotensive pregnancy. British Journal of Obstetrics and Gynaecology 93: 145–155

Abdul-Karim R, Assali N S 1961 Pressor response to angiotonin in pregnant and non-pregnant women. American Journal of Obstetrics and Gynecology 82: 246–251

Abdul-Karim R W, Rizk P T 1970 The effect of oxytocin on renal hemodynamics, water and electrolyte excretion. Obstetrical and Gynecological Survey 25: 805–813

Abitbol M M 1969 Weight gain in pregnancy. American Journal of Obstetrics and Gynecology 104: 140–156

Abitbol M M 1977 Hemodynamic studies in experimental toxemia of the dog. Obstetrics and Gynecology 50: 293–298

Adams E M, MacGillivray I 1961 Long-term effect of pre-eclampsia on blood pressure. Lancet ii: 1373–1375

Altura B M, Altura B T 1981 Magnesium ions and contraction of vascular smooth muscles: relationships to some vascular diseases. Federation Proceedings 40: 2672–2679

Arias F, Mancilla-Jimenez R 1976 Hepatic fibrinogen deposits in pre-eclampsia. New England Journal of Medicine 295: 578–582

Assali N S, Kaplan S, Oighenstein S, Suyemoto R 1953 Hemodynamic effects of 1-hydrazinophthalazine in human pregnancy; results of intravenous administration. Journal of Clinical Investigation 32: 922–930

Assali N S, Holm L W, Parker H R 1964 Systemic and regional hemodynamic alterations in toxemia. Circulation 29, 30 (suppl II): 53–57

Augensen K, Bergsjo P 1984 Maternal mortality in the Nordic countries 1970–1979. Acta Obstetricia et Gynecologica Scandinavica 63: 115–121

Baillie T W 1963 Vasopressor activity of ergometrine maleate in anaesthetised parturient women. British Medical Journal 1: 585–588

Baird D 1977 Epidemiological aspects of hypertensive pregnancy. Clinics in Obstetrics and Gynaecology 4: 531–548
Baird D, Thomson A M, Billewicz W Z 1957 Birthweights and placental weights in pre-eclampsia. Journal of Obstetrics and Gynaecology of the British Commonwealth 64: 370–372
Beaudry P H, Sutherland J M 1960 Birth weights of infants of toxemic mothers. Journal of Pediatrics 56: 505–509
Beaufils M, Uzan S, Donsimoni R, Colau J C 1985 Prevention of pre-eclampsia by early antiplatelet therapy. Lancet i: 840–842
Beck D W, Menezes A H 1981 Intracerebral hemorrhage in a patient with eclampsia. Journal of the American Medical Association 246: 1442–1443
Beeson J H, Duda E E 1982 Computed axial tomography scan demonstration of cerebral edema in eclampsia preceded by blindness. Obstetrics and Gynecology 60: 529–532
Benedetti T J, Carlson R W 1979 Studies of colloid osmotic pressure in pregnancy induced hypertension. American Journal of Obstetrics and Gynecology 135: 308–311
Benedetti T J, Cotton D B, Read J C, Miller F C 1980 Hemodynamic observations in severe pre-eclampsia with a flow-directed pulmonary artery catheter. American Journal of Obstetrics and Gynecology 136: 465–470
Bhose L 1964 Postpartum eclampsia. American Journal of Obstetrics and Gynecology 89: 898–902
Bing R F, Smith A J 1981 Plasma and interstitial volumes in essential hypertension: relationship to blood pressure. Clinical Science 61: 287–293
Bis K A, Waxman B 1976 Rupture of the liver associated with pregnancy: a review of the literature and report of two cases. Obstetrical and Gynecological Survey 31: 763–773
Blair R G 1963 Phaeochromocytoma and pregnancy. Journal of Obstetrics and Gynaecology of the British Commonwealth 70: 110–119
Boneu B, Fournie A, Sie P, Grandjean H, Bierme R, Pontonnier G 1980 Platelet production time, uricemia and some hemostasis tests in pre-eclampsia. European Journal of Obstetrics, Gynecology and Reproductive Biology 11: 85–94
Bonnar J 1975 The blood coagulation and fibrinolytic systems during pregnancy. Clinics in Obstetrics and Gynaecology 2: 321–343
Bonnar J, McNicol G P, Douglas A S 1969 Fibrinolytic enzyme system and pregnancy. British Medical Journal 3: 387–389
Brain M C, Dacie J V, Hourihane D O'B 1962 Microangiopathic haemolytic anaemia: the possible role of vascular lesions in pathogenesis. British Journal of Haematology 8: 358–374
Brosens I 1964 A study of the spiral arteries of the decidua basalis in normotensive and hypertensive pregnancies. British Journal of Obstetrics and Gynaecology 71: 222–230
Brosens I A, Robertson W B, Dixon H G 1972 The role of the spiral arteries in the pathogenesis of pre-eclampsia. In Wynn R M (ed) Obstetrics and gynecology annual. Appleton Century-Crofts, New York, pp 177–191
Brosens I, Dixon H G, Robertson W B 1977 Fetal growth retardation and the arteries of the placental bed. British Journal of Obstetrics and Gynaecology 84: 656–663
Broughton Pipkin F, Hunter J C, Turner S R, O'Brien P M S 1982 Prostaglandin E_2 attenuates the pressor response to angiotensin II in pregnant subjects but not in nonpregnant subjects. American Journal of Obstetrics and Gynecology 142: 168–176
Browne F J, Dodds G H 1942 Pregnancy in the patient with chronic hypertension. Journal of Obstetrics and Gynaecology of the British Empire 49: 1–17
Burstein R, Blumenthal H T, Soule S D 1957 Histogenesis of pathological processes in placentas of metabolic diseases of pregnancy. I. Toxemia and hypertension. American Journal of Obstetrics and Gynecology 74: 85–95
Butler N R, Bonham D G 1963 Toxemia in pregnancy. Perinatal mortality. E. and S. Livingstone, Edinburgh, pp 87–100
Byrom F B 1954 Pathogenesis of hypertensive encephalopathy and its relation to the malignant phase of hypertension. Experimental evidence from the hypertensive rat. Lancet ii: 201–211
Campbell D M, MacGillivray I 1985 Pre-eclampsia in second pregnancy. British Journal of Obstetrics and Gynaecology 82: 131–140
Campbell S, Pearce J M F, Hackett G, Cohen-Overbeek T, Hernandez C 1986 Qualitative assessment of uteroplacental blood flow: early screening test for high-risk pregnancies. Obstetrics and Gynecology 68: 649–653
Cavanagh D, Rao P S, Tsai C C, O'Connor T C 1977 Experimental toxemia in the pregnant primate. American Journal of Obstetrics and Gynecology 128: 75–85
Chamberlain G V P, Lewis P J, DeSwiet M, Bulpitt J J 1978a How obstetricians manage hypertension in pregnancy. British Medical Journal i: 626–629
Chamberlain G V P, Philipp E, Howlett B, Masters K 1978b British births 1970. Heinemann, London, pp 80–107
Chapman K, Karimi R 1973 A case of post partum eclampsia of late onset confirmed by autopsy. American Journal of Obstetrics and Gynecology 117: 858–861
Chesley L C 1939 The variability of proteinuria in the hypertensive complications of pregnancy. Journal of Clinical Investigation 18: 617–620
Chesley L C 1976 Blood pressure, edema and proteinuria in pregnancy. Progress in Clinical Biology Research 7: 249–268
Chesley L C 1978a Hypertensive disorders in pregnancy. Appleton-Century-Crofts, New York, pp 157–162
Chesley L C 1978b Hypertensive disorders of pregnancy, Appleton-Century-Crofts, New York, p 34
Chesley L C 1978c Hypertensive disorders in pregnancy, Appleton-Century-Crofts, New York, p 210
Chesley L C 1984 Habitus and eclampsia. Obstetrics and Gynecology 64: 315–318
Chesley L C, Annitto J E 1943 A study of salt restriction and of fluid intake in prophylaxis against pre-eclampsia in patients with water retention. American Journal of Obstetrics and Gynecology 45: 961–971
Chesley L C, Annitto J E 1947 Pregnancy in the patient with hypertensive disease. American Journal of Obstetrics and Gynecology 53: 372–381
Chesley L C, Cooper D W 1986 Genetics of hypertension in pregnancy: possible single gene control of pre-eclampsia and eclampsia in the descendants of eclamptic women. British Journal of Obstetrics and Gynaecology 93: 898–908
Chesley L C, Williams L O 1945 Renal glomerular and tubular functions in relation to the hyperuricaemia of pre-eclampsia and eclampsia. American Journal of Obstetrics and Gynecology 50: 367–375
Chesley L C, Annitto J E, Jarvis D G 1947 A study of the interaction of pregnancy and hypertensive disease. American Journal of Obstetrics and Gynecology 53: 851–863
Chesley L C, Annitto J E, Cosgrove R A 1968 The familial factor in toxemia of pregnancy. Obstetrics and Gynecology 32: 303–311
Chesley L C, Annitto J E, Cosgrove R A 1976 The remote prognosis of eclamptic women. Sixth periodic report. American Journal of Obstetrics and Gynecology 124: 446–459
Chester E M, Agamanolis D P, Banker B Q, Victor M 1978 Hypertensive encephalopathy: a clinicopathologic study of 20 cases. Neurology 28: 928–939
Chun D, Braga C, Chow C, Lok L 1964 Clinical observations on some aspects of hydatidiform moles. Journal of Obstetrics and Gynaecology of the British Commonwealth 71: 180–184
Claireaux A E 1961 Perinatal mortality in toxaemia of pregnancy. Pathologia et Microbiologica 24: 607–621
Clark S L, Greenspoon J S, Aldahl D, Phelan J P 1986 Severe pre-eclampsia with persistent oliguria: management of hemodynamic subsets. American Journal of Obstetrics and Gynecology 154: 490–494
Clarke E, Murphy E A 1956 Neurological manifestations of malignant hypertension. British Medical Journal ii: 1319–1326
Cloeren S E, Lippert T H 1972 Effect of plasma expanders in toxemia of pregnancy. New England Journal of Medicine 278: 1356–1357
Cockburn J, Moar V A, Ounsted M, Redman C W G 1982 Final report of study on hypertension during pregnancy: the effects of specific treatment on the growth and development of the children. Lancet i: 647–649
Coden J 1972 Phaeochromocytoma in pregnancy. Journal of the Royal Society of Medicine 65: 863
Cohn J N 1967 Blood pressure measurement in shock. Journal of the American Medical Association 199: 972–976
Collins R, Yusuf S, Peto R 1985 Overview of randomised trials of diuretics in pregnancy. British Medical Journal 290: 17–23
Cooper D W, Liston W A 1979 Genetic control of severe pre-eclampsia. Journal of Medical Genetics 16: 409–416

Corkill T F 1961 Experience of toxaemia control in Australia and New Zealand. Pathologia et Microbiologica 24: 428–434
Crawford D M 1941 Plasma uric acid and urea findings in eclampsia. Journal of Obstetrics and Gynaecology of the British Empire 48: 60–72
Cree J E, Meyer J, Hailey D M 1973 Diazepam in labour: its metabolism and effect on the clinical condition and thermogenesis of the newborn. British Medical Journal 4: 251–255
Davey D A, MacGillivray I 1986 The classification and definition of the hypertensive disorders of pregnancy. Clinical and Experimental Hypertension B5: 97–133
Davies A M 1971 Georgraphical epidemiology of the toxemias of pregnancy. Israel Journal of Medical Sciences 7: 753–821
Davies A M, Czaczkes J W, Sadovsky E, Prywes R, Weiskopf P, Sterk V V 1970 Toxemia of pregnancy in Jerusalem I. Epidemiological studies of a total community. Israel Journal of Medical Sciences 6: 253–266
Davies M H, Wilkinson S P, Hanid M A et al 1980 Acute liver disease with encephalopathy and renal failure in late pregnancy and the early puerperium: a study of 14 patients. British Journal of Obstetrics and Gynaecology 87: 1005–1014
Dennis E J, Smythe C M, McIver F A, Howe H G 1963 Percutaneous renal biopsy in eclampsia. American Journal of Obstetrics and Gynecology 87: 364–371
Denson K W E 1977 The ratio of factor VIII-related antigen and factor VIII biological activity as an index of hypercoagulability and intravascular clotting. Thrombosis Research 10: 107–119
Department of Health and Social Security 1986 Report on confidential enquiries into maternal deaths in England and Wales 1979–1981. HMSO, London, pp 13–21
De Souza S W, John R W, Richards B 1976 Studies on the effect of maternal pre-eclamptic toxaemia on placental weight and on head size and birth weight of the newborn. British Journal of Obstetrics and Gynaecology 83: 292–298
De Wolf F, Brosens I, Renaer M 1980 Fetal growth retardation and the maternal arterial supply of the human placenta in the absence of sustained hypertension. British Journal of Obstetrics and Gynaecology 87: 678–685
Dieckmann W J, Michel H L 1973 Vascular-renal effects of posterior pituitary extracts in pregnant women. American Journal of Obstetrics and Gynecology 33: 131–137
Dixon H G, McClure Browne J C, Davey D A 1963 Choriodecidual and myometrial blood-flow. Lancet ii: 369–373
Donchin Y, Amirav B, Sahar A, Yarkoni S 1978 Sodium nitroprusside for aneurysm surgery in pregnancy. British Journal of Anaesthesia 50: 849–851
Douglas J T, Shah M, Lowe G D O, Belch J J F, Forbes C D, Prentice C R M 1982 Plasma fibrinopeptide A and beta-thromboglobulin in pre-eclampsia and pregnancy hypertension. Thrombosis and Haemostasis 47: 54–55
Duffus G, MacGillivray I 1968 The incidence of pre-eclamptic toxaemia in smokers and non-smokers. Lancet i: 994–995
Duffus G M, Tunstall M E, Condie R G, MacGillivray I 1969 Chlormethiazole in the prevention of eclampsia and the reduction of perinatal mortality. Journal of Obstetrics and Gynaecology of the British Commonwealth 76: 645–651
Duffus G M, MacGillivray I, Dennis K J 1971 The relationship between baby weight and changes in maternal weight, total body water, plasma volume, electrolytes and proteins and urinary oestriol excretion. Journal of Obstetrics and Gynaecology of the British Commonwealth 78: 97–104
Eden T W 1922 Eclampsia: a commentary on the reports presented to the British Congress of Obstetrics and Gynaecology. Journal of Obstetrics and Gynaecology of the British Empire 29: 386–401
Edouard L, Alberman E 1980 National trends in the certified causes of perinatal mortality, 1968 to 1978. British Journal of Obstetrics and Gynaecology 87: 833–838
Eisenbud E, LoBue C C 1976 Hypocalcemia after therapeutic use of magnesium sulfate. Archives of Internal Medicine 136: 688–691
Elliott J P, O'Keeffe D F, Greenberg P, Freeman R K 1979 Pulmonary edema associated with magnesium sulfate and betamethasone administration. American Journal of Obstetrics and Gynecology 134: 717–719
Everett R B, Worley R J, MacDonald P C, Gant N F 1978 Effect of prostaglandin synthetase inhibitors on pressor response to angiotensin II in human pregnancy. Journal of Clinical Endocrinology and Metabolism 46: 1007–1010.
Fadel H E, Northrop G, Misenhimer R H 1976 Hyperuricaemia in pre-eclampsia. American Journal of Obstetrics and Gynecology 125: 640–647
Felding C F 1969 Obstetric aspects in women with histories of renal disease. Acta Obstetricia et Gynecologica Scandinavica 48 (suppl 2): 1–43
Fidler J, Bennett M J, De Swiet M, Ellis C, Lewis P J 1980 Treatment of pregnancy hypertension with prostacyclin. Lancet ii: 31–32
Fidler J, Smith V, Fayers P, De Swiet M 1983 Randomised controlled comparative study of methyl dopa and oxprenolol for the treatment of hypertension in pregnancy. British Medical Journal 286: 1927–1930
Fisher E R, Pardo V, Paul R, Hayashi T T 1969 Ultrastructural studies in hypertension. IV. Toxemia of pregnancy. American Journal of Pathology 55: 109–131
Fisher K A, Ahuja S, Luger A, Spargo B, Lindheimer M 1977 Nephrotic proteinuria with pre-eclampsia. American Journal of Obstetrics and Gynecology 129: 643–646
Fitzgerald T B, Clift A D 1958 Foetal loss in pregnancy toxaemia. Lancet i: 283–286
Fletcher A P, Alkjaersig N K, Burstein R 1979 The influence of pregnancy upon blood coagulation and plasma fibrinolytic enzyme function. American Journal of Obstetrics and Gynecology 134: 743–751
Forman J B, Sullivan R L 1952 The effects of intravenous injections of ergonovine and methergine on the post partum patient. American Journal of Obstetrics and Gynecology 63: 640–644
Fox E J, Sklar G J, Hill C H, Villanueva R, King B D 1977 Complications related to the pressor response. Anesthesiology 47: 524–525
Freis E D, Kenny J F 1948 Plasma volume, total circulating protein and available fluid abnormalities in pre-eclampsia and eclampsia. Journal of Clinical Investigation 27: 283–289
Freis E D, Rose J A, Higgins T F, Finnerty F A, Kelly R T, Partenope E A 1953 The hemodynamic effects of hypotensive drugs in man IV. 1 — Hydrazinophthalazine. Circulation 8: 199–204
Fullerton W T, Hytten F E, Klopper A I, McKay E 1965 A case of quadruplet pregnancy. Journal of Obstetrics and Gynaecology of the British Commonwealth 72: 791–796
Gaitz J P, Bamford C R 1982 Unusual computed tomographic scan in eclampsia. Archives of Neurology 39: 66
Gallery E D M, Hunyor S N, Gyory A Z 1979 Plasma volume contraction: a significant factor in both pregnancy-associated hypertension (pre-eclampsia) and chronic hypertension in pregnancy. Quarterly Journal of Medicine 48: 593–602
Gallery E D M, Ross M R, Gyory A Z 1985 Antihypertensive treatment in pregnancy: analysis of different responses to oxprenolol and methyldopa. British Medical Journal 291: 563–566
Gant N F, Daley G L, Chand S, Whalley P J, MacDonald P C 1973 A study of angiotensin II pressor response throughout primigravid pregnancy. Journal of Clinical Investigation 52: 2682–2689
Gant N F, Madden J D, Siiteri P K, MacDonald P C 1975 The metabolic clearance rate of dehydroisoandrosterone. III. The effect of thiazide diuretics in normal and future pre-eclamptic pregnancies. American Journal of Obstetrics and Gynecology 123: 159–163
Garden A, Davey D A, Dommisse J 1982 Intravenous labetalol and intravenous dihydralazine in severe hypertension in pregnancy. Clinical and Experimental Hypertension [B] 1: 371–383
Gedekoh R H, Hayashi T T, MacDonald H M 1981 Eclampsia at Magee Women's Hospital 1970–1980. American Journal of Obstetrics and Gynecology 140: 860–866
Giese J 1964 Acute hypertensive vascular disease. 1. Relation between blood pressure changes and vascular lesions in different forms of acute hypertension. Acta Pathologica et Microbiologica Scandinavica 62: 481–496
Giles C, Inglis T C M (1981) Thrombocytopenia and macrothrombocytosis in gestational hypertension. British Journal of Obstetrics and Gynaecology 88: 1115–1119
Girard H, Brun J-L, Muffat-Joly M 1971 An angiographic study of the sensitivity to epinephrine of the uterine arteries of the guinea pig: a comparison with angiotensin. American Journal of Obstetrics and Gynecology 111: 687–691
Goldby F S, Beilin L J 1972 Relationship between arterial pressure and the permeability of arterioles to carbon particles in acute hypertension in the rat. Cardiovascular Research 6: 384–390

Goldfinger S, Klinenberg J R, Seegmiller J E 1965 Renal retention of uric acid induced by infusion of beta-hydroxybutyrate and acetoacetate. New England Journal of Medicine 272: 351–355

Goodlin R C 1983 Safety of sodium nitroprusside. Obstetrics and Gynecology 62: 270

Goodlin R C, Cotton D B, Haesslein H C 1978 Severe edema-proteinuria-hypertension gestosis. American Journal of Obstetrics and Gynecology 132: 595–598

Graham C, Goldstein A 1980 Epidural analgesia and cardiac output in severe pre-eclampsia. Anaesthesia 35: 709–712

Greenwood P A, Lilford R J 1986 Effect of epidural analgesia on maximum and minimum blood pressures during the first stage of labour in primigravidae with mild/moderate gestational hypertension. British Journal of Obstetrics and Gynaecology 93: 260–263

Grimes D A, Ekbladh L E, McCartney W H 1980 Cortical blindness in pre-eclampsia. International Journal of Gynecology and Obstetrics 17: 601–603

Groenendijk R, Trimbos J B M J, Wallenburg H C S 1984 Hemodynamic measurements in pre-eclampsia: preliminary observations. American Journal of Obstetrics and Gynecology 150: 232–236

Gruenwald P 1966 Growth of the human fetus. II. Abnormal growth in twins and infants of mothers with diabetes, hypertension or isoimmunisation. American Journal of Obstetrics and Gynecology 94: 1120–1132

Harley J M G 1966 Pregnancy in the chronic hypertensive woman. Proceedings of the Royal Society of Medicine 39: 835–838

Hauch E, Lehmann K 1934 Investigations into the occurrence of eclampsia in Denmark during the years 1918–1927. Acta Obstetricia et Gynecologica Scandinavica 14: 425–481

Hayashi T 1956 Uric acid and endogenous creatinine clearance studies in normal pregnancy and toxemias of pregnancy. American Journal of Obstetrics and Gynecology 71: 859–870

Heller P J, Scheider E P, Marx G F 1983 Pharolaryngeal edema as a presenting symptom in pre-eclampsia. Obstetrics and Gynecology 62: 523–524

Henrich W L, Cronin R, Miller P D, Anderson R J 1977 Hypertensive sequelae of diazoxide and hydralazine therapy. Journal of the American Medical Association 237: 264–265

Hibbard L T 1973 Maternal mortality due to acute toxemia. Obstetrics and Gynecology 42: 263–270

Hibbard B M, Rosen M 1977 The management of severe pre-eclampsia and eclampsia. British Journal of Anaesthesia 49: 3–9

Hodgkinson R, Husain F J, Hayashi R H 1980 Systemic and pulmonary blood pressure during caesarean section in parturients with gestational hypertension. Canadian Anaesthetists' Society Journal 27: 385–394

Horne C H W, Howie P W, Goudie R B 1970 Serum alpha$_2$-macro-globulin, transferrin, albumin and IgG levels in pre-eclampsia. Journal of Clinical Pathology 23: 514–516

Howie P W, Prentice C R M, Forbes C D 1975 Failure of heparin therapy to affect the clinical course of severe pre-eclampsia. British Journal of Obstetrics and Gynaecology 82: 711–717

Hughes E C 1972 Hypertensive states of pregnancy — classification. In Obstetric–gynecologic terminology. Davis, Philadelphia pp 422–423

Hytten F E, Paintin D B 1963 Increase in plasma volume during normal pregnancy. Journal of Obstetrics and Gynaecology of the British Commonwealth 70: 402–407

Iams J D, Semchyshyn S, O'Shaughnessy R, Moynihan V, Zuspan F 1980 Blood pressure response in hypertensive pregnancies treated with cortisol. Clinical and Experimental Hypertension 2: 923–932

Jacobs M 1984 Mechanism of action of hydralazine on vascular smooth muscle. Biochemical Pharmacology 33: 2915–2919

Jeffcoate T N A, Scott J S 1959 Some observations on the placental factor in pregnancy toxemia. American Journal of Obstetrics and Gynecology 77: 475–489

Jellinek E H, Painter M, Prineas J, Russell R R 1964 Hypertensive encephalopathy with cortical disorders of vision. Quarterly Journal of Medicine 33: 239–256

Johansson B, Strandgaard S, Lassen N A 1974 On the pathogenesis of hypertensive encephalopathy. Circulation Research 34 (suppl 1): 167–171

Johnson T, Clayton C G 1957 Diffusion of radioactive sodium in normotensive and pre-eclamptic pregnancies. British Medical Journal 1: 312–314

Jones H M R, Cummings A J 1978 A study of the transfer of alpha-methyldopa to the human fetus and newborn infant. British Journal of Clinical Pharmacology 6: 432–434

Jouppila R, Jouppila P, Hollmen A 1980 Laryngeal oedema as an obstetric anaesthesia complication: case reports. Acta Anaesthesiologica Scandinavica 24: 97–98

Jouppila P, Jouppila R, Hollmen A, Koivula A 1982 Lumbar epidural analgesia to improve intervillous blood flow during labour in severe pre-eclampsia. Obstetrics and Gynecology 59: 158–161

Jouppila P, Kirkinen P, Koivula A, Ylikorkala O 1985 Effects of dihydralazine infusion on the fetoplacental blood flow and maternal prostanoids. Obstetrics and Gynecology 65: 115–118

Joyce D N, Kenyon V G 1972 The use of diazepam and hydralazine in the treatment of severe pre-eclampsia. Journal of Obstetrics and Gynaecology of the British Commonwealth 79: 250–254

Kaulhausen H, Oney T, Leyendecker G 1982 Inhibition of the renin–aldosterone axis and of prolactin secretion during pregnancy by L-dopa. British Journal of Obstetrics and Gynaecology 89: 483–488

Kaunitz A M, Hughes J M, Grimes D A, Smith J C, Rochat R W, Kafrissen M E 1985 Causes of maternal mortality in the United States. Obstetrics and Gynecology 65: 605–612

Killam A, Dillard S., Patton R, Pederson P 1975 Pregnancy-induced hypertension complicated by acute liver disease and disseminated intravascular coagulation. American Journal of Obstetrics and Gynecology 123: 823–828

Kincaid-Smith P, McMichael J, Murphy E A 1958 The clinical course and pathology of hypertension with papilloedema (malignant hypertension). Quarterly Journal of Medicine 27: 117–153

Kirby J C, Jaindl J J 1984 Cerebral CT findings in toxemia of pregnancy. Radiology 151: 114

Kirkendall W M, Feinleib M, Freis E D, Mark A L 1981 Recommendations for human blood pressure determination by sphygmomanometers. Sub-committee of the AHA postgraduate education committee. Hypertension 3: 510A–519A

Kuzniar J, Piela A, Skret A, Szmigiel Z B, Zaczek T 1982 Echocardiographic estimation of hemodynamics in hypertensive pregnancy. American Journal of Obstetrics and Gynecology 144: 430–437

Ladner C, Brinkman C R, Weston P, Assali N S 1970 Dynamics of uterine circulation in pregnant and nonpregnant sheep. American Journal of Physiology 218: 257–263

Lean T H, Ratnam S S, Sivasamboo R 1968 The use of chlordiazepoxide in patients with severe pregnancy toxaemia. Journal of Obstetrics and Gynaecology of the British Commonwealth 75: 853–855

Leather H M, Humphreys D M, Baker P, Chadd M A 1968 A controlled trial of hypotensive agents in hypertension in pregnancy. Lancet ii: 488–490

Ledingham J G G, Rajagopalan B 1979 Cerebral complications in the treatment of accelerated hypertension. Quarterly Journal of Medicine 48: 25–41

Lewis P J, Boyland P, Friedman L A, Hensby C N, Downing I 1980 Prostacyclin in pregnancy. British Medical Journal 280: 1581–1582

Lichtenstein M J, Rose G, Shipley M 1986 Distribution and determinants of the difference between diastolic phase 4 and phase 5 blood pressure. Journal of Hypertension 4: 361–363

Liebowitz H A 1984 Cortical blindness as a complication of eclampsia. Annals of Emergency Medicine 13: 365–367

Liley A W 1970 Clinical and laboratory significance of variations in maternal plasma volume in pregnancy. International Journal of Obstetrics and Gynecology 8: 358–362

Lin M-S, McNay J L, Shepherd A M M, Musgrave G E, Keeton T K 1983 Increased plasma norepinephrine accompanies persistent tachycardia after hydralazine. Hypertension 5: 257–263

Lindberg B S, Sandstrom B 1981 How Swedish obstetricians manage hypertension in pregnancy. A questionnaire study. Acta Obstetricia et Gynecologica Scandinavica 60: 327–331

Lindheimer M D, Katz A I 1985 Hypertension in pregnancy. New England Journal of Medicine 313: 675–680

Lindheimer M D, Spargo B H, Katz A I 1974 Eclampsia during the 16th week of gestation. Journal of the American Medical Association 230: 1006–1008

Linton A L, Gavras H, Gleadle R I et al 1969 Microangiopathic haemolytic

anaemia and the pathogenesis of the malignant hypertension. Lancet i: 1277–1282
Lipshitz P J 1971 The clinical and biochemical effects of excess magnesium in the newborn. Pediatrics 47: 501–509
Lipson A, Hsu T-H, Sherwin B, Geelhoed G W 1978 Nitroprusside therapy for a patient with a phaeochromocytoma. Journal of the American Medical Association 239: 427–428
Little W A 1960 Placental infarction. Obstetrics and Gynecology 15: 109–130
Long R G, Scheuer P J, Sherlock S 1977 Pre-eclampsia presenting with deep jaundice. Journal of Clinical Pathology 30: 212–215
Long P A, Abell D A, Beischer N A 1980 Fetal growth retardation and pre-eclampsia. British Journal of Obstetrics and Gynaecology 87: 13–18
Lopez-Espinoza I, Dhar H, Humphreys S, Redman C W G 1986 Urinary albumin excretion in pregnancy. British Journal of Obstetrics and Gynaecology 93: 176–181
Lopez-Llera M, Linares G R, Horta J L H 1976 Maternal mortality rates in eclampsia. American Journal of Obstetrics and Gynecology 124: 149–155
Lowe C R 1961 Toxaemia and pre-pregnancy weight. Journal of Obstetrics and Gynaecology of the British Commonwealth 68: 622–627
Lumbers E R 1970 Peripheral vascular reactivity to angiotensin and noradrenaline in pregnant and non-pregnant women. Australian Journal of Experimental Biology and Medical Science 48: 493–500
Lunell N O, Nylund L, Lewander R, Sarby B 1982 Acute effect of an anti-hypertensive drug, labetalol, on uteroplacental blood flow. British Journal of Obstetrics and Gynaecology 89: 640–644
Lunell N O, Lewander R, Nylund L, Sarby B, Thornstrom S 1983 Acute effect of dihydralazine on uteroplacental blood flow in hypertension during pregnancy. Gynecologic and Obstetric Investigation 16: 274–282
MacGillivray I 1958 Some observations on the incidence of pre-eclampsia. Journal of Obstetrics and Gynaecology of the British Commonwealth 65: 536–539
MacGillivray I 1961 Hypertension in pregnancy and its consequences. British Journal of Obstetrics and Gynaecology 68: 557–569
MacGillivray I 1967 The significance of blood pressure and body water changes in pregnancy. Scottish Medical Journal 12: 237–245
MacGillivray I 1982 Pregnancy hypertension — is it a disease? In: Sammour M B, Symonds E M, Zuspan F P, El-Tomi N (eds) Pregnancy hypertension. Ain Shams University Press, Cairo, pp 1–15
MacGillivray I, Rose G A, Rowe B 1969 Blood pressure survey in pregnancy. Clinical Science 37: 395–407
Manning F A, Platt L D, Sipos L 1980 Antepartum fetal evaluation: development of a fetal biophysical profile. American Journal of Obstetrics and Gynecology 136: 787–795
Maqueo M, Azuela J C, de la Vega M D 1964 Placental pathology in eclampsia and pre-eclampsia. Obstetrics and Gynecology 24: 350–356
Maxwell M H, Waks A U, Schroth P C, Karam M, Dornfeld L P 1982 Error in blood-pressure measurement due to incorrect cuff size in obese patients. Lancet ii: 33–35
McCall M L 1953 Cerebral circulation and metabolism in toxemia of pregnancy. Observations on the effects of veratrum viride and Apresoline (1-hydrazino-phthalazine). American Journal of Obstetrics and Gynecology 66: 1015–1030
McCubbin J H, Sibai B M, Abdella T N, Anderson G D 1981 Cardiopulmonary arrest due to acute maternal hypermagnesaemia. Lancet i: 1058
McKay D G 1972 Hematologic evidence of disseminated intravascular coagulation in eclampsia. Obstetrical and Gynecological Survey 27: 399–417
McKay D G, Merrill S J, Weiner A E, Hertig A T, Reid D E 1953 The pathologic anatomy of eclampsia, bilateral renal cortical necrosis, pituitary necrosis, and other acute fatal complications of pregnancy, and its possible relationship to the generalised Shwartzman phenomenon. American Journal of Obstetrics and Gynecology 66: 507–539
McKenna P, Shaw R W 1979 Hyponatremic fits in oxytocin-augmented labours. International Journal of Gynecology and Obstetrics 17: 250–252
McLane C M, Kuder K 1943 Severe pre-eclampsia. American Journal of Obstetrics and Gynecology 46: 549–557
Mengert W E, Tacchi D A 1961 Pregnancy toxemia and sodium chloride. American Journal of Obstetrics and Gynecology 81: 601–605
Moore M P, Redman C W G 1983 Case-control study of severe pre-eclampsia of early onset. British Medical Journal 287: 580–583
Moore T R, Key T C, Reisner L S, Resnik R 1985 Evaluation of the use of continuous lumbar epidural anesthesia for hypertensive pregnant women in labour. American Journal of Obstetrics and Gynecology 152: 404–412
Mordes J P, Wacker W E 1978 Excess magnesium. Pharmacological Reviews 29: 253–300
Mordes J P, Swartz R, Arky R A 1975 Extreme hypermagnesemia as a cause of refractory hypotension. Annals of Internal Medicine 83: 657–658
Morris J A, O'Grady J P 1979 Volume expansion in severe edema-proteinuria-hypertension gestosis. American Journal of Obstetrics and Gynecology 135: 276
Morrison R, Crawford J, Macpherson M, Heptinstall S 1985 Platelet behaviour in normal pregnancy, pregnancy complicated by essential hypertension and pregnancy induced hypertension. Thrombosis and Haemostasis 54: 607–611
Mule J G, Tatum H J, Sawyer R E 1957 Nitrogenous retention in patients with toxemia of pregnancy — an unusual complication of salt restriction. American Journal of Obstetrics and Gynecology 74: 526–537
Naeye R L, Friedman E A 1979 Causes of perinatal death associated with gestational hypertension and proteinuria. American Journal of Obstetrics and Gynecology 133: 8–10
Nelson T R 1955a A clinical study of pre-eclampsia. Part II. Journal of Obstetrics and Gynaecology of the British Empire 62: 58–66
Nelson T R 1955b A clinical study of pre-eclampsia. Part I. Journal of Obstetrics and Gynaecology of the British Empire 62: 48–57
Newsome L R, Bramwell R S, Curling P E 1986 Severe pre-eclampsia: hemodynamic effects of lumbar epidural anesthesia. Anesthesia and Analgesia 65: 31–36
Oian P, Maltau J M, Noddeland H, Fadnes H O 1985 Oedema-preventing mechanisms in subcutaneous tissue of normal pregnant women. British Journal of Obstetrics and Gynaecology 92: 1113–1119
Oian P, Lande K, Kjeldsen S E et al 1986 Enhanced platelet release reaction related to arterial plasma adrenaline and blood pressure in pre-eclampsia. British Journal of Obstetrics and Gynaecology 93: 548–553
Overgaard J, Skinhoj E 1975 A paradoxical cerebral hemodynamic effect of hydralazine. Stroke 6: 402–404
Page E W 1972 On the pathogenesis of pre-eclampsia and eclampsia. Journal of Obstetrics and Gynaecology of the British Commonwealth 79: 883–894
Palomaki J F, Lindheimer M D 1970 Sodium depletion simulating deterioration in a toxemic pregnancy. New England Journal of Medicine 282: 88–89
Pickering G 1968 In High blood pressure. J and A Churchill, London, pp 1–5
Pirani B B K, Campbell D M, MacGillivray I 1973 Plasma volume in normal first pregnancy. Journal of Obstetrics and Gynaecology of the British Commonwealth 80: 884–887
Pollak V E, Nettles J B 1960 The kidney in toxemia of pregnancy: a clinical and pathologic study based on renal biopsies. Medicine 39: 469–526
Porapakkham S 1979 An epidemiologic study of eclampsia. Obstetrics and Gynecology 54: 26–30
Pritchard J A 1955 The use of the magnesium ion in the management of eclamptogenic toxemias. Surgery, Gynecology and Obstetrics 100: 131–140
Pritchard J A, Stone S R 1967 Clinical and laboratory observations on eclampsia. American Journal of Obstetrics and Gynecology 99: 754–765
Pritchard J A, Pritchard S A 1975 Standardised treatment of 154 consecutive cases of eclampsia. American Journal of Obstetrics and Gynecology 123: 543–549
Pritchard J A, Weisman R, Ratnoff O D, Vosburgh G J 1954 Intravascular hemolysis, thrombocytopenia and other hematologic abnormalities associated with severe toxemia of pregnancy. New England Journal of Medicine 250: 89–98
Pritchard J A, Cunningham F G, Mason R A 1976 Coagulation changes in eclampsia: their frequency and pathogenesis. American Journal of Obstetrics and Gynecology 124: 855–864
Raab W, Schroeder G, Wagner R, Gigee W 1956 Vascular reactivity and electrolytes in normal and toxemic pregnancy. Journal of Clinical Endocrinology 16: 1196–1216

Raftery E B, Ward A P 1968 The indirect method of recording blood pressure. Cardiovascular Research 2: 210–218
Rakoczi I, Tallian F, Bagdany S, Gati I 1979 Platelet life-span in normal pregnancy and pre-eclampsia as determined by a non-radioisotope technique. Thrombosis Research 15: 553–556
Ram C V S, Kaplan N M 1979 Individual titration of diazoxide dosage in the treatment of severe hypertension. American Journal of Cardiology 43: 627–630
Redman C W G 1980 Treatment of hypertension in pregnancy. Kidney International 18: 267–278
Redman C W G 1984 Hypertension in pregnancy. In: De Swiet M (ed) Medical disorders in obstetric practice. Blackwell, Oxford, pp 149–191
Redman C W G 1987 The definition of pre-eclampsia. In: Sharp F, Symonds E M (eds) Hypertension in pregnancy. Perinatology Press, New York, pp 3–17
Redman C W G, Jefferies M 1988 A revised definition of pre-eclampsia Lancet i: 809–812
Redman C W G, Beilin L J, Bonnar J 1976a Renal function in pre-eclampsia. Journal of Clinical Pathology 10 (suppl): 91–94
Redman C W G, Beilin L J, Bonnar J, Wilkinson R H 1976b Plasma-urate measurements in predicting fetal death in hypertensive pregnancy. Lancet i: 1370–1373
Redman C W G, Beilin L J, Bonnar J, Ounsted M K 1976c Fetal outcome in trial of antihypertensive treatment in pregnancy. Lancet ii: 753–756
Redman C W G, Allington M J, Bolton F G, Stirrat G M 1977a Plasma beta-thromboglobulin in pre-eclampsia. Lancet ii: 248
Redman C W G, Beilin L J, Bonnar J 1977b Treatment of hypertension in pregnancy with methyldopa: blood pressure control and side effects. British Journal of Obstetrics and Gynaecology 84: 419–426
Redman C W G, Denson K W E, Beilin L J, Bolton F G, Stirrat G M 1977c Factor VIII consumption in pre-eclampsia. Lancet ii: 1249–1252
Redman C W G, Bonnar J, Beilin L J 1978 Early platelet consumption in pre-eclampsia. British Medical Journal 1: 467–469
Robertson E G 1971 The natural history of oedema during pregnancy. Journal of Obstetrics and Gynaecology of the British Commonwealth 78: 520–529
Robertson W B, Brosens I, Dixon H G 1967 The pathological response of the vessels of the placental bed to hypertensive pregnancy. Journal of Pathology and Bacteriology 93: 581–592
Robinson M 1958 Salt in pregnancy. Lancet i: 178–181
Robson R H, Vishwanath M C 1982 Nifedipine and beta-blockade as a cause of cardiac failure. British Medical Journal 284: 104
Rodda R, Denny-Brown D 1966 The cerebral arterioles in experimental hypertension. I The nature of arteriolar constriction and its effects on the collateral circulation. American Journal of Pathology 49: 53–76
Rotton W N, Sachtleben M R, Friedman E A 1959 Migraine and eclampsia. Obstetrics and Gynecology 14: 322–330
Rovinsky J J, Jaffin H 1965 Cardiovascular hemodynamics in pregnancy I. Blood and plasma volumes in multiple pregnancy. American Journal of Obstetrics and Gynecology 193: 1–15
Rubin P C, Butters L, Clark D M et al 1983 Placebo-controlled trial of atenolol treatment of pregnancy-associated hypertension. Lancet i: 431–434
Rush R W, Keirse M J N C, Howat P, Baum J D, Anderson A B M, Turnbull A C 1976 Contribution of preterm delivery to perinatal mortality. British Medical Journal 2: 965–968
Samuels B 1960 Postpartum eclampsia. Obstetrics and Gynecology 15: 748–752
Schenker J G, Chowers I 1971 Pheochromocytoma and pregnancy. Obstetrical and Gynecological Survey 26: 739–747
Scher J, Hailey D M, Beard R W 1972 The effects of diazepam on the fetus. Journal of Obstetrics and Gynaecology of the British Commonwealth 79: 635–638
Schramm M 1979 Prophylactic anticoagulation in the management of recurrent pre-eclampsia and fetal death. Australia and New Zealand Journal of Obstetrics and Gynaecology 19: 230–232
Sejeny S A, Eastham R D, Baker S R 1975 Platelet counts during normal pregnancy. Journal of Clinical Pathology 28: 812–813
Seligman S A 1971 Diurnal blood-pressure variation in pregnancy. British Journal of Obstetrics and Gynaecology 78: 417–422
Semchyshyn S 1981 Gastrointestinal hemorrhage in puerperium of pre-eclamptic patients who received glucocorticoid therapy. American Journal of Obstetrics and Gynecology 139: 217–218
Sheehan H L, Lynch J B 1973a Pathology of toxaemia in pregnancy. Churchill Livingstone, Edinburgh, pp 328–330
Sheehan H L, Lynch J P 1973b Pathology of toxaemia in pregnancy. Churchill Livingstone, Edinburgh, pp 413–453
Sheehan H L, Lynch J P 1973c Pathology of toxaemia in pregnancy. Churchill Livingstone, Edinburgh, pp 384–397
Sheehan H L, Lynch J P 1973d Pathology of toxaemia in pregnancy. Churchill Livingstone, Edinburgh, pp 340–383
Sheehan H L, Lynch J P 1973e Pathology of toxaemia in pregnancy. Churchill Livingstone, Edinburgh, pp 328–339
Sheehan H L, Lynch J P 1973f Pathology of toxaemia in pregnancy. Churchill Livingstone, Edinburgh, pp 524–553
Sibai B M, McCubbin J H, Anderson G D, Lipshitz J, Dilts P V 1981 Eclampsia. I Observations from 67 recent cases. Obstetrics and Gynecology 58: 609–613
Simanowitz M D, MacGregor W G, Hobbs J R 1973 Proteinuria in pre-eclampsia. Journal of Obstetrics and Gynaecology of the British Commonwealth 80: 103–108
Slater R M, Wilcox F L, Smith W D et al 1987 Phenytoin infusion in severe pre-eclampsia. Lancet i: 1417–1420
Smith J H, Anand K J S, Cotes P M et al 1988 Antenatal fetal heart rate variation in relation to the respiratory and metabolic status of the compromised fetus. British Journal of Obstetrics and Gynaecology 95: 980–989
Solanki D L, Blackburn B C 1985 Spurious thrombocytopenia during pregnancy. Obstetrics and Gynecology 65: 14S–17S
Spargo B, McCartney C P, Winemiller R 1959 Glomerular capillary endotheliosis in toxemia of pregnancy. Archives of Pathology 68: 593–599
Stempel J E, O'Grady J P, Morton M J, Johnson K A 1982 Use of sodium nitroprusside in complications of gestational hypertension. Obstetrics and Gynecology 60: 533–538
Stewart A, Hewitt D 1960 Toxaemia of pregnancy and obesity. Journal of Obstetrics and Gynaecology of the British Empire 67: 812–818
Strandgaard S, Olesen J, Skinhoj E, Lassen N A 1973 Autoregulation of brain circulation in severe arterial hypertension. British Medical Journal 1: 507–510
Strauss R G, Keefer J R, Burke T, Civetta J M 1980 Hemodynamic monitoring of cardiogenic pulmonary edema complicating toxemia of pregnancy. Obstetrics and Gynecology 55: 170–174
Stubbs T M, Lazarchik J, Van Dorsten J P, Cox J, Loadholt C B 1986 Evidence of accelerated platelet production and consumption in nonthrombocytopenic pre-eclampsia. American Journal of Obstetrics and Gynecology 155: 263–265
Studd J W W, Blainey J D, Bailey D E 1970 Serum protein changes in the pre-eclampsia–eclampsia syndrome. Journal of Obstetrics and Gynaecology of the British Commonwealth 77; 796–801
Suonio S, Saarikoski S, Tahvanainen K, Paakkonen A, Olkkonen H 1986 Acute effects of dihydralazine mesylate, furosemide, and metoprolol on maternal hemodynamics in pregnancy-induced hypertension. American Journal of Obstetrics and Gynecology 155: 122–125
Svensson A, Andersch B, Hansson L 1984 Hypertension in pregnancy. Analysis of 261 consecutive cases. Acta Medica Scandinavica 693: (suppl) 33–39
Talledo O E, Chesley L C, Zuspan F P 1968 Renin-angiotensin system in normal and toxemic pregnancies III. Differential sensitivity to angiotensin II and norepinephrine in toxemia of pregnancy. American Journal of Obstetrics and Gynecology 100: 218–221
Tarazi R C, Dustan H P, Bravo E L, Niarchos A P 1976 Vasodilating drugs: contrasting haemodynamic effects. Clinical Science 51: 575S–578S
Tatum H J, Mule J G 1956 Puerperal vasomotor collapse in patients with toxemia of pregnancy — a new concept of the etiology and a rational plan of treatment. American Journal of Obstetrics and Gynecology 71: 492–501
Templeton A, Campbell D 1979 A retrospective study of eclampsia in the Grampian region 1965–1977. Health Bulletin 37: 55–59
Tepperman H M, Beydoun S N, Abdul-Karim R W 1977 Drugs affecting myometrial contractility in pregnancy. Clinical Obstetrics and Gynecology 20: 423–445
Thien Th, Koene R A P, Schijf Ch, Pieters G F F M, Eskes T K A B, Wijdeveld P G A B 1980 Infusion of diazoxide in severe hypertension

during pregnancy. European Journal of Obstetrics, Gynecology and Reproductive Biology 10: 367–374
Thomson A M, Hytten R E, Billewicz W Z 1967 The epidemiology of edema during pregnancy. Journal of Obstetrics and Gynaecology of the British Commonwealth 74: 1–10
Tillmann Hein H A 1984 Cardiorespiratory arrest with laryngeal oedema in pregnancy-induced hypertension. Canadian Anaesthetists Society Journal 31: 210–212
Tominaga T, Page E W 1966 Accommodation of the human placenta to hypoxia. American Journal of Obstetrics and Gynecology 94: 679–685
Trudinger B J, Cook C, Giles W B, Connelly A, Thompson R S 1987 Umbilical artery flow velocity waveforms in high-risk pregnancy. Randomised controlled trial. Lancet i: 188–190
Tygart S G, McRoyan D K, Spinnato J A, McRoyan C J, Kitay D Z 1986 Longitudinal study of platelet indices during normal pregnancy. American Journal of Obstetrics and Gynecology 154: 883–887
Underwood P, Hester L L, Lafitte T, Gregg K V 1965 The relationship of smoking to the outcome of pregnancy. American Journal of Obstetrics and Gynecology 91: 270–276
Valentine B H, Baker J L 1977 Treatment of recurrent pregnancy hypertension by prophylactic anticoagulation. British Journal of Obstetrics and Gynaecology 84: 309–311
Van Dongen P W J, Eskes T K A B, Martin C B, Van't Hoff M A 1980 Postural blood pressure differences in pregnancy. American Journal of Obstetrics and Gynecology 138: 1–5
Vardi J, Fields G A 1974 Microangiopathic hemolytic anemia in severe pre-eclampsia. American Journal of Obstetrics and Gynecology 119; 617–622
Vinall P E, Simeone F A 1981 Cerebral autoregulation: an in vitro study. Stroke 12: 640–642
Vink G J, Moodley J 1982 The effect of low-dose dihydralazine on the fetus in the emergency treatment of hypertension in pregnancy. South African Medical Journal 62: 475–477
Vink G J, Moodley J, Philpott R H 1980 Effect of dihydralazine on the fetus in the treatment of maternal hypertension. Obstetrics and Gynecology 55: 519–522
Vosburgh G J 1976 Blood pressure, edema and proteinuria in pregnancy–edema relationships. Progress in Clinical and Biological Research 7: 155–168
Wainscott G, Sullivan F M, Volans G N, Wilkinson M 1978 The outcome of pregnancy in women suffering from migraine. Postgraduate Medical Journal 54: 98–102
Wallenburg H C S Van Kessel P H 1978 Platelet lifespan in normal pregnancy as determined by a nonradioisotopic technique. British Journal of Obstetrics and Gynaecology 85: 33–36
Wallenburg H C S, Hutchinson D L 1979 A radioangiographic study of the effects of the catecholamines on uteroplacental blood flow in the rhesus monkey. Journal of Medical Primatology 8: 57–65
Wallenburg H C S, Dekker G A, Makovitz J W, Rotmans P 1986 Low-dose aspirin prevents pregnancy-induced hypertension and pre-eclampsia in angiotensin-sensitive primigravidae. Lancet i: 1–3
Walters W A W 1966 Effects of sustained maternal hypertension on fetal growth and survival. Lancet ii: 1214–1217
Walters B N J, Redman C W G 1984 Treatment of severe pregnancy-associated hypertension with the calcium antagonist nifedipine. British Journal of Obstetrics and Gynaecology 91: 330–336
Walters B N J, Thompson M E, Lee A, De Swiet M 1986 Blood pressure in the puerperium. Clinical Science 71: 589–594
Wardle E N, Wright N A 1973 Role of fibrin in a model of pregnancy toxemia in the rabbit. American Journal of Obstetrics and Gynecology 115: 17–26
Watson D l, Sibai B M, Shaver D C, Dacus J V, Anderson G D 1983 Late postpartum eclampsia: an update. Southern Medical Journal 76: 1487–1489
Weinstein L 1982 Syndrome of hemolysis, elevated liver enzymes, and low platelet count: a severe consequence of hypertension on pregnancy. American Journal of Obstetrics and Gynecology 142: 159–167
Wentworth P 1967 Placental infarction and toxemia of pregnancy. American Journal of Obstetrics and Gynecology 99: 318–326
Whitelaw A 1981 Maternal methyldopa treatment and neonatal blood pressure. British Medical Journal 283: 471
Wiggers C J 1956 Dynamic patterns induced by compression of an artery. Circulation Research 4: 4–7
Wightman H, Hibbard B M, Rosen M 1978 Perinatal mortality and morbidity associated with eclampsia. British Medical Journal 2: 235–237
Willocks J, Moir D 1968 Epidural analgesia in the management of hypertension in labour. Journal of Obstetrics and Gynaecology of the British Commonwealth 75: 225–228
Zabriskie J R 1963 Effect of cigaret smoking during pregnancy. Study of 2000 cases. Obstetrics and Gynecology 21: 405–411
Zinaman M, Rubin J, Lindheimer M D 1985 Serial plasma oncotic pressure levels and echoencephalography during and after delivery in severe pre-eclampsia. Lancet i: 1245–1247
Zuspan F P, Nelson G H, Ahlquist R P 1964 Epinephrine infusions in normal and toxemic pregnancy. American Journal of Obstetrics and Gynecology 90: 88–96

37

Michael de Swiet

Cardiovascular problems in pregnancy

Cardiovascular disease in pregnancy is a worrying condition for the obstetrician. Even excluding hypertensive disease (considered in Chapter 36), cardiovascular disease and specifically heart disease has an appreciable maternal mortality (10 per 100 000 in the most recent Report on Confidential Enquiries into Maternal Deaths Series; (Department of Health and Social Security 1982). If the presence of a heart murmur is considered indicative of heart disease, the majority of women are at risk, for as many as 90% have systolic murmurs in pregnancy. Yet the prevalance of heart disease in pregnancy in the west is probably no more than 1%.

In this chapter we will consider, as they refer to pregnancy the physiology of the cardiovascular system, the epidemiology of heart disease, the general management of patients with heart disease and certain specific conditions. For further reviews see de Swiet (1984), Elkayam & Gleicher (1982) and Sullivan & Ramanathan (1985).

THE PHYSIOLOGY OF THE CARDIOVASCULAR SYSTEM IN PREGNANCY

During pregnancy, oxygen consumption at rest increases by about 50 ml/min, i.e. from 300 to 350 ml/min. The oxygen is used by the fetus and other contents of the developing uterus, and to support the increased metabolic rate of the mother. Arterial blood is fully saturated. The only ways in which the mother can increase the supply of oxygen to peripheral tissues are either to increase the quantity of oxygen removed from the blood (increased arteriovenous oxygen difference) or to increase the delivery of oxygenated blood to the tissues (increased cardiac output). The pregnant woman chooses the latter course and, as in so many other physiological adaptations to pregnancy, overcompensates for the increased load, so that cardiac output increases to such an extent that arteriovenous oxygen difference decreases from 100 ml/l in the non-pregnant state to 80 ml/l in pregnancy.

The 40% increase in cardiac output from 3.5 to 6.0 l/min occurs early in pregnancy; at least two-thirds of the increase has occurred by the end of the first trimester. It has generally been believed that the increased cardiac output was maintained until the end of pregnancy, and that any fall in cardiac output at the end of pregnancy was associated with measurements made in the supine position, in which the uterus obstructs the vena cava and decreases venous return. More recent studies made with non-invasive techniques have challenged this concept (Rubler et al 1977, James et al 1985, Davies et al 1986). Although there have been methodological problems with some of these studies (de Swiet & Talbert 1986, it is possible that there is a fall in cardiac output towards the end of pregnancy, even in patients lying in the left lateral position. It has also been suggested that the uterus can obstruct the vena cava even in the erect position, causing hypotension and changes in the fetal heart rate (Schneider et al 1984).

It is not clear to what extent myocardial contractility increases in pregnancy independently of the increase in preload and decrease in afterload. However, echocardiographic studies show an increase in the speed of circumferential shortening (Rubler et al 1977), which would suggest some increase in contractility.

Most studies have been performed at rest. Cardiac output rises still further on exertion and in labour. Each uterine contraction will increase cardiac output by about 20% (Ueland & Hansen 1969) by increasing preload (increased venous return). The pain of contractions is another important contributing factor. Cardiac output does increase on exercise in pregnancy, but as pregnancy progresses, the increase gets smaller. Limitation of venous return is a probable reason (Morton et al 1985). Although heart rate increases by about 10% in pregnancy, this is not sufficient

Table 37.1 The prevalence (percentage) of various forms of congenital heart disease in pregnancy

	Ohio[1] (*n* = 125)	Queensland[2] (*n* = 93)	Dublin[3] (*n* = 74)	Connecticut[4] (*n* = 482)	Leicester[5] (*n* = 73)
Patent ductus arteriosus	24	27	9	22	11
Atrial septal defect	29	26	38	14	22
Pulmonary stenosis	4	12	6	10*	11
Ventricular septal defect	22	14	13	20	16
Tetralogy of Fallot	4	4	13	8†	8
Coarctation of the aorta	10	6	6	12	7
Aortic valve diseasse	3	4	6		7
Mitral valve disease				7	14
Other	2	2		7	4
Unclassified	5	5			

[1]Copeland et al (1963); [2]Neilson et al (1970); [3]Sugrue et al (1981); [4]Whittemore et al (1982); [5]MacNab and MacAfee (1985).

* Includes all pregnancies where mother had obstruction to right ventricular outflow.
† Expressed as percentage of all 233 mothers who became pregnant (some had more than one pregnancy).

to account for the 40% increase in cardiac output and so there is also an increase in stroke volume.

In normal pregnancy, blood pressure does not rise and, indeed, usually falls in the second trimester. The increased cardiac output is therefore accommodated by a decrease in peripheral resistance. Although some of these effects are probably caused by increased oestrogen levels, other mechanisms must be implicated since maximal oestrogen stimulation does not cause such large changes as are seen in pregnancy (Slater et al 1986). It is very likely that prostanoids also contribute. Further support for active vasodilatation in pregnancy comes from the refractoriness to angiotensin infusion, as measured by a relative lack of pressor response to angiotensin infusion in normal pregnancy compared to the non-pregnant state (Gant et al 1973). This effect of pregnancy has also been associated with prostanoids and, in particular, prostacyclin.

Cardiac output also increases in pregnancy because of the increased preload caused by increased circulating blood volume. Blood volume rises very early in pregnancy; the total increase is about 40%, and this rise is maintained until delivery (Hytten & Paintin 1963).

It is not known how rapidly the circulation returns to the prepregnant state after delivery. Since it may take 3 months for blood pressure to return to the prepregnancy value, other cardiovascular indices may regress over an equally long timescale.

The rise in cardiac output and associated vasodilatation in pregnancy cause changes in the circulation which may mimic heart disease. Heart rate increases and it is likely that arrhythmias are more common in pregnancy. Pulse volume is increased. Jugular venous pressure waves are more prominent, though the height of the venous pressure is not increased in pregnancy. Heart size increases and displacement of the apex beat by up to 1 cm from the mid-clavicular line should not be considered abnormal. The first heart sound is loud; there is often a very prominent third heart sound and an ejection systolic murmur up to grade 3/6 in intensity is heard over the whole praecordium in up to 90% of pregnant women. Venous hums — continuous murmurs usually audible in the neck which can be modified by stethoscope pressure — may also be heard in pregnancy.

In addition, oedema is very common in pregnancy, and usually does not indicate heart disease.

NATURAL HISTORY

Prevalance of heart disease

The prevalence and incidence of all heart disease in pregnancy varies between 0.3% (MacNab & MacAfee 1985) and 3.5% (Mendelson 1956). The figures vary because of differences in the prevalence of heart disease in different communities at different times. Thus rheumatic heart disease is becoming less common and congenital heart disease is proportionately more important. In addition, diagnostic criteria change, so that, for example, most cases of mitral valve abnormality are now thought to be congenital rather than rheumatic. It is also likely that we will see a change in the pattern of congenital heart disease in pregnancy following the increase in paediatric cardiac surgery which occurred between 1965 and 1975.

In all series, the dominant lesion in rheumatic heart disease has been mitral stenosis. In 1048 patients with rheumatic heart disease reported from Newcastle, Szekely et al (1973) found dominant mitral stenosis in 90%, mitral regurgitation in 6.6%, aortic regurgitation in 2.5% and aortic stenosis in 10%.

At present, the experience of congenital heart disease in pregnancy is limited to relatively simple defects. Five representative series are shown in Table 37.1. Although the total numbers in each series are very different, the overall pattern is similar. The most common lesions are atrial septal defect and patent ductus arteriosus, which account for about 50% of cases, followed by ventricular septal defect, pulmonary stenosis and Fallot's tetralogy which together contribute another 20%. In the more modern series from Dublin and

Connecticut, we see the effect of surgery, as more women with patent ductus arteriosus and atrial septal defect have had these corrected in earlier life and are now childbearing.

Maternal mortality

Although sporadic fatalities will be seen in all forms of heart disease in pregnancy, maternal mortality is most likely in those conditions where pulmonary blood flow cannot be increased (Jewett 1979). This occurs because of obstruction, either within the pulmonary blood vessels or at the mitral valve. The situation is documented clearly in Eisenmenger's syndrome, where up to now there has been no effective treatment, and where the maternal mortality is between 30 and 50% (Morgan Jones & Howitt 1965, Gleicher et al 1979.) An elevation in pulmonary vascular resistance is also seen in primary pulmonary hypertension in which the reported maternal mortality is 40–50% (Morgan Jones & Howitt 1965, McCaffrey & Dunn 1974, Tsou et al 1984).

In contrast, in women with Fallot's tetralogy in which pulmonary vascular resistance is normal, the reported maternal mortality varies between 4 and 20% (Jacoby 1964, Morgan Jones & Howitt 1965). Furthermore, the figure of 20% is only based on one maternal death in five pregnancies reported by Jacoby. The Connecticut series (Whittemore et al 1982) shows how good the results can be with obsessional care, since in 482 pregnancies from 233 women, including 8 mothers with Eisenmenger's syndrome, there were no maternal deaths.

In Ehlers–Danlos syndrome, the arterial and classical forms have also been associated with a high mortality due to arterial dissection and bleeding (Barabas 1967, Pearl & Spicer 1981, Rudd et al 1983).

In rheumatic heart disease, maternal mortality can now be very low. Szekely et al (1973) report 26 mortalities (about 1%) in 2856 pregnancies complicated by rheumatic heart disease between 1942 and 1969. Half of the deaths were due to pulmonary oedema, which became much less common once mitral valvotomy was freely available. These authors reported no maternal deaths in about 1000 pregnancies occurring after 1960. Rush et al (1979) also reported a maternal mortality of 0.7% in 450 mothers with rheumatic heart disease in South Africa.

There is no evidence that a well managed pregnancy is detrimental to the long term health of the woman with heart disease, providing she survives pregnancy itself. Chesley (1980) has reported a group of 38 patients with 51 pregnancies occurring after they were diagnosed as having severe heart disease. These were compared with a group of 96 women with equally severe rheumatic heart disease who did not have any pregnancies after diagnosis. The mean survival time (14 years) was no less and, in fact, was greater in the group that did have further pregnancies, compared to the group that did not (12 years).

Fetal outcome

The fetal outcome among those whose mothers have rheumatic heart disease in pregnancy is usually good and little different from that in those who do not have heart disease (Rush et al 1979, Sugrue et al 1981). However, the babies are likely to be lighter at birth (Ueland et al 1972) by about 200 g, as reported in the study of Ho et al (1980).

In the five series of patients with congenital heart disease in pregnancy cited in Table 37.1, there was no excess fetal mortality, except in the group with cyanotic congenital heart disease. Here the babies are generally growth-retarded (Batson 1974, Whittemore et al 1982), and the fetal loss including abortion may be as high as 45% (Copeland et al 1963, Batson 1974 Gleicher et al 1979, Whittemore et al 1982). This is hardly surprising, in view of the inefficient mechanisms of placental exchange which cannot compensate for maternal systemic hypoxaemia. It is likely that the fetus dies because of inadequate oxygen supply or because of immaturity (Gleicher et al 1979) which may be iatrogenic.

Of great importance is the prevalence of congenital heart disease in the infants of mothers who themselves have congenital heart disease; this prevalence varies according to series from 3 to 14% (Nora 1978, Whittemore et al 1982). This compares with a prevalence of 1% in the general population (Nora 1978). The highest prevalence was in infants whose mothers had outflow obstruction, particularly left-sided. Most congenital abnormalities were represented in the infants; in about one-half, the child had the same abnormality as the mother.

MANAGEMENT

If possible, all women with heart disease attending one maternity hospital should be managed in a combined obstetric/cardiac clinic by one obstetrician and one cardiologist. In this way, the number of visits the patient makes to the hospital is kept to a minimum, and the obstetrician and cardiologist obtain the maximum experience in the management of relatively rare conditions.

History

As in all forms of medicine, the history is the most important single factor in the assessment of a patient who may have heart disease. In developed countries, most patients know whether they have heart disease. Even in developing countries it is very unusual though not unknown to have haemodynamically significant heart disease with no symptoms.

The most frequent symptom of heart disease in pregnancy is breathlessness. This can be difficult to assess because it is a variable feature of all pregnancies (Milne et al 1978); it is therefore important to consider whether the woman was breathless before she became pregnant. Syncope occurs in severe aortic stenosis, hypertrophic cardiomyopathy or subaortic stenosis, Fallot's tetralogy and Eisenmenger's syndrome; it is also a feature of normal pregnancy. Syncope, like chest pain, may occur because of dysrhythmias. The pregnant woman may also be aware of the dysrhythmia as a feeling of palpitations. Chest pain is usually a feature of ischaemic disease which is uncommon in pregnancy; chest pain may also occur in severe aortic stenosis, or, more commonly in pregnancy, in hypertrophic cardiomyopathy.

Physical signs

As noted above, the hyperdynamic circulation of pregnancy causes alterations in the cardiovascular system which mimic heart disease. Thus 20% of patients originally thought to have rheumatic heart disease may have none at all, following a reassessment performed up to 30 years later (Gleicher et al 1979). The changes which occur in the cardiovascular system associated with normal pregnancy have already been considered. Any other murmurs or additional heart sounds should be considered to be significant. Particular difficulty occurs with systolic murmurs, since they are so common in pregnancy. Those that are significant are:

1. Pansystolic murmurs of ventricular septal defect, mitral regurgitation or tricuspid regurgitation;
2. Late systolic murmurs of mitral regurgitation, mitral valve prolapse or hypertrophic cardiomyopathy;
3. Ejection systolic murmurs louder than grade 3/6 of aortic stenosis;
4. Ejection systolic murmurs which vary with respiration in pulmonary stenosis;
5. Ejection systolic murmurs associated with other abnormalities, e.g. ejection clicks — valvar pulmonary and aortic stenosis.

In addition, an assessment of the patient's cardiac status should also include the signs of heart failure: whether the patient is cyanosed or has finger-clubbing, the presence of pulse deficits and other peripheral signs of endocarditis such as splinter haemorrhages.

Investigations

Chest radiography

The chest radiograph is unhelpful in the diagnosis of minor degrees of heart disease but will, of course, show typical changes in those who have haemodynamically significant heart pathology. Patients with normal hearts show slight cardiomegaly, increased pulmonary vascular markings and distension of the pulmonary veins.

Electrocardiography

In pregnancy, T wave inversion in lead III, S-T segment changes and Q waves, which would usually be considered pathological, occur frequently. In pregnancy, therefore, the electrocardiograph is more helpful in the diagnosis of dysrhythmias than in the demonstration of a structural abnormality of the heart.

Echocardiography

Recent studies have shown that the majority of structural cardiac abnormalities can be detected by echocardiography. This is the investigation of choice in pregnancy, since there is no radiation hazard, and because of the detailed information available in skilled hands. Nevertheless, echocardiography is still a relatively new investigation, and more studies are required of its clinical application in patients with heart disease in pregnancy.

Clinical management

The nature and severity of the heart lesion should first be assessed in the combined clinic. In practice, many patients will have no evidence of any lesion at all and no further follow-up will be required. Some may only have a mild lesion with no haemodynamic problems, such as congenital mitral prolapse which has such an excellent prognosis (Rayburn & Fontana 1981) that again, no further follow-up is necessary. The remainder will have a condition with real or potential haemodynamic implications. These women must first be assessed as to the need for termination, if seen early enough in pregnancy, and secondly, as to the need for surgery. In patients with well managed heart disease, these assessments would have been made before the patient became pregnant.

Because of the mortality statistics indicated above, Eisenmenger's syndrome and primary pulmonary hypertension are absolute indications for termination of pregnancy. Very rarely, termination may also be indicated in patients with such severe pulmonary disease that they have pulmonary hypertension. In all other cases, the decision whether the pregnancy should continue depends on an individual assessment of the risk of pregnancy compared to the patient's desire to have children.

In general, the indications for surgery in pregnancy are similar to those in the non-pregnant state: failure of medical treatment with either intractable heart failure or intolerable symptoms. However, because of the bad reputation of severe mitral stenosis in pregnancy, mitral valvotomy is performed relatively commonly in patients with suitable heart valves, whereas open heart surgery is only performed with reluctance because of worries about the fetus (Zitnik et al 1969). More recent studies suggest that these worries about fetal survival are not justifiable, at least in the short term (Eilen et al 1981, Becker 1983). Possible long-term effects on the development of the child are unknown.

Antenatal care

After the initial assessment of the pregnant woman, the remainder of medical management during pregnancy is associated with avoiding, if possible, those factors which increase the risk of heart failure, and the vigorous treatment of any heart failure if it occurs. Risk factors for heart failure in pregnancy include infections (particularly urinary tract infection), hypertension (both pregnancy-associated and pregnancy-induced), obesity, multiple pregnancy, anaemia, the development of arrhythmias and, very rarely, hyperthyroidism. The increase in cardiac output in twin pregnancy, which is about 30% greater than in singleton pregnancy, is achieved by increasing heart rate and contractility rather than by increasing venous return. This suggests that cardiac reserve is particularly compromised in multiple pregnancy (Veille et al 1985).

Treatment of heart failure

The principles of treatment of heart failure in pregnancy are the same as in the non-pregnant state.

Digoxin The indications for the use of digoxin are to control the heart rate in atrial fibrillation and some other supraventricular tachycardias, and, when given acutely in heart failure, to increase the force of contraction. Dosage requirements of digoxin are the same in pregnancy as in the non-pregnant state. Both digoxin (Rogers et al 1972) and digitoxin (Okita et al 1956) cross the placenta, producing similar drug levels in the fetus to those seen in the mother (Rogers et al 1972; Saarikosi 1976). Digoxin enters the umbilical circulation within 5 minutes of intravenous administration to the mother (Saarikosi 1976). In general, there is no evidence that therapeutic levels of digoxin in the mother affect the neonatal electrocardiograph (Rogers et al 1972) or cause any harm to the fetus. However, although therapeutic drug levels in the mother do not harm the fetus, toxic levels do.

There may be a place for prophylactic digoxin therapy in selected women who are not in heart failure. This is most likely to be of value in those at risk from developing atrial fibrillation, i.e. those with rheumatic mitral valve disease with an enlarged left atrium, and possibly those who have paroxysmal atrial fibrillation or frequent atrial ectopic beats. However, this form of treatment has not been subjected to formal clinical trial, and there is certainly no case for digitalization of all women with heart disease in pregnancy. Digoxin is also secreted in breast milk, but since the total daily excretion in the mother with therapeutic blood levels should not exceed 2 μg (Levy et al 1977), this too is unlikely to cause any harm to the neonate, unless it suffers from some other disorder predisposing to digitalis toxicity, such as hypokalaemia.

Diuretic therapy Frusemide is the most commonly used and rapidly acting loop diuretic for the treatment of pulmonary oedema. In congestive cardiac failure where speed of action is not so important, oral thiazides are normally used in the first instance, although the extra potency of the loop diuretics may be necessary in a minority of cases. The use of thiazide in late pregnancy is not associated with any significant salt or water depletion in the neonate (Andersen 1970).

There are no risks with the use of diuretics for the treatment of heart failure specific to pregnancy, but, as in the non-pregnant state, hypokalaemia is an important complication in the woman who may also be taking digoxin. Treatment of pulmonary oedema should also include opiates such as morphine, which reduces anxiety and decreases venous return by causing venodilatation, and also aminophylline if there is associated bronchospasm. Life-threatening pulmonary oedema that does not respond to drug therapy may be helped by mechanical ventilation. If this is successful, and in other cases which do not respond to medical treatment, cardiac surgery should be considered if the patient has a potentially operable lesion.

Dysrhythmias

Most dysrhythmias that require treatment are due to ischaemic heart disease, which usually presents in women after their childbearing years and is rare in pregnancy. Therefore, there is limited experience in the treatment of dysrhythmias during pregnancy. Nevertheless, the problem does exist, particularly in patients who have non-ischaemic abnormalities of cardiac-conducting tissue, such as are believed to occur in the Wolff–Parkinson–White, Lown–Ganong–Levine (Carpenter & Decuir 1984) and Long Q-T syndromes (Bruner et al 1984). Furthermore, paroxysmal atrial tachycardia is said to occur more frequently in pregnancy than in the non-pregnant state (Szekely & Snaith 1953).

The antidysrhythmic drugs used most frequently in pregnancy are digoxin, quinidine and beta-adrenergic blocking agents, in particular propranolol, oxprenolol and atenolol. The indications for the use of these drugs are unaltered by pregnancy. Although there are isolated case reports of intrauterine growth retardation, acute fetal distress in labour and hypoglycaemia in the newborn in patients taking beta-adrenergic blocking agents, these have not been confirmed in clinical trials of oxprenolol used for treating hypertension in pregnancy. It would seem reasonable, therefore, to use propranolol or oxprenolol in both the acute and long-term treatment of supraventricular and ventricular tachycardia in pregnancy.

Quinidine is used to maintain or induce sinus rhythm in patients either after DC conversion or when taking digoxin. It is well tolerated in pregnancy and has only minimal oxytocic effect. There is much less experience with other antidysrhythmic drugs such as verapamil, diltiazem, amiodarone or disopyramide. The use of disopyramide has been associated with hypertonic uterine activity on one occasion (Leonard et al 1978). Therefore disopyramide should be used in pregnancy with caution. The long-term risks of phenytoin are well known. However, this drug is only likely to be used in the acute treatment of dysrhythmias, particularly those induced by digitalis intoxication. Procainamide has also been used successfully to abolish atrial fibrillation in pregnancy (Szekely & Snaith 1974). Pitcher et al (1983) have reported the successful use of amiodarone in pregnancy in one case of resistant atrial tachycardia, with no obvious adverse effects in the fetus. The cord blood levels were only 10–25% of maternal plasma levels, even after therapy 3 weeks before delivery. Amiodarone contains substantial quantities of iodine, but neonatal thyroid function was normal. On the basis of this one report, it would seem reasonable to use amiodarone for resistant arrhythmias in late pregnancy that cannot be treated in any other way. Amiodarone and verapamil have been successfully used for the intrauterine treatment of fetal supraventricular tachycardia (Rey et al 1985).

DC conversion for tachyarrhythmias is safe in pregnancy and does not harm the fetus (Finlay & Edmunds 1979).

The difficulty arises in considering long-term prophylactic treatment with antidysrhythmic drugs which have not been extensively used in pregnancy. Here each case must be considered on its own merits, paying particular attention to the frequency and severity of the attacks of dysrhythmia. A single short episode of supraventricular tachycardia associated with no other symptoms does not require prophylactic treatment. Frequent attacks of ventricular tachycardia associated with syncope would require prophylaxis whatever the outcome in the fetus.

Anticoagulant therapy is a major problem in the management of patients with heart disease in pregnancy and is considered in the section on artificial heart valves, below.

Labour

Heart disease per se is not an indication for induction of labour; indeed, the risks of failed induction and of possible sepsis are relative contraindications. Nevertheless, these risks are slight, and induction should not be withheld if it is necessary for obstetric reasons. Furthermore, in complicated cases requiring optimal medical support, induction near term may be justified to plan delivery in daylight hours.

Fluid balance necessitates careful and expert attention during labour in women with significant heart diasease. Many women in labour are given copious quantities of intravenous fluid and if they have normal hearts, can cope with the resultant increase in circulating blood volume. Patients with heart disease cannot, however, and may easily develop pulmonary oedema. This effect is exacerbated by the tendency to use crystalloid intravenous fluids which decrease the colloid osmotic pressure of plasma by about 5 mmHg over the course of labour (Gonik et al 1985).

Some centres are gaining increasing experience in the use of elective central catheterization (Swan–Ganz technique) to measure right atrial pressure, wedge pressure (indirect left atrial pressure) and cardiac output in labour in patients with heart disease. There is no doubt that this technique facilitates a more rational use of fluid therapy, diuretics and inotropes. Preliminary results also suggest that measurement of central venous pressure alone is so misleading as an index of left ventricular filling pressure that it should not be used for this purpose (although it is still invaluable in managing patients with bleeding problems). The technique of Swan–Ganz catheterization is quite difficult, however, and has a significant morbidity. Therefore, it should only be used in centres where there is sufficient experience.

Women with heart disease are also particularly sensitive to the effects of aortocaval compression by the gravid uterus when lying in the supine position. Marked hypotension can develop, causing maternal and fetal distress. The risk of this complication developing is even greater after epidural anaesthesia (Ueland et al 1968).

Most patients with heart disease do have quite rapid, uncomplicated labours, particularly if they are taking digoxin (Weaver & Pearson 1973). In the majority, analgesia is best given by epidural anaesthesia since it is an effective analgesic which also decreases cardiac output, by causing peripheral vasodilation and decreasing venous return, and reduces heart rate. However, epidural anaesthesia is inadvisable in Eisenmenger's syndrome and contraindicated in hypertrophic cardiomyopathy.

Most obstetric emergencies arising in labour, including the need for Caesarean section, can be managed using epidural anaesthesia. If this is not available, however, or if elective Caesarean section is advised, general anaesthesia probably causes less haemodynamic derangement than epidural anaesthesia. But there are few adequate comparisons of these forms of anaesthesia in comparable patients, and much depends on the skill and preference of the anaesthetist.

In women with heart disease, it seems sensible to keep the second stage of labour short in order to decrease maternal effort, but there is obviously no advantage in performing forceps delivery in a woman who would deliver easily by herself.

The use of oxytocic drugs in the third stage of labour is much debated. The theoretical disadvantage is that ergometrine and Syntocinon will cause a tonic contraction of the uterus, expressing about 500 ml of blood into a circulation whose capacitance has also been reduced by associated venoconstriction. The associated rise in left atrial pressure (Fig. 37.1), which averages 10 mmHg in patients with mitral stenosis, may be quite sufficient to precipitate pulmonary oedema. However, the management of postpartum haemorrhage in a patient with heart disease is not easy. Syntocinon should be used in all patients in the third stage, unless they are in failure, since it has less effect on blood vessels than ergometrine and can be given by intravenous infusion, which can be accompanied by intravenous frusemide.

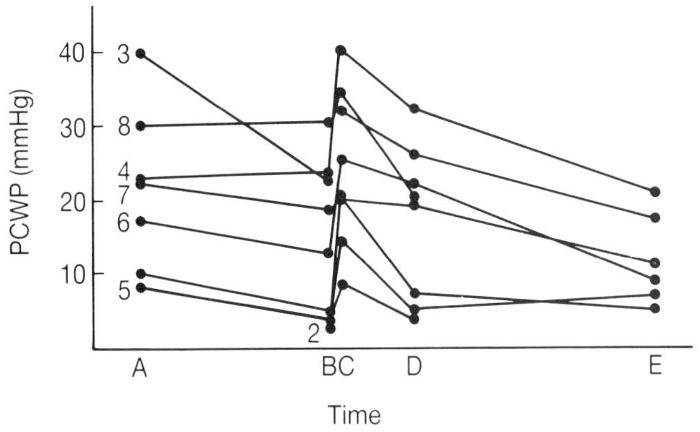

Fig. 37.1 Intrapartum alterations in pulmonary capillary wedge pressure (PCWP) in eight patients with mitral stenosis. A = First-stage labour; B = second-stage labour, 15–30 min before delivery; C = 5–15 min postpartum; D = 4–6 h postpartum; E = 18–20 h postpartum. From Clark e t al (1985), with permission.

Endocarditis and its prevention in pregnancy

The Report on Confidential Enquiries into Maternal Deaths in England and Wales (Department of Health and Social Security 1982) shows that there have been 10 such deaths from endocarditis in England and Wales between 1970 and 1975. However, the case for antibiotic prophylaxis in labour has not been proven. There are several large series of women with heart disease in pregnancy in whom no antibiotics were given and in whom no endocarditis was observed (Fleming 1977; Sugrue et al 1981). Yet, the data in the Confidential Enquiries into Maternal Deaths series suggests that women are at increased risk from endocarditis in pregnancy. What is not clear from these reports is whether the endocarditis was contracted during labour and therefore potentially preventable by antibiotics, or whether it arose at some other time. Until more details are available, the author continues to use antibiotic prophylaxis—ampicillin 500 mg i.m. and gentamicin 80 mg i.m. three injections given every 8 hours at the onset or induction of labour (Durack 1975). The woman who is penicillin-sensitive receives one intravenous injection of vancomycin 500 mg (Durack 1975).

SPECIFIC CONDITIONS OCCURRING DURING PREGNANCY

Acquired heart disease

Chronic rheumatic heart disease

As already indicated, this form of heart disease has been commonest in pregnancy in the UK and still is in many parts of the world. By far the most important lesion is mitral stenosis, which may be the only lesion or the dominant abnormality amongst several others. Women with mitral stenosis are particularly likely to develop pulmonary oedema in pregnancy because of the increase in cardiac output, the increase in heart rate preventing ventricular filling and the increase in pulmonary blood volume. Mitral stenosis is the lesion that is most likely to require treatment for pulmonary oedema or heart failure and also to require surgery during pregnancy. The haemodynamic changes associated with labour in patients with mitral stenosis have been documented by Swan–Ganz catheterization. Women entering labour with a wedge pressure (indirect left atrial pressure) less than 14 mmHg are unlikely to develop pulmonary oedema (Clark et al 1985).

Mitral regurgitation puts a volume load on the left atrium and left ventricle, but it does not cause pulmonary hypertension until late in the condition, and heart failure is rare in pregnancy; it occurs usually in older women.

Rheumatic aortic valve disease is much less common in women than in men, and much less common than mitral valve disease in pregnancy. Severe aortic regurgitation causes pulmonary oedema; aortic stenosis may be associated with chest pain, syncope and sudden death, but aortic valve disease is usually not severe enough to be a problem in pregnancy. Severe aortic stenosis has a 17% maternal mortality (Arias & Pineda 1978).

Disease of the tricuspid valve almost never occurs in isolation. Also, tricuspid valve disease rarely requires specific treatment; the patient improves when the rheumatic disease of the other valves is treated, either medically or surgically.

Pregnancy in women with artificial heart valves

Anticoagulation is the major problem in this group. Those who have successful isolated aortic or mitral valve replacements usually have near normal cardiac function and do not incur haemodynamic problems in pregnancy (Oakley 1983). Even those with multiple valve replacements usually have sufficient cardiac reserve for a successful pregnancy (Andrinopoulos & Arias 1980).

The problem of anticoagulation is shown in Table 37.2. The combined fetal morbidity and mortality rates varied between 31 and 50% in women who were anticoagulated with warfarin compared with 4–9% in those who were not anticoagulated. The long-term outlook is not as good for women with artificial heart valves as for those with tissue valves and the latter also fare better in pregnancy.

For conditions such as pulmonary embolism, subcutaneous heparin is safer than warfarin (see Chapter 64). There appears to be less maternal bleeding and less fetal risk of congenital abnormalities such as chrondrodysplasia punctata or optic atrophy. However, where there is a risk of systemic thromboembolism as with artificial heart valves, subcutaneous heparin treatment does not seem to be adequate; indeed there are reports of Starr Edwards aortic and Björk–Shiley mitral valves that have thrombosed during pregnancy when the mothers were either managed with subcutaneous heparin (Bennett & Oakley 1968, McLeod et al 1978) or were not anticoagulated (Chen et al 1982). There is no ideal

Table 37.2 Fetal outcome of oral anticoagulation in pregnancy in mothers with artificial heart valves

	Hammersmith[1]	Dublin[2]	Hong Kong[3]	Barcelona[4]
Number of pregnancies	39	18	41	46
Number anticoagulated (fetal mortality and morbidity % of those anticoagulated)	15 (53)	18 (50)	30 (40)	42 (31–38)*
Causes of fetal mortality and morbidity (% of those anticoagulated)				
Abortion	3 (20)	8 (44)	10 (33)	12 (21–29)*
Perinatal deaths	4 (27)	0 (0)	0 (0)	2 (0–5)*
Fetal malformation	1 (7)	1 (5)	2 (7)	2 (0–5)*
Number not anticoagulated (fetal mortality and morbidity % of those not anticoagulated)	24 (4)	0	11 (9)	3 (?–?)*

[1]Oakley & Doherty (1976); [2]O'Neill et al (1982); [3]Chen et al (1982); [4]Javares et al (1984).

* Not stated which of the fetal losses etc. were in the anticoagulated group so possible range is given.

solution to this problem. Even though the risk of fetal malformations may persist after 16 weeks' gestation (Shaul & Hall 1977), warfarin should be used from before conception until about 37 weeks' gestation, because subcutaneous heparin does not give adequate protection. Furthermore, subcutaneous heparin therapy has the risk of bone demineralization (de Swiet et al 1983), while the risks of warfarin therapy have probably been over-estimated (Chong et al 1984). Alternative approaches to management in early pregnancy are to use intravenous heparin given by a Hickman catheter (Nelson et al 1984), or through a heparin lock (Pearson 1984) or to use high-dose continuous subcutaneous infusion of heparin (Rabinovici et al 1987), in all cases aiming to achieve a heparin level (protamine sulphate neutralization test; Dacie 1975) of 0.4–0.6 u/ml. Such treatment, which ideally should be given from before conception, must be considered experimental at present and is unlikely to suit all patients.

At 37 weeks, when the risk of fetal bleeding associated with labour in patients treated with warfarin seems to be too great, the patient should be admitted to hospital and given continuous intravenaous heparin to produce a heparin level of 0.4–0.6 u/ml, as assayed by protamine sulphate neutralization (Dacie 1975). Heparin does not cross the placenta and therefore will not cause bleeding in the fetus. It is believed that the clotting system of the fetus will return to normal after warfarin has been withheld for 1 week. At that time maternal heparin therapy should be reduced to give a heparin level of less than 0.4 u/ml and labour should be induced. If the woman inadvertently goes into labour while taking warfarin, she should be given vitamin K to reverse the action of warfarin in the fetus and started on heparin therapy as above. In extreme cases vitamin K has been given intramuscularly to the fetus in utero by transamniotic injection (Larsen et al 1978).

After delivery, because of the risk of maternal postpartum haemorrhage, the patient should continue to receive heparin for 7 days, when warfarin may be recommenced. This is not a contraindication to breastfeeding, since insignificant quantities of warfarin are secreted in breast milk (Orme et al 1977). However, Dindevan is excreted in breast milk (Eckstein & Jack 1970); women taking it should not breastfeed.

Myocardial infarction

Myocardial infarction is rare in pregnancy (1 in 10 000 gravidas or less) and in young women in general. Most cases occur in women aged 30–40 years. About 40% of women die in pregnancy or within 1 week of delivery. However, infarction occurring in the first two trimesters has a lower mortality (23%) than that occurring in the last trimester (45%; Hawkins et al 1985). Successful outcomes have been reported following cardiac arrest (Stokes et al 1984) and the development of left ventricular aneurysm in pregnancy (Roberts et al 1983). In contrast to myocardial infarction during pregnancy, infarction in the puerperium occurs in younger, often primigravid women. Their pregnancies have frequently been complicated by pre-eclampsia (Beary et al 1979). The precise mechanism of myocardial infarction is open to speculation in all patients. Women have a particularly high incidence of coronary spasm, and atypical mechanisms seem to be common in pregnancy. Patients with myocardial infarction occurring in the puerperium are most likely to have spasm or coronary artery thrombosis unassociated with atherosclerotic narrowing. Another possible cause is primary dissection of the coronary arteries.

The diagnosis of myocardial infarction in pregnancy is made on the basis of chest pain, with possible pericardial friction rub and fever supported by the typical changes in the electrocardiogram. Moderate elevations of the white cell count and erythrocyte sedimentation rate are seen in normal pregnancy, when the level of lactic acid dehydrogenase may also be raised (Stone et al 1960). However, elevation of serum glutamic acid transaminase level would indicate myocardial infarction in the appropriate clinical setting (Stone et al 1960). During the puerperium even this enzyme will not be helpful, because it is liberated by the involuting uterus.

It is difficult to be dogmatic about management, for there is little experience and the pathology may be diverse. It would be sensible to treat the initial episode in a coronary care unit, with conventional opiate analgesics and medication for complications such as dysrhythmias. Because of the possibility of coronary spasm, nitroglycerine or other vasodilators should be used early in women with continuing pain. Once delivery has occurred, there is a good case for coronary arteriography. The angiographic demonstration of coronary embolus would be an indication for anticoagulation, but otherwise the benefits of anticoagulation in myocardial infarction unassociated with pregnancy do not seem great enough to justify the considerable extra risks imposed on the pregnancy (Borchgrevnik et al 1968). Spontaneous vaginal delivery should be allowed unless there are good obstetric reasons for interfering. Epidural anaesthesia should be used because of its efficacy as an analgesic and in reducing cardiac output by reducing preload. As in other cases of heart disease, the second stage should be limited by forceps delivery. Syntocinon infusion should be used rather than ergometrine in the third stage, since ergometrine is more likely to cause coronary artery spasm.

There is no evidence that pregnancy specifically predisposes women to myocardial infarction. Unless it is thought that the woman has had a coronary embolus, pregnancy should not be discouraged in patients who have had myocardial infarction in the past.

Cardiomyopathy in pregnancy

Cardiomyopathy may arise de novo during pregnancy, and there is probably at least one form of cardiomyopathy (peripartum cardiomyopathy) that is specific to pregnancy. Alternatively, any form of cardiomyopathy due to other causes may complicate pregnancy.

Hypertrophic obstructive cardiomyopathy

The most common of these other causes is hypertrophic obstructive cardiomyopathy or subaortic stenosis. The cause is not known but the pathological features are hypertrophy and disorganization of cardiac muscle, particularly that of the left ventricular outflow tract. Women present with chest pain, syncope, arrhythmias or the symptoms of heart failure. They should not be allowed to become hypovolaemic, since this too increases the risk of obstruction of the left ventricular outflow tract. Particular care should be taken to give adequate fluid replacement if there is antepartum haemorrhage and also in avoiding postpartum haemorrhage. During labour, those with hypertrophic obstructive cardiomyopathy should not have epidural anaesthesia, since this causes relative hypovolaemia by increasing venous capacitance in the lower limbs. Beta-blocking drugs are often used in women with symtoms (Oakley et al 1979) and should be considered safe in pregnancy (see Chapter 36).

Peripartum cardiomyopathy

For reviews of this important condition see Stuart (1968), Homans (1985) and Julian & Szekely (1985). The woman

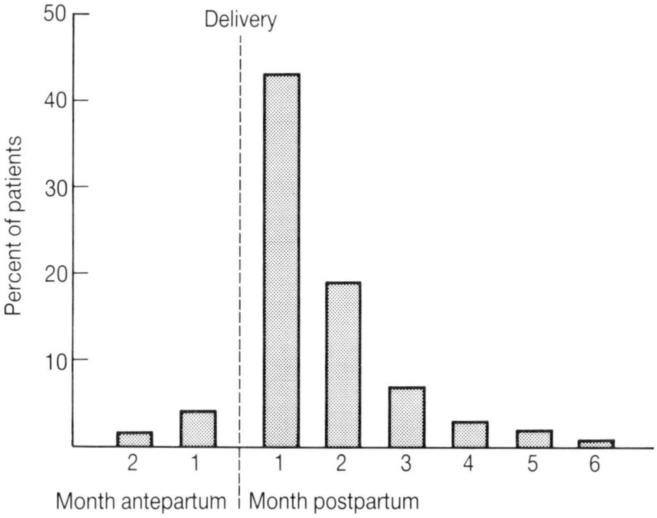

Fig. 37.2 Onset of peripartum cardiomyopathy in relation to time of delivery. From Homans (1985), with permission.

usually presents with heart failure, which is usually right-sided, either at the end of pregnancy or more commonly in the puerperium (Fig. 37.2). There is no predisposing cause for the heart failure and the heart is grossly dilated. The diagnosis is made by excluding all other causes of right and left ventricular dysfunction. Patients tend to be multiparous, black, relatively elderly and socially deprived. Pregnancy has often been complicated by hypertension. Pulmonary, peripheral and particularly cerebral embolization are major causes of morbidity and mortality. Apart from conventional antifailure treatment, these women should also receive anticoagulant therapy until heart size has returned to normal, and they have no further dysrhythmias. If they recover from the initial episode, the long-term prognosis is good, but the condition may recur in future pregnancies, particularly if there is evidence of even subclinical left ventricular dysfunction.

The pathogenesis is unknown; immunological (Rand et al 1975), nutritional and infective (Melvin et al 1982) aetiologies have been proposed.

A specific form of peripartum cardiac failure occurs in the Hausa tribe in northern Nigeria (Davidson & Parry 1978). The peak incidence is 4 weeks postpartum. During this period, for up to 40 days after delivery, the Hausa woman spends 18 h/day lying on a mud bed, heated so that the ambient temperature reaches 40°C. She also increases her sodium intake to 450 mmol/day by eating *kanwa* salt from Lake Chad. Many are hypertensive, but the condition regresses rapidly with diuretic and digoxin therapy. The contribution of hypertension to the heart failure is debated (Sanderson 1977), but this would seem an extreme example of the instability of the cardiovascular system in the first few weeks of the puerperium interacting with the particular susceptibility of West Africans to dilated cardiomyopathy (Lancet Editorial 1985).

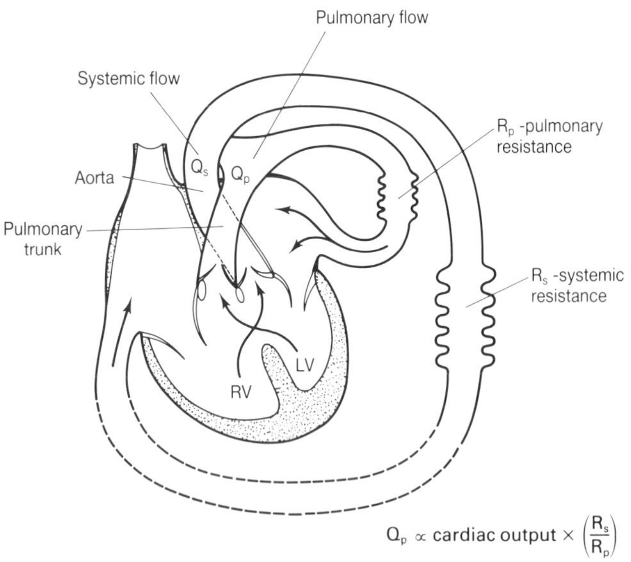

Fig. 37.3 Pulmonary (Q_p) and systemic (Q_s) blood flows and resistances (R_p, R_s) in Eisenmenger's syndrome associated with ventricular septal defect. From de Swiet & Fidler (1981), with permission.

Congenital heart disease

Eisenmenger's syndrome

Eisenmenger's syndrome has a very high maternal mortality, particularly if there is superimposed pre-eclampsia. Only recently has there been any form of surgical treatment—heart and lung transplantation—and that must be considered experimental.

Most of those with Eisenmenger's syndrome who die do so in the puerperium. Although death may be occasionally sudden, due to thromboembolism, this is unusual. More frequently, these women die due to a slowly falling systemic PO_2 with associated decrease in cardiac output. It is likely that this is due to a change in the shunt ratio whereby pulmonary blood flow decreases at the expense of systemic flow (Fig. 37.3).

What can be offered to the pregnant woman with Eisenmenger's syndrome? Unfortunately, abortion would appear to be the answer. The maternal mortality associated with abortion is only 7% in comparison to 30% for continuing pregnancy (Gleicher et al 1979). However, if she decides to continue with pregnancy, prophylactic anticoagulation, probably with subcutaneous heparin, should be offered, because of the risk of systemic and pulmonary thromboembolism. Labour should not be induced unless there are good obstetric reasons. Induced labour carries a higher risk of Caesarean section, which is associated with a particularly high maternal mortality in Eisenmenger's syndrome (Gleicher et al 1979).

There is controversy concerning the place of epidural anaesthesia for the management of labour. Although epidural anaesthesia could decrease the shunt ratio by decreasing systemic vascular resistance, this is not invariable (Midwall et al 1978). On balance, an elective epidural anaesthetic carefully administered at the beginning of labour is probably preferable to emergency epidural or general anaesthesia needed if a sudden decision is made to perform instrumental delivery (Gleicher 1979).

If the woman does become hypotensive with increasing cyanosis and decreasing cardiac output, high inspired oxygen concentrations will decrease pulmonary vascular resistance, increasing the pulmonary blood flow and increasing peripheral oxygen saturation (Midwall et al 1978). In addition, alpha-sympathomimetic agents, such as phenylephrine, methoxamine and noradrenaline, will increase systemic resistance and thus divert blood to the lungs (Devitt & Noble 1980). However, drugs such as tolazoline, phentolamine, nitroprusside and isoprenaline, which have been used to decrease pulmonary vascular resistance in other clinical situations, probably should not be given since they will also decrease the systemic vascular resistance. The same problem may occur with dopamine and beta-sympathomimetic drugs which have been given to increase cardiac output.

Coarctation of the aorta and Marfan's syndrome

In both these conditions, the maternal risk is of dissection of the aorta associated with the hyperdynamic circulation of pregnancy and possibly with an increased risk of medial degeneration due to the hormonal environment of pregnancy (Konishi et al 1980). Although earlier studies had indicated a high maternal mortality, they date from the period before surgery was available for correction of severe cases. There were no maternal deaths among 83 patients studied from 1960 (Deal & Wooley 1973). Only those who already have evidence of dissection should have the coarctation repaired in pregnancy. Any upper limb hypertension should be treated aggressively with antihypertensive drugs. If there is gross widening of the ascending aorta, suggesting intrinsic disease, the woman should be delivered by elective Caesarean section to reduce the risk of dissection associated with labour.

In Marfan's syndrome there is also a risk of dissection of the aorta. Dilatation of the aorta to more than 40 mm (determined echocardiographically) is the limit at which pregnancy is contraindicated (Pyeritz 1981). As in coarctation of the aorta, any associated hypertension should be treated aggressively and delivery should be by Caesarean section if there is evidence of aortic disease.

Congenital heart block

This usually presents no problem in pregnancy. Although part of the normal response to pregnancy includes an increase in heart rate to increase the cardiac output, this is not obligatory. There are many records of successful pregnancy among those with heart block (Ginns & Holinrake 1970, Szekely & Snaith 1974). Presumably, they are able to increase stroke volume sufficiently to cope with the increased demands of pregnancy. A few are unable to increase cardiac output sufficiently at the end of pregnancy or during labour (Bowman & Millar-Craig 1980). Therefore, women with heart block who are not paced, or those in whom there is any possibility of pacemaker failure, should be managed in obstetric units where there is access to pacing facilities.

CONCLUSIONS

Heart disease in pregnancy remains a worrying problem for the obstetrician because of those women (very much in the minority) who are at risk. Future advances will help us to define this minority with more precision and optimize management strategies for these patients.

REFERENCES

Andersen J B 1970 The effect of diuretics in late pregnancy on the new born infant. Acta Paediatrica Scandinavica 59: 659–663
Andrinopoulos G C, Arias F 1980 Triple heart valve prosthesis and pregnancy. Obstetrics and Gynecology 55: 762–764
Ardias F, Pineda J 1978 Aortic stenosis and pregnancy. Journal of Reproductive Medicine 20: 229–232
Barabas A P 1967 Heterogeneity of the Ehlers–Danlos syndrome: description of three clinical types and a hypothesis to explain the basic defect(s). British Medical Journal 2: 612–613
Batson G A 1974 Cyanotic congenital heart disease and pregnancy. British Journal of Obstetrics and Gynaecology 81: 549–553
Beary J F, Sumner W R, Bulkley B H 1979 Postpartum acute myocardial infarction: a rare occurrence of uncertain etiology. American Journal of Cardiology 43: 158–160
Becker R M 1983 Intracardiac surgery in pregnant women. Annals of Thoracic Surgery 36: 453–458
Bennett G G, Oakley C M 1968 Pregnancy in a patient with a mitral valve prosthesis. Lancet i: 616–619
Borchgrevink C F, Bjerkelund C, Abrahamsen A M et al 1968 Longterm anticoagulant therapy after myocardial infarction in women. British Medical Journal 2: 571–574
Bowman P R, Millar-Craig M W 1980 Congenital heart block and pregnancy: a further case report. Journal of Obstetrics and Gynaecology 1: 98–99
Bruner J P, Barry M J, Elliott J P 1984 Pregnancy in a patient with idiopathic long QT syndrome. American Journal of Obstetrics and Gynecology 149: 690–691
Carpenter R J, Decuir P 1984 Cardiovascular collapse associated with oral terbutaline tocolytic therapy. American Journal of Obstetrics and Gynecology 148: 821–823
Chen W W C, Chan C S, Lee P K, Wang RYC, Wong V C W 1982 Pregnancy in patients with prosthetic heart valves: an experience with 45 pregnancies. Quarterly Journal of Medicine 51: 358–365
Chesley L C 1980 Severe rheumatic cardiac disease and pregnancy: the ultimate prognosis. American Journal of Obstetrics and Gynecology 136: 552–558
Chong M K B, Harvey D, de Swiet M 1984 Follow-up study of children whose mothers were treated with warfarin during pregnancy. British Journal of Obstetrics and Gynaecology 91: 1070–1073
Clark S L, Phelan J P, Greenspoon J, Aldahl D, Horenstein J 1985 Labor and delivery in the presence of mitral stenosis: central hemodynamic observations. American Journal of Obstetrics and Gynecology 152: 984–1088
Copeland W E, Wooley C F, Ryan J M, Runco V, Levin H S 1963 Pregnancy and congenital heart disease. American Journal of Obstetrics and Gynecology 86: 107–110
Dacie J 1975 Practical haematology. Churchill Livingstone, Edinburgh, pp 413–414
Davidson N McD, Parry E H O 1978 Peri-partum cardiac failure. Quarterly Journal of Medicine 47: 431–461
Davies P, Francis R I, Docker M F, Watt J M, Selwyn Crawford J 1986 Analysis of impedance cardiography longitudinally applied in pregnancy. British Journal of Obstetrics and Gynaecology 93: 717–720
Deal K, Wooley C F 1973 Coarctation of the aorta and pregnancy. Annals of Internal Medicine 78: 706–710
Department of Health and Social Security 1982 Report on confidential enquiries into maternal deaths in England and Wales 1976–1978. Her Majesty's Stationery Office, London
de Swiet M 1984 Heart disease in pregnancy. In: de Swiet M (ed) Medical disorders in obstetric practice. Blackwell Scientific Publications, Oxford, pp 116–148
de Swiet M, Fidler J 1981 Heart disease in pregnancy: some controversies. Journal of the Royal College of Physicians 15: 183–186
de Swiet M, Talbert D G 1986 The measurement of cardiac output by electrical impedance plethysmography in pregnancy. Are the assumptions valid? British Journal of Obstetrics and Gynaecology 93: 721–726
de Swiet M, Dorrington Ward P, Fidler J et al 1983 Prolonged heparin therapy in pregnancy causes bone demineralisation (heparin-induced osteopenia). British Journal of Obstetrics and Gynaecology 90: 1129–1134
Devitt J H, Noble W H 1980 Eisenmenger's syndrome and pregnancy. New England Journal of Medicine 302: 751
Durack D T 1975 Current practice in prevention of bacterial endocarditis. British Heart Journal 37: 478–481
Eckstein H, Jack B 1970 Breast feeding and anticoagulant therapy. Lancet i: 672–673
Eilen B, Kaiser I H, Becker R M, Cohen M N 1981 Aortic valve replacement in the third trimester of pregnancy: case report and review of the literature. Obstetrics and Gynecology 57: 119–121
Elkayam U, Gleicher N 1982 Cardiac problems in pregnancy. Diagnosis and management of maternal and fetal disease. Alan R Liss, New York
Finlay A Y, Edmunds V 1979 DC cardioversion in pregnancy. British Journal of Clinical Practice 33: 88–94
Fleming H A 1977 Antibiotic prophylaxis against infective endocarditis after delivery. Lancet i: 144–145
Gant N F, Daley G L, Chand S, Whalley P J, MacDonald P C 1973 A study of angiotensin II pressor response throughout primigravid pregnancy. Journal of Clinical Investigation 52: 2682–2689
Ginns H M, Holinrake K 1970 Complete heart block in pregnancy treated with an internal cardiac pacemaker. Journal of Obstetrics and Gynaecology of the British Commonwealth 77: 710
Gleicher N, Midwall J, Hochberger D, Jaffin H 1979 Eisenmenger's syndrome and pregnancy. Obstetrical and Gynecological Survey 34: 721–741
Gonik B, Cotton D, Spillman T, Abouleish E, Zavisca F 1985 Peripartum colloid osmotic pressure changes: effects of controlled fluid management. American Journal of Obstetrics and Gynecology 151: 812–815
Hawkins G D V, Wendel G D, Leveno K J, Stoneham J 1985 Myocardial infarction during pregnancy: a review. Obstetrics and Gynecology 65: 139–147
Ho P C, Chen T Y, Wong V 1980 The effect of maternal cardiac disease and digoxin administration on labour, fetal weight and maturity at birth. Australian and New Zealand Journal of Obstetrics and Gynaecology 20: 24–27
Homans D C 1985 Peripartum cardiomyopathy. New England Journal of Medicine 312: 1432–1436
Hytten F E, Paintin D B 1963 Increase in plasma volume during normal pregnancy. Journal of Obstetrics and Gynaecology of the British Commonwealth 70: 402–407
Jacoby W J 1964 Pregnancy with tetralogy and pentalogy of Fallot. American Journal of Cardiology 14: 866–873
James C F, Banner T, Levelle P, Caton D 1985 Noninvasive determination of cardiac output throughout pregnancy. Anesthesiology 63: A434
Javares T, Coto E C, Maiques V, Rincon A, Such M, Caffarena J M 1984 Pregnancy after heart valve replacement. International Journal of Cardiology 5: 731–739
Jewett J F 1979 Pulmonary hypertension and pre-eclampsia. New England Journal of Medicine 301: 1063–1064
Julian D G, Szekely P 1985 Peripartum cardiomyopathy. Progress in Cardiovascular Diseases 27: 223–240

Konishi Y, Tatsuta N, Kumada K et al 1980 Dissecting aneurysm during pregnancy and the puerperium. Japanese Circulation Journal 44: 726–732
Lancet Editorial 1985 Dilated cardiomyopathy in Africa. Lancet i: 557–558
Larsen J F, Jacobsen B, Holm H H Pedersen J F, Mantoni M 1978 Intrauterine injection of vitamin K before the delivery during anticoagulant treatment of the mother. Acta Obstetricia et Gynecologica Scandinavica 57: 227–230
Leonard R F, Braun T E, Levy A M 1978 Initiation of uterine contractions by disopyramide during pregnancy. New England Journal of Medicine 299: 84
Levy M, Grait L, Laufer N 1977 Excretion of drugs in human milk. New England Journal of Medicine 297: 789
MacNab G, MacAfee C A J 1985 A changing pattern of heart disease associated with pregnancy. Journal of Obstetrics and Gynaecology 5: 139–142
McCaffrey R M, Dunn L J 1974 Primary pulmonary hypertension in pregnancy. Obstetrical and Gynecological Survey 19: 567
McLeod A A, Jennings K P, Townsend E R 1978 Near fatal puerperal thrombosis on Björk-Shiley mitral valve prosthesis. British Heart Journal 40: 934–937
Melvin K R, Richardson P J, Olsen E G J, Daly K, Jackson G 1982 Peripartum cardiomyopathy due to myocarditis. New England Journal of Medicine 307: 731–734
Mendelson C L 1956 Disorders of the heart beat during pregnancy. American Journal of Obstetrics and Gynecology 72: 1268–1301
Midwall J, Jaffin H, Herman M V, Kuper Smith J 1978 Shunt flow and pulmonary haemodynamics during labor and delivery in the Eisenmenger syndrome. American Journal of Cardiology 42: 299–303
Milne J A, Howie A D, Pack A I 1978 Dyspnoea during normal pregnancy. British Journal of Obstetrics and Gynaecology 85: 260–263
Morgan Jones A, Howitt G 1965 Eisenmenger syndrome in pregnancy. British Medical Journal 1: 1627–1631
Morton M J, Paul M S, Campos G R, Hart M V, Metcalfe J 1985 Exercise dynamics in late gestation: effects of physical training. American Journal of Obstetrics and Gynecology 152: 91–97
Neilson G, Galea E G, Blunt A 1970 Congenital heart disease and pregnancy. Medical Journal of Australia 1: 1086–1088
Nelson D M, Stempel L E, Fabri P J, Talbert M 1984 Hickman catheter use in a pregnant patient requiring therapeutic heparin anticoagulation. 149: 461–462
Nora J J 1978 The evolution of specific genetic and environmental counselling in congenital heart diseases. Circulation 57: 205–213
Oakley C M 1983 Pregnancy in patients with prosthetic heart valves. British Medical Journal 286: 1680–1682
Oakley C M, Doherty P 1976 Pregnancy in patients after valve replacement. British Heart Journal 38: 1140–1148
Oakley G D G, McGarry K, Limb D G, Oakley C M 1979 Management of pregnancy in patients with hypertrophic cardiomyopathy. British Medical Journal 1: 1749–1750
Okita G T, Plotz E J, Davis M E 1956 Placental transfer of radioactive digitoxin in pregnant woman and its fetal distribution. Circulation Research 4: 376–380
O'Neill H, Blake S, Sugrue D, MacDonald D 1982 Problems in the management of patients with artificial heart valves during pregnancy. British Journal of Obstetrics and Gynaecology 89: 940–943
Orme M l'E, Lewis P J, de Swiet M et al 1977 May mothers given warfarin breast-feed their infants? British Medical Journal 1: 1564–1565
Pearl W, Spicer M 1981 Ehlers–Danlos syndrome. Southern Medical Journal 74: 80–81
Pearson J N 1984 Outpatient intravenous heparin. American Journal of Obstetrics and Gynecology 149: 108
Pitcher D, Leather H M, Storey G C A, Holt D W 1983 Amiodarone in pregnancy. Lancet ii: 597–598
Pyeritz R E 1981 Maternal and fetal complications of pregnancy in the Marfan syndrome. American Journal of Medicine 71: 784–790
Rabinovici J, Mani A, Barkai G, Hod H, Frenkel Y, Mashiach S 1987 Long-term ambulatory anticoagulation by constant subcutaneous heparin infusion in pregnancy. British Journal of Obstetrics and Gynaecology 94: 89–91
Rand R J, Jenkins D M, Scott D G 1975 Maternal cardiomyopathy of pregnancy causing stillbirth. British Journal of Obstetrics and Gynaecology 82: 172–175
Rayburn W F, Fontana M E 1981 Mitral valve prolapse and pregnancy. American Journal of Obstetrics and Gynecology 14: 9–11
Rey E, Duperron L, Gauthier R, Lemay M, Grignon A, LeLorier J 1985 Transplacental treatment of tachycardia-induced fetal heart failure with verapamil and amiodarone: a case report. American Journal of Obstetrics and Gynecology 153: 311–312
Roberts A D G, Low R A L, Rae A P, Hillis W S 1983 Left ventricular aneurysm complicating myocardial infarction occurring during pregnancy. Case report. British Journal of Obstetrics and Gynaecology 90: 969–970
Rogers M E, Willerson J T, Goldblatt A, Smith T W 1972 Serum digoxin concentrations in the human fetus, neonate and infant. New England Journal of Medicine 287: 1010–1013
Rubler S, Prabod Kumar M D, Pinto E R 1977 Cardiac size and performance during pregnancy estimated with echocardiography. American Journal of Cardiology 40: 534–540
Rudd N L, Nimrod C, Holbrook K A, Byers P H 1983 Pregnancy complications in type IV Ehlers–Danlos syndrome. Lancet i: 50–53
Rush R W, Verjans M, Spracklen F H N 1979 Incidence of heart disease in pregnancy. A study done at Peninsular Maternity Services Hospital. South African Medical Journal 55: 808–810
Saarikoski S 1976 Placental transfer and fetal uptake of 3H-digoxin in humans. British Journal of Obstetrics and Gynaecology 83: 879–884
Sanderson J E 1977 Oedema and heart failure in the tropics. Lancet ii: 1159–1161
Schneider K T M, Bollinger A, Huch R 1984 The oscillating 'vena cava syndrome' during quiet standing — an unexpected observation in late pregnancy. British Journal of Obstetrics and Gynaecology 91: 766–780
Shaul W L, Hall J G 1977 Multiple congenital anomalies associated with oral anticoagulants. American Journal of Obstetrics and Gynecology 127: 191–198
Slater A J, Gude N, Clarke I J, Walters W A W 1986 Haemodynamic changes in left ventricular performance during high-dose oestrogen administration in transsexuals. British Journal of Obstetrics and Gynaecology 93: 532–538
Stokes I M, Evans J, Stone M 1984 Myocardial infarction and cardiac output in the second trimester followed by assisted vaginal delivery under epidural anaesthesia at 38 weeks gestation. Case report. British Journal of Obstetrics and Gynaecology 91: 197–198
Stone M L, Lending M, Slobody L B, Mestern J 1960 Glutamine oxalacetic transaminase and lactic acid dehydrogenase in pregnancy. American Journal of Obstetrics and Gynecology 80: 104
Stuart K L 1968 Cardiomyopathy of pregnancy and the puerperium. Quarterly Journal of Medicine 37: 463–478
Sugrue D, Blake S, MacDonald D 1981 Pregnancy complicated by maternal heart disease at the National Maternity Hospital, Dublin, Ireland, 1969 to 1978. American Journal of Obstetrics and Gynecology 139: 1–6
Sullivan J M, Ramanathan K B 1985 Management of medical problems in pregnancy — severe cardiac disease. New England Journal of Medicine 313: 304–309
Szekely P, Snaith L 1953 Paroxysmal tachycardia in pregnancy. British Heart Journal 15: 195
Szekely P, Snaith L 1974 Heart disease and pregnancy. Churchill Livingstone, Edinburgh
Szekely P, Turner R, Snaith L 1973 Pregnancy and the changing pattern of rheumatic heart disease. British Heart Journal 35: 1293–1303
Tsou E, Waldhorn R E, Kerwin D M, Katz S, Patterson J A 1984 Pulmonary venoocclusive disease in pregnancy. Obstetrics and Gynecology 64: 281–284
Ueland K, Hansen J M 1969 Maternal cardiovascular dynamics. II Posture and uterine contractions. American Journal of Obstetrics and Gynecology 103: 1–7
Ueland K, Gills R, Hansen J M 1968 Maternal cardiovascular dynamics. I. Cesarean section under subarachnoid block anesthesia. American Journal of Obstetrics and Gynecology 100: 42–53
Ueland K, Novy M J, Metcalfe S 1972 Hemodynamic responses of patients with heart disease to pregnancy and exercise. American Journal of Obstetrics and Gynecology 113: 47–59
Veille J C, Morton M J, Burry K J 1985 Maternal cardiovascular adaptations to twin pregnancy. American Journal of Obstetrics and Gynecology 153: 261–263

Weaver J B, Pearson J F 1973 Influence on time of onset and duration of labour in women with cardiac disease. British Medical Journal 2: 519–520
Whittemore R, Hobbins J C, Engle M A 1982 Pregnancy and its outcome in women with and without surgical treatment of congenital heart disease. American Journal of Cardiology 50: 641–651
Zitnik R S, Brandenburg R O, Sheldon R, Wallace R B 1969 Pregnancy and open heart surgery. Circulation 39 (suppl): 257

38

Elizabeth A. Letsky

Coagulation defects in pregnancy

HAEMOSTASIS AND PREGNANCY

Healthy haemostasis depends on normal vasculature, platelets, coagulation factors and fibrinolysis. These act together to confine the circulating blood to the vascular bed and arrest bleeding after trauma. Normal pregnancy is accompanied by dramatic changes in the coagulation and fibrinolytic systems. There is a marked increase in some of the coagulation factors, particularly fibrinogen. Fibrin is laid down in the uteroplacental vessel walls and fibrinolysis is suppressed. These changes, together with the increased blood volume, help to combat the hazard of haemorrhage at placental separation, but play only a secondary role to the unique process of myometrial contraction which reduces the blood flow to the placental site. They also produce a vulnerable state for intravascular clotting, and a whole spectrum of disorders involving coagulation occur in complications of pregnancy, falling into two main groups—thromboembolism (see Ch. 64) and bleeding due to disseminated intravascular coagulation (DIC). To make more understandable the measures taken to deal with these obstetric emergencies, a short account follows of haemostasis during pregnancy and how it differs from that in the non-pregnant state.

VASCULAR INTEGRITY

It is not known how vascular integrity is normally maintained but it is clear that the platelets have a key role to play because conditions in which their number is depleted or their function is abnormal are characterized by widespread spontaneous capillary haemorrhages. It is thought that the platelets in health are constantly sealing microdefects of the vasculature, with mini fibrin clots being formed and the unwanted fibrin being removed by a process of fibrinolysis. Generation of prostacyclin appears to be the physiological mechanism which protects the vessel wall from excess deposition of platelet aggregates, and explains the fact that contact of platelets with healthy vascular endothelium is not a stimulus for thrombus formation (Moncada & Vane 1979).

Prostacyclin is an unstable prostaglandin first discovered in 1976. It is the principal prostanoid synthesized by blood vessels, a powerful vasodilator and potent inhibitor of platelet aggregation. Moncada & Vane (1979) have proposed that there is a balance between the production of prostacyclin by the vessel wall, and the production of the vasoconstrictor and powerful aggregating agent thromboxane by the platelet. Prostacyclin prevents aggregation at much lower concentrations than are needed to prevent adhesion, therefore vascular damage leads to platelet adhesion but not necessarily to aggregation and thrombus formation.

When injury is minor, small platelet thrombi form and are washed away by the circulation as described above, but the extent of the injury is an important determinant of the size of the thrombus—and of whether or not platelet aggregation is stimulated. Prostacyclin synthetase is abundant in the intima and progressively decreases in concentration from the intima to the adventitia, whereas the proaggregating elements increase in concentration from the subendothelium to the adventitia. It follows that severe vessel damage or physical detachment of the endothelium will lead to the development of a large thrombus as opposed to simple platelet adherence.

There are several conditions in which the production of prostacyclin could be impaired, thereby upsetting the normal balance. Deficiency of prostacyclin production has been suggested in platelet consumption syndromes such as haemolytic uraemic syndrome and thrombotic thrombocytopenic purpura (Lewis 1982). Prostacyclin production has been shown to be reduced in fetal and placental tissue from pre-eclamptic pregnancies, and the current role of prostacyclin in pathogenesis of this disease and potential for treatment in hypertension of pregnancy is undergoing active investigation.

Platelets are produced in the bone marrow by the megakaryocytes and have a lifespan of 9–12 days. At the end of their normal lifespan the effete cells are engulfed by cells of the reticuloendothelial system and most damaged platelets are sequestered in the spleen.

There have been conflicting reports concerning the platelet count during normal pregnancy. A review of publications over the past 25 years (Sill et al 1985) revealed a majority consensus (of six) suggesting a small fall in the platelet count towards term during normal pregnancy; two publications suggested that there is no change and one early, probably inaccurate, study documented a rise. However, few of these studies obtained data on a longitudinal basis and in none of them was a within-patient analysis performed.

Until recently platelet counts have been performed manually in a haemocytometer, calculating the number of platelets per cubic millimetre in anticoagulated blood samples. This is time-consuming and had to be requested as a separate investigation and was only asked for in those patients giving concern. Now that automated platelet counting is part of the profile offered by most electronic whole blood counters, platelet counts are part of the routine estimation whenever a full blood count is requested, and more information is available about the platelet count in normal, uncomplicated pregnancy. It is becoming clear that in any series if mean values for platelet concentration are analysed throughout pregnancy there may well be a downward trend (Fay et al 1983), but individual responses vary; within-patient longitudinal studies show no change or a fall or even a slight rise, but all values are within the normal accepted range outside pregnancy (Sill et al 1985). There is probably no significant change in the count in normal uncomplicated, healthy pregnancy even towards term (Fenton et al 1977, Sill et al 1985, Beal & de Masi 1985).

There appears to be more evidence suggesting that there is an increased platelet turnover and low-grade platelet activation as pregnancy advances, with a larger proportion of younger platelets with a greater mean platelet volume (Fay et al 1983, Sill et al 1985). However, other studies have shown no significant difference in platelet lifespan between non-pregnant and healthy pregnant women (Wallenberg & Van Kessel 1978, Rakoczi et al 1979).

Most investigators agree that low-grade chronic intravascular coagulation within the uteroplacental circulation is a part of the physiological response of all women to pregnancy. This is partially compensated and it is not surprising that the platelets should be involved at some level, even in healthy pregnancy.

One study (Lewis et al 1980) demonstrated significantly more aggregated platelets in a small number of women during late pregnancy and the puerperium compared with non-pregnant controls. In another more recent study, patients with a normal pregnancy were compared with non-pregnant controls (O'Brien et al 1986). They were shown to have a significantly lower platelet count and an increase in circulating platelet aggregates. In vitro the platelets were shown to be hypoaggregable. This was interpreted as suggesting platelet activation during pregnancy causing platelet aggregation and followed by exhaustion of platelets (O'Brien et al 1986).

Earlier publications suggesting that there was no evidence of changes in platelet function (Shaper et al 1968) or differences in platelet lifespan (Rakoczi et al 1979, Romero & Duffy 1980) between healthy non-pregnant and pregnant women must be re-evaluated in the face of more recent investigations, but it is clear that normal pregnancy has little significant effect on the screening parameter usually measured, namely the platelet count.

The problem remains in defining completely normal pregnancy. Certain disease states specific to pregnancy have profound effects on platelet consumption lifespan and function. For example, a decrease in platelet count has been observed in pregnancies with fetal growth retardation (Redman et al 1978) and the lifespan of platelets is shortened significantly even in mild pre-eclampsia.

Arrest of bleeding after trauma

An essential function of the haemostatic system is a rapid reaction to injury which remains confined to the area of damage. This requires control mechanisms which will stimulate coagulation after trauma, and limit the extent of the response. The substances involved in the formation of the haemostatic plug normally circulate in an inert form until activated at the site of injury, or by some other factor released into the circulation which will trigger intravascular coagulation.

Local response

Platelets adhere to collagen on the injured basement membrane, which triggers a series of changes in the platelets themselves, including shape change and release of adenosine diphosphate and other substances. Adenosine diphosphate release stimulates further aggregation of platelets, which triggers the coagulation cascade, and the action of thrombin leads to the formation of fibrin which converts the lone platelet plug into a firm, stable wound seal. The role of platelets is of less importance in injury involving large vessels, because platelet aggregates are of insufficient size and strength to breach the defect. The coagulation mechanism is of major importance here, together with vascular contraction.

COAGULATION SYSTEM

The end-result of blood coagulation is the formation of an insoluble fibrin clot from the soluble precursor fibrinogen

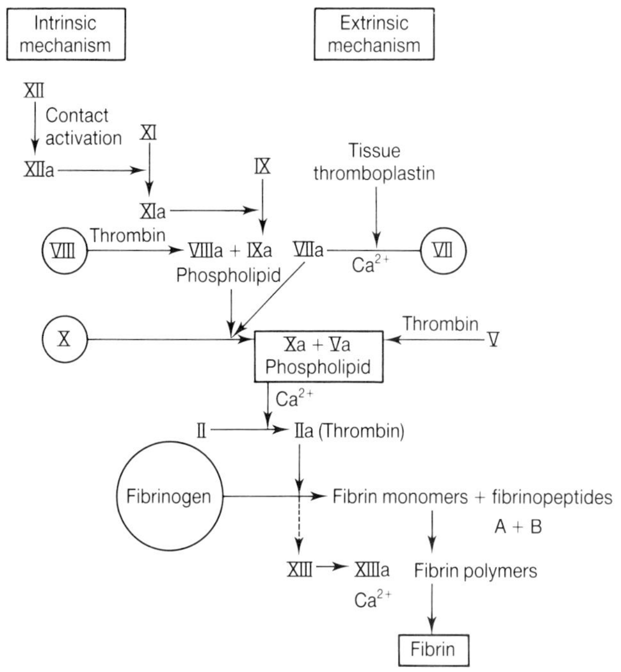

Fig. 38.1 The factors involved in blood coagulation and their interactions. The circled factors show significant increases in pregnancy.

in the plasma. This involves a complex interaction of clotting factors, and a sequential activation of a series of proenzymes which has been termed the coagulation cascade (Fig. 38.1).

When a blood vessel is injured, blood coagulation is initiated by activation of factor XII by collagen (intrinsic mechanism) and activation of factor VII by thromboplastin release (extrinsic mechanism) from the damaged tissues. Both the intrinsic and extrinsic mechanisms are activated by components of the vessel wall and both are required for normal haemostasis. Strict divisions between the two pathways do not exist and interactions between activated factors in both pathways have been shown. They share a common pathway following the activation of factor X.

The intrinsic pathway (or contact system) proceeds spontaneously and is relatively slow, requiring 5–20 minutes for visible fibrin formation. All tissues contain a specific lipoprotein, thromboplastin (particularly concentrated in lung and brain), which markedly increases the rate at which blood clots. The placenta is also very rich in tissue factor; tissue factor produces fibrin formation within 12 seconds. The acceleration of coagulation is brought about by bypassing the reactions involving the contact (intrinsic) system (see Fig. 38.1).

Normal pregnancy is accompanied by major changes in the coagulation system, with increases in levels of factors VII, VIII and X, and a particularly marked increase in the level of plasma fibrinogen (Bonnar 1981, Fig. 38.1), which is probably the chief cause of the accelerated erythrocyte sedimentation rate observed in pregnancy. The effect of pregnancy on the coagulation factors can be detected from about the third month of gestation, and the amount of fibrinogen in late pregnancy is at least double that of the non-pregnant state (Bonnar 1981).

Blood coagulation is strictly confined to the site of tissue injury in normal circumstances. Powerful control mechanisms must be at work to prevent dissemination of coagulation beyond the site of trauma.

THE NATURALLY OCCURRING ANTICOAGULANTS

Mechanisms that limit and localize the clotting process at sites of trauma are critically important to protect against generalized thrombosis, and also to prevent spontaneous activation of those powerful procoagulant factors which circulate in normal plasma.

In recent years, in the investigation of healthy haemostasis, emphasis has been switching from the factors which promote clotting to those that prevent generalized and spontaneous activation of these factors. It is not appropriate to give an account of the complex interactions and biochemistry of all of these factors here. Only those of major importance in haemostasis and relevance to pregnancy will be mentioned. The balance of procoagulant and inhibitory factors is discussed in a review by Lammle & Griffin (1985).

Antithrombin III (ATIII) is considered to be the main physiological inhibitor of thrombin and factor Xa. It is well known that heparin greatly enhances the reaction rate of enzyme ATIII interaction and this is the rationale for the use of small-dose heparin as prophylaxis in patients at risk of thromboembolic phenomena postoperatively, in pregnancy and the puerperium. An inherited deficiency of ATIII is one of the few conditions in which a familial tendency to thrombosis has been described.

ATIII is synthesized in the liver. Its activity is low in cirrhosis and other chronic diseases of the liver, as well as in protein-losing renal disease, DIC and hypercoagulable states. The commonest cause of a small reduction in ATIII is use of oral contraceptives and this has been shown to be related to the oestrogen content.

During pregnancy there appears to be little change in ATIII levels but some decrease at parturition and an increase in the puerperium (Hellgren & Blomback 1981), but there must be increased synthesis in the antenatal period to maintain normal mean levels in the face of an increasing plasma volume.

Protein C, thrombomodulin, protein S

Protein C inactivates factors V and VIII in conjunction with its cofactors thrombomodulin and protein S. Protein C is a vitamin K-dependent anticoagulant synthesized in the liver. To exert its effect it has to be activated by an endothelial cell cofactor termed thrombomodulin. The importance of

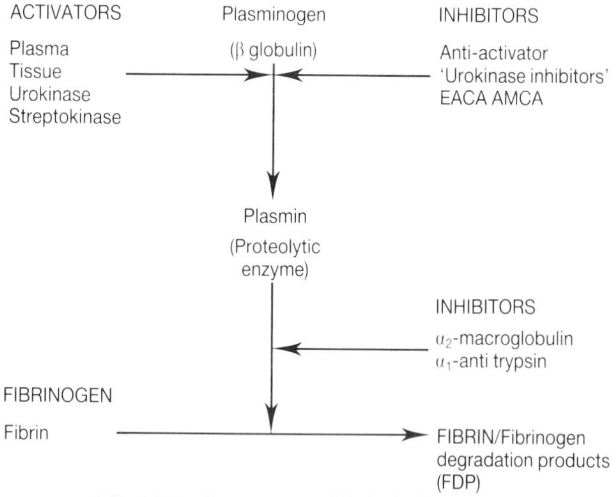

Fig. 38.2 Components of fibrinolytic system.

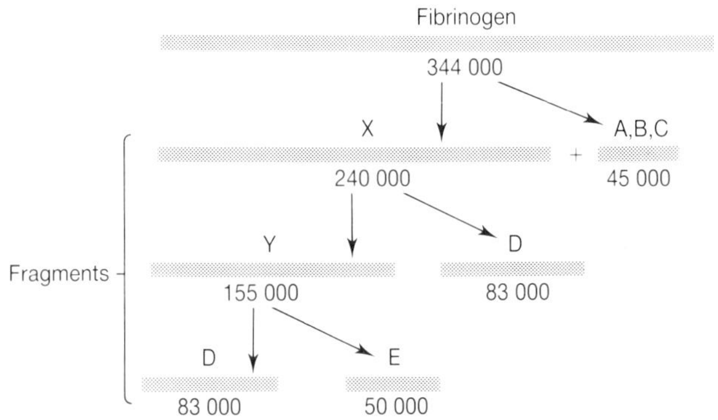

Fig. 38.3 Fibrin degradation products produced by degradation of fibrinogen by plasmin. Molecular weights are shown.

the protein C thrombomodulin protein S system is exemplified by the absence of thrombomodulin in the brain where the priority for haemostasis is higher than for anticoagulation.

Many kindreds with a deficiency or a functional deficit of protein C with associated recurrent thromboembolism have been described. Purpura fulminans neonatalis is the homozygous expression of protein C deficiency with severe thrombosis and neonatal death.

Protein S, also a vitamin K-dependent glycoprotein, acts as a cofactor for activated protein C by promoting its binding to lipid and platelet surface, thus localizing the reaction. Several families have been described with protein S deficiency and thromboembolic disease.

Data on protein C and protein S levels in healthy pregnancy are sparse. One study showed a significant reduction in functional protein S levels during pregnancy and the puerperium (Comp et al 1986). More recently, 14 patients followed longitudinally throughout gestation and postpartum showed a rise of protein C within the normal non-pregnant range during the second trimester. In contrast, free protein S fell from the second trimester onwards but remained within the confines of the normal range (Warwick et al 1989).

Although the investigation of natural anticoagulants has only just begun, the system has grown in complexity as our knowledge increases. There is little doubt that in the near future more components will be recognized which will allow a better and more thorough understanding of the mechanisms underlying the control of the delicate balance between procoagulant and anticoagulant factors which results in a healthy haemostatic system (Salem 1986).

Fibrinolysis

Fibrinolytic activity is an essential part of the dynamic interacting haemostatic mechanism, and is dependent on plasminogen activator in the blood (Fig. 38.2). Fibrin and fibrinogen are digested by plasmin, a proenzyme derived from an inactive plasma precursor plasminogen.

Increased amounts of activator are found in the plasma after strenuous exercise, emotional stress, surgical operations and other trauma. Tissue activator can be extracted from most human organs, with the exception of the placenta. Tissues especially rich in activator include the uterus, ovaries, prostate, heart, lungs, thyroid, adrenals and lymph nodes. Activity in tissues is concentrated mainly around blood vessels; veins show greater activity than arteries. Venous occlusion of the limbs will stimulate fibrinolytic activity, a fact which should be remembered if tourniquets are applied for any length of time before blood is drawn for measurement of fibrin degradation products.

The inhibitors of fibrinolytic activity are of two types—antiactivators (antiplasminogens) and the antiplasmins. Inhibitors of plasminogen include epsilon amino caproic acid (EACA) and tranexamic acid. Aprotinin (Trasylol) is another antiplasminogen which is commercially prepared from bovine lung.

Platelets, plasma and serum exert a strong inhibitory action on plasmin. Normally plasma antiplasmin levels exceed levels of plasminogen and hence the levels of potential plasmin; otherwise we would dissolve away our connecting cement! When fibrinogen or fibrin is broken down by plasmin, fibrin degradation products are formed: these comprise the high molecular weight slip products X and Y, and smaller fragments A, B, C, D and E (Fig. 38.3). When a fibrin clot is formed 70% of fragment X is retained in the clot; Y, D and E are retained to a somewhat lesser extent. Therefore serum, even under normal circumstances, may contain small amounts of fragment X and larger amounts of Y, D and E. All of these components have antigenic determinants in common with fibrinogen and will be recognized by antifibrinogen antisera. It is important to be aware of this when examining blood for the presence of fibrin degradation products as confirmation of excess fibrinolytic activity (e.g. in DIC). Blood should be taken by clean venepuncture and the tourniquet should not be left on too long. The blood should be allowed to clot in the presence of an antifibrinolytic agent such as EACA to stop the process of fibrinolysis which would otherwise continue in vitro.

Plasma fibrinolytic activity is decreased during pregnancy, remains low during labour and delivery and returns to normal within 1 hour of delivery of the placenta (Bonnar et al 1970). The rapid return to normal systemic fibrinolytic activity following delivery of the placenta and the fact that the placenta has been shown to contain inhibitors which block fibrinolysis, suggest that inhibition of fibrinolysis during pregnancy is mediated through the placenta.

SUMMARY OF CHANGES IN HAEMOSTASIS IN PREGNANCY

The changes in the coagulation system in normal pregnancy are consistent with a continuing low-grade process of coagulant activity. Using electron microscopy, fibrin deposition can be demonstrated in the intervillous space of the placenta and in the walls of the spiral arteries supplying the placenta (Sheppard & Bonnar 1974). As pregnancy advances, the elastic lamina and smooth muscle of these spiral arteries are replaced by a matrix containing fibrin. This allows expansion of the lumen to accommodate an increasing blood flow and reduces the vascular resistance of the placenta. At placental separation during normal childbirth, a blood flow of 500–800 ml/min has to be staunched within seconds, or serious haemorrhage will occur. Myometrial contraction plays a vital role in securing haemostasis by reducing the blood flow to the placental site. Rapid closure of the terminal part of the spiral artery will be further facilitated by the structural changes within the walls. The placental site is rapidly covered by a fibrin mesh following delivery. The increased levels of fibrinogen and other coagulation factors will be advantageous to meet the sudden demand of haemostasis components.

The changes also produce a vulnerable state for intravascular clotting and a whole spectrum of disorders involving coagulation occur in complications of pregnancy (Letsky 1985).

DISSEMINATED INTRAVASCULAR COAGULATION

The changes in the haemostatic system and the local activation of the clotting system during parturition carry with them a risk not only of thromboembolism (see Ch. 64) but also of DIC. This results in consumption of clotting factors and platelets, leading in some cases to severe, particularly uterine and sometimes generalized, bleeding (Talbert & Blatt 1979).

The first problem with DIC is in its definition. It is never primary, but always secondary to some general stimulation of coagulation activity by release of procoagulant substances into the blood (Fig. 38.4). Hypothetical triggers of this process in pregnancy include the leaking of placental tissue fragments, amniotic fluid, incompatible red cells or bacterial products into the maternal circulation. There is a great spectrum of manifestations of the process of DIC (Table 38.1), ranging from a compensated state with no clinical manifestation but evidence of increased production and breakdown of coagulation factors, to the condition we all fear of massive uncontrollable haemorrhage with very low concentrations of plasma fibrinogen, pathological raised levels of fibrin degradation products and variable degrees of thrombocytopenia.

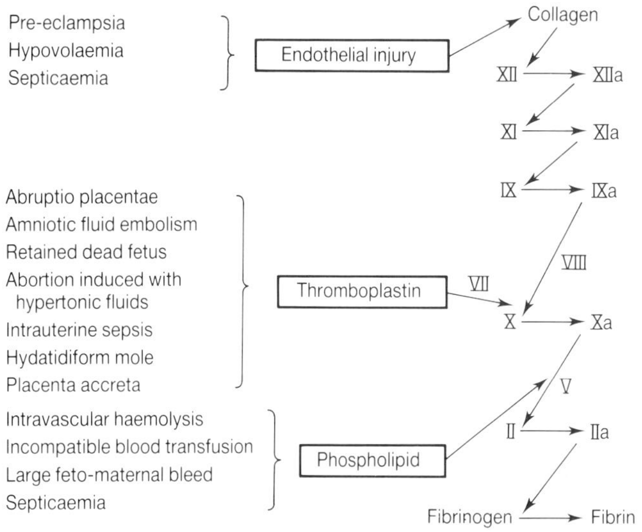

Fig. 38.4 Trigger mechanisms of disseminated intravascular coagulation during pregnancy. Interactions occur in many of these obstetric complications.

Another confusing entity is that there appears to be a transitory state of intravascular coagulation during the whole of normal labour, maximal at the time of birth (Gilabert et al 1978, Stirling et al 1984, Wallmo et al 1984).

Fibrinolysis is stimulated by DIC, and the fibrin degradation products resulting from the process interfere with the formation of firm fibrin clots. Thus a vicious circle is established, resulting in further disastrous bleeding (Fig. 38.5). Fibrin degradation products also interfere with myometrial function and possibly cardiac function and therefore in themselves aggravate both haemorrhage and shock.

Obstetric conditions classically associated with DIC include abruptio placentae, amniotic fluid embolism, septic abortion and intrauterine infection, retained dead fetus, hydatidiform mole, placenta accreta, pre-eclampsia and eclampsia and prolonged shock from any cause (see Fig. 38.4).

Despite the advances in obstetric care and highly developed blood transfusion services, haemorrhage still constitutes a major factor in maternal mortality and morbidity. There have been many reports concerning small series of patients or individual patients with coagulation failure during pregnancy. However, no significant controlled trials of

Table 38.1 Spectrum of severity of DIC: its relationship to specific complications in obstetrics

	Severity of DIC	In vitro findings	Obstetric condition commonly associated
Stage 1	Low-grade compensated	FDP ↑ Increased soluble fibrin complexes Increased ratio factor VIIIRAg/factor VIII	 Pre-eclampsia Retained dead fetus
Stage 2	Uncompensated but no haemostatic failure	As above, plus fibrinogen ↓ platelets ↓ factors V and VIII ↓	 Small abruptio Severe pre-eclampsia
Stage 3	Rampant with haemostatic failure	Platelets ↓↓ Gross depletion of coagulation factors, particularly fibrinogen FDP ↑	Abruptio placentae Amniotic fluid embolism Eclampsia

DIC = disseminated intravascular coagulation; FDP = fibrin degradation products.
Rapid progression from stage 1 to stage 3 is possible unless appropriate action is taken.

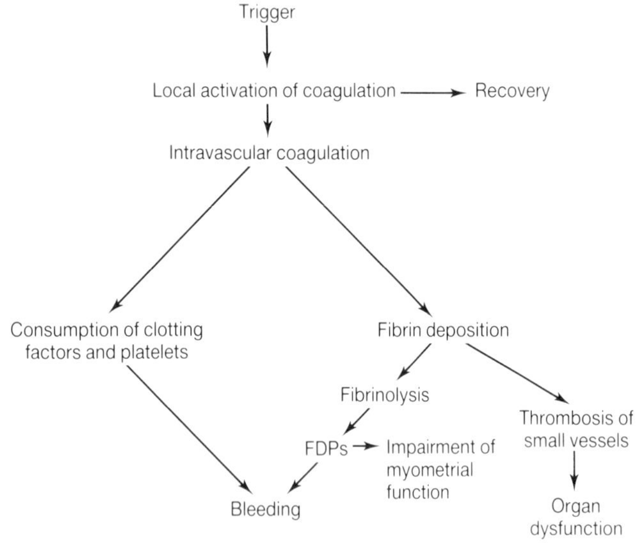

Fig. 38.5 Stimulation of coagulation activity and its possible consequences. FDPs = fibrin degradation products.

the value of the many possible therapeutic measures have been carried out. This is mainly because no one person or unit is likely to see enough cases to randomize patients into groups in which the numbers would achieve statistical significance. Also the complex and variable nature of the conditions associated with DIC, which are often self-correcting and treated with a variety of measures, make it impossible to make an objective assessment of the published reports.

HAEMATOLOGICAL MANAGEMENT OF THE BLEEDING OBSTETRIC PATIENT

The management of the bleeding obstetric patient is an acute and frightening problem. There is little time to think and there must be in every unit a planned practice decided on by haematologist, physician, anaesthetist, obstetrician and nursing staff to deal with this situation whenever it arises. This should be read by all junior staff and attention should be drawn to it frequently, for when the emergency occurs there is little time for leisurely perusal. Good reliable communication between the various clinicians, nursing, paramedical and laboratory staff is essential.

It is imperative that the source of bleeding, often an unsuspected uterine or genital laceration, should be located and dealt with. Prolonged hypovolaemic shock, or indeed shock from any cause, may also trigger off DIC and this may lead to haemostatic failure and further prolonged haemorrhage.

The management of haemorrhage is virtually the same whether the bleeding is caused or augmented by coagulation failure or not. The clinical condition usually demands urgent treatment and there is no time to wait for results of coagulation factor assays or sophisticated tests of the fibrinolytic system activity for precise definition of the extent of haemostatic failure, although blood can be taken for this purpose and analysed at leisure once the emergency is over.

Simple rapid tests, recommended below, will establish the competence or otherwise of the haemostatic system. In the vast majority of obstetric patients, coagulation failure results from a sudden transitory episode of DIC triggered by a variety of conditions (Fig. 38.4).

As soon as there is any concern about a patient bleeding from any cause, venous blood should be taken and delivered into a set of bottles kept in an emergency pack with a set of laboratory request forms previously made out which only require the patient's name and identification number added to them.

In order to avoid testing artefacts it is essential that the blood is obtained by a quick, efficient non-traumatic technique. Thromboplastin release from damaged tissues may contaminate the specimen and alter the results. This is likely to occur if difficulty is encountered in finding the vein, if the vein is only partly canalized and the flow is slow, or if there is excessive squeezing of tissues and repeated attempts to obtain a specimen with the same needle. In such circumstances the specimen may clot in the tube in spite

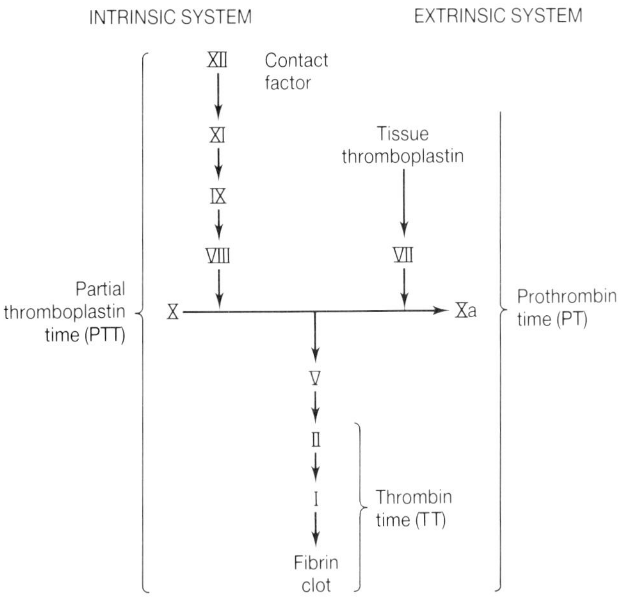

Fig. 38.6 In vitro screening tests of coagulation competence and their relationship to the systems involved.

of the presence of anticoagulant, or the coagulation times of the various tests will be altered and not reflect the true situation in vivo. The platelets may aggregate in clumps and give a falsely low count, be it automated or manual.

Heparin characteristically prolongs the partial thromboplastin time and thrombin time out of proportion to the prothrombin time. As little as 0.05 units of heparin per ml will prolong the coagulation test times. It is customary, though not desirable, to take blood for coagulation tests from lines which have been washed through with fluids containing heparin to keep them patent. It is almost impossible to overcome the effect on the blood passing through such a line, however much blood is taken and discarded before obtaining a sample for investigation. It is strongly recommended that blood is taken from another site not previously contaminated with heparin.

Any blood taken into a glass tube without anticoagulant will clot within a few minutes and natural fibrinolysis will continue in vitro. Unless the blood is taken into a fibrinolytic inhibitor such as EACA, a falsely high level of fibrin in degradation products will be found which bears no relationship to fibrinolysis in vivo. Similarly, leaving a tourniquet on too long before taking the specimen will stimulate local fibrinolytic activity in vivo.

Useful rapid screening tests for haemostatic failure include the platelet count, partial thromboplastin time or accelerated whole-blood clotting time (which tests intrinsic coagulation), prothrombin time (which tests extrinsic coagulation), thrombin time and estimation of fibrinogen (Fig. 38.6).

The measurement of the products of plasmin digestion of fibrinogen or fibrin provides an indirect test for fibrinolysis. Fibrin degradation products can be detected in several ways. They interfere with the production of fibrinogen by thrombin and will prolong the thrombin time. The most sensitive methods are immunological.

In practice the most rapid assessment of fibrin degradation products in the circulation is to add particles coated with fibrinogen antibody (raised in rabbits) to dilutions of the patient's serum taken into EACA to prevent in vitro fibrinolysis. In obstetric practice the measurement of fibrin degradation products is usually part of the investigation of suspected acute or chronic DIC. In the acute situation raised fibrin degradation products only confirm the presence of DIC, but are not diagnostic and once the specimen is taken the laboratory measurement should be delayed until after the emergency is over, so that skilled laboratory workers can be performing a much more valuable service in providing results of coagulation screening tests and blood and blood products suitable for transfusion. Of the tests of coagulation, probably the thrombin time, an estimation of the thrombin clottable fibrinogen in a citrated sample of plasma, is the most valuable overall rapid screen of haemostatic competence of coagulation factors. The thrombin time of normal plasma is adjusted in the laboratory to 10–15 seconds, and the fibrin clot formed is firm and stable. In the most severe forms of DIC there is no clottable fibrinogen in the sample, and no fibrin clot appears even after 2–3 minutes. Indication of severe DIC is obtained usually by a prolonged thrombin time with a friable clot which may dissolve on standing owing to fibrinolytic substances present in the plasma.

Prolongation of the thrombin time is observed not only with depleted fibrinogen but in conditions where fibrin degradation products are increased, and even traces of heparin will significantly prolong the time it takes for a clot to be formed. A crude but valuable rapid estimation of the fibrinogen level is obtained by a titre of the thrombin time test.

There is no point whatsoever in the obstetrician, anaesthetist or nursing staff wasting time trying to perform bedside whole-blood clotting tests. Whole-blood clotting normally takes up to 7 minutes and should be performed in clean tubes in a 37°C water bath with suitable controls. It furnishes little information of practical value and only creates more panic. The valuable hands at the bedside are of more use doing the things they are trained to do in this emergency situation rather than wasting time performing a test which is time-consuming, of little value or significance unless performed under strict control conditions, and which will not contribute anything to management. The alerted laboratory worker will be able to provide significant results within half an hour at the most of receiving the specimen in the laboratory.

The tests referred to above are straightforward and should be available from any routine haematology laboratory. It is not necessary to have a high-powered coagulation laboratory to perform these simple screening tests to confirm or refute a diagnosis of DIC.

Treatment of severe haemorrhage must include prompt and adequate fluid replacement in order to avoid renal shutdown. If effective circulation is restored without too much delay, fibrin degradation products will be cleared from the blood mainly by the liver, which will further aid restoration of normal haemostasis. This is an aspect of management which is often not appropriately emphasized (Pritchard 1973).

Plasma substitutes

There is much controversy about which plasma substitute to give to any bleeding patient. The remarks which follow are very much slanted towards the supportive laboratory management of acute haemorrhage from the placental site and should not be taken to apply to those situations in which hypovolaemia may be associated with severe hypoproteinaemia, such as occurs in septic peritonitis, burns and bowel infarction. The choice lies between simple crystalloids, such as Hartmann's solution or Ringer's lactate, and artificial colloids, such as dextran, hydroxyethyl starch and gelatin solution or the very expensive preparations of human albumin (albuminoids). If crystalloids are used, two or three times the volume of estimated blood loss should be administered because the crystalloid remains in the vascular compartment for a shorter time than colloids if renal function is maintained.

The infusion of plasma substitutes, i.e. plasma protein, dextran, gelatin and starch solutions, may result in adverse reactions. Although the incidence of severe reactions is rare, they are diverse in nature, varying from allergic urticarial manifestations and mild fever to life-threatening anaphylactic reactions due to spasm of smooth muscle, with cardiac and respiratory arrest (Doenicke et al 1977).

Dextrans adversely affect platelet function, may cause pseudoagglutination and interfere with interpretation of subsequent blood grouping and cross-matching tests. They are, therefore, contraindicated in the woman who is bleeding due to a complication associated with pregnancy where there is a high chance of there being a serious haemostatic defect already. Dextrans are also associated with allergic anaphylactoid reactions. The anaphylactoid reactions accompanying infusion of dextrans are probably related to IgG and IgM antidextran antibodies which are found in high concentrations in all patients with severe reactions.

Albuminoids are thought to be associated less with anaphylactoid reactions but they may be particularly harmful when transfused in the shocked patient by contributing to renal and pulmonary failure, adversely affecting cardiac function and further impairing haemostasis (Cash 1981).

Many studies have suggested that the best way to deal with hypovolaemic shock initially is by transfusing simple balanced salt solutions (crystalloid) followed by red cells and fresh frozen plasma (Carey et al 1970, Moss 1972, Virgilio et al 1979). More recent work (Hauser et al 1980) has challenged this approach and suggests that albumin-containing solutions are superior to crystalloids for volume replacement in postoperative shocked patients with respiratory insufficiency. This aspect of management of shocked patients with blood loss will remain controversial pending the results of further clinical trials.

In many hospitals nowadays, the derivatives of gelatin (Haemaccel or Gelofusine) are the first-line fluids in resuscitation. They have a half-life of 8 years and can be stored at room temperature. They are iso-oncotic and do not interfere with platelet function or subsequent blood grouping or cross-matching. Renal function is improved when they are administered in hypovolaemic shock. They are generally considered to be non-immunogenic and do not trigger the production of antibodies in man, even on repeated challenge. The reactions which occur related to Haemaccel infusion are thought to be due to histamine release (Lorenz et al 1976), the incidence and severity of reactions being proportional to the extent of histamine release. There have been a few rare reports of severe reactions with bronchospasm and circulatory collapse and there has been one report of a fatality (Freeman 1979). Nevertheless, whatever substitute is used it is only a stopgap until suitable blood component therapy can be administered.

The use of whole blood and component therapy

Whole blood may be the treatment of choice in coagulation failure associated with obstetric disorders (Phillips 1984), but whole fresh blood is not generally available in the UK nowadays, because there is insufficient time to complete hepatitis surface antigen, human immunodeficiency virus antibody and blood grouping tests before it is released from the transfusion centre. To release it earlier than the usual 18–24 hours would increase the risk of transmitting viral B hepatitis and acquired immune deficiency syndrome (AIDS). Serologically incompatible transfusions, syphilis, cytomegalovirus and Epstein–Barr virus are examples of other infections which may be transmitted in fresh blood. Their viability diminishes rapidly on storage at 4°C. These infections, particularly in immunosuppressed or pregnant patients, can be particularly hazardous. Apart from the hazards of giving whole blood which is less than say 6–24 hours old, its use in the UK today represents a serious waste of vitally needed components required for patients with specific isolated deficiencies (Boulton & Letsky 1985). The use of fresh frozen plasma followed by bank red cells provides all the components, apart from platelets, which are present in whole fresh blood and allows the plasma from the freshly donated unit to be used to make the much needed blood components.

Plasma component therapy

Fresh frozen plasma (FFP) contains all the coagulation factors present in plasma obtained from whole blood within

6 hours of donation. Frozen rapidly and stored at −30°C, the factors are well preserved for at least 1 year. Plasma stored at −20°C does degenerate and should be used within 6 months of preparation.

Freeze-dried plasma is prepared by pooling blood donations prior to dispensing and freezing and hence there is an increased risk of transmitting hepatitis and AIDS. Also this product is deficient in factors V and VIII. The advantage is it can be stored in the dark below 25°C for up to 8 years. It can be of value in providing colloid in the management of surgical or traumatic haemorrhage.

Concentrated fibrinogen should not be used in obstetric haemorrhage associated with DIC. The depletion of fibrinogen in these conditions is well known but undue importance is attributed to this lack of fibrinogen, which is part of a general consumptive coagulopathy. FFP provides abundant fibrinogen, together with factors V and VIII which are also depleted and the coagulation inhibitor ATIII.

Concentrated fibrinogen prepared from pooled donations carries a greater risk of subsequent hepatitis and AIDS. Administration has been shown to result in a sharp fall in levels of ATIII, suggesting that the concentrates may aggravate intravascular coagulation (Bonnar 1981) by adding fuel to the fire. The concept of feeding the fire by giving FFP to a patient who has DIC has not been proved. Although sometimes ineffective, such therapy has not been shown to do any harm (Sharp 1977).

Platelets, an essential haemostatic component, are not present in FFP and their functional activity rapidly deteriorates in stored blood. The platelet count reflects both the degree of intravascular coagulation and the amount of bank blood transfused. A patient with persistent bleeding and a very low platelet count (less than $20 \times 10^9/l$) may be given concentrated platelets, although they are seldom required in addition to FFP to achieve haemostasis. Indeed it has been suggested that platelet transfusions are more likely to do harm than good in this situation since most concentrates contain some damaged platelets which might in themselves provide a fresh trigger or mediator of DIC in the existing state (Sharp 1977). A spontaneous recovery from the coagulation defect is to be expected once the uterus is empty and well contracted, provided that blood volume is maintained by adequate replacement monitored by central venous pressure and urinary output.

Problems arise when bleeding is difficult to control and the woman has a low haemoglobin before blood loss, but this is unusual at term in a well managed obstetric patient.

Red cell transfusion

Cross-matched blood should be available within 40 minutes of the maternal specimen reaching the laboratory. If the woman has had normal antenatal care and carries her co-operation card her blood group will be known. There is a good case for giving uncross-matched blood of her group should the situation warrant it, provided that blood has been properly processed at the transfusion centre. If the blood group is unknown, uncross-matched group O rhesus-negative blood may be given if necessary. By this time laboratory screening tests of haemostatic function should be available. If these prove to be normal, but vaginal bleeding continues, the cause is nearly always trauma or bleeding from the placental site due to failure of the myometrium to contract. It is imperative that the source of bleeding, often an unsuspected uterine or genital laceration, should be located and dealt with. Prolonged hypovolaemic shock or indeed shock from any cause may also trigger DIC and this may lead to haemostatic failure and further prolonged haemorrhage.

Stored whole blood, even under optimal conditions, undergoes certain deleterious changes. The oxygen affinity of red cells increases. Plasma ionic concentrations of potassium and hydrogen increase but these changes are not significant until after 4 days of shelf-life. Platelets deteriorate rapidly within the first 24 hours and after 72 hours they have lost all haemostatic function.

The activity of the labile coagulation factors V and particularly factor VIII decrease within the first 24 hours of donation. After 6 days' storage microaggregates of platelets, white cells and fibrin form.

If the blood loss is replaced only by stored bank blood which is deficient in the labile clotting factors V and VIII and platelets, then the circulation will rapidly become depleted in these essential components of haemostasis even if there is no DIC initially as the cause of haemorrhage. It is advisable to transfuse 1 unit of fresh frozen plasma for every 4–6 units of bank red cells administered.

SAG-M blood

The concept of removing all the plasma from a unit of blood and replacing it with a crystalloid solution has now become routine procedure in the UK in many regional blood transfusion centres so that maximum use of a donated unit can be made.

The process involves centrifuging the anticoagulated unit of whole blood, removing all the plasma and resuspending the packed red cells in 100 ml of sodium chloride, adenine, glucose and mannitol—so-called SAG-M. The resulting unit of packed red cells has better flow properties than plasma-reduced blood and is very suitable for top-up transfusion, but contains practically no protein and no coagulation factors whatsoever. It is not ideal to transfuse in an obstetric emergency or any situations of massive rapid blood loss, but if this is all that is available on site at the time, then the following guidelines should be followed.

The regional transfusion centres do not recommend the use of any more than 4 units of SAG-M blood, but in an emergency after the first 4 units of SAG-M red cells, 1 unit of plasma protein fraction should be given for every 2 units of SAG-M blood in order to maintain plasma oncotic pressure. FFP should be considered after 8 units of SAG-M red cells have been transfused. In an obstetric emergency FFP should have been administered long before this. Most hospital blood banks are provided with a mixture of SAG-M and citrated whole blood or plasma-reduced red cells. Whole blood or plasma-reduced red cells is always available on request to the regional transfusion centre.

It seems sensible in any event, whatever the cause of bleeding, to change the initial plasma substitute and transfuse 2 units of FFP once it has thawed, while waiting for compatible blood to be available.

Finally, citrate used as an anticoagulant in transfused blood may complex calcium ions. Some centres recommend giving one ampoule (10 ml) of 10% calcium gluconate slowly over 10 minutes for every 6 units of blood infused. It seems more sensible to check calcium levels routinely with the other electrolytes and treat only if indicated.

A spontaneous recovery from the coagulation defect is to be expected once the uterus is empty and well contracted, provided that blood volume is maintained by adequate replacement monitored by central venous pressure and urinary output.

Clinicians may be helped in the decision of which replacement fluid to give in an obstetric emergency with the knowledge that very few bleeding patients die from lack of circulating red cells, the oxygen-carrying moiety of the blood. Death in the majority of cases results from hypovolaemia leading to poor tissue perfusion. Every effort should be made to maintain a normal blood volume and restoration of red cell mass can be delayed until suitable compatibility tests have been performed and bleeding is at least partially controlled (Marshall & Bird 1983).

The single most important component of haemostasis at delivery in normal circumstances is contraction of the myometrium stemming the flow from the placental site. All the clotting factors and platelets in the world will not stop haemorrhage if the uterus remains flabby. Vaginal delivery will make less severe demand on the haemostatic mechanism than delivery by Caesarean section which requires the same haemostatic competence as any other major surgical procedure. Should DIC be established with the fetus in utero, rather than to embark on heroic surgical delivery, it is better to wait for spontaneous delivery if possible, or to stimulate vaginal delivery, avoiding soft-tissue damage.

DIC IN CLINICAL CONDITIONS

In vitro detection of low-grade DIC

Rampant uncompensated DIC results in severe haemorrhage with characteristic findings in vitro dealt with above. However, low-grade DIC does not usually give rise to any clinical manifestations although the condition is a potentially hazardous one for both mother and fetus.

Many in vitro tests have been claimed to detect low-grade compensated DIC and space does not allow an account of all of these.

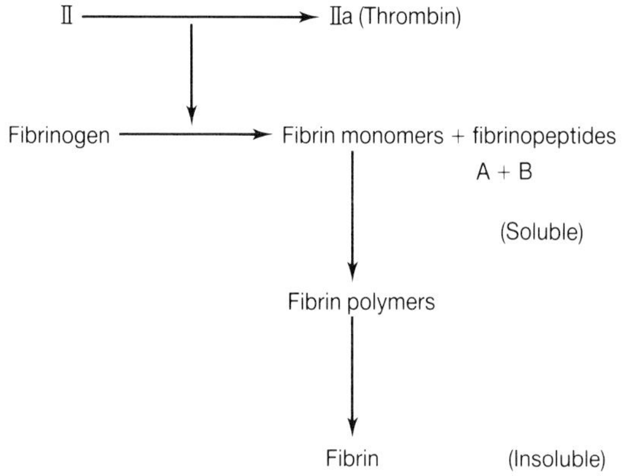

Fig. 38.7 Generation of soluble complexes during the conversion of fibrinogen to insoluble fibrin.

Fibrin degradation products

Estimation of fibrin degradation products will give some indication of low-grade DIC if these are significantly raised when fibrinogen, platelets and screening tests of haemostatic function appear to be within the normal range.

Soluble fibrin complexes

The action of thrombin on fibrinogen is crucial in DIC. Thrombin splits two molecules of fibrinopeptide A and two molecules of fibrinopeptide B from fibrinogen. The remaining molecule is called a fibrin monomer and polymerizes rapidly to fibrin (Fig. 38.3). Free fibrinopeptides in the blood are a specific measure of thrombin activity and high levels of fibrinopeptide A have been shown to be associated with compensated DIC in pregnancy (Wallmo et al 1984).

Soluble fibrin complexes made up of fibrin–fibrinogen dimers are increased in conditions of low-grade DIC (Aznar et al 1982). These complexes are generated during the process of thrombin generation and the conversion of soluble fibrinogen to insoluble fibrin (Fig. 38.7). Levels of soluble fibrin complexes are increased in patients with severe pre-eclampsia and with a retained dead fetus (Hafter & Graeff 1975).

Factor VIII

During normal pregnancy the levels of both factor VIII-related antigen (factor VIIIRAg) and factor VIII coagulation activity (factor VIIIC) rise concomitantly (Whigham et al 1979, Fournie et al 1981). An increase in the ratio of factor VIIIRAg to factor VIIIC has been observed in conditions accompanied by low-grade DIC whether associated with pregnancy or not. An increase in the ratio has been observed in pregnancy with a retained dead fetus and with pre-eclamp-

Table 38.2 Factor VIII molecular complex

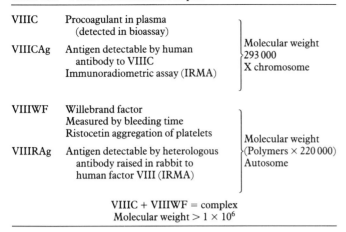

VIIIC	Procoagulant in plasma (detected in bioassay)	Molecular weight 293 000 X chromosome
VIIICAg	Antigen detectable by human antibody to VIIIC Immunoradiometric assay (IRMA)	
VIIIWF	Willebrand factor Measured by bleeding time Ristocetin aggregation of platelets	Molecular weight (Polymers × 220 000) Autosome
VIIIRAg	Antigen detectable by heterologous antibody raised in rabbit to human factor VIII (IRMA)	

VIIIC + VIIIWF = complex
Molecular weight $> 1 \times 10^6$

sia (Caires et al 1984) without any alteration in the simple screening tests of haemostatic function previously described.

The stages in the spectrum of severity of DIC (see Table 38.1) are not strictly delineated and there may be rapid progression from low-grade compensated DIC as diagnosed by paracoagulation tests described above, to the rampant form with haemostatic failure.

There now follows an account of the obstetric conditions most commonly associated with DIC, the past rationale for specific measures as well as those being used at present to manage haemostatic failure optimally.

Abruptio placentae

Premature separation of the placenta or abruptio placentae is a well-known cause of coagulation failure in most obstetric units. Many of the problems which confront the attendant in this situation are common to other conditions associated with DIC in pregnancy, therefore this will be used as the central focus of discussion of some of the controversial methods of management.

Abruptio placentae may occur in apparently healthy women with no clinical warning or may be in association with established pre-eclampsia. It is possible that clinically silent placental infarcts may predispose to placental separation by causing low-grade abnormalities of the haemostatic system such as increased factor VIII consumption and raised fibrin degradation products (Redman 1979).

There is a great spectrum in the severity of the haemostatic failure in this condition (Gilabert et al 1985) which appears to be related to the degree of placental separation. Only 10% of patients overall with abruptio placenta show significant coagulation abnormalities (Naumann & Weinstein 1985). In some cases of a small abruptio, there is a minor degree of failure of haemostatic processes and the fetus does not succumb (Table 38.1). When the uterus is tense and tender and no fetal heart can be heard, the separation and retroplacental bleeding are extensive. No guide to the severity of the haemorrhage or coagulation failure will be given by the amount of vaginal bleeding. Often there is no external vaginal blood loss, even when the placenta is completely separated, the fetus is dead, the circulating blood is incoagulable and there is up to 5 litres of concealed blood loss resulting in hypovolaemic shock.

Haemostatic failure may be suspected if there is persistent oozing at the site of venipuncture or bleeding from the mucous membranes of the mouth or nose. Simple rapid screening tests will confirm the presence of DIC. There will be a low platelet count, greatly prolonged thrombin time, low fibrinogen and raised fibrin degradation products, due to secondary fibrinolysis stimulated by the intravascular deposition of fibrin (Estelles et al 1980). The mainstay of treatment is to maintain the circulating blood volume. This not only prevents renal shutdown and further haemostatic failure caused by hypovolaemic shock, but helps clearance of fibrin degradation products which in themselves act as potent anticoagulants. It has also been suggested that fibrin degradation products inhibit myometrial activity; serious postpartum haemorrhage in women with abruptio placentae was found to be associated with high levels of fibrin degradation products (Basu 1969, Sher 1977). High levels of fibrin degradation products may also have a cardiotoxic effect.

If the fetus is dead the aim should be prompt vaginal delivery avoiding soft-tissue damage. Once correction of hypovolaemia is underway, measures to speed up delivery should be instituted. Amniotomy, or if this fails, prostaglandin or oxytocin stimulation can be used. There is no evidence that the use of oxytocic agents aggravates thromboplastin release from the uterus (Bonnar 1978).

Following emptying of the uterus, myometrial contraction will greatly reduce bleeding from the placental site and spontaneous correction of the haemostatic defect usually occurs shortly after delivery if the measures recommended above have been taken. However, postpartum haemorrhage is a frequent complication and is the commonest cause of death in abruptio placentae (Department of Health and Social Security 1982).

In cases where the abruptio is small and the fetus is still alive, prompt Caesarean section may save the baby if vaginal delivery is not imminent. FFP, bank red cells and platelet concentrates should be available to correct the potentially severe coagulation defect in the maternal circulation.

In rare situations where vaginal delivery cannot be stimulated and haemorrhage continues, Caesarean section may be indicated even in the presence of a dead fetus. In these circumstances normal haemostasis should be restored as far as possible by the administration of FFP and platelet concentrates, if necessary, as well as red cells before surgery is undertaken.

Despite extravasation of blood throughout the uterine muscle its function is not impaired and good contraction will follow removal of fetus, placenta and retroperitoneal clot. Hysterectomy should be avoided as delayed internal bleeding may occur. Regional anaesthesia or analgesia is contraindicated. Expansion of the lower limb vascular bed resulting from regional block can add to the problem of uncorrected hypovolaemia, plus in the presence of haemostatic failure there is the additional hazard of bleeding into the epidural space (Bonnar 1981).

In recent years, heparin has been used to treat all kinds of DIC, whatever their cause. There is, however, no objective evidence to demonstrate that its use in abruptio placentae has decreased morbidity and mortality, although anecdotal reports continue to suggest this (Thragarajah et al 1981). Very good results have been achieved without the use of heparin (Pritchard 1973). Its use, with an intact circulation, would be sensible and logical to break the vicious circle of DIC, but in the presence of already defective haemostasis with a large bleeding placental site, it may prolong massive local and generalized haemorrhage (Feinstein 1982).

Treatment with an antifibrinolytic agent such as tranexamic acid (Cyclokapron) or Trasylol can result in blockage with fibrin of small vessels in vital organs such as the kidney or brain. It is therefore contraindicated, although Bonnar (1981) suggests that delayed severe and prolonged haemorrhage from the placental site several hours post-delivery may respond to antifibrinolytic therapy if all other measures fail.

It has been suggested (Sher 1977, Sher & Statland 1985) that aprotinin (Trasylol) may be helpful in the management of abruptio placentae, particularly in those cases with uterine inertia associated with high levels of fibrin degradation products. There is a high incidence (1.5%) of abruptio placentae in the obstetric admissions (18 000 per annum) at the Groote Scheur Obstetric Unit, Cape Town, South Africa, where the first study was carried out.

Intravenous administration of Trasylol in eight patients with abruptio placentae and uterine inertia together with other prompt supportive measures resulted in a rapid re-coordination of uterine activity as well as a steady fall in serum fibrin degradation product levels and a progressive rise in platelet count. The selection of the drug Trasylol as opposed to tranexamic acid depended on its alleged anticoagulant activity in addition to its well known antifibrinolytic properties. An anticoagulant effect would make it a less hazardous agent in view of intravascular deposition of fibrin in vital organs and particularly useful in the management of haemorrhage due to DIC. However in vitro studies indicate that very high concentrations are required to have any anticoagulant effect (Amris & Hilden 1968). Another study (Prentice et al 1970) showed that high concentrations of Trasylol in vitro appeared to inhibit only the contact phase of coagulation and the authors concluded that Trasylol would be a relatively weak anticoagulant in doses liable to be achieved in vitro. It would of course have no direct effect on the extrinsic coagulation pathway which is activated in the course of DIC due to abruptio placentae. However, Nordstrom and colleagues (1968) showed that DIC in dogs, induced by injection of thromboplastin, was partially inhibited if they were treated prophylactically with Trasylol. In recent years, obstetricians appear unconvinced of the benefits of Trasylol in the treatment of DIC and abruptio placentae, judging by many published reports.

Prompt supportive measures alone, maintaining central venous pressure and replacing blood loss together with essential coagulation factors, will of course result in reduction in fibrin degradation products. This will improve myometrial function and contribute to the return of healthy haemostasis.

One patient with recurrent abruptio placentae successfully treated with the fibrinolytic inhibitor tranexamic acid has been reported (Astedt & Nilsson 1978). Investigations in this woman suggested abnormally increased fibrinolytic activity in the 26th week of her third pregnancy. The previous two pregnancies had been complicated by abruptio placentae associated with a neonatal death and a stillbirth respectively. The intravenous administration of tranexamic acid following a small vaginal bleed resulted in restoration of normal coagulation status and the bleeding stopped; oral administration was continued. Another small bleed occurred at 33 weeks' gestation, treated again with intravenous tranexamic acid. The eventual successful outcome of this pregnancy was attributed by the authors to the use of this agent but many other variables may have been involved.

Amniotic fluid embolism

Amniotic fluid embolism is very rare but one of the most dangerous and untreatable conditions in obstetrics. The incidence has been estimated as between 1 in 8000 and 1 in 80 000 in various reports (Morgan 1979) but the latter figure is probably nearer the true incidence. During the triennium 1979–1981 in England and Wales, 18 histologically confirmed and 6 suspected fatal cases occurred associated with 1 942 859 maternities. This gives an incidence of fatal amniotic fluid embolism of approximately 1 in 81 000 (Department of Health and Social Security 1986). The maternal mortality is very high—over 80% in most reports. An excellent review of 272 cases in the English literature reported that only 39 survived, giving a mortality rate of 86% (Morgan 1979). Amniotic fluid embolism is the most common cause of death in the immediate postpartum period (Herbert 1982).

Amniotic fluid embolism is said to occur most frequently in elderly multiparous patients with large babies at or near term following a short tumultuous labour associated with the use of uterine stimulants. However, the review quoted (Morgan 1979) did not substantiate this statement. The most recent Report on Confidential Enquiries into Maternal Deaths in England and Wales (Department of Health and Social Security 1986) confirmed that there were higher rates of mortality at older ages and higher parity but the relationship between violent contractions and rapid labour was less apparent.

There have been some reports of this complication of pregnancy occurring in different situations: in young primiparous women (Morgan 1979), during the second trimester (Meier & Bowes 1983), in women undergoing legally induced terminations (Guidotti et al 1981), after evacuation of a missed abortion (Stromme & Fromke 1979) and even after deliberate termination of pregnancy (Cates et al 1981).

The passage of amniotic fluid into the maternal circulation is thought to occur through the endocervical veins, the normal placental site, through uterine trauma at Caesarean section or if the uterus ruptures. Torn fetal membranes is a prerequisite of amniotic fluid embolism. Lethal amniotic fluid embolism is most commonly associated with small tears in the uterus, cervix or vagina which have not totally disrupted the wall (Rushton & Dawson 1982). This is not surprising since a complete tear would allow amniotic fluid to escape into the peritoneal cavity or the vagina.

The clinical features associated with amniotic fluid embolism are respiratory distress, cyanosis, cardiovascular collapse, haemorrhage and coma. Although coagulation failure occurs rapidly the presenting clinical feature is sudden extreme shock with cyanosis due to an almost complete shutdown of the pulmonary circulation, followed by the onset of intractable uterine bleeding. The coagulation abnormalities are ascribed to the thromboplastic activity of amniotic fluid (Courtney & Allington 1972, Yaffe et al 1977). Massive intravascular coagulation occurs and consumption of the clotting factors can be almost total (Bonnar 1981). Platelet fibrin thrombi are formed and trapped within the pulmonary blood vessels. Profound shock follows, accompanied by respiratory distress and cyanosis. There is a high mortality at this stage from a combination of respiratory and cardiac failure; if the mother survives long enough the effect of massive intravascular coagulation will invariably follow with bleeding from venepuncture sites and severe haemorrhage from the placental site after delivery (Gregory & Clayton 1973).

Until recently confirmation of diagnosis could only be made at autopsy by finding histological evidence of amniotic fluid and fetal tissue within the substance of the maternal lungs, with or without identification of the portal of entry in the placenta or uterine wall (Rushton & Dawson 1982). It is therefore difficult to assess the value of therapeutic measures suggested in the few reports which have appeared of successful management of a clinical syndrome diagnosed clinically as amniotic fluid embolism (Skjodt 1965, Bonnar 1973, Chung & Merkatz 1973, Resnik et al 1976).

More recent techniques of diagnosis include detection of squamous cells and lanugo hair on cytological examination of blood aspirated through a Swan–Ganz catheter and detection of squamous cells in maternal sputum (Herbert 1982). A recent report (Dolyniuk et al 1983) describes a case in which the diagnosis of amniotic fluid embolism was made using these techniques and the patient survived. In a 19-year-old primigravida acute respiratory failure developed following Caesarean section; fragments of vernix caseosa were identified in a pulmonary artery blood sample obtained through a Swan–Ganz catheter. The patient received intensive supportive care and recovered completely.

The management of cardiorespiratory failure associated with amniotic fluid embolism must be carefully planned. This condition is similar to pulmonary embolism but there is also profound haemorrhage; too rigorous attempts at maintenance of the circulation, as recommended above for other conditions associated with DIC, may result in cardiac failure. There should be careful monitoring of the central venous pressure to avoid cardiac overload; the object is to sustain the circulation while the intravascular thrombin in the lungs is cleared by the naturally stimulated intense fibrinolytic response of the endothelium of the pulmonary vessels.

Measures to stimulate uterine contractions to reduce blood loss from the placental site are important in maintaining the blood volume. If bleeding from the placental site can be controlled by stimulation of uterine contraction then the logical treatment is carefully monitored transfusion of FFP and packed red cells, with heparin administration and, if indicated, positive pressure ventilation (Bonnar 1981). It is obviously essential that a competent intensive care unit should be immediately available for any obstetric service to deal promptly with this rare but often lethal complication of pregnancy.

Retention of dead fetus

The question of intrauterine fetal death and haemostatic failure has been reviewed by Romero et al (1985). There is a gradual depletion of maternal coagulation factors following intrauterine fetal death and the changes are not usually detectable in vitro until after 3–4 weeks (Hodgkinson et al 1964). Thromboplastic substances released from the dead tissues in the uterus into the maternal circulation are thought to be the trigger of DIC in this situation, which occurs in about one-third of patients who retain the dead fetus for more than 4–5 weeks (Pritchard 1959). There is depletion of fibrinogen, factor VIII and platelets, together with elevation of fibrin degradation products. Gross increase of soluble fibrin–fibrinogen complexes amounting to 25% of the total fibrinogen in association with a dead fetus has been described (Hafter & Graeff 1975). Around 80% of pregnant women will go into spontaneous labour within 3 weeks of intrauterine fetal death. Problems arising from defective haemostasis are much less common with this situation in modern obstetric practice because labour is induced promptly following diagnosis of fetal death before clinically significant coagulation changes have developed.

Rupture of the membranes is recommended once induced labour is established in such patients, as there is a risk of precipitate labour and amniotic fluid embolism has been known to occur (Bonnar 1978).

If the screening tests previously described indicate that there is defective haemostasis the coagulation factors should be restored to normal before delivery is attempted. Where the circulation is intact heparin is the logical treatment to interrupt the activation of the coagulation systems. Intravenous infusion of 1000 iu heparin hourly for up to 48 hours is usually sufficient to restore the number of platelets and the levels of fibrinogen and factors V and VIII to normal (Bonnar 1978). The heparin should then be discontinued and onset of labour stimulated. There should be a plentiful supply of compatible red cells and FFP prepared to treat any haemorrhage at placental separation promptly. If the patient goes into spontaneous labour while heparin is being administered the infusion should be stopped. It is not necessary to neutralize the heparin with protamine sulphate unless the patient is bleeding. There is no rational basis for the use of fibrinolytic inhibitors in the management of the patient with coagulation failure associated with a retained dead fetus. The increased fibrinolytic activity is secondary to DIC and the defective haemostasis will be corrected by the powerful anticoagulant effect of heparin in the presence of an intact circulation before the onset of labour.

Retained dead fetus and living twin

The occurrence of single fetal death in a preterm multiple pregnancy poses unique therapeutic dilemmas. Prolongation of the pregnancy could result in life-threatening maternal haemostatic failure. Termination of the pregnancy for maternal indications would result in the birth of an immature infant. The incidence of this problem is unknown but is likely to be observed more frequently with the advent of widespread use of ultrasound in obstetrics. In addition, on occasion selective termination of the life of the affected twin is being offered in situations where only one fetus has been shown to be affected with a genetic disorder.

A report of the successful prolongation of pregnancy with the spontaneous death in utero of one of the twins at 26 weeks' gestation has been published by Romero et al (1986). The patient was treated with intravenous heparin and the reversal of the consumption coagulopathy resulted in the uneventful prolongation of pregnancy for 8 weeks, by which time the fetus had achieved lung maturity.

Abortion

Changes in haemostatic components consistent with DIC have been demonstrated in patients undergoing abortion induced with hypertonic solutions of saline and urea (Stander et al 1971, Spivak et al 1972, Van Royen 1974, MacKenzie et al 1975, Grundy & Craven 1976).

The stimulus appears to be the release of tissue factor into the maternal circulation from the placenta which is damaged by the hypertonic solutions. DIC has been described in association with late dilatation and evacuation procedures (Davis 1972), and also in association with prostaglandin and oxytocin methods (Savage 1982).

The risk of DIC was increased five times in women receiving oxytocin while undergoing induced saline abortions (Cohen & Ballard 1974), but in another study the risk of DIC in women given urea plus prostaglandin or oxytocin was only one-quarter of that for women receiving saline alone (Burkman et al 1977). The resulting haemorrhage may be massive and has resulted in maternal deaths. Prompt restoration of blood volume and transfusions with red cells and FFP as described above should resolve the situation which, once the uterus is empty, is self-limiting.

A unique case of DIC associated with chronic ectopic pregnancy has been reported (Collier & Birrell 1983).

Intrauterine infection

The interactions of sepsis and coagulation in obstetrics have been reviewed by Beller (1985).

Endotoxic shock associated with septic abortion, antepartum or postpartum intrauterine infection can trigger DIC in pregnancy and the puerperium (Steichele & Herschlein 1968, Graeff et al 1978). Infections with Gram-negative micro-organisms is the usual finding. Fibrin is deposited in the microvasculature owing to endothelial damage by the endotoxin, and secondary red cell intravascular haemolysis with characteristic fragmentation, so-called microangiopathic haemolysis, is characteristic of the condition.

The patient is usually alert and flushed with a rapid pulse and low blood pressure. Transfusion, unlike in other obstetric emergencies complicated by DIC, has little or no effect on the hypotension. Some few centres in Europe have used heparinization in the management of septic abortion and have claimed a decrease in mortality (Bonnar 1978). In the situation where the uterus is empty and contracted and there is no undue risk of severe bleeding from the placental site with evidence of a consumptive coagulopathy, heparin may be useful as part of the management of this hazardous emergency (Clarkson et al 1969).

Elimination of the uterine infection remains the most important aspect of management; claims that therapy with heparin has significantly decreased maternal mortality in septic abortions are in doubt (Beller & Uszynski 1974) and use of heparin remains controversial (Beller 1985).

Purpura fulminans

This rare complication of infection sometimes occurs in the puerperium, precipitated by Gram-negative septicaemia.

Extensive haemorrhage occurs into the skin in association with DIC. The underlying mechanism is unknown but there appears to be an acute activation of the clotting system resulting in the deposition of fibrin thrombi within blood vessels of the skin and other organs (McGibbon 1982). The extremities and face are usually involved first; the purpuric patches have a jagged and erythematous border, which can be shown histologically to be the site of a leukocytoclastic vasculitis. Rapid enlargement of the lesions, which become necrotic and gangrenous, is associated with shock tachycardia and fever. Without treatment the mortality rate is high and among those who survive digit or limb amputation may be necessary. The laboratory findings are those of DIC with leukocytosis. In this situation treatment with heparin should be started as soon as the diagnosis is apparent, to prevent further consumption of platelets and coagulation factors. It should always be remembered, however, that bleeding from any site in the presence of the defective coagulation factors will be aggravated by the use of heparin.

Survival in purpura fulminans is currently much improved because of better supportive treatment for the shocked patient and effective control of the triggering infection, together with heparin therapy.

Acute fatty liver of pregnancy

This is a rare complication of pregnancy and it is included in this section because it is often, if not always, associated with variable degrees of DIC, which contributes significantly to its morbidity and mortality (Feinstein 1982, Laursen et al 1983). First identified by Sheehan (1940) as a separate entity, there are now about 90 patients documented in the English literature (Burroughs et al 1982) and probably less than 150 cases in the world literature (Hague et al 1983). The salient histological factors on which the diagnosis is ultimately based are the presence of fat in small vacuoles in centrilobular hepatocytes while a ring of normal hepatocytes remains around the portal systems without any evidence of cellular necrosis (Davies et al 1980). Renal failure with tubular necrosis is a common association (Rushton & Dawson 1982). The aetiology of this rare condition remains unknown.

Clinical presentation is typically during the last trimester with sudden onset of malaise, nausea, repeated vomiting and abdominal pain followed by jaundice. Haematemesis often occurs (Burroughs et al 1982) and is part of a bleeding diathesis due to thrombocytopenia, consumption coagulopathy and defects of coagulation factor synthesis (Lancet Editorial 1983).

The fetus is usually stillborn and, following delivery, the mother lapses into deeper coma associated with progressive hepatic and renal failure. The maternal mortality is between 75 and 85% and the fetal mortality is around 85% (Burroughs et al 1982). There are some few reports of this condition presenting in the puerperium (Lancet Editorial 1983).

Diagnosis during life has usually been made in the past on clinical grounds alone because the severe coagulation defect precludes liver biopsy. Even at post-mortem the acute fatty liver may well go undiagnosed unless the liver is carefully examined histologically using specific stains. An apparently normal liver to naked-eye inspection may show severe fatty infiltration on microscopic examination (Lancet Editorial 1983).

Proteinuria, hypertension and oedema are frequent accompanying features (Burroughs et al 1982) but pre-eclampsia is a much more common complication of pregnancy than acute fatty liver of pregnancy. Thus, with the possibility of the missed histological diagnosis, the validity of statistics concerning the incidence of acute fatty liver of pregnancy must be questioned. The most recent Confidential Enquiries into Maternal Deaths in England and Wales (Department of Health and Social Security 1986) attributed 36 deaths to hypertensive diseases of pregnancy of which 16 were associated with cerebral haemorrhage, cerebral oedema, DIC and hepatorenal failure, all of which are well recognized features of acute fatty liver of pregnancy. In the same period only six deaths were attributed to liver disorders. The distinction between eclampsia and acute fatty liver of pregnancy may not be as clear as has been previously assumed: they may represent different clinical expressions of the same underlying disorder, and deaths due to acute fatty liver of pregnancy may have been underestimated.

Most observers agree that prompt delivery of the fetus offers the best chance of survival for both mother and child. Both Caesarean section and induction of labour led to a lower than expected maternal and fetal mortality in a series of 12 patients reported from the Royal Free Hospital (Burroughs et al 1982). This being so, early accurate diagnosis would seem to be a prerequisite for improving survival of both mother and child.

There should be a high order of suspicion when nausea and vomiting occur late in pregnancy, particularly if accompanied by abdominal pain and heartburn and associated with twins. This combination warrants immediate admission to hospital for investigation and observation. Further studies are required to establish the value of liver function tests, uric acid levels, amino acid profiles and examination of the blood film to achieve an early diagnosis of acute fatty liver of pregnancy. Biopsy of the liver obtained before delivery would be valuable in establishing the diagnosis but is often precluded because of the severe haemostatic defect.

At present the clinical problem of acute fatty liver of pregnancy remains that of early diagnosis since prompt delivery seems to be the specific management which limits progression of the disease and decreases both maternal and fetal mortality.

Summary on DIC

As emphasized, DIC is always a secondary phenomenon and the mainstay of management is therefore to remove the initiating stimulus if possible.

With rampant DIC and haemorrhage, recovery will usually follow delivery of the patient provided the blood volume is maintained and shock due to hypovolaemia is prevented. An efficiently acting myometrium post-delivery will stem haemorrhage from the placental site. Measures taken to achieve a firm contracted uterus will obviously contribute one of the most important factors in preventing continuing massive blood loss from the placental site.

It is of interest that the maternal mortality of DIC associated with placental abruption is less than 1% (Pritchard & Brekken 1967), whereas that associated with infection and shock is 50–80% (Mant & King 1979). The mortality rate reported in series of patients with DIC due to various aetiologies is 50–85% and the wide variation probably reflects the mortality rate of the underlying disorder, not of DIC per se (Feinstein 1982). There is no doubt that the major determinant of survival is our ability to identify the underlying trigger and manage it successfully.

ACQUIRED PRIMARY DEFECTS OF HAEMOSTASIS

Thrombocytopenia

The commonest platelet abnormality encountered in clinical practice is thrombocytopenia. During the hundred years since platelets were first described, an increasing understanding of their role in haemostasis and thrombosis has taken place. At the same time there have been dramatic reductions in maternal and fetal mortality, but maternal thrombocytopenia remains a difficult management problem during pregnancy and can have profound effects on fetal and neonatal well-being. The causes and management of maternal and fetal thrombocytopenia have been reviewed by Colvin (1985). Emphasis here will be laid on those conditions which cause particular diagnostic and management problems in obstetric practice.

A low platelet count is seen most frequently in association with DIC, as already described. Sometimes severe megaloblastic anaemia of pregnancy is accompanied by thrombocytopenia, but the platelet count rapidly returns to normal after therapy with folic acid (Bonnar 1981). Toxic depression of bone marrow megakaryocytes in pregnancy can occur in association with infection, certain drugs and alcoholism. Neoplastic infiltration may also result in thrombocytopenia. Probably the single most important cause of isolated thrombocytopenia is autoimmune thrombocytopenic purpura (AITP), which is a disease primarily of young women in their reproductive years (McMillan 1981).

Autoimmune thrombocytopenia

Due to its common occurrence in women during the childbearing years, AITP is one of the most frequently encountered haematological disorders in pregnancy apart from anaemia. The diagnosis used to be made when severe thrombocytopenia was found to be associated with normal or increased numbers of megakaryocytes in the bone marrow. There are now more reliable tests for demonstrating the responsible IgG antibody (Hegde et al 1977, Van Leeuwen et al 1981). The antibody is directed against and coats the platelet, which is rapidly removed from the circulation by the reticuloendothelial system. It is possible with these new tests to distinguish between IgG antibodies which can cross the placenta and IgM antibodies which do not (Van Leeuwen et al 1981), and also to identify platelet-bound antibody and the more dangerous free IgG antibody in the maternal plasma (Hegde et al 1981, Cines et al 1982).

Much of the published literature (Territo et al 1973, Carloss et al 1980, Terao et al 1981) consists of retrospective analyses of women suffering from AITP, managed throughout pregnancy without the advantage of tests which identify specific platelet autoantibodies. However, since there are still centres where these laboratory investigations are not freely available, diagnosis and management may have to be planned without their aid. The direct antiglobulin test (Coombs' test) and tests to exclude systemic lupus erythematosus, such as anti-DNA antibodies and antinuclear factor, must be done in all patients who present with immune thrombocytopenia as this may be the first manifestation of a more generalized autoimmune disease.

The IgG platelet autoantibody may cross the placenta and cause immune destruction of fetal platelets. Hegde (1985) has analysed the reported cases in the literature from 1950 to 1983 and suggests an overall prevalence of neonatal thrombocytopenia of 52%, with significant morbidity in 12%. The incidence increases to 70% of deliveries if maternal platelet counts are less than $100 \times 10^9/l$ at term and the probability of fetal thrombocytopenia increases with the severity of maternal thrombocytopenia.

However, even in the asymptomatic mother with relatively high platelet counts ($>100 \times 10^9/l$) there appears to be an incidence of thrombocytopenia in roughly 20% of infants (Hegde 1985). These risk factors are modified further by previous maternal splenectomy. In this situation the incidence of neonatal thrombocytopenia and morbidity is increased even if the mother has a normal platelet count (Carloss et al 1980). A study of 41 pregnancies in 38 patients with AITP from Canada (Kelton et al 1982) showed that the maternal platelet count was not related to the platelet count in the fetus, but that maternal platelet-associated antibody was predictive of infant platelet count. The maternal platelet count should be checked regularly during pregnancy and if it falls below $20 \times 10^9/l$ then steroids are indicated. These should be tapered to the lowest dose that provides safe platelet counts (Carloss et al 1980, McMillan 1981). It has been suggested (Hegde 1985) that high doses of steroids to elevate platelet counts at or near term may increase the transplacental passage of IgG antibody and thus expose the fetus to greater risk of severe thrombocytopenia and should, if possible, be avoided.

Splenectomy during pregnancy should be avoided because an appreciable maternal mortality rate has been reported (10%) which does not exist outside pregnancy (Bell 1977). Splenectomy also predisposes to premature labour, and the fetal loss rate is high.

Because the IgG antibody will cross the placenta, the major

risk to the fetus is that of intracranial bleeding during delivery. If there is any question that a vaginal delivery will be difficult because of cephalopelvic disproportion and premature delivery, elective Caesarean section should be carried out. It has also been recommended by several authors (see Carloss et al 1980) that if the maternal platelet count is less than $100 \times 10^9/l$, indicating active AITP, Caesarean section should be performed. McMillan (1981) states that this is indicated if the spleen is absent, regardless of platelet count. If, however, one has access to reliable reproducible platelet antibody tests, and no appreciable IgG platelet-bound or free maternal autoantibody can be demonstrated, this rule need not apply.

If an easy vaginal delivery is expected in a term baby this should present no more risk of intracranial bleeding than does a Caesarean section. It should be remembered that a Caesarean section in the presence of maternal thrombocytopenia carries considerable risk of haemorrhage from incisions (not from the placental site, which is protected by normal myometrial contraction). Although transfused platelets will have a short life in the maternal circulation due to the antibody, they will help to achieve haemostasis of the wound, and should be standing by for the mother at delivery, but should only be given if she bleeds excessively. This has never occurred in the author's experience, however low the platelet count. The unnecessary transfusion of platelet concentrates in the absence of haemostatic failure may stimulate more autoantibody and increase the severity of maternal thrombocytopenia. Whatever the mode of delivery, maternal soft-tissue damage should be avoided as far as possible.

A method for direct measurement of the fetal platelet count in scalp blood obtained transcervically prior to or early in labour has been described (Scott et al 1980). The authors recommend that Caesarean section should be performed in all cases where the fetal platelet count is less than $50 \times 10^9/l$. This approach is more logical than a decision about the mode of delivery based on the maternal platelet count and splenectomy status, but it is not without risk and demands urgent action on the results obtained. We have found that if reliable platelet antibody tests are available and have been performed throughout the antenatal period, the decision concerning the need for Caesarean section and its timing can be taken at leisure; this can be based on a rational assessment of disease activity and the risk to the mother and fetus.

The recent introduction of intravenous infusion of immunoglobulin in the management of AITP has made the difficult decision regarding delivery much easier. It is known that intravenous administration of monomeric polyvalent human IgG in doses greater than that produced endogenously prolongs the clearance time of immune complexes by the reticuloendothelial system. It is thought that in AITP such a prolongation of clearance of IgG-coated platelets by the reticuloendothelial system results in an increase in the number of circulating platelets, but the mechanism is as yet unknown.

The successful use of high-dose intravenous IgG in the treatment of childhood AITP in the early 1980s led to its adoption in the management of severe cases of maternal AITP in pregnancy. Used in the recommended doses of 0.4 mg/kg for 5 days by intravenous transfusion it results in a consistent and predictable response in platelet count in over 80% of reported cases. Platelets begin to rise on about the fourth day of infusion and peak about 5 days later; remission lasts for about 3 weeks. Most patients achieve a platelet count within the normal range, some rise to safe but still thrombocytopenic levels and a very few fail to respond or have an extremely sluggish response. It will be clear within 5 or 6 days if the patient is the rare non-responder.

IgG given intravenously can cross the placenta and should provoke an identical response in the at-risk fetus, but this has never been proven (Tchernia et al 1984, Hegde 1985, Lavery et al 1985). Anecdotal reports of the value of intravenous IgG in the management of AITP in pregnancy have appeared in the literature but so far no large series have been published (Newland et al 1984, Tchernia et al 1984, Davies et al 1986). One of the first reports of successful outcome using this therapy comes from the UK (Morgenstern et al 1983). The authors suggested that if infusion is started 10–14 days before the expected date of delivery, benefits should be threefold:

1. Vaginal delivery will be safe.
2. The neonatal platelet count should be normal.
3. An instrumental delivery with its potential for soft-tissue trauma or even a Caesarean section, if necessary, may be undertaken without the hazard of maternal bleeding.

Hegde (1985) recommends the use of IgG as described above in all patients with platelet counts of less than 75–100 $\times 10^9/l$. However, the cost is very high (£2500 or more for one 5-day course) and at this hospital non-symptomatic women with platelet counts of $50–70 \times 10^9/l$ have delivered babies with normal platelet counts and needed no supportive therapy even to cover Caesarean section. Also at Queen Charlotte's Hospital for Women we have had a severely thrombocytopenic baby born to a woman who was a partial responder to intravenous IgG and who had received several 5-day courses before delivery. More recent reports suggest that the transplacental effect of intravenous IgG is not reliable (Davies et al 1986). There is no doubt about the value of intravenous IgG in selected cases of severe and particularly non-steroid responsive pregnant women with AITP, but its indiscriminate use in moderately severe cases would have to be shown to improve dramatically both maternal and fetal outcome to justify the high cost.

No active measures need to be taken in the infant with non-symptomatic thrombocytopenia once delivery is negotiated successfully, unless surgery is necessary or other trauma is inflicted. The platelet count in the newborn may fall further in the first few days of life, in spite of static or falling maternally derived antibody, perhaps because of the development of the neonatal splenic circulation and more efficient removal of IgG-coated platelets.

The platelet count usually rises to normal levels within the first month of life, but occasionally thrombocytopenia persists for up to 12 or even 16 weeks. Intravenous hydrocortisone and platelet transfusion can be used in more severely thrombocytopenic infants with evidence of skin and mucosal bleeding.

Even without the introduction of more recent aids to diagnosis of activity of disease and before the discovery of the effects of intravenous IgG, the maternal death rate had fallen from 8–9% in 1950 to virtually zero. The outlook for the fetus, which previously had a death rate of up to 26%, is also much more promising (Epstein et al 1950, Terao et al 1981).

Thrombocytopenia and systemic lupus erythematosus

Systemic lupus erythematosus is frequently complicated by thrombocytopenia but this is seldom severe: less than 5% of cases have platelet counts below $30 \times 10^9/l$ during the course of the disease (Hughes 1979). Thrombocytopenia is often the first presenting feature and may outdate any other manifestations by months or even years. Such patients are often labelled as suffering from AITP, unless appropriate additional tests are carried out. Platelet-associated IgG is often found on testing but it is not clear whether this is due to antiplatelet antibody, immune complexes or both. The management of isolated thrombocytopenia associated with systemic lupus erythematosus in pregnancy does not differ substantially from that of AITP but immunosuppressive therapy should not be reduced or discontinued during pregnancy (Varner et al 1983). However, the main management problem of systemic lupus erythematosus and pregnancy is the complication of the variably present in vitro lupus anticoagulant and its paradoxical association with in vivo thromboembolism and recurrent mid-trimester abortion.

Alloimmune thrombocytopenia

If fetal platelets carry paternally derived antigens which the mother lacks, she may produce antibodies against the fetal platelets in a manner similar to that observed in rhesus D sensitization. Approximately 98% of the population is positive for the platelet antigen PLA1. If a woman is PLA1-negative she may produce anti-PLA1 antibodies which can cause quite severe thrombocytopenia in the fetus and newborn. The documented incidence is low—approximately 1–2 per 10 000 births—but these babies appear to be at far greater risk than those born to mothers with AITP and the perinatal mortality and morbidity are estimated at between 25 and 35%. The children of first pregnancies are often affected (Surainder et al 1981).

Unless the presence of maternal platelet antibodies or neonatal thrombocytopenia has been detected in a previous pregnancy, there are no prenatal clues to fetal thrombocytopenia because the maternal platelet count is absolutely normal. Unlike the fetus exposed to maternal autoimmune platelet antibodies, serious, apparently spontaneous, bleeding may occur in utero weeks before term (Zulneraitis et al 1979). Neonatal deaths, due mainly to intracranial haemorrhage, have occurred in 14% of documented cases. Those who survive may be severely handicapped. The serious haemostatic defect observed in this condition in contrast to that seen in AITP has been attributed to a functional defect of the PLA1-positive platelet when exposed to specific PLA1 antibody. Once the PLA1 site is interfered with the platelet has a serious defect of adherence and aggregation similar to that seen in the inherited condition thrombasthenia or Glanzmann's disease. Non-specific coating of platelets with IgG as in AITP does not interfere with their haemostatic function.

PLA1 antibodies cannot be demonstrated in all cases so other platelet antigens may be involved rarely. In recent years improved techniques for detecting platelet-associated IgG, platelet antigens and free antibodies in the serum have helped to identify this condition and separate it more clearly from AITP (Kelton et al 1980).

The clinical diagnosis of alloimmune purpura depends on the combination of congenital thrombocytopenia, normal maternal platelet count, negative history of maternal AITP and no evidence in the infant of any systemic disease such as infection or malignancy.

If the diagnosis is made for the first time at birth or shortly thereafter the recommended management is to give washed maternal platelets and if this is done the specificity of the platelet antibody need not be determined. Both steroids and high-dose intravenous IgG may have a place in management (see Colvin 1985). Random donor platelets may be tried in an emergency, but they are usually ineffective (Kelton et al 1980). However, the usual situation is one in which the mother has produced alloimmune antibodies with anti-PLA1 specificity in a previous pregnancy which were identified in the routine investigation of thrombocytopenia in the neonate. In this case PLA1-negative platelets from pre-selected blood bank donors should be used to treat and prevent any bleeding at delivery. The principles surrounding management of delivery are the same as for AITP.

The main additional problem with alloimmune antibodies is the risk of serious intracranial bleeding and neurological damage in utero before delivery. Antenatal diagnosis of an at-risk fetus has been reported (Daffos et al 1984). Cord sampling at 32 weeks revealed thrombocytopenia. At 37 weeks an intrauterine transfusion of PLA1-negative platelets was given followed by Caesarean section.

Recently at Queen Charlotte's Maternity Hospital we have successfully managed a fetus with a platelet count of $20 \times 10^9/l$ at 26 weeks' gestation with weekly intrauterine PLA1-negative platelet transfusions; a normal baby was delivered at 34 weeks (Nicolini et al 1988). Management of a previous similar case with platelet transfusions starting at 34 weeks resulted in delivery of a baby who had no thrombocytopenia or bleeding but had intracranial cysts, presumably due to bleeds sustained before treatment was started in utero. This infant is now severely handicapped (De Vries et al 1988).

Early antenatal diagnosis and pre-delivery prophylactic platelet transfusions appear to be the only answer for these severely affected cases if serious morbidity is to be avoided.

Pre-eclampsia and platelets

Thrombocytopenia can occur in association with pre-eclampsia and its severity seems to be related directly to disease activity. The mechanism appears to be multifactorial and may result from a selective intravascular consumption of platelets without significant fibrinogen consumption, as postulated in thrombotic thrombocytopenic purpura (see below), or it may be part of the picture of DIC. Data are accumulating toward the premise that there is a subset of patients with pre-eclampsia at high risk for multiple organ failure. Now that most centres have electronic automated platelet counting facilities, thrombocytopenia is becoming an important simple differentiating parameter in the categorization and management of the high-risk pregnant patient.

In a study of pregnancy outcome in 303 cases with severe pre-eclampsia (Sibai et al 1984), 51 patients (17%) had thrombocytopenia. It was clear on analysis of these 303 cases that early identification of thrombocytopenia was a valid indicator of increasing severity of disease and warranted both screening for it and aggressive intervention when present. Liver enzyme abnormalities were rarely observed in the absence of thrombocytopenia. The whole question of pathogenesis of pre-eclampsia and DIC relationship to the HELLP syndrome and management of these complex conditions is discussed in detail in Chapter 36.

Thrombotic thrombocytopenic purpura (TTP) and haemolytic uraemic syndrome (HUS)

These conditions share so many features that they should probably be considered as one disease with pathological effects confined largely to the kidney in HUS and more generalized in TTP.

Although these conditions occur extremely rarely in the non-pregnant woman they are relatively common in pregnancy. HUS usually presents in the postpartum period with renal failure.

The diagnosis of TTP is based on the typical clinical pentad of fever, microangiopathic haemolytic anaemia, thrombocytopenia, neurological symptoms and renal abnormalities (Bukowski 1982). Symptoms can be quite variable but fluctuating neurological abnormalities and haemorrhagic manifestations of thrombocytopenia predominate. The disease is usually rapidly progressive and fatal. In this very rare and often fatal complication of pregnancy there is the possibility that DIC may play a pathogenic role in TTP and this has been the subject of speculation by many authors. Evidence of a true consumptive coagulopathy is absent in most patients. The levels of fibrinogen and the labile coagulation factors V and VIII are usually within the normal range. The most consistent abnormalities appear to be the presence of fibrin degradation products and a prolonged thrombin time. Laboratory evidence of DIC is minimal and when present is probably secondary to severe intravascular haemolysis (Bukowski 1982, de Swiet 1985).

An essential requisite of the pathogenesis is damage to the wall of small vessels. There is no doubt that local intravascular coagulation contributes to the vascular damage. In HUS the hyaline material laid down on basement membranes and occluding glomerular arterioles is rich in fibrin and in TTP the occluding material in arterioles and capillaries is also rich in fibrin, but laboratory and clinical evidence of DIC has only rarely been documented in association with TTP (Atlas et al 1982, Ingram et al 1982). It has been shown that plasminogen activator is absent from the walls of occluded vessels in TTP but whether this is primary or secondary is not clear. There is heightened platelet aggregability of platelets from normal donors (Lian et al 1979). It was suggested therefore that the plasma of patients with TTP lacked an inhibitor which allowed intravascular platelet aggregation leading to widespread microvascular damage. Remission was induced and the defect corrected by administration of FFP (Lian et al 1979). It has been proposed by several groups that the missing inhibitor of platelet aggregation in TTP stimulates the production of prostacyclin (Remuzzi et al 1978), but whether this deficiency is cause or effect is still not clear (de Swiet 1985). Circulating prostacyclin levels were low in all four cases studied by Machin et al (1981) and in a further two cases from Italy prostacyclin synthesis-stimulating factors were found to be low (Stratta et al 1983). Some patients fail to remit on simple plasma infusions but respond to plasmapheresis or after exchange transfusion and it has been suggested that soluble immune complexes are responsible for vascular damage leading to organ dysfunction.

Because HUS and TTP are sometimes associated with systemic lupus erythematosus and related disorders, it has been suggested that the reticuloendothelial system may have an important role to play. The capacity of the reticuloendothelial system to clear potentially damaging substances such as immune complexes, soluble fibrin monomer complexes (SFMC) and platelet microaggregates is greatly reduced during the course of such conditions (Ingram et al 1982).

Possibly the most crucial problem when dealing with TTP is to establish a correct diagnosis (Atlas et al 1982). The condition can be confused with severe pre-eclampsia and abruptio placentae, especially if DIC is also triggered, although evidence of DIC is not often associated with TTP.

Unlike acute fatty liver of pregnancy there is no evidence that prompt delivery favourably affects the course of HUS or TTP. Most clinicians would recommend delivery if these conditions present in late pregnancy to enable the mother to be treated vigorously without fear of harming the fetus. If the conditions present before the fetus is viable, the patient will have to be treated and the fetus left to take its own chances (de Swiet 1985).

The management of TTP remains difficult and not always successful since the aetiology and pathogenesis are poorly understood. Once the correct diagnosis has been made the management of TTP is the same in principle whether the patient is pregnant or not. The fetus is involved only in as far as it may suffer from placental insufficiency but it is not directly involved in the disease process. The logical approach is to give FFP as a source of the missing inhibitory factor and an antiplatelet agent which will not interfere with prostacyclin production, such as dipyridamole or low-dose aspirin, to reduce platelet aggregability (Ingram et al 1982).

If these measures fail, infusions of prostacyclin or plasmapheresis and exchange transfusion may be tried. If all these measures fail, steroids, immunosuppressants and splenectomy are usually tried but their value is not clear from the few reports in the literature (Atlas et al 1982, Ingram et al 1982).

There are only isolated recent reports of the efficacy of modern treatment of TTP during pregnancy (Davies 1984). Atlas and colleagues (1982) successfully treated a primigravida with intrauterine fetal death at 20 weeks using repeated plasmapheresis. FFP and dipyridamole were used to treat two women in pregnancy in Italy (Stratta et al 1983). Although both women made a full recovery, both lost the fetus. This led the authors to speculate that some form of endothelial injury, damaging the fetoplacental microvasculature and leading to haemolysis and thrombocytopenia, could result in the haemolytic abortion syndrome and be responsible for recurrent unexplained miscarriages. The similarity between TTP and HUS may be of great importance in the light of the successful management of HUS in pregnancy using prostacyclin infusions (Webster et al 1980), although more recent reports of its use have been disappointing (Machin 1984).

Factor VIII antibody

An inhibitor of antihaemophilic factor is a rare cause of haemorrhage in previously healthy postpartum women (O'Brien 1954, Marengo Rowe et al 1972, Voke & Letsky 1977, Coller et al 1981, Reece et al 1982). There are fewer than 50 documented cases in the literature (Voke & Letsky 1977, Reece et al 1982). Women who may have had this type of haemorrhagic disorder were first reported in the late 1930s and the nature of the defect was first reported in 1946, when the plasma of two such patients was shown not only to resemble haemophilic plasma but to have an inhibitory effect on normal clotting. In the late 1960s it was demonstrated that these inhibitors of factor VIII were immunoglobulins, as are the factor VIII antibodies found in treated haemophiliacs (for references see Voke & Letsky 1977). Of the postpartum coagulation defects of this type reported, nearly all were found on in vitro testing to be directed against factor VIII. Only two were found to be anti-factor IX antibodies.

Aetiology. The aetiology of antibodies to factor VIII is complex. The appearance of anti-VIIIC in non-haemophilic individuals is usually attributed to an autoimmune process, or in postpartum women to isoimmunization. However, no difference between maternal and fetal factor VIII has been demonstrated and neutralization of both maternal and fetal factor VIII by the antibody is similar.

There is at present no definite experimental evidence that factor VIII antigen allotypes exist. If the bleeding tendency is to be explained, the antibody formed by stimulation of the maternal immune system by fetal factor VIII has to cross-react with maternal factor VIII. One would expect such an antibody to reappear after some of the subsequent pregnancies (by analogy with rhesus sensitization), but relapses have not been reported. Assuming that these inhibitors are IgG antibodies, they are likely to cross the placenta and persist for several weeks in the neonate, as do anti-rhesus or antiviral antibodies. However, although factor VIII antibody and low levels of factor VIIIC have been found in neonates born to mothers with antibody, there have been no case reports of haemorrhagic problems in their offspring.

The variable nature of this disorder argues in favour of a more complex pathogenesis. There is an association between factor VIII antibodies and autoimmune disorders such as rheumatoid arthritis and systemic lupus erythematosus. There is also a well known alteration of immune reactivity in normal pregnancy. These observations suggest that a likely explanation of postpartum factor VIII antibodies is that of a temporary breakdown in the mother's tolerance to her own factor VIII (or factor IX). This rare disorder resembles other autoimmune states in its variable onset and duration, its varying severity and in the fact that its aetiology is still a mystery (Voke & Letsky 1977).

Clinical manifestations. The patient usually presents within 3 months of delivery with severe bleeding, extensive painful bruising, bleeding from the gastrointestinal or genitourinary tract and occasional haemarthroses. The reported confirmed cases presented in a period of 3 days to 17 months postpartum. The factor VIII antibody is associated with life-threatening haemorrhage at various sites, not necessarily related to parturition.

Diagnosis of factor VIII antibody. The diagnosis is established on the basis of characteristic laboratory findings. The prothrombin time and thrombin time are normal but the partial thromboplastin time is very long. The partial thromboplastin time is not corrected by the addition of normal plasma or factor VIII.

The potency of the antibody is determined by an assay in which the ability of concentrations of the patient's plasma to destroy factor VIIIC is observed, the result being expressed in units per millilitre. The unit is defined as that quantity of antibody contained in undiluted patient's plasma which will destroy 0.5 iu VIIIC in 4 hours at 37 °C.

Management. Any woman who develops such an antibody should be under the care of an expert coagulation unit. Treatment of the acute bleeding episode is difficult because conventional amounts of factor VIII may merely enhance antibody formation and fail to control the bleeding. Immunosuppressive agents in combination with corticosteroid have been suggested to reduce the antibody production and there are reports of a decrease or disappearance of the antibody in response to treatment (Coller et al 1981).

In one reported case (Reece et al 1982) after failure of factor VIII concentrate and fresh plasma, improvement in the clinical status was achieved by administration of an anti-inhibitor coagulation complex (Autoplex), a preparation of pooled fresh plasma containing precursors and activated clotting factors. The mechanism of action of Autoplex is unknown. It does not suppress or destroy the inhibitor but seems to control the acute haemorrhage diathesis (Reece et al 1982).

The natural history is for the antibody to disappear gradually, usually within 2 years. Women should be advised to avoid further pregnancy until coagulation is back to normal, although in the one documented case where conception occurred in the presence of clinically active antibody, the antibody disappeared during the course of the pregnancy (Voke & Letsky 1977).

GENETIC DISORDERS OF HAEMOSTASIS

It is important to recognize these uncommon conditions not only because the morbidity and mortality they cause in the sufferer is almost completely preventable by correct diagnosis and treatment, but also because carriers of the most devastating of these conditions, particularly the X-linked haemophilias, can be identified and prenatal diagnosis offered if couples at risk so desire.

However, because of the profound changes in haemostasis during normal pregnancy it is desirable to establish a correct diagnosis with appropriate family studies and DNA analysis where relevant, before conception, so that appropriate management, and in conditions where DNA prenatal diagnosis is feasible, chorionic villus sampling can be planned in advance.

Severe congenital disorders of haemostasis are nearly always apparent early in life so that they will have been diagnosed before the obstetrician has to deal with the patient. Milder forms may go unrecognized until adult life and are more of a diagnostic challenge.

Patients with thrombocytopenia or platelet function abnormalities suffer primarily from mucosal bleeding with epistaxes, gingival and gastrointestinal bleeding and menorrhagia. Bleeding occurs immediately after surgery or trauma and may not occur at all if primary haemostasis can be achieved with suturing.

In contrast patients with coagulation disorders typically suffer deep muscle haematomata and haemarthroses. Bleeding after trauma or surgery may be immediate or delayed. A history of previous vaginal deliveries without undue bleeding does not exclude a significant coagulopathy because of the increase in coagulation factors, particularly factor VIII, which occurs during normal pregnancy and the fact that powerful uterine contractility is the most important haemostatic factor at parturition.

Complete laboratory evaluation of a patient giving a history of easy bleeding or bruising is time-consuming and expensive and a history of significant previous haemostatic challenges should be obtained. For example, a patient who has undergone tonsillectomy without transfusion or special treatment and lived to tell the tale cannot possibly have an inherited haemostatic disorder.

Of more relevance perhaps is any history of dental extractions where haemorrhage can occur with both platelet disorders and coagulopathies. If prolonged bleeding has occurred and particularly if blood transfusion has been required, then a high index of suspicion of a congenital haemorrhagic disorder is justified. In such cases, even if initial laboratory screening tests—partial thromboplastin time, prothrombin time, platelet count and bleeding time—are normal, the diagnosis should be vigorously pursued in consultation with an expert haematologist.

The most common congenital coagulation disorders are von Willebrand's disease, factor VIII deficiency (haemophilia A) and factor IX deficiency (haemophilia B). Less common disorders include factor XI deficiency, abnormal or deficient fibrinogen and deficiency of factor XIII (fibrin-stabilizing factor). All other coagulation factor disorders are extremely rare. The most frequent disorders of platelet function are von Willebrand's disease and storage pool disease.

Von Willebrand's disease

Von Willebrand's disease is the most frequent of all inherited haemostatic disorders with an overt disease incidence of more than 1 in 10 000, similar to that of haemophilia A. Because subclinical forms of the disorder are common, the total incidence of von Willebrand's disease is actually greater than that of haemophilia. In contrast to haemophilia (an X-linked condition), von Willebrand's disease has an autosomal inheritance and equal incidence in males and females and therefore is the most frequent genetic haemostatic disorder encountered in obstetric practice.

Nature of the defect

Von Willebrand's disease is a disorder of the von Willebrand factor portion of the human factor VIII complex. Factor VIII circulates as a complex of two proteins of unequal size. There is a low molecular weight portion (VIIIC), which promotes coagulation, linked to a large multimer known as von Willebrand factor (VIIIWF). The larger VIIIWF, under autosomal control, serves as a carrier for VIIIC, coded for on the X-chromosome. The complex is found in the circulation as polymers of varying size. VIIIWF is the major protein in plasma which promotes platelet adhesion by forming a bridge between the subendothelial collagen and a specific receptor on the platelet membrane. Reduction in VIIIWF usually leads to comparable decrease in VIIIC activity.

There are subgroups of von Willebrand's disease based on qualitative and quantitative changes in the multimers of the factor VIII complex (see Caldwell et al 1985).

Clinical features

Clinical manifestations of the disease are primarily those of a platelet defect, namely spontaneous mucous membrane or skin bleeding and prolonged bleeding following trauma or surgery. There are also manifestations of a coagulation defect due to VIIIC activity reduction. The most frequent problem encountered in the non-pregnant female is menorrhagia which may be quite severe. Patients with mild abnormalities may be asymptomatic and the diagnosis made only after excessive haemorrhage has followed trauma or related to surgery. The severity of the disorder does not run true within families and fluctuates from time to time in the same individual.

Treatment

Several treatments in von Willebrand's disease are in current use, the choice depending on the severity and type of the disease and on the clinical setting. The aim is to correct the platelet and coagulation disorder by achieving normal levels of factor VIII coagulant activity and a bleeding time within the normal range. The key feature in treatment is substitution with plasma concentrates containing functional von Willebrand's factor and VIIIC. In less severe cases the vasopressin analogue I-desamino-8-arginine-vasopressin (DDAVP) has been used with success. Contraceptive hormones have been used with success in the treatment of menorrhagia in von Willebrand's disease (Holmberg & Nilsson 1985). Aspirin and related anti-inflammatory drugs should not be used in von Willebrand's disease as they will further compromise platelet function.

The main treatment in von Willebrand's disease was replacement therapy with cryoprecipitate or FFP. The latter is efficient, but large volumes may be required to secure haemostasis. In obstetric practice, however, this does not usually cause any problems when covering delivery. Cryoprecipitate was the product of choice to cover cold surgery. Factor VIII concentrates were not used in the management of von Willebrand's disease because, in commercial preparations, the factor promoting platelet adhesion may be lost and because of the increased risk of transmitting infection. Newer preparations of factor VIII concentrate now retain some platelet promoting activity and have the added advantage on being heat-treated and therefore sterile. They now no longer carry the hazard of transmitting HIV and other viral infections.

DDAVP has been shown to cause release of von Willebrand's factor from endothelial cells where it is synthesized and stored. It is particularly effective in mildly affected patients and may in some cases replace the use or need for blood products in patients undergoing surgery. Toxicity associated with use of this product has been trivial. Occasional patients experience flushing and dizziness (Holmberg & Nilsson 1985). The theoretical risk of water intoxication and hyponatraemia due to a vasopressive effect has not been observed using the current dosage schedules. The recommended dose is an intravenous infusion of 0.3 μg/kg DDAVP given over 30 minutes up to a total dose of 15–25 μg. This may be repeated every 12–24 hours (Linkler 1986). In patients with severe von Willebrand's disease, DDAVP has no effect and replacement therapy must be used.

Von Willebrand's disease and pregnancy

A rise in both factor VIIIC and von Willebrand's factor is observed in normal pregnancy. Patients with all but the severest forms of von Willebrand's disease show a similar but variable rise in both these factors, although there may not be a reduction in the bleeding time (Caldwell et al 1985, Chediak et al 1986, Conti et al 1986).

After delivery, normal women maintain an elevated factor VIIIC level for at least 5 days. This is followed by a slow fall to baseline levels over 4–6 weeks. The duration of factor VIII activity postpartum in women with von Willebrand's disease seems to be related to the severity of the disorder. Women with more severe forms of the condition may have a rapid fall in factor VIII procoagulant and platelet haemostatic activity. They are then at risk of quite severe secondary postpartum haemorrhage.

Published reports of 33 pregnancies in 22 women showed abnormal bleeding in 27% at the time of abortion, delivery or postpartum (Conti et al 1986). The general consensus is that the most important determinant for abnormal haemorrhage at delivery is a low factor VIIIC plasma level. The vast majority of women will have increased their factor VIIIC production to within the normal range (20–150%) by late gestation and although cryoprecipitate should be standing by at delivery it will probably not be needed to achieve haemostasis.

While there is virtually no place for DDAVP in obstetric

practice it is valuable in the management of women with von Willebrand's disease undergoing gynaecological surgery.

The haemophilias

The haemophilias are inherited disorders associated with reduced or absent coagulation factors VIII or IX with an incidence of around 1 in 10 000 in developed countries (Jones 1977). The most common is haemophilia A which is associated with deficiency of factor VIII; about one-sixth of the 3000–4000 cases in Britain today have a condition known as Christmas disease due to a lack of coagulation factor IX (haemophilia B). Clinical manifestations of the two conditions are indistinguishable; symptoms and signs are variable and depend on the degree of the lack of the coagulation factors concerned. Severe disease with frequent spontaneous bleeding (particularly haemarthroses) is associated with clotting factor levels of 0–1%. Less severe disease is found in subjects with clotting factors of 1–4%. Spontaneous bleeding and severe bleeding after minor trauma are rare even in cases with coagulation factor levels between 5 and 30%; the danger is that the condition may be clinically silent but during the course of major surgery or following trauma, such subjects behave as if with the severest forms of haemophilia. Unless the defect is recognized and replacement of the lacking coagulation factor replaced, such patients will continue to bleed. The inheritance of both haemophilias is X-linked—recessive—being expressed in the male and carried by the female.

The risks in pregnancy for a female carrier of haemophilia are twofold:

1. She may, by process of Lyonization, have a very low factor VIII or IX level which puts her at risk of excessive bleeding, particularly following a traumatic or surgical delivery.
2. Fifty per cent of her sons will inherit haemophilia and 50% of her daughters will be carriers like herself.

This has important implications now that prenatal diagnosis of these conditions is possible.

Management of haemophilia in pregnancy

On average female carriers of haemophilia do not have clinical manifestations but in rare individuals in whom the factor VIIIC or IX levels are unusually low (10–30% of normal), abnormal bleeding may occur after trauma or surgery (Lusher & McMillan 1978). It is important to identify carriers prior to pregnancy, not only to provide genetic counselling but so that appropriate provision can be made for those cases with pathologically low coagulation factor activity. Fortunately the level of the deficient factor tends to increase during the course of pregnancy, as in normal women. There have been anecdotal reports of female homozygotes for haemophilia A who have negotiated pregnancy successfully (Lusher & McMillan 1978). Haemorrhage postpartum does not appear to be a consistent feature, particularly if delivery is by the vaginal route at term with little or no soft-tissue damage. The effect of pregnancy on factor VIIIC levels in these rare cases has not been studied.

If the factor VIII level remains low in carriers of haemophilia, heat-treated factor VIII concentrates should be given to cover delivery.

DDAVP has been shown to be of benefit in patients with mild haemophilia, as with von Willebrand's disease (see above). However, the storage pools of factor VIII released during treatment may become exhausted and tachyphylaxis does occur (Linkler 1986). There are no controlled studies concerning the use of DDAVP during pregnancy and its safety and efficacy in obstetric practice remain to be determined.

The effects of DDAVP on uterine contractability could limit its use, although it has been employed in the management of diabetes insipidus in pregnancy with no harm to the fetus (Caldwell et al 1985). However, as pointed out previously, if the stimulus of pregnancy has not raised the level of factor VIII as expected in mild haemophilia, it is unlikely that DDAVP will do so.

A clinical problem is more likely in carriers of factor IX deficiency (Christmas disease) than in women with factor VIII deficiency (Levin 1982). In the exceptionally rare situations where factor IX level is very low and remains low during pregnancy, the patient should be managed with FFP to cover delivery and for 3–4 days postpartum. This is preferable to factor IX concentrates which are prepared from multiple donations and contain factors II, VII and X as well as factor IX and therefore carry a much greater thrombogenic hazard adding to the innate risk of thromboembolism in pregnancy. These patients should be managed in a unit with access to expert advice, 24-hour laboratory coagulation service and immediate access to the appropriate plasma components required for replacement therapy.

Factor XI deficiency (plasma thromboplastin antecedent (PTA) deficiency). This is a rare coagulation disorder which is less common than the haemophilias but more common than the very rare inherited deficiencies of the remaining coagulation factors. It is inherited as an autosomal recessive, predominantly in Ashkenazi Jews and both men and women may be affected. Usually only the homozygotes have clinical evidence of a coagulation disorder, though occasionally carriers may have a bleeding tendency. It is a mild condition in which spontaneous haemorrhages and haemarthroses are rare but the danger lies in the fact that profuse bleeding may follow major trauma or surgery if no prophylactic plasma is given. Indeed it is often diagnosed late in life following surgery in an individual who was unaware of a serious haemostatic defect. The diagnosis is made by finding a prolonged partial thromboplastin time, with a low factor XI level in a coagulation assay system but in which all other coagulation tests are normal. Management consists of replacement with FFP to treat bleeding and for prophylaxis before and after surgery. In a known case of PTA deficiency it would be wise to cover parturition with plasma.

Fortunately the condition rarely causes problems either during pregnancy and labour or in the child; in particular, prolonged bleeding at ritual circumcision is not usual. There is therefore, no justification in screening routinely for this condition in the mother, fetus or neonate.

The effective haemostatic level of factor XI is approximately 25% and factor XI has a half-life of around 2 days. To cover surgery or delivery, women can be treated with FFP in an initial dose of 20 ml/kg, followed by a maintenance dose of 5 ml/kg daily until primary healing is established.

Genetic disorders of fibrinogen (factor I). Fibrinogen is synthesized in the liver, has a molecular weight of 340 000 and circulates in plasma at a concentration of 300 mg/dl. Both quantitative and qualitative genetic abnormalities are described.

Afibrinogenaemia or hypofibrinogenaemia. These are rare autosomal recessive disorders resulting from reduced fibrinogen synthesis. Most patients with hypofibrinogenaemia are heterozygous.

Congenital hypofibrinogenaemia has been associated with recurrent early miscarriages and with recurrent placental abruption (Ness et al 1983).

Afibrinogenaemia is characterized by a lifelong bleeding tendency of variable severity. Prolonged bleeding after minor injury and easy bruising are frequent symptoms. Menorrhagia can be very severe. Spontaneous deep tissue bleeding and haemarthroses are rare, but severe bleeding can occur after trauma or surgery and several patients have suffered intracerebral haemorrhages. In afibrinogenaemia all screening tests of coagulation are prolonged, but corrected by addition of normal plasma or fibrinogen. A prolonged bleeding time may be present. The final diagnosis is made by quantitating the concentration of circulating fibrinogen.

Plasma or cryoprecipitate may be used as replacement therapy to treat bleeding, cover surgery or delivery. The in vivo half-life of fibrinogen is between 3 and 5 days. Initial replacement should be achieved with 25 ml plasma/kg and daily maintenance with 5–10 ml/kg for 7 days.

Dysfibrinogenaemia. Congenital dysfibrinogenaemia is an autosomal dominant disorder. In contrast to patients with afibrinogenaemia, patients with this disorder are often symptom-free. Some have a bleeding tendency; others have been shown to have thromboembolic disease. The diagnosis is made by demonstrating a prolonged thrombin time with a normal immunological fibrinogen level.

Affected women like those with hypofibrinogenaemia may have recurrent spontaneous abortion or repeated placental abruption (Ness et al 1983).

Factor XIII deficiency (fibrin-stabilizing factor deficiency)

This is an autosomal recessive disorder classically characterized by bleeding from the umbilical cord during the first few days of life and later by ecchymoses, prolonged post-traumatic haemorrhage and poor wound healing. Bleeding is usually delayed and characteristically of a slow oozing nature. Cases of intracranial haemorrhage have been described in a significant proportion of reported cases. Spontaneous recurrent abortion with excessive bleeding occurs in association with factor XIII deficiency (Kitchens & Newcomb 1979). All standard coagulation tests are normal. Diagnosis of severe factor XIII deficiency is made by the clot solubility test. Normal fibrin clots will not dissolve when incubated overnight in 5 mol/l urea solutions, whereas the unstable clots formed in the absence of factor XIII will be dissolved.

Since factor XIII has a half-life of 6 days to 2 weeks and only 5% of normal factor XIII levels is needed for effective haemostasis, patients can be treated with FFP in doses of 5 ml/kg repeated every 3 weeks. Using this therapy, pregnancy has progressed safely to term in a woman who had previously suffered repeated abortions. Because of the high incidence of intracranial haemorrhage, replacement therapy is recommended for all individuals known to have factor XIII deficiency (Kitchens & Newcomb 1979).

Other plasma factor disorders. Congenital deficiencies of factors II, V, VII and X are extremely rare and the reader is referred to Caldwell et al's review of hereditary coagulopathies in pregnancy for an account of their diagnosis and special management problems (Caldwell et al 1985).

REFERENCES

Amris C J, Hilden M 1968 Anticoagulant effects of Trasylol: in vitro and in vivo studies. Annals of the New York Academy of Sciences 146: 612–694

Astedt B, Nilsson I M 1978 Recurrent abruptio placentae treated with the fibrinolytic inhibitor tranexamic acid. British Medical Journal i: 756–757

Atlas M, Barkai G, Menczer J, Houlu N, Lieberman P 1982 Thrombotic thrombocytopenic purpura in pregnancy. British Journal of Obstetrics and Gynaecology 89: 476–479

Aznar J, Gilabert J, Estelles A, Fernandez M A, Villa P, Aznar J A 1982 Evaluation of the soluble fibrin monomer complexes and other coagulation parameters in obstetric patients. Thrombosis Research 27: 691–701

Basu H K 1969 Fibrinolysis and abruptio placentae. Journal of Obstetrics and Gynaecology of the British Commonwealth 76: 481–496

Beal D W, de Masi A D 1985 Role of the platelet count in the management of the high-risk obstetric patient. Journal of the American Osteopathic Association 85: 252–255

Bell W R 1977 Hematologic abnormalities in pregnancy. Medical Clinics of North America 61: 1–165

Beller F K 1985 Sepsis and coagulation. Clinical Obstetrics and Gynecology 28: 46–52

Beller F K, Uszynski M 1974 Disseminated intravascular coagulation in pregnancy. Clinical Obstetrics and Gynecology 17: 264–278

Bonnar J 1973 Blood coagulation and fibrinolysis in obstetrics. Clinics in Haematology 2: 213–233

Bonnar J 1978 Haemorrhagic disorders during pregnancy in perinatal

coagulation. In: Hathaway W E, Bonnar J (eds) Monographs in neonatology. Grune & Stratton, New York
Bonnar J 1981 Haemostasis and coagulation disorders in pregnancy. In: Bloom A L, Thomas D P (eds) Haemostasis and thrombosis. Churchill Livingstone, Edinburgh, pp 454–471
Bonnar J, Prentice C R M, McNicol G P, Douglas A S 1970 Haemostatic mechanism in uterine circulation during placental separation. British Medical Journal 2: 564–567
Boulton F E, Letsky E 1985 Obstetric haemorrhage: causes and management. Clinics in Haematology 14: 683–728
Bukowski R M 1982 Thrombotic thrombocytopenic purpura. Progress in Haemostasis and Thrombosis 6: 287–337
Burkman R T, Bell W R, Atizenza M F, King T M 1977 Coagulopathy with midtrimester induced abortion. Association with hyperosmolar urea administration. American Journal of Obstetrics and Gynecology 127: 533–536
Burroughs A K, Seong N G, Dojcinoov D M, Scheuer P J, Sherlock S V P 1982 Idiopathic acute fatty liver of pregnancy in 12 patients. Quarterly Journal of Medicine 51: 481–497
Bydder G M, Kreel L, Chapman R W G, Harry D, Sherlock S 1980 Accuracy of completed tomography in diagnosis of fatty liver. British Medical Journal 281: 1042–1044
Caires D, Arocha-Pinango C L, Rodriguez S, Linares J 1984 Factor VIII R:Ag/Factor VIII:C and their ratio in obstetrical cases. Acta Obstetricia et Gynecologica Scandinavica 63: 411–416
Caldwell D C, Williamson R A, Goldsmith J C 1985 Hereditary coagulopathies in pregnancy. Clinical Obstetrics and Gynecology 28: 53–72
Carey L C, Cloutier C T, Lowery B D 1970 The use of balanced electrolyte solution for resuscitation. In: Fox Nahas (ed) Body fluid replacement in the surgical patient. Grune & Stratton, New York
Carloss H W, McMillan R, Crosby W H 1980 Management of pregnancy in women with immune thrombocytopenia purpura. Journal of the American Medical Association 244: 2756–2758
Cash J 1981 Blood replacement therapy. In: Bloom A L, Thomas D P (eds) Haemostasis and thrombosis. Churchill Livingstone, Edinburgh
Cates W Jr, Boyd C, Halvorson-Boyd G I, Holck S, Gilchrist T F 1981 Death from amniotic fluid embolism and disseminated intravascular coagulation after a curettage abortion. American Journal of Obstetrics and Gynecology 141: 346–348
Chediak J R, Alban G M, Maxey B 1986 Von Willebrand's disease and pregnancy: management during delivery and outcome of offspring. American Journal of Obstetrics and Gynecology 155: 618–624
Chung A F, Merkatz I R 1973 Survival following amniotic fluid embolism with early heparinization. Obstetrics and Gynecology 42: 809–814
Cines D B, Dusak B, Tomaski A, Mennuti M, Schreiber A D 1982 Immune thrombocytopenic purpura and pregnancy. New England Journal of Medicine 306: 826–831
Clarkson A R, Sage R E, Lawrence J R 1969 Consumption coagulopathy and acute renal failure due to Gram negative septicaemia after abortion. Complete recovery with heparin therapy. Annals of Internal Medicine 70: 1191–1199
Cohen E, Ballard C A 1974 Consumptive coagulopathy associated with intra-amniotic saline instillation and the effect of intravenous oxytocin. Obstetrics and Gynecology 43: 300–303
Coller B S, Hultin M B, Homer L W et al 1981 Normal pregnancy in a patient with a prior post-partum factor VIII inhibitor: with observations on pathogenesis and prognosis. Blood 58: 619–624
Collier C B, Birrell W R S 1983 Chronic ectopic pregnancy complicated by shock and disseminated intravascular coagulation. Anaesthesia in Intensive Care II: 246–248
Colvin B T 1985 Thrombocytopenia. Clinics in Haematology 14: 661–681
Comp P C, Thurnau G R, Welsh J, Esmon C T 1986 Functional and immunologic protein S levels are decreased during pregnancy. Blood 68: 881–885
Conti M, Mari D, Conti E, Muggiasca M L, Mannuci P M 1986 Pregnancy in women with different types of von Willebrand disease. Obstetrics and Gynecology 68: 282–285
Courtney L D, Allington M 1972 Effect of amniotic fluid on blood coagulation. British Journal of Haematology 29: 353–356
Daffos F, Forest E R, Muller J Y et al 1984 Prenatal treatment of allo-immune thrombocytopenia. Lancet ii: 632
Davies G E 1984 Thrombotic thrombocytopenia in pregnancy with maternal survival. British Journal of Obstetrics and Gynaecology 91: 396–398
Davies M H et al 1980 Acute liver disease with encephalopathy and renal failure in late pregnancy and the early puerperium. A study of 14 patients. British Journal of Obstetrics and Gynaecology 87: 1003–1014
Davies S V, Murray J A, Gee H, Giles H McC 1986 Transplacental effect of high-dose immunoglobulin in idiopathic thrombocytopenia (ITP). Lancet i: 1098–1099
Davis G 1972 Midtrimester abortion. Late dilation and evacuation and DIC. Lancet ii: 1026
Department of Health and Social Security 1982 Report on confidential enquiries into maternal deaths in England and Wales 1976–78. Report on health and social subjects 26. Her Majesty's Stationery Office, London
Department of Health and Social Security 1986 Report on confidential enquiries into maternal deaths in England and Wales 1979–81. Report on health and social services no. 29. Her Majesty's Stationery Office, London
de Swiet M 1985 Some rare medical complications of pregnancy. British Medical Journal 290: 2–4
De Vries L S, Connell J, Bydder G M et al 1988 Recurrent intracranial haemorrhages in utero in an infant with allo-immune thrombocytopenia. British Journal of Obstetrics and Gynaecology 95: 299–302
Doenicke A, Grote B, Lorenz W 1977 Blood and blood substitutes in management of the injured patient. British Journal of Anaesthesia 49: 681–688
Dolyniuk M, Oriel E, Vania H, Karlman R, Tomich P 1983 Rapid diagnosis of amniotic fluid embolism. Obstetrics and Gynecology 61: 28S–30S
Epstein R D, Longer E L, Conbey J T 1950 Congenital thrombocytopenia purpura. Purpura haemorrhage in pregnancy and the newborn. American Journal of Medicine 9: 44–56
Estelles A, Aznar J, Gilabert J 1980 A quantitative study of soluble fibrin monomer complexes in normal labour and abruptio placentae. Thrombosis Research 18: 513–519
Fay R A, Hughes A D, Farron N T 1983 Platelets in pregnancy: hyper-destruction in pregnancy. Obstetrics and Gynecology 61: 238–240
Feinstein D I 1982 Diagnosis and management of disseminated intra-vascular coagulation: the role of heparin therapy. Blood 60: 284–287
Fenton V, Saunders K, Cavill I 1977 The platelet count in pregnancy. Journal of Clinical Pathology 30: 68–69
Ferris T F, Erdson P B, Dunhill M S, Lee M R 1969 Toxaemia of pregnancy in sheep: a clinical physiological and pathological study. Journal of Clinical Investigation 48: 1643–1655
Fournie A, Monrozies M, Pontonnier G, Boneu B, Bierne R 1981 Factor VIII complex in normal pregnancy, pre-eclampsia and fetal growth retardation. British Journal of Obstetrics and Gynaecology 88: 250–254
Freeman M 1979 Fatal reaction to Haemaccel. Anaesthesia 34: 341–343
Gilabert J, Aznar J, Parilla J, Reganon E, Vila V, Estelles A 1978 Alteration in the coagulation and fibrinolysis system in pregnancy, labour and puerperium, with special reference to a possible transitory state of intravascular coagulation during labour. Thrombosis and Haemostasis 40: 387–396
Gilabert J, Estelles A, Aznar J, Galbis M 1985 Abruptio placentae and disseminated intravascular coagulation. Acta Obstetricia et Gynecologica Scandinavica 64: 35–39
Goodlin R C 1984 Acute fatty liver of pregnancy. Acta Obstetricia et Gynecologica Scandinavica 63: 379–380
Graeff H, Ernst E, Bocaz J A 1978 Evaluation of hypercoagulability in septic abortion. Haemostasis 5: 285–294
Gregory M G, Clayton E M J 1973 Amniotic fluid embolism. Obstetrics and Gynecology 42: 236–244
Grundy M F B, Craven E R 1976 Consumption coagulopathy after intra-amniotic urea. British Medical Journal ii: 677–678
Guidotti R J, Grimes D A, Cates W Jr 1981 Fatal amniotic fluid embolism during legally induced abortion. United States, 1972–1978. American Journal of Obstetrics and Gynecology 141: 257–261
Hafter R, Graeff H 1975 Molecular aspects of defibrination in a reptilase treated case of 'dead fetus syndrome'. Thrombosis Research 7: 391–399
Hague W M, Fenton D W, Duncan S L B, Slater D N 1983 Acute fatty liver of pregnancy. Journal of the Royal Society of Medicine 76: 652–661
Hauser C J, Shoemaker W C, Turpin I, Goldberg S J 1980 Oxygen

transport responses to colloids and crystalloids in critically ill surgical patients. Surgica Gynecologica Obstetrica 159: 181–186
Hegde U M 1985 Immune thrombocytopenia in pregnancy and the newborn. British Journal of Obstetrics and Gynaecology 92: 657–659
Hegde U M, Gordon-Smith E C, Worrlledge S M 1977 Platelet antibodies in thrombocytopenic patients. British Journal of Haematology 56: 191–197
Hegde U M, Bowes A, Powell D K, Joyner M V 1981 Detection of platelet bound and serum antibodies in thrombocytopenia by enzyme linked assay. Vox Sanguinis 41: 306–312
Hellgren M, Blomback M 1981 Blood coagulation and fibrinolysis in pregnancy, during delivery and in the puerperium. Gynecologic Obstetric Investigation 12: 141–154
Hellgren M, Hagnevik K, Robbe H, Bjork O, Blomback M, Eklund J 1983 Severe acquired antithrombin III deficiency in relation to hepatic and renal insufficiency and intrauterine fetal death in late pregnancy. Gynecologic Obstetric Investigation 16: 107–118
Herbert W N P 1982 Complications of the immediate puerperium. Clinical Obstetrics and Gynecology 25: 219–232
Hodgkinson C R, Thompson R J, Hodari A A 1964 Dead fetus syndrome. Clinics in Obstetrics and Gynaecology 7: 349–358
Holmberg L, Nilsson I M 1985 Von Willebrand disease. Clinics in Haematology 14: 461–488
Hughes G R V 1979 Systemic lupus erythematosus in connective tissue diseases. Blackwell Scientific Publications, Oxford
Ingram G I L, Brozovic M, Slater N G P 1982 Thrombotic thrombocytopenic purpura. In: Bleeding disorders—investigation and management. Blackwell Scientific Publications, Oxford
Jones P 1977 Developments and problems in the management of haemophilia. Seminars in Haematology 14: 375–390
Kelton J C, Blanchette V S, William E W 1980 Neonatal thrombocytopenia due to passive immunisation. Prenatal diagnosis and distinction between maternal platelet alloantibodies and autoantibodies. New England Journal of Medicine 302: 1401–1403
Kelton J C et al 1982 The prenatal prediction of thrombocytopenia in mothers with clinically diagnosed immune thrombocytopenia. American Journal of Obstetrics and Gynecology 144: 449–454
Kitchens C S, Newcomb T F 1979 Factor XIII. Medicine 58: 413–429
Lammle B, Griffin J H 1985 Formation of the fibrin clot: the balance of procoagulant and inhibitory factors. In: Ruggeri Z M (ed) Coagulation disorders. WB Saunders, London, pp 281–342
Lancet Editorial 1983 Acute fatty liver of pregnancy. Lancet i: 339
Laursen B, Mortensen J Z, Frost L, Hansen K B 1981 Disseminated intravascular coagulation in hepatic failure treated with antithrombin III. Thrombosis Research 22: 701–704
Laursen B, Frost L, Mortensen J Z, Hansen K B, Paulsen S M 1983 Acute fatty liver of pregnancy with complicating disseminated intravascular coagulation. Acta Obstetricia et Gynecologica Scandinavica 62: 403–407
Lavery J P, Koontz W L, Liu Y K, Howell R 1985 Immunologic thrombocytopenia in pregnancy: use of antenatal immunoglobulin therapy: case report and review. Obstetrics and Gynecology 66: 41S–43S
Letsky E A 1985 Coagulation problems during pregnancy. Current Reviews in Obstetrics and Gynaecology, vol 10, Churchill Livingstone, Edinburgh
Levin J 1982 Disorders of blood coagulation and platelets. In: Barrow G N, Ferris T F (eds) Medical complications during pregnancy, 2nd edn. WB Saunders, London, pp 70–73
Lewis P J 1982 The role of prostacyclin in pre-eclampsia. British Journal of Hospital Medicine 62: 1048–1052
Lewis P J, Boylan P, Friedman L A, Hensman C N, Downing I 1980 Prostacyclin in pregnancy. British Medical Journal 280: 1581–1582
Lian E C, Harkness D R, Byrnes J J, Wallach H, Nunez R 1979 Presence of a platelet aggregating factor in the plasma of patients with thrombotic thrombocytopenic purpura (TTP) and its inhibition by normal plasma. Blood 53: 333–338
Liebman H A, McGehee W G, Patch M J, Feinstein D I 1983 Severe depression of antithrombin III associated with disseminated intravascular coagulation in women with fatty liver of pregnancy. Annals of Internal Medicine 98: 330–333
Linkler C A 1986 Congenital disorders of haemostasis. In: Laros R K (ed) Blood disorders in pregnancy. Lea & Febiger, Philadelphia, p 160
Lorenz W, Doenicke A, Messmer K et al 1976 Histamine release in human subjects by modified gelatin (Haemaccel) and dextran: an explanation for anaphylactoid reactions observed under clinical conditions. British Journal of Anaesthesia 48: 151–165
Lusher J M, McMillan C W 1978 Severe factor VIII and IX deficiency in females. American Journal of Medicine 65: 637
Machin S J 1984 Thrombotic thrombocytopenic purpura. British Journal of Haematology 56: 191–197
Machin S J, Defrey N G, Vermylen J, Willoughby M L N 1981 Prostacyclin deficiency in thrombotic thrombocytopenic purpura (TTP) and the haemolytic uraemic syndrome (HUS). British Journal of Haematology 49: 141–142
MacKenzie I Z, Sayers L, Bonnar J et al 1975 Coagulation changes during second trimester abortion induced by intra-amniotic prostaglandin E_{2+} and hypertonic solutions. Lancet ii: 1066–1069
Mant M J, King E G 1979 Severe acute disseminated intravascular coagulation. A reappraisal of its pathophysiology, clinical significance and therapy, based on 47 patients. American Journal of Medicine 67: 557–563
Marengo Rowe A J, Murff G, Leveson J E, Cook J 1972 Haemophilia-like disease associated with pregnancy. Obstetrics and Gynecology 40: 56–64
Marshall M, Bird T 1983 Blood loss and replacement. Edward Arnold, London
McGibbon D H 1982 Dermatological purpura. In: Ingram G I C, Brozovic M, Slater N G P (eds) Bleeding disorders—investigation and management. Blackwell Scientific Publications, Oxford
McMillan R 1981 Chronic idiopathic thrombocytopenic purpura. New England Journal of Medicine 304: 1135–1147
Meier P R, Bowes W A 1983 Amniotic fluid embolus-like syndrome presenting in the second trimester of pregnancy. Obstetrics and Gynecology 61 (suppl 3): 31S–34S
Moncada M D, Vane J R 1979 Arachidonic acid metabolites and the interactions between platelets and blood-vessel walls. New England Journal of Medicine 300: 1142–1147
Morgan M 1979 Amniotic fluid embolism. Anaesthesia 34: 20–32
Morgenstern G R, Measday B, Hegde U M 1983 Auto-immune thrombocytopenia in pregnancy. New approach to management. British Medical Journal 287: 584
Moss G 1972 An argument in favour of electrolyte solutions for early resuscitation. Surgical Clinics in North America 52: 3–17
Naumann R O, Weinstein L 1985 Disseminated intravascular coagulation—the clinician's dilemma. Obstetrical and Gynecological Survey 40: 487–492
Ness P M, Budzynski A Z, Olexa S A et al 1983 Congenital hypofibrinogenemia and recurrent placental abruption. Obstetrics and Gynecology 61: 519–523
Newland A C, Boots M A, Patterson K G 1984 Intravenous IgG for autoimmune thrombocytopenia in pregnancy. New England Journal of Medicine 310: 261–262
Nicolini U, Rodeck C, Kochenour N, Greco P, Fisk N, Letsky E 1988 In utero platelet transfusion for alloimmune thrombocytopenia. Lancet ii: 506
Nordstrom S, Blomback B, Blomback M, Olsson P, Zettequist E 1968 Experimental investigations on the antithromboplastic and antifibrinolytic activity of Trasylol. Annals of the New York Academy of Sciences 146: 701–714
O'Brien J R 1954 An acquired coagulation defect in a woman. Journal of Clinical Pathology 7: 22–25
O'Brien W F, Saba H I, Knuppel R A, Scerbo J C, Cohen G R 1986 Alterations in platelet concentration and aggregation in normal pregnancy and pre-eclampsia. American Journal of Obstetrics and Gynecology 155: 486–490
Phillips L P 1984 Transfusion support in acquired coagulation disorders. Clinics in Haematology 13: 137–150
Prentice C R M, McNicol G P, Douglas A 1970 Studies on the anticoagulant action of aprotinin (Trasylol). Thrombosis et Diathesis Haemorrhagica 24: 265–272
Pritchard J A 1959 Fetal death in utero. Obstetrics and Gynecology 14: 573–580
Pritchard J A 1973 Haematological problems associated with delivery, placenta abruption, retained dead fetus and amniotic fluid embolism. Clinics in Haematology 2: 563–580
Pritchard J A, Brekken A L 1967 Clinical and laboratory studies on severe abruptio placentae. American Journal of Obstetrics and Gynecology 57: 681–695

Rakoczi I, Tallian F, Bagdan Y S, Gati I 1979 Platelet lifespan in normal pregnancy and pre-eclampsia as determined by a non-radioisotope technique. Thrombosis Research 15: 553–556
Redman C W G 1979 Coagulation problems in human pregnancy. Postgraduate Medical Journal 55: 367–371
Redman C W G, Bonnar J, Bellin C 1978 Early platelet consumption in pre-eclampsia. British Medical Journal 1: 467–469
Reece A, Fox H E, Rapoport F 1982 Factor VIII inhibitor: a cause of severe postpartum haemorrhage. American Journal of Obstetrics and Gynecology 144: 985–987
Remuzzi G, Misiani R, Marchesi D et al 1978 Haemolytic-uraemic syndrome. Deficiency of plasma factor(s) regulating prostacyclin activity? Lancet ii: 871–872
Resnik R, Swartz W H, Plumer M H I, Bernirske K, Stratthaus M E 1976 Amniotic fluid embolism with survival. Obstetrics and Gynecology 47: 395–398
Romero R, Duffy T P 1980 Platelet disorders in pregnancy. Clinics in Perinatology 7: 327–348
Romero R, Copel J A, Hobbins J C 1985 Intrauterine fetal demise and hemostatic failure: the fetal death syndrome. Clinical Obstetrics and Gynecology 28: 24–31
Romero R, Duffy T, Berkowitz R L, Change E, Hobbins J C 1986 Prolongation of a preterm pregnancy complicated by death of a single twin in utero and disseminated intravascular coagulation. New England Journal of Medicine 310: 772–774
Rushton D I, Dawson I M P 1982 The maternal autopsy. Journal of Clinical Pathology 35: 909–921
Salem H H 1986 The natural anticoagulants. In: Chesterman C N (ed) Thrombosis and the vessel wall. Clinics in Haematology 15: 371–391
Savage W 1982 Abortion: methods and sequelae. British Journal of Hospital Medicine 27: 364–384
Schultz J, Adamson J, Workman W, Norman T 1983 Fatal liver disease after intravenous administration of tetracycline in a high dose. New England Journal of Medicine 269: 999–1004
Scott J R, Cruickshank D P, Kochenou R M D, Pitkin R M, Warenski J C 1980 Fetal platelet counts in the obstetric management of immunologic thrombocytopenia purpura. American Journal of Obstetrics and Gynecology 136: 495–499
Shaper A G, Kear J, MacIntosh D M, Kyobe J, Njama D 1968 The platelet count, platelet adhesiveness and aggregation and the mechanism of fibrinolytic inhibition in pregnancy and the puerperium. Journal of Obstetrics and Gynaecology of the British Commonwealth 75: 433–441
Sharp A A 1977 Diagnosis and management of disseminated intra-vascular coagulation. British Medical Bulletin 33: 265–272
Sheehan H 1940 The pathology of acute yellow atrophy and delayed chloroform poisoning. Journal of Obstetrics and Gynaecology of the British Empire 47: 49–62
Sheppard B L, Bonnar J 1974 The ultrastructure of the arterial supply of the human placenta in early and late pregnancy. Journal of Obstetrics and Gynaecology of the British Commonwealth 81: 497–511
Sher G 1977 Pathogenesis and management of uterine inertia complicating abruptio placentae with consumption coagulopathy. American Journal of Obstetrics and Gynecology 129: 164–170
Sher G, Statland B E 1985 Abruptio placentae with coagulopathy: a rational basis for management. Clinical Obstetrics and Gynecology 28: 15–23
Sibai B M, Spinnato J A, Watson D L, Hill G A, Anderson G D 1984 Pregnancy outcome in 303 cases with severe pre-eclampsia. Obstetrics and Gynecology 64: 319–325
Sill P R, Lind T, Walker W 1985 Platelet values during normal pregnancy. British Journal of Obstetrics and Gynaecology 92: 480–483
Skjodt P 1965 Amniotic fluid embolism—a case investigated by coagulation and fibrinolysis studies. Acta Obstetricia et Gynecologica Scandinavica 44: 437–457
Spivak J L, Sprangler D B, Bell W R 1972 Defibrination after intra-amniotic injection of hypertonic saline. New England Journal of Medicine 287: 321–323
Stander R W, Flessa H C, Glueck H C et al 1971 Changes in maternal coagulation factors after intraamniotic injection of hypertonic saline. Obstetrics and Gynecology 37: 321–323
Steichele D F, Herschlein H J 1968 Intravascular coagulation in bacterial shock. Consumption coagulopathy and fibrinolysis after febrile abortion. Medizinische Welt 1: 24–30
Stirling Y, Woolf L, North W R S, Seghatchian M J, Meade T W 1984 Haemostasis and normal pregnancy. Thrombosis in Haematology 52: 176
Stratta P, Canavese C, Bussolino P, Mansueto M G, Gagliardi G, Vercellone A 1983 Haemolytic abortive syndrome. Lancet i: 424–425
Stromme W B, Fromke V L 1979 Amniotic fluid embolism and disseminated intravascular coagulation after evacuation of missed abortion. Obstetrics and Gynecology 52: 76S–80S
Surainder S Y, Bellar B, Choudry A, Chilis T J, Rao S 1981 Isoimmune thrombocytopenia: co-ordinated management of mother and infant. Obstetrics and Gynecology 57: 124–128
Talbert I M, Blatt P M 1979 Disseminated intravascular coagulation in obstretrics. Clinics in Obstetrics and Gynecology 22: 889–900
Tchernia G, Dreyfus M, Laurian Y, Derycke M, Merica C, Kerbrat G 1984 Management of immune thrombocytopenia in pregnancy: response of infusions of immunoglobulins. American Journal of Obstetrics and Gynecology 148: 2225–2226
Terao T et al 1981 Pregnancy complication by idiopathic thrombocytopenia purpura. Journal of Obstetrics and Gynecology 2: 1–10
Territo M, Finkelstein J, Oh O 1973 Management of autoimmune thrombocytopenia in pregnancy and the neonate. Obstetrics and Gynecology 41: 579–582
Thragarajah S, Wheby M S, Jarn R, May H V, Bourgeois J, Kitchin J D 1981 Disseminated intravascular coagulation in pregnancy. The role of heparin therapy. Journal of Reproductive Medicine 26: 17–24
Van Leeuwen E F, Helmerhorst F M, Engelfriet C P, Von Dem Borne A E G Kr 1981 Maternal autoimmune thrombocytopenia and the newborn. British Medical Journal 283: 104
Van Royen E A 1974 Haemostasis in human pregnancy and delivery. MD thesis, University of Amsterdam
Varner M W, Meehan R T, Syrop C H, Strottmann M P, Goplerud C P 1983 Pregnancy in patients with systemic lupus erythematosus. American Journal of Obstetrics and Gynecology 145: 1025–1037
Virgilio R W K, Rice C L, Smith D E et al 1979 Crystalloid versus colloid resuscitation: is one better? Surgery 85: 129–139
Voke J, Letsky E 1977 Pregnancy and antibody to factor VIII. Journal of Clinical Pathology 30: 928–932
Wallenberg H C S, Van Kessel P H 1978 Platelet lifespan in normal pregnancy as determined by a non-radioisotopic technique. British Journal of Obstetrics and Gynaecology 85: 33–36
Wallmo L, Karlsson K, Teger-Nilsson A-C 1984 Fibrinopeptide and intravascular coagulation in normotensive and hypertensive pregnancy and parturition. Acta Obstetricia et Gynecologica Scandinavica 63: 637–640
Warwick R, Hutton R A, Goff L, Letsky E, Heard M 1989 Changes in protein C and free protein S during pregnancy and following hysterectomy. Journal of the Royal Society of Medicine (in press)
Weber F L, Snodgrass P J, Powell D E, Rao P, Huffman S L, Brady P G 1979 Abnormalities of hepatic mitochondrial urea-cycle, enzyme activities and hepatic ultrastructure in acute fatty liver of pregnancy. Journal of Laboratory and Clinical Medicine 94: 27–41
Webster J, Rees A J, Lewis P J, Hensby C N 1980 Prostacyclin deficiency in haemolytic uraemic syndrome. British Medical Journal 281: 271
Whigham K A E, Howie P W, Shaf M M, Prentice C R M 1979 Factor VIII related antigen and coagulant activity in intrauterine growth retardation. Thrombosis Research 16: 629–638
Yaffe H, Eldor A, Hornshtein E, Sadovsky E 1977 Thromboplastin activity in amniotic fluid during pregnancy. Obstetrics and Gynecology 50: 454–456
Zulneraitis E L, Young R S K, Krishanmoorthy K S 1979 Intracranial haemorrhage in utero as a complication of isoimmune thrombocytopenia. Journal of Pediatrics 95: 611–614

39

Michael Brudenell

Diabetic pregnancy

INTRODUCTION

Banting & Best published their first paper on the discovery of insulin in 1922 and revolutionized the management of insulin-dependent diabetes, a condition which up to that time had been invariably fatal. Diabetic pregnancy pre-insulin had a very high maternal and fetal mortality. There were 10 pregnancies among 650 diabetic women attending the Joselin Clinic between 1898 and 1917: of these two were terminated, two babies were stillborn, two women died undelivered and only four women were delivered of a live-born child. Even as late as 1922 Joselin could only describe 108 cases of diabetic pregnancy with a perinatal mortality rate of 440 per 1000 births. Once insulin was available maternal mortality in diabetic pregnancy fell sharply but perinatal mortality remained high and was still in the region of 400 per 1000 by the 1940s. Since that time, however, perinatal mortality has fallen steadily with increasingly good control of maternal diabetes and a better understanding of the problems of the fetus.

CARBOHYDRATE METABOLISM IN PREGNANCY

Hormonal changes occur in pregnancy which profoundly affect carbohydrate metabolism. The levels of oestrogen and progesterone, human placental lactogen, free cortisol and prolactin rise progressively as pregnancy advances. Of these a number, notably human placental lactogen and cortisol, are insulin antagonists and so insulin resistance develops in the mother as the pregnancy advances, and is most marked in the last trimester. In response to this change the normal woman produces an increased amount of insulin to keep carbohydrate metabolism stable. In normal pregnancy the increased insulin production counters the rise in insulin resistance and blood glucose levels are kept within a very narrow range of between 4 and 6 mmol/l during much of every 24 hours.

As a result of the hormonal changes carbohydrate metabolism in pregnancy undergoes characteristic changes. The fasting level of glucose is significantly lower than normal from the 10th week until the 16th week when there is a slow but significant rise up to 32 weeks. Thereafter the fasting level falls again slowly so that at term it is not significantly different from the non-pregnant level (Baird 1986). The peak levels of glucose after a carbohydrate load are higher than normal, especially after the 20th week. In response to an intravenous injection of glucose the rate of disappearance of glucose is increased in early pregnancy and returns to a normal level in late pregnancy. The insulin response to oral or intravenous glucose is substantially increased during the third trimester of pregnancy. In the second half of pregnancy, especially during the third trimester, there is an increase in insulin resistance with a slight deterioration in glucose tolerance and the hypoglycaemic effect of intravenous insulin is less. Pregnancy-onset gestational diabetes is most commonly seen at this time.

Animal experimental work suggests that the increased insulin action on carbohydrate metabolism in early human pregnancy is reduced in later pregnancy so as to provide ample glucose to the fetus at a time when its growth is maximal and its preferential utilization of this substance reaches a peak. The extent to which blood glucose levels are kept within a relatively narrow range cannot be matched when the mother is diabetic, no matter how good the diabetic control may be.

FETOMATERNAL BLOOD GLUCOSE RELATIONSHIPS

Glucose crosses the placenta by a process of facilitated diffusion and the fetal blood glucose level follows closely the maternal level. The glucose transport mechanism protects the fetus from excessively high levels becoming saturated by maternal blood glucose levels of 10 mmol/l or more so that the fetal blood glucose level peaks at 8–9 mmol/l. This ensures that in normal pregnancy the fetus is not overstimulated by postprandial peaks in the maternal blood glucose levels. In diabetic pregnancy although the protective action of the placental barrier persists, higher levels of glucose in the fetus will occur in response to maternal hyperglycaemia.

Glycosuria

Glycosuria is common in pregnancy, starting within 6 weeks of the last menstrual period. The mean excretion rate of glucose per 24 hours is 76 mg in the pregnant woman and a minority of women secrete significantly larger amounts of glucose, up to 1 g or more in 24 hours, in the last 4 weeks of pregnancy. There is a tendency for glycosuria to increase as pregnancy advances but there is a great deal of diurnal and day-to-day variation in excretion rate. There is no constant relationship between urinary and blood glucose levels. The reason for this is that the increase in glucose excretion in pregnancy is complex but is mainly due to an increased glomerular filtration rate and a diminished ability by the proximal and perhaps the distal renal tubules to absorb glucose. The hormonal basis for these changes is confirmed by the fact that they decline rapidly after delivery, as does glucose excretion.

Lipid metabolism

Every aspect of lipid metabolism is affected by pregnancy, particularly free fatty acids, triglycerides, phospholipids and cholesterol. The plasma level of free fatty acids falls from early to mid-pregnancy and thereafter shows a significant rise. The same is true of the plasma level of glycerol. This is in keeping with the accumulation of body fat that occurs during the anabolic phase of pregnancy (first two trimesters). In the catabolic phase of pregnancy (last trimester) raised free fatty acid and glycerol levels are available as fuel to the maternal tissues to offset the increasing diversion to the rapidly growing fetus of glucose and amino acids. Free fatty acids and glycerol levels fall postpartum, followed by a rise during breastfeeding, presumably to allow similar diversion of the ingested maternal nutrients for the synthesis of breast milk.

As with free fatty acids, glycerol and triglycerides, plasma levels of cholesterol and phospholipid are increased in pregnancy. The increase in the latter two substances accounts for the predisposition of the pregnant woman to gall stones, especially as there is a relative reduction in the excretion of bile acids (O'Sullivan et al 1975). The significance of changes of lipid metabolism in pregnancy is not clear, but they are mediated by hormonal changes and fit into the general pattern of an increase in storage of glycogen and fat in most maternal tissues during the anabolic first two trimesters of pregnancy followed by the mobilization of fuel for the benefit of both mother and fetus in the catabolic third trimester (Kalkhoff et al 1979).

Table 39.1 Classification of diabetes mellitus and other types of glucose intolerance (from the National Diabetes Data Group 1979)

Diabetes mellitus*	Insulin-dependent (IDD) or type 1 Non-insulin-dependent (NIDD) or type 2 Secondary diabetes with obesity without obesity
Diabetes with reduced glucose tolerance	
Gestational diabetes	
Prior abnormal glucose tolerance†	
Potentially abnormal glucose tolerance†	

* Based on fasting hyperglycaemia or an abnormal glucose tolerance test.
† May be part of the natural history of diabetes. No alteration in carbohydrate metabolism.

DIABETES MELLITUS DEFINED

Diabetes mellitus is a clinical syndrome characterized by hyperglycaemia due to a deficiency or diminished effectiveness of insulin. The metabolic disturbances affect the metabolism of carbohydrate, protein, fat, water and electrolytes. The deranged metabolism depends on the loss of insulin activity in the body, in many cases eventually leading to cellular damage, especially to vascular endothelial cells in the eye, kidney and nervous system. Diabetes mellitus is not a single disease but a group of diseases.

The classification of diabetes mellitus suggested by the National Diabetes Data Group in 1979 is generally accepted (Table 39.1). The three main clinical types of interest to the obstetrician are insulin-dependent diabetes (IDD or type 1), non-insulin-dependent diabetes (NIDD or type 2) and gestational diabetes.

Table 39.2 Diagnostic glucose concentrations (from World Health Organization 1980)

Diagnosis	Venous blood (mmol/l)	Capillary whole blood (mmol/l)	Venous plasma (mmol/l)
Diabetes mellitus*			
Fasting	≥ 7.0	≥ 7.0	≥ 8.0
2-h blood glucose	≥10.0	≥11.0	≥11.0
Impaired glucose tolerance			
Fasting	< 7.0	< 7.0	< 8.0
2-h blood glucose	≥ 7.0 − <10.0	≥ 8.0 − <11.0	≥ 8.0 − <11.0

* In the absence of diabetic symptoms an abnormal 1-h level is required in addition to the 2-h figure to confirm the diagnosis of diabetes mellitus.

The diagnosis of diabetes mellitus

In a patient with symptoms, the diagnosis of diabetes mellitus is established by a raised fasting blood glucose level of 8 mmol/l or more or 11 mmol/l or more after food. A fasting level of less than 6 mmol/l usually excludes the diagnosis of diabetes. When the fasting level is between 6 and 8 mmol/l a glucose tolerance test (GTT) should be performed. Although there are variations of oral GTTs and an extensive literature on intravenous GTTs, the 75 g oral GTT, as advocated by the World Health Organization (WHO 1980) is likely to become the most widely used in the future and has the virtue of simplicity in interpretation. A standard load of 75 g of glucose in 250 ml of water is given after an overnight fast following 3 days of adequate carbohydrate intake (greater than 250 g/day). Blood samples are taken before and at 1 and 2 hours after the load. The test distinguishes between normal, diabetes mellitus and impaired glucose tolerance (IGT). The latter has particular relevance in pregnancy, since some women with IGT in early pregnancy may progress to diabetes in late pregnancy (Table 39.2).

Non-insulin-dependent diabetes (NIDD)

The majority of all diabetics are non-insulin-dependent but NIDD is less common in the childbearing age group than among older women. There is an association between obesity and NIDD which is more common in fat than thin women. Obesity is associated with insulin insensitivity and glucose tolerance improves with weight loss. However, most obese women are not diabetic and many NIDD women are not obese, so the exact role of obesity in the pathogenesis of NIDD is uncertain.

There is a heriditary element in NIDD; 25% of NIDD patients have a first-degree family history of the disease and nearly all identical twins with NIDD have a similarly affected co-twin. Certain racial groups have a tendency to NIDD, especially those of Indian origin. The NIDD woman has few symptoms and is not prone to ketosis but in pregnancy the management needs to be just as careful as for IDD if perinatal losses are to be avoided.

Insulin-dependent diabetes (IDD)

This type of diabetes occurs most often in young adults; the prevalence rate is about 0.2% in whites under the age of 30. It is unusual in newborn children but the incidence increases with increasing age to reach a peak at 11–14 years. Thereafter, the incidence declines slowly to a plateau of about eight per 100 000 (Lernmark 1985). Shortly after the diagnosis of IDD has been made, inflammatory cells are found infiltrating and surrounding the islets of Langerhans. There is a marked decrease in the number of beta cells.

A number of factors are involved in the aetiology of IDD: genetic determinants involve certain human leukocyte antigens (HLA) on chromosome 6 (Cudworth & Woodrow 1976), especially HLA-DR3 and DR4 which are associated with an increased incidence of IDD. Given that these genetic markers indicate an increased susceptibility to diabetes for the individuals concerned, there are a number of possible initiators of the disease, including environmental factors and viruses such as the coxsackie B4 and rubella and chemicals such as streptozocin and certain rodenticides. IDD patients have a cellular and humoral autoimmunity to pancreatic β cells. The current hypothesis as to the cause of the IDD is that a combination of specific antigen molecules with an invading antigen, virus, bacteria or chemical triggers the formation of effector cells which cross-react with the islet beta cells. When sufficient of these are destroyed IDD is precipitated (Lernmark 1985).

Gestational diabetes and impaired glucose tolerance in pregnancy

Traditionally gestational diabetes was a term applied to women who became diabetic during pregnancy and reverted to normal thereafter. Recently the term has been applied to women who become diabetic in pregnancy regardless of whether or not they return to normal once the pregnancy is over. Many women who develop diabetes in pregnancy do revert to normal postpartum but some do not and the two groups may differ in epidemiological terms, representing two distinct populations. For this reason Essex & Pyke (1978) preferred to use the term diabetes diagnosed in pregnancy. From the obstetrician's point of view the distinction between the two groups is probably academic for if a woman becomes truly diabetic in pregnancy, i.e. a gestational diabetic in modern parlance, the pregnancy is at once at risk, regardless of the eventual postpartum maternal status and there is, at present, no clear evidence that the course of the pregnancy is affected by whether or not the patient remains diabetic postpartum or reverts to normal.

The definition of diabetes proposed by the WHO and outlined earlier in this chapter is acceptable to most diabetic physicians and obstetricians, as is the proposal for an intermediate group of individuals whose carbohydrate metabolism does not constitute gestational diabetes but is not entirely normal. Impaired glucose tolerance (IGT) has the merit of being factual and of identifying a group of women who may progress to gestational diabetes as the pregnancy advances or who may remain with impairment of carbohydrate metabolism until the end of the pregnancy, reverting to normal thereafter. The significance of IGT to the obstetrician has been much debated but providing it remains within the WHO criteria, it seems unlikely that it will have any adverse effect on the clinical course of the pregnancy. The true gestational diabetic is a different proposition: her risks are similar to those of established diabetics and she must be treated with or without insulin depending on the severity of the diabetes and managed in the combined diabetic–antenatal clinic if fetal loss is to be avoided.

Potential abnormality of glucose tolerance

Certain groups of women are more likely to develop diabetes mellitus at some time during their life than normal and are labelled potential diabetics. From the obstetrician's point of view the risk that these individuals will develop gestational diabetes or impaired glucose tolerance in pregnancy is low but the risk factors remain useful criteria in clinical screening where routine screening of the whole antenatal population is not carried out. The risk factors that are important to the obstetrician are given below.

Family history

Genetic factors play a part in the development of diabetes although the exact mode of inheritance is not established. Approximately 1% of all offspring of IDD parents may be expected to develop the disease themselves — an incidence of between 5 and 10 times greater than that of a child with non-diabetic parents. A history of IDD in the father is of greater predictive value than in the mother and even greater when a sibling is diabetic. A family history in grandparents is less significant. If both parents are diabetic the incidence of diabetes in the offspring rises, depending upon the age at which the parents became diabetic. The greatest risk of the offspring developing diabetes occurs when one or both parents developed the disease before the age of 40. Even so, not more than 25% of their children will become diabetic and the figure is lower in children of parents with diabetes of late onset. The extent to which a positive family history makes an individual a potential diabetic will therefore vary with circumstances (Pyke 1968).

Previous heavy babies

The incidence of babies weighing 4.5 kg or more is about 1.5% of all births. Among the children of women who later develop diabetes the rate is much higher, varying in different reports from 4 to 31% (Pyke 1962). A tendency to bear heavy babies may precede the development of clinical diabetes by many years. There is no clearcut evidence to support the idea that the proportion of heavy babies increases as the time of diagnosis draws near, suggesting that genetic factors are more important than environmental factors, particularly maternal hyperglycaemia.

Table 39.3 Classification of diabetic mothers and perinatal mortality rates (PMR) 1981–1985 (proportions of group in parentheses)

	IDD	NID	Total	PHR
Group 1 Gestational	1	29	30 (16%)	0/30 (0‰)
Group 2 Established	116	17	133 (70%)	0/133 (0‰)
Group 3 Established with complications	27	0	27 (14%)	2/27 (74‰)
Total	144 (75%)	46 (25%)	190 (100%)	2 (10‰)

Obesity

Women who are obese (weight exceeding 90 kg) have a greater tendency to become diabetic in later life than non-obese women.

CLASSIFICATION OF SEVERITY OF DIABETES IN PREGNANCY

In general terms the more severe the diabetes the greater the risk of maternal complications in pregnancy and perinatal mortality and morbidity. Severity in this context is measured by the presence of diabetic vascular complications and by the duration of the diabetes. Traditionally the classification used is that of White (1965) but this now seems unnecessarily complicated. At King's College Hospital since 1971 a classification based on the severity of vascular complications has been used instead of White's classification. There are three groups:

Group 1 Diabetes diagnosed during pregnancy (synonymous with gestational diabetes in most modern publications).
Group 2 Established diabetes with less than six microaneurysms seen on ophthalmoscopy.
Group 3 Established diabetes with more than six microaneurysms or proliferative retinopathy and/or nephropathy.

This simple classification indicates the distribution of diabetic pregnancies by severity of maternal disease in a given population and the effect which severity has on clinical outcome, particularly perinatal mortality. The distribution of diabetic mothers, insulin-dependent and non-insulin-dependent, at King's College Hospital in 1981–1985 is shown in Table 39.3.

THE EFFECT OF DIABETIC COMPLICATIONS ON PREGNANCY OUTCOME

Diabetes is associated with an increased incidence of vascular disease. Diabetic vasculopathy develops to a variable extent and over a variable period of time in many diabetics. Diabetic retinopathy, diabetic vascular disease and neuropathy are common in diabetics but tend to develop late and are not adversely affected by pregnancy. However diabetic symptoms increase the risk of perinatal mortality and morbidity when they are present (see Table 39.3).

Diabetic retinopathy is the most easily documented diabetic vascular lesion. Background retinopathy follows a benign course during pregnancy and does not require treatment but proliferative retinopathy may require treatment with an argon laser. Diabetic nephropathy is commonly associated with hypertension and the pregnancy may be complicated by intrauterine growth retardation. The series reported by Kitzmiller et al (1981) and Jovanovic & Jovanovic (1984) indicate that the outlook for the fetus in diabetic pregnancy with nephropathy is good as long as hypertension and significant renal impairment are absent at the outset of the pregnancy. Most patients show an increase in proteinuria during pregnancy and have a stable or falling creatinine clearance. These changes return to prepregnancy levels after delivery.

Several cases of diabetic pregnancy following renal transplantation have been reported (Penn et al 1980, Grenfell et al 1986). It should be borne in mind that the long-term prospects for patients with diabetic renal disease are not generally good and many will require renal transplantation or long-term dialysis when the disease has progressed. Ischaemic heart disease is occasionally seen. One case has been reported of an IDD woman who had a pregnancy following a coronary artery bypass operation for coronary artery disease (Reece et al 1986).

SCREENING TESTS FOR IMPAIRED GLUCOSE TOLERANCE AND GESTATIONAL DIABETES

The problem with screening tests in pregnancy is that they tend to be time-consuming and expensive. Their use can only be justified if they have a significant detection rate. On this ground antenatal screening tests for diabetes can be justified if resources permit but they are not likely to make a big impact on perinatal mortality and morbidity rates since the incidence of otherwise undetectable gestational diabetes is likely to be small.

The object of the screening test is to detect asymptomatic gestational diabetes and women with IGT. Because of the unreliability of urinary glucose estimations and the traditional stigmata of potential diabetes (a close family history or a previous heavy baby) a screening test should be based on blood glucose estimation. The most effective screening test is a full GTT at or about 30 weeks, but this would be too costly and time-consuming in practice. A random blood glucose estimation on the other hand is simple and may easily be combined with other routine antenatal blood tests.

Table 39.4 Screening for gestational diabetes and IGT

Random tests (mmol/l)	Preprandial	Postprandial
USNDD group (plasma)	⩾5.8	⩾6.7
Lind (venous blood)	⩾5.8	⩾6.4
50 g oral glucose load	*1-h level*	
O'Sullivan (venous blood)	⩾8.3	
Gillmer (venous blood)	⩾7.7	

Allowance must be made when interpreting the results of random testing for the time of the last meal. Lind & McDougall (1972) adopted such a screening test dividing the patients up into two groups: those who had eaten within 2 hours of the blood samples being taken and those who had had their last meal more than 2 hours previously. A blood glucose level of 6.4 mmol/l or more for the former, or 5.8 mmol/l for the latter, was taken as indicating the need for a full oral GTT. About 1% of the antenatal population was picked out by these criteria at 28 weeks and of these about half had some impairment of glucose tolerance with the full oral GTT.

O'Sullivan & Mahan (1964) screened using blood glucose estimations on whole blood measured 1 hour after oral ingestion of 50 g of glucose. A level of greater than 8.3 mmol/l was taken to be positive and the full GTT then carried out. Gillmer et al (1980) had suggested 7.7 mmol/l as the critical level. Screening of all patients in one antenatal clinic over a year by estimating plasma glucose 1 hour after oral ingestion of 50 g of glucose and taking a plasma glucose level of greater than 7.7 mmol/l identified 74 out of 948 women. Sixty-eight of those were given an oral GTT and 14 (1.5% of the study population) were found to have IGT. The screening tests listed in Table 39.4 are likely to pick out between 1 and 1.5% of the population screened as having some degree of IGT.

Clearly no ideal method of screening for impairment of carbohydrate metabolism in pregnancy is currently available. Clinicians running busy antenatal clinics may feel unable to add to the load of clinic staff by instituting an additional blood test or tests. In such situations reliance must be placed on the detection of glycosuria, clinical symptoms of diabetes, hydramnios and excessive fetal growth, especially in the last trimester (Table 39.5). Blood glucose measurements are reserved for these suspicious cases. This approach will fail to detect most cases of IGT and some women with true gestational diabetes. Whether this will significantly affect a unit's overall perinatal mortality or morbidity will depend on the general standards of antenatal, intrapartum and paediatric neonatal care. Where these standards are high the impact will probably be negligible.

Table 39.5 Clinical criteria for doing a GTT

1.	Potential diabetics
2.	Obesity: over 20% of ideal weight for height
3.	Glycosuria on two or more occasions, especially if the morning postprandial specimen examined
4.	Previous congenital abnormality, unexplained stillbirth or neonatal death
5.	Hydramnios in current pregnancy
6.	Previous gestational diabetes
7.	Developing fetal macrosomia

Many clinicians will, however, wish to employ some method of antenatal screening for carbohydrate intolerance and should use either random or post-glucose load blood glucose estimations depending on their available resources. The simplest and cheapest approach is to do a random blood glucose estimation between 28 and 30 weeks and define a level for the population being screened above which an oral GTT will be performed. This level will probably be between two and three standard deviations above the mean random level. Lind's method is an example of how this screening test can be applied in practice (Lind & McDougall 1972), and if used at 28–30 weeks only is unlikely to impose too great a burden on even the busiest antenatal clinic staff, whilst at the same time detecting a majority of women showing IGT and all true gestational diabetics. If economies have to be made in even such a simple screening method then excluding those under 25 years old is reasonable and will only result in a very few cases being missed.

Glycosylated haemoglobin

Haemoglobin A (HbA) constitutes about 90% of the haemoglobin of adults and infants above the age of 6 months (Gabbay et al 1977). Glycosylation of haemoglobin occurs as a two-stage process. The first is a rapid and reversible non-enzymatic attachment between the glucose molecule and the N-terminal amino group of the chains of the beta haemoglobin molecule (Schiff base linkage) and to a lesser extent the N-terminal groups in the alpha chains and the N group in epsilon lysine (Gabbay et al 1979). The second is the Amadori rearrangement leading to the formation of a stable ketoamine linkage HbA_1. This comprises HbA_{1a}, HbA_{1b} and HbA_{1c}, and these together with HbA_2 and HbF make up the remaining 10%. Of the total haemoglobin, HbA_{1c}, may comprise up to 4%. The level of HbA_1 is raised in diabetes, reflecting diabetic control over the previous 2 or 3 months. During rapid changes of diabetic control, the labile fraction, which is thought to be the Schiff base, reflects transient rather than long-term changes which occur throughout the lifespan of the red cell.

Since glycosylated haemoglobin measurement in the first trimester will give retrospective assessment of diabetic control at this critical time in development, various studies have examined HbA_1 at this stage (Fig. 39.1).

It was observed (Leslie et al 1978) that three out of five women with high glycosylated haemoglobin measurements at presentation had babies with congenital malformations including hemivertebrae, neural tube defects and congenital heart disease. This led to a multicentre trial in the UK. Out of 168 women with an $HbA_1 < 12\%$, three had babies with major malformations (1.8%). In 62 women with $HbA_1 > 12\%$, there were four babies with major malformations (6.8%; Stubbs et al 1987). The trial also showed that the two groups had similar miscarriage rates: 20/168 had an $HbA_1 < 12\%$ (12%) and 7/62 had an $HbA_1 > 12\%$ (11%). Two other studies have reported a high incidence of miscarriage — 26% (Wright et al 1983) and 30% (Miodovnik et al 1984). In the former series HbA_1 was found to be significantly higher in those who aborted spontaneously. Ylinen et al (1984) in Finland looked at 142 pregnancies and found that the incidence of major malformation rose progressively with increasing levels of HbA_1 (between the 6th and 15th weeks) rising to an incidence of 23.5% in 17 pregnancies with an initial $HbA_1 > 10\%$.

Table 39.6 shows the congenital abnormalities seen in diabetic pregnant patients at King's College Hospital between 1981 and 1985 and indicates that most were associated with raised levels of HbA_1.

Figure 39.1 shows HbA_1 levels in two women with IDD. One was well controlled throughout pregnancy and had a normal delivery of a normal-sized baby. The other had a high level of HbA_1 at the start of the pregnancy; her diabetes

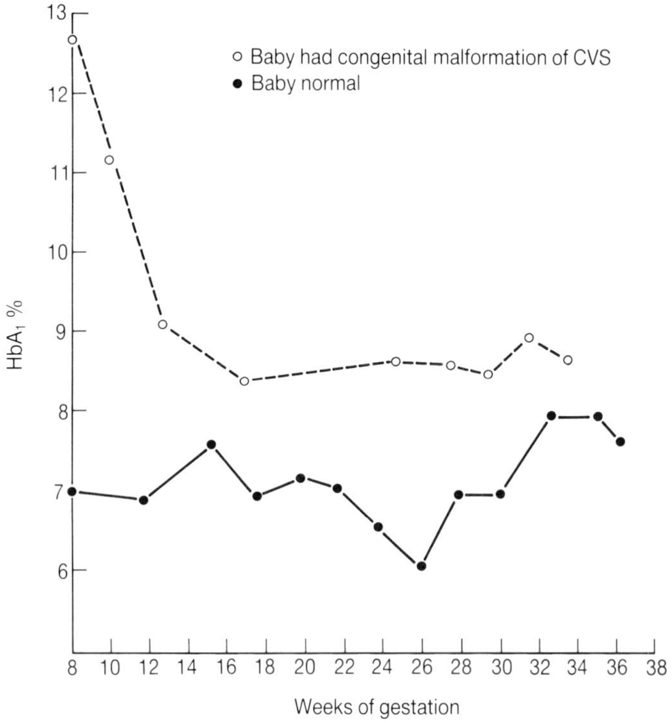

Fig. 39.1 HbA_1 levels in two women with IDD. One was well controlled throughout pregnancy and had a normal baby. The other had a high level of HbA_1 initially and the baby had a congenital cardiac lesion (truncus arteriosus).

Table 39.6 HbA_1 in first trimester and major congenital malformations: King's College Hospital 1981–1985

HbA_1 (%)	Congenital malformations
8.9	Microcephaly
11.0	Absent radius, deformed thumbs
	Hemivertebrae
11.6	Caudal regression
12.3	Truncus arteriosus
12.4	Microcephaly
13.8	Multiple (including exomphalos)

HbA_1 levels of six severely congenital malformed babies born to diabetic mothers at King's College Hospital.

Table 39.7 Major congenital abnormalities in diabetic pregnancies at King's College Hospital 1971–1985

System/abnormality	Number
Central nervous system	11
Skeletal	10
Cardiac	9
Alimentary	3
Caudal regression	2
Multiple abnormalities	2
Hypoplastic lungs	1
Potter's syndrome	1
Total	39

Prevalence = 39/545 = 7.2%.

was quickly brought under control and the HbA_1 was lowered and remained lowered for the rest of the pregnancy. Sadly, however, the baby had a truncus arteriosus which was not detected at the 18-week fetal anomaly scan.

Glycosylated haemoglobin may also be of value as a postpartum screen for unrecognized diabetes where there has been macrosomia (Steel et al 1981). HbA_1 has been found to increase in anaemia (Brooks et al 1980) and to be decreased in chronic renal failure (Dandona et al 1979). The latter is probably related to the shortened lifespan of erythrocytes, with the result that those in circulation have a relatively short time to glycosylate haemoglobin. The same applies to haemolytic disease.

Maternal HbA_1 correlation with birthweight

Birthweight ratio (birthweight divided by the 50th centile birthweight for gestational age) did not correlate with cord or maternal HbA_1 at delivery in one series (Worth et al 1983) and was explained by relatively tight control of maternal diabetes towards the end of pregnancy. There have been conflicting reports about the correlation of maternal HbA_1 with birthweight or birthweight ratio. Stubbs et al (1981), Fadel et al (1981), Miller et al (1981), O'Shaughnessy et al (1979), Poon et al (1981) and Sosenko et al (1982) did not find such a correlation but others have found a link between third-trimester HbA_1 and relative birthweight (Widness et al 1978, Ylinen et al 1981). Russell et al (1984) and Knight (1983) found near normal HbA_1 levels in macrosomic pregnancy.

HbA_1 estimation has proved a valuable additional aid to good control and when elevated in early pregnancy serves as a warning to the obstetrician to be on the look-out for major congenital abnormality.

LUNG FUNCTION IN THE INFANTS OF DIABETIC MOTHERS

Maternal diabetes if badly controlled retards the maturation of the fetal lung cells and delays the production of surfactant. The mechanism is that fetal hyperinsulinaemia consequent upon maternal hyperglycaemia inhibits the production of surfactant by the fetal lung cells. The occurrence of respiratory distress in the infants of diabetic mothers has fallen sharply since the introduction of strict control of maternal diabetes. In a strictly controlled diabetic pregnancy fetal lung maturation at 37 weeks and thereafter is no different from in a non-diabetic pregnancy (Tyden et al 1984). When delivery occurs between 32 and 37 weeks respiratory complications are more likely to occur but if maternal diabetic control has been good severe respiratory distress is uncommon. When control has been poor, delivery before 37 weeks, but especially before 32 weeks, is likely to be complicated by respiratory distress and in such cases estimation of surfactant levels, i.e. the lecithin:sphingomyelin (L:S) ratio and the detection of phosphatidylglycerol provides an accurate prognostic guide and in selective cases indicates the need for postponing delivery until corticosteroids can be given to the mother to accelerate fetal lung maturation. An L:S ratio of >2 and/or the presence of phosphatidylglycerol in the amniotic fluid indicate that fetal lungs are sufficiently mature to avoid respiratory distress in the baby.

CONGENITAL ABNORMALITY IN DIABETIC PREGNANCY

Congenital abnormality is now the most important contributor to perinatal mortality and morbidity in diabetic pregnancy. It is now accepted that the diabetic woman is three to four times more likely to have a congenitally malformed baby than her non-diabetic counterpart (Malins 1979, Fuhrmann et al 1983). This is in accord with our experience at King's College Hospital (see Table 39.7, which also lists the range of abnormalities). Table 39.8 illustrates the contribution which fatal congenital malformations have made to perinatal mortality during the years 1951–1985. To the clinician, the interest lies in two aspects: what causes the abnormalities, and can good diabetic control decrease the incidence of abnormality?

Table 39.8 Diabetic pregnancies at King's College Hospital 1951–1985

	No.	Perinatal deaths	Fatal congenital malformations	TOP for congenital malformations
1951–60	318	72	6 (8%)	—
1961–70	389	39	5 (13%)	—
1971–80	352	13	6 (46%)	5
1981–85	193	2	2 (100%)	3

The cause of congenital abnormality in diabetic pregnancy

The most important time for organogenesis is the first 7 weeks of intrauterine life and it is during this period that abnormal carbohydrate metabolism might cause abnormality (Mills et al 1979). In the female rat with streptozocin-induced diabetes, pregnancy results in a high incidence of congenital abnormality, especially visceral eversion and incomplete ossification of the sacrum (Deuchar 1979). The latter anomaly is particularly significant in diabetes.

So far it has not been possible to identify the exact cause of the abnormalities. Experimental ketoacidosis in mice causes chromosomal abnormalities with and without manifest deformities (Enricho & Ingalls 1968) so the effect of maternal diabetes may be on the chromosomes of the oocyte or the pre- or postimplantation embryo. Once the embryo is implanted and starts to develop, a direct effect on the process of organogenesis is possible. Since most pregnant diabetic women do not become ketoacidotic in early pregnancy, hyperglycaemia seems the most likely culprit.

Goldman et al (1985) proposed that hyperglycaemia causes a functional deficiency of arachidonic acid at a critical stage of organogenesis and have shown experimentally that supplementation of the diet of rats and mice exerts a protective effect against the teratogenic action of hyperglycaemia in vivo (rat) and in vitro (mouse animal models).

The effect of good diabetic control on the incidence of abnormality

There is good evidence that abnormality occurs less frequently in well controlled diabetics (Pedersen 1979, Fuhrmann et al 1983) and it has long been recognized that diabetic mothers with vascular complications, i.e. severe diabetics, are more prone to have abnormal babies (Baker et al 1981).

The emergence of HbA_1 estimation as a means of judging diabetic control retrospectively has shed further light on the question of the effect of hyperglycaemia on fetal development in the first trimester. Since HbA_1 levels reflect to some extent the blood glucose concentrations during the preceding 4–8 weeks it is not surprising that those patients with a low HbA_1 level at 12 weeks' gestation have a lower risk of having an abnormal baby than those with a high level.

Preventing congenital abnormality in diabetic pregnancy

All diabetic women should be made aware of the need for prepregnancy counselling so as to ensure that their diabetes is well controlled from the very start of the pregnancy. Diabetic clinics, physicians and obstetricians seeing non-diabetic women should take the opportunity to press this point (Watkins 1982). In dealing with those women who report to the clinic when already pregnant, those who are most at risk should be recognized; they include the badly controlled, the long-standing IDD with vascular complications and those women who have previously had an abnormal baby. A high HbA_1 level (>12%) during the first 12 weeks or at the 12th week should alert the obstetrician since it is highly likely that such high levels are associated with an increased risk of abnormality. The risks are relative however, and as indicated above, the majority of women with badly controlled diabetes and high HbA_1 levels in early pregnancy will have normal babies — the incidence in both cases is, however, increased.

Detecting congenital abnormalities

Ultrasound scanning has made possible early detection of congenital abnormality and the opportunity to offer the mother a termination if the abnormality is severe. It has been suggested that delayed fetal growth in very early pregnancy (between 7 and 14 weeks) may indicate fetal abnormality (Pedersen & Mølsted-Pedersen 1981). All diabetic women should have a full fetal anomaly scan done at 18–20 weeks with the possibility of increased fetal abnormality borne very much in mind, especially where earlier HbA_1 levels have been high.

Caudal regression syndrome (caudal dysplasia syndrome)

This congenital abnormality, described by Hohl in 1852, is rare and consists of absence of vertebrae from any level below T10 and the consequent deformities. If the sacrum is missing (sacral agenesis) the transverse diameter of the pelvis is reduced, the buttocks are flattened and there is muscular atrophy in the legs. There may be dislocation of the hips, talipes, spina bifida, renal anomalies and urinary and faecal incontinence. Lesser degrees of abnormality of the lower limbs not amounting to true caudal regression are also seen. The caudal regression syndrome is akin to rumplessness in chickens. This abnormality occurs as a hereditary condition or spontaneously. More interestingly it can be produced experimentally in white leghorn chickens by injecting insulin into the incubating eggs. This suggests that either insulin itself or the hypoglycaemia produced by it may be teratogenic. This observation does not fit in with clinical experience which, as noted above, does not implicate either insulin or hypoglycaemia in the aetiology of congenital abnormality in women with IDD. Nevertheless, it is of some interest because although the caudal regression syndrome

Table 39.9 Obstetric causes of perinatal death

	1951–1970	1971–1985
Birth trauma	9	0
Pre-eclampsia	9	0
Antepartum haemorrhage	4	2
Acute hydramnios	4	0
Intrauterine growth retardation	3	0
Intrapartum asphyxia	3	0
Rhesus incompatibility	2	0
Unexplained	8	0

does not only occur in IDD, its incidence in diabetic pregnancy does seem to be considerably higher.

The estimates of incidence of caudal regression syndrome in diabetic pregnancy vary widely but it is probably of the order of one in 1000 (Leny & Maier 1964). This level accords with the experience of King's College Hospital in recent years. Any woman who is not diagnosed as being diabetic giving birth to a baby showing caudal regression syndrome should have a GTT.

The combined approach of prevention and early detection of congenital abnormality and selected termination in diabetic pregnancy should ensure a decrease in congenital abnormality as a cause of perinatal mortality and morbidity.

PERINATAL MORTALITY IN DIABETIC PREGNANCY

The high perinatal mortality seen in diabetic pregnancy 30 years ago has diminished sharply to the present time, as shown in Table 39.8. This table also illustrates the changing pattern of perinatal mortality. Deaths from obstetric causes (Table 39.9), mainly birth trauma, pre-eclampsia, antepartum haemorrhage and acute hydramnios, were relatively common in the early years but have completely disappeared latterly with better obstetric care. Fetal death as a result of diabetic ketoacidosis in the mother has shown a similar decline, as has perinatal death from respiratory distress. Unexplained late intrauterine death, the classic problem of diabetic pregnancy, has also fallen sharply and no deaths from this cause occurred at King's College Hospital in the 1981–1985 quinquennium. It seems likely that these unexplained late intrauterine deaths in late diabetic pregnancy are due to fetal anoxia. Although the delivery of blood to the intervillous space is normal in uncomplicated diabetic pregnancy, blood flow through the intervillous space is slowed and transfer of oxygen to the fetal circulation is impaired. HbA_{1c}, often raised in badly controlled diabetes, has an increased affinity for oxygen so when levels of HbA_1 in the maternal blood are high the release of oxygen to the fetal circulation is further reduced. The placenta and especially the fetal consumption of oxygen are increased in the presence of hyperinsulinaemia. This combination of factors leads occasionally to a fatal degree of fetal hypoxia. Proof that the diabetic fetus may be hypoxic is suggested by some preliminary studies of PO_2 levels on samples of fetal blood obtained by cordocentesis but further work needs to be done before hypoxia can be finally identified as the cause of this type of fetal loss.

Only congenital abnormalities continue to pose problems. Indeed the only two deaths that occurred in this latter quinquennium were from serious congenital abnormalities which had not been diagnosed antenatally.

MATERNAL MORTALITY IN DIABETIC PREGNANCY

A general fall in maternal mortality for all pregnancies is reflected in the fall in maternal mortality for diabetic pregnancy, so that it is now extremely rare for a diabetic woman to die as a result of pregnancy. This contrasts sharply with the maternal mortality figures in the pre-insulin era; these were as high as 45% in the 66 diabetic pregnancies reported by Williams in 1909. There was only one maternal death in diabetic pregnancy at King's College Hospital from 1971 to 1986 and this occurred in a patient with advanced diabetic nephropathy who died from renal failure 11 months after successful delivery. Of the seven maternal deaths in diabetic pregnancy reported in the Reports on Confidential Enquiries into Maternal Deaths in England and Wales (1976–1981), three resulted from infection, one from myocardial infarction, one from severe hypoglycaemia, one from pulmonary embolus and one from cardiac arrest of unknown origin during induction of anaesthesia prior to Caesarean section. In all seven cases diabetic control was less than optimal — an important practical point in the management of diabetic pregnancy.

MEDICAL MANAGEMENT OF DIABETIC PREGNANCY

Prepregnancy care

Diabetic women who plan to become pregnant should ensure that their diabetes is as well controlled as it can be in order to reduce the risk of congenital abnormality. Diabetic women with vascular complications should also discuss fully the implications of pregnancy with the diabetic physician and, in the case of retinopathy, may need to have appropriate local treatment.

Patients attending for prepregnancy advice should have a complete physical examination to confirm their fitness for pregnancy and their routine blood glucose and urine tests, as well as an HbA_1 estimation. Based on the results of these investigations appropriate adjustments may need to be made to diet and insulin to ensure tight control of the maternal diabetes. For women with NIDD the importance of sticking closely to diet in order to keep blood glucose levels as near normal as possible may need to be emphasized.

Women who are not doing home monitoring of blood glucose levels should be encouraged to do so using either a glucose oxidase stick alone or a glucose meter. The results of these tests should be recorded and kept, so that at the next diabetic clinic visit the diabetic physician can confirm that control is good. Patients are advised to maintain blood glucose readings between 5 and 10 mmol as far as possible and an HbA_1 preferably below 10% and not above 12%. A simple prepregnancy advice sheet to diabetic women who are planning to become pregnant, which is also relevant when they do achieve a pregnancy, is helpful.

The obstetrician's contribution to prepregnancy care

The obstetrician should also see diabetic women planning to become pregnant in order to deal with any anxieties they may have about the pregnancy. The importance of keeping a menstrual calendar should be emphasized so that pregnancy can be accurately dated. When infertility is a problem, suitable investigations can be undertaken. Rubella status, blood pressure and weight need to be checked and the patient who smokes should be discouraged from doing so.

The advantages of prepregnancy care

It is hard to quantify the advantages of prepregnancy care but the strong impression is that those women who have had prepregnancy care do better in pregnancy. Steel (1985) reported a higher incidence of congenital abnormality in women who did not attend the prepregnancy care clinic. This was due to the fact that non-attenders were more likely to be poorly motivated and, consequently, badly controlled. Fuhrmann et al (1983) reported a significant reduction in congenital abnormality from 7.5% in 292 diabetic women seen after 8 weeks' gestation to 0.8% in 128 diabetic women seen whilst planning a pregnancy and before conception actually occurred. Prepregnancy care is the most important aspect of the management of diabetic pregnancy and holds out the best hope for reducing the number of congenital abnormalities.

Pregnancy

Medical management of diabetic pregnancy is based on diet alone or diet and insulin, depending on the type of the maternal diabetes. Oral hypoglycaemic agents are not recommended for the patient who is planning a pregnancy unless she is unable to control her diabetes adequately with diet alone or to use insulin where diet is not adequate. In developing countries oral hypoglycaemics may have an important role to play but in developed countries insulin is preferable when diet alone is not sufficient.

Diet

Proper diet is an essential part of the management of all pregnant diabetic women, including gestational diabetics and those with IGT. It is important that pregnant women do not become hungry and an increased allowance of carbohydrate to meet the extra energy requirements of pregnancy may be needed. An increase in dietary fibre is helpful since it exerts a flattening effect on the postprandial rise of blood glucose concentration (Eastwood & Kay 1979). An experienced dietitian should supervise the patient's diet and it will be necessary to take note of the patient's ethnic requirements. In Asian communities it has been shown that in many groups diet consists of a low carbohydrate and high fat content and appropriate adjustments will have to be made although it is not always an easy task to restructure eating habits in these patients.

Insulin

There are no advantages in any particular type of insulin. All are now purified at a single strength of 100 u/ml. There has been a trend towards using monocomponent or human insulin preparations but there are no special advantages to the patient and there is no indication for changing patients from an established insulin regime using one species of insulin to another species. Instances of insulin allergy or resistance are extremely rare.

The majority of women with IDD require insulin injections at least twice daily. The best regime uses a mixture of short-acting (soluble) and medium-acting (isophane or insulin zinc suspensions) insulin mixed in the syringe and given 20–30 minutes before the main morning and evening meals. The proportions and amounts of each type of insulin are determined by trial and error, by examining blood glucose profiles measured by the patients themselves and when they attend hospital. Self-monitoring of blood glucose levels by patients is an important aspect of diabetic care during pregnancy and all patients should now undertake some form of blood glucose measurement. When unacceptable swings of blood glucose occur they do so more frequently during the middle of the night or at noon, when hypoglycaemia may be a problem, and during the 2 hours after breakfast when hyperglycaemia is often seen. The splitting of the twice-daily double-mix regime, giving the soluble insulin alone before the main evening meal and the medium-acting insulin before the bedtime snack, may improve matters (Peacock et al 1979).

Continuous subcutaneous insulin is a technique which can achieve even better control than conventional insulin regimes in some patients but adequate control cannot be obtained by intermittent subcutaneous injection. It is unsuitable for women whose difficulty with diabetic control arises from their personal problems rather than an intrinsic problem arising from the diabetes itself. The method does require very careful control and complete co-operation on the part of the patient.

When IDD develops acutely during pregnancy — a comparatively rare occurrence — soluble insulin is used two or three times daily initially, with the medium-acting insulin being added as the diabetes comes under control. Women with NIDD whose diet alone has failed to give adequate control will also need insulin during pregnancy. In these patients it is often sufficient to use a single dose of medium-acting insulin starting with approximately 10 u/day.

First trimester

Although the insulin requirement increases later in pregnancy it does not do so in the first trimester. Hypoglycaemia at this stage is common especially if the insulin dose is inappropriately increased and may result in part from anorexia and be due to normal pregnancy nausea and vomiting.

Second and third trimesters

The degree of co-operation on the part of the pregnant woman and the enthusiasm of her diabetic physician are key factors in achieving the necessary tight control of diabetes during the second and third trimesters of pregnancy. The insulin dose increases steadily, especially after the 28th week. Most patients learn how to make their own adjustments to the insulin dose to maintain a control between visits to hospital but it is important that they are able to contact the hospital in any case of doubt. The increase in insulin requirement varies considerably from a negligible amount to two or three times normal requirements. Sometimes there is a small decrease in the last few weeks of pregnancy; this is not in itself an ominous feature. The need for high insulin dosage ceases abruptly at the time of delivery, when it is important to reduce the dose to its prepregnancy level immediately, otherwise profound hypoglycaemia will develop. The aim of control is to keep preprandial blood glucose levels between 5 and 6 mmol/l and the HbA_1 below 8%.

Labour

Labour, and any acute situation arising during pregnancy (e.g. severe infection) calls for a change to intravenous insulin and glucose to ensure close control at these critical times. The intravenous insulin infusion should be started as soon as labour is established or in the early morning if labour is to be induced electively. An infusion pump enables fine adjustments to be made and is the best method of administration. Soluble insulin is diluted in normal saline — 1 unit of insulin per 1 ml of saline — and is delivered initially at 1 u/h. Blood glucose is kept within the range 3–6 mmol and, in general, small variations of insulin rate in the range of 0.5–2 u/h are sufficient to achieve this. Along with the intravenous insulin an intravenous infusion of 5% glucose is maintained at 1 litre every 8 hours; oral feeding is discontinued during the whole of the labour. The same regime is employed when delivery is by elective Caesarean section; insulin and glucose infusions are commenced 2 hours prior to the time of the operation.

OBSTETRIC MANAGEMENT OF DIABETIC PREGNANCY

Early pregnancy

There is an increased risk of miscarriage in early pregnancy as well as the increased risk of congenital fetal abnormality; both these risks are reduced sharply by good diabetic control, especially if this has been achieved prior to conception. Early attendance at the combined diabetic–antenatal clinic should ensure that diabetic control is optimal and also give the obstetrician an opportunity to confirm that the pregnancy is proceeding normally. Early ultrasound scan establishes the maturity of the pregnancy and the size of the embryo as well as detecting early failure of embryonic development or growth abnormality.

Combined diabetic–antenatal clinic

Essential to good management of diabetic pregnancy is the combined diabetic–antenatal clinic where both diabetic physician and obstetrician work together in the same clinic seeing the pregnant woman together. Free communication between the doctors involved and the patient herself greatly increases understanding and ensures the best possible patient co-operation. Specialized diabetic–antenatal clinics in hospitals with intensive special care baby units are a feature of many regions of the UK and the results obtained in such units are usually better than those in isolated units where the numbers of cases seen do not give enough experience to either obstetrician or diabetic physician to be confident in the handling of the complex problems that may arise during the course of the pregnancy and labour.

Routine antenatal care

The routine obstetric antenatal care of the patient does not differ greatly from that of the non-diabetic patient. Diagnostic ultrasound is important but routine clinical observation remains very important.

The use of ultrasound in diabetic pregnancy

Diagnostic ultrasound plays an important part in the management of diabetic pregnancy. Before 12 weeks the object of the early pregnancy scan is to establish maturity and the well-being of the embryo as well as detecting gross abnormality. The diagnosis of maturity of the pregnancy is based on crown–rump length. Pedersen (1979) found that crown–

rump lengths were, on average, 5.4 days smaller than those in non-diabetics of the same age. A number of factors affect fetal growth in early pregnancy and it is always wise to confirm maturity at a later stage by biparietal diameter and femur length measurements. Early fetal growth delay may result from poor diabetic control or may be associated with a congenital abnormality.

At 18–20 weeks detailed anomaly scans are an essential part of the antenatal care of all pregnant diabetics and are particularly important in those women whose diabetic control in the first trimester, as indicated by blood glucose levels and/or HbA_1 estimations at 12 weeks, has been bad. From 24 weeks onwards the task of the ultrasonographer in a diabetic pregnancy is to detect the development of fetal macrosomia which may occur even though maternal diabetes is impeccably controlled. Evidence of fetal macrosomia can be obtained by serial measurements of the fetal abdominal and head circumference starting at 24 weeks and continuing at 2-weekly intervals until delivery. Developing macrosomia is evident by 32–34 weeks and is an indication that the maternal diabetes may be affecting fetal growth. Macrosomia may, of course, occur in the absence of maternal diabetes but it is wise to assume that macrosomia developing in a pregnant diabetic woman is due to the maternal diabetes and check that diabetic control is satisfactory. If the maternal diabetes is not well controlled then urgent steps must be taken to correct it. Where diabetic control is satisfactory the obstetrician can only observe and plot the developing macrosomia by the evidence of serial ultrasound scan but can time the planning and mode of delivery from this point of view.

Ultrasound is also helpful in late pregnancy in observing fetal movements and can form part of the biophysical profile used to evaluate fetal well-being. Ultrasound can also be used to study blood flow on the fetal and maternal sides of the placenta, using a duplex pulse Doppler system. This is particularly of value where diabetic pregnancy is complicated by uterine growth retardation but does not seem to be of any particular help in normal diabetic pregnancy or diabetic pregnancy complicated by developing fetal macrosomia.

MATERNAL OBSTETRIC COMPLICATIONS IN PREGNANCY

There are three important obstetric complications in diabetic pregnancy: pre-eclampsia, polyhydramnios and preterm labour.

Pre-eclampsia

Pre-eclampsia, often severe, was a common occurrence in diabetic pregnancy and a cause of perinatal mortality in the past. More recently it has become much less common and there have been no perinatal deaths due to pre-eclampsia at King's College Hospital from 1971 to 1985. Broughton Pipkin et al (1982) showed that in diabetic pregnancy the plasma renin and aldosterone concentrations were higher than in non-diabetic pregnancy and the plasma renin substrate is lower. Plasma angiotensin too showed a strong inverse relationship to serum sodium and was directly proportional to blood glucose concentrations. These differences from normal may contribute to the raised incidence of hypertension in diabetic pregnancy and explain why good control leads to a lower incidence.

In the UK Diabetic Pregnancy Survey (Brudenell 1982) the overall incidence of pre-eclampsia in established diabetics was 14.4% but there was no increase in perinatal mortality in these patients, so that although pre-eclampsia remains a more common occurrence in diabetic than in non-diabetic pregnancy, it does not present a particular problem in antenatal care, since it is detected and managed as in non-diabetic pregnancy. In view of the findings of Broughton Pipkin et al (1982) it is reasonable to assume that better control of maternal diabetes leads to a lower incidence of pre-eclampsia.

Polyhydramnios

Polyhydramnios complicates 25% of pregnancies in established diabetics included in the UK Diabetic Pregnancy Survey (Brudenell 1982). Severe acute polyhydramnios which was responsible for perinatal deaths in the past is not now seen but the development of any degree of polyhydramnios during the course of diabetic pregnancy is an indication to look closely at the level of diabetic control, since there is a definite clinical relationship between mean glucose levels and polyhydramnios. It is likely that fetal hyperglycaemia resulting from maternal hyperglycaemia leads to fetal polyuria and hence polyhydramnios. Patients who seem to be developing polyhydramnios quickly should be admitted to hospital for more closely supervised diabetic control and extra rest. This will often halt the progress of developing polyhydramnios and postpone the onset of preterm labour, which may otherwise complicate it.

Preterm labour

Preterm labour, i.e. labour starting prior to the completion of the 37th week of pregnancy, is more common in diabetic than in non-diabetic pregnancy. It occurred in 17% of diabetic patients at King's College Hospital in recent times. When it occurs it is usually associated with polyhydramnios and hence the chances that it will occur are reduced if maternal diabetes is well controlled. The management of preterm labour calls for fine judgement on the part of the obstetrician.

Management of preterm labour

In general if pregnancy has reached 32 weeks no attempt should be made to stop the labour. If, however, preterm labour begins with spontaneous rupture of membranes unaccompanied by uterine contractions, a sample of liquor should be obtained either by vaginal collection or ultrasound-directed amniocentesis to assess the maturity of the fetal lungs. If the fetal lungs are immature, as judged by the L:S ratio and the presence or absence of phosphatidylglycerol, a course of dexamethasone 4 mg 8-hourly for 48 hours should be given to accelerate lung function. In all cases of preterm labour with ruptured membranes a sample of liquor obtained by amniocentesis or vaginal swab should be sent for bacteriological examination and the patient meanwhile started on amoxycillin to counter the risk of intrauterine infection, especially by beta-haemolytic streptococci.

Preterm labour with intact or ruptured membranes before 32 weeks should generally be stopped unless it is clear that the labour is fully established, as evident by the strength and frequency of the contractions and by cervical dilatation. Beta-agonists such as salbutamol or ritodrine to inhibit uterine contractions and corticosteroids to accelerate lung function tend to cause hyperglycaemia and subsequent ketoacidosis so that, if they are used, it should be in conjunction with an intravenous infusion of soluble insulin to keep blood glucose levels within the normal range of 3–5 mmol/l. A glucose level should be estimated every hour and the plasma potassium every 2 hours. An intravenous 5% glucose drip may be needed to counteract transient hypoglycaemia and intravenous potassium supplements up to 100 mmol/24 h should be given, if necessary, to maintain normal potassium levels. The maternal pulse rate and blood pressure are taken hourly and a continuous cardiotocographic trace taken of the fetal heart. This regime is continued for 48 hours.

Thereafter, if the membranes are ruptured, no further attempts should be made to inhibit labour and delivery should be allowed to occur vaginally or, in some cases, by Caesarean section. If the membranes are intact and the contractions have been successfully inhibited, the beta-agonist infusion is slowly scaled down over the succeeding 48 hours. The insulin infusion should be continued at the appropriate rate until the beta-agonist is discontinued, the dose being adjusted according to blood glucose levels. Preterm labour often recurs after successful inhibition and the regime may have to be reinstated.

If preterm labour has been successfully inhibited in these cases with intact membranes an amniocentesis should be performed to obtain a liquor sample to assess further fetal lung maturity. A mature fetal lung should encourage the obstetrician to abandon attempts to inhibit preterm labour if it threatens again. If the pregnancy proceeds, a repeat course of corticosteroids should be given at 10-day intervals after the first until 32 weeks. With regard to delivery, Caesarean section should be considered unless labour and vaginal delivery seem likely to be straightforward. In the presence of added complications such as severe pre-eclampsia, unstable presentation or malpresentation or an increased risk of intrauterine infection, a Caesarean section should generally be performed but each case needs to be considered individually.

Late pregnancy admission to hospital

In well controlled uncomplicated diabetic pregnancy antenatal care can follow a normal pattern up to full term. Where complications arise during the last several weeks, e.g. difficulty in diabetic control or developing polyhydramnios or pre-eclampsia, admission to hospital is advisable so that diabetic control can be kept closely supervised and fetal well-being monitored. Patients whose serial ultrasound scans show developing fetal macrosomia should also be admitted. Diabetic control may be better at home than in hospital (Stubbs et al 1980), but this is only true with well motivated patients who make regular checks of their own blood glucose levels. Less intelligent or less well motivated patients are likely to be better controlled in hospital.

Monitoring of fetal well-being in late pregnancy

When the patient is admitted to hospital because of complications, biophysical tests are commonly employed to assess fetal well-being. Biochemical tests, e.g. estimations of oestriol and placental lactogen levels in maternal serum, were employed formerly but have been largely replaced now by biophysical testing which relies on the recording of fetal movements by the patient and observations by regular ultrasound scan and on antenatal fetal cardiotocography. Any abnormality in the cardiotocograph calls for a full fetal biophysical profile, and if there is any doubt about fetal well-being immediate delivery is called for by induction of labour or by Caesarean section. A normal biophysical profile is helpful in providing reassurance to the clinician and to the patient that a conservative policy with regard to delivery can be continued.

DELIVERING THE INFANT OF A DIABETIC MOTHER

Apart from preterm labour and unless complications occur indicating earlier delivery, diabetic patients are not nowadays delivered before 37 weeks and in well controlled uncomplicated diabetes with normal fetal growth pregnancy is allowed to proceed to 40 weeks. Once the patient has reached full term it is the present policy at King's College Hospital to induce labour or, if indicated, deliver the patient by Caesarean section. It is not felt desirable at present to allow a diabetic pregnancy to continue beyond full term since experience of the management of diabetic pregnancy beyond established ultrasound-confirmed full term is extremely limited and the risk of unexplained intrauterine death probably still exists in these patients.

Table 39.10 Indications for planned Caesarean section

Previous Caesarean section
Malpresentation
Disproportion
Severe pre-eclampsia
Age 35 or over
Long history of infertility
Diabetic complications

Table 39.11 Indications for induction of labour

Uncomplicated diabetes at 40 weeks
Developing fetal macrosomia
Pre-eclampsia and hypertension
Diabetic complications

Planned Caesarean section

Every effort should be made to avoid complicated, difficult or prolonged labour in diabetic women. Planned Caesarean section will therefore be appropriate in a number of cases and will usually be performed between 38 and 40 weeks. Of the indications shown in Table 39.10, disproportion is probably the most important in modern practice since the prevalence of macrosomia means that the risk of disproportion and difficult vaginal delivery is always present in diabetic pregnancy. Birth trauma has often featured in diabetic deliveries in earlier series (Stallone & Ziel 1974) and was a major cause of perinatal mortality at King's College Hospital in 1951–1970. If macrosomia has been detected by serial ultrasound scanning it is likely that dystocia will result, serious consideration must be given to a planned Caesarean section.

The management of planned Caesarean section

The obstetric management is no different from that in non-diabetic pregnancy. Either general anaesthesia or epidural analgesia is appropriate. The use of the latter facilitates control of maternal diabetes pre- and immediately postoperatively since the patient is able to take carbohydrate by mouth. Intravenous insulin and glucose will often be preferred by the diabetic physician if general anaesthesia is used and in any complicated case this is the best way of ensuring good control throughout the perioperative period.

Induction of labour

The indications for the induction of labour are shown in Table 39.11. The indication for the induction of labour in diabetic pregnancy has changed during the past decade, reflecting the growing confidence obstetricians have in managing the well controlled patient and the diminishing risk of unexplained intrauterine death up to full term. Uncomplicated diabetes per se therefore does not normally constitute an indication to induce labour.

Full-term uncomplicated diabetes

Once the diabetic woman reaches full term labour should be induced. Cordocentesis studies at King's College Hospital indicate that the diabetic fetus is often hypoxic in utero. Postmaturity is likely to make this worse and may lead occasionally to intrauterine death. There is, however, no substantial clinical evidence to support this view but, for the present, it seems a reasonable compromise and the result of its application to diabetic pregnancy at King's is satisfactory in terms of perinatal mortality and morbidity.

Developing fetal macrosomia

A baby that is growing excessively as judged by serial ultrasound scans is clearly being affected by the maternal diabetes and becoming hyperinsulinaemic. Induction of labour at 38 weeks seems reasonable then since a considerable increase in body size and weight may occur in the last 2 weeks. By inducing the patient at 38 weeks the possible risk of late unexplained intrauterine death in the remaining 2 weeks of the pregnancy is also avoided.

Pre-eclampsia and hypertension

The indications for induction for pre-eclampsia and hypertension in diabetic women are the same as for non-diabetic women. In the case of essential hypertension in diabetic pregnancy (pregnancy-associated hypertension) there may be a degree of intrauterine growth retardation which can be, to some extent, masked by the macrosomia-inducing effect of the mother's diabetes. The timing of induction for hypertension will depend on the progress of the condition and on the fetus. As long as the blood pressure does not rise significantly above the early pregnancy readings, there is no proteinuria and the fetal parameters of growth and well-being are satisfactory, induction is not indicated but a rise in blood pressure, especially if proteinuria develops or if there is a definite falling off in the fetal growth pattern, indicates the need for induction or, in some cases, the need for elective Caesarean section.

Diabetic microvasculopathy

Diabetic retinopathy or nephropathy are not thought generally to be made worse by pregnancy or by labour but in the case of nephropathy pre-eclampsia is more likely to be superimposed on pregnancy and induction, therefore, may be indicated for this reason.

Obstetric management of induced labour

Induction of labour can be achieved by the use of a single prostaglandin pessary (PGE_2 3 mg) inserted into the posterior fornix; when contractions are established and the cervix starts to dilate, this is followed by a simple forewater rupture. If necessary, labour contractions are augmented by the cautious use of intravenous oxytocin, taking great care to avoid hyperstimulation. Continuous fetal heart monitoring using an external ultrasound sensor or a fetal scalp electrode and, if indicated, fetal scalp blood sampling are an essential part of the management of diabetic labour because of an increased risk of fetal distress (Brudenell 1978). Epidural analgesia has much to commend it but there is no objection to any of the alternative forms of analgesia commonly used in labour.

Spontaneous labour

When labour starts spontaneously it is managed in the same way as induced labour, except that the need for augmentation is less likely.

Delivery

When labour progresses normally and the baby is not macrosomic, spontaneous vaginal delivery can be confidently expected. However, the obstetrician will often be called upon to decide whether or not to terminate a labour by operative delivery. Delay in progress in the first or second stages, fetal distress or difficulty in controlling the maternal diabetes — a rare occurrence nowadays — all indicate the need to expedite delivery. Caesarean section will often be the method of choice but, when the patient is fully dilated, if an easy forceps delivery can be carried out this is preferable. A difficult forceps delivery, bearing in mind that the baby may be big if not actually macrosomic, should be avoided because of the risk of shoulder dystocia and birth trauma. A very careful assessment of the patient in the operating theatre with preparations made for immediate Caesarean section is often helpful. In this circumstance a tentative attempt at forceps delivery can be made and if easy vaginal delivery is effected this is clearly desirable; otherwise immediate recourse should be made to Caesarean section. A competent neonatal paediatrician should always be present when a diabetic patient is delivered so that paediatric care of the baby can be started immediately after birth.

Mode of delivery

The actual mode of delivery at King's College Hospital in the years 1970–1985 is shown in Table 39.12. The overall Caesarean section rate remains higher than in non-diabetic pregnancy and this is true for both primigravidae and multigravidae, although the rate for primigravidae is less than the overall rate because of the influence which repeat Caesarean section has on the multigravidae rate. Given the problems of diabetic pregnancy and labour a delivery by Caesarean section is a small price to pay by those women whose diabetic and obstetric complications make labour more hazardous for the fetus than normal.

Table 39.12 Mode of delivery of diabetic mothers at King's College Hospital

	1971–1980	1981–1985
Spontaneous onset followed by vaginal delivery	41 (12%)	33 (17%)
Induction followed by vaginal delivery	132 (38%)	60 (31%)
Induction followed by Caesarean section	45 (13%)	30 (16%)
Spontaneous onset followed by Caesarean section	11 (3%)	23 (12%)
Planned Caesarean section	123 (34%)	47 (24%)

The anticipation of the problems in labour is an essential part of all antenatal care but this is especially true of diabetic pregnancy when a decision to perform a planned rather than an emergency Caesarean section will relieve the patient as well as the obstetric and diabetic team of a great deal of anxiety. The same readiness to perform an emergency Caesarean section when labour is not progressing satisfactorily is an equally important part of the management of the pregnant diabetic.

Judgement

With careful monitoring in both pregnancy and labour the overall rate of Caesarean section should fall, and especially steadily in primigravidae.

THE INFANT OF THE DIABETIC MOTHER

The characteristic appearance of the infant of the diabetic mother as described by Farquhar (1959) is well known. The tomato baby is most often associated with a diabetic pregnancy where maternal control has been bad, but may occur where maternal care has been good. The management of all infants of diabetic mothers, whether presenting characteristic appearance or not, calls for expert neonatal care.

Neonatal morbidity

The neonatal morbidity in these infants has changed considerably over the past 20 years and many now have a normal and uncomplicated neonatal course. Most will not require to be admitted to a special care baby unit.

Asphyxia

Asphyxia is more common in the infant of the diabetic mother. About one-third of all cases require intubation, although this figure includes a number of preterm and other compromised infants. Acidosis (pH < 7.20) is seen in about 10% and may require intravenous sodium bicarbonate.

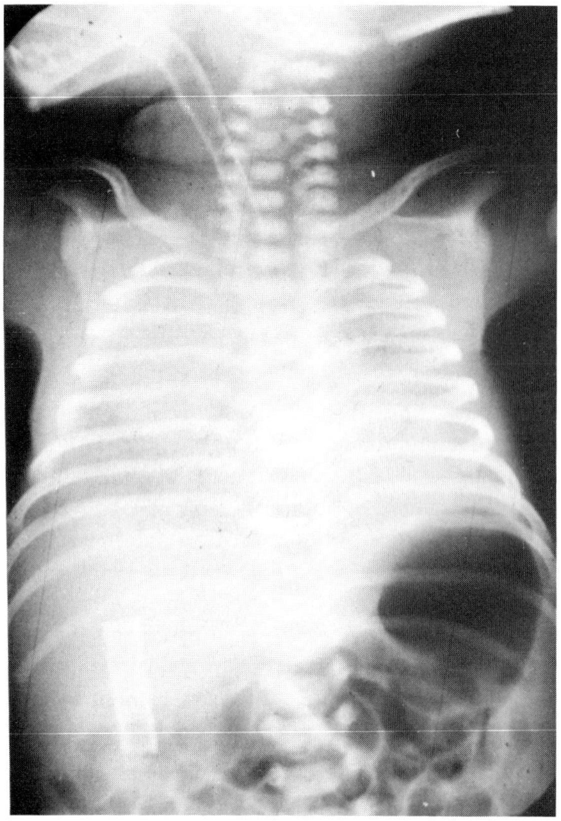

Fig. 39.2 RDS showing a typical air bronchogram.

Respiratory distress syndrome (RDS)

The importance of RDS as a cause of perinatal mortality and morbidity has diminished sharply in recent times, although it remains a hazard for the preterm infant of the diabetic mother. The infant of a well controlled diabetic mother delivered after 37 weeks is unlikely to develop RDS (Fig. 39.2). Diagnosis is made by the typical air bronchogram appearance on chest X-ray. Prompt raising of the ambient oxygen concentration is called for. Only the very premature infant of a diabetic mother is likely to succumb to this cause given good modern neonatal paediatric care.

Hypoglycaemia

Blood glucose levels of <1.1 mmol/l occur more frequently in the infant of a diabetic mother. The lowest levels are seen in the first hour of life, after which the concentration begins to rise. Hypoglycaemia is more commonly seen in macrosomic babies or after birth asphyxia. Hypoglycaemia is usually asymptomatic in these infants, but apnoea attacks, hypertonia, extreme excitability and frank convulsions may occur. The condition results from hyperinsulaemia which is in turn a reflection of maternal hyperglycaemia. Whether hyperinsulaemia is the sole cause of neonatal hypoglycaemia in such babies is debated, but it is probably the major factor. Hypoglycaemia is best prevented by early breastfeeding. The blood glucose levels should be measured at 2 and 4 hours after birth. If the level is <2.5 mmol/l on both occasions intravenous glucose is commenced and continued until a sustained rise in glucose levels is obtained.

Hypocalcaemia and hypomagnesaemia

Neonatal hypocalcaemia (serum <1.65 mmol/l) and hypomagnesaemia (serum magnesium <0.62 mmol/l) are more common in these babies. Hypocalcaemia may lead to increased neuromuscular excitability, causing apnoeic spells and fits. If the levels are low, intravenous calcium gluconate 5% (50–100 mg/kg) is given.

Polycythaemia

Polycythaemia is more common in infants of diabetic mothers. It seems likely to be a response to intrauterine fetal anoxia. The increased maternal levels of HbA_1 may cause a degree of fetal anoxia and account for some decrease in the transfer of oxygen across the placenta. It seems unlikely that this is the sole explanation however. Polycythaemia is less of a problem in those pregnancies where maternal diabetic control has been good. If the haematocrit is more than 65% (20 g% of Hb) during the first 8 hours after birth venesection is recommended, with 10% of the infant's blood volume being removed. The red cells are centrifuged off and the plasma replaced.

Jaundice

Hyperbilirubinaemia may result from neonatal polycythaemia. Like polycythaemia it is much less common nowadays. Other contributors to hyperbilirubinaemia are bruising, including cephalhaematoma following a traumatic delivery and sepsis. Jaundice is of course more likely to occur in premature babies and in those who have had respiratory distress. A careful check on the level of bilirubin in these newborn babies is necessary and phototherapy or, rarely, exchange transfusion is carried out as required.

Birth trauma

Birth trauma results from a difficult vaginal delivery often because of fetal macrosomia. In general, difficult vaginal delivery has no place in the modern management of diabetic pregnancy. Macrosomia should be diagnosed by routine antenatal ultrasound scanning and, where disproportion exists, the baby delivered by planned Caesarean section. Birth trauma is a rare cause of perinatal mortality and morbidity in modern obstetric practice.

The long-term outlook for infants of diabetic mothers

The infants of diabetic mothers have a greater than average chance of developing diabetes in later life, but the actual risk is of the order of 1% as against 0.1% in infants of mothers who are not diabetic. A study by Persson (1986) found that 2 (3%) of 73 such children had developed diabetes in the first 10 years of life. Macrosomic babies tend to become obese and obesity may then be associated with abnormal glucose tolerance, but the majority of these babies, macrosomic or otherwise, usually exhibit normal physical development. Mental development is also usually normal, although there is a risk of neurological abnormality where prolonged neonatal hypoglycaemia occurs (Gamsu 1978).

BREASTFEEDING FOR THE DIABETIC MOTHER

Breastfeeding should be encouraged in diabetic women, as in non-diabetic women. In a survey by Whichelow & Doddridge (1983) it was found that three-quarters of the diabetic mothers at King's College Hospital were breastfeeding at 6 weeks. Those babies who were encouraged to suckle within 12 hours of delivery were more likely to be weaned later than those put to the breast after that time. An increase in the dietary allowance of carbohydrate by 50 g as a contribution for the extra 600 calories per day needed for lactation is essential. This increase is usually taken in the form of an extra pint of milk daily and two extra carbohydrate portions taken at tea and dinner. Insulin requirements do not on the whole alter during lactation. It is clear then that all diabetic mothers should be encouraged to breastfeed; this aim can usually be achieved by early suckling and an appropriate increase in the maternal carbohydrate intake.

FAMILY PLANNING AND THE DIABETIC WOMAN

For the average diabetic woman who wishes to have children a small family should be the aim. The problem of managing her diabetes and the possibility that long-term vascular complications will at some stage further impair her health make pregnancy and the addition of children to her life much more of a burden than for the non-diabetic woman. Family planning for the diabetic woman should result in a planned family and in the timing of conception in order to ensure that it occurs at a time when diabetic control is optimal. Diabetic women should aim to have their children as early as possible in their reproductive lives since the vascular complications of diabetes are more likely to arise after some years.

The traditional methods of contraception – sheath and contraceptive diaphragm — are appropriate for a woman who is well motivated toward family planning and has a caring partner. They offer a reasonable degree of safety from unplanned pregnancy with no risk of complications.

The intrauterine contraceptive device is a safer option and although it has certain disadvantages it has the important advantage that once placed in position the woman and her partner need take no further contraceptive measures. It is not suitable as a method of contraception for a nulliparous woman unless no alternative method can be used. The risk of intrauterine infection does not seem to be greater in well controlled diabetic women and a reported higher failure rate among diabetic intrauterine contraceptive device users (Steel & Duncan 1980) has not been borne out by experience or by subsequent papers (Thiery 1982).

The combined oral contraceptive pill is the most effective contraceptive method available, but has a slight but definite risk of causing venous thromboembolism; it is this complication rather than its minor effects on carbohydrate lipid metabolism which gives the greatest cause for concern in diabetic women, particularly amongst those known to have vascular disease or hypertension. Adjustment of insulin dosage may be required but the majority of diabetic women suffer no disturbance of diabetic control when taking the pill. Diabetic women who wish to use the pill should be examined carefully for evidence of microvasculopathy and hypertension and should be encouraged to lose weight if they are obese. They should also be strongly discouraged from smoking. True gestational diabetics, i.e. those who revert to the non-diabetic state after pregnancy, do nevertheless often have some impairment of glucose tolerance and should also avoid the combined pill.

When diabetic women do opt for oral contraception the low-dose triphasic pill or the progesterone-only pill should be advised. The progesterone-only pill is not associated with increased risk of venous thromboembolism and from this point of view is suitable for the diabetic woman. It does sometimes cause irregular menstrual periods with intermenstrual spotting and has a higher failure rate than the combined pill. The failure rate can be kept to acceptably low levels if the patient takes the pill without fail every day, starting immediately after delivery; it is useful if the patient is breastfeeding. If it proves successful, it can be continued thereafter.

To the average non-pregnant diabetic woman who wishes to use oral contraception a low-dose triphasic preparation with its regularity of menstrual periods and very low failure rate is probably the pill of choice but the progesterone-only pill is a valuable alternative.

Laparoscopic sterilization is an easily performed gynaecological procedure with a low failure rate (one in 500 cases). It offers the diabetic woman who has completed her family the most satisfactory long-term solution to family planning problems and should be freely available. It is best performed 6 weeks postpartum and the patient can usually be dealt with on a day-case basis. Sterilization at the time of Caesarean section is an option which should be discussed with diabetic patients during the antenatal period and generally will only be applicable to those women having planned repeat Caesarean sections. Vasectomy may be an appropriate alternative to female sterilization in some cases, but only if the male partner is certain he will not want to bear more children under any circumstances.

REFERENCES

Baird J D 1986 Some aspects of metabolism and hormonal adaptation to pregnancy. Acta Endocrinologica (suppl) 277: 11–18

Baker L, Egler J M, Klein S H, Goldman A S 1981 Meticulous control of diabetes during organogenesis prevents congenital lumbo-sacral defects in rats. Diabetes 30: 955–959

Banting F G, Best C H 1922 The internal secretion of the pancreas. Journal of Laboratory and Clinical Medicine 7: 1–5

Brooks A P, Metcalfe J, Day J L, Edwards M S 1980 Iron deficiency and glycosylated haemoglobin A_1. Lancet ii: 141

Broughton Pipkin F, Hunter J C, Oats J J N, O'Brien P M S 1982 The renin angiotensin system in normal and diabetic pregnancy. In: Sammour M B, Symonds E M, Zuspan F P, El Tomi N (eds) Pregnant hypertension. Ain Sham University Press, Cairo, pp 185–192

Brudenell M 1978 Delivering the baby of a diabetic mother. Proceedings of the Royal Society of Medicine 71: 207–211

Brudenell M 1982 Obstetric complications in the antenatal period in diabetic pregnancy. Results of UK Diabetic Pregnancy Survey (Beard R W & Lowy C (eds)) presented at RCOG scientific meeting 1982

Cudworth A G, and Woodrow J C 1976 Genetic susceptibility in diabetes mellitus: analysis of the HLA association. British Medical Journal 2: 1333–1336

Dandona P, Freedman D, Moorhead F J 1979 Glycosylated haemoglobin in chronic renal failure. British Medical Journal i: 1183–1184

Deuchar E M 1979 Experimental evidence relating fetal abnormalities to diabetes. In: Sutherland H W, Stowers J M (eds) Carbohydrate metabolism in pregnancy and the newborn. Springer Verlag, Berlin, pp 519–522

Eastwood M A, Kay R M 1979 An hypothesis for the action of dietary fibre along the gastrointestinal tract. American Journal of Clinical Nutrition 32: 364–367

Enricho A, Ingalls T M 1968 Chromosomal anomalies in the embryos of diabetic mice. Archives of Environmental Health 16: 316–325

Essex N, Pyke D A 1978 Management of maternal diabetes in pregnancy. In: Sutherland H W, Stowers J M (eds) Carbohydrate metabolism in pregnancy and the newborn. Springer Verlag, Berlin, pp 357–368

Fadel H E, Reynolds A, Stallings M, Abraham E C 1981 Minor (glycosylated) hemoglobins in cord blood of infants of normal and diabetic mothers. Journal of Obstetrics and Gynaecology 139: 397–402

Farquhar J W 1959 The child of the diabetic woman. Archives of Disease in Childhood 34: 76–96

Fuhrmann K, Reiher H, Semmler K, Fischer F, Fischer M, Glockner E 1983 Prevention of congenital malformations in infants of insulin-dependent diabetic mothers. Diabetes Care 6: 219–223

Gabbay K H, Hasty K, Breslow J L, Ellison R C, Bunn H F, Fallop P M 1977 Long term blood glucose control in diabetes mellitus. Journal of Clinical Endocrinology and Metabolism 44: 859–864

Gabbay K H, Sosenko J M, Banuchi C A, Mininsohn M J, Fluckiger R 1979 Glycosylated hemoglobins: increased glycosylation of hemoglobin A in diabetic patients. Diabetes 28: 337–340

Gamsu H R 1978 Neonatal morbidity in infants of diabetic mothers. Proceedings of the Royal Society of Medicine 71: 211–221

Gillmer M D G, Oakley N W, Beard R W et al 1980 Antenatal screening for diabetes mellitus by random blood glucose sampling. British Journal of Obstetrics and Gynaecology 87: 377–382

Goldman A S, Baker L, Piddington R, Marx B, Harold R, Egler J 1985 Hyperglycaemia induced teratogenesis is mediated by a functional deficiency of arachidonic acid. Proceedings of the National Academy of Sciences (USA) 82: 8227–8231

Grenfell A, Bewick M, Brudenell M et al 1986 Diabetic pregnancy following renal transplantation. Diabetic Medicine 3: 177–179

Jovanovic R, Jovanovic L 1984 Obstetric management when normoglycaemia is maintained in diabetic pregnant women with vascular compromise. American Journal of Obstetrics and Gynecology 149: 617–623

Kalkhoff R, Kissebah A H, Hak Joong K 1979 Lipid metabolism during normal pregnancy. In: Merkatz K R, Adam P A J (eds) The diabetic pregnancy; a perinatal perspective. Grune & Stratton, New York, pp 10–17

Kitzmiller J L, Brown E R, Phillipe M 1981 Diabetic nephropathy and perinatal outcome. American Journal of Obstetrics and Gynecology 141: 741–751

Knight A 1983 Concerning macrosomy in diabetic pregnancy. Lancet ii: 1431

Leny W, Maier W 1964 Congenital malformations and maternal diabetes. Lancet ii: 1124

Lernmark A 1985 Causes of insulin dependent diabetes. Medicine International 13: 535–538

Leslie R D G, Pyke D A, John P N, White J M 1978 Haemoglobin A_1 in diabetic pregnancy. Lancet ii: 958–959

Lind T, McDougall A N 1972 Antenatal screening for diabetes mellitus by random blood glucose sampling. British Journal of Obstetrics and Gynaecology 112: 213–220

Malins J 1979 Fetal anomalies related to carbohydrate metabolism: the epidemiological approach. In: Sutherland H W, Stowers J M (eds) Carbohydrate metabolism in pregnancy and the newborn. Springer Verlag, Berlin, pp 229–246

Miller E, Hare J W, Cloherty J P et al 1981 Elevated maternal haemoglobin A_{1c} in early pregnancy and major congenital anomalies in infants of diabetic mothers. New England Journal of Medicine 304: 1331–1334

Mills J L, Baker L, Goldman A S 1979 Malformations in infants of diabetic mothers occur before the 7th gestational week. Implications for treatment. Diabetes 28: 292–293

Miodovnik M, Lavin J P, Knowles H C et al 1984 Spontaneous abortion among insulin-dependent diabetic women. American Journal of Obstetrics and Gynecology 150: 372–376

National Diabetes Data Group 1979 Classification and diagnosis of diabetes mellitus and other categories of glucose tolerance. Diabetes 28: 1039–1057

O'Shaughnessy R, Cuss J, Zuspan F P 1979 Glycosylated hemoglobins and diabetes mellitus in pregnancy. American Journal of Obstetrics and Gynecology 135: 783–790

O'Sullivan J M, Mahan D H 1964 Criteria for the oral glucose tolerance test in pregnancy. Diabetes 13: 278

O'Sullivan G C, Walker K, Bondar G F 1975 Effects of pregnancy on bile acid metabolism. Surgical Forum 26: 442–444

Peacock I, Hunter J C, Walford S et al 1979 Self-monitoring of blood glucose in diabetic pregnancy. British Medical Journal 2: 1333–1336

Pedersen J 1979 Congenital malformations in newborns of diabetic mothers. In: Sutherland H W, Stowers J M (eds) Carbohydrate metabolism in pregnancy and the newborn. Springer Verlag, Berlin, pp 264–276

Pedersen J F, Mølsted-Pedersen L 1981 Early fetal growth delay detected by ultrasound marks increased risk of congenital malformation in diabetic pregnancy. British Medical Journal 283: 269–271

Penn K, Makowski E L, Harris P 1980 Parenthood following renal transplantation. Kidney International 18: 221–233

Persson B 1986 Long term morbidity in the offspring of diabetic mothers. Acta Endocrinologica (Copenhagen) (suppl) 277: 150–155

Poon P, Turner R C, Gillmer M D G 1981 Glycosylated fetal haemoglobin. British Medical Journal 283: 469

Pyke D A 1962 Pre-diabetes. In: Pyke D A (ed) Disorders of carbohydrate metabolism. Pitman, London

Pyke D A 1968 Aetiology of diabetes mellitus. In: Oakley W G, Pyke D A, Taylor K W (eds) Clinical diabetes. Blackwell, Oxford, pp 220–221

Reece E A, Eagan J F X, Constan D R et al 1986 Coronary artery disease in diabetic pregnancies. American Journal of Obstetrics and Gynecology 154: 150–151

Report on Confidential Enquiries into Maternal Deaths in England and Wales 1979–1981 (1986) HMSO, London

Russell G, Farmer G, Lloyd D et al 1984 Macrosomia despite well-controlled diabetic pregnancy. Lancet i: 283–284

Sosenko J M, Kitsmiller J L, Fluckiger R et al 1982 Umbilical cord glycosylated hemoglobin in infants of diabetic mothers: relationships to neonatal hypoglycaemia macrosomia and cord serum C-peptide. Diabetes Care 5: 566–570

Stallone L A, Ziel H K 1974 Management of gestational diabetes. American Journal of Obstetrics and Gynecology 119: 1191–1194

Steel J, Duncan L J P 1980 Contraception for insulin dependent diabetics. Diabetes Care 3: 557

Steel J M 1985 The prepregnancy clinic. Practical Diabetes 2(6): 8–10

Steel J M, Thomson P, Johnstone F et al 1981 Glycosylated haemoglobin concentrations in mothers of large babies. British Medical Journal 282: 1357–1358

Stubbs S M, Brudenell J M, Pyke D A, Watkins P J, Stubbs W A, Alberti

K G M M 1980 Management of the pregnancy diabetic: home or hospital, with or without glucose meters. Lancet i: 1122
Stubbs S M, Leslie R D G, John P N 1981 Fetal macrosomia and maternal diabetic control in pregnancy. British Medical Journal 282: 439–440
Stubbs S M, Doddridge M, John P N, Steel J M, Wright A D 1987 Haemoglobin A_1 and congenital malformations. Diabetic Medicine 4: 156–159
Thiery M 1982 Intra-uterine contraceptive devices for diabetics. Lancet ii: 883
Tyden O, Berne C, Eriksson U J et al 1984 Fetal maturation in strictly controlled diabetic pregnancy. Diabetes Research 1: 131–134
Watkins P J 1982 Congenital malformations and blood glucose control in diabetic pregnancy. British Medical Journal 284: 1357–1358
Whichelow M J, Doddridge M C 1983 Lactation in diabetic women. British Medical Journal 287: 649–650
White P 1965 Pregnancy and diabetes, medical aspects. Medical Clinics of North America 49: 1015
Widness J A, Schartz H C, Thompson D et al 1978 Haemoglobin A_{1c} (glycohaemoglobin) in diabetic pregnancy: an indicator of glucose control and fetal size. British Journal of Obstetrics and Gynaecology 85: 812–817
World Health Organization Expert Committee on Diabetes 1980 Second report. WHO Technical Report Series 646, Geneva
Worth R, Ashworth L, Home P et al 1983 Glycosylated haemoglobin in cord blood following normal and diabetic pregnancies. Diabetologia 25: 482–485
Wright A D, Nicholson H O, Pollock A, Taylor K G, Betts S 1983 Spontaneous abortion and diabetes mellitus. Postgraduate Medical Journal 59: 295–298
Ylinen K, Hekali R, Teramo K 1981 Haemoglobin A_{1c} during pregnancy of insulin dependent diabetics and healthy controls. Journal of Obstetrics and Gynaecology 1: 223–228
Ylinen K, Aula P, Stenman U-H et al 1984 Risk of minor and major fetal malformations in diabetics with high haemoglobin A_{1c} values in early pregnancy. British Medical Journal 289: 345–346

40

Alan G. Amias

Abdominal pain in pregnancy

INTRODUCTION

All pregnant women experience abdominal pain from time to time and much of the discussion that takes place in antenatal clinics is centred on abdominal symptoms of one sort or another. Minor aches and pains are expected and accepted by women and their attendants as normal features of the pregnant state, being usually attributed to the combined effects of displacement and direct pressure on neighbouring structures by the enlarging uterus, stretching of the abdominal wall and peritoneum and the discomfort and muscular spasm associated with nausea and vomiting.

A more specific and traditional explanation for lower abdominal and groin pain in the first half of pregnancy is spasm of the round ligaments, though such a diagnosis should be made only by exclusion (Glassman 1959, Graber 1974a). This topic is discussed in a presentation of 30 personal cases and a review of the sparse literature by Glassman (1959) who speculates on the function of the hypertrophied round ligaments during pregnancy and labour and the probable causation of pain and spasm in their muscular component.

Apart from such familiar discomforts which are usually mild and transient, uterine activity is the commonest cause of progressive abdominal pain in pregnancy and the recognition of the onset of abortion or normal labour is the first step in differential diagnosis. The distinction between physiological and pathological causes of pain requires a high degree of clinical awareness on the part of the obstetrician, who is usually the first on the scene and will often have the advantage of prior knowledge of the patient and her pregnancy.

The causes of significant abdominal pain in pregnancy include most of the major complications of the pregnancy itself as well as all of the general abdominal conditions which may affect women of childbearing age. In attempting to arrive at a diagnosis Alders' sign (1951) may be of help in differentiating between pain and tenderness of genital or extragenital origin. The source of pain is located by palpation with the patient lying flat. She is then turned on her left side with the examining hand still in position. If the pain shifts to the left it is likely to originate in the uterus or adnexa but if there is no change the source is probably extragenital (e.g. appendicitis).

Whilst no coverage of such a wide topic can be exhaustive, this chapter concentrates on those disorders, some common, some rare, in which abdominal pain is the first or main symptom and in which differential diagnosis may present special problems. It thus excludes conditions such as inflammatory bowel disease and primary disorders of the liver which are likely to have been diagnosed before pregnancy; abortion, ectopic pregnancy and renal disease (other than stone) which are discussed elsewhere; and relative rarities such as diaphragmatic hernia, myocardial infarction and pneumonia, in which abdominal pain is an associated rather than a primary symptom.

UTERINE CAUSES

Abruptio placentae

Abruptio placentae (accidental antepartum haemorrhage) is the most serious and potentially catastrophic cause of uterine pain in late pregnancy. It results in loss of the fetus in 30–60% of cases (Notelowitz et al 1979) and is still an occasional if diminishing cause of maternal death (Department of Health and Social Security (DHSS) 1986a). It occurs in about 1 in 80 to 1 in 200 pregnancies (Hurd et al 1983) and is four times commoner in multiparae than primigravidae (Donald 1979a). Despite its traditional association with hypertensive states its aetiology remains obscure. It is the commonest cause of coagulation failure in obstetric practice (Letsky 1984).

The immediate pathology is haemorrhage between placenta and uterine wall, which may range in severity from minor retroplacental bleeding to a complete separation of the entire placental surface with effusion of blood into the uterine muscle (Couvelaire uterus). The clinical manifestations and their gravity are a reflection of the amount of bleeding and also the extent to which blood remains entrapped within the uterus (concealed haemorrhage) rather than appearing externally (revealed haemorrhage). This in turn relates to the degree of atony of the uterine muscle.

Typically there is a clinical triad of abdominal pain, uterine rigidity and vaginal bleeding, though painless abruption is described with a posterior fundal placenta when the patient may only complain of vaginal bleeding and backache (Notelowitz et al 1979, Hurd et al 1983). On the other hand there may be a complete separation of the placenta with several litres of incoagulable blood concealed within the uterus and no external bleeding at all (Letsky 1984).

The classical presentation is the admission to hospital of a multigravida in late pregnancy with acute abdominal pain, shock, a woody-hard uterus and a dead fetus. The amount of external bleeding is variable and may bear little relationship to the extent of circulatory collapse. This should alert the obstetrician to the diagnosis, which is usually clear enough with a major abruption, though lesser degrees may provide diagnostic pitfalls. Even in the classic case confusion may arise in distinguishing the condition from a ruptured uterus — especially if there is an abdominal scar — or an extrauterine catastrophe such as acute appendicitis with peritonitis, a perforated viscus or acute intestinal obstruction in which secondary spasm and rigidity of the uterus are likely to occur.

Minor placental separations which are unlikely to kill the fetus are accompanied by relatively mild abdominal pain and localized tenderness. Such cases have to be distinguished from degeneration or torsion in a uterine fibroid, rupture of a vein on the surface of the uterus and the effects of direct abdominal trauma, whether deliberate or accidental. The diagnosis, especially of relatively minor placental abruption, has been revolutionized by ultrasonography. Yiu-Chiu & Chiu (1982) and Grannum (1983) have described the ultrasonic feature of retroplacental haemorrhage which produces a transonic or complex collection; the echogenicity depends on the degree of organization of blood clot. In some cases a retroplacental haematoma does not form and blood may dissect under the chorion to form an echo-free or complex collection behind an elevated chorionic plate. Other details may be commended to specialist ultrasonographers but Yiu-Chiu & Chiu (1982) warn that the investigation may be unhelpful despite profuse external bleeding, especially if there is no appreciable accumulation in the uterus. In such cases a negative ultrasound examination cannot preclude the diagnosis of abruption.

In the acute phase ultrasound is equally valuable in assessing the state of the fetus. The patient is ill, anxious, shocked and in great pain. The woody-hard, tense uterus makes clinical assessment of the fetus impossible and although a large abruption will almost certainly result in fetal death this is not always so. If ultrasound can confirm a fetal circulation prompt Caesarean delivery may save the child.

In all major cases the immediate priorities of management are to restore and maintain the blood volume, to empty the uterus and to anticipate coagulation failure which will develop in one-third to one-half of cases of severe abruption (Pritchard & Brekken 1967, Taylor 1979).

The replacement of blood volume is the most urgent primary measure mainly by whole blood transfusion augmented by SAG suspended red cells, fresh frozen plasma and, if appropriate, plasma expanders and plasma concentrates. A central venous pressure line is mandatory (DHSS 1986a). The most useful blood investigations include platelet counts, serum fibrinogen levels and measurement of fibrin degradation products as well as thrombin, prothrombin and partial thromboplastin times (Taylor 1979). Pritchard & Brekken (1967) found that 38% of cases of severe abruption developed significant hypofibrinogenaemia but were unlikely to do so beyond 8 h after the onset. This suggests that early anticipation is the key to management and that an experienced haematologist should be involved in the care of the patient at the first opportunity (DHSS 1986a).

The management of coagulation failure is fully discussed in Chapter 38.

Although obstetricians are aware of the association between placental abruption and hypertension it is common experience that most cases occur without warning. Blair (1973) found 26 patients with hypertensive disorders amongst 189 cases of abruptio placentae — an incidence of 19.6% or twice that of the general obstetric population, but still leaving 80% of cases unassociated. From the opposite standpoint, Abdella et al (1984) studied the occurrence of abruption within each hypertensive category. The incidence was highest amongst cases of eclampsia (23.6%) but low for patients with chronic hypertension (10%) and pre-eclampsia (2.3%).

Uncertainty about the role of pre-existing hypertension in the aetiology of abruptio placentae can lead to difficulties in the initial assessment of a patient with antepartum haemorrhage, as shock and hypovolaemia may obscure an underlying hypertensive condition especially in a patient seen for the first time. Similarly, a normal blood pressure on admission may be the effect of profound but underestimated blood loss in a patient with chronic hypertension — hence the vital importance of central venous pressure monitoring.

In most cases of severe abruption the fetus will already be dead when the patient is first seen and once the blood volume has been restored steps must be taken to hasten delivery. Often, despite the apparent uterine atony, vaginal examination reveals that the cervix is dilating and labour is well advanced. Otherwise induction is carried out by amniotomy and oxytocin infusion (Letsky 1984). Emptying

Table 40.1 Maternal death rates from placental abruption in England and Wales (from DHSS 1982a, 1986a)

Years	Death rates from abruption per million maternities
1952–1954	38
1964–1966	10.4
1979–1981	1.04

the uterus with evacuation of the concealed retroplacental blood clot usually results in rapid recovery and reduces the likelihood or mitigates the severity of coagulation failure.

Maternal death rates from placental abruption have fallen steadily in England and Wales since Confidential Enquiries were started in 1952 (Table 40.1). None the less, perinatal mortality remains in the region of 50% and has led to a re-appraisal of traditional conservative management in favour of earlier recourse to Caesarean section in selected cases (Blair 1973, Hurd et al 1983). Modern techniques of maternal and fetal monitoring and imaging should permit the diagnosis of placental abruption in any patient with vaginal bleeding in the third trimester who also has uterine pain or hypertonus and evidence of fetal distress. If the maternal condition is satisfactory and the fetus is estimated to weigh over 1500 g, abdominal delivery should not be delayed as the timespan between the onset of fetal distress and fetal death is very short (Hurd et al 1983). Rarely, there is no alternative to Caesarean section even when the fetus is known to be dead if attempts at vaginal delivery are unsuccessful and the patient is losing ground.

At operation the classical Couvelaire uterus may be found with ecchymoses on the surface and frank bleeding into the uterine muscle, which has a characteristic dark purple appearance. After delivery of the child and removal of the placenta and accumulated haematoma, the soggy blotting paper consistency of the uterus may prevent immediate retraction, so that massage and compression with hot packs are usually required for a few moments. The return of uterine tone is often surprisingly rapid.

In all cases of placental abruption postpartum haemorrhage has to be anticipated as a consequence of uterine atony and coagulation failure. The early restoration of blood volume, in addition to its circulatory function, also helps to clear fibrin degradation products which apart from acting as potent anticoagulants may also inhibit myometrial activity (Basu 1969, Letsky 1984).

After delivery whole blood and oxytocin or prostaglandin infusions should be maintained until uterine retraction is adequate and bleeding minimal.

Rupture of the uterus

Consideration of ruptured uterus as a cause of abdominal pain in pregnancy follows logically upon a discussion of placental abruption, as the clinical picture is similar with varying degrees of pain, vaginal bleeding, uterine tenderness and shock. A previous uterine scar is the dominant single precipitating factor accounting for over half of the cases in published series (Garnet 1964, Cavanagh et al 1965, Schrinsky & Benson 1978). Horowitz et al (1981) state that 'an abruptio placentae in a patient with a uterine scar is probably a ruptured uterus' and Jones (1974) quotes Moir's legendary wisdom in advising that 'an abdominal section should be performed if the features of concealed accidental haemorrhage are not clearly defined or typical'.

It is traditional teaching that the classical Caesarean scar is the main culprit predisposing to uterine rupture in a subsequent pregnancy at a rate 10 times that of a lower segment scar (4% compared with 0.4%). This figure is convenient but open to question. Cavanagh et al (1965) rate the likelihood of a classical rupture as twice that of a lower segment scar and Donald (1979b) quotes a series of 43 ruptures of previous Caesarean scars in Dublin between 1950 and 1964 with an incidence of 1.4% following lower segment section and 6.4% after the classical operation.

Owing to the relative rarity of ruptured uterus (1/1000–1/2500 cases; Garnet 1964, Cavanagh et al 1965, Schrinsky & Benson 1978, Donald 1979b), substantial series have either been collated from several sources (e.g. Garnet 1964) or extend back over many years (e.g. Felmus et al 1953, Schrinsky & Benson 1978) during which clinical obstetric practice will have altered in a number of ways but principally in the abandonment of classical section in favour of the lower segment approach. Thus although the classical scar is undoubtedly the weaker, the lower segment scar figures with relative prominence as a cause of uterine rupture in published series. Cavanagh et al (1965) discuss 24 cases of ruptured scar between 1954 and 1963, of which 15 were classical and nine lower segments scars. Sheth (1969) in the same decade found 21 classical and eight lower segment ruptures and Schrinsky & Benson (1978), reviewing a series of 47 ruptures over 25 years, found that the classical scar was responsible for 16 cases and the lower segment for nine.

The data of Schrinsky & Benson also cast doubt on the traditional view that by and large the classical scar is more likely to rupture in late pregnancy and the lower segment scar during labour (Table 40.2). It can be seen that the timing of scar rupture is virtually identical for each site and the figures underline the need for vigilance antenatally as well as in labour in all pregnancies following Caesarean section.

Complacency about the relative safety of the lower uterine incision may be misplaced, in view of the current preference for abdominal delivery for the very premature infant especially when presenting by the breech. It must be doubtful whether an incision in a uterus of less than 30 weeks' gestation — albeit placed as low as possible — can be said not to encroach upon the upper segment. Furthermore there are some who advocate a low vertical incision in such circumstances and even when a planned transverse incision is made there are occasions when a vertical extension may be

Table 40.2 Timing of 47 cases of uterine rupture (Schrinsky & Benson 1978)

	Pre-labour	Labour
Classical scar	8	8
Lower segment scar	4	5
Unscarred	3*	19

* Including 1 cornual pregnancy.

unavoidable, especially if the after-coming head is trapped. The consequence of such practices for a future pregnancy are still unknown but the possibility of dehiscence either before or during labour must be borne in mind.

Table 40.2 also demonstrates the relative rarity of rupture of the unscarred uterus during pregnancy compared with its predominance during labour. When spontaneous rupture of the apparently intact uterus does occur before labour it tends to be a more catastrophic event than scar dehiscence (Felmus et al 1953, Lalos et al 1977, Schrinsky & Benson 1978). The subsequent discovery of chronic inflammatory changes and myometrial degeneration at the rupture site may draw attention to the weakening effect of previous trauma from a post-abortum curettage or manual removal of the placenta, but only in retrospect (Lalos et al 1977). Deaths from spontaneous rupture of the uterus of unknown cause at 14 and 18 weeks' gestation are documented in the Reports on Confidential Enquiries into Maternal Deaths in England and Wales 1973–1975 and 1976–1978 (DHSS 1979, 1982b) and as a stark reminder that previous myomectomy is not risk-free, the 1982 Report describes the death of a primigravida aged 41 from massive fundal rupture at 16 weeks' gestation; the woman had undergone elective myomectomy 10 months earlier.

Despite such rare catastrophes in early pregnancy and uncommon disasters from ruptured cornual pregnancies (Graber 1974a), rupture of the uterus is predominantly an event of the third trimester due no doubt to the rapid growth and stretching of the uterine wall at that time. Spontaneous rupture is almost always complete (Cavanagh et al 1965), involving the full thickness of the uterine wall with corresponding massive haemorrhage and shock. The need for immediate rescuscitation and laparotomy is rarely in doubt and hysterectomy after delivery of the baby is the safest and probably the only course in most cases (Garnet 1964, Sheth 1969, Taylor 1969).

Scar dehiscence, on the other hand, is incomplete (occult) in at least 25% of cases (Cavanagh et al 1965) and may range in presentation from a chance discovery at elective repeat Caesarean section (Garnet 1964), through minor warning symptoms of pain and tenderness, to the fully developed picture of a rapidly progressive abdominal emergency. Most Caesarean section scars are relatively avascular and the clinical severity of the rupture will depend on its site, the length of the tear and its proximity to the placental bed. In the occult form the peritoneal surface is not breached and, if not entirely silent, the rupture manifests itself as local intermittent discomfort which may be mistaken for early labour or a small placental abruption. At a more advanced stage and with complete rupture the symptoms and signs will be correspondingly more intense with increasing pain, variable vaginal bleeding and in some cases a sensation of bursting or 'something giving way' (Jones 1974).

Schrinsky & Benson (1978), Donald (1979b) and Horowitz et al (1981) have drawn attention to the similarity of the clinical picture of ruptured uterus with that of placental abruption in view of the uterine pain and tenderness commonly accompanied by evidence of fetal distress or death. Distinguishing signs of rupture may be uterine asymmetry due to the development of a broad ligament haematoma, easily palpable fetal parts and an unusual high transverse lie of the fetus (Lalos et al 1977, Taylor 1977a). Ultrasound scanning may be of considerable help in the differential diagnosis, by excluding an abruptio placentae.

At laparotomy for ruptured scar both fetal and uterine salvage are much more likely than after rupture of a uterus not previously scarred. The chance of fetal survival relates to the degree of interference with the placental circulation, which may be minimal with silent or occult rupture and total if the scar is situated over the placental site. The overall perinatal mortality for uterine rupture is in the region of 50%.

Whereas 85% of spontaneous ruptures require hysterectomy, at least two-thirds of cases of ruptured scar are amenable to repair by suture; this should be the first choice for young patients and those of low parity (Reyes-Ceja et al 1969, Sheth 1969).

Uterine fibroids

Uterine fibroids, the commonest of gynaecological tumours, are not infrequently found in association with pregnancy. The incidence varies between 0.5 and 5%, being highest in women over 30 and in the Afro-Caribbean population. If not already suspected clinically, fibroids will be discovered during early ultrasound scanning and their progress — innocuous in the vast majority — may be charted by this means (Winer-Muram et al 1983). In the natural course of events fibroids enlarge and soften with the growth and increased vascularity of the uterus and may be less easy to palpate as the pregnancy advances. The increase in size is due to oedema as well as hypertrophy and during the second trimester when growth is particularly rapid the blood supply may become precarious, especially if the lesion is large and subserous or pedunculated (Barter & Parks 1958, Graber 1974a, Donald 1979c). The previous symptomless tumour is now a potential cause of acute abdominal pain from red degeneration or torsion or a combination of both.

Red degeneration in a fibroid (necrobiosis) tends to occur in the second half of pregnancy or in the puerperium. Thrombosis in the capsular vessels is followed by venous engorgement and a local inflammatory reaction (Jones 1974). The patient will complain of acute abdominal pain and vomiting and may develop a low grade pyrexia. The principal signs are exquisite localized peritoneal tenderness over the surface of the fibroid accompanied by marked leukocytosis (Taylor 1984). Diagnosis will present little difficulty in a patient known to have fibroids and the possibility of such a complication argues for regular antenatal ultrasound monitoring of lesions found early in pregnancy (Winer-Muram et al 1983).

Unless there is serious doubt about the diagnosis the treatment of red degeneration is medical rather than surgical. The patient is managed with bedrest, sedation and analgesia. Taylor (1984) recommends the application of abdominal ice-packs 2-hourly to help resolution of the condition — usually a matter of 4–7 days (Graber 1974a). Rarely, laparotomy may be required if the symptoms worsen or fail to improve and the possibility of an unconnected acute surgical condition such as appendicitis or torsion of an ovarian cyst cannot be ruled out. A pedunculated fibroid may have undergone torsion and secondary degeneration and such a situation provides the sole indication for myomectomy during pregnancy as it is a relatively simple matter to ligate and divide a narrow pedicle. In all other circumstances once the diagnosis of red degeneration has been confirmed the abdomen should be closed (Jones 1974, Graber 1974a, Donald 1979c).

Torsion of the uterus

Axial rotation of the uterus, usually to the right, is a normal physiological change observed in over 80% of pregnancies (Smith 1975); usually this is of the order of 30–40° (Nowosielski & Henderson 1960, Graber 1974a) but very rarely this natural rotation progresses beyond 90° to produce subacute or acute torsion of the uterus — an uncommon but serious cause of abdominal symptoms in mid and late pregnancy. In the majority of cases there is a predisposing cause such as a fibroid or congenital anomaly producing asymmetry of the uterus, an adnexal mass or a history of pelvic surgery (Taylor 1985). In 10–20% of cases, often the most sudden and catastrophic, no pre-existing uterine or pelvic pathology is found (Mitchell & Garrett 1960).

The clinical picture is of abdominal pain of increasing severity, usually in the third trimester and sometimes heralded by earlier unexplained episodes of discomfort. Signs of shock rapidly develop and may become profound. The uterus is tender and tense, leading to a preliminary diagnosis of concealed antepartum haemorrhage in many cases, but the asymmetry of the uterus may be noticed and the thickened cord-like round ligament is sometimes palpable obliquely across the abdomen in the direction of the torsion (Nowosielski & Henderson 1960, Caughey et al 1965). If the patient is already known to have a fibroid or a uterine abnormality a change in the position of the tumour or non-gravid horn may be detected on vaginal examination (Mitchell & Garrett 1960). Acute retention of urine usually occurs and attempted catheterization may reveal a twisted vaginal canal and displacement of the urethra (Smith 1975).

Despite these indicators the true diagnosis is rarely made before laparotomy when the torsion, most commonly of about 180°, will be discovered by finding the posterior surface of the uterus presenting in the wound (Mitchell & Garrett 1960, Taylor 1985). The best procedure is to perform a Caesarean section; this usually means untwisting the uterus first but Taylor (1985) finds no objection to an incision in the posterior uterine wall if this seems the safest way of extracting the baby, after which the torsion can be rectified.

OVARIAN CAUSES

Ovarian tumours

In the modern era of antenatal care the unexpected presentation of an ovarian lesion as an abdominal emergency is relatively rare. As with fibroids, ovarian enlargement should be detected in early pregnancy by clinical examination and ultrasonography. The majority of such swellings will prove to be follicular or luteal and most will disappear spontaneously as pregnancy advances. Ovarian lesions over 5 cm in diameter which persist beyond the first trimester should be electively removed between the 14th and 16th weeks of pregnancy. The choice of this gestational window in time will avoid interference with a functioning corpus luteum on the one hand and prevent complications from a neglected ovarian tumour on the other.

Using strict diagnostic criteria, the incidence of ovarian tumours in association with pregnancy is no higher than 1 in 800 to 1 in 1000 cases (Tawa 1964, Chung & Birnbaum 1973, White 1973) but operations on the ovary form a large proportion of surgical procedures carried out on pregnant women. Levine & Diamond (1961) reviewing 50 major operations in pregnancy found 22 cases of ovarian cyst — the commonest single lesion—and Saunders & Milton (1973) in a study of 74 laparotomies in pregnancy (of which 26 were negative) reported 19 patients with ovarian cysts and 14 with appendicitis—the two largest groups.

Elective procedures in the second trimester following the earlier discovery of an ovarian swelling account for most operations on the ovary in pregnancy but acute abdominal complications, including torsion, rupture and haemorrhage requiring emergency laparotomy, form a sizeable though widely divergent proportion of published cases. Tawa (1964), reviewing 62 ovarian tumours in pregnancy of which 25 were dermoid cysts and 12 cystadenomas, noted eight complications demanding immediate surgical intervention — an incidence of 13% compared with 18% in other series. Malkasian et al (1967) in a general study of 612 cystic teratomas stated that dermoid cysts formed 22–48.5% of ovarian neoplasms in association with pregnancy. All the cases of acute rupture in the study series occurred in pregnancy or labour, giving an incidence of rupture of 15.8% during pregnancy compared with 1.3% for the series as a whole.

Confirming the prevalence of dermoid cysts (27%) and cystadenomas (24%) amongst a series of 164 ovarian tumours in pregnancy, Beischer et al (1971) found that no less than 78 (47%) had undergone torsion by the time of diagnosis or had produced abdominal symptoms sufficient to warrant laparotomy. This high proportion of complications is counterbalanced by a review of 100 neoplasms in pregnancy by Novak et al (1975), who noted that most of the lesions were asymptomatic and remained undiagnosed unless presenting as an acute abdomen, which occurred in five cases only. Hermann & Simon (1983) quoted an incidence of torsion of between 10 and 15% of patients with ovarian cysts in pregnancy and McGowan (1983) noted that 25% of all cases of torsion of the adnexa occurred in association with pregnancy.

Consideration of published work to date leads to the conclusion that between 10 and 20% of patients with ovarian lesions in pregnancy are likely to develop complications requiring urgent laparotomy.

Torsion of an ovarian cyst in pregnancy is more likely to occur during the phase of rapid uterine growth between the 8th and 16th weeks and also in the early puerperium when intra-abdominal relationships have dramatically altered (McGowan 1964, 1983). The onset may be sudden with acute lower abdominal pain, nausea and vomiting and signs of shock. The pain, either constant or colicky, is accompanied by guarding, rigidity and rebound tenderness mimicking acute appendicitis or ruptured tubal pregnancy. The presence of a tense, tender lower abdominal or pelvic mass will aid the diagnosis but may be difficult to distinguish from the enlarged uterus in the acute condition. If the torsion is unrelieved haemorrhage and necrosis will lead to secondary rupture of the cyst wall with signs of increasing shock and spreading peritoneal irritation.

The clinical picture will be less dramatic if the torsion of the ovarian pedicle is incomplete. Recurrent abdominal symptoms of dull, intermittent lower quadrant pain may be difficult to evaluate unless the patient is already known to have an ovarian lesion. Peritoneal irritation may produce abdominal distension and signs of ileus, suggesting an intestinal lesion such as subacute obstruction. Graber (1974b) has argued that the peritoneal reaction around a cyst which has undergone a minimal degree of torsion may prevent the normal drawing up of the adnexa out of the pelvis as the pregnancy advances resulting in obstruction during labour.

The difficulties of diagnosis due to confusion with other abdominal disorders are illustrated by McGowan's contention (1983) that torsion of the adnexa is rarely diagnosed before surgical intervention and, more specifically, in the series of 74 laparotomies in pregnancy reported by Saunders & Milton (1973), 19 patients were found to have ovarian cysts of which 12 had been correctly predicted before operation. Of the other seven patients the preoperative diagnosis was ectopic pregnancy in six and fibroids in one. Conversely, laparotomy with negative findings was performed for suspected ovarian swelling in another six patients. Fifteen of the operations were carried out in the first trimester and although only 7 of the 19 patients had an acute complication (three torsion, two rupture, two haemorrhage), this series exemplifies the problem of antenatal abdominal diagnosis.

If laparotomy is carried out before irreversible changes in the ovarian pedicle have occurred, the operation of choice is to rectify the torsion and perform an ovarian cystectomy. Steps should also be taken to stabilize the ovary by anchoring it to adjacent tissues and by plicating the ovarian ligament. If the case is one of haemorrhage or rupture without torsion a similar attempt should be made to conserve the ovary by excising the damaged area, removing redundant tissue and reconstituting the ovarian capsule. When it is clear that the ovary is damaged beyond recall salpingo-oophorectomy must be carried out.

The possibility of encountering an ovarian cancer at the time of laparotomy in pregnancy, though remote in view of the age group concerned, must not be overlooked. Jubb (1963), Beischer et al (1971), Chung & Birnbaum (1973) and McGowan (1983) all report an incidence of malignancy of up to 5% of ovarian tumours in pregnancy with an average of about 2% in published series. Within this small population dysgerminoma is prominent; although it is a rare ovarian tumour, forming only 3.5% of primary ovarian malignancies (Pece 1964), 85% occur in young girls and women under the age of 30 (McGowan 1983). The diagnosis of 15–20% of dysgerminoma is first made in pregnancy or the puerperium and the tumour represents 25–35% of all ovarian cancer associated with pregnancy (Karlen et al 1979).

Malignancy should be suspected in any case of ovarian rupture, especially in the absence of torsion as a precipitating factor. Other signs of malignancy should be sought, as in the non-pregnant woman, and salpingo-oophorectomy performed if the diagnosis is not in doubt. Inspection and wedge biopsy of the opposite ovary must be part of the procedure. Management beyond the emergency stage will depend on the gestational age, the stage of the disease and the wishes of the patient and is not further considered here (see Chapter 43).

Apart from its importance in cases of suspected malignancy, inspection of the opposite tube and ovary should be undertaken in all cases of adnexal pathology not only to rule out a contralateral lesion but also to carry out a prophylactic stabilization in the rare instance of torsion of the normal Fallopian tube in pregnancy (Goplerud & Hanson 1965, Chambers et al 1979).

ALIMENTARY CAUSES

Appendicitis

Acute appendicitis makes an appropriate centrepiece in a review of the causes of abdominal pain in pregnancy as the condition demonstrates the general problems of diagnosis and management of the acute abdomen under altered physiological conditions. Because of both the proximity of the appendix to the uterus and adnexa and the opportunity for diagnostic confusion, appendicitis forms a bridge between disorders of genital and extragenital origin. Appendicitis accounts for over 60% of non-gynaecological conditions requiring laparotomy during pregnancy (Saunders & Milton 1973, Griffen 1974, Weingold 1983) and is the commonest general surgical emergency encountered (Levine & Diamond 1961, McCorriston 1963, Hermann & Simon 1983).

The Report on Confidential Enquiries into Maternal Deaths in England and Wales 1979–1981 (DHSS 1986b) describes the death of a patient from a ruptured appendix abscess on the day after the spontaneous delivery of a stillborn child at 35 weeks' gestation. She had attended hospital with abdominal pain twice before labour but was allowed to go home. To quote the report: 'Her case illustrates the difficulty of diagnosing appendicitis in pregnancy.'

The seriousness of appendicitis in pregnancy is apparent from the fact that, although the incidence is no greater than in the non-pregnant woman and is distributed equally between the three trimesters, the mortality of the disease in pregnancy is still four to five times that in the general population and is 10 times higher in the second half of pregnancy than in the first (Black 1960, Saunders & Milton 1973, Babaknia et al 1977). The evidence suggests that the basic disease process of appendicitis in pregnant women is no more fulminant than at other times (Black 1960, Finch & Lee 1974, Weingold 1983) but that delay in diagnosis—especially in the third trimester—allows the condition to reach an advanced stage before the patient comes to operation. The physiological changes of pregnancy which are the principal cause of the diagnostic delay also contribute to the severity of the condition by encouraging extension rather than localization of the inflammatory process (Black 1960, Saunders & Milton 1973, Finch & Lee 1974, Hermann & Simon 1983).

Finch & Lee (1974) compared 56 cases of acute appendicitis in pregnancy with matched non-pregnant controls and noted a significant difference in the operative findings (Table 40.3). In addition to noting the greater severity of the disease found at operation in pregnancy, Finch & Lee also pointed out that only 4 cases of perforation were found amongst 45 operations carried out before the 26th week, but of the 11 cases in late pregnancy 6 had perforated by the time of laparotomy.

Confirmation of the high incidence of perforation amongst pregnant woman with appendicitis compared with others, and its clustering in the later stages, is provided by the experience of O'Neill (1969a), Babaknia et al (1977), Gomez & Wood (1979) and Masters et al (1984). Accepting an incidence of perforation with appendicitis in the general population of about 10% of cases, its occurrence in pregnancy appears to be in the region of 15–20%.

Table 40.3 Acute appendicitis: comparison of operative findings in pregnant and non-pregnant women (Finch & Lee 1974)

State of appendix	Pregnant		Non-pregnant	
Acutely inflamed	29		44	
Gangrenous	17	48%	6	21%
Perforated	10		6	
Total	56		56	

Table 40.4 Maternal and fetal loss in 373 cases of appendicitis in pregnancy and the puerperium (Black 1960)

	Maternal mortality		Fetal loss
First trimester	0	1.9%	12.5
Second trimester	3.9		15.7
Third trimester	10.9	11.2%	20
abour	16.7		
Puerperium	0		

Maternal mortality = 4.6%; fetal loss = 17%

Babaknia et al (1977), in a review of 333 confirmed cases of appendicitis in pregnancy, reported 70 perforations (21%); 41 occurred in the group of 233 cases in the first and second trimesters—an incidence of 17.6%—and 29 amongst the 100 cases presenting in the third trimester or in association with labour. In a comparable study of 250 cases from nine published series, Weingold (1983) found 39 cases of perforation (15.6%) with a similar preponderance in late pregnancy.

The adverse effects of late diagnosis and perforation are clearly demonstrated by comparing the risk of maternal death and of perinatal loss in different circumstances. Black (1960) reported a maternal mortality rate of 4.6% and a perinatal loss of 17% amongst 373 cases of appendicitis in pregnancy and the puerperium (Table 40.4).

In the series of Babaknia et al (1977) there were no maternal deaths and a perinatal mortality rate of 1.5% amongst 263 cases of uncomplicated appendicitis but within the group of 70 patients with perforated appendix there were three deaths (4.3%) and a perinatal mortality rate of 35.7%.

Although the percentage figures for perinatal mortality vary widely between published series, an overall fetal loss of between 5 and 10% for localized appendicitis rises to over 30% with perforation and peritonitis. The increase in perinatal mortality with appendicitis in late pregnancy is a reflection of the severity of the disease and the higher likelihood of perforation in the third trimester rather than the gestational age in itself (Saunders & Milton 1973, Finch & Lee 1974, Griffen 1974).

The lesson that emerges from this accumulated experience is that early diagnosis of appendicitis in pregnancy is the key to a successful outcome. With localized disease, promptly treated, the risk to a pregnant patient is minimal and no greater than at other times. Similarly, uncomplicated appendicitis does not appear to jeopardize fetal survival, even with operation in the first trimester when the quoted fetal loss compares favourably with the background rate for spontaneous abortion.

Diagnosis in the first trimester should present little difficulty. The uterus does not yet encroach upon the abdominal cavity and the appendix remains in its normal position in the right iliac fossa. The most universal symptoms of abdominal pain and tenderness over the site of the appendix should not be overlooked provided that accompanying symptoms and signs of nausea, vomiting and distension are not dismissed as normal pregnancy features. The differential diagnosis, especially if the patient is not known to be pregnant, includes urinary tract infection, salpingitis and ectopic gestation. Many such cases will first be seen by a general surgeon and will undergo immediate laparotomy; those falling into gynaecological hands may have the benefit of a preliminary laparoscopy. Either way, the diagnosis will be confirmed or refuted and the condition treated at an early stage.

With advancing pregnancy, major changes within the abdominal cavity may obscure the classical picture of acute appendicitis and lead to serious delay in diagnosis. As demonstrated by the barium studies of Baer et al (1932), the appendix migrates upwards and laterally as the uterus enlarges and also rotates in an anticlockwise direction so that by late pregnancy the tip points towards the costal margin (Fig. 40.1). In addition, the enlarging uterus draws the abdominal wall forwards so that the appendix becomes a relatively posterior structure which is no longer in close contact with the parietal peritoneum — reminiscent of a retrocaecal or retroileal position in the non-pregnant woman.

These changes are reflected in the altered physical signs of appendicitis in the second half of pregnancy, with less clearcut localization of pain and tenderness to the right lower abdomen, less rebound tenderness, guarding and rigidity, and a tendency for symptoms to be referred to the paraumbilical and subcostal regions (Black 1960, Finch & Lee 1974). Nevertheless, the classical symptom of periumbilical pain shifting to the right iliac fossa remains the commonest presentation of appendicitis in pregnancy at any stage (Jones 1974, Babaknia et al 1977, Masters et al 1984).

The differential diagnosis encompasses all causes of abdominal pain in mid and late pregnancy, including premature labour, placental abruption, adnexal torsion, cholecystitis, pancreatitis and pyelonephritis. The last of these is a common cause of confusion because right loin pain and tenderness with pyuria may be present with late pregnancy

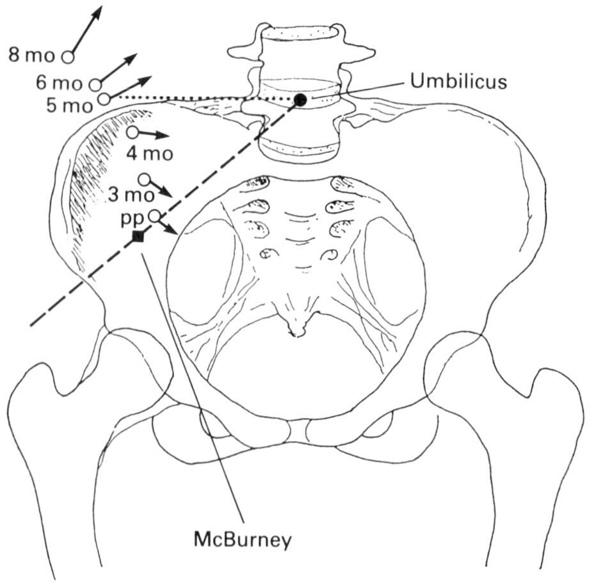

Fig. 40.1 Migration of the appendix in pregnancy (Baer et al 1932). pp = prepregnancy.

appendicitis — due to irritation of the adjacent renal pelvis — and infection of the urinary tract is a frequent complication of pregnancy in any case. A catheter specimen of urine should be examined in all doubtful cases (Black 1960, O'Neill 1969a, Babaknia et al 1977) and a diagnosis of pyelonephritis only accepted if bacteriuria and pyuria are both present. No account can be taken of body temperature in the diagnosis of appendicitis as it remains normal or is only slightly raised in two-thirds of cases (McCorriston 1963, Hermann & Simon 1983). The white blood count is similarly unhelpful as a leukocytosis of between $10 \times 10^9/l$ and $15 \times 10^9/l$ is normal in late pregnancy.

A detailed knowledge of diagnostic differences is less important than a constant awareness of the possibility of appendicitis in any pregnant woman with unexplained abdominal symptoms. Nausea and vomiting persisting beyond 20 weeks must be regarded with suspicion (Kammerer 1979) and, as in many clinical situations, a careful history will lead towards the diagnosis even before the patient is examined. A history of recurrent abdominal pain before pregnancy is not uncommon (Black 1960, Jones 1974).

Suspected appendicitis in pregnancy is *par excellence* an opportunity for co-operation between general surgeon and obstetrician, neither of whom will have encountered the two conditions together very frequently. The incidence of appendicitis in pregnancy is between 1 in 1000 and 1 in 2000 cases (McCorriston 1963, Finch & Lee 1974, Hermann & Simon 1983) and the likelihood of pregnancy amongst women admitted with appendicitis is of the order of 2% (Baer et al 1932, Jones 1974). The general surgeon needs to be conscious of the positional changes of the appendix and also of the unusual laxity of the abdominal wall in pregnancy and the obstetrician must be aware that the uterus may become tense, tender and woody-hard as a result of peritonitis or be activated into premature labour by any extrauterine abdominal pathology.

The danger resulting from delay in operating for acute appendicitis in pregnancy has been demonstrated but it is equally clear that laparotomy on suspicion, even if a normal appendix is found, carries minimal risk for patient and fetus and is a vastly preferable alternative. By adopting such a policy a correct preoperative diagnosis of between 60 and 75% can none the less be achieved, comparing favourably with rates of between 70 and 85% in the general population (O'Neill 1969a, Saunders & Milton 1973, Griffen 1974).

At operation the surgeon must be prepared to encounter more widespread disease than may be clinically suspected. Spread of the infection, especially in late pregnancy, is encouraged by the upward displacement of the appendix from the pelvis and by limitation of mobility of the omentum due to the enlarging uterus, which also interferes with localization of the inflammatory process by its intermittent muscular activity. Increased local vascularity leading to more rapid lymphatic drainage also hinders localization of the infection (Black 1960, Saunders & Milton 1973, Finch & Lee 1974). Preoperative correction of dehydration and electrolyte imbalance is vital.

Laparotomy is performed through a muscle-splitting incision centred over the site of maximum tenderness (Jones 1974, Babaknia et al 1977, Weingold 1983). Access will be improved and handling of the uterus minimized by tilting the patient 30° to the left, which also avoids caval compression (McCorriston 1963, Finch & Lee 1974). This approach provides adequate exposure and allows exploration of the right side of the abdominal cavity without having to displace the uterus by retraction. The incision can be extended by cutting the muscle if necessary. In the first trimester, if the diagnosis is in real doubt a paramedian incision is justified but such an approach could lead to serious difficulty in late pregnancy (Finch & Lee 1974).

Appendicectomy with or without drainage is the procedure of choice. If an appendix abscess is found the site is drained with a view to re-operation at a later date. A normal appendix should be removed to avoid confusion in the future.

The place of Caesarean section during an operation for appendicitis in pregnancy has been debated in the literature. The consensus view is that with uncomplicated appendicitis the uterus should be left intact even if the patient is on the verge of labour as subsequent progress towards vaginal delivery is unimpaired (Black 1960, Jones 1974, Babaknia et al 1977). A difference of opinion emerges over the correct management if general peritonitis is present; O'Neill (1969a) and Jones (1974), amongst others, argue for operative delivery because labour is likely to follow within 48 hours and stillbirth is a common result. Gomez & Wood (1979) take the opposite view that Caesarean section in the presence of widespread peritonitis is fraught with danger and should never be contemplated. Babaknia et al (1977) refer to the possibility of Caesarean hysterectomy under exceptional circumstances.

It seems clear that a decision to perform Caesarean section at the time of laparotomy for appendicitis will only be taken in the rarest of circumstances and for the most pressing obstetric indications.

Intestinal obstruction

Intestinal obstruction is a rare event in pregnancy and also an elusive diagnosis because the classical symptoms of abdominal pain, vomiting and constipation are common complaints and liable to be overlooked or passed off as normal discomforts of the pregnant state. The vague and non-descript picture in the early stages of a bowel obstruction coupled with the natural reluctance of doctors and patient to contemplate surgical exploration may lead to serious delay in diagnosis and treatment to the detriment of mother and child (DHSS 1982c). As with appendicitis, awareness of the possibility is the first step towards timely diagnosis. In this respect the sudden acute event — which then becomes a question of differential diagnosis — holds less potential danger than the insidious presentation of obstruction of the bowel, which should be considered if the apparently innocuous discomforts of early pregnancy do not resolve or appear for the first time in the later weeks of gestation, especially if the patient has an abdominal scar (Taylor 1977b).

The incidence of intestinal obstruction in pregnancy varies widely in published reports but probably lies within the range of 1 in 3000 to 1 in 6000 maternities (Morris 1965, O'Neill 1970, Pratt et al 1981, Davis & Bohon 1983). A rising incidence in recent years (Morris 1965, Hill & Symmonds 1976) has been attributed to the larger number of laparotomies performed in general, and thus a greater potential pool of cases of obstruction from adhesions. Hill & Symmonds (1976) noted that in the 1920s adhesions accounted for only 7% of hospital admissions with obstruction whereas half a century later the figure was 60%. Amongst pregnant women with obstruction the commonest preceding operations are appendicectomy (40–50%) and gynaecological procedures such as ovarian cystectomy (30–40%; Jones 1974, Hill & Symmonds 1976, Davis & Bohon 1983). Morris (1965) drew attention to the particular risks of operations for ectopic gestation and McCorriston (1963) to the sometimes forgotten dangers of previous classical Caesarean section. The possibility of adhesions from earlier episodes of pelvic inflammatory disease must not be overlooked as a focus for obstruction, even in the absence of an abdominal scar.

Next in frequency to adhesions, volvulus of the small or large bowel accounts for about 25% of cases of obstruction during pregnancy with the sigmoid colon the most common site (Lazaro et al 1968, Beck 1973, Jones 1974). Predisposing to volvulus are an elongated sigmoid loop, a narrow mesentery and a short distance between the points of fixation to the posterior abdominal wall (Hammouda 1967, Pratt et al 1981). Adhesions are often found at the site of torsion of a volvulus and are probably the primary cause of many cases of volvulus and thus of most cases of intestinal obstruction in pregnancy (Beck 1973). Volvulus of the caecum and right side of the colon arises in a similar manner to sigmoid volvulus (Pratt et al 1981) and small bowel volvulus also occurs, although it is a comparative rarity (Wanetick et al 1975).

Pratt et al (1981) state that caecal volvulus, though rare in general, accounts for between 25 and 44% of cases of volvulus in pregnancy and thus appears to be a commoner condition at such a time than in other circumstances. Contributing factors in addition to those mentioned above include distension of the right colon by faeces and gas, increased muscular activity and changes in intraperitoneal relationships, especially associated with labour and delivery, as well as hypermobility of the ileocaecal region due to failure of lateral peritoneal fixation during the period of development. In the case reported by Pratt et al (1981), laparotomy 2 days after Caesarean section revealed a partial malrotation of the small bowel, absence of the ligament of Treitz, agenesis of the left kidney and a redundant sigmoid colon. A right hemicolectomy was performed and the patient made a good recovery.

Other, though uncommon, causes of intestinal obstruction in pregnancy include intussusception, external hernias and neoplasms of the bowel in descending order of frequency and in direct contrast with the incidence in the general population amongst whom incarcerated or strangulated hernia and bowel cancer are common presentations (Hill & Symmonds 1976, Davis & Bohon 1983).

Intestinal obstruction is rare in early pregnancy, the incidence rising in the fourth and fifth months after the uterus has become an abdominal organ with distortion and stretching of pre-existing adhesions (Morris 1965). Over 50% of cases of obstruction occur in the third trimester (Wanetick et al 1975; Kammerer 1979) at a time when the fetal head is entering the pelvis and perhaps reinforcing the changing relationships in the abdominal cavity. At this time also the sheer bulk of the uterus can be a cause of obstruction to the large bowel from external pressure without any additional predisposing factor (Jones 1974). As with torsion of ovarian cysts, intestinal obstruction may also be precipitated by the rapid and major intra-abdominal changes that occur immediately after delivery (O'Neill 1970, Beck 1973, Hermann & Simon 1983).

Abdominal pain is the commonest symptom of intestinal obstruction in pregnancy, occurring in over 80% of cases (Morris 1965). It may be vague and diffuse, constant and unremitting or periodic and colicky (Hill & Symmonds 1976, Davis & Bohon 1983). If intermittent, an interval of 4–5 minutes is characteristic of small bowel obstruction and 10–15 minutes if the obstruction is lower down (Hill & Symmonds 1976). A severe and steady pain is suggestive of strangulation, especially if accompanied by rebound tenderness and rigidity which are unusual with mechanical obstruction unless gangrene and perforation are imminent (Jones 1974, Davis & Bohon 1983).

Vomiting is the second cardinal symptom of obstruction of the bowel but though an early feature of high level lesions, it may be delayed or absent with closed loop obstruction unless strangulation occurs, when persistent vomiting is the rule (Morris 1965). Morris also warned that there may be a delay in the resumption of vomiting after the first attack even when there is complete obstruction. With such a common symptom of pregnancy the character of the vomiting is significant requiring investigation if it appears after the first trimester, if it is continuous and if the material is dark green or faeculent (Jones 1974).

Constipation completes the classical triad of symptoms of intestinal obstruction and is an early complaint in most cases, but the patient may have several bowel actions after she has developed a high-level obstruction (Morris 1965, Davis & Bohon 1983) and diarrhoea may occur with strangulation (Lazaro et al 1968). Eventually the constipation is total, despite enemas.

Clinical examination of the abdomen in late pregnancy is hampered by the enlarged uterus and laxity of the abdominal wall which will obscure the gaseous distension characteristic of large bowel obstruction and volvulus and also mask the presence of an abdominal mass (Hill & Symmonds 1976). Both of these physical signs may be revealed only after delivery (Morris 1965, Jones 1974). Abdominal tenderness — an ominous sign in obstruction, suggesting bowel necrosis — may be ascribed to a uterine lesion such as placental abruption as the involved intestine is concealed posteriorly (Lazaro et al 1968). This is a situation when Alders' sign may be of great help. Percussion of the abdomen is a neglected art amongst obstetricians; it can be invaluable, especially if volvulus is suspected and auscultation may detect the increase in bowel sounds characteristic of obstruction or the silence of secondary paralytic ileus.

Apart from concealed antepartum haemorrhage, acute pancreatitis and cholecystitis are the main conditions to be considered in the differential diagnosis but potentially the most serious error is to confuse the intermittent colic of small bowel obstruction with the onset of normal labour (Hammouda 1967, Griffen 1974, Simmons & Luck 1984). Uterine monitoring should prevent this mistake but it must never be forgotten that the two conditions could coexist, as labour can be precipitated by the acute abdomen and, conversely, a latent obstruction may become complete during the course of spontaneous labour. If there is any suspicion of intestinal obstruction erect and supine abdominal X-rays should be ordered. These are not always helpful but may clinch the diagnosis if a volvulus is present (Jones 1974).

Malkasian et al (1959) have described the successful reduction of a sigmoid volvulus in late pregnancy by decompression with a rectal tube but this option is rarely applicable and early laparotomy in suspected intestinal obstruction regardless of the stage of the pregnancy is the safest course for mother and child (Hill & Symmonds 1976). Preoperative attention to fluid and electrolyte balance is essential to combat maternal shock, which is often present as a consequence of delay in diagnosis in late pregnancy (Kammerer 1979). An ample vertical incision is required depending on the suspected site of the obstruction and the appropriate surgery to the bowel carried out as in a non-pregnant patient (Davis & Bohon 1983). Occasionally a Caesarean section is required in order to gain adequate access to the surgical field (Beck 1973, Hermann & Simon 1983) but if division of adhesions, correction and stabilization of a volvulus or bowel resection can be performed without disturbing the pregnancy this is preferable. The subsequent course of labour, even within a few days of major surgery, can be quite straightforward (Hill & Symmonds 1976, Taylor 1977b).

The maternal mortality from intestinal obstruction in pregnancy varies between 10 and 20% and the fetal loss between 30 and 50% (Kammerer 1979). Such unacceptable statistics will be improved by early diagnosis on suspicion, close attention to biochemical stabilization and laparotomy without delay.

Carcinoma of the colon and rectum

As may be expected from the age group concerned, cancer of the bowel is extremely rare in association with pregnancy, accounting for no more than 5% of cases of intestinal obstruction in pregnant women (Morris 1965, Jones 1974). In the absence of obstruction the onset is insidious with vague abdominal pain and distension, cramps, constipation and rectal bleeding (O'Leary et al 1967, Girard et al 1981). Being such a rarity the diagnosis is often delayed but should be considered in any patient with colonic symptoms, especially if there are factors predisposing to malignancy such as chronic ulcerative colitis and familial polyposis, which usually do appear in the obstetric age group (Green et al 1975).

Peptic ulcer

Complications of peptic ulcer are rarely seen in pregnancy and the majority of women with a pre-existing ulcer experience a remission of symptoms (Clark 1953). Peptic ulcer arising for the first time during a pregnancy is extremely uncommon in the UK. These facts are partly explained by reduced gastric activity and acid secretion — a probable effect of circulating hormones on the gastric mucosa and also of a rise in plasma histaminase of placental origin blocking acid production from the parietal cells (Becker-Andersen & Husfeldt 1971, Hermann & Simon 1983). However, the main reasons for symptomatic improvement during pregnancy are probably a more careful diet, closer medical supervision and adequate rest (Jones et al 1969, Fagan & Chadwick 1984a).

The rarity of ulcer complications during pregnancy may delay diagnosis but they should be anticipated if a patient known to have an ulcer does not obtain the expected relief of her symptoms as pregnancy continues. Ulcer perforation and haemorrhage can occur — usually in the third trimester — and require appropriate resuscitation and urgent laparotomy. The evidence for perforation is usually clearcut, with acute epigastric or substernal pain, a rigid silent abdomen and clinical shock. Due to the laxity of the abdominal muscles the rigidity may not be as board-like as in the non-pregnant patient but the diagnosis is rarely in doubt. Ulcer haemorrhage will manifest itself by haematemesis and increasing signs of circulatory collapse depending on the amount of internal bleeding.

Although suture of perforated ulcer during pregnancy had previously been described, Burkitt (1961) reported the first emergency gastrectomy for what he described as an 'enormous perforation' of a duodenal ulcer at 31 weeks' gestation. Subsequently Becker-Andersen & Husfeldt (1971) reviewed 31 perforations and 30 cases of ulcer haemorrhage during pregnancy, 17 of the perforations were treated conservatively with a fatal outcome in all cases, whereas the 14 patients receiving surgery all recovered. This consisted of simple closure in 13 cases — two with Caesarean section — and partial gastrectomy in one case. Only 3 infants were lost amongst the surgical group compared with 11 in the group treated conservatively. Similarly, surgical treatment is preferable to conservative measures in the management of upper gastrointestinal haemorrhage. In Becker-Andersen & Husfeldt's series 7 of 16 patients treated without operation died, compared with 2 deaths amongst 14 patients treated surgically, mainly by partial gastrectomy. Surgical treatment of ulcer haemorrhage was also safer for the fetus than conservative management though the difference in perinatal mortality was not as clearcut as with perforation.

The superiority of surgical over medical treatment for the rare complications of peptic ulceration during pregnancy is evident from the above review and from other publications (Jones et al 1969, Jones 1974, Hermann & Simon 1983, Fagan & Chadwick 1984a). Caesarean section may occasionally be indicated at the time of surgery during the third trimester either for fetal distress or to gain easier access to the operative field, especially if gastrectomy rather than simple closure of a perforation is to be undertaken (Jones et al 1969, Fagan & Chadwick 1984a).

Cholecystitis

In contrast with the rarity of peptic ulceration during pregnancy, symptoms from gallbladder disease are relatively common. Next to appendicectomy cholecystectomy is the most frequent non-gynaecological abdominal operation performed on pregnant women (O'Neill 1969b, Simon 1983) at a rate of 1–6 cases in 10 000 pregnancies (Hill et al 1975, Kammerer 1979). More than half of the patients have symptoms dating from before the pregnancy and, contrary to traditional teaching, are usually of normal weight (Hill et al 1975).

Pregnancy encourages the formation of gallstones as a result of stasis in the biliary tract and increased secretion of lithogenic bile (Printen & Ott 1978, Fagan & Chadwick 1984b). Biliary stasis is demonstrated by reduced motility of the gallbladder wall, an increase in gallbladder volume during fasting and also in the residual volume after food (Braverman et al 1980, Simon 1983). During pregnancy there is a rise in the cholesterol saturation in the bile and, conversely, a reduction in the total bile acid pool — in particular of chenodeoxycholic acid — and this alteration in the proportions of cholesterol and bile acids predisposes the pregnant woman to an increase in the size of existing stones or the formation of new cholesterol stones (Printen & Ott 1978, Simon 1983). These changes in the composition of bile and in gallbladder function are probably due to the rise in circulating oestrogens and progesterone during pregnancy but doubt remains as to whether there is a true increase in the frequency of cholelithiasis and cholecystitis in pregnancy compared with a matched non-pregnant population (Hill et al 1975, Kammerer 1979, Hermann & Simon 1983).

The clinical features of gallbladder disease in pregnancy are no different from those in non-pregnant women. The patient complains of sharp stabbing or a constant pain in the epigastrium and right subcostal region radiating to the right shoulder or loin (Printen & Ott 1978, Simon 1983). These symptoms are usually accompanied by nausea and vomiting. Jaundice is unusual as stones in the common duct account for only 5% of cases of jaundice in pregnant women (Kammerer 1979, Fagan & Chadwick 1984b). Cases are evenly distributed throughout pregnancy and are relatively easy to diagnose in the early weeks in view of the probable past history of similar attacks, the radiation of the pain and the appropriate costal tenderness on inspiration (Murphy's sign). From mid-pregnancy onwards anatomical changes make the clinical picture less clearcut and liable to confusion with appendicitis which, being a far commoner condition, is the most important differential diagnosis. Other rarer possibilities to be considered are acute peptic ulceration, pancreatitis, myocardial infarction and pneumonia (Printen & Ott 1978, Simon 1983).

Cholangiography, with its radiation hazards, has now been largely replaced by ultrasound in the diagnosis of gallbladder disease in pregnancy. Ultrasound can confirm or refute the presence of gallstones with a high degree of accuracy (Anderson et al 1976).

The management of gallbladder disease in pregnancy is largely medical with a view to definitive surgery at some time after delivery. The patient is treated with bedrest, sedation, nasogastric suction and intravenous fluids. Antibiotics are sometimes required but the use of chenodeoxycholic acid to dissolve gallstones is contraindicated, certainly in early pregnancy, whilst doubt exists about its safety for the developing fetus (Kammerer 1979, Fagan & Chadwick 1984b). Cholecystectomy, postponed if possible to the second trimester, is indicated in the presence of obstruction to the common duct, cholangitis, pancreatitis and empyema of the gallbladder or if the condition fails to improve on conservative treatment (Hill et al 1975, Printen & Ott 1978, Hermann & Simon 1983). Laparotomy is also mandatory if there is doubt about the diagnosis and appendicitis cannot be ruled out.

Pancreatitis

Acute pancreatitis is a rare occurrence in pregnancy but being a serious condition with a high morbidity and mortality it must be considered in the differential diagnosis of upper abdominal pain in a pregnant patient. The incidence varies between 1 in 1000 and 1 in 11 000 pregnancies (Corlett & Mishell 1972, Wilkinson 1973, Thomason et al 1980) with an average figure of about 1 in 4000 deliveries (Jouppila et al 1974, McKay et al 1980). The aetiology is discussed by Berk et al (1971) who noted the relatively low incidence of alcoholism as an associated factor amongst pregnant women compared with non-pregnant patients and, conversely, the high incidence of gallstones in cases of pancreatitis in pregnancy. The use of thiazide diuretics appears as a significant precipitating factor in reviews of cases of acute pancreatitis in pregnancy (Berk et al 1971, Corlett & Mishell 1972, Wilkinson 1973) but should cease to be relevant as such substances are now much less used in modern antenatal management (Griffen 1974). Stasis in the biliary tract, already discussed in the aetiology of gallstones in pregnancy, may be an effect of progesterone producing hypotonia in the bile ducts and allowing reflux of bile along the pancreatic duct (Jouppila et al 1974, Fagan & Chadwick 1984b). A similar effect might be produced by bouts of vomiting in severe pre-eclampsia, causing a rise of intra-abdominal pressure leading to disruption of pancreatic ducts and release of enzymes (Berk et al 1971, Fagan & Chadwick 1984b).

Acute pancreatitis usually occurs in late pregnancy or soon after delivery. The clinical picture is no different from that in a non-pregnant patient but is liable to be overlooked because nausea, vomiting and abdominal discomfort are common symptoms. Repeated vomiting is characteristic and may be treated as hyperemesis gravidarum, but the stage of pregnancy and the increasing epigastric pain and tenderness should raise suspicions of the true diagnosis (Jones 1974). Ultrasonography is a safe and highly reliable technique for the diagnosis of pancreatic as well as biliary disease in pregnancy (Anderson et al 1976, McKay et al 1980) and has replaced contrast radiology of the biliary tract. The discovery of gallstones as a cause of the pancreatitis — probable in 40–50% of cases — allows the option of early cholectystectomy to be considered in mid-pregnancy if the pancreatitis has unusually occurred in the first or second trimesters or as a planned procedure soon after delivery (McKay et al 1980).

Although an elevated serum amylase level is recorded in many cases of acute pancreatitis in pregnancy and is a valuable diagnostic test (Corlett & Mishell 1972), false negative results may occur if the blood is taken 24–72 hours after the attack or in acute haemorrhagic pancreatitis with massive necrosis (Wilkinson 1973). For this reason Fagan & Chadwick (1984b) recommend the measurement of the ratio of renal clearance of amylase to creatinine as diagnostically more valuable than the serum ratios of these substances. Strickland et al (1984) have found that serum amylase levels may be as high as 150 iu/l in normal pregnant women but are unrelated to gestational age and not accompanied by a rise in serum amylase isoenzyme activity in normal women. They thus infer that the serum amylase activity remains the single most useful diagnostic test for pancreatitis in pregnant as well as non-pregnant patients.

The management of acute pancreatitis in pregnancy is identical with that in the non-pregnant patient and is based on the objectives of the prevention and treatment of shock; suppression of pancreatic activity; relief of pain; prevention and treatment of infection; and diagnosis and treatment of surgical complication (Wilkinson 1973). Fagan & Chadwick (1984b) throw doubt on the use of nasogastric suction which, although traditional, is of no proven value and may even cause a rise in serum amylase levels. These authors also itemize the various therapeutic agents used as inhibitors of pancreatic secretion, including anticholinergic drugs, steroids, prostaglandins, glucagon, cimetidine and trypsin inhibitors, none of which are of proven benefit although all have been associated with clinical improvement in individual cases (Berk et al 1971, Corlett & Mishell 1972, Wilkinson 1973, Jouppila et al 1974, McKay et al 1980, Thomason et al 1980).

As with many medical complications of pregnancy, neither early induction of labour nor therapeutic abortion influences the course of the disease and delivery should not be hastened unless there are adequate obstetric indications (Wilkinson 1973, Jouppila et al 1974, McKay et al 1980).

RENAL AND URETERIC COLIC

The quoted incidence of urinary calculus in association with pregnancy ranges from 1 in 300 to 1 in 3800 deliveries, with a probable average occurrence of about 1 in 1500 pregnancies (Strong et al 1978, Lattanzi & Cook 1980, Gabert & Miller 1985). This is the same incidence as in the general population (Klein 1984); similarly, calcium stones predominate whilst uric acid and cystine stones are only found in 10% of cases (Gabert & Miller 1985). Urinary calculi, particularly when sited in the kidney or renal pelvis, may be silent during pregnancy and only come to light during postnatal investigation or recurrent or resistant urinary infection, especially when due to *Proteus mirabilis* or *Pseudomonas aeruginosa* (Meares 1978).

Nevertheless, renal or ureteric colic may occur as a dramatic and acute incident predominantly in the second and third trimesters and, interestingly, more frequently in multiparous than in primigravid patients — possibly an effect of age (Lattanzi & Cook 1980, Klein 1984). Unlike the pain of pyelonephritis, which may be difficult to distinguish from that due to other lesions — particularly when right-sided — urinary colic is relatively easy to differentiate and the diagnosis is usually correctly made, especially in patients with a history of a recent or recurrent urinary infection (Cumming & Taylor 1979).

The majority of patients present with acute loin pain upon which abdominal colic is superimposed and there is usually associated tenderness in the costovertebral angle and in the abdomen, mainly towards the lower quadrant. Stones occur on the left and right sides with equal frequency despite the predominance of stasis and urinary tract dilatation on the right side during pregnancy (Lattanzi & Cook 1980, Klein 1984). Although gross haematuria is uncommon microscopic haematuria with or without an active urinary infection is present in the majority (Klein 1984). Despite an admirable clinical reluctance to expose the fetus to X-radiation during pregnancy, such an examination is eminently justified when a stone is suspected, particularly for patients with resistant urinary infections associated with persistent pain (Strong et al 1978). The investigation judiciously performed as a modified intravenous urogram with one film taken at 20 minutes will clinch the diagnosis in the majority, as 90% of stones contain calcium (Meares 1978, Strong et al 1978, Cumming & Taylor 1979).

Due presumably to the physiological dilatation of the ureters there is a 50% rate of spontaneous passage of urinary calculi in pregnancy (Strong et al 1978, Cumming & Taylor 1979, Lattanzi & Cook 1980). Thus, if the diagnosis is not in doubt, conservative management is justified and if surgical treatment has to be entertained this can usually be postponed until after delivery, assuming that in the meantime the urine can be kept essentially sterile by appropriate and continuous antibacterial treatment (Meares 1978, Lattanzi & Cook 1980, Klein 1984). Fortunately, open-access surgery is becoming rapidly obsolete in the field of urology with the development of closed urethral lithotrity for bladder stones and the increasing accessibility of the interior of the ureter by means of the ureterorenoscope for removal of stones (and tumours). Pressure in the pelvis or the kidney can be relieved by the procedures of percutaneous nephrolithotomy with extracorporeal shock-wave lithotripsy (Wickham 1987). Such developments, apart from the last, may well have a place for the small number of patients who require urgent surgical relief of urinary tract obstruction before the pregnancy is over, though none has yet been evaluated for such a purpose.

INTRA-ABDOMINAL HAEMORRHAGE

Haematoma of the rectus abdominis muscle

Bleeding into the rectus muscle and haematoma formation from rupture of a branch of the inferior epigastric artery may occur after a bout of coughing or without obvious trauma in late pregnancy, producing acute abdominal symptoms and signs of spreading subperitoneal haemorrhage (Shepherd 1982a). A large unilateral painful swelling develops behind the rectus muscle; it may be confused with a twisted ovarian cyst, degenerating fibroid, rupture of the uterus or concealed accidental haemorrhage (Jones 1974). The swelling is often visible and is acutely tender. Depending on its position it may appear to be directly subcutaneous or as deeply situated as the uterus. The diagnosis may only become obvious on abdominal exploration when the rectus sheath is incised and the haematoma evacuated (Shepherd 1982a).

Hepatic rupture

Spontaneous rupture of the liver, a rare complication of severe pre-eclampsia or eclampsia, is an occasional cause of major abdominal haemorrhage in late pregnancy or the immediate puerperium. Though an extremely uncommon condition, sporadic case reports have accumulated in the literature and have been comprehensively reviewed by Bis & Waxman (1976) who found 89 published cases and added 2 of their own. Recent case reports and shorter reviews by Hibbard (1976), Baumwol & Park (1976), Nelson et al (1977) and Golan & White (1979) supplement Bis & Waxman's study and allow a picture to emerge of the typical presentation of hepatic rupture in pregnancy.

The patient is over 30, multiparous and almost invariably suffering from pregnancy-induced hypertension. The onset is usually sudden and dramatic with severe epigastric or right upper abdominal pain radiating to the back and shoulder rapidly followed by signs of intraperitoneal bleeding and peripheral circulatory failure. The diagnosis is rarely made before laparotomy, undertaken in most cases for presumed abruptio placentae or rupture of the uterus as the fetal and maternal conditions deteriorate (Simon 1983).

The typical findings at operation or autopsy are of rupture of a subcapsular haematoma, predominantly of the right lobe of the liver and usually confined to the anterior and upper surfaces of the lobe (Bis & Waxman 1976). It is presumed that the periportal necrosis following fibrin deposition in the hepatic sinusoids and arterioles in severe pre-eclampsia and eclampsia results in areas of microscopic haemorrhage beneath Glisson's capsule; this may produce distension and right upper abdominal tenderness but these usually resolve after delivery. In rare cases however these areas of scattered haemorrhage enlarge and coalesce to produce a subcapsular haematoma (Baumwol & Park 1976, Nelson et al 1977). Enlargement of the haematoma and rupture may be precipitated by vomiting, an eclamptic fit, contractions of the uterus during labour and by disseminated intravascular coagulation. In addition the reduction of intra-abdominal pressure when the peritoneum is incised may produce a sudden catastrophic increase in bleeding from the liver substance (Golan & White 1979).

The treatment of hepatic rupture depends on the operative findings. Immediate compression of the hepatic artery and portal vein allows some respite to explore the damage and also to deliver the child by Caesarean section. Methods of controlling the bleeding include evacuation of the haematoma and simple pressure, packing, direct ligation of bleeding vessels, deep hepatic sutures and, if unavoidable, lobectomy (Herbert & Brenner 1982, Simon 1983).

Bis & Waxman (1976) report a maternal mortality of 59% and a fetal loss of 62% in their review of 91 cases of hepatic rupture in pregnancy. Improved survival for mother and infant can be achieved by earlier diagnosis of subclinical hepatic damage in patients with pre-eclampsia, using ultrasound and by modern methods of circulatory support and surgical repair (Herbert & Brenner 1982).

Epigastric pain in pre-eclampsia

The epigastric pain and tenderness traditionally associated with fulminating pre-eclampsia probably represents a prodromal phase leading in the direction of hepatic rupture, though such a catastrophic outcome is exceptional. The mechanism is a matter for speculation but is likely to be initially similar, with deposition of fibrin thrombi in and around the hepatic sinusoids and associated haemorrhagic necrosis leading to subcapsular bleeding and thus distension of the liver to a greater or lesser degree (Nelson et al 1977, Sommer et al 1979). Only if the necrosis becomes confluent and extensive is rupture likely to occur. Otherwise presumably small areas of haemorrhage and necrosis resolve and the upper abdominal pain, which may wax and wane in intensity, eventually disappears as the patient recovers.

Rupture of utero-ovarian veins

Haemorrhage from veins on the surface of the uterus, though rare, may confront the obstetrician as an unexpected cause of acute abdominal pain and collapse during pregnancy. Hodgkinson & Christensen (1950) have reviewed 75 reported cases of ruptured utero-ovarian veins in pregnancy since 1902, including three of their own patients. Haemorrhage was intraperitoneal, with generalized signs of peritoneal irritation, or retroperitoneal producing an enormous haematoma, loin pain and severe shock. The mortality was 50%. In most cases the diagnosis was made at autopsy with the discovery of torn varicosities on or near the uterus. Possibly a rise of venous pressure in the already dilated vascular network was precipitated by uterine action or other muscular activity, including lifting, defecation and coitus, though in many cases the reason for such a catastrophic event would only be speculative.

This subject was reviewed again by Finch (1956), reporting the spontaneous rupture of a uterine varix at 28 weeks' gestation and more recently by Cordiner et al (1973) and by Estep & Dettling (1974), both of whose patients survived after massive haemorrhage from ruptured uterine veins at 29 and 37 weeks' gestation, though the infants were stillborn.

Arterial haemorrhage

The overall reduction in maternal mortality in recent years throws into relative prominence uncommon causes of maternal death. The Report on Confidential Enquiries into Maternal Deaths in England and Wales 1976–1978 and 1979–1981 (DHSS 1982d, 1986c) include nine cases of ruptured abdominal aneurysm amongst 651 maternal deaths during pregnancy or the puerperium (1.4%). Three arose from the splenic artery and one each from the hepatic and renal arteries. There were four cases of dissecting aortic aneurysm, one of which was associated with Marfan's syndrome.

Splenic artery aneurysms, which are two to four times as common in women than men (O'Grady et al 1977, Hermann & Simon 1983) figure most prominently in the literature of ruptured abdominal aneurysms in pregnancy (Macfarlane & Thorbjarnarson 1966, Gibbens & Heath 1974, O'Grady et al 1977, Barrett & Caldwell 1981). The aetiology of rupture of splenic artery aneurysms in pregnancy is discussed by O'Grady et al (1977) who noted that 20% of all reported ruptures have occurred in pregnant women, the majority in the third trimester. Gibbens & Heath (1974), noting a maternal mortality of 69% and a fetal mortality of 97% in published reports, presented the first case of maternal and fetal survival in Britain and the third recorded in the literature. In the study of O'Grady et al (1977), which included the fourth case of dual survival, in none of the 90 cases previously reported was an accurate diagnosis made until laparotomy. All survivors had undergone ligation of the aneurysm and splenectomy.

Although the clinical presentation of acute abdominal pain and increasing signs of shock is common to all forms of intraperitoneal bleeding, splenic artery aneurysm rupture may be preceded by a history of recurrent left upper abdominal discomfort (Schug & Rankin 1965). Ring-like calcification in the splenic area on abdominal X-ray would suggest the diagnosis, though such an investigation is unlikely to be ordered in the circumstances.

Depending on the location of the aneurysm, bleeding may at first be restricted to the lesser sac with initial shock and temporary recovery as partial tamponade occurs (Schug & Rankin 1965, O'Grady et al 1977). Later secondary rupture through the foramen of Winslow in minutes or days will produce more catastrophic intraperitoneal haemorrhage, presenting the picture of double rupture (Schug & Rankin 1965, Gibbens & Heath 1974). The latent period might allow time for preliminary rescuscitation whilst urgent preparations for laparotomy are made.

Control of haemorrhage from a ruptured splenic artery aneurysm involves ligation of the splenic artery in continuity proximal to the site of bleeding, isolation of the splenic pedicle and splenectomy (Shepherd 1982b, Hermann & Simon 1983). The assistance of an experienced abdominal or vascular surgeon should be sought if time permits, as the exposure of the hilum of the spleen is likely to be hampered by the profuse haemorrhage from an unfamiliar source and by the presence of the gravid uterus. As the majority of cases occur in late pregnancy delivery of the child by Caesarean section will be required to permit adequate exploration of the upper abdomen.

REFERENCES

Abdella T N, Sibai B H, Hays J M, Anderson G D 1984 Relationship of hypertensive disease to abruptio placentae. Obstetrics and Gynecology 63: 365–370

Alders N 1951 A sign for differentiating uterine from extra-uterine complications of pregnancy and puerperium. British Medical Journal 2: 1194–1195

Anderson J M, Lee T G, Nagel N 1976 Ultrasonic diagnosis of nonobstetric disease in pregnancy. Obstetrics and Gynecology 48: 359–362

Babaknia A, Parsa H, Woodruff J D 1977 Appendicitis during pregnancy. Obstetrics and Gynecology 50: 40–44

Baer J L, Reis R A, Arens R A 1932 Appendicitis in pregnancy with changes in position and axis of the normal appendix in pregnancy. Journal of the American Medical Association 98: 1359–1364

Barrett J M, Caldwell B H 1981 Association of portal hypertension and ruptured splenic artery aneurysm in pregnancy. Obstetrics and Gynecology 57: 255–257

Barter R H, Parks J 1958 Myomas in pregnancy. Clinical Obstetrics and Gynecology 1: 519–533

Basu H K 1969 Fibrinolysis and abruptio placentae. Journal of Obstetrics and Gynaecology of the British Commonwealth 76: 481–496

Baumwol M, Park W 1976 An acute abdomen: spontaneous rupture of liver during pregnancy. British Journal of Surgery 63: 718–720

Beck W W 1973 Intestinal obstruction in pregnancy. Obstetrics and Gynecology 43: 374–378

Becker-Andersen H, Husfeldt V 1971 Peptic ulcer in pregnancy: report of 2 cases of surgically treated bleeding duodenal ulcer. Acta Obstetricia et Gynecologica Scandinavica 50: 391–395

Beischer N A, Buttery B W, Fortune B W, Macafee C A J 1971 Growth and malignancy of ovarian tumours in pregnancy. Australian and New Zealand Journal of Obstetrics and Gynaecology 11: 208–220

Berk J E, Smith B H, Akrawi M M 1971 Pregnancy pancreatitis. American Journal of Gastroenterology 56: 216–226

Bis K A, Waxman B 1976 Rupture of the liver associated with pregnancy: a review of the literature and report of 2 cases. Obstetrical and Gynecological Survey 31: 763–773

Black W P 1960 Acute appendicitis in pregnancy. British Medical Journal 1: 1938–1941

Blair R G 1973 Abruption of the placenta. Journal of Obstetrics and Gynaecology of the British Commonwealth 80: 242–245

Braverman D Z, Johnson M L, Kern F 1980 Effects of pregnancy and contraceptive steroids on gallbladder function. New England Journal of Medicine 302: 362–364

Burkitt R 1961 Perforated peptic ulcer in late pregnancy. British Medical Journal 2: 938–939

Caughey A F, Higuera J G, Mohajer R 1965 Torsion of the normal pregnant uterus. Report of a case. Obstetrics and Gynecology 26: 344–345

Cavanagh D, Membery J H, McLeod A G W 1965 Rupture of the gravid uterus: an appraisal. Obstetrics and Gynecology 26: 157–164

Chambers J T, Thiagarajah S, Kitchin J D 1979 Torsion of the normal fallopian tube in pregnancy. Obstetrics and Gynecology 54: 487–489

Chung A, Birnbaum S J 1973 Ovarian cancer associated with pregnancy. Obstetrics and Gynecology 41: 211–214

Clark D H 1953 Peptic ulcer in women. British Medical Journal 1: 1254–1257

Cordiner J W, Low R A L, McKay Hart D, Smith I S 1973 Spontaneous haemoperitoneum in pregnancy due to rupture of a uterine vein. Journal of Obstetrics and Gynaecology of the British Commonwealth 80: 940–941

Corlett R C, Mishell D R 1972 Pancreatitis in pregnancy. American Journal of Obstetrics and Gynecology 113: 281–290

Cumming D C, Taylor P J 1979 Urologic and obstetric significance of urinary calculi in pregnancy. Obstetrics and Gynecology 53: 505–508

Davis M R, Bohon C J 1983 Intestinal obstruction in pregnancy. Clinical Obstetrics and Gynecology 26: 832–841

Department of Health and Social Security 1979 Report on Confidential Enquiries into Maternal Deaths in England and Wales 1973–1975. HMSO, London, pp 88–92

Department of Health and Social Security 1982a Report on Confidential Enquiries into Maternal Deaths in England and Wales 1976–1978. HMSO, London, p 26

Department of Health and Social Security 1982b Report on Confidential Enquiries into Maternal Deaths in England and Wales 1976–1978. HMSO, London, pp 88–95

Department of Health and Social Security 1982c Report on Confidential Enquiries into Maternal Deaths in England and Wales 1976–1978. HMSO, London, pp 120–121

Department of Health and Social Security 1982d Report on Confidential Enquiries into Maternal Deaths in England and Wales 1976–1978. HMSO, London, p 116

Department of Health and Social Security 1986a Report on Confidential Enquiries into Maternal Deaths in England and Wales 1979–1981. HMSO, London, pp 22–29

Department of Health and Social Security 1986b Report on Confidential Enquiries into Maternal Deaths in England and Wales 1979–1981. HMSO, London, p 103

Department of Health and Social Security 1986c Report on Confidential Enquiries into Maternal Deaths in England and Wales 1979–1981. HMSO, London, p 101

Donald I 1979a Abruptio placentae. In: Practical obstetric problems. Lloyd Luke, London, pp 455–479

Donald I 1979b Uterine rupture. In: Practical obstetric problems. Lloyd Luke, London, pp 795–804

Donald I 1979c Fibroids and pregnancy. In: Practical obstetric problems. Lloyd Luke, London, pp 263–268

Estep E, Dettling J J 1974 Spontaneous rupture of vein of gravid uterus. Obstetrics and Gynecology 43: 573–575

Fagan E A, Chadwick V S 1984a Disorders of gastrointestinal tract, pancreas and hepato-biliary system. In: de Swiet M (ed) Medical disorders in obstetric practice. Blackwell Scientific Publications, Oxford, pp 276–277

Fagan E A, Chadwick V S 1984b Disorders of gastrointestinal tract, pancreas and hepato-biliary system. In: de Swiet M (ed) Medical disorders in obstetric practice. Blackwell Scientific Publications, Oxford, pp 322–325

Felmus L B, Pedowitz P, Nassberg S 1953 Spontaneous rupture of the apparently normal uterus during pregnancy: a review. Obstetrical and Gynecological Survey 8: 155–172

Finch D R A, Lee E 1974 Acute appendicitis complicating pregnancy in the Oxford region. British Journal of Surgery 61: 129–132

Finch T V 1956 Spontaneous rupture of a uterine varix at 28 weeks pregnancy. American Journal of Obstetrics and Gynecology 72: 1189–1190

Gabert H A, Miller J M 1985 Renal disease in pregnancy. Obstetrical and Gynecological Survey 40: 449

Garnet J D 1964 Uterine rupture during pregnancy: an analysis of 133 patients. Obstetrics and Gynecology 23: 898–905

Gibbens D, Heath D 1974 Ruptured aneurysm of splenic artery in pregnancy. British Medical Journal 4: 103–104

Girard R M, Lamarche J, Baillot R 1981 Carcinoma of the colon associated with pregnancy: report of a case. Diseases of the Colon and Rectum 24: 473–475

Glassman O 1959 Spasm of the round ligaments in pregnancy. New York State Journal of Medicine 59: 1541–1545

Golan A, White R G 1979 Spontaneous rupture of the liver associated with pregnancy. South African Medical Journal 56: 133–136

Gomez A, Wood M 1979 Acute appendicitis during pregnancy. American Journal of Surgery 137: 180–183

Goplerud C P, Hanson G E 1965 Torsion of adnexa in pregnancy: report of 2 cases. Obstetrics and Gynecology 25: 209–212

Graber E A 1974a Surgery of the uterus in pregnancy. In: Barber H R K, Graber E A (eds) Surgical diseases in pregnancy. W B Saunders, Philadelphia, pp 375–395

Graber E A 1974b Ovarian tumors in pregnancy. In: Barber H R K, Graber E A (eds) Surgical diseases in pregnancy. W B Saunders, Philadelphia, pp 428–439

Grannum P A 1983 Ultrasound examination of the placenta. Clinics in Obstetrics and Gynaecology 10: 459–473

Green L K, Harris R E, Massey F M 1975 Cancer of the colon during pregnancy: a review of the literature and report of a case associated with ulcerative colitis. Obstetrics and Gynecology 46: 480–483

Griffen W O 1974 Surgery of the gastro-intestinal tract in pregnancy. In: Barber H R K, Graber E A (eds) Surgical diseases in pregnancy. W B Saunders, Philadelphia, pp 85–93

Hammouda A A 1967 Acute intestinal obstruction during pregnancy: a brief review and report of 2 cases. Australian and New Zealand Journal of Obstetrics and Gynaecology 7: 101–103

Herbert W N P, Brenner W E 1982 Improved survival with liver rupture complicating pregnancy. American Journal of Obstetrics and Gynecology 142: 530–534

Hermann G, Simon J S 1983 Nonobstetric abdominal surgery. In: Abrams R S, Wexler P (eds) Medical care of the pregnant patient. Little, Brown, Boston, pp 219–227

Hibbard L T 1976 Spontaneous rupture of the liver in pregnancy: a report of 8 cases. American Journal of Obstetrics and Gynecology 126: 334–338

Hill L M, Symmonds R E 1976 Small bowel obstruction in pregnancy: a review and report of 4 cases. Obstetrics and Gynecology 49: 170–173

Hill L M, Johnson C E, Lee R A 1975 Cholecystectomy in pregnancy. Obstetrics and Gynecology 46: 291–293

Hodgkinson C P, Christensen R C 1950 Haemorrhage from ruptured utero-ovarian veins during pregnancy. American Journal of Obstetrics and Gynecology 59: 1112–1117

Horowitz B J, Edelstein S W, Lippman L 1981 Once a caesarean . . . always a caesarean. Obstetrical and Gynecological Survey 36 (suppl): 592–598

Hurd W W, Miodovnik M, Hertzberg V, Lavin J P 1983 Selective management of abruptio placentae; a prospective study. Obstetrics and Gynecology 61: 467–473

Jones P J 1974 The acute abdomen in pregnancy and the puerperium. In: Emergency abdominal surgery in infancy, childhood and adult life. Blackwell Scientific, Oxford, pp 598–620

Jones P F, McEwan A B, Bernard R M 1969 Haemorrhage and perforation complicating peptic ulcer in pregnancy. Lancet ii: 350–352

Jouppila P, Mokka R, Larmi T K I 1974 Acute pancreatitis in pregnancy. Surgery, Gynecology and Obstetrics 139: 879–882

Jubb E D 1963 Primary ovarian cancer in pregnancy. American Journal of Obstetrics and Gynecology 85: 345–354

Kammerer W S 1979 Nonobstetric surgery during pregnancy. Medical Clinics of North America 63: 1157–1164

Karlen J R, Akbari A, Cook W A 1979 Dysgerminoma associated with pregnancy. Obstetrics and Gynecology 53: 330–335

Klein E A 1984 Urologic problems of pregnancy. Obstetrical and Gynecological Survey 39: 605–615

Lalos O, Lundstrom P, Probst F P 1977 Spontaneous rupture of the uterus in the third trimester with a living fetus expelled into the abdominal cavity. Acta Obstetricia et Gynecologica Scandinavica 56: 153–156

Lattanzi D R, Cook W A 1980 Urinary calculi in pregnancy. Obstetrics and Gynecology 56: 462–466

Lazaro E J, Das P B, Abraham P V 1968 Volvulus of the sigmoid colon complicating pregnancy. Obstetrics and Gynecology 33: 553–557

Letsky E 1984 Abruptio placentae. In: de Swiet M (ed) Medical disorders in obstetric practice. Blackwell Scientific Publications, Oxford, pp 82–83

Levine W, Diamond B 1961 Surgical procedures during pregnancy. American Journal of Obstetrics and Gynecology 81: 1046–1052

Macfarlane J R, Thorbjarnarson B 1966 Rupture of splenic artery

aneurysm during pregnancy. American Journal of Obstetrics and Gynecology 95: 1025–1037
Malkasian G D, Welch J S, Hallenbeck G A 1959 Volvulus associated with pregnancy: a review and a report of 3 cases. American Journal of Obstetrics and Gynecology 78: 112–124
Malkasian G D, Dockerty M B, Symmonds R E 1967 Benign cystic teratomas. Obstetrics and Gynecology 29: 719–725
Masters K, Levine B A, Gaskill H V, Sirinek K R 1984 Diagnosing appendicitis during pregnancy. American Journal of Surgery 148: 768–771
McCorriston C C 1963 Nonobstetrical abdominal surgery during pregnancy. American Journal of Obstetrics and Gynecology 86: 593–599
McGowan L 1964 Torsion of the uterine adnexa. American Journal of Surgery 108: 811–814
McGowan L 1983 Surgical diseases of the ovary in pregnancy. Clinical Obstetrics and Gynecology 26: 843–852
McKay A J, O'Neill J, Imrie C W 1980 Pancreatitis, pregnancy and gallstones. British Journal of Obstetrics and Gynaecology 87: 47–50
Meares E M 1978 Urologic surgery during pregnancy. Clinical Obstetrics and Gynecology 21: 907–920
Mitchell P R, Garrett W J 1960 The diagnosis of acute torsion of the pregnant uterus. Journal of Obstetrics and Gynaecology of the British Empire 67: 654–658
Morris E D 1965 Intestinal obstruction and pregnancy. Journal of Obstetrics and Gynaecology of the British Commonwealth 72: 36–44
Nelson E W, Archibald L, Albo D 1977 Spontaneous hepatic rupture in pregnancy. American Journal of Surgery 134: 817–820
Notelowitz M, Bottoms S F, Dase D F, Leichter P J 1979 Painless abruptio placentae. Obstetrics and Gynecology 53: 270–272
Novak E R, Lamrrou C D, Woodruff J D 1975 Ovarian tumors in pregnancy. An ovarian tumor registry review. Obstetrics and Gynecology 46: 401–406
Nowosielski P F, Henderson H 1960 Axial torsion of the pregnant uterus. American Journal of Obstetrics and Gynecology 80: 272–273
O'Grady J P, Day E J, Toole A L, Paust J C 1977 Splenic artery aneurysm rupture in pregnancy: a review and case report. Obstetrics and Gynecology 50: 627–630
O'Leary J A, Pratt J H, Symmonds R E 1967 Rectal carcinoma and pregnancy: a review of 17 cases. Obstetrics and Gynecology 30: 862–868
O'Neill J P 1969a Surgical conditions complicating pregnancy 1. Acute appendicitis—real and simulated. Australian and New Zealand Journal of Obstetrics and Gynaecology 9: 94–99
O'Neill J P 1969b Surgical conditions complicating pregnancy 2. Diseases of the gall bladder and pancreas. Australian and New Zealand Journal of Obstetrics and Gynaecology 9: 249–252
O'Neill J P 1970 Surgical conditions complicating pregnancy 3. Intestinal obstruction and miscellaneous conditions. Australian and New Zealand Journal of Obstetrics and Gynaecology 10: 10–16
Pece G 1964 Dysgerminoma of the ovary in pregnancy (report of a case and review of the literature). Obstetrics and Gynecology 24: 768–773
Pratt A T, Donaldson M D, Evertson L R, Yon J L 1981 Cecal volvulus in pregnancy. Obstetrics and Gynecology 57 (suppl): 37S–40S
Printen K J, Ott R A 1978 Cholecystectomy during pregnancy. American Surgeon 44: 432–434
Pritchard J A, Brekken A L 1967 Clinical and laboratory studies on severe abruptio placentae. American Journal of Obstetrics and Gynecology 97: 681–700
Reyes-Ceja L, Cabrera R, Insfran E, Herrera-Casso F 1969 Pregnancy following previous uterine rupture. Obstetrics and Gynecology 34: 387–389
Saunders P, Milton P J D 1973 Laparotomy during pregnancy: an assessment of diagnostic accuracy and fetal wastage. British Medical Journal 3: 165–167
Schrinsky D C, Benson R C 1978 Rupture of the pregnant uterus: a review. Obstetrical and Gynecological Survey 33: 217–232
Schug J, Rankin R P 1965 Rupture of a splenic artery aneurysm in pregnancy: report of a survivor and review of the literature. Obstetrics and Gynecology 25: 717–723
Shepherd J A 1982a Rupture of the rectus abdominis muscle in pregnancy. In: Management of the acute abdomen. Oxford University Press, Oxford, p 318
Shepherd J A 1982b Rupture of splenic artery aneurysms in pregnancy. In: Management of the acute abdomen. Oxford University Press, Oxford, pp 253–254
Sheth S S 1969 Suturing the tear as treatment in uterine rupture. American Journal of Obstetrics and Gynecology 105: 440–443
Simmons S C, Luck R J 1984 Surgical disorders. In: Brudenell M, Wilds P L (eds) Medical and surgical problems in obstetrics. Wright, Bristol, pp 283–296
Simon J A 1983 Biliary tract disease and related surgical disorders during pregnancy. Clinical Obstetrics and Gynecology 26: 810–821
Smith C A 1975 Pathological uterine torsion: a catastrophic event in late pregnancy. American Journal of Obstetrics and Gynecology 123: 32–33
Sommer D G, Greenway G D, Bookstein J J, Orloff M J 1979 Hepatic rupture with toxaemia of pregnancy: angiographic diagnosis. American Journal of Roentgenology 132: 455–456
Strickland D M, Hauth J C, Widdish J, Strickland K, Perez R 1984 Amylase and isoamylase activities in serum of pregnant women. Obstetrics and Gynecology 63: 389–391
Strong D W, Murchison R J, Lynch D F 1978 The management of ureteral calculi during pregnancy. Surgery, Gynecology and Obstetrics 146: 604–608
Tawa K 1964 Ovarian tumors in pregnancy. American Journal of Obstetrics and Gynecology 90: 511–516
Taylor E S 1969 Editorial comment. Obstetrical and Gynecological Survey 25: 225
Taylor E S 1977a Editorial comment. Obstetrical and Gynecological Survey 32: 710–711
Taylor E S 1977b Editorial comment. Obstetrical and Gynecological Survey 32: 662
Taylor E S 1979 Editorial comment. Obstetrical and Gynecological Survey 34: 381–382
Taylor E S 1984 Editorial comment. Obstetrical and Gynecological Survey 39: 93–94
Taylor E S 1985 Editorial comment. Obstetrical and Gynecological Survey 40: 81
Thomason J L, Sampson M B, Farb H F, Spellacy W N 1980 Pregnancy complicated by concurrent primary hyperparathyroidism and pancreatitis. Obstetrics and Gynecology 57 (suppl): 34S–36S
Wanetick L H, Roschen F P, Dunn J M 1975 Volvulus of the small bowel complicating pregnancy. Journal of Reproductive Medicine 14: 82–83
Weingold A B 1983 Appendicitis in pregnancy. Clinical Obstetrics and Gynecology 26: 801–809
White K C 1973 Ovarian tumors in pregnancy. American Journal of Obstetrics and Gynecology 116: 544–550
Wickham J E A 1987 The new surgery. British Medical Journal 295: 1581–1582
Wilkinson E J 1973 Acute pancreatitis in pregnancy: a review of 98 cases and a report of 8 new cases. Obstetrical and Gynecological Survey 28: 281–303
Winer-Muram H T, Muram D, Gillieson M S, Ivey B J, Muggah H F 1983 Uterine myomas in pregnancy. Canadian Medical Association Journal 128: 949–950
Yiu-Chiu V, Chiu L 1982 Sonographic features of placental complications in pregnancy. American Journal of Roentgenology 138: 879–885

41

Rosalinde Hurley

Infections in pregnancy

Table 41.1 Scrutiny for infectious disease at booking

History taking

General examination, especially heart, lungs and genital tract
Serological testing of booking blood*

1. for treponemal disease (TPHA, VDRL)
2. for markers of hepatitis B virus
3. for rubella immune status
4. for toxoplasma immune status†
5. for HTLV-III antibody‡

*It is important that booking serum should be stored by the laboratory until after the birth of the baby.
†In some European countries.
‡In high-risk patients, with maternal consent.

GENERAL CONSIDERATIONS

Pregnancy and the puerperium

Any of the acute or chronic specific infectious diseases may be contracted during the course of pregnancy or the puerperium, and conception may occur in women already subject to infection. The coexistence of pregnancy may aggravate the risk to maternal life of the more serious of these diseases, some of which constitute a hazard to the fetus and the newborn. Fetal death may result from contagion since some viruses, bacteria and protozoa are able to cross the placental barrier, or it may be caused by placental insufficiency, hyperpyrexia or maternal exhaustion and toxaemia. The newborn may contract a transmissible disease from close contact with an infected mother shortly after birth, or as a result of maternal infection, may be born in a sickly and marasmic condition and soon succumb to intercurrent infection. In the early part of the puerperium parturient women are peculiarly susceptible to serious infections of the genital tract and childbed fever has always been one of the most important causes of maternal death.

Although serious microbial disease is well controlled in the UK, mothers of young children, particularly of those at school, are exposed to the specific infectious diseases of childhood and in addition to the common upper respiratory tract infections may contract mumps, chickenpox, measles, rubella, scarlet fever, acute bacterial tonsillitis, whooping cough, dysentery or viral diarrhoeas. As young adults the mothers may contract toxoplasmosis or poliomyelitis. Some of these diseases have important consequences in obstetric practice but all pose a problem if the mother's antenatal condition necessitates admission to an obstetric unit, since isolation may be required.

The venereal diseases may be contracted at any time during pregnancy or the puerperium and those that could have fatal or crippling effects on the fetus are tested for during the antenatal period. Routine serological tests for syphilis are performed during pregnancy usually at the first visit together with other booking tests (Table 41.1).

The other venereal diseases — gonorrhoea, chancroid, granuloma inguinale and lymphogranuloma venereum — are sought during pregnancy at the routine antenatal clinical examination by eliciting the medical and social history, by physical examination and by appropriate laboratory tests.

There is some evidence that pregnancy may act as a cofactor, accelerating the development of the acquired immune deficiency syndrome (AIDS) in those with HIV (HTLV–III) disease. Signs of opportunistic infection may be paramount in the presentation and should alert the clinician to the diagnosis. Exacerbation of caries and dental sepsis occurs during pregnancy and women with valvular disease of the heart are at risk of infective endocarditis if dental surgery is necessitated, as well as at parturition. Endocarditis in pregnancy is discussed by Hurley (1977).

Pregnancy may occur during the course of a chronic infection, or chronic infection may first be diagnosed during pregnancy. Its detection is one of the purposes of the general medical examination made at the first antenatal visit.

While no infection is peculiar to pregnancy, the incidence of some seems to be increased in pregnant as compared with non-pregnant women. Infections of the urinary tract are common complications and emphasis is placed on their early diagnosis and treatment. The incidence of vulvovaginitis is increased in pregnancy and is occasioned largely by infections with members of the genus *Candida*, the fungi of thrush. The other important cause of vaginitis in pregnancy is the protozoan parasite *Trichomonas vaginalis*. Vaginosis associated with *Gardnerella vaginalis* is of less consequence; this microbe is sought under defined conditions, such as the presence of clue cells in the smear, or if other pathogens cannot be isolated.

The most notorious of the acute infections associated with the puerperium is infection of the genital tract, which formerly accounted for the majority of infectious deaths in pregnancy and the puerperium and is still the most important cause of maternal death from infection in obstetric practice in the UK. Inflammation and suppuration of the lactating breast may occur and urinary tract infections are fairly frequent. Women who have been subjected to surgery may develop bronchopneumonia or wound infections. All are common causes of elevation of the temperature in the lying-in period.

Fever during pregnancy or the puerperium is likely to be infectious in origin, although drug or serum fever, fever associated with malignant or thromboembolic disease, haemolytic disease or metabolic disorder may have to be considered in its differential diagnosis. Acute febrile illnesses of less than 2 weeks' duration are amongst the most frequent occurrences in medical practice; many are self-limiting, perhaps viral in origin, and definitive aetiological diagnosis is seldom made. However, prolonged febrile illnesses in which the diagnosis remains obscure for weeks or months do occur and in some patients fever is the dominant sign or symptom. Before diagnosis is established this condition is called pyrexia or fever of unknown (or uncertain) origin, although the term should be reserved for patients who have had episodes of fever in excess of 38°C for a prolonged period of at least 3 weeks and who have been investigated for at least 1 week. The causes of fever during pregnancy are discussed by Hurley (1984).

The newborn is peculiarly prone to certain infections and is less able to localize them than the adult. Conversely, it is immune to some other infections and immunity continues for several months after birth. The immunological status of the newborn is the result of two systems: the first is active and depends on the infant's own capacity to develop immunity; the second is passive and derived from the transfer of maternal antibody during gestation. Immunity in the neonatal period to diseases like mumps and measles is the consequence of transferred immunity from the mother. The infant is temporarily immune from certain diseases if the mother has suffered from them or is herself immune; transferred virus antibodies may confer on the child an immunity that lasts 6–12 months, although antibodies to bacterial antigens do not persist as long.

Infections such as rubella, cytomegalic inclusion disease, toxoplasmosis and listeriosis may be disseminated and fatal in the newborn, while rarely so in the adult. Bacteria such as *Flavobacterium meningosepticum* cause meningitis in the newborn but are never isolated as pathogens in adults. The newborn infant therefore demonstrates a proclivity towards severe infections with organisms which in the adult are usually of low virulence or even non-pathogenic (e.g. some staphylococci) and is also at risk from the tendency of microbial diseases to disseminate, with fatal consequences.

The response of adults to antigen stimulation consists of production of IgM, followed quickly by production of IgG. The pattern of response in the newborn is different; IgM is elaborated as a first response, but this persists for several weeks before IgG is elaborated. The fetus elaborates IgM in response to antigen exposure in utero and detection of specific antibody in the IgM fraction of cord blood is the most useful of the diagnostic tests for congenital infections such as rubella or syphilis. Elevation of the non-specific IgM level to 18 mg/100 ml is regarded by many as indicative of intrauterine infection and is used as a screening test in sickly or debilitated infants.

The reasons for the poor response of the newborn to certain infections are not clearly understood but there is some evidence that in addition to the physiological dysglobulinaemia mentioned above, the cellular response to infection varies in the newborn and the phagocytes are less active. There is a lack of antigen-presenting macrophages.

Prematurity and low birthweight are not only prejudicial peripartum events but also predispose to serious bacterial infections with high mortality rates (neonatal sepsis). Minor sepsis of skin or conjunctivae is common. The most frequent cause of minor sepsis in the UK is *Staphylococcus aureus*. Meningitis and septicaemia may be caused by *Escherichia coli* or by other Gram-negative bacteria, including *Pseudomonas aeruginosa*, or by streptococci particularly those of Lancefield group B. The aetiology of severe forms of epidemic diarrhoea of the newborn is still disputed. Occasionally salmonella are isolated, or pathogenic *E. coli*, while other cases may have a viral aetiology.

Host–parasite interactions

With respect to microbial disease, the term immunity embraces the whole array of states that may exist between the host and indigenous or exogenous microbes — states that range from complete susceptibility with evolution of fulminant life-threatening disease to commensalism.

The indigenous flora comprise many genera and species of bacteria and to a lesser extent some of the yeasts. These commensals occupy as their habitats ecological niches determined by the physiological characteristics of the micro-organism, by local chemical and physical properties of the host and, to some extent, by the nature of other microbes inhabiting the locale. Specific nutritional requirements are supplied either by the host or by adjacent microbes and the population is kept in check by limitation of nutrients or the inhibitory effects of bacterial metabolites such as hydrogen peroxide. Environmental pH, itself brought about in part through bacterial metabolism, is clearly important, for few microbes are able to thrive at extremes of pH. By and large, commensal microbes are not pathogenic. Some, however, are members of pathogenic genera and while not exerting a harmful effect in their customary habitat, will do so if they gain ingress into the tissues of the host. Others may cause localized disease through possession of properties such as bacterial adherence and toxin production.

The integrity of anatomical and physiological barriers is important in preventing microbial disease for breaches of the integument occasioned by injury or disease provide important portals of entry for pathogenic bacteria. Intact skin and mucous membranes bar entry, the skin through its thick keratinized layer and through the pH-reducing secretions of sweat and sebacous glands while there are special mechanisms in the conjunctiva (tears); in the respiratory tract (mucus secretion, action of ciliated cells, alveolar macrophages); in the gastrointestinal tract (gastric acidity, enzymic and bile salt activity mucus, secretory IgA, peristalsis) and in the genitourinary tract (flushing action of urine, vaginal secretions). Although the vagina is heavily colonized the cervical mucus prevents ingress of microbes and the uterus is practically sterile. Human amniotic fluid contains a zinc-dependent low molecular weight antibacterial polypeptide as well as effective concentrations of lysosyme, low concentrations of immunoglobulins and beta-lysin.

In order to produce disease pathogenic microbes must be capable of entering and colonizing host tissue and then of causing local or systemic damage. They must, therefore, be capable of overcoming host resistance either by specific aggressive mechanisms or by taking advantage of local or general impairment of function. Once the integument has been penetrated possibly through a breach in its surface, by the elaboration of bacterial adhesions, destruction of surface epithelium occurs by toxic substances, or through ingestion by epithelial cells. Then the pathogen is able to resist defence mechanisms by interfering with non-specific mechanisms such as leukocyte chemotaxis, the inflammatory response and the action of phagocytes. Further it can spread through enzymes such as hyaluronidase and collagenase or agents such as fibrinolysin or haemolysin.

Host resistance depends on innate (genetic) as well as environmental factors and is engineered by non-specific as well as specific (immune) mechanisms. The principal mechanism of protection against invading micro-organisms is the immune system which is characterized by three attributes—specificity, memory and recognition of self-antigens. Its function is to protect against foreign substances. The immune status of individuals may be innate or acquired. Innate immunity is genetically or constitutionally determined and is not a function of cells of the immune system or of specific antibody, but the result of physiological, biochemical or anatomical differences principally between species. There is well defined species immunity exemplified in man by the species-specificity of microbes such as *Neisseria meningitidis*, *Treponema pallidum* and the measles (rubeola) virus, which naturally infect only man, while other species are resistant. Racial immunity also exists; a well known example is the resistance of blacks with sickle cell anaemia to disease caused by *Plasmodium falciparum*. The most outstanding example of innate immunity as it applies to obstetrics is the relative inability of *Brucella abortus* to cause abortion in man although it causes contagious abortion in cattle, formerly of considerable economic consequence in Europe. The special predilection of *B. abortus* for the reproductive system of cattle is due in part to the high concentration of erythritol, a growth-promoting substance for the microbe, in the bovine placenta and seminal vesicles; this situation is not found in man in whose tissues erythritol concentrations are low. Body temperature is an important mechanism of innate immunity. With few exceptions the optimum temperature for growth of human pathogens is around 37°C.

Immunity is acquired either passively or actively. Naturally acquired passive immunity follows the transfer of immune antibody of the IgG class from mother to fetus by the transplacental route and the ingestion of IgA antibody in colostrum. Artificially acquired passive immunity follows injection of immune products such as antitoxins, antisera or immune globulin from the same or a different species.

Prevention of hospital-acquired sepsis in maternity units

Virtually all fatal or serious infections and most superficial infections arising in the puerperium and in the later newborn period of infants born at term are preventable.

The control of communicable sepsis begins at the admission desk. A series of simple questions on admission together with ascertainment of the body temperature will quickly define those patients likely to have or to be incubating infectious disease. These patients should be admitted to the isolation ward or room and delivered in isolation with full protective nursing until the laboratory tests and clinical findings establish that they are free from contagious disease. Staff with frankly septic lesions should not be allowed to remain on duty in vulnerable areas of the hospital and those with febrile illness, sore throats or other respiratory tract infections or diarrhoea should be sent off duty until the laboratory reports indicate that they are not harbouring dangerous communicable pathogens. Patients who develop purulent lesions or streptococcal or other communicable disease

Table 41.2 Control of methicillin-resistant *Staphylococcus aureus* (MRSA)

Screening on admission and isolation of patients transferred from affected hospitals
Isolation of infected or colonized* patients in single rooms
Staff in contact to wear gloves and protective clothing and practise rigorous hand hygiene with disinfectant
Bacteriological screening of staff and patients in contact with the affected
Use of topical antiseptics and/or pseudomonic acid to carriage sites
Restriction on inter-ward movements of staff and patients
Terminal disinfection of affected areas with phenolic disinfectant
Marking of affected patients' notes, especially on transfer

*This is only feasible if the strain is not endemic.

should be immediately isolated and nursing procedures appropriate to the suspected infection invoked.

About 20% of hospital-acquired infections are attributable to *Staphylococcus aureus*, which is the most frequent cause of postoperative wound sepsis and which, together with *Escherichia coli* and *Streptococcus pneumoniae*, accounts for the majority of bacteraemias occurring in inpatients. Since 1976 multiple antibiotic-resistant strains (resistant also to methicillin, an isoxazolyl penicillin stable to beta-lactamase) have re-emerged, causing outbreaks of infection in the UK, USA, Australia and Eire (Shanson 1986). Most of those affected in the UK were merely colonized or had minor septic complications but some developed moderately severe or fatal infections. Methicillin-resistant *Staph. aureus* (MRSA) has spread in many hospitals in south-east Britain. Although these strains seem less virulent than those prevalent in the 1950s, they none the less represent a serious threat of nosocomial sepsis. The most important route of spread is the introduction of a colonized or infected patient from another hospital since epidemic MRSA exhibits the dangerous feature of spreadability, being transmitted between patients by hands or contaminated clothing of staff. Disposable gloves and scrupulous hand hygiene with antiseptics reduce the chance of spread.

If an outbreak is not brought under control quickly the strain is likely to become endemic in the hospital population. Patients transferred from hospitals where MRSA is endemic should be bacteriologically screened on admission and isolated until results of culture are repeatedly negative. General measures for control are shown in Table 41.2 and the control of infection officer, usually a consultant microbiologist, assisted by the control of infection nurse, should keep epidemiological records. Sanderson (1986) outlines general measures of control.

Some central areas of the hospital, such as the operating theatres, theatre and central sterile supply departments, pharmacy, hospital kitchen and central feed kitchen, are of vital importance since if hygiene, antisepsis or asepsis in these areas are faulty, it may prove disastrous in remote wards and units. Regular checks should be made on equipment used for sterilizing, for aseptic assembly or for pasteurizing and the premises inspected for general cleanliness. In these areas the air may be sampled by settle plates or by a slit sampler. While the sale of cows' milk is subject to statutory regulation in the UK, no such control is exercised over the sale of human milk. Maternity units must therefore remedy this statutory omission and insist on aseptic techniques for the collection of expressed breast milk, that bacteriological tests for cleanliness and safety are made and that the milk is carefully processed and correctly stored before use.

Baby incubators particularly repay bacteriological monitoring. It is sound practice to establish whether they are free of dangerous pathogens before babies are placed in them and to monitor them by sterility tests on any humidifier fluid used and by swabbing the interior chamber while in use. If gross contamination of the walls of the chamber is detected or the humidifier fluid ceases to be sterile the incubator should be taken out of use and decontaminated before retesting.

Periodic checks on disinfectant fluids in use on wards and on stored sterile water are also worthwhile. Some disinfectants deteriorate on exposure and water will not remain sterile when exposed to the atmosphere or stored in an unsealed container.

In general, two disinfectants should suffice for the majority of uses. One for coarse disinfection procedures for large inanimate surfaces and one for disinfection of the person or of impedimenta coming into contact with the person. Phenolic disinfectants are suitable for the former use and the various preparations of chlorhexidine are suitable for the latter since the disinfectant is versatile and completely free of toxic effect. Betadine iodine, isopropyl alcohol and other skin disinfectants all have their proponents and where there is risk of viral transmission glutaraldehyde is useful. Hypochlorites have disadvantages but as they are suitable for domestic use instruction in their uses is often given to nursing mothers. Gaseous disinfectants may be required in particular circumstances. Chemical disinfectants should not be used where adequate physical methods are available. Disposable and prepacked sterilized articles have undoubtedly reduced the risks of nosocomial infections.

The microbial flora of the newborn infant and female genital tract

The origin of the different organisms in the infant is the immediate environment. During passage through the birth canal the skin and mucous membranes become contaminated with organisms from the mother and microbes are proliferating in the infant's alimentary tract within a few hours. It may also acquire microbes from the wider external environment. If these are virulent and the baby is disadvantaged by prematurity or low birthweight, neonatal sepsis may arise, being early onset in type with microbes derived from the maternal genital tract and late onset with those derived from the environment. The infant's mouth becomes colonized within a few days of birth and the main source of the colonizing organisms is the maternal vagina. At birth, the intestine may contain only a few bacteria but is rapidly colonized. The flora of the breastfed infant consists largely of anaerobes such as *Lactobacillus* and *Bacteroides* (about 99%) but coliforms are also present. After weaning the flora resembles that of the adult. The upper respiratory tract is colonized soon after birth particularly after close contact with the mother at the first feed.

The vulva and vestibulum of the newborn are sterile; organisms appear in 7–8 hours. The commonest aerobic organisms are staphylococci, diphtheroids, enterococci, coliform bacilli and yeasts. Many anaerobes also occur. The vagina of the newborn is sterile and organisms appear in 12–14 hours. Staphylococci, enterococci and diphtheroids appear at first but are replaced in 2–3 days by an almost pure culture of Döderlein's bacilli. At this time the vaginal secretion is acid and glycogen is demonstrable in the vaginal epithelium. The occurrence of glycogen appears to be due to the presence of oestrogens derived from the maternal circulation. Soon this is excreted in the urine and the vaginal secretion becomes alkaline. Thereafter, until puberty, the secretion remains alkaline and staphylococci, streptococci other than *Streptococcus pyogenes*, coliforms and diphtheroid bacilli predominate.

At puberty, glycogen is again deposited in the vaginal wall, the secretion becomes acid and Döderlein's bacilli and corynebacteria are re-established as the predominant organisms. The flora is mixed and streptococci, coliforms and fungi are present. The streptococci of the vagina are varied and *Str. faecalis* (Lancefield group D) is common. Lancefield groups C, B, F and G occur but are less frequent. Other streptococci are also found. *Mycoplasma* can be demonstrated occasionally. In addition to these, numbers of Gram-negative rods, not all members of the Enterobacteriaceae, are encountered and some Gram-variable coccobacilli (*Gardnerella*) are found.

The distribution of microbes isolated from the posterior fornices of pregnant women is shown in Table 41.3 (Hurley et al 1974). The incidence of large colony mycoplasmas in pregnant women according to several authors ranges from 23 to 71% for T-mycoplasmas and from 4 to 39% for *Mycoplasma hominis*. de Louvois et al (1974) also noted an incidence of 51.6% T-mycoplasmas and of 11.7% *M. hominis* in infertile women.

After the menopause, oestrogenic activity decreases, glycogen is not deposited in the vaginal epithelium, the vaginal secretions are less acid and cocci are said to predominate amongst the vaginal flora. Many of the endogenous microbes isolated from the vagina during pregnancy are members of pathogenic genera. Some may be implicated in puerperal sepsis and others in chorioamnionitis and neonatal sepsis. Occasionally microbes are isolated that are not part of the resident flora; their presence may indicate disease of the genital tract. Those microbes exogenous to the genital tract are shown in Table 41.4.

Large numbers of bacteria occur in human milk but if

Table 41.3 Flora of lower genital tract in 280 unselected pregnant women

Organism	% Incidence
Corynebacteria	84
Lactobacilli	82
Staphylococcus epidermidis	66
Micrococci	37
Faecal streptococci	34
Microaerophilic and anaerobic streptococci	22
Escherichia coli	19
Candida albicans	17
Mycoplasma hominis	11
Beta-haemolytic streptococci	9
Group B	5
Group C	<1
Groups F and G	<1
Not groupable	3
Gram-variable coccobacilli	7
Proteus mirabilis	6
Bacteroides species	5
Staphylococcus aureus	5
Non-haemolytic streptococci	4
Torulopsis glabrata	4
Trichomonas vaginalis	3
Neisseria species (*pharyngis* and *catarrhalis*)	1
Klebsiella aerogenes	<1
Pseudomonas aeruginosa	<1
Sought but not isolated	
Lancefield group A streptococci	Nil
Clostridium perfringens	Nil
Neisseria gonorrhoea	Nil
Listeria monocytogenes	Nil
Haemophilus species	Nil
Not sought	
Viruses, chlamydia, T-strain mycoplasmas	

Table 41.4 Abnormal pathogenic flora* of the female genital tract

Lancefield group A streptococci
Streptococcus pneumoniae
Clostridium perfringens
Clostridium tetani
Corynebacterium diphtheriae
Mycobacterium tuberculosis
Treponema pallidum
Neisseria gonorrhoeae
Neisseria meningitidis
Haemophilus ducreyi
Haemophilus influenzae
Chlamydia trachomatis
Schistosoma mansoni
Schistosoma haematobium
Enterobius vermicularis
Cytomegalovirus
Rubella virus, or vaccine virus
Herpes hominis

*Being either exogenous flora, or encountered with frequency of less than 1 in 250.

it is collected under strictly aseptic conditions the plate count should not exceed 2500 organisms per ml. Micrococci, diphtheroids, occasional coliforms, staphylococci, non-haemolytic streptococci and anaerobic lactobacilli are isolated and the milk of healthy nursing mothers delivered in hospital often contains appreciable numbers of *Staphylococcus aureus*.

Some commensals of man belong to the category of microbes that pathologists describe as opportunistic. Lacking genuinely invasive powers, they only occasionally exert a hostile effect on their hosts, usually when general or local resistance is lowered as a consequence of debilitating disease, trauma, haemorrhage or other conditions, or in consequence of a particular physiological state such as being newly born or pregnant. When such microbes cause disease localized to body areas where they are usually or often demonstrable as commensals, the assignment to them of a pathogenic role cannot be inferred simply from the cultural findings. The staphylococci are normal denizens of the skin, conjunctiva, nasopharynx, vagina and the alimentary tract. Their demonstration in these sites is to be expected. None the less, the newborn is especially prone to skin or conjunctival sepsis caused by staphylococci. Occasionally re-examination of available evidence and prospective studies may lead pathologists to a reversal of formerly held opinions on the normal habitat of certain microbes. *Streptococcus pyogenes* was once regarded as part of the normal flora of the vagina before the work of Lancefield provided a means for epidemiologists to establish it as an exogenous microbe. Today no one is able to say for certain whether the Lancefield group B streptococcus (*Str. agalactiae*) is endogenous or exogenous to the vagina. In view of the increasing number of reports of serious neonatal infection associated with this streptococcus it is important that the point should be resolved. *Candida albicans* was long deemed part of the normal flora of the vagina and its isolation from this site was regarded as insufficient evidence to substantiate a diagnosis of candida vaginitis. However, Carroll et al (1973) showed firstly that only direct examination of the vagina reveals the presence or absence of vaginitis which may not be deduced from a history of pruritus or discharge and secondly, that isolation of *C. albicans* coincides with active or recently treated vaginitis in 84% of cases and with other signs or symptoms of morbidity in a further 14%. They concluded that *C. albicans* is not part of the normal flora of the healthy vagina during pregnancy, that its presence indicates morbidity and that it should be eliminated promptly by use of appropriate antimycotic agents to prevent it leading to chronic vaginitis which is stubborn and refractory to treatment. Clearly, the proof that an organism, normally commensal in a given site, is responsible for disease in that particular site cannot rest solely on demonstration of the microbe but must be interpreted in conjunction with the clinical findings and the results of other laboratory tests. The reaction of the host to the microbe must be shown to be abnormal since the presence of the microbe is not.

NON-SPECIFIC INFECTIONS OCCURRING IN PREGNANCY

Urinary tract infections

Urinary tract infections are common in women, particularly during pregnancy, labour and the puerperium. Infections of all grades of severity are encountered and any part of the urinary tract may be involved. Infections range from mild urethritis through cystitis and pyelitis to pyelonephritis. They are considered in Chapter 42.

Puerperal sepsis and wound infections

Puerperal sepsis includes a series of febrile disorders of the lying-in period that share the common aetiology of being wound infections of the genital tract. Puerperal sepsis may occur after delivery or abortion and is occasioned by several genera of pathogenic bacteria, of which the most notorious and dangerous are *Clostridium* and *Streptococcus*. In the great majority of fatal cases, the microbes are introduced from without, and such infections are preventable. In general, endogenous microbes, harboured in the vagina, such as *Enterobacteriaceae* and *Staphylococcus* cause less severe forms of sepsis. Puerperal sepsis is discussed in Chapter 63.

Other wound infections

The organism most frequently found in septic wounds in gynaecological and obstetric practice is *Staph. aureus*, followed by coliform bacilli and *Proteus* spp. and streptococci, including *Str. pyogenes*, *Str. faecalis* and anaerobic cocci. Infection with *Pseudomonas aeruginosa* may also occur.

Opinions differ on the relative importance of the operating theatre and the ward as the place of infection and this probably differs from hospital to hospital. Certainly the hands of the surgeon, the body of a member of the operating team, fomites surrounding the patient such as blankets, air sucked into the theatre from other parts of the hospital and the patient's own skin may be the source of infection. Inexpert and clumsy surgery is undoubtedly a contributory factor.

Septic abortion and shock

The availability of contraceptive techniques and legislation on abortion has led to diminution in the number of women with septic abortion but the diagnosis should be suspected in every febrile woman who is bleeding in the first trimester of pregnancy. In the majority of cases the cervical os is open and there is evidence of the passage of the products of conception. High spiking fevers and the presence of hypotension are bad prognostic signs. Pelvic examination with assessment of uterine size is important for most serious infections follow attempts to terminate pregnancy in women beyond the 12th week of gestation. As in puerperal sepsis following delivery, extension of the infection beyond the uterus is attended by correspondingly grave risks for the patient. Plain X-rays of the abdomen with the patient both in the supine and the upright positions may demonstrate the presence of intraperitoneal or myometrial gas. Exploratory laparotomy may be required. Myometrial gas suggests *Clostridium welchii (perfringens)* infection and operative intervention may be required. Foreign bodies, such as intrauterine contraceptive devices, may require removal.

Many patients respond successfully to curettage and antibiotic therapy or even to antibiotic therapy alone. Many antibiotics have been used but the most favoured regimen is a combination of intravenous penicillin and metronidazole with intramuscular aminoglycoside in high dosage. The blood pressure and urinary output should be measured at regular intervals and antibiotic concentrations should be assayed.

The microbes causing septic abortion are similar to those causing postdelivery sepsis, but non-sporing anaerobes such as *Bacteroides fragilis* may be implicated more frequently, and with Gram-negative aerobes such as *Escherichia coli* and *Klebsiella* spp., are related to endotoxic shock. The onset of bacteraemia is accompanied by fever, rigors, nausea, vomiting, diarrhoea and prostration. Tachycardia, tachypnoea, hypotension — usually with cool, pale extremities and often with peripheral cyanosis — oliguria and mental confusion are added to the development of septic shock. The haematological manifestations of shock and the renal complications have been considered by Letsky (1984) and Davison (1984).

CHORIOAMNIONITIS

Chorioamnionitis (Charles & Hurry 1983) may be a major factor in the aetiology of preterm labour, contributing to perinatal mortality from prematurity. Prolonged rupture of the membranes is associated with a high incidence of chorioamnionitis and known to predispose to neonatal sepsis.

Inflammation of the fetal membranes arises in consequence of an ascending infection by microbes colonizing the lower genital tract and may result in infection of the amniotic fluid and thence the fetus. Most intrauterine infections are thought to arise in this way; the transplacental or haematogenous routes are relatively unimportant. The inflammatory reaction begins within the umbilical cord vessels or the large vessels of the chorionic plate. Leukocytes migrate, traverse the vessel walls and spread to the mesenchyme, involving the subamniotic zone of the placenta as well as the membranes and the umbilical cord. Spread of infected material to the amniotic sac may occur and fetal infection may result through swallowing or gasping or by haematogenous spread from infected fetal vessels.

Evidence favours the spread of infection through intact membranes, initiated in some cases by coitus (Naeye & Peters 1980) since seminal fluid facilitates the passage of micro-organisms through cervical mucus. Fetal membranes weakened by infection are more likely to rupture. Thus infection may precede as well as follow premature rupture of membranes.

Chorioamnionitis occurs more frequently than neonatal sepsis and is often clinically silent, being diagnosed from macroscopic and histological examination of the placenta, membranes and cord. Since these have usually been delivered through the heavily colonized vagina, bacteriological examination is unrewarding. The organisms most commonly isolated from inflamed membranes are *Escherichia coli*, staphylococci and streptococci. Clinical featues in the mother include fever, leukocytosis and fetid vaginal discharge, sometimes accompanied by uterine tenderness. Rupture of membranes is invariably present.

Infection of the amniotic fluid may produce the amniotic fluid syndrome of chorioamnionitis, intrauterine and fetal lung infection (Blanc 1959). Congenital pneumonia may occur. Poor nutrition with lowering of the amniotic fluid antibacterial zinc-dependent polypeptide, may contribute to the high incidence of premature births and amniotic fluid infection in women from low socioeconomic groups. Chorioamnionitis is an important predisposing cause of neonatal sepsis. Following infection of the respiratory tree from amniotic fluid, infection of the middle ear and paranasal sinuses may occur. The onset of respiration extends the infection to the pulmonary alveoli and systemic spread may occur.

NEONATAL SEPSIS

Septicaemia and meningitis

In terms of survival and lack of crippling sequelae, the prognosis for babies of low or very low birthweight has altered completely in the last four decades. The virtual certainty of death in 1945 has been replaced by an expected survival rate in specialist centres of 30–50% for those weighing less than 1000 g and of 85% for those weighing between 1000 and 1500 g. Paradoxically, the improvement has increasingly led to more cases of neonatal septicaemia and meningitis: infection rates are between five and 100 times higher in those of low birthweight. Neonatal meningitis is less common than septicaemia and the data reported by Remington & Klein (1983) suggest overall figures of 1.8/1000 births for septicaemia and of 0.2/1000 births for meningitis, as well as rates of 13.3 and 2.6/1000 for those of birthweight less than 2500 g, and 74.5 and 18.6/1000 for those of birthweight less than 1000 g.

Both diseases have high mortality rates which again are inversely proportional to birthweight. Thus Hurley & de Louvois (1981) recorded an overall mortality of 40.1% for septicaemia, rising to 62.5% in those born weighing less than 1000 g and to 83% in those in whom meningitis supervened, as it did in six of their 27 treated cases. All available evidence suggests that neonatal meningitis is consequent on bloodstream infection since the primary site of invasion is the bloodstream with spread to meninges in 25–30% of cases. The term sepsis neonatorum or neonatal sepsis is used for both septicaemia and meningitis.

Neonatal septicaemia is a clinical syndrome characterized by signs of systemic infection and confirmed by a positive blood culture in the first 4 weeks of life. Although some commentators have distinguished primary septicaemia from septicaemia secondary to congenital anomalies, surgical procedures or debility, for epidemiological reasons it is more practical to consider neonatal sepsis in terms of early- and late-onset disease. The cardinal distinction between the two types lies in the source of the infection which in the former is the birth canal and in the latter, the environment.

Early-onset disease occurs in the first week of life as fulminant systemic illness in babies who are usually premature and of low birthweight and who have been born to women who have had abnormal pregnancies and deliveries. Premature and prolonged rupture of the membranes with premature labour, obstetric complications leading to operative or instrumental delivery, maternal or fetal distress, haemorrhage, maternal anaemia or intercurrent illness and peripartum fever are factors that should alert the neonatologist to the potential development of serious infection. The causal bacteria of early-onset sepsis are derived from the birth canal and acquired either by ascending infection in intrauterine life or during passage through the birth canal. Transplacental transmission rarely occurs but the child may be born with a true congenital bacteraemia. The bacteria associated with early-onset sepsis are usually indigenous to the maternal congenital tract but rarely, adventitious microbes such as beta-haemolytic streptococci (Lancefield group A) or *Clostridium perfringens* are isolated. The mortality rate of early-onset sepsis is high and lies between 20 and 50%.

Late-onset disease occurs after the first week of life. There are fewer prejudicial maternal peripartum events but the babies are often afflicted by congenital malformations or illness or other disease. The microbes responsible are usually those disseminated in the infant's environment, epidemiologically reflecting the distribution of pathogens at large in the particular nursery or intensive care baby unit. *Pseudomonas aeruginosa*, *Staphylococcus aureus* and *Klebsiella aerogenes* are examples of such pathogens. Group B streptococci and *Escherichia coli* are causally related both to early- and late-onset disease. Mortality is lower in late-onset neonatal sepsis: between 10 and 20%. It is often difficult to determine the precise time of onset of neonatal sepsis in babies who are weak and marasmic from birth, but the diagnosis must be considered in almost every sick newborn infant.

While it is often difficult in practice to distinguish the type of infection in individual babies, disease of late onset, originating from microbes disseminated in the environment of the susceptible newborn, must be regarded as iatrogenic and preventable by the imposition of rigorous standards of hygiene, antisepsis and asepsis. It is becoming more difficult to control, however, due to the importation of seriously ill babies, often colonized with bacteria foreign to the host centre, into special care baby units which are already overloaded and overworked from the amount of care needed for low birthweight babies. Neonatal sepsis accounts for at least 20% of all referrals of sick babies to special units. Such babies constitute an infectious hazard; necropsy studies at Queen Charlotte's Maternity Hospital showed that 80% of those with septicaemia harbour the microbe in the bronchial tree from whence during life, it may contaminate the attendant's hands and clothing, adjacent fomites, or the larger environment of the special care unit. Terminal septicaemia, whether treated or not, may thus contribute to late-onset sepsis. Dying infected babies should be nursed in isolation.

Meningitis is more frequent in the first month of life than in any other month. It is frequently undiagnosed and may not be suspected until autopsy.

The microbial aetiology of neonatal septicaemia and meningitis is similar. Most accounts, including the first systematic study of septicaemia by Silverman & Homan (1949), attest the pre-eminence of *Escherichia coli* and other Gram-negative rods as causative bacteria. In the past, *Str. haemolyticus*, often consequent on puerperal sepsis, seems to have caused the majority of reported cases. Davies (1971) fully discussed the source and pathogenesis of bacterial infection in the newborn and chronicled the changing pattern of sepsis, alluding to the falling incidence of staphylococcal disease and the prominence of Gram-negative rods as causes of serious infection. Many studies in the 1960s from the USA emphasized the increasing frequency of Gram-negative rod sepsis (Gluck et al 1966, McCracken & Shinefield 1966). The group B streptococcus is also an important cause, recognised by Siegel & McCracken (1981) as the predominant pathogen in most American nurseries and together with *Escherichia coli*, accounting for 60% of all cases. The relative incidence of the causal microbes varies in different parts of the world. Recent reports from the UK show similar ratios of 7:1 and 10:1 for Gram-negative rods, principally *E. coli* and group B streptococci, respectively. Amongst the rare causes of neonatal and early infantile sepsis are *Pasteurella multocida*, *Flavobacterium meningosepticum*, *Haemophilus influenzae* and *Vibrio fetus* (now *Campylobacter*). *Neisseria meningitidis* is a rare cause although it does occur in early infancy, as does *N. gonorrhoeae*. *Candida* septicaemia is well known. Epidemics of neonatal sepsis have been associated with *Citrobacter koseri*, *Achromobacter*, *Listeria monocytogenes* and *Hansenula anomala* (Murphy et al 1986).

Fatal viral infection is rare in the newborn period and life-threatening disease is overwhelmingly of bacterial origin. Only five cases came to necropsy in 58 160 births in our hospital over a 17-year period. Disseminated candidosis is also rare; six cases were encountered over the same period.

Meningoencephalitis may be caused by *Toxoplasma gondii* and by the viruses of rubella and of cytomegalic inclusion disease, as well as by those of herpes simplex, zoster, poliomyelitis, mumps and chickenpox. Coxsackieviruses also affect the central nervous system.

SPECIFIC INFECTIONS

Trichomoniasis

The protozoan parasite *Trichomonas vaginalis*, a pear-shaped, motile organism, is accepted as an aetiological agent of vaginitis. An extremely similar organism, *T. hominis*, inhabits the gastrointestinal tract. Nowadays *T. vaginalis* is a less frequent cause of vaginitis than species of *Candida*. Up to 6% of pregnant women develop vaginitis with a *Trichomonas*:yeast ratio of 1:3 and an incidence of simultaneous infection with yeasts and trichomonads of the order of 0.8%.

The infection is diagnosed when motile trichomonads are demonstrated in the vaginal discharge and the patient has symptoms. The discharge is greenish yellow, frothy and irritant, with a musty odour.

The organism is recognized by its characteristic jerky movements in wet preparations. The vaginal secretion should be examined microscopically with low magnification and then with the 1/6-inch lens. Films stained with Leishman, Giemsa or Papanicolaou's technique may also be used to demonstrate the parasite. Cultural methods are available. Metronidazole is curative when administered both to the patient and her sexual partner.

The infection is most frequently encountered in women of reproductive age and is sexually transmitted. Studies have failed to show that it is transmitted to the newborn and it is not associated with adverse effects on the growing fetus.

Candidosis

The fungi that cause candidosis belong to the genus *Candida*, a genus of dimorphic fungi reproducing by budding but capable of filamentous growth. While some eight species are pathogenic in man, only *C. albicans*, the principal member of the genus and *C. glabrata* (formerly called *Torulopsis glabrata*) are commonly associated with vaginal thrush.

Candida species are widely spread in nature, principally as commensals in the gastrointestinal tracts of birds and animals. Numerous surveys attest to the predominant incidence of *C. albicans*, which can be found in the vaginas of up to 36% of pregnant women and up to 16% of non-pregnant women. Yeast-like fungi, predominantly *C. albicans*, have been found in the mouths of up to 54% of children aged 2–6 weeks. The organisms are rarely harboured on the skin. In spite of their occurrence as commensals, infection by these organisms can still on occasion be exogenous — in the vagina as the result of unclean instrumentation and in the mouths of babes as a result of contaminated teats or bottles. Conjugal infection can also occur. Thus although usually endemic, vaginal candidosis and thrush can occur in epidemic form.

Pregnancy and diabetes predispose to thrush vaginitis as does administration of some broad-spectrum antibiotics. Multiparous are more often infected than nulliparous women. The incidence of vaginal yeasts rises in pregnancy but there is general agreement that the number is greatly diminished after parturition, possibly as a consequence of the cleansing effect of the lochia. The overall incidence of vaginal thrush in pregnant women is about 16%. The incidence is highest in the third trimester and in the summer months. In non-pregnant women, the incidence is higher in the summer months and exacerbations occur in the premenstrual period. *Candida* vulvovaginitis rarely occurs in little girls but is fairly frequent after the menopause. Although typically white and curd-like, the discharge may be thick and often highly acid in the acute stages; vulvitis is a concomitant feature.

The diagnosis of candidosis is made on clinical grounds but positive culture is required for confirmation. The criteria for diagnosis include the observation of plaques or of cheesy debris in the vagina; signs of vaginitis or vulvovaginitis accompanied by isolation of fungus, or isolation of the fungus alone which in 84% of instances is associated with the first two criteria. Clinically, the disease is characterized by pruritus and discharge.

Polyene antifungal antibiotics such as nystatin or amphotericin B are effective in vaginal thrush, as are drugs of the imidazole group. The cure rate with specific drugs in vaginal candidosis is of the order of 90% although more than one course may have to be given. Currently, dissatisfaction is expressed by many gynaecologists and genitourinary physicians with schedules of therapy since a small but appreciable number of women suffer from long-standing thrush which is refractory to treatment.

Syphilis

Although it has declined in incidence, syphilis is the most notorious of the congenital infections; the ready transmissibility of *Treponema pallidum* to the fetus led Stokes et al (1944) to include this feature in their definition of the disease. Syphilis appeared to be under some measure of control in the late 1960s and early 1970s but since then there has been a rise in the number of cases of infectious syphilis throughout the world. Transmission of spirochaete to the fetus is always from the infected mother since direct transmission to the fetus via spermatozoa does not occur. Traditionally it is held that infection of the fetus does not occur before the fourth month of pregnancy and that it is most likely after the sixth month, since this accords with observed pathological change in the fetus. The Langhans' cells of the early placenta are thought to be impenetrable by the spirochaete. Infection involves the placenta with haematogenous spread, resulting in widespread involvement of fetal tissues.

The risk to the fetus varies with the stage of untreated syphilis in the mother. In general, the outcome of earlier pregnancies will be miscarriages or stillbirths and subsequently, living syphilitic children will be born. After many years healthy non-infected children may be born. This sequence of events is called Kassowitz' law but according to Catterall (1979) it seldom occurs. More usually miscarriages alternate with stillbirths or live syphilitic children and healthy babies may be born between two infected babies. Fiumara et al (1952) assessed the risk to the fetus according to the stage of untreated syphilis in the mother. In primary or secondary syphilis the risk of transmission approaches 100% and normal full-term infants are not to be expected. Some 50% are born prematurely or die in the perinatal period and 50% have congenital syphilis. The risk is lower in early and late latent syphilis; in the former 20% will be normal infants and in the latter 70%.

The clinical manifestations of congenital syphilis have been well described (Ingall & Norins 1976; Catterall 1979) and can be considered in three groups. Those of *early infectious syphilis* include skin rashes (syphilitic pemphigus or rashes typical of secondary syphilis), mucus patches (snuffles), hepatosplenomegaly, lymphadenopathy, osteochondritis (pseudoparalysis of Parrot) and meningovascular syphilis. Definitive diagnosis is based on dark ground microscopy; lesions of the skin and mucous membranes are teeming with spirochaetes. Serological tests establish a presumptive diagnosis, particularly if specific IgM is demonstrable in the infant's blood.

The *late, non-infectious manifestations of congenital syphilis* occur after the second year of life, most commonly between the ages of 7 and 15. Interstitial keratitis is the most common of these lesions but nerve deafness, Clutton's joints, gummata and neurosyphilis may all occur.

The *stigmata of congenital syphilis* are occasioned by structural abnormalities consequent on fetal infection and include Parrot's nodes, frontal bossing and the 'hot cross bun' skull, saddle nose, high arched palate, bulldog facies and anomalies of secondary dentition (Hutchinson's teeth and Moon's molars). Hutchinson's triad (interstitial keratitis, Hutchinson's teeth and eighth nerve deafness) is pathognomonic of congenital syphilis. The diagnosis of late congenital syphilis can be confirmed by serological tests in the majority of instances.

Congenital syphilis can be prevented and its prevention is one of the aims of antenatal care. Serological tests for treponemal disease should be made on serum taken at the booking visit; retesting later in pregnancy may also be advisable. In the UK those with serological evidence of treponemal disease should be referred to the care of a genitourinary physician; Ingall & Norins (1976) state the guidelines that should be followed by American physicians.

Gonorrhoea

This is an acute, specific infectious disease, usually transmitted during sexual intercourse and characterized in adults primarily by invasion of the genitourinary tract although secondary disturbances may complicate its course. In women the disease begins with an acute urethritis, infection of Skene's ducts and spread to the cervix. After a few days it becomes subacute and the infection may spread to Bartholin's glands, the bladder, the Fallopian tubes and the pelvic peritoneum. Unless treated promptly the infection becomes chronic, resulting in Bartholin cyst or abscess, chronic cervicitis, chronic salpingo-oophoritis and occasionally through bloodstream dissemination, in arthritis, tenosynovitis or ophthalmia. Rarely the disease is disseminated and fatal from the beginning. Venereal warts affecting the thighs and labia are probably of viral aetiology but are often associated with gonorrhoea.

In neonates, gonococcal ophthalmia which is rare in adults, is the most common manifestation of infection. Vulvovaginitis also occurs in infants, spreading by contact with imperfectly sterilized fomites such as napkins, and assuming epidemic proportions in institutions. The gonococcus is not, however, the only cause of epidemic vulvovaginitis; it can also be caused by streptococci or staphylococci.

The diagnosis depends in the main on demonstration of the parasite and in acute infections with typical signs and symptoms direct examination of a Gram-stained smear will often show the characteristic kidney- or bean-shaped Gram-negative intracellular diplococci. However, these may be concealed by a heavy flora of commensal organisms and the resemblance of some of these to *Neisseria gonorrhoeae* may give rise to difficulty. Experience is needed in identifying *N. gonorrhoeae* in stained films. Wherever possible cultures must be made. In chronic cases the gonococcus is less easy to demonstrate and to cultivate and specimens sent to the laboratory must be taken from the sites most likely to be the seat of chronic infection, such as Bartholin's glands and the cervical glands. Fluid withdrawn from joint lesions and pus from chronically inflamed Fallopian tubes are frequently sterile. The gonococcus is extremely susceptible to drying and care must be taken with swabs sent to distant laboratories; these swabs should be placed in transport medium. Procaine penicillin or ampicillin with probenecid, or spectinomycin, co-trimoxazole or cefuroxime are used in treatment. Penicillin-resistance occurs in some strains.

Chlamydial infections

Evidence has accumulated that isolates from lymphogranuloma venereum, trachoma, inclusion conjunctivitis and milder infections of the genital tract are related, justifying their inclusion in the genus *Chlamydia*. *Chlamydia trachomatis* has been isolated from various clinical conditions including non-specific urethritis, cervicitis and Reiter's disease.

The chlamydiae are a group of organisms lying between bacteria and viruses which do not grow on artificial media but can be propagated in fertile eggs and by tissue culture. The inclusion bodies associated with *C. trachomatis* contain glycogen and stain with iodine. The organisms can be serotyped and those isolated from the genital tract and eye in the UK are serotypes D, E, F and G. *C. trachomatis* is an important cause of non-specific infection of the genital tract and its role in pelvic inflammatory disease is established. The agent is sensitive to sulphonamides, tetracycline and erythromycin. The latter is the agent of choice for treating chlamydial cervicitis during pregnancy.

Toxoplasmosis

Toxoplasmosis is probably unique amongst the parasitic diseases of man in that its congenital form was recognized before the postnatally acquired form of infection. Although the reported incidence of the congenital disease in the UK is not as high as in France, it exceeds that of congenital syphilis. There is little difference in the prevalence rates between sexes although the disease is clearly more important and more frequently diagnosed in women of childbearing age. There are few data from which to derive morbidity, mortality or case fatality rates.

Serological surveys show that infection with the protozoan parasite *Toxoplasma gondii* is common and widespread in man. The organism is an obligatory intracellular parasite, elongated or sickle-shaped and approximately $3-4 \times 6-7\ \mu m$. The coccidian parasite exists in three forms — the trophozoite, the tissue cyst and the cat-associated oocyst. The latter two are the principal forms implicated in transmission. It is therefore reasonable to advise pregnant women to avoid the consumption or handling of raw meat and to wear gloves if it is necessary for them to handle cat litter. Of great importance in obstetrics is the fact that infection can be passed congenitally from mother to fetus, in some species through several generations. The disease may be acquired during intrauterine life if the mother is first infected during pregnancy.

Illness is a rare accompaniment of this common infection and the best known manifestation of acquired toxoplasmosis is lymphadenopathy, which may be accompanied by the presence of glandular fever-like cells in the blood. The disease affects both sexes and the peak incidence is between 25 and 35 years.

Although placental transmission has been demonstrated in chronically infected mice, in humans congenital infection is believed to follow primary infection and the prognosis for subsequent pregnancies is good. The risk to the fetus appears to be related to the gestational age at which primary maternal infection occurs, with transmission being less likely in the first trimester but if it does occur, resulting in more severe disease. Infection leading to stillbirth or neonatal death, or to survival with ocular and cerebral involvement, occurs only in the offspring of mothers who acquire primary infection in the first or second trimester.

Although transmission rates as high as 33% have been reported following primary maternal infection, 72% of the infected newborn were spared overt clinical infection. Such asymptomatic infants may suffer no serious consequences or may later develop chorioretinitis, blindness, strabismus, hydrocephaly or microcephaly, cerebral calcification, psychomotor or mental retardation, epilepsy, or deafness. Children known to have had congenital toxoplasmosis must therefore be kept under observation for months or years.

The available data are insufficient to support or to refute the hypothesis that *T. gondii* causes malformations during the period of organogenesis. The infected infant should be treated with spiramycin or pyrimethamine/sulphonamide and folinic acid. There is some evidence that treatment of the mother who has an acute attack in pregnancy with spiramycin decreases the fetal risk.

T. gondii may be isolated from ventricular or cerebrospinal fluid, blood, lymph node or other tissue. Mice or multimammate rats are inoculated by the intracerebral, intraperitoneal or subcutanous routes and left for 6–8 weeks. Their sera are tested for antibodies and finally after killing, a saline emulsion of brain is examined for *Toxoplasma* cysts. Fertile hen's eggs or tissue cultures may be inoculated but these methods are less sensitive. The histological appearance of excised lymph nodes may suggest toxoplasmosis.

Serological tests include the cytoplasm-modifying (dye) test of Sabin and Feldman, complement fixation, haemagglutination and fluorescence inhibition. The interpretation of serological tests can be very difficult as latent infection is so common. Demonstration of a rising titre or the presence of specific IgM antibody indicates active infection. When it is not possible to demonstrate a rise a dye test titre of 1:1000 is probably reliable evidence of current infection.

The risk to the fetus of primary maternal toxoplasmosis is of the order of 50%, some 15% in the first trimester and 70% in the third. In early gestational life abortion is the likely outcome. Since 1975 in Austria, all women have been screened for *Toxoplasma* antibody during pregnancy (Aspock 1985). If seroconversion (primary infection) occurs the mother is treated. Spiramycin is used if infection occurs in the first trimester; otherwise pyrimethamine and sulphametoxydiazine are given. It is believed that congenital infection has been reduced by 50–70% in consequence of these measures. Prenatal diagnosis of toxoplasmosis was discussed by Desmonts et al (1985). The results of a 20-year follow-up of those with congenital toxoplasmosis demonstrated that subclinical infection at birth could have severe consequences and persuaded Koppe et al (1986) that women should be screened before marriage and during pregnancy.

In the UK, screening for *Toxoplasma* antibodies is not routinely performed during pregnancy because the incidence of infection is low.

Listeriosis

Listeria monocytogenes is one of few pathogens that can form colonies at 4°C and it can survive in nature in hay, straw and earth for many months. It has been isolated from many species of domestic birds, insects and crustaceans. The infective cycle is probably based on its survival in soil or vegetation, multiplication in silage, establishment of carrier or diseased state in animals or fowls, and for man, growth in food derived from these sources and consumed after inadequate heating. Its localization in the genital tracts of many vertebrates and its transmission to the fetus characterize its importance in obstetrics. A large outbreak of listeriosis occurred in 1981 in the Atlantic provinces of Canada, including many perinatal cases, and was attributed to cabbage fertilized with infected sheep manure. Of 25 cases of maternal and perinatal listeriosis in Nova Scotia, 17 infants were born alive although five died; there were three stillbirths and five spontaneous abortions.

Characteristically, infection in pregnant women is associated with two or more febrile episodes. The first, recognized in retrospect as the primary infection, is associated with malaise, headache, fever, backache, pharyngitis, conjunctivitis, diarrhoea and abdominal or loin pain. The condition may be diagnosed as pyelonephritis since the kidneys may be involved in the listeric process but the true nature of the infection will be recognized if the often slowly growing *L. monocytogenes* is actively sought in cultures of blood and of other sites, such as the genital tract and urine. Resolution of fever may occur if antibacterial therapy has been given but relapse is likely. Within 1–20 days of delivery, often of an infected premature baby, there is a further febrile episode regarded as a manifestation of reinfection from the placenta. In about 40% of cases fever is not marked at any time; the disease presents as an influenza-like illness or is completely unremarked by the patient. There is a suggestion that recurrent or persistent genital listeric infection may be a cause of habitual abortion in man as in domestic or wild animals. Due to difficulties in isolation of the microbe and until recently in the performance and interpretation of serological tests, the aetiological diagnosis may be difficult to substantiate in abortion.

The incidence of listeric infection in the perinatal period in the UK is about 1 in 20 000 births and in the USA in the early 1980s about 3.7 in 1 000 000 population. Neonatal septicaemia may occur in epidemic form in cattle and epidemics in man have been reported from East Germany and New Zealand. Cross-infection in neonatal units has also occurred.

Listeric infection of the newborn occurs in two forms. The early-onset type results from infection in utero, whether by the haematogenous transplacental route or following the inhalation of contaminated amniotic fluid, and is manifest as septicaemia within 2 days of birth. There is meconium staining of the amniotic fluid and the usually prematurely born infant has signs of respiratory distress and sometimes a rash. The late form of the disease presents predominantly as a meningoencephalitis, sometimes with slow hydrocephalus developing after the fifth day. This type may be transmitted from the environment. About one-quarter to one-third of babies with early-onset disease are born dead; necropsy demonstrates typical appearances of granulomatosis infantiseptica with miliary microabscesses and granulomata in the liver, spleen, adrenal glands, lungs, pharynx, gastrointestinal tract, central nervous system and skin. The disease is more frequent in continental Europe than in the British Isles and *L. monocytogenes* is thought to rank third after *Escherichia coli* and the group B streptococcus as a cause of neonatal sepsis in France. Mortality rates of 90% used to be recorded for infantile listeriosis but given early diagnosis and prompt treatment with bactericidal agents in high dosage, an overall mortality of 50% is more likely. If a surviving infant is more than 36 weeks of gestation at birth there are likely to be adverse sequelae. Combination therapy with ampicillin and gentamicin is the treatment of choice.

VIRAL DISEASES

Some viral diseases in pregnancy are important because of the deleterious effects they may have on the developing fetus and in the newborn. The main complications of these diseases are shown in Table 41.5. Only major diseases will be discussed here.

Rubella

Although more severe disease may occur in adults, rubella is a mild infection characterized by a generalized rash which may be preceded by catarrh and enlargement of the posterior cervical lymph nodes. Constitutional disturbance is slight and complications apart from those affecting the fetus in utero are uncommon. The brief and evanescent rash of rubella starts as a faint macular erythema which first involves the face and neck, spreads rapidly to the trunk and extremities and disappears from one site even as the next becomes involved. The eruption has vanished by the third day and sometimes does not occur at all. The rash of rubella is traditionally regarded as characteristic but similar rashes may be caused by other viruses. The incubation period is usually 17–18 days. Patients are infectious during the last week of the incubation period and for about a week after the disappearance of the rash.

The incubation period, the date of known contact, the degree of contact and the duration of infectivity are all factors that must be considered by the pathologist and obstetrician when interpreting the results of serological tests for rubella in early pregnancy. An accurate history is of paramount importance. The disease is rarely acquired by children under the age of 6 months except by the intrauterine route and it is also rare in persons over 40 years old.

Rubella virus is carried in the nasopharynx and the disease is spread by droplets emanating from persons in the last week of the incubation period or who have had the rash

Table 41.5 Viral infections during pregnancy implicated in fetal or neonatal disease

Virus	Potential effect on mother	Potential effect on fetus or newborn
Coxsackie A	Herpangina, hand, foot and mouth disease; myocardiopathy	
Coxsackie A_9		?Gastrointestinal defects
Coxsackie B	Often unnoticeable; aseptic meningitis; Bornholm disease	Myocarditis–meningoencephalitis; neonatal sepsis
B_2 and B_4		?Urogenital anomalies
B_3 and B_4		?Cardiovascular lesions
Cytomegalovirus	Usually asymptomatic but sometimes moderate to high fever in primary infection	Chronic infection; acute disease; late-onset sequelae
ECHO virus	Rash of $ECHO_9$ may resemble rubella; maternal disease may mimic appendicitis or abruptio placentae, as in other enterovirus infections	Neonatal sepsis
Hepatitis A and B	Flu-like illness; chills and high fever; constitutional symptoms and jaundice; increased severity in pregnancy	Prematurity; neonatal hepatitis; vertical transmission of hepatitis B virus
Herpes simplex	Oral or genital infection; more severe in pregnancy	?Abortion; ?prematurity; fatal disseminated infections (HSV2 > HSV1); congenital malformations
HIV	Acceleration of disease	Vertical transmission; infantile disease; central nervous system malformations
Influenza	Increased mortality in pandemics	?Increased fetal mortality; ???congenital malformations; ?increase in childhood leukaemia
Lymphocytic choriomeningitis	Meningitis/meningoencephalitis	Congenital disease
Measles	May be complicated by pneumonia and CCF; more severe and may be fatal	Probably increased mortality; congenital measles
Mumps	No special effect	Increased fetal mortality; ?endocardial fibroelastosis
Poliomyelitis	Increased severity and mortality	Fetal death; neonatal disease
Polyoma	Asymptomatic	?Increased risk of jaundice
Rubella	No special effect	Fetal death; chronic persisting infection; congenital malformations
Varicella-zoster	Often more severe; maternal death	Neonatal chickenpox; probable specific congenital defects
Vaccinia and variola	Increased severity and mortality	Fetal death; intrauterine or neonatal disease
Venezuelan and western equine encephalomyelitides	Meningoencephalitis	Neonatal encephalitis

HSV = herpes simplex virus; HIV = human immunodeficiency virus; CCF = chronic congestive failure

7–14 days previously. Susceptible people who wish to work in units where they will contact women in the first trimester of pregnancy should be actively encouraged to accept rubella vaccine, as should susceptible women contemplating pregnancy, for example those attending infertility clinics.

The disease is often clinically inapparent because there is no rash. In the UK over 80% of women of childbearing age have serological evidence of past rubella infection and are immune. This percentage is rising as those who have been immunized in early adolescence enter their childbearing years. Serologically demonstrable reinfection is possible but viraemia is not detectable in such cases and in its absence the products of conception should remain uninfected. Susceptibility or immunity to rubella cannot be adduced from evidence of the past history and must be based on serological examination.

Before laboratory diagnosis was possible rubella was diagnosed on clinical grounds, as are the majority of cases today. Not all rubella-like rashes are caused by the rubella virus however, and recourse to a diagnostic virology laboratory should be made wherever feasible . During pregnancy this must always be done because of the serious consequences of misdiagnosis. The presence of a transient arthralgia as the rash begins to fade, which occurs in 60–70% of postpubertal females, supports the clinical diagnosis of rubella.

Rubella in pregnancy is uncommon. The attack rate overall is approximately 1 in 1000 pregnancies rising to 22 in 1000 during epidemics. It is probably less infectious than measles or varicella and the chance of contracting it from brief or casual exposure is small. The risk is five times greater when the contact is within the family group than when the contact is outside it, which emphasizes the importance of eliciting an accurate history of the nature of the contact during pregnancy.

Maternal virus is transmitted to the fetus transplacentally and maternal viraemia is postulated as the factor essential for the genesis of fetal infection. Rubella causes spontaneous abortion and stillbirth; the incidence is about double that in control populations — 10% compared with 5%. The virus produces an antimitotic effect upon infected cells which leads to retardation in cell division and results in major malformations if it occurs during a critical phase of organogenesis. Chronic infection may persist throughout gestation and may cause further damage. The perinatal mortality rate varies from 110 to 290 per 1000 total births (Horstmann et al 1965, Banatvala 1971).

Prospective studies have shown that when rubella is acquired in early pregnancy the incidence of congenital malformations varies from 15 to 35%. If it is acquired during the first month of gestation, the incidence of defects may approach 50–60% and such defects may be multiple. Thereafter the incidence of malformations declines until by the 16th week it is about 5%. Even if infection is acquired after the first trimester, up to the 31st week, the babies may show evidence of intrauterine infection since, when followed up for 2–3 years, poor communicative ability, poor physical growth and developmental retardation may be noted.

It is important that babies born to women known to have had rubella even late in pregnancy should be regularly surveyed for physical or other defects before reaching school age. Congenitally infected children may themselves act as vectors of infection. At 6 months of age, 20–30% of them may still be excreting virus from the nasopharynx and even at 1 year of age, 7–9% still do so. Susceptible women of childbearing age who nurse or attend such children should be protected by vaccination.

The diagnosis of rubella in pregnancy is established by serological tests. Since rubella antibodies persist indefinitely, antibody detected within 14 days of contact when the contact date is certain indicates that the patient has previously had rubella. If serum can be obtained during the acute phase of the illness paired sera are examined to detect a significant rise in antibody. If serum cannot be obtained during the acute phase or if only one sample is available but the duration of pregnancy necessitates rapid diagnosis, the presence of rubella-specific IgM, which does not usually persist for more than 2 months, indicates active or recent infection. Serological tests made on patients presenting well after the incubation period are difficult to interpret, although the presence of high titres may suggest the diagnosis.

Virus isolation is a lengthy and exacting procedure and is not usually feasible in pregnancy when rapid diagnosis is desirable. At birth, congenitally infected infants generally have high rubella antibody levels which persist for longer than would be expected if such antibody was maternally derived — that is, longer than 4–6 months. Rubella-specific IgM can usually be detected during the first year of life and since the IgM class of immunoglobulins cannot cross the placenta the presence of this antibody in cord blood indicates intrauterine infection. Virus may be detected in the nasopharynx, urine and stools.

Protective antibodies, whether acquired in response to a naturally occurring infection or in response to vaccine, persist and afford clinical protection of an extremely high order. It is therefore desirable that vaccine should be offered to girls before they reach childbearing years. There is a case for also giving an effective rubella vaccine to mature women as 15–20% are susceptible to rubella, gamma globulin offers no appreciable protection and subclinical infection is common. Rubella vaccine is now offered on a national basis to young children in the UK. It may also be offered to mature women provided they are advised to avoid pregnancy for at least 3 months. The puerperium offers a good opportunity for vaccination in women who are susceptible but have not yet completed their families. The menstrual period is also said to offer a good opportunity.

Women who are to be offered vaccine in the puerperium are usually tested for susceptibility by appropriate serological tests on serum obtained at booking. The baseline value obtained then is also useful if they are exposed to a rubella-like illness later in pregnancy. The suggestion that termination of pregnancy should be offered to those who are inadvertently vaccinated just before or during early pregnancy is not supported by clinical observations, although the theoretical risk that the vaccine is itself teratogenic remains and vaccine virus can cross the placenta.

Cytomegalovirus infections

Cytomegalovirus is a member of the herpesvirus group; these viruses are characterized by their tendency to cause latent as well as acute infections. Cytomegalovirus is probably transmitted in urine and saliva, requiring close and prolonged contact. Up to 12% of healthy women excrete virus during pregnancy and it is possible that pregnancy enhances susceptibility to infection or reactivation of virus. However, about half the female population in the western hemisphere are without antibody by the time they reach childbearing years and as the highest seroconversion rate occurs between the ages of 15 and 35, the chances of primary infection coinciding with pregnancy are high.

Since 0.5–3% of newborn infants excrete virus, congenital infection is by no means rare. The majority of babies excreting virus escape serious disease or even outward signs of infection although in the past it was thought that intrauterine infection invariably resulted in central nervous system damage in a high proportion of cases. The outcome of primary infection during pregnancy probably depends upon its virulence and duration. Peckham et al (1983) noted an incidence of 3 per 1000 of the congenital infection in 14 789 pregnancies. A total of 7% of the 42 infected babies were seriously handicapped; 33% had minor or transient problems and 60% were unscathed. Sixty-seven per cent were born to women who had developed primary infection during pregnancy.

Infection during pregnancy may cause abortion or congenital defects and late in pregnancy it may cause severe fetal disease with stillbirth, either preterm or at term. The child may be born alive, often of low birthweight, only to die in the neonatal period with fulminating disease of which the extraneural symptoms are jaundice, often with hepatosplenomegaly, thrombocytopenic purpura, choroidoretinitis and anaemia. Others may develop symptoms after an apparently normal neonatal period. A number show spasticity, microcephaly and mental retardation. Hydrocephalus, optic atrophy and epilepsy have also been reported.

Herpes simplex

Herpes virus hominis infection of the female genital tract is the most common viral disease in gynaecology and the most common cause of ulcerative lesions of the female genital tract in England. Many cases are asymptomatic. More than 90% of the genital infections are caused by type 2 virus while the majority of infections of the oral mucosa, cornea and brain are caused by type 1. With the prevalence of oral sex, type 1 genital infections are becoming more frequent. Primary genital infection is caused most frequently by venereal contact but non-venereal infection has been described. After initial infection the condition can be reactivated by temperature change, emotional trauma, premenstrual tension, menstruation and the use of oral contraceptives.

Clinically apparent infections of the vulva or perineum may be accompanied by pain, burning, malaise, ulceration, inguinal adenopathy and fever but infections of the cervix and those high in the vagina produce few subjective symptoms. Vesicular vulvovaginitis is not the main feature of the infection and 50% or more of all genital herpes infections may be asymptomatic. Asymptomatic infections of the vulva are rare but cervical lesions may present as diffuse cervicitis with multiple tiny superficial ulcers or more rarely as a necrotizing cervicitis resembling squamous carcinoma.

There is some evidence that the virus may be transmitted transplacentally but most neonatal infections are caused by type 2 virus which is probably transmitted during the second stage of labour and more often in consequence of primary infection rather than recurrence. The incidence of disseminated herpes is greater among premature infants. The liver and adrenals are involved, with focal coagulative necrosis as the characteristic lesion. The virus may be recovered from many organs and infection of the central nervous system may be the dominant clinical feature. The diagnosis can be made clinically if typical vesicular eruption of the skin occurs during the first week of life but about half the infants who go on to develop disseminated infection do not have vesicles in the early stages of the disease. Diagnosis is confirmed by examination of cells scraped from the base of local lesions by electron or light microscopy. The virus may be cultured within 2–4 days.

If virus is known to be present in the genital tract at or near term Caesarean section should be considered and the case for section is strengthened if lesions are present. There is no real evidence that Caesarean section reduces the probability of neonatal disease unless it is performed within 4 hours of rupture of membranes. Monif and Hardt (1984) discuss the management of herpetic vulvovaginitis during pregnancy, basing it on the recommendations of the American Academy of Pediatrics (Committee on Fetus and Newborn 1980). Repeated viriculture is not favoured in the UK (Kelly 1988).

Varicella-zoster

Women of childbearing age are rarely affected by varicella-zoster virus since most are already immune as a result of childhood infection. Abortion and intrauterine infection resulting in disseminated disease have been reported. If maternal infection occurs near or at term neonatal chickenpox presents at birth or within the first 2–3 weeks of life, depending on the interval between maternal infection and birth.

The fetus may be infected in the early weeks of pregnancy and still survive to term; brain damage is the main feature. Cerebral complications and pneumonitis are common in neonatal chickenpox although generalized rash and local eruption along a dermatome may be seen, as in zoster. Early treatment with immunoglobulins may be of value in the case of women with chickenpox in early pregnancy and immunoglobulin may be administered prophylactically to the offspring of women who have varicella at or about term. The mortality rate of neonatal varicella is variously reported as 0–23%. Zoster immune globulin should be given to newborn babies exposed within 5 days of delivery.

Congenital malformation (varicella embryopathy) may follow maternal varicella-zoster infection in the first trimester of pregnancy. The syndrome is characterized by fetal growth retardation, aplasia and scarring of a limb, neurological damage or eye abnormalities and is fully described by Brunell (1984). The magnitude of the risk is not known but is believed to be less than one in a hundred.

Hepatitis

Pregnant women may contract hepatitis A or B or non-A non-B. Of these, hepatitis B is the most likely. Because of the risk of vertical transmission, which plays a major part in maintaining a reservoir of virus in nature, hepatitis B has been most studied during pregnancy. Women who have HBeAg and/or DNA polymerase are more likely to transmit hepatitis B virus than those who are seronegative for these markers.

Other than non-A non-B hepatitis, which is associated with a mortality rate of the order of 20%, viral hepatitis in the USA and Europe is not associated with increased risks to the mother and does not result in fetal death or anomaly. However, acute maternal infection with hepatitis B virus may result in neonatal hepatitis and the risk is dependent

Table 41.6 Risks of hepatitis B virus transfer from mother to child (from Mowat 1980)

Mother HBsAG-positive	Infant infection rate
Acute hepatitis 3 months before to 1 month after delivery	80–90%
Acute hepatitis in early pregnancy	10–30%
Asymptomatic carrier mother	10%
HBeAg-positive	90%
HBeAg-negative	30%
HBeAg-negative, HBeAg-positive	0%

on the trimester in which maternal infection occurs, being highest at or about term.

The risks of hepatitis B transmission from mother to child are shown in Table 41.6. Infants born to hepatitis B carriers or HBsAg-positive mothers should be protected by active and passive immunization, particularly if the mothers are e-antigen positive, or lack anti-e antibody. Three intramuscular doses of 0.5 ml vaccine are given together with hepatitis B immune globulin.

Acquired immune deficiency syndrome (AIDS)

This syndrome is the late effect of a lymphocytopathic retrovirus named as human T-lymphotropic virus III (HTLV-III) or more recently as human immunodeficiency virus (HIV). The virus is transmitted sexually, predominantly by anal intercourse and traumatic sexual practices, particularly in homosexual males although it can be transmitted heterosexually. It is also transmitted by blood-to-blood contact, especially through the shared syringes and needles used by intravenous drug abusers. Its importance in obstetrics is twofold: firstly pregnancy may aggravate the course of the disease and secondly the disease is transmissible from mother to fetus.

Fever, weight loss, diarrhoea and lymphadenopathy are the major presenting signs of AIDS together with pneumonia, thrombocytopenic purpura and others. Opportunist infections include amongst the viruses cytomegalovirus (pulmonary, central nervous system or gastrointestinal involvement) and herpes simplex virus (mucocutaneous, pulmonary, gastrointestinal or disseminated disease). Progressive multifocal leukoencephalopathy (papovavirus-induced) may occur. Overwhelming bacterial sepsis may be associated inter alia with *Salmonella* or *Mycobacteria*, especially *M. avium intracellulare*. As with other conditions associated with severe immune defects, candidosis is frequent and infections by *Aspergillus* species, *Cryptococcus* and other fungi occur. Dissemination or extensive local involvement by parasites including *Toxoplasma gondii*, *Cryptosporidium*, *Strongyloides* and *Pneumocystis carinii* is frequent.

Tumours other than Kaposi's sarcoma especially Hodgkin's and non-Hodgkin's lymphomas are also associated, together with squamous carcinoma of the rectum and other tumours. Other disorders such as enteropathy and progressive encephalopathy or myelopathy may also occur. The latter seems to be separate from the immune deficiency. Neurological manifestations are reviewed by Carne & Adler (1986).

The cytopathic virus is a retrovirus of the subfamily Lentiviridae, a group of viruses rapidly lethal to the domestic animals they infect (Seale 1985). It attacks T-cell subsets as well as macrophages and cells throughout the brain. In a proportion of infected persons, infection with virus after an incubation period of 15–57 months as determined in recipients of infected blood, or of 4.5 years with a range of 2.6–14.2 years as more recently calculated, causes symptoms of AIDS (12%) or AIDS-related complex (48%; Weber et al 1986). It is calculated that the proportion developing AIDS will increase with time.

The route of spread is similar to that of hepatitis B virus — by sexual transmission especially by homosexual anal intercourse, by blood-to-blood contact through transfusion of whole blood or blood components, by semen and by maternal–fetal or neonatal transmission. Certain groups of individuals are thus at high risk. These include homosexual or bisexual males, recipients of unscreened or untreated blood or blood products, intravenous drug abusers and those whose consorts have AIDS or are HIV-antibody positive. Preventive measures include education of the public in safer sex, guidance to health care personnel from the Department of Health and Social Security (1985a,b 1986a), donor selection and antibody screening for blood donors (Barbara et al 1986) and for potential semen donors (Department of Health and Social Security 1986b).

Transplacental transmission of HIV occurs in early pregnancy (Jovaisas et al 1985, Sprecher et al 1986). Abnormal development in such fetuses includes growth failure, a prominent box-like forehead, wide-set eyes, short nose and patulous lips (Marion et al 1986). Children of infected mothers probably acquired the infection in utero but may also acquire it from maternal blood at birth or postnatally or from breast milk. The risk of transmission is not known but may be as high as 65% in children of mothers who have already given birth to an infected child (Centers for Disease Control 1985). It is considerably less in those born to mothers who are antibody positive but not ill (Lancet 1988).

As the AIDS epidemic gains ground in the UK there is a case for screening those in high-risk categories for antibody to the virus. A positive test denotes exposure to the virus and because the infection persists, probably for life, it is presumptive evidence of infectiousness (Curran et al 1985). If screening tests are to be undertaken during pregnancy, maternal consent for counselling will be required. Obstetricians who need to advise mothers with AIDS of the risk of vertical transmission will find help from a useful Royal College of Obstetricians and Gynaecologists document on the subject of AIDS in children (Hudson 1987). Termination of pregnancy would have to be considered.

CONCLUSIONS

Life-threatening microbial disease is currently in the UK rare in pregnant and parturient women. With advances in paediatric intensive care, the emphasis on serious infections has shifted to the unborn or recently born child, particularly if the latter is of low, or very low birthweight. Great advances have been made in the prevention of congenitally acquired infections, notably through the introduction of rubella virus vaccine.

As knowledge of microbial pathogens increases, newly recognized disease entities emerge or older observations are re-emphasized. Such are the apparent adverse effects on the fetus of Lyme disease (Markowitz et al 1986) the role of *Chlamydia psittaci* of ovine origin and of *Streptococcus milleri* in spontaneous abortion (Roberts et al 1967, Johnson et al 1985, MacGowan & Terry 1987), fetal distress associated with *Cryptosporidium* infection (Dale et al 1987), maternal and fetal death caused by *Pasteurella multocida* (Rasaiah et al 1986) and hydrops fetalis associated with human parvovirus infection (Anand et al 1987, Thurn 1988). Many of these infections are currently receiving intense study. Some will remain rarities; others may be important as causes of maternal and fetal morbidity or mortality.

REFERENCES

Anand A, Gray E S, Brown T et al 1987 Human parvovirus infection in pregnancy and hydrops fetalis. New England Journal of Medicine 316: 183–186

Aspock H 1985 Toxoplasmosis in prenatal and perinatal infections. WHO, Geneva

Banatvala J E (ed) 1971 Current problems in clinical virology. Churchill Livingstone, Edinburgh

Barbara J A J, Contreras M, Hewitt P 1986 AIDS: a problem for the transfusion service? British Journal of Hospital Medicine 36: 18–184

Blanc W A 1959 Amniotic infection syndrome: pathogenesis, morphology and significance in circumnatal mortality. Clinics in Obstetrics and Gynaecology 2: 704–734

Brunell P A 1984 Fetal and neonatal varicella–zoster infections. In: Amstey M S (ed) Virus infections in pregnancy. Grune & Stratton, New York

Carne C A, Adler M W 1986 Neurological manifestations of human immunodeficiency virus infection. Lancet 293: 462–463

Carroll C J. Hurley R, Stanley V C 1973 Criteria for diagnosis of candida vulvovaginitis in pregnant women. Journal of Obstetrics and Gynaecology of the British Commonwealth 80: 258–263

Catterall R D 1979 Venereology and genitourinary medicine, 2nd edn. Hodder & Stoughton, London

Centers for Disease Control 1985 Recommendations for assisting in the prevention of perinatal transmission of human T-lymphotropic virus type III/lymphadenopathy associated virus and acquired immunodeficiency syndrome. Communicable Disease Center: Mortality and Morbidity Weekly Reports 34: 721–726, 731–732

Charles D, Hurry D J 1983 Chorioamnionitis. In: Charles D (ed) Clinics in obstetrics and gynaecology, vol 10. W B Saunders, London

Committee on Fetus and Newborn, Committee on Infectious Diseases 1980 Perinatal herpes simplex virus infections. Pediatrics 66: 142

Curran J W, Morgan W M, Hardy A M, Jaffe H W, Darrow W W, Dowdle W R 1985. The epidemiology of AIDS: current status and future prospects. Science 229: 1352–1357

Dale B A S, Gordon G, Thomson R, Urquhart R 1987 Perinatal infection with cryptosporidium. Lancet i: 1042–1043

Davies P A 1971 Bacterial infection in the fetus and newborn. Archives of Disease in Childhood 46: 1–27

Davison J 1984 Renal disease. In: de Swiet M (ed) Medical disorders in obstetric practice. Blackwell Scientific Publications, Oxford

de Louvois J, Blades M, Harrison R F, Hurley R, Stanley V C 1974 Frequency of mycoplasmas in fertile and infertile couples. Lancet i: 1073

Department of Health and Social Security 1985a Acquired immune deficiency syndrome AIDS. General information for doctors. DHSS, London

Department of Health and Social Security 1985b Acquired immune deficiency syndrome AIDS. Information for doctors concerning the introduction of the HTLV–III antibody test. DHSS, London

Department of Health and Social Security 1986a Acquired immune deficiency syndrome AIDS. Guidance for surgeons, anaesthetists, dentists and their teams in dealing with patients infected with HTLV-III. DHSS, London

Department of Health and Social Security 1986b Acquired immune deficiency syndrome AIDS. Guidance for doctors and AI clinics concerning AIDS and artificial insemination. DHSS, London

Desmonts G, Forestier F, Thulliez P H et al 1985 Prenatal diagnosis of congenital toxoplasmosis. Lancet i: 500–504

Fiumara N J, Bleming W L, Downing J G, Good F L 1952 The incidence of prenatal syphilis at the Boston City Hospital. New England Journal of Medicine 247: 48

Gluck L, Wood H F, Fousek M D 1966 Septicemia of the newborn. Pediatric Clinics of North America 13: 1131–1148

Horstmann D M, Banatvala J E, Riordan J R et al 1965 Maternal rubella syndrome in infants. American Journal of Diseases of Children 110: 408

Hudson C (ed) 1987 Report of the subcommittee on problems associated with AIDS in relation to obstetrics and gynaecology. Royal College of Obstetrics and Gynaecology, London

Hurley R 1977 Heart disease, parturition and antibiotic prophylaxis In: Lewis P (ed) Therapeutic problems in pregnancy. MTP Press, Lancaster

Hurley R 1984 Fever and infectious diseases In: de Swiet M (ed) Medical disorders in obstetric practice. Blackwell Scientific Publications, Oxford

Hurley R, de Louvois J 1981 Bloodstream infections and perinatal mortality. Journal of Clinical Pathology 34: 271–276

Hurley R, Stanley V C, Leask B G S, de Louvois J 1974 Microflora of the vagina during pregnancy In: Skinner F A, Carr J G (eds) The normal microbial flora of man. Academic Press, London

Ingall D, Norins L 1976 Syphilis. In: Remington J S, Klein J O (eds) Infectious diseases of the fetus and newborn infant. W B Saunders, London

Johnson F W A, Matheson B A, Williams H et al (1985) Abortion due to infection with *Chlamydia psittaci* in a sheep farmer's wife. British Medical Journal 290: 592–594

Jovaisas E, Koch M A, Schafer A, Stauber M, Lowenthal D 1985 LAV/HTLV-III in 20-week fetus. Lancet ii: 1129

Kelly J 1988 Genital herpes during pregnancy. British Medical Journal 297: 1146–1147

Koppe J G, Loewer-Sieger D H, de Roever-Bonnet 1986 Results of a 20 year follow-up of congenital toxoplasmosis. Lancet i: 254–256

Lancet 1988 Vertical transmission of HIV. Lancet ii: 1057–1058

Letsky E 1984 Haemostasis and haemorrhage In: de Swiet M (ed) Medical disorders in obstetric practice. Blackwell Scientific Publications, Oxford

MacGowan A P, Terry P B 1987 *Streptococcus milleri* and second trimester abortion. Journal of Clinical Pathology 40: 292–293

Marion R W, Wiznia A A, Hutcheon R G, Rubinstein A 1986 Human T-cell lymphotropic virus type III (HTLV-III) embryopathy. A new dysmorphic syndrome associated with intrauterine HTLV-III infection. American Journal of Diseases of Children 140: 638–640

Markowitz L E, Steere A C, Benach J L, Slade J D, Broom C V 1986 Lyme disease during pregnancy. Journal of the American Medical Association 255: 3394–3396

McCracken G H, Shinefield H R 1966 Changes in the pattern of neonatal septicaemia and meningits. American Journal of Diseases of Children 112: 33–39

Monif G R G, Hardt N S 1984 Management of herpetic vulvovaginitis in pregnancy In: Amstey M S (ed) Virus infection in pregnancy. Grune & Stratton, New York

Mowat A P 1980 Viral hepatitis in infancy and childhood. In: Sherlock S (ed) Virus hepatitis. W B Saunders, London

Murphy N, Damjanovi C V, Hart C A, Buchanan C R, Whittaker R,

Cooke R W I 1986 Infection and colonisation of neonates by *Hansenula anomala*. Lancet i: 291–293
Naeye R L, Peters E C 1980 Causes and consequences of premature rupture of fetal membranes. Lancet i: 192–194
Peckham C S, Chin K S, Coleman J C et al 1983 Cytomegalovirus infection in pregnancy: preliminary findings from a prospective study. Lancet ii: 352
Rasaiah B, Otero J G, Russell I J et al 1986 *Pasteurella multocida* septicaemia during pregnancy. Canadian Medical Association Journal 135: 1369–1372
Remington J S, Klein J O (eds) 1983 Infectious diseases of the fetus and newborn infant, 2nd edn. W B Saunders, London
Roberts W, Grist N R, Giroud P 1967 Human abortion associated with infection by ovine abortion agent. British Medical Journal 4: 37
Sanderson P J 1986 Staying one jump ahead of resistant *Staphylococcus aureus*. British Medical Journal 293: 573–574
Seale J 1985 AIDS virus infection: prognosis and transmission. Journal of the Royal Society of Medicine 78: 613–615
Shanson D C 1986 Staphylococcal infections in hospital. British Journal of Hospital Medicine 35: 312–320
Siegel J D, McCracken G H Jr 1981 Sepsis neonatorum. New England Journal of Medicine 1: 642–647
Silverman W A, Homan W E 1949 Sepsis of obscure origin in the newborn. Pediatrics 3: 157–176
Sprecher S, Soumenkoff G, Puissant F, Degueldre M 1986 Vertical transmission of HIV in 15-week fetus. Lancet ii: 288
Stokes J H, Beerman H, Ingraham N R Jr (eds) 1944 Modern clinical syphilology, 3rd edn. W B Saunders, London
Thurn J 1988 Human parvovirus B19: historical and critical review. Reviews of Infectious Diseases 10: 1005–1011
Weber J N, Wadsworth J, Rogers L A et al 1986 Three year prospective study of HTLV-III/LAV infection in homosexual men. Lancet i: 1179

W. Dunlop and J. M. Davison

Urinary tract in pregnancy

INTRODUCTION

Few aspects of maternal physiology change more profoundly during pregnancy than those affecting the urinary tract. An understanding of these changes is of fundamental importance since abnormalities must be assessed against basal values inappropriate for the non-pregnant state. For these reasons, a brief account of the most significant alterations in renal physiology must be considered before discussing urinary disorders which may complicate pregnancy.

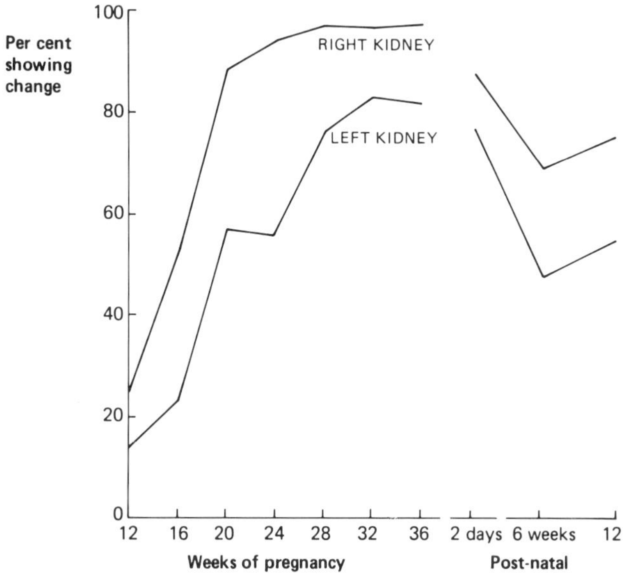

Fig. 42.1 Changes throughout pregnancy in percentage incidences for both kidneys of stasis and hydronephrosis with or without clubbing. Derived from the nephrosonographic data of Cietak & Newton (1985a).

PREGNANCY-INDUCED ALTERATIONS IN THE URINARY TRACT

Pregnancy is associated with substantial dilatation of the urinary tract (Bailey & Rolleston 1971, Roberts 1976, Peake et al 1983). By the third trimester some 97% of women show evidence of stasis or hydronephrosis (Cietak & Newton 1985a). Dilatation is more pronounced on the right than the left at all stages of pregnancy (Fig. 42.1), perhaps because of the customary dextrorotation of the uterus. Nephrosonographic studies suggest that renal parenchymal volumes also increase during pregnancy (Cietak & Newton 1985b), probably the result of increases in intrarenal fluid predominantly (Davison & Lindheimer 1980). It appears that a 70% increment has occurred by the beginning of the third trimester but that there may be a slight reduction during the latter weeks of pregnancy (Cietak & Newton 1985b). These anatomical changes relate to the physiological changes in renal function in pregnancy.

Renal haemodynamics

By the second trimester, renal blood flow (assessed indirectly as effective renal plasma flow) has increased (Sims & Krantz 1956), probably by as much as 70–80% (Davison & Dunlop 1984). During the third trimester a significant reduction has been described (Dunlop 1981). This cannot be attributed solely to the effects of maternal posture (Dunlop 1976, Ezimokhai et al 1981), although posture may have a substantial effect upon the results of investigations during late pregnancy (Chesley & Sloan 1984, Baird et al 1966). Since renal blood flow is one of the most important influences on the rate of filtration by the kidney, substantial increases in glomerular filtration rate occur during pregnancy (Bonsnes & Lange 1950, Davison & Hytten 1974). However the 50% increase is rather less than renal blood flow (Dunlop 1981); in consequence the filtration fraction, the proportion of renal plasma flow filtered at the glomerulus, decreases during early pregnancy (Davison & Dunlop 1980).

In clinical practice, it is convenient to assess the glomerular filtration rate by means of the creatinine clearance, usually over a 24-hour period in order to ensure reasonable accuracy. Serial investigations of groups of healthy women suggest that this has increased by 45% by the eighth week of pregnancy (6 weeks after conception; Davison & Noble 1981); this increase is maintained throughout the second trimester (Davison & Hytten 1974) but a significant and consistent decrease in values equivalent to the non-pregnant occurs during the last weeks of pregnancy (Davison et al 1980). Since the renal clearance of a substance bears a reciprocal relationship to its plasma concentrations, plasma creatinine concentration falls during early pregnancy but rises progressively during the third trimester. During pregnancy significant renal impairment may be present in women who have plasma concentrations of creatinine within the normal non-pregnant range, but on the other hand, increases in plasma creatinine concentrations (or decreases in creatinine clearance) during the third trimester of pregnancy may not imply pathological changes.

Tubular function

Few constituents of the urine are excreted at the same rate as they are filtered at the glomerulus. Some substances, such as hippurate derivatives, are actively secreted into the urine but most are partially reabsorbed during passage through the nephron. In many cases of apparent tubular reabsorption a degree of secretion by the kidney is also present, although it is difficult to determine the relative contributions of these two processes in human subjects. Virtually no reliable information is available about the changes associated with human pregnancy.

Glucose is so avidly reabsorbed by the kidney that none is detectable by routine clinical testing in the urine of healthy non-pregnant individuals. However, during normal pregnancy, glucose excretion increases soon after conception (Davison 1974, Davison & Dunlop 1980). Excretion rates may be as much as 10 times those of non-pregnant women (20–100 mg/day) and there is marked variability both within and between days, the pattern bearing no demonstrable relationship to blood sugar concentrations. Some two-thirds of apparently healthy pregnant women will exhibit glycosuria to a degree conventionally considered clinically significant on repeated urinalysis (Lind & Hytten 1972); conversely, not all women with impaired glucose tolerance during pregnancy are significantly glycosuric on routine testing (Lind 1975). Glycosuria does not therefore provide reliable information about carbohydrate metabolism during pregnancy.

The extent to which glycosuria is provoked by pregnancy bears a significant relationship to the extent to which glucose is reabsorbed from the glomerular filtrate, not only during pregnancy but also in the same subjects in the non-pregnant state (Davison & Hytten 1975, Davison & Dunlop 1984). It has been suggested that this phenomenon may be related to unsuspected renal tubular damage caused by previous urinary tract infections (Davison & Dunlop 1980, Davison et al 1984). Within a week of delivery, glucose excretion has returned to non-pregnant patterns (Davison & Lovedale 1974). This is almost certainly due to the reduction of the glomerular filtration rate, for defects in glucose reabsorption can still be demonstrated by appropriate infusion protocols in women who have previously been severely glycosuric (Davison & Dunlop 1984).

Changes in glomerular filtration rate are also partly responsible for the increased renal clearances of other urinary constituents and for reductions in their circulating concentrations. Of particular note in clinical practice are urea and uric acid, both of which decrease considerably during the first trimester of pregnancy (Davison & Dunlop 1984, Lind et al 1984). However, during late pregnancy, the circulating concentrations of uric acid tend to increase. Part of this increase may reflect decreasing glomerular filtration (Davison et al 1980) but there is also convincing evidence of altered renal handling. Renal reabsorption of uric acid decreases significantly during early pregnancy and rises gradually towards non-pregnant values thereafter (Dunlop & Davison 1977).

The distal renal tubule is actively concerned with volume homeostasis. Once again there is evidence of substantial change in this area of physiology during human pregnancy. Total body water increases by between 6 and 8 litres and there is a net retention of some 900 mmol of sodium (Nolten & Ehrlich 1980). Although plasma osmolality is markedly reduced (by about 10 mosmol/l) from the early weeks of pregnancy (Davison et al 1981), it is not associated with the water diuresis which would occur in the non-pregnant individual. While the process of osmoregulation is effective during pregnancy, there must be important changes in the osmotic thresholds which trigger control mechanisms, such as the sensation of thirst and the release of the antidiuretic hormone, arginine vasopressin (Davison et al 1988).

These substantial alterations in physiological norms affect the interpretation of disordered renal function during pregnancy. A brief account of the changes of greatest clinical significance is provided in Table 42.1.

INFECTION OF THE URINARY TRACT

Definitions

The analysis of urine specimens during pregnancy is especially likely to be hampered by contamination at the time of collection with bacteria from urethra, vagina or perineum. This problem can be overcome by suprapubic aspiration of bladder urine (McFadyen et al 1973), but this inconvenient procedure is distasteful to most patients and obstetricians. Another approach is to use the number of colony counts obtained upon culture of a fresh midstream urine

Table 42.1 Physiological changes in common indices of renal function associated with human pregnancy: mean value (±1 standard deviation)

Measurement	Units	Non-pregnant	Early pregnancy	Late pregnancy	Source
Effective renal plasma flow	ml/min	480 (72)	841 (144)	771 (175)	1
Glomerular filtration rate					
Inulin clearance	ml/min	105 (24)	163 (19)	169 (22)	2
24-h creatinine clearance	ml/min	94 (8)	136 (11)	114 (10)	3, 4
Plasma					
Creatinine	μmol/l	77 (10)	60 (8)	64 (9)	5
Urea	mmol/l	4.3 (0.8)	3.0 (0.7)	2.8 (0.7)	5
Uric acid	μmol/l	246 (59)	189 (48)	269 (56)	6
Osmolality	mosmol/kg	288 (2.5)	278 (2.0)	280 (2.0)	7, 8

Sources: 1. Dunlop 1981; 2. Davison & Hytten 1974; 3. Davison & Noble 1981; 4. Davison et al 1980; 5. Lind, unpublished observations; 6. Lind et al 1984; 7. Davison et al 1981; 8. Davison et al 1988.

specimen (Cohen & Kass 1967) collected by a clean-catch technique involving anteroposterior swabbing of the vulva with water or a soap solution (not antiseptic) at least three times before starting micturition. True bacteriuria may then be defined as more than 100 000 bacteria of the same species per millilitre of urine, present in two consecutive specimens. Bacteriuria is frequently associated with discomfort on voiding, urgency and increased frequency of micturition but these symptoms are common in pregnancy even in the absence of urinary tract infection. Conversely, asymptomatic (covert) bacteriuria, in which true bacteriuria is present without subjective evidence of urinary tract infection, may be of considerable clinical significance.

Bacteriuria originating from the upper urinary tract is more likely to recur and requires more rigorous surveillance and treatment (Fairley et al 1966). Numerous techniques have been used to investigate this problem (Lindheimer & Katz 1981) without great success. The identification of antibody-coated bacteria in urine (Mundt & Polk 1979) seemed promising but its precise value remains controversial (Gargan et al 1983).

Pathogenesis

Bacteria originating in the large bowel probably colonize the urinary tract transperineally. By far the commonest infecting organism is *Escherichia coli*, responsible for 75–90% of bacteriuria during pregnancy. The pathogenic virulence of this organism, which is not the most plentiful in faeces, appears to derive from a number of factors, including resistance to vaginal acidity, rapid division in urine, adherence to cells and the production of chemicals which decrease ureteric peristalsis and inhibit phagocytosis (McFadyen 1986). Other organisms frequently responsible for urinary tract infection include *Klebsiella*, *Proteus*, coagulase-negative staphylococci and *Pseudomonas* (Elder et al 1971).

Although potential pathogens and the conditions predisposing to urinary tract infection are present in most pregnant women, only a small minority develop bacteriuria. Susceptible women may differ immunologically from those who resist infection: they are less likely to express antibody to the O antigen of *E. coli* on the vaginal epithelium (Stamey et al 1978) and display less effective leukocyte activity against the organism (Mitchell et al 1970).

Asymptomatic bacteriuria

About 5% of young women are susceptible to bacteriuria. This is approximately the proportion found to be bacteriuric on routine screening during pregnancy (Whalley 1967). Of those found to be non-bacteriuric on screening, only 1.5% develop bacteriuria later in pregnancy. However, since the number of women in the initially uninfected group greatly exceeds the number with initial bacteriuria, this small percentage contributes substantially to the total population of pregnant women with urinary tract infection, accounting for some 30% of cases (Fig. 42.2). Asymptomatic bacteriuria has been implicated in several complications of pregnancy, including low birthweight, fetal loss, pre-eclampsia and maternal anaemia (Kass 1962). Several of these apparent relationships may have resulted from inaccuracies in matching cases and controls (Beard & Roberts 1968) and none is supported by more recent studies (Gilstrap et al 1981, Davison et al 1984).

Not all untreated bacteriuric women develop symptoms of acute urinary tract infection during pregnancy and those found to have sterile urine when screened at antenatal booking will later contribute substantially to the pool of symptomatic women. Some therefore argued that screening programmes are not cost-effective (Lawson & Miller 1973, Campbell-Brown et al 1987). Chng & Hall (1982) found that as a predictor of symptomatic urinary infection, bacteriuria had a specificity of 89% but a sensitivity of only 33% and a false positive rate of almost 90%. However, their population was screened only by a single urine test an unusually high prevalence (11.8%) of bacteriuria was detected. Interestingly, they suggested that women with a history of previous urinary tract infection and current bacteriuria were 10 times more likely to develop symptoms during pregnancy than women without either feature.

Most obstetricians still treat asymptomatic bacteriuria. The agent chosen must not only be effective against the organism identified but also acceptable for use during pregnancy. Ampicillin and cephalosporins are commonly prescribed but

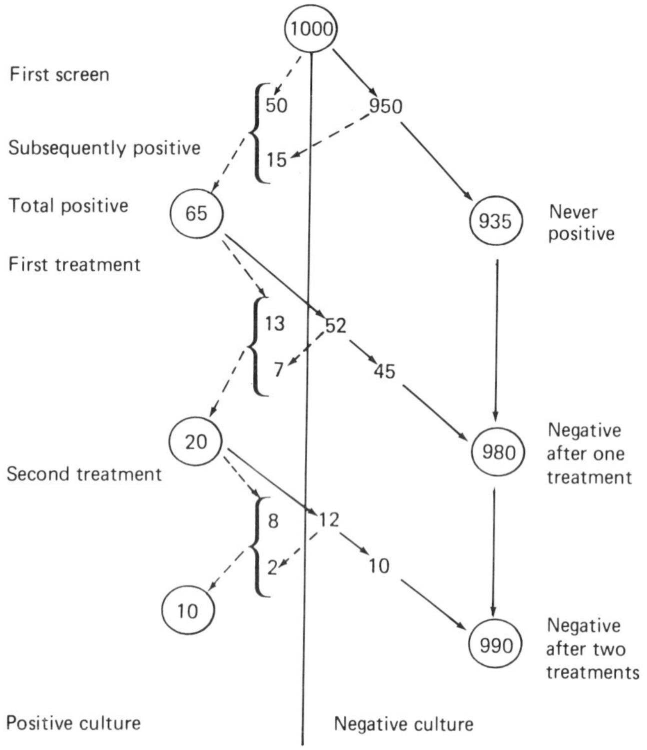

Fig. 42.2 Approximate outcome of screening and treatment for asymptomatic bacteriuria in 1000 women during pregnancy. Continuous arrows represent a change from positive to negative culture; interrupted arrows represent change towards positive culture. The 6.5% total positive rate comprises 5.0% positive on first culture and 1.5% subsequently positive. The first course of treatment produces a negative culture in 80% of bacteriuric women, but 15% of these develop recurrent bacteriuria. Second and subsequent courses of treatment produce negative cultures in only 40% of remaining bacteriuric women.

short-acting sulphonamides may be equally effective. However, sulphonamides should be avoided during the last few weeks of pregnancy since they competitively inhibit the binding of bilirubin to albumin and can increase the risk of neonatal hyperbilirubinaemia. Nitrofurantoin, which often causes nausea, may not be readily tolerated by pregnant women and should also be avoided during late pregnancy because of the risk of haemolysis due to deficiency of erythrocyte phosphate dehydrogenase in the newborn. The tetracyclines are not recommended during pregnancy because they predispose to dental staining in the child and (rarely) to acute fatty liver in the mother.

A 2-week course of therapy is usually adequate. Recurrent infection is common, however, affecting some 30% of bacteriuric women; after two courses of treatment about 15% will continue to have positive urinary cultures (Fig. 42.2). Recurrence may be due either to relapse, when the same organism is found within 6 weeks of the initial infection, or to reinfection, when a different organism is detected more than 6 weeks after treatment. Treatment during pregnancy has little effect on the subsequent prevalence of bacteriuria (Brumfitt 1981), nor does persistent bacteriuria in women with normal urinary tracts contribute to chronic renal disease. Some 20% of bacteriuric women have some abnormality of the urinary tract (Fowler & Pulaski 1982), but in most this is minor and not clearly related to the disease. Postpartum intravenous urography is probably best reserved for bacteriuric women with a history of acute symptomatic infections before or during pregnancy, for those in whom bacteriuria is difficult to eradicate or for those in whom there is postpartum recurrence of disease (Davison & Lindheimer 1985).

Symptomatic urinary tract infection

In the series of Chng & Hall (1982) 11.8% of bacteriuric women developed symptoms of urinary tract infection during pregnancy, whereas only 3.2% of women with sterile urine at initial screening did so. In the pregnant population as a whole, the incidence of symptoms was 4%. The upper urinary tract appears to be involved in a substantial proportion of cases: other workers estimate that acute pyelonephritis occurs in 1–2% of pregnancies, making it the most common renal complication of pregnancy (Davison & Lindheimer 1985).

Acute pyelonephritis classically presents as a febrile illness associated with loin pain and vomiting, but there is considerable individual variation. The differential diagnosis includes other urinary tract pathology such as renal calculus or acute hydronephrosis (which can be recognized on ultrasound scanning or limited excretory urography), other causes of pyrexia such as respiratory tract infection, viraemia or toxoplasmosis (appropriate serological screening should be performed) and other causes of acute abdominal pain such as acute appendicitis, biliary colic, gastroenteritis, necrobiosis of a uterine fibroid or abruption of the placenta (Cunningham et al 1987). Acute pyelonephritis is associated with an increased incidence of premature labour and possibly also with intrauterine growth retardation or fetal death. The glomerular filtration rate may be reduced at the time of an acute episode during pregnancy (Whalley et al 1975) in contradistinction to the usual lack of impairment of renal haemodynamics in non-pregnant patients.

Women with acute pyelonephritis should be managed in hospital. On admission, a midstream urine sample should be obtained, together with blood cultures in severely ill patients, but it will usually be necessary to begin antibiotic treatment before microbiological results are available. The chosen antibiotic must achieve high concentrations both in blood and in renal parenchyma. Ampicillin and the cephalosporins are widely favoured but an aminoglycoside such as gentamicin may be of value in the acutely ill patient. The intravenous route of administration is preferred until pyrexia resolves, when oral therapy may be substituted. Antibiotic therapy should be continued for at least 1 month after an episode of acute pyelonephritis; thereafter urine culture should be arranged at each antenatal visit.

CHRONIC RENAL DISEASE

There are conflicting views regarding pregnancy in women with renal disease (Katz & Lindheimer 1985). The majority view is that, with the exception of certain specific disease entities such as systemic lupus erythematosus, renal polyarteritis nodosa, scleroderma, perhaps IgA nephropathy, membranoproliferative glomerulonephritis and reflux nephropathy, the obstetric outcome is usually successful provided renal function is at most moderately compromised and hypertension is absent or minimal. In general, pregnancy does not have an adverse effect on the natural history of the renal disease (Davison et al 1985a).

Renal dysfunction and its obstetric implications

It is inadvisable to assess renal function by plasma creatinine levels alone, as an individual may lose up to 50% of renal function, be symptom-free and still have a deceptively normal plasma creatinine level. Although a plasma creatinine of 75 μmol/l and a urea of 4.5 mmol/l, would be acceptable in non-pregnant subjects; they are suspect in pregnant women (Table 42.1).

The ability to conceive and sustain a viable pregnancy is reduced more by the degree of functional impairment than by the nature of the underlying renal lesion. Fertility is diminished as renal function falls. When prepregnancy plasma creatinine and urea levels exceed 275 μmol/l and 10 mmol/l respectively, normal pregnancy is rare. There are exceptions and successes have been documented in women with moderate to severe disease, including some treated by chronic ambulatory peritoneal dialysis as well as by haemodialysis (Hensel et al 1982, Registration Committee of the European Dialysis and Transplant Association 1980).

Prepregnancy counselling

Ideally, pregnancy is probably best restricted to women whose prepregnancy plasma creatinine levels are 200 μmol/l or less and whose diastolic blood pressure is 90 mmHg or less. Some clinicians recommend that pregnancy should not be undertaken if blood creatinine exceeds 135 μmol/l (Bear 1978). Whatever level is chosen, it should be recognized that degrees of impairment which do not cause symptoms or appear to disrupt homeostasis in non-pregnant individuals can certainly jeopardize pregnancy. The question has to be asked: 'Is pregnancy advisable?' (Table 42.2). In a woman with chronic renal disease who wishes to have a family, the sooner she conceives the better because in some, renal function will decline as they get older.

Table 42.2 Prepregnancy assessment: Is pregnancy advisable?

Factors to be considered
Type of chronic renal disease (see Table 42.6)
General health considerations
Diastolic blood pressure <90 mmHg
Renal function
Plasma creatinine <250 μmol/l
Plasma urea <10 mmol/l
Presence or absence of proteinuria
Review of all drug therapy

Effect of renal disease on pregnancy versus effect of pregnancy on renal disease

Clinicians do not always have the opportunity to counsel women with chronic renal disease before pregnancy. A patient with suspected or known renal disease often presents with pregnancy as a *fait accompli* and then the question is: 'Should pregnancy continue?' (Table 42.3). In view of the radically different obstetric and long-term outlooks in women with different degrees of renal insufficiency (Abe et al 1985, Davison et al 1985b), it is important to consider the impact of pregnancy by categories of renal functional status prior to conception (Table 42.4).

Table 42.3 Antenatal assessment: Should pregnancy continue?

Factors to be considered
Type of chronic renal disease (see Table 42.6)
General health considerations
Gestational age
Effect of pregnancy on blood pressure
Effect of pregnancy on renal function or plasma biochemistry
Review of all drug therapy
Past obstetric history

Table 42.4 Prepregnancy assessment: categories of renal functional status

Classification	Plasma creatinine (μmol/l)
Intact or mildly impaired renal function	≤125
Moderate renal insufficiency	≥125
Severe renal insufficiency	≥250

Intact or mildly impaired renal function with minimal hypertension

Women with chronic renal disease but normal or only mildly decreased renal function at conception usually have a successful obstetric outcome and pregnancy does not adversely affect the course of their disease (Katz et al 1980, Surian et al 1984, Hayslett 1985). Some authors suggest that this statement, although generally correct, should be tempered somewhat in lupus nephropathy, membranoproliferative glomerulonephritis and perhaps IgA and reflux nephropathies, which may be adversely affected by intercurrent pregnancy (Becker et al, 1985). When renal disease is detected or suspected for the first time during pregnancy (often because proteinuria or hypertension is first detected at the booking antenatal examination), it is usually surmised that renal function had been satisfactorily maintained until pregnancy brought an underlying mild lesion to clinical expression (Lindheimer & Katz 1987).

In most women with renal disease the glomerular filtration rate increases during pregnancy, but the increases are usually less than those in normal pregnant women. Increased proteinuria is the most common effect of pregnancy in chronic renal disease, occurring in almost 50% of pregnancies (although rarely in women with chronic pyelonephritis), and can be massive (often exceeding 3 g in 24 hours), frequently leading to nephrotic oedema. Between pregnancies and during long-term follow-up, hypertension, renal functional abnormalities and proteinuria are less common and less severe. When renal failure does supervene, it usually reflects the inexorable course of a particular renal disease.

Moderate renal insufficiency

Prognosis has to be more guarded when renal function is moderately impaired before pregnancy (plasma creatinine 125–250 μmol/l but the number of cases reported is still small. In one series, renal morbidity often occurred early in pregnancy; five of 11 developed serious deterioration in renal function culminating in terminal renal failure several months postpartum (Kincaid-Smith et al 1980). Because of this experience and the fact that deterioration was also seen in an occasional patient with apparently stable renal function, these investigators are rather pessimistic about pregnancy in women with either mild or moderate renal disease.

Another study of the influence of pregnancy on chronic renal disease specifically examined the influence of the level of kidney function before pregnancy or when first seen in pregnancy (Bear 1976). No immediate loss of renal function could be detected in 29 patients whose plasma creatinine levels were less than 170 μmol/l. In four of eight patients whose initial plasma creatinine level was above 180 μmol/l, however, there was a further significant increase in plasma creatinine during pregnancy, which was complicated in virtually every case. Four patients in this group progressed to end-stage renal failure within 18 months of delivery. These and other workers have emphasized that uncontrolled hypertension is a very important factor in the overall deterioration (Imbasciati et al 1984, Hou et al 1985, Jungers et al 1986).

We generally recommend that pregnancy is best avoided in women who have lost 50% of their kidney function but recent studies question this. Hou et al (1985) recorded a successful obstetrical outcome in 92% of the pregnancies in 22 women with plasma creatinine levels of 190–300 μmol/l whose pregnancies were allowed to go beyond the second trimester. Many of these patients had hectic blood pressure and in 25% there was an accelerated decline in renal function. Thus, although fetal survival is now improved in such women, maternal risks, especially complications of poorly controlled hypertension, preclude encouraging such women to conceive or continue pregnancies which are already in progress.

Severe renal insufficiency

Most women in this category (plasma creatinine >250 μmol/l) are amenorrhoeic or anovulatory (Lim 1987). The likelihood of conceiving, let alone having a normal pregnancy and delivery, is therefore low but not impossible. As data on such patients are very limited, it is difficult to evaluate whether pregnancy has an adverse effect on their disease (Hou 1987). In our opinion the risk of maternal complications (severe pre-eclampsia or bleeding) is greater than the probability of a successful obstetric outcome.

Antenatal assessment

Patients should be seen at 2-week intervals until 32 weeks' gestation and weekly thereafter. Routine serial antenatal observations should be supplemented by:

1. assessment of 24-hour creatinine clearance and protein excretion;
2. careful monitoring of blood pressure for early detection of hypertension and assessment of its severity;
3. early detection of pregnancy-induced hypertension (pre-eclampsia);
4. assessment of fetal size, development and well-being;
5. early detection of asymptomatic bacteriuria or urinary tract infection.

Renal function

If renal function deteriorates, reversible causes should be sought, such as urinary tract infection, subtle dehydration, or electrolyte imbalance, occasionally precipitated by inadvertent diuretic therapy. Near term, a 15–20% decrement in function, which affects plasma creatine minimally, is permissible. Failure to detect a reversible cause of a significant decrement is reason to end the pregnancy by elective delivery. When proteinuria occurs and persists but blood pressure is normal and renal function is preserved the pregnancy can be allowed to continue.

Blood pressure

Most of the specific risks of hypertension appear to be mediated through superimposed pre-eclampsia. There is still controversy about the incidence of pre-eclampsia in those women with pre-existing renal disease. The diagnosis cannot be made with certainty on clinical grounds alone, because hypertension and proteinuria may be manifestations of the underlying renal disease. Treatment with hypertension usually awaits diastolic pressure >110 mmHg (see Chapter

Table 42.5 Renal disease and pregnancy: improvements in perinatal mortality over the past four decades

Renal disease	1950s	1960s	1970s	1980s
Mild				
Preterm delivery	8%	10%	19%	25%
Perinatal mortality	18%	15%	7%	<5%
Moderate				
Preterm delivery	15%	21%	40%	52%
Perinatal mortality	58%	45%	23%	10%

These estimates are based on studies reviewed in Davison et al (1985a, b) and do not include cases of systemic lupus erythematosus.

36), but many would treat women with underlying renal disease more aggressively, believing this preserves function.

Fetal surveillance and timing of delivery

Serial assessment of fetal well-being is essential because renal disease can be associated with intrauterine growth retardation and, when complications do arise, the judicious moment for intervention is influenced by fetal status. Current management should minimize intrauterine fetal death as well as neonatal morbidity and mortality (Table 42.5). Regardless of gestational age, most babies weighing 1500 g or more survive better in a special care nursery than in a hostile intrauterine environment. Delivery before 38 weeks may be necessary if there are signs of impending intrauterine fetal death, if renal function deteriorates substantially, if uncontrollable hypertension supervenes or if eclampsia occurs.

Problems with particular renal diseases

Specific problems are associated with particular renal diseases (Table 42.6). The crux of the clinical situation is the balance between maternal prognosis and fetal prognosis — the effect of pregnancy on that disease and the effect of that disease on pregnancy. This balance is influenced by factors such as the degree of renal insufficiency, the presence or absence of hypertension as well as the type of disease.

Acute and chronic glomerulonephritis

The acute disease is very rare as a complication of pregnancy and it can be mistaken for pre-eclampsia. The prognosis of chronic glomerulonephritis during pregnancy is hard to evaluate primarily because most reports are poorly documented, often failing to list the degree of functional impairment, the blood pressure prior to conception and the histological characteristics of the glomerulonephritis. One view is that most glomerular diseases are aggravated because of the hypercoagulable state that accompanies pregnancy, and patients are more prone to superimposed pre-eclampsia or hypertensive crises earlier in pregnancy (Fairley et al 1973). Our experience is that renal function decreases most often in patients with diffuse glomerulonephritis in whom hypertension is invariably both more common and severe; nonetheless, most of the pregnancies are successful (Katz et al 1980).

Hereditary nephritis, an uncommon disorder which may first manifest itself or exacerbate during pregnancy, is a variant of hereditary nephritis in which the patient has disordered platelet morphology and function. Pregnancy in women with this disorder has been successful from a renal viewpoint, but their pregnancies can be complicated by bleeding problems.

Pyelonephritis (tubulointerstitial disease)

The prognosis of pregnancy in women with chronic pyelonephritis seems similar to that of patients with glomerular disease in that its outcome is most favourable in normotensive patients with adequate renal function. Disease of an infectious nature has a propensity to exacerbate during pregnancy, and may be minimized if the patient is well hydrated and rests frequently, positioned in lateral recumbency (ureteral obstruction by the enlarged uterus probably does not occur in this position). It has been suggested that patients with this condition are more prone to hypertensive complications during pregnancy, but in our experience they have a more benign antenatal course than women with glomerular disease.

Polycystic renal disease

This entity may remain undetected during pregnancy, but careful questioning of pregnant women for a history of familial problems and the use of ultrasonography may lead to earlier detection. These patients do well when functional impairment is minimal and hypertension absent, which is often the case during childbearing years. They do, however, have an increased incidence of hypertension late in pregnancy, when their pregnancies are compared with those of sisters unaffected by this autosomal dominant disease.

Diabetic nephropathy

Because many patients have been diabetic since childhood, they probably already have microscopic changes in their kidneys. During pregnancy, diabetic women have an increased prevalence of bacteriuria and may be more susceptible to symptomatic urinary tract infection. They also have an increased frequency of peripheral oedema and pre-eclampsia. Most women with diabetic nephropathy demonstrate the normal increments in renal function, and pregnancy does not accelerate deterioration of diabetic nephropathy (Kitzmiller et al 1981, Hayslett & Reece 1987).

Systemic lupus erythematosus

Systemic lupus erythematosus is a relatively common disease; its predilection to childbearing age makes the coinci-

Table 42.6 Effects of pregnancy on established chronic renal disease

Renal disease	Effects
Chronic glomerulonephritis	Usually no adverse effect in the absence of hypertension. One view is that glomerulonephritis is adversely affected by the coagulation changes of pregnancy. Urinary tract infections may occur more frequently
Chronic pyelonephritis	Bacteriuria in pregnancy can lead to exacerbation
Polycystic disease	Functional impairment and hypertension, usually minimal in childbearing years
Diabetic nephropathy	No adverse effect on the renal lesion, but there is increased frequency of infection, oedema, and/or pre-eclampsia
Systemic lupus erythematosus	Controversial; prognosis most favourable if disease in remission >6 months prior to conception. Steroid dosage should be increased postpartum
Periarteritis nodosa	Fetal prognosis is dismal and maternal death often occurs
Scleroderma	If onset during pregnancy then there can be rapid overall deterioration. Reactivation of quiescent scleroderma may occur postpartum
Permanent urinary diversion	Might be associated with other malformations of the urogenital tract. Urinary tract infection common during pregnancy. Renal function may undergo reversible decrease. No significant obstructive problem but Caesarean section often needed for abnormal presentation
After nephrectomy, solitary and pelvic well tolerated	Might be associated with other malformations of urogenital tract. Pregnancy dystocia rarely occurs with a pelvic kidney
Urolithiasis	Infections can be more frequent, but ureteral dilatation and stasis do not seem to affect natural history

dence of systemic lupus erythematosus and pregnancy an important clinical problem (Grimes et al 1985). The profound disturbance of the immunological system in systemic lupus erythematosus, the complicated immunology of pregnancy, the multiple organ involvement and the complex clinical picture are just a few reasons for the vast literature (Mor-Yosef et al 1984).

There are differing opinions regarding the effects of pregnancy on lupus nephropathy. Transient improvements, no change, and a tendency to relapse have all been reported. Decisions regarding the status of the disease, as well as the assessment of the importance of having a baby to the patient and her partner, should be made on an individual basis. The majority of pregnancies succeed, especially when the maternal disease is in sustained, complete clinical remission for at least 6 months prior to conception. This applied even if the patient had severe pathological changes in her original renal biopsy and heavy proteinuria in the early stages of her disease. Continued signs of disease activity or increasing renal dysfunction certainly reduce the likelihood of an uncomplicated pregnancy (Jungers et al 1982). Lupus nephropathy may sometimes become manifest during pregnancy and when accompanied by hypertension and renal dysfunction in late pregnancy may be mistaken for pre-eclampsia. Some patients have a definite tendency to relapse, occasionally severely in the puerperium, and therefore it is prudent to prescribe or increase the use of steroids at this time (Leikin et al 1986).

Placental transmission of lupus serum factors (perhaps the so-called LE-anticoagulant) can occur (Lancet Editorial 1984). Although the LE-anticoagulant was first described in patients with systemic lupus erythematosus, it has since been observed in patients with other conditions and even in patients without any identifiable disorder (Hughes 1983, Lubbe et al 1984). Intrauterine death is common in women with circulating LE-anticoagulant, and it is known that the placentas in such cases show extensive thrombotic and arteriosclerotic changes. Because treatment with steroids and aspirin can lead to successful pregnancies, it is important to screen for LE-anticoagulant in all women with systemic lupus erythematosus in order to identify this particular cohort, and perhaps also in women with a history of recurrent intrauterine death or thrombotic episodes.

An increased incidence of congenital cardiac anomalies has been described in the offspring of women with systemic lupus erythematosus and other maternal connective tissue disease, even when maternal pathology appears quiescent (Singsen et al 1985). This association appears to be related to the transplacental passage of a maternal antibody to soluble tissue ribonucleoprotein. This maternal antibody (anti-Ro (SS-A)) is detectable in almost all cases of isolated congenital complete heart block (Scott et al 1983). The prevalence of anti-Ro(SS-A) in patients with systemic lupus erythematosus is 25–30%, where it may also have other untoward associations, particularly recurrent abortion. Paradoxically, the mother's heart is usually unaffected, even though the antibody is present in her system at a higher concentration than in the fetus. The fetal heart may therefore be more vulnerable to antibody-mediated damage than the mature heart, or it may possess phase-specific antigens (Taylor et al 1986). Alternatively, blocking maternal antibodies of the IgA or IgM class (not transferred to the fetus) could prevent an IgG antibody causing maternal damage.

Interestingly, maternal lupus may become apparent, clinically and serologically, many years after the birth of a baby with heart block (Kasinath & Katz 1982).

Periarteritis nodosa

In contrast to lupus nephropathy, the outcome of pregnancy in women with renal involvement due to periarteritis nodosa is very poor, largely because of the associated hypertension which is frequently of a malignant nature (Mor-Yosef et al 1984). Although a few successful gestations have been reported, in most cases fetal prognosis is dismal and many pregnancies have ended with maternal deaths. This may merely reflect the nature of the disease itself, but it must nevertheless be taken into consideration when making a decision to go on with a pregnancy. It appears that therapeutic termination of pregnancy (as an alternative form of management) has less risk to the mother (Nagey et al 1983).

Scleroderma

The combination of pregnancy and scleroderma is unusual because this infrequent disease occurs most often during the fourth and fifth decades and because patients with scleroderma tend to be relatively infertile. Whenever scleroderma has its onset during pregnancy, there is a greater tendency for deterioration. Even after an uneventful and successful pregnancy reactivation may occur in the puerperium (Smith 1982).

Most maternal deaths have involved rapidly progressive scleroderma with pulmonary complications and infection.

Permanent urinary diversion

Permanent urinary diversion is still used in the management of patients with congenital lower urinary tract defects; but since the introduction of self-catheterization for neurogenic bladders, its use in this group has declined in these patients. The most common complication of pregnancy is urinary infection, ranging from asymptomatic bacteriuria to severe pyelonephritis (Barrett & Peters 1983). Preterm labour occurs in 20% and there is some evidence that the use of prophylactic antibiotics throughout pregnancy reduces the incidence of this complication.

Renal function during pregnancy may decline, usually related to underlying infection or intermittent obstruction. With an ileal conduit, elevation and compression by the expanding uterus can cause outflow obstruction whereas with a ureterosigmoid anastomosis, actual ureteral obstruction may occur. The changes usually reverse after delivery.

The mode of delivery is dictated by obstetric factors and not the presence of the urinary diversion. Abnormal presentation mainly accounts for a Caesarean section rate of 25%, but of course minor genital tract abnormalities may contribute. Vaginal delivery is safe for women with either an ileal conduit or an ureterosigmoid anastomosis if one bears in mind that in the latter group, continence is dependent on an intact anal sphincter, which should be protected during vaginal delivery with an adequate mediolateral episiotomy.

Solitary kidney

Some patients have either a congenital absence of one kidney or marked unilateral hypoplasia. The majority that we know about, however, have had a previous nephrectomy because of pyelonephritis with abscess or hydronephrosis, unilateral tuberculosis, congenital abnormalities or tumour (Klein 1984). When counselling women with a single kidney, one should know the indication for and the time since the nephrectomy. In patients who had an infectious or structural renal problem sequential prepregnancy investigation is needed for detection of any persistent infection.

There is no difference whether the right or left kidney remains as long as it is located in the normal anatomical position: if function is normal and stable, women with this problem seem to tolerate pregnancy well despite the superimposition of increases in glomerular filtration rate on the already hyperfiltering nephrons. Ectopic kidneys, usually pelvic, are more vulnerable to infection and are associated with decreased fetal salvage, probably because of an association with other malformations of the urogenital tract. If infection occurs in a solitary kidney during pregnancy and does not quickly respond to antibiotics, then termination may have to be considered for preservation of renal function.

Urolithiasis

The prevalence of urolithiasis in pregnancy ranges from 0.3 to 0.35 per 1000 women (Coe et al 1978). Renal and uteric calculi are one of the most common causes of non-uterine abdominal pain severe enough to necessitate hospital admission during pregnancy. When there are complications that need surgical intervention, pregnancy should not be a deterrent to intravenous urography, although there may be valid reluctance on the part of the clinician to consider radiological reinvestigation. Recently it was proposed that specific clinical criteria should be met before the undertaking of an intravenous urogram, as follows:

1. microscopic haematuria;
2. recurrent urinary tract symptoms;
3. sterile urine culture when pyelonephritis is suspected.

The presence of two of these criteria points to a diagnosis of calculi in approximately 50% of gravidas, and an intravenous urogram is advised (Miller & Kakkis 1982).

Management should be conservative in the first instance, consisting primarily of adequate hydration, appropriate antibiotic therapy and pain relief with systemic analgesics (Maikranz et al 1987). The use of continuous segmental epidural block (T11 and L2) has been advocated, an approach that has long been used in non-pregnant patients with ureteric colic and which may even favourably influence spontaneous passage of the calculi. When the block is carefully confined to the relevant segments for pain relief, the patient micturates without difficulty, moves without assistance, and is at lower risk from thromboembolic problems than a drowsy patient immobilized in bed with pain, nausea and vomiting (Maikranz et al 1987).

Nephrotic syndrome

The most common cause of nephrotic syndrome in late pregnancy is pre-eclampsia (Fisher et al 1981). This form has a poorer fetal prognosis than pre-eclampsia with less heavy proteinuria, but the maternal prognosis is similar. Other causes of nephrotic syndrome in pregnancy include proliferative or membranoproliferative glomerulonephritis, lipid nephrosis, lupus nephropathy, hereditary nephritis, diabetic nephropathy, renal vein thrombosis, amyloidosis and secondary syphilis. Some of these conditions do not respond to, and may even be seriously aggravated by steroids, serving to emphasize the importance of establishing a tissue diagnosis before initiating steroid therapy.

The term nephrotic syndrome denotes the triad of heavy proteinuria, hypoalbuminaemia and generalized oedema, often associated with hyperlipidaemia. Since most of its manifestations derive from the excessive loss of protein in the urine, a more liberal definition is often used by nephrologists. This includes any renal disease characterized by proteinuria in excess of 3.5 g/24 h in the absence of depressed glomerular filtration rate. The prognosis of this syndrome is usually determined by the nature of the underlying glomerular problem. Of course, the most common cause of nephrotic syndrome in late pregnancy is pre-eclampsia (Fisher et al 1981).

If renal function is adequate and hypertension is absent, there should be few complications during pregnancy. Several of the physiological changes occurring during pregnancy may, however, simulate aggravation or exacerbation of the disease. For example, increments in renal haemodynamics as well as increase in renal vein pressure may enhance protein excretion. Levels of serum albumin usually decrease by 5–10 g/l during normal pregnancy, and the further decreases that can occur in the nephrotic syndrome may enhance the tendency toward fluid retention. Despite oedema, diuretics should not be given, because these patients have a decreased intravascular volume and diuretics could compromise uteroplacental perfusion or aggravate the increased tendency to thrombotic episodes.

Table 42.7 Renal disease and pregnancy: renal functional status, complications and outcome

	Disease severity		
Prospects	Mild	Moderate	Severe
Pregnancy complications	22%	41%	84%
Successful obstetric outcome	95%	90%	47%
Long-term sequelae	<5%	25%	53%

These estimates are based on data reviewed in Davison et al (1985a,b) and do not include cases of systemic lupus erythematosus.

Questions that patients ask

Patient expectation is higher than ever. The questions are usually quite simple. 'Is pregnancy advisable? Will the pregnancy be complicated? Will I have a live and healthy baby? Will I come to long-term term harm?' (Table 42.7).

For any patient a balance must be struck between pregnancy outcome and the impact pregnancy has in the long term. Crucial determinants are the functional status of the kidneys at conception, the presence or absence of hypertension, and the nature of the renal lesion. If a patient wants to know if pregnancy will have a successful outcome, the answer is a qualified yes, provided her renal dysfunction is minimal. If dysfunction is moderate, there is still a fair chance that pregnancy will succeed, but the risks are much greater than in normal pregnancy. These statements have to be tempered somewhat in certain nephropathies which appear to have a more problematical outcome during pregnancy. This is most true of collagen disorders affecting the kidney. Pregnancy outcome in the presence of focal glomerular sclerosis, reflux nephropathy, IgA nephropathy and mesangioproliferative glomerulonephritis is disputed.

Pregnancy does not adversely affect the natural history of the underlying renal lesion if kidney dysfunction is minimal and hypertension is absent at conception, again with the exception of certain collagen disorders. An important factor to be considered in long-term prognosis is the sclerotic effect that hyperfiltration might have in the residual (intact) glomeruli in kidneys of patients with moderate renal insufficiency, which could cause further progressive loss of renal function. Similarly, the compensatory changes in a woman with a single kidney are another form of hyperfiltration which might over many years lessen the lifespan of that kidney. At the centre of this hypothesis is the implication that increases in glomerular pressure or glomerular plasma flow lead to sclerosis within the glomerulus (Brenner et al 1982), a concept that certainly cannot be ignored, since a pregnant woman with renal disease, like any healthy pregnant woman, experiences months of physiological hyperfiltration as part of the overall maternal adaptation to pregnancy. It seems unlikely, however, that there are any long-term sequelae in normal pregnancy (Baylis & Rennke 1985) but clearly this whole area awaits further assessment.

RENAL TRANSPLANT PATIENTS

After transplantation, renal and endocrine functions return rapidly and normal sexual activity invariably ensues. About one in 50 women of childbearing age with a functioning renal transplant becomes pregnant. A total of 40% of all conceptions do not go beyond the initial trimester largely due to spontaneous or therapeutic abortions. Over 90% of pregnancies that do continue past the first trimester end successfully (Davison 1987). Over 1500 pregnancies are on record in women with a renal allograft, but of course many pregnancies, successful and unsuccessful, go unreported.

There is a report of a transplant performed with the surgeons unaware that the recipient was in the second trimester of pregnancy (Burleson et al 1983). The fact that mother, baby and kidneys came to no harm does not negate the importance of contraception counselling for all renal failure patients and the exclusion of pregnancy prior to transplantation.

Counselling and clinical considerations

The return of fertility and the possibility of conception in women of childbearing age who have transplants dictate appropriate counselling for all such patients. Contraceptive advice should be routine. Couples who want a child should be encouraged to discuss all the implications, including the harsh realities of maternal prospects of survival. All involved must appreciate the possibility that the woman may not live to participate in the long-term care of her child.

Prepregnancy guidelines

Individual centres formulate their own specific guidelines, but certain basic considerations cannot be ignored. Most advise that it is best to wait 18 months to 2 years post-transplant. This has turned out to be good advice because by then the patient will certainly have recovered from the major surgery and any sequelae, graft function will have stabilized and immunosuppression will be at maintenance levels (Davison et al 1985c). Thus potential teratogenic and suppressive effects and the risks of low birthweight or small-for-dates babies will be minimal.

A suitable set of guidelines is given here, bearing in mind that these criteria are only relative indications:

1. good general health for about 2 years since transplantation;
2. stature compatible with good obstetric outcome;
3. no proteinuria;
4. no significant hypertension;
5. no evidence of graft rejection;
6. no evidence of pelvicalyceal distension on a recent intravenous urogram;
7. stable renal function plasma creatinine of 200 μmol/l or less;
8. drug therapy reduced to maintenance levels: prednisone, 15 mg/day or less and azathioprine, 2 mg/kg body weight/day or less. Safe doses of cyclosporin A have not yet been established because of limited clinical experience (Flechner et al 1985).

Antenatal assessment

Pregnant renal transplant patients must be considered at high risk (Table 42.8). Antenatal care should be hospital-based and supplemented with attention to renal function surveillance, blood pressure control, bone disease, anaemia, detection of any infection (however trivial) and assessment of fetal well-being. Serial immunological surveillance, as yet in its infancy and of unknown value, has also been used to assess progress in pregnancy.

Table 42.8 Pregnancy in renal allograft recipients: antenatal watchpoints

Serial surveillance of renal function
Hypertension or pre-eclampsia
Graft rejection
Maternal infection
Fetal surveillance: intrauterine growth retardation
Premature rupture of membranes
Preterm labour
Decision of timing and method of delivery
Effects of drugs on fetus and neonate

Graft rejection

Serious rejection episodes occur in 9% of pregnant renal allograft recipients where pregnancy is beyond the second trimester (Davison & Lindheimer 1984). This incidence of rejection is no greater than that expected for non-pregnant allograft recipients, but it might be considered high because it is generally assumed that the privileged immunological state of pregnancy benefits the transplant. Furthermore, there are reports of reduction or cessation of immunosuppressive therapy during pregnancy without rejection episodes.

Whether pregnancy influences the course of subclinical chronic rejection, a problem present in most recipients, is unknown. No factors consistently predict which patients will develop rejection during pregnancy. There may also be a non-immune contribution to chronic graft failure due to the damaging effect of hyperfiltration through remnant nephrons, perhaps even exacerbated during pregnancy (Feehally et al 1986).

Difficulties can arise in distinguishing rejection from acute pyelonephritis, recurrent glomerulopathy, possibly severe pre-eclampsia and even cyclosporin A nephrotoxicity. Renal biopsy, which can be undertaken safely during pregnancy, might be necessary for definitive diagnosis. Ultrasonography alone may be very helpful because alterations in the echogenicity of the renal parenchyma and the presence of an indistinct corticomedullary boundary are indications of rejection (Levzow 1982).

Immunosuppressive therapy is usually maintained at prepregnancy levels, but adjustments may be needed if maternal leukocyte or platelet counts decrease. When white blood cell counts are maintained within physiological limits for pregnancy, the neonate is usually born with a normal blood count (Davison et al 1985c). Azathioprine liver toxicity has been noted occasionally during pregnancy and responds to dose reduction (Campos et al 1984). The most sensitive method of monitoring azathioprine dosage is measurement of red blood cell 6-thioguanine nucleotide. This metabolite of both azathioprine and 6-mercaptopurine is the best index of bioavailability (Lennard et al 1984).

At present there are only a few published reports of (non-complicated) pregnancies in patients taking cyclosporin A (Lewis et al 1983). It is supposedly more effective than conventional immunosuppression, but evaluations are urgently needed in pregnancy because numerous adverse effects are attributed to this drug in non-pregnant transplant recipients, including renal and hepatic toxicity, tremor, convulsions and neoplasia (Annals of Internal Medicine Editorial 1983, Lancet Editorial 1983).

Renal function

The better the renal function before pregnancy the more satisfactory the obstetrical outcome (Davison 1985), although one study indicates that increments in glomerular filtration rate in pregnancy are highest in women with lowest initial glomerular filtration rate (Tegzess et al 1985). In patients with satisfactory renal function before pregnancy, there may be a decline in glomerular filtration rate as well as appearance of significant proteinuria during the third trimester. These are usually transient and normal function returns postpartum. Permanent impairment of renal function is seen occasionally, especially where compromised prior to conception.

Hypertension

There is a 30% incidence of pre-eclampsia but, since the diagnosis is usually made by clinical criteria, it may be incorrect. In the absence of a renal biopsy, it may be difficult to distinguish pre-eclampsia from rejection and even recurrent glomerulopathy. Blood uric acid levels and 24-hour urinary protein excretion are often well above the norms for pregnancy in normotensive pregnant transplant patients. Increased values do not necessarily signify pre-eclampsia or herald its onset. Furthermore, although many of the hypertensive syndromes occurring in pregnant transplant recipients are quite severe, there is only one report of a patient in whom the condition progressed rapidly to eclampsia (Williams & Jelen 1979). Incidentally, a subsequent pregnancy was normotensive and uneventful (Williams & Johnstone 1982).

Timing and method of delivery

The factors previously discussed in relation to chronic renal disease also apply here. Timing depends on balancing fetal intrauterine jeopardy against neonatal morbidity and mortality, bearing in mind the mother's well-being at all times.

The transplanted kidney very rarely produces mechanical dystocia during labour and does not sustain mechanical injury during vaginal delivery. Caesarean section is usually necessary only for purely obstetrical reasons. Regardless of the route of delivery, steroids must be augmented. Prophylactic antibiotics should be used for any surgical procedure, however trivial; for example, episiotomy.

Table 42.9 Neonatal problems in offspring of renal allograft recipients

Preterm delivery/small for gestational age
Respiratory distress syndrome
Depressed haematopoiesis
Lymphoid/thymic hypoplasia
Adrenocortical insufficiency
Septicaemia
Cytomegalovirus infection
Hepatitis B surface antigen carrier state
Congenital abnormalities
Immunological problems
Reduced lymphocyte phytohaemagglutin-reactivity
Reduced T-lymphocyte
Reduced immunoglobulin levels
Chromosome aberrations in lymphocytes

Neonatal problems

There are hazards for the newborn (Table 42.9). Preterm delivery occurs in 50% and intrauterine growth retardation in at least 20%. Although there are no frequent or predominant congenital anomalies, one or more complications occur in about 40% of babies including respiratory distress syndrome, adrenocortical insufficiency, thrombocytopenia, leukopenia, cytomegalovirus and other infection, as well as development of hepatitis B surface antigen (HB Ag) carrier state (Davison et al 1985b).

Infectious hepatitis

These patients may have been exposed to multiple transfusions when on haemodialysis, and some may carry hepatitis B virus. Whereas women developing acute hepatitis in late pregnancy or within 2 months after delivery often transmit HB Ag to their offspring, the risk to children of asymptomatic carriers is much lower, and antigenicity is most likely to occur in infants whose mothers were also HB Ag-positive (Beasley et al 1983, Lil et al 1986).

When HB Ag is transmitted to the baby, the antigen invariably disappears within a few weeks after birth, only to be found later in life if active infection develops. This suggests that many HB Ag-positive neonates have been infected with their mother's blood or vaginal secretions at delivery and that this maternally acquired antigen is cleared before a fresh infection is contracted (alternatively, it may incubate outside the blood system). Further evidence of perinatal infection is that most cord blood specimens are HB Ag-negative or have very low AB Ag titres, even among infants who become HB Ag carriers.

Without prophylaxis, a high percentage of infants of HB Ag-positive mothers become carriers within 2–3 months of birth — an interval that again suggests that infection first occurred during labour or delivery. Furthermore, if infection occurs during pregnancy, immunoprophylaxis initiated at birth would be unlikely to prevent acquisition of the carrier state by the infant (Flewett 1986). However, hepatitis B immune globulin (HBIG) or hepatitis B virus vaccine

(HBVV) given within a few hours of birth is highly effective in reducing the HB Ag carrier state in 50–70% of infants, but not if administration is delayed beyond 48 hours. HBIG and HBVV combined are highly effective in preventing perinatal transmission of HB Ag infection. Over 90% of infants born to HB Ag-positive carrier mothers are protected — a much better rate than achieved with either HBIG or HBVV alone. Most of the remaining 10% who become carriers, despite combined therapy, are presumed to have had in utero infections that were already established at birth.

Breastfeeding

As there are substantial benefits to breastfeeding and it can be argued that the baby has already been exposed to azathioprine and its metabolites throughout pregnancy and that their concentrations in mothers' milk are minimal, then breastfeeding should be allowed. Little is known, however, about the quantities of azathioprine and its metabolites in breast milk and about which levels are biologically trivial or substantial (Fagerholm et al 1980). Even fewer data are available about cyclosporin A in breast milk except that levels are usually greater than those in a simultaneously taken blood sample (Flechner et al 1985). Until these many uncertainties are resolved, breastfeeding should not be encouraged.

Long-term assessment

Azathioprine can cause transient gaps and breaks in the chromosomes of leukocytes. These defects may take almost 2 years to disappear spontaneously but in tissues not yet studied these anomalies may not be as temporary. The sequelae could be eventual development of malignancies in affected offspring or abnormalities in the reproductive performance in the next generation. There are some disturbing animal observations. For instance, fertility problems affect the female offspring of mice that have received low doses of 6-mercaptopurine, the major metabolite of azathioprine (equivalent to 3 mg/kg, Reimers & Sluss 1978). These offspring subsequently prove sterile, or if they conceive, have smaller litters and more dead fetuses than do unexposed dams. Thus, exposure in utero may not affect otherwise normal females until they embark on their reproductive careers.

Maternal follow-up after pregnancy

General outlook

The long-term impact, in terms of general well-being and renal prognosis, is difficult to quantify. The consensus is that it is safest to wait 2 years after transplantation before becoming pregnant. Pregnancy does occasionally and sometimes unpredictably cause irreversible declines in renal function. A recent study, however, based on a comparison of very small groups of renal cadaver transplant recipients who did and did not become pregnant, concluded that pregnancy had no effect on graft function or survival (Whetam et al 1983).

Contraception

Oral contraceptives can produce subtle changes in the immune system, but this does not necessarily contraindicate their use. Low-dose oestrogen–progestogen preparations can be prescribed, although some authorities avoid them because of the possibility of causing or aggravating hypertension or further increasing the incidence of thromboembolism. If oral contraceptives are prescribed, careful and frequent surveillance is needed.

An intrauterine contraceptive device (IUCD) may aggravate menstrual problems, which in turn, may obfuscate signs and symptoms of abnormalities of early pregnancy, such as threatened abortion or ectopic pregnancy. The increased risk of pelvic infection associated with the IUCD makes this method worrisome in an immunosuppressed patient. In any case, the efficacy of these devices may be reduced by immunosuppressive and anti-inflammatory agents, possibly due to modification of the leukocyte response (Buhler & Papiernik 1983). Nevertheless, many patients request this method. Careful counselling and follow-up are essential.

Gynaecological problems

Long-term immunosuppression increases the risk of developing malignancy a hundred-fold. This is probably due to loss of immune resistance, chronic immunosuppression allowing tumour proliferation or prolonged antigenic stimulation of the reticuloendothelial system. The genital tract is an important site for cancer (Halpert et al 1986). Reports of cervical change range from cellular atypia to invasive squamous cell carcinoma. Carcinoma of the vulva has also been noted in young patients. Regular pelvic examinations and cervical cytology are essential in these women. Lastly, unusual malignancies have been reported and include reactivation of latent choriocarcinoma (Lelievre et al 1978) and metastases from occult choriocarcinoma in a cadaver kidney (Manifold et al 1983).

REFERENCES

Abe S, Amagasaki Y, Konishi K et al 1985 The influence of antecedent renal disease on pregnancy. American Journal of Obstetrics and Gynecology 153: 508–514

Annals of Internal Medicine Editorial 1983 Cyclosporin nephrotoxicity. Annals of Internal Medicine 99: 851–854

Bailey R R, Rolleston G L 1971 Kidney length and ureteric dilatation in the puerperium. Journal of Obstetrics and Gynaecology of the British Commonwealth 78: 55–61

Baird D T, Gason P W, Doig A 1966 The renogram in pregnancy. American Journal of Obstetrics and Gynecology 95: 597–603

Barret R J, Peters W A 1983 Pregnancy following urinary diversion. Obstetrics and Gynaecology 62: 582–586

Baylis C, Rennke H G 1985 Renal hemodynamics and glomerular morphology in repetitively pregnant aging rats. Kidney International 28: 140–145

Bear R A 1976 Pregnancy in patients with renal disease: study of 44 cases. Obstetrics and Gynecology 48: 13–18
Bear R A 1978 Pregnancy in patients with chronic renal disease. Canadian Medical Association Journal 18: 663–665
Beard R W, Roberts A P 1968 Asymptomatic bacteriuria during pregnancy. British Medical Bulletin 24: 44–48
Beasley R P, Hwang L-U, Lee G Y 1983 Prevention of perinatally transmitted hepatitis B virus infections with hepatitis B immune globulin and hepatitis B vaccine. Lancet ii: 1099–1102
Becker G J, Fairley K F, Whitworth J A 1985 Pregnancy exacerbates glomerular disease. American Journal of Kidney Disorders 6: 266–272
Bonsnes R W, Lange W A 1950 Inulin clearance during pregnancy. Federation Proceedings 9: 154–158
Brenner B M, Meyer T W, Hostetter T H 1982 Dietary protein intake and the progressive nature of kidney disease: the role of hemodynamically mediated glomerular injury in the pathogenesis of progressive glomerular sclerosis in aging, renal ablation and intrinsic renal disease. New England Journal of Medicine 307: 652–659
Brumfitt W 1981 The significance of symptomatic infection in pregnancy. Contributions to Nephrology 25: 23–29
Buhler M, Papiernik E 1983 Successive pregnancies in women fitted with intrauterine devices who take anti-inflammatory drugs. Lancet i: 483
Burleson R L, Sunderji S G, Aubry R H et al 1983 Renal allo-transplantation during pregnancy. Transplantation 36: 334–335
Campbell-Brown M, McFadyen I R, Seal D V, Stephenson M L 1987 Is screening for bacteriuria in pregnancy worthwhile? British Medical Journal 294: 1579–1582
Campos H, Kreiss H A, Rioux P et al 1984 Azathioprine withdrawal in renal transplant recipients. Transplantation 38: 29–31
Chesley L C, Sloan D M 1964 The effect of posture on renal function in late pregnancy. American Journal of Obstetrics and Gynecology 89: 754–759
Chng P K, Hall M H 1982 Antenatal prediction of urinary tract infection in pregnancy. British Journal of Obstetrics and Gynaecology 89: 8–11
Cietak K A, Newton J R 1985a Serial qualitative maternal nephro-sonography in pregnancy. British Journal of Radiology 58: 399–404
Cietak K A, Newton J R 1985b Serial quantitative maternal nephro-sonography in pregnancy. British Journal of Radiology 58: 405–413
Coe F L, Parks J H, Lindheimer M D 1978 Nephrolithiasis during pregnancy. New England Journal of Medicine 298: 324–326
Cohen S N, Kass E H 1967 A simple method for quantitative urine culture. New England Journal of Medicine 277: 176–180
Cunningham F G, Lucas M J, Hankins G D V 1987 Pulmonary injury complicating antepartum pyelonephritis. American Journal of Obstetrics and Gynecology 156: 797–807
Davison J M 1974 Changes in renal function and other aspects of homeostasis in early pregnancy. Journal of Obstetrics and Gynaecology of the British Commonwealth 71: 1003
Davison J M 1985 The effect of pregnancy on renal function in renal allograft recipients. Kidney International 27: 74–79
Davison J M 1987 Renal transplantation and pregnancy. American Journal of Kidney Diseases 9: 374–380
Davison J M, Dunlop W 1980 Renal hemodynamics and tubular function in normal human pregnancy. Kidney International 18: 152–161
Davison J M, Dunlop W 1984 Changes in renal hemodynamics and tubular function induced by normal human pregnancy. Seminars in Nephrology 4: 198–207
Davison J M, Hytten F E 1974 Glomerular filtration during and after pregnancy. Journal of Obstetrics and Gynaecology of the British Commonwealth 81: 588–595
Davison J M, Hytten F E 1975 The effect of pregnancy on the renal handling of glucose. Journal of Obstetrics and Gynaecology of the British Commonwealth 82: 374–381
Davison J M, Lindheimer M D 1980 Changes in renal haemodynamics and kidney weight during pregnancy in the unanaesthetised rat. Journal of Physiology, London 301: 129–136
Davison J M, Lindheimer M D 1984 Pregnancy in women with renal allografts. Seminars in Nephrology 4: 240–251
Davison J M, Lindheimer M D 1985 Pregnancy and the kidney: an update. In: R M Pitkin, F J Zlantnik (eds) The yearbook of obstetrics and gynecology. Year Book Medical Publishers, Chicago, pp 55–83
Davison J M, Lovedale C 1974 The excretion of glucose during normal pregnancy and after delivery. Journal of Obstetrics and Gynaecology of the British Commonwealth 81: 30–34
Davison J M, Noble M C B 1981 Serial changes in 24 hour creatinine clearance during normal menstrual cycles and the first trimester of pregnancy. British Journal of Obstetrics and Gynaecology 88: 10–17
Davison J M, Dunlop W, Ezimokhai M 1980 24 hour creatinine clearance during the third trimester of normal pregnancy. British Journal of Obstetrics and Gynaecology 87: 106–109
Davison J M, Vallotton M B, Lindheimer M D 1981 Plasma osmolality and urinary concentration and dilution during and after pregnancy: evidence that lateral recumbency inhibits maximal urinary concentrating ability. British Journal of Obstetrics and Gynaecology 88: 472–479
Davison J M, Sprott M S, Selkon J B 1984 The effect of covert bacteriuria in schoolgirls on renal function at 18 years and during pregnancy. Lancet ii: 651–655
Davison J M, Katz A I, Lindheimer M D 1985a Obstetric outcome and longterm renal prognosis. Clinics in Perinatology 12: 497–519
Davison J M, Katz A I, Lindheimer M D 1985b Pregnancy in women with renal disease and renal transplantation. Proceedings of the European Dialysis and Transport Association and European Renal Association 22: 439–459
Davison J M, Dellagrammatikas H, Parkin J M 1985c Maternal azathioprine therapy and depressed haemopoiesis in the babies of renal allograft recipients. British Journal of Obstetrics and Gynaecology 92: 233–239
Davison J M, Shiells E A, Philips P R et al 1988 Serieal evaluation of vasopressin release and thirst in human pregnancy: role of human chorionic gonadotrophin in the osmoregulatory changes of gestation. Journal of Clinical Investigation 81: 798–806
Dunlop W 1976 Investigations into the influence of posture on renal plasma flow and glomerular filtration rate during late pregnancy. British Journal of Obstetrics and Gynaecology 83: 17–23
Dunlop W 1981 Serial changes in renal haemodynamics during normal human pregnancy. British Journal of Obstetrics and Gynaecology 88: 1–9
Dunlop W, Davison J M 1977 The effect of normal pregnancy upon the renal handling of uric acid. British Journal of Obstetrics and Gynaecology 84: 13–21
Elder H A, Santsmarina B A G, Smith S et al 1971 The natural history of asymptomatic bacteriuria during pregnancy: the effect of tetracycline on the clinical course and outcome of pregnancy. American Journal of Obstetrics and Gynecology 111: 441–462
Ezimokhai M, Davison J M, Philips P R et al 1981 Non-postural serial changes in renal function during the third trimester of normal human pregnancy. British Journal of Obstetrics and Gynaecology 88: 465–471
Fagerholm M I, Coulan C G, Moyer T P 1980 Breast feeding after renal transplantation. 6-Mercaptopurine content of human breast milk. Surgical Forum 31: 447–449
Fairley K F, Bond A G, Adey F 1966 The site of infection in pregnancy bacteriuria. Lancet i: 939–941
Fairley K F, Whitworth J A, Kincaid-Smith P 1973 Glomerulonephritis: II. In: Kincaid-Smith P, Mathew T H, Becker E L (eds) Glomerulo-nephritis and pregnancy. New York, John Wiley, pp 997–1011
Feehally J, Bennett S E, Harris K P G et al 1986 Is chronic renal transplant rejection a non-immunological phenomenon? Lancet ii: 486–488
Fisher K, Luger A, Spargo B H et al 1981 Hypertension in pregnancy: Clinical–pathological correlations and remote prognosis. Medicine 60: 267–274
Flechner S M, Katz A R, Rogers A J et al 1985 The presence of cyclosporine in body tissues and fluids during pregnancy. American Journal of Kidney Diseases 5: 60–63
Flewett T H 1986 Can we eradicate hepatitis B? British Medical Journal 293: 404
Fowler J E, Pulaski E T 1982 Excretion urography, cystography and cystoscopy in the evaluation of women with urinary tract infection. New England Journal of Medicine 304: 462–464
Gargan R A, Brumfitt W, Hamilton-Miller J M T 1983 Antibody-coated bacteria in urine: criterion for a positive test and its value in defining a higher risk of treatment failure. Lancet ii: 704–706
Gilstrap L C, Leveno K J, Cunningham F G et al 1981 Renal infection and pregnancy outcome. American Journal of Obstetrics and Gynecology 141: 709–716
Grimes D A, Le Bolt S A, Grimes K R et al 1985 Systemic lupus

erythematosus and reproductive function: a case control study. American Journal of Obstetrics and Gynecology 153: 179–186
Halpert R, Fruchter R G, Sedlis A et al 1986 Human papillomavirus and lower genital neoplasia in renal transplant patients. Obstetrics and Gynecology 68: 251–258
Hayslett J P 1985 Pregnancy does not exacerbate primary glomerular disease. American Journal of Kidney Disorders 6: 273–277
Hayslett J P, Reece E A 1987 Managing diabetic pregnancy. Clinical Obsterics and Gynecology 1: 939–954
Hensel A, Pauls A, von Herrath D et al 1982 Successful hemodialysis for acute renal failure in late pregnancy. American Journal of Nephrology 2: 98–101
Hou S 1987 Peritoneal and hemodialysis in pregnancy. Clinical Obstetrics and Gynecology 1: 1009–1025
Hou S H, Grossman S D, Madias N E 1985 Pregnancy in women with renal disease and moderate renal insufficiency. American Journal of Medicine 78: 185–194
Hughes G R V 1983 Thrombosis, abortion, cerebral disease and the lupus anticoagulant. British Medical Journal 287: 1088–1089
Imbasciati E, Pardi G, Bozetti P et al 1984 Pregnancy in women with chronic renal failure. Proceedings of the 4th World Congress of the International Society for the Study of Hypertension in Pregnancy: 78
Jungers P, Dougados M, Pelissies C et al 1982 Lupus nephropathy and pregnancy. Archives of Internal Medicine 142: 771–776
Jungers P, Forget D, Henry-Amar M et al 1986 Chronic kidney disease and pregnancy. Advances in Nephrology 15: 103–141
Kasinath B S, Katz A I 1982 Delayed maternal lupus after delivery of offspring with congenital heart block. Archives of Internal Medicine 142: 2317
Kass E H 1962 Pyelonephritis and bacteriuria. Annals of Internal Medicine 56: 46–53
Katz A I, Lindheimer M D 1985 Does pregnancy aggravate primary glomerular disease. American Journal of Kidney Diseases 6: 261–265
Katz A I, Davison J M, Hayslett J P et al 1980 Pregnancy in women with kidney disease. Kidney International 28: 192–206
Kincaid-Smith P, Whitworth J A, Fairley K F 1980 Mesangial IgA nephropathy in pregnancy. Clinical and Experimental Hypertension 2: 821–838
Kitzmiller J L, Brown E R, Phillipe M et al 1981 Diabetic nephropathy and perinatal outcome. American Journal of Obstetrics and Gynecology 141: 741–751
Klein E A 1984 Urologic problems of pregnancy. Obstetrical and Gynecological Surveys 39: 605–615
Lancet Editorial 1983 Cyclosporin and neoplasia. Lancet i: 1083
Lancet Editorial 1984 Lupus anticoagulant. Lancet i: 1157–1158
Lawson D H, Miller A W F 1973 Screening for bacteriuria in pregnancy: a critical reappraisal. Archives of Internal Medicine 132: 904–908
Leikin J B, Arof H M, Pearlman L M 1986 Acute lupus pneumonitis in the postpartum period: a case history and review of the literature. Obstetrics and Gynecology 68: 298–318
Lelievre R, Ribet M, Gosselin B et al 1978 Chorio-carcinoma après transplantation. Journal of Urological Nephrology (Paris) 84: 345–346
Lennard L, Brown C B, Fox M et al 1984 Azathioprine metabolism in kidney transplant recipients. British Journal of Clinical Pharmocology 18: 693–700
Levzow B L 1982 The appearance of renal transplant rejection with ultrasound. Medicine and Ultrasound 6: 43–52
Lewis G J, Lamont C A R, Lee H A et al 1983 Successful pregnancy in a renal transplant recipient taking cyclosporin A. British Medical Journal 286: 603
Lil L, Sheng M H, Tong S P 1986 Transplacental transmission of hepatitis B virus. Lancet ii: 872
Lim V S 1987 Reproductive function in patients with renal insufficiency. American Journal of Kidney Diseases 9: 363–367
Lind T 1975 Changes in carbohydrate metabolism during pregnancy. Clinics in Obstetrics and Gynaecology 2: 395–412
Lind T, Hytten F E 1972 The excretion of glucose during normal pregnancy. Journal of Obstetrics and Gynaecology of the British Commonwealth 79: 961–965
Lind T, Godfrey K A, Otum H et al 1984 Changes in serum uric acid concentrations during normal pregnancy. British Journal of Obstetrics and Gynaecology 91: 128–132
Lindheimer M D, Katz A I 1981 In: Brenner B M, Rector F C Jr (eds) The kidney. W B Saunders, Philadelphia, pp 1762–1815
Lindheimer M D, Katz A I 1987 Gestation in women with kidney disease: prognosis and management. Clinical Obstetrics and Gynecology 1: 921–967
Lubbe W F, Butler W S, Palmer S J et al 1984 Lupus anticoagulant in pregnancy. British Journal of Obstetrics and Gynaecology 91: 357–363
Maikranz P, Coe F L, Parks J, Lindheimer M D 1987 Nephrolithiasis in pregnancy. American Journal of Kidney Diseases 9: 354–358
Manifold I H, Champion A E, Goepel J R et al 1983 Pregnancy complicated by gestational trophoblastic disease in a renal transplant recipient. British Journal of Medicine 287: 1025–1026
McFadyen I R 1986 Urinary tract infection in pregnancy. In: Andreucci V E (ed) The kidney in pregnancy. Martinus Nijhoff, Boston, pp 195–229
McFadyen I R, Eknyn S J, Gardner N H N et al 1973 Bacteriuria of pregnancy. Journal of Obstetrics and Gynaecology of the British Commonwealth 80: 385–405
Miller D R, Kakkis J 1982 Prognosis, management and outcome of obstructive renal disease in pregnancy. Journal of Reproductive Medicine 27: 199–201
Mitchell G W, Jacobs A A, Haddad V et al 1970 The role of the phagocyte in host–parasite interactions. XXV. Metabolic and bactericidal activities of leukocytes from pregnant women. American Journal of Obstetrics and Gynecology 108: 804–813
Mor-Yosef S, Navot D, Rabinowitz R et al 1984 Collagen disease in pregnancy. Obstetrical and Gynecological Surveys 39: 67–83
Mundt K A, Polk B F 1979 Identification of urinary tract infections by antibody-coated bacteria assay. Lancet ii: 1172–1175
Nagey D A, Fortier K J, Linder J 1983 Pregnancy complicated by periarteritis nodosa: induced abortion as an alternative. American Journal of Obstetrics and Gynecology 147: 103–105
Nolten W E, Ehrlich E N 1980 Sodium and mineralocorticoids in normal pregnancy. Kidney International 18: 162–172
Peake S L, Roxburgh H B, Langlois S 1983 Ultrasonic assessment of hydronephrosis of pregnancy. Radiology 128: 167–170
Registration Committee of the European Dialysis and Transplant Association 1980 Successful pregnancies in women treated by dialysis and kidney transplantation. British Journal of Obstetrics and Gynaecology 87: 839–845
Reimers T J, Sluss P M 1978 6-Mercaptopurine treatment of pregnant mice: effects on second and third generations. Science 201: 65–67
Roberts J 1976 Hydronephrosis of pregnancy. Urology 8: 1–5
Scott J S, Maddison P J, Taylor P V et al 1983 Connective-tissue disease, antibodies to ribonucleoprotein and congenital heart block. New England Journal of Medicine 309: 209–212
Sims E A H, Krantz K E 1956 Serial studies of renal function throughout pregnancy and the puerperium in the normal woman. Journal of Clinical Investigation 37: 1764–1774
Singsen B H, Akhter J E, Weinstein M M et al 1985 Congenital complete heart block and SSA antibodies: obstetric implications. American Journal of Obstetrics and Gynecology 152: 655–658
Smith C A 1982 Progressive systemic sclerosis and post-partum renal failure complicated by peripheral gangrene. Journal of Rheumatology 9: 455–460
Stamey T A, Wehner N, Mihara G et al 1978 The immunologic basis of recurrent bacteriuria: role of cervicovaginal antibody in enterobacterial colonization of the introital mucosa. Medicine (Baltimore) 57: 47–56
Surian M, Imbasciati E, Cosci P et al 1984 Glomerular disease and pregnancy: a study of 123 pregnancies in patients with primary and secondary glomerular diseases. Nephron 36: 101–105
Taylor P V, Scott J S, Gerlis L M et al 1986 Maternal antibodies against fetal cardiac antigens in congenital complete heart block. New England Journal of Medicine 315: 667–672
Tegzess A M, Meijer S, Visser G H et al 1985 Improvements of renal function during pregnancy in patients with a cadaveric allograft. Proceedings EDTA-ERA 22: 503–507
Whalley P J 1967 Bacteriuria of pregnancy. American Journal of Obstetrics and Gynecology 97: 723–738
Whalley P J, Cunningham F G, Martin F G 1975 Transient renal

dysfunction associated with acute pyelonephritis of pregnancy. Obstetrics and Gynaceology 46: 174–179

Whetam J C G, Cardelle C, Harding M 1983 Effect of pregnancy on graft function and graft survival in renal cadaver transplant patients. American Journal of Obstetrics and Gynecology 145: 193–197

Williams P F, Jelen J 1979 Eclampsia in a patient who had had a renal transplant. British Medical Journal 2: 972

Williams P F, Johnstone M 1982 Normal prgnancy in renal transplant recipient with a history of eclampsia and intrauterine death. British Medical Journal 285: 1535

43

Albert Singer

Malignancy and premalignancy of the genital tract in pregnancy

Malignancy of the genital tract in pregnancy presents the clinician with not only diagnostic and therapeutic problems but also those of an emotional nature. Decisions have to be made which cause much anguish to patient and doctor alike. The problem increases when one has to accommodate the varied and diverse opinions that exist about the effect of pregnancy on the genital cancer and the results of the interaction of pregnancy and genital cancer. Unfortunately, decisions are frequently based on emotion rather than on objective scientific data.

With the continuing reduction in maternal mortality due to improved antenatal care and the advances in intrapartum therapeutic management, the role of cancer as a cause of maternal morbidity and mortality is relatively increased. Even so the prevalance of genital cancer in pregnancy is still preceded by breast cancer, lymphoma and malignant melanoma. Pregnancy presents a unique opportunity during which to detect premalignant disease, especially of the cervix; these lesions are now increasing at a rapid rate in many countries. Their easy recognization by cytology and colposcopy and the high rate of success in their eradication makes it imperative that they should be recognized and treated.

This review will cover only pelvic neoplasms; those of an extrapelvic nature, such as breast, have been comprehensively reviewed elsewhere (Barber 1981, DiSaia & Creasman 1984, Monaghan 1986a). Cervical lesions are by far the most common of all pelvic neoplasms in pregnancy and their premalignant and malignant stages will be described. Lesions within the ovaries, vagina and vulva, although very uncommon, will also be considered.

CERVICAL NEOPLASIA

Cervical neoplasia is a preventable disease, as long as its premalignant stages are diagnosed and treated. These stages are dysplasia or carcinoma in situ, or more correctly cervical intraepithelial neoplasia (CIN). There is a marked increase in the prevalence of CIN lesions worldwide with a corresponding increase in cervical cancer (Peto 1986). There is also an ominous increase in the rate of premalignant and malignant lesions in women aged under 35 (Draper & Cook 1983). The mortality in this group is also increasing (Hall & Monaghan 1983, Ward et al 1985). This being so there needs to be an increasing awareness of these premalignant stages so that their malignant potential can be removed at an early stage.

Premalignant disease of the cervix

Cervical intraepithelial neoplasia (CIN)

Natural history of CIN in pregnancy. It is now accepted that a proportion — possibly as high as one-third — of premalignant cervical lesions will progress to malignancy (McIndoe et al 1984). It is still difficult to assess which lesions will progress and so all must be regarded as potentially malignant. Confusion also exists about the effect of pregnancy on these lesions, but there is at present no convincing evidence to suggest that CIN converts to cancer as a result of pregnancy (Singer & Kirkup 1980, DiSaia & Creasman 1984). This concept forms the basis of the conservative approach to CIN during pregnancy. It has been shown that the mild form of CIN (CIN 1) can progress to a more severe form (CIN 3) over a very short period in the non-pregnant state but it is not known if this progression is also accelerated during pregnancy (Campion et al 1986). Even if this were so there would still be no reason for treating the milder lesions, CIN 1 and CIN 2, during pregnancy.

Aetiology. It seems that the major factor involved in the aetiology of CIN is the human papilloma wart virus (HPV) (Singer & McCance 1985, Doll 1986). Evidence comes from

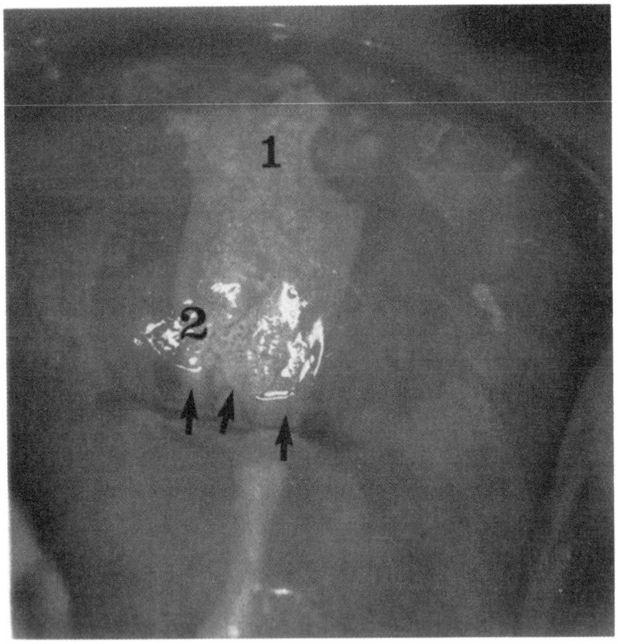

Fig. 43.1 Premalignant lesion. A colpophotograph (× 10) of a 22-year-old woman in her 10th week of pregnancy with an abnormal cytological smear (class 3) showing an area of atypical epithelium extending from the ectocervix (1) into the endocervical canal (2). The upper extent of the lesion is arrowed. Eversion of the endocervix has occurred, making it easy to visualize this upper extent. Biopsy revealed moderate to severe dysplasia (CIN 2–3).

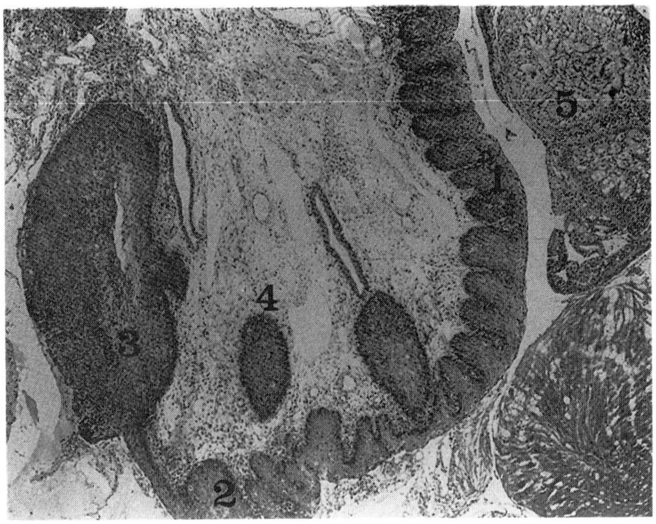

Fig. 43.2 Biopsy specimen: CIN 3 (carcinoma in situ) with gland crypt involvement. This specimen shows the presence of severe dysplasia and carcinoma in situ (CIN 3) at (1) and (2) with extension into glandular crypts (3). The latter appearance is easily confused with that of early invasive disease, especially where a segment of CIN has been isolated because of the plane of section of the specimen. It is purely an extension of CIN into a glandular crypt, as seen at (4). However, no breach of the basement membrane, which would suggest early invasive cancer, has occurred in any part of this section. Typical changes of pregnancy, i.e. microglandular hyperplasia, are seen at (5).

the detection of genomic material from the type 16 wart virus in 90% of cervical lesions and 50–70% of CIN lesions (McCance et al 1985) as well as the overwhelming epidemiological data (Doll 1986) associating male and female clinical wart viral lesions with genital tract neoplasia (Campion et al 1985). This means that any signs of clinical wart virus disease in the genital tract during pregnancy would indicate that this woman was at risk for the development of neoplasia in these areas. This being so, she must be investigated in order to exclude the presence of such lesions.

Diagnosis by cytology. Exfoliative cytology should be relied upon as the major screening technique for cervical neoplasia detection in pregnancy. It should be used at the first antenatal visit in association with a thorough inspection of the cervix. This should be done before and after the procurement of the cytological sample to detect any contact bleeding produced by taking the smear.

The report of any cellular abnormalties in the sample, such as dyskaryosis or malignant cells, should be an indication for referral to a colposcopy clinic. Colposcopy relies upon the magnified illumination of the cervical epithelium and allows a gynaecologist to manage the pregnant woman objectively (Fig. 43.1). The gynaecologist can immediately detect any abnormal epithelium and differentiate this with accuracy from possible early invasive (malignant) disease (Benedet et al 1977, Ostegard & Nieberg 1979, Fowler et al 1980).

The management of the patient with an abnormal cervical smear in pregnancy is conservative, relying principally on the use of colposcopy to exclude invasive cancer; thereafter the lesion is left to be treated after pregnancy. The author and others (Singer & Kirkup 1980, Lees & Singer 1982, Shingleton & Orr 1983, DiSaia & Creasman 1984) have described a conservative regime which involves:

1. Colposcopic differentiation between premalignant or malignant disease.
2. Colposcopically directed biopsy of any atypical epithelium.
3. Sampling by wedge biopsy under general anaesthetic of any lesions considered at colposcopy to be suggestive of invasive disease, no matter how early (Lees & Singer 1982).
4. Only by procuring a significant amount of tissue can the pathologist determine the existence of any early invasive disease; differentiation from physiological changes in the pregnant cervical epithelium can be difficult (Fig. 43.2).
5. The employment of cone biopsy if any suggestion of microinvasion exists on either the wedge or the colposcopically directed punch biopsy. When cone biopsy is indicated it is performed under general anaesthesia; great care is required because of the extremely friable nature of the tissue.

Diagnosis by colposcopy in the presence of abnormal smear. The cervix in pregnancy undergoes a number of physiological changes; these include eversion of the squamocolumnar

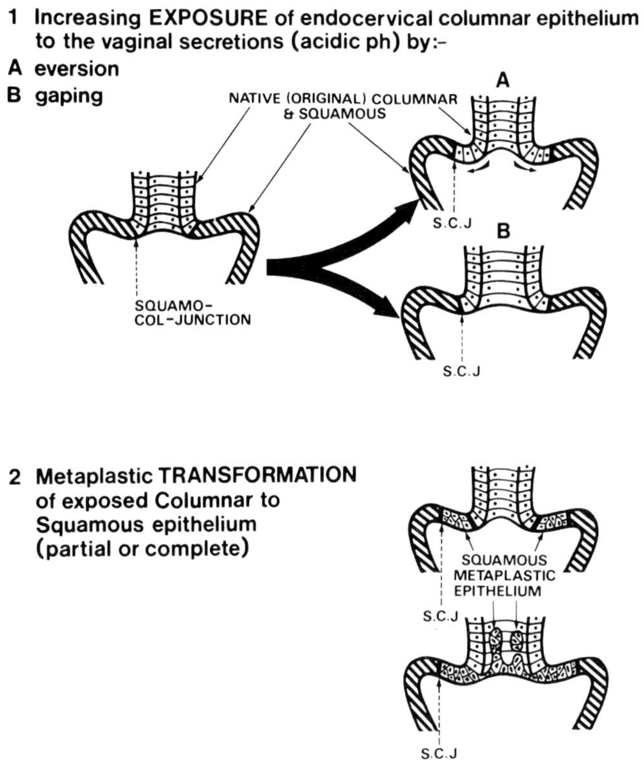

Fig. 43.3 Physiological mechanisms operating in the cervix during pregnancy. From Singer (1976).

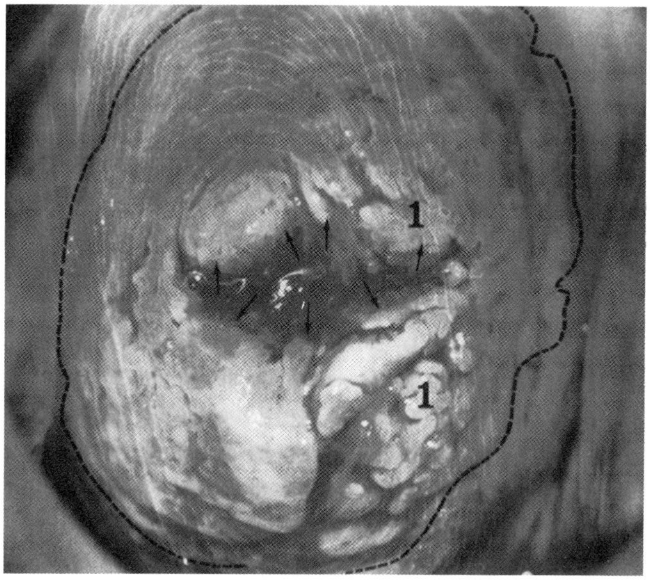

Fig. 43.4 Premalignant lesion. Colpophotograph (× 10) of a 24-year-old woman with a class 3 smear at 12 weeks of pregnancy. An area of atypical epithelium (white epithelium) exists within the broken line and its upper extent is easily seen and is arrowed. No suspicion exists colposcopically of early invasive cancer. A punch biopsy will be taken from the two areas (1) which show the most atypical change.

junction in the primipara and opening or gaping of the endocervix in the multipara (Fig. 43.3). These processes, which are associated with a general increase in vascularity of the area, aid in the detection of atypical epithelium which may harbour a premalignant lesion. These lesions are rendered more accessible by the eversion process and the increased vascularity, which produces a darker background colour of the cervix, thereby accentuating the colour difference between the pale atypical epithelium and the surrounding tissue (Fig. 43.1, 43.4). This makes their recognition more simple and any subsequent biopsy under colposcopic vision is extremely accurate.

Diagnosis by colposcopically directed biopsy. Once the atypical epithelium has been seen, most clinicians recommend biopsy under colposcopic vision although with the increased vascularity there is always a theoretical risk of excessive bleeding after biopsy. However, many authors have testified to the low risk of substantial bleeding after this procedure, and of the low risk of abortion (Talebean et al 1976, Ostegard & Nieberg 1979, Fowler et al 1980, Shingleton & Orr 1983). By employing colposcopy with associated biopsy these authors had no patient who had an undetected invasive cancer during pregnancy.

The biopsy should be taken with great care using sharp and relatively atraumatic biopsy forceps. The author employs Patterson colon biopsy forceps for this procedure (Fig. 43.5) with the immediate application of an astringent agent to the biopsy site — either a silver nitrate or ferric subsulphate solution (Fig. 43.6). A tampon is inserted afterwards as an added haemostat (Fig. 43.7).

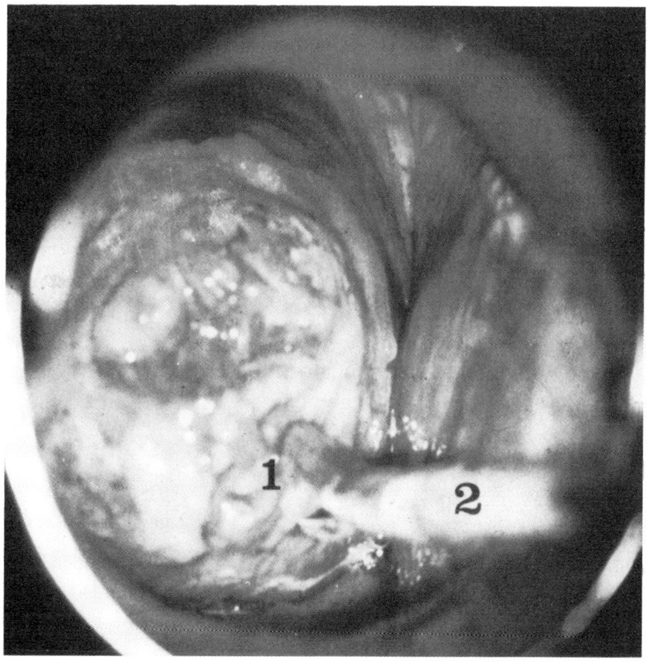

Fig. 43.5 Biopsy procedure. A punch biopsy is about to be taken by the forceps (Patterson's colon forceps; 2) of one of the atypical areas (1) as seen in the patient in Figure 43.4. No anaesthesia is needed.

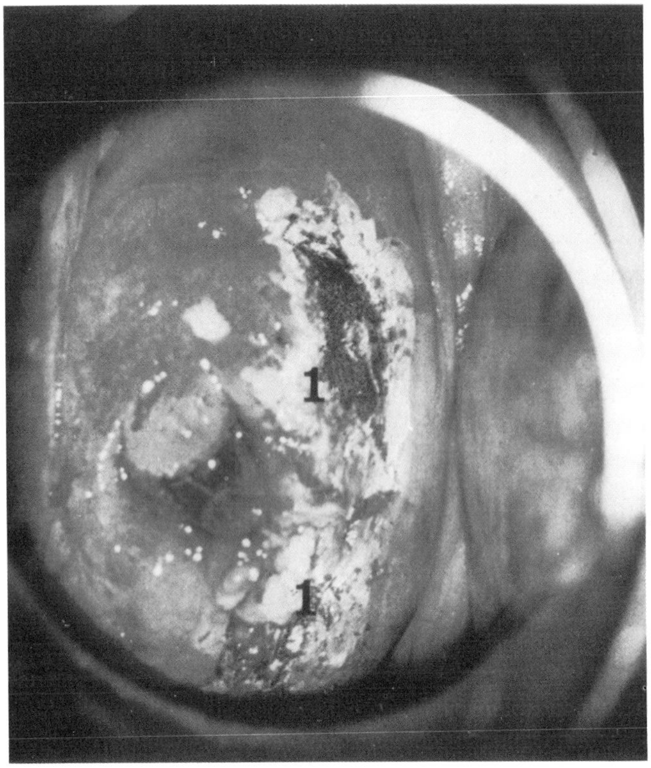

Fig. 43.6 Post-biopsy haemostasis. Biopsies have been taken at (1) and haemostasis has been achieved by the local application of silver nitrate.

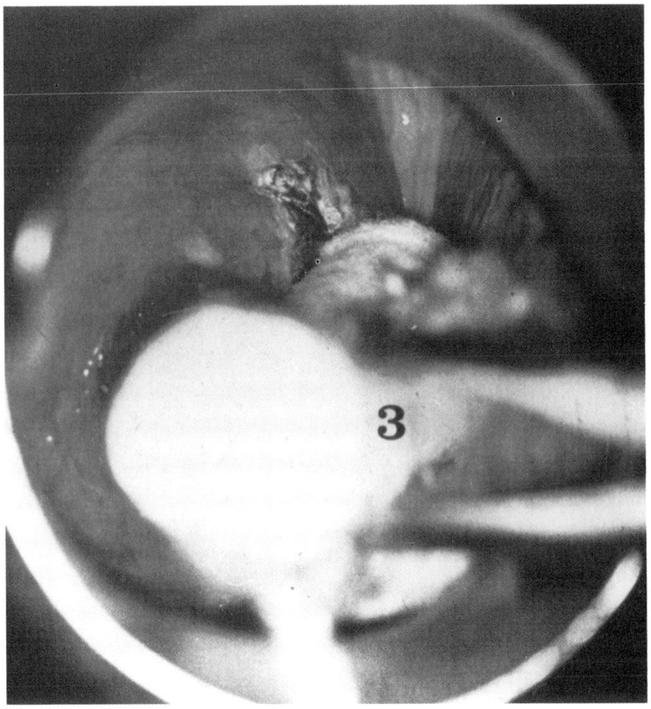

Fig. 43.7 Tampon insertion. Although haemostasis has been achieved, a pressure tampon (3) is being inserted for 6–8 h to achieve further protection. It is placed over the biopsy sites. In cases in which bleeding persists after silver nitrate application, it is suggested that a pressure tampon should be applied for 4–6 min in the first instance; if this is successful a tampon can be inserted for 6–8 h, as in this case.

Colposcopic recognition of CIN without biopsy. In the past some authors did not advocate routine biopsy of the atypical epithelium, reserving it instead for those lesions in which they considered that a more severe form of CIN probably existed (Singer & Kirkup 1980, Lees & Singer 1982). However, the differentiation between premalignant and possibly early invasive disease by colposcopy should only be made by an experienced colposcopist. It is now the author's recommendation that punch biopsy should be performed on all areas of atypical epithelium seen on the cervix during pregnancy. If there are, however, reservations about biopsy (e.g. a threatened miscarriage), then colposcopic assessment only would be acceptable.

Treatment of CIN and early invasion

If punch biopsy shows presence of CIN. If colposcopic impression or punch biopsy suggests the presence of CIN, then a conservative non-intervention regime is undertaken. Repeat colposcopy should be performed between 24 and 34 weeks of pregnancy and repeated between 8 and 12 weeks postpartum. Treatment by local destruction is then arranged, assuming that the lesion is still CIN. Usually cryosurgery, diathermy under anaesthesia or the versatile CO_2 laser can be used. This can be delayed till the third or fourth postpartum month. It is the author's regime to postpone treatment in this manner since before this time the cervix is still highly vascular and the risk of haemorrhage during the healing period is high.

If colposcopy suggests early invasion. If the colposcopist suspects the presence of early invasive disease at the initial colposcopic examination, there are two management options. A punch biopsy of the lesion can be taken and if it is shown to be of early invasion, i.e. microinvasive cancer, the colposcopist can resort to cone biopsy. This necessity has arisen in between 1 and 2% of cases screened by the technique of colposcopy and punch biopsy during pregnancy (De-Petrillo et al 1975, Fowler et al 1980).

The second option, favoured by the author, is to take a wedge biopsy of the area believed to be at risk of containing an area of early invasive disease (Lees & Singer 1982). This avoids performing a more extensive cone biopsy with all the significant complications entailed in that procedure. Figure 43.8 shows the procedure, which entails a wedge-shaped removal of tissue under general anaesthetic and the resuture of the defect with uninterrupted sutures. A tocolytic agent is given to cover the potential effect of the procedure in stimulating uterine contractions.

If colposcopic biopsy shows early invasion. The finding of early invasion in colposcopic biopsy should be followed by a cone biopsy. It is only by obtaining a portion of tissue that objective decisions can be made about conservative, medical management during the remainder of the pregnancy. Obviously if early invasion is found on a wedge biopsy, cone biopsy is again indicated. This can be undertaken within 2 weeks.

Cone biopsy in pregnancy. Cone biopsy in pregnancy is a formidable procedure with risks of haemorrhage and of spontaneous abortion. However, despite these risks and other lesser complications, approximately 80% of those women having conization in pregnancy will deliver term infants with a fetal salvage rate of 90% (Shingleton & Orr 1983a).

In contrast to conization in the non-pregnant woman, residual disease is more likely following the procedure in pregnancy. This is because of the conservative nature of the operation and probably results from the clinician's fears of harming the gestation. This makes the follow-up of these patients very important, especially if an early microinvasive lesion has been found.

Because of the friable and vascular nature of the cervix various modifications of the technique of conization have been adopted to reduce haemorrhage. These include:

1. The use of special clamps applied around the cervix, i.e. the Simmon's cervical clamp.
2. Injection of vasopressin solution directly into the cervical tissue.
3. Insertion of haemostatic sutures. Many use two lateral sutures at 10 and 2 o'clock, inserted to ligate the lateral cervical arteries (Monaghan 1986a). Di Saia & Creasman (1984a) describe the use of six haemostatic sutures evenly distributed around the cervix close to the vaginal reflection (Fig. 43.9). These have the effect of reducing blood flow and everting the squamocolumnar junction, thereby facilitating the performance of a shallow cone with minimal invasion of the endocervical canal. It is claimed that this procedure produces a coin-like specimen rather than a typical cone, with thereapeutic benefits (Fig. 43.10).

Management of the early invasive lesion. If early invasion is found in the cone biopsy specimen then certain questions must be asked of the pathologist. It is only when all these questions have been answered that a conservative course of management can be considered. These questions are:

1. Is the line of excision clear?
2. What is the depth of invasion?
3. Is there any confluence in the invasive pattern of the growth into the underlying stroma?
4. What is the width of invasion and the presence or absence of vascular channel involvement?

Depth of invasion is the mainstay of the diagnosis of microinvasion. Controversy surrounds its exact limits; 3 mm or less seems to be the level associated with a risk of metastasis. If the involvement of disease is less than 3 mm and the margins of resection are clear, it seems reasonable to allow the pregnancy to progress. Deeper than 3 mm and conservatism should give way to the more radical approach of Wertheim's hysterectomy and lymphadenectomy.

The limits of resection being clear indicate conservative management. If the ectocervical margin is involved colposcopy will resolve the dilemma, while an involved endocervical limit indicates either repeat biopsies under coloposcopic vision or further deeper conization.

The width of invasion indirectly determines the volume of the disease. Lesions up to 10 mm wide may be treated conservatively if other parameters, such as the depth of invasion, confluence and lack of capillary lymphatic space involvement, are within limits for conservative therapy.

Confluence in the pattern of invasion and vascular channel involvement tend to suggest a risk of developing metastic disease (Shingleton & Orr 1983). However, controversy still exists on this point (Roche & Norris 1975).

Cervical cancer in pregnancy

Incidence

The true incidence of cervical cancer in pregnancy is difficult to assess, especially as many reports include patients treated both antepartum and up to 2–18 months postpartum. Shingleton & Orr (1983), in a review of the prevalence of invasive cancer in pregnancy, showed that 0.02–0.4% of pregnancies are complicated by coexisting disease. This means that the chance of finding an invasive lesion in pregnancy ranges from 1 in 250 to 1 in 5000. Conversely, between 0.1 and 7.6% of cervical cancer patients are pregnant at the time of diagnosis. Depending on the duration of postpartum follow-up, it appears that postpartum patients comprise 0.03–6.9% of patients with cervical cancer. As Shingleton & Orr (1983) point out, studies with a shorter postpartum interval present a lower incidence than those with longer postpartum follow-up.

Age range

In a number of large series age ranges from 19 to 46 years with a mean of 33 years (Creasman et al 1970, Shingleton & Orr 1983). In the series by Creasman et al, the age at diagnosis of the cancer had no influence on the prognosis of the lesion when correlated for stage. The same applies when parity is considered; increasing parity does not adversely affect prognosis when stage of disease is standardized.

Symptoms and signs at presentation

Between one-third and two-thirds of women with invasive lesions in pregnancy are asymptomatic (Shingleton & Orr 1983). About one-half of these are detected by a Papanicolaou smear. Of those with symptoms, vaginal bleeding seems to be the most common, occurring in some 5–85% of women; vaginal discharge presents in only 8–20%. Pain is a very rare presenting symptom.

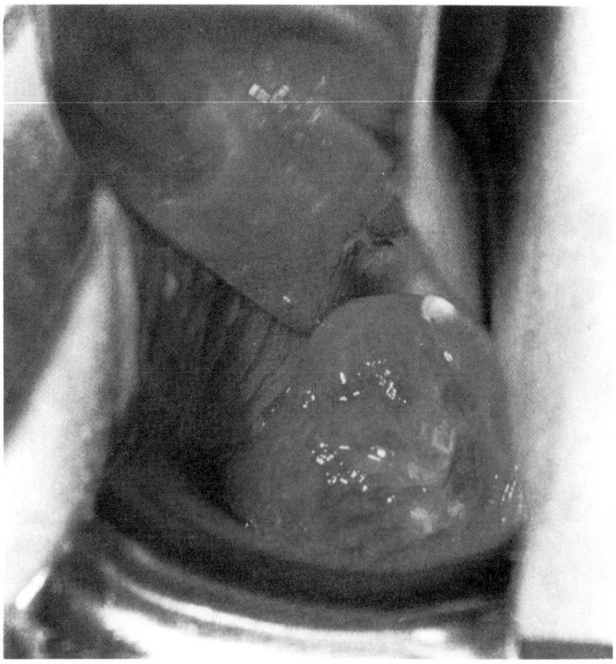

Fig. 43.8a Preclinical cervical lesion. Colposcopy of the cervix of a 32-year-old woman, para 2, with a class 4–5 smear in early pregnancy revealed atypical epithelium extending over the ectocervix and into the posterior region of the endocervix. The latter area was regarded by the colposcopist as suspicious of early invasive cancer and so warranted a wedge biopsy. Fig. 43.8a shows the cervix with no apparent clinically abnormal features.

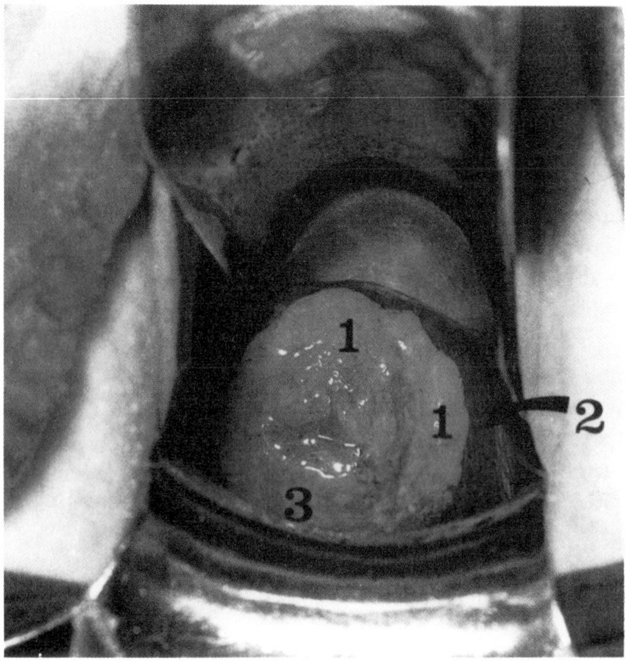

Fig. 43.8b The outline and extent of the atypical epithelium (1) after the application of Schiller's iodine solution; normal tissues absorb the iodine solution and stain brown as seen as (2). The area containing the colposcopically suspicious lesion is at (3).

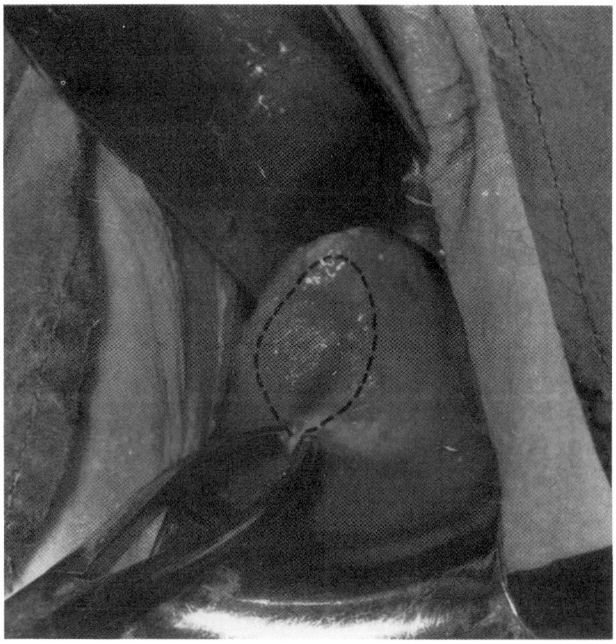

Fig. 43.8c Excision of the suspicious area. Two ellipitical incisions (dashed lines) are made — one on the right (Fig. 43.8d) and one on the left so as to encompass the whole of the atypical area. The incision is carried 2 cm into the stroma so that the area of tissue removed is adequate for pathological assessment. Care must be taken not to abrade or damage the tissue during excision.

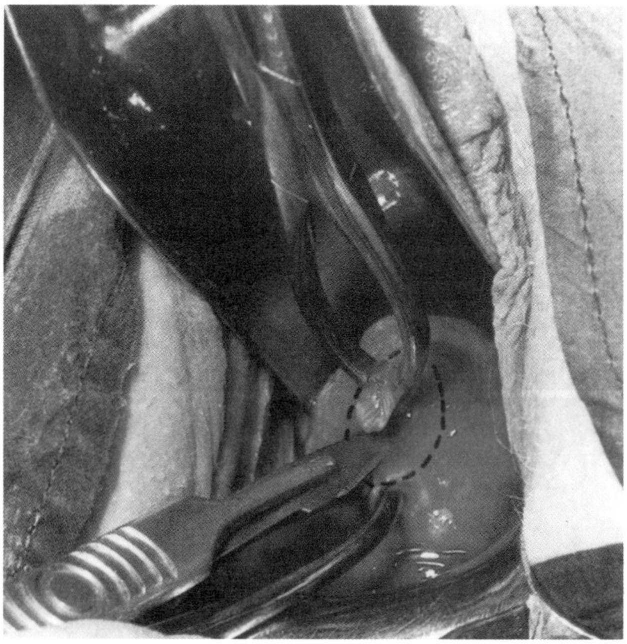

Fig. 43.8d The area after the tissue has been removed.

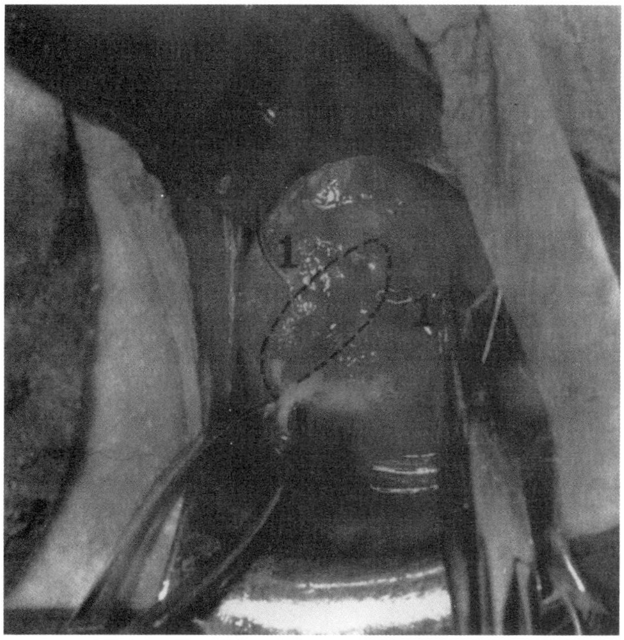

Fig. 43.8e Resuture of biopsy site. The outline of the biopsy can be clearly seen in Fig. 43.8e (dashed line). It is closed with interrupted sutures of 000 suture material. Occasionally, if bleeding is excessive, a figure-of-eight haemostatic suture has to be inserted instead of the simple interrupted suture. In this figure the first suture is inserted (1).

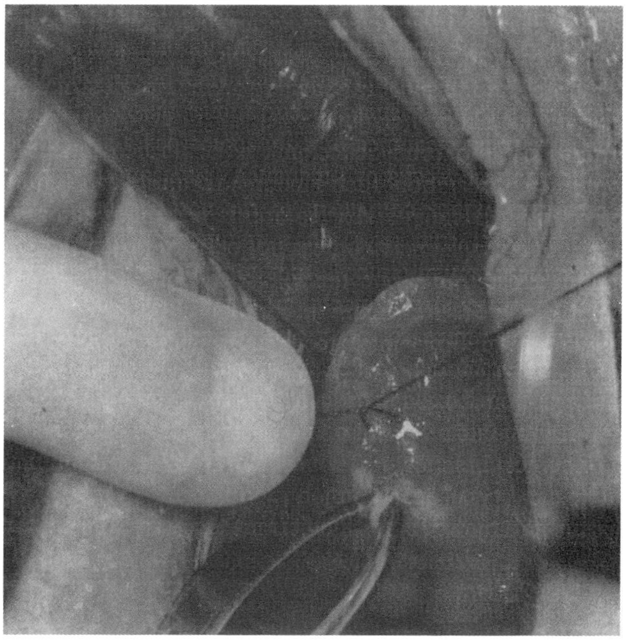

Fig. 43.8f The first suture being tied. Only one other suture was necessary to produce complete closure and haemostasis.

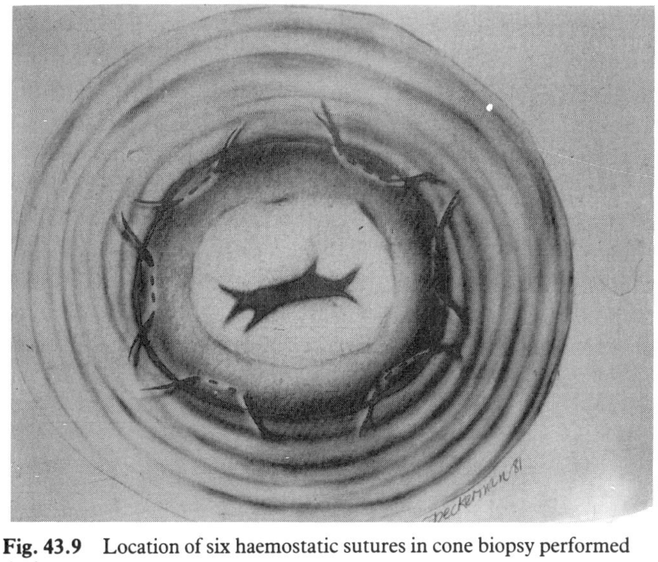

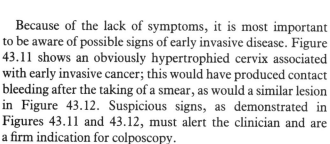

Fig. 43.9 Location of six haemostatic sutures in cone biopsy performed during pregnancy.

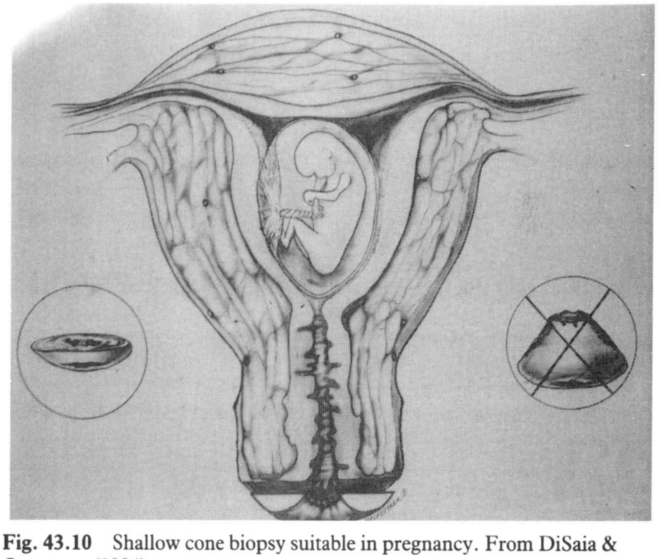

Fig. 43.10 Shallow cone biopsy suitable in pregnancy. From DiSaia & Creasman (1984).

Because of the lack of symptoms, it is most important to be aware of possible signs of early invasive disease. Figure 43.11 shows an obviously hypertrophied cervix associated with early invasive cancer; this would have produced contact bleeding after the taking of a smear, as would a similar lesion in Figure 43.12. Suspicious signs, as demonstrated in Figures 43.11 and 43.12, must alert the clinician and are a firm indication for colposcopy.

Colposcopy in pregnancy must always include adequate visualization of the endocervix looking for an early invasive lesion, as seen in Figures 43.13 and 43.14; Figure 43.14 shows an early invasive lesion only discovered because the endocervical canal was visualized.

Treatment

Once a diagnosis of cervical cancer has been made by histological examination of biopsy tissue, certain lines of treatment are open to the clinician. However, before these can be described it is important to consider two important points:

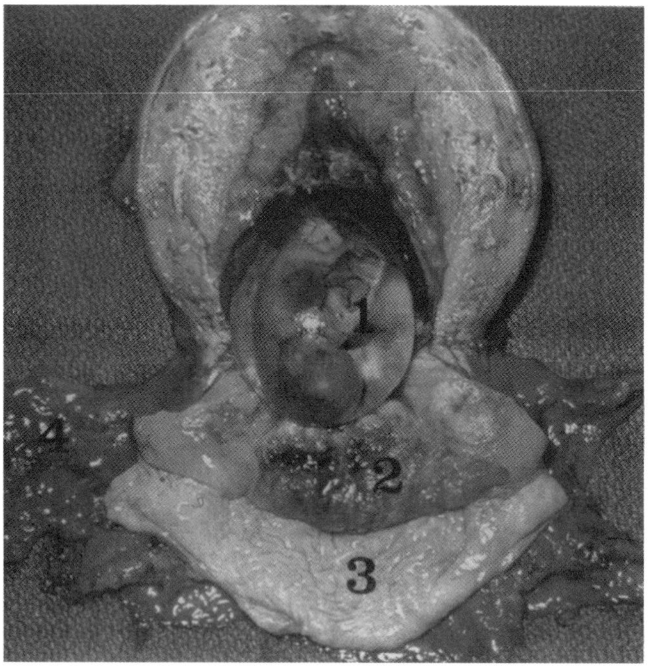

Fig. 43.11 Radical surgery (Wertheim's hysterectomy) specimen of an early pregnancy (1) in conjunction with a stage 1 cervical cancer (2). A substantial amount of vagina (3) and parametrial tissue (4) has been removed.

1. What effect would delay in treatment have on the invasive lesion?
2. What effect would vaginal delivery have on the prognosis?

Delay in instituting treatment is a controversial topic. It would seem reasonable to delay treatment of a radical nature in those lesions diagnosed after 24 weeks of gestation until fetal viability is obtained. Is this a safe procedure? The answer seems to be yes. Certainly with microinvasive carcinoma or even early clinical invasive cancer, the literature suggests that delays of up to 16 or 17 weeks after an early biopsy or wedge diagnostic procedure, and before more radical treatment, did not seem to influence adversely either the pregnancy outcome or the cancer therapy (Prem et al 1966, Boutselis 1972, Thompson et al 1975, Lee et al 1981). However, Dudan et al (1973) express some reservations about leaving such lesions and report progression of the disease in eight patients with early clinical disease in these circumstances.

Considering the literature objectively it appears that in patients with clinical stage 1B disease confined to the cervix it is reasonable to delay therapy to improve the chances of fetal viability. Survival rates at 28 weeks are approximately 75% and nearly 90% at 32 weeks. Accurate assessment of fetal maturity can be done as early as 26 weeks and steroids given to induce fetal lung maturity. Under these conditions it is possible to delay treatment to about 32 weeks. Patients with disease discovered earlier than 24 weeks however are treated by interruption of the pregnancy and definitive therapy.

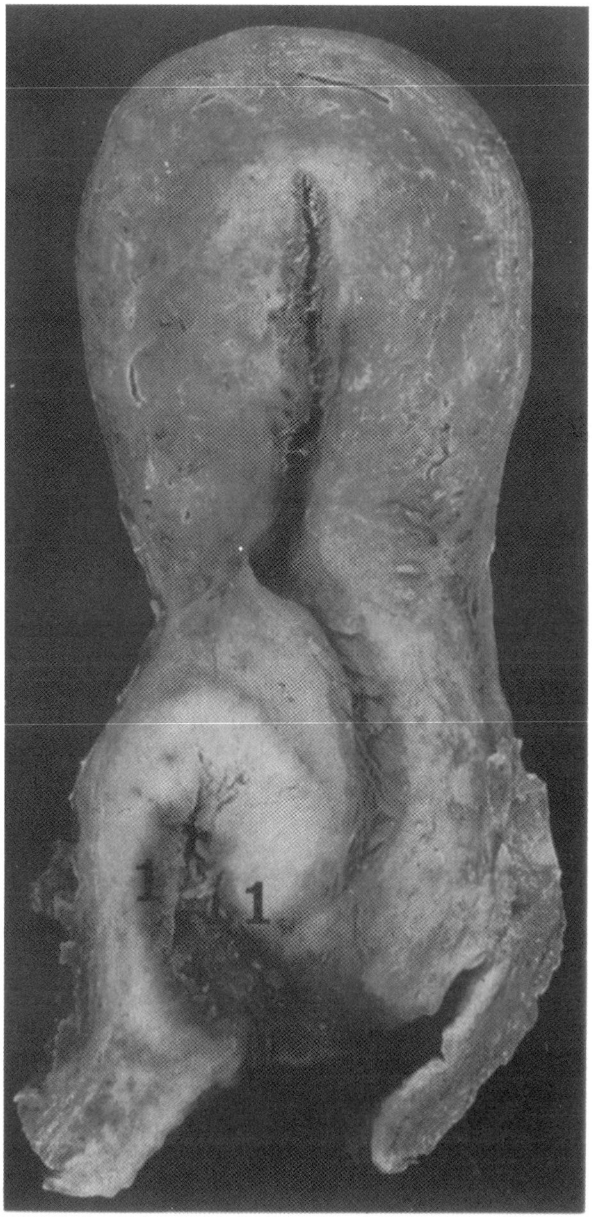

Fig. 43.12 Invasive cervical cancer (1) diagnosed at 15 weeks postpartum. It had already metastasized to the pelvic lymph nodes. It was considered erroneously to be a preclinical lesion during pregnancy and presented with a class 3 smear.

The effect of delivery also does not seem to affect prognosis adversely. Theoretically it is assumed that cancer cells may be disseminated into the circulation during vaginal delivery of a woman with cervical cancer. This, associated with the increased chance of excessive bleeding, has deterred obstetricians from undertaking vaginal delivery but these assumptions are not correct. Among patients with all stages of cervical cancer the survival rate following vaginal delivery (419 women) was not different from that following abdominal delivery (115 patients), being 52.9% compared with 46.1% (Shingleton & Orr 1983). In patients with stage 1

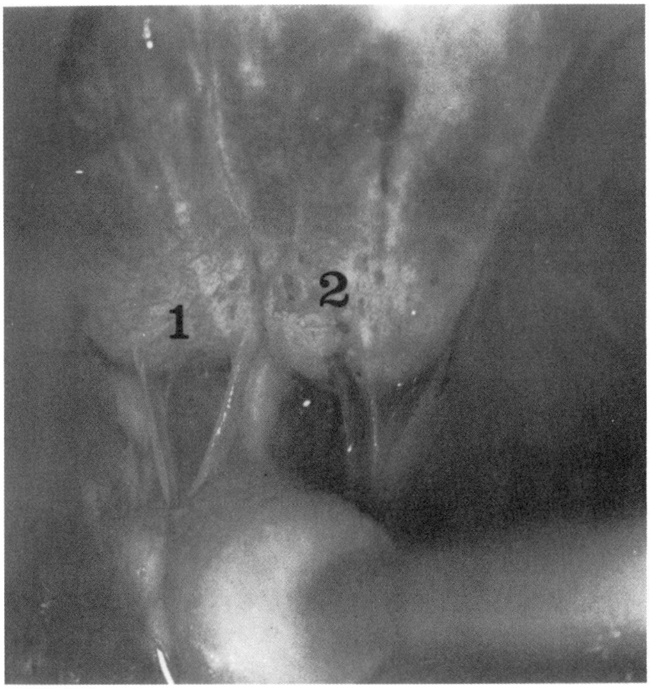

Fig. 43.13 Suspicion of early invasive lesion. A colpophotograph (× 20) of a 38-year-old woman, para 4, with a class 4–5 smear at 18 weeks' gestation. A small swab stick opens up the endocervical canal into which the atypical epithelium extends. The upper limit of this tissue cannot be seen. The epithelium at (1) and (2) was regarded as suspicious of early invasive cancer by the colposcopist and because of this and the non-visualization of the upper extent, a wedge biopsy was undertaken. This showed the presence of carcinoma in situ (CIN 3) involving gland crypts but no early invasive cancer.

disease the collected results indicate that following vaginal delivery 80.5% of treated patients are survivors while 71.6% of treated patients survive after abdominal delivery (Shingleton & Orr 1983). It seems that the fear of cancer cell spread with vaginal delivery is largely theoretical.

Recommended therapy

For very early invasive disease (microinvasion). Once the diagnosis of microinvasion has been made by cone biopsy then it seems reasonable to delay treatment until after delivery has been accomplished. Re-evaluation should be performed at 6 weeks postpartum. If at that stage residual disease exists then further conization in women desirous of future pregnancies or even hysterectomy may be considered.

Clinical stage 1B, cancer when presenting before 24 weeks. As discussed above, delay until fetal viability is reached is not recommended under 24 weeks' gestation. Treatment can be by surgery or by radiotherapy. There is little to choose between these from survival results. Shingleton & Orr (1983) summarized 15 studies where either method or a combination had been used in women with stage 1B disease. For surgery, the 5-year or more survival was 89% compared with 87% for radiotherapy and 82% for combined treatment. Some authors prefer surgery (Shingleton & Orr 1983)

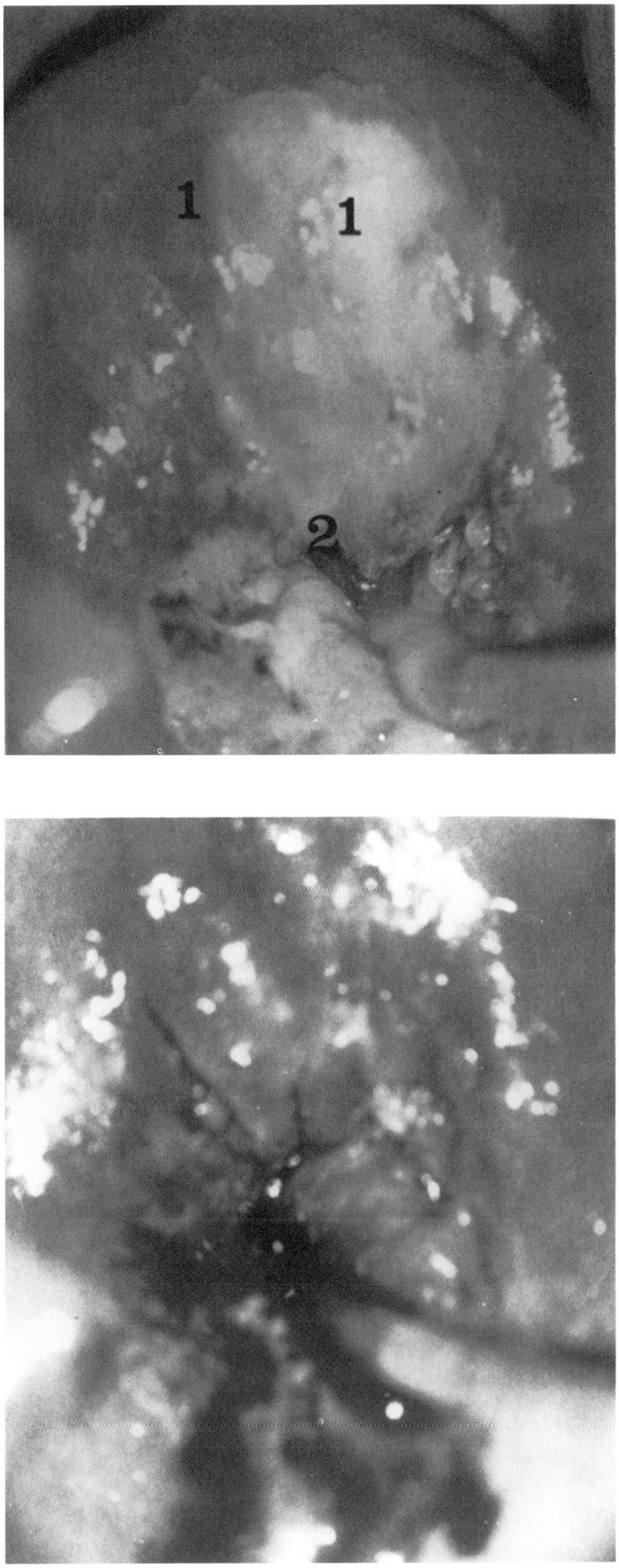

(a)

(b)

Fig. 43.14 (a) Early invasive (clinical) cancer in endocervical canal. Colpophotographs (× 10) of a 34-year-old woman, para 4. The epithelium extends on to the ectocervix at (1) and into the endocervical canal at (2). A swab stick attempts to open the canal to visualize the upper extent. (b) Bleeding is produced as the swab stick passes into the endocervix.

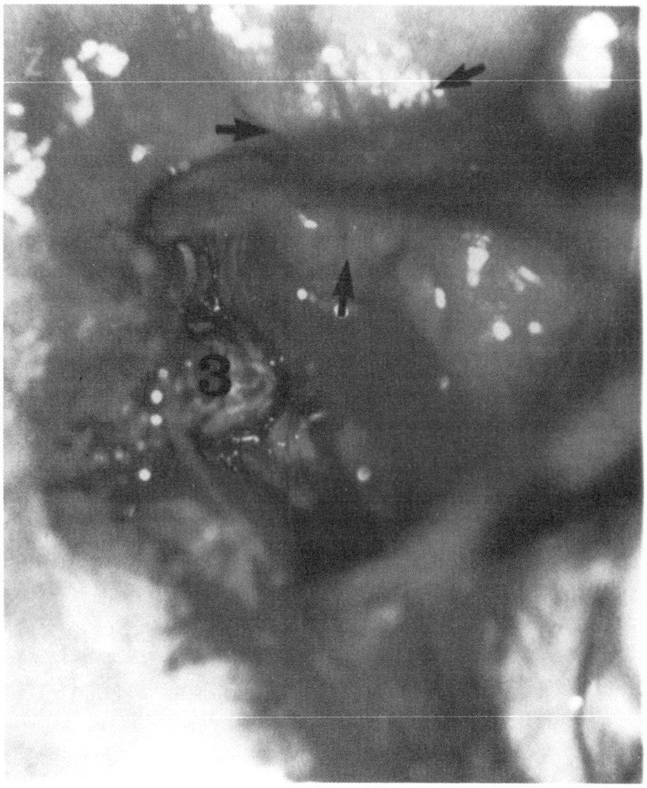

Fig. 43.14c A pair of Desjardins forceps (used for viewing the endocervical canal) opens the endocervix to show an early clinical invasive cancer at (3). The extent of the associated premalignant lesion is arrowed. This shows the importance of proper visualization of the upper extent of the atypical epithelium; if that is not seen, then the presence of early invasive cancer, as in this case, cannot be excluded.

whilst others prefer radiotherapy (DiSaia & Creasman 1984). Their regimen is as follows: patients begin with whole-pelvis irradiation. Spontaneous abortion usually occurs during therapy and so treatment is completed with intracavity radium or caesium applications.

If spontaneous abortion does not occur by completion of the external beam therapy, as occurs commonly after the 16th week of gestation, then a modified radical hysterectomy without pelvic lymphadenectomy is performed to remove the remaining central neoplasm.

This technique delivers potentially curative doses of radiation to pelvic lymph glands with metastatic foci. A dose of 45 Gy is normally given to the whole pelvis and if abortion occurs then a dose of 60 Gy can be given by internal sources. The surgery removes adequate amounts of paracervix and parametrium as well as the upper vagina. Some units perform hysterotomy on those who have not aborted and follow this by conventional intracavity irradiation delivered within 1 or 2 weeks.

There seems to be no advantage in inducing abortion prior to initiation of radiotherapy. Creasman et al (1970) showed that over 70% of abortions occurred prior to the patient receiving 40 Gy of external therapy, while Bosch & Marcial (1966) reported that 16 of 17 patients aborted spontaneously within 3–6 weeks. Prem et al (1966) also stated that the time from starting treatment to spontaneous abortion was shorter in the first trimester (29 days) than in the second trimester (38 days).

Clinical stage 1B cancer when presenting after 24 weeks. Therapy should be delayed until viability is reached. At this stage delivery can be accomplished either vaginally or by Caesarean section. If the latter is chosen then a Wertheim radical hysterectomy with pelvic lymphadenectomy is undertaken at the same time. If irradiation is chosen then it is started when the abdominal incision has healed.

Whole pelvic irradiation using 50–60 Gy can be used, followed by the application of internal sources using a dose of up to 40–50 Gy.

Clinical stage 2B/3B cancer when presenting before 24 weeks. Radiation is normally given to the whole pelvis up to a dose of 50 Gy. When spontaneous abortion occurs a further dose of 50 Gy can be given in the form of internal sources. If no abortion occurs then surgical evaluation is performed, after which 50 Gy is given by internal sources. DiSaia & Creasman (1984) suggested that if abortion does not occur then a radical hysterectomy with pelvic lymph node removal can be undertaken.

Clinical stage 2B/3B cancer when presenting after 24 weeks. At this stage radiotherapy is given after Caesarean section: 50 Gy is given to the whole pelvis and this is followed by the same dose via internal sources.

Factors influencing survival

Two factors significantly influence survival:

1. Clinical stage of lesion when diagnosed.
2. Stage of gestation when the lesion is discovered.

Clinical stage of lesion when diagnosed. Five-year survival is dependent purely on the stage at which the cancer is detected. It seems from a collection of cases by Hacker et al (1982) that the stage 1B survival rate is 74.5%, followed by stage 2 at 47.8% and 3/4 stages at 16.2%. Surprisingly, stage 1 results are comparable to the results in non-pregnant women but for the more advanced stages, the prognosis is poorer than for the non-pregnant woman, i.e. (55 compared with 47% for stage 2 and 28 compared with 16% for stages 3/4).

Stage of gestation when lesion is diagnosed. When all four stages of cervical cancer are assessed together, there are gross differences in survival according to the time in pregnancy when diagnosis is made. Hacker et al (1982) in a review of 896 cases showed that for those diagnosed in the first trimester the 5-year survival rate was 69%; for second-trimester diagnosis it was 63%; for the third trimester it was 52% and 46% in the postpartum period, with an overall survival rate of 51%.

However, if the results are broken down by stage then

it can be seen that there is no difference in survival for stage 1 and stage 2 disease patients seen in any of the three trimesters or postpartum. Shingleton & Orr (1983) quote 5-year survival rates for stage 1 in the first trimester of 84%, 89% in the second and 77% in the third trimester. Postpartum survival was 77%. More advanced disease is usually found in the latter stages of pregnancy and probably accounts for the poorer survival figures in the stages.

OVARIAN CANCER

Ovarian tumours are an uncommon accompaniment of pregnancy; when they occur their presence is usually revealed as a consequence of a complication, such as torsion, haemorrhage or rupture of the cyst. Although ovarian cysts in pregnancy occur in from 1 in 80 to 1 in 300 pregnancies (Grimes 1954, Eastman & Hellman 1966), some authors compute the prevalence of ovarian cancer in pregnancy as between 1 in 8000 to 1 in 20 000 deliveries (Barber 1981, DiSaia & Creasman 1984); the chance of a malignant transformation is in the region of 2–5%.

Pathology

Follicular and corpus luteum cysts are the most common type in pregnancy, followed by the cystic teratoma and mucinous cystadenoma. Beischer (1971) reported that only about 2.5% of these latter lesions were malignant. Germ cell tumours are not uncommon considering the young age of the population. In the young patient the most likely tumours are the germ cell tumours such as endodermal sinus tumours, immature embryonal carcinoma teratomas and dysgerminomas. Fortunately these tumours, when they occur in pregnancy, are usually benign. Epithelial tumours are more common in the older pregnant patient, i.e. around 40.

Presentation

Symptoms

Complication of ovarian tumour mass usually alerts the obstetrician to the presence of a lesion. Torsion is not uncommon; 10–15% of all ovarian tumours in pregnancy undergo this complication. The most common stage for torsion is between 8 and 16 weeks, corresponding to the time of the most rapid uterine growth. Acute abdominal symptoms such as pain, nausea and vomiting may occur (see Chapter 40).

Signs

Although some ovarian tumours may present without signs the majority are suspected as a result of palpated ovarian enlargement. Within the pelvis such enlargements must be differentiated from a pedunculated uterine fibroid, retroverted gravid uterus, congenital uterine abnormality, such as a rudimentary uterine horn, or even a pelvic kidney. As the uterus enlarges the pelvic tumour becomes an abdominal mass and may be difficult to diagnose; it may go undetected.

Investigations

The use of ultrasonography is of value in the diagnosis of ovarian neoplasia. However, when an ovarian mass presents in an advanced stage of labour then full diagnosis can only be made after removal.

Treatment

Surgery

The removal of the ovarian neoplasm is the object of treatment but the extent of removal will usually depend upon the type of lesion and the extent of disease.

If the lesion is found during an exploratory laparoscopy for an adnexal mass, the surgeon's first responsibility is to make a correct evaluation of the extent of disease, by correct staging.

Stage 1A lesions, that is those confined to the ovaries with no ascites, may be treated conservatively by unilateral salpingo-oophorectomy. However, strict limits must be set before this technique can be adopted. These are:

1. Only for stage 1A lesions.
2. Young women of low parity.
3. Normal pelvis otherwise.
4. No obvious invasion of capsule, lymphatics or mesoverium; no adhesions.
5. Opposite ovary clear of disease as seen at a wedge biopsy done at the same time.

The early staging of the condition should be promptly confirmed after operation by:

1. Lesions well differentiated histologically.
2. Negative peritoneal cavity washings.
3. Negative omental biopsy.

Probable excision of the other ovary once childbearing has been completed should be considered. A meticulous follow-up must go on for many years, by regular ultrasound and the use of tumour markers.

Patients with more advanced disease are not suitable for such a conservative approach and total hysterectomy with bilateral salpingo-oophorectomy is preferred.

Adjuvant chemotherapy

Chemotherapy plays an important part in management of many of the highly malignant germ cell tumours, excepting the dysgerminomas. Combined chemotherapy has improved survival rates as well as allowing continuation of childbearing capacity and, in certain instances, even of the pregnancy during which such a lesion has been found. There is a dilemma when such lesions are discovered early in the first or second trimester of pregnancy. In these conditions the patient and her advisers have to decide whether to continue the pregnancy until viability is reached and then institute chemotherapy; it is well known that such tumours grow rapidly and the best response to chemotherapy is in those cases where chemotherapy is started soon after surgery. There is controversy on this point and DiSaia & Creasman (1984) feel that delay by with-holding therapy is not warranted. However, it has not yet been proven by large studies that delay in starting therapy is detrimental.

There is also controversy about giving therapy during pregnancy. In general, all chemotherapeutic agents are potential teratogenic agents, but there have been no large studies showing increased malformation rates in women treated in the second or third trimester with the standard agents.

The dysgerminomas: a special case

These tumours constitute a special group. They show a very good response to surgery especially in stage 1 disease but a lack of response to chemotherapy. There is usually a marked sensitivity to radiation.

In stage 1A, dysgerminoma can be treated by unilateral salpingo-oophorectomy. If the pathology is suspected at operation, it is also recommended that pelvic lymph node sampling should be performed, especially on the side of the tumour since these tumours metastasize unilaterally.

Dysgerminomata also present commonly in pregnancy with complications. Karlen (1979), reviewing 27 cases, showed that torsion and partial infarction occurred commonly with obstetric complications in half the patients; these are associated with a high perinatal mortality rate.

Recurrence rates of between 10 and 30% are quoted, with recurrence usually in the first 2 years (Karlen 1979, DiSaia & Creasman 1984).

Rare ovarian tumours

These are mainly the granulosa-theca tumours, and the Sertoli–Leydig cell tumours. They have a low malignant potential and as they occur in younger patients, conservative management is indicated.

VULVAR MALIGNANCY

Vulvar carcinoma in pregnancy is extremely rare, as the peak age of occurrence is in the 60–70-year age group. However, the premalignant stage of the disease, vulval intraepithelial neoplasia (VIN), is seen in younger women in increasing numbers. This increase is linked to the dramatic rise in wart viral lesions in the genital tract; the aetiology of vulval precancer and cancer seem to be related to the HPV (human papilloma virus).

Diagnosis

Premalignant lesions

These usually present with few clinical signs except occasional white patches around the labia minora and on the fourchette. The use of the colposcope is invaluable; after application of acetic acid 5%, the limits of many clinically suspicious lesions can be defined. Many are multifocal. The symptom of presentation in many women is pruritus; it is important therefore to examine the vulva of these women with the colposcope. A small punch biopsy of the affected area will confirm the diagnosis.

Malignant lesions

Suspicious signs, such as fissuring, ulceration or raised areas, should be submitted to biopsy. This should be of sufficient size to allow the pathologist to determine the degree of invasion into stroma, the basic histopathological pattern, the degree of lymphocytic reaction and the confluence and permeation or penetration of capillary–lymphatic spaces.

Treatment

Premalignant lesions

Lesions with proven in situ carcinoma (VIN 3) can be safely left until the puerperium for treatment. The natural history of these lesions has yet to be determined. Treatment can be by either local surgical removal or, more effectively, by carbon dioxide laser.

Malignant lesions

The size and site of the tumour determine the mode of treatment (Hacker et al 1984, Monaghan 1986b).

Early invasive disease. In these lesions the biopsy has shown the depth of penetration to be no more than 1 mm. In this case wide local excision is adequate.

Stage 1 disease (2 cm diameter). Especially with laterally placed tumours, a radical vulvectomy with ipsilateral groin node dissection through a separate incision is adequate (Monaghan 1986b). Where the lesion encroaches on the midline, a lateral groin node dissection through a separate incision is added to the radical vulvectomy.

Lesions greater than 4 cm diameter. For these larger lesions a pelvic node dissection is added to the groin node dissection and both groins should be dissected *en bloc* in direct continuity with the radical vulvectomy.

Monaghan (1986b) believes that management in this way does not significantly affect the pregnancy; this is the case even when a pelvic node dissection is performed. Delivery may be per vaginam unless there is an intruding introital lesion.

Timing of surgical treatment

If diagnosed up to 36 weeks of gestation, treatment can be performed during pregnancy; after that it can be left until the puerperium.

Delivery route

If the vulvar wound has healed there seems to be no contra-indication to vaginal delivery.

Acknowledgements

The author wishes to thank Dr Ian Duncan for Figures 43.3 and 43.12. Figures 43.9 and 43.12 are from Creasy and Resnick (1987).

REFERENCES

Barber H R K 1981 Malignant disease in pregnancy. In: Coppleson M (ed) Gynecologic oncology, 1st edn. Churchill Livingstone, Edinburgh, pp 795–806
Beischer H A 1971 Growth and malignancy of ovarian tumours in pregnancy. Australian and New Zealand Journal of Obstetrics and Gynaecology 11: 208–214
Benedet J L, Boyes D A, Nichols T 1979 Colposcopic evaluation of pregnant patients with abnormal cytology. British Journal of Obstetrics and Gynaecology 84: 517–519
Bosch A, Marcial V A 1966 Carcinoma of the uterine cervix associated with pregnancy. American Journal of Roentgenology 96: 92–96
Boutselis J G 1972 Intraepithelial cancer of the cervix associated with pregnancy. Obstetrics and Gynecology 40: 657–666
Campion M J, Singer A, Clarkson P K, McCance D J 1985 Increased risk of cervical neoplasia in consorts of men with penile condylomata acuminata. Lancet i: 943–945
Campion M J, Cuzick J, McCance D, Singer A 1986 Progressive potential of mild cervical atypia. Lancet ii: 237–240
Creasman W T, Rutledge F, Fletcher G 1970 Carcinoma of the cervix associated with pregnancy. Obstetrics and Gynecology 36: 495–498
Creasy R K, Resnick R 1987 Maternal fetal medicine. Principles and practice. W B Saunders, Philadelphia
De-Petrillo A D, Townsend D E, Morrow C P, Lickrish C M, Disaia P, Roy M 1975 Colposcopic evaluation of the abnormal Pap test in pregnancy. American Journal of Obstetrics and Gynecology 121: 441–445
DiSaia P J, Creasman W 1984 Cancer in pregnancy. In: Disaia P J, Creasman W T (eds) Clinical gynecologic oncology, 2 edn. C V Mosby, St Louis, pp 428–443
Doll R 1986 Implications of epidemiological evidence for future progress. In: Peto R, Zur Hausen H (eds) Viral aetiology of cervical cancer. 21: Banbury report, Cold Spring Harbor Laboratory New York, 321
Draper G J, Cook G A 1983 Changing pattern of cervical cancer rates. British Medical Journal 287: 510–512
Dudan R C, Yon J L, Ford J H, Averette H 1973 Carcinoma of the cervix in pregnancy. Gynaecologic Oncology 1: 283–289
Eastman N J, Hellman L M 1966 Ovarian tumours in pregnancy. In: Eastman N J, Hellman L M (eds) Williams obstetrics, 13th edn. Appleton Century Croft, New York, p 732
Fowler W C, Walton L A, Edelman D A 1980 Cervical intraepithelial neoplasia in pregnancy. Southern Medical Journal 73: 1180–1185
Grimes W H 1954 Ovarian cysts in pregnancy. American Journal of Obstetrics and Gynecology 65: 594
Hacker N F, Berek J S, Lagasse L D, Charles E H, Savage E W, Moore J G 1982 Carcinoma of the cervix associated with pregnancy. Obstetrics and Gynecology 59: 735–746
Hacker N F, Berek J S, Lagasse L D, Nieberg R K, Leuchter R S 1984 Individualisation of treatment of stage 1 squamous cell vulvar carcinoma. Obstetrics and Gynecology 63: 155–162
Hall S W, Monaghan J M 1983 Invasive carcinoma of the cervix in young women. Lancet ii: 731–733
Karlen J R 1979 Dysgerminomas associated with pregnancy. Obstetrics and Gynecology 53: 330–334
Lee R B, Neglia W, Park W C 1981 Cervical carcinoma in pregnancy. Obstetrics and Gynecology 58: 584–589
Lees D H, Singer A 1982 Management of cervical neoplasia in pregnancy. In: Lees D H, Singer A (eds) A colour atlas of gynaecological surgery, 1st edn. Wolfe Medical, London, p 147
McCance D J, Clarkson P K, Dyson J L, Walker P G, Singer A 1985 Human papilloma virus types 6 and 16 in multifocal neoplasias of the female genital tract. British Journal of Obstetrics and Gynaecology 92: 1093–1101
McIndoe W A, McLean M R, Jones P R 1984 The invasive potential of carcinoma in situ of cervix. Obstetrics and Gynecology 64: 451–454
Monaghan J 1986a Management of cancers complicating pregnancy. In: Monaghan J (ed) Bonney's gynaecological surgery, 9th edn. Baillière Tindall, London, pp 235–240
Monaghan J 1986b Vulvar carcinoma in pregnancy. British Journal of Obstetrics and Gynaecology 93: 985–986
Ostegard D R, Nieberg R K 1979 Evaluation of abnormal cervical cytology during pregnancy with colposcopy. American Journal of Obstetrics and Gynecology 124: 756–758
Peto R 1986 Geographic patterns and trends. In: Peto R, Zur Hausen H (eds) Viral aetiology of cervical cancer. 21: Banbury report, Cold Spring Harbor Laboratory, New York pp 3–16
Prem K A, Makowski E L, McKelvey J L 1966 Carcinoma of the cervix associated with pregnancy. American Journal of Obstetrics and Gynecology 95: 99–108
Roche W D, Norris H G 1975 Microinvasive carcinoma of the cervix. Cancer 36: 180–186
Shingleton H M, Orr J W 1983 Cancer complicating pregnancy. In: Shingleton H M, Orr J W (eds) Cancer of the cervix, diagnosis and treatment, Churchill Livingstone, Edinburgh, pp 193–206
Singer A 1976 Cervix during pregnancy. In: Jordan J, Singer A (eds) The cervix. Saunders, London, pp 105–125
Singer A, Kirkup W 1980 Colposcopy in the management of the pregnant patient with abnormal cervical cytology. British Journal of Obstetrics and Gynaecology 87: 322–326
Singer A, McCance D 1985 The wart virus and genital neoplasia — a causal or casual association. British Journal of Obstetrics and Gynaecology 92: 1083–1085
Talebean F, Krumholz B A, Shayon A, Mann L I 1976 Colposcopic evaluation of patients with abnormal smears during pregnancy. Obstetrics and Gynecology 47: 693–696
Thompson J D, Capito T A, Franklin E W, Dale E 1975 The surgical management of cervical cancer in pregnancy. American Journal of Obstetrics and Gynecology 121: 853–863
Ward B G, Shepherd J H, Monaghan J M 1985 Occult advanced cervical cancer. British Medical Journal 290: 1301–1302

SECTION 6

Normal Labour

44

Ann Oakley

The labouring mother

In modern industrial societies the last 100 years have brought enormous changes in the reproductive roles of women in general, and in the management of childbirth in particular. Average family size has decreased substantially — between 1840 and 1980 fertility (live births per 1000 women aged 15–44) fell by almost half (Macfarlane & Mugford 1984). The losses that women incurred during the Victorian era in the world of paid work and civil rights have been largely recovered. In 1984, 41% of the labour force in the UK were women. Although this percentage is not much higher than it was in the 1880s, it hides a large change in the proportion of married women employed — while 1 in 10 held a job in 1911 (Klein 1965), 6 in every 10 did so in 1980. In 1980, 52% of women with dependent children were in the labour force — 27% of those with children aged 4 or under (Martin & Roberts 1984).

Accompanying these changes has been an increased social emphasis on sex equality, though in many ways the social and economic positions of men and women remain different. For example, in 1980 average earnings of women in full-time work were 59% of men's (Martin & Roberts 1984). Other social changes have profoundly affected the reproductive roles of women. There has been a very large rise in the number of one-parent families: from 474 000 in 1961 to 975 000 in 1981 (National Council for One-Parent Families 1983). One consequence of the economic recession of the 1980s is that some 28% of the population in Britain now lives in poverty (Mack & Lansley 1985). Whereas in the 1970s the elderly formed the largest group in poverty, that group is now families with children and especially female-headed one-parent families (Department of Health and Social Security 1983). There has also been a growing awareness of the different needs and situations of different ethnic groups.

These facts form the backdrop against which women's experiences of obstetric care need to be seen. As far as childbirth is concerned, the greatest change that has occurred over the last century is that reproduction has become a medical specialty and its control has been removed from the community and from women and is now vested with medical professionals instead.

One consequence of this transformation is that the point of view of mothers themselves may be forgotten. Thus it has become necessary to articulate and make visible their perspective — an exercise which is considerably aided by two important 20th-century social movements — feminism and the consumer movement in health care.

MOTHERS AND THE MEDICALIZATION OF CHILDBIRTH

In the 19th century doctors played a minor role in the care of pregnant women. This was partly because medical care was expensive and most people could not afford it, but there were other important reasons. Before the era of laboratory pregnancy tests and ultrasound scanning, it was difficult for doctors and midwives to diagnose pregnancy. The morality of the time made clinical examination of the patient difficult; it was rarely done, and when it was the textbooks advised the doctor to keep his eyes on the ceiling (Smith 1979). The lack of specialist medical knowledge about childbearing forced practitioners to rely antenatally almost wholly on life-style advice — healthy babies would be secured if the mother slept with the window open, ate meat sparingly and occupied her mind with pleasant thoughts. Until the late 19th century and even early 20th century, a popular therapy for reproductive problems was bloodletting, based on the old Hippocratean theory of pregnancy as a state of plethora, in which the body contained too much blood (Oakley 1984). Nevertheless the predominant view was that pregnancy was not in itself a pathological condition but 'a natural physiological state' (Johnstone 1913).

Prior to the modern obstetric era, most women would never have seen a doctor in pregnancy, and most had their babies with the help of midwives—either the trained or untrained variety. As one historian has put it: 'It is not generally realized that until the seventeenth century, midwifery in England had been a strictly non-medical lay craft which was quite marginal to the existing framework of medical practice and medical training, and medical corporate control ... No medical licences were granted in midwifery and the care of women in labour was in no sense a medical responsibility' (Versluysen 1981). For centuries the main requirement for the office of midwife in Europe was that the woman should be married, of mature age and a mother herself (Donnison 1977). Even after the state intervened to regulate the work of midwives, untrained but experienced (bona fide) midwives were allowed to continue practising. It was not until 1947 that the roll of the Central Midwives Board in England no longer contained names of women admitted under the bona fide practice clause.

This practice of women caring for women in childbirth was part of a long tradition of women's community health care (Oakley 1976). In preindustrialized Europe and colonial America, ordinary people turned to the *good woman*, *cunning woman* or *wise woman* for help with illness. Healing the sick and caring for the dependent was part of women's domestic role. Women's domestic knowledge embraced the recognition and use of pain-killers, digestive aids, anti-inflammatory agents, ergot, belladonna and digitalis; it was within this context that lay midwifery flourished (Clark 1968, Chamberlain 1981).

The story of the male medical takeover of childbirth is relatively well known. At its centre is the apocryphal story of the Chamberlen family who, in the 17th century, negotiated their way into upper-class homes with a magic box containing forceps, blindfolded the labouring woman and locked the door in order to guard their technological secret. Although some medical historians have argued that the invention of the obstetric forceps was the single most important factor in the successful medicalization of midwifery, this would appear to be largely wishful thinking. Even contemporary proponents of the forceps contended that they were needed in only some 0.1–0.2% of cases (Smellie 1752, Bland 1781). Without effective antiseptics forceps carried a high risk of untreatable—sometimes fatal—infection.

In reality the aspiring male midwives of the 18th and 19th centuries were not popular with labouring women or with doctors. Women were afraid of instruments and unhappy about permitting male access to their bodies during birth. Male midwives not only used the technology of the forceps, but also carried out destructive surgery of the fetus in obstructed labour, which did not increase their appeal as childbirth attendants (though it was undoubtedly sometimes useful). At one end of the social continuum the male midwife William Smellie paid his working-class clients for the privilege of delivering them and allowing his male apprentices to watch (Glaister 1894). At the other end of the spectrum, upper-class households paid physicians to hang around outside the labour room, in case they were needed, thereby preventing them from any access to knowledge of normal labour. Midwifery was stereotyped as women's work and so those men who wanted to enter it had to contend with the dismissive attitudes of the medical profession, who regarded midwifery as something doctors ought not to get themselves embroiled in. In line with this attitude hospital-based physicians and surgeons refused to admit maternity patients to hospital at all. Labouring women were placed with small children, the insane, those infected with venereal disease, and the dying and incurable as categories of people whose claim to medical importance was so tenuous that they were said to have no place in hospital at all.

Table 44.1 Labour and delivery in 1818 (from Granville 1819)

Normal* % (n)	Abnormal† % (n)	Total % (n)
96.7 (619)	3.3 (21)	100 (640)

* Defined as 'terminated without the slightest interference, by nature alone' (84% of these labours took 12 hours or less).
† 'When nature becomes passive ... and the assistance either of the *hand* or instruments, is absolutely necessary to terminate the labour' (in 38% of these 21 deliveries instruments were used—1.3% of the grand total of all deliveries).

This was an important factor in the development of the early lying-in hospitals in the 18th century; gaining control over client preferences by hospitalizing them was much more of an influential factor in the increasing medicalization of childbirth than the invention of the forceps. One of the explicit aims behind the founding of the early maternity institutions was that medical men ought to be able to gain more experience of normal deliveries. The lying-in hospitals provided hospitalized delivery for poor women. Table 44.1 shows some figures for deliveries during 1818 at one of the early dispensaries providing maternity care. The physician–accoucheur of the Westminster General Dispensary was an unusual man, Augustus Bozzi Granville, who had been present when Laennec had first demonstrated his use of the stethoscope in 1816. Granville's analysis of midwifery at the Westminster General Dispensary showed that the bulk of labours were normal, and instruments were used in little more than 1% of all deliveries.

It is very hard to know how labouring women felt about the care available to them during these years of fundamental changes in the management of childbirth. Granville himself was of the opinion, in 1819, that 'however distressed the poor mother may be, she will always prefer her own habitation, and the unbought, soothing cares of her own family, during her time of trial, to the spacious ward, and the precise attention of a hired matron and strange nurses' (Granville 1819). He also noted 'a decided aversion amongst lying-in women, against the interference of the Accoucheur, and the use of the most harmless instruments'. At this time the mother's risk of dying in childbirth was probably around 1 in 200. Puerperal fever accounted for about 40% of these deaths (Farr 1885). Infant mortality was around 150 per 1000 livebirths throughout the 19th century (incomplete registration makes it impossible to compile an accurate figure for stillbirths and other perinatal deaths). Death of mother and child was therefore a real risk, but we cannot assume that women necessarily approached childbirth with fatalism or great fear, because cultural attitudes to birth were not the same then as they are now.

If hospitals were needed by the obstetrical specialists to build up their knowledge and control of clients, they had, by the late 19th century, a particular attraction for women also: they offered the possibility of pain relief in labour. Midwives delivering babies at home had no analgesia to offer mothers until R. J. Minnitt at Liverpool Maternity Hospital designed a portable apparatus for delivering gas and air in 1932. This fact may have been partly responsible for the move among middle-class mothers to have babies in hospital in the early decades of the 20th century, a move which was associated with the unusual epidemiological picture of higher social class temporarily going hand-in-hand with higher maternal mortality (Registrar-General 1930).

Place of delivery was first documented by the British Registrar-General in 1927, when 15% of all livebirths occurred in institutions: he thought the main reason for hospital birth was lack of home facilities. By 1954 the figure for institutional deliveries was 64% and in that year, whatever mothers thought, the British Medical Journal was still able to declare that 'the proper place for the confinement is the patient's own home' (British Medical Journal Editorial 1954). By 1960 the proportion of babies delivered in institutions had risen by only 1% since 1954 and this, not coincidentally, was the year in which one of Britain's most energetic consumer pressure groups in the maternity care field was born: the Association for Improvements in Maternity Services (AIMS), originally named the Society for the Prevention of Cruelty to Pregnant Women.

CONSUMERS' REVOLT?

Table 44.2 compares the objectives of AIMS when it was first founded with those formulated 21 years later in 1981. It is apparent that interpreting the rights of women to make choices in childbirth in 1960 meant an emphasis on hospital delivery: in its early years AIMS campaigned to increase the number of hospital maternity beds, because at the time there was a demand by women for them. By 1981 the emphasis had shifted to an increase in community care. Midwives remained important. The research called for on analgesia and psychological aspects of childbirth in 1960 became, in 1981, a demand for attention to diet as a component of good maternity care. Financial support for childbearing women has emerged as a priority.

Table 44.2 Aims of AIMS 1960–1981

1960	1981
More money for the NHS, especially hospital maternity services	Midwife control of maternity care for low-risk women
More midwives, and improvements in their working conditions	Antenatal care for low-risk women to be community-based
More home helps (for home births)	Antenatal care to include evaluation and information related to mother's diet
No woman in labour should be left alone against her will	Nutritional assistance for women with poor diets
More research on pain relief and the psychology of childbirth	Increase in the maternity grant to be given to all pregnant women

The rise of groups such as AIMS, the National Childbirth Trust (NCT), the Maternity Alliance and a host of others has given prominence to the maternal (and parental) point of view. Collectively they have provided a voice for what is incorrectly dubbed the 'consumer's perspective' (Stacey 1976). Although many women belong to these organizations, many do not; membership is likely to be weighted towards the informed middle classes, which means that these pressure groups cannot be assumed to speak for all women. Having said that, it is of course necessary to query the assumption that all women share a single viewpoint on any specific issue, such as analgesia or position in labour, or more generally as to the overall management of childbirth. There is no reason to assume this. Women having babies do not form a homogeneous group (Riley 1977). In the same way not all obstetricians are in agreement about how to treat women in childbirth — there is a wide range of attitudes and great variation in clinical practice.

Consumer groups in the maternity care field have nevertheless stressed certain themes, and continue to do so. From a historical viewpoint the existence of these organizations is a response to the situation that had evolved by the mid 20th century — one in which control of childbirth had passed into the hands of the professionals. It became necessary for those using the maternity services to reclaim their own rights to have a voice in the shaping of these services. Comparing the situation in Britain with that in other countries, it appears that protest of this kind is much more likely to happen when services have been increasingly centralized in hospital and there has been an erosion of community care (Houd & Oakley 1986), hence the AIMS appeal for more community-based care (Table 44.2). For example, in some northern European countries such as Sweden and Finland, antenatal care remains community-based and there are few organizations of client groups. Conversely, countries with fee-for-service private health care systems such as the USA seem to make client protest more likely.

The consumers' revolt in childbirth has everywhere emphasized the same key themes: the right to information, the right to choose, respect for social and psychological aspects of childbearing and for the integrity and privacy and individuality of childbearing women and their families, and pregnancy and birth as normal physiological events. Over the last 10 years there has also been increasing stress on the need for obstetric procedures to be properly evaluated for effectiveness and safety before they enter routine practice. These themes are closely intermeshed, as is evident in the following editorial entitled 'Safety first?' from a 1984 edition of the AIMS newsletter:

> Our health care, like other aspects of our lives, has been fragmented, specialised and with increasing specialisation comes loss of an overall vision of purpose. Pregnancy and birth have been removed from the continuum of normal women's health care; pregnancy is regarded as an abnormal state and the line between the abnormal and the pathological is very thin. Obstetricians' responses to pregnancy and birth are conditioned by their training: they specialise in the abnormal, and seek to discover and cure the pathological. The more tests and procedures that are deemed necessary in their searching, the more reason there is to believe that pregnancy is indeed fraught with danger. The more interventions that become accepted as standard practice, the further we move away from the baseline of a truly normal birth—a strong, healthy woman giving birth to a strong, healthy child.
>
> Much of the data needed for a thorough evaluation of many procedures is not even collected, far less published in an accessible form for prospective parents. If it is 'all for your own good', it should be demonstrably so. (AIMS Editorial 1984.)

Two other factors have contributed to the assertiveness of organizations such as AIMS. One is the women's movement, which has entailed an emphasis on appropriate health care for women, and the other is medical sociology, which, as an academic-based discipline, has sought (among many other enterprises) to highlight the social within medicine (Stacey & Homans 1978).

As a result of these forces, there are now systematic data which can be marshalled to answer questions about what women want in obstetric care—bearing in mind, naturally, the need to be sceptical about the formulation of the question itself. Although it is tempting to regard these data as new, the omission from obstetric data of the childbearing woman's point of view is a relatively recent development. Many of the government reports on maternity care published in the first half of this century, for instance, gave a good deal of prominence to women's experiences and attitudes and stressed the desirability of considering the implications for the maternity services of the social and economic position of women (see Ministry of Health 1927). If one compares the three national birth surveys carried out in 1946, 1958 and 1970 (Joint Committee 1948, Butler & Bonham 1963, Chamberlain et al 1978), it is clear that the first of these was sensitive to these issues in a way in which the later two were not. (For example, in 1946 there was concern about the costs of childbearing to women, about women's views of their care and the relationship between household work and pregnancy outcome.)

Table 44.3 Preferences for place of birth in the next pregnancy (from Cartwright 1979)

	Place of birth in the last pregnancy	
	Home birth (%)	Hospital birth (%)
Prefer same as last time	91	83
Prefer not to have same as last time	9	15
Other comment	—	2
Number of mothers (=100%)	97	2083

The rest of this chapter will explore some of what is known about the point of view of mothers in relation to specific topics in the maternity care debate today. The following will be considered: place of birth, delivery personnel, natural childbirth, analgesia, induction of labour, instrumental delivery, Caesarean section, monitoring in labour, client–professional communication, and mother–infant bonding.

PLACE OF BIRTH

Where do women want to have their babies? This is a complicated question, because it lacks meaning in the abstract. People's wants are the outcome of many factors, including their own personalities and psychologies, the information they have about different options and the long-term implications of settling for one option rather than another, and the pressures on them to want certain things. On the whole people want what they have. If they did not do so, society would be in a constant state of flux and change. To want something very different requires a vision of an alternative, and most people's daily lives do not encourage visions.

These generalizations apply to maternity care. But given this generally conservative impulse, a number of statements can be made on the basis of available surveys about women's preferences for place of delivery. Table 44.3, which is taken from Ann Cartwright's national study of induction, certainly shows that most women would prefer the place of delivery in which their last child was born. This applies both to the group whose last baby was born in hospital and to the group who had a home birth. But the table also shows a preference for a second home birth in the group who have already experienced one, which is considerably stronger than the preference expressed for a second hospital delivery among women whose last baby was delivered in hospital. Whereas 9% of women who had a home birth last time said they would not want one again, 15% of those who had a hospital birth last time would not choose to repeat this. Cartwright also asked the women in the sample who had had one baby at home and one in hospital to compare their experiences; 76% preferred it at home and 15% in hospital—the remainder had no preference (Cartwright 1979).

Table 44.4 Reactions to pain relief (from O'Brien 1978)

	Hospital birth (%)	Home birth (%)
First given pain relief at right time	69	82
Given enough pain relief	72	87
On balance, felt glad about what they had	74	87
Number given pain relief	1730	60

Table 44.5 Average cost per birth by place of delivery (from Stilwell 1979)

	Home (£)	GP/Hospital (£)	Consultant unit (£)
Public sector costs	196.69	216.87	241.02
Family costs	60.67	53.80	89.15
Total	257.36	270.67	330.17

Reviewing studies of preferences for place of birth, Macintyre (1977) has shown that the proportion of women who would like to have a baby at home is always higher than the proportion booked to do so. The preference for home delivery appears to rise with parity and also with the experience of home delivery. The best evidence for this latter point is Goldthorpe & Richman's (1974) study of unintended home delivery due to a strike by hospital ancillary staff. The sample consisted of 65 women who had their babies at home because of the strike, although they had been booked for hospital delivery. When told that they could not have their babies as planned, 22% of the women said they felt pleased, 40% did not mind, and 38% were disappointed or very disappointed. However, after having the baby, 80% said they wanted to have their next baby at home, and this was independent of whether the labour at home had been easy or difficult (Goldthorpe & Richman 1974).

Preferences for place of birth, even if comprehensive information can be obtained about them, are fairly meaningless unless we can also find out what it is about a home or hospital delivery that renders it attractive. From a policy point of view, this is important information. Going back to the Cartwright survey, some of its findings are suggestive. Comparing home and hospital experiences, it was found that labour lasted a significantly shorter time at home, fewer women were left alone during labour and significantly fewer had episiotomies. In the home group, 76% of husbands were present at the birth compared with 30% in hospital. Of the mothers at home, 57% held their babies as long as they wanted, compared with 29% in hospital. Table 44.4 shows reactions to pain relief. Again, the home birth group seem to do better, perhaps because it is easier for women to receive individualized care at home. This is reflected in the findings relating to communication between mothers and their attendants. Mothers in home and hospital groups were equally likely to have had worries during their labour and to have discussed these worries with someone. But those at home were more likely to say that the person they talked to was helpful (89% compared with 59% of the hospital group). Overall, 44% of the home group as against 34% of the hospital group said labour and delivery had been pleasurable experiences (O'Brien 1978).

The economic costs to the mother and the family of maternity care are frequently forgotten in debates about the best form of care. In 1979 Stilwell calculated the average cost per birth of home, general practitioner unit and consultant unit deliveries (Table 44.5). The cost of a home delivery is lower than the other two options, although the family costs are actually lowest for a general practitioner unit delivery.

Women having babies are people with a variety of other roles and responsibilities. Commonly they have households to run and other children to look after. These considerations may push some women towards hospital delivery, where they will be able to have a temporary break from these responsibilities and others towards home, so that they can continue to assume them. However none of these reasons may apply, and one important issue remains to be mentioned: safety.

Safety is a concept that can be interpreted in many ways. It has at least two dimensions: physical and psychological. In thinking about the idea of safety we often split these two meanings, but to do so is really nonsensical because the psyche and the soma are closely related. There is a vast body of evidence demonstrating that stress is bad for successful reproduction and that psychologically felt stress has physiological manifestations in childbearing women (Oakley et al 1982). It is difficult to attach a precise value to findings such as the white coat effect—the impact on fetal heart rates of physicians' arrival in the labour room (Myers 1979), but the links between the mother's environment and her behaviour are none the less real.

Whereas the supposedly superior physical safety of hospital delivery is constantly emphasized, the greater psychological safety of home birth is a message that emerges clearly from women's accounts of having a baby at home (Kitzinger 1979). In part this is because the chances of maternal psychological stress are generally lower at home, and this, as Richards has pointed out in a discussion of the risks of hospital delivery, is related to the fact that:

> the mother's attendants are visitors in her home; she is not staying temporarily in the institution *they* run. This means that many of the procedures and routines that a mother is forced to accept by social pressures in hospital are avoided in the home. At home social relationships are not influenced by the demands of a large bureaucratic structure dominated by an ethos of technical efficiency; instead they result from the needs and wishes of the individuals concerned. This is a point of overwhelming importance . . . (Richards 1979).

It is not an invariable rule that what benefits the mother also benefits the baby. However, it is undoubtedly true that it is easier for mother and baby to feel close after the birth when both are in their own home: the phenomenon of mother–infant bonding could only have been discovered as a necessity under conditions of near universal hospital delivery.

As well as emphasizing the enhanced psychological safety of home birth, consumer groups in the childbirth field have of course also tangled with the epidemiologists and statisticians on the question of comparative perinatal mortality rates at home and in hospital. In doing so, they have made the point that many parents wish to be informed about the relative risks of different places of birth and are intelligent enough to understand the basic statistical arguments. It is the case that no one has yet successfully proved that hospital birth is a physically safer alternative for most mothers and babies (Campbell & Macfarlane 1987). It is equally clear that many obstetricians do not regard home delivery as a sensible option, though perhaps few would go so far as to say, along with the President of the American College of Obstetricians and Gynecologists (ACOG) in 1979, that: 'home delivery is the earliest form of child abuse' (ACOG 1979). On the contrary, it is worth noting that when a select committee in Britain investigated the topic of violence in the family in 1977, one of its recommendations was for more home deliveries, since this was seen to facilitate the making of a good mother–baby relationship, thereby making child abuse less likely (Select Committee on Violence in the Family 1977).

As Alberman wrote in 1977:

> the opportunity to examine the relative safeties of home and hospital delivery without bias has been lost . . . as is the case with so many innovations . . . the rapid expansion of hospital confinement was carried out without regard to well-planned trials, and now, with a confinement rate of over 94% it is too late for such trials to be performed . . . In addition, a true comparison of home versus institutional delivery will never be achieved until it is possible to study outcomes such as the long-term quality of births in terms of physical, psychological and mental health, the benefit to the mother of relief of pain or anxiety, the long-term benefit in terms of incidence of complications such as prolapse or urinary incontinence, and other similar measures (Alberman 1977).

In this situation, the fact that some women are asking for the right to choose where they have their babies hardly seems unreasonable. Surveys show that the maternity services function in such a way that relatively few women are able to exercise choice about where they have their antenatal care or their babies. In a study carried out in London in the mid 1970s, 58% of the women interviewed were simply told by their general practitioners where they would have their babies and 61% were given no choice about shared or hospital-only antenatal care (Oakley 1981). In the Cartwright study (1979) the women who were happy about their initial booking for delivery were asked: 'Did you feel you had a choice about this?' A total of 87% of women who had their babies at home said yes, compared with 56% of those who had their babies in hospital (O'Brien 1978).

WHO SHOULD DELIVER?

In Britain in 1985 a midwife was the senior person present at 76% of births. There is very little information available about women's preferences for attendants during labour and delivery. Perhaps the first preference is that there should be *someone* there: many complaints in the 1950s and 1960s highlighted the loneliness of labouring mothers in hospitals where staff were too busy or not sufficiently sensitive to stay with the mother during labour. Continuous support during labour is not irreconcilable with high-technology obstetrics. For example, the policy pioneered by O'Driscoll at the National Maternity Hospital in Dublin combines active management of labour with the provision of a personal nurse (O'Driscoll & Meagher 1980).

A second commonly stated preference is for the birth attendant to be someone the mother already knows. When the mother delivers in hospital this is not very likely to happen: the London study already referred to found that 75% of the women had never seen the person who delivered their baby before. As one of the women said:

> It was *horrific* that the midwife and the pupil midwife who were there I'd never seen in my life before and I've never seen them again since. And yet they were *the* people in about the most vital and powerful experience of my life so far (Oakley 1981).

In historical and cross-cultural terms this is an unusual situation (Mead & Newton 1967). Whilst it may be reassuring to feel that the person helping the mother to deliver the baby is technically expert, yet the impact of a familiar deliverer is likely to be considerable.

A Know-your-Midwife (KYM) scheme conducted in London recently looked at the effect of continuity of care on labour and delivery, and found some interesting differences. One group of women (the KYM group) were looked after throughout the pregnancy, labour and the postnatal period by a team of four midwives. The other group received the standard pattern of hospital care. The KYM group were less often admitted to hospital antenatally than the control group; they used less analgesia in labour although they had longer labours; they had more normal deliveries; were more likely to deliver in an alternative position; they found motherhood easier and were more satisfied with their care than women in the control group (Flint & Poulengris 1987).

These findings are consistent with other evidence showing that midwifery care leads to more normal results for low-risk women than specialist care (Runnerstrom 1969). On these grounds, those women who want a normal labour and delivery should prefer care by midwives; however, nothing is simple in the maternity care field, and a preference for doctors may often be expressed. This is congruent with the professional claim that obstetricians are the people who know best how to secure healthy babies, which is itself part of the medicalization of life we are all socialized to accept (McKeown 1979).

The question of who should be with the labouring mother

Table 44.6 Percentage of patients who experienced perinatal problems during labour and delivery (from Klaus et al 1986)

Problems	No support ($n = 249$) (%)	Support ($n = 168$) (%)
Caesarean section	17	7 ($P < 0.01$)
Meconium staining	18	13
Asphyxia	3	2
Oxytocin	13	2 ($P < 0.001$)
Analgesia	4	1
Forceps	3	1
Other	1	1
Total	59	27 ($P < 0.001$)

was tackled in a different way by Sosa and his colleagues in a randomized controlled trial (RCT) carried out in Guatemala some years ago. In this study, women randomized to the intervention group received the support of a lay companion throughout labour, whereas the control group (as in the KYM scheme) received the standard pattern of care. There were impressive differences in some labour and delivery variables in favour of the supported group (Sosa et al 1980). A more recent application of this approach by Klaus et al (1986) resulted in the findings shown in Table 44.6. All the differences in the incidence of perinatal problems were in favour of the supported group. As Table 44.6 shows, the findings for the comparative incidence of Caesarean section and oxytocin and the overall incidence of problems were statistically significant. Another finding not shown in the table was that mean duration of labour was significantly shorter in the supported group (7.7 versus 15.5 hours; $P < 0.001$).

NATURAL CHILDBIRTH?

Both natural and technological forms of childbirth are capable of breeding their own orthodoxies. The modern conflict between users and providers of maternity care is often seen as centring on this notion of the natural as opposed to the unnatural medicalized, technological version of childbirth. There is a sense in which this is clearly true, and it is the sense in which medical services and therapies have the status of a cultural accretion. Human beings invented them, but they did not invent childbirth. The impact of this on women having babies is sometimes to make them believe in childbirth as an unnatural activity because it, like illness, has become the province of hospitals and doctors (Oakley 1977).

The equation between the unnatural and the medicalized derives its meaning from the very fact that pregnancy and birth are taken to hospitals and doctors, just as are other forms of illness. While this is clearly appropriate for those mothers and fetuses who develop problems, many consumer groups contend that it is not appropriate care for most mothers and fetuses, because it enhances the risk of complications arising. This was the substance of one of the early books in the present alternative childbirth movement—Suzanne Arms' 'Immaculate Deception' (1975). Arms argues that women have been deceived by obstetricians into believing in an unobtainable ideal—the no-risk birth. They have been co-opted by the obstetrical establishment into accepting a hospitalized and interventionist management of childbirth whereby a structure said to minimize the risks of childbearing actually inflates these risks by leading to iatrogenic complications.

Anthropologists point out that no human society provides for childbirth as a purely natural event. Everywhere childbirth is defined and hedged about with rules, rituals and prescriptions dictating how labouring women, their families and helpers should behave (Ford 1945). The stereotype of primitive childbirth as an unattended birth behind a bush describes an event 'as rare and remarkable as an American birth taking place in a taxi cab' (Mead & Newton 1967). Most importantly, the lack of modern medical facilities and therapies does not necessarily mean an attitude of non-interference; for example, herbs may be used to accelerate labour, abdominal stimulation, including external version, may be used, and manual removal of the placenta is by no means unknown (Oakley 1982).

In modern obstetric practice, the question is often asked whether women really want natural childbirth. This issue causes heated reactions on both sides. Obstetricians condemn women's viewpoints as cranky, whimsical and dangerous and women object that obstetricians are trying to frighten them into submission. It may be objected (by obstetricians) that they should not have to contend with something called 'The Good Birth Guide'; neurosurgeons, after all, do not have to grapple with 'The Good Neurosurgery Guide'. Total lack of comprehension may be expressed about instances such as the mother whose pregnancy was initiated by in vitro fertilization but who chose to have her baby at home and whose baby died during the second stage of labour: how could someone be so foolish as to risk such a precious hard-won pregnancy through the selfish desire for a familiar place of birth? (Francis 1985).

One explanation of these patterns is the fact that by and large women and obstetricians do have different perspectives on childbirth. A pooled analysis of data from two research projects in York and London showed that obstetricians and mothers see the nature, context, control and criteria of success of childbirth differently. These differences in the frames of reference of the two groups are responsible for at least some of the conflicts that develop (Graham & Oakley 1981).

Is there any systematic evidence about the proportion of women who support natural (i.e. non-interventionist) childbirth? No research has exclusively and directly tackled this question, but partial answers can be gleaned from a variety of sources. Macintyre (1981) approached this question by asking how the women in her Scottish study felt about the prospect of intervention during labour or delivery; her findings are shown in Table 44.7. Negative feelings were

Table 44.7 Women's feelings at 34 weeks' gestation about intervention during labour or delivery (from Macintyre 1981)

Feelings	% Women ($n = 45$)
Positive feelings about intervention	2
Accepting or indifferent	58
Negative feelings	36
Not asked	4
Total	100

Table 44.8 Planning for childbirth—choices about procedures by social class (from Nelson 1983)

	Percentage of women who wanted each procedure*	
	Working class (%)	Middle class (%)
Shave	20	20
Enema	42	46
Labour medication	57	11
Delivery medication	58	17
ARM†	59	4
Episiotomy	64	62
Fetal monitoring	90	55
Hold baby at birth	92	97

* Calculated on number in each group who expressed a choice. Total number of subjects in study = 322.
† Artificial rupture of membranes.

expressed by a third of the women; a very small proportion said they felt positively about the prospect.

In Cartwright's study of induction (1979), the main reason women gave for not wanting an induction was that they wanted the baby to come naturally. A study of British Asian women in Warwickshire found that 48% of mothers expressed a desire that nature would determine the timing and mode of birth. This desire was voiced most strongly by women who had experienced an unwelcome level of medical intervention in a previous birth. The chief reasons given for preferring a natural birth were twofold: firstly, that women who had had induced labours with epidural analgesia and perhaps an instrumental delivery tended to feel they had not really given birth; secondly, they were concerned that elective delivery led to a disturbed mother–child relationship (Homans 1980). In London in the mid 1970s, 96% of a sample of women interviewed before delivery said they would prefer a labour and delivery without medical intervention because such a birth would be more natural. Specifically, 73% said they would not like to have an induction on these grounds — but 21% of these women did experience an induction (Oakley 1981).

It is commonly said that the desire for natural childbirth is limited to middle-class women, and it may also be objected that some women actually campaign for medical interventions. The latter point is undoubtedly true — indeed, it follows from the point made earlier, that not all women want the same kind of birth experience. The question of social class is more complex. In a study done in New England, Nelson (1983) found that there were two client models of childbirth; both were in competition with the medical model. Table 44.8 shows some dimensions of the two client models identified in this study. Quite large differences exist between the two groups with respect to medication, artificial rupture of membranes (ARM) and fetal monitoring, but not for the other procedures shown in the table. Nelson summed up the differences thus:

> The working class women . . . favoured intervention because they thought it could bring the product easily, quickly and safely. The middle class women favoured a process which entailed safety (as they defined it) and personal participation, but excluded medical intervention in a natural process (Nelson 1983).

As Nelson points out, the preferences of working-class women in such settings may reflect inhibition, due to a feeling of not being able to control the birth process. In addition, middle-class women may have access to more information about childbirth. But account must also be taken of the fact that the social and economic position of the two groups is different. Working-class women have children younger, have more accidental pregnancies and more limited material resources for childbearing. The pursuit of natural childbirth requires time, money and assertiveness, and will not be pursued at all unless it is seen to be a priority. It is clear that some women do not see it as a priority.

PAIN: THE CURSE OF WOMEN?

There are many views on the subject of pain in childbirth. How much pain do women feel? How much should they feel? What are the best methods for relieving pain? Who should determine how much pain relief should be available? From a biblical position, the pain of childbirth is part of the meaning of womanhood. A more recent rendering of this is its psychoanalytic reworking, according to which masochism is to be regarded as a feminine personality trait. As an editorial in the British Medical Journal (1973) put it: 'The assumption that man is born to suffer and that woman is born to suffer more than man is found in the earliest human literature'. However, there is a continuum of views on the matter of pain in childbirth. There are those who say that relaxation and information are the main analgesics necessary; others assert that every appropriate modern analgesic method should be applied to its relief. Care-providers and their clients are divided on this topic, and a political ideology such as feminism is compatible with opposing points of view.

There is surprisingly little research directly tapping the views of labouring women about pain. In 1982, 1000 women delivering at Queen Charlotte's Maternity Hospital were asked to grade the pain they felt in labour on a linear analogue scale (Morgan et al 1982). Those who had felt the most pain were mothers who had not received any analgesia and those who felt the least were those who had been given an epidural.

Table 44.9 Pain relief and induced and spontaneous labours (from Cartwright 1979)

	Induced labours (%)	Labours starting spontaneously (%)	All labours (%)
Pain relief			
None	11	21	19
Epidural/spinal anaesthesia	9	4	5
Other injection	72	62	64
Inhalant analgesia	4	6	5
Other	4	6	5
Amount of pain relief			
Enough	70	73	72
Would have liked more	7	7	7
Too much	9	7	8
Mixed views/other	14	13	13
Number of labours	522	1599	2134

One in three mothers experienced more pain than they had expected and this proportion was the same in all analgesic groups (Morgan et al 1982). Other surveys provide similar kinds of information although, unfortunately, there has been no standard way of eliciting the information, so it is difficult to make direct comparisons between different studies. Cartwright (1979) looked at pain relief in her study of induction: Table 44.9 gives data for her study according to whether the labour was induced or not, and for all labours. About one in four women said that they had not been given the right amount of pain relief. It is important to note that a drug or procedure given to alleviate pain may have other physical effects for the mother: thus Cartwright found that the proportion of women who felt sick or were sick during labour was considerably higher for the epidural than for any other group.

Surveys using smaller samples demonstrate some of the regional and subcultural differences in attitudes to pain and pain relief. A study carried out in Oxford found that 26% of women assessed their labour pain as greater and 65% as less than expected: for 9% it was as they had expected (Ounstead & Simons 1979). Macintyre's prospective interview study of married primigravidae in Aberdeen found that the overall experience of childbirth, in which pain was a prominent component, was worse than expected for one in three mothers, but also better than expected for one in three; the rest had no particular expectations, were not able to remember them, or found the experience similar to what they had expected (Macintyre 1981). Two of the comments quoted by Macintyre were:

(It's) totally different. It's really, well, it's a pain you can never realise until you have it yourself . . . it's something that you don't realise until you have a baby of your own.

and

Well, with having an epidural I couldn't really say if it was worse than I expected because I was hoping to have a normal delivery.

The picture with respect to pain and its relief during labour is considerably more complicated than it may at first appear. An important consideration is that different analgesic experiences are associated with different rates of intervention, and both analgesic and intervention experiences are combined in the mothers' recollections.

In the Queen Charlotte's survey, for example, 11% of the mothers having no analgesia had their labours induced, and 1% had an assisted delivery, compared with a 35% induction and 51% assisted delivery rate in the epidural group (Morgan et al 1982). Secondly, satisfaction with childbirth, including feelings about the amount of pain experienced and relieved, evolves over time. It is necessary to know not only how mothers feel immediately or soon after delivery, but also what they make of the experience months or years later. The Queen Charlotte's study showed that the proportion of mothers dissatisfied with the experience of childbirth 1 year later was lowest in the no analgesia group, and highest in the miscellaneous combinations group, and at a point in between for the group of women who had had epidurals alone or in combination with another method.

There are also methods aside from medical ones for relieving labour pain. Fear, as described by Grantly Dick-Read (1942) and others, can lead to pain; thus the alleviation of fear by information and relaxation may directly affect pain. Contrary to some of its claims, however, there is no evidence that childbirth preparation classes on their own have an appreciable effect (Enkin 1982). There is some evidence that childbirth preparation classes reduce the need for analgesia, though they do not necessarily have all the dramatic effects claimed for them. Other relaxation strategies such as music may be seen as helpful: the music of Barry Manilow (in this context said to be relaxing) became fashionable in 1984 as an aid to childbirth by Caesarean section (Guardian 4 April 1984). Flynn et al (1978) found that ambulation in labour reduced the need for analgesia and had other effects, including higher Apgar scores and a reduced need for augmentation of labour with oxytoxic drugs.

The pain of childbirth may be different in important ways from other types of pain — in having the achievable end-product of a baby, for example — yet important connections can be made between its experience and management and those of other types of pain. For example, giving information to surgical patients has been shown to reduce postoperative pain (Janis 1985). It is known that individual pain thresholds vary, and although some health professionals and others may tend to see patterned differences between social groups in terms of attitudes to pain, at least for the British population, the notion that people in lower social classes have a high perception of pain and a greater prevalence of neuroticism has been shown to be false (Larson & Mercer 1984).

ELECTIVE DELIVERY

The present wave of consumer criticism in obstetrics was provoked by concern in the mid 1970s about rising induction rates (Gillie & Gillie 1974) and the same wave is now riding the tide of critical attitudes towards rising Caesarean section rates (Maternity Alliance 1983). The issues involved in induction of labour and Caesarean section relate both to what may be seen as the prevention of natural childbirth, and to the unwarranted promotion of medical and technological control, unwarranted in the sense that high induction and Caesarean section rates may carry more hazards than they provide benefits for mothers and babies.

Induction

It is clear from studies of women's attitudes that a number of different components are involved. The main ones are pain, medical interventions associated with induction, and patterns of interaction and communication with medical staff. Overall, induction appears to mean more pain for mothers, more medical interventions and a less satisfying mode of staff–patient communication.

In an NCT study of women attending NCT antenatal classes, 64% of the multiparae who had the opportunity to compare their induced labour with a previous non-induced one reported induction as worse because of its greater pain and discomfort (Kitzinger 1975). On the same basis of a comparison with previous labours, the mothers in Cartwright's (1979) study found induction more painful than a spontaneous labour. Stewart's (1979) survey of attitudes to induction in women delivering in the Nuneaton Maternity Hospital found that in 45% of induced patients the pain of labour was greater than they had expected; the same figure was reported in the study of Lewis et al (1975) which also contained a control group of women having spontaneous labours: 33% of the spontaneous group said the pain of labour had exceeded their expectations.

The question of the degree of pain felt is, of course, intimately linked to the question of the degree of pain relief offered and accepted. All available studies concur in the conclusion that women whose labours are induced receive more pain relief. In the retrospective study by Yudkin et al (1979) 32% of a spontaneous onset group of 200 women received no pain relief or Entonox (nitrous oxide and oxygen) only, as against only 6% in an induced group of a further 200 women—findings not dissimilar from those of the NCT report (Kitzinger 1975); 49% of inductions were accompanied by epidural analgesia, while the figure was 14% for the spontaneous group.

In Stewart's (1979) study, twice as many women who were induced had epidurals. The increased use of analgesic drugs with induction is likely to have negative effects on the baby (Richards 1977, 1979) and induced labours tend to be shorter than those that begin spontaneously (Cartwright 1979). Indeed, shortening the length of labour sometimes appears to be a carrot held out by obstetricians to women to persuade them of the advantages of induced labour specifically, and the active management of labour in general. According to the active management of labour policy, as advocated and practised by O'Driscoll, it is important to assure women that their babies will be born within a definite time period 'because the prospect of prolonged labour is often a cause of serious concern' (O'Driscoll & Meagher 1980). In fact no one appears to have asked women which of the two alternatives they would prefer: a shorter more painful labour or a longer, possibly less painful one.

In many places routine fetal heart rate monitoring is practised in all induced labours. The women in Cartwright's national sample (1979) who had their babies in 1975 reported a rate of electronic fetal heart rate monitoring of 32% for induced and 17% for spontaneous labours; the sample in the study by Yudkin et al (1979) of women delivering in Oxford in the same year yielded rates of 65 and 19% respectively. The procedures involved in attaching scalp electrodes to the fetus are experienced by some women as painful (Oakley 1981) but maternal reactions to continuous fetal heart rate monitoring have in general received scant investigation. Of more than 500 articles on this topic published between 1970 and 1980, only two considered maternal attitudes. The following range of reactions was reported in one of these:

> The monitor was seen as a protector, sometimes with quasi-magical powers; as an extension of their own bodies; as an aid to communication; as an extension of the baby; as a distraction; as an aid to recognising the onset of contractions; as a mechanical monster; as a competitor for the husband's attention—or the midwife's, or the doctor's—as a facilitator of husband participation in labour and as a source of anxiety (Lumley & Astbury 1980).

A more recent randomized controlled trial of electronic fetal heart rate monitoring compared mothers' views of this technique with their views about intermittent auscultation: the electronically monitored women experienced more restriction of movement and were not more reassured by this method of monitoring than women exposed to the traditional alternative (Garcia et al 1985a).

It is not entirely clear why induced labours attract more epidurals. Are epidurals administered more often in these cases because women request them, because medical staff expect an induced labour to be more painful and advise the mother accordingly, or because it is more convenient to organize an epidural at the same time as the other procedures required for an induction? Another possibility is that the greater use of epidurals in induced labour may be the consequence of a more general attitude to intervention among obstetricians, so that those who favour induction are also likely to favour epidurals. Obstetricians regard epidurals as increasing their job satisfaction—and that of midwives; though most midwives in fact hold the view that this is not so (Cartwright 1979).

The more common use of epidural analgesia in induced

as opposed to spontaneous labours is part of the explanation of the higher rate of instrumental delivery associated with induced labours (Cartwright 1979, Yudkin et al 1979). Cartwright found differences in the incidence of instrumental delivery according to whether or not the husband was present (a higher rate characterized the husband-present group), and she suggests that 'possibly husbands agitate for something to be done — or possibly forceps are occasionally used as a reason for asking the husband to leave?' Yudkin et al (1979) present the following interpretation:

> It could be that the high rate of forceps deliveries among the induced women reflects not so much the inability of these women to deliver spontaneously, but rather the close attention of the supervising obstetrician. Having started a woman's labour electively and closely followed it through to full dilation with fetal monitoring the obstetrician may well feel that he can ensure a successful delivery by intervening in the second stage as well.

Kirke (1975), in one of the very few studies of consumer attitudes carried out by doctors, reports that 'almost three quarters of those who had forceps deliveries said they either did not mind or were pleased about it, and one quarter were disappointed because they had wanted a natural birth'. It is difficult to know how to regard those who were pleased at having a forceps delivery. Would they have been very pleased if they had been offered a Caesarean section instead? Without some assessment of the meaning of the use of techniques like these for the mothers the recording of simple votes is not very illuminating. A randomized controlled trial designed to compare the consequences for mothers and babies of the vacuum extractor versus forceps found that women allocated to vacuum extraction reported less pain at delivery, but had more worries about their babies (Garcia et al 1985b).

There is some evidence that, not unreasonably, and as is the case with fetal monitoring (Starkman 1976), instrumental deliveries are more positively evaluated by mothers when they are seen as a solution to real obstetric problems rather than as a routine procedure (Oakley 1981). The same probably holds for episiotomy, a procedure which has become more common in recent years, and which appears to be considerably more painful and problematic for mothers than is usually recognized (Kitzinger 1981).

In a leading article on induction in labour in 1976, the British Medical Journal attempted to disentangle the main points emerging from the media debate on induction. The article took the view that since induction was only practised by clinicians 'in good faith for the good of the mother and the baby' its misrepresentation in the media must be 'disquieting evidence that doctors were not adequately communicating their intentions to their patients' (British Medical Journal Editorial 1976).

Lack of information and inadequate discussion are certainly major themes in the studies that have been done of women's attitudes to induction. The most detailed data on this are given by Cartwright (1979). Only 57% of women whose labours were induced had discussed induction at all in pregnancy. Two out of five said they would have liked more information about it. Whereas middle-class women were more likely to have discussed induction beforehand, working-class women were more likely to feel deprived of adequate information about pregnancy and birth in general. The more middle-class sample described in the NCT report appear to have had a similar experience: only 56% of the induced group had discussed induction.

The situation with respect to induction is a prime example of that described by Friedson as liable to promote overt conflict between doctor and patient. Friedson (1975) notes that 'the very nature of professional practice seems to stimulate the patient on occasions to be especially wary and questioning'. In the first place, professional knowledge is never complete, and procedures applied to parents may eventually turn out to be incorrect or hazardous; professional knowledge tends to disregard the validity of the patient's definitions of her condition. Secondly, there is the tendency towards the routinization of cases that constitute clinical material, so that patients become mere instances of a class, each individual instance being considered the same as every other in its class. Given that the variation between different practitioners and institutions in induction rates is a matter of relatively public knowledge, and that hazards of the procedure are fairly openly discussed, it is hardly surprising that many women feel these days that induction of labour is not a purely clinical matter to be left to obstetricians, but one in which they themselves should be able to exercise choice. Indeed, 81% of the women in Cartwright's study indicated that in circumstances where a doctor was uncertain about what clinical course to adopt in their case, they would like the situation explained to them so that they could choose what should be done. This is surely a very important point. Despite the fact that four-fifths of mothers would prefer to be involved in the decision-making process, only a third of those whose labours were induced felt they had had any kind of choice.

The desire of many women to take part in decisions about induction does not necessarily mean that they are opposed to induction. As Ounsted & Simons (1979) somewhat provocatively phrase it: 'in addition to those women who insist on natural childbirth at all costs, there appears to be another group who may exert pressure on their obstetricians to induce labour in the absence of clear-cut medical reasons'. Although 6% of Cartwright's sample had tried to arrange not to have an induction, 2% recorded an attempt to have one. Both adequate discussion of induction beforehand and good emotional support from medical staff during labour and delivery contribute to relatively comfortable experiences of induction (Kitzinger 1975, Cartwright 1979). Attitudes and reactions to childbirth are, in this sense, a function of many different variables, including women's prior experiences of birth and obstetric care, their confidence (or lack of it) in their body's ability to labour spontaneously, and

Table 44.10 Preferences for induction in the next labour (from Cartwright 1979)

	Labour last time	
	Induced (%)	Not induced (%)
Prefer same as last time	17	93
Prefer not to have same as last time	78	5
Other comments	5	2
Number of mothers (=100%)	552	1593

Table 44.11 Preferences for epidural analgesia in the next labour (from Cartwright 1979)

	Analgesia in the last labour	
	Epidural (%)	No epidural (%)
Prefer same as last time	63	82
Prefer not to have same as last time	34	13
Other comments	3	5
Number of mothers (=100%)	110	2053

the degree of unpredictability their social circumstances are able to support concerning the time of birth. Tables 44.10 and 44.11 from Cartwright's study show the same pattern as Table 44.3: the proportions of women who would prefer the same pattern of care for their next baby as they had for the last one are highest for the natural alternative in each case, i.e. no induction, no epidural, home birth.

No study has been done to date on the specific topic of women's attitudes to post-term pregnancy, although there is evidence that such pregnancy may often be experienced as 'tedious, frustrating and uncomfortable' (Cartwright 1979). The issue of elective induction of labour also involves the matter of a correct expected date of delivery; many mothers feel quite strongly about the negotiation of this as an area in which they possess personal knowledge (Oakley 1981). From the point of view of obstetricians exercising control over the timing of women's deliveries, the development and routine application of ultrasonic scanning have, of course, been extremely important; this is yet another field in which maternal attitudes have not been adequately investigated.

Caesarean section

More research has been done in the USA than in the UK on the social and psychological costs of a Caesarean section (Marieskind 1979). It is interesting to note that a Consensus Development Task Force set up in 1979 by the National Institutes of Health to examine Caesarean childbirth numbered a sociologist and a psychologist among its members; one of its assignments was to consider the 'psychological effects of Caesarean delivery on the mother, infant and family' (Shearer 1981).

It is significant that the operation of Caesarean section is referred to in a different way from other forms of abdominal surgery; it is not called an operation, or surgery, but a section. Following this terminology, while it is accepted among surgeons that depression is a common consequence of major surgery, especially if it is carried out as an emergency procedure, the same assumption is not made about a Caesarean section. Many of the psychological consequences of surgery in general also apply to Caesarean section. These include a temporary response of emotional relief and elation at having survived the operation, worry about the mutilating effects of the operation on the body and its attractiveness to others, and a long drawn-out period of physical and psychological discomfort (Janis 1958). It is worth noting that the kinds of demands that the care of the newborn may make involve activities that are likely to be forbidden to any patient on a surgical ward for some days (if not weeks) after abdominal surgery. It is presumably factors of this kind that account for the association between an admission to a psychiatric hospital in the first 90 days after childbirth and a Caesarean delivery (Kendell et al 1981).

In one British study, Trowell (1978) compared 16 mothers who had emergency Caesarean sections under general anaesthetic with a control group of spontaneously vaginally delivered women. All were having first babies and the babies weighed over 2.49 kg (5.5 lb) and were not admitted to a special care unit. No sections were performed for pressing obstetric reasons. At 1 month, observations showed that mothers who had had a Caesarean section looked more but smiled less at their babies and the Caesarean babies were rated as being more tense. Striking differences emerged from the questioning of the mothers. Those who had had sections more often remembered birth as a bad experience, expressed doubts about their capacity to care for the baby and were depressed or anxious. As the author comments:

> These women had expected a normal vaginal delivery and had prepared themselves for this. They tended to feel a failure as a woman, unable to have a normal delivery and angry with the baby for not 'coming out', and there was some anger towards the hospital, although at the same time, an acknowledgement of the crisis that had occurred and a belief that the hospital had saved their and their baby's lives. Perhaps because of these feelings the Caesarean mothers were more anxious and apprehensive about parenthood and its responsibilities (Trowell 1978).

These sorts of attitudes were still present at a year, with the mothers who had had a Caesarean section more likely to describe motherhood in negative terms, more likely to delay responding to their child's crying and reporting a late age at which they first felt their child responded to them as a person. The group of mothers who had had a Caesarean section expressed more anger in their handling of their children by shouting, smacking and losing their tempers. There were indications that the babies born by Caesarean section had a slower motor development (age of sitting unaided), and some interaction measures from the observations showed continuing differences between the groups. The groups in this study are small and as the author herself emphasizes, it was intended to be a pilot study.

Another study comparing perceptions of childbirth among socially similar groups of women having Caesarean and vaginal deliveries found a generalized loss of self-esteem among the former mothers (Marut & Mercer 1979).

The profound effects that can follow a Caesarean section are recognized among women, and one of the more striking developments in recent years has been the growth of self-health groups offering support to mothers. The very existence of these groups is, of course, a clear indication of the psychological and social needs for support which women who have undergone these procedures may feel. As with induction there are situations in which some women prefer an elective delivery by Caesarean section to a vaginal one. Section rates are very high among private patients (Richards 1979) which may in part reflect a movement of women who request Caesarean sections into the private sector where they may be more likely to get them on demand.

In conclusion, out of this discussion of specific topics from the general viewpoint of the labouring mother, certain key themes emerge about women's perspectives on the management of childbirth today. These themes are:

1. *Control:* who should be in control of labour and delivery — the health professional or the mother? What is the appropriate time perspective for measuring success-delivery and its immediate aftermath at one extreme, or the long-term development of the child at one extreme and the family on the other?
2. *Evaluation:* have obstetric procedures been systematically evaluated and has this evaluation represented the consumer's perspective within it?
3. *Success:* how is the success of childbearing to be measured? What relative weighting should be given to hard versus soft measures of outcomes: mortality and physical morbidity versus depression and dissatisfaction, for example?
4. *Communication:* what kind of communication marks the interaction of the labouring mother with those who care for her? In particular, to what extent are information and support of mothers by health professionals part of this communication?

This chapter ends with a brief consideration of each of these themes.

WHOSE BABY IS IT ANYWAY?

This is the title of an editorial in the Lancet in 1980 which considered professional responses to women's assertion of the right to make informed choices about childbirth. The editorial observed that there is a spectrum of response — from the declared goal of seeking to help parents to free themselves of dependence on the medical profession, through to condemning the consumer protest as dangerous faddism.

However professionals respond, it remains true that it is the mother who is having the baby and who will live with the consequences of the management of her particular childbirth for the rest of her life. Whereas professionals might wish to control childbirth (Beazley 1975) so, on the whole, do mothers; at least, they wish to remain in control within the parameters of what that means to them (Humenick 1981). To have a feeling of control is not the same as having a labour and delivery free of medical intervention. Much more important is the extent to which a woman feels that her own wishes have been respected.

COMMUNICATION: THE GOLDEN RULE

In order to respect the wishes of the labouring mother, it is a prerequisite for those caring for her to find out how she approaches birth and her own role in it. There is a substantial literature on communication problems in obstetric and midwifery practice: much of the debate within consumer groups concerns what is wrong with the way professionals relate to childbearing women, and what can be done about it. There is not enough communication; staff treat mothers as cases and not as individuals; they offer patronizing reassurance when what has been asked for is information, and so forth. Richards (1981) has drawn attention to one dimension of communication failure as perceived by mothers:

> Characteristic of many conversations between doctor and mother is the use of that peculiar 'we' by the doctor. 'We would not want to do anything that might jeopardise the baby'. In one way there is the correct implication that everyone is, or should be united in the wish to see the mother delivered safely of a healthy baby. But, especially if the mother does not sound too keen to submit to whatever is being proposed, there is also an implicit message that it is only the doctor who has the true interests of mother or, more especially, the child at heart. It is a patronising and paternalistic 'we' that is often used. There is the hint that the mother is not only an incompetent vessel for her baby (labours are only safe in retrospect) but that she may be selfishly uncaring and not doing what is best for her baby (Richards 1981).

Under the busy and understaffed conditions of many care-settings today, it is often difficult for staff to convey an attitude of caring and sensitivity to each mother's preferences and status as a person. Also, medical and midwifery training contain very little in the way of lessons in human interaction. Medical ideologies proscribe, rather than prescribe, involvement with the patient, and this may mean that emotional distance between mother and professionals is felt to be preferable.

These difficulties have led to the suggestion from at least one childbirth activist that what is needed is verbal disarmament: mothers must practise techniques of verbally disarming professionals in order to get across their point of view to them. Thus, for example, the following remark of an obstetrician:

> I find your wish for a home birth selfish and irresponsible. You are just looking for a fulfilling experience for yourself and not thinking about your baby

might be countered by the mother saying:

> I am sorry you find it necessary to say such things, doctor. *Pause*. I want you to know that it will damage our relationship (Wright 1983).

Whether or not such suggestions are being taken up by women using the maternity services today, there is clearly enormous scope for improving professional–client communication.

A HEALTHY BABY OR A GOOD EXPERIENCE?

Within the medical model of childbirth, there is an overwhelming emphasis on mortality and its avoidance and on physical morbidity. Within the social model of childbirth on the one hand, more holistic criteria of success are stressed: the mother's experience of birth is part of this, as is her emotional condition during the early years and months of motherhood, her relationship with the baby, the baby's long-term development and the whole nexus of relationships—the nuclear family, the extended family, the household—into which the baby is born.

The conflict between these two ways of assessing success in childbirth is evident in the question above, which poses a healthy baby and a good experience as opposing aims. If the consumer movement in maternity care has succeeded in saying anything loudly and clearly then it is surely this: that a healthy baby and a good experience are, for the majority of mothers, not different goals, but the same one. This message is brought out most sharply in the literature on mother–infant bonding which has stressed the fact that childbirth does not end with the delivery of the baby; a relationship, begun prenatally, has to be forged between mother and neonate, and in the forging of this relationship obstetric procedures either may or may not help. Table 44.12 shows the association between some such procedures and breastfeeding as one indicator of the mothers' and babies' relationships with one another. Mothers who have Caesarean deliveries and any type of analgesia or anaesthesia in labour and whose babies go into special care are more likely than other mothers to have stopped breastfeeding within 2 weeks of delivery. Of course these factors are inter-related but the statistical analysis showed that any factor causing a delay of more than 4 hours between delivery and the first breastfeed was likely to jeopardize the success of breastfeeding (Martin & Monk 1982). It is obvious that what obstetricians do may have long-term effects, especially when the link between early feeding and adult health is considered (Faulkner 1980). When childbirth is not successful and a perinatal death occurs, then the behaviour of obstetricians and paediatricians is not necessarily less important. Seeing and touching the dead baby are often important, and it is rare for those parents who have done so to regret it, while fantasies about the dead child's appearance may be a real obstacle to grieving for those who are not given this opportunity (Stringham et al 1982).

Table 44.12 Proportion of mothers who had stopped breastfeeding within 2 weeks by type of delivery, analgesia or anaesthesia and baby's postpartum care (from Martin & Monk 1982)

	Proportion (%) of mothers who had stopped breastfeeding within 2 weeks in England and Wales ($n = 2499$)
Delivery type	
Normal	19
Forceps/vacuum	19
Caesarean section	28
All mothers	19
Analgesia/anaesthesia	
Nothing	11
Gas and air	20
Injection (excluding epidural)	20
Epidural	22
General anaesthetic	28
All mothers	19
Baby's care	
No special care	18
Special care	23
All babies	19

EVALUATION

As Haggerty (1980) has commented in relation to early interventions designed to improve mother–infant bonding: 'there are no quick fixes for parenting difficulties arising from generational inadequacies and poverty'. Thus while some professional attempts to improve bonding may be relatively successful, the total amount of variance attributable to such interventions is small compared to that explained by background social characteristics (2–3% versus 10–25%). Doctors and other health professionals are, fortunately, not gods.

One meaning of evaluation is therefore an attempt to assess the boundaries of obstetric care in its claim to expertise in childbearing. Another meaning, which runs through many of the points made in this chapter about the experiences of mothers, is to locate these experiences more centrally within studies designed to answer questions about the effectiveness and safety of specific therapies and procedures. What is effective and safe physiologically may not be so psychosocially, and vice versa. There is no doubt that at least part of the recent critique highlighting the experiences of labouring mothers themselves has concerned the anxiety women can feel about being subjected to procedures which have not been shown to be effective. Like the dormouse and the doctor in A. A. Milne's poem of that name, women and those who care for them in labour are engaged in a dispute about the kind of scenario that is good for health. Whereas the doctor took the view that chrysanthemums were what the dormouse needed, the dormouse himself felt that geraniums and delphiniums were better. In the end, the dormouse gave up, closed his eyes and resigned himself merely to dreaming about what he wanted. There is, however, no sign that women are likely to do that.

REFERENCES

ACOG 1979 American College of Obstetricians and Gynecologists Newsletter, 4 May

Alberman E 1977 Facts and figures. In: Chard T, Richards M (eds) Benefits and hazards of the new obstetrics. Spastics International Publications, London

Arms S 1975 Immaculate deception. Bantam Books, New York

Beazley J 1975 The active management of labor. American Journal of Obstetrics and Gynecology 122: 161–168

Bland R 1781 Some calculations from the Midwifery Reports of the Westminster General Dispensary, London

British Medical Journal Editorial 1954 24(4): 54

British Medical Journal Editorial 1976 1: 729

Butler N R, Bonham D 1963 Perinatal mortality. E & S Livingstone, Edinburgh

Campbell R, Macfarlane A 1987 Where to be born? The debate and the evidence. National Perinatal Epidemiology Unit, Oxford

Cartwright A 1979 The dignity of labour. Tavistock, London

Chamberlain G, Howlett B, Philipp E, Masters K 1978 British births 1970. Obstetric care. Heinemann, London

Chamberlain M 1981 Old wives' tales. Virago, London

Clark A 1968 The working life of women in the seventeenth century. Frank Cass, London

Department of Health and Social Security 1983 Low income families 1981. DHSS, London

Dick-Read G 1942 Childbirth without fear. Heinemann, London

Donnison J 1977 Midwives and medical men. Heinemann, London

Enkin M 1982 Antenatal classes. In: Enkin M, Chalmers I (eds) Effectiveness and satisfaction in antenatal care. Spastics International Medical Publications, London

Farr W 1885 Vital statistics. Edward Stanford, London

Faulkner F 1980 Prevention in childhood of health problems in adult life. WHO, Geneva

Flint C, Poulengris P 1987 The 'know your midwife' report. Private publication, 49 Peckerman's Wood, London SE26 6RZ

Flynn A M, Kelly J, Hollins G, Lynch P F 1978 Ambulation in labour. British Medical Journal 2: 591–593

Ford C S 1945 A comparative study of human reproduction. Yale University Publications in Anthropology no 32, New York

Francis H H 1985 Obstetrics: a consumer-oriented service? Journal of Maternal and Child Health March: 69–72

Friedson E 1975 Dilemmas in the doctor–patient relationship. In: Cox C, Mead A (eds) A sociology of medical practice. Collier–Macmillan, London

Garcia J, Corry M, MacDonald D, Elbourne D, Grant A 1985a Mothers' views of continuous electronic fetal heart rate monitoring and intermittent auscultation in a randomized controlled trial. Birth 12: 79–85

Garcia J, Anderson J, Vacca A, Elbourne D, Grant A, Chalmers I 1985b Views of women and their medical and midwifery attendants about instrumental delivery using vacuum extraction and forceps. Journal of Psychosomatic Obstetrics and Gynaecology 4: 1–9

Gillie L, Gillie O 1974 The childbirth revolution and the vital first hours. Sunday Times 13 October, 20 October

Glaister J 1894 Dr W Smellie and his contemporaries. James Nackhose, Glasgow

Goldthorpe W O, Richman J 1974 Maternal attitudes to unintended home confinement. Practitioner 212: 845

Graham H, Oakley A 1981 Competing ideologies of reproduction: medical and maternal perspective on pregnancy. In: Roberts H (ed) Women, health and reproduction. Routledge & Kegan Paul, London

Granville A B 1819 A report of the practice of the midwifery at the Westminster General Dispensary during 1818. Burgess and Hill, London

Haggerty R J 1980 Damn the simplicities. Pediatrics 66: 323–324

Homans H 1980 Pregnant in Britain: a sociological approach to Asian and British women's experiences. PhD thesis, University of Warwick

Houd S, Oakley A 1986 Alternative perinatal services. In: Phaff J M L (ed) Perinatal health services in Europe: searching for better childbirth. Croom Helm, London

Humenich S S 1981 Mastery: the key to childbirth satisfaction? A review. Birth and the Family Journal 8: 79–90

Janis I 1958 Psychological stress: psychoanalytic and behavioural studies of surgical patients. John Wiley, New York

Johnstone R W 1913 A textbook of midwifery. Adam & Charles Black, London

Joint Committee of the Royal College of Gynaecologists and the Population Investigation Committee 1948 Maternity in Great Britain. Oxford University Press, Oxford

Kendell R E, Rennie D, Clarke J A, Dean C 1981 The social and obstetric correlates of psychiatric admissions in the puerperum. Psychological Medicine 11: 341–350

Kirke P 1975 The consumer's view of the management of labour. In: Beard R, Brudenell M, Dunn P, Fairweather D (eds) The management of labour. Proceedings of the 3rd study group of the RCOG. RCOG, London

Kitzinger S 1975 Some mothers' experiences of induced labour. NCT, London

Kitzinger S 1979 Birth at home. Oxford University Press, Oxford

Kitzinger S (ed) 1981 Episiotomy. NCT, London

Klaus M H, Kennell J H, Robertson S S, Sosa R 1986 Effects of social support during parturition on maternal and infant morbidity. British Medical Journal 293: 585–587

Klein V 1965 Britain's married women workers. Routledge & Kegan Paul, London

Lancet Editorial 1980 Whose baby is it? i: 1284–1285

Larson A G, Mercer D 1984 The who and why of pain: analysing social class. British Medical Journal 288: 883–886

Lewis B V, Rana S, Crook E 1975 Patient response to induction. Lancet i: 1197

Lumley J, Astbury J 1980 Birth rites. Sphere Books, Melbourne

Macfarlane A, Mugford M 1984 Birth counts: statistics of pregnancy and childbirth. HMSO, London

Macintyre S 1977 The management of childbirth: a review of sociological research issues. Social Science and Medicine 11: 477–484

Macintyre S 1981 Expectations and experiences of first pregnancy. Report on a prospective interview study of married primigravidae in Aberdeen. Occasional paper no 5. University of Aberdeen, Aberdeen

Mack J, Lansley S 1985 Poor Britain. Allen & Unwin, London

Marieskind H I 1979 An evaluation of Caesarean section in the United States. Report submitted to the US Department of Health, Education and Welfare

Martin J, Monk J 1982 Infant feeding 1980. OPCS Social Survey Division, HMSO, London

Martin J, Roberts C 1984 Women and employment: a lifetime perspective. HMSO, London

Maternity Alliance 1983 One birth in nine—trends in Caesarean sections since 1978. Maternity Alliance, London

Marut J S, Mercer R T 1979 The Caesarean birth experience. Nursing Research 28: 260–266

McKeown T 1979 The role of medicine. Basil Blackwell, Oxford

Mead M, Newton N 1967 Cultural patterning of perinatal behaviour. In: Richardson S A, Guttmacher A F (eds) Childbearing—its social and psychological aspects. Williams and Wilkins, Baltimore

Ministry of Health 1927 The protection of motherhood (by Campbell J M). Reports on Public Health and Medical Subjects no 48. HMSO, London

Morgan B, Bulpitt C, Clifton P, Lewis P J 1982 Effectiveness of pain relief in labour: survey of 1000 mothers. British Medical Journal 285: 689–690

Myers R E 1979 Maternal anxiety and fetal death. In: Zichella Pancheri L (ed) Psychoneuroendocrinology in reproduction. North Holland iomedical Press, Elsevier, Holland
National Council for One-Parent Families 1983 One parent families. NCOPF, London
Nelson M K 1983 Working class women, middle class women and models of childbirth. Social Problems 30: 285–296
Oakley A 1976 Wisewoman and medicine man: changes in the management of childbirth. In: Mitchell J, Oakley A (eds) The rights and wrongs of women. Penguin, Harmondsworth
Oakley A 1977 Cross-cultural practices. In: Chard J, Richards M (eds) Benefits and hazards of the new obstetrics. Spastics International Medical Publications, London
Oakley A 1981 From here to maternity. Penguin, Harmondsworth
Oakley A 1982 Obstetric practice: cross-cultural comparisons. In: Stratton P (ed) Psychobiology of the human newborn. Wiley, New York
Oakley A 1984 The captured womb: a history of the medical care of pregnant women. Basil Blackwell, Oxford
Oakley A, Macfarlane A, Chalmers I 1982 Social class, stress and reproduction. In: Rees A R, Purcell H (eds) Disease and the environment. John Wiley, Chichester
O'Brien M 1978 Home and hospital: a comparison of the experiences of mothers having home and hospital confinements. Journal of the Royal College of General Practitioners 28: 460–466
O'Driscoll K, Meagher D 1980 Active management of labour. WB Saunders, London
Ounstead M, Simons C 1979 Maternal attitudes to their obstetric care. Early Human Development 3: 201–204
Registrar-General 1930 Decennial supplement on occupational mortality. HMSO, London
Richards M P M 1977 The induction and acceleration of labour: some benefits and complications. Early Human Development 1: 3–17
Richards M P M 1978 A place of safety? An examination of the risks of hospital delivery. In: Kitzinger A, Davis J A (eds) The place of birth. Oxford University Press, Oxford
Richards M P M 1979 Perinatal morbidity and mortality in private obstetric practice. Journal of Maternal and Child Health September: 341–345
Richards M P M 1981 Whose choice in childbirth? Unpublished paper presented at National Childbirth Trust Silver Jubilee Conference, 10 October 1981
Riley E D M 1977 What do women want? The question of choice in the conduct of labour. In: Chard T, Richards M P M (eds) Benefits and hazards of the new obstetrics. Spastics International Medical Publications, London
Runnerstrom L R 1969 The effectiveness of nurse-midwifery in a supervised hospital environment. American College of Nurse Midwives Bulletin 14: 40
Select Committee on Violence in the Family 1977 Violence to children, vol 1. HMSO, London
Shearer E 1981 National Institutes of Health consensus development task force on Caesarean childbirth. The process and the result. Birth and the Family Journal 8: 25–30
Smellie W 1752 A treatise on the theory and practice of midwifery. London
Smith F B 1979 The people's health 1830–1910. Croom Helm, London
Sosa R, Kennell, Klaus M, Robertson S 1980 The effect of a supportive companion on perinatal problems, length of labour and mother–infant interaction. New England Journal of Medicine 303: 597–600
Stacey M 1976 The health service consumer: a sociological misconception. In: Stacey M (ed) The sociology of the National Health Service. Monograph no 22. University of Keele, Staffordshire
Stacey M, Homans H 1978 The sociology of health and illness: its present state, future prospects and potential for health research. Sociology 12: 281–307
Starkman M 1976 Psychological responses to the use of the fetal monitor during labour. Psychosomatic Medicine 38: 269–277
Stewart P 1979 Patients' attitudes to induction and labour. British Medical Journal ii: 749–752
Stilwell J A 1979 Relative costs of home and hospital confinement. British Medical Journal 2: 257–259
Stringham J G, Riley J H, Ross A 1982 Silent birth: mourning a stillborn baby. Social Work July: 322–327
Trowell J 1978 The effects of obstetric procedures on the mother/child relationship. A pilot study of emergency Caesarean section. Unpublished paper. Department for Children and Parents, Tavistock Clinic, London
Versluysen J C 1981 Midwives, medical men and 'poor women labouring of child'—lying-in hospitals in eighteenth century London. In: Roberts H (ed) Women, health and reproduction. Routledge & Kegan Paul, London
Wright M 1983 Verbal disarmament. New Generation 1: 8–9
Yudkin P, Frumar A M, Anderson A B M, Turnbull A C, Yudkin P 1979 A retrospective study of the induction of labour. British Journal of Obstetrics and Gynaecology 86: 257–263

45

Donald Gibb

The measurement of uterine action

Measurement forms the basis of all scientific work; observations are quantified by measurement. Parameters such as height, weight and fetal heart rate are measured easily. Uterine contractions, the clinical manifestation of uterine action, are more difficult. Measurement requires methods of detection, recording and quantification. The human uterus contracts intermittently throughout reproductive life; this chapter is concerned primarily with its action during expulsion of the fetus at the end of pregnancy. At this stage the uterus is large, appearing like a balloon filled with fluid and solid parts, consequently being more accessible to examination and observation. The contracting uterus is to a large extent autonomous with limited hormonal and neural control mechanisms. An electrical impulse spreads from cell to cell causing depolarization of the membrane resulting in calcium ion flux, an essential prerequisite for contraction of myofibrils. Calcium is transported into the cells as well as being passively released from sarcoplasmic reticulum, mitochondria, plasma membrane and surface vesicles. Contraction of segments of the uterus occurs which, when co-ordinated, results in rising intrauterine pressure and progressive expulsion of the fetus through the only exit from its confined space: the uterine cervix and the birth canal.

In clinical practice contractions are detected and recorded as the manifestation of uterine action. In research several methods have been used for the detection of contractions while external and internal tocography are used in clinical practice. Tocometry is the measurement of a contraction; tocography is its record which permits sequential analysis and measurement. External tocography is generally adequate and used most frequently whilst internal tocography provides valuable additional information in difficult cases.

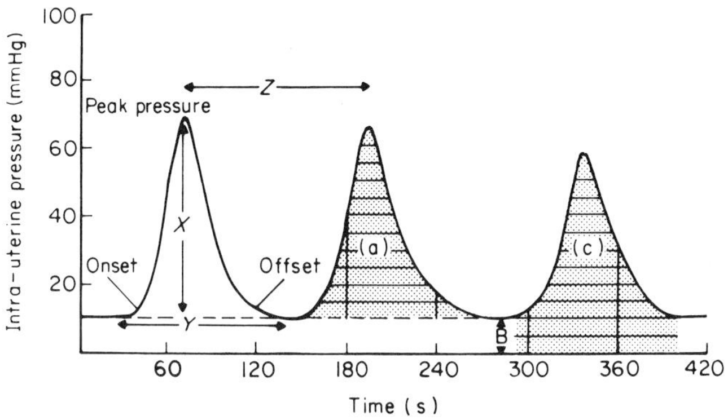

Fig. 45.1 Record of palpated contractions on partogram.

TERMINOLOGY OF UTERINE CONTRACTIONS

The elements of uterine contractions are shown in Figure 45.1. The duration measured depends on identification of the beginning (onset) and the end (offset). A sensitive device records a contraction for a longer duration than a palpating hand does. The amplitude (active pressure) is the difference between basal and peak pressure. The basal pressure (basal tone) is the resting pressure between contractions. The frequency is the number of contractions in a fixed time period, usually 10 minutes. This may vary because of irregularity of contractions. Irregularity of timing is reflected in changes in frequency while irregularity of shape is termed incoordination. There is no absolute definition of incoordination; however, significant changes in shape, varying amplitude, merging of contractions (coupling, tripling) and failure to return to basal pressure may all be seen.

EXTERNAL METHODS

A hand placed between the umbilicus and uterine fundus is most commonly used to observe uterine contractions. A

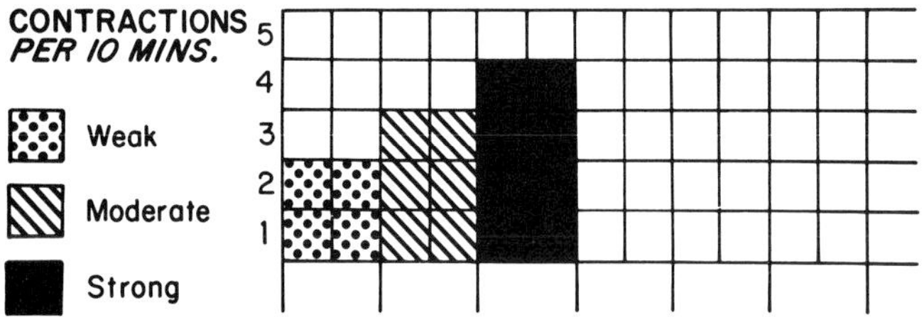

Fig. 45.2 Terminology of uterine contractions.

sensation of hardening and forward movement of the abdominal wall is felt. Braxton Hicks contractions are felt in this way and indeed Braxton Hicks (1872) used observation of contractions early in pregnancy to confirm the diagnosis. Palpation may provoke a reflex contraction, making delineation of the fetal parts more difficult. When this occurs the observer should desist from examining for a short time and then recommence. Such contractions should not be misinterpreted as meaning the patient is in labour. They are often painless and may be localized, non-propagating and not leading to significant rises in intrauterine pressure. Palpation of contractions permits a crude estimate of their duration and frequency but reveals little information about amplitude. There is no permanent record but a shaded-box method may be used on the labour record indicating the observer's subjective estimate of strength, duration and frequency (Fig. 45.2).

External tocography

Schaffer (1896) was the first person to employ an external method of recording uterine contractions. Ruebsamen (1913) used an instrument applied externally to the abdominal wall to observe uterine behaviour. The apparatus consisted of a device of known weight suspended from a frame by means of cord and pulleys so as to rest on the abdominal wall covering the uterus. This was connected mechanically to a recording drum. It was not very sensitive and was affected by gross artefacts due to movement of the patient. Most of Ruebsamen's observations concerned the effects of drugs given after delivery and the method was unsuitable for use in the first and second stages of labour. Dodeck (1932) devised a system incorporating a plunger applied to the maternal abdomen linked to a recording tambour by a pneumatic system. With this he studied the effects of 12 different drugs on the human uterus at term. Moir (1935) used a modification of the apparatus in which the method of recording was hydraulic. Mechanical and electromechanical recorders then appeared, with Murphy (1947) popularizing the Lorand tocograph. This was a mechanical clockwork instrument in which the plunger projected a fixed distance from the base; this plunger was placed directly on to the subject's anterior abdominal wall and held in place by a belt.

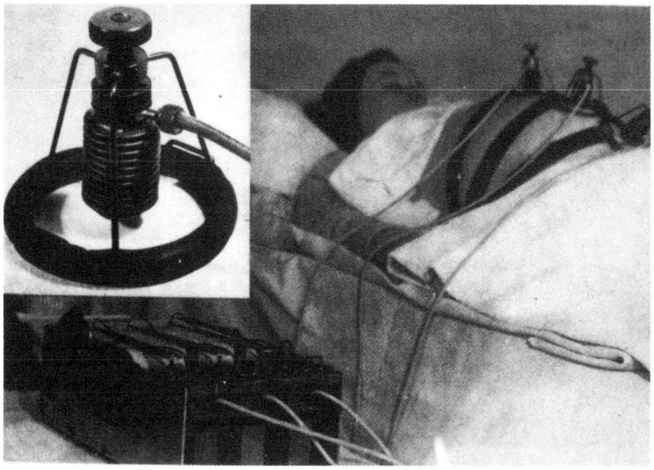

Fig. 45.3 Embrey's equipment.

The introduction of electromechanical devices simplified the use of the previously cumbersome equipment. Reynolds et al (1948) exploited this with the introduction of a multichannel strain gauge tocodynamometer. They documented uterine activity in three separate zones of the uterus at the same time and related this to the progress of labour. Progress in labour was associated with strong intermittent contractions in the fundus rising quickly to a maximum and being of relatively long duration. In contrast the contractions in the mid-portion of the uterus were less intense and shorter. They found the lower uterine segment to be inactive throughout the first stage of labour and proposed that cervical dilatation is the result of diminishing physiological activity from the fundus to the lower segment — the important concept of fundal dominance.

Embrey (1955) reported from Oxford on a new multichannel external tocograph (Fig. 45.3). This was similar to Reynolds's equipment except that it depended on a hydraulic system to transmit the impulse. The aim was to produce a simple yet efficient, robust, easily operated machine requiring little supervision and capable of recording uterine contractions in all cases. This purpose was revolutionary because until that time all devices had been used for research purposes only and had not been employed clinically.

Smyth (1957) introduced the guard ring tocodynamometer. This instrument differed from previous devices. It was a flat disc with an outside ring and an inner circular pressure-sensing area. The deflection of a spring mounted on the guard ring supporting the central measuring area was taken as a measure of force on the central area. This deflection was calibrated to measure intra-amniotic pressure. The instrument must be applied to the patient over a fluid-filled part of the uterus. The pressure must be sufficient to flatten the abdominal surface into contact with the guard ring. It requires quite a firm application with a tight band round the maternal abdomen. With very careful adjustment and placement it was claimed that this instrument actually measured intrauterine pressure accurately. It has since been used successfully by Bell (1981, 1983) in the assessment of patients at risk of preterm labour. When the membranes are still intact a non-invasive technique is required and this is appropriate. Prediction of preterm labour by quantifying uterine activity could form part of a comprehensive approach to reduce mortality and morbidity from preterm birth.

The technology for recording uterine contractions developed pari passu with that for recording the fetal heart. Gunn & Wood (1953) presented a paper to the Royal Society of Medicine on the amplification and recording of fetal heart sounds. Fetal heart rate monitors as we know them did not become commercially available until the late 1960s. Miniaturization of electronics permitted both cardio- and toco-recording equipment to be placed in a single mobile box and mass-produced at reasonable cost. The recent generation of fetal monitors incorporates a tocograph of guard ring type. Telemetric internal and external tocography permitting assessment of contractions in a mobile patient is now available.

Lacroix (1968) described the use of the parturiograph. This comprised a hollow gas-filled plastic-domed transducer applied to the maternal abdomen by adjustable straps. This was connected by a gas-filled system transmitting pressure to a recording device. Comparison of parturiographic and intrauterine pressure tracings revealed similar contraction patterns with respect to configuration, frequency and resting pressure. However, only 60–90% of intrauterine pressure was measured. None the less it was suggested that such continuous monitoring identified abnormal uterine contractility and thus was a useful guide for regulation of oxytocin infusion and the facilitation of the management of abnormal labour. This method did not become widely used.

Clinical experience shows that external tocography does have its limitations. The guard ring tocograph requires a tight and somewhat uncomfortable application to the pregnant abdomen to permit its accurate use. A significant proportion of patients are restless or have a thick adipose anterior abdominal wall which precludes proper placement and adjustment. It is uncommon to find a technically perfect external tocographic tracing on every patient in the labour ward: whether it is necessary is discussed elsewhere. An undesirable result of external tocography is undue attention paid by staff and patient alike to each contraction as it appears in late prelabour or early labour. Even regular contractions may be painless, not resulting in cervical changes and should not be misinterpreted as diagnostic of the onset of labour. These should be described as prelabour contractions; the term false labour should be discarded.

INVASIVE METHODS

More direct access to uterine function than that permitted by external methods has been attempted by many workers. Assessment of intrauterine pressure has been extensively studied. However, the preceding electrical events are of some interest. Csapo et al (1963, Csapo & Takeda 1965) placed separated electrodes in the myometrium of pregnant rabbits together with an intra-amniotic probe to measure intrauterine pressure. During pregnancy before labour the electrical activity showed a lack of transmission, irregularity and lack of synchrony. The active pressure was low, associated with a slow rise and a prolonged time of propagation from the activity at one electrode to another. During labour activity at each electrode occurred synchronously; active pressure was much higher with a more rapid rise of a quadratic nature. The potential propagation time and the time of pressure rise shortened at the same rate; the ratio remained constant, indicating that the rate of pressure rise was controlled by the rate of propagation. This work is consistent with the later work of Garfield & Hayashi (1981), showing the formation of gap junctions seen under the electron microscope as gestation proceeds to the time of labour. Such gap junctions are thought to facilitate propagation of the electrical impulse. Csapo distinguished between the propagating synchronic activity and the asynchronic local activity. This also raises the possibility that some forms of external tocograph may suggest good contractions when the area of the uterus under the sensor is active, but this may be local non-propagating activity. This work suggests that the intrauterine pressure reflects the conduction characteristics of the uterus to a considerable degree. Dill & Maiden (1946) attempted to record changes in electrical potential with uterine contractions using external devices without success. External electromyography of the uterus is difficult because of the many possible sources of artefact, such as movement of the patient, respiratory movement, abdominal wall muscle activity, abdominal organ activity, electrocardiogram of the mother and skin potentials. All these affect the signal to noise ratio adversely.

Access to the human uterus before or during labour is difficult but Sakaguchi & Nakajima (1970) inserted bipolar needle electrodes through the os 10–25 cm along the posterior wall of the gravid uterus. During labour they recorded bursts of action potentials initially poorly synchronized with contractions. With progression of labour good synchronization developed. Wolfs & Van Leeuwen (1979) confirmed these observations using a linear array of 10 electrodes inserted on a wire 30 cm into the uterus between the membranes and myometrium. Such a device produces fascinating data for physiological studies but would not be acceptable in clinical practice.

INTRAUTERINE PRESSURE

There are two laws of physics governing the pressure within a closed spheroid: those of Laplace and Pascal.

The law of Laplace states that the pressure (P) is equal

to twice the wall thickness (W) divided by the radius (R) multiplied by the wall tension (T).

$$P = \frac{(2W)T}{(R)}$$

P and T are in balance at all times and at a given T the size of P becomes a function of R. If this law were directly applicable to the uterus then if R is known, T and P may be calculated from each other. However, the Laplace theorem was originally aimed at the description of behaviour of non-living matter. The tension (T) of living muscle increases with increasing radius because of increased excitability, conduction and contractility. The thickness of uterine wall also changes. The quantification of T and P cannot therefore be made by mathematical manipulation but it must be based on direct measurement. Direct measurement of wall tension is not feasible.

Is pressure measured at one point within the uterus representative of its overall function? The law of Pascal states that pressure is equal and uniform at all points throughout a fluid-filled space. The space must be continuous and closed. After membrane rupture it might be suspected that neither the law of Laplace nor Pascal applies on account of leakage from the space. During active leakage measurements are inaccurate but when the descending head completely prevents the leakage of amniotic fluid, as is usually the case in the second half of labour, then measurements are relevant. Does oligohydramnios lead to difficulties in measurement of intrauterine pressure? It seems not to do so because if there is a space in which to insert a probe it must be filled with fluid, however little, and a pressure value is produced.

Internal tocography: detection and recording

The history of internal tocography is longer than that of external methods, going back to the work of Schatz in the late 19th century (Schatz 1872). He inserted a balloon on the end of a catheter into the pregnant uterus. Polaillon (1880) passed a rubber air balloon just inside the cervix with less success. Westermark (1893) measured pressures accurately but did not record the changes continuously. Bourne & Burn (1927) introduced a rubber bag into the uterus in the form of a hollow disc. This was attached to the end of a gum elastic catheter. Rubber tubing was attached to this and filled with water to transmit the impulse. The pressure was recorded by an ink writing point on a revolving drum driven by clockwork (Fig. 45.4). Prior to insertion the patient was anaesthetized, placed in the lithotomy position and the vagina prepared with iodine. Using a speculum to prevent contact between the bag and vaginal wall, the bag was passed through the cervix and insinuated between the internal os and the membranes and gently pushed into the uterus to a distance of 8 inches (20 cm) above the os.

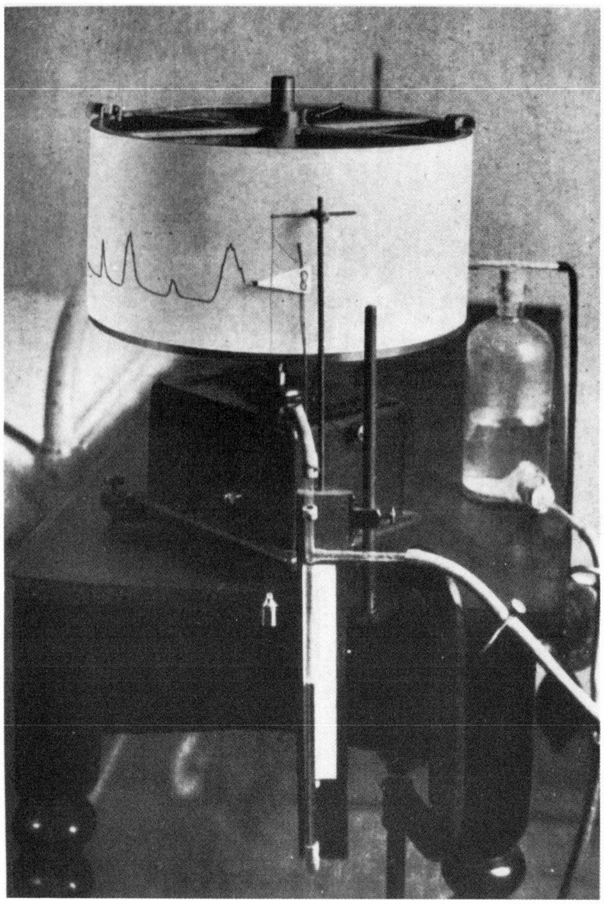

Fig. 45.4 Bourne & Burns' (1927) revolving drum.

In no case did the membranes rupture or the placenta become detached. This was an extraovular balloon method and was used to study the effect of drugs on the uterus in labour. Incidentally, the observation was made by Bourne & Burn that during the first 15 or 20 minutes after insertion there was usually an increase in contraction due to the stimulant effect of the bag and of the waning of the effects of the anaesthetic. This observation has been made by later workers (Gibb et al 1984) and is consistent with release of oxytocic substances during manipulation. This must be borne in mind after any manipulation of the lower segments during vaginal examination. In a well primed uterus this effect may in itself be enough to augment labour.

Caldeyro Barcia and colleagues in Uruguay undertook fundamental work on uterine activity from 1948 onwards. They passed intrauterine catheters through the anterior wall at all stages of pregnancy, sometimes sequentially in individual patients. Caldeyro Barcia & Poseiro (1960) documented the progressive development of contractions until delivery of the baby. They used a transabdominal fluid-filled catheter. A second catheter was passed into the urinary bladder to measure vesical pressure. The abdominal pressure is equal to the vesical pressure when the contents of the urinary bladder are less than 20 ml. Subtraction of abdominal pressure permits the assessment of true intrauterine pressure. Caldeyro Barcia et al (1950) used external receptors on the abdominal wall to record local contractility, relating this information to intra-amniotic pressure. This was taken a step further with the introduction of tiny rubber balloons into various parts of the interstitium of uterine muscle (Caldeyro Barcia & Alvarez 1952). These balloons were compressed by contractions of the surrounding muscle and the pressure recorded by an electromanometer. The results were consistent with those of Reynolds et al (1948), showing lack of synchronization of the spread of contractions in abnormal labours. They also demonstrated the high resting basal pressure of a patient with polyhydramnios and the frequent contractions and high basal pressure of a patient suffering from placental abruption.

Few investigators could justify the degree of invasion necessitated by the techniques of the Montevideo group and certainly such studies are unlikely to be repeated today because of ethical constraints. Williams & Stallworthy (1952) working in Oxford described the use of a polythene tube passed through the cervix into the amniotic sac. This intra-amniotic open-ended fluid-filled catheter technique was reported as simple, accurate and safe. At that time such developments were stimulated by the increasing use of oxytocic drugs during prolonged labour. Theobald et al (1948) had administered the first Pituitrin drip in Bradford in 1948.

Csapo (1970) considered the use of an extraovular open catheter filled with fluid. He found this simple technique to be grossly inaccurate, probably because of the entry of air into the open catheter and insufficient fluid transmission. Lack of a fluid pool around the catheter tip is also important: this can only be created and sustained with difficulty. This difficulty is resolved by a micro balloon placed on the end of the catheter (extraovular microballoon method). Such a system generates tracings indistinguishable from a trans-abdominal intra-amniotic device. There is no more than 0.7 ml fluid in the balloon. Such a device requires skill and experience in the placement of the catheter, freeing of the system of air, control of fluid leakage and the avoidance of membrane rupture. Csapo and co-workers were well satisfied with this device not only in research but also for monitoring labour. They believed there was no interference with normal physiology, no placental detachment or infection and accidental rupture of the membranes during placement occurred in less than 3% of subjects.

In 1970 Csapo reported preliminary work using a micro-transducer mounted on the end of a catheter and placed in an extra-amniotic position. This produced identical recordings to an extraovular micro balloon. Until the 1970s intrauterine pressure recording was usually performed using the transcervical intra-amniotic approach with a fluid-filled catheter (Turnbull 1957, Hon & Paul 1973, Huey et al 1976, Miller et al 1976). These devices had to be flushed to maintain continuity of the fluid column and were prone to blockage with vernix, blood clot or fetal parts (Odendaal et al 1976). Such complications are dangerous because falsely low values in a subject requiring oxytocin augmentation might lead to over-stimulation. In the late 1970s a few reports appeared of fetal and placental damage associated with their use (Nuttall 1978, Trudinger & Pryse Davies 1978). The incidence of such complications is not obvious for two reasons. They are probably under-reported and the total number of intrauterine catheter insertions (the denominator) is not known. Several institutions use such devices without problems. Only a small minority of obstetric units in the UK undertake intrauterine pressure monitoring at all.

In 1978 Steer et al introduced the Sonicaid Gaeltec catheter tip pressure transducer, shown in Figure 45.5a. This is an intra-amniotic device and will not produce recordings from an extra-amniotic site for reasons already referred to. It is easy to use and after removal from its storage tube attached to the fetal monitor (Fig. 45.5b), requires to be wiped, dried with a gauze swab and inserted through the ruptured membranes. Simple calibration is undertaken beforehand. The Gaeltec catheter is compatible with modern fetal monitors. These devices are not associated with any increased risk of infection and there have been no reports of complications from their use. They are fragile and expensive but if properly handled should last for more than 100 insertions and be as cost-effective as a fluid-filled system.

Svenningsen & Jensen (1986) have reported the use of a fibreoptic pressure transducer mounted on the end of a solid catheter. The principle of this device is that a light impulse is passed down the catheter to a pressure-sensitive membrane from which it returns by a different channel, having been altered by the pressure. This does produce reliable results but is in an early stage of development.

Internal tocography: measurement

Developments in the measurement of uterine activity have progressed at the same time as developments in recording techniques. Although Smyth (1957) claimed accuracy in recording actual intrauterine pressure with external techniques, this generally only reveals duration of contractions and frequency with a rather poor subjective impression of amplitude. The technical difficulties of obtaining clean tocographic recordings by this method have already been mentioned. Accurate measurements of uterine action, especially in the labouring subject, have only been made using intrauterine transducers.

Average intensity (active pressure, amplitude) of contractions has been most commonly used. Alvarez & Caldeyro Barcia (1950) considered the average intensity of contractions in the first stage of labour to range between 30 and 60 mmHg. If the average intensity was below 25 mmHg labour progressed slowly and if below 15 mmHg it rarely progressed at all. They observed the frequency to be generally between three and five contractions per 10 minutes and

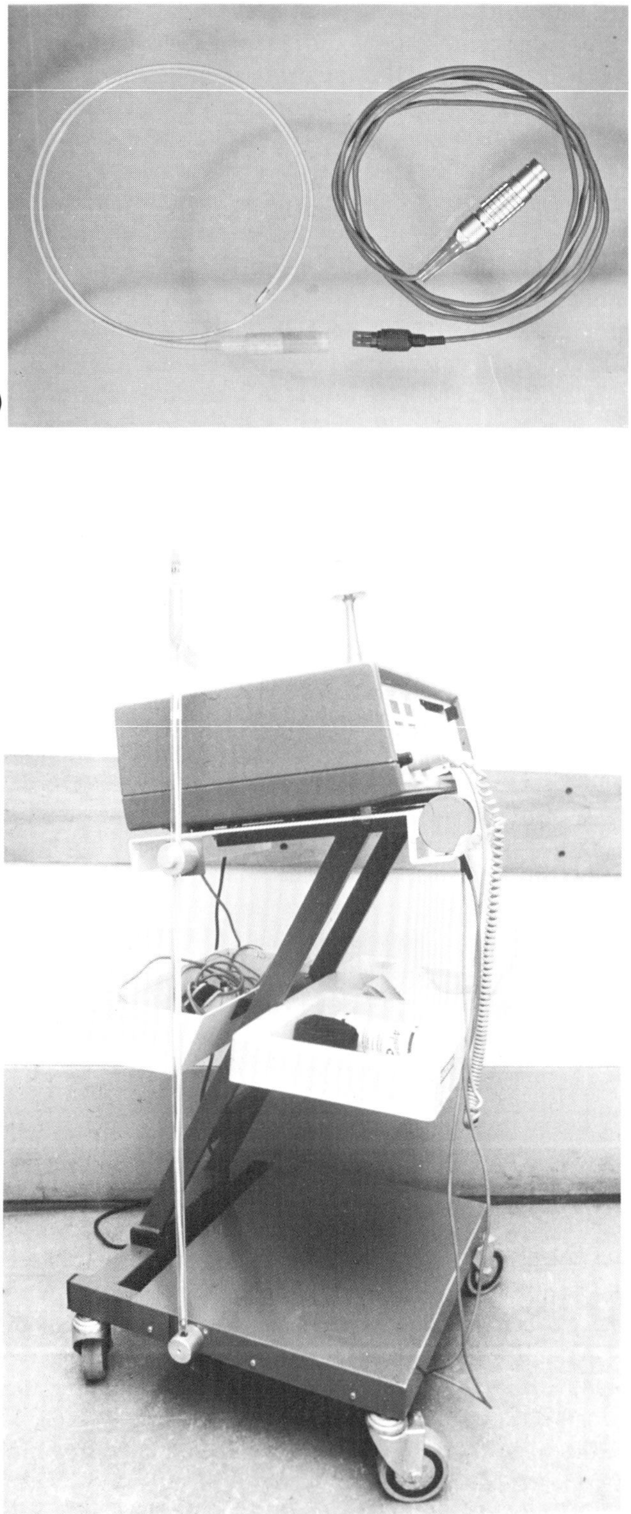

Fig. 45.5 (a) Gaeltec catheter; (b) Gaeltec catheter in storage tube, attached to monitor.

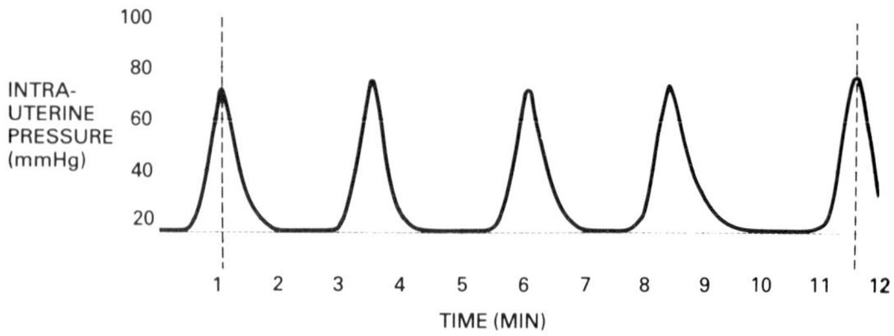

FREQUENCY OF CONTRACTIONS: 4 in 10.5 MIN = 3.8 in 10 MIN

MEAN ACTIVE PRESSURE: 60 mmHg

MONTEVIDEO UNITS: MEAN ACTIVE PRESSURE × FREQUENCY
= 3.8 × 60
= 228 MONTEVIDEO UNITS PER 10 MIN

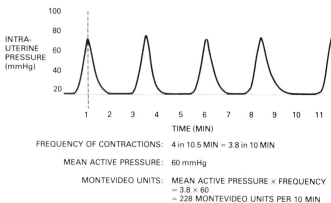

Fig. 45.6 Montevideo units.

considered the normal range to be between two and six. They did not document the duration of contractions. This may have been because of difficulties in identifying the end of a contraction. The upstroke of a contraction is rather steep and its beginning can be easily identified. The downstroke is less steep, especially in its terminal part. Often in a trace of normal labour the subsequent contraction begins before the pressure has subsided to the precontraction baseline. A more major degree of this is coupling and a greater degree becomes incoordination. For the same reason it may be difficult to identify basal pressure (basal tone) and this may be stated to be within a range (8–12 mmHg). The problems of recognizing basal pressure exactly have been referred to at the end of the preceding section.

The shape of contractions will vary according to the paper speed of the machine. In the UK cardiotocography is generally performed at a paper speed of 1 cm/min but in the USA speeds of 2 or even 3 cm/min are common. This results in contractions appearing to be of longer duration than they are. Pressure tends to rise more abruptly in the first part of a contraction and fall more slowly later (Fig. 45.1). It becomes clear that referring to several elements of contractions sequentially makes comparison difficult. Caldeyro Barcia et al (1957) wished to relate overall activity to duration of pregnancy and labour. They therefore devised Montevideo units named after the city where they worked. Montevideo units are the product of average active pressure multiplied by frequency in a 10-minute period (Fig. 45.6). They produced a series of reference values for this during pregnancy and labour (Fig. 45.7). At that time this could only be calculated retrospectively and the information was not available during labour when it would have been of diagnostic and therapeutic value. Dehart et al (1977) later devised an on-line recording system. This system did not allow for duration of contractions. Montevideo units are only useful when one of the parameters is changing but less so when both are changing, especially in opposite directions. El-Sahwi et al (1967) added the mean duration of the contraction to the multiplication, devising Alexandria units. This only increased the complexity further and did not find favour.

Bourne & Burn had suggested in 1927 that the area described by the writing point of the tocograph above the line

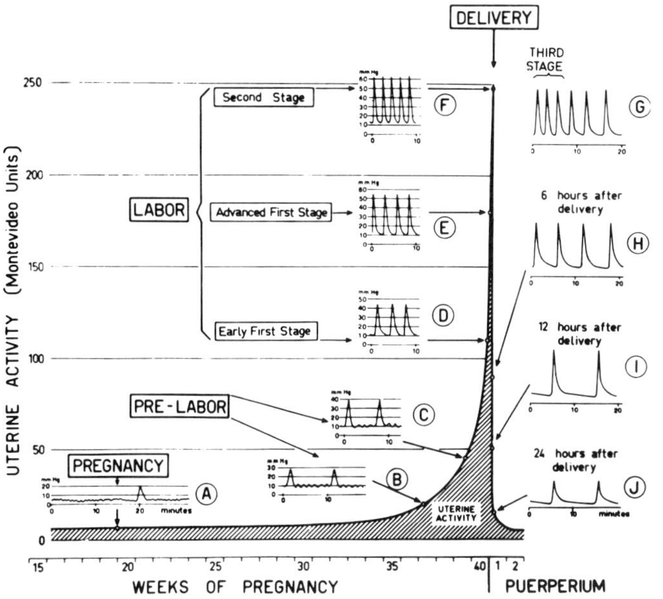

Fig. 45.7 Caldeyro Barcia diagram. From Caldeyro Barcia et al (1957).

of zero pressure was proportional to the work done by the uterus. This concept was used by Hon & Paul (1973) when they devised uterine activity units. The total contraction area (TCA; Fig. 45.1) is the area above zero enclosed by the contraction curve. This had to be divided into units and Bourne & Burn decided that one uterine activity unit (1 UAU) would be the area enclosed by a pressure of 1 mmHg for 1 minute. This is also called 1 Torr minute. Advances in technology permitted this to be available on-line whilst labour was in progress. It is evident that the area under basal pressure accounts for a substantial part of the total. Significant changes in active contractions might therefore be submerged by this large unchanging area. It might also be considered that in terms of the dynamic process of labour pressure below basal pressure may not play such an active part.

Seitchik & Chatkoff (1975, 1977) opted to study the waveform of contractions. They digitized the waveform and derived its slope in mmHg/s. Each contraction was divided into four components. They observed that oxytocin-stimulated contractions differed from prostaglandin-stimulated contractions or spontaneous contractions in that they showed a disproportionately rapid rise in pressure. They suggested that the ratio of amplitude to the rate of pressure rise identified the myometrial response to oxytocin earlier than amplitude or Montevideo units. This ratio is a more sensitive dose–response indicator which changes little with increasing doses once a steady state is reached. These observations suggest that the ratio of amplitude to rate of intrauterine pressure rise may be a useful measure for monitoring oxytocin therapy.

In the trend towards Système International (SI) units Steer (1977) used the Pascal SI Unit of pressure instead of mmHg

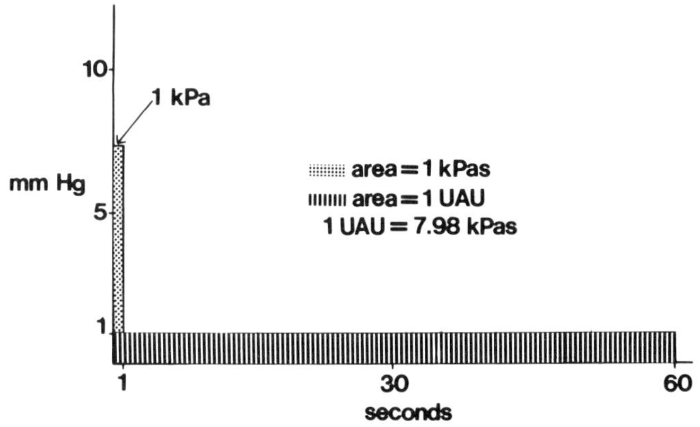

Fig. 45.8 1 kPas compared with 1 UAU.

(1 kPa = 7.52 mmHg). One kilopascal of pressure existing over a duration of 1 second is 1 kPa second. This measure of active area under the pressure curve must be quantified over a period of time. The time intervals used are kilopascal seconds per 15 minutes (kPas/15 min). This quantity is termed the uterine activity integral (UAI). As uterine activity units (UAU) are traditional units depending on mmHg, and kPas are SI units, there is a direct relationship between them as shown in Figure 45.8 (1 UAU = 7.98 kPas). It should be emphasized that UAU are computed from total contraction area and kPa from active contraction area.

TOTAL UTERINE ACTIVITY — CERVICAL AND PELVIC TISSUE RESISTANCE

Rossavik (1978) proposed that a certain total uterine activity in labour was needed to overcome cervical and pelvic tissue resistance. He calculated the uterine work as the product of active pressure in kilopascals and the duration of contractions in seconds and called it the total uterine impulse. He showed a positive correlation between total uterine impulse (and hence resistance) between 5 and 10 cm cervical dilatation and the frequency of operative vaginal deliveries, especially in nulliparae.

Arulkumaran et al (1985) used such a concept but calculated cumulative UAI values throughout the induced labours reported by Gibb et al (1985). This was termed the total uterine activity (TUA). Nulliparae with a poor cervical score required the greatest TUA: 60 000 kPas between induction and delivery, whilst nulliparae with a good score and multiparae with a poor score required 30 000 kPas and multiparae with a good score required the least — about 15 000 kPas. These differences were all statistically significant; women having a Caesarean section were excluded from the analysis. These values are entirely consistent with the theory that the uterus has to generate enough activity to overcome the cervical and pelvic tissue resistance presented to it. In induced labour, if the TUA exceeds the value expected for the relevant parity and cervical score, the possibility of cephalopelvic disproportion, malposition or failed induction of labour should be considered. If there is borderline feto-placental function, it may be possible to effect delivery with lower uterine activity values over a longer period of time.

Further work is required to elaborate the prognostic value of cumulative uterine activity in difficult labours. It may be that limits could be set for individual patients when a trial of labour is deemed complete. Time spent in abnormal labour is time of high risk to the fetus.

INCOORDINATION

Incoordination of uterine action is a descriptive term for contractions recorded on a tocograph showing a degree of irregularity of shape, timing, merging of contractions and often a rise in basal pressure. Contrary to popular belief, most labours show some degree of incoordination, especially in the earlier stages. This may or may not be associated with poor progress in labour. Turnbull (1957), recognizing the difficulty in measuring regularity, classified the pattern of contractions into three types, with type 1 the most regular and type 3 the most irregular. He found a significant proportion of normal labours manifested contractions classified as type 2 and type 3 patterns. In fact no correlation could be found between the degree of regularity and the duration of labour.

Effer et al (1969) devised an index of uterine arrhythmia which objectively and quantitatively represents the irregularity of uterine contractile rhythm. This involved calculating coefficients of variation of intervals between peak pressure of contractions. They found an intrinsic pattern of irregularity which each individual assumes once labour is established. This pattern does not change remarkably during the remainder of the labour. Schulman & Romney (1970) also remarked on the degree of individual variability of contractions and pointed out that the uterus, being smooth muscle, would be expected to behave like other such organs. Each contraction may be initiated by a different cell and it is known that every smooth muscle cell is a potential pacemaker. A pacemaker cell has never been demonstrated directly, either by electrophysiological techniques or by histological study. Gibb et al (1984) also noted the recurrence of irregular patterns throughout an individual labour. Excitation impulses travel from cell to cell and each uterus has its preferred pathway. None of this denies the concept of fundal dominance in normal labour suggested by Reynolds et al (1948). The implications for area measurement of a series of contractions showing incoordination are important because the UAI will tend to be high under these circumstances and should be interpreted with care.

CLINICAL APPLICATION

Should uterine contractions be recorded and measured routinely? Should internal or external tocography be used? These simple questions have not yet been answered.

When labour progress is normal and the fetal heart rate is normal, anything more than simple information about the contractions is unnecessary. External tocography is not essential. However some form of external assessment, preferably by simple palpation, should be retained so that the importance of contractions in the labour process is not forgotten. Some women find the abdominal belt and external transducer uncomfortable; its placement should certainly not be used to justify immobilizing the woman in a dorsal position. Timing of contractions, whether by external or internal tocography, becomes more important when periodic fetal heart rate changes in the form of decelerations are present. Obesity or excessive restlessness indicates a need for internal tocography.

The prime purpose of internal tocography is to obtain more information about the nature of contractions in abnormal labour and to observe the effect of treatment with oxytocin. Uncertainty about the nature of contractions after treatment may lead to failed labour because of inadequate dose of oxytocin or fetal compromise because of an excessive dose. What are normal contractions in labour? Normal contractions are those that lead to progressive dilatation of the cervix and descent of the presenting part. They are variable in quantity but generally proceed from two in every 10 minutes, 40 second duration, of weak strength at the onset of labour, to a regular frequency of four or five in every 10 minutes, 60 seconds long and of greater strength during the expulsive phase.

The other problem in abnormal labour is quantifying the three variables sequentially. A method of computation of the area under the tocographic curve appears to answer this problem, although due considerations should be made of the effect of co-ordination. Normal ranges have been constructed for UAI in a dilatation-specific manner according to parity (Fig. 45.9, 45.10, Arulkumaran et al 1984, Gibb et al 1984). Although these were constructed for normal Singaporean Chinese women, there appear to be no significant racial variations. Whilst physical characteristics and disease may have different incidences in different racial groups, physiology does not differ.

There are three situations where some express reservations about the use of oxytocin in abnormal labour: labour with a previous uterine scar, breech presentation and grand multiparity. The concern has been that if the contractions are already adequate then the use of oxytocin may lead to complications. Intrauterine pressure measurement is an ideal device for ensuring this is not the case. The author advises the use of an intrauterine catheter in these circumstances and such practice is followed in our unit with great satisfaction.

The other situation where we use the procedure is during

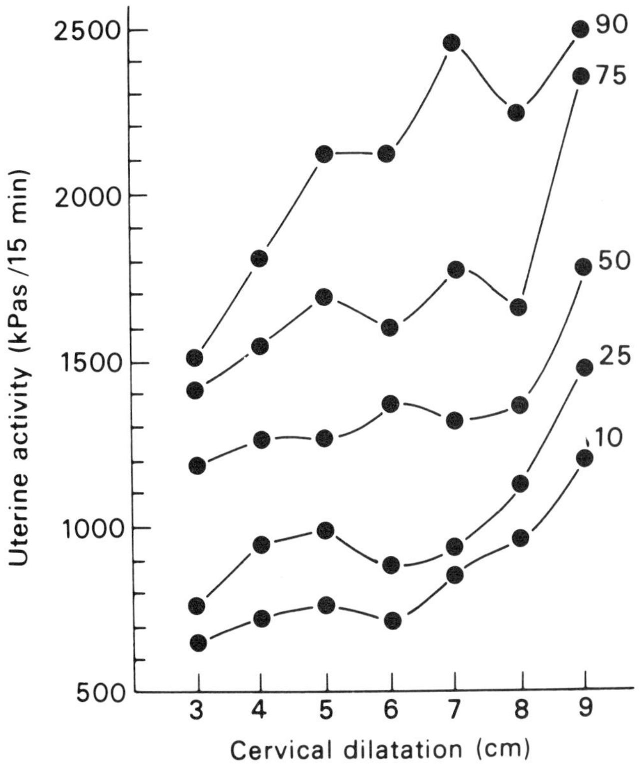

Fig. 45.9 UAI percentiles in spontaneous nulliparous labour related to cervical dilatation. From Gibb et al (1984).

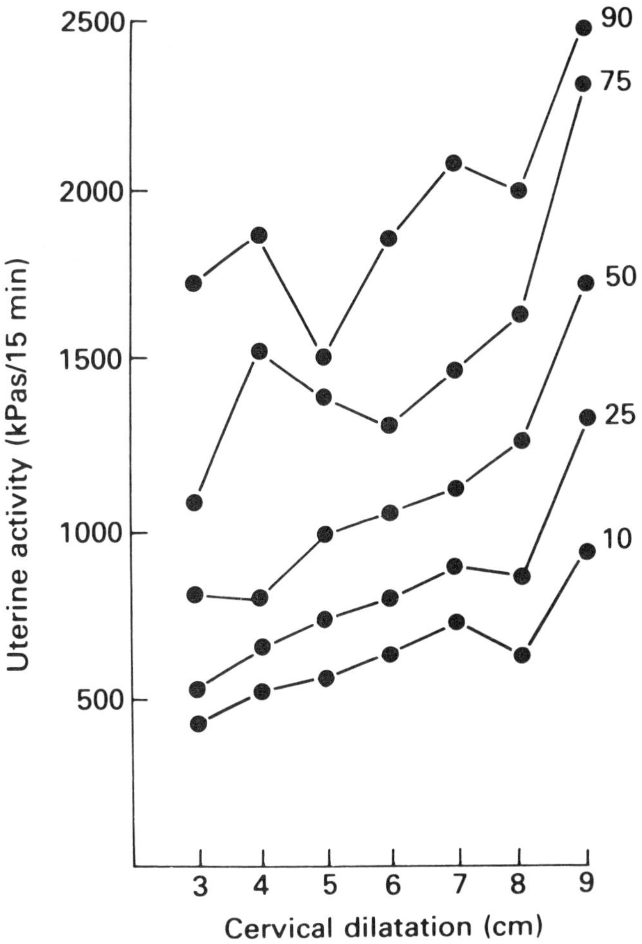

Fig. 45.10 UAI percentiles in spontaneous multiparous labour related to cervical dilatation. From Arulkumaran et al (1984).

induction or augmentation of labour even when the above conditions do not exist. A fair proportion of inductions and augmentations will not prove difficult and a most useful functional differentiation of significant difficulty is when the dose rate exceeds 12 mu/min oxytocin (when a litre bottle containing 4 units of oxytocin is replaced by one containing 8 units). Escalation of dose up to this level is reasonable with careful external assessment of contractions. In this period many women, especially multiparae, will have become well established in good labour and some will have delivered. When this is not the case, progressive time spent in abnormal difficult labour leads to cumulative fetal and maternal compromise. In an endeavour to limit this, accurate assessment of contractions becomes necessary. The correct dose of oxytocin can be achieved in optimal time and a well conducted trial of labour completed. Should this culminate in Caesarean section, the indication will be clear, the operation will be performed sooner rather than later, and the baby in the best condition.

Many operators are familiar with the dilemma of the delayed late first stage and second stage of labour when there is an epidural anaesthetic used. It is the author's experience that many of these women have poor contractions; this can be proven by internal tocography. Forceps should not be applied too early but effective second-stage augmentation with oxytocin should be administered if necessary, using pressure measurement as a guide. This often leads to further descent and rotation, culminating in normal delivery or at least produces the best conditions for a safe assisted delivery; the head is delivered from a lower level.

The rationale for contraction monitoring is quite different from that for electronic fetal heart monitoring. There is no justification for routine internal contraction monitoring. Any methods should be used selectively and their application correctly appreciated. Facilities have to be provided and a need assessed. Assuming certain characteristics of women and practice, a computation may be made and no more than 15% of patients are likely to require this technique in an average labour ward.

In King's College Hospital (London) labour ward during 1987 5.6% of labouring mothers had an intrauterine pressure catheter. From a postal survey we found that at least 40% of hospitals in England and Wales have a facility for intrauterine pressure monitoring; some hospitals use it more often but most use it rather infrequently.

CURRENT STATUS

There is general agreement that the best way to record uterine contractions for measurement is by an intrauterine pressure-sensing device mounted on a solid catheter and placed in an intra-amniotic position. What is not clear is the optimal way to process these data for clinical application. Steer et al (1984) compared the uterine activity integral (UAI) with the more traditional measures of frequency, active pressure and Montevideo units. They found that UAI is the measure which shows the closest correlation with rates of cervical dilatation in the active phase of spontaneous labour.

Average pressure and frequency of contractions have been used most commonly in assessment and Arulkumaran et al (1986) have shown that labour can be induced as easily and safely using frequency rather than UAI as a guide. This is certainly the practice in the USA. Medical staff familiar with the UAI concept find it easy to use as it gives immediately available values.

Unless great care is exercised, introduction of new systems of measurement, especially to computerize on-line labour care (Henry et al 1979, Tromans et al 1982) will serve only to depersonalize the labour experience further and add to the complexity of management. The technological imperative should not be allowed to dominate and submerge the important advances in the understanding of uterine activity which can contribute to improvements in intrapartum care.

REFERENCES

Alvarez H, Caldeyro R 1950 Contractility of human uterus recorded by new methods. Surgery, Gynecology and Obstetrics 91: 1–13

Arulkumaran S, Gibb D M F, Lun K C, Heng S H, Ratnam S S 1984 The effect of parity on uterine activity in labour. British Journal of Obstetrics and Gynaecology 91: 843–848

Arulkumaran S, Gibb D M F, Ratnam S S, Lun K C, Heng S H 1985 Total uterine activity in induced labour — an index of cervical and pelvic tissue resistance. British Journal of Obstetrics and Gynaecology 92: 693–697

Arulkumaran S, Ingemarsson J, Ratnam S S 1986 Oxytocin titration to achieve preset active contraction area values does not improve the outcome of induced labour. British Journal of Obstetrics and Gynaecology 94: 242–248

Bell R 1981 Measurement of spontaneous uterine activity in the antenatal patient. American Journal of Obstetrics and Gynecology 140: 713–715

Bell R 1983 The prediction of preterm labour by recording spontaneous antenatal uterine activity. British Journal of Obstetrics and Gynaecology 90: 884

Bourne A, Burn J H 1927 The dosage and action of pituitary extract of the ergot alkaloids on the uterus in labour, with a note on the action of adrenaline. Journal of Obstetrics and Gynaecology of the British Empire 34: 249–272

Braxton Hicks J 1872 On the contractions of the uterus throughout pregnancy; their physiological effects and their value in the diagnosis of pregnancy. Transactions of the Obstetric Society XIII: 216–231

Caldeyro Barcia R, Alvarez H 1952 Abnormal uterine action in labour. Journal of Obstetrics and Gynaecology of the British Empire 59: 646–656

Caldeyro Barcia R, Poseiro J J 1960 Physiology of uterine contractions. Clinical Obstetrics and Gynecology 3: 386–408

Caldeyro Barcia R, Alvarez H, Reynolds S R M 1950 A better understanding of uterine contractility through simultaneous recording with an internal and a seven channel external method. Surgery, Gynecology and Obstetrics 91: 641–650

Caldeyro Barcia R, Sica-Blanco Y, Poseiro J J et al 1957 A quantitative study of the action of synthetic oxytocin on the human uterus. Journal of Pharmacology and Experimental Therapeutics 121: 18–31

Csapo A 1970 The diagnostic significance of the intrauterine pressure. Part I. Obstetrical and Gynecological Survey 25: 403–432

Csapo A I, Takeda H 1965 Effect of progesterone on the electric activity and intra uterine pressure of pregnant and parturient rabbits. American Journal of Obstetrics and Gynecology 91: 221–231

Csapo A I, Takeda H, Wood C 1963 Volume and activity of the parturient rabbit uterus. American Journal of Obstetrics and Gynecology 85: 813–835

Dehart W R, Laros R K, Witting W C, Work B A 1977 System for computing Montevideo units for monitoring progress of labour. IEEE Transactions on Biomedical Engineering 24: 94–101

Dill L V, Maiden R M 1946 The electrical potentials of the human uterus in labour. American Journal of Obstetrics and Gynecology 52: 719–734

Dodeck S M 1932 A new method for graphically recording the contractions of the parturient human uterus. Surgery, Gynecology and Obstetrics 55: 45–67

Effer S B, Bertola R P, Vrettos A, Caldeyro-Barcia R 1969 Quantitative study of the regularity of uterine contractile rhythm in labour. American Journal of Obstetrics and Gynecology 105: 909–915

El-Sahwi S, Gaafar A A, Toppozada H K 1967 A new unit for evaluation of uterine activity. American Journal of Obstetrics and Gynecology 98: 900–903

Embrey M P 1940 External hysterography. A graphic study of the human parturient uterus and the effect of various therapeutic agents on it. Journal of Obstetrics and Gynaecology of the British Empire 47: 371–390

Embrey M P 1955 A new multichannel external tocograph. Journal of Obstetrics and Gynaecology of the British Empire LXII: 1–5

Garfield R E, Hayashi R H 1981 Appearance of gap junctions in the myometrium of women during labour. American Journal of Obstetrics and Gynecology 140: 254–260

Gibb D M F, Arulkumaran S, Lun K C, Ratnam S S 1984 Characteristics of uterine activity in nulliparous labour. British Journal of Obstetrics and Gynaecology 91: 220–227

Gibb D M F, Arulkumaran S, Ratnam S S 1985 A comparative study of methods of oxytocin administration for induction of labour. British Journal of Obstetrics and Gynaecology 92: 688–692

Gunn A L, Wood M C 1953 The amplification and recording of foetal heart sounds. Proceedings of the Royal Society of Medicine 46: 85–91

Henry M J, McColl D D F, Crawford J W, Patel N 1979 Computing techniques for intra partum physiological data reduction. Journal of Perinatal Medicine 7: 209–214

Hon E H, Paul R H 1973 Quantitation of uterine activity. Obstetrics and Gynecology 43: 368–370

Huey J R, Al Hadjiev A, Paul R H 1976 Uterine activity in the multiparous patient. American Journal of Obstetrics and Gynecology 126: 682–686

Lacroix G E 1968 Monitoring labour by an external tokodynamometer. American Journal of Obstetrics and Gynecology 101: 111–119

Miller F C, Yeh S Y, Schifrin B S, Paul R H, Hon E H 1976 Quantitation of uterine activity in 100 primiparous patients. American Journal of Obstetrics and Gynecology 124: 398–405

Moir C 1935 The merits and demerits of oxytocic drugs in the post partum period. Proceedings of the Royal Society of Medicine 28: 1654–1666

Murphy D P 1947 Uterine contractility in pregnancy. J B Lippincott, Philadelphia, pp 3–6

Nuttall I D 1978 Perforation of a placental fetal vessel by an intrauterine pressure catheter. British Journal of Obstetrics and Gynaecology 85: 573–574

Odendaal H J, Neves Dos Santos L M, Henry M J, Crawford J W 1976 Experiments in the measurement of intrauterine pressure. British Journal of Obstetrics and Gynaecology 83: 221–224

Polaillon P 1880 Archives de Physiologie 2: 1. Cited in Bourne & Burn 1927

Reynolds S R M, Hellman L M, Bruns P 1948 Patterns of uterine contractility in women during pregnancy. Obstetrical and Gynecological Survey 3: 629–646

Ruebsamen W 1913 W Munchener Medizinische Wochenschrift. 1913 LX 627, Cited in Embrey 1940

Rossavik I K 1978 Relation between total uterine impulse, method of delivery and one-minute apgar score. British Journal of Obstetrics and Gynaecology 85: 847–851
Sakaguchi M, Nakajima A 1970 Electrical activity of the human uterus in labour. American Journal of Obstetrics and Gynecology 108: 992–993
Schaffer O 1896 Experimentele Untersuchungen uber Wehenthatigkeit. Berlin, 1896. Cited in Embrey 1940
Schatz F 1872 Archiv für Gynäkologie iii: 58–144. Cited in Bourne & Burn 1927
Schulman H, Romney S L 1970 Variability of uterine contractions in normal human parturition. Obstetrics and Gynecology 36: 215–221
Seitchik J, Chatkoff M L 1975 Intrauterine pressure waveform characteristics in hypocontractile labour before and after oxytocin administration. American Journal of Obstetrics and Gynecology 123: 426–434
Seitchik J, Chatkoff M L, Hayashi R H 1977 Intrauterine pressure waveform characteristics of spontaneous and oxytocin or prostaglandin induced active labour. American Journal of Obstetrics and Gynecology 127: 223–227
Smyth C N 1957 The guard ring tocodynamometer. Absolute measurement of intra-amniotic pressure by a new instrument. Journal of Obstetrics and Gynaecology of the British Empire 64: 59–66
Steer P J 1977 The measurement and control of uterine contractions. In: Beard R W, Campbell S (eds) The current status of fetal heart rate monitoring and ultrasound in obstetrics. Royal College of Obstetricians and Gynaecologists, London, pp 48–60
Steer P J, Carter M C, Gordon A J, Beard R W 1978 The use of cathetertip pressure transducers for the measurement of intrauterine pressure in labour. British Journal of Obstetrics and Gynaecology 85: 561–566
Steer P J, Carter M C, Beard R W 1984 Normal levels of active contraction area in spontaneous labour. British Journal of Obstetrics and Gynaecology 91: 211–219
Svenningsen L, Jensen O 1986 Application of fibre optics to the clinical measurement of intrauterine pressure in labour. Acta Obstetricia et Gynecologica Scandinavica 65: 551–555
Theobald G W, Graham A, Campbell J, Gange P D, Driscoll W J 1948 The use of post pituitary extract in physiological amounts in obstetrics. British Medical Journal 2: 123–127
Tromans P M, Sheen M A, Beazley M 1982 Feto-maternal surveillance in labour: a new approach with an on line microcomputer. British Journal of Obstetrics and Gynaecology 89: 1021–1030
Trudinger B J, Pryse Davies J 1979 Fetal hazards of the intrauterine pressure catheter: five case reports. British Journal of Obstetrics and Gynaecology 85: 567–572
Turnbull A C 1957 Uterine contractions in normal and abnormal labour. Journal of Obstetrics and Gynaecology of the British Empire 66: 321–333
Westermark J 1893 Skand. Arch. f. Physiol. IV 331. Cited in Bourne & Burn 1927
Williams E A, Stallworthy J A 1952 A simple method of internal tocography. Lancet i: 330–332
Wolfs G M J A, Van Leeuwen M 1979 Electromyographic observations on the human uterus during labour. Acta Obstetricia et Gynecologica Scandinavica (suppl) 90: 1–61

46

Alec Turnbull and A. López Bernal

Physiology and biochemistry of labour

Successful parturition involves the establishment of regular and effective uterine contractions and the ripening and dilatation of the cervix. Control of the onset of human labour remains a mystery (see Ch. 12) but recent advances in reproductive biochemistry have greatly increased our understanding of the mechanism of cervical softening in preparation for labour, and the factors that increase uterine contractility. In this chapter we review the functional anatomy of the human uterus, the biochemical basis of cervical ripening and myometrial contractility and the factors that may predict the onset of term and preterm labour.

FUNCTIONAL ANATOMY OF THE UTERUS

The uterus is a remarkable organ because, after implantation of the blastocyst, it remains quiescent for several months, allowing the growth of the fetus. However, at term it must be able to perform considerable mechanical work to expel its contents through the birth canal. The uterus is primarily formed by bundles of smooth muscle separated by connective tissue (collagen and elastin). The distribution of these components varies throughout the organ. There is a gradual fall in the smooth muscle content from the fundus to the cervix, but even at the lower end of the cervix muscle accounts for 10–30% of the tissue (Schwalm & Dubrauszky 1966). In the non-pregnant uterus the collagen concentration in the cervix is about 50% higher than in the fundus and corpus uteri, but this difference decreases towards the end of gestation (Ekman et al 1986). There are several smooth muscle layers across the uterus. The innermost layers contain mainly longitudinal fibres and the outermost layers have both longitudinal and circular bundles. The middle layers contain the vascular supply with muscle fibres forming a multidirectional mesh. The interaction between smooth muscle and connective tissue allows the uterus to expand considerably during pregnancy to accommodate the growing fetus and to develop strong, coordinated and effective contractions at the time of delivery.

The innervation of the uterus is autonomic. Both adrenergic and cholinergic nerves are present and are more abundant in the cervix than in the fundus (Owman et al 1967). There are also sensory fibres. The adrenergic response of the uterus can be both excitatory (alpha-adrenergic) and inhibitory (beta-adrenergic). It is not known to what extent uterine activity is modulated physiologically by the autonomic nervous system; the onset and progress of labour appears to be normal in paraplegic women and in women with bilateral lumbar sympathectomy, suggesting that hormonal control is more important than neural control. Clinically, beta-adrenergic agonists have been extensively used to stop contractions in preterm labour but such drugs are associated with cardiovascular side-effects.

BIOCHEMICAL CHANGES DURING CERVICAL RIPENING

Cervical ripening is characterized by softening, effacement and dilatation. The consistency of the cervix becomes softer in preparation for labour and its shape changes from a cylindrical structure 2–3 cm long, to a wide-funnelled canal with very thin edges. This softening of the cervical canal is called effacement and in primigravida is normally completed before the beginning of cervical dilatation, although in multipara effacement and dilatation occur at the same time. The cause of these changes is not completely understood but results from a combination of structural changes in the cervix and the pressure exerted by the membranes or the fetal presenting part.

Structure of the cervix

The cervix is composed largely of fibrous connective tissue but there are also smooth muscle cells, fibroblasts, blood vessels, epithelium and mucous glands. At term, water accounts for 90% of its weight. The cervical connective tissue is made up of collagen fibres and elastin which are separated by the ground substance (van der Rest 1980). The collagen molecules (tropocollagen) are arranged in a staggered longitudinal way to form the typical striated fibrils. Tropocollagen molecules consist of three polypeptides packed in a triple helix with short, non-helical telopeptides at both ends. The ground substance is composed mainly of proteoglycans. These are made up of a number of glycosaminoglycans connected to a protein core. Glycosaminoglycans are acid mucopolysaccharides and some have sulphate groups which make these molecules highly hydrophilic. Proteoglycans are arranged around the collagen fibres and may modify the water content and the mechanical properties of the cervix. The most important glycosaminoglycan in the human cervix is dermatan sulphate which has a high affinity for collagen (Uldbjerg et al 1983a).

The softening of the cervix during pregnancy is due to striking changes in the connective tissue (Danforth 1983). Although most of the changes described here refer to the cervix, it must be borne in mind that the corpus and fundus uteri also contain a high proportion of connective tissue and that similar changes occur there and are partly responsible for uterine compliance. Compared with the non-pregnant uterus, the concentration of collagen (measured as hydroxyproline, an aminoacid typical of collagen) in cervical tissue during pregnancy is decreased by more than 50% (Uldbjerg et al 1983b). Furthermore, towards term the number of intermolecular collagen cross-links decreases, making collagen more soluble and easy to digest. The collagenolytic activity of the human cervix increases towards term (Kitamura et al 1980) and this may contribute to endogenous collagen breakdown and cervical ripening. Collagen can be cleaved by both collagenase, which originates in the fibroblasts, and by leukocyte elastase (Uldbjerg et al 1983c).

There are also important changes in the ground substance. The concentration of sulphated glycosaminoglycans is markedly decreased in the late pregnant cervix compared with the non-pregnant state. Another important glycosaminoglycan, hyaluronic acid, is significantly decreased in the cervix of pregnant, compared with non-pregnant women (Uldjberg et al 1983c).

Control of cervical ripening

Cervical ripening is thought to be under hormonal control. In rodents, relaxin of ovarian or decidual origin has an important physiological role in cervical softening, but a similar role has not been proved in higher mammals. Plasma levels of relaxin in women are highest in early pregnancy (12–16 weeks) and decline towards term (Eddie et al 1986). However, some success has been reported with the pharmacological use of purified porcine relaxin for the ripening of the human cervix at term (MacLennan et al 1986). Oestrogens regulate the biosynthesis of glycosaminoglycans in several tissues and may be involved in the connective tissue changes in the human cervix in pregnancy, but the use of oestrogens or oestrogen precursors, such as dehydroepiandrosterone-sulphate, to ripen the cervix in pregnant women has been very limited. By contrast, the use of prostaglandin E_2 (PGE_2) in the form of vaginal gels or pessaries (Calder et al 1977, MacKenzie & Embrey 1977) in patients with an unfavourable cervix is now routine practice in many hospitals and the results are generally very good. It is likely that PGE_2 has a physiological role during cervical ripening because it is produced by the cervix itself and by the neighbouring fetal membranes and decidua (Ellwood et al 1980). PGE_2 is thought to increase the collagenolytic activity of cervical tissue but has little effect on the metabolism of proteoglycans (Uldbjerg et al 1983a). The importance of local factors in cervical ripening is emphasized by experiments in sheep where, despite surgical transection of the cervix in late pregnancy, with loss of vascular and mechanical connections with the uterus, cervical softening still occurred in labour (Ledger et al 1985).

BIOCHEMICAL CONTROL OF MYOMETRIAL CONTRACTILITY

While many important questions remain to be answered, progress in understanding the biochemical events leading to smooth muscle contraction and relaxation has been enormous in recent years. We will summarize here the structural and functional components of the uterus and the most important aspects of the signal transduction mechanisms that translate hormone-receptor interactions on cell membranes into regulatory changes in myometrial cells.

Structure of the myometrium

Myometrial cells are embedded in a matrix of collagen fibres which facilitate transmission of the contractile forces generated in the individual myometrial cells. The cytoplasm of uterine smooth muscle cells is largely occupied by the myofilaments actin and myosin, which are not organized as in striated muscle, but occur in long random bundles throughout the muscle cells (Marsten & Smith 1985). Myosin has both a structural role and a catalytic effect, converting the chemical energy of ATP into the mechanical energy of muscle contraction. Myosin consists of two heavy and four light polypeptide chains; the two heavy chains form a globular head where the ATPase sites are located and where actin and myosin interaction occurs. The light chains attached to the globular head are the sites of calcium binding and phosphorylation.

Myometrial contractility

The contractile forces of labour are generated by the interaction of actin and myosin in myometrial cells. The two filaments slide past each other during contractions as the myosin heads and actin molecules form reversible cross-bridges. The actin–myosin interaction is regulated by the level of intracellular calcium ions. Activation of smooth muscle cells occurs when free intracellular calcium concentrations reach 10^{-6} M, and when the levels are reduced to 10^{-7}–10^{-8} M the cells relax (Carsten & Miller 1987). A well-accepted theory is that calcium, in combination with calmodulin, activates the enzyme myosin kinase which phosphorylates a 20 K light chain of myosin. Phosphorylated myosin interacts with actin and causes contractions. When calcium levels decrease, calmodulin dissociates from myosin light chain kinase, and the enzyme becomes inactive. Myosin light chain is then dephosphorylated by a phosphatase and relaxation occurs. The activity of myosin light chain kinase is also regulated by a cAMP-dependent protein kinase. The phosphorylated form of the enzyme cannot bind the calcium–calmodulin complex and relaxation occurs because myosin is dephosphorylated (Carsten & Miller 1987).

Part of the calcium required for the activation of myometrial cells comes from outside, through calcium channels in the cell membrane. The so-called calcium channel blockers, such as nifedipine, block the entry of calcium into the cells and so decrease uterine activity (Nonomura & Ebashi 1980). However, most of the calcium necessary for contractions comes from intracellular stores, i.e. the sarcoplasmic reticulum. In the presence of ATP, calcium is actively stored in the sarcoplasmic reticulum and this causes muscle relaxation. In the human pregnant myometrium this process is inhibited by prostaglandins (PGE_2 and $PGF_{2\alpha}$) and oxytocin (Carsten & Miller 1987). These hormones increase the availability of free intracellular calcium and hence stimulate uterine activity. Progesterone promotes calcium uptake by the sarcoplasmic reticulum and so induces relaxation. It may also do so by inhibiting cAMP catabolism.

Hormone receptors and second messengers

The precise mechanism controlling intracellular calcium levels is not known but appears to be under hormonal control. It is in this area where recent advances in cellular biology have greatly improved our knowledge of uterine function. Many hormones interact with cell surface receptors and modulate cell function through the generation of second messengers. Two major second messenger pathways have been established, and others are likely to emerge in the next few years. One group of receptors control cells by influencing adenylate cyclase activity—either stimulating or inhibiting cAMP formation. Stimulatory and inhibitory receptors are coupled to the adenylate cyclase through different GTP-dependent proteins, known respectively as Gs and Gi proteins (Michell 1987). As described above, increasing cAMP levels leads to smooth muscle relaxation and this is thought to be the mechanism of action of betamimetic agents and, possibly, progesterone.

However, prostaglandins (PGE) which contract the uterus also increase cAMP levels. The role of cAMP in the myometrium is so far controversial. It is not clear whether cAMP increases the uptake of calcium by the sarcoplasmic reticulum, but it seems well established that cAMP activates a protein kinase that phosphorylates and inactivates myosin light chain kinase. This inhibits myosin light chain phosphorylation and prevents actin–myosin interaction.

A second major receptor pathway involves the hydrolysis of phosphatidylinositol, a phospholipid component of the cell membrane, by a specific phospholipase C. As with adenylate cyclase, control of phospholipase C activity by receptors requires intermediary G proteins (Michell 1987). In the uterus, the hydrolysis of phosphatidylinositol 4,5-bisphosphate (PIP_2) produces two compounds with unique intracellular messenger functions. The water-soluble fragment, inositol 1,4,5-trisphosphate (IP_3), diffuses into the cell and reaches the endoplasmic reticulum where it binds to its own receptors and triggers a rapid release of calcium (Hashimoto et al 1986). The lipid fragment, 1,2-diacylglycerol (1,2-DAG), activates protein kinase C which can phosphorylate various proteins and modify cell function (Berridge 1984). In addition, DAG can be metabolized further to release arachidonic acid, the precursor for prostaglandin synthesis.

It has recently been shown that in the human pregnant myometrium oxytocin activates PIP_2 hydrolysis and IP_3 generation (Schrey et al 1986, López Bernal, unpublished observations). It is therefore possible that IP_3 provides the link between oxytocin-receptor binding, intracellular calcium release and uterine muscle contraction (Fig. 46.1). Furthermore, prostaglandins produced from DAG-generated arachidonic acid could also release calcium from the sarcoplasmic reticulum and potentiate the effect of IP_3 (Carsten & Miller 1987). This model is attractive because it brings together the actions of oxytocin and prostaglandins into one single mechanism of myometrial contractility. Oxytocin and prostaglandins also interact by a similar mechanism in human decidua. Oxytocin releases arachidonic acid and stimulates prostaglandin production in decidual cells (Fuchs & Fuchs 1984, Wilson et al 1988), possibly through phosphatidylinositol breakdown (Schrey et al 1987), and prostaglandins, in turn, sensitize the tissue to the action of oxytocin.

PROGRESS OF LABOUR

The function of the uterus during labour is to develop enough progressive force to deliver the fetus through the birth canal. The three major variables in this process are the degree of myometrial contractility, the size and presentation of the fetus and the resistance of the cervix and other pelvic structures. The progress of labour can be divided

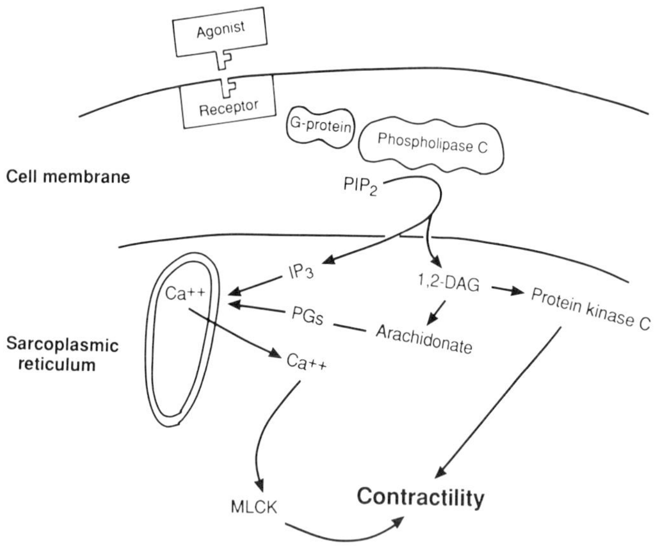

Fig. 46.1 Simplified diagram of agonist-stimulated myometrial contractility. The action of oxytocin on the human pregnant myometrium is believed to fit this model. PIP_2 = phosphatidylinositol 4,5-bisphosphate; IP_3 = inositol 1,4,5-trisphosphate; 1,2-DAG = Diacyglycerol; PGs = Prostaglandins; MLCK = Myosin light chain kinase.

into three stages: the first stage, from the onset of regular contractions until full cervical dilatation; the second stage, when voluntary expulsion efforts by the mother are often superimposed to the uterine contractions; and the third stage, from the delivery of the fetus to the delivery of the placenta. The first stage was classically divided into a latent phase, from the onset of regular contractions to a cervical dilatation of about 2–3 cm, and the active phase, from 3 cm to full cervical dilatation (Friedman 1954). In practice, the first stage of labour is measured from the time of admission in labour, when objective assessment of cervical dilatation can be initiated. Uterine activity during labour was first studied quantitatively by Caldeyro Barcia and his group in Montevideo (1957). They devised the Montevideo unit which is the product of the average intensity of the contractions in millimetres of mercury by the frequency in a 10-minute period. As described in Chapter 45, nowadays the best way to correlate the rate of cervical dilatation during the active phase of labour with uterine activity is by integrating the intrauterine pressure area over a period of time. This measurement is called the uterine activity integral (UAI) and is expressed in SI units in kilopascal seconds per 15 minutes (kPa.s/15 min).

It has been estimated (Arulkumaran et al 1985) that a minimum UAI of 450 kPa.s/15 min is required for normal progress of labour, and the calculated cumulative total uterine activity varies between 15 000 kPa.s and 60 000 kPa.s depending on parity and initial cervical score. Fairlie et al (1988) have quantitated uterine activity (kPa.s) in the first and second stage of labour; their mean figures for primigravidae were 21 000 kPa.s for the first stage and 12 600 kPa.s for the second stage. The corresponding values in parous women were significantly lower — 10 400 kPa.s and 4000 kPa.s respectively. These authors express uterine activity as mean active pressure (MAP), that is the activity integral (in kPa.s) divided by the time (in seconds) over which the pressure is integrated. The advantage of MAP (in kPa.s) over the UAI (kPa.s/15 min) is that the measurement is not restricted to 15-minute intervals. In practice, these measurements are easily convertible. MAP in the first stage of labour (Fairlie et al 1988) averages 1.5 kPa in multiparous and 1.2 kPa in parous women and rises to about 3 kPa in the second stage in both groups of women.

In normal primigravidae the mean duration of the first stage of labour, taken from the time of admission to hospital, is 5.6 hours, with almost 90% of women being delivered within 10 hours of admission (Duignam 1985). The rate of cervical dilatation in primigravidae is about 1.3 cm/h between 1 and 5 cm and 2.5 cm/h between 5 and 10 cm (Duignam 1985). These rates are significantly faster in multiparous women.

Several chapters in this book are dedicated to the management of labour and its complications (Chs 51–62). However, we will briefly refer here to the physiology of the third stage of labour.

The third stage of labour begins with the delivery of the fetus and involves separation and expulsion of the placenta and fetal membranes. Within a few minutes of delivery, the uterus contracts vigorously thus reducing the area of attachment of the placenta, which separates through the decidual layer and is usually delivered by controlled cord traction. The factors controlling the third stage of labour are not well understood but prostaglandins appear to have a major role. Sellers et al (1982) measured the peripheral plasma concentrations of oxytocin and 13,14-dihydro-15-oxo-prostaglandin $F_{2\alpha}$ (PGFM) during labour and in the immediate puerperium. The findings showed that PGFM levels reached a maximum 5 minutes after delivery, before placental separation was detected clinically. The large increase in PGFM levels was not accompanied by changes in oxytocin concentrations. Hence, it seems likely that this surge in prostaglandins contributes to the expulsion of the placenta and fetal membranes, in the same way that intrauterine prostaglandin release is necessary for the normal progress of labour (see Ch. 12). The successful use of prostaglandins or their analogues for the management of intractable postpartum haemorrhage supports the concept that prostaglandins are involved in the third stage of labour.

PREDICTION OF PRETERM LABOUR

The pregnant uterus, unlike other smooth muscle organs, only expels its contents after a period of time which is constant for each species. The duration of human pregnancy is more variable than in some other species, with only about 50% of women being delivered within seven days of the calculated date, with 27% before the 40th week and 23%

in the 42nd week or later (Walker 1962). Preterm delivery (delivery before 37 weeks) accounts for less than 7% of all pregnancies; yet, when congenital lethal abnormalities are excluded (Rush et al 1976, Hernández-García 1988), it carries a perinatal mortality rate 20 times greater than term delivery. Due to the high incidence of perinatal mortality and morbidity in preterm delivery (see Ch. 51), the prevention of preterm labour is a major aim of modern obstetrics. While total prevention seems impossible, for this would require the elimination of every complication of pregnancy (hypertension, multiple pregnancies, antepartum haemorrhage, infection, etc.), there is no doubt that improved methods of predicting the onset of term and especially preterm labour would have a great impact on neonatal outcome.

Measurement of uterine contractility in pregnancy

Surprisingly little is known about the relationship between uterine contractility in pregnancy and gestational age at the onset of labour. Caldeyro Barcia (1959), who made direct measurements of amniotic pressure, showed that spontaneous activity was low until the 30th week of gestation and then gradually increased in late pregnancy. The increased contractility associated with spontaneous labour at term developed suddenly and increased rapidly to delivery.

Anderson & Turnbull (1968) measured spontaneous uterine contractility and oxytocin sensitivity in patients prior to therapeutic abortion in the second trimester. Uterine activity was measured directly via a transabdominal catheter recording amniotic fluid pressure. Up to the 18th week of pregnancy no spontaneous uterine contractions were recorded in any patient studied, irrespective of age or parity; however, from the 20th week onwards uterine activity was always present. Furthermore, there was a sudden increase in the sensitivity of the uterus to the intravenous infusion of oxytocin soon after the 20th week of gestation (Fig. 46.2).

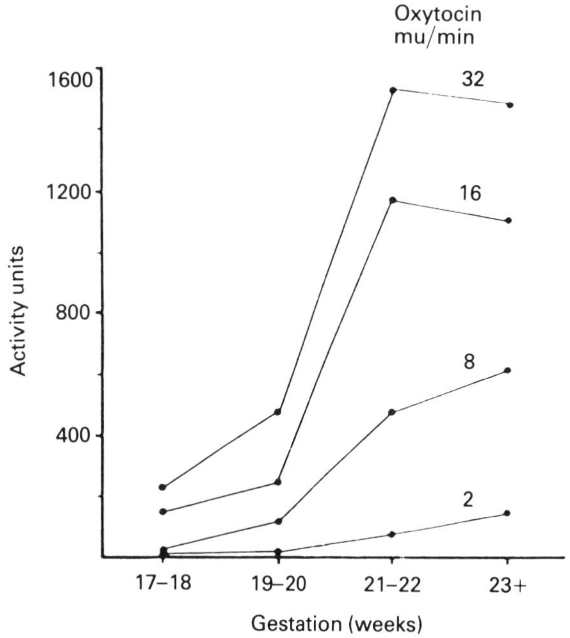

Fig. 46.2 Mean uterine response in activity units to oxytocin infusion (2, 8, 16 and 32 mu/min) in mid-pregnancy. From Anderson & Turnbull (1968), with permission.

Turnbull & Anderson (1969) extended these studies to the second half of human pregnancy. They made external recordings of contractions for 1 hour every 2 weeks from the 28th week to the onset of labour and related their findings to the duration of pregnancy at spontaneous labour. All patients had normal pregnancies, with no doubt about the menstrual dates, and subsequent labour was of spontaneous onset, the product of contraction intensity and frequency was expressed as activity units.

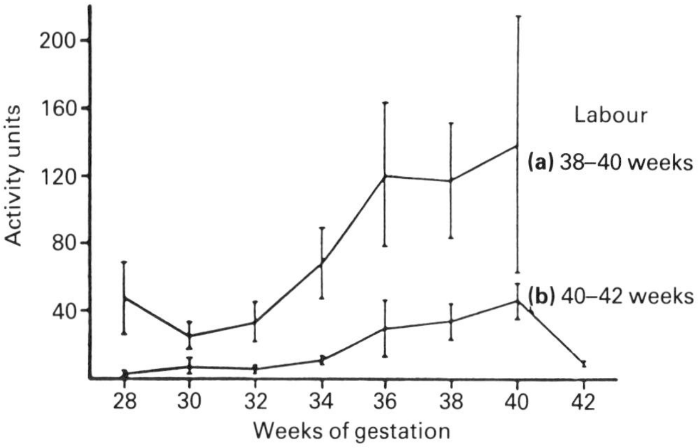

Fig. 46.3 Mean and standard error of uterine activity units from the 28th week of pregnancy in two groups of 14 patients in whom the spontaneous onset of labour was (**a**) between 38 and 40 weeks and (**b**) between 40 and 42 weeks. After Turnbull & Anderson (1968).

As Figure 46.3 shows, in women in whom labour began at 38–40 weeks (up to 15 days before term) consistently high levels of uterine activity were found from the 28th week onwards; uterine activity rose steeply between 32 and 36 weeks' gestation but then little more before the onset of labour. In women in whom labour did not commence until 40–42 weeks (up to 11 days after term), uterine activity was generally low during pregnancy (Fig. 46.3). In women in whom an intensive study of uterine contractility was made daily for 1 hour for an average of 14 days before the spontaneous onset of labour, no progressive increase in uterine contractility was found as the onset of labour approached; 24 hours before labour there was still no warning of its impending onset in terms of increased uterine contractility. Katz et al (1986) measured antepartum uterine activity in ambulatory patients expecting different data from those of studies in recumbent patients. However, their findings were comparable with those reported by other investigators who monitored prelabour uterine contractions with conventional stationary monitors; 50% of women with normal pregnancies have a high level of uterine activity but do not deliver

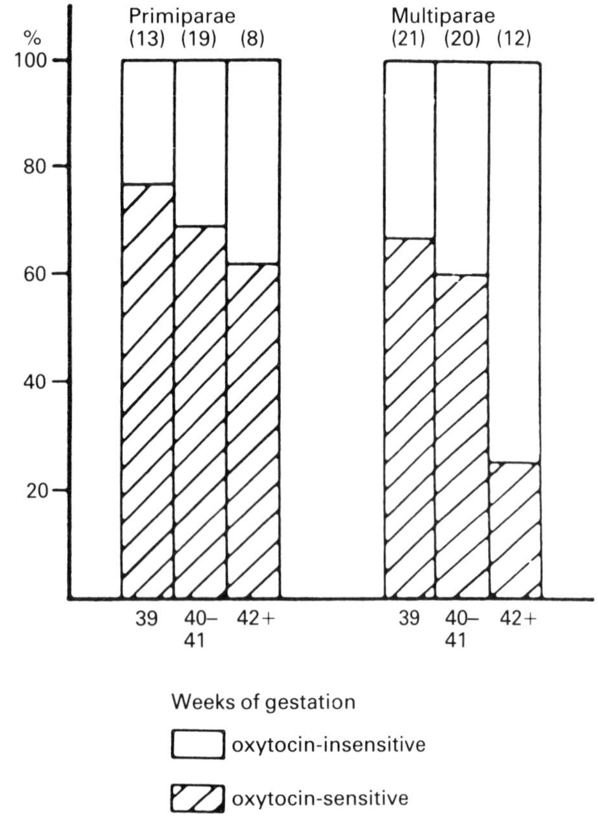

Fig. 46.4 The percentage of primiparae and multiparae sensitive to oxytocin before induction of labour up to the 39th week, at 40th and 41st week and at the 42nd week or later. The number of patients in each group is shown at the top of each column. After Turnbull & Anderson (1968).

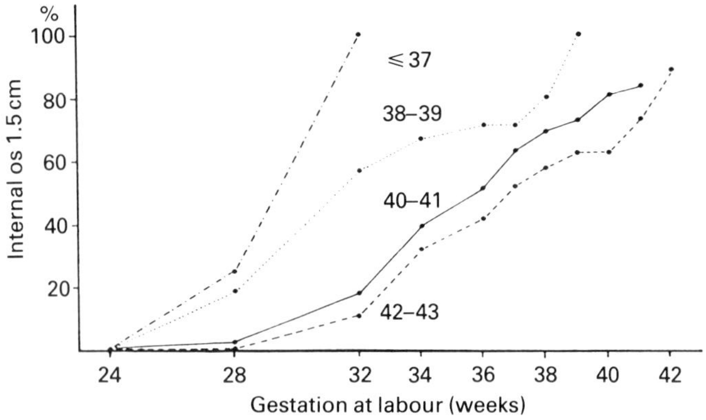

Fig. 46.5 Cumulative percentage of primigravidae in whom the internal cervical os admitted 1.5 cm from the 24th week of pregnancy, in relation to gestation at labour. After Anderson & Turnbull (1969).

until 38 weeks or later. Hence, it is difficult to distinguish them from the much smaller group of women actually destined to deliver preterm.

Turnbull & Anderson (1968) measured uterine oxytocin sensitivity in women immediately before surgical induction of labour, and as Figure 46.4 shows, oxytocin sensitivity is clearly lower in women being induced for prolonged pregnancy at 42 weeks or more, especially multiparous women. These findings are in accord with the results in Figure 46.3, which show that in pregnancy destined to be prolonged, uterine contractility is low, while in pregnancy likely to end before term, uterine contractility is much greater. Since oxytocin sensitivity is related to spontaneous uterine contractility, the former group would be likely to show lower oxytocin sensitivity.

Caldeyro Barcia & Sereno (1981), using intrauterine catheters, also noted that the response of the uterus to oxytocin increased as pregnancy advanced, reaching a maximum value between 32 and 36 weeks. Later, Takahashi et al (1980) confirmed these findings with oxytocin challenge tests, using external tocodynamometry, and showed that oxytocin sensitivity was significantly increased in women who went into spontaneous labour before 38 weeks and decreased in those who started labour after 42 weeks' gestation.

Overall, the available data indicate that there is a clear increase in uterine contractility in pregnant women in the second half of human pregnancy, especially from 32 to 36 weeks, but measurement of uterine contractility is not a reliable parameter for predicting the spontaneous onset of labour. Nevertheless, the increased sensitivity to oxytocin in women who go on to deliver after spontaneous preterm labour suggests that oxytocin hypersensitivity might be implicated in the aetiology of uncomplicated preterm labour. It is of interest that preliminary studies show that uncomplicated preterm labour can be stopped with oxytocin antagonists (Åkerlund et al 1987). The increase in the sensitivity of the human uterus to oxytocin with advancing gestation and in preterm labour is probably the result of increased oxytocin receptor concentrations (Fuchs & Fuchs 1984) and maturation of the signal transduction mechanism (Fig. 46.1), together with the increases in the functional and catalytic proteins necessary for the contractile process, and gap junction formation (Ch. 12).

Cervical dilatation and length of gestation

Anderson & Turnbull (1969) investigated the relationship between the state of the cervix and uterine contractility during pregnancy, in relation to gestational age at spontaneous labour. They investigated healthy primigravidae with 'certain' menstrual data, with single fetuses presenting by the vertex. Dilatation of the external and internal os and the length of the cervical canal were assessed by vaginal examination at various intervals from the 24th week of pregnancy onwards. Uterine activity was measured in the same women with an external tocodynamometer over 1 hour at the 36th week and expressed as activity units. In some women, biopsies from the anterior cervical lip were taken immediately following completion of the third stage of labour and the amount of collagen in the cervix (measured as hydroxyproline) was estimated.

Figure 46.5 shows the cumulative percentage of patients

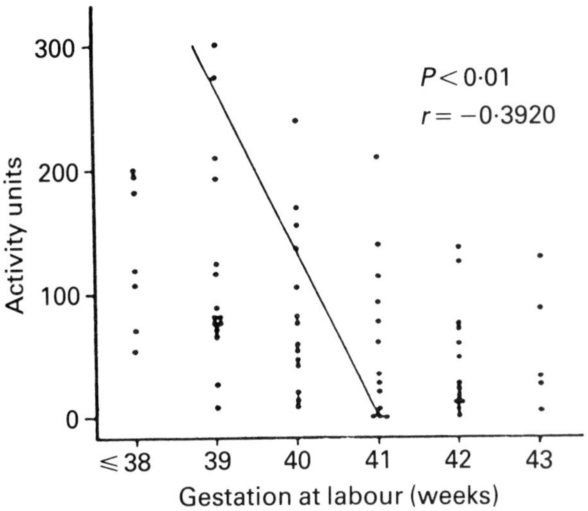

Fig. 46.6 Level of uterine activity units in primigravidae at the 36th week of pregnancy in relation to gestation at labour. After Anderson & Turnbull (1969).

in whom the internal cervical os was dilated to 1.5 cm at various intervals from the 24th week of pregnancy, in relation to the subsequent onset of labour. It can be clearly seen that differences in cervical dilatation depend on the gestation at subsequent spontaneous labour. For example, at the 32nd week the internal os admitted 1.5 cm in 100% of those who subsequently delivered before 38 weeks, but only in 10% of those who delivered after the 41st week. Conversely, of primigravidae with a closed cervix at 32 weeks, only 17% were later delivered before the 40th week, and in 32% pregnancy continued until the 42nd week or later whereas of primigravidae whose internal os at 32 weeks admitted 1.5 cm, labour later started spontaneously before the 40th week in 67% and after 42 weeks or more in only 8%.

There was a highly significant negative correlation ($r =$ 0.39, $P < 0.01$) between the activity of the uterus at the 36th week of pregnancy and gestation at the subsequent onset of labour (Fig. 46.6). Uterine contractility related to the ripeness of the cervix only in some circumstances; for example, in women in whom the fetal head had engaged by the 36th week and in whom the internal os had been 1.5 cm dilated for at least 4 weeks, uterine activity at 36 weeks was 107 ± 25 activity units; if the cervix had remained closed, the level of uterine activity was only 66 ± 15.

There was no relationship between the amount of hydroxyproline in the cervix obtained after delivery of the baby and the clinical state of the cervix before labour started, activity of the uterus at the 36th week, the gestation at the onset of labour or the length of labour. This lack of correlation between the clinical assessment of the cervix and the concentration of cervical hydroxyproline suggests that, as mentioned earlier, dissociation rather than dissolution of cervical collagen fibres may be responsible for effacement and dilatation of the cervix in late pregnancy (Ellwood & Anderson 1981).

In summary, the results of Turnbull & Anderson (1968) suggested that although dilatation of the internal os after the 28th week of pregnancy was related to the time of onset of labour, it was not possible consistently to identify cases in which labour would commence so early as to be pathological and endanger the baby, even if there was additional information about the level of uterine activity. Nevertheless, Leveno et al (1986) reported recently that in women between 26 and 30 weeks' gestation with a cervical dilatation of 2 or 3 cm, the incidence of delivery before 34 weeks was 27%, compared with only 2% in women with less than 1 cm cervical dilatation. They concluded that early third trimester cervical examination could be an important adjunct in identifying women at risk for preterm labour. Papiernik et al (1986), in a large series of women examined at least once before 37 weeks' gestation, found the relative risk for preterm delivery to be approximately four times greater if the maternal os was opened 1 cm or more. Almost one-quarter of the 4.4% of the population found to have this dilatation of the internal cervical os between 25 and 28 weeks' gestation experienced preterm birth.

Oestrogens and progesterone

Turnbull et al (1967) investigated the relationship between urinary oestriol, oestrone and pregnandiol at the 34th and 37th weeks of gestation in relation to the subsequent onset of labour in healthy primigravidae having a normal pregnancy. Urinary oestriol was measured because it was shown that, by midpregnancy, 70% of maternal oestriol excretion is derived from fetal precursors. Oestrone production involves the fetus, but to a lesser extent than oestriol, while pregnandiol, the excretion product of progesterone, is an entirely placental product.

As shown in Figure 46.7, there was a significant negative correlation between oestriol excretion at 34 weeks and gestation at the subsequent onset of labour. The correlation was reversed for oestrone, i.e. the higher the urinary oestriol excretion and the lower the oestrone at the 34th week, the nearer in time was delivery (Fig. 46.8). There was no correlation between urinary pregnandiol and gestation at delivery. By the 37th week there was still a significant negative correlation between oestriol excretion and gestation at the onset of labour. As described in Chapter 12, these findings were interpreted as suggesting a rapid rate of oestrogen metabolism within the fetoplacental unit by a fetus whose delivery was reasonably imminent, thus supporting the concept of a fetal contributory role in timing the onset of human labour. More recently, Darne et al (1987) have reported that salivary oestriol : progesterone ratios (salivary steroids represent the free, not protein bound, steroid fraction in plasma) in late pregnancy increased markedly before spontaneous labour and might predict preterm labour. Subsequently, however,

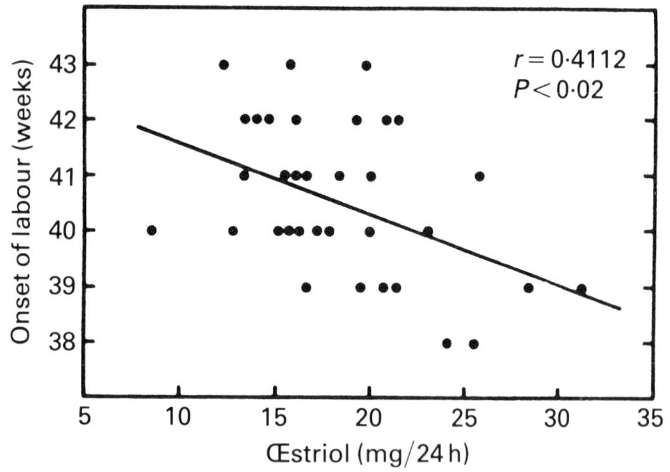

Fig. 46.7 Urinary oestriol excretion at the 34th week of pregnancy in relation to gestation at onset of labour. From Turnbull et al (1967), with permission.

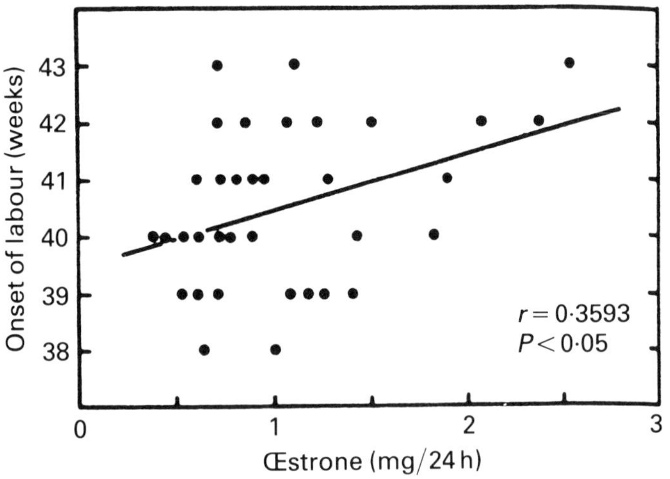

Fig. 46.8 Urinary oestrone excretion at the 34th week of pregnancy in relation to gestation at onset of labour. From Turnbull et al (1967), with permission.

Lewis et al (1987) failed to confirm this, using similar methodology although in a much smaller number of women.

The placenta synthesizes a number of peptides resembling hypothalamic and pituitary hormones, both in structure and function. These include thyrotrophin releasing hormone (TRH), luteinizing hormone releasing hormone (LHRH), growth hormone releasing hormone (GHRH) and corticotrophin releasing factor (CRF), as well as ACTH, hCG, hPL and others. CRF is a 41-amino acid peptide originally isolated from sheep hypothalami which stimulates the release of ACTH from the anterior pituitary, which in turn stimulates cortisol secretion from the adrenal gland. CRF has recently been measured by several groups in maternal plasma in the second half of gestation as a predictive test for the onset of labour (Sasaki et al 1987, Goland et al 1986, Campbell et al 1987). Wolfe et al (1988), using a direct two-site

Table 46.1 Levels of corticotrophin-releasing factor (CRF) (pg/ml) in normal and complicated pregnancies. After Wolfe et al (1988)

Patients	Gestational age (weeks)			
	< 28	30–32	34–36	38–40
Normal pregnancies *n* (48–83)	20	60	351	1126
Twin pregnancies *n* (3–12)	87*	505*	1935*	1597
Diabetic pregnancies *n* (15–61)	26	141	522	1126
Pregnancy induced hypertension *n* (14–45)	68†	840†	1253†	1896†
Pre-term labour *n* (10–14)	86†	320†	1198†	—

Results are median values of CRF (pg/ml) in unextracted maternal plasma. *n* = number of samples, *P* value * < 0.01 † < 0.001.

immunoradiometric assay, which depends on the use of two antibodies directed to opposite ends of CRF-41 and consequently detects only intact molecules and not peptide fragments, found that CRF values in normal pregnancy rose dramatically in the third trimester from a median of 20 pg/ml at 28 weeks to 1320 pg/ml at 40 weeks (Table 46.1). The median value in labour was 1732 pg/ml, but there was no progressive rise during the course of labour. CRF levels were elevated in twin pregnancies, in women with pregnancy-induced hypertension and in women admitted in preterm labour or with premature rupture of the membranes and who delivered before 37 weeks (Table 46.1). The elevated levels of CRF in some women weeks before the onset of preterm labour raises the possibility of its clinical application for the prediction of preterm labour. Prospective controlled studies of the value of maternal CRF estimation for the prediction of preterm labour could be of great interest.

Another placental product which could become a potential marker to predict the spontaneous onset of term and preterm labour is pregnancy-associated major basic protein (MBP). This protein, isolated from human placenta, is chemically identical to the major basic protein in eosinophils. Preliminary data from Coulam et al (1987) show that MBP rises steeply in maternal plasma from 35 to 40 weeks' gestation. In women with idiopathic preterm labour, increases in MBP began 3–4 weeks prior to delivery thus raising the possibility of its clinical use to identify women at risk of preterm labour.

Fetal breathing movements

As pointed out earlier, preterm birth will only be prevented when every complication of pregnancy has been resolved. Several surveys in Britain (summarized by Turnbull 1988) show that neonatal mortality is relatively low in idiopathic or uncomplicated preterm labour compared with complicated preterm labour. Our data from Oxford (López Bernal et al 1988) show that uncomplicated preterm labour tends to occur around 32–34 weeks, when the chances of good-quality neonatal survival are very high. However, preterm labour complicated by chorioamnionitis or antepartum haemorrhage tends to occur at least 4 weeks earlier, and neonatal mortality is much higher because the newborns are extremely premature. The prevention of preterm labour complicated with chorioamnionitis may well require aggressive management (MacGregor 1988) with potent and safe anti-inflammatory drugs, antibiotics and prostaglandin synthesis inhibitors, especially those with additional inhibitory effects on myometrial prostaglandin receptors (Rees et al 1988).

However, when the outcome of uncomplicated preterm labour is now so good, it is essential that medical intervention in preterm labour should be clearly indicated and should do no harm. Castle & Turnbull (1983) pioneered the use of real-time ultrasound scanning of fetal breathing movements (FBM) for the diagnosis of preterm labour. The fetus makes intermittent breathing movements during the second half of pregnancy and the frequency of FBM diminishes considerably 24 to 36 hours before the onset of labour in both man (Boddy et al 1979) and sheep (Dawes 1973). The mechanism behind the inhibition of fetal breathing with approaching labour is not known, but experiments in sheep show that it is related to the fall in placental progesterone output before labour (Parkes et al 1988), but it is possible that a rise in fetal plasma prostaglandin levels may also be involved.

The diagnosis of preterm labour can be difficult, since in 50% of women admitted with intact membranes and without haemorrhage it actually subsides and the pregnancy may continue towards term (Anderson 1981). In other cases, however, premature labour is associated with potentially dangerous complications, and early delivery is the safest both for mother and baby. Castle & Turnbull (1983) demonstrated that if, in women admitted in uncomplicated preterm labour, FBM were demonstrable for at least 20 seconds within 1 hour, labour would subside and the pregnancy continue in the great majority of cases. If, however, FBM were undetectable in 1 hour, labour was likely to progress to delivery. These findings have been confirmed by several groups (Boylan et al 1985, Jaschevatzky et al 1986, Augustsson & Patel 1987, Bessinger et al 1987). Of course, this chapter is not concerned with the management of preterm labour, which is dealt with in Chapter 51, but these observations illustrate a practical application of how knowledge of fetal physiology relates to the progression of labour.

CONCLUSIONS

Successful parturition results from the establishment of intermittent but regular and effective uterine contractions and the ripening and dilatation of the cervix. The control of uterine contractility is not completely understood but oxytocin and prostaglandins play prominent roles (see Ch. 12). Second messenger pathways involving phosphoinositide hydrolysis in myometrial cell membranes may provide the link between oxytocin–prostaglandin interactions and the stimulation of uterine contractility.

Cervical ripening results from a decrease in collagen cross-links and by changes in the glycosaminoglycans of the ground substance.

In human pregnancy, the uterus appears to be quiescent during most of the first 20 weeks. From the 28th week onwards, uterine contractions of approximately 5–10 mmHg amniotic fluid pressure can be recorded and occur at a frequency of 1–5 per hour.

During the last 8–10 weeks of pregnancy, there is a gradual increase in uterine contractility but the rate of increase is related to the gestation at which labour ultimately commences. In women whose labour starts between 38 weeks and full term, uterine activity rises steeply between 32 and 36 weeks and remains at a high level thereafter; if labour is to start after term, between 40 and 42 weeks, there is relatively little uterine activity during pregnancy.

Neither the spontaneous contractility of the uterus nor its sensitivity to oxytocin within the last few weeks, days or even hours of pregnancy clearly forecasts the impending onset of labour.

In primigravidae, cervical dilatation and effacement during pregnancy relate to the time in gestation at which labour will start. At 32 weeks, for example, the internal cervical os was 1.5 cm dilated in all women who were subsequently delivered before the 38th week but in only 10% of women who delivered after the 41st week.

During first pregnancies, cervical dilatation and effacement are closely related to the level of uterine contractility. Changes in the biochemical state of the cervix seem to be less important in detecting these changes than uterine contractility since the concentration of hydroxyproline in the cervix did not relate to gestation at labour, nor to the physical state of the cervix during pregnancy.

In normal primigravidae, the higher the urinary oestriol and the lower the oestrone at both the 34th and 37th week, the nearer was delivery. There was no association between pregnandiol secretion at 34 or 37 weeks and gestation at delivery. These findings provide indirect support for the concept that the fetus makes some contribution to the timing of the onset of human labour. Measurements of corticotrophin releasing factor (CRF) and major basic protein (MBP) in maternal plasma may help to predict the spontaneous onset of term and preterm labour, and real time ultrasound assessment of fetal breathing movements is useful for the early diagnosis of impending premature labour.

In Chapter 12 the evidence is reviewed that the onset of human labour does not depend on activation of the fetal pituitary–adrenal axis, as occurs in the sheep and other ruminants. Nevertheless, the relationship between maternal oestrogen excretion and labour onset suggests that some aspect of human fetal physiology, related to oestriol excretion, influences the evolution of increasing uterine contractility, cervical dilatation and the onset of labour.

REFERENCES

Agustsson P, Patel N B 1987 The predictive value of fetal breathing movements in the diagnosis of preterm labour. British Journal of Obstetrics and Gynaecology 94: 860–863

Åkerlund M, Strömberg P, Hauksson A et al 1987 Inhibition of uterine contractions of premature labour with an oxytocin analogue. Results from a pilot study. British Journal of Obstetrics and Gynaecology 94: 1040–1044

Anderson A B M 1981 Second thoughts on stopping preterm labour. In: Studd J (ed) Progress in Obstetrics and Gynaecology, vol 1, pp 125–138

Anderson A B M, Turnbull A C 1968 Spontaneous contractility and oxytocin sensitivity of the human uterus in mid-pregnancy. Journal of Obstetrics and Gynaecology of the British Commonwealth 75: 271–277

Anderson A B M, Turnbull A C 1969 Relationship between length of gestation and cervical dilatation, uterine contractility and other factors during pregancy. American Journal of Obstetrics and Gynecology 105: 1207–1214

Arulkumaran S, Gibb D M F, Ratnam S S, Kun K C, Heng S H 1985 Total uterine activity in induced labour — an index of cervical and pelvic tissue resistance. British Journal of Obstetrics and Gynaecology 92: 693–697

Berridge M J 1984 Inositol trisphosphate and diacylglycerol as second messengers. Biochemical Journal 220: 345–360

Bessinger R E, Compton A A, Hiyashi R H 1987 The presence or absence of fetal breathing movement as a predictor of outcome in preterm labor. American Journal of Obstetrics and Gynecology 157: 753–757

Boddy K, Dawes G S, Robinson J 1979 In: Gluck L (ed) Intrauterine fetal breathing movements, Modern Perinatal Medicine. Medical Year Book, Chicago, pp 381–390

Boylan P, O'Donovan P, Owen O J 1985 Fetal breathing movements and the onset of labor. A prospective analysis of 100 cases. Obstetrics and Gynecology 66: 517–520

Calder A A, Embrey M P, Tait T 1977 Ripening of the cervix with extra amniotic prostaglandin E_2 in viscous gel before induction of labour at term. British Journal of Obstetrics and Gynaecology 84: 264–268

Caldeyro Barcia R 1959 Uterine contractility in obstetrics. Proceedings of the Second International Congress of Gynecology and Obstetrics, vol 1, Montreal, p 65

Caldeyro Barcia R, Sereno J A 1981 The response of the human uterus to oxytocin throughout pregnancy. In: Caldeyro Barcia R, Heller H (eds) Oxytocin. Pergamon, Oxford, p 177

Caldeyro Barcia R, Sica-Blanco Y, Poseiro J J et al 1957 A quantitative study of the action of synthetic oxytocin on the pregnant uterus. Journal of Pharmacology and Experimental Therapeutics 121: 18–31

Campbell E A, Linton E A, Wolfe C D A, Scraggs P R, Jones M T, Lowry P J 1987 Plasma corticotrophin-releasing hormone concentrations during pregnancy and parturition. Journal of Clinical Endocrinology and Metabolism 64: 1054–1059

Carsten M E, Miller J D 1987 A new look at uterine muscle contraction. American Journal of Obstetrics and Gynecology 157: 1303–1315

Castle B M, Turnbull A C 1983 The presence or absence of fetal breathing movements predicts the outcome of preterm labour. Lancet ii: 471–473

Coulam C B, Wasmoen T, Creasy R, Siiteri P, Gleich G 1987 Major basic protein as a predictor of preterm labor: a preliminary report. Clinical Journal of Obstetrics and Gynecology 156: 790–796

Danforth D N 1983 The morphology of the human cervix. Clinical Obstetrics and Gynecology 26: 7–13

Darne J, McGarrigle H H G, Lachelin G C L 1987 Saliva oestriol, oestradiol, oestrone and progesterone levels in pregnancy: spontaneous labour at term is preceded by a rise in the saliva oestriol: progesterone ratios. British Journal of Obstetrics and Gynaecology 94: 227–235

Dawes G S 1973 Fetal physiology and the onset of labour. Memoirs of the Society in Endocrinology 20: 25–36

Duignam N 1985 Active management of labour. In: Studd J (ed) The management of labour, Blackwell Scientific, Oxford, pp 146–158

Eddie L W, Bell R J, Lester A et al 1986 Radioimmunoassay of relaxin in pregnancy with an analogue of human relaxin. Lancet i: 1344–1346

Ekman G, Malmström A, Uldbjerg N, Ulmsten U 1986 Cervical collagen: an important regulator of cervical function in term labor. Obstetrics and Gynecology 67: 633–636

Ellwood D A, Anderson A B M 1981 The cervix in pregnancy and labour. Churchill Livingstone, Edinburgh, p 273

Ellwood D A, Mitchell M D, Anderson A B M, Turnbull A C 1980 The in vitro production of prostanoids by the human cervix during pregnancy: preliminary observations. British Journal of Obstetrics and Gynaecology 87: 210–214

Fairlie F M, Phillips G F, Andrews B J, Calder A A 1988 An analysis of uterine activity in spontaneous labour using a microcomputer. British Journal of Obstetrics and Gynaecology 95: 57–64

Friedman E A 1954 The graphic analysis of labor. American Journal of Obstetrics and Gynecology 68: 1568–1575

Fuchs A R, Fuchs F 1984 Endocrinology of human parturition: a review. British Journal of Obstetrics and Gynaecology 91: 948–967

Goland R S, Wardlaw S L, Stark R I, Brown L S, Frantz A G 1986 High levels of corticotrophin releasing hormone immunoreactivity in maternal and fetal plasma during pregnancy. Journal of Clinical Endocrinology and Metabolism 63: 1199–1203

Hashimoto T, Hirata M, Itoh T, Kanmura Y, Kuriyama H 1986 Inositol 1,4,5-trisphosphate activates pharmacomechanical coupling in smooth muscle of the rabbit mesenteric artery. Journal of Physiology 370: 605–618

Hernández-Garcia J M, De la Fuente P, Puyol P, Sotelo M T et al 1988 Mortalidad perinatal. Estudio de la repercusión de diversos factores. Clinical Investigation in Gynecology and Obstetrics 15: 199–212

Jaschevatzky O, Ellenbogen A, Anderman S, Frisch L, Moy Y, Grunsten S 1986 The predictive value of fetal breathing movements in the outcome of premature labour. British Journal of Obstetrics and Gynaecology 93: 1256–1258

Katz M, Gill P J, Newman R B 1986 Detection of preterm labor by ambulatory monitoring of uterine activity for the management of oral tocolysis. American Journal of Obstetrics and Gynecology 154: 1253–1256

Kitamura K, Ito A, Mori Y 1980 The existing forms of collagenase in the human uterine cervix. Journal of Biochemistry (Tokyo) 87: 753–760

Ledger W L, Webster M, Harrison L P, Anderson A B M, Turnbull A C 1985 Increase in cervical extensibility during labor induced after isolation of the cervix from the uterus in pregnant ewes. American Journal of Obstetrics and Gynecology 115: 397–402

Leveno K J, Cox K, Roark M L 1986 Cervical dilatation and prematurity revisited. Obstetrics and Gynecology 68: 434–435

Lewis P R, Galvin P M, Short R V 1987 Salivary oestriol and progesterone concentrations in women during late pregnancy, parturition and the puerperium. Journal of Endocrinology 115: 177–181

López Bernal A, Hansell D J, Khong T Y, Keeling J W, Turnbull A C 1988 Marked differences in gestational age and prostaglandin E production by the fetal membranes in unexplained preterm labour compared with complicated preterm labour associated with chorioamnionitis (submitted for publication)

MacLennan A H, Green R C, Grant P, Nicolson R 1986 Ripening of the human cervix and induction of labor with intracervical purified porcine relaxin. Obstetrics and Gynecology 68: 598–601

MacKenzie I Z, Embrey M P 1977 Cervical ripening with intravaginal prostaglandin E_2 gel. British Medical Journal ii: 1381–1384

Marsten J B, Smith C W J 1985 The thin filaments of smooth muscles. Journal of Muscle Research and Cell Motility 6: 669–708

McGregor J A 1988 Prevention of preterm birth: new initiatives based on microbial-host interactions. Obstetrics and Gynecological Survey 43: 1–14

Michell R H 1987 How do receptors at the cell surface send signals to the cell interior? British Medical Journal 295: 1320–1323

Nonomura Y, Ebashi S 1980 Calcium regulatory mechanism in vertebrate smooth muscle. Biomedical Research 1: 1–12

Owman C H, Rosengren E, Sjöberg N O 1967 Adrenergic innervation of the human female reproductive organs: a histochemical and chemical investigation. Obstetrics and Gynecology 30: 763–773

Papiernik E, Bouyer J, Collin D, Winisdoerffer G, Dreyfus J 1986 Precocious cervical ripening and preterm labor. Obstetrics and Gynecology 67: 238–252

Parkes M J, Moore P J, Hanson M A 1988 The effects of inhibition of 3β-hydroxysteroid dehydrogenase activity and steroid replacement on breathing movements and electrocortical activity in sheep fetuses in utero. Proceedings of the 15th Annual Meeting of the Society for the Study of Fetal Physiology, Cairns, Australia, p 28

Rees C M P, Cañete Soler R, López Bernal A, Turnbull A C 1988 Effect

of fenamates on prostaglandin E receptor binding. Lancet ii: 541–542
Rush R W, Keirse M J N C, Howat P, Baum J J, Anderson A B M, Turnbull A C 1976 Contribution of pre-term delivery to perinatal mortality. British Medical Journal ii: 965–966
Sasaki A, Shinkawa O, Margioris A N et al 1987 Immunoreactive corticotropin releasing hormone in human plasma during pregnancy, labor and delivery. Journal of Clinical Endocrinology and Metabolism 64: 224–229
Schrey M P, Read A M, Steer P J 1986 Oxytocin and vasopressin stimulate inositol phosphate production in human gestational myometrium and decidua cells. Bioscience Reports 6: 613–619
Schrey M P, Read A M, Steer P J 1987 Stimulation of phospholipid hydrolysis and arachidonic acid mobilisation in human uterine decidua cells by phorbol ester. Biochemical Journal 246: 705–713
Schwalm H, Dubrauszky V 1966 The structure of the musculature of the human uterus-muscles and connective tissue. American Journal of Obstetrics and Gynecology 94: 391–404
Sellers S M, Hodgson H T, Mitchell M D, Anderson A B M, Turnbull A C 1982 Raised prostaglandin levels in the third stage of labor. American Journal of Obstetrics and Gynecology 144: 209–212
Takahashi K, Diamond F, Bieniarz T, Yen H, Burd L 1980 Uterine contractility and oxytocin sensitivity in preterm, term and post-term pregnancy. American Journal of Obstetrics and Gynecology 136: 774–779
Turnbull A C 1988 The early diagnosis of impending premature labour. European Journal of Obstetrics and Gynaecology (in press)
Turnbull A C, Anderson A B M 1968 Uterine contractility and oxytocin sensitivity during human pregnancy in relation to the onset of labour. Journal of Obstetrics and Gynaecology of the British Commonwealth 75: 278–288
Turnbull A C, Anderson A B M, Wilson G R 1967 Maternal urinary oestrogen excretion as evidence of a fetal role in determining gestation at labour. Lancet ii: 627–629
Uldbjerg N, Ekman G, Herltoft P, Malmström A, Ulmsten U, Wingerup L 1983a Human cervical connective tissue and its reaction to prostaglandin E_2. Acta Obstetricia et Gynecologica Scandinavica Supplement 113: 163–166
Uldbjerg N, Ulmsten U, Ekman G 1983b The ripening of the human uterine cervix in terms of connective tissue biochemistry. Clinical Obstetrics and Gynecology 26: 14–26
Uldbjerg N, Ekman G, Malmström A, Olsson K, Ulmsten U 1983c Ripening of the human uterine cervix related to changes in collagen, glycosaminoglycans and collagenolytic activity. Clinical Journal of Obstetrics and Gynecology 147: 662–666
van der Rest M 1980 Collagen and its metabolism. In: Naftolin F, Stubblefield P (eds) Dilatation of the cervix. Raven, New York, pp 61–78
Walker J 1962 In: Baird D (ed) Combined textbook of obstetrics and gynaecology, 7th edn. Livingstone, Edinburgh, p 159
Wilson T, Liggins G C, Whittaker D J 1988 Oxytocin stimulates the release of arachidonic acid and prostaglandin $F_{2\alpha}$ from human decidual cells. Prostaglandins 35: 771–780
Wolfe C D A, Patel S P, Linton E A et al 1988 Plasma corticotrophin-releasing factor (CRF) in abnormal pregnancy. British Journal of Obstetrics and Gynaecology 95: 1003–1006

47

John Malvern

The clinical management of labour

During the past two decades in the UK there has been no medical subject that has captured such publicity as that of the management and mismanagement of labour (British Medical Journal Leading Article 1986, Dyer 1986). This topic, highlighted, usually inaccurately, by extremists has thrust itself into newsprint and on to the television screen almost daily. It has become a major theme of medical litigation, even reaching the House of Lords (Times Law Report 1980) and on occasions has led to banner-waving marches. As a result, division and dissension have arisen between midwives, obstetricians and natural childbirth enthusiasts. Cliques have developed and the pregnant mother has become more than a little disillusioned.

Despite the great heat created by the controversies of domiciliary confinement, liberal induction and the over- or underuse of monitoring and Caesarean sections, a significant degree of re-examination of certain rigid intrapartum practices has been stimulated; this has led to the modification of labour ward management and the humanizing of childbirth.

AIMS OF INTRAPARTUM CARE

1. To deliver a normal, healthy, well oxygenated, mature baby without trauma.
2. To assist a mentally prepared mother to enjoy the experience of childbirth, avoid unnecessary delay, pain or trauma and prevent the development of dehydration and infection.
3. To provide the mother and, if possible, the father with a relaxed, pleasant environment in a site staffed by competent midwives and obstetricians capable of establishing a reassuring rapport. In addition, to ensure that full technical back-up facilities are immediately at hand for monitoring. These must include immediately available anaesthetic, paediatric and pathological services, in case complications arise.

To satisfy these aims a fine balance must be struck between the high technologists and the naturalists. At one end of the spectrum is the cold, clinical, intensive care approach, with close monitoring as a theme, where the earliest detectable deviation from the norm will require prompt action, while at the other end there is the 'let us leave it all entirely to nature' approach, where supervision is misinterpreted as a form of interference.

Since it is impossible always to predict the development of a sudden intrapartum problem, even in a low-risk pregnancy, it is essential to reduce domiciliary obstetrics to a minimum and to sweeten the pill of hospitalization by encouraging visits to the various hospital departments in the antenatal period, by providing birth rooms; by the increased involvement of community midwives and general practitioners and an increased emphasis on early discharge from hospital within 12–24 hours.

THE MANAGEMENT OF LABOUR

The management of labour does not start on arrival at the hospital, nor with the onset of uterine contractions, but starts during the antenatal period with preparatory education. This ensures that the woman knows what to expect, when to ring up the hospital, when to come in, and what to bring with her. At the same time antenatal instruction should try to dispel the fears arising from the tales she may have heard of the horrific experiences of her relatives, friends and neighbours, as well as possible untoward memories of a previous pregnancy. In more enlightened centres the woman is becoming involved in the formulation of a desired personal birth plan.

The arrival at hospital

This should be both welcoming and reassuring, to allay the woman's natural anxieties. Admission should be conducted with calm efficiency, by both midwives and doctors and a full explanation given of their findings and plans for subsequent care. Nothing is more demoralizing than being abandoned alone in a cubicle with increasingly powerful labour pains and being uncertain about what will happen next.

Immediately before the admitting doctor and midwife see the woman, they should study the hospital antenatal notes and the shared-care co-operation card to form a full picture of the past history. The potential risks and possible management should have been outlined with discussed comments about the conduct of labour and the method of delivery.

General assessment

Certain features may be obvious at once and the speed of action determined accordingly, since admissions cover a spectrum of patients in all stages of labour as well as prelabour.

The recognition of labour

It can be difficult to establish the time of onset of labour and to differentiate between true and false labour. True labour is characterized by regular contractions of increasing frequency and intensity, radiating from the fundus to the lower abdomen and sometimes the back, as well as evidence of cervical thinning and dilatation. In false labour, the contractions tend to be irregular, milder and more constant in intensity, often occurring only in the lower abdomen. The loss of the bloodstained mucus plug, suggesting cervical opening, is an inconsistent sign and may have been caused by antenatal cervical assessment.

Health of the mother

The psychological and physical health of the mother should be established at an early stage. The severity of and her response to uterine contractions should be particularly noted. At the same time basic observations of temperature, blood pressure, pulse, recent urinary output and bowel activity should be enquired about. If possible, a simple dipstick urinalysis for sugar and protein should be performed.

Assessment of the fetus

Abdominal palpation should assess the overall size which should be correlated with the maturity, by history or previous ultrasound estimates. The presentation and degree of descent of the presenting part into the pelvic brim should be ascertained; this may be ascertained in fifths of the head engaged (Crichton 1974). The presence and position of the fetal heart should be auscultated initially with a Pinard stethoscope and later by external cardiotocography to ascertain the nature of the heart rate trace and its response to fetal movements and uterine contractions.

Assessment of uterine activity

The frequency, duration and intensity of uterine contractions should be determined initially by palpation and later by external tocography. This may be done in conjunction with the preliminary fetal heart monitoring.

Assessment by vaginal examination

Aseptic technique is required, particularly if there is evidence of membrane rupture. The vulva and introitus should be cleansed with chlorhexidene solution and cream. The following information should be sought and charted, so that subsequent assessments can be correlated with this baseline.

1. *Bony pelvis*. The size of the pelvic cavity and outlet should be assessed digitally to exclude any previously unsuspected disproportion. The station of the presenting fetal part can be related to bony landmarks: the number of centimetres above or below the ischial spines is noted.
2. *Orientation of the fetus*. This can be determined by palpation per vaginam of the sutures of the head if the presentation is cephalic and of the buttocks or feet if a breech. The amount of moulding and caput formation are determined, as well as how closely the presenting part is applied to the cervix. In addition, any malpresentation or prolapse of the umbilical cord should be excluded.

Assessment of the cervix

The cervical features alter during the course of labour, and so are helpful in determining progress. These include dilatation of the cervix (in centimetres), the degree of effacement or thickness (in percentages), the degree of softness or consistency and the anterior or posterior position of the cervix in relation to the presenting part.

Assessment of the vulva and vagina

This involves some determination of the rigidity of the musculature and the presence of scarring from previous surgery or trauma. In the second stage of labour this may lead to delay of descent and possible tearing. The admitting obstetrician should inspect the labia and introitus for signs of infection, e.g. herpetic ulceration.

Assessment of liquor

The fore or hind compartments of amniotic fluid may be released following rupture of the membranes as a gush, a trickle, or just a dampness, which on occasions may be confused with urine or vaginal discharge. It then becomes important to establish the nature of this fluid loss, as prolonged rupture of the membranes is associated with an increased incidence of intrauterine infection and an increased fetomaternal morbidity (Lebherz et al 1963, Fayez et al 1978). Often the amniotic fluid can be identified visually by the use of a sterile speculum, but nitrazine-soaked cotton on an applicator stick, which is pH-sensitive, changes from orange to blue in contact with the alkaline amniotic fluid and remains an unaltered orange colour in the acidic media of upper vaginal secretions. Unfortunately, false positive results are encountered in the presence of semen, alkaline urine, trichomonal vaginitis, certain soaps and antiseptics as well as blood, and occasionally false negative results are obtained when the membranes have been ruptured for a long period of time. Several studies have shown that the accuracy is over 90% and that it is a simple and practical procedure (Friedman & McElin 1969, Mills & Garrioch 1977). Other techniques for identifying amniotic fluid such as nile blue sulphate, diamine oxidase and prolactin do not seem to be superior in the accuracy of their results.

However, an important finding is the green discoloration of meconium-stained liquor, which indicates that there has been at some time relaxation of the fetal anal sphincter, which may be a sign of hypoxia (Walker 1954, 1959, Desmond et al 1957, Krebs et al 1980, Starks 1980) and thus will require a more intensive monitoring of the fetal well-being and precautionary steps to be taken to avoid bronchial aspiration at the time of delivery. Nevertheless, meconium-stained liquor is not an absolute sign of fetal distress and was only found to be associated with fetal acidaemia in 9% of cases by Coltart et al (1969). Conversely, its absence cannot be considered a reassuring sign as some hypoxic premature fetuses fail to relax their anal sphincters and thick or scanty liquor may easily be obstructed by the presenting part, preventing its recognition.

The above information should now be noted and entered on to a partogram (see Fig. 47.8b), so that the subsequent monitoring of mother and baby in labour can be graphically portrayed and any deviation from the norm readily seen and, if necessary, acted upon at an early stage (Philpott & Castle 1972, Studd 1973).

Management plan

A plan of management should now be formulated, so that the woman, midwives and doctors on the labour ward are fully aware of the proposed line of action. This must include the intensity of fetal monitoring required, the need to modify uterine activity, when to rupture the membranes and the type of analgesia or anaesthesia appropriate, if any.

THE FIRST STAGE OF LABOUR

General management

Pubic hair shaving and enemas cause more misery than benefit, although clipping of excessively long hair and encouragement to defecate, with or without the help of glycerin suppositories in early labour, may be of value.

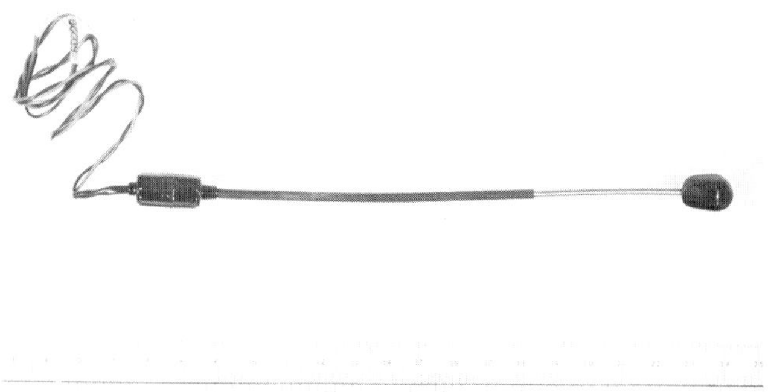

Fig. 47.1 Surgicraft Copeland reusable scalp electrode.

Food consumption should be avoided as gastric motility is diminished by analgesics such as pethidine and vomiting is more likely, with potential risks of aspiration and Mendelson's syndrome, if general anaesthetic is later required (Mendelson 1946). The mouth can be moistened by drinking small volumes of water or sucking ice. As a precautionary measure against the acid inspiration syndrome, the administration of ranitidine, 50 mg intramuscularly or 150 mg orally every 6 hours is recommended, and is superior to antacids in reducing gastric pH (Johnston et al 1982, McAuley et al 1984).

Ambulation is recommended, particularly in low-risk women in early labour, as it encourages fetal descent into the pelvis, diminishes pain by allowing the mother to adopt varying postures and is a useful form of occupational therapy (Stewart & Calder 1984). However, the woman should have her own room in the labour ward; here she can deposit her possessions and return to rest on a soft bed whenever she wishes.

Monitoring

The welfare of the fetus in labour is determined primarily by the measurement of the fetal heart rate, which reflects the oxygenation of the brain stem centres (Dawes 1968). The fetus in a higher risk category, such as one who is growth-retarded or one who has an abnormal tracing on admission in labour, should have intensive continuous assessment of the fetal heart. Thus the baseline pattern and the response to uterine contractions can be graphically monitored, using either an external ultrasound monitor, or a direct pick-up of fetal electrical signals from scalp clip (Hon 1968; Fig. 47.1, 47.2). The fetus should be considered to have entered a higher risk category and be monitored continuously if the pattern of uterine activity is found to be excessive or is altered by stimulants such as oxytocin. Similarly, if the placental bed perfusion is altered by cardiovascular

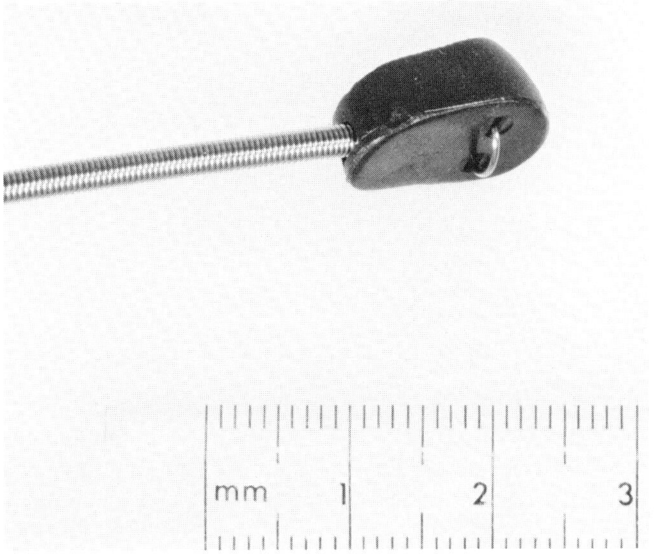

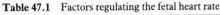

Fig. 47.2 Magnification of closed clip of scalp electrode.

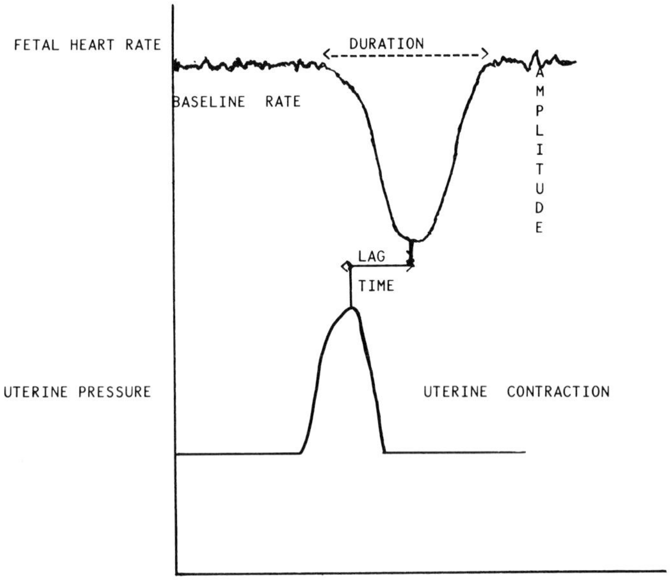

Fig. 47.3 Diagrammatic representation of a late deceleration.

Table 47.1 Factors regulating the fetal heart rate

Slowing factors	Accelerating factors
Vagal parasympathetic tone	Sympathetic tone
Sympathetic block	Vagal block (e.g. atropine)
Reduced fetal oxygenation	Maternal pyrexia, dehydration
Myocardial damage by local anaesthesia	Early hypoxia

Table 47.2 Definitions of fetal heart recording

Term used	Definition
Baseline fetal heart rate	Rate recorded between contractions
Baseline variations	Interval between R waves of continuous ECG complexes normally $>\pm5$ beats / min
Lag time	Time interval between peak of uterine contraction and lowest point of fetal heart deceleration
Early deceleration	Commences with onset of uterine contraction
Late deceleration	Onset >30 s after onset of uterine contractions
Variable deceleration	No constant relationship to onset of a uterine contraction

changes in the mother, as sometimes occurs in vena caval compression or epidural anaesthesia, continuous monitoring is wise.

On the other hand, babies in the lower risk category need not be so intensively supervised (Neutra et al 1978, Havercamp et al 1979, Klein et al 1983, MacDonald et al 1985), provided that auscultation with a Pinard stethoscope takes place immediately after the end of a contraction for about 15–30 seconds every 30 minutes in early labour and every 10–15 minutes towards the end of the first stage. This allows the woman greater mobility and freedom from the technology of electronic machinery with its wires and belts.

Recognition of fetal distress

Fetal heart rate monitoring is only of value when abnormalities are recognized and acted upon. In normal circumstances the fetal heart rate is in the range of 120–160 beats/minute, and there is a baseline variation of greater than 5 beats caused by response to vagal tone, sympathetic stimulae and catecholamines in a well oxygenated, sensitive brain stem (Table 47.1). Conversely, loss of baseline variability (less than 5 beats) is recognized by a flattening of the trace. Although this is sometimes associated with a preterm fetus who is asleep, and can be caused by certain drugs, such as diazepam, morphine and phenothiazine, it is more often associated with a blunting of the activity and sensitivity of the brain stem associated with hypoxia.

Fetal tachycardia (greater than 160 beats / min) may sometimes be associated with maternal pyrexia and dehydration, but can also be a sign of fetal distress (Tipton & Shelley 1971), particularly when associated with loss of baseline variation (Table 47.2; Fig. 47.3). Bradycardia (less than 120 beats / min) may reflect increased vagal tone, and this may sometimes arise following elevation of intracranial pressure caused by head compression during a uterine contraction (Fig. 47.4), so that the deceleration coincides with tightening of the uterine musculature (type I or type II early deceleration: the nomenclature, type I or type II deceleration, is now obsolete). In contrast, a late deceleration, developing some 30 seconds after the peak of the uterine contraction, is an indication of fetal hypoxia, and the degree and duration

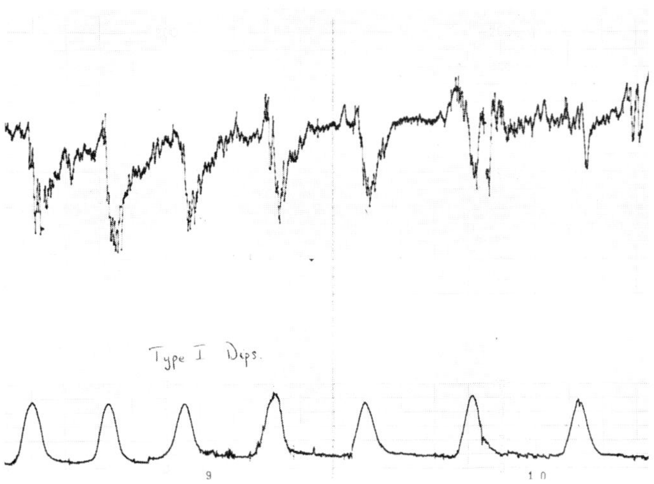

Fig. 47.4 Cardiotocographic tracing showing type I decelerations.

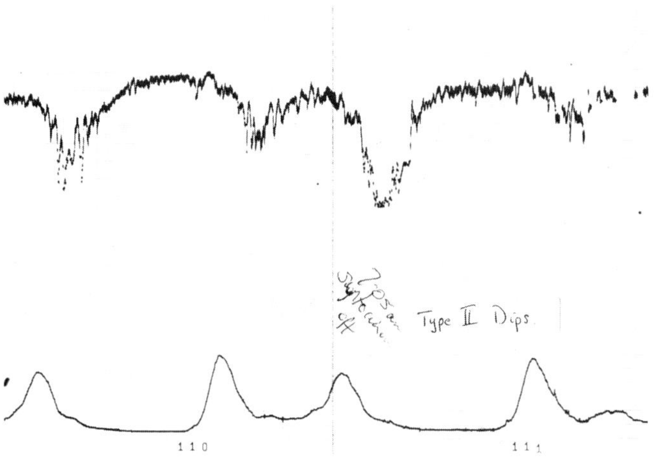

Fig. 47.5 Cardiotocographic tracing showing type II late decelerations.

of bradycardia reflects its severity (Hon 1958, 1959, 1962, 1968, Hon & Lee 1963; Fig. 47.5).

Variable decelerations, both in degree and in their relationships to the uterine contractions, may be seen in association with umbilical cord compression around the limbs or by the presenting part.

If cardiotocographic patterns indicate that the fetus may be hypoxic, it becomes essential to find the cause and to locate the site of interruption for oxygen from the outside air passing through the maternal lungs into her circulation, across the uterine wall into the placental bed and along the umbilical cord. The maternal blood pressure should be assessed and the obstetrician should ensure that the maternal posture is not causing vena caval compression, that the myometrium is not in spasm, there are no signs of abruption, and that the umbilical cord is not being compressed. Treatment may involve giving the mother oxygen by facemask; placing her in the left lateral position; stopping uterine stimulants such as oxytocin, and possibly giving uterine relaxants systemically or by inhalation, such as ritodrine hydrochloride or salbutamol. A vaginal examination is peformed to ensure that the cord is not presenting and that the patient is not further advanced in labour than was expected. If the signs of fetal distress are not so severe as to demand immediate delivery, then the significance of the abnormal fetal heart trace pattern and the severity of the hypoxia, if present, can be determined by measurement of the fetal pH in a sample of blood obtained from the fetal scalp. Acidaemia is caused by the accumulation of lactic acid which forms when glucose is broken down through the anaerobic Embden–Meyerhof pathway.

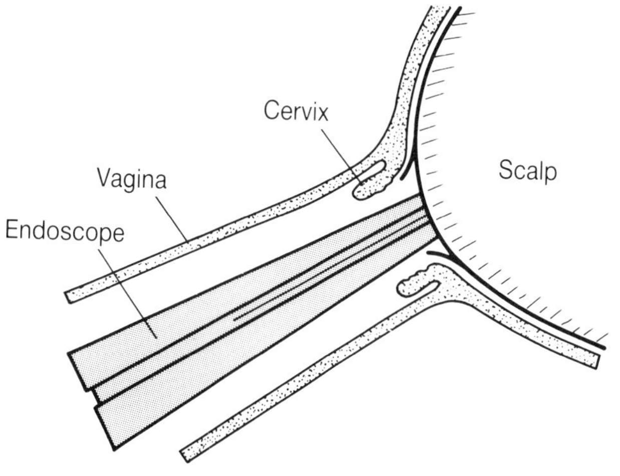

Fig. 47.6 Diagram of fetal blood sampling.

Fetal pH

The technique, initially described by Saling & Schneider (1967), involves visualizing the fetal skin by an amnioscope, passed through the dilated cervix after membrane rupture. Hyperaemia is induced using ethyl chloride spray, the fetal skin is smeared with silicone gel to encourage the formation of blood globules, and the skin punctured with a special guarded bleed; 0.4 ml of fetal blood can then be aspirated through a pre-heparinized capillary tube (Fig. 47.6, 47.7).

A pH level of less than 7.2 requires immediate delivery of the fetus, while one of 7.2–7.25 requires the test to be repeated within half an hour. A pH level greater than 7.25 needs re-evaluation only if the fetal heart trace pattern fails to improve.

Progress in labour

This is partly determined by:

1. The size of the fetus and the attitude (degree of flexion) of the presenting part.

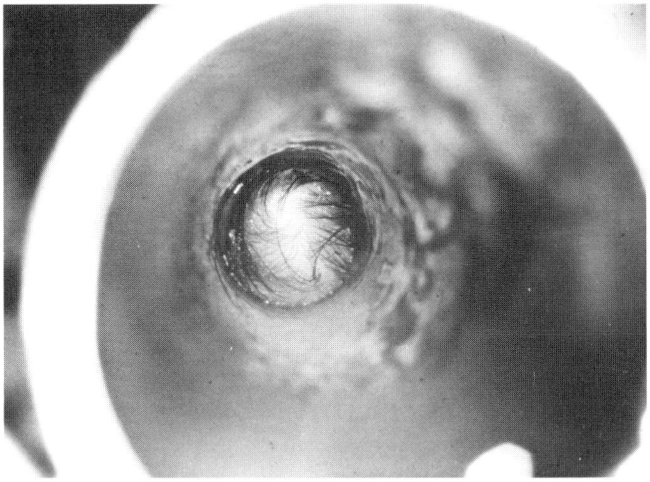

Fig. 47.7 Fetal scalp seen down amnioscope.

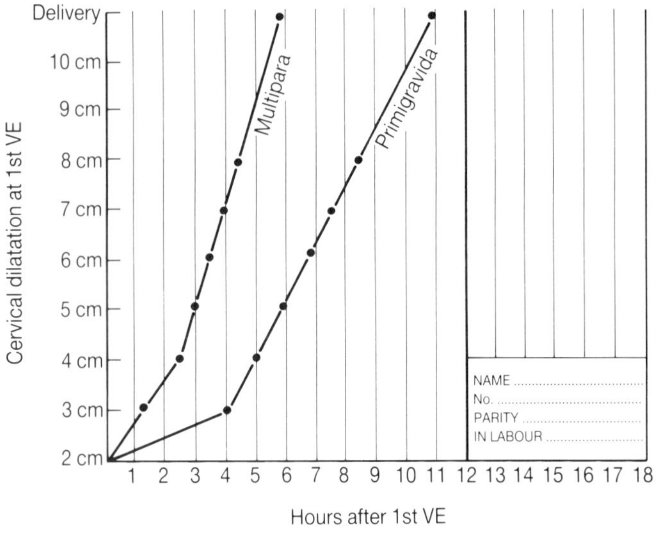

Fig. 47.8a Partograph showing cervical dilatation time curve in a normal multipara and primigravida in study at Queen Charlotte's Maternity Hospital (Beazley & Kurjak 1972).

2. The size of the pelvis and its ability to increase its diameters by sacroiliac and pubic symphyseal movement.
3. The distensibility, thickness and softness of the collagen of the cervix.
4. The strength and frequency of the uterine contractions.

The best indicators of progress are the rate of alteration of cervical diameter and the speed of the descent of the presenting part into the pelvis. Studies by Friedman (1955) noted that the cervical dilatation time curve in primigravid women is characteristically sigmoid in shape. The curve can be divided into a latent and an active phase. The former is the time taken to reach 3 cm dilatation from the onset of labour; effacement occurs during this time. The active phase is between 3 and 9 cm and dilatation takes place at the rate of 3 cm/h. In some women there is an additional deceleration phase in which the pace is slightly slower, during dilatation of the last centimetre of the first stage of labour.

Since this original work similar studies have been carried out, with the development of graphic representation of what constitutes normal labour in a primigravida (Beazley & Kurjak 1972, Philpott & Castle 1972, Studd 1973, Duignan et al 1975; Fig. 47.8a). These have become incorporated into partograms (Fig. 47.8b); their use commences on hospital admission in labour. With the help of a stencil, the relevant part of the sinusoidal curve of Friedman, based on the first noted cervical dilatation, can be pencilled on to the graph. Thus deviation from a normal primigravid labour, based on the experience of the above workers, can easily be seen and steps taken to determine and treat the cause (Fig. 47.8b).

The active management of labour

The augmentation or acceleration of uterine contractions was dramatically demonstrated in the study of 1000 primigravidae at the National Maternity Hospital, Dublin (O'Driscoll et al 1969, 1970, 1973). It was considered that cephalopelvic disproportion had in the past been over-diagnosed and amniotomy, followed by oxytocin infusion could be used to stimulate the progress of normal labour at an early stage. Cephalopelvic disproportion was found in less than 1%, the Caesarean section rate was 4%, and all patients were delivered within 24 hours.

It is recommended therefore that primigravidae in labour should be examined at least every 4 hours in order to assess the cervical dilatation and descent of the presenting part, and that this information should be plotted on a partogram, to compare the woman's progress with that of a group of normal primigravidae. If this appears to be less than that of the ideal labour, then consideration should be given to augmentation of contractions by intravenous oxytocin.

Artificial rupture of the membranes

Deliberate rupture of the membranes during the latent phase of labour does not alter its progress in any way. It is potentially dangerous if the presenting part lies high within the pelvic inlet or if the lie is unstable for umbilical cord prolapse becomes a risk. In addition, the cervix is not so uniformly pressed upon by the presenting part and a potential communication for infection is opened up between the vagina and the uterine cavity (Caldeyro-Barcia et al 1974). However, it may become essential to monitor the baby carefully using a scalp electrode. The incidental finding of meconium staining of the amniotic fluid indicates a need for continuous monitoring of the fetus. Some studies also suggest early amniotomy shortens the length of labour (O'Driscoll et al 1969, Stewart et al 1982).

During the active phase of labour, forewater amniotomy encourages further descent of the head on to the cervix, leading to more rapid dilatation. Provided the presenting part has descended, an Amnihook may be used to advantage.

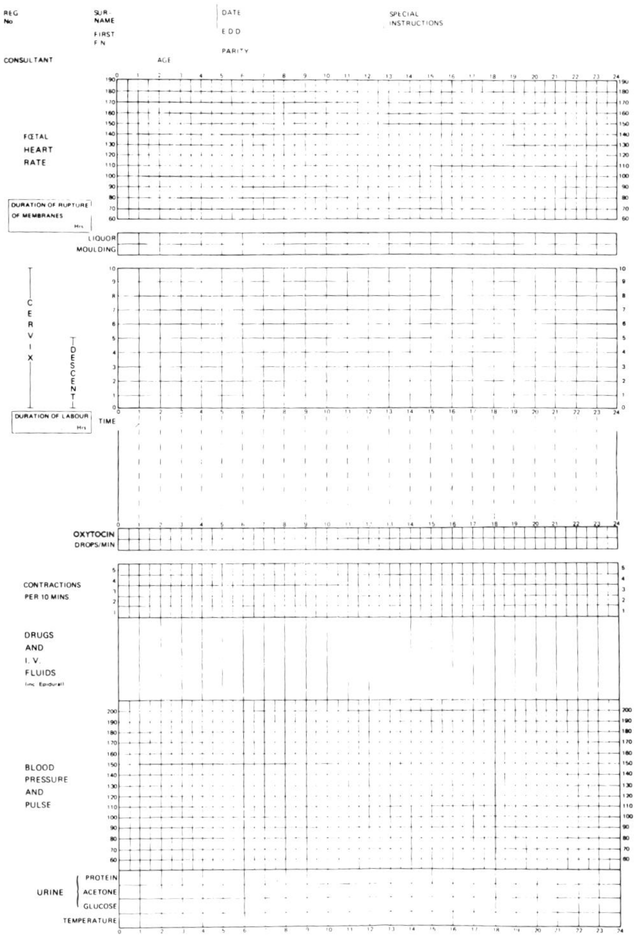

Fig. 47.8b Partogram used at Queen Charlotte's Maternity Hospital (after Studd 1973).

Pain relief

Many factors contribute to the appreciation of labour pains by the mother. Antenatal relaxation classes and team training of husband and wife to try to control pain is of enormous value. Equally useful is the personalized supervision and exhortation of a midwife. The details of the various forms of analgesia are discussed in Chapter 49.

Oral analgesics are usually worthless, except in very early prelabour. The parenteral use of pethidine has to be judged carefully to prevent excessive narcosis to the mother, which could curtail her co-operation in the second stage and cause respiratory depression of the newborn. Epidural anaesthesia in good hands can provide total abdominopelvic anaesthesia and is ideal for performing forceps deliveries and Caesarean sections. It may be associated with a temporary reduction in the strength of uterine contractions. It can also cause peripheral vasodilatation in the lower limbs; this must be counteracted with a parenteral infusion of Hartmann's solution to avoid hypotension. Epidural anaesthesia also leads to immobilization of the woman, loss of the sensation of bladder filling and of distension of the pelvic floor. This last feature may be a particular problem in primigravidae, who have a higher instrumental delivery rate, as their pelvic musculature is rigid and requires a fuller awareness of pressure for efficient bearing down.

There is no doubt that many women receive initial benefit from the use of transcutaneous electrical nerve stimulation (TENS), which is not harmful to the fetus or dangerous to the mother.

Monitoring the general health of the mother

Maternal temperature, pulse and blood pressure should be assessed every 1 or 2 hours. The temperature may become elevated in association with intrauterine infection and dehydration. When there has been prolonged rupture of the membranes — greater than 12 hours — swabs should be taken from the vagina and sent for culture. The prophylactic use of antibiotics should be considered to reduce intrapartum and puerperal morbidity with mother and infection in the newborn child. The pulse and blood pressure should be noted at more frequent intervals if the woman has high blood pressure from pre-eclampsia or is hypotensive because of epidural anaesthesia or haemorrhage.

The state of hydration should be determined by general examination of the tongue and the turgidity of the soft tissues. An assessment of the urinary output is made with examination of urine specific gravity and the presence of ketonuria. However, parenteral administration of fluids such as Hartmann's solution should only be considered where dehydration is obvious and the anticipated time of delivery is still a long way off. Such fluids are essential in transporting oxytocin when labour is being augmented and as a prophylactic measure prior to insertion of an epidural catheter for continuous anaesthesia.

Urinary output may be reduced if there is urethral obstruction by the presenting part. It is thus important that the mother's suprapubic region should be examined at frequent intervals, particularly when parenteral fluids are being administered. An enlarged bladder is not only associated with suprapubic aching discomfort, but also with a diminution in the frequency and strength of uterine contractions.

THE SECOND STAGE OF LABOUR

Onset

The imminence of full dilatation of the cervix may be recognized by the development of a desire to defecate or bear down in association with the peaks of uterine contractions. This stimulus is from stretching of the levator ani muscles by the presenting part, and is thus more a feature of the station of the presenting part rather than of the dilatation of the cervix. Stewart (1984) showed how two-thirds of women, regardless of parity, pushed before full dilatation, 20% were pushing with the cervix fully dilated, and 12%

had the urge to bear down some 5–15 minutes after full dilatation. The exact time of onset of the second stage is not easy to determine; further, with the increase in use of epidural anaesthesia which diminishes or abolishes any sensation in the pelvic floor, the diagnosis of full dilatation is made late. Often it is dependent on the physical findings of anal dilatation and perineal stretching and a marked descent of the scalp clip electrode. These are all signs of descent of the presenting part rather than of dilatation. Hence the real diagnosis of full dilatation can only be made by vaginal examination.

Duration

The time interval between full dilatation of the cervix and birth of the baby depends on:

1. The size of the presenting part, its orientation, its degree of flexion and its ability to mould.
2. The size of the mid-cavity and outlet of the pelvis and the rigidity of the musculature of the pelvic floor and perineum.
3. The strength of the uterine contractions, the ability of the woman to increase her intra-abdominal pressure with pushing and how she can direct her efforts towards a relaxed pelvic floor.

Investigation into the normal length of the second stage depends on the criterion determining the exact time of its onset. Most studies would suggest that in primigravidae it lasts about 40 minutes, and in multigravidae about 13–19 minutes (Duignan et al 1975, Cardozo et al 1982, Gibb et al 1982, Stewart 1984).

Management

Vaginal examination is essential to confirm full dilatation of the cervix and to determine the station and orientation of the presenting part. Fetal heart rate monitoring should be more intensive, either by auscultation immediately after each contraction or by a scalp electrode, since fetal head compression and umbilical cord traction from a cord wrapped around the neck of the baby become more likely as the head descends through the pelvic outlet (Fig. 47.9).

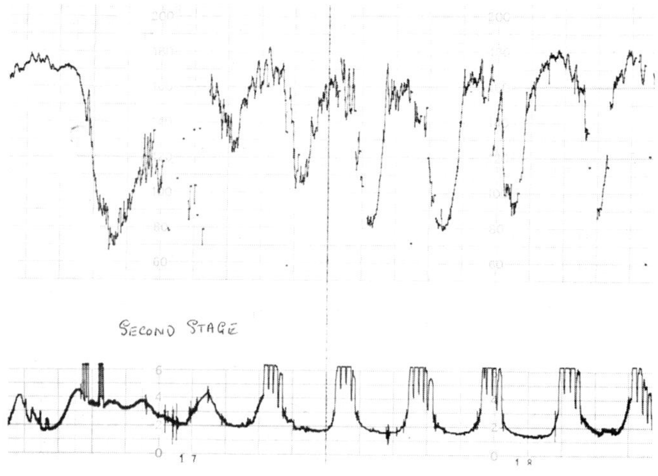

Fig. 47.9 Cardiotocographic tracing in the second stage showing late decelerations.

Posture

The position of the mother in the final phase of childbirth varies from the vertical to the horizontal, from the supine to the prone, as well as from hospital to hospital, decade to decade and country to country (Russell 1982). In practical terms, the aim is to find a position which allows the mother, to focus her intra-abdominal pressure on the pelvic floor with the greatest efficiency and in reasonable comfort. The position chosen must allow the attendant midwife or doctor reasonable access to the baby as it is being delivered. As it is not always possible to satisfy both criteria equally, a compromise has to be struck.

During the second stage there are two phases of descent: the first phase is when the presenting part descends from the mid-cavity region on to the pelvic floor and underneath the subpubic arch. Bearing down in the squatting position, which maximizes the size of the pelvic outlet, or propped up on the delivery bed at 60°, are probably the more efficient postures. However, in the second phase of crowning, when the baby's head is extended upwards beyond the subpubic arch stretching the vulva and perineum, the direction of push is closer to the horizontal. Hence the woman lying at an angle of 30°, or even in a lithotomy position, allows a more efficient angle of thrust when she pushes, as well as good access to the introitus and perineum for the controlled delivery in turn of the baby's head and shoulders.

Delivery of the baby's head

Crowning is said to take place when the widest part of the baby's head passes through the introitus. At this stage, to avoid intracranial trauma, the aim should be to deliver the head as slowly as possible, by encouraging the mother to curtail her expulsive efforts to panting only.

Immediately following delivery of the head, the nuchal region should be examined with a finger to exclude the presence of umbilical cord, which is said to occur in about one in four of all cephalic deliveries. If coils of the cord are too tight to allow them to be looped over the head, then they should be clamped and divided before delivery of the baby's body. Simultaneously the oropharnyx can be aspirated to avoid the inhalation of amniotic fluid debris, and after the head has undergone realignment with the long axis of the baby following its rotation on the pelvic floor (restitution), the anterior shoulder can be initially drawn downwards and backwards to pass under the pubic symphysis.

Following that further traction in an upwards direction will usually result in the easy delivery of the rest of the body.

Episiotomy

This is a subject in which not only musculature but also opinion is divided. There is no doubt that excessive stretching of the perineal musculature leads to neuropraxia and subsequently impaired reinnervation (Snooks et al 1985a, b). Similarly, excessive tearing of the vaginal wall and perineum should be deplored, for repair is often difficult; in inexpert hands repair is quite often imperfect, leading to the development of a rectovaginal haematoma in the short term and of dyspareunia in the long term. On the other hand, the use of episiotomy should not become routine in every delivery, because quite often, when the baby is not large and when the vaginal and perineal tissues are not rigid, it is possible to avoid both cutting and tearing in this region. However, if just before crowning the introitus is tight, thinning and starting to split, a vertical midline incision in the perineum increases the diameter of the outlet, is easier to resuture and causes less bruising than the mediolateral incision (Beynon 1974, Coates et al 1980). If it appears that such an incision is likely to extend, the episiotomy should be redirected obliquely laterally at the lower end of the vertical incision, in order to avoid the anal sphincter and rectum.

THE THIRD STAGE OF LABOUR

Although there is a tendency for the attendants to relax after the delivery of the child, careful vigilance is essential during the 10-minute interval between the delivery of the baby and the expulsion of the placenta and its membranes.

Clamping of the cord

If there has been fetal distress, meconium staining of the amniotic fluid or evidence of an unreactive baby likely to have a low Apgar score, the cord should be clamped immediately and the baby resuscitated; amniotic fluid is aspirated from the oropharynx and oxygen is administered. If the baby is active and cries immediately on delivery however, clamping of the cord can be deferred to allow the transfer of blood from the placenta to the fetus, which should be held below the level of the introitus (Yao & Lind 1969). Prolonged deferment of cord clamping provides no great advantage to the newborn who in subtropical climates is likely to become cold: it does not hasten expulsion of the placenta.

Delivery of the placenta

Parenteral administration of Syntometrine (oxytocin 5 u/ml with ergometrine 500 μg), when given intramuscularly at the time of delivery of the anterior shoulder, causes a sustained contraction of the uterus within 2.5 minutes lasting up to about 3 hours. It encourages the separation of the placenta from the uterine wall and reduces the chances of postpartum haemorrhage to the order of 1%. However, such a pharmacological preparation may induce vomiting in almost half the women and 10 units of oxytocin may be an acceptable alternative in the first instance, although the blood loss is slightly higher (Moodie & Moir 1976).

After the baby has been treated by oropharyngeal aspiration, is wrapped up and presented to the mother, the obstetrician or midwife should be preparing for the delivery of the placenta. The border of the left hand is placed on the abdominal wall at the level of the fundus, the umbilical cord grasped with the right hand and kept under gentle tension. Placental separation is indicated when the uterus contracts the fundus becomes globular, a small gush of blood flows from the vagina and the umbilical cord lengthens. Once these signs are recognized, the hand should be placed just below the fundus of the uterus and the mother encouraged to increase her abdominal pressure. The umbilical cord can then be drawn down gently, delivering the placenta and its membranes. The uterus can then be massaged to stimulate contraction and reduce bleeding.

The placenta should be inspected to ensure that there is no cotyledon missing and that the membranes are complete. The umbilical vessels should also be inspected since the absence of an umbilical artery is associated with fetal anomalies (Bernischke & Brown 1955), and blood can be taken in rhesus-negative mothers to determine the blood group of the baby, as well as the haemoglobin, bilirubin and direct Coombs' test.

Assessment of trauma to the genitalia

Following delivery of the placenta, the vagina, introitus and perineum should be carefully inspected to determine if any injury has occurred during the course of childbirth. Ideally this should be performed in the lithotomy position, particularly if there has been an instrumental delivery as cervical and upper vaginal tears can be missed without careful inspection in a good light.

Cervical tears should be repaired if they are extensive or bleeding. The cervix is held gently with ovum forceps and the tear repaired with locking 2/0 chromic catgut sutures from the apex of the tear down to the external os.

In closing vaginal lacerations, the apex should first be identified and the tear repaired from above downwards: any dead space should be obliterated to prevent paravaginal and pararectal haematomata. Repair of the perineum and lower vagina requires infiltration with 10 ml of 1% lignocaine unless an epidural anaesthetic is already in place. The perineal and pelvic floor musculature should be realigned to restore normal anatomy using either 2/0 chromic catgut or Dexon. Midline tears and episiotomies can be closed with continuous sutures, a deeper layer closing the musculature and a subcuticular layer approximating the skin edges.

More extensive lesions require interrupted sutures in the perineal musculature. Where there has been a third-degree tear, it is essential to identify and close the tear in the rectal mucosa with interrupted catgut, then identify the divided portions of the external sphincter and approximate them with interrupted catgut sutures before closing the perineal musculature.

The volume of blood loss should be assessed, although measurement may be inaccurate because urine, faeces, amniotic fluid and cleaning solution are all mixed on the drapes, kidney dishes and on the floor. Nevertheless, an effort should be made to calculate it to help with maternal management during the puerperium. The baby should be inspected in front of the mother to reassure her that it is normal and it should then be weighed so that the information can be passed to the mother and her friends and relatives as soon as possible.

Finally, the notes and the partogram should be completed and checked by a senior obstetrician to ensure that all details of the labour have been entered fully, for future reference.

REFERENCES

Beazley J M, Kurjak A 1972 Influence of a partograph on the active management of labour. Lancet ii: 348–351

Bernischke K, Brown W H 1955 Vascular anomaly of the umbilical cord: the absence of one umbilical artery in the umbilical cord of normal and abnormal fetuses. Obstetrics and Gynecology 6: 399–404

Beynon C L 1974 Midline episiotomy as a routine procedure. British Journal of Obstetrics and Gynaecology of the British Commonwealth 81: 126–130

British Medical Journal Leading Article 1986 The lessons from the Savage enquiry. British Medical Journal 293: 285–286

Caldeyro Barcia R, Schwarz R, Belran et al 1974 Adverse perinatal effects of early amniotomy during labour. In: Gluck L (ed) Modern perinatal medicine. Year Book Medical, Chicago, pp 431–442

Cardozo L D, Gibb D M F, Studd J W W, Vasant R V, Cooper D J 1982 Predictive value of cervimetric labour patterns in primigravidae. British Journal of Obstetrics and Gynaecology 89: 33–38

Coates P M, Chan K K, Wilkins M, Beard R J 1980 A comparison between midline and mediolateral episiotomies. British Journal of Obstetrics and Gynaecology 87: 408–412

Coltart T M, Trickey N R, Beard R W 1969 Fetal blood sampling, practical approach to management of fetal distress. British Medical Journal i: 342–346

Crichton D 1974 Establishing the level of the fetal heart. South African Medical Journal 48: 784–787

Dawes G S 1968 Labour and delivery. In: Fetal and neonatal physiology. Year Book Medical, Chicago, pp 117–124

Desmond M, Moore J, Lindley J E, Brown C A 1957 Meconium staining of the amniotic fluid: the marker of fetal hypoxia. Obstetrics and Gynecology 9: 91–103

Duignan N M, Studd J W W, Hughes A 1975 The characteristics of labour in different racial groups. British Journal of Obstetrics and Gynaecology 82: 593–601

Dyer C 1986 The Savage case. British Medical Journal 292: 476, 549, 613, 686, 753–754

Fayez J A, Hasan A, Jonas H S, Miller G L 1978 The management of premature rupture of the membranes. Obstetrics and Gynecology 52: 17–21

Friedman E A 1955 Primigravid labour — a graphostatistical analysis. Obstetrics and Gynecology 6: 567–589

Friedman M L, McElin T W 1969 Diagnosis of ruptured fetal membranes: clinical study and review of the literature. American Journal of Obstetrics and Gynecology 104: 544–550

Gibb D M F, Cardozo L D, Studd J W W, Magos A L, Cooper D J 1982 The outcome of spontaneous labour in multigravidae. British Journal of Obstetrics and Gynaecology 89: 708–711

Havercamp A D, Orleans M, Langendorfer M, McFee J, Murphy J, Thompson H E 1979 A controlled trial of the differential effects of intrapartum monitoring. American Journal of Obstetrics and Gynecology 134: 399–412

Hon E H 1958 The electronic evaluation of the fetal heart rate — preliminary report. American Journal of Obstetrics and Gynecology 75: 1215–1230

Hon E H 1959 The fetal heart rate patterns preceding death in utero. American Journal of Obstetrics and Gynecology 78: 47–56

Hon E H 1962 Electronic evaluation of the fetal heart rate — fetal distress, a working hypothesis. American Journal of Obstetrics and Gynecology 83: 333–353

Hon E H 1968 An atlas of fetal heart rate patterns. Harty Press, Newhaven, Connecticut

Hon E H, Lee S T 1963 Electronic evaluation of the fetal heart rate. American Journal of Obstetrics and Gynecology 87: 814–826

Johnston J R, McCaughey W M, Moore J, Dundee J W 1982 Cimetidine as an oral antacid before elective Caesarean section. Anaesthesia 37: 26–32

Klein M, Lloyd I, Redman C R, Bull M, Turnbull A C 1983 A comparison of low risk pregnant women booked for delivery in two systems of care: shared care (consultant) and integrated general practice unit — labour and delivery, management and neonatal outcome. British Journal of Obstetrics and Gynaecology 90: 123–128

Krebs H B, Petres R E, Dunn L J, Jordaan H, Segreti A 1980 Intrapartum fetal heart rate monitoring. American Journal of Obstetrics and Gynecology 137: 936–943

Lebherz T B, Hellman L D, Madding R, Anctil A, Arje S L 1963 Double blind study of premature rupture of the membranes. American Journal of Obstetrics and Gynecology 87: 218–225

McAuley D M, Moore J, Dundee J W, McCaughey W 1984 Oral ranitidine in labour. Anaesthesia 39: 433–438

Macdonald D, Grant A, Sheridan-Pereira M, Boylan P, Chalmers I 1985 The Dublin randomized controlled trial of intrapartum fetal heart rate monitoring. American Journal of Obstetrics and Gynecology 152: 524–539

Mendelson C L 1946 The aspiration of stomach contents into the lungs during obstetric anaesthesia. American Journal of Obstetrics and Gynecology 52: 191–205

Mills A M, Garrioch D B 1977 Use of nitrazine yellow swab test in the diagnosis of ruptured membranes. British Journal of Obstetrics and Gynaecology 87: 138–140

Moodie J E, Moir D D 1976 Ergometrine, oxytocin and extradural analgesia. British Journal of Anaesthesia 48: 571–574

Neutra R R, Fienberg S E, Greenland S, Friedman E A 1978 Effect of fetal monitoring on neonatal death rate. New England Journal of Medicine 299: 324–326

O'Driscoll K, Jackson R J A, Gallagher J T 1969 Prevention of prolonged labour. British Medical Journal ii: 470–480

O'Driscoll K, Jackson R J A, Gallagher J T 1970 Active management of labour and cephalo-pelvic disproportion. Journal of Obstetrics and Gynaecology of the British Commonwealth 77: 385–389

O'Driscoll K, Stronge J M, Minogue M 1973 Active management of labour. British Medical Journal iii: 135–137

Philpott R H, Castle W M 1972 Cervicographs in the management of labour in primigravidae. Journal of Obstetrics and Gynaecology of the British Commonwealth 79: 592–602

Russell J G B 1982 The rationale of primitive delivery positions. British Journal of Obstetrics and Gynaecology 89: 712–715

Saling E, Schneider D 1967 Biochemical supervision of the fetus during labour. Journal of Obstetrics and Gynaecology of the British Commonwealth 74: 799–811

Snooks S J, Henry M M, Swash M 1985a Faecal incontinence due to external anal sphincter division in childbirth is associated with damage to the innervation of the pelvic floor musculature: a double pathology. British Journal of Obstetrics and Gynaecology 92: 824–828

Snooks S J, Badenoch D F, Tiptaft R C, Swash M 1985b Perineal nerve damage in genuine stress incontinence — an electrophysiological study. British Journal of Urology 57: 422–426
Starks G C 1980 Correlation of meconium-stained amniotic fluid, early intrapartum fetal pH and Apgar scores as predictors of perinatal outcome. Obstetrics and Gynecology 56: 604–609
Stewart K S 1984 The second stage. In: Studd J W W (ed) Progress in obstetrics and gynaecology. Churchill Livingstone, Edinburgh, pp 197–216
Stewart P, Calder A A 1984 Posture in labour: patients' choice and its effect on performance. British Journal of Obstetrics and Gynaecology 91: 1091–1095
Stewart P, Kennedy J H, Calder A A 1982 Spontaneous labour: when should the membranes be ruptured? British Journal of Obstetrics and Gynaecology 89: 39–43
Studd J W W 1973 Partograms and normograms in the management of primigravid labour. British Medical Journal 4: 451–484
Times Law Report 1980 Whitehouse v Jordan and another. 18 December
Tipton R H, Shelley T 1971 An index of fetal welfare in labour. Journal of Obstetrics and Gynaecology of the British Commonwealth 78: 702–706
Walker J 1954 Fetal anoxia. Journal of Obstetrics and Gynaecology of the British Empire 61: 162–180
Walker J 1959 Fetal distress. American Journal of Obstetrics and Gynecology 77: 94–107
Yao A C, Lind J 1969 Effect of gravity on placental transfusion. Lancet ii: 505–508

Philippa Cardale

The midwife's role in the management of normal labour

The law about the provision of maternity services has developed to emphasize the interests of the child against those of the mother (Eekelaar & Dingwall 1984). In the course of this process, legislation has limited the range of those upon whom the mother may call for assistance in childbirth to a small professional group, consisting of a registered medical practitioner, a registered midwife and those training for either of these professions.

The activities of the midwife are defined by the United Kingdom Central Council for Nursing, Midwifery and Health Visiting in the Midwives Rules and the Midwives Code of Practice (UKCC 1986a,b). The Code of Practice states that the midwife:

> must be able to give the necessary supervision care and advice to women during pregnancy, labour and the post partum period, to conduct deliveries on her own responsibility and to care for the newborn and the infant. This care includes preventative measures, the detection of abnormal conditions in mother and child, the procurement of medical assistance and the execution of emergency measures in the absence of medical help.

In addition to these activities the midwife provides the mother with emotional support and participates in programmes of parenthood preparation for the mother and her partner, which include providing information about the process of childbirth.

If there is any deviation from the normal course of events, the midwife is responsible for referral to medical assistance. For labours in hospital, the arrangements for referral are normally clearly established. If a labour is conducted at home, the midwife refers to the general practitioner (GP) with whom the mother has booked for maternity care (who may differ from her usual GP). If the woman is unable to book maternity care with a GP, the midwife has a duty to inform the supervisior of midwives and call upon any doctor who is on call for emergency work. The midwife also has a duty to inform her supervisor if a mother insists on home delivery, despite advice to the contrary, or if the mother refuses to accept the attendance of a medical practitioner when the midwife considers it necessary.

The Midwives Code of Practice (UKCC 1986b) states that 'each midwife as a practitioner of midwifery is accountable for her own practice in whatever environment she practises.' It requires that the introduction of any new practices calling for new midwifery skills should invoke her responsibility for undertaking appropriate preparation in developing and maintaining those skills. In the management of normal labour the midwife is required to be aware of new developments and findings in midwifery as well as obstetric practice and to be able to explain her practice within the context of current knowledge and clinical developments.

Labour ward policies are being introduced increasingly to many units; these are intended to form a protocol of guidelines and recommendations for the management of certain clinical situations. Such policies are normally drawn up by a multidisciplinary forum after consultation with staff to whom they may apply; they are regularly updated to reflect current knowledge and practice. Such policy statements may be helpful in outlining current good practice or the listing of detailed requirements for the management of less common and high-risk cases. However they should not and cannot override a decision made by a midwife based on her clinical judgement or the mother's wishes (Royal College of Midwives 1987).

Midwives are required to maintain records of their observations, care and any treatment initiated; these records will contain details of the mother's wishes or requests that deviate from the midwives' proposed practice and of communications with other health professionals, including the timing of any such communication. These records will need to meet the requirements of the health authority which employs the midwife or, if she is in independent practice, to meet the needs of the local supervising authority (UKCC 1986a). In view of the Congenital Disabilities (Civil Liabilities) Act 1976 which enables a child to claim damages up to the age of 21 years, records must therefore be kept for that period and midwives are responsible for ensuring that this is done.

The organization of midwives who provide care for women in labour has changed over the last 50 years; it has been influenced largely by the changing trend from home to hospital delivery and the fragmentation of care given by midwives now based in rotation on antenatal wards, clinics, labour wards, postnatal wards and special care baby units. Such fragmentation does not occur for those midwives practising in the community.

More recently and in response to consumer demands for better continuity of care, a number of initiatives based on organizing midwifery care on a team basis have been set up. The organization has involved teams of not more than eight midwives working together and providing the total midwifery care for a specific group of low-risk women through pregnancy, labour and the puerperium. The demands on the administration of such schemes are great but the outcome in terms of consumer and midwives' satisfaction has been well documented. The *Know Your Midwife* scheme (Flint 1987) reports that mothers receiving this care experienced less waiting time, saw fewer unfamiliar faces, had fewer antenatal admissions, requested less analgesia in labour and had less intervention.

These initiatives are still in the early stages of evaluation. From the interests and advantages already demonstrated it appears likely that the trend towards providing more care on this basis will continue in the UK.

PREPARATION FOR CHILDBIRTH

Fifty years ago Grantly Dick-Read (1942) described the fear–tension–pain syndrome. He suggested:

> the most important contributory cause of pain in otherwise normal labour is fear and that the tension and pain which can follow this fear can establish a vicious circle which mounts and so disturbs the physiological process of childbirth, that increased intervention is necessitated and outcome affected.

Increasingly, women have also sought to be better informed about the process of childbirth, including the reasons for different forms of intervention, types of management and choice of pain relief. Enkin (1971) in a well conducted trial reported that those women who attended preparation classes for childbirth were less likely to require intervention, used less analgesia and were more satisfied with their experience of childbirth than those who were unable to attend.

The facility of antenatal classes to prepare women and their partners for pregnancy, childbirth and parenthood is now widely established in health districts, hospitals and in health centres. The aim of these classes to inform women of the events which might occur during childbirth, to eliminate or reduce fear associated with the unknown and the unexpected and to teach methods of relaxation which can be adopted in labour to reduce tension.

Midwives play a principal role in the provision of such classes, which may be conducted in association with other health professionals such as health visitors, physiotherapists, obstetricians and dieticians. The classes for mothers or couples generally provide more than mere information on the process of labour. Normal pregnancy and complications in the antenatal period, parenting and care of the baby are discussed; they also provide opportunities for women to meet others expecting babies at the same time.

The classes are generally organized on a weekly basis, as a series of 5–10 sessions. They are sited in hospitals or health centres. Alternative or complementary courses may also be run on a voluntary basis by individuals or by organizations such as the National Childbirth Trust. The arrangements for these classes vary from one centre to another but are frequently planned so that part of the time is devoted to teaching relaxation methods and part to information-giving, questions and discussion. Information about labour includes recognition of the onset of labour, how and when to contact the midwife and the best use of time in early labour.

The physiological changes that occur during the first, second and third stages of labour are described and the course of events of a normal labour and delivery are discussed with the variation and expectations of the length of labour. The methods of pain relief available are described. These will obviously vary according to the intended place of delivery; the advantages and limitations of the different methods are discussed. The complications of labour and delivery are discussed in general terms also, together with the range of possible interventions which may be necessary. This includes the need for induction or acceleration of labour and situations which warrant continuous fetal heart rate monitoring. The occasions in which intravenous infusions may be necessary, episiotomies, forceps, vacuum extraction and Caesarean section deliveries are also considered. Mothers are informed about the care of the baby after delivery and arrangements for its examination. They are advised about the appearance of the baby at delivery.

Most courses of classes are open for partners to attend but since many classes are held during the day, specific sessions for the fathers and complete courses designed for couples are increasingly being held in the evenings.

As a result of the information given by midwives through such classes and articles in the media, women now tend to be better informed and participate more in the decisions made over choices of labour and delivery than in the past. Many women find that preparing a birth plan or written list of their preferred type of care — which can be discussed with the midwife and obstetrician during the antenatal period and is then kept with the rest of her records — is a useful way of communicating her wishes to her birth attendant and will remain permanently on record regardless of the changes in shift or on-call rota of midwives during her labour and postnatal period (see Ch. 47).

MIDWIFERY CARE AT THE ONSET OF LABOUR

The mother is normally advised to contact the midwife (either the one on duty at the hospital or her community midwife, depending on the system of care provided) when she recognizes that her labour is well established. The midwife and mother then discuss whether or not it is an appropriate time for the woman to come into hospital or be seen at home by the midwife.

There are a number of factors which influence these decisions. Certain signs such as the forewater rupture of membranes are sufficient indications on their own for a woman to be admitted to the delivery suite; however, if the woman describes only the onset of regular contractions, the decision is taken in the context of other factors. The woman's family, geographical circumstances and her own feelings need to be taken into account, and the midwife balances the advantages and disadvantages for each woman of staying at home with the anticipated course of her labour in the following hours.

The woman's parity affects the decision and a woman with a history of particularly short labours will already be aware of the need to obtain professional help quickly. In second or subsequent labours, generally expected to be shorter than the first, a woman may recognize established labour more readily (as opposed to Braxton Hicks contractions) and may feel able to delay contacting the midwife. In her first labour, however, a woman may feel prompted to contact the midwife sooner.

The midwife will also need to consider the distance that a woman has to travel, if she is having a hospital delivery, and her facilities for transport to the unit.

For the mother who appears more than usually anxious about her symptoms and forthcoming labour, the reception, advice and discussion given by the midwife over the telephone may be particularly beneficial in preparing her for admission. If the mother is experiencing mild, albeit regular and frequent contractions, the midwife, after visiting the mother and assessing the situation, may advise her to stay at home, keeping active, or perhaps making herself a warm drink or relaxing in a bath. If the early part of labour is slow and protracted, the mother will almost certainly feel more relaxed and cope better with the contractions in a familiar setting, in which time will pass more quickly and in which she can continue to undertake small activities.

The incidence of false labours already experienced by this mother and any events occurring in the antenatal period which put the woman at higher risk for complications in her labour should also be considered by the midwife, together with the frequency, duration and strength of contractions. In the past, the nature of contractions has often been described to mothers for use as a rule of thumb as to whether or not she is in established labour and should come into hospital. But contractions by themselves do not always provide the best criteria.

For many women who have reached 40 weeks of pregnancy or beyond, the humiliation of being admitted in false labour at a time which has already become frustrating can be extremely demoralizing. For the midwife caring for such cases it can be equally so. The midwife's role therefore is principally to review the psychological, physical, and professional needs of each woman and advise her to transfer to hospital at the optimum time. Each woman will be different.

The atmosphere of the labour ward and attitude of the midwife at her admission may be the woman's first impression of the delivery service. A calm and confident welcome and approach with a full explanation of all procedures can do much to relax the woman and offset the inevitable element of an unfamiliar, clinical setting. Once the mother has talked about the onset of labour, the midwife obtains her maternity records (and reviews with the obstetrician on duty any events or complications that have occurred antenatally) and any birth plans or requests that may have been discussed during her pregnancy. If antenatal care has been provided as part of a team approach or community delivery scheme, the background of the woman's pregnancy and attitude to the labour will be clear and the woman more confident that her particular needs and wishes will be met. If not, the mother will be seeking reassurance that she will receive some continuity of care in terms of the philosophy and attitudes of her attendants. For a few mothers this anxiety may be great and an early reassurance that the mother and midwife are full partners in care needs to be stressed as soon as possible.

In many cases the mothers' partner is present and provides great support for her during labour. He is generally aware of her hopes and expectations for childbirth and the midwife will include him in discussion. The partner may feel overawed and threatened by the hospital setting; enabling him to feel at ease and included in his partner's care is important to the atmosphere of the labour and the woman's ability to relax.

Increasingly mothers are now admitted into all-purpose delivery rooms where what used to be the admission room, first-stage room and second-stage room are combined in one. The midwife takes the woman straight into this room which is prepared with the minimum of technical equipment on view and in which the mother is encouraged to bring her own items such as pictures, cushions, and beanbags to create as familiar a setting as possible. The mother remains in this room until a few hours after her delivery.

As soon as possible after admission the midwife will want to ensure that the mother and fetus are showing no adverse signs to the onset of labour and to establish the progress that has been made up to that time. The mother's temperature, pulse and blood pressure are recorded and the fetal heart rate measured, usually with a Pinard's stethoscope or Doppler ultrasound. In many normal labours the midwife may prefer to record the fetal heart rate continuously, using an electronic monitor for 15–20 minutes initially, to establish that normal variability and acceleration patterns are present (see Ch. 47). An abdominal examination confirms the findings in late pregnancy of the lie and presentation of the fetus; a vaginal examination confirms the state of the membranes and colour of the amniotic fluid, changes in the cervix, descent and position of the presenting part and moulding. The strength of contractions, their duration and frequency are measured during these procedures.

At one time, midwives routinely gave women a pubic shave and enema on admission in labour. Both procedures are unnecessary and unpleasant for the mother; however in cases where a woman reports having been constipated, she is offered a suppository.

Throughout these recordings the mother is encouraged by the midwife, who talks through the examination, explaining her findings and their significance. Despite many hours of painful contractions, this may be the first knowledge the mother has of the effect that they have had on her labour.

The trained midwife is perfectly capable of assessing a woman in early labour but many units, fearing possible legal repercussions, expect a junior doctor also to assess the newly admitted woman. This is a matter of opinion and tact is needed by both groups of professionals to avoid clashes and apparently divergent opinions being offered to the couple.

None of these procedures need restrict the mother if she feels happier moving around and remaining active. The midwife can help by rearranging the furniture and enable the mother to use her own cushions, the chair or floor if she prefers at this stage. The mother continues to wear her own nightclothes for as long as she wishes.

With labour progressing normally, the midwife continues to observe the mother, noticing how she copes with the contractions and reminding her to empty her bladder regularly, take small drinks or snacks and providing reassurance and encouragement.

MIDWIFERY MANAGEMENT IN THE FIRST STAGE OF LABOUR

In the first stage of labour and particularly in the early part, the midwife, mother and her partner have the opportunity of discussing more easily the couple's expectations and wishes for childbirth. The midwife may feel it appropriate to express reservations about any wishes which may be more hazardous in the event of complications arising, and suggest that such wishes may need to be discussed again. She also explains that except in the case of major emergencies (when a very short time could affect the outcome) an explanation of any complication, proposed change in management or medical intervention will be given and discussed fully if it is necessary. But in the event of labour progressing normally, the mother will be reassured to know that the midwife both knows and understands her wishes, which she will feel less able to convey as labour progresses.

In the early phase of labour the mother may find that she can easily adopt the controlled breathing and relaxation techniques that she has practised in the antenatal period. However, she may find that the frequency of contractions has been such that she has not had time to concentrate sufficiently on these, and the midwife provides support by reminding the couple of the techniques in a calm and confident way. If the mother has not attended classes at all, the midwife may need to demonstrate the breathing and relaxation technique and to concentrate her attention completely on the woman; she shows the woman's partner how to help her into comfortable positions, whether on the bed, floor or chair and how to massage her back during episodes of backache.

Observations of the maternal and fetal conditions and the progress of labour are continued and the clinical findings are recorded on a partogram. This style of labour record enables the midwife to recognize more readily any deviations in observations from the normal as well as concurrent changes in several observations; the recording of such observations is also simpler and less time-consuming (see Ch. 47). Quarter-hourly observations are made of the maternal pulse and fetal heart rate together with the strength, duration and frequency of contractions. Maternal blood pressure and temperature are recorded intermittently.

The progress in labour is also estimated by vaginal examination, the findings of which are drawn on the partogram; changes in cervical effacement, descent and position of the presenting part and observations of the degree of moulding, caput and the drainage of amniotic fluid or meconium are recorded. The frequency of performing vaginal examination is determined by the events occurring in the mother's labour, but will normally be carried out at least every 4 hours. A suspected delay in the progress of labour or any complications, spontaneous rupture of membranes or decision to administer analgesia would be sufficient indication of the need to carry out an examination earlier than this. The fetal heart rate is auscultated after the examination.

Continuous fetal heart rate monitoring by means of an electrode attached to the fetal scalp or abdominal ultrasound may be instigated for high-risk labours, or carried out intermittently for periods of 15–20 minutes about every 2 hours in normal labour. Although the benefits of such monitoring in normal labour in all women are currently disputed, a recent trial of its use in the low-risk fetus showed no association between its use and long-term effects on the neonate (Grant 1986). Many midwives prefer to carry out recordings on this basis in normal labours, particularly midwives who were trained and practised when monitoring was widely used.

In most cases a woman will be aware of the types of analgesia available and may have made some decisions in the antenatal period about those which she thinks would be most appropriate should the need arise. In some cases, a mother may have a passionate wish to avoid analgesic drugs altogether. Generally her partner will be aware of her wishes and support her in achieving these. However, it is only once the labour is progressing and the contractions are effective that the mother will consider putting her earlier decisions into practice; the midwife advises her of the limitations of these decisions as she assesses her progress in labour. If she wishes to change her mind, the midwife has an important role to play in reinforcing the decision, so that the mother does not feel she has failed by deviating from her original thinking.

Throughout the labour the mother continues to need to be reminded to empty her bladder and to take small quantities of fluids — light soup, hot and cold drinks — in whatever form she prefers.

MANAGEMENT OF THE SECOND STAGE

Towards the end of the first stage of labour, the midwife begins to observe the early indications of descent of the head on to the perineum: anal pouting, bulging of the perineum and gaping of the vulva. In many cases the midwife may be alerted by the mother starting to grunt and stating that she has to push, as the first indications of full dilatation. The midwife may observe a transitional stage in which there is a change in the frequency of contractions and apparent slowing of the labour. Confirmation that the cervix is fully dilated must be made by vaginal examination; it is important to note the position of the presenting part by definition of the sutures and fontanelles at this examination to confirm rotation and anticipate the method of delivery.

As the second stage continues, the midwife continues to explain her findings and their significance in terms of the progress in labour.

Once the presenting part has descended on to the perineum, or before, if the mother feels compelled, she should start to bear down. If a woman has had pain relief from an epidural, the midwife may suggest delaying pushing until its effects have somewhat worn off so that the urge to push is stronger. In the absence of fetal or maternal distress there is no urgency for the mother to start pushing.

Observations of maternal pulse and blood pressure are continued more frequently during the second stage once the mother has started pushing. The fetal heart rate is monitored between each contraction to ensure that deceleration during a contraction returns quickly to the baseline.

The woman may have adopted various positions during labour but most frequently resorts to the dorsal position for delivery — either on a bed or chair. Alternative positions may be preferred; for example, squatting, on all fours, or in the left or right lateral position. In whichever position the mother decides to deliver, the midwife ensures that delivery is facilitated by the mother's legs being well open, by the midwife being in a position in which she can observe and monitor progress easily and continue to encourage and communicate easily with the mother and her partner.

As the second stage progresses, the midwife stays with the mother, preparing her equipment and a sterile field for the delivery; a second midwife (perhaps a student) will normally be available at this time. As the vertex becomes visible at the vulva and by the time that crowning of the head takes place, it is essential that the mother's attention is concentrated on the midwife and that she listens to her description of progress and the need for the mother to control her pushing. The midwife supports the perineum at crowning of the head and advises the woman when to pant with contractions or to push between contractions until the perineum has thinned out, allowing the head to deliver slowly in a controlled manner. There is rarely a need for episiotomy unless rapid delivery is required because of fetal distress. If it is indicated, however, the midwife infiltrates the perineum with local analgesia and performs a mediolateral incision.

With delivery of the head, the midwife ensures that the cord is not tight around the baby's neck. If it is, she slips the cord over the head; occasionally it is so tight that it has to be clamped and cut before delivery of the rest of the baby.

With the following contraction the mother normally pushes the baby out. The midwife assists delivery of the anterior shoulder first, followed by the posterior shoulder and the remainder of the body on to the mother's abdomen or into her arms until the cord is cut. Her immediate questions will be — boy or girl, and is the baby all right?

MANAGEMENT OF THE THIRD STAGE

There are three methods of management of the third stage of labour. The management used most frequently is active management in which prophylactic intramuscular injection of 1 ml of Syntometrine (5 units of oxytocin and 0.5 mg ergometrine maleate) is administered by the accompanying midwife at the time of delivery of the anterior shoulder of the baby.

The umbilical cord is clamped shortly after delivery and with the contraction of the uterus, controlled traction is applied to deliver the placenta while the other hand is cupped across the mother's abdomen supporting the uterus from beneath. This management has been standard practice for many years and is frequently included in a labour ward policy, discussed earlier; it is implemented with the intention of reducing the incidence of postpartum haemorrhage.

However some suggest that this intervention may have undesired effects on the mother and necessitates not one but a number of further interventions which interfere with the mother and baby (Inch 1985). In certain cases, and generally if a specific request has been made by the mother, the midwife may adopt a management of the third stage in which separation of the placenta is allowed to occur spontaneously, the placenta is delivered and Syntometrine is then administered.

Finally physiological management may be adopted; the baby is delivered and nursed at the same level as the uterus, the placenta separates and is then delivered without the use of oxytocic drugs and the cord is then clamped, tied and severed. The signs of separation of the placenta which the midwife waits to observe are hardening of the fundus of the uterus and lengthening of the cord associated with a spurt of blood.

The blood clots and loss from the vaginal tract are collected into a bowl during this stage to aid in the estimation of the total blood loss. As soon as possible after delivery of the placenta the vaginal tract, vulva and perineum are carefully examined to assess the need for sutures; if this is necessary the midwife may perform this herself if she is proficient or she may assess this with a midwifery colleague or an obstetrician.

The placenta, membranes and cord are examined by the midwife to detect abnormalities and identify areas of the membranes from which placental tissue may appear to be missing and may therefore have been retained in the uterus.

The few hours after delivery are sometimes referred to as the fourth stage of labour. The mother normally remains in the delivery room for at least an hour after delivery, during which time she remains under close observation by the midwife. The maternal temperature, pulse and blood pressure are taken and intermittent checks are made to ensure that the uterus remains well contracted and blood loss is not excessive.

During this time the mother will be offered a drink and have the opportunity to wash and rest with her new family.

CARE OF THE NEWBORN BABY

Unless the mother has requested otherwise the baby is normally delivered into her arms. The midwife's responsibilities continue to include care of the newborn baby although in practice a second midwife is usually available and present to initiate resuscitation if necessary, to assess the baby's condition and help the mother hold her baby.

If antenatal factors or events in labour suggest that resuscitation procedures may be necessary for the child, a paediatrician will be alerted and called prior to delivery. However the midwife is also responsible and will initiate these procedures if delivery takes place before his arrival or if indication for resuscitation presents unexpectedly.

Mucus extraction may be necessary at the moment of birth and can be carried out while the baby is in the mother's arms. If meconium has been detected in labour, mucus suction is initiated prior to delivery of the thorax.

As soon as possible, moisture is removed from the baby's skin using a towel. Another towel should be placed over the baby to prevent loss of heat through evaporation. The baby's cot and linen will have been warmed by a heater during the second stage of labour.

Help is given to the new mother in holding and getting to know her baby by the midwife who at the same time observes the baby's condition and discusses this with the parents. The Apgar score (an assessment of the baby's colour, heart rate, respirations, reflex irritability and muscle tone) is universally carried out and recorded by the midwife at 1 and 5 minutes and enables a systematic check of the adaption of the baby's different systems to newborn life.

As soon as possible a full examination of the baby is made and its head circumference and length are measured. Examination aims to identify any major or minor abnormalities of development. It includes inspection and feeling the skull formation, sutures and fontanelles. The setting of the ears and eyes is observed and the hard and soft palate palpated. The chest and abdomen are inspected and the length of the spine felt. The external genitalia and movement of limbs are inspected and the digits are counted.

After asking the sex of the baby the mother will always want to know whether her baby is normal. Explaining to her that babies do not have to cry at birth and including her in the examination by suggesting that she also feels the spine, counts the toes and examines the facial features can be reassuring.

The practice of bathing babies after delivery remains controversial and is under continued discussion. Pressure to avoid this practice from those — mainly paediatricians — who have observed too many newborn infants become suddenly chilled, is now being balanced by the arguments that blood and body fluid should be washed from the skin as soon as possible. The midwife will weigh up these options with the wishes of the mother who generally prefers to have traces of blood removed. If the midwife decides to wash the baby she will find it necessary to prepare a corner of the delivery room with an overhead or additional heater and bath the baby quickly or in such a way to conserve body heat.

While the baby is being dressed its temperature and pulse are recorded and labels placed on a wrist and an ankle. The midwife should show these labels to the mother before attaching them to the baby and check the spelling of the baby's name, and that the mother's hospital number is correct. Two labels are always attached in case one slips off. The midwife will also observe whether meconium or urine is passed during this period. Vitamin K 1 mg is normally administered to all newborn babies.

Nowadays most women plan to breastfeed their babies. For this group, it is advantageous for the baby to be suckled within the first hour, which is generally while the mother is in the delivery room (Salariya et al 1978). Women who feed their babies at this time find that the infant has a strong instinct to suck, and they are filled with confidence at future feeds; they are subsequently less likely to give up, and they breastfeed for longer than those who delay the first feed (De Chateau et al 1977). The midwife may encourage the mother to offer the baby the breast and may demonstrate the correct way of fixing the baby. While she does this she also reminds the mother of the special qualities of breast milk; large quantities of fluid are provided at the beginning of the feed, known as the foremilk, while there is a high-calorie intake from the hindmilk at the end of the feed. The midwife will also reassure the mother that the baby will take all the milk it requires. The mother generally finds great satisfaction in this method of feeding.

As soon as possible after delivery and completion of examination and observations, the midwife ensures that all the records have been completed and are correct. In the hospital, these will include the individual case notes and the labour ward register; in the community different case notes may be used while the independent midwife practitioner keeps her own register of cases. A further responsibility is the notification of birth; in theory this is the responsibility of the father or, failing him, of anyone present at the delivery or shortly afterwards; in practice this is normally undertaken by the midwife and must be carried out within 36 hours.

The midwife will have notified her intention to practise to the local supervising authority when starting employment within a health authority or booking a woman for delivery. However if this was an unforeseen case, the midwife must provide notification within 72 hours of the delivery or attendance.

After delivery the clearing and tidying away of equipment takes time; in hospital as soon as the midwife sees fit, after an hour or two, she arranges for the mother and baby to be transferred to a postnatal ward. If the midwife is involved in providing care on a team basis, she may continue the care in this setting but otherwise it will be undertaken by the postnatal ward midwife. In any event the midwife will accompany the mother and baby on to the postnatal ward to ensure a careful and full handover.

If the mother has delivered at home, she will continue to be visited by the same midwife or another community midwife.

DEVIATIONS FROM THE NORM

Low-risk cases and normal deliveries are the domain of the midwife and she is generally the sole trained attendant. The British Birth Survey (1977) reported that the midwife was the most senior person present at 76% of deliveries. In addition she remains the key person in the care of those women who are at high risk or who develop complications during the course of their labour. In many cases when the midwife requires the help of medical care or treatment, the obstetric input may be transient and the midwife may continue the management and remain the most senior professional at delivery. When major complications are present, the midwife is required to supply nursing duties, prepare equipment and assist during procedures. She also has an important role in supporting the mother during the labour and during any interventions. It is rare that a midwife is not present at delivery.

Although the midwife's role has always been in the care of the low-risk mother, the extent of that role in terms of the minor procedures has varied over the years. More recently, her competences have been extended to include undertaking the application of a fetal scalp clip for fetal heart rate monitoring, insertion of an interuterine catheter and suturing of the perineum (Robinson et al 1983). She has always been required to carry out any procedures in an emergency such as a breech or forceps delivery.

The midwife's most important function however is to be with the woman and to provide preparation and support, detect any deviations from the normal and assist at her delivery. Trust is needed between the midwife and mother or parents and a close relationship can be established, one which generally has to be established quickly and in which the midwife needs to have immediate impact. It is the ability that a midwife has to provide this as well as her professional care that may have the greatest influence on the woman's experience of her childbirth.

REFERENCES

Chamberlain G, Philipp E, Howlett B, Masters K 1977 British births 1970, vol 2. Heinemann Medical, London
De Chateau P, Homberg H, Jacobsson K, Winberg J 1977 A study of factors promoting and inhibiting lactation. Developmental Medicine and Child Neurology 19: 575–584
Dick-Read G 1942 Childbirth without fear 1974 Pan Books, London
Ekelaar J M, Dingwall R W J 1984 Some legal issues in obstetric practice. Journal of Social Welfare Law, September: 258–270
Enkin M W, Smith S L, Dermer S W, Emmet J O 1972 An adequately controlled study of the effectiveness of PPN training. In: Morris N (ed) Psychosomatic Medicine in Obstetrics and Gynaecology
Flint C, Poulengris P 1987 The 'know your midwife' report. Private publication, 49 Peckerman's Wood, London SE26 6RZ
Grant A 1986 Some answers to questions raised about the Dublin trial. Birth 13: 255–256
Inch S 1985 Management of the third stage — another cascade of intervention. Midwifery 1: 114–122
Royal College of Midwives 1987 Towards a healthy nation. Royal College of Midwives, London
Robinson S, Golden J, Bradley S 1983 A Study of the role and responsibilities of the midwife. Chelsea College Nursing Education Research Unit report no 1. HMSO, London
Salariya E M, Easton P M, Cater J I 1978 Duration of breast feeding after early initiation and frequent feeding. Lancet ii: 1141–1143
UKCC 1986a A midwives' code of practice for midwives practising in the United Kingdom. United Kingdom Central Council for Nursing, Midwifery and Health Visiting, London
UKCC 1986b Handbook of midwives' rules. United Kingdom Central Council for Nursing, Midwifery and Health Visiting, London

49

Michael Harmer and Michael Rosen

Analgesia and anaesthesia

INTRODUCTION

The knowledge that it is possible to alleviate the pain of labour dates far back. Early Chinese writings describe the use of opiates and soporifics during childbirth, whilst in the Middle Ages they seemed to depend more upon self-administration of alcoholic drinks. However in some groups of people the relief of childbirth pain was considered evil and had led to the execution of those attempting to help the mother, a practice which fortunately is no longer in fashion. The first recognized obstetric anaesthetic, using ether, was administered by Dr James Young Simpson in 1847 but perhaps it was not until John Snow in 1853 administered chloroform to Queen Victoria for the birth of Prince Leopold that obstetric anaesthesia and analgesia gained respectability.

Following the early work on nitrous oxide, it was first used as an obstetric analgesic by Klikowitsch in 1881. Nitrous oxide later became widely available with the introduction of the Minnitt apparatus in 1934 which delivered a mixture of nitrous oxide in air. In 1961 the currently used 50:50 mixture of nitrous oxide and oxygen was described by Tunstall. While nitrous oxide has been in use, other inhalational agents (trichloroethylene and methoxyflurane) have been available, administered in air via drawover vaporizers.

The use of systemic analgesics in labour was not seen until 1902 when von Steinbuchel introduced the combination of morphine and scopolamine. In 1940, pethidine was first used and has remained the most common systemic analgesic in obstetric practice in the UK to this day.

The earliest use of local anaesthetics in labour dates from 1910 when Stiasny applied cocaine to the vagina and vulva. Although spinal subarachnoid analgesia had first been performed in 1885, it was not until 1928 that Pitkin popularized its use in obstetric practice. Lumbar epidural analgesia was described by Dogliotti in the 1940s but continuous lumbar epidural analgesia only became popular in the UK in the late 1960s.

Whilst the provision of general anaesthesia in obstetrics has a degree of inherent risk, due in part to the changes in maternal physiology consequent upon pregnancy, the provision of analgesia in labour should be absolutely safe. The long-standing methods of intermittent inhalation of analgesic agents and the use of intermittent intramuscular injections of narcotic analgesics have shown themselves in millions of pregnancies to be safe procedures. Newer techniques, which have the advantage of providing better quality of analgesia, must also prove themselves as safe. Therefore, concern must be expressed that epidural analgesia has been associated with more than one maternal death (Department of Health and Social Security 1982).

One major limiting factor in the provision of widespread totally safe obstetric analgesia and anaesthesia is that despite recommendations to the contrary (Social Services Committee Second Report 1980), small maternity units without emergency anaesthetic cover persist. In addition the same report recommended that consultant anaesthetic sessions should be allocated for all maternity units delivering more than 1000 women a year, that anaesthetic services should be readily available in all units and that an epidural service should be available in all consultant obstetric units. To date, these recommendations have not been fulfilled throughout the country, as illustrated by a survey of obstetric anaesthetic services in Yorkshire (MacDonald & Webster 1986). This was also shown in the recent national survey of facilities available at the place of birth prepared by the National Birthday Trust (Chamberlain & Gunn 1987). This report highlighted some grave deficiencies in the anaesthetic service. It is a sad fact that the shortage of obstetric anaesthetists may mean that not all women will be able to benefit equally from the methods of analgesia described in this chapter.

NON-PHARMACOLOGICAL METHODS

Psychophysical methods

Psychoprophylaxis is often wrongly considered as a simple distraction technique when in fact it is far more widely based and includes full education of the mother and awareness of the events that she may encounter during labour. The total package consists of antenatal preparation and education along with the development of various techniques of relaxation. In preparation for labour the mother requires careful explanation of events that may happen and, hopefully, allaying of fear. This form of instruction has formed part of the basis of *natural childbirth* as first introduced by Dick-Read in the 1930s (Dick-Read 1944). Fundamental to this philosophy is the belief that pain is the result of fear and misinterpretation of sensations associated with uterine contractions. If the mother learns how to relax fully and how to dissociate herself from the episode of contraction, labour can become an enjoyable experience. To this end a self-distraction technique, such as drumming out a pattern or tune, is taught to the mother. Whilst some may scorn the aims of natural childbirth, it is prudent to remember that a relaxed and fully prepared mother is likely to be easier to manage should problems arise in labour.

The greatest value of psychoprophylaxis is in the early stages of labour when it can be most beneficial, but it is seldom satisfactory for the whole of labour. Studies on the efficacy of psychoprophylaxis are often difficult to compare with other approaches but one well conducted study has been reported (Scott & Rose 1976). Two matched groups were compared; one had attended a full course of psychoprophylaxis classes based on the Lamaze method (Lamaze 1956) whilst the other had not. The results showed that the prepared group had a higher frequency of spontaneous vaginal delivery which possibly related to the lower rate of epidural block employed in this group. In other aspects — length of labour, Apgar scores and incidence of fetal distress — there was no difference between the groups. In UK hospitals, where a wide range of pain relief methods is available, less than 5% of mothers use only psychophysical techniques. This compares with the more than 50% of mothers who attend parentcraft classes. More mothers might attend such classes and perhaps have greater success with psychophysical methods if they were held at times more convenient for the working mother and her partner.

Hypnosis

Hypnosis is helpful in a small minority of patients but the reported success rate has varied from 23 to 59% amongst selected subjects of successful relief of pain during labour (Moya & James 1960, Davidson 1962, Gross & Posner 1963). Analgesics were required during delivery in most of the mothers in two of these studies (Moya & James 1960, Gross & Posner 1963). The major problem is that for a high success rate a great deal of time is required to be spent on hypnosis in the antenatal period.

Acupuncture

Although this technique has been of value in the management of certain painful conditions, particularly chronic pain, what little evidence there is available suggests that it has only limited efficacy for the pain of labour. Wallis et al (1974) found that even when an experienced acupuncturist was employed, the technique failed to give pain relief in 19 of 21 cases so treated. Another study using electroacupuncture (Abouleish & Depp 1975) found the method time-consuming and restrictive and the analgesia to be inconsistent and unpredictable.

Transcutaneous nerve stimulation (TNS)

This technique involves the application of a variable electrical stimulus to the skin at the site of pain and is based upon the gate theory of pain control of Melzack & Wall (1965). There is great or considerable relief of labour pain in 20–24% of mothers and about 60% have slight relief (Robson 1979, Stewart 1979). It is said to be most helpful for backache. A controlled study of two parity groups comparing TNS and a placebo (Harrison et al 1986) showed that in terms of pain relief there was no difference between the groups. However, mothers did find the apparatus reassuring and the study concludes that TNS may have a part to play in short labour. TNS is an attractive method as it is simple to use and easily applied by a machine.

Audioanalgesia

The use of white sound as a form of dissociation has been reported by one or two enthusiasts (Burt & Korn 1964, Barbe & Sattenspiel 1965) as helpful during labour but not appropriate for use during delivery.

Abdominal decompression

The technique of abdominal decompression as a method of reducing the pain of labour was introduced by Heyns (1959). The apparatus required is large and cumbersome. The hypothesis for its efficacy rests upon the contention that if the muscles of the anterior and posterior abdominal walls are held in a state of contraction, the pregnant uterus is flattened and excessive contraction of the upper segment of the uterus leads to pain. If the excessive tone in the abdominal walls is reduced, pain should be reduced also. There have been conflicting reports of the technique's success (Scott & Loudon 1960) and its failure (Shulman & Birnbaum 1966). The claim that abdominal decompression improves the acid–base status and oxygenation of the fetus has been denied (Newman & Wood 1967). As a technique it would seem to have little place in modern practice.

INHALATION ANALGESIA

Until 1983 when the Central Midwives Board withdrew approval for the use of trichloroethylene by unsupervised midwives there were three agents available for use: nitrous oxide, trichloroethylene and methoxyflurane. The withdrawal of approval for the use of trichloroethylene and other factors discussed later have also tended toward a diminution in the use of methoxyflurane.

Nitrous oxide

Nitrous oxide has been in use as an obstetric analgesic since it was first used by Klikowitsch in 1881. It became more widely used with the introduction of the Minnitt apparatus (1934) which delivered a mixture of nitrous oxide in air but there was always unease about its use in this apparatus as mixtures containing as little as 10% oxygen could be produced. In addition there were reports of machines in use that delivered even lower concentrations of oxygen (Cole & Nainby-Luxmore 1962). In the early 1960s the currently available 50:50 mixture of nitrous oxide and oxygen (Entonox) was described by Tunstall (1961). The apparatus (which is not available in the USA) consists of a gas cylinder containing 50% nitrous oxide and 50% oxygen as a preprepared mixture and a demand valve. The composition of the gas in the cylinder remains constant throughout the time when the cylinder is in use. The one exception to this is that if the contents of the cylinder are allowed to cool below −7°C the constituent gases separate. This would lead to pure oxygen being available initially until it was exhausted, when pure nitrous oxide would be delivered. Temperatures of −7°C are not exceptional in some parts of the British Isles (Crawford et al 1967) and recommendations have been made on the storage and use of Entonox cylinders based on the advice of Medical Research Council committee which considered the problem (Cole et al 1970).

Entonox is employed as a self-administered intermittent inhalation which, if used in the correct manner, can lead to acceptable levels of analgesia. It takes some 20–30 seconds of Entonox inhalation to achieve effective blood concentrations of nitrous oxide, so it is important that pain is anticipated and inhalation started when the contraction is first felt. In the first stage of labour, where the initial part of the contraction is not always very painful, it may be tempting for the mother to wait until the pain is fully established before using the Entonox. However, if she breathes Entonox early she has an effective blood concentration of nitrous oxide when the peak of the contraction occurs. Delay in utilization is one of the major reasons for dissatisfaction with inhalational analgesia. The problem of this lag period before analgesia is achieved can be partly overcome by continually breathing a low concentration of Entonox as a background so that intermittent inhalation takes less time to reach the peak concentration, and is therefore more effective (Davies et al 1978, Arthurs & Rosen 1981).

One factor that influences the use of the Entonox apparatus is that about 30% of mothers have a horror of anaesthetic masks. A simple mouthpiece provides an acceptable alternative to over 95% of mothers with no loss of efficacy (Dolan & Rosen 1975).

The effectiveness of Entonox in preventing the pain of labour is of approximately the same order as pethidine. This has been stated by Beazley et al (1967) as 23% total success but 40% total failure. Other studies on the efficacy of nitrous oxide have produced similar results (Report to the Medical Research Council 1970, Holdcroft & Morgan 1974). It should be possible for 80% of mothers to obtain substantial benefit from inhalational analgesia when properly managed by the midwife.

Trichloroethylene

Although trichloroethylene no longer has approval by the Central Midwives Board for use by unsupervised midwives, it would be wrong to make no mention of its use in obstetric analgesic practice. It was introduced as an alternative to nitrous oxide which at that time was administered via the Minnitt apparatus. It was approved for use by the unsupervised midwife in two temperature-compensated vaporizers, the Emotril (*E*pstein, *M*acintosh, *O*xford, *Tril*ene) and the Tecota (*Te*mperature *co*mpensated *t*richloroethylene *a*ir) which produced a concentration of 0.35 or 0.5% trichloroethylene in air within a narrow range.

The uptake, distribution and elimination of trichloroethylene are slow in comparison with nitrous oxide and analgesia does not occur until about 4 minutes of inhalation (Dundee & Moore 1960). However, because elimination is also slow it allows the development of a resting level of analgesia, sometimes accompanied by drowsiness. The quality of analgesia achieved is similar to Entonox.

Since the introduction of Entonox there has been a steady decline in the use of trichloroethylene and Central Midwives Board approval was withdrawn in 1983. It may still be useful in situations where cost is a major factor or Entonox is unavailable.

Methoxyflurane

Methoxyflurane has solubility characteristics which allow a slow build-up and slow elimination of the agent in a similar way to trichloroethylene. This should lead to a resting blood concentration of methoxyflurane which is not markedly below that required for good analgesia. Methoxyflurane is administered as a 0.35% mixture in air delivered from an automatically temperature-compensated drawover vaporizer, the Cardiff inhaler (Jones et al 1971). Higher concentrations had been investigated but led to too great an incidence of side-effects (Major et al 1967). Reservations were expressed about the possibility of renal damage associated with its use but most authorities deny any renal damage when it is used at a concentration of 0.35% (Rosen et al 1972, Creasser et al 1974). Although from solubility characteristics there would appear to be a possibility of methoxyflurane accumulation in the tissues, this is slight during intermittent inhalation (Latto et al 1972). Use of methoxyflurane has declined since the British Standards Institution found it was no longer feasible annually to test Cardiff inhalers and is largely limited to regions having their own reliable and accountable servicing arrangements.

Enflurane

Enflurane in a 1% concentration in air has been shown to be more effective than Entonox for obstetric analgesia during labour (McGuinness & Rosen 1984). However there was an incidence of excessive drowsiness associated with these levels of analgesia.

NARCOTIC ANALGESICS

Pethidine

The mainstay of systemically administered analgesics has been pethidine since its introduction into obstetric practice in the 1940s. The reason for the popularity of pethidine has been ascribed to the fact that it is less soporific than the alternatives of morphine or heroin. The standard method of administration is for the labouring mother to receive a dose of pethidine (100–150 mg), given intramuscularly. The onset of analgesia takes some 10–15 minutes, which may partly be due to variable uptake characteristics of pethidine following intramuscular injection (Austin et al 1980). This dose of pethidine is normally repeated as necessary every 3–4 hours. In modern obstetric practice it is rare for a mother to receive more than two doses. Due to its side-effects of nausea and vomiting, it is best administered with an antiemetic. There is now a tendency to move to using lower doses (pethidine 50 mg) repeated as necessary.

Placental transfer of pethidine is extensive with fetal blood levels averaging about 70% of those in maternal blood; depressant effects on neurobehavioural functions and feeding in the neonate persist for 48 hours (Wiener et al 1979).

The effectiveness of intermittently administered intramuscular pethidine was studied by Beazley et al (1967) who revealed that less than 25% of mothers so treated had pain-free labour whilst 40% had not experienced any relief.

Other analgesics

Pentazocine

When pentazocine was first introduced it was considered to be non-dependent but this has been shown not to be true. However it is free of the strict prescribing restrictions imposed upon drugs such as pethidine and morphine. It was also claimed to have a lower incidence of nausea and vomiting (Moore et al 1970). In clinical practice it is usually administered in a similar manner to pethidine but given in doses of 50–60 mg. A major drawback is hallucinogenic side-effects.

Meptazinol

Meptazinol, a partial agonist analgesic, is also free of strict prescribing restrictions. Given intramuscularly, it was initially believed to be equipotent with pethidine (Paymaster 1977) but administered intravenously by a patient-controlled method was only half as potent as pethidine (Slattery et al 1981). It has also been said to have less respiratory-depressant effects than pethidine but this has been questioned (Slattery et al 1983). Meptazinol may have less respiratory-depressant effects on the neonate than pethidine, as Nicholas & Robson (1982) found more babies with Apgar scores greater than 8 in mothers receiving meptazinol than those receiving pethidine. This effect could be associated with the elimination half-life of meptazinol in the newborn which is 3.4 hours (Jackson & Robson 1983), as compared to pethidine which is 22.7 hours (Caldwell et al 1978). However a high degree of nausea and vomiting — an uncomfortable side-effect — may limit its use.

Patient-controlled analgesia

The effect of biological variation on a fixed dose schedule for pain relief by the intramuscular route leads to many dissatisfied mothers. Administration of small doses of drug intravenously should enable titration to an adequate level of analgesia. Scott (1970) used an infusion of dilute pethidine administered intravenously by a simple patient-controlled clamp on the infusion line to control labour pain in a problem mother. A more sophisticated approach was developed by Evans et al (1976a) — a patient-activated syringe pump, the Cardiff Palliator, which includes electronic controls. Other alternative machines have since become available. Most devices incorporate safety features designed to avoid the possibility of overdose and have shown great promise in obstetric units, particularly those unable to provide a full epidural service (Harper et al 1983). The effectiveness of patient-controlled analgesia is greater than standard intramuscular injection (Evans et al 1976a, Robinson et al 1980). Such apparatus shows wide variation in the demand by mothers for analgesics, indicating the necessity for a system which will allow for considerable interindividual variation.

Epidural and spinal opiates

In recent years morphine receptors in the spinal cord have been identified. Morphine and other analgesic drugs placed in the epidural space have been shown to produce good pain relief in the postoperative period. Trials in obstetrics, however, have shown great variability in effectiveness (Skjoldebrand et al 1982). Many factors have been proposed to explain the non-effectiveness in obstetrics, including the type of pain associated with labour and the site of morphine receptors involved in uterine pain. Single injections of opiates into the subarachnoid space have been effective in obstetric practice (Scott et al 1980) but the technique has a potential problem of late-onset respiratory depression.

Opiate antagonists

A major concern with any narcotic agent used in labour is that respiratory depression will result in the neonate. It is believed that if narcotic analgesics have been given to the mother within 2 hours of delivery, neonatal depression is more likely. However this is by no means an unbreakable rule. The use of patient-controlled analgesia up to delivery has not been associated with problems of respiratory depression in the newborn (Evans et al 1976a).

The only narcotic antagonist now acceptable for use in obstetrics is naloxone which is a pure narcotic antagonist. It is not advisable to administer naloxone to the mother before delivery as this would terminate analgesia, but it is best administered to the infant as necessary at birth. The intravenous dose of naloxone for rapid reversal of respiratory depression in the neonate is 40 μg (Evans et al 1976b). Administered intramuscularly in a 200 μg dose, it produces reversal within a few minutes (Wiener et al 1977). Pethidine has been shown to have long-term depressant effects on feeding and neurobehavioural status and naloxone has been shown to prevent or considerably diminish such effects (Wiener et al 1977, 1979). No adverse effects have been reported in the use of naloxone in these dosages in the newborn.

CONDUCTION ANALGESIA

Local anaesthesia

The increased use of local anaesthesia, especially for epidural analgesia, for pudendal block and for infiltration is a major development in obstetric practice in the last two decades. It is essential therefore to review the toxicity and side-effects of local anaesthetics in both the mother and the fetus.

Effects on the mother

The most serious side-effects affect the central nervous system. Moderate overdose may only lead to drowsiness but severe overdose will cause a convulsion or even a series of convulsions. The possibility of a local anaesthetic as the cause of a convulsion should always be considered. Whilst central nervous system effects are the most likely following overdose, serious cardiovascular responses also occur. They consist of bradycardia and hypertension which may be followed by cardiac arrest, especially if an inadvertent intravenous injection of bupivacaine has been administered. Local anaesthetics affect the heart by blocking sodium channels and hence slowing conduction. Whilst the heart tolerates lignocaine well (it is used as an antiarrhythmic), Clarkson et al (1984) found that bupivacaine appears to cause a prolonged blockade. Such toxicity is further enhanced by existing acidosis, hypoxia or hypercarbia (Thigpen et al 1983).

Table 49.1 Safe doses and concentrations of local anaesthetics

Drug used	Dose/concentration
Lignocaine	
With adrenaline	500 mg (7 mg/kg)
Without adrenaline	200 mg (3 mg/kg)
For infiltration	0.25–0.5%
For nerve block	1–2%
Prilocaine	
With adrenaline	600 mg
Without adrenaline	400 mg
For infiltration	0.25–0.5%
For nerve block	1%
Bupivacaine	
Without adrenaline	150 mg (2 mg/kg)
For infiltration	0.25%
For nerve block	0.25–0.5%

The exact doses of local anaesthetic which are toxic is not agreed but the following figures may act as a guideline to safe dosage (Table 49.1).

Side-effects from local anaesthetics are much more likely to occur if the dose of drug is inadvertently injected intravenously. They rarely occur as a result of repeated administration, particularly if doses are only given when the analgesic effect of the preceding dose has worn off.

Effects on the fetus

Local anaesthetics can indirectly affect the fetus by blocking sympathetic activity and causing hypotension in the mother, leading to a reduction in placental blood flow. All local anaesthetics cross the placental barrier and can have direct effects upon the fetus. Changes in beat-to-beat variability have been reported following injection of local anaesthetic into the mother's epidural space (Lavin et al 1981, Abboud et al 1982). These changes, due to the uptake of drug into the fetal myocardium, are not considered to be of great importance. The most serious toxic reactions are associated with misplaced injections of local anaesthetics, such as into the fetal scalp during perineal infiltration (Kim et al 1979).

There has been much interest in the long-term effects on the fetus of local anaesthetics. These studies are based upon changes in neurobehavioural patterns. Lignocaine or mepivacaine cause a slight diminution of responsiveness and muscle tone persisting for more than a week after delivery (Tronick et al 1976), whilst bupivaciane was not considered to have these problems (Scanlon et al 1976). Other work

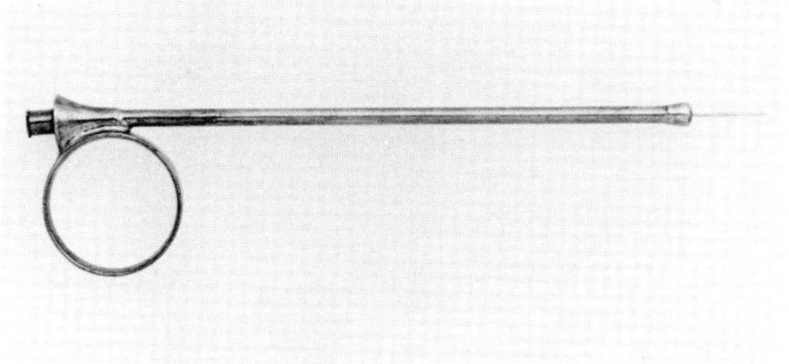

Fig. 49.1 Pudental block needle.

shows that, depending upon the dose, bupivacaine causes similar neurobehavioural changes to the other local anaesthetic agents (Wiener et al 1979). Overall, the effects of local anaesthetics on the fetus are minor and appear to be of little clinical importance.

Infiltration with local anaesthetic

The most commonly administered form of local anaesthesia is infiltration of the perineum with a local anaesthetic such as lignocaine prior to performing an episiotomy incision at the time of delivery. Large amounts of local anaesthetic are not necessary, therefore side-effects from this block are rare so long as misplaced or intravenous injections are avoided.

Nerve blocks

Only two nerve blocks are commonly used: the pudendal nerve block and the paracervical block.

Pudendal nerve block

Pudendal nerve block is almost always used to facilitate operative vaginal delivery and is performed by the obstetrician. The nerve is blocked in or close to the pudendal canal on the lateral wall of the ischiorectal fossa where it is closely associated with the pudendal artery and vein. There are two methods of performing bilateral pudendal block: via the transvaginal or the transperineal approach.

Transvaginal approach. This is performed with the mother in the lithotomy position. A pudendal block needle (Fig. 49.1) some 12.5 cm in length is attached to a 20 ml syringe containing local anaesthetic solution. The needle is placed along the second and third fingers of one hand and introduced carefully into the vagina. The region of the ischial spine is palpated with the tips of the fingers and the needle advanced through the vaginal wall immediately behind the ischial spine to a depth of about 1.25 cm, with the needle passing through the sacrospinous ligament. Following aspiration to check that the needle is not in a vein, an injection of 10 ml of local anaesthetic solution is made. The procedure is repeated on the other side.

Transperineal approach. This is only used when the presenting part of the fetus is too low to permit the use of the transvaginal approach. An unguarded needle is inserted through the perineal skin at a point halfway between the fourchette and the ischial tuberosity. Two fingers of the other hand are placed within the vagina and the ischial spine is identified and the needle advanced until its point lies just behind the ischial spine. After careful aspiration, 10 ml of local anaesthetic solution is injected. The procedure is repeated on the other side.

Paracervical block

Paracervical block can be of value in the first stage of labour. It is performed by inserting a special sheathed needle 1–2 cm through the epithelium of each lateral fornix of the vagina and depositing 5–10 ml of local anaesthetic solution into each paracervical region. This is a highly vascular area and an inadvertent intravascular injection is possible. It provides successful analgesia in approximately 80% of mothers (Belfrage & Floberg 1983).

Paracervical block enjoyed a period of popularity but as a single-shot technique, analgesia lasts only 1 hour, though the duration of action has been extended by the use of catheter techniques. Doubts have been expressed concerning the safety of paracervical block for the fetus. In the first few minutes after initiating a block a high incidence of fetal bradycardia associated with a falling pH and oxygen tension has been seen (Baxi et al 1979). These changes have been investigated by Cibils (1976) who demonstrated that if local anaesthetic solution at a concentration similar to that attained during paracervical block is applied to a segment of uterine artery it causes marked vasoconstriction. So fetal asphyxia may be caused by a reduction in uteroplacental blood flow secondary to uterine artery vasoconstriction. It has been suggested that the block should be administered in well spaced stages in order to minimize these effects (Van Dorsten et al 1981). This complication has led to a marked diminution of its use worldwide, although its success and simplicity might justify reinvestigation.

Subarachnoid (spinal) block

The use of a subarachnoid (or spinal) injection of local anaesthetic has been widely used for anaesthesia in the second stage of labour. Its use in the first stage of labour is limited by the fact that it is usually a single injection and therefore of limited duration. Continuous spinal block maintained by intermittent injection via a catheter is practised in some centres but it is perhaps best avoided because of its potential complications. A low spinal anaesthetic (a saddle block) may be achieved by injecting a small amount of local anaesthetic (10 mg bupivacaine) prepared as a hyperbaric solution into the subarachnoid space with the mother sitting up. This produces good anaesthesia for operative vaginal delivery or removal of retained placenta. The use of a more extensive spinal anaesthetic has been advocated as a simple and rapid-onset method of providing anaesthesia for Caesarean section. However the quality of block obtained has been shown to be very variable (Shnider 1970). Others have expressed concern that excessively high blocks can occur with standard doses of local anaesthetic (Bembridge et al 1986). Spinal anaesthesia should still be considered as an alternative to epidural in a mother in whom general anaesthesia is contra-indicated.

Epidural block

The epidural (extradural) space, which contains arteries, veins, lymphatics and fat, extends from the foramen magnum to the sacrococcygeal membrane. It is the space between the dura mater internally and the bony vertebral canal externally (Fig. 49.2). Anteriorly the bony vertebral canal is bounded by the posterior ligament of the vertebrae and posteriorly by the ligamentum flavum covering the vertebral laminae. The lateral aspect of the epidural space is limited by the vertebral pedicles and between these the intervertebral foramina.

When local anaesthetic is injected into the epidural space it penetrates the dural cuffs surrounding the nerves and blocks the fully formed spinal nerves. In addition, there is evidence of spread of local anaesthetic into the cerebrospinal fluid, though the importance of this is questionable. However, it is accepted that, for effective anaesthesia, the local anaesthetic must gain direct access to the appropriate spinal nerve in the vicinity of the intervertebral foramen.

The nerve supply involved in the pain of labour is derived from two distinct areas which require to be blocked. In the first stage of labour, nerves from T10 to L1 must be blocked, whilst the lower sacral nerves (S2–5) are involved in the second stage of labour. For this reason optimal positioning of mothers for epidural block is important to achieve best results as labour progresses.

The epidural space can be approached from two directions: through the sacrococcygeal membrane (the caudal approach) or between two adjacent vertebral spines. The lumbar region is usually selected to allow blockade to an adequate level with the added safety factor that the spinal cord normally stops at L1–2, although any convenient spinous space can be utilized.

Any deficiency of coagulation is a contraindication to epidural block. Women with disseminated intravascular coagulation following placental abruption or severe pre-eclampsia, thrombocytopenia or who are anticoagulated should not receive an epidural block.

Caudal epidural block

The caudal epidural space is accessible through the sacrococcygeal membrane found at the lower end of the sacral vertebrae where the posterior laminae are not fused. The membrane is located by careful palpation in the midline down the back of the sacrum. At the lower end of the sacrum a gap is appreciated which can be likened to palpating the space between the knuckles of the clenched hand. Once located, suitable preparation of the skin and superficial infiltration with local anaesthetic should be performed. The caudal epidural block is usually a single-shot procedure and a disposable 20 gauge needle may be used.

The needle is inserted pointing slightly cephalad through the sacrococcygeal membrane until it abuts against the posterior aspect of the sacral vertebrae (Fig. 49.3). The needle is then slightly withdrawn and turned in a much more cepha-

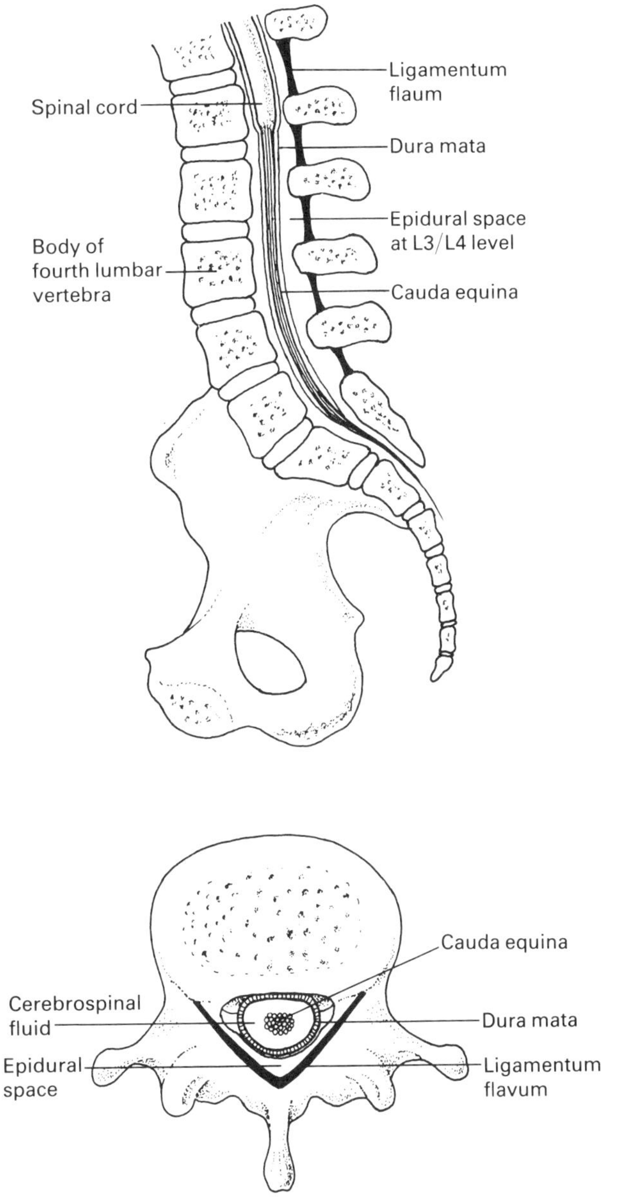

Fig. 49.2 Anatomy of the epidural space in the lumbosacral region. From Crawford (1984).

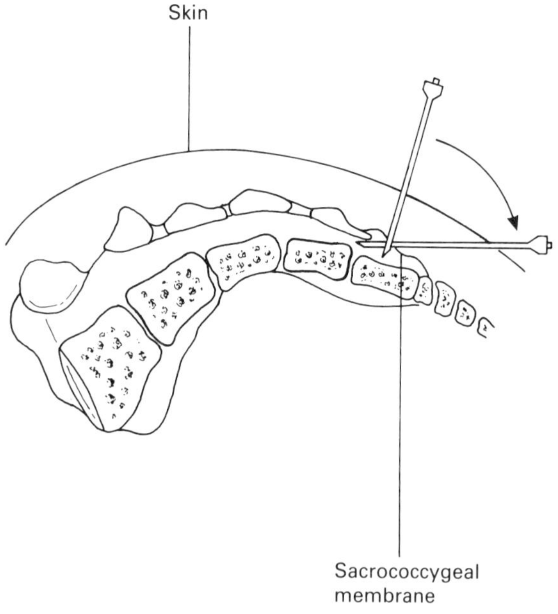

Fig. 49.3 Insertion of needle for caudal anaesthesia. From Cotton (1985).

lad direction so that the hub of the needle lies in the natal cleft when the needle can easily be advanced up the sacral canal for a distance of 1–2 cm. A syringe should be attached to the needle and careful aspiration carried out. If blood is present, the procedure to this point should be repeated. If clear fluid is obtained it can be assumed that the dural sac extends below its normal level of S2 and has been pierced. In this case the procedure is best abandoned. If there is no aspiration of liquid, 1–2 ml of air should be injected through the needle with the fingers of the operator's other hand placed lightly over the sacral hiatus. If injection is easy and no crepitus is felt, the needle is in position and local anaesthetic may be administered through it in increments of about 50 mg lignocaine or 20 mg bupivacaine.

A continuous technique can be used via the caudal approach using a suitable needle and catheter but this has no advantages over the lumbar region. As a single injection it is of more value in the second stage of labour. To achieve a block high enough to relieve first-stage pain a large volume of local anaesthetic has to be used.

Although this is a simple technique it is not without complications. Inadvertent dural puncture can occur due to wide variability in the distance between the upper limit of the sacral hiatus and the lower extremity of the dural sac, which may range from 16 to 75 mm (Trotter 1947). If during initial insertion the needle is inadvertently advanced too far and passed through the sacrococcygeal joint it may pierce the rectum, which in itself would not be a great problem, but it may also enter the fetal head if it is pressed on to the perineum at the same time. This complication has been reported on several occasions, and in two reports led to fetal death (Finster et al 1965, Sinclair et al 1965). Referring to this complication, Bonica (1970) suggests that caudal block should not be initiated after the presenting part has descended to the perineum whilst Moore (1966) in addition advocates that a rectal examination of the mother should always be performed before solution is injected in order to ensure that the needle has not penetrated deep to the sacrum.

Continuous lumbar epidural block

It is important to bear in mind that one cannot guarantee that an epidural will be successful, a fact that should be explained to the mother before the procedure is embarked upon. It is equally important to differentiate for the mother between sensation and pain, for in an ideal epidural uterine contraction should be felt without pain. In addition to analgesia some degree of motor paralysis is inevitable.

The epidural space is most commonly approached by the lumbar route. An epidural in labour is normally inserted with the mother in the lateral position as this is most comfortable. It is also possible in the sitting position, which can be particularly advantageous in the obese in allowing better identification of bony landmarks. The approach to the epidural space is usually in the midline although a more lateral approach has been advocated (Carrie 1977) to avoid trauma to the ligaments of the spine and to run less risk of dural puncture.

Prior to initiation of the epidural block an intravenous infusion of Hartmann's solution is set up to ensure circulatory preloading during siting of the epidural cannula. Preloading should be cautious in mothers at risk of fluid overload. Fetal heart rate and maternal blood pressure are recorded before the procedure and at regular intervals, particularly after a subsequent top-up dose of local anaesthetic has been given. Full resuscitation facilities for the mother must always be closely available.

The mother is usually turned into the left lateral position and her back aligned with the edge of the bed or trolley. Her back should be flexed only as far as is comfortable. The operator, after a full scrub-up, dons sterile gown and gloves. The skin is cleaned carefully over the lower thoracic and lumbar region and the area towelled up. The skin, subcutaneous tissue and supraspinous ligament are infiltrated with local anaesthetic. The most commonly used epidural needle is a Tuohy (Fig. 49.4); this is advanced through the ligaments to reach the ligamentum flavum. These needles have an internal diameter equivalent to 16 gauge and will allow a catheter to be threaded through.

Once the ligamentum flavum has been reached a technique needs to be employed to identify accurately the epidural space. The basis behind such techniques is that the pressure in the epidural space is normally negative and so will suck in a small drop of fluid at the needle hub or will deflate a small balloon attached at the hub (Mackintosh balloon). However the most commonly used technique relies upon the loss of resistance to injected air. Using a freely moving syringe containing a small amount of air, it is not possible

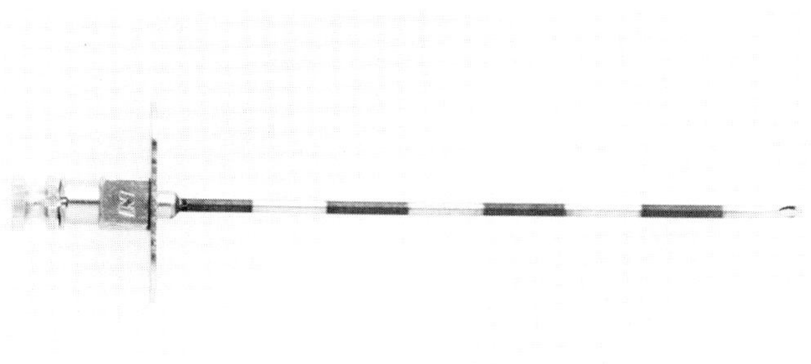

Fig. 49.4 A winged Tuohy epidural needle.

to inject whilst the needle tip is in the ligament but injection becomes easy when the epidural space is entered.

A test for loss of resistance is made with each incremental insertion of the Tuohy needle through the ligamentum flavum. When the ligamentum flavum is punctured it is often possible to sense a slight click at the same time as loss of resistance to injection occurs. Careful aspiration through the needle confirms that the dura mater has not been punctured; if any fluid is aspirated it can be assumed to be cerebrospinal fluid and the needle should be withdrawn and resited in a different interspace. If there is no fluid aspirated, a fine catheter is threaded down the needle into the epidural space.

The catheter employed for epidural block may have a single end-hole or a number of side-holes. In the case of the side-hole catheter, this should be inserted 3 cm into the epidural space for most reliable results (Kumar et al 1985) whilst only 2 cm of an end-hole catheter should be inserted (Gough et al 1986). If problems are encountered in passing the catheter through the needle it is important that the catheter should never be pulled back as it can be severed by the needle tip.

Once the catheter is satisfactorily sited, the puncture site is sprayed with antibiotic and an occlusive dressing applied. A bacterial filter is attached to the hub of the catheter and a small test dose of local anaesthetic is injected (15 mg bupivacaine). This small test dose is intended to confirm that the catheter has not penetrated the dura mater. If there is no sign of nerve blockade after 5 minutes, it is safe to inject the first full dose of local anaesthetic to produce the epidural block. An initial dose of 10 ml of 0.5% bupivacaine is usual and depending upon its effectiveness, the dose is adjusted in volume or concentration in future top-ups. In addition to misplacement of the catheter in the subarachnoid space it is also possible for it to be passed intravascularly; some feel that the test dose should contain adrenaline which if accidently injected intravascularly will produce maternal tachycardia.

Contraindications to epidural block

The contraindications of epidural block may be considered as either absolute or relative.

Absolute contraindications. The first absolute contraindication is when the mother refuses permission for the epidural. The second is when there is sepsis in the lumbosacral region involving the area through which the epidural needle will pass. Although an absolute contraindication, this is extremely rare. Thirdly, epidural block is absolutely contraindicated when there is any condition that will lead to a maternal coagulopathy. The fear is that blood vessels may be traumatized as the catheter or needle is inserted and continuing haemorrhage into the epidural space may cause spinal cord compression.

Obstetric conditions that predispose to coagulopathy include moderate or severe pre-eclampsia, placental abruptions, prolonged retention of products of conception, recent spontaneous abortion and thrombocytopenia. If it is deemed necessary or desirable to use epidural analgesia in any mother in these groups, it is essential that coagulation studies should confirm normal clotting. Such tests must have been performed immediately (less than 30 minutes) before commencement of the procedure.

The use of anticoagulants (but not low-dose heparin: Minihep) should be considered an absolute contraindication to epidural analgesia. If it is necessary to give anticoagulants to a mother with an epidural in situ a period of 30 minutes should pass after insertion of the catheter in order to ensure that any traumatized vessel has time to seal.

In any mother with coagulopathy, whether of pathological or therapeutic origin, it is also important that normal coagulation is present prior to the withdrawal of the catheter as damage can also be caused.

Maternal hypotension and active substantial haemorrhage must be considered temporary absolute contraindications. If an epidural is to be used after such occurrences it is important to consider the effects that haemorrhage may have on coagulation and the guidelines mentioned above should be followed.

Relative contraindications. Chronic central nervous system disease has traditionally been considered a relative contraindication on the grounds that progressive neurological disease may be unpredictable, leading to relapse at any time. If a relapse coincides with the use of an epidural there could be a dispute over the possibility of damage having been caused by the epidural. It is therefore a relative contraindication on litigation grounds. It is advisable in any mother with such disease to explain the situation at length (and document the explanation) prior to embarking upon epidural analgesia.

The importance placed on the relative contraindication group will vary from unit to unit depending upon the experience and availability of staff. Many mothers classed in the relative contraindication group can be managed successfully and safely in well equipped and staffed units whilst units only recently beginning to offer an epidural service should perhaps consider anything apart from the normal mother as an absolute contraindication until staff and facilities have been fully developed.

Complications of epidural block

In a review of maternal complications of epidural analgesia for labour (Crawford 1985), covering some 27 000 lumbar epidurals, there were 9 potentially life-threatening complications, of which only 3 caused real concern for the mother's safety.

Complications can be considered as problems associated with the siting of the catheter and those associated with the use of epidural block. In general if a problem is encountered in inserting the epidural needle and catheter, the attempt should be abandoned and another attempt made at a different interspace.

Aspiration of blood. Blood may be aspirated through the needle or catheter from a traumatized epidural vein. If blood is continually aspirated it must be assumed that the catheter lies in a vein and it should be removed and resited.

Dural puncture. The needle may be accidently advanced through the dura mater into the cerebrospinal fluid (CSF). In order to avoid the development of low CSF pressure, it is important to prevent fluid leaking out of the epidural needle. If dural puncture has occurred the needle should be withdrawn and resited at a different interspace. If a catheter is sited in a new interspace, there does not appear to be any substantial entry of local anaesthetic through the puncture hole into CSF. However, a dural tap leads to problems in labour and the postdelivery period from CSF leakage through the puncture hole. In such a case it is advisable to avoid any raised CSF pressure during labour and therefore assisted delivery may be advantageous.

In the postdelivery period headaches are a common complication occurring in 70% of dural taps (Crawford 1972). These are best treated with an epidural drip consisting of an infusion of Hartmann's solution into the epidural space through a bacterial filter. In addition, sitting and standing in the immediate postdelivery period should be discouraged. Liquid paraffin is useful to prevent excessive straining at defecation, which may aggrevate the leak of CSF. If symptoms continue after the use of these procedures then an epidural blood patch should be performed (Crawford 1980). This consists of injecting 15–20 ml of freshly taken blood from the patient into the epidural space. This appears to be safe and generally does not interfere with any subsequent epidural (Abouleish et al 1975). However, one case has been reported in which it was found to be impossible to extend a block — administered 3 years subsequent to blood patching — above the L2 level (Rainbird & Pfitzner 1983). The authors of this last report postulate that the organized clot following blood patching may have led to fibrous tethering of the dura to the wall of the spinal canal, hence interferring with local anaesthetic spread.

Sympathetic block. The most common finding after initiation of epidural block is a fall in maternal blood pressure. In general, if the fall in systolic blood pressure is greater than 20 mmHg some effective action should be taken. Normally the drip rate of the intravenous Hartmann's infusion is increased and the possibility of aortocaval compression excluded. If the fall in blood pressure does not respond to these simple measures, a vasopressor may be administered — usually ephedrine in increments of 5 mg repeated as necessary. Ephedrine is used as it causes less effect on uterine blood flow than other sympathomimetics (Ralston et al 1974).

Inadvertent subarachnoid block (total spinal). The migration of epidural catheters is possible with consequent inadvertent subarachnoid injection of a large dose of local anaesthetic. In the authors' unit the epidural, inserted by an anaesthetist, is always topped up by an anaesthetist, although this is not usual in the UK. Possibly in very small units which offer an epidural service this may also happen. After an injection of a large volume of local anaesthetic into the subarachnoid space a widespread spinal block will occur with cardiovascular and respiratory collapse; full resuscitation measures must be employed promptly to support ventilation and circulation.

Partial block. A unilateral block is a not infrequent result of the initial injection of local anaesthetic. It can usually be corrected by having the mother lie on the unblocked side whilst another dose is injected. If the problem persists the catheter has probably been advanced too far and withdrawal by 2–3 cm may overcome the problem. If the initial block is confined to a single nerve root this suggests that the catheter has passed into or through a paravertebral foramen and slight withdrawal of the catheter will frequently correct the situation. A missed segment occurs in about 6–7% of epidurals and is persistent throughout labour in 1.5% (Ducrow 1971, Bromage 1972). It typically involves the first lumbar nerve root and can often be relieved by varying the mother's position and the drug concentration.

Top-up doses and infusions

Good continuous analgesia is only possible by ensuring top-up doses of local anaesthetic are given promptly as pain returns. The United Kingdom Central Council for Nursing, Midwifery and Health Visiting has authorized the administration of top-up doses by experienced midwives as long as certain criteria are fulfilled:

1. that the ultimate responsibility for such a technique should be clearly stated to rest with the doctor;
2. that written instructions regarding the dose are provided;
3. that in all cases the dose given by a midwife should be checked by one other person;
4. that the initial dose through the catheter should be given by the doctor;
5. that the instructions should be given by the doctor as to the posture of the patient at the time of injection, observation of blood pressure and measures to be taken in the event of any side-effects;
6. that the midwife should have been thoroughly instructed

in the technique so that the doctor concerned is satisfied as to her ability.

In addition the anaesthetist should be on the premises whenever an epidural is in use; a person capable of resuscitating the mother must also be in the labour ward.

It is important to note the pattern of return of pain as this allows optimal positioning of the mother prior to top-up and hence the best quality block can be obtained.

The use of an intermittent top-up regime requires regular doses at intervals of about 2 hours, the average labour requiring between three and six top-ups. There has recently been interest in the use of epidural infusions of local anaesthetics to reduce this need. Bupivacaine infusions at different concentrations have been reported (Glover 1977, Evans & Carrie 1979). More recent work (Li et al 1985) has shown that using a 0.125% solution of bupivacaine at 10 ml/h, the median interval between top-ups is extended from 145 to 245 minutes. At higher flow rates there is little additional effect. In primigravid mothers, 69% require none or only one top-up of 8–10 ml of 0.25% bupivacaine as compared to 32% in mothers not receiving an infusion. At this infusion rate, if the epidural catheter were to migrate into the subarachnoid space it would take about 2 hours or more to have a significant effect upon breathing and therefore 1–2-hourly sensory testing at the T5–6 level would ensure the safe use of this technique. Such sensory testing can be accurately determined by the midwife using an ice cube. These techniques show promise in reducing the need for intermittent top-up injections.

Epidural analgesia and delivery

The characteristics of the second stage of labour and delivery are altered by the provision of an epidural. There will be a reduction in pelvic floor tone which may reduce the ability of the presenting part to rotate to the anteroposterior position. There will be a reduction in lower abdominal muscle power which will affect maternal expulsive effort. The degree that these are affected will depend upon the amount of motor blockade produced by the epidural. With full sensory loss, the bearing-down reflex will be lost but this should not influence the mother's ability to bear down.

The combination of these effects is to attenuate the interval between full dilatation of the cervix and delivery. This should not be considered hazardous as evidence suggests that mothers with epidurals have less fatigue and acidosis and in consequence there is less fetal acidosis (Pearson & Davies 1974).

Overall the incidence of forceps delivery should not be higher in mothers having an epidural if ample time is allowed for the presenting part to move down the birth canal. However if a forceps delivery is considered advantageous, the quality of analgesia achieved with an epidural allows for easy instrumentation.

GENERAL ANAESTHESIA

Important principles

General anaesthesia for obstetric procedures is still a significant cause of morbidity and mortality. The reasons for this are multifactorial and beyond the scope of this chapter but there are two aspects that are of particular interest and concern to the obstetrician: maternal starvation and antacid therapy and aortocaval compression.

Maternal starvation and antacid therapy

In the emergency situation it is not always possible to be certain of the amount of stomach contents present when general anaesthesia needs to be induced. In elective Caesarean section it is traditional to starve mothers for several hours and this increases, rather than diminishes, the likelihood that gastric contents will be highly acidic. In either case it is important that adequate antacid should be administered to the mother. The standard antacid in regular use in most obstetric units was magnesium trisilicate mixture BPC but the continued use of this has been called into question by experimental evidence suggesting that particulate antacids can cause severe damage to lung parenchyma (Gibbs et al 1979). Although this work was performed on dogs there is some clinical experience of aspiration of a mixture of magnesium hydroxide and aluminium hydroxide (Bond et al 1979). Many advocate the use of sodium citrate as an alternative antacid; when administered 10–47 minutes before elective section it has been shown to raise the intragastric pH to a safe level (Gibbs et al 1982).

The H_2-receptor blockers, cimetidine and ranitidine, have been widely investigated as a means of reducing gastric acid production. Cimetidine must be administered 90–150 minutes before induction of anaesthesia to ensure that the stomach pH is at a safe level (Johnson et al 1983). If given intravenously it must be administered about 45–60 minutes before (McCaughey et al 1981). Ranitidine has a longer action than cimetidine but timing is still critical. For elective procedures, oral ranitidine given preoperatively has been shown to be safe.

In addition to the problems of gastric acid production, it is important to remember that preoperative and intrapartum starvation may lead to dehydration.

Perhaps of even greater importance than the selection of antacid employed is the experience of the anaesthetist and the assistance available at induction of anaesthesia. A recurring feature of Confidential Enquiries into Maternal Mortality (Department of Health and Social Security 1986) is that the combination of an inexperienced anaesthetist with a poor standard of assistance is often associated with maternal death from anaesthesia.

Aortocaval compression

There is now general appreciation of the danger to both mother and fetus from aortocaval compression. It has been shown (Crawford et al 1973) that there is less likelihood of maternal and fetal acidosis if the mother is transported from the ward to the operating theatre in the lateral position. In addition, oxygen should be administered during such transit.

It is not possible within a single chapter to cover in depth all aspects of obstetric analgesia and anaesthesia. If further information is required, the reader should consult one of a number of standard books on obstetric anaesthesia, such as Crawford (1984) and Moir & Thorburn (1986).

REFERENCES

Abboud T K, Khoo S S, Miller F, Doan T, Henriksen E M 1982 Maternal, fetal and neonatal responses after epidural anaesthesia with bupivacaine, 2-chloroprocaine or lidocaine. Anesthesia and Analgesia 61: 638

Abouleish E, Depp R 1975 Acupuncture in obstetrics. Anesthesia and Analgesia 54: 83

Abouleish E, Wadhwa R K, De La Vega S, Tan R N, Uy N T L 1975 Regional analgesia following epidural blood patch. Anesthesia and Analgesia 54: 634

Arthurs G J, Rosen M 1981 Acceptability of continuous nasal nitrous oxide during labour — a field trial in six maternity hospitals. Anaesthesia 36: 384

Austin K L, Stapleton J V, Mather L E 1980 Multiple intramuscular injections: a major source of variability in analgesic response to meperidine. Pain 8:47

Barbe D P, Sattenspiel E 1965 Audioanalgesia in labor and delivery. Obstetrics and Gynecology 25: 683

Baxi L V, Petrie R H, James L S 1979 Human fetal oxygenation following paracervical block. American Journal of Obstetrics and Gynecology 135: 1109

Beazley J M, Leaver E P, Morewood J H M, Bircumshaw J 1967 Relief of pain in labour. Lancet i: 1033

Belfrage P, Floberg J 1983 Obstetrical paracervical block with chloroprocaine or bupivacaine. Acta Obstetricia et Gynecologica Scandinavica 62: 245

Bembridge M, MacDonald R, Lyons G 1986 Spinal anaesthesia with hyperbaric lignocaine for elective caesarian section. Anaesthesia 41: 906

Bond V K, Stoelting R K, Gupta C D 1979 Pulmonary aspiration syndrome after inhalation of gastric fluid containing antacids. Anesthesiology 51: 452

Bonica J J 1970 Lumbar epidural versus caudal anesthesia. In: Shnider S M (ed) Obstetrical anesthesia. Williams & Wilkins, Baltimore

Bromage P R 1972 Unblocked segments in epidural analgesia for relief of pain in labour. British Journal of Anaesthesia 44: 676

Burt R K, Korn G W 1964 Audioanalgesia in obstetrics. American Journal of Obstetrics and Gynecology 88: 361

Caldwell J, Walkie L A, Notarianni L J et al 1978 Maternal and neonatal disposition of pethidine in childbirth — study using quantitative gas chromatography–mass spectrometry. Life Science 22: 587

Carrie L E S 1977 The paramedian approach to the epidural space. Anaesthesia 32: 670

Chamberlain G, Gunn P 1987 Birthplace. Report of the National Birthday Trust national survey. John Wiley, Chichester

Cibils L A 1976 Response of human uterine arteries to local anaesthetics. American Journal of Obstetrics and Gynecology 126: 202

Clarkson C W, Hondeghem L, Matsubara T et al 1984 Possible mechanism of bupivacaine toxicity: fast inactivation block with slow diastolic recovery. Anesthesia and Analgesia 63: 199

Cole P V, Nainby-Luxmore R C 1962 The hazards of gas and air in obstetrics. Anaesthesia 17: 505

Cole P V, Crawford J S, Doughty A G et al 1970 Specifications and recommendations for nitrous oxide/oxygen apparatus to be used in obstetric analgesia. Anaesthesia 25: 317

Cotton B R 1985 Obstetric anaesthesia. In: Smith G, Aitkenhead A R (eds) Textbook of Anaesthesia. Churchill Livingstone, Edinburgh, pp 407–418

Crawford J S 1972 The prevention of headache consequent upon dural puncture. British Journal of Anaesthesia 44: 588

Crawford J S 1980 Experiences with epidural blood patch. Anaesthesia 35: 513

Crawford J S 1984 Principles and practice of obstetric anaesthesia, 5th edn. Blackwell Scientific Publications, Oxford

Crawford J S 1985 Some maternal complications of epidural analgesia for labour. Anaesthesia 40: 1219

Crawford J S, Ellis D B, Hill D W, Payne J P 1967 Effects of cooling on the safety of premixed gases. British Medical Journal 2: 138

Crawford J S, Burton M, Davies P 1973 Anaesthesia for section: further refinements of a technique. British Journal of Anaesthesia 45: 726

Creasser C W, Stoelting R K, Krishna G, Peterson C 1974 Methoxyflurane metabolism and renal function after methoxyflurane analgesia during labor and delivery. Anesthesiology 41: 62

Davidson J A 1962 An assessment of the value of hypnosis in pregnancy and labour. British Medical Journal 2: 951

Davies J M, Willis B A, Rosen M 1978 Entonox analgesia in labour. A pilot study to reduce the delay between demand and supply. Anaesthesia 33: 545

Department of Health and Social Security 1982 Report on Health and Social Subjects 26. Report on Confidential Enquiries into Maternal Deaths in England and Wales 1976–1978. HMSO, London

Department of Health and Social Security 1986 Report on Health and Social Subjects 29. Report on Confidential Enquiries into Maternal Deaths in England and Wales 1979–1981. HMSO, London

Dick-Read G 1944 Childbirth without fear. Heinemann, London

Dolan P F, Rosen M 1975 Inhalation analgesia in labour: facemask or mouthpiece. Lancet ii: 1030

Ducrow M 1971 The occurrence of unblocked segments during continuous lumbar epidural analgesia. British Journal of Anaesthesia 43: 1172

Dundee J W, Moore J 1960 Alterations in response to somatic pain associated with anaesthesia. IV. Effect of sub-anaesthetic concentration of inhalational agents. British Journal of Anaesthesia 32: 453

Evans K R L, Carrie L E S 1979 Continuous epidural infusion of bupivacaine in labour. Anaesthesia 34: 310

Evans J M, Rosen M, MacCarthy J, Hogg M I J 1976a Apparatus for patient-controlled administration of intravenous narcotics during labour. Lancet i: 17

Evans J M, Hogg M I J, Rosen M 1976b Reversal of narcotic depression in the neonate by naloxone. British Medical Journal 2: 1098

Finster M, Poppers P J, Sinclair J C, Morishima H O, Daniel S S 1965 Accidental intoxication of the fetus with local anesthetic drug during caudal anesthesia. American Journal of Obstetrics and Gynecology 92: 922

Gibbs C P, Schwartz D J, Wynne J W, Hood C I, Kuck E J 1979 Antacid pulmonary aspiration in the dog. Anesthesiology 51: 380

Gibbs C P, Spohr L, Schmidt D 1982 The effectiveness of sodium citrate as an antacid. Anesthesiology 57: 44

Glover D J 1977 Continuous epidural analgesia in the obstetric patient: a feasibility study using a mechanical infusion pump. Anaesthesia 32: 499

Gough J D, Johnston K R, Harmer M 1986 Kinking of epidural catheters. Anaesthesia 41: 1060

Gross H N, Posner N A 1963 Evaluation of hypnosis for obstetric delivery. Medical Journal of Australia 43: 819

Harper N J N, Thomson J, Brayshaw S A 1983 Experience with self-administered pethidine with special reference to the general practitioner obstetric unit. Anaesthesia 38: 52

Harrison R F, Woods T, Shore M, Mathews G, Unwin A 1986 Pain relief in labour using transcutaneous electrical nerve stimulation (TENS). A TENS/TENS placebo controlled study in two parity groups. British Journal of Obstetrics and Gynaecology 93: 739

Heyns O S 1959 Abdominal decompression in the first stage of labour. Journal of Obstetrics and Gynaecology of the British Empire 66: 220

Holdcroft A, Morgan M 1974 Assessment of the analgesic effect in labour of pethidine and 50% nitrous oxide in oxygen (Entonox). Journal of Obstetrics and Gynaecology of the British Commonwealth 81: 603

Jackson M B A, Robson P J 1983 Preliminary clinical and pharmacokinetic experiences in the newborn with meptazinol as compared to pethidine as an obstetric analgesic. Postgraduate Medical Journal 59 (suppl 1): 47
Johnson J R, Moore J, McCaughey W et al 1983 Use of cimetidine as an oral antacid in obstetric anesthesia. Anesthesia and Analgesia 62: 720
Jones P L, Molloy M J, Rosen M 1971 The Cardiff Penthrane inhaler. A vaporiser for the administration of methoxyflurane as an obstetric analgesic. British Journal of Anaesthesia 43: 190
Kim W Y, Pomerace J J, Miller A A 1979 Lidocaine intoxication in a newborn following local anesthesia for episiotomy. Pediatrics 64: 643
Kumar C M, Dennison B, Lawler P G P 1985 Excessive dose requirements of local anaesthetic for epidural analgesia. How far should an epidural catheter be inserted? Anaesthesia 40: 1100
Lamaze F 1956 Qu'est ce que l'accouchement sans douleur, 1st edn. La Farandale, Paris
Latto I P, Rosen M, Molloy M J 1972 Absence of accumulation of methoxyflurane during intermittent self-administration for pain relief in labour. British Journal of Anaesthesia 44: 391
Lavin J P, Samuels S V, Miodovnik M, Holroyde J, Loon M, Joyce T 1981 The effects of bupivacaine and chloroprocaine as local anesthetic for epidural anesthesia on fetal heart rate monitoring patterns. American Journal of Obstetrics and Gynecology 141: 717
Li D F, Rees G A D, Rosen M 1985 Continuous extradural infusion of 0.0625% or 0.125% bupivacaine for pain relief in primigravid labour. British Journal of Anaesthesia 57: 264
MacDonald R, Webster D C S 1986 Obstetric anaesthetic services in the Yorkshire region. British Medical Journal 293: 431
Major V, Rosen M, Mushin W W 1967 Concentration of methoxyflurane for obstetric analgesia by self-administered intermittent inhalation. British Medical Journal 4: 767
McCaughey W, Howe J P, Moore J, Dundee J W 1981 Cimetidine in elective caesarian section. Anaesthesia 36: 167
McGuinness C, Rosen M 1984 Enflurane as an analgesic in labour. Anaesthesia 39: 24
Melzack R, Wall P D 1965 Pain mechanism: a new theory. Science 150: 971
Minnitt R J 1934 Self-administered analgesia for the midwifery of general practice. Proceedings of the Royal Society of Medicine 27: 1313
Moir D D, Thorburn J 1986 Obstetric anaesthesia and analgesia, 3rd edn. Baillière Tindall, London
Moore D C 1966 Caudal anesthesia in obstetrics. New England Journal of Medicine 274: 749
Moore J, Carson R M, Hunter R J 1970 A comparison of the effects of pentazocine and pethidine administered during labour. Journal of Obstetrics and Gynaecology 77: 830
Moya F, James L S 1960 Medical hypnosis for obstetrics. Journal of the American Medical Association 174: 2026
Newman J W, Wood E C 1967 Abdominal decompression and foetal blood gases. British Medical Journal 3: 368
Nicholas A D G, Robson P J 1982 Double blind comparison of meptazinol and pethidine in labour. British Journal of Obstetrics and Gynaecology 89: 31
Paymaster N J 1977 Analgesia after operation — a controlled comparison of meptazinol, pentazocine and pethidine. British Journal of Anaesthesia 49: 1139
Pearson J F, Davies P 1974 The effect of continuous lumbar epidural analgesia upon fetal acid–base status during the second-stage of labour. Journal of Obstetrics and Gynaecology of the British Commonwealth 81: 975
Rainbird A, Pfitzner J 1983 Restricted spread of analgesia following epidural blood patch. Case report with a review of possible complications. Anaesthesia 38: 481
Ralston D H, Shnider S M, DeLorimar A A 1974 Effects of equipotent ephedrine, metaraminol, mephentamine and methoxamine on uterine blood flow in the pregnant ewe. Anesthesiology 40: 354
Report to the Medical Research Council of the committee on nitrous oxide and oxygen analgesia in midwifery 1970 Clinical trials of different concentration of oxygen and nitrous oxide for obstetric analgesia. British Medical Journal 1: 709
Robinson O, Rosen M, Evans J M, Revill S I, David H, Rees G A D 1980 Self-administered intravenous and intramuscular pethidine: controlled trial in labour. Anaesthesia 35: 763
Robson J E 1979 Transcutaneous nerve stimulation for pain relief in labour. Anaesthesia 34: 357
Rosen M, Latto I P, Asscher A W 1972 Kidney function after methoxyflurane analgesia during labour. British Medical Journal 1: 81
Scanlon J W, Ostheimer G W, Lurie A D, Brown W U, Weiss J B, Alper M H 1976 Neurobehavioral responses and drug concentrations in newborns after maternal epidural anesthesia with bupivacaine. Anesthesiology 45: 400
Scott J S 1970 Obstetric analgesia. A consideration of labor pain and a patient-controlled technique for its relief with meperidine. American Journal of Obstetrics and Gynecology 106: 959
Scott D P, Loudon J D O 1960 A method of abdominal decompression in labour. Lancet i: 1181
Scott J R, Rose N B 1976 Effect of psychoprophylaxis (Lamaze preparation) on labor and delivery in primipara. New England Journal of Medicine 294: 1205
Scott P V, Bowen F E, Cartwright P et al 1980 Intrathecal morphine as sole analgesic during labour. British Medical Journal 2: 351
Shnider S M 1970 Anesthesia for elective Cesarian section. In: Shnider S M (ed) Obstetrical anesthesia. Williams & Wilkins, Baltimore
Shulman H, Birnbaum S J 1966 Evaluation of abdominal decompression during first stage of labor. American Journal of Obstetrics and Gynecology 95: 421
Sinclair J C, Fox H A, Lentz J F, Fuld C L, Murphy J 1965 Intoxication of the fetus by a local anesthetic. A newly recognised complication of maternal caudal anesthesia. New England Journal of Medicine 273: 1173
Skjoldebrand A, Garle M, Gustafsson L L, Johansson H, Lunell N O, Rane A 1982 Extradural pethidine with and without adrenaline during labour: wide variation in effect. British Journal of Anaesthesia 54: 415
Slattery P J, Harmer M, Rosen M, Vickers M D 1981 A comparison between meptazinol and pethidine given intravenously on demand in the management of postoperative pain. British Journal of Anaesthesia 53: 927
Slattery P J, Harmer M, Rosen M, Vickers M D 1983 Comparison of the respiratory depressant effects of IV meptazinol and pethidine. British Journal of Anaesthesia 55: 245P
Social Services Committee Second Report 1980 Perinatal and neonatal mortality. HMSO, London
Stewart P 1979 Transcutaneous nerve stimulation as a method of analgesia in labour. Anaesthesia 34: 361
Thigpen J W, Kotelko D M, Shnider S M et al 1983 Bupivacaine cardiotoxicity in hypoxic–acidiotic sheep. Anesthesiology 59: A204
Tronick E, Wise S, Als H, Adamson R, Scanlon J, Brazelton T B 1976 Regional obstetric anesthesia and newborn behaviour. Effect over the first 10 days of life. Pediatrics 58: 94
Trotter M 1947 Variations of the sacral canal: their significance in the administration of caudal analgesia. Current Researches in Analgesia and Anesthesia 26: 192
Tunstall M E 1961 Use of a fixed nitrous oxide and oxygen mixture from one cylinder. Lancet ii: 964
Van Dorsten J P, Miller F C, Yeh S-Y 1981 Spacing the injection interval with paracervical block: a randomised study. Obstetrics and Gynecology 58: 696
Wallis L, Shnider S M, Palahnuik R J, Spivey H T 1974 An evaluation of acupuncture analgesia in obstetrics. Anesthesiology 41: 506
Wiener P C, Hogg M I J, Rosen M 1977 Effects of naloxone on pethidine-induced neonatal depression. British Medical Journal 2: 228
Wiener P C, Hogg M I J, Rosen M 1979 Neonatal respiration, feeding and neurobehavioural state. Effects of intrapartum bupivacaine, pethidine and pethidine reversed by naloxone. Anaesthesia 34: 996

SECTION 7

Abnormal Labour

50

Lindsay S. Alger and M. Carlyle Crenshaw

Preterm labour and delivery of the preterm infant

During the past 20 years developed countries have seen a steady decline in the neonatal mortality rate. Since prematurity is the leading cause of perinatal morbidity and mortality, it is disappointing to realize that this improvement has been accomplished without any significant reduction in the delivery of very low birthweight infants (Lee et al 1980). Preterm delivery has assumed even greater prominence as advances in the fields of infectious disease, genetics, neonatology and paediatric surgery have reduced morbidity from other causes. Despite the considerable optimism of the obstetrical community, it is apparent that pharmacological inhibition of preterm labour, cervical cerclage, prolonged bedrest and nutritional assistance have not resulted in a major reduction in preterm delivery. To accomplish this will require a comprehensive programme of identification of the patient at risk, prevention of labour onset, early detection of excessive uterine activity and eradication of existent contractions.

DEFINITION, INCIDENCE AND CONSEQUENCES

Preterm labour is defined as the occurrence of regular contractions productive of cervical change (dilatation or effacement) prior to 37 completed weeks of gestation from the first day of the last menstrual period (Anderson 1977). Pregnancies terminating before 20 weeks of gestation are considered abortions in the USA. In the UK, an abortion is a delivery of a dead baby before the 28th week of gestation. Therefore in the USA the terms preterm labour and preterm birth assume a lower limit for gestational age of 20 weeks but in the UK dead babies are not stillbirths until 28 weeks. Since gestational age is often difficult to ascertain, many statistics refer to birthweight of between 500 and less than 2500 g. However, this results in the inclusion of many term infants with retarded growth and the exclusion of preterm infants of greater birthweight. The very low birthweight infant is defined as weighing less than 1500 g. This typically corresponds to a gestation of less than 32 weeks but the severely growth-retarded term infant will be included as well. A system of reporting which combines the objective measure of birthweight in addition to the more subjective assessment of gestational age appears most useful.

The incidence of preterm birth is dependent on many factors and varies from one country to another and institution to institution. In developed countries reported rates generally vary between 5 and 9% (Rush et al 1976, Chase 1977, New Zealand Health Statistics Report 1978). Because the diagnosis of preterm labour is harder to define, rates are unavailable, although undoubtedly greater than those for preterm birth.

As many as 85% of the neonatal deaths occurring in structurally normal infants can be attributed to preterm delivery (Rush et al 1976). In addition to the increased risk of developing early complications such as respiratory distress syndrome, intraventricular haemorrhage, patent ductus ateriosus and necrotizing enterocolitis, many of the survivors will be permanently handicapped. Preterm and low birthweight infants subsequently demonstrate lower IQ scores and a higher incidence of neurological abnormalities, learning disabilities, chronic pulmonary disease and visual deficits (Kitchen et al 1982, Astbury et al 1983, McCormick 1985). These consequences are both emotionally and financially draining for the family of the preterm infant. Prolonged hospitalization can disrupt parent–infant bonding. A recent estimate of the financial burden concluded that each survivor weighing 600–699 g at birth costs society 10 times the amount required for the surviving 800–899 g infant (Walker et al 1984). It is unclear whether the lifetime earnings of such

Table 50.1 Risk factors associated with preterm labour

Maternal characteristics
Age under 15 or over 35
Race
Weight
Smoking
Coitus
Psychosocial stresses
Socioeconomic factors
Social class
Occupation (heavy or stressful work)
Lack of antenatal care
Unmarried
Past reproductive history
Previous preterm delivery
Second-trimester spontaneous abortion
Congenital uterine anomalies
Leiomyomata
Asherman's syndrome
Maternal in utero diethylstilboesterol exposure
Previous pregnancy bleeding
Present pregnancy complications
Multiple gestation
Polyhydramnios
Fetal congenital anomalies
Fetal growth retardation
Placenta praevia
Placental abruption
Other pregnancy bleeding
Incompetent cervix
Preterm rupture of the membranes
Maternal illness
Retained intrauterine device
Iatrogenic
Genital tract infections
Neisseria gonorrhoeae
Group B beta-haemolytic streptococci
Chlamydia trachomatis
Bacteroides sp. and other anaerobes
Trichomonas vaginalis
Mycoplasmas
Rubella
Herpes
Cytomegalovirus
Varicella

extremely small infants can be expected to exceed the costs of their initial and long-term medical care.

Epidemiology and risk factors

The aetiology of preterm labour is only partially understood since multiple factors may play a role either singly or in combination. While further clarification of the mechanism of initiation of both term and preterm labour is sought, several epidemiological associations and risk factors have been recognized (Table 50.1). The identification of risk factors for preterm birth is essential for developing intervention programmes designed to reduce the incidence of preterm delivery. Known risk factors may be grouped under five headings: maternal characteristics, socioeconomic factors, past reproductive history, present pregnancy complications and genital tract infections. A sixth category, unknown causes, still accounts for greater than one-third of all cases. Although associated with preterm labour, there is no evidence that maternal and socioeconomic epidemiological factors actually cause preterm labour.

Maternal characteristics

Age. The incidence of preterm delivery is lowest for patients between 25 and 29 years of age and highest for those under age 15 or those having their first child over age 35 (Frederick & Anderson 1976, Baird 1977, Hardy & Mellitts 1977).

Race. In the USA, preterm delivery occurs twice as often in black women compared to white, even after controlling for socioeconomic factors (Chase 1977, Garn et al 1977). Pregnancies resulting from inter-racial marriages achieve a greater gestational age than those of black couples (Garn & Bailey 1977).

Weight. Prepregnancy weight of less than 50 kg is associated with a threefold increase in the preterm delivery rate compared to prepregnancy weight greater than 57 kg (Frederick & Anderson 1976). Height has also been reported to affect gestational age at delivery, with shorter women more likely to deliver preterm. However, when height and weight are examined simultaneously, it appears that only weight is related to preterm birth.

Habits. Maternal smoking decreases birthweight and increases the incidence of preterm birth in direct proportion to the number of cigarettes smoked (Meyer & Tonascia 1977). There is an increased incidence of abruptio placentae, placenta praevia and premature rupture of the membranes, especially when more than 20 cigarettes per day are smoked. Although ethanol and narcotic abuse may also be correlated with prematurity, these associations have not been clearly delineated. Coitus during the second half of pregnancy has been reported to increase risk, although this is controversial (Wagner et al 1976, Naeye 1979). Possible mechanisms include the effects of seminal prostaglandins locally, the triggering of uterine contractions from orgasm, or the deposition of infectious agents adjacent to the products of conception. Maternal employment, particularly in a physically demanding or emotionally stressful job, has been reported in some studies, but not all, to be correlated with increased risk of preterm labour (Mamelle et al 1984, Murphy et al 1984). Other psychosocial stresses may play a role, perhaps through the release of endogenous catecholamines which could increase uterine irritability (Newton & Hunt 1984).

Socioeconomic factors

Examining the worldwide variations in the incidence of preterm delivery, Boldman & Reed (1977) observed that: 'income, food supplies, sanitation, industrialization, education, urbanization, social customs, and the medical care system interact with each other' to influence prematurity rates.

Social class. Data from the Obstetrical Statistical Cooperative from the years 1970–1976 in the USA indicate that, for both whites and non-whites, public ward patients are at greater risk for delivering preterm than are private patients (Kaltreider & Kohl 1980). Both paternal and maternal occupation may be correlated since labourers have the highest incidence, professionals a lower rate and farmers the lowest incidence of all (Baird 1977). Lack of antenatal care is also associated with increased risk with the lowest rate reported for patients registering for care in the first trimester (Kaltreider & Kohl 1980). The economically disadvantaged woman, who often has additional risk factors, is particularly likely to benefit from medical care (Moore et al 1986).

Marital status. The risk of preterm delivery among white unmarried gravidas is almost double that of their married counterparts (Frederick & Anderson 1976, Chase 1977, Kaltreider & Kohl 1980). Although the relationship is less striking for black women, Chase reported that low birthweight infants occurred more frequently in illegitimate pregnancies regardless of maternal age or race.

Past reproductive history

Previous preterm delivery. The reported risk of recurrent preterm labour following one previous preterm birth varies between 17 and 50% but is generally considered to be about 35% (Keirse et al 1978, Bakketeig & Hoffman 1981). The risk increases with each subsequent preterm birth and may be as high as 70% following two or more preterm deliveries.

Previous abortion. Although second-trimester spontaneous abortions or stillbirths are risk factors for a subsequent preterm birth (Rush 1979), first-trimester pregnancy loss does not appear to be predictive (Keirse et al 1978). Older reports described an increased risk following repeated first-trimester induced abortions, but with the current use of laminaria and atraumatic cervical dilatation, this no longer holds true (Keirse et al 1978, Linn et al 1983).

Uterine abnormalities. Congenital uterine anomalies (e.g. bicornuate, didelphic or unicornuate uteri; Heinonen et al 1982), intramural or submucosal leiomyomata (Muran et al 1980), and Asherman's syndrome (Forssman 1965) decrease the likelihood of carrying a pregnancy to term. The T-shaped uterus associated with in utero exposure to diethylstilboesterol (DES) is also a factor (Stillman 1982). Incompetence of the cervix, a rare condition, whether congenital or secondary to trauma or cervical conization, predisposes to preterm birth rather than preterm labour in the strict sense.

Previous pregnancy bleeding. Patients with a prior history of antepartum bleeding from a placenta praevia or placental abruption are at increased risk of recurrence, and hence of preterm birth (Crenshaw et al 1973, Bakketeig & Hoffman 1981).

Present pregnancy complications

Uterine overdistension. Both multiple gestations and polyhydramnios are independently associated with preterm labour (Rush et al 1976, Kirbinen & Jouppila 1978). Monozygous twins are at higher risk than dizygous twins, primarily due to an increased rate of premature rupture of membranes and induction of labour for fetal indications (MacGillivray et al 1982; see Chapter 34). Preterm delivery occurs in 30–40% of pregnancies complicated by polyhydramnios (Kirbinen & Jouppila 1978).

Congenital anomalies. The fetus with multiple congenital anomalies, central nervous system anomalies, or renal agenesis is at increased risk. These pregnancies are often associated with intrauterine growth retardation and it is possible that the fetus stressed by placental insufficiency produces a hormonal milieu conducive to labour onset.

Antepartum haemorrhage. Whether due to placenta praevia, abruptio placenta, threatened abortion in early pregnancy or antepartum bleeding with a normally implanted placenta, antepartum haemorrhage is associated with an increased incidence of preterm birth (Turnbull 1977).

Maternal illness. Almost any severe maternal disease may be associated with preterm delivery, if for no other reason than indicated obstetric intervention. Iatrogenic factors play a large role in the prematurity associated with diabetes mellitus — polyhydramnios and congenital anomalies also contribute — chronic hypertension or renal disease. Many illnesses such as asthma, heart disease, hepatitis, cholestasis, hyperthyroidism, Cushing's disease, hyperparathyroidism, and severe anaemia may also be associated with spontaneous preterm labour. Systemic infection such as bacterial pneumonia, acute pyelonephritis or appendicitis may release endotoxins. In experimental studies, endotoxins stimulate myometrial activity (Creasy 1984). Asymptomatic bacteriuria in the absence of renal involvement does not appear to increase risk (Kincaid-Smith 1968).

Miscellaneous. A retained intrauterine device increases the likelihood of preterm labour (Tatum et al 1976) as does fetal death. Unfortunately, preterm delivery may result when elective repeat Caesarean section or labour induction are performed after inaccurate determination of gestational age. Preterm rupture of the membranes precedes preterm labour in one-third of cases. In this situation it is the aetiology of the membrane rupture which is the true cause of the preterm labour.

Genital tract infections

Several observations support the hypothesis that maternal genital tract infection frequently plays an aetiological role in preterm premature membrane rupture:

1. Similar demographic risk factors (such as youth and low socioeconomic status) are associated with both preterm

delivery and an increased incidence of sexually transmitted infections.
2. Seasonal variations in coital frequency parallel the variations in amniotic fluid infection and perinatal mortality with all three incidences peaking in the spring (Naeye 1980).
3. Clinical and histologically documented chorioamnionitis occurs more frequently in association with preterm deliveries (Russell 1979).
4. More mothers and infants are likely to develop early-onset infectious sequelae following a preterm delivery compared with a term delivery.
5. Empiric treatment of patients in preterm labour with erythromycin increases the chances of successful labour inhibition (McGregor et al 1986a).
6. Direct sampling of amniotic fluid using amniocentesis demonstrates pathogenic micro-organisms in a significant proportion of patients in preterm labour or with preterm rupture of the membranes. Bacteria may be recovered in 20–30% of such samples compared with 2–4% of fluid specimens from uncomplicated third-trimester pregnancies (Garite et al 1979, Bobitt et al 1981).
7. A large number of studies demonstrate on association between specific organisms and preterm delivery. Organisms linked to prematurity include *Neisseria gonorrhoeae* (Edwards et al 1978), group B streptococcus (Regan et al 1981), Bacteroides sp. (and perhaps other anaerobes; Minkoff et al 1984), *Trichomonas vaginalis* (Minkoff et al 1984), *Chlamydia trachomatis* (Martin et al 1982, Alger et al 1988), and possibly mycoplasmas. Several viruses including rubella, herpes, cytomegalovirus, smallpox, and chicken pox have been implicated (Remington & Klein 1983).

Theoretically, there is good reason to suggest that infection can initiate preterm delivery. Several investigators have postulated that term labour is initiated by the activation of amniotic and chorionic phospholipase A_2 which hydrolyses the phospholipids in the placental membranes, producing an increase in free arachidonic acid and the synthesis of prostaglandins. Bejar et al (1981) have found that:

1. human amnion contains the same concentration of arachidonic acid in early pregnancy as at term (significantly higher than that in the chorion);
2. the micro-organisms commonly associated with prematurity and perinatal infections possess phospholipase A_2 activities several times higher than that of the membrane phospholipase A_2;
3. the most common bacteria found in the cervix and vagina have low specific activities;
4. bacteria such as *Bacteroides fragilis*, *Peptostreptococcus*, *Fusobacterium*, or *Gardnerella vaginalis* which have been cultured from amniotic fluid in cases of premature labour have the highest specific activities. Bejar et al hypothesize that bacteria infecting the cervix may penetrate through the chorion to the amnion with proteolytic enzymes. These bacteria may thus trigger premature labour as they synthesize and release enzymes that could split arachidonic acid from the membranes.

DIAGNOSIS OF PRETERM LABOUR

It is frequently difficult to diagnose preterm labour and early prodromal labour may not be distinguishable from false labour except in retrospect. Perhaps half of all women presenting preterm with regular uterine contractions are in false labour, as evidenced by the efficacy of placebo treatment in achieving reduction of their symptoms. Frequency, regularity, or discomfort of contractions does not readily distinguish true preterm labour from false labour, nor does the period of time over which contractions persist. In order to prevent unnecessary pharmacological intervention with its attendant side-effects, evidence of cervical change is required prior to making the diagnosis and initiating therapy. It is equally important to determine whether the pregnancy is truly preterm.

Patients with intact membranes who present with little or no cervical change are observed at bedrest avoiding the dorsal supine position. Intravenous hydration is initiated; this may improve uterine blood flow and reduce myometrial activity. The infusion of water inhibits the release of antidiuretic hormone, and perhaps oxytocin as well (Niebyl et al 1978). Preterm labour may be preceded by a prodromal phase which is reversible following these simple, non-specific measures. However, these women still remain at high risk for developing subsequent preterm labour which will require more elaborate treatment (Valenzuela et al 1983).

External tocographic and fetal heart rate monitoring is begun. The cervix is assessed at regular intervals by the same examiner for evidence of effacement or dilatation. Preterm labour is diagnosed if there is documented cervical change or if on initial evaluation the cervix is at least 2 cm dilated or 80% effaced. Such initial findings are probably the result of uterine activity and further cervical change might preclude successful labour inhibition. It is unusual for cervical change to occur when the interval between contractions is greater than 8 minutes. Therefore, the most frequently used definitions of preterm labour stipulate a contraction frequency of 4 in 20 minutes or 6–8 in 1 hour, but there must be associated cervical change.

When the gestational age is uncertain, a determination must be made whether the small fetus is in fact preterm or rather a mature but growth-retarded fetus. It may be detrimental to maintain the growth-retarded fetus in an adverse intrauterine environment. Even if the initial ultrasound evaluation is performed in the third trimester, it is of some use and is non-invasive. Determination of the head–abdomen circumference ratio and amniotic fluid volume may aid in the diagnosis of growth retardation but can be misleading in cases of symmetrical growth retardation.

When in doubt, amniocentesis can be useful for although it cannot distinguish a term from a preterm fetus, it can establish the presence of pulmonary maturity and, therefore, identify those fetuses not requiring labour inhibition. In addition, analysis of amniotic fluid for evidence of infection may allow early detection of chorioamnionitis. Amniocentesis is performed after the initiation of tocolytic therapy in order to reduce the chance of membrane rupture. Tocolysis is continued pending the results of the studies.

Table 50.2 Contraindications to inhibition of preterm labour

Absolute contraindications
Fetal death
Fetal congenital anomaly incompatible with life
Chorioamnionitis
Fetal complications requiring immediate delivery
Maternal complications requiring immediate delivery
Relative contraindications
Fetal growth retardation
Fetal distress
Pre-eclampsia
Vaginal bleeding (placenta praevia, abruption)
Cervix more than 4 cm dilated

MANAGEMENT

Initial patient evaluation

Once the diagnosis of preterm labour is established, a search for the aetiology should be undertaken since failure to identify a treatable condition could sabotage attempts to inhibit labour. A midstream urine specimen should be examined by microscope and sent for culture to rule out bacteriuria. Presumptive evidence of infection by urinalysis warrants antibiotic therapy pending culture results. The association of lower genital tract infection with preterm labour requires a sterile speculum examination to be performed and cervical cultures obtained for group B streptococci, *Neisseria gonorrhoeae* and *Chlamydia trachomatis*. Positive culture results necessitate prompt institution of appropriate antibiotics. Although empiric treatment with erythromycin of women presenting in preterm labour has been reported to improve the chances of successful prolongation of pregnancy (McGregor et al 1986a), it is generally recommended that antibiotic therapy should be reserved for a proven infection. Culture evidence of herpes might alter intrapartum management but it has not been determined whether obtaining such cultures routinely is cost-effective.

If the patient is febrile, a source of infection should be sought and appropriate antibiotic therapy initiated. If the source is obscure or chorioamnionitis is suspected, amniocentesis should be performed and an unspun drop of fluid examined microscopically for bacteria. In cases of true chorioamnionitis, attempts at labour inhibition do not result in any significant prolongation of pregnancy (Gravett et al 1986).

A complete history and physical examination are necessary to determine whether there are any maternal or fetal contraindications to tocolytic therapy. Although the upper limit of gestational age for preterm labour is defined as 37 weeks, labour inhibition beyond 35 weeks is usually not warranted unless there is uncertainty regarding gestational age (Korenbrot et al 1984). Attempts to achieve any further reduction in morbidity after this time are not cost-effective although individual cases may benefit from delaying labour until 37 weeks' gestation (Konte et al 1986).

There are few absolute contraindications to the use of tocolytic drugs (Table 50.2). While several conditions are associated with increased risk, judicious tocolysis with careful monitoring of both mother and fetus may be undertaken if the risks of preterm delivery appear to outweigh the risks of tocolysis. In selected cases, even the patient with pre-eclampsia may be a candidate for tocolysis in order to gain an additional 48 hours during which time corticosteroids may be administered to promote pulmonary maturation. Conditions such as maternal diabetes or cardiac disease may influence the selection of tocolytic agent since the beta-adrenergic agonists, in contrast to magnesium sulphate, may exacerbate existing abnormalities.

Severe bleeding from a placenta praevia or placental abruption contraindicates the use of any agent which will increase vascular instability, but, in milder forms, tocolysis may help to prevent further placental separation. The chances of successfully prolonging pregnancy are greatly reduced if the cervix is already more than 4 cm dilated at the initiation of the tocolytic therapy and it is likely that the fetus will deliver with high systemic levels of the agent present. An attempt at tocolysis may be warranted for the very preterm infant where a week's prolongation may improve perinatal outcome. The guidelines are no substitute for individualized patient care.

PHARMACOLOGICAL INHIBITION OF LABOUR

The physiology and regulation of normal labour, including the mechanism of myometrial smooth muscle contractility, are discussed in Chapter 45. The pharmacological agents most commonly used to inhibit labour act at different points in this contraction pathway and therefore may be associated with different side-effects. It is difficult to compare their relative efficacies and none is universally successful.

The tocolytics currently in use are beta-adrenergic agonists, magnesium sulphate, calcium channel blockers, prostaglandin synthetase inhibitors, as well as various miscellaneous agents. Ethanol also possesses tocolytic activity but has been supplanted by more effective agents with fewer side-effects.

Table 50.3 Beta-adrenergic physiological effects

$Beta_1$-receptor effects	$Beta_2$-receptor effects
↑ Heart rate	↓ Vascular tone
↑ Stroke volume	↓ Mean arterial pressure
↑ Cardiac output	↓ Uterine activity
↑ Lipolysis, ketones	↓ Bronchiolar tone
↑ Intracellular potassium	↑ Glycogenolysis, hyperglycaemia
↓ Bowel motility	↑ Insulin release
	↑ Lactate
	↑ Renin

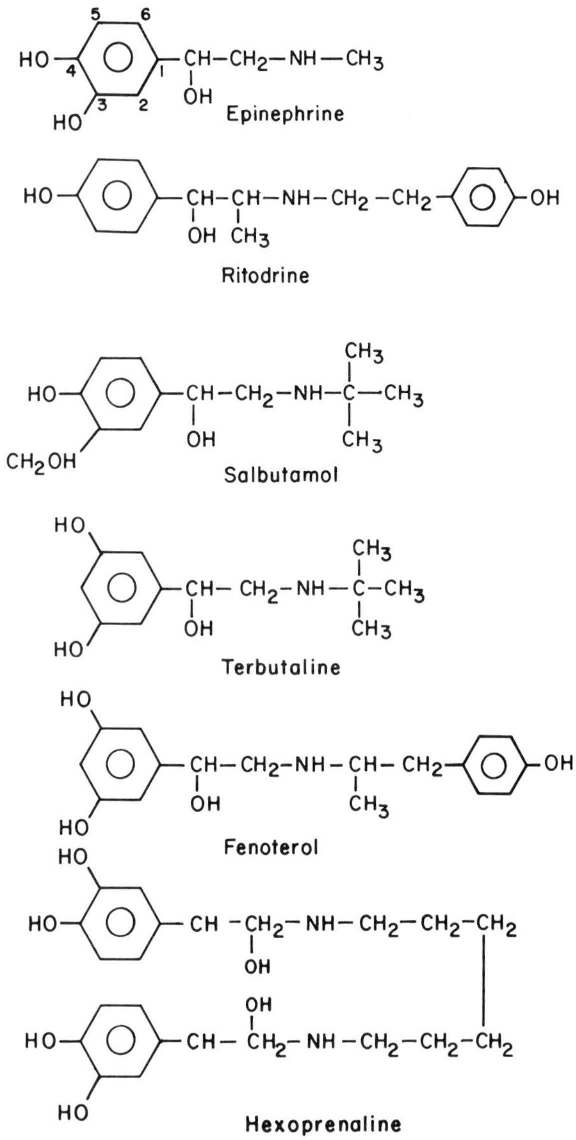

Fig. 50.1 Chemical structure of adrenaline (epinephrine) and related beta-adrenergic drugs used for tocolysis. Activity is related to large alkyl substitutions on the ethylamine side chain and hydroxyl groups at the 3 or 5 position of the benzene ring.

The woman in false labour whose contractions persist may respond to sedatives and narcotics. However, there is no evidence that these agents are effective in inhibiting true preterm labour. If the fetus is delivered in the next few hours, these medications can result in neonatal depression. Mild sedation may occasionally be indicated to alleviate maternal anxiety which, understandably, often accompanies preterm labour.

Beta-adrenergic agonists

Mechanism of action

The smooth muscle-relaxing properties of the beta-adrenergic agonists is derived from their interaction with $beta_2$-adrenergic receptor sites on myometrial cell membranes. The agonist–receptor complex activates the enzyme adenylate cyclase, resulting in an increase in the intracellular concentrations of cyclic adenosine monophosphate (cAMP; Roberts 1984). The increase in cAMP activates a protein kinase which causes both a phosphorylation of membrane proteins in the sarcoplasmic reticulum responsible for reducing the intracellular concentration of calcium and an inhibition of myosin light-chain kinase activity which prevents the actin–myosin interaction necessary for smooth muscle contraction. The trophoblast also has $beta_2$ receptors and in this tissue cAMP increases progesterone production (Caritis et al 1983).

Efficacy

There are no pure $beta_2$ stimulants. All of the beta-adrenergic agonists have both $beta_1$ and $beta_2$ effects (Table 50.3) and the efficacy of a given agent is generally limited by the severity of its associated cardiovascular $beta_1$ effects. Isoxsuprine was the first beta-adrenergic agent used for inhibition of premature labour (Hendricks 1964), followed by the introduction of orciprenaline (Baillie et al 1970). Controlled trials have demonstrated their efficacy in delaying delivery compared to placebo but significant maternal hypotension and tachycardia are associated with their use.

These agents have been replaced by a second generation of $beta_2$-selective drugs which include: salbutamol, fenoterol, hexoprenaline, ritodrine and terbutaline. Most, but not all, trials with these agents have shown them to be successful in delaying delivery for more than 7 days. In individual studies differing efficacies have been reported. The currently available data do not consistently indicate superior efficacy or safety for any one of these agents.

In theory, $beta_2$ activity is increased by hydroxyl groups in the 3 and 5 positions of the benzene ring and by the extent of the alkyl substitutions on the amino group of the ethylamine side chain (Fig. 50.1). At equipotent uterine inhibitory doses hexoprenaline has significantly less effect on the maternal heart rate than most beta-mimetics (Lipshitz & Baillie 1976).

Table 50.4 Maternal side-effects of the beta-agonist tocolytic agents

Palpitations	Nausea, bloating
Arrhythmias	Paralytic ileus
Myocardial ischaemia	Tremor
Pulmonary oedema	Restlessness, agitation
Anaemia	Rash
Glucose intolerance	Elevated transaminase levels
Hypokalaemia	

Side-effects

Maternal side-effects of the beta-adrenergic agonists are listed in Table 50.4. Alterations in the cardiovascular response are the most pronounced with at least one-third of patients experiencing mild palpitations. Vascular beta$_2$-receptor stimulation produces vasodilation, hypotension, and a compensatory tachycardia. With the use of the newer beta-mimetics, systolic blood pressure may actually rise slightly due to an increase in cardiac output but the fall in diastolic blood pressure is greater, resulting in a slight reduction in mean arterial pressure (Lipshitz & Baillie 1976, Bieniarz 1977). In addition, despite predominant beta$_2$-receptor activity there is residual beta$_1$ activity resulting in direct cardiac effects. Cardiac arrhythmias (Merkatz et al 1980), myocardial ischaemia (Benedetti 1983) and pulmonary oedema (Hawker 1984) have been reported with the use of these agents. Premature ventricular and nodal contractions are the most frequent arrhythmias arising but atrial fibrillation has been described. Myocardial ischaemia is usually localized to the subendocardial region and is the result of decreased myocardial perfusion secondary to a reduction in both diastolic perfusion pressure and length of diastole. Creatine phosphokinase isoenzyme confirmation of mycardial damage has not been documented (Ying & Tejani 1982) however and similar electrocardiogram findings can be seen in asymptomatic patients (Hendricks et al 1986).

The mechanism responsible for the generation of pulmonary oedema is uncertain. A high output state, pulmonary capillary endothelial leaks and fluid retention secondary to increased renin levels have been suggested as playing a role. However, in the majority of cases there is no evidence of left ventricular failure on echocardiography or by Swan–Ganz catheter evaluation (Philipsen et al 1981). Risk factors for the development of pulmonary oedema include multiple gestation, fluid overload, anaemia and prolonged duration of maternal tachycardia. Pulmonary oedema does not usually develop within the first 24 hours of therapy. Intravenous administration of physiological saline solutions contributes to fluid overload and decreased colloid oncotic pressure. Although in the majority of reported cases patients received corticosteroids as well, the agents used have negligible mineralocorticoid activity and their apparent association with the development of pulmonary oedema may be coincidental. Certainly, pulmonary oedema can still occur in their absence.

Another consequence of the stimulation of the renin aldosterone system is a dilutional anaemia resulting from plasma volume expansion. On average there is a 15% fall in haematocrit. Acute cerebral ischaemic episodes have been reported in patients with a previous history of migraine headaches (Rosen et al 1982).

Maternal metabolic effects are the result of beta$_2$-receptor stimulation which increases cAMP production. In the liver this promotes hepatic glycogenolysis and hence maternal hyperglycaemia. In the pancreas cAMP increases insulin secretion but insulin levels rise, largely as a direct response to hyperglycaemia (Cano et al 1985). In most patients there is a transient modest increase in blood glucose levels which is of little consequence, rarely exceeding 180 mg/dl. Since glucose levels peak 3–6 hours after the initiation of therapy and return towards baseline within 24 hours without therapy, exogenous insulin is usually unnecessary (Young et al 1983). Ketoacidosis has been reported in the insulin-dependent diabetic who is inadequately monitored (Thomas et al 1977b, Mordes et al 1982). Simultaneous administration of insulin via calibrated infusion pump will provide glucose control allowing the use of beta-agonists in the diabetic maternity patient. Prolonged oral therapy is usually not associated with abnormal carbohydrate metabolism (Mordes et al 1982) but some patients on terbutaline will exhibit persistent altered glucose tolerance (Main EK et al 1987). Lactate produced by increased muscle glycogenolysis is usually insufficient to produce acidosis.

Transient hypokalaemia with serum potassium levels falling on average to a nadir of 2.7 mmol may occur as a result of redistribution of potassium from the extracellular to the intracellular compartment. This is partially due to hyperinsulinaemia but is possibly a consequence of direct beta-adrenoceptor stimulation as well (Cano et al 1985). Urinary excretion and total body potassium remain unchanged. The electrocardiogram appears to be unaltered and there are no reports of adverse effects (Thomas et al 1977a). Since potassium levels return to normal without therapy within 24 hours, potassium supplementation is unnecessary (Young et al 1983).

Women may complain of tremor, palpitations or chest tightness. Nausea, bloating, and, rarely, paralytic ileus may develop (Robertson et al 1981). Restlessness, agitation, and anxiety are not uncommon. Rash and elevation of serum liver transaminase levels are infrequent occurrences (Lotgering et al 1986).

Fetal and neonatal effects

Fetal and neonatal side-effects depend on the agent used and the interval from discontinuation of therapy to delivery. All of the agents, by producing maternal hyperglycaemia, may be associated with neonatal hypoglycaemia. Ritodrine crosses the placenta in humans, although fetal levels are lower than maternal levels (Gandar et al 1980). Fetal tachycardia results and this is seen with terbutaline administration as well. In animal studies fenoterol transfer is minimal (Meissner & Klostermann 1976), while hexoprenaline does not appear to cross the placenta, perhaps because it is not fat-soluble (Lipshitz et al 1982).

A possible beneficial fetal side-effect is a reduction in respiratory distress syndrome with the use of ritodrine or terbutaline, but this is not well documented in humans. Neonatal hypoglycaemia, hypocalcaemia, ileus, hypotension and death have been reported with the use of isoxsuprine in two retrospective studies, particularly when used in the extremely preterm gestation with a short interval from loading dose to delivery (Brazy & Pupkin 1979, Epstein et al 1979). Only hypoglycaemia has been noted with the use of other agents. Multiple prospective trials as well as follow-up series in exposed children up to age 4 have demonstrated no significant adverse short- or long-term effects (Freysz et al 1977, Creasy 1984).

Administration

The patient is placed in a left lateral, tilt, recumbent position and an intravenous line is inserted. Baseline maternal heart rate, blood pressure and respiratory rate are determined. The fetal heart rate and uterine activity are continuously monitored. Initial therapy is administered via a calibrated intravenous infusion pump. Intravenous fluids low in salt, such as half-strength normal saline initially, followed by 5% dextrose in water (in the absence of significant hyperglycaemia), are preferred.

The drug infusion is introduced as a separate infusion into the main intravenous line at the point of entry closest to the arm. The initial infusion rate is the lowest recommended for the selected agent. The dosage is increased every 10–20 minutes by increasing the infusion rate until uterine activity is inhibited to less than one contraction every 15 minutes, or when adverse maternal effects occur. As contractions begin to space out the infusion rate is increased less frequently. Further increase in dosage is often unnecessary once contractions are 10 minutes apart because uterine activity may continue to decline while the same infusion rate is maintained. A maternal heart rate greater than 140 beats/min or any other unacceptable side-effect requires a reduction in dose. The recommended maximum dosage of the drug is used as a guideline but may be exceeded on an individual basis when a patient demonstrates less sensitivity to the drug, as evidenced by a lack of side-effects.

During therapy maternal vital signs, uterine contractions, and fetal heart rate should be recorded every 15 minutes until a maintenance dose has been established and then every 30 minutes for the duration of intravenous administration. Once effective tocolysis has been achieved, intravenous infusion is maintained for an additional 12–24 hours depending upon the difficulty encountered in initially inhibiting contractions. The infusion rate may be tapered during this time as long as uterine activity remains inhibited. During this time maternal intake and output are monitored, blood studies are reassessed at 12-hour intervals and the patient is periodically examined for evidence of uterine tenderness or pulmonary oedema.

Following this maintenance period, the infusion rate is gradually reduced at half-hour intervals until the maternal heart rate decreases to 100 beats/min. Subcutaneous or intramuscular administration followed by oral therapy is then initiated and the intravenous infusion discontinued 30 minutes later. Alternatively, oral therapy may directly follow intravenous therapy. It is unreasonable to expect successful conversion to oral therapy unless uterine activity remains inhibited at intravenous infusion rates which result in serum levels comparable to those achieved with oral administration. Normally this occurs at the lowest recommended infusion rate for the agent. Occasionally, long-term intravenous tocolysis for several weeks will be necessary because recurrent contractions prevent switching to oral therapy (Hill et al 1985).

Magnesium sulphate

Mechanism of action

For many years it has been recognized that magnesium sulphate inhibits myometrial contractility since clinical use of magnesium for the treatment of pre-eclampsia frequently resulted in decreased uterine activity as a side-effect. The exact mechanism of its action is uncertain. Magnesium decreases the frequency of depolarization and uncouples depolarization from the contraction in isolated muscle strips in vitro (Harbert et al 1969). This suggests that magnesium competes with calcium for entry into the cell at depolarization. There is less intracellular free calcium available to participate in the actin–myosin interaction of smooth muscle contraction. Hypocalcaemia resulting from increased urinary excretion further decreases available intracellular calcium.

Efficacy

Magnesium levels of 5–8 mg/dl are necessary to inhibit uterine activity. Uterine activity does not subside in most cases until levels are above 5 mg/dl while patients become lethargic when levels exceed 8 mg/dl (Hollander et al 1987). However, levels as high as 11 mg/dl, a level exceeding recommended therapeutic levels, do not guarantee labour inhibition (McCubbin et al 1981).

A comparison trial of magnesium sulphate and ethanol demonstrated that magnesium sulphate was superior to ethanol, but only marginally effective if the cervix was more than 1 cm dilated (Steer & Petrie 1977). The maintenance dose of 2 g/h used in this study could result in subtherapeutic levels. In another comparison trial with a small number of patients, magnesium sulphate appeared as effective as terbutaline and was associated with fewer adverse cardiovascular effects (Miller et al 1982). Administration of magnesium sulphate at constant infusion rates greater than 2 g/h improves the chances for successful labour inhibition. Titrating infusion rates to clinical response, Elliott (1983) was able to achieve prevention of delivery for at least 48 hours in 62% (53/85) patients with cervical dilatation of 3–5 cm and intact membranes. Delivery was successfully delayed in 31% (5/16) of patients with cervical dilatation of 6 cm or greater.

Long-term intravenous magnesium sulphate tocolysis has been employed successfully for as long as 13 weeks where therapy with intravenous ritodrine failed to halt uterine contractions (Wilkins et al 1986). Additional comparative studies are necessary to determine whether magnesium sulphate or a beta-mimetic is the intravenous tocolytic of choice but magnesium sulphate is preferred by some for those with diabetes mellitus, hyperthyroidism, or possible cardiovascular complications. The use of magnesium sulphate in combination with a beta-adrenergic agent may be more effective than using either agent alone (Hatjis et al 1984) although this approach is controversial, since side-effects may be increased (Ferguson et al 1984). In general, when the initially selected agent fails to inhibit labour, the alternative agent is substituted rather than added after searching carefully for an underlying aetiology which could explain the failure of tocolysis.

Side-effects

In contrast to ritodrine, magnesium sulphate does not cause a significant decrease in maternal diastolic blood pressure or increase in maternal and fetal heart rates although a mild maternal tachycardia and reduction in mean arterial pressure may be associated with bolus infusion (Cotton et al 1984a). In the rhesus monkey, magnesium sulphate increases uterine and placental blood flow while ritodrine results in a decrease in placental blood flow (Thiagarajah et al 1985). Magnesium sulphate may therefore be the agent of choice if there is the possibility of placental insufficiency.

Magnesium sulphate administration causes peripheral vasodilation. The woman may experience uncomfortable warmth and a flushing sensation. Nausea, headache, dizziness, chest tightness, and lethargy can occur. Pulmonary oedema has been observed in patients who also received corticosteroids (Elliott 1983). Maternal temperature falls on the average by 0.5°C potentially obscuring evidence of early intra-amniotic infection (Parsons et al 1987). Magnesium levels of 15–18 mg/dl depress respiration and higher levels can produce cardiac arrest. However, as long as deep tendon reflexes remain present, the patient is not at risk for these complications. Calcium gluconate is an effective antidote. Magnesium is contraindicated in patients with myasthenia gravis and should be used with caution, if at all, in patients with renal failure if drug accumulation is to be avoided.

Neonatal depression has been reported following prolonged intravenous therapy with high doses close to delivery. Respiratory and motor depression have been observed in infants with umbilical cord magnesium concentrations greater than 4 mg/dl (Lipsitz & English 1967). However, in the majority of infants there is no significant alteration in neurological state or Apgar scores (Green et al 1983).

Dosage and administration

An initial loading dose of 4 g is administered intravenously over 20 minutes followed by a maintenance dose of 4 g/h by constant infusion. If uterine contractions are successfully inhibited, the maintenance dose is tapered to 2 g/h and continued for 12–24 hours. Intravenous therapy is then discontinued but since there is no practical oral form of magnesium sulphate, the woman receives beta-adrenergic agents orally. If there is no initial response, the magnesium sulphate infusion rate is gradually increased by 0.5 g every 30 minutes until tocolysis is achieved or to a maximum dose of 6 g/h. Women can be maintained on high doses for only a relatively short period of time before the serum magnesium level becomes excessive (greater than 8 mg/dl). The patient's deep tendon reflexes are checked prior to each increase in dosage and serum magnesium levels are ascertained frequently. The infusion rate is tapered as necessary to maintain an acceptable serum magnesium level. Failure to achieve tocolysis despite a serum magnesium level of 7–8 mg/dl suggests an underlying process such as chorioamnionitis or placental abruption.

Prostaglandin synthetase inhibitors

Mechanism of action

Prostaglandins, specifically $PGF_{2\alpha}$ and PGE_2, play a dual role in preterm labour. These compounds are probably the final pathway for smooth muscle contraction. At the same time, PGE_2 induces biochemical changes in cervical collagen which facilitate cervical dilatation. A group of enzymes called collectively prostaglandin synthetases act to convert free arachidonic acid to prostaglandin. Indomethacin, the agent tested most extensively as a tocolytic agent, when administered orally or rectally acts specifically and reversibly to inhibit the cyclo-oxygenase enzyme necessary for conversion of arachidonic acid. Addition of indomethacin to human myometrial strips in vitro abolishes spontaneous contractions (Garrioch 1978). Aspirin is best avoided as a tocolytic agent since it may be associated with maternal or fetal peripartum bleeding (Stuart et al 1982).

Efficacy

Indomethacin can prolong pregnancy beyond term in the rhesus monkey but this is often associated with staining of the skin and umbilical cord as well as oligohydramnios (Novy 1978). The use of indomethacin as a tocolytic agent in humans was first reported by Zuckerman et al (1974) who studied 50 women in preterm labour. Contractions were inhibited in 40 with an average delay in delivery of 7 weeks. Wiqvist et al (1978) used indomethacin to arrest labour successfully in 6 women who failed to respond to beta-agonists. There was a concomitant reduction in plasma metabolites of PGF_2 which were initially as high as those of normal patients at term. Similarly, Niebyl et al (1980) found that a 24-hour course of indomethacin was significantly more effective than placebo in inhibiting preterm labour in 15 women. They also noted a reduction of PGF_2 metabolites.

Side-effects

By inhibiting synthesis of prostanoids including prostaglandins, prostacyclins and thromboxanes, indomethacin might be expected to produce a wide variety of effects. Few side-effects have been reported with the use of indomethacin for tocolysis. On rare occasions, postpartum haemorrhage has been observed (Reiss et al 1976). Gastrointestinal side-effects can be minimized by giving the drug with meals.

Indomethacin crosses the placenta freely. Although no adverse fetal effects were reported in any of the above studies, the patency of the fetal ductus arteriosus is maintained by circulating prostaglandins. Indomethacin theoretically might result in closure of the ductus arteriosus in utero. There are case reports of narrowing of the fetal ductus arteriosus and persistent fetal circulation (primary pulmonary hypertension) but these have generally occurred when indomethacin was used for prolonged periods, in high doses, or close to term (Csaba et al 1978, Goudie & Dossetor 1979).

Oligohydramnios, thought to be secondary to a decrease in fetal urine excretion, has also been described in association with perinatal death (Dudley & Hardie 1985). Reassuringly, two recent studies out of a total of 213 infants exposed in utero to indomethacin for periods in general of less than 48 hours, failed to find a single case of premature ductal closure, persistent fetal circulation, or any other adverse effect (Dudley & Hardie 1985, Niebyl & Witter 1986).

Indomethacin appears to be an extremely effective agent. When used for short periods of time at less than 34 weeks' gestation in the absence of maternal infection, bleeding disorders, or renal or peptic ulcer disease, initial evidence suggests that it is safe for both mother and fetus. It cannot be recommended for general use until further clinical trials are completed. However, in selected cases where alternative agents have failed, a short course of therapy may be warranted despite the uncertain risks.

Calcium channel blockers

A diverse group of drugs, which includes nifedipine and verapamil, inhibit the influx of calcium ions through voltage-dependent channels in the cell membrane. The reduction in cytoplasmic, free calcium inhibits smooth muscle contractility. In an uncontrolled trial, nifedipine successfully prevented delivery for 3 days in all of 10 women in preterm labour (Forman et al 1981). Flushing and a modest increase in heart rate were the only reported side-effects. Hypotension can occur secondary to vasodilation. Side-effects appear to be greater for verapamil than for nifedipine. The combination of a calcium channel blocker and a beta-agonist may prove particularly effective and is currently under investigation.

Miscellaneous

Diazoxide, an antihypertensive agent, has uterine-relaxant activity and has been used successfully to inhibit labour in humans. The drug may cause significant hypotension and has diabetogenic effects. It has not gained popularity as a tocolytic agent. Similarly, aminophylline possesses mild tocolytic properties but is less useful than the previously mentioned agents.

Pregnenolone sulphate, an immediate precursor of placental progesterone, has been reported in small trials to inhibit uterine activity. Progesterone decreases the concentration of myometrial oxytocin and alpha-adrenergic receptors, reduces local synthesis of $PGF_{2\alpha}$ and myometrial sensitivity to exogenous prostaglandin perfusion, and inhibits the appearance of intracellular gap junctions. The tocolytic effect of oral micronized progesterone was not as intense or as rapid as that of beta-mimetics in a double-blind study of 57 women, of whom 29 received a single oral dose of 400 mg progesterone (Erny et al 1986). But it was sufficient in 80% of cases to stop premature labour without any detectable side-effects. Because it selectively inhibits alpha-adrenergic receptors progesterone may permit a reduction in the effective dose of beta-mimetics when both agents are used in combination, thus reducing side-effects. Progesterone use is currently generally limited to prophylaxis against preterm labour rather than for the treatment of established labour.

Ethanol

Ethanol was the first widely used tocolytic agent and several clinical trials have demonstrated its ability to inhibit uterine activity. Ethanol acts both centrally and peripherally. Centrally, it suppresses release of antidiuretic hormone and oxytocin from the posterior pituitary. Peripherally, uterine response to both endogenous and exogenous oxytocin is reduced. Ethanol also inhibits contractions induced by PGE_2. The administration of ethanol requires constant supervision because of its many associated side-effects. These include intoxication, vomiting, restlessness, disorientation, and hangover. Maternal lactic acidosis and dehydration are potential complications. Most serious of all, aspiration may occur if the sleepy woman vomits. Ethanol freely crosses the placenta but neonatal depression is only occasionally encountered and in most studies has not been considered a significant problem. In one trial comparing ethanol and ritodrine, there was a higher incidence of neonatal death and respiratory distress in the group receiving ethanol (Lauerson et al 1977).

GLUCOCORTICOIDS TO PROMOTE FETAL PULMONARY MATURATION

The corticosteroids have numerous and diverse physiological effects. In the human fetus glucocorticoids produce an increase in alveolar surfactant which is associated with an increase in the lecithin:sphingomyelin (L:S) ratio in amniotic fluid. The exact mechanism of action of steroids is speculative, but specific steroid receptor sites exist in the cytoplasm and nucleus of lung cells. After entering the nucleus the receptor–steroid complex initiates synthesis of mRNAs which are translated in the cytoplasm to increase synthesis of phosphatidylcholine. Steroids may also promote release of surfactant from type II alveolar cells. Current evidence indicates that antenatal steroid administration reduces the frequency of respiratory distress syndrome (RDS). The relative efficacy of a given steroid depends upon its ability to cross the placenta and its receptor affinity.

Liggins & Howie (1972) were the first to report that there was a significant reduction in the incidence of RDS lasting up to 7 days following completion of steroid therapy for infants born prior to 34 weeks' gestation and for whom delivery was delayed for at least 24 hours. Reports of more than 25 studies, including at least six prospective, randomized controlled trials, have been published in which attempts were made to duplicate the work of Liggins & Howie. Although many of these studies had methodological errors of varying magnitude, almost all have confirmed a beneficial effect of exogenously administered steroids in reducing the complications associated with RDS.

A more recent multicentre, double-blind trial conducted by the National Institutes of Health in the USA confirmed a general reduction in RDS in the treated group (Avery et al 1986). This beneficial effect did not extend to cases involving the presence of multiple pregnancy or premature rupture of membranes, although a trend towards reduction in RDS was noted in the latter case. Interestingly, this study could not document any benefit for the male fetus, although approximately half of published trials do report benefit to both sexes. Early trials did not evaluate the efficacy of steroids in the extremely premature infant of less than 28 weeks' gestation, but more recent non-randomized comparisons indicate increased survival for infants receiving steroids (Worthington et al 1983). Since infants of less than 28 weeks do survive, it is reasonable to expect that such infants have sufficient pulmonary maturation to enable them to respond to steroids.

Evidence in the literature reporting the effects of steroid administration following preterm rupture of the membranes is inconclusive. There is some support for the postulate that rupture of the membranes acts as a stressor to initiate an outpouring of endogenous fetal steroids which act directly on pulmonary enzyme systems. Such an effect could mask any potential benefits of exogenous steroid administration. While several prospective randomized studies comparing steroid treatment and timed delivery at 48 hours to expectant management have found no benefit from steroids (Garite et al 1981), other studies which followed both groups expectantly have noted a decrease in RDS in the group receiving steroids. A reduction in the incidence of intraventricular haemorrhage has also been noted (Morales et al 1986).

Despite evidence of the efficacy of steroids in preventing RDS in most situations, and possibly, necrotizing enterocolitis, bronchopulmonary dysplasia, and patent ductus arteriosus as well (Avery et al 1986), many institutions have preferred to avoid their use out of concern for potential complications. From a maternal standpoint, steroids adversely affect glucose utilization, aggravating the diabetogenic effects of the beta-agonists used for tocolysis. The risk of infection may be increased (Taeusch et al 1979), and on a theoretical basis, wound healing might be impaired although as yet this remains undocumented. When used in combination with a tocolytic agent, it is possible that the patient is at increased risk for developing pulmonary oedema.

From the standpoint of the fetus or infant, some reports suggest an increased risk of neonatal sepsis. Taeusch and co-workers (1979) diagnosed serious infection in 13% of infants whose mothers received dexamethasone for treatment of preterm rupture of the membranes, while only 6% of infants whose mothers did not receive steroids became infected. The majority of studies have noted no increase in either maternal or fetal infection. Since animal models have demonstrated a runting effect with impaired growth of brain, heart, liver, kidney, and adrenals, there has been some concern regarding the long-term risks for treated infants (Mosier et al 1979). However, the animal studies have used pharmacological doses of steroids for extended treatment periods. When the Liggins protocol for betamethasone administration is used, the fetus is exposed to corticoid levels which do not exceed the physiological stress level spontaneously achieved by infants developing RDS who have not received steroids. Long-term follow-up of human infants up to 6 years post-treatment has failed to demonstrate neurological or developmental sequelae following antepartum steroid administration (MacArthur et al 1982, Avery et al 1986).

The regimen most commonly used in the USA is betamethasone, 12 mg administered intramuscularly and repeated in 24 hours. If membranes are intact and the threat of delivery remains, many physicians administer a repeat course 7 days later for the fetus of less than 32 weeks' gestation or which has evidence of pulmonary immaturity in amniotic fluid L:S ratios. By 1 week the drug has been cleared and any beneficial effects of the initial course of treatment are no longer apparent, but it is uncertain whether there may be cumulative adverse effects. RDS is not eliminated by steroid therapy and investigations are currently evaluating the value of thyroxine and its analogues or prolactin in the prevention of RDS.

Phenobarbital

Intraventricular haemorrhage occurs in 30–60% of very low birthweight infants. The majority of haemorrhages are grades I and II and are well tolerated. More severe haemorrhages are associated with major neurological sequelae. Administration of phenobarbital to the infant immediately after birth has been reported to decrease the incidence and severity of intraventricular haemorrhage (Donn et al 1981, Bedard et al 1984). Proposed mechanisms by which phenobarbital exerts its beneficial effects include a decrease in the cerebral metabolic rate, decreased intracranial pressure, inhibition of catecholamine release, decreased cerebral blood flow and enzyme induction.

Postnatal administration will not prevent antepartum haemorrhage. A recent prospective, randomized trial of combined antepartum and postpartum phenobarbital administration reported a significant reduction in severe intraventricular haemorrhage and neonatal mortality in infants whose mothers received phenobarbital prior to delivery as compared to infants who were not treated until after delivery (Morales & Koerten 1986). If these findings are confirmed, antepartum phenobarbital therapy may be indicated in the management of preterm labour prior to 34 weeks.

OUTPATIENT MANAGEMENT

Successful management of preterm labour requires long-term surveillance and tocolytic therapy since there is a significant risk of recurrence throughout the remainder of the gestation. Oral therapy will reduce the numbers of women requiring repeated intravenous courses (Creasy et al 1980a). Once the frequency of uterine contractions has been inhibited to less than 1 per 15-minute period with the intravenous administration of the selected tocolytic agent, the infusion rate is maintained for 12–24 hours depending upon the difficulty of achieving initial tocolysis. If side-effects are excessive, the infusion rate is tapered as necessary to reduce these to an acceptable level while maintaining effective tocolysis. Attempts to wean the patient rapidly from parenteral administration frequently result in resumption of uterine activity and repeated cycles of intravenous followed by oral therapy.

Subsequent to this maintenance period, the infusion rate is gradually reduced at hourly intervals over several hours until the heart rate decreases to 100 beats/min. This allows for a smooth transition to oral therapy without an abrupt drop in circulating drug levels, since oral dosage regimens are similarly designed to maintain the maternal pulse at 100–110 beats/min.

The most widely used agents for oral therapy are the beta-agonists. There is no practical oral form of magnesium sulphate which would permit therapeutic levels to be achieved and prolonged use of indomethacin has not been studied. Ritodrine 10–20 mg is administered every 2–6 hours depending on maternal heart rate, uterine activity and side-effects. An agent with a longer half-life, such as terbutaline, may offer the advantage of less frequent dosing but if the uterus remains inactive, administration of any of the agents may be limited to the patient's waking hours, allowing her to sleep at night undisturbed. A double-blind randomized comparison between oral terbutaline and ritodrine demonstrated that terbutaline is significantly more effective for preventing a recurrence of labour (Caritis et al 1984). Since it is also less expensive it is the authors' preferred oral agent. The intravenous infusion is discontinued 30 minutes after the initial dose. If labour resumes despite oral therapy, repeated courses of intravenous therapy may be employed provided the woman still satisfies the selection criteria.

In the absence of diabetes or conditions affecting potassium exchange, outpatient monitoring of blood sugars and serum electrolytes is unnecessary. The patient is assessed weekly to determine the maternal heart rate and assess the cervix for evidence of change. Although rare, symptoms suggesting cardiac or pulmonary decompensation require prompt evaluation. The woman is instructed to restrict her activities. As the pregnancy progresses, in the absence of recurrent uterine contractions, she may gradually progress from bedrest to resumption of moderate activity levels. Intercourse, orgasm and nipple stimulation should be avoided. Therapy is discontinued at 36–37 weeks' gestation. Although the patient may theoretically develop tachyphylaxis (Casper & Lye 1986) and indeed there is little evidence to support the effectiveness of oral agents after the first week of therapy, as long as the patient remains mildly tachycardic she can be expected to derive benefit.

MANAGEMENT OF ADVANCED PRETERM LABOUR

Preterm labour may progress despite maximal therapy or the patient may present in advanced labour, precluding successful labour inhibition. In such situations decisions must be made as to how best to accomplish delivery. Ideally, the delivery should be performed at a facility equipped to care for the preterm infant since transferring the neonate postdelivery reduces the chances for a successful outcome (Paneth et al 1982). Central to management of delivery is the determination of fetal gestational age and hence the potential for survival.

In recent decades outcome for preterm neonates delivered in a tertiary care setting has improved such that survival rates for infants weighing over 1000 g (or over 28 weeks' gestation) are approximately 90% (Worthington et al 1983, Milligan et al 1984). Survival rates for babies weighing between 750 and 1000 g (26–28 weeks' gestation) exceed 60% (Milligan et al 1984, Yu et al 1984). In addition, the majority of survivors born without congenital defects or chronic fetal infection will not have severe mental retardation or other major handicaps.

Until recently, few infants delivered prior to 26 weeks' gestation survived and it has been suggested that resuscitation of these infants is not a good investment of medical resources. However, new studies indicate that in selected centres, as many as 20–40% of infants delivered at 24–25 weeks' gestation survive (Dillon & Egan 1981, Milligan et al 1984, Milner & Beard 1984). Some reports indicate that these survivors are no more likely to have major handicaps than infants born at 26–28 weeks' gestation, since 'the fragility of the organism is such that death, not damage will result' (Milligan et al 1984). Of surviving infants weighing less than 800 g, only 20% will exhibit major neurological handicaps (Hirata et al 1983, Milligan et al 1984, Yu et al 1984), although greater numbers do demonstrate learning disabilities or hyperactivity.

Precise determination of gestational age is frequently impossible, with errors of as much as 2 weeks a not infrequent occurrence. In order to avoid non-intervention in cases subsequently found to involve a salvageable fetus, it is prudent to provide intensive care during and after birth for any infant of 24 weeks' gestational age or greater until it can be determined that the infant is previable or has major anomalies.

Once it is apparent that labour cannot be inhibited, the first step in management is to discontinue the use of all tocolytic medications. As described previously, these agents produce a variety of fetal side-effects which can depress the newborn and complicate resuscitative efforts. To ensure the best outcome, it is important that birth asphyxia should be avoided. In animal models, hypoxia causes the disappearance of lamellar bodies and surfactant from the lung (Schaefer et al 1964). Lecithin synthesis is impaired by acidosis. In the human, birth asphyxia predisposes to the development of RDS and intracranial haemorrhage. Infants with decreased fetal heart rate variability antepartum are also more likely to die from RDS (Martin et al 1974).

Low maternal serum oestradiol and progesterone levels are common in patients in premature labour, suggesting that placental dysfunction may be a common component of this pregnancy complication (Cousins et al 1977). The preterm infant does demonstrate a relatively high incidence of late deceleration fetal heart rate patterns. Continuous fetal heart rate monitoring allows prompt diagnosis of asphyxia and significantly reduces neonatal mortality in the fetus weighing less than 1500 g (Bowes et al 1980). Interpretation of heart rate recordings from the preterm infant is the same as that for term infants (Zanini et al 1980), although the baseline heart rate may be somewhat higher and the variability reduced in the very preterm infant. Heart rates above 170 beats/min are unexpected at any gestation and require investigation. Fetal scalp blood sampling should be performed to confirm fetal compromise suggested by the heart rate tracing.

While a traumatic delivery is particularly hazardous for the preterm infant, this does not mean that Caesarean section is the preferred route of delivery. At present, the evidence that Caesarean section of the preterm vertex infant improves perinatal outcome is insufficient to recommend its routine use (Olshan et al 1984, Kitchen et al 1985). Caesarean section after the onset of labour does not prevent central nervous system bleeding in these infants (Tejani et al 1984). Vaginal delivery may have some advantages since amniotic fluid is more completely expressed from the fetal lungs as the chest is compressed at delivery, perhaps facilitating lung expansion. In addition, the placental transfusion that occurs at delivery may be greater with the vaginal route. However, in specific situations which might require a prolonged induction in the presence of a rigid, unyielding cervix, Caesarean section may be preferable.

Both prolonged and precipitous labour are particularly hazardous to the preterm infant. Oxytocin use should be carefully monitored to prevent hyperstimulation. Vaginal examinations should be performed sparingly because the preterm gestation is especially prone to infection. Arguments persist over the relative merits of spontaneous vaginal delivery versus outlet forceps delivery to protect the fragile preterm head, but all agree that a generous episiotomy is indicated to reduce head compression and sudden decompression at the time of delivery. It is doubtful that forceps delivery generally produces less trauma (Schwartz et al 1983) and may possibly be harmful (O'Driscoll et al 1981). Forceps should not be used to extract the fetus before the head reaches the pelvic floor. Currently available forceps intended for use on the preterm infant were not designed for the very low birthweight infant. Although studies are lacking, the potential risks associated with use of the vacuum extractor in the very low birthweight infant argue against its use. A neonatologist must be present at the delivery and be prepared to resuscitate the infant immediately if necessary.

As yet, there are no controlled prospective trials to indicate that the preterm breech infant should be delivered by Caesarean section. Several retrospective reports suggest that Caesarean section is the safest route of delivery, especially for the fetus weighing less than 1500 g or presenting as a footling breech (Goldenberg & Nelson 1977, Duenhoelter et al 1979, Main et al 1983). In general, these studies have been plagued by confounding variables such as biased allocation of infants assumed to be previable to the vaginal delivery group. Other studies have not demonstrated an advantage for Caesarean section (Bodmer et al 1986) but until the results of prospective randomized, controlled studies become available the authors prefer to deliver the infant expected to weigh between 800 and 1500 g by Caesarean section. It is presently unclear whether the increased maternal morbidity associated with Caesarean section is justified for infants weighing less than 800 g, although head entrapment is most likely to occur in this group.

Since major congenital anomalies occur more frequently in premature breech babies, careful sonographic evaluation to exclude lethal defects is advisable before proceeding with surgery. Selection of the type of low-segment uterine incision is dependent upon whether or not there is a well developed lower uterine segment. Although in many cases a transverse incision is feasible, it is inconsistent to perform a surgical procedure to avoid fetal trauma only to have the fetal head trapped by an unyielding narrow incision in a poorly developed lower segment.

In recent years Caesarean section has been recommended for delivery of all preterm twin gestations in which twin A is non-vertex (Chervenak et al 1985). However, there are no controlled trials to support this recommendation. Electronic fetal heart monitoring allows the continuous assessment of fetal well-being for both infants simultaneously. In the event of fetal distress, immediate Caesarean section can be performed. If twin A meets the criteria for singleton vaginal breech delivery (weight approaching 2500 g, flexed head, adequate maternal pelvis), then the same consideration for vaginal breech delivery should be accorded the twin fetus as is given the singleton. The phenomenon of locked twins is extremely rare, occurring once in 1000 twin gestations (Khunda 1972), but the obstetrician must be prepared to proceed immediately with Caesarean section if the diagnosis is suspected intrapartum.

If twin A is in vertex presentation and twin B is breech, vaginal delivery is planned. Immediately after delivery of twin A, external version (possibly under sonographic guidance) may be attempted. Short-term intravenous tocolysis may facilitate this procedure. If this is not immediately successful, delivery may be achieved by breech extraction or by allowing the woman to continue labour with an assisted breech delivery. Although some obstetricians prefer to perform a Caesarean section, there is little evidence that this will improve outcome for twin B (Acker et al 1982). An anaesthetist (or anaesthesiologist in the USA) should be in attendance for all twin deliveries.

Anaesthesia

Parenteral narcotics and sedatives have a depressant effect on the preterm infant and should be used sparingly if at all. Although general anaesthesia may be preferred when uterine relaxation is needed for intrauterine manipulation of the fetus, usually conduction anaesthesia is the method of choice. Continuous epidural anaesthesia can be used mostly when the appropriate precautions for preventing maternal hypotension are taken. Epidural anaesthesia is particularly useful for avoiding premature maternal expulsive efforts and helps to reduce outlet resistance from the perineal musculature.

PRETERM RUPTURE OF THE MEMBRANES

Rupture of the fetal membranes occurring after 20 weeks and prior to 37 completed weeks of gestation is referred to as preterm rupture of the membranes. Uterine contractions may or may not be present. This entity accounts for 30% of preterm deliveries. Although many of the conditions associated with preterm labour are also associated with preterm rupture of the membranes it is usually impossible to identify the aetiology in a given patient. Factors implicated in the development of preterm rupture of the membranes include focal thinning of the membranes (Artal et al 1976); reduced elasticity as a result of strain hardening from repetitive stresses (uterine contractions; Toppozada et al 1970, Lavery et al 1982); local flaws in the chorion as a result of biochemical alterations in the supporting connective tissue (Artal et al 1979b, Lavery et al 1982, Hills & Cotton 1984, Kanayama et al 1985); nutritional and dietary factors such as inadequate ascorbic acid intake (Wideman et al 1964), copper or zinc deficiency (Artal et al 1979a) and smoking (Meyer & Tonascia 1977); sexual activity (Naeye & Ross 1982); cervical incompetence; pregnancy-related conditions such as multiple gestation, polyhydramnios, or a marginal cord insertion (Brody & Frenkel 1953); and falls in the barometric pressure.

Infection has been implicated in many cases. Indirect evidence suggesting that infection antedates preterm rupture of the membranes is provided by the observation that histologically apparent amniotic fluid infections are two-to-three-fold more common when the fetal membranes rupture just before labour starts than when they rupture just after the onset of labour (Naeye & Peters 1980). Further, amniotic fluid samples from patients with preterm rupture of the membranes are more frequently colonized with pathogens than are samples from patients without preterm rupture of the membranes (Cotton et al 1984b, Zlatnik et al 1984). Many organisms replicate in the fetal membranes, releasing proteolytic enzymes or causing cell death (McGregor et al 1986b). Varner et al (1985), investigating the effect of group B streptococcal infection on the human amnion using a transmission electron microscope, have shown a progressive decrease in desmosome counts and alterations of the basement membrane.

Patients with a history of preterm rupture of the membranes constitute a high-risk group since one out of five subsequent pregnancies will be similarly affected (Naeye 1982).

Diagnosis

The woman's report of onset of fluid leakage may be valuable for determining the time of membrane rupture and the character of the fluid, but it may also be erroneous. It is important to verify objectively all reports of membrane rupture by a properly performed sterile speculum examination. Fluid may be seen escaping spontaneously through the cervical os or after application of fundal pressure. When gross flow is not seen, diagnostic accuracy can be improved by placing the patient in a semi-upright position for 20 minutes to allow further escape and pooling of amniotic fluid in the vaginal vault. Confirmation of amniotic fluid leakage can be obtained by testing the pH of vaginal secretions from the posterior fornix with nitrazine paper. Amniotic fluid has a slightly alkaline pH of 7–7.5 which causes nitrazine paper to change from yellow to a blue colour but if there is contamination with blood, urine, lubricants, or antiseptic solutions, false positive results will occur. Microscopic examination of the vaginal secretions which have been smeared on to a glass slide and allowed to air-dry might reveal an arborization or ferning pattern if amniotic fluid is present. The posterior vault, not the cervix, must be sampled in order to prevent contamination with mucus which can produce false positive results. The combination of these two tests yields a correct diagnosis in 95% of cases (Smith 1976). A reduction in amniotic fluid volume seen on ultrasound evaluation is supportive but not diagnostic of preterm rupture of the membranes.

If the diagnosis remains uncertain, the question can be resolved by injecting 1 ml of indigo carmine dye into the amniotic fluid by amniocentesis, placing a sterile tampon in the vagina and inspecting it several hours later for evidence of blue. This procedure is rarely necessary and entails the slight risk of producing the very condition one is trying to diagnose. Although generally not available, testing of vaginal secretions for the presence of alpha-fetoprotein using a latex agglutination technique or a colorimetric monoclonal antibody test has been described (Rochelson et al 1983, 1987). These tests appear to be more sensitive and specific than either fern or nitrazine testing in preterm rupture of the membranes. They are not affected by urine or semen but can give false positive results in the presence of maternal blood in the fluid being tested.

Initial management

As in the case of preterm labour, a culture from the cervix should be obtained at the time of initial sterile speculum examination. If sufficient amniotic fluid is present in the vaginal vault, collection of an aliquot allows assessment of fetal pulmonary maturity from the presence of phosphatidylglycerol, or by determining the L:S ratio. In most cases both of these tests have provided accurate results for vaginal amniotic fluid samples although, rarely, the L:S ratio may be altered by the presence of blood or meconium. Test results may indicate which women are candidates to receive steroids but in general do not alter management for the fetus of less than 33–34 weeks' gestation.

Inspection of the cervix through the non-invasive sterile speculum will give an estimate of cervical dilatation, effacement, position, and exclude gross prolapse of the umbilical cord. Digital examination of the cervix is avoided until it has been decided to proceed with labour and delivery. Otherwise, digital examination may introduce bacteria into the lower uterine segment, increasing the risk of chorioamnionitis (Schutte et al 1983). It rarely provides sufficient additional information to alter management plans based on visual inspection of the cervix (Munson et al 1985).

An ultrasound evaluation is useful for assessing fetal age and presentation. The role of amniocentesis in preterm rupture of the membranes for determining occult amniotic fluid infection remains undefined but if performed, should be done under ultrasound guidance. Many women will have insufficient amniotic fluid to permit amniocentesis. Some with negative amniotic fluid studies will still develop chorioamnionitis. Some women who have positive Gram stains or cultures do not develop clinical infection and on occasion, the fetus may gain significant additional time in utero if the physician does not attempt to terminate the pregnancy. Other indicators of chorioamnionitis should be sought, such as maternal fever, maternal or fetal tachycardia, uterine tenderness, contractions, foul vaginal discharge, or a leukocytosis with a shift in the differential to the polymorpho-nuclear leukocyte.

Subsequent management

There is considerable controversy regarding the optimal management of patients with preterm rupture of the membranes. This is because prevention of the two major complications associated with this condition, infection and prematurity, requires divergent management plans. Once the membranes are ruptured, they no longer serve as a barrier to the ascent of infectious agents. Loss of amniotic fluid reduces the inherent antibacterial activity present in the intra-amniotic cavity. This activity is proportional to gestational age (Shlievert et al 1975), perhaps in part explaining the increase in infectious complications associated with decreasing gestational age at membrane rupture. The longer the latent period from membrane rupture to the onset of contractions, the greater the maternal and fetal infectious morbidity (Burchell 1964, Gunn et al 1970, Schreiber & Benedetti 1980). Fetal mortality from infection also increases with latent periods greater than 24 hours. An aggressive management scheme calling for early induction or augmentation of labour would reduce the risk of infection.

Counterbalancing these considerations is concern for the complications associated with prematurity, which include RDS, intraventricular haemorrhage and necrotizing enterocolitis. To minimize these risks, a conservative management plan which allows intrauterine development to continue for as long as possible is indicated. The majority of perinatal deaths in cases of premature rupture of the membranes are due to RDS, not neonatal sepsis (Taylor et al 1961).

Other variables such as cervical inducibility and the specific patient population must be considered. An inner-city hospital population may be at sufficiently high risk for infectious morbidity and mortality that conservative management would be inappropriate in most cases. The management plans must take all of these factors into account, assigning relative weights on an individual basis.

The chances of a successful pregnancy outcome following preterm rupture of the membranes prior to 24 weeks' gestation are low, but intact survivors do occur (Taylor & Garite 1984, Beydoun & Yasin 1986). In a series of 53 pregnancies with preterm rupture of the membranes between 16 and 25 weeks' gestation, 25% of the infants survived (Taylor & Garite 1984). Although maternal infectious complications were frequent, they did not produce long-term sequelae. Therefore, depending upon the patient's wishes after thorough discussion of risks and benefits, either immediate pregnancy termination or expectant management is acceptable.

Patients presenting after 24 and prior to 34 weeks' gestation are placed at strict bedrest and undergo monitoring for evidence of uterine contractions, fetal distress, or sepsis. Variable decelerations seen on cardiotocography may indicate an occult cord prolapse. If a non-stress test is reactive and there is no evidence of labour or infection, the woman is observed.

Pending amniotic fluid pulmonary maturity test results, the patient is given an initial dose of betamethasone. This is particularly controversial since, unlike the situation in preterm labour where there is general agreement that steroids reduce the risk of RDS, with preterm rupture of the membranes there are almost as many studies reporting no benefit from steroid administration as there are describing improvement in outcome. The most likely explanation for the less pronounced effect of steroids in this situation is that preterm rupture of the membranes itself provides a stress which stimulates production of endogenous steroids causing accelerated fetal lung maturation. An increased L:S ratio has been found in fluid from patients with preterm rupture of the membranes for greater than 24 hours (Verder et al 1978). Although there are conflicting reports, the preponderance of evidence supports the contention that premature rupture of the membranes promotes pulmonary maturity but it certainly does not guarantee protection from RDS. The location and size of the amniotic fluid leak may influence the degree to which this process is stimulated. Since it is impossible to determine whether or not there has been sufficient stimulus to endogenous steroid production at the time of initial patient presentation, in the absence of amniotic fluid studies demonstrating pulmonary maturity a repeat dose of betamethasone is administered in 24 hours. Subsequent courses of steroids are not indicated.

If contractions supervene during the initial 48 hours of observation, as may be expected in approximately half of patients, tocolytic agents are instituted, provided there is no evidence of infection. These agents are discontinued 48 hours after the initial dose of betamethasone or, if steroids are not used, 48 hours after membrane rupture. Labour can be an early sign of chorioamnionitis and continued use of tocolytics might prevent recognition of infection until it becomes serious. There are as yet no studies available to indicate whether prolonging tocolysis beyond 48 hours might improve outcome for the very preterm infant of less than 28 weeks' gestation where the problems of prematurity are paramount. A small prospective randomized study of 42 patients with premature rupture of the membranes between 25 and 43 weeks' gestation found that administration of oral ritodrine until the onset of labour significantly prolonged the mean latent period (Levy & Warsof 1985). Almost one-half of the treated patients had a latent period of more than 1 week without an increase in infectious complications compared to 14% of controls, suggesting that prolonged tocolysis may be beneficial.

Lung maturity does not mean fetal maturity. A preterm infant without RDS may still develop serious complications such as necrotizing enterocolitis, intracerebral bleeding or hyperbilirubinaemia. For most institutions, prior to 34 weeks of gestation the complications of prematurity outweigh the risks of infection and, therefore, a policy of expectant management with close observation for evidence of infection is justified. However, when premature rupture of the membranes occurs at less than 28 weeks of gestation such a policy, although appropriate, does result in a higher incidence of complications related to lack of adequate volumes of amniotic fluid. Positional foot deformities, congenital dislocation of the hips and hypoplastic lungs are all seen more frequently (Nimrod et al 1984).

White blood cell counts with a differential count are initially obtained every 12 hours. Vital signs and temperature are taken every 4 hours. Elevated C-reactive protein levels may herald intra-amniotic infection (Evans et al 1980) but they are non-specific and may be elevated by betamethasone administration. After 48 hours, surveillance may be modified such that a complete blood count is obtained daily and cardiotocography weekly. Although daily fetal heart rate checks might on occasion detect an occult prolapsed cord, the fetus would remain unmonitored for the vast majority of the time. Therefore, careful auscultation of the fetal heart rate at 4-hour intervals is more useful and practical. However, preliminary evidence suggests that daily cardiotocography may help to predict infectious complications (Vintzileos et al 1986).

If fluid leakage stops and this is confirmed on repeated sterile speculum examination, the patient may be sent home with precautions against intercourse, douching or using tampons. Rarely, a motivated patient with a stable home situation and adequate transportation to the hospital may be followed as an outpatient despite continued fluid leakage.

The patient takes her own temperature three times a day while a visiting nurse or midwife can obtain daily blood counts. This is reasonable when findings suggest a high amniotic fluid leak and there is little risk of infection.

After 34 weeks' gestation, the neonatal mortality is sufficiently low that the risk of cord prolapse and infection assume greater importance. In the presence of a favourable cervix labour induction is generally warranted, although some investigators feel that continued expectant management is preferable even at term (Kappy et al 1979). When the cervix is unfavourable induction attempts may fail, resulting in a high incidence of Caesarean section. Since the antimicrobial properties of amniotic fluid increase and neonatal infectious morbidity decreases as term approaches, it remains unsettled as to whether the fetal risks of continued expectant management are sufficient to justify the increased maternal morbidity resulting from a policy of active intervention in such cases. Allowing a latent period of 24 hours to elapse might provide for further pulmonary maturation and cervical ripening (whether spontaneous or facilitated by prostaglandin application), thus improving the chances for successful vaginal delivery.

Once a diagnosis of chorioamnionitis is made, delivery should be accomplished expeditiously in all cases. Generally, this may be accomplished by the vaginal route. Variable fetal heart decelerations commonly accompany labour after preterm rupture of the membranes. Saline amnioinfusion has been used successfully to abolish this pattern by restoring fluid volume and relieving cord compression (Nageotte et al 1985). Caesarean section is reserved for the usual obstetrical indications, since perinatal outcome is not improved and maternal morbidity is increased when infection is the sole indication for this procedure. Unless delivery is imminent, broad-spectrum antibiotics in high doses should be started immediately.

Prophylactic antibiotics

In an attempt to reduce the infectious complications associated with preterm rupture of the membranes, prophylactic antibiotics have been administered intravenously, vaginally, and even by intra-amniotic catheter. Regardless of route of administration, multiple studies have concluded that prophylactic antibiotics decrease the incidence of maternal puerperal infectious morbidity. However, such infections are relatively uncommon and benign even without prophylaxis and respond rapidly to therapeutic regimens initiated at the onset of symptoms.

Whether or not antibiotics reduce neonatal infectious morbidity is unsettled. Creatsas et al (1980) have demonstrated that levels of ampicillin and gentamycin can be achieved in the amniotic fluid and fetal circulation after maternal intravenous administration which are adequate to be effective against a high proportion of infecting pathogens. There are isolated reports of successful antibiotic cure of overt chorioamnionitis which has allowed the pregnancy to continue (Monif 1983). Using ampicillin alone, Miller et al (1980) found a marked reduction in both maternal and infant infection.

Other investigators have not noted such a beneficial effect and are concerned that prophylactic use of antibiotics may mask the earliest clinical signs of intrauterine infection, thus exposing the infant to an infected environment for a longer period of time. There is general agreement, however, that prophylactic antibiotics are indicated in the event of a Caesarean section. In addition, evidence is mounting in support of the use of prophylactic ampicillin, pending cervical culture results, specifically to prevent early onset group B beta-haemolytic streptococcal infection in the neonate. Antepartum intravenous administration of ampicillin dramatically reduces the incidence of infant colonization and maternal postpartum fever in women known to be vaginal carriers delivering preterm (Boyer & Gotoff 1986). Until rapid diagnostic methods are perfected which would permit identification of maternal streptococcal colonization upon presentation with either premature rupture of the membranes or preterm labour, Minkoff & Mead (1986) advocate antibiotic treatment in labour of all patients whose admission culture results are unavailable. This is a more cost-effective alternative to antenatal screening of the total obstetric population.

PREVENTION OF PRETERM LABOUR

Many who present in preterm labour have already progressed to the point where labour inhibition is no longer feasible. In order to prevent these preterm births, which result from failure of the woman to recognize the early signs of preterm labour rather than a failure of tocolytic agents or contraindications to their use, the high-risk patient must first be identified and then educated as to the early signs and symptoms of preterm labour. Identification of the high-risk woman might also allow modification of risk factors through alterations in lifestyle, health practices, or the use of prophylactic tocolytic agents.

Several risk-scoring systems based upon epidemiological indices and observed cervical changes have been proposed. All emphasize the importance of previous reproductive history as the major predictor of future obstetric outcome, and hence are more accurate in identifying the multigravida at risk. Using a modification of Papiernik's system in a New Zealand population, Creasy et al (1980b) were able to identify 77% of the multigravidae who delivered preterm but only 31% of the primigravidae. Other investigators applying this scoring system to an indigent American population found it failed to identify accurately women who delivered before term (Main DM et al 1987). All systems fail to identify at least 25–35% of patients who deliver preterm while identifying many high-risk women who never develop preterm labour. To achieve greater precision, biochemical or biophysical markers must be developed. However, thus far, serial measurements of serum or plasma progesterone, oestradiol and prostaglandin levels have proved unrewarding (Mitchell et al 1978, Block et al 1984).

Modifications in lifestyle which may help prevent preterm labour include cessation of smoking and proper nutrition. Reduction in psychological stresses may also be advantageous. Screening for cervical colonization with *Neisseria gonorrhoeae*, group B streptococcus and *Chlamydia trachomatis* is reasonable although there are no studies indicating whether eradication of these organisms will reduce the incidence of preterm labour. Similarly, routine urinary screening to allow identification and treatment of asymptomatic bacteria is warranted. The usefulness of prophylactic bedrest for a portion of each day in preventing preterm labour in singleton gestations remains unproven, as does avoidance of sexual intercourse. Although effective treatment for cervical incompetence, cerclage has not been demonstrated to be an efficacious prophylactic measure in women at risk for preterm labour. Recently, it has been suggested that early preterm labour may be identified in ambulatory high-risk women by using a home tocodynamometer (Katz et al 1986).

There is presently no accepted pharmacological method for the prevention of preterm labour. Long-term oral administration of beta-agonists has been demonstrated to decrease the recurrence rate of preterm labour but the usefulness of prophylactic beta-adrenergic treatment in singleton gestation has not been documented with controlled prospective studies. One prospective but non-blind trial in a small number of twin gestations found prophylactic oral terbutaline increased gestational age and birthweight at delivery (O'Leary 1986), confirming a previous study (Tamby Raja et al 1978). In order to be effective, these drugs likely must be administered in sufficiently high doses to cause a mild maternal tachycardia. Since present screening systems are inaccurate, many patients not truly at risk would unnecessarily experience the side-effects of these drugs over a considerable period of time. Johnson et al (1979) found that weekly injections of 17-alpha-hydroxyprogesterone caproate were effective in preventing preterm labour but these results have not been obtained in all studies (Hauth et al 1983). The efficacy of this regimen remains uncertain.

Currently, the most useful approach appears to be education of the high-risk obstetric patient about the early signs of preterm labour and the necessity of seeking prompt medical treatment. Symptoms may be subtle and often may occur in normal pregnancies. It is the change in symptoms which should prompt evaluation. Early signs of preterm labour are:

1. Changes in Braxton Hicks contractions from an irregular pattern to a more regular pattern or an increase in frequency to greater than one every 10 minutes.
2. Mild abdominal cramping. Cramps may be reminiscent of menstrual cramps or gastrointestinal distress with the urge to defecate.
3. Low backache experienced as a change in character from that previously present.
4. Pelvic pressure.
5. An increase in the amount of vaginal discharge or a change in its character, particularly if it becomes blood-tinged or mucoid.

The patient should also be taught to recognize uterine contractions as a tightening or hardening of the fundus followed by relaxation. It should be emphasized that contractions do not have to be painful to initiate preterm labour. Should contractions occur as frequently as one every 10 minutes for a period of 1 hour, the patient should immediately seek medical attention. Using a programme of patient and staff education, self-detection of early contractions and weekly evaluations of the cervix by medical personnel for evidence of change, Creasy and associates were able to reduce the incidence of preterm delivery in a middle-class population by 50% (Herron et al 1982). In an inner-city indigent population this approach was not successful (Main et al 1985).

It is clear that the diverse aetiology of preterm delivery will require a multifaceted approach to achieve substantial reductions in prematurity. A programme which is successful in one population may have little use in another group of women. However, the success of all programmes ultimately depends upon women receiving timely prenatal care.

REFERENCES

Acker D, Lieberman M, Holbrook R H et al 1982 Delivery of the second twin. Obstetrics and Gynecology 59: 710

Alger L S, Lovchik J C, Hebel J R et al 1988 The association of *Chlamydia trachomatis*, *Neisseria gonorrhoeae* and group B streptococci with preterm rupture of membranes and pregnancy outcome. American Journal of Obstetrics and Gynecology 159: 397

Anderson A B M 1977 Pre-term labour: definition. In: Anderson A B M et al (eds) Proceedings of the fifth study group of the Royal College of Obstetricians and Gynaecologists. Royal College of Obstetricians and Gynaecologists, London

Artal R, Sokol R J, Neuman M et al 1976 The mechanical properties of prematurely and non-prematurely ruptured membranes: methods and preliminary results. American Journal of Obstetrics and Gynecology 125: 655

Artal R, Burgeson R, Fernandez F J, Hobel C J 1979a Fetal and maternal copper levels in patients at term with and without premature rupture of membranes. Obstetrics and Gynecology 53: 5

Artal R, Burgeson R E, Hobel C J, Hollister D 1979b An in vitro model for the study of enzymatically mediated biochemical changes in the chorioamniotic membranes. American Journal of Obstetrics and Gynecology 133: 365

Astbury J, Orgill A, Bajuk B, Yu V 1983 Determinants of developmental performance of very low-birthweight survivors at 1 and 2 years of age. Developmental Medicine and Child Neurology 25: 709

Avery M E, Aylward G, Creasy R K et al 1986 Update on prenatal steroids for prevention of respiratory distress. American Journal of Obstetrics and Gynecology 155: 2

Baillie P, Mechan P P, Tyack A J 1970 Treatment of premature labour with orciprenaline. British Medical Journal 4: 154

Baird D 1977 Epidemiologic patterns over time. In: Reed D M, Stanley

F J (eds) The epidemiology of prematurity. Urban and Schwarzenberg, Baltimore, Maryland, p 3

Bakketeig L S, Hoffman H J 1981 The epidemiology of preterm birth: results from a longitudinal study of births in Norway. In: Elder M G, Hendricks C H (eds) Preterm labor. Butterworths International Medical Reviews, London, p 17

Bedard M P, Shankaran S, Slovis T L et al 1984 Effect of prophylactic phenobarbital on intraventricular hemorrhage in high risk infants. Pediatrics 73: 435

Bejar R, Curbelo V, Davis C, Gluck L 1981 Premature labor II. Bacterial sources of phospholipase. Obstetrics and Gynecology 57: 479

Benedetti T J 1983 Maternal complications of parenteral beta-sympathomimetic therapy for premature labor. American Journal of Obstetrics and Gynecology 145: 1

Beydoun S N, Yasin S Y 1986 Premature rupture of membranes before 28 weeks: conservative management. American Journal of Obstetrics and Gynecology 155: 471

Bieniarz J 1977 Cardiovascular effects of beta-adrenergic agonists. In: Anderson A B M et al (eds) Proceedings of the fifth study group of the Royal College of Obstetricians and Gynaecologists. Royal College of Obstetricians and Gynaecologists, London

Block B S B, Liggins G C, Creasy R K 1984 Preterm delivery is not predicted by serial plasma estradiol or progesterone concentration measurements. American Journal of Obstetrics and Gynecology 150: 716

Bobitt J R, Hayslip C C, Damato J D 1981 Amniotic fluid infection as determined by trans-abdominal amniocentesis in patients with intact membranes in premature labor. American Journal of Obstetrics and Gynecology 140: 947

Bodmer B, Benjamin A, McLean F H, Usher R H 1986 Has use of cesarean section reduced risks of delivery in the preterm breech presentation? American Journal of Obstetrics and Gynecology 154: 244

Boldman R, Reed D M 1977 Worldwide variations in low birthweight. In: Reed D M, Stanley F J (eds) The epidemiology of prematurity. Urban and Schwarzenberg, Baltimore, Maryland, p 39

Bowes W A, Gabbe S G, Bowes C 1980 Fetal heart rate monitoring in premature infants weighing 1500 gm or less. American Journal of Obstetrics and Gynecology 137: 791

Boyer K M, Gotoff S P 1986 Prevention of early-onset neonatal group B streptococcal disease with selective intrapartum chemoprophylaxis. New England Journal of Medicine 314: 1665

Brazy J E, Pupkin M J 1979 Effects of maternal isoxsuprine administration on preterm infants. Journal of Pediatrics 94: 444

Brody S, Frenkel D A 1953 Marginal insertion of the cord and premature labor. American Journal of Obstetrics and Gynecology 65: 1305

Burchell R C 1964 Premature rupture of the membranes. American Journal of Obstetrics and Gynecology 88: 251

Cano A, Tovar I, Parilla J J, Abad L 1985 Metabolic disturbances during intravenous use of ritodrine: increased insulin levels and hypokalemia. Obstetrics and Gynecology 65: 356

Caritis S N, Hirsch R P, Zeleznik A J 1983 Adrenergic stimulation of placental progesterone production. Journal of Clinical Endocrinology and Metabolism 56: 969

Caritis S N, Toig G, Heddinger L A, Ashmead G 1984 A double-blind study comparing ritodrine and terbutaline in the treatment of preterm labor. American Journal of Obstetrics and Gynecology 150: 7

Casper R F, Lye S J 1986 Myometrial desensitization to continuous but not to intermittent β-adrenergic agonist infusion in the sheep. American Journal of Obstetrics and Gynecology 154: 301

Chase H C 1977 Time trends in low birth weight in the United States, 1950–1974. In: Reed D M, Stanley F J (eds) The epidemiology of prematurity. Urban and Schwartzenberg, Baltimore, Maryland, p 17

Chervenak F A, Johnson R E, Youcha S 1985 Intrapartum management of twin gestation. Obstetrics and Gynecology 65: 119

Cotton D B, Gonik B, Dorman K F 1984a Cardiovascular alterations in severe pregnancy-induced hypertension: acute effects of intravenous magnesium sulfate. American Journal of Obstetrics and Gynecology 148: 162

Cotton D B, Hill L M, Strassner H T et al 1984b Use of amniocentesis in preterm labor with ruptured membranes. Obstetrics and Gynecology 63: 38

Cousins L M, Hobel C J, Chang R J et al 1977 Serum progesterone and estradiol-17 B levels in premature and term labor. American Journal of Obstetrics and Gynecology 127: 612

Creasy R K 1984 Preterm labor and delivery. In: Creasy R K, Resnik R (eds) Maternal–fetal medicine. Principles and practice. WB Saunders, Philadelphia, p 415

Creasy R K, Golbus M S, Laros R K et al 1980a Oral ritodrine maintenance in the treatment of preterm labor. American Journal of Obstetrics and Gynecology 137: 212

Creasy R K, Gummer B A, Liggins G C 1980b A system for predicting spontaneous preterm birth. Obstetrics and Gynecology 55: 692

Creatsas G K, Pavlatos M, Kaskarelis D 1980 Ampicillin and gentamycin in the treatment of fetal intrauterine infection. Journal of Perinatal Medicine 8: 13

Crenshaw C, Jones D E D, Parker R T 1973 Placenta previa: a survey of 20 years' experience with improved perinatal survival by expectant therapy and cesarean delivery. Obstetrical and Gynecological Survey 28: 461

Csaba I F, Sulyok E, Erth T 1978 The relationship of maternal treatment with indomethacin to persistence of fetal circulation syndrome. Journal of Pediatrics 92: 484

Dillon W, Egan E 1981 Aggressive obstetric management in late second trimester deliveries. Obstetrics and Gynecology 58: 685

Donn S M, Roloff D W, Goldstein G W 1981 Prevention of intra-ventricular haemorrhage in preterm infants by phenobarbitone. Lancet ii: 215

Dudley, D K L, Hardie M J 1985 Fetal and neonatal effects of indo-methacin used as a tocolytic agent. American Journal of Obstetrics and Gynecology 151: 181

Duenhoelter J H, Wells C E, Reisch J S 1979 A paired controlled study of vaginal and abdominal delivery of the low birth weight breech fetus. Obstetrics and Gynecology 54: 310

Edwards L E, Barrada M I, Hamann A A, Hakanson E Y 1978 Gonorrhea in pregnancy. American Journal of Obstetrics and Gynecology 132: 637

Elliott J P 1983 Magnesium sulfate as a tocolytic agent. American Journal of Obstetrics and Gynecology 147: 277

Epstein M F, Nichols E, Stubblefield P G 1979 Neonatal hypoglycemia after beta-sympathomimetic tocolytic therapy. Journal of Pediatrics 94: 449

Erny R, Pigne A, Prouvost C et al 1986 The effects of oral administration of progesterone for premature labor. American Journal of Obstetrics and Gynecology 154: 525

Evans M I, Hajj S N, Devoe L D et al 1980 C-reactive protein as a predictor of infectious morbidity with premature rupture of membranes. American Journal of Obstetrics and Gynecology 138: 648

Ferguson J E, Hensleigh P A, Kredenster D 1984 Adjunctive use of magnesium sulfate with ritodrine for preterm labor tocolysis. American Journal of Obstetrics and Gynecology 148: 166

Forman A, Andersson K E, Ulmsten U 1981 Inhibition of myometrial activity by calcium antagonists. Seminars in Perinatology 5: 288

Forssman L 1965 Posttraumatic intrauterine synechiae and pregnancy. Obstetrics and Gynecology 26: 710

Frederick J, Anderson A B M 1976 Factors associated with spontaneous preterm birth. British Journal of Obstetrics and Gynaecology 83: 342

Freysz H, Willard D, Lehr A, Misser J 1977 A long-term evaluation of infants who receive a beta-mimetic drug while in utero. Journal of Perinatal Medicine 5: 94

Gandar R, de Zoeten L W, van der Schoot J B 1980 Serum level of ritodrine in man. European Journal of Clinical Pharmacology 17: 117

Garite T J, Freeman R K, Linzey E M, Braley P 1979 The use of amniocentesis in patients with premature rupture of membranes. Obstetrics and Gynecology 54: 226

Garite T J, Freeman R K, Linzey E M et al 1981 Prospective randomized study of corticosteroids in the management of premature rupture of the membranes and the premature gestation. American Journal of Obstetrics and Gynecology 141: 508

Garn S M, Bailey S M 1977 Genetics of maturation processes. In: Falkner F, Tanner J M (eds) Human growth. Plenum Press, New York

Garn S M, Shaw H A, McCabe K D 1977 Effects of socioeconomic status and race on weight-defined and gestational prematurity in the United States. In: Reed D M, Stanley F J (eds) The epidemiology of pre-maturity. Urban and Schwartzenberg, Baltimore, Maryland, p 127

Garrioch D B 1978 The effect of indomethacin on spontaneous activity in the isolated human myometrium and on the response to oxytocin and prostaglandin. British Journal of Obstetrics and Gynaecology 85: 47

Goldenberg R J, Nelson K G 1977 The premature breech. American Journal of Obstetrics and Gynecology 127: 240
Goudie B M, Dossetor J F B 1979 Effect on the fetus of indomethacin given to suppress labor. Lancet ii: 1187
Gravett M C, Hummel D, Eschenbach D, Holmes K K 1986 Preterm labor associated with subclinical amniotic fluid infection and with bacterial vaginosis. American Journal of Obstetrics and Gynecology 67: 229
Green K W, Key T C, Coen R, Resnik R 1983 The effects of maternally administered magnesium sulfate on the neonate. American Journal of Obstetrics and Gynecology 146: 29
Gunn G L, Mishell D R, Morton D G 1970 Premature rupture of membranes: a review. American Journal of Obstetrics and Gynecology 106: 469
Harbert G M, Cornell G W, Thornton W N 1969 Effect of toxemia therapy on uterine dynamics. American Journal of Obstetrics and Gynecology 105: 94
Hardy J B, Mellits E D 1977 Relationship of low birth weight to maternal characteristics of age, education, and body size. In: Reed D M, Stanley F J (eds) The epidemiology of prematurity. Urban and Schwarzenberg, Baltimore, Maryland, p 105
Hatjis C G, Nelson L H, Meis P J, Swain M 1984 Addition of magnesium sulfate improves effectiveness of ritodrine in preventing premature delivery. American Journal of Obstetrics and Gynecology 150: 142
Hauth J C, Gilstrap L C, Brekken A L, Hauth J M 1983 The effect of 17-alpha-hydroxyprogesterone caproate on pregnancy outcome in an active-duty military population. American Journal of Obstetrics and Gynecology 146: 187
Hawker F 1984 Pulmonary oedema associated with $beta_2$-sympathomimetic treatment of premature labour. Anaesthesiology and Intensive Care 12: 143
Heinonen P K, Saarikoski S, Pystynen P 1982 Reproductive performance of women with uterine anomalies. Acta Obstetricia et Gynecologica Scandinavica 61: 157
Hendricks C H 1964 The use of isoxsuprine for the arrest of premature labor. Clinical Obstetrics and Gynecology 7: 687
Hendricks S K, Keroes J, Katz M 1986 Electrocardiographic changes associated with ritodrine-induced maternal tachycardia and hypokalemia. American Journal of Obstetrics and Gynecology 154: 921
Herron M, Katz M, Creasy R K 1982 Evaluation of a preterm birth prevention program. Preliminary report. Obstetrics and Gynecology 59: 452
Hill W C, Katz M, Kitzmiller J L, Gill P J 1985 Continuous long-term intravenous β-sympathomimetic tocolysis. American Journal of Obstetrics and Gynecology 152: 271
Hills B A, Cotton D B 1984 Premature rupture of membranes and surface energy: possible role of surfactant. American Journal of Obstetrics and Gynecology 149: 896
Hirata T, Epcar J, Wash A et al 1983 Survival and outcome of infants 501 to 750 gm: 6-year experience. Journal of Pediatrics 102: 741
Hollander D I, Nagey D A, Pupkin M J 1987 Magnesium sulfate and ritodrine hydrochloride: a randomized comparison. American Journal of Obstetrics and Gynecology 156: 631
Johnson J W C, Lee P A, Zachary A S et al 1979 High risk prematurity—progestin treatment and steroid studies. Obstetrics and Gynecology 54: 512
Kaltreider D F, Kohl S 1980 Epidemiology of preterm delivery. Clinical Obstetrics and Gynecology 23: 17
Kanayama N, Terao T, Kawashima Y et al 1985 Collagen types in normal and prematurely ruptured amniotic membranes. American Journal of Obstetrics and Gynecology 153: 899
Kappy K A, Cetrulo C L, Knuppel R A et al 1979 Premature rupture of the membranes: a conservative approach. American Journal of Obstetrics and Gynecology 134: 655
Katz M, Newman R B, Gill P G 1986 Assessment of uterine activity in ambulatory patients at high risk of preterm labor and delivery. American Journal of Obstetrics and Gynecology 154: 44
Keirse M J N C, Rush R W, Anderson A B M, Turnbull A C 1978 Risk of preterm delivery in patients with previous pre-term delivery and/or abortion. British Journal of Obstetrics and Gynaecology 85: 81
Khunda S 1972 Locked twins. Obstetrics and Gynecology 39: 453
Kincaid-Smith P 1968 Bacteriuria and urinary infection in pregnancy. Clinical Obstetrics and Gynecology 11: 533
Kirbinen P, Jouppila P 1978 Polyhydramnion. A clinical study. Annales Chirurgiae et Gynaecologiae Senniae 67: 117
Kitchen W, Yu V Y H, Orgill A A et al 1982 Infants born before 29 weeks gestation: survival and morbidity at 2 years of age. British Journal of Obstetrics and Gynaecology 89: 887
Kitchen W, Ford G W, Doyle L W et al 1985 Cesarean section or vaginal delivery at 24 to 28 weeks' gestation: comparison of survival and neonatal and 2-year morbidity. Obstetrics and Gynecology 66: 149
Konte J M, Holbrook R H Jr, Laros R K, Creasy R K 1986 Short-term neonatal morbidity associated with prematurity and the effect of a prematurity prevention program on expected incidence of morbidity. American Journal of Perinatology 3: 283
Korenbrot C C, Aalto L H, Laros R K 1984 The cost effectiveness of stopping preterm labor with beta-adrenergic treatment. New England Journal of Medicine 310: 691
Lauerson N H, Merkatz I R, Tejani N et al 1977 Inhibition of premature labor: a multicenter comparison of ritodrine and ethanol. American Journal of Obstetrics and Gynecology 127: 837
Lavery J P, Miller C E, Knight R D 1982 The effect of labor on the rheologic response of chorioamniotic membranes. Obstetrics and Gynecology 60: 87
Lee K-S, Paneth N, Gartner L et al 1980 Neonatal mortality: an analysis of the recent improvement in the United States. American Journal of Public Health 70: 15
Levy D L, Warsof S L 1985 Oral ritodrine and preterm premature rupture of membranes. Obstetrics and Gynecology 66: 621
Liggins G C, Howie R N 1972 A controlled trial of antepartum glucocorticoid treatment for prevention of the respiratory distress syndrome in premature infants. Pediatrics 50: 515
Linn S, Schoenbaum S C, Monson R R et al 1983 The relationship between induced abortion and outcome of subsequent pregnancies. American Journal of Obstetrics and Gynecology 146: 136
Lipshitz J, Baillie P 1976 The uterine and cardiovascular effects of $beta_2$-selective sympathomimetic drugs administered as an intravenous infusion. South African Medical Journal 50: 1973
Lipshitz J, Broyles K, Whybrew W D 1982 Placental transfer of ^{14}C-hexoprenaline. American Journal of Obstetrics and Gynecology 142: 313
Lipsitz P J, English I C 1967 Hypermagnesemia in the newborn infant. Pediatrics 40: 856
Lotgering F K, Huikeshoven F J M, Wallenburg H C S 1986 Elevated serum transaminase levels during ritodrine administration. American Journal of Obstetrics and Gynecology 155: 390
MacArthur G, Howie R, Dezoete J, Elkins J 1982 School progress and cognitive development of 6-year-old children whose mothers were treated antenatally with betamethasone. Pediatrics 70: 99
MacGillivray I, Campbell D M, Samphier M, Thompson B 1982 Preterm deliveries in twin pregnancies in Aberdeen. Acta Geneticae Medicae et Gemellologiae 31: 207
Main D M, Main E K, Maurer M M 1983 Cesarean section versus vaginal delivery for the breech fetus weighing less than 1500 grams. American Journal of Obstetrics and Gynecology 146: 580
Main D M, Gabbe S G, Richardson D, Strong S 1985 Can preterm births be prevented? American Journal of Obstetrics and Gynecology 151: 892
Main D M, Richardson D, Gabbe S G et al 1987 Prospective evaluation of a risk scoring system for predicting preterm delivery in black inner city women. Obstetrics and Gynecology 69: 61
Main E K, Main D M, Gabbe S G 1987 Chronic oral terbutaline tocolytic therapy is associated with maternal glucose intolerance. American Journal of Obstetrics and Gynecology 157: 644
Mamelle N, Laumon B, Lazar P 1984 Prematurity and occupational activity during pregnancy. American Journal of Epidemiology 119: 309
Martin C M, Siassi B, Hon E H 1974 Fetal heart rate patterns and neonatal death in low birth weight infants. Obstetrics and Gynecology 44: 503
Martin D H, Koutsky L, Eschenbach D A et al 1982 Prematurity and perinatal mortality in pregnancies complicated by maternal *Chlamydia trachomatis* infection. Journal of the American Medical Association 247: 1585
McCormick M 1985 The contribution of low birth weight to infant mortality and childhood morbidity. New England Journal of Medicine 312: 82
McCubbin J H, Sibai G M, Abdella T M et al 1981 Cardiopulmonary arrest due to acute maternal hypermagnesaemia (letter). Lancet i: 1058
McGregor J A, French J I, Reller L B et al 1986a Adjunctive erythromycin

treatment for idiopathic preterm labor: results of a randomized, double-blinded, placebo-controlled trial. American Journal of Obstetrics and Gynecology 154: 98

McGregor J A, Lawellin D, Franco-Buff A et al 1986b Protease production by microorganisms associated with reproductive tract infection. American Journal of Obstetrics and Gynecology 154: 109

Meissner J, Klostermann H 1976 Distribution and diaplacental passage of infused ^{3}H-fenoterol hydrobromide (Partusisten) in the gravid rabbit. International Journal of Clinical Pharmacology and Biopharmacology 13: 27

Merkatz I R, Peter J B, Barden T P 1980 Ritodrine hydrochloride. A beta-mimetic agent for use in preterm labor. II. Evidence of efficacy. Obstetrics and Gynecology 56: 7

Meyer M B, Tonascia J A 1977 Maternal smoking, pregnancy complications, and perinatal mortality. American Journal of Obstetrics and Gynecology 128: 494

Miller J M, Brazy J E, Gall S A et al 1980 Premature rupture of the membranes. Maternal and neonatal infectious morbidity related to betamethasone and antibiotic therapy. Journal of Reproductive Medicine 25: 173

Miller J M, Keane M W D, Horger E O III 1982 A comparison of magnesium sulfate and terbutaline for the arrest of premature labor. Journal of Reproductive Medicine 27: 348

Milligan J E, Shennan A T, Hoskins E M 1984 Perinatal intensive care: where and how to draw the line. American Journal of Obstetrics and Gynecology 148: 499

Milner R, Beard R 1984 Limit of fetal viability. Lancet i: 1079

Minkoff H, Mead P 1986 An obstetric approach to the prevention of early onset group B beta-hemolytic streptococcal sepsis. American Journal of Obstetrics and Gynecology 154: 973

Minkoff H L, Grunebaum A N, Schwarz R H et al 1984 Risk factors for prematurity and premature rupture of membranes: a prospective study of the vaginal flora in pregnancy. American Journal of Obstetrics and Gynecology 150: 965

Mitchell M D, Flint A P, Bibby J et al 1978 Plasma concentration of prostaglandins during late human pregnancy: influence of normal and preterm labour. Journal of Clinical Endocrinology 46: 947

Monif G R 1983 Recurrent chorioamnionitis and maternal septicemia: a case of successful in utero therapy. American Journal of Obstetrics and Gynecology 146: 334

Moore T R, Origel W, Key T C, Resnik R 1986 The perinatal and economic impact of prenatal care in a low-socioeconomic population. American Journal of Obstetrics and Gynecology 154: 29

Morales W J, Koerten J 1986 Prevention of intraventricular hemorrhage in very low birth weight infants by maternally administered phenobarbital. Obstetrics and Gynecology 68: 295

Morales W J, Diebel N D, Lazar A J, Zadrozny D 1986 The effect of antenatal dexamethasone administration on the prevention of respiratory distress syndrome in preterm gestations with premature rupture of the membranes. American Journal of Obstetrics and Gynecology 154: 591

Mordes D, Kreutner K, Metzger W, Colwell J 1982 Dangers of intravenous ritodrine in diabetic patients. Journal of the American Medical Association 248: 973

Mosier H P Jr, Dearden L C, Tanner S M et al 1979 Disproportionate organ growth in the fetus after betamethasone administration. Pediatric Research 13: 486

Munson L A, Graham A, Koos B J, Valenzuela G J 1985 Is there a need for digital examination in patients with spontaneous rupture of the membranes? American Journal of Obstetrics and Gynecology 153: 562

Muran D, Gillieson M, Walters J H 1980 Myomas of the uterus in pregnancy: ultrasonographic follow-up. American Journal of Obstetrics and Gynecology 138: 16

Murphy J, Dauncey M, Newcombe R et al 1984 Employment in pregnancy: prevalence, maternal characteristics, perinatal outcome. Lancet i: 1163

Naeye R L 1979 Coitus and associated amniotic-fluid infections. New England Journal of Medicine 301: 1198

Naeye R L 1980 Seasonal variations in coitus and other risk factors, and the outcome of pregnancy. Early Human Development 4: 61

Naeye R L 1982 Factors that predispose to premature rupture of the fetal membranes. Obstetrics and Gynecology 60: 93

Naeye R L, Peters E C 1980 Causes and consequences of premature rupture of fetal membranes. Lancet i: 192

Naeye R L, Ross S 1982 Coitus and chorioamnionitis: a prospective study. Early Human Development 6: 91

Nageotte M P, Freeman R K, Garite T J, Dorchester W 1985 Prophylactic intrapartum amnioinfusion in patients with preterm premature rupture of membranes. American Journal of Obstetrics and Gynecology 153: 557

Newton R W, Hunt L 1984 Psychosocial stress in pregnancy and its relation to low birth weight. British Medical Journal 288: 1191

New Zealand Health Statistics Report 1978

Niebyl J R, Witter F R 1986 Neonatal outcome after indomethacin treatment for preterm labor. American Journal of Obstetrics and Gynecology 155: 747

Niebyl J R, Blake D A, Johnson J W C, King T M 1978 Pharmacologic inhibition of premature labor. Obstetrical and Gynecological Survey 33: 507

Niebyl J R, Blake D A, White R D et al 1980 The inhibition of premature labor by indomethacin. American Journal of Obstetrics and Gynecology 136: 1014

Nimrod C, Varela-Gittings F, Machin G et al 1984 The effect of very prolonged membrane rupture on fetal development. American Journal of Obstetrics and Gynecology 148: 540

Novy M J 1978 Effects of indomethacin on labor, fetal oxygenation and fetal development in rhesus monkeys. Advances in Prostaglandin and Thromboxane Research 4: 285

O'Driscoll K, Maegher D, MacDonald D, et al 1981 Traumatic intracranial haemorrhage in firstborn infants and delivery with obstetric forceps. British Journal of Obstetrics and Gynaecology 88: 577

O'Leary J A 1986 Prophylactic tocolysis of twins. American Journal of Obstetrics and Gynecology 154: 904

Olshan A F, Sky K K, Luthy D A et al 1984 Cesarean birth and neonatal mortality in very low birth weight infants. Obstetrics and Gynecology 64: 267

Paneth N, Kiely J, Wallenstein S et al 1982 Newborn intensive care and neonatal mortality in low-birth-weight infants. New England Journal of Medicine 307: 149

Parsons M T, Owens C A, Spellacy W N 1987 Thermic effects of tocolytic agents: decreased temperature with magnesium sulfate. Obstetrics and Gynecology 69: 88

Philipsen T, Erikson P S, Lynggard F 1981 Pulmonary edema following ritodrine–saline infusion in premature labor. Obstetrics and Gynecology 58: 304

Regan J A, Chao S, James L S 1981 Premature rupture of membranes, preterm delivery, and group B streptococcal colonization of mothers. American Journal of Obstetrics and Gynecology 141: 184

Reiss U, Atad J, Reuinstein I et al 1976 The effect of indomethacin in labour at term. International Journal of Gynaecology and Obstetrics 14: 369

Remington J T, Klein J O 1983 Infectious diseases of the fetus and newborn infant, 2nd edn. WB Saunders, Philadelphia

Roberts J M 1984 Current understanding of pharmacologic mechanisms in the prevention of preterm birth. Clinical Obstetrics and Gynecology 27: 592

Robertson P A, Herron M, Katz M, Creasy R K 1981 Maternal morbidity associated with isoxsuprine and terbutaline tocolysis. European Journal of Obstetrics, Gynecology and Reproductive Biology 11: 317

Rochelson B L, Richardson D A, Macri J N 1983 Rapid assay — possible application in the diagnosis of premature rupture of the membranes. Obstetrics and Gynecology 62: 414

Rochelson B L, Rodke G, White R et al 1987 A rapid colorimetric AFP monoclonal antibody test for the diagnosis of preterm rupture of the membranes. Obstetrics and Gynecology 69: 163

Rosen K A, Featherstone H J, Benedetti T J 1982 Cerebral ischemia associated with parenteral terbutaline use in pregnant migraine patients. American Journal of Obstetrics and Gynecology 143: 405

Rush R W 1979 Incidence of pre-term delivery in patients with previous preterm delivery and/or abortion. South African Medical Journal 56: 1085

Rush R W, Keirse M J N C, Howat P et al 1976 Contribution of preterm delivery to perinatal mortality. British Medical Journal 2: 965

Russell P 1979 Inflammatory lesions of the human placenta: I. Clinical significance of acute chorioamnionitis. American Journal of Diagnostic Gynecology and Obstetrics 1: 127

Schaefer K F, Avery M E, Bensch K 1964 Time course of changes in

surface tension and morphology of alveolar epithelial cells in CO_2 induced hyaline membrane disease. Journal of Clinical Investigation 43: 2080
Schreiber J, Benedetti T 1980 Conservative management of preterm rupture of the fetal membranes in a low socioeconomic population. American Journal of Obstetrics and Gynecology 136: 92
Schutte M F, Treffers P E, Kloosterman G J, Soepatmi S 1983 Management of premature rupture of membranes: the risk of vaginal examination to the infant. American Journal of Obstetrics and Gynecology 146: 395
Schwartz D B, Miodovnik M, Lavin J P 1983 Neonatal outcome among low birth weight infants delivered spontaneously or by low forceps. Obstetrics and Gynecology 62: 283
Shlievert P, Larson B, Johnson W, Galask R P 1975 Bacterial growth inhibition by amniotic fluid. III. Demonstration of the variability of bacterial growth inhibition by amniotic fluid with a new plate-count technique. American Journal of Obstetrics and Gynecology 122: 809
Smith R 1976 A technic for the detection of rupture of the membranes. A review and preliminary report. Obstetrics and Gynecology 48: 172
Steer C M, Petrie R H 1977 A comparison of magnesium sulfate and alcohol for the prevention of premature labor. American Journal of Obstetrics and Gynecology 129: 1
Stillman R J 1982 In utero exposure to diethylstilbesterol: adverse effects on the reproductive tract and reproductive performance in male and female offspring. American Journal of Obstetrics and Gynecology 142: 905
Stuart M J, Gross S J, Elrad H et al 1982 Effects of acetylsalicylic-acid ingestion on maternal and neonatal homeostasis. New England Journal of Medicine 307: 909
Taeusch H W, Frigoletto F, Kitzmiller J et al 1979 Risk of respiratory distress syndrome after prenatal dexamethasone treatment. Pediatrics 63: 64
Tamby Raja R, Atputhrajah V, Salman Y 1978 Prevention of prematurity in twins. Australian and New Zealand Journal of Obstetrics and Gynaecology 18: 179
Tatum H J, Schmidt F H, Jain A K 1976 Management and outcome of pregnancies associated with Copper-T intrauterine contraceptive device. American Journal of Obstetrics and Gynecology 126: 869
Taylor J, Garite T J 1984 Premature rupture of membranes before fetal viability. Obstetrics and Gynecology 64: 615
Taylor E S, Morgan R L, Bruns P D et al 1961 Spontaneous premature rupture of the fetal membranes. American Journal of Obstetrics and Gynecology 82: 1341
Tejani N, Rebold B, Tuck S et al 1984 Obstetric factors in the causation of early periventricular–intraventricular hemorrhage. Obstetrics and Gynecology 64: 510
Thiagarajah S, Harbert G M, Bourgeois F J 1985 Magnesium sulfate and ritodrine hydrochloride: systemic and uterine hemodynamic effects. American Journal of Obstetrics and Gynecology 153: 666
Thomas D J B, Dove A F, Alberti K G M M 1977a Metabolic effects of salbutamol infusion during premature labour. British Journal of Obstetrics and Gynaecology 84: 497
Thomas D J B, Gill B, Brown P, Subbs W A 1977b Salbutamol-induced diabetic keto-acidosis. British Medical Journal 2: 1152
Toppozada M K, Sallam N A, Gaafar A A, El-Kashlan K M 1970 Role of repeated stretching in the mechanism of timely rupture of the membranes. American Journal of Obstetrics and Gynecology 108: 243
Turnbull A C 1977 Aetiology of pre-term labour. In: Anderson A B M et al (eds) Proceedings of the fifth study group of the Royal College of Obstetricians and Gynaecologists. Royal College of Obstetricians and Gynaecologists, London, p 56
Valenzuela G, Cline S, Hayashi R H 1983 Follow-up of hydration and sedation in the pretherapy of premature labor. American Journal of Obstetrics and Gynecology 147: 396
Varner M N, Turner J W, Petzold C R, Galask P P 1985 Ultrastructural alterations of term human amnion epithelium following incubation with group B beta-hemolytic streptococci. American Journal of Immunology and Microbiology 8: 27
Verder H, Fonseca J, Falck L et al 1978 Lecithin/sphingomyelin ratio in eight cases of premature rupture of the membranes. Danish Medical Bulletin 25: 218
Vintzileos A M, Campbell W A, Nochimson S J, Weinbaum P J 1986 The use of the nonstress test in patients with premature rupture of the membranes. American Journal of Obstetrics and Gynecology 155: 149
Wagner N N, Butler J C, Sanders J P 1976 Prematurity and orgasmic coitus during pregnancy: data on a small sample. Fertility and Sterility 27: 911
Walker D, Feldman A, Vohr B, Oh W 1984 Cost-benefit analysis of neonatal intensive care for infants weighing less than 1000 grams at birth. Pediatrics 74: 20
Wideman G L, Baird G H, Bolding O T, 1964 Ascorbic acid deficiency and premature rupture of fetal membranes. American Journal of Obstetrics and Gynecology 88: 592
Wilkins I A, Goldberg J D, Phillips R N et al 1986 Long-term use of magnesium sulfate as a tocolytic agent. Obstetrics and Gynecology 67 (suppl): 38
Wiqvist N, Kjellmer I, Thiringer K et al 1978 Treatment of premature labor by prostaglandin synthetase inhibitors. Acta Biologica Medica 37: 923
Worthington D W, Davis L E, Grausz J P, Sobocinski K 1983 Factors influencing survival and morbidity with very low birth weight delivery. Obstetrics and Gynecology 62: 550
Ying Y-K, Tejani N A 1982 Angina pectoris as a complication of ritodrine hydrochloride therapy in premature labor. Obstetrics and Gynecology 60: 385
Young D C, Toofanian A, Leveno K J 1983 Potassium and glucose concentrations without treatment during ritodrine tocolysis. American Journal of Obstetrics and Gynecology 145: 105
Yu V, Orgill A, Bajuk B, Astbury J 1984 Survival and 2-year outcome of extremely preterm infants. British Journal of Obstetrics and Gynaecology 91: 640
Zanini B, Paul R H, Huey J R 1980 Intrapartum fetal heart rate: correlation with scalp pH in the preterm fetus. American Journal of Obstetrics and Gynecology 136: 43
Zlatnik F J, Cruikshank D P, Petzold C R, Galask R P 1984 Amniocentesis in the identification of inapparent infection in preterm patients with premature rupture of the membranes. Journal of Reproductive Medicine 29: 656
Zuckerman H, Reiss U, Rubinstein I 1974 Inhibition of human premature labor by indomethacin. Obstetrics and Gynecology 44: 787

51

Michael M. Dooley and John Studd

Prolonged pregnancy

> There can no more be an 'exact' time for gestation than an 'exact' height or an 'exact' weight for everyone or exact rate of urinary secretion, gastric digestion or (for that matter) cerebration (Wrigley 1958).

The approach to prolonged pregnancy in the UK has been, to some experts, out of step with clinical practice in other parts of Europe and the USA and has now been greatly modified into a more conservative one. The reports of 30 years ago indicated a considerably increased perinatal mortality for the postmature fetus but, as a knowledge of fetal pathology and methods of assessing fetal health have developed, the current debate concerns the added risk, if any, to normal postmaturity or, to use the currently accepted term, prolonged pregnancy.

Since the turn of the century a considerable volume of material has been published concerning the effects on both mother and child when pregnancy extends beyond the calculated expected date of delivery. Divided opinion on the management of prolonged pregnancy has caused considerable concern and confusion to those involved in clinical decisions. The pendulum swings between the dated belief of Ballantyne (1902); 'the postmature infant . . . can with difficulty be born alive' to that of Cardozo et al (1986): 'prolonged pregnancy is a variant of normal and should be treated as such'.

Precise knowledge of the age of the fetus is imperative for ideal obstetric management, being important not only for the health of mother and infant but also for the legal rights of those directly involved. The length of human pregnancy is variable. Beyond what gestation, if any, is the fetus in jeopardy? Does placental ageing, as a primary cause for placental insufficiency, exist? Is the fetus compromised more commonly with prolonged pregnancies? At what stage beyond the expected date of confinement does interruption of pregnancy improve the prognosis? How can we assess the correct time for interference? These questions are important and will be considered in this chapter.

DEFINITION

The International Federation of Gynecology and Obstetrics (FIGO 1982) which quotes World Health Organization (WHO) recommendations from 1967 and 1976, defines prolonged pregnancy as a pregnancy lasting '42 completed weeks or more (294 days or more)'. This differs from an earlier FIGO (1980) definition which defines post-term pregnancy as: 'a pregnancy that is calculated to have proceeded beyond the end of the 42nd week (i.e. more than 294 days)'. The discrepancy of 1 day may seem of little clinical importance but it is important to be clarified in any statistical comparisons; further, many interventions actually take place on the 294th day and so prompt deliveries would be included in the new definition but excluded from the former.

Postmaturity or prolonged pregnancy?

Confusion exists between the terms postmaturity and prolonged pregnancy. The latter has the clear definition, as has been described. Postmaturity, on the other hand, is associated with the clinical state in which the fetus shows signs of intrauterine malnutrition (see Table 51.1). Clifford (1954) described the postmaturity syndrome as the undernourished fetus suffering because of placental ageing and dysfunction. A wider definition of postmaturity suggested by Kloosterman (1979) includes 'every fetus that dies before or during labour or shows signs of severe fetal distress during a normal labour; whereas its development and degree of maturity would have guaranteed survival, as a healthy individual, if it had been brought into the outer world at a slightly earlier date'.

Table 51.1 Features of the postmaturity syndrome (Gibb 1985)

Absence of vernix caseosa
Absence of lanugo hair
Abundant scalp hair
Long fingernails
Dry, cracked desquamated skin
Body length increased in relation to body weight
Alert and apprehensive facies
Meconium staining of skin and membranes

HISTORICAL PERSPECTIVE

Historical evidence exists which demonstrates that there is no 'exact time for gestation' with a documented case of a woman being pregnant for 476 days giving birth to a boy weighing 13 lb (5.8 kg) in 1883. Her last menstrual period (LMP) was on 17 July 1882 with an expected date of delivery of 24 April 1883. In May 1883 she had some labour pains and these continued on and off for the next few months. In September 1883 the cervix admitted two fingers and in November 1883 she went into spontaneous labour with the forceps delivery of a male infant (Ferguson et al 1982).

Comparing prolonged human pregnancy with certain mammalian pregnancies, Mills (1970) proposed the term fetal hibernation, to be applied to cases in which there was evidence of retarded fetal growth followed by resumption of normal development. This hypothesis, based on clinical estimations of uterine size and the duration of amenorrhoea, was rejected by Campbell et al (1970) who stressed how unreliable uterine palpation is in the estimation of fetal growth, size and maturity.

DURATION OF PREGNANCY AND INCIDENCE OF PROLONGED PREGNANCY

Not only is there dispute amongst clinicians about the duration of normal pregnancy but other disciplines use different starting points and care must be taken when comparisons are made. Embryologists and reproductive biologists use ovulatory age or fertilization age while clinicians calculate the estimated date of delivery from the LMP.

It is surprising that modern obstetricians still support Naegele's rule, which adds 280 days (9 calendar months plus 7 days; Naegele 1812) to the LMP, for it was introduced when ovulation was thought to follow soon after menstruation. This idea was rejected when it was realized that Orthodox Jewish women, who are barred from intercourse at this time, were extremely fertile. However Naegele's rule has stood the test of time with many studies supporting the findings (Table 51.2). More accurate methods of determining time of ovulation and even actual conception are now available and data from these studies provide more concrete evidence on the duration of normal gestation.

There remains some debate as to the duration of normal pregnancy. In any scientific work a fixed definition is required, if only to compare results. Prolonged pregnancy may be physiologically normal and the FIGO definition of 294 or more days could, when there is appropriate evidence, be changed.

Table 51.2 Average duration of pregnancy in the literature

Author	Method of assessment	Duration from LMP (days)
Naegele (1812)		180
Cary (1948)	Artificial insemination	285 (271 days from conception)
Kortenoever (1950)	History of LMP	282
Stewart (1952)	Basal body temperature	280–284 (266–270 days from conception)
Park (1968)	History of LMP	287–289
Guerrero & Florex (1969)	Basal body temperature	280
Nakano 1972	History of LMP	278.5

LMP = last menstrual period.

LEGAL IMPLICATIONS

Not only is the most precise possible knowledge of the fetus imperative for ideal obstetric care but there is also a legal aspect to the problem. The plaintiff is usually the supposed father who is disputing paternity on the ground that he had no opportunity to cohabit with his wife within usually accepted limits of pregnancy duration.

In Gaskill v Gaskill (Times Law Reports 1921) the petitioner, Mr Gaskill, a soldier at the time, gave evidence that on 4 October 1918 he had sexual intercourse with his wife for the last time. He left for Salonika on 12 October and did not return to England until September 1919. On 1 September 1919 his wife gave birth to a child, the lapse of time since the husband's departure being 331 days. Dr Munroe, the doctor in charge, stated that the child weighed around 11 lb and the labour was prolonged. The only evidence of adultery was the abnormal length of pregnancy and an extract from the judgment by the Lord Chancellor summarizes the case:

> No other fact or circumstances has been deduced which in the slightest degree casts any reflection upon the chastity or modesty of the respondent who has on oath denied adultery. I can only find her guilty if I come to the conclusion that it is impossible, having regard to the present state of medical knowledge and belief, that the petitioner can be the father of the child. In these circumstances I accept the evidence of the respondent and find that she has not committed adultery and accordingly dismiss the petitioner.

A more recent trend of medicolegal work is observed by Freeman (see Elliott & Flaherty 1984) who reported that in the USA approximately 40% of obstetric malpractice cases involve post-term pregnancies.

Table 51.3 Methods of assessment for gestational age

History	
Last menstrual period	
Symptoms of pregnancy	
	Nausea
	Breast tenderness
	Cravings etc.
Quickening	
On examination	
Uterine size	
	Hegar's sign
Fundal height	
Investigation	
Beta human chorionic gonadotrophin	
Ultrasound	
	Gestational sac
	Crown–rump length
	Biparietal diameter
	Femur length
	Head circumference
	Abdominal circumference

DIAGNOSIS OF PROLONGED PREGNANCY

In order to provide appropriate care accurate dating is essential. Although sophisticated equipment is often available the important role of basic symptoms and signs must not be forgotten (Table 51.3).

History and examination

Anderson et al (1981a) stated that the date of the woman's LMP is the best clinical predictor for the date of confinement; prediction of actual day of delivery in women with known dates of LMP was not improved with ultrasound. It was these cases with sure dates which were used in the early days of sonography to develop the normograms. A total of 71% of women were found to be able to recall the LMP exactly; 25% could provide an approximate date and in up to 4% this date was completely unknown. This differs from Campbell (1974), who reported a 40% incidence of suspect menstrual histories and in other studies there is up to a 45% incidence (Warsof et al 1983). Wenner & Young (1974) found that one-third of their study group of patients had a non-specific date of LMP; reviewing the findings of other authors, between 14 and 58% of patients have an uncertain LMP. Basal body temperature charts or other signs and symptoms of ovulation, including mittelschmerz, which has been demonstrated to be a preovulatory rather than postovulatory symptom (O'Herlihy et al 1980), may also be of help. Information on menstrual patterns, ovulation induction agent use or recent discontinuation of hormonal contraceptive agents will be beneficial.

Using LMP, quickening, fetal heart tones first audible with an unamplified stethoscope, the uterus at the level of the umbilicus and fundal height measurement, Anderson et al (1981b) developed a more comprehensive approach to the problem of gestational age (Table 51.4). In patients with a known LMP, additional information did not improve the prediction of delivery date; however, if the LMP was uncertain or unknown, averaging the predicted delivery dates by several clinical examinations provided a prediction of delivery date as precise as if the LMP had been known. This may be of particular value late in pregnancy when ultrasound is not a good tool for estimating gestational age and the clinical data recorded in the antenatal notes may become the main basis for estimating gestational age.

Table 51.4 Mean observed intervals to delivery date for last menstrual period (LMP) and obstetric landmarks (data from 418 patients; Anderson et al 1981b)

	Mean interval to delivery date (days)	Standard deviation (days)
Known LMP	284.2	14.6
Quickening	156.3	18.0
Fetal heart tones first audible	136.2	17.0
Uterus at the umbilicus	140.8	14.9

Quickening, defined as the date when the patient first feels fetal movement for three consecutive days, is of limited value. Traditionally quickening is said to occur sometime between 16 and 20 weeks after the onset of the hMP. In a prospective study of 200 patients, O'Dowd & O'Dowd (1985) concluded that the range of quickening is wide; 15–22 weeks for primigravidae and 14–22 weeks for multigravidae. Quickening is of limited value in assessing and estimating gestational age and the main value of knowing when quickening occurs may be to answer the inevitable question: 'When will I feel my baby move?'

Due to wide biological variations, neither bimanual nor abdominal examination is sufficiently accurate to be useful in the estimation of gestational age. Serial estimations of fundal height with their results plotted graphically may be of benefit in detection of growth retardation.

Investigations

Hormones, with the advantage of being relatively non-invasive and inexpensive, have been extensively investigated with regard to the role they may play in the estimation of gestational age. However due to a wide variation in the biological norm the initial optimism has not been supported.

Rapid enzyme immunoassay kits for the beta subunit of human chorionic gonadotrophin (hCG) are available and can detect an early pregnancy before the missed menstrual period. Lagrew et al (1983) measured quantitative levels of hCG in patients of less than 60 days' gestation and observed only a 3.5 day mean difference between predicted and actual gestation.

Ultrasound scanning has now become the best method of backing up history and physical examination information. Measurement of the gestational sac diameter was the first to be described but may sometimes be inaccurate because of inclusion of the yolk sac. Weiner (1981) has concluded that the definitive sonographic diagnosis of intrauterine pregnancy requires the demonstration of fetal heart motion which can only be detected at 49 days of gestational age, or at approximately the time of peak hCG levels (10 000–20 000 ng / ml).

Ultrasonic measurement of crown–rump length can be used to predict accurately the expected date of delivery. Drumm et al (1976) demonstrated that fetal crown–rump length can be correlated accurately with reliable menstrual data and known date of ovulation with a range of ±3 days. In a later study (Drumm 1977) the crown–rump length was found to be better than biparietal diameter and as good as a reliable menstrual history in predicting the time of spontaneous onset of labour. Earlier than 9 weeks the greatest problem in crown–rump length measurement lies in knowing whether the maximum longitudinal diameter of the fetus has actually been measured.

At around 12 weeks the fetus develops a kyphosis and crown–rump length measurement loses accuracy and the biparietal diameter, femur length, head circumference and abdominal circumference become more relevant. The accuracy of pregnancy dating from 12–20 weeks by ultrasound is probably just as good as that done earlier. However, waiting until 16–20 weeks is prudent because without significant loss of accuracy it is the gestation when the majority of other prenatal diagnostic studies are performed and with more fetal and placental anatomy appreciated, congenital abnormalities may be detected. The routine use of ultrasound early in pregnancy to estimate gestational age has been demonstrated to reduce significantly the incidence of prolonged pregnancy due to more accurate dating (Eik-Nes et al 1984).

In the third trimester prediction of gestational age without prior information is more difficult. In the past, radiological detection of fetal femoral and tibial epiphyses was used to confirm a clinical assessment of fetal maturity. The distal femoral epiphysis can first be detected between the 35th and 40th week and by term is present in 95% of fetuses. The proximal tibial epiphysis appears between the 37th and 42nd week and by term is present in 75% of cases.

Amniotic fluid sampling has been used to confirm fetal maturity. Measurement includes fetal fat-filled cells, amniotic creatinine and lecithin : sphingomyelin ratios. These have fallen out of favour due not only to the invasive nature of sample collection, but also to the development of alternative methods of assessment.

AETIOLOGY

Although prolonged pregnancy is often within normal limits, several studies have attempted to identify aetiological factors.

Seasonal variation

Pronounced seasonal variations in the length of pregnancy have been demonstrated by Boe (1951), with pregnancy being distinctly longer in the summer than the winter months, with an average difference of 2.5–4 days.

Improved living standards

The hypothesis that improved living standards may lead to postmaturity was raised with the knowledge that poor nutrition leads to prematurity. Boe (1951) found that since 1900 there has been tendency for the average duration of pregnancy and size of babies to be increased but only to a minor degree. During the starvation that followed the occupation of Norway, the duration of pregnancy was not appreciably shortened although birthweights tended to fall.

Hereditary and racial factors

Prolonged pregnancy tends to recur in successive pregnancies in the same woman, and the condition often runs in families. Surveys have shown (Barron & Vessey 1966, Tuck et al 1983) a significantly shorter mean length of gestation and lower frequency of pregnancies continuing beyond 42 weeks' gestation in black than in white women. This difference has not been observed in Asian women (Bissenden et al 1981, Tuck et al 1983).

Hormonal influence

Oestrogen and cortisol play a role in the initiation of labour. A defect in the pituitary adrenal axis may be of importance in prolonged pregnancy and occurs with anencephaly. However, there is at present little evidence of endocrinological defects in the majority of prolonged pregnancies except in a small number of cases with placental sulphatase deficiency and congenital adrenal hyperplasia.

Placental ageing

> When the embryo has matured, the maternal organism can no longer adequately supply nutrient; then movement becomes violent. In its search for more nutrition than is available, the child moves and it seeks freedom. This seldom is later than the tenth month . . . for in every species a time must come when the nutritive balance is lessened and exhausted (Hippocrates; see Petersen 1946).

Earlier belief in the ageing placenta has been dispelled by Fox (1979) who has demonstrated that there are no morphological features of the term or post-term placenta, at either light or electron microscope level, which can be considered as a manifestation of ageing. Recent studies have also demonstrated that total placental DNA rises in a linear fashion beyond the 40th week of gestation (Fox 1983), and the placenta grows, at a decreased growth rate, during the later stages of pregnancy. The placenta is somewhat like the liver in that once it has reached its optimal size it shows little evidence of cell replication but retains a latent potential for growth activity. Fetal growth continues, though at a reduced velocity, after 38 weeks of pregnancy (Gruenwald 1967) and babies delivered at 42 weeks are nearly three times as likely to weigh over 4000 g as those delivered between term and 41 weeks (Boyd et al 1983).

SIGNIFICANCE OF PROLONGED PREGNANCY

Fetal implications

The yardstick for fetal care is perinatal mortality and Clifford (1954) demonstrated the classical U-shaped curve of perinatal mortality with the nadir at 270–289 days. Perinatal mortality rate was demonstrated to be significantly increased in postmature infants but only in primigravidae and not multigravidae. Earlier, Ballantyne & Browne (1922) suggested that postmaturity was dangerous and induction of labour should be performed at or soon after term. Browne revised his position in 1957, when he studied hospital reports from 20 hospitals with a very large variation in the frequency of induction of labour for prolonged pregnancy; no significant difference in mortality rates was found. Clayton (1941) noted an increase in perinatal mortality but no change occurred when analysis was restricted to babies who died for no apparent cause.

The 1958 survey of the National Birthday Trust (NBT) reviewed by McClure Browne (1963) showed very significant increases in perinatal mortality after 42 weeks of completed gestation. However the significance of oligohydramnios, intrauterine growth retardation, glucose intolerance and other causes of fetal compromise was not appreciated and antenatal tests of fetal well-being were not available. Other reports (Dawkins et al 1961) emphasized the association of hypertension in the postmature pregnancy with perinatal death; however, uncomplicated postmaturity was rarely associated with death.

The NBT study of birth in Britain in 1958 was reviewed by Butler & Bonham (1963) who reported that the lowest perinatal mortality rate was at 40 weeks; by 44 weeks of gestation the rate had risen more than threefold. At 41 weeks the perinatal mortality rate was almost the same as at 40, but by 42 weeks it had doubled. Performing the same calculations from the 1970 NBT nationwide survey of births in Britain, Chamberlain et al (1978) showed the influence of postdates had changed since 1958: the perinatal mortality rate was lower at 41–42 weeks than at 39–40 weeks and at 43+ weeks was just over twice that at 39–40 weeks.

A retrospective study of perinatal mortality in term (37–41 weeks) and post-term (>42 weeks) pregnancies delivered at the National Maternity Hospital, Dublin, between 1974 and 1981, showed that the perinatal mortality, exclusive of lethal malformation, was 5.0 per 1000 at 37–42 weeks and 9.4 per 1000 after 42 weeks (Crowley et al 1984).

The arguments will continue. The increase in perinatal mortality which may exist can be reduced with careful monitoring and selective intervention, with the majority of prolonged-pregnancy infants expected to have an uncomplicated perinatal course (Paterson et al 1970, Schneider et al 1978).

Intrapartum implications

Miller & Read (1981) and Klapholz & Friedman (1977) documented no increased incidence of fetal distress in postdates infants in labour, differing from Freeman et al (1981) and Schneider et al (1978) who demonstrated a significant increase. An increase of meconium in the post-term fetus in labour may be secondary to the presence of a more dominant vagal system rather than an actual increase in intrauterine insults (Zwerdling 1967, Miller & Read 1981). Meconium still remains a problem and extra caution must be exercised with the combination of meconium and fetal distress, which leads to a particularly poor outcome. The incidence of the meconium aspiration syndrome has been reduced by adequate suction of the respiratory tract at delivery (Carsons et al 1976). Prolonged pregnancy is also associated with oligohydramnios; not only may this indicate poor placental reserve but cord compression is more likely.

Neonatal implications

Congenital malformations are increased by 50% in post-term pregnancies (Vorherr 1975) with an eightfold increase in the incidence of anencephaly (Zwerdling 1967); this is associated with failure of the natural onset of labour to occur.

Infants born at term have been compared to those born post-term in a study by Field et al (1977). The post-term, postmature infants had more perinatal complications and lower motor scores at birth. At 8 months their daily motor scores were similar to those of control infants but their mental scores were lower. They also had more illness and feeding and sleep disturbances; however, long-term follow-up was not performed. An earlier study of 400 000 births found an increase in perinatal mortality, fetal distress, birth injury, meconium aspiration and congenital malformations in the postdates infant (Zwerdling 1967). Follow-up showed a continued increase of mortality among infants up to 2 years of age, although at 5 years no difference in mortality rates was noted between babies born at term and those postdates.

The influence of prolonged pregnancy on infant development at 1 and 2 years of age following otherwise uncomplicated pregnancies with meticulous dating was investigated by Shime et al (1986). At 1 and 2 years the general IQ, physical milestones and intercurrent illness of normal infants and those of prolonged pregnancies were found to be not significantly different.

Maternal implications

On the maternal side, many iatrogenic problems exist. Incorrect counselling regarding the expected date of delivery may create unnecessary anxiety for the mother and father if delivery does not occur at the determined date. Often social circumstances are geared around a fixed date and great disruption occurs if delivery is late. The temptation to induce with no valid medical indication occurs and avoidable problems develop. The increased Caesarean section rate in patients being induced with low Bishop's score greatly increases the maternal risk. Freeman et al (1981) found the incidence of Caesarean section rose from 13.6% at term to 25.6% in the post-term group, although with improved methods of induction this may not be as significant. Correct advice during the first trimester as to the incidence and the significance of postdates may often help to overcome these problems.

ANTENATAL CARE

No exact date for the onset of labour should be given and if no exact date is given then management of the condition can vary from patient to patient (Wrigley 1958).

The management of postdate pregnancy remains one of the most controversial areas in modern obstetric practice. The two management policies that predominate are elective and selective induction of labour.

Elective induction

Intervention involved jumping from the frying pan of postmaturity into the fire of induction of labour (Gibberd 1958).

Induction at term was adopted in the UK after the work by Walker (1954) demonstrated fetal oxygen tension decreased as the length of gestation increased after term. Bancroft-Livingston & Neill (1957) utilized spectrophotometric techniques and failed to establish such a relationship. They pointed out the limitations in the experimental method employed by Walker. McClure Browne (1963) studied 16 986 pregnancies, demonstrated an increased fetal morbidity after 42 weeks and suggested induction at 42 weeks. There was an associated morbidity with such a policy but the morbidity from routine induction equalled that of non-intervention.

Knox et al (1979), Hauth et al (1980) and Gibb et al (1982) have shown that routine induction at 42 weeks does not improve neonatal outcome. The reason for this may be due to one of several factors. Firstly, there is an associated increase in morbidity with no benefit being derived by post-date patients with delayed ovulation or poor historians who have not actually gone postdates. Secondly, most fetuses despite going post-term are not compromised. Thirdly, with any method of induction there is always the possibility of failure and the associated morbidity and mortality.

Several studies have shown an increase in the Caesarean section rate associated with routine induction (Vorherr 1975, Gibb et al 1982). Cardozo et al (1986) failed to demonstrate

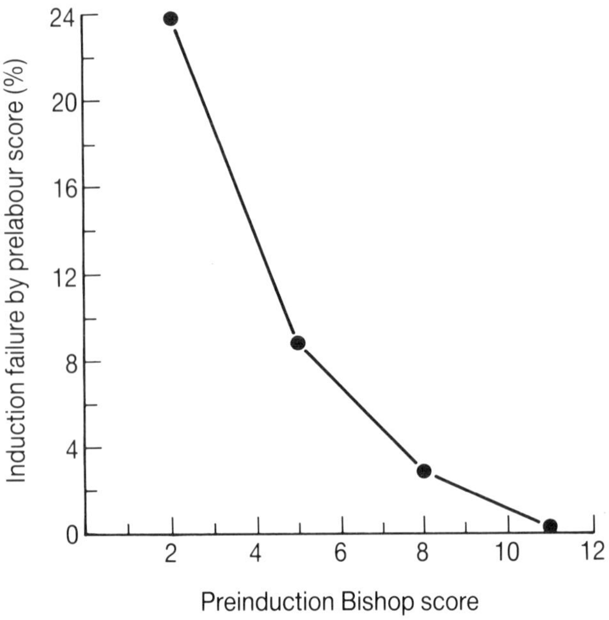

Fig. 51.1 The relationship of the Bishop score to the chances of successful outcome (after Friedman 1966).

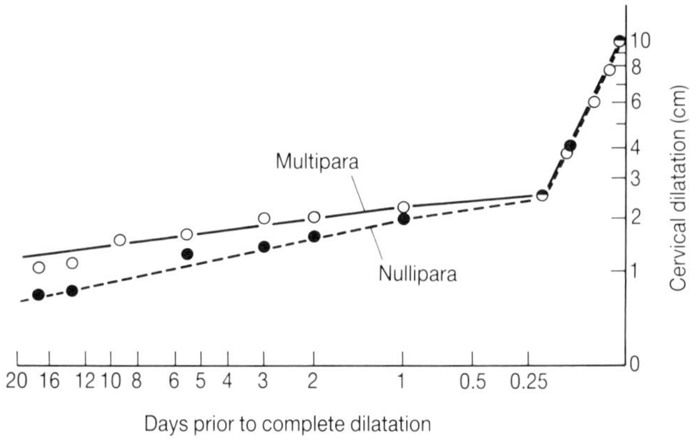

Fig. 51.2 The development of cervical ripening (after Hendricks et al 1970).

an increased Caesarean section rate but this was felt to be due to an improved induction protocol using prostaglandin pessaries rather than to new evidence.

Harris et al (1983) found that in a group of well documented 42-week pregnancies, the mean cervical Bishop score was 3.6 and only 8.2% had a Bishop score of >7; they concluded that among patients with prolonged pregnancy, the cervix tends to be unfavourable for induction. This supports many clinicians' impressions and refutes the notion that if the cervix is not favourable the dates must be wrong. As can be seen by Figure 51.1 (Friedman et al 1966), a low Bishop score is associated with an increased failure rate; this explains why routine attempts at induction when the patient has reached 42 weeks' gestation are often unsuccessful (Hauth et al 1980). It has been shown that cervical ripen-

Table 51.5 Methods to assess fetal well-being

Clinical
Fetal growth
Palpation
Maternal abdominal circumference
Symphysis fundal height
Fetal kick chart
Amniotic fluid volume by palpation
Biophysical
Ultrasonic growth (serial scans)
Biparietal diameter
Fetal abdominal circumference
Fetal femur length
Ultrasound
Liquor volume
Fetal tone
Fetal breathing
Fetal movement
Doppler blood flow
Cardiotocography
Rate
Variability
Reactivity
Biochemical
Oestriol

ing is a slow gradual development (Hendricks et al 1970; Fig. 51.2) and thus unless the situation warrants intervention it is wise to delay, with careful observation, awaiting natural ripening and spontaneous labour.

Cervical ripening with prostaglandins is helpful but Beck & Clayton (1982) have suggested that prostaglandin pessaries should be used with caution as there is a possibility of placental insufficiency. The fetus should be monitored with cardiotocography for about 20 minutes before insertion of the pessaries and at least 40 minutes afterwards. In an attempt to encourage physiological cervical ripening, Elliott & Flaherty (1984) advocated breast stimulation, which was shown to be of some benefit. However, patient compliance was poor.

Antenatal surveillance and selective induction

Carefully obtained historical and physical examination remains the cornerstone of appropriate obstetric care (Hertz et al 1978).

Various protocols have been evaluated in an attempt to screen for those pregnancies at higher risk for fetal morbidity and mortality. Testing methods must be reasonably cost-effective, acceptable to the patient, reliable and should minimize unnecessary intervention. The emerging attitude to natural childbirth has put a shadow of suspicion on unnecessary induction, giving extra momentum towards a conservative approach. Some means of identifying the fetus in jeopardy is required. The fear that something may go wrong is often present in the patient, her immediate family and the doctor. This can be significantly overcome by constant supervision, accurate education, monitoring and positive motivation.

Antenatal fetal well-being can be assessed by several methods (Table 51.5). To date there appears no single ideal method to assess fetal reserve. The availability of these tests varies according to the area in which one is working and obviously is affected by any financial restraints. There is no area in which good clinical judgement cannot be made.

Clinical assessment of fetal growth

Abdominal palpation, although limited, can be of benefit in detecting fetal growth retardation. Belizan et al (1978) and Quaranta et al (1981) have demonstrated the value of symphysis fundal height. Fundal height should be measured from the fundus of the uterus to the top of the symphysis pubis, with the tape measure lying in contact with the skin of the abdominal wall. The measurement at the fundus should be made by gentle pressure on the tape, at right angles to the abdominal wall.

Oligohydramnios, which may be suspected clinically, has been associated with a statistically significant increase in fetal acidosis, meconium aspiration and low Apgar scores (Crowley 1980).

The recognition that reduction or cessation in maternally perceived fetal movement may precede fetal death by a day or longer (Sadousky & Yaffe 1973) led to the development of the Cardiff Count-to-Ten Kick Chart (Pearson & Weaver 1978). This has now become a most popular and inexpensive method of evaluating fetal health.

Biophysical assessment of fetal well-being

Measurement of amniotic fluid by ultrasound has been reported (Crowley et al 1984) with reduced amniotic fluid being diagnosed when no single vertical pool measures more than 30 mm. Patients with reduced amniotic fluid had a statistical increase in meconium-stained amniotic fluid and growth-retarded babies and were more likely to require delivery by Caesarean section for fetal distress.

Fetal heart rate testing for assessment in prolonged pregnancy is helpful as it is safe, inexpensive, readily available, rapid, non-invasive and easy to interpret. The fetal cardiovascular system has considerable reserve; changes in fetal heart rate pattern often occur only in response to serious deterioration in health and assessment should then be performed at least twice weekly in the prolonged pregnancy. A reactive trace can be defined according to the criteria proposed by Everston & Paul (1978) and simplified by Everston et al (1979) as good variability (range >5 beats/min, frequency >2 cycles/min), two accelerations of fetal movements in 20 minutes and no decelerations. A reactive trace is a good index of fetal health at the time of the assessment. In a more recent survey (Granados 1984) the non-stress test was the most commonly used test to assess fetal well-being after 42 weeks. Several studies (Klapholz & Friedman 1977, Homburg et al 1979, Keegan & Paul 1980, Freeman et al 1981, Gibb et al 1982, Cario 1984) have indicated that care-

Table 51.6 Biophysical profile

Parameter	Score 2	Score 0
Amniotic fluid volume	>1 cm pocket in two perpendicular planes	<1 cm pocket in two perpendicular planes
Fetal movement	Three or more gross body movements in 30 minutes	Two or less gross body movements in 30 minutes
Fetal breathing movements (FBM)	At least 30 seconds of sustained FBM in 30 minutes	Less than 30 seconds of FBM in 30 seconds
Fetal tone	One episode of limb motion from flexion to extension to flexion in a rapid motion	No evidence of flexion movement or fetal movement
Fetal reactivity	Two or more fetal heart rate accelerations of 15 beats/min for 15 seconds with fetal movements in 40 minutes	Less than two accelerations in 40 minutes

After Manning et al (1981)

fully monitored pregnancies carried beyond 42 weeks are not associated with an increased perinatal morbidity or mortality rate.

Fetal growth can be monitored via serial scanning or a biophysical profile can be performed as described by Manning et al (1981) (Table 51.6). Combined observations of five fetal biophysical variables (qualitative amniotic fluid volume, fetal movement, breathing, tone and reactivity) are made. This method can be used effectively to screen and manage a high-risk population.

Johnson et al (1986) reviewed 307 consecutive post-term pregnancies assessed by biophysical profile scoring. Twice-weekly scores differentiated accurately normal fetuses from those at risk of intrauterine hypoxia. When the profile score was normal, waiting for spontaneous labour resulted in healthy neonates and a much lower Caesarean section rate (15 compared with 42% for prophylactic induction).

The application of Doppler ultrasound examination of umbilical artery flow velocity has provoked much interest. Flow velocity wave forms are simple to record and there are very definite differences between the wave forms of normal and high-risk pregnancies, with a reduction in the diastolic flow velocity in the latter group. The availability of Doppler studies has been demonstrated to improve obstetrical decision-making (Trudinger et al 1987).

Biochemical assessment of fetal well-being

Biochemical assessment has emerged to be of limited value. Human placental lactogen and oestriol levels will fall with decreasing placental function but the tests are prone to a high false negative and false positive result, and this makes them a poor method of primary surveillance. With the need for serial assessment and the delay obtaining results the role of this test is in decline.

INTRAPARTUM CARE

Despite the utilization of antepartum fetal heart rate testing, other biophysical evaluation and clinical inspection, intrapartum problems still remain a contributor to perinatal mortality and morbidity.

The most prudent course of action in dealing with a post-term woman in labour is to treat her as one would treat any other labouring woman, individualizing according to need, maintaining appropriate vigilance and intervening when required, with the selected use of fetal scalp pH. Some fetuses will have enough fetal reserve for normal antepartum health but will exceed that reserve with the greater stress of labour. Lagrew & Freeman (1986) have demonstrated an increase in fetal distress in postdate pregnancies and concluded they should all be electronically monitored from the onset of labour to delivery. In the presence of thick meconium or oligohydramnios, sampling of fetal scalp blood is indicated even with a normal fetal heart rate pattern. Oligohydramnios increases the likelihood of compression of the umbilical cord and subsequent vagal activation induces gastrointestinal peristalsis and release of meconium. Meconium occurs in 25–43% of postdate labours (Zwerdling 1967, Schneider et al 1978, Miller & Read 1981, Yeh & Read 1982). Chest compression combined with proper endotracheal suction for meconium beyond the vocal cords after delivery will help to eliminate cases of severe meconium aspiration syndrome. Measurement of umbilical cord gases at delivery will be beneficial in order to document the neonatal status and guide future management.

Oligohydramnios has been significantly associated with fetal distress, in part attributed to umbilical cord compression (Leveno et al 1984). Gabbe et al (1977) induced and then relieved cord compression by removing and then replacing amniotic fluid in rhesus monkeys. Miyazaki & Taylor (1983) reported relief of both variable and prolonged decelerations by infusing saline solution into the uterus during labour in humans.

Two German studies (Holtorff & Schmidt 1966, Schussling & Radzuweit 1968) found the prevalence of uterine inertia in labour occurring in prolonged pregnancy to be twice that reported in labour occurring at term. This has not been confirmed by Cardozo et al (1986) who found the prevalence of abnormal labour patterns was similar in the prolonged pregnancy group to the term pregnancy group. A total of 25% of post-term infants are greater than 4000 g (Lagrew & Freeman 1986) and anticipation of dystocia, notably of the shoulders, becomes important.

FUTURE DEVELOPMENTS

Research with careful clinical studies into improved techniques of antenatal surveillance will continue. Effective cervical ripening agents, including prostaglandin and relaxin, continue to be developed for those patients with low Bishop's score who require delivery. Following Miyazaki & Taylor's work (1983) the intra-amniotic infusion of saline in patients with ruptured membranes may decrease intrapartum cord compression (Lagrew & Freeman 1986).

CONCLUSIONS

> Induction . . . should be accepted as a necessary burden limited to a small number of cases in which conditions are favourable (O'Driscoll & Meagher 1980).

Prolonged pregnancy is not as dangerous as many would believe and routine induction of labour has not proved to be of benefit. Social considerations often weigh as heavy as medical ones and elective post-term induction is usually an unnecessary intervention carried out for convenience (Bergsjo 1985).

With good antenatal surveillance and selective induction of labour the delivery of a healthy infant need not be put at jeopardy. With adequate patient education, early clarification of dates and good clinical acumen, the management of the post-term pregnancy may be guided between the Charybdis of unnecessary intervention and the Scylla of intrauterine hypoxia.

Management of prolonged pregnancy begins in the first antenatal clinic by a truthful explanation of estimated date of delivery. Prevention of the iatrogenically caused anxiety of being past the time to be born is one of the hurdles that must be overcome.

With the introduction of more elaborate methods of monitoring fetal well-being, we can help to reassure not only many mothers but also doctors that there may indeed be no exact length of gestation nor any compulsion to induce labour in normal prolonged pregnancy.

REFERENCES

Anderson H F, Johnson T R B, Barclays M L, Flora J D 1981a Gestation age assessment. 1. Analysis of individual clinical observations. American Journal of Obstetrics and Gynecology 139: 173–177

Anderson H F, Johnson T R B, Flora J D, Barclay M L 1981b Gestational age assessment II. Prediction from combined clinical observation. American Journal of Obstetrics and Gynecology 140: 770–774

Ballantyne J W 1902 The problem of the postmature infant. Journal of Obstetrics and Gynaecology of the British Empire II: 521–554

Ballantyne J W, Browne F J 1922 Problems of fetal post-maturity and prolongation of pregnancy. Journal of Obstetrics and Gynaecology of the British Empire 29: 177–238

Bancroft-Livingston G, Neill D W 1957 Studies in prolonged pregnancy. Journal of Obstetrics and Gynaecology of the British Empire 64: 498

Barron S L, Vessey M P 1966 Birth weight of infants born to immigrant women. British Journal of Preventative and Social Medicine 20: 127–134

Beck I, Clayton J K 1982 (letter) Hazards of prostaglandin pessaries in postmaturity. Lancet 28: 16

Belizan J M, Villar J, Nardin J C, Malamud J, Sainz de Vicuna 1978 Diagnosis of intrauterine growth retardation by a simple clinical method: measurement of uterine height. American Journal of Obstetrics and Gynecology 131: 643–646

Bergsjo P 1985 Post-term pregnancy. In: Studd J (ed) Progress in obstetrics and gynaecology, vol 5. Churchill Livingstone, Edinburgh, pp 121–133

Bissenden J G, Scott P H, Hallum J, Mansfield H N, Scott P, Wharton B A 1981 Racial variations in tests of fetoplacental function. British Journal of Obstetrics and Gynaecology 88: 109–114

Boe F 1951 Variations in the duration of pregnancy and in the weight of newborn infants. Acta Obstetricia et Gynecologica Scandinavica 30: 247–255

Boyd M E, Usher R H, McLean F H 1983 Fetal macrosomia: prediction, risks, proposed management. Obstetrics and Gynecology 61: 715–722

Browne F J 1957 Foetal postmaturity and prolongation of pregnancy. British Medical Journal 1: 851–855

Butler N R, Alberman E D 1969 Perinatal problems. Second report of the 1958 British Perinatal Mortality Survey. Under the auspices of the National Birthday Trust Fund. E & S Livingstone, Edinburgh

Campbell S 1974 The assessment of fetal development by diagnostic ultrasound. Clinics in Perinatalology 1: 507–519

Campbell S, Underhill R A, Beazley J M 1970 Fetal hibernation. Lancet i: 468

Cardozo L, Fysh J, Pearce J M 1986 Prolonged pregnancy: the management debate. British Medical Journal 293: 1059–1063

Cario G M 1984 Conservative management of prolonged pregnancy using fetal heart rate monitoring only: a prospective study. British Journal of Obstetrics and Gynaecology 91: 23–30

Carsons B S, Losey R W, Bowes W A, Simmons M A 1976 Combined obstetric and pediatric approach to prevent meconium aspiration syndrome. American Journal of Obstetrics and Gynecology 126: 712–715

Cary W H 1948 Results of artificial inseminations with an extramarital specimen (semi-adoption). American Journal of Obstetrics and Gynecology 56: 727–732

Chamberlain G, Philipp E, Howlett K, Masters K (eds) 1978 British births 1970, vol 2, Obstetric care. Heinemann Medical, London

Clayton S G 1941 Fetal mortality in postmaturity. Journal of Obstetrics and Gynaecology of the British Empire 48: 450–460

Clifford S H 1954 Postmaturity — with placental dysfunction. Clinical syndrome and pathological finding. Journal of Pediatrics 44: 1–13

Crowley P 1980 Non quantitative estimation of amniotic fluid volume in the suspected prolonged pregnancy. Journal of Perinatal Medicine 8: 249–251

Crowley P, O'Herlihy C, Boylan P 1984 The value of ultrasound measurement of amniotic fluid volume in the management of prolonged pregnancies. British Journal of Obstetrics and Gynaecology 91: 444–448

Dawkins M J R, Martin J D, Spector W G 1961 Intrapartum asphyxia. Journal of Obstetrics and Gynaecology of the British Commonwealth 68: 604–610

Drumm J E 1977 The prediction of delivery date by ultrasonic measurement of fetal crown rump length. British Journal of Obstetrics and Gynaecology 74: 1–5

Drumm J E, Clinch J, MacKenzie G 1976 The ultrasonic measurement of fetal crown rump length as a method of assessing gestational age. British Journal of Obstetrics and Gynaecology 83: 417–421

Eik-Nes S H, Okland O, Aure J C, Ulstein M 1984 Ultrasound screening in pregnancy: a randomised controlled trial. Lancet i: 1347

Elliott J P, Flaherty J F 1984 The use of breast stimulation to prevent post date pregnancy. American Journal of Obstetrics and Gynecology 149: 628–632

Everston L R, Paul R H 1978 Antepartum fetal heart rate testing: the non-stress test. American Journal of Obstetrics and Gynecology 132: 895–900

Everston L R, Gauthier R J, Schifrin B S, Paul R H 1979. Antepartum fetal heart rate testing. 1. Evolution of the non-stress test. American Journal of Obstetrics and Gynecology 133: 29–33

Ferguson I L C F, Taylor R W, Watson M 1982 Records and curiosities in obstetrics and gynaecology. Baillière Tindall, London

Field T M, Dabiri C, Hallock N, Shuman H H 1977 Developmental effects

of prolonged pregnancy and the postmaturity syndrome. Journal of Pediatrics 90: 836–839
FIGO 1980 International classification of diseases: update. International Journal of Gynaecology and Obstetrics 17: 634–640
FIGO 1982 Report of the committee following a workshop on monitoring and reporting perinatal mortality and morbidity. FIGO standing committee on perinatal mortality. International Federation of Gynecology and Obstetrics. Chameleon Press, London, p 78
Fox H 1979 The placenta as a model for organ ageing. In: Beaconsfield P, Villee C (eds) Placenta — a neglected experimental animal. Pergamon Press, Oxford, pp 351–378
Fox H 1983 Placental pathology. In: Studd J (ed) Progress in obstetrics and gynaecology, vol 3. Churchill Livingstone, Edinburgh, pp 47–56
Freeman R K, Garite T J, Mondanlou H, Dorchester W, Rommall C, Devaney M 1981 Post date pregnancy: utilization of contraction stress testing for primary fetal surveillance. American Journal of Obstetrics and Gynecology 140: 128–135
Friedman E A, Niswander K R, Bayonet-Rivera N P, Sachtleben M R 1966 Relations of prelabor evaluation in inducibility and the course of labor. Obstetrics and Gynecology 28: 495–501
Gabbe S G, Ettinger B B, Freeman R K, Makrhn C B 1977 Umbilical cord compression associated with amniotomy: laboratory observations. American Journal of Obstetrics and Gynecology 26: 353–355
Gibb D 1985 Prolonged pregnancy. In: Studd J (ed) The management of labour. Blackwell Scientific Publications, London, pp 108–122
Gibb D M F, Cardozo L D, Studd J W W, Cooper D J 1982 Prolonged pregnancy: is induction of labour indicated? A prospective study. British Journal of Obstetrics and Gynaecology 89: 292–925
Gibberd G F 1958 The choice between death from post maturity and death from induction of labour. Lancet i: 64–66
Granados J L 1984 Survey of the management of postterm pregnancy. Obstetrics and Gynecology 63: 651–653
Gruenwald P 1967 Growth of the human fetus. In: McLaren A (ed) Advances in reproductive physiology, vol 2. Logos Press, London, pp 279–309
Guerrero R, Florex P E 1969 Duration of pregnancy. Lancet ii: 268–269
Harris B A, Huddleston J F, Sutlitt G, Perlis H W 1983 The unfavourable cervix in prolonged pregnancy. Obstetrics and Gynecology 62: 171–174
Hauth J C, Goodman M T, Gilskap L C, Gilskap J E 1980 Post term pregnancy I. Obstetrics and Gynecology 56: 467–469
Hendricks C H, Brenner W E, Kraus G 1970 Normal cervical dilatation pattern in late pregnancy and labor. American Journal of Obstetrics and Gynecology 106: 1065–1082
Hertz R H, Sokol R J, Knoke J D, Rosen M G, Chik L, Hirsch V J 1978 Clinical estimation of gestational age: rules for avoiding preterm delivery. American Journal of Obstetrics and Gynecology 131: 395–402
Holtorff J, Schmidt H 1966 Die verlangerte Schwangerschaft und ihr Einfluss auf das Schicksal des Kindes. Zentralblatt für Gynaekologie 88: 441–449
Homburg R, Ludomirski A, Insler V 1979 Detection of fetal risk in postmaturity. British Journal of Obstetrics and Gynaecology 86: 759–764
Johnson J M, Harman C R, Lange I R, Manning F A 1986 Biophysical profile scoring in the management of the post term pregnancy — an analysis of 307 patients. American Journal of Obstetrics and Gynecology 154: 269–273
Keegan K A, Paul R H 1980 Antepartum fetal heart rate testing IV: the non stress test as a primary approach. American Journal of Obstetrics and Gynecology 136: 75–80
Klapholz H, Friedman E A 1977 Incidence of intrapartum fetal distress with advancing gestational age. American Journal of Obstetrics and Gynecology 127: 405–407
Kloosterman G J 1979 Epidemiology of postmaturity. In: Keirse M J N C, Anderson A B M, Bennebroek Gravenhorst J P (eds) Human parturition. Martinas Nijoff, The Hague, pp 247–261
Knox G E, Huddleston J F, Flowers C E, Eubanks A, Sutliffe G 1979 Management of prolonged pregnancy: results of a prospective randomised trial. American Journal of Obstetrics and Gynecology 134: 376–384
Kortenoever M E 1950 Pathology of pregnancy: pregnancy of long duration and post mature infant. Obstetrical and Gynecological Survey 5: 812–814
Lagrew D C, Freeman R K 1986 Management of post date pregnancy. American Journal of Obstetrics and Gynecology 154: 8–13
Lagrew D C, Wilson E A, Jawad M J 1983 Determination of gestational age by serum concentration of human chorionic gonadotrophin. Obstetrics and Gynecology 61: 37–40
Leveno K J, Quirk J G, Cunningham F G et al 1984 Prolonged pregnancy I. Observations concerning the causes of fetal distress. American Journal of Obstetrics and Gynecology 150: 465–473
Manning F A, Baskett T F, Morrison I, Lange I 1981 Fetal biophysical profile scoring: a prospective study in 1184 high risk patients. American Journal of Obstetrics and Gynecology 140: 289–294
McClure Browne J C 1963 Postmaturity. American Journal of Obstetrics and Gynecology 85: 573–582
Miller F C, Read J A 1981 Intrapartum assessment of the postdate fetus. American Journal of Obstetrics and Gynecology 141: 516–520
Mills W G 1970 Fetal hibernation? Lancet i: 334–336
Miyazaki F S, Taylor N A 1983 Saline amnioinfusion for relief of variable or prolonged decelerations. A preliminary report. American Journal of Obstetrics and Gynecology 146: 670
Naegele F C 1812 Erfahrung und Abhandlungen des weiblichen. Geslechter, Mannheim
Nakano R 1972 Post term pregnancy. Acta Obstetricia et Gynecologica Scandinavica 51: 217–222
O'Dowd M J, O'Dowd T M 1985 Quickening — a reevaluation. British Journal of Obstetrics and Gynaecology 92: 1037–1039
O'Driscoll K, Meagher D 1980 Active management of labour, 1st edn. W B Saunders, Philadelphia, p 172
O'Herlihy C, Robinson H P, de Crespigny L J 1980 Mittelschmerz is a preovulatory symptom. British Medical Journal 280: 986
Park G L 1968 The duration of pregnancy. Lancet ii: 1388–1389
Paterson P J, Dunstan M K, Trickey N R A, Beard R W 1970 A biochemical comparison of the mature and postmature fetus and newborn infant. Journal of Obstetrics and Gynaecology of the British Commonwealth 77: 390–397
Pearson J F, Weaver J B 1978 Fetal activity and fetal wellbeing: an evaluation. British Medical Journal 1: 1305–1307
Petersen W F 1946 Hippocratic wisdom. Charles C Thomas, Springfield, Illinois, p 31
Quaranta P, Currell R, Redman C W, Robinson J S 1981 Prediction of small for dates infants by measurement of symphysis–fundal height. British Journal of Obstetrics and Gynaecology 88: 113–119
Sadousky E, Yaffe H 1973 Daily fetal movement recording and fetal prognosis. Obstetrics and Gynecology 41: 845–850
Schneider J M, Olson R W, Curet L B 1978 Screening for fetal and neonatal risk in post date pregnancy. American Journal of Obstetrics and Gynecology 131: 473–478
Schussling G, Radzuweit H 1968 Ubertragung in der Schwangerschaft. Zentralblatt für Gynaekologie 49: 143–147
Shime J, Librach C L, Gare D J, Cook C 1986 Influence of prolonged pregnancy on infant development at 1 and 2 years of age. A prospective controlled study. American Journal of Obstetrics and Gynecology 154: 341–345
Stewart H L 1952 Duration of pregnancy and postmaturity. Journal of the American Medical Association 148: 1079–1083
Times Law Reports 1921 Gaskill v Gaskill. 12 August, p 977
Trudinger B J, Cook C M, Giles W B, Connelly A, Thompsom R S 1987 Umbilical artery flow velocity waveforms in high risk pregnancy. Randomised controlled trial. Lancet i: 188–190
Tuck S M, Cardozo L D, Studd J W W, Gibb D M, Cooper D J 1983 Obstetric characteristics in different racial groups. British Journal of Obstetrics and Gynaecology 90: 892–897
Vorherr H 1975 Placental insufficiency in relation to post term pregnancy and fetal postmaturity. Evaluation of fetoplacental function; management of the post term gravida. American Journal of Obstetrics and Gynecology 123: 67–103
Walker J 1954 Fetal anoxia. Journal of Obstetrics and Gynaecology of the British Empire 61: 162–180
Warsof S L, Pearce J M, Campbell S 1983 The present place of routine ultrasound screening. Clinics in Obstetrics and Gynaecology 10: 445–458
Weiner C P 1981 The pseudogestational sac in ectopic pregnancy. American Journal of Obstetrics and Gynecology 139: 959–961

Wenner W, Young E B 1974 Nonspecific date of last menstrual period. An indication of poor reproductive outcome. American Journal of Obstetrics and Gynecology 120: 1071–1079
Wrigley A J 1958 Postmaturity. Lancet i: 1167–1168
Yeh S Y, Read J A 1982 Management of post term pregnancy in a large obstetric population. Obstetrics and Gynecology 60: 282–287
Zwerdling M A 1967 Factors pertaining to prolonged pregnancy and its outcome. Pediatrics 40: 202–212

P. J. Steer

Abnormal uterine action

Uterine action in labour is variously considered to be abnormal if it falls into one of the following categories:

1. *Hypotonic:* too little.
2. *Hypertonic:* too much.
3. *Incoordinate:* abnormal in pattern.
4. *Inefficient:* not associated with progressive cervical dilatation.

Of these, the first, third and fourth are often associated. Incoordinate contractions (irregular in shape and timing) are probably of no significance unless they are also hypotonic (Turnbull 1957, Seitchik & Chatkoff 1977). Hypertonic uterine action is a special case and will be considered separately.

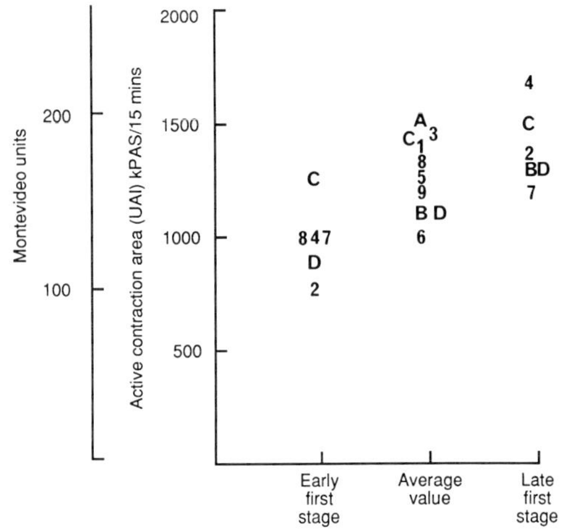

Fig. 52.1 Normal levels of uterine activity in spontaneous labour. 1 = Zambrana et al (1960); 2 = Poseiro & Noriega-Guerra (1961); 3 = Cibils & Hendricks (1965); 4 = El Sahwi et al (1967); 5 = Krapohl et al (1970); 6 = Mendez-Bauer et al (1975); 7 = Pontonnier et al (1975); 8 = Lindmark & Nilsson (1977); 9 = Flynn et al (1978); A = Cowan et al (1982); B = Steer et al (1984); C = Gibb et al (1984); D = Arulkumaran et al (1984).

THE NORMAL LEVEL OF UTERINE ACTIVITY IN LABOUR

Uterine action cannot be categorized as hypotonic or hypertonic without knowledge of the normal levels of uterine action; there is no precise agreement about these. Variations will depend to a considerable extent on the population studied. The rate of cervical dilatation in labour is directly proportional to the level of uterine action (i.e. higher levels of uterine activity are associated with higher rates of cervical dilatation; Steer et al 1984). Hence, the selection for study of women progressing rapidly in labour (often described arbitrarily as normal) is likely to result in a higher mean level of observed uterine activity than if a total unselected population sample is studied. The rate of cervical dilatation is also inversely proportional to the resistance to progress, a hypothetical concept which involves pelvic and fetal size, presentation, and consistency of the soft tissues and cervix (Rossavik 1978, Arulkumaran et al 1985, Steer et al 1985). For any particular level of uterine activity, the higher the resistance, the slower is the rate of cervical dilatation. Therefore, if women are short and have large babies so that their resistance to progress is high, for a particular rate of cervical dilatation they will have a higher level of uterine activity than women with a low resistance, for example, grand multiparae (Al-Shawaf et al 1987). Thus to enable true comparison of results, researchers should quote values of uterine action in relation to groups specified in terms of parity, height, birthweight and rate of cervical dilatation. Most reported studies lack this type of information and thus are difficult to compare with each other. However, despite their lack of precise comparability, a number of important conclusions can be drawn from the reported data (Fig. 52.1).

Firstly, uterine action increases by about 50% as labour progresses. Secondly, mean uterine activity levels fall somewhere between 1000 and 1500 kPas/15 min or 130–200 Montevideo units; see Ch. 45). Most studies give a similar distribution around the mean value such that the 10th percentile is about 700 kPas/15 min and the 90th percentile is about 1800 kPas/15 min. By analogy with other distributions (such as birthweight) where the 10th and 90th percentiles are used as the boundaries of normality, it seems reasonable to designate levels <700 kPas/15 min as hypotonic and >1800 kPas/15 min as hypertonic.

The individual components of uterine activity

The three terms used to describe the main components of a uterine contraction are basal tonus, active pressure (peak pressure above basal tonus) and frequency. The shape of the contraction can also be described.

The reported range of normal baseline tonus varies from 0.8 to 2.6 kPa (5–20 mmHg) depending on the measuring technique used (external pressure transducer connected to a fluid-filled intrauterine catheter or internal catheter-tipped pressure transducer) and the position of the transducer relative to the upper level of amniotic fluid within the uterus (Ch. 45). Values greater than 3 kPa are likely to represent hypertonus and will compromise maternal blood flow into the placenta, resulting in fetal hypoxia.

The rate of cervical dilatation is more closely related to the mean active pressure of contractions than any of the other variables (Richardson et al 1978). Active pressure needs to be at least 2 kPa to produce progressive cervical dilatation and contractions are most efficient above 3.5 kPa (Caldeyro et al 1950). Mean active pressure averaged over the active phase of labour is approximately 5 kPa (SD 1.3): 40 mmHg, SD 10), rising to 6.3 kPa in the late first stage (Alvarez & Caldeyro 1950, Krapohl et al 1970, Pontonnier et al 1975, Steer et al 1984). Fetal oxygen supply, on the other hand, is related more to the frequency and duration of contractions and to basal tonus (Martin 1965, Brotanek et al 1969, Morishima et al 1975, Novy et al 1975). The mean frequency averaged over the active phase of labour is 4/10 minutes (SD 1.1), rising to a mean of about 5/10 minutes in the late first stage (Alvarez & Caldeyro 1950, Krapohl et al 1970, Pontonnier et al 1975, Steer et al 1984). The duration of contractions however is remarkably constant throughout labour in any particular individual, normally ranging between 70 and 90 seconds (Krapohl et al 1970, Pontonnier et al 1975).

HYPOTONIC UTERINE ACTIVITY

Most cases of slow progress in labour are associated with hypotonic uterine activity and are therefore likely to respond to oxytocics (Steer et al 1985). This suggests that in most cases there is not an inherent defect in the ability of the uterus to contract but that uterine contractility is at an early stage of its evolution. Such a conclusion is supported by the report of Hemminki et al (1985) who showed that 83% of women progressing slowly in labour subsequently developed normal levels of uterine activity when managed expectantly (ambulation was encouraged) rather than being given oxytocics. A similar evolution of activity is seen in women progressing slowly in labour and nursed in the lateral recumbent position with epidural anaesthetic rather than being ambulant (Bidgood & Steer 1987).

However, in a few cases, hypotonic uterine activity fails to respond to oxytocics. It has long been suggested that in some cases this is due to the suppression of uterine activity by the autonomic nervous system. Bourne & Burn noted in 1927 that 'the effect of emotion appears to be to delay the uterine contractions in labour', and since they considered one of the main effects of emotion to be the stimulation of the sympathetic nervous system, they investigated the effects of injections of adrenaline into labouring patients. They demonstrated that the intravenous injection of 5 minims of adrenaline produced complete cessation of uterine contractions for 12 minutes, following which the contractions began again. They also observed that the administration of hypnotics to the labouring mother sometimes produced a marked increase in uterine activity. They suggested that 'the augmentor action of hypnotics such as chloral may in part be due to the depression by these hypnotics of inhibitory impulses passing from the brain centres of anxious or emotional patients to the uterus by way of the sympathetic supply'.

The inhibitory effects of adrenaline on uterine activity were confirmed by Kaiser & Harris (1950). They monitored uterine activity with the Reynolds multichannel tocodynamometer. In large doses (such as to have unacceptably severe side-effects) adrenaline stimulated the uterus. However, in lower concentrations which had no demonstrable systemic effect, they found that adrenaline was 'strikingly inhibitory' to uterine activity. They also noted that 'in difficult labour there is a state of emotional stress which may well induce excessive secretion of endogenous adrenaline'. They considered that the disordered patterns of uterine activity involved in inertial labour resembled in many respects that induced by exogenous adrenaline. 'Systemic sedation and nerve-conduction blocks may in some cases shorten the length of labour by allaying apprehension'.

A similar theme was pursued by Arthur & Johnson (1952). They compared the outcome in 22 cases of prolonged labour treated with caudal anaesthesia with 26 controls. The mean duration of labour in the test group was 51 hours with a 14% Caesarean section rate, compared with 66 hours and a 50% Caesarean section rate in the controls. They attributed the difference to an improvement in uterine activity produced by the analgesia. Similar claims have been made for epidural anaesthesia (Moir & Willocks 1967).

Caldeyro-Barcia et al have claimed that an improvement in incoordinate activity can be produced by spinal anaesthesia (Caldeyro et al 1950) and also by hypnotic sleep (Caldeyro-Barcia & Alvarez 1952).

Jeffcoate (1963) recommended the use of intravenous morphine or pethidine to treat incoordinate uterine activity, and reported an example of improvement in the pattern of uterine activity and the rate of cervical dilatation following an intravenous infusion of pethidine.

An illustrative example of the apparent augmentor action of a hypnotic observed by the author is shown in Figure 52.2. A primigravida was admitted to the labour ward complaining of painful contractions, one every 3 minutes. A vaginal examination revealed ruptured membranes, and a cervix that was fully effaced but only 2 cm dilated. A further examination 4 hours later showed the cervix to be only 3 cm dilated and because of the slow progress an oxytocin infusion was commenced. Four hours later the infusion rate had reached 12 mu/min, without any obvious effect on uterine activity or cervical dilatation. External tocography showed apparently normal contractions (Fig. 52.2a). In view of the lack of progress, the oxytocin infusion rate was increased again, reaching 20 mu/min after a further 4 hours. At this point the cervix had reached only 5 cm dilatation and an intrauterine catheter was inserted. This showed the typical pattern of incoordinate uterine activity (Fig. 52.2b). Instead of a contraction wave originating at the pacemaker site (which is usually one or other uterine cornu) and propagating progressively down the uterus towards the cervix (fundal dominance; Caldeyro et al 1950), various parts of the uterus contract independently at irregular intervals (Caldeyro et al 1950). An external tocograph placed over a particular part of the uterus may show a deflection indistinguishable from a normal contraction whenever that part contracts. However, the intrauterine pressure reflects the sum of activity in the whole uterus, and therefore shows the weak and irregular pressure rises which occur when the muscle fibres of the uterus fail to act in unison.

Because oxytocin had manifestly failed to correct the abnormal contraction pattern, a hypnotic dose of pethidine (150 mg) was administered intramuscularly. By about an hour later (Fig. 52.2c), the contractions had improved to such an extent that a fetal bradycardia developed and the oxytocin had to be turned off. Uterine activity continued at a normal level without further oxytocic stimulation (Fig. 52.2d), and a normal delivery occurred 6 hours later.

Mitrani et al (1975) hypothesized that since adrenaline exerts its suppressive effect on uterine activity via the uterine muscle beta-receptors, a beta-blocker such as propranolol could be used to treat incoordinate activity. They treated 10 primigravidae in dysfunctional labour with intravenous propranolol at the rate of 1 mg/min for 4 minutes. The authors observed a marked increase in uterine activity in all cases; in two cases there was tachysystole with hypertonus sufficient to produce fetal bradycardia. This interesting observation has never been repeated, nor have systematic studies of the effect of hypnotics on dysfunctional labour been car-

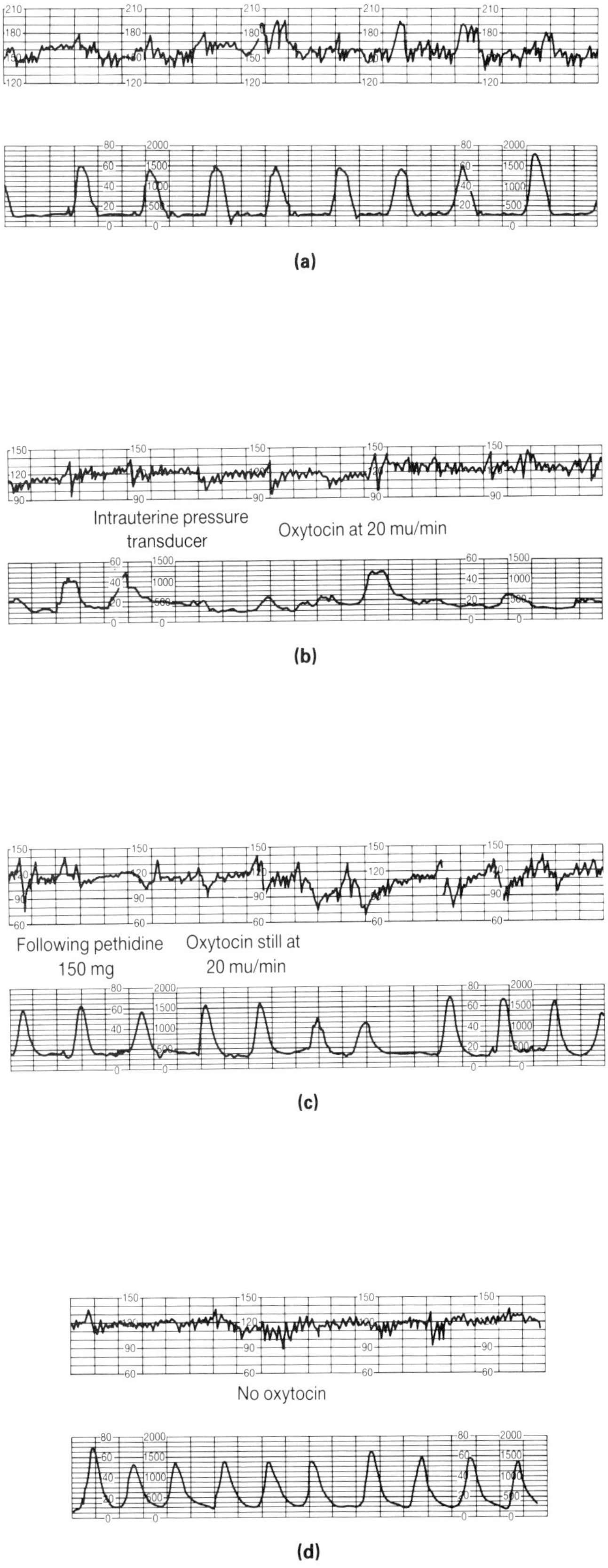

Fig. 52.2 An example of hypotonic incoordinate labour, resistant to oxytocin infusion but apparently responding to maternal sedation with pethidine.

ried out using modern techniques for recording uterine activity. This partly reflects the difficulty of studying a relatively uncommon event, and partly the current emphasis on oxytocics as the primary treatment for dysfunctional labour. This latter emphasis can largely be attributed to the work of O'Driscoll and his colleagues at the National Maternity Hospital in Dublin. For example, O'Driscoll et al wrote in 1969:

> no distinction was made in the present series between hypotonic and hypertonic uterine activity and oxytocin proved equally effective in both circumstances. This is completely at variance with the experience of Jeffcoate, who found that oxytocin often makes matters worse when given in labour complicated by incoordinate activity. It is our experience that the correct treatment of incoordinate action is to increase the rate of oxytocin infusion and not the dose of analgesic drugs.

The resolution of this dispute awaits further study.

HYPERTONIC UTERINE ACTIVITY

Spontaneous uterine hypercontractility without placental abruption is rare, probably occurring in not more than 1 in 3000–4000 pregnancies. Most cases of hypoxia in labour are due to intrauterine growth retardation with consequent inability of the fetus to withstand the normal stress of labour, rather than excessive uterine activity (Lissauer & Steer 1986). Nonetheless, cases of excessive uterine activity without obvious causes are sometimes seen. There is no evidence that an unusually high active pressure of contractions (i.e. above 12 kPa) is associated with any clinical problem; an increase in any of the other three contraction variables above normal levels, however, may lead to problems with fetal oxygen supply.

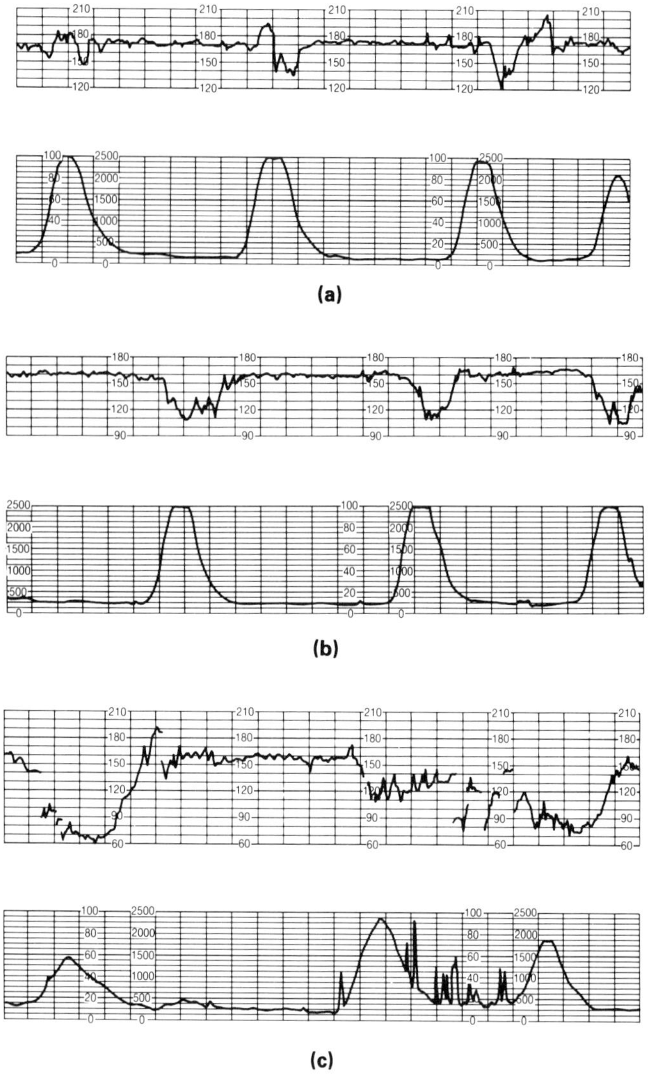

Fig. 52.3 An example of spontaneous uterine hypercontractility—prolonged duration of contractions.

Duration

Figure 52.3 illustrates a case of spontaneous labour where the duration of contractions averaged 120 seconds. Frequency and baseline tone were normal. Figure 52.3a shows small decelerations synchronous with contractions which became larger 2 hours later (Fig. 52.3b). After a further 2 hours (Fig. 52.3c) the decelerations became prolonged and a fetal blood sample showed a pH of 7.15. Delivery was effected by Caesarean section as the cervix was still only 6 cm dilated. Frequency and basal tonus remained normal throughout.

Frequency

Figure 52.4 illustrates a case of spontaneous labour where contraction frequency became excessive without obvious cause (the traces illustrated form a continuous sequence). Contraction frequency was normal initially (Fig. 52.4a) but as contractions increased to six every 10 minutes, early fetal heart rate (FHR) decelerations appeared (Fig. 52.4b). As the frequency increased to seven every 10 minutes, the decelerations became larger (Fig. 52.4c). Eventually intrauterine pressure failed to return to a normal tonus between contractions and a persistent fetal bradycardia developed (Fig. 52.4d). A slow intravenous infusion of salbutamol (150 μg) was given with immediate reduction in the frequency and active pressure of contractions, and recovery of the FHR. The contractions then continued to be normal until the second stage (Fig. 52.4e), when some mild hypertonus recurred. However, a healthy infant was born after only 15 minutes in the second stage.

Hypertonic uterine action with placental abruption

Placental abruption occurs in about 1 in 100 pregnancies, and is severe enough to kill the fetus in one in every 8 cases (Pritchard et al 1985). Death may occur due to extensive

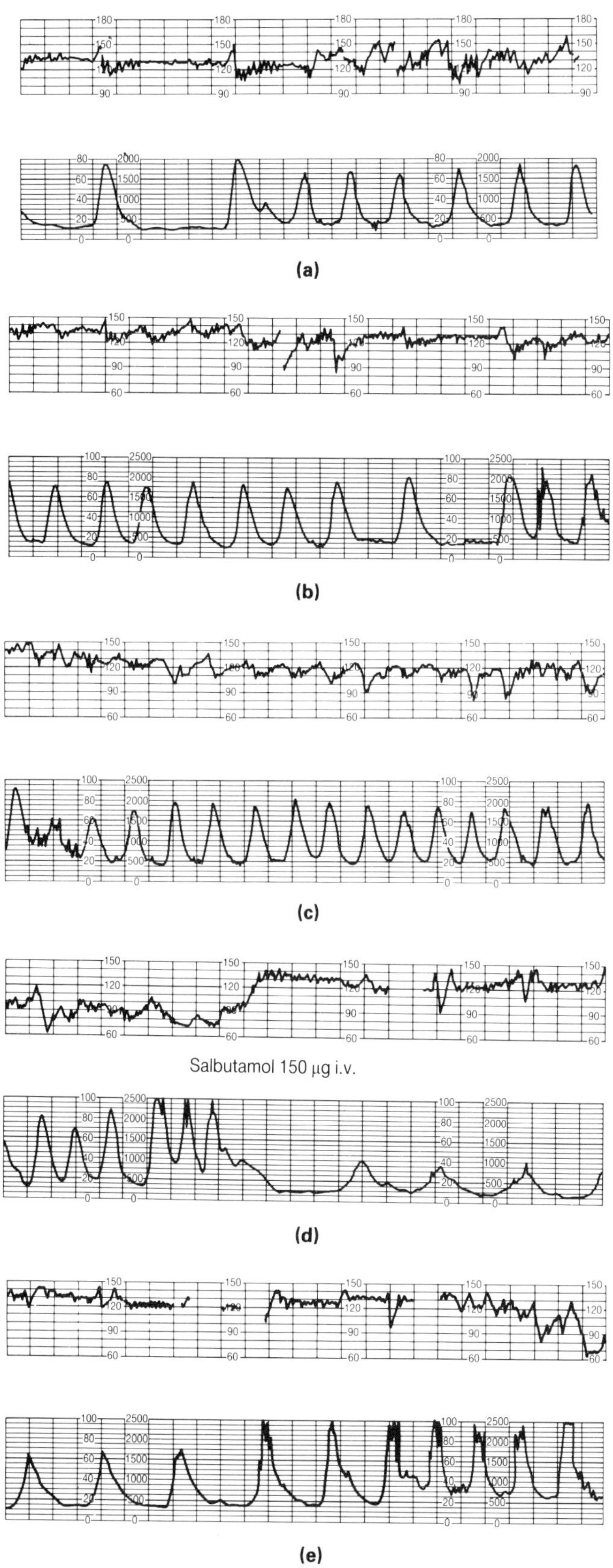

Fig. 52.4 An example of spontaneous uterine hypercontractility—excessive frequency of contractions.

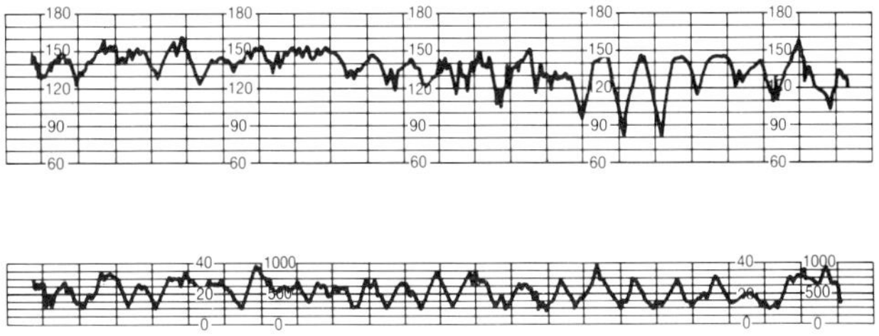

Fig. 52.5 Uterine hypercontractility associated with placental abruption, recorded with an external tocodynamometer.

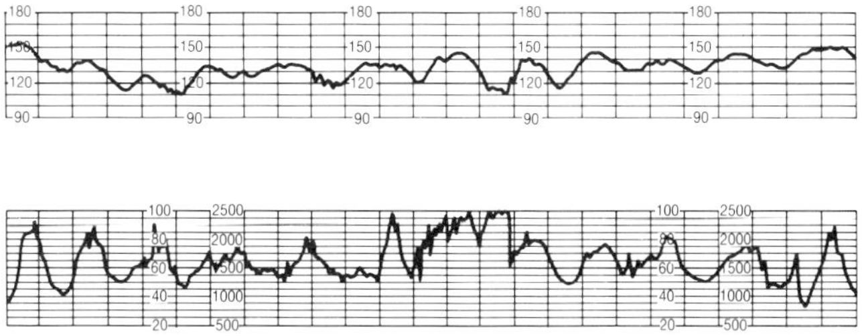

Fig. 52.6 Uterine hypercontractility associated with placental abruption, recorded with a catheter-tip pressure transducer.

placental separation but in many cases the excessive uterine activity produced by the massive release of prostaglandins from the disrupted decidua is also a major factor. Odendaal in 1976 drew attention to the high mean frequency of contractions seen in association with abruption. Mean contraction frequency recorded in 37 studied cases was 7.9 in 10 minutes, with some occurring as often as 16 in 10 minutes.

The importance of excessive contraction frequency as a sign in the diagnosis of abruption was emphasized by Saunderson & Steer in 1978. They pointed out that the high frequency of contractions meant that associated late decelerations could be misinterpreted as increased baseline variability, or a reduced baseline rate with accelerations. Such a case is shown in Figure 52.5. The contractions were recorded with an external tocodynamometer, so true baseline tone is not shown. In the initial half of the tracing, without careful synchronization of the FHR changes with the contractions it would be easy to interpret it as showing a baseline FHR of 125 beats/min with frequent accelerations. In the latter half of the tracing, however, the reduced baseline variability and the increasing amplitude of the late decelerations make the correct diagnosis more obvious. Figure 52.6 shows a similar case with intrauterine pressure recording, using a Gaeltec catheter-tipped pressure transducer (Ch. 45). The initial baseline tone is set rather high, at 25 mmHg; however, the subsequent rise of baseline tone by 25 mmHg to 50 mmHg, the abnormal contraction pattern, and the excessive frequency of contractions are all typical of abruption. The FHR is grossly abnormal, with loss of variability and late decelerations. The baby was delivered by emergency

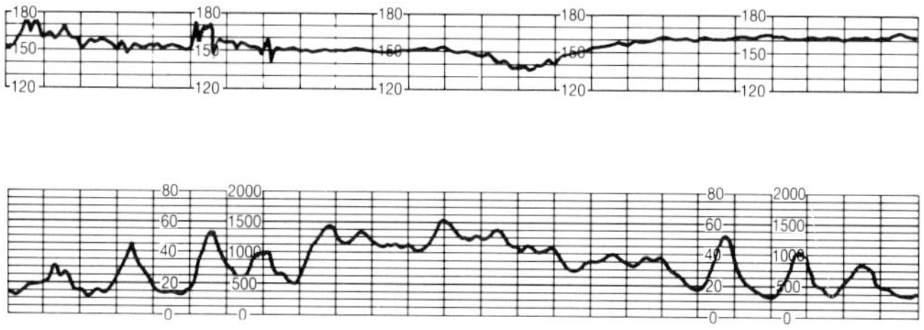

Fig. 52.7 Uterine hypercontractility associated with oxytocin infusion—acute hyperstimulation.

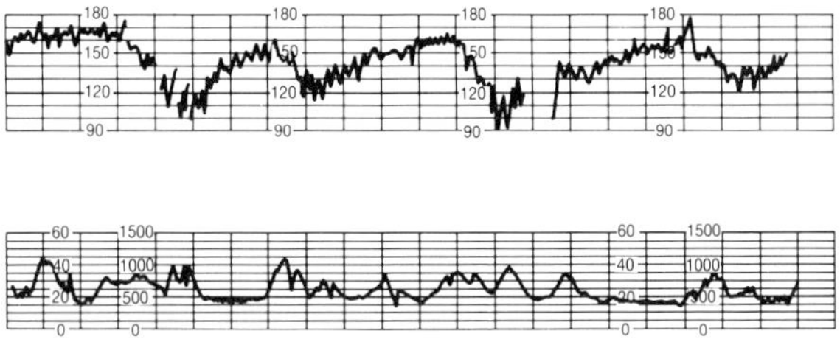

Fig. 52.9 Uterine hypercontractility associated with vaginal prostaglandin administration.

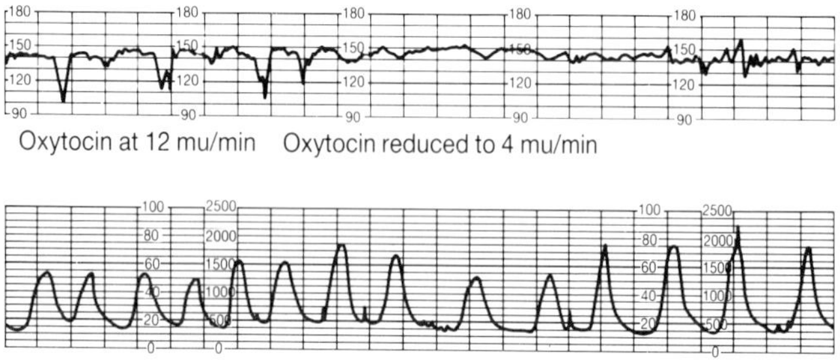

Fig. 52.8 Uterine hypercontractility associated with oxytocin infusion—chronic hyperstimulation; restoration of normal contraction pattern with reduction in oxytocin infusion rate.

Caesarean section with a cord artery pH of 6.98; however, it made a good long-term recovery.

Hyperstimulation with oxytocics

One of the commonest causes of uterine hyperactivity in modern clinical practice is the use of oxytocics. Bourne & Burn warned against the careless use of oxytocin in 1927 and Liston & Campbell echoed their warnings in 1974. Fuchs reported in 1985 that incorrect use of oxytocin was causing more lawsuits in the USA than anything else in obstetrics.

An obvious example of oxytocin-induced hypertonus is shown in Figure 52.7. However, the effects of hyperstimulation may be more subtle. Figure 52.8 shows the tracing of a woman who was having her labour induced. Oxytocin had been increased over the first 90 minutes to 12 mu/min. This dose produced satisfactory uterine activity and it was maintained at this level for the next 2.5 hours. However, as labour proceeded, the uterus became more sensitive to the oxytocin and the frequency of contractions gradually increased until at the beginning of the tracing shown it had reached seven in 10 minutes. The FHR showed loss of variability with late decelerations, indicating fetal hypoxia. Fortunately the hyperstimulation was recognized, and the infusion rate was reduced to 4 mu/min. Over the next 15 minutes the frequency subsided to a more normal five in 10 minutes and the FHR returned to normal. The tracing also illustrates the reduced active pressure associated with excessive contraction frequency; the active pressure rose from 4 kPa (30 mmHg) to 8 kPa (60 mmHg) as the frequency fell.

Prostaglandin administration is also associated with abnormal uterine action (Felmingham et al 1976, Sutton & Steer 1979, Lamb 1981). Figure 52.9 shows the excessively frequent and incoordinate contractions which occurred following the vaginal administration of a 2.5 mg prostaglandin E_2 pessary used to induce labour. Large late decelerations demonstrated the resulting fetal hypoxia and emergency delivery by Caesarean section was necessary.

INEFFICIENT UTERINE ACTIVITY

By definition, any level or type of uterine activity which does not produce progressive cervical dilatation is inefficient. Some workers prefer this term to expressions such as hypotonic, incoordinate, and hypertonic. However, the cervix may fail to dilate despite apparently normal contractions, because of cephalopelvic disproportion or cervical dystocia. Some authorities recommend the use of oxytocics in this situation, despite the risk of uterine hyperstimulation (British Medical Journal Leading Article 1972) but this is a controversial issue and more properly considered in Chapter 54. More recently some workers have noted a rise in the plasma concentrations of the metabolites of prostaglandin $F_{2\alpha}$ in labour associated with progressive cervical dilatation; this rise was not observed even in the presence of apparently normal contractions if cervical dilatation did not occur (Fuchs et al 1983, Weitz et al 1986). The significance of this observation is not yet clear.

ABNORMAL UTERINE ACTION AND POSTURE IN LABOUR

Williams (1952) was the first worker to demonstrate clearly that the supine position in labour can be associated with the development of abnormal uterine action. In the case he reported, uterine activity with the parturient in the sitting position was normal, with a contraction frequency of three in 10 minutes and an active pressure of 5.3 kPa (40 mmHg). When the woman was allowed to lie supine, the contraction frequency rose to 6.4 in 10 minutes and the active pressure fell to 2.1 kPa (16 mmHg). A similar example recorded by the author is shown in Figure 52.9. The change in pattern is abrupt and dramatic. In this case the FHR continues unaffected, but in some cases the increase in contraction frequency is associated with signs of hypoxia. Caldeyro-Barcia et al reported in 1960 that similar changes could be observed in 94% of women in spontaneous labour, and in 76% of those in oxytocin-induced labour. The mechanism by which the supine position can produce abnormal uterine action in this way is completely unknown.

THE MANAGEMENT OF ABNORMAL UTERINE ACTION

The key to appropriate management is the recognition of the category of abnormality. It is particularly important to recognize promptly hypertonic uterine activity, as it is potentially harmful to the fetus. In addition, the diagnosis of uterine hyperactivity may be the first clue to a diagnosis of placental abruption.

Placental abruption

Abruptio placentae is not only likely to have serious implications for the fetus because of interference with placental gaseous exchange, but it can also have major consequences for the mother (particularly blood loss leading to shock, and coagulopathy: see Chs 32 and 38). In severe cases, with lower abdominal pain and vaginal bleeding or the signs of shock (pallor, sweating, tachycardia and hypotension) the diagnosis may be obvious, but in the early stages of abruption the possibility is all too easily overlooked. For example, the lower abdominal pain and uterine irritability may be misattributed to a urinary tract infection.

In any pregnant woman, the occurrence of spontaneous uterine contractions with a frequency exceeding 1 every 2 minutes should lead one to consider the diagnosis of placental abruption.

In addition, the mother may give a history of continuous lower abdominal pain, or backache, which persists between contractions. She may give a history of bleeding per vaginam; this may be quite slight and is sometimes only elicited on direct questioning. Examination is likely to show uterine tenderness, which is often localized but in severe cases will spread to include the entire uterus.

Cardiotocography has an important place in the early diagnosis of abruption, because it facilitates recognition of tachysystolia (excessively frequent contractions). In addition, the interference with placental perfusion which occurs in abruption often causes fetal hypoxia, resulting in abnormal fetal heart rate patterns. In their early stages, these abnormalities (such as loss of variability and shallow late decelerations) are not readily detectable using the Pinard stethoscope. Because of their subtlety it is important that the cardiotocography should be performed carefully, with particular attention to the placement of the external tocodynamometer (contraction transducer). Ideally the mother should be in the semi-Fowler position, sitting up at about 60° to the horizontal, supported by pillows, with the tocodynamometer sited firmly in the midline about 12 cm below the fundus of the uterus. If the mother is lying on her side, then the tocodynamometer should be placed in a similar position but displaced about 10 cm towards the upper side. Only tachysystolia is demonstrable using an external contractions transducer, since neither baseline tone nor amplitude of contractions can be measured in absolute terms using commercially available tocodynamometers. The demonstration of raised baseline tone requires the insertion of an intrauterine catheter. Ideally this should have a catheter-tipped pressure transducer. This is because the maximum error in measurement of baseline tone using this type of catheter is about 2 kPa (15 mmHg) due to variations in hydrostatic pressure at different points within the uterus. In contrast, if a fluid-filled catheter with external pressure transducer is used, unless the transducer is placed carefully at the same level as the uterus, very large offsets in measured baseline tone can occur, making the assessment of true baseline tone unreliable.

Once the diagnosis of abruption has been made, management depends on whether the fetus remains in good condition and upon the state of the cervix. If the mother's condition is satisfactory and if the FHR remains normal then conservative management can proceed with continuing and continuous monitoring of maternal condition, uterine activity and FHR.

If the fetus is sufficiently mature and the cervix is favourable, an induction of labour by artificial rupture of the membranes is probably advisable in case there is a further and larger abruption later on. If the FHR is abnormal or if there is any concern over the mother's condition, immediate delivery is the only safe treatment. Caesarean section will often be the method of choice, particularly if the cervix is unfavourable or if the FHR abnormality is severe.

Attempts to suppress uterine activity with tocolytics such as ritodrine or salbutamol should never be made in the presence of placental abruption for raised intrauterine tone limits the inflow of blood into the uterus and if the tone is reduced, it may precipitate further catastrophic intrauterine bleeding. In addition, if the mother is developing tachycardia and hypotension, these will be exacerbated by tocolytics. This is in contrast to the situation with antepartum haemorrhage due to placenta praevia, where the bleeding is not restricted by raised intrauterine tone but instead is often provoked by uterine contractions. In this situation tocolytics can be used relatively safely and often result in the cessation of bleeding. However, the same caveats about the use of tocolytics in placentae praevia apply with respect to maternal condition; they should not be used if tachycardia and hypotension suggest haemodynamically significant blood loss.

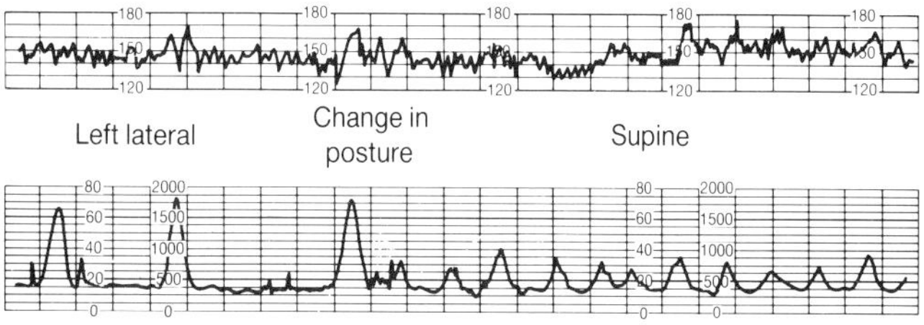

Fig. 52.10 The production of an abnormal uterine contraction pattern by the supine position.

Uncomplicated tachysystolia

If abruption can be ruled out as a cause of excessive uterine contractions, then tocolytics can be used with advantage to reduce the level of uterine action to within normal limits. They are particularly useful as an emergency measure if hypercontractility is secondary to an oxytocic such as prostaglandin E_2, whose action cannot easily be terminated. Oxytocin has a short half-life in the blood; if hyperstimulation occurs with oxytocin use, it is usually sufficient to discontinue the infusion. The effect will wear off within 5–10 minutes.

Inadequate uterine activity

This is usually diagnosed initially because of a slow rate of cervical dilatation. The rate of dilatation below which progress is designated slow varies from one obstetric unit to another but in the UK usually lies between 1 cm an hour and 1 cm every 2 hours. About 75% of slow labours are due to inadequate levels of uterine activity (Steer et al 1985) and most of these will respond effectively to intravenous oxytocin infusion at a rate between 2 and 8 mu / min (techniques for augmentation of labour are covered fully in Ch. 55). Ideally such infusion should be monitored by intrauterine pressure measurement, particularly in women of high parity, in those with a uterine scar and in those where the fetus is known to be at particular risk (e.g. small-for-gestational-age). If intrauterine pressure monitoring is not available, then contraction frequency should not be stimulated beyond one contraction every 2 minutes, and the rate of infusion should be reduced by half as soon as there is any sign of abnormality of the FHR, and reduced further if the abnormality persists.

INCOORDINATE UTERINE ACTION

There is no need to treat incoordinate uterine action so long as the FHR and the rate of cervical dilatation remain normal. As previously mentioned, the role of oxytocin in the management of incoordinate activity where both overall levels of activity and rates of cervical dilatation are low remains controversial. The author's experience is that the cervical dilatation rate increases in parallel with any increase in uterine activity, even if that uterine activity appears incoordinate. It therefore seems appropriate to use oxytocin infusion in the first instance, and in many cases improvement in the level of uterine activity and the rate of cervical dilatation will occur. Prostaglandins are not recommended as they have an inherent tendency to produce incoordinate uterine contractions and may make the situation worse. If, however, there is a poor response to oxytocin, further measures may be tried. It must be emphasized that at the present time there are no firm scientific data to support the use of these measures.

Firstly, the posture of the woman should be adjusted; while the supine position should always be avoided any other position in which uterine activity improves should be maintained. If this is not effective then adequate analgesia must be ensured. This will usually be a regional block such as an epidural anaesthetic. This not only produces an improvement in uterine activity but also provides analgesia, which is important in prolonged labour; if the mother is comfortable and fetal condition is satisfactory, it may be possible to wait long enough so that even a slow rate of cervical dilatation will result in a vaginal delivery. Care should be taken to continue observing FHR and uterine contractions as the anaesthetic is administered, particularly if an oxytocin infusion is being given; if the uterus suddenly becomes more sensitive and there is hypertonus, fetal hypoxia may result. If there is also hypotension from the epidural (despite preloading the circulation with fluid) the effect on the fetus can be catastrophic. If there is still no improvement in the overall level of uterine activity, then sedation with 150 mg pethidine may be tried as a last resort. At the present time there is insufficient evidence on which to recommend the use of beta-blockers such as propranolol.

CONCLUSIONS

The main categories of abnormal uterine action are hypotonic (too little), hypertonic (too much), incoordinate (abnormal in pattern) and inefficient (not associated with progressive cervical dilatation).

The main priority in dealing with hypertonic activity is to decide whether it is due to placental abruption. If not, it may be treated with tocolytics.

None of the other abnormalities matters as long as fetal condition is satisfactory and the cervix is dilating at an adequate rate. If the cervix is dilating at less than 1 cm every 2 hours then ideally intrauterine pressure measurement should be undertaken and oxytocin infusion commenced if activity is deficient; the dose rate should be titrated against response. Persistent incoordinate action associated with poor progress should be treated initially with regional anaesthesia and subsequently with sedation if poor progress persists.

If neither of these treatments is effective and delivery cannot be anticipated within a reasonable time (depending on maternal and fetal condition) then delivery by Caesarean section is indicated.

REFERENCES

Al-Shawaf T, Al-Moghvaby S, Akiel A 1987 Normal levels of uterine activity in primigravidae and women of high parity in spontaneous labour. Journal of Obstetrics and Gynaecology 8: 18–23

Alvarez H, Caldeyro R 1950 Contractility of the human uterus recorded by new methods. Surgery, Gynecology and Obstetrics 91: 1–13

Arthur H R, Johnson G T 1952 Continuous caudal anaesthesia in the management of cervical dystocia. Journal of Obstetrics and Gynaecology of the British Empire 59: 372–377

Arulkumaran S, Gibb D M F, Lun K C, Heng S H, Ratnam S S 1984 The effect of parity on uterine activity in labour. British Journal of Obstetrics and Gynaecology 91: 843–848

Arulkumaran S, Gibb D M F, Ratnam S S, Lun K C, Heng S H 1985 Total uterine activity in induced labour—an index of cervical and pelvic tissue resistance. British Journal of Obstetrics and Gynaecology 92: 693–697

Bidgood K A, Steer P J 1987 Randomised control study of oxytocin augmentation of labour. British Journal of Obstetrics and Gynaecology 94: 512–517

Bourne A, Burn J H 1927 The dosage and action of pituitary extract and the ergot alkaloids on the uterus in labour, with a note of the action of adrenaline. Journal of Obstetrics and Gynaecology of the British Empire 34: 249–272

British Medical Journal Leading Article 1972 Active management of labour. British Medical Journal 4: 126

Brotanek V, Hendricks C H, Yoshida T 1969 Changes in uterine blood flow during uterine contractions. American Journal of Obstetrics and Gynecology 103: 1108–1116

Caldeyro R, Alvarez H, Reynolds S R M 1950 A better understanding of uterine contractility through simultaneous recording with an internal and seven channel external method. Surgery, Gynecology and Obstetrics 91: 641–650

Caldeyro-Barcia R, Alvarez H 1952 Abnormal uterine action during labour. Journal of Obstetrics and Gynaecology of the British Empire 59: 648–654

Caldeyro-Barcia R, Noriega-Guerra L, Cibils L A et al 1960 Effect of position changes on the intensity and frequency of uterine contractions during labour. American Journal of Obstetrics and Gynecology 80: 284–290

Cibils L A, Hendricks C H 1965 Normal labour in vertex presentation. American Journal of Obstetrics and Gynecology 91: 385–395

Cowan D B, Van Middlekoop A, Philpott R H 1982 Intrauterine pressure studies in African nulliparae: normal labour progress. Journal of Obstetrics and Gynaecology of the British Empire 89: 364–369

El-Sahwi S, Gaafar A A, Toppozada H K 1967 A new unit for evaluation of uterine activity. American Journal of Obstetrics and Gynecology 98: 900–903

Felmingham J E, Oakley M C, Atlay R D 1976 Uterine hypertonus after induction of labour with prostaglandin E_2 tablets. British Medical Journal 1: 586

Flynn A M, Kelly J, Hollins G, Lynch P F 1978 Ambulation in labour. British Medical Journal ii: 591–593

Fuchs F 1985 Cautions on using oxytocin for inductions. Contemporary Obstetrics and Gynecology 24: 13–14

Fuchs A-R, Goeschen K, Husslein P, Rasmussen A B, Fuchs F 1983 Plasma concentrations of oxytocin and 13,14-dihydro-15-keto-prostaglandin F_{2alpha} in spontaneous and oxytocin-induced labour at term. American Journal of Obstetrics and Gynecology 147: 497–507

Gibb D M F, Arulkumaran S, Lun K C, Ratnam S S 1984 Characteristics of uterine activity in nulliparous labour. British Journal of Obstetrics and Gynaecology 91: 220–227

Hemminki E, Lenck M, Saariksoki S, Henriksson L 1985 Ambulation versus oxytocin in protracted labour: a pilot study. European Journal of Obstetrics, Gynecology and Reproductive Biology 20: 199–208

Jeffcoate T N A 1963 Physiology and mechanism of labour. In: Claye A, Bourne A (eds) British obstetric and gynaecological practice. Heinemann Medical, London, pp 145–183

Kaiser I H, Harris J S 1950 The effect of adrenalin on the pregnant human uterus. American Journal of Obstetrics and Gynecology 59: 775–784

Krapohl A J, Myers G G, Caldeyro-Barcia R 1970 Uterine contractions in spontaneous labour. American Journal of Obstetrics and Gynecology 106: 378–387

Lamb M P 1981 Prostaglandins in obstetrics. British Medical Journal 282: 1398

Lindmark G, Nilsson B A 1977 A comparative study of uterine activity in labour induced with prostaglandin F_{2alpha} or oxytocin, and in spontaneous labour. Acta Obstetricia et Gynecologica Scandinavica 56: 87–94

Lissauer T J, Steer P J 1986 The relationship between the need for neonatal resuscitation, abnormal cardiotocograms in labour and cord blood gas measurements. British Journal of Obstetrics and Gynaecology 93: 1060–1066

Liston W A, Campbell A J 1974 Dangers of oxytocin induced labour to fetuses. British Medical Journal 3: 606–607

Martin C B 1965 Uterine blood flow and placental circulation. Anesthesiology 26: 447–459

Mendez-Bauer C, Arroyo J, Garcia Ramos C et al 1975 Effects of standing position on spontaneous uterine contractility and other aspects of labour. Journal of Perinatal Medicine 3: 89–100

Mitrani A, Oettinger M, Abinader E G, Sharf M, Klein A 1975 Use of propranolol in dysfunctional labour. British Journal of Obstetrics and Gynaecology 82: 651–655

Moir D D, Willocks J 1967 Management of incoordinate uterine action under continuous epidural anaesthesia. British Medical Journal 3: 396–400

Morishima H O, Daniel S S, Richards R T, James L S 1975 The effect of increased maternal paO_2 upon the fetus during labour. American Journal of Obstetrics and Gynecology 123: 257–264

Novy M J, Thomas C L, Lees M H 1975 Uterine contractility and regional blood flow responses to oxytocin and prostaglandin E_2 in pregnant rhesus monkeys. American Journal of Obstetrics and Gynecology 122: 419–433

Odendaal H J 1976 The frequency of uterine contractions in abruptio placentae. South African Medical Journal 50: 2129–2131

O'Driscoll K, Jackson R J A, Gallagher J T 1969 Prevention of prolonged labour. British Medical Journal 2: 447–480

Pontonnier G, Puech F, Granjean H, Rolland M 1975 Some physical and biochemical parameters during normal labour. Biology of the Neonate 26: 159–173

Poseiro J J, Noriega-Guerra L 1961 Dose response relationships in uterine effects of oxytocin infusions. In: Caldeyro-Barcia R, Heller H (eds) Oxytocin. Pergamon Press, Oxford

Pritchard J A, MacDonald P C, Gant N F 1985 Placental abruption. In: Williams obstetrics. Appleton-Century-Crofts, Norwalk, Connecticut, pp 395–407

Richardson J A, Sutherland I A, Allen D W 1978 A cervimeter for continuous measurement of cervical dilatation in labour—preliminary results. British Journal of Obstetrics and Gynaecology 85: 178–184

Rossavik I K 1978 Relation between total uterine impulse, method of delivery and 1 minute Apgar score. British Journal of Obstetrics and Gynaecology 85: 847–851

Saunderson P R, Steer P J 1978 The value of cardiotocography in abruptio placentae. British Journal of Obstetrics and Gynaecology 85: 796–797

Seitchik J, Chatkoff M L 1977 Intrauterine pressure waveform characteristics of successful and failed first stage labour. Gynecological Investigation 8: 246–253

Steer P J, Carter M C, Beard R W 1984 Normal levels of active contraction area in spontaneous labour. British Journal of Obstetrics and Gynaecology 91: 211–219

Steer P J, Carter M C, Beard R W 1985 The effect of oxytocin infusion on uterine activity levels in slow labour. British Journal of Obstetrics and Gynaecology 92: 1120–1126

Sutton M, Steer P J 1979 Induction of labour. British Medical Journal 3: 671

Turnbull A C 1957 Uterine contractions in normal and abnormal labour. Journal of Obstetrics and Gynaecology of the British Empire 64: 321–333
Weitz C M, Ghodgaonker R B, Dubin N H, Niebyl J R 1986 Prostaglandin F metabolite concentration as a prognostic factor in preterm labour. Obstetrics and Gynecology 67: 496–499
Williams E A 1952 Abnormal uterine action during labour. Journal of Obstetrics and Gynaecology of the British Empire 59: 635–641
Zambrana M A, Gonzalez-Panizza V H, Santiso-Galvez R, Garcia De Paz H, Fernandez R, Arellano-Hernandez G 1960 Relacion de la contractilidad espontanea del utero con el progreso del parto. In: Third Uruguayan Congress of Obstetrics and Gynecology 3: 354. Cited in: Greenhill J P (ed) Obstetrics, 3rd edn. WB Saunders, Philadelphia, pp 281, 304

53

James Clinch

Abnormal fetal presentations and positions

In late pregnancy and during the early stages of labour a favourable presentation and position is one where the baby's head is entering the mother's pelvis with the occiput directed towards the side wall or some point between it and the symphysis pubis. The subsequent labour and delivery should be a normal physiological function requiring no obstetric intervention. Unfortunately, in some women either the presentation or the position is not normal and this may lead to complications requiring special management and occasionally operative treatment.

A considerable amount of difficulty arises from the shape of the human birth canal. When eye contact became a most important tool for the developing hominid as she descended from the trees (Morgan 1972), she started to walk with an upright stance. The subsequent development of the gluteal and thigh muscles led to thickening and strengthening of the bones of the pelvis and forward curvature of the lower half of the sacrum. Eye contact during intercourse required a forward facing procreation tract so that the vagina gradually turned at a right angle to the brim of the pelvis and to the uterus itself. Delivery of a child came to mean not only pushing it through a rigid bony canal, the entrance to which was wider from side to side while the exit was larger from front to back, but negotiation of a right-angled bend half way down the canal followed by traversing strong perineal muscles designed more for keeping things in than letting them out (Stewart 1984a; Fig. 53.1).

These changes were accompanied by an increase in the size of the human brain required to develop and utilize the skills which humans need to remain the dominant animal (Moore 1970), so that as the pelvis was becoming less suitable for delivery the most important part of the infant increasingly came to have more difficulty fitting through it.

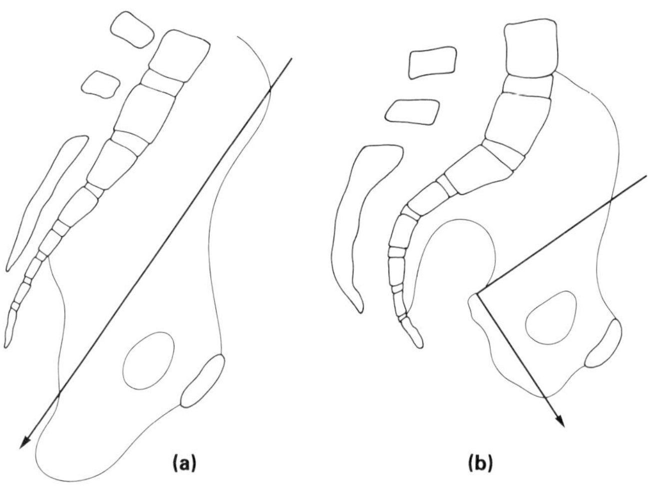

Fig. 53.1 (**a**) Gorilla pelvis showing straight birth canal. (**b**) Human pelvis showing birth canal with right-angle turn.

These disadvantages are normally overcome by what are known as the mechanics of labour. The bigger parts of the baby, such as the head, shoulders, and breech, enter the pelvis with their largest diameters running transversely. They rotate as they descend so that the same diameters leave the pelvis in an anterior–posterior direction. Because the spine is inserted into the back of the skull, pressure directed along it will make the head flex (Fig. 53.2). Thus, before labour commences or in its early stages the occipito-frontal diameter of the head is in the transverse diameter of the pelvis. As it descends it quickly flexes so that the occipito-frontal diameter becomes the suboccipito-bregmatic, identical in length with the biparietal diameter at 9.5 cm. These form a circle to apply pressure equally all round the cervix, resulting in a reflex arc which stimulates fundal contractility and subsequently more downward pressure. When the head reaches the gutter formed by the levator muscles deep in the pelvis, the occiput, which is larger than the sinciput, is funnelled forwards to present at the vulval opening. With

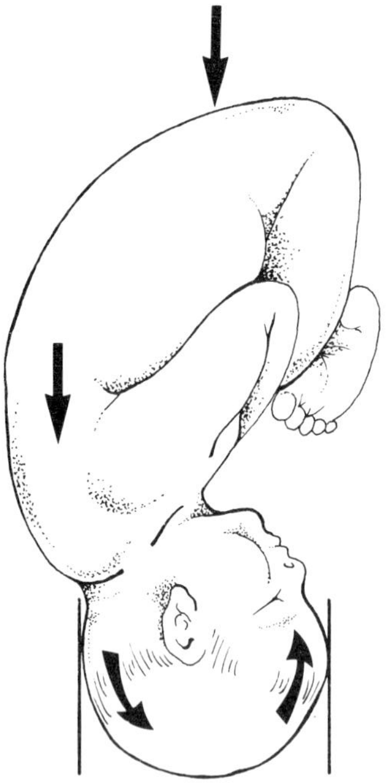

Fig. 53.2 Fundal pressure directed down fetal spine promotes flexion rather than extension of head.

further downward pressure it can emerge from the larger of the two diameters at the pelvic outlet, finally extending as it does so.

Subsequent restitution and external rotation of the head are merely reflections of the remainder of the baby coming through the pelvis but are not important as the largest part of it has by now delivered.

Using these mechanics most babies negotiate the pelvis safely. However, in a small number of cases the presentation is not cephalic or if it is, it rotates the wrong way in mid-pelvis, extending instead of flexing and these mechanisms cannot apply. Such problems form the basis of this chapter. It is written from a western European perspective where it is tempting to manage them by delivering the baby abdominally. This solution is not always available in the less well developed areas of the world and even in more advanced countries the tendency to treat every complication by Caesarean section has been criticized because, however straightforward for the baby, it is a major procedure for the mother (Chalmers 1984, Gilstrap et al 1984, Yudkin & Redman 1986).

This chapter concentrates on the function of the mother delivering her baby and does not dwell on the different pelvic shapes. Fetal size in utero is related to the height of the mother. Thus, tall women should have large pelves and be capable of delivering large babies while smaller women with smaller pelves should have correspondingly lighter infants. Antenatal X-rays of the pelvis may label a small woman as having a contracted pelvis and lead to unnecessary interference. Radiology should be restricted to those with breech presentation or after delivery in patients who have had an unexpectedly difficult birth for no obvious reason (Joyce et al 1975, O'Brien and Cefalo 1982, Floberg et al 1987).

DEFINITIONS

The definitions used in this chapter are as follows.

The *attitude* of the fetus describes the relationship between the fetal head and limbs to the trunk. Usually this is one of flexion.

The *lie* of the fetus is its relationship to the long axis of the uterus. This can be longitudinal, oblique or transverse.

The *presentation* is that part of the fetus presenting in the lower pole of the uterus or at the pelvic brim.

The *presenting part* is that part of the presentation which lies immediately inside the internal os.

The *position* defines the relationship of the presentation or the presenting part to the maternal pelvis.

The *denominator* is that part of the presentation or the presenting part which denotes the position. For a cephalic presentation with the vertex as the presenting part, the denominator is the occiput. With a face as the presenting part it is the chin and for a breech it is the sacrum.

It is important to distinguish between presentation and presenting part. For example, a patient can have a cephalic presentation with the brow or the face as a presenting part: it is incorrect to refer to these as brow or face presentations.

It is also incorrect to write vertex as the presentation on abdominal palpation. It is the presenting part at the commencement of most labours before the head has flexed.

OCCIPITO-POSTERIOR POSITIONS OF THE HEAD

Occiputo-posterior position means that the occiput, the denominator for the position of the head, points posteriorly in the pelvis, either directly at the sacrum (direct occipito-posterior) or to one side of it in the region of the sacroiliac joints (oblique occiputo-posterior). This may be the case during the antenatal period, or at any time in labour right up to delivery. Because the head rotates during labour, discussion about these positions has to include women in whom the occiput points sideways (occipito-lateral, occipito-transverse). It is accepted that 10–20% of cephalic presentations enter labour with the occiput directed posteriorly (Myerscough 1982). Some rotate to occipito-anterior so that by the time of delivery, only 5% remain occipito-posterior or have arrested in the occipito-lateral position while attempting to turn towards the front.

There are several possible causes for the abnormal position. Braxton Hicks contractions may not be strong enough to push the head into the brim and make it flex prior to the onset of labour. Conversely the fact that the head is

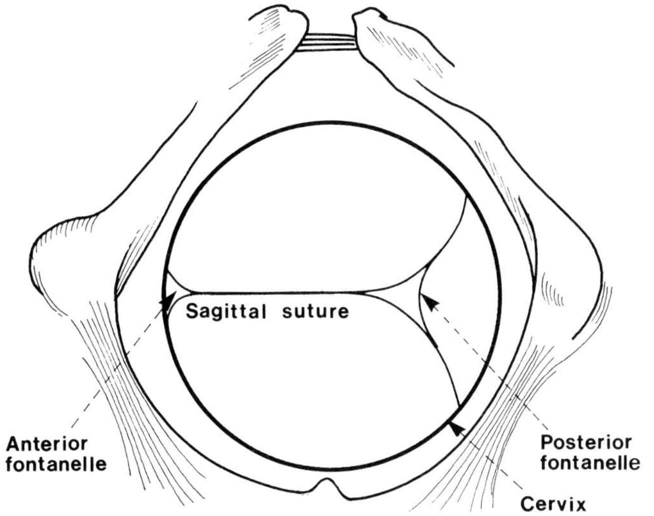

Fig. 53.3a Flexed head presenting as a circle to the cervix. Biparietal diameter 9.5 cm; suboccipito-bregmatic diameter also 9.5 cm.

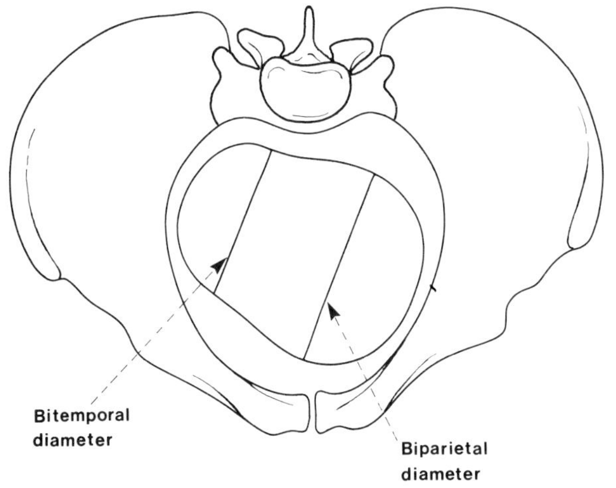

Fig. 53.4a Left occipito-anterior position. Biparietal diameter (9.5 cm) lying between the sacroiliac joint and the summit of the symphysis pubis. Bitemporal diameter (8.5 cm) occupies the smaller sacrocotyloid dimension.

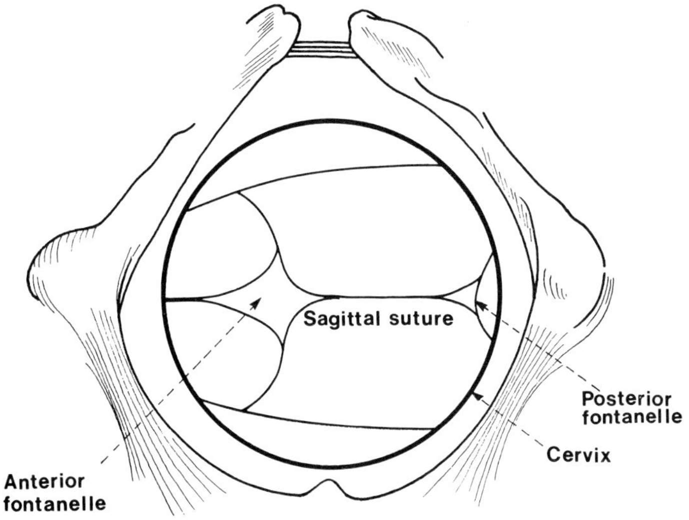

Fig. 53.3b Deflexed head presenting a rectangular surface to the cervix. Biparietal diameter 9.5 cm; occipito-frontal diameter 11.5 cm.

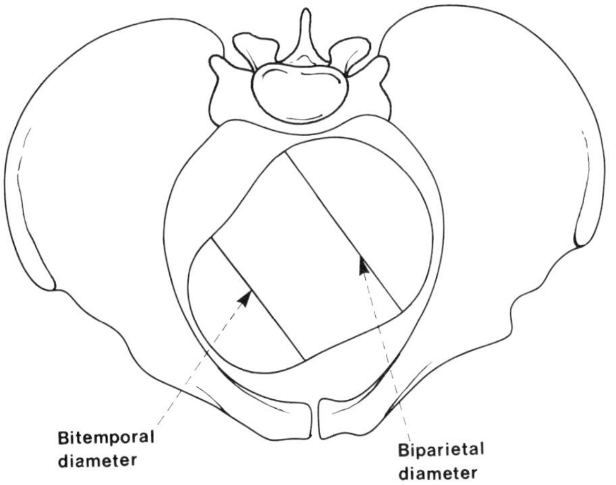

Fig. 53.4b Left occipito-posterior position. Biparietal diameter squeezed into the sacrocotyloid while the bitemporal has excess space.

extended presents a rectangular-shaped outline to the lower segment so that the stimulus to fundal contractility may be irregular and incomplete (Fig. 53.3b). In late pregnancy, attempts by the uterus to turn the baby's head and shoulders may be impeded by the latter catching on to the mother's lower lumbar spine and sacral promontory. Hypertonus in the fetus can prevent the normal flexed attitude in utero.

The babies of women with either anthropoid or android pelves are more likely to be occipito-posterior. The former is very uncommon but is usually large; the baby presents directly occipito-posterior for the whole labour and delivers easily in that position. Viewed from above, the more commonly found android pelvis is triangular in shape with the apex at the symphysis pubis so that the larger part of the fetal head finds more room in the back of the pelvis and turns into the sacral curve as it descends (Holmberg et al 1977, Stewart 1984b).

Whatever the precise aetiology, the fact that the baby's spine is juxtaposed to the mother's means that downward pressure along the spine is more likely to extend the head than flex it, thus increasing the diameters presented to the pelvic brim. In addition, since the head is rarely directly occipito-posterior, the biparietal, its largest transverse diameter, will be trying to squeeze through the space between the sacral promontory and the pectineal line while the smaller bitemporal measurement will have all the space available from the sacroiliac joint to the back of the symphysis pubis (Fig. 53.4). Uterine contractility is adversely affected because the cervix is not stimulated correctly by the rectangular surface presented by the extended head (Fig. 53.3b). When the occiput eventually meets the pelvic floor it may fail to rotate to the front partly because of the long way it has to travel, through three-eighths of a circle, and partly because the posterior shoulder remains caught on the wrong side of the mother's sacral promontory. In many cases the

Table 53.1 Mode of delivery of 1384 babies presenting as occipito-posterior or with deep transverse arrest at full dilatation at Coombe Hospital, Dublin, 1971–1977

Mode of delivery	Percentage
Spontaneous occipito-posterior	22
Forceps occipito-posterior	21
Manual rotation/forceps	20
Kiellands forceps	17
Vacuum extraction	16
Caesarean section	2

head rotates through 45° and can go no further, eventually ending up as deep transverse arrest. Some turn the same distance but posteriorly and become persistent occipito-posterior positions. Neither delivers or can be delivered as easily as a well-flexed head in the normal occipito-anterior position. Thus, progress of labour is marred by misapplication of the head to the cervix, the largest transverse diameter of the head trying to pass through the smallest diameter of the pelvic brim and the tendency of the head to deflex and present bigger and bigger diameters as it descends in the pelvis. In a small number of cases this extension continues so that first the baby's brow and then its face becomes the presenting part.

The resultant trend towards prolonged labour possibly with operative delivery increases morbidity for both mother and child. Table 53.1 shows that in the Coombe Hospital, Dublin, between 1971 and 1977, of 1384 children who were occipito-posterior or arrested in the transverse position at full dilatation of the cervix, only 22% had a spontaneous vaginal delivery. The rate was exactly the same in 1984. Phillips & Freeman (1974) in a retrospective review of 552 cases which were born vaginally reported an operative delivery rate of 66% with 22% requiring rotation. There was more puerperal pyrexia and so many episiotomies extended posteriorly that the authors recommended never using a midline technique. Friedman et al (1977) examined 656 children aged between 3 and 4 years and found that a history of prolonged labour and mid-forceps either together or independently had an adverse effect on subsequent intelligence.

The diagnosis of an occipito-posterior position can be suspected antenatally on abdominal palpation. With the baby lying on its back when the mother is examined, its flexed legs mean that the maximum protrusion of the maternal abdomen viewed from the side is well above the umbilicus with a sharp fall down to the xyphi sternum and a gentle slope towards the symphysis pubis (Fig. 53.5). The head will feel smaller because the sinciput is anterior and the back may be difficult to palpate clearly.

Management of the occipito-posterior position

There is no point in attempting to alter the position during the antenatal period as many correct themselves once labour starts; most cases are not diagnosed until labour is well established and some may have arisen only in its early stages.

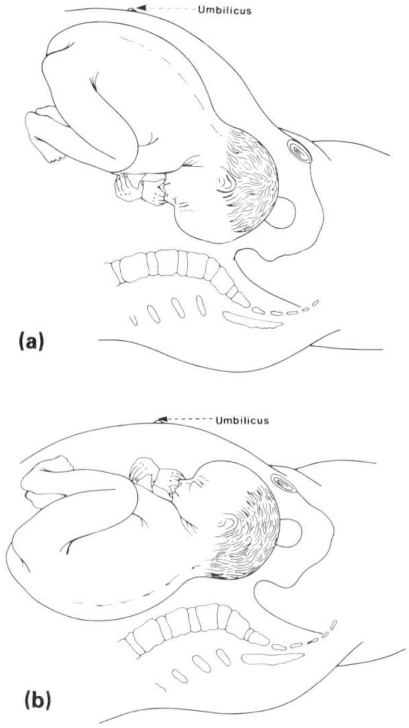

Fig. 53.5 Lateral view of abdomen near term. (**a**) Occipito-anterior position: maternal umbilicus at summit of abdominal swelling. (**b**) Occipito-posterior with umbilicus inferior to summit.

However, it is important to emphasize that because the condition may be associated with incoordinate uterine action, the cervix is most unlikely to be ripe if induction is being considered.

Once labour is underway some cases of occipito-posterior position progress quickly and either rotate to occipito-anterior spontaneously or deliver as face to pubes before the malposition has been diagnosed. These cause no problem apart from a tendency towards perineal damage. Most cases come to light because of failure to progress in labour and in units where active management is practised a vaginal examination quickly reveals the abnormal position. It is essential that such examinations are thorough and produce as much information as possible. Abnormal positions often develop moulding and caput formation as labour progresses and it is easier to define the suture lines on the fetal skull in the early stages.

The degree of deflexion of the fetal head is also noted and not only should the bony pelvis be assessed but the thickness and elasticity of the maternal soft tissues may be relevant to subsequent attempts at operative delivery. Application of the cervix to the presenting part is assessed, especially during a contraction. If it is not well applied, then uterine contractility is inadequate, however much discomfort the patient is having. Observations as to the colour of the amniotic fluid and whether the cord can be palpated are also important. A vaginal examination which merely states the dilatation of the cervix and the station of the head is not sufficient for the management of complicated cases and has no place in a good unit. Such limited information could have been obtained by rectal examination, which is much quicker.

Having made the diagnosis of occipito-posterior it is important to remember that while the position of the head may slow its descent down the birth canal there is no reason why the cervix should not become fully dilated provided the labour is managed actively. A rate of 1 cm/h (as in patients with an occipito-anterior position) must be anticipated; Syntocinon should be administered in sufficient doses if this does not occur spontaneously. There is considerable doubt as to how much of the drug may be necessary. Gibb et al (1984) found that Chinese primigravidae in Singapore required much higher intrauterine pressures to achieve progress than was found by either Seitchik & Castillo (1983) or Steer and his colleagues (1985a), who felt that intrauterine pressures above 1500 kPa/15 min caused uterine hyperstimulation and fetal distress. Steer et al (1985b) also recommended the use of a closed loop system which Gibb et al (1985) found not to be as effective as manually controlled infusion. Arulkumaran and his co-workers (1985), writing about induction of labour, again used higher doses, stressing the importance of maternal soft tissue resistance.

For labour wards which do not have the benefit of catheter-tipped transducers and for the sake of simplicity it seems that the quantity of oxytocic required is that which is sufficient to dilate the cervix without causing more than 4 contractions in 10 minutes or fetal distress. Since it takes 40 minutes for the level of plasma oxytocin to peak, there is no point in increasing the infusion rate more quickly (Seitchik et al 1984). Both oxytocin and glucose can cause neonatal and maternal hyponatraemia so normal saline should be used as an infusion base (Singhi et al 1985). The fetus must be continuously monitored and the mother is an ideal candidate for an epidural, although a labouring woman does not always appreciate the analgesia provided (Morgan et al 1982). There is no need to give glucose intravenously to combat ketosis if the labour appears slow (Dumoulin & Foulkes 1984). Maternal dehydration can be dealt with by intravenous saline (Morton et al 1985). Indeed, if dehydration occurs the obstetrician in charge must question the preceding management of the case and make certain that labour advances more quickly.

With this approach every cervix should become fully dilated. In some, the head will have descended to the pelvic floor and deliver spontaneously either with the occiput anterior or in the direct occiput posterior position. The latter may require a large enough episiotomy to prevent excess tearing of the perineum. Provided that some progress is being made and the baby's heart rate and pH remain normal, patience and care will result in a spontaneous delivery for many women. However, if the head remains high a full reassessment of the case is essential. If the pelvis appears smaller than was first thought; if the antenatal records imply that the baby always felt large; if the mother is small or even if the father is tall (Pritchard et al 1983), then there may be a degree of disproportion even without an abnormal position. There is no point in doing pelvimetry as even with a large pelvis, failure of the head to descend to a level where forceps or vacuum extraction can be safely applied will result in abdominal delivery (Bottoms et al 1987). In such instances the operator must not feel in any way that labour has been wasted.

If none of these applies, an increase in the amount of oxytocin may effect further descent or rotation of the head. This is especially so if an epidural is in situ. Goodfellow et al (1983) have shown that the oxytocin surge stimulated by dilatation of the upper vagina is suppressed by conduction analgesia. Allowing the epidural to wear off neither shortens the second stage nor reduces the incidence of forceps delivery (Phillips & Thomas 1983), but instituting an infusion (Kirwan 1983) or increasing the dose (Bates et al 1985) may improve progress. Despite the finding of Smith et al (1982) that delayed pushing in the second stage did not lessen the need for instrumental delivery, Maresh et al (1983) reported exactly the opposite. They also stated that the resultant prolongation of the second stage had no adverse effect on mother or child, which concurred with Cohen's view (1977) that there was no point in having time limits for the second stage. Nevertheless, most obstetricians would agree with Kadar et al (1986) that the prospect of a normal delivery after 3 hours in the second stage is most unlikely.

For some women a change of position may be helpful. Despite the inconsistent findings of many workers, most of whom have concentrated on the effects of ambulation in the first stage of labour—Dunn (1978), Flynn et al (1978) and Lupe & Gross (1986) feel an upright posture helps while McManus & Calder (1978a,b), Williams et al (1980), Calvert et al (1982) and Stewart & Calder (1984) all feel it makes no difference—squatting, semi-squatting, lying on the side or sitting in a birth chair may enable the woman who feels the urge to push to do so more effectively than lying on her back even when propped up with pillows. Failure of any of these measures will lead to operative vaginal delivery.

Operative vaginal delivery

This must start with careful palpation of the abdomen. If any part of the head can be felt above the symphysis pubis its station in the pelvis is higher than may have appeared to be the case on vaginal examination, usually because of moulding or caput or both. While such a finding is not an absolute contraindication to vaginal delivery it acts as a warning not to persist if the first attempt is unsuccessful.

The woman is put into the lithotomy position with both buttocks slightly over the edge of the bed. If vaginal examination shows the head to be directly occipito-posterior and low in the pelvis, a direct application of a Neville Barnes-type forceps with the aid of a suitable episiotomy and gentle traction should deliver the baby. However, if the head fails to descend it will be necessary to rotate it manually, with straight forceps or by means of a vacuum extractor. This will also be the case if the head is in the oblique occipito-posterior position or is arrested at mid-cavity in the deep transverse position.

The lower birth canal must be suitably anaesthetized. Depending on the procedure undertaken, pudendal block may be adequate but in many who do not already have an epidural in place, a single-shot caudal may be inserted quickly, making certain that a wedge is placed under one of the patient's buttocks when she is returned to the lithotomy position.

Manual rotation of the head

This involves the operator's hand grasping the sinciput and rotating it towards the sacrum. An alternative method is to insert the hand alongside the head, turning the head with pressure from the palmar surface of the fingers. Placing the fingertips in the suture lines may help, as does an abdominal hand pulling the anterior shoulder of the baby in the appropriate direction.

It is simpler if the operator uses the right hand for rotation so that once the head has been turned the first blade of the forceps can be applied immediately. The left hand is then inserted quickly along the right side of the pelvic wall in an effort to hold the head in its new position while the right blade is put in place. Correct application means that the handles will close easily with the operator rechecking the suture lines before using any traction. Non-closure demands that the blades should be removed and the vaginal assessment repeated.

Insertion of a hand alongside the baby's head leaves even less room in the pelvis, so to effect rotation it may be necessary to push the head into the upper pelvis or even out of the pelvis, which will turn a low- or mid-cavity forceps into a high-forceps and this is not recommended. Ideally, the operator should have slim fingers which can fit around the head without displacing it upwards: unfortunately, this attribute often goes with weak hands so that those best shaped for the manoeuvre are not always strong enough to carry it out. For these reasons manual rotation should be restricted to cases where the head is obliquely posterior low in the pelvis and easily turned to direct occipito-posterior for delivery in that position.

Forceps rotation

Forceps have the advantage that the blades are thinner than human fingers so that the operator keeps the head low when applying them. In the direct or oblique occipito-posterior position the blades of a Keillands-type of instrument can be applied directly. Rotation is then performed with one hand while the index finger of the other is kept on the sagittal suture to make certain it is turning with the forceps. Rotation may be helped by either pulling down or pushing up the head a centimetre or two and since there is no pelvic curve the handles of the forceps must always be directed more posteriorly than with axis traction forceps. In the direct occipito-posterior position, rotation can be either clockwise or anticlockwise, usually towards the side on which the back has been palpated abdominally. With an obliquely posterior head the rotation is towards the side on which the occiput already is. In both cases it is important to remember that if rotation in one direction is unsuccessful it is worth trying to turn the forceps the other way.

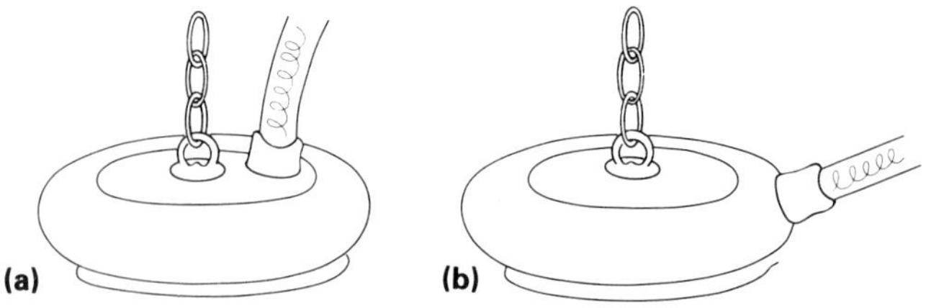

Fig. 53.6 Vacuum extractor cups: (**a**) for application to well-flexed head; (**b**) for application to deflexed head or occipito-posterior position.

As soon as the occipito-anterior position is attained the same forceps are used to effect delivery. Removing them and reapplying ordinary traction forceps not only risks increased trauma to the maternal tissues but the head may turn back in the process.

For those who feel that the head in deep transverse arrest is better allowed to rotate at its own level than at one chosen by the operator, Barton's forceps may be more suitable (Ch. 56). A sharp angle makes the posterior blade easier to apply than Keillands and rotation occurs spontaneously as traction is applied (Parry-Jones 1968).

Vacuum extractor

This instrument has the advantage that it occupies no space to the side of the baby's head. When properly applied, it actually flexes the baby's head, reducing one of the diameters presenting to the pelvic outlet from the occipito-frontal to the smaller suboccipito-bregmatic. In addition, with traction the head can rotate to whichever position enables it to be delivered most easily. The largest possible cup must be used—one with the traction apparatus separate from the air tubing, which is inserted into the top of the cup for flexed heads but into the side for those which are deflexed (Fig. 53.6). The cup is applied as far back as possible on the occiput. The direction of traction is usually downwards but must be varied slightly to achieve the best descent, while the thumb and finger of the operator's other hand are kept on the cup to help it stay well applied and to assess rotation.

Soft vacuum cups have been advocated because of their lack of trauma to the fetal scalp but a more important factor is the method of traction. O'Neil et al (1981) have designed a cup with a flat disc on the top which rotates through 360° and to which is attached a half ring. Pulling the ring in any direction exerts traction through the centre of the vacuum surface, avoiding any tendency for one edge of the cup to lift off the scalp. Once rotation to the anterior position has been achieved the head usually delivers easily. If it emerges without rotating the attendant has to accept that this was the most suitable position for that particular head.

If the cup comes off during rotation or traction, a more experienced operator may be permitted one more attempt, using either a larger cup or changing to forceps, provided the new position of the head is easily ascertainable. If this is not the case or further attempts fail, Caesarean section will be indicated.

Forceps or vacuum extraction?

O'Driscoll et al (1981), pointing out that in their institution intracranial trauma with cephalic presentation only occurred when forceps had been applied, caused considerable worry about the place of instrumental vaginal delivery in modern obstetrics. Cyr et al (1984) found that mid-forceps with epidural was the main cause of neonatal trauma while Chiswick & James (1979) and Chiswick (1980) reported an unacceptable level of neurological deficit in babies delivered by Keillands forceps. Yet Healy et al (1982), Cardozo et al (1983) and Traub et al (1984) reported that Keillands were just as safe for the baby as Caesarean section, while Dierker and his co-workers (1986) reported that at 2 years of age babies delivered by mid-cavity forceps were equally fit as those who had undergone abdominal delivery. Paintin (1982) will not do rotational forceps if there is any fetal distress while Moolgaoker et al (1979), Dyack (1980) and Goodlin (1986) have attempted to reduce fetal trauma by using blades modified to lessen compression of the fetal head. Kadar & Romero pointed out in 1983 that patients who underwent mid-cavity forceps for their first delivery have a sixfold increase in operative procedures for their second, implying that some will have suffered from a minor degree of cephalopelvic disproportion.

None of these reports, including Drife (1983), considered seriously the replacement of all forms of rotation by use of the vacuum extractor. Yet Greis et al (1981), Vacca et al (1983), and Berkus et al (1985) all showed that the vacuum caused considerably less maternal trauma than forceps while having no adverse effect on the neonate. Berkus and his colleagues showed later (1986) that this was true even if the vacuum failed and Caesarean section had to be undertaken. Halme & Ekbladh pointed out in 1982 how much easier it was to instruct trainees in the use of the vacuum extractor, stating that it was safer than mid-cavity forceps. In one of his earlier papers (1968), Chalmers employed it in 224 cases of direct occipito-posterior position: 70% of these rotated to occipito-anterior, the remainder delivering face to pubes. Of 189 patients with deep transverse arrest, only 9 made a face-to-pubes exit. He pointed out the advantage of the head being able to rotate to its most advantageous position rather than being forcibly turned by the operator.

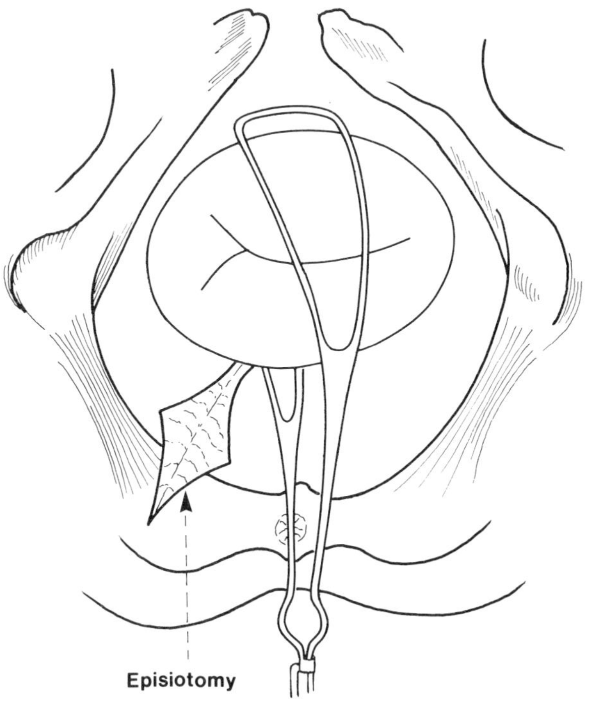

Fig. 53.7 Rotation forceps. With clockwise rotation the posterior blade will pass through the episiotomy, risking extension. In this case the incision should have been made on the left side of the perineum.

In summary, it would appear that for arrested malpositions a modern vacuum extractor has distinct advantages over obstetric forceps. However, it is vitally important before attempting any vacuum delivery that the equipment should be inspected thoroughly by the operator before each application. Regular checks must be made to see that the pressure gauges are accurate, that the air tubing is intact and that there are no leaks from it or other parts of the machine (Ch. 57).

Two further points should be emphasized in connection with operative delivery for abnormal cephalic positions—relating to episiotomy and failed forceps delivery.

Episiotomy

Because the head is extended the episiotomy may need to be larger than for an occipito-anterior position. With instrumental delivery there is a temptation to do the episiotomy prior to inserting either the forceps or the vacuum in order to make the application easier. This should be avoided: failure to effect the delivery and subsequent Caesarean section means the patient will have an unnecessary wound in her perineum. In addition, until one knows which way the head will rotate it is impossible to be sure whether the episiotomy is better done on the right or the left side. If the head is right occipito-transverse and rotation forceps are applied with the aid of a right mediolateral episiotomy (Fig. 53.7), clockwise rotation will drag the posterior blade across the episiotomy site with the risk of extending it and causing

Table 53.2 Failed forceps: eventual mode of delivery at Coombe Hospital, Dublin, 1971–1977

Mode of delivery	Number
Vacuum extraction	9
Caesarean section	43

severe trauma. The operator should aim to reserve the incision until vaginal delivery is certain, by which stage even a midline incision may be adequate.

Episiotomy discomfort worries many puerperal women more than anything else (Reading et al 1982) and great care should be taken in its performance and repair. Midline incisions are easier to suture but unfortunately are not less painful than mediolateral ones (Coats et al 1980). A subcuticular repair (Isager-Sally et al 1986) with polyglycolic suture material (Roberts & McKay Hart 1983, Grant 1986) is better than other techniques.

Failed forceps delivery

No surgeon likes a procedure to fail but it is important to remember that a forceps delivery which requires a strong pull is occasionally followed by shoulder dystocia. Benedetti & Gabbe (1978), along with Acker and his colleagues (1985, 1986), have shown that secondary arrest or a prolonged second stage with mid-cavity forceps is a warning sign for this complication. While in theory it can be overcome by a variety of manoeuvres (Harris 1984, Carter 1986, Gross et al 1987), including replacement of the head and later Caesarean section (Sandberg 1985), in practice fetal mortality and morbidity are high.

If rotation cannot be achieved, if a large vacuum cup properly applied comes off, or if firm one-handed traction with forceps applied to a head in the direct occipito-anterior position fails to deliver the baby, Caesarean section must be undertaken. Table 53.2 shows that in the years 1971 to 1977 at the Coombe Hospital, Dublin, there were 52 cases of failed operative vaginal delivery—49 with forceps and 3 with the vacuum extractor. Forty of these were primigravidae. In 9 of the cases where forceps were not successful, a vacuum extraction was, but 43 women required Caesarean section.

With foresight, operative deliveries which look as though they may be difficult can be done in an operating theatre with everything prepared to proceed to Caesarean section (Lowe 1987), but any maternity unit which never has a failed operative delivery is under-reporting its cases or doing traumatic vaginal deliveries.

FACE AND BROW PRESENTING PARTS

These two abnormal presenting parts may be considered together as they are similar in many respects. Cruikshank & Cruikshank (1981) quote an incidence of 1 in 500 for the face and 1 in 1500 for the brow as presenting parts. The chin is the denominator when the face is presenting but traditionally there is no such marker for a brow; it is thought that the large occipito-mental diameter can never pass through a pelvis and therefore no mechanism is necessary. The diameters of a face are the normal biparietal (9.5 cm) and the submento-bregmatic, which is the same as the occipito-frontal of a deflexed vertex (11.5 cm). However, labour can be more difficult than with an extended head because the facial bones do not mould as satisfactorily as parietal ones; if the chin rotates posteriorly, then the large area of skull comprising the vertex and the occiput cannot follow the face out under the symphysis. Both conditions are due to hyperextension of the fetal neck, usually cases of occipito-posterior position which extend first into a brow and then into a face either before labour but usually as labour is progressing. Abnormalities such as anencephaly or tumours of the fetal neck may also be associated.

The principal complication for the mother is that of operative delivery, often Caesarean section. For the baby there exists the danger of the presenting part attempting to mould adequately enough to fit through the pelvis and therefore straining the intracranial membranes with resultant intracranial haemorrhage. The excess oedema of eyelids, nose, lips and cheeks found when the face presents looks spectacular but resolves quickly. Vaginal operative delivery must be done by someone experienced to avoid causing damage to these organs.

Diagnosis is suspected on palpation when the head will be high or will feel larger than normal with a sharp angulation between the fetal back and the occiput. Often an ultrasound scan or X-ray is done to exclude abnormality and shows the unusual presenting part. Most cases appear for the first time in labour, when vaginal examination will demonstrate the root of the nose and the two orbital ridges of a brow, or the nose, the mouth and the two orbital hollows of a face. Confirmation by a senior colleague is often of value: these cases are rare and occasionally the mouth can be mistaken for the anal orifice.

Management of face and brow

There is no point in attempting to correct the abnormality prior to the onset of labour, the advent of which will hopefully lead to the head flexing and the vertex becoming the presenting part. If there is an over-riding requirement to deliver the baby, elective Caesarean section is usually a wiser choice than inducing labour with the high presenting part, even if the cervix is suitable.

Once labour starts it should be managed in the normal fashion until full dilatation. Seeds & Cefalo (1982) pointed out that many brows convert to a vertex or a face and most faces are mento-anterior. The cervix should be expected to dilate at 1 cm/h and Syntocinon may be used to achieve this, remembering that many of these patients are multiparous and the abnormal presenting part can lead to obstructed labour and rupture the uterus. Thus if after 1 hour of contractions which have been considered adequate there is no increase in dilatation of the cervix or alteration in the presenting part, such as a brow turning to a face or a face descending in the pelvis, it is safer to deliver the baby by Caesarean section. At full dilatation, management will be determined by the size of the pelvis. If it is small, the presenting part will remain high and Caesarean section will be needed. If large, as is often the case, the presenting part will descend below the spines and may come to vaginal delivery.

Face presentation may be encouraged to deliver spontaneously provided that the chin is already anterior or is rotating forwards. Should it be mento-posterior, it is usually high in the pelvis and although rotation forceps can be successfully applied, most operators will opt for Caesarean section as the wiser choice. However, Cruikshank & Cruikshank (1981) report a section rate of only 15% in a review of 2373 faces with 72% requiring low-forceps and only 12% needing mid-forceps.

Manipulations such as Thorn's manoeuvre for turning a brow into a vertex do work but the complication is so rare that few people have much experience of their use. Provided the head is engaged, it is possible to treat a forward-facing brow as an exaggerated occipito-posterior position. It can be flexed with a vacuum cup or by applying a Neville Barnes forceps with the handles held very posteriorly at first and then brought forwards.

Most experienced obstetricians and midwives have seen babies delivered brow first with no untoward effects but there are no references in the literature to this being an acceptable procedure. The author has personally applied a 4-cm vacuum cup to a brow which delivered with one gentle pull. The baby was subsequently found to weigh 3750 g.

TRANSVERSE LIE

A transverse lie involves the long axis of the fetus lying at right angles to the uterus. The incidence is 2% early in the third trimester but only 0.3% at term. Most cases have no obvious aetiology and are presumably due to laxity of the abdominal musculature in a multiparous patient. However, this must not be assumed until pelvic tumours such as placenta praevia, fibroids and ovarian cysts have been excluded, along with fetal malformations, including twins. Rarely the cause is an abnormal uterus with the baby fixed in a transverse lie, its back pointing towards the lower segment. Antenatal diagnosis is usually easy with two poles of the fetus felt on either side of the abdomen. Ultrasound must be done to exclude the various abnormalities already mentioned. Vaginal examination is contraindicated for fear of disturbing a possibly low-lying placenta.

Once labour starts the diagnosis is made in the same manner but vaginal examination can confirm the lie by feeling a shoulder or the baby's ribs. The shoulder can feel like the breech, hence the importance of having the facility to do ultrasound scans in the delivery suite.

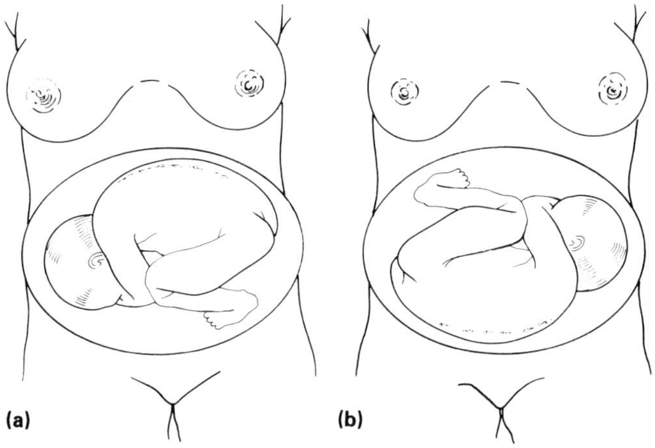

Fig. 53.8 Transverse lie. **(a)** Baby facing pelvis: pushing down the head produces flexion and makes version easy. **(b)** Baby facing maternal diaphragm: pushing down the head extends the fetal spine and makes version difficult.

Management

Provided the gestational age has been confirmed, a persistently transverse or unstable lie should be managed conservatively until 37 weeks' gestation. At that stage external cephalic version may be done and repeated at each antenatal visit until the presentation is cephalic. This is easier to perform if the baby is facing downwards (Fig. 53.8a) than if it is facing upwards (Fig. 53.8b) but should always be attempted. As the volume of amniotic fluid diminishes nearer term the uterus may close down on the fetus and hold it in a longitudinal lie. The mother must be given strict instructions to come into hospital if there is any sign of labour and many units will feel happier if they can admit her 2 or 3 weeks before term for daily observation.

There are three methods of managing these cases after 37 weeks—conservative, stabilizing induction, and elective Caesarean section.

The conservative approach involves keeping the mother in hospital in the hope that the lie will straighten either before labour or when it starts. This is expensive and disruptive to the patient's family life; there is no guarantee that the membranes will not rupture spontaneously with cord prolapse and death of the baby before an emergency Caesarean section can be undertaken.

Stabilizing induction is done by first converting the lie to a cephalic presentation, starting an oxytocin infusion and having a midwife sitting with the patient and checking the lie frequently. Once the head enters the pelvic brim the membranes are ruptured and the infusion continued. Edwards & Nicholson (1969) produced excellent results with this approach but while it works well with patients of low parity, in the grand multipara the tendency is for the membranes to rupture spontaneously before the head enters the brim and the lie then becomes oblique or reverts to transverse as the amniotic fluid drains out. Elective Caesarean section is the safest route for the baby provided it is mature. For the mother it is a major procedure but may be safer than the emergency operation necessary if either of the other modes of management is unsuccessful.

If the transverse lie is first diagnosed in labour, placenta praevia and fetal abnormality must be excluded by ultrasound, which can also sometimes demonstrate a cord in the lower segment (Lange et al 1985). Provided these other complications are not present, external version to a longitudinal lie may be attempted between contractions. The bladder is kept empty with an indwelling catheter and if the fetus remains longitudinal a normal labour is anticipated. Vaginal examination is done when the membranes rupture to exclude cord prolapse; cord prolapse or failure of the fetus to stabilize will demand immediate Caesarean section. If the diagnosis is not suspected until after the membranes have ruptured the uterus will be wrapped tightly around the baby, making abdominal palpation more difficult. Careful vaginal examination will reveal an arm, a shoulder or some ribs, all of which can be mistaken for a breech presentation. Immediate Caesarean section is essential to prevent ruptured uterus in all cases where the baby is alive and in most where it is dead.

Internal version is contraindicated even with a live fetus and intact membranes, because while the cervix may appear fully dilated, once the procedure ruptures the membranes the uterus will clamp down on the baby and the cervix will then be found to be only 6 or 7 cm dilated with subsequent entrapment of the aftercoming head.

Transverse lie in labour is most commonly found with a second twin. This differs from a singleton pregnancy in that the cervix has already been fully dilated and will not start to close down for 20 or 30 minutes. The fetal lie is checked or corrected abdominally and with rupture of the membranes, maternal effort and possibly an oxytocin infusion will push the presenting part into the pelvis and the baby will deliver. With any signs of fetal distress, internal version and then breech extraction are permissible. Helped by suitable analgesia and occasionally general anaesthesia a hand pushes up the membranes, grasps a foot and pulls it down through the membranes, tearing them as it emerges. It is important not to release amniotic fluid before grasping the foot as the uterus clamps down on the baby and by the time the foot is located attempts to turn the baby can harm it and rupture the uterus.

A compound presentation is uncommon, and is diagnosed in labour by vaginal examination. Most cases have a limb beside the fetal head. Provided the latter is descending with contractions the head usually pushes its way past the limb and labour continues normally. A high unstable presentation should be managed as for transverse lie, with repeated vaginal examinations to exclude cord prolapse and monitor alterations in the presentation.

BREECH PRESENTATION

The incidence of breech presentation varies with fetal maturity. Scheer & Newbar (1976) report a 16% incidence at 32 weeks, falling to 7% at 38 weeks and 5% at 40 weeks. Thus it should not be considered abnormal until late in pregnancy and causes no problems unless premature labour intervenes. Nearer term a breech presentation is due to something preventing spontaneous version. Fianu & Vaclavinkova (1978) stated that 78% of breech babies had cornual implantations of the placenta, compared with 4% of cephalic presentations, although Luterkort et al (1984) contested this. Where there is no such obvious pathology the lesion would appear to lie in the infant's inability to kick itself around. Thus any baby born after a breech delivery must be suspected of having some neurological impairment of its lower limbs until proved otherwise.

Faber-Nijolt and his colleagues (1983) felt that the mild neurological dysfunction found after breech birth was not always due to the vaginal delivery while O'Connell & Keane (1985) have described several inherent differences in breech babies. Torgrim & Bakke (1986) reported that breech babies have shorter cords than cephalic-presenting babies, but whether this is due to their lack of mobility or whether the short cord actually prevents them turning in utero is not clear.

The mechanism of breech labour involves the bitrochanteric diameter (9.25 cm) entering the pelvis in the transverse plane, rotating in mid-cavity and presenting at the pelvic outlet in the anterior–posterior diameter. The buttocks deliver in this position and then the whole body rotates to allow the shoulders to do exactly the same. Delivery of the anterior shoulder occurs as the head enters the pelvis in the transverse diameter, hopefully flexed as much as possible. Internal rotation then occurs so that the chin appears at the perineum, followed by the face, and then flexion allows the remainder of the skull to leave the pelvis. Thus there are no difficulties about the mechanics: the problem of a vaginal delivery is that the largest and least compressable part of the baby comes out last.

Because of the irregular outline of the breech, spontaneous rupture of the membranes may be followed by cord prolapse. This is not always as serious as in a cephalic presentation because the soft breech is less likely to compress the cord, although the cord may still go into spasm and cause acute fetal hypoxia. The ill-fitting breech can also be associated with slower labour but this appears to happen only in multiparous women (Clinch & Matthews 1985). The classical complication at the end of labour is that caused by the bitrochanteric diameter being smaller than the biparietal, so that the breech and the lower limbs can fit through a cervix or pelvis which is not sufficiently large for the aftercoming head.

The small baby is unlikely to have bony problems but as the head is relatively larger than in the mature baby it may be caught in a partially dilated cervix, causing acute asphyxia. This can happen to the larger baby, especially if a foot pressing on the maternal rectum causes the mother to push before full dilatation.

In both premature and mature babies the skull does not have sufficient time to mould when passing through the pelvis; Wigglesworth & Husemeyer (1977) have shown the danger of damage to the occipital bone which increases the possibility of intracranial haemorrhage. Nevertheless, most premature breeches suffer more from the complications of immaturity than the actual mode of delivery and good management in labour rarely allows a mature breech to get into trouble.

Diagnosis in the antenatal period should be made by abdominal palpation and if the presentation persists, ultrasound to exclude fetal abnormality and demonstrate the placental site will confirm it. Occasionally, vaginal examination in labour reveals a previously unsuspected case.

Management of breech presentation has traditionally distinguished between primigravid and multigravid mothers. While this is correct in virtually every other type of obstetric complication, it is of little value in breech because most cases are really side-effects of premature labour. Small breeches suffer from immaturity as well as from the mode of delivery and should therefore be considered separately from larger babies. A dividing line of 37 weeks is convenient to take because until that gestation no active measures are needed on account of the presentation.

Management of the preterm breech in labour

The incidence of breech presentation in babies born before 37 weeks is approximately 15%. They are not a cohesive group. Some mothers arrive with ruptured membranes or a small antepartum haemorrhage but few contractions, and yet are found a few hours later with the cervix fully dilated and a bearing-down sensation, having had no obvious labour. Others labour, but at 6 or 7 cm push the small limbs and body through the cervix, which remains insufficiently stretched to allow passage of the aftercoming head.

On admission to the delivery suite the mother's chart should be checked to see that fetal abnormality has been ruled out. Even if this is the case ultrasound must be employed to confirm it, to exclude a low-lying placenta, to make an estimate of fetal weight, and possibly to assess the presence or absence of fetal breathing which may give some indication of whether labour is likely to proceed (Besinger et al 1987). Both O'Driscoll (1977) and Anderson (1981) have reported that in up to 80% of cases where the mother thinks she is in premature labour contractions cease spontaneously and the pregnancy continues. Therefore immediate vaginal examination is contraindicated: it may introduce infection leading to chorioamnionitis or premature rupture of the membranes if these are still intact (Iams et al 1987, Sbarra et al 1987).

Nevertheless, the baby must be monitored by external techniques as in some cases the cord will be in the lower segment of the uterus and virtually prolapsed. Should contractions persist or the membranes rupture, vaginal examination may be undertaken in the expectation that the baby is going to be delivered. To prevent the mother pushing before full dilatation an epidural or caudal block should always be utilized (David & Rosen 1976, Crawford 1985). This will also relax the pelvic floor, reducing pressure on the fetal head when it passes through as well as facilitating any vaginal manoeuvre which may become necessary.

The actual delivery is the same as for a mature breech but there is some evidence that a caul delivery is better for the baby than rupturing the membranes (Goldenberg & Nelson 1984). The infant must be handled particularly gently, with a paediatrician present for the birth. Should the cervix clamp down on the head, rapid infusion of a tocolytic may relax it somewhat but this is not always available so the head should be flexed with one hand abdominally and the middle finger of the vaginal hand in the baby's mouth. Turning the baby into the transverse diameter may make it easier to deliver through the cervix. If this is unsuccessful, scissors with the intracervical blade guarded by a finger are used to incise the cervix at 4 and 8 o'clock. The previously described manoeuvre should then deliver the head. The edges of the cervical incisions are grasped with sponge-holding forceps and are usually easy to suture as the cervix hangs down into the vagina.

Caesarean section for preterm breech

Whether preterm vaginal breech delivery has any place was first questioned by Ingemarsson and his colleagues in 1978. They showed that babies delivered by Caesarean section between 1975 and 1977 had a better outlook than those born vaginally between 1971 and 1974. Other writers concurred (Duenhoelter et al 1979, Weaver 1980, Kauppila et al 1981) but Crowley and Hawkins (1980), in a review of 11 papers, indicated that while babies weighing between 1000 and 1500 g did better, the prognosis for smaller ones was not improved by an abdominal approach. Further confirmation of this soon appeared (Lamont et al 1983, Main et al 1983, Yu et al 1984, Morales & Koerten 1986). On the other hand, Cox et al (1982) found that increasing the use of Caesarean section, whatever the fetal size, carried no advantage. Olshan and his colleagues (1984) agreed, partly because their series included babies weighing 700–1500 g. Kitchen and co-workers had stated in 1982 that abdominal delivery for very small breech babies did not reduce long-term handicap and in 1985, describing infants born between 24 and 28 weeks' gestation, showed no statistical difference between the two modes of delivery. Both Rayburn et al (1983) and Effer et al in the same year came to the conclusion that the side-effects of immaturity were far more important than the mode of delivery, while Myers & Gleicher (1987) in a review of the critical factors involved in breech delivery concluded that a clearcut case had not yet been made for elective Caesarean section in any particular group of premature breech babies.

However, Canadian workers (Bodmer et al 1986) felt that since head entrapment killed 7 out of 55 premature breech babies born between 25 and 28 weeks's gestation, perhaps Caesarean section should be undertaken for all babies weighing less than 1000 g. Karp and his colleagues (1979) had already tried to distinguish between the various types of presenting part and felt that small footling breeches should always be delivered by Caesarean section, but that those with extended legs could be allowed a trial of labour.

At present it would seem sensible to consider Caesarean section in babies thought to weigh between 1000 and 1500 g, allowing the others to progress in labour and always remembering how difficult it can be to assess fully a premature breech baby in early labour.

Reporting from a hospital where the policy is to utilize abdominal delivery, Westgren et al (1985a) remarked that many cases advanced so quickly that it was not possible to estimate the baby's weight before delivery was imminent. Admitting that the study was retrospective, they had difficulty in showing that Caesarean section produced a statistically better result but reported that 25% of the deaths in the vaginally delivered group were due to head entrapment.

Management of the mature breech baby

If by 37 weeks the malpresentation persists, external cephalic version should be attempted. There is no point in considering the procedure before this gestation in view of the possibility of spontaneous version occurring. Kasule and his colleagues (1985) showed that version at various stages after 30 weeks produced no significant difference in the ultimate vaginal breech delivery, Caesarean section or perinatal mortality rates between those in whom version was attempted and controls. On the other hand several groups of workers have shown that version in the last 3 weeks of pregnancy results in a lower incidence of Caesarean section (Van Dorsten et al 1981, Hofmeyer 1983, Brocks et al 1984, Phelan et al 1985, Morrison et al 1986). All of these employed tocolytics. Dyson et al (1986) give details of dosage and point out that either ritodrine or terbutaline can be used.

The same factors which are thought to prevent spontaneous version also make external cephalic version more difficult. These are primigravidity, extended legs and firm abdominal muscles (Westgren et al 1985b) but even so, after the 37th week spontaneous version will result in only one-third of the number of cephalic presentations at term which will follow use of the external cephalic procedure (Hofmeyer et al 1986). Ferguson & Dyson (1985) even use version with tocolysis after labour has commenced. Their paper describes 22 term breeches in labour. Attempted version failed in 7 with ruptured membranes, but succeeded in 11 of the remaining cases, of whom 10 had spontaneous vaginal deliveries.

In an extensive review Savona-Ventura (1986) agrees with the concept of attempting version late in pregnancy. He reminds the reader that many authors have reported transient fetal heart irregularities after the procedure but points out that if more serious complications arise the baby is mature enough to be delivered immediately. He also points out that while there is no significant fall in perinatal mortality as a result of version, it does lower neonatal morbidity and reduces the maternal morbidity associated with Caesarean section.

An active policy of version with tocolysis cannot yet be justified in women with a history of antepartum haemorrhage, hypertension or previous Caesarean section, but there is nothing to stop them using Elkins' manoeuvre. Elkins (1982) describes 71 women with confirmed breech presentation after the 37th week of gestation. All were instructed to adopt the knee–chest position for 15 minutes every 2 hours of waking time for 5 days. A total of 65 babies underwent spontaneous version and all had normal vaginal deliveries. Of the 6 who failed to turn, 2 had low-lying placentas, 2 had unusually short cords and one mother had a bicornuate uterus. All 6 underwent Caesarean section: there were no perinatal deaths in either group and no evidence of side-effects or complications from the manoeuvre.

After the baby has been turned, patients who are rhesus-negative will need anti-D immunoglobulin. All mothers must then be seen weekly to ascertain that the cephalic presentation persists. If it does not, it must be accepted that the baby is unable to tolerate being head-down and is best left as a breech. Whatever happens it is important to monitor the baby in labour, as doing the version may well have wrapped the cord around its neck or body, which can subsequently cause problems.

Management of the persistent breech presentation

Failure of version means that a decision must be made as to whether a breech presentation should be delivered by elective Caesarean section or allowed to go into labour. During the 1970s Caesarean section was being used increasingly: in the Coombe Hospital, Dublin, it rose for breeches from 11% in 1971 to 50% in 1978. However, in 1978 Collea and his colleagues pointed out that 37% of mothers sectioned for breech experienced significant morbidity, including 10% with intraoperative complications. In 1982 Green et al reported that a Caesarean section rate increase from 22% to 94% produced no significant improvement for breech babies either in the short or long term. A review by Russell (1982) lamented the increased Caesarean section rate without giving concrete alternatives. Gimovsky et al (1983), in a preliminary report of a randomized study, recommended that the section rate should not exceed 50%, while a year later Watson and Benson produced an overall abdominal delivery rate of 36%. Despite this trend towards vaginal delivery, Flanagan and colleagues (1987) found it necessary to perform elective Caesarean section on 68% of 623 term breeches. To resolve such conflicting views it is suggested that the practising clinician should assess every mature breech in a series of simple steps, as described below.

Abdominal palpation, done by an experienced obstetrician, may occasionally indicate that the infant is so large that elective Caesarean section is justified. Ultrasound, after excluding abnormality, should be used to estimate the fetal weight. If this is more than 4000 g, again a Caesarean section may be indicated. The fetal attitude is also important and even with a small baby, extension of the head is an unfavourable finding. Westgren et al (1981) reported an incidence of 7.4% neck extension in a series of breeches. There was a 22% incidence of neurological problems in these babies if delivered vaginally, but none after Caesarean section. They advocated abdominal delivery if the neck was extended to any degree.

Ballas et al (1978) had already made the same point, defining four grades of deflexion. They felt that section was required only in those where the angle between the cervical and thoracic spine was greater than 90°. Mention has already been made of the head of a breech baby differing from one delivered with a cephalic presentation; it is important when doing ultrasound not to diagnose retarded intrauterine growth on the basis of biparietal measurements, which Kasby & Poll (1982) have shown to be relatively smaller in the breech than in a baby presenting head first.

X-ray pelvimetry should be used in patients not so far chosen for elective section, even if they have had a previous vaginal delivery of a good-sized baby. Ridley et al (1982) have shown that neonates whose mothers underwent a radiological assessment of their pelvis were fitter than those in whom this was not done, whatever the eventual route of delivery.

The simplest method is a standing lateral X-ray of the pelvis; Gimovsky et al (1985), along with Adam and his co-workers (1985), have shown that digital radiography is more accurate than conventional techniques and, like computerized tomography, results in less fetal and maternal irradiation (Kopelman et al 1986). Presumably magnetic resonance imaging will be used in the future, which may prove interesting as the pelvic dimensions will probably be slightly larger if the patient is lying down.

Whatever method is used it is essential that a picture should be seen by the obstetrician in charge. While the radiologist will give accurate measurements, the shape of the pelvis must be taken into consideration. A well-curved sacrum supplies a large pelvic cavity but if the upper anterior surface is flat, any part of the baby negotiating the brim has to pass down a tunnel, as opposed to slipping between two narrow points. On occasion, the anterior surfaces of the first and second sacral vertebrae are so prominent that they actually produce funnelling in the upper pelvis (Fig. 53.9). To a lesser extent, the size of the sacrosciatic notch will indicate pelvic adequacy. Should any of these unfavourable features be present or if the anterior–posterior diameter of either the inlet or the outlet is less than 11.5 cm, Caesarean section may be indicated.

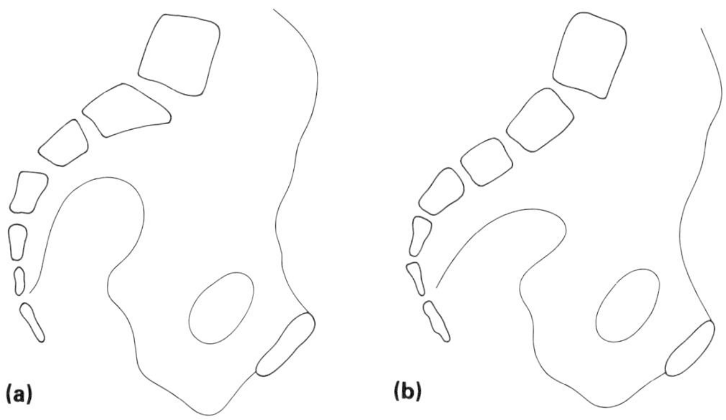

Fig. 53.9 Lateral view of pelves with identical inlet measurements. However, (**a**) has a good sacral curve so that once the brim is negotiated there is adequate space, while (**b**) has a straight sacrum so the head has to travel to mid-cavity before there is extra space.

Using more extensive radiology, Westin (1977) has described a scoring system for calculating which breech babies will require elective Caesarean section. This will appeal to some units. On the other hand, Clinch & Matthews (1985) have pointed out that while the procedures mentioned here will select approximately 25% of breeches for section before labour, even if they fail to pick out a baby who is too large for vaginal delivery this usually leads to lack of progress in labour and an intrapartum section without adverse effects. Thus it is safe to allow a trial of labour in term breeches provided it is competently supervised, and that the unit in which it takes place is adequately equipped and staffed so that if it fails, the fact that the subsequent section is undertaken on an emergency rather than an elective basis is unlikely to increase maternal morbidity or mortality (Bingham & Lilford 1987).

Inducing labour prematurely in an attempt to achieve a smaller baby would have to be done so early in the pregnancy that the chances of successful induction would be much reduced. Induction for other reasons is not totally contraindicated but most obstetricians would regard two pregnancy complications as a reason for Caesarean section.

Management of labour in the mature breech

Once labour commences cervical dilatation and descent of the breech should be plotted on a partogram, as with a cephalic presentation. Vaginal examination is done to exclude cord prolapse and to confirm whether the breech is flexed or extended, while a monitoring clip is attached to the buttock. Rupture of the membranes along with an oxytocin infusion is permissible in a fully assessed patient, provided the procedures are used to accelerate a dilatory labour in its early stages rather than to drive an over-sized breech through the pelvis (Beazley et al 1975). As with premature breeches, epidural anaesthesia both relieves pain and prevents the mother pushing involuntarily before full dilatation. Failure of the cervix to dilate at a standard rate or of the breech to descend should be accepted as indicating that the baby is larger (or the pelvis smaller) than the prelabour assessment had implied, and Caesarean section will be required. There is no need to encourage maternal efforts immediately the cervix is fully dilated but once she does start pushing, failure of the breech to descend should lead to section rather than breech extraction. The bitrochanteric diameter is usually a little smaller than the biparietal; if the former does not pass easily through the pelvis, neither will the latter.

Provided labour progresses satisfactorily preparation should be made for an assisted breech delivery. This involves a standard forceps trolley on which there is also a sterile razor and a scalpel with a no. 1 blade. The mother is in the lithotomy position with a wedge under one side of the buttocks if she has an epidural. If not, it will be necessary to infiltrate the perineum and preferably do a pudendal block once the breech has descended on to it. Episiotomy is essential but is reserved until the fetal anus has appeared at the vulva. Once done, maternal effort should deliver the baby's buttocks and, with flexed legs, the lower limbs. With extended legs the operator will have to flex each knee joint separately, pushing it to the side of the baby so that the foot pops out.

The mother is encouraged to bear down until the trunk up to the scapula becomes visible. Cord pulsation is checked and a small loop pulled down to prevent a tight cord impeding further progress. The mother is asked to push again and the shoulders should deliver one at a time, along with the arms folded over the chest.

Failure of the shoulders to deliver is dealt with by lifting up the baby's legs and trunk, which enables a finger to reach an elbow joint; flexing it, and delivering it across the chest. This is repeated for the other side. Gentle rotation of the fetal trunk at the same time will assist this manoeuvre. Rarely, the baby's abdomen is facing the operator: if so, the trunk is turned and as the mother pushes, one shoulder will deliver under the symphysis with further rotation producing the other. With extended arms it is necessary to slide an index finger along the baby's scapula over the shoulder and down into the antecubital fossa to deliver the elbow between the body and the side of the vulva. These manoeuvres virtually always deliver the shoulders.

If case selection has been good, at this stage the baby's head may start to appear without any further effort on the operator's part. He or she should attempt to apply forceps to control the speed of delivery but if this is not possible

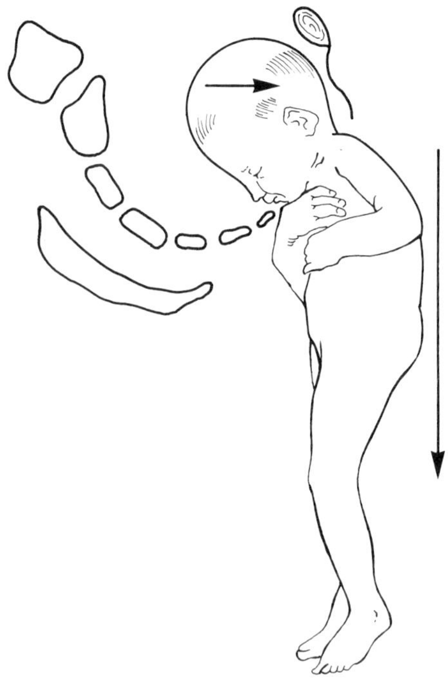

Fig. 53.10 Trunk of breech allowed to hang. Traction on fetal spine will extend not flex the head. Contrast this with Figure 53.2.

the legs may be swung out and up in a Burns Marshall manoeuvre, keeping the vulva completely covered with the other hand. It is essential that the baby's legs should be kept vertically in the air and the weight taken off the cervical spine. Hyperextension of the neck with the body being held over the mother's abdomen will occlude the vertebral arteries and can lead to necrosis of the cervical cord. Excess weight on the cervical spine will either have the same effect or dislocate the baby's neck. The operator's vulval hand can then be opened slowly to allow first the baby's face and then the remainder of the head to deliver. The latter should be supported while the operator sits down with the baby across his or her knee.

Should maternal effort not push down the head, more assistance is needed as the occiput must be low enough in the pelvis to hinge around the back of the symphysis and not be caught above it. Simply permitting the baby to hang may delay progress: the manoeuvre can cause extension rather than flexion of the head as the head swivels on an axis through the biparietal eminences (Fig. 53.10). Therefore, while the baby is hanging feet down, the operator must insert two fingers behind the symphysis pubis to push up an anterior lip of cervix which is often dragged down by the occiput and will slow its final descent (Fig. 53.11). This will also tend to flex the head, an action which can be further assisted either by some suprapubic pressure or by renewed maternal effort or by both. Once the hair line is visible the head is delivered. The baby's feet are grasped and, using as much traction as required to keep the body straight and take weight off its neck, they are swung outwards and

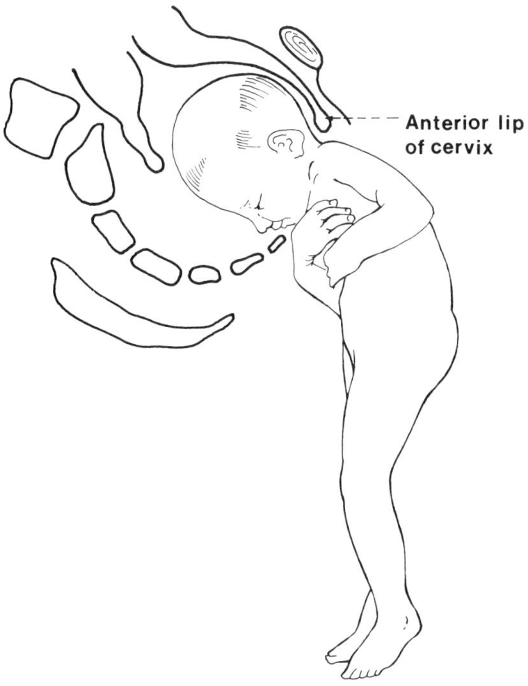

Fig. 53.11 Hanging breech. Anterior lip of cervix pulled down by occiput must be pushed up before forceps can be applied.

upwards to be held by an assistant, using a towel to make certain they do not slip. The operator then applies a Neville Barnes forceps and delivers the head slowly, sucking out the mouth as soon as it can be seen and remembering that the final part of the head only appears as the face flexes on to the chest.

Problems

Shoulder dystocia rarely occurs without extended arms; this has usually been caused by traction on the fetus early in the delivery. The body is pulled down leaving the arms behind rather than the uterus pushing down the whole fetus in a flexed attitude. Often the arms can be brought down as already described but lack of success means that Lovset's manoeuvre will be required. The classical procedure comprises three rotations but the fewer done the better, as each involves traction and rotation of the whole body. The baby must be held by the thighs—never by the trunk—and the operator must wrap the legs in a towel so that they do not slip when gripped.

Should the head not enter the pelvis after the shoulders have delivered, the baby's body must be turned sideways and suprapubic pressure used to flex the head and push it into the pelvis. This may be helped on occasions by the vaginal hand inserting a finger into the baby's mouth to flex it. Both these actions also make the head descend if it has entered the pelvis but is still not low enough to apply forceps.

Continued failure of the head to engage is the sole indication for symphysiotomy. The technique is described by Hartfield (1973), Philpott (1980) and Gebbie (1982), although the latter points out that in a mature baby, if the head is not going to fit through the pelvis the buttocks too should be obstructed. With proper predelivery assessment the technique will never be necessary, nor should such bizarre measures as replacing the body of the baby and proceeding to Caesarean section, as described by Iffy et al (1986), although their case probably succeeded only because the uterus was still distended by the second twin. Such potential disasters emphasize the importance of delivery suites having the facilities available to make rapid assessment in unbooked or unsuspected breech deliveries (Davis & Brunfield 1984).

Mauriceau Smellie Veit is favoured by some obstetricians for routine delivery of the head. While a finger in the mouth may cause flexion, traction on the cervical spine will do the opposite. Combined, they can draw the base of the skull away from the vault, stretching the falx cerebri and producing a perfect way of tearing the tentorium cerebelli as well as causing brachial plexus injuries. The manoeuvre is best avoided. On the other hand, inexperienced operators can forget that unlike a conventional forceps application, a breech delivery means that the smallest part of the baby's skull appears at the vulva first with the large parietal area at the back of the pelvis. Thus, if the forceps handle is straightened out too soon after insertion of the blade, the distal part of the blade will dig into the side of the baby's head and it will not be possible to lock the handles. The tip must be kept pointed at the sacrum for as long as possible, which means that the guiding hand has to be inserted well into the vagina until the tip has passed round the occiput. Properly trained obstetricians can manage this: those taught simply to open the labia (Fig. 53.12) will find the correct application virtually impossible.

Caesarean section for abnormal positions and presentations

Abdominal delivery for fetal malposition or malpresentation often takes place at the end of a long labour and may technically be more difficult than with a normal presentation. Although there is no need to use any of the more complicated extraperitoneal approaches which are occasionally suggested (Wallace et al 1984), there should always be someone experienced scrubbed up in theatre; the operating table must be tilted laterally or a simple wedge inserted under the mother's right buttock (Endler & Donath 1985) and a paediatrician skilled in neonatal resuscitation should be present. Several other points are worth emphasizing.

Occipito-posterior positions

However high the head feels on vaginal examination, at Caesarean section it can be difficult to extricate from the pelvis and an assistant must be scrubbed up ready to push it up

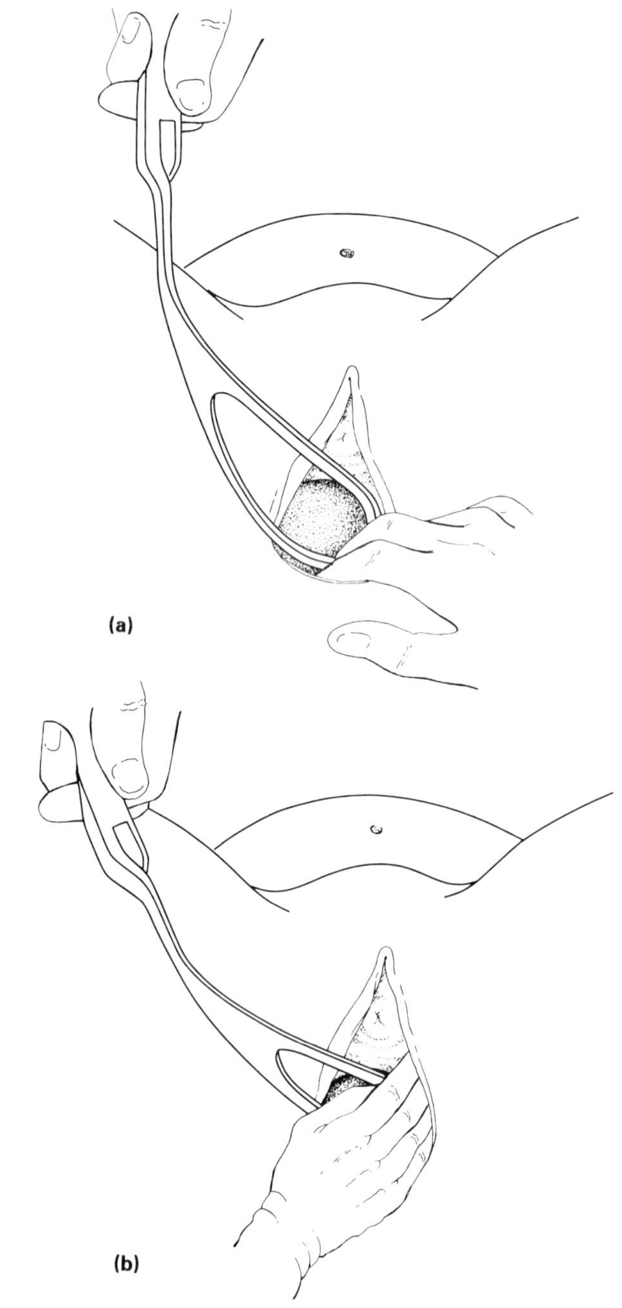

Fig. 53.12 Application of forceps. (**a**) Incorrect method. As the handle is straightened the tip of the blade will catch on the side of the baby's head, thus preventing application. (**b**) Correct method. The hand must be inserted alongside the fetal head to guide the tip around the head.

vaginally. It must be assumed that the lower segment of the uterus will be thin and may tear readily. Therefore the surgeon should make the uterine incision fairly high in the lower segment so that if it does extend downwards the subsequent repair will be easier. He or she should aim to insert a hand around the side of the baby's head and deliver it slowly out of the pelvis before bringing it anteriorly through the wound. In this way the head is flexed, with the chin going on to the baby's chest. Tears arise because the chin catches on the upper edge of the wound and as the face, followed by the brow, the vertex, and finally the occiput deliver, the lower edge is stretched to allow passage of these large diameters and often splits. Such lacerations are never easy to repair and occasionally involve the base of the bladder. The same comments apply to face and brow presenting parts, where the diameters may be even larger and, especially with the brow, the labour may have become obstructed, leading to excess thinning of the lower segment and occasionally a constriction ring.

Transverse lie

With intact membranes the operator has the choice of looking for the baby's head and steering it quickly into the incision as the uterus clamps down when the amniotic fluid rushes out. In practice, a limb appears in the incision: usually this is an arm. It should be replaced quickly, a leg grasped and the baby extracted as a breech. Many operators choose a breech delivery as a first option, pushing the membranes in front of the operating hand, finding a limb, palpating its lower end to make certain it is a foot and withdrawing it through the incision just as the amniotic fluid starts to escape.

With a transverse lie and already ruptured membranes the lower segment of the uterus will be so narrow that a conventional incision would not be large enough for any baby. The anaesthetist should be asked to give a rapid dose of a uterine relaxant for 2 or 3 minutes (Akamatsu 1975, Maduska 1981). Jovanovic (1985) has made the point that if the uterine incision is enlarged by cutting rather than tearing, with the extremes of the incision pointing upwards rather than laterally, then not only will the aperture be larger but any extension will go upwards rather than downwards and be easier to repair. Should these measures not be successful the operator has no choice but to proceed to enlarge the incision vertically from its middle point, making an inverted T incision. To avoid the possibility of this, many obstetricians regard transverse lie with ruptured membranes as almost the sole remaining indication for the classical operation. Here, the bladder should be pushed down and the incision brought as far as possible into the lower segment and only extended upwards as needed.

In all cases the inside of the uterus must be inspected to exclude an abnormality such as a small septum or a fibroid which might have caused the transverse lie. This is carefully noted in the patient's chart for future reference, along with inspection of the ovaries and tubes, to rule out other tumours which may have had the same effect.

Premature breech

If the baby is very small the lower segment may not have formed. Although Haesslein & Goodlin (1979) proposed solving this problem by using a classical incision, most other workers do not agree with them. Westgren et al (1982) advocated a bolus of uterine relaxant, probably terbutaline, just before opening the uterus, although Westgren later modified this when writing with Paul in 1985, suggesting that the lower segment should be carefully examined and in some cases a vertical incision performed. Hobel & Oakes (1980) thought that halothane at the induction of anaesthesia was best for all small section babies. Schutterman & Grimes (1983), reviewing 416 breeches of all gestations allocated randomly to transverse or low vertical incisions, found no advantages for low vertical incisions.

It would appear that the normal lower segment transverse incision, with an added uterine relaxant in some cases, is satisfactory for breech section. Whatever incision is used the baby must be delivered as gently as with the vaginal approach: forceps are essential for the aftercoming head. In order that no part of the baby is caught in the abdominal wound the incision should be sufficiently big to take the beak of a large, not just a small, Doyen retractor.

Section for mature breech should produce no technical difficulties but forceps are advisable for controlling delivery of the aftercoming head. The remarks made earlier about not hyperextending or placing too much weight on the cervical spine apply equally forcibly.

THE NEWBORN BABY

All babies born after abnormal presentations or positions require a thorough paediatric examination even if the delivery was spontaneous and however well they may appear at the time. The unusual moulding due to the abnormal position of the head or the speed of this moulding may cause intracranial lesions. Some will have had operative vaginal deliveries which, however easy they may seem to the attendant, are more traumatic for the fetus. Above all, there is always the suspicion that the malpresentation or the malposition has been due to some abnormality in the fetus. This is especially so in the case of the breech baby. Many of these will be premature and paediatric assessment will be routine in any case.

In the mature breech, it should be assumed until proved otherwise that some inherent defect in the baby prevented it from turning a somersault in utero; one looks forward to studies assessing whether those in whom external version has been successful suffer from the same disabilities.

Above all, it is important to be aware that not all neonatal deficiencies are due to the mode of delivery or to incorrect obstetrical management in labour. Illingworth (1985) stressed that most cases of cerebral palsy or mental subnormality follow a normal pregnancy and delivery: to ascribe brain damage solely to events occurring during labour is too simplistic.

THE FUTURE

Abnormal presentations and positions will continue to arise in obstetrical practice. It is essential that labour ward routines should be constantly updated to counteract the adverse effects of abnormal presentations on both mother and child. Fetal assessment by cardiotocography and pH estimations is accepted, but Modanlou and his coworkers (1982) feel that it is important to establish the relationship between the whole baby and the maternal pelvis. The authors point out that the average fetal size is increasing and that more effort should be made to diagnose macrosomia at term. Knowledge of the chest circumference and its ratio to head size should reduce the incidence of shoulder dystocia and contribute to a fall in the number of difficult vaginal deliveries. All labours are trials: one looks forward to the day when the result can be forecast accurately in every labouring woman.

REFERENCES

Acker D B, Sachs B P, Friedman E A 1985 Risk factors for shoulder dystocia. Obstetrics and Gynecology 66: 762–768

Acker D B, Sachs B P, Friedman E A 1986 Risk factors for shoulder dystocia in the average-weight infant. Obstetrics and Gynecology 67: 614–618

Adam P, Alberge Y, Castellano S, Kassab M, Escude V 1985 Pelvimetry by digital radiography. Clinical Radiology 36: 327–330

Akamatsu T J 1975 Anaesthesia for Caesarean section. Clinics in Obstetrics and Gynaecology 2: 647–659

Anderson A B M 1981 Second thoughts on stopping labour. In: Studd J (ed) Progress in obstetrics and gynaecology, vol I. Churchill Livingstone, Edinburgh, pp 125–138

Arulkumaran S, Gibb D M F, Ratnam S S, Lun K C, Heng S H 1985 Total uterine activity in induced labour—an index of cervical and pelvic tissue resistance. British Journal of Obstetrics and Gynaecology 92: 693–697

Ballas S, Toaff R, Jaffa A J 1978 Deflexion of the fetal head in breech presentation. Incidence, management, and outcome. Obstetrics and Gynecology 52: 653–655

Bates R G, Helm C W, Duncan A, Edmonds D K 1985 Uterine activity in the second stage of labour and the effect of epidural analgesia. British Journal of Obstetrics and Gynaecology 92: 1246–1250

Beazley J M, Banovic I, Feld M S 1975 Maintenance of labour. BritishMedical Journal 2: 248–250

Benedetti T J, Gabbe S G 1978 Shoulder dystocia. A complication of fetal macrosomia and prolonged second stage of labor with midpelvic delivery. Obstetrics and Gynecology 52: 526–529

Berkus M D, Ramamurthy R S, O'Connor P S, Brown K, Hayashi R H 1985 Cohort study of silastic obstetric vacuum cup deliveries: I. Safety of the instrument. Obstetrics and Gynecology 66: 503–509

Berkus M D, Ramamurthy R S, O'Connor P S, Brown K J, Hayashi R H 1986 Cohort study of silastic obstetric vacuum cup deliveries. II. Unsuccessful vacuum extraction. Obstetrics and Gynecology 68: 662–666

Besinger R, Compton A, Hayashi R 1987 The presence of fetal breathing movements as a predictor of outcome in preterm labour. American Journal of Obstetrics and Gynecology 157: 753–757

Bingham P, Lilford R J 1987 Management of the selected term breech presentation: assessment of the risks of selected vaginal delivery versus caesarean section for all cases. Obstetrics and Gynecology 69: 965–977

Bodmer B, Benjamin A, McLean F H, Usher R H 1986 Has caesarean section reduced the risks of delivery in the preterm breech presentation? American Journal of Obstetrics and Gynecology 154: 244–250

Bottoms S F, Hirsch V J, Sokol R J 1987 Medical management of arrest

disorders of labor: a current overview. American Journal of Obstetrics and Gynecology 156: 935–939
Brocks V, Philipsen T, Secher N J 1984 A randomized trial of external cephalic version with tocolysis in late pregnancy. British Journal of Obstetrics and Gynaecology 91: 653–656
Calvert J P, Newcombe R G, Hibbard R M 1982 An assessment of radiotelemetry in the monitoring of labour. British Journal of Obstetrics and Gynaecology 89: 285–291
Cardozo L D, Gibb D M F, Studd J W W, Cooper D J 1983 Should we abandon Kielland's forceps? British Medical Journal 287: 315–317
Carter V 1986 Another technique for resolution of shoulder dystocia. American Journal of Obstetrics and Gynecology 154: 964
Chalmers I 1984 Trends and variations in the use of caesarean delivery. In: Clinch J, Matthews T (eds) Perinatal Medicine. MTP Press, Lancaster, p 145
Chalmers J A 1968 The management of malrotation of the occiput. Journal of Obstetrics and Gynaecology of the British Commonwealth 75: 889–891
Chiswick M L 1980 Forceps delivery—neonatal outcome. In: Beard R W, Paintin D B (eds) Outcome of obstetric intervention in Britain. RCOG, London, pp 33–41
Chiswick M L, James D K 1979 Kielland's forceps: association with neonatal morbidity and mortality. British Medical Journal 1: 7–9
Clinch J, Matthews T 1985 The obstetric management of the mature breech. In: Clinch J, Matthews T (eds) Perinatal medicine. MTP Press, Lancaster, pp 213–217
Coats P M, Chan K K, Wilkins M, Beard R J 1980 A comparison between midline and mediolateral episiotomies. British Journal of Obstetrics and Gynaecology 87: 408–412
Cohen W R 1977 Influence of the duration of second stage labor on perinatal outcome and puerperal morbidity. Obstetrics and Gynecology 49: 266–269
Collea J V, Rabin S C, Weghorst G R, Quilligan E J 1978 The randomized management of term frank breech presentation: vaginal delivery versus cesarean section. American Journal of Obstetrics and Gynecology 131: 186–195
Cox C, Kendall A C, Hommers M 1982 Changed prognosis of breech-presenting low birthweight infants. British Journal of Obstetrics and Gynaecology 89: 881–886
Crawford J S 1985 Lumbar epidural analgesia for labour and delivery: a personal view. In: Studd J (ed) The management of labour. Blackwell Scientific Publications, Oxford, pp 226–234
Crowley P, Hawkins D F 1980 Review: premature breech delivery—the caesarean section debate. Journal of Obstetrics and Gynaecology 1: 2–6
Cruikshank D P, Cruikshank J E 1981 Face and brow presentation: a review. Clinical Obstetrics and Gynecology 24: 333–351
Cyr R M, Usher R H, McLean F H 1984 Changing patterns of birth asphyxia and trauma over 20 years. American Journal of Obstetrics and Gynecology 148: 490–498
David H, Rosen M 1976 Perinatal mortality after epidural analgesia. Anaesthesia 31: 1054–1059
Davis R O, Brunfield C G 1984 The use of real-time ultrasound in the management of obstetric emergencies. Clinical Obstetrics and Gynecology 27: 68–77
Dierker L J, Rosen M G, Thompson K, Lynn P 1986 Midforceps deliveries: long-term outcome of infants. American Journal of Obstetrics and Gynecology 154: 764–766
Drife J O 1983 Kielland or Caesar? British Medical Journal 287: 309–310
Duenhoelter J H, Wells E, Reich J S, Santos-Ramos R, Jimenez J M 1979 A paired controlled study of vaginal and abdominal delivery of low birth weight breech fetus. Obstetrics and Gynecology 54: 310–313
Dumoulin J G, Foulkes J E 1984 Ketonuria during labour. British Journal of Obstetrics and Gynaecology 91: 97–98
Dunn P M 1978 Posture in labour. Lancet i: 496–497
Dyack C 1980 Rotational forceps in midforceps delivery. Obstetrics and Gynecology 56: 123–126
Dyson D C, Ferguson J E, Hensleigh P 1986 Antepartum external version under tocolysis. Obstetrics and Gynecology 67: 63–68
Edwards R L, Nicholson H O 1969 The management of the unstable lie in late pregnancy. Journal of Obstetrics and Gynaecology of the British Commonwealth 76: 713–718
Effer S B, Saigal S, Rand C et al 1983 Effect of delivery method on outcomes in the very low-birth weight breech infant: is the improved survival related to cesarean section or other perinatal care maneuvers? American Journal of Obstetrics and Gynecology 145: 123–128
Elkins V H 1982 Procedure for turning breech. In: Enkin M, Chalmers I (eds) Effectiveness and satisfaction in antenatal care. Spastic International Medical Publishers, London, p 216
Endler G C, Donath R W 1985 Inflation device to prevent aortocaval compression during pregnancy. Anesthesia and Analgesia 64: 1015–1016
Faber-Nijholt R, Huisjes H J, Touwen B C L, Fidler V J 1983 Neurological follow-up of 281 children born in breech presentation: a controlled study. British Medical Journal 286: 9–12
Ferguson J E, Dyson D C 1985 Intrapartum external cephalic version. American Journal of Obstetrics and Gynecology 152: 297–298
Fianu S, Vaclavinkova V 1978 The site of placental attachment as a factor in the aetiology of breech presentation. Acta Obstetricia et Gynecologica Scandinavica 57: 371–372
Flanagan T A, Mulchahey K M, Korenbrot C C, Green J R, Laros R K 1987 Management of term breech presentation. American Journal of Obstetrics and Gynecology 156: 1492–1502
Floberg J, Belfrage P, Ohlsen H 1987 Influence of pelvic outlet capacity on labor. A prospective pelvimetry study of 1429 selected primiparae. Acta Obstetricia et Gynecologica Scandinavica 66: 121–126
Flynn A M, Kelly J, Hollins G, Lynch P F 1978 Ambulation in labour. British Medical Journal 2: 591–593
Friedman E A, Sachtleben M R, Bresky P A 1977 Dysfunctional labor. American Journal of Obstetrics and Gynecology 127: 779–783
Gebbie D 1982 Symphysiotomy. Clinics in Obstetrics and Gynaecology 9: 663–683
Gibb D M F, Arulkumaran S, Lun K C, Ratnam S S 1984 Characteristics of uterine activity in nulliparous labour. British Journal of Obstetrics and Gynaecology 91: 220–227
Gibb D M F, Arulkumaran S, Ratnam S S 1985 A comparative study of methods of oxytocin administration for induction of labour. British Journal of Obstetrics and Gynaecology 92: 688–692
Gilstrap L C, Hauth J C, Toussaint S 1984 Cesarean section: changing incidence and indications. Obstetrics and Gynecology 63: 205–208
Gimovsky M L, Wallace R L, Schifrin B S, Paul R H 1983 Randomised management of non frank breech presentation at term: a preliminary report. American Journal of Obstetrics and Gynecology 146: 34–40
Gimovsky M L, Willard K, Neglio M, Howard T, Zerne S 1985 X-ray pelvimetry in a breech protocol: a comparison of digital radiography and conventional methods. American Journal of Obstetrics and Gynecology 153: 887–888
Goldenberg R L, Nelson K G 1984 The unanticipated breech presentation in labor. Clinical Obstetrics and Gynecology 27: 95–105
Goodfellow C F, Hull M G R, Swaab D F, Dogterom J, Buijs R M 1983 Oxytocin deficiency at delivery with epidural analgesia. British Journal of Obstetrics and Gynaecology 90: 214–219
Goodlin R C 1986 Modified manual rotation in midpelvic delivery. Obstetrics and Gynecology 67: 128–130
Grant A 1986 Repair of episiotomies and perineal tears. British Journal of Obstetrics and Gynaecology 93: 417–419
Green J F, McLean F, Smith L P, Usher R 1982 Has an increased cesarean section rate for term breech delivery reduced the incidence of birth asphyxia, trauma, and death? American Journal of Obstetrics and Gynecology 142: 643–648
Greis J B, Bierniarz J, Scommegna A 1981 Comparison of maternal and fetal effects of vacuum extraction with forceps or cesarean deliveries. Obstetrics and Gynecology 57: 571–577
Gross S J, Shime J, Farin D 1987 Shoulder dystocia: predictors and outcome. American Journal of Obstetrics and Gynecology 156: 334–336
Haesslein H C, Goodlin R C 1979 Delivery of the tiny newborn. American Journal of Obstetrics and Gynecology 134: 192–197
Halme J, Ekbladh L 1982 The vacuum extractor for obstetric delivery. Clinical Obstetrics and Gynecology 25: 167–175
Harris B A 1984 Shoulder dystocia. Clinical Obstetrics and Gynecology 27: 106–111
Hartfield V J 1973 A comparison of the early and late effects of subcutaneous symphysiotomy and of lower segment caesarean section. Journal of Obstetrics and Gynaecology of the British Commonwealth 80: 508–514
Healy D L, Quinn M A, Pepperell R J 1982 Rotational delivery of the fetus: Kielland's forceps and two other methods compared. British Journal of Obstetrics and Gynaecology 89: 501–506

Hobel C J, Oakes G K 1980 Special considerations in the management of preterm labor. Clinical Obstetrics and Gynecology 23: 147–164
Hofmeyr G J 1983 Effect of external cephalic version in late pregnancy on breech presentation and caesarean section rate: a controlled trial. British Journal of Obstetrics and Gynaecology 90: 392–399
Hofmeyr G J, Sadan O, Myer I G, Galal K C, Simko G 1986 External cephalic version and spontaneous version rates: ethnic and other determinants. British Journal of Obstetrics and Gynaecology 93: 13–16
Holmberg N G, Lilieqvist B, Magnusson S, Segerbrand E 1977 The influence of the bony pelvis in persistent occiput posterior position. Acta Obstetricia et Gynecologica Scandinavica 66: (suppl) 49–54
Iams J D, Clapp D H, Contos D A, Whitehurst R, Ayers L, O'Shaughnessy R W 1987 Does extra-amniotic infection cause preterm labor? Gas–liquid chromatography studies of amniotic fluid in amnionitis, preterm labour, and normal controls. Obstetrics and Gynecology 70: 365–368
Iffy L, Apuzzio J J, Cohen-Addad N, Zwolska-Demczuk B, Francis-Lane M, Olenczak J 1986 Abdominal rescue after entrapment of the aftercoming head. American Journal of Obstetrics and Gynecology 154: 623–624
Illingworth R S 1985 A paediatrician asks—why is it called birth injury? British Journal of Obstetrics and Gynaecology 92: 122–130
Ingemarsson I, Westgren M, Svenningsen N W 1978 Long-term follow-up of preterm infants in breech presentation delivered by caesarean section. Lancet ii: 172–175
Isager-Sally L, Legarth J, Jacobsen B, Bostofte E 1986 Episiotomy repair—immediate and long-term sequelae. A prospective randomised study of three different methods of repair. British Journal of Obstetrics and Gynaecology 93: 420–425
Jovanovic R 1985 Incisions of the pregnant uterus and delivery of low-birth weight infants. American Journal of Obstetrics and Gynecology 152: 971–974
Joyce D N, Giwa-Osagie F, Stevenson G W 1975 Occasional survey: role of pelvimetry in active management of labour. British Medical Journal 4: 505–507
Kadar N, Romero R 1983 Prognosis for future childbearing after midcavity instrumental deliveries in primigravidas. Obstetrics and Gynecology 62: 166–170
Kadar N, Cruddas M, Campbell S 1986 Estimating the probability of spontaneous delivery conditional on time spent in the second stage. British Journal of Obstetrics and Gynaecology 93: 568–576
Karp L E, Doney J R, McCarthy T, Meis P J, Hall M 1979 The premature breech: trial of labor or Cesarean section? Obstetrics and Gynecology 53: 88–92
Kasby C B, Poll K 1982 The breech head and its ultrasound significance. British Journal of Obstetrics and Gynaecology 89: 106–110
Kasule J, Chimbira T H K, Brown I McL 1985 Controlled trial of external cephalic version. British Journal of Obstetrics and Gynaecology 92: 14–18
Kauppila O, Gronroos M, Aro P, Aittoniemi P, Kuoppala M 1981 Management of low birth-weight breech delivery: should Cesarean section be routine? Obstetrics and Gynecology 57: 289–294
Kirwan P 1983 Oxytocin and the second stage of labour. Irish Journal of Medical Science 152: 201–202
Kitchen W H, Yu V Y H, Orgill A A et al 1982 Infants born before 29 weeks' gestation: survival and morbidity at 2 years of age. British Journal of Obstetrics and Gynaecology 89: 887–891
Kitchen W, Ford G W, Doyle L W et al 1985 Cesarean section or vaginal delivery at 24 to 28 weeks' gestation: comparison of survival and neonatal and 2-year morbidity. Obstetrics and Gynecology 66: 149–157
Kopleman J N, Duff P, Karl R T, Schipul A H, Read J A 1986 Computed tomographic pelvimetry in the evaluation of breech presentation. Obstetrics and Gynecology 68: 455–458
Lamont R F, Dunlop P D M, Crowley P, Elder M G 1983 Spontaneous preterm labour and delivery at under 34 weeks' gestation. British Medical Journal 286: 454–457
Lange I R, Manning F A, Morrison I, Chamberlain P F, Harman C R 1985 Cord prolapse: is antenatal diagnosis possible? American Journal of Obstetrics and Gynecology 151: 1083–1085
Lowe B 1987 Fear of failure: a place for the trial of instrumental delivery. British Journal of Obstetrics and Gynaecology 94: 60–66
Lupe P J, Gross T L 1986 Maternal upright posture and mobility in labor—a review. Obstetrics and Gynecology 67: 727–734
Luterkort M, Persson P, Weldner B 1984 Maternal and fetal factors in breech presentation. Obstetrics and Gynecology 64: 55–59
Maduska A L 1981 Inhalation analgesia and general anesthesia. Clinical Obstetrics and Gynecology 24: 619–633
Main D M, Main E K, Maurer M M 1983 Cesarean section versus vaginal delivery for the breech fetus weighing less than 1500 grams. American Journal of Obstetrics and Gynecology 146: 580–584
Maresh M, Choong K H, Beard R W 1983 Delayed pushing with lumbar epidural analgesia in labour. British Journal of Obstetrics and Gynaecology 90: 623–627
McManus T J, Calder A A 1978a Upright posture and the efficiency of labour. Lancet i: 72–74
McManus T J, Calder A A 1978b Posture in labour. Lancet i: 1041
Modanlou H D, Komatsu G, Dorchester W, Freeman R K, Bosu S K 1982 Large-for-gestational-age neonates: anthropometric reasons for shoulder dystocia. Obstetrics and Gynecology 60: 417–423
Moolgaoker A S, Ahamed S O S, Payne P R 1979 A comparison of different methods of instrumental delivery based on electronic measurements of compression and traction. Obstetrics and Gynecology 54: 299–309
Moore R 1970 Evolution. Life Nature Library. Time–Life International (Nederland), NV, p 165
Morales W J, Koerten J 1986 Obstetric management and intraventricular hemorrhage in very-low-birth-weight infants. Obstetrics and Gynecology 68: 35–40
Morgan B 1972 The descent of woman. Souvenir Press, London, pp 21–42
Morgan B M, Bulpitt C J, Clifton P, Lewis P J 1982 Occasional survey: analgesia and satisfaction in childbirth (the Queen Charlotte's 1000 mother survey). Lancet ii: 808–811
Morrison J C, Myatt R E, Martin J N et al 1986 External cephalic version of the breech presentation under tocolysis. American Journal of Obstetrics and Gynecology 154: 900–903
Morton K E, Jackson M C, Gillmer M D G 1985 A comparison of the effects of four intravenous solutions for the treatment of ketonuria during labour. British Journal of Obstetrics and Gynaecology 92: 473–479
Myers S A, Gleicher N 1987 Breech delivery: why the dilemma? American Journal of Obstetrics and Gynecology 156: 6–10
Myerscough P R 1982 Occipitoposterior positions of the vertex. In: Munro Kerr's operative obstetrics, 10th edn. Baillière Tindall, London, pp 50–60
O'Brien F, Cefalo R C 1982 Evaluation of X-ray pelvimetry and abnormal labor. Clinical Obstetrics and Gynecology 25: 157–164
O'Connell P, Keane A 1985 The term breech: subsequent growth and development. In: Clinch J, Matthews T (eds) Perinatal medicine. MTP Press, Lancaster, p 219
O'Driscoll K 1977 Discussion. In: Anderson A, Beard R, Brudenell M, Dunn P M (eds) Preterm labour. RCOG, London, pp 369–370
O'Driscoll K, Meagher D, MacDonald D, Geoghegan F 1981 Traumatic intracranial haemorrhage in firstborn infants and delivery with obstetric forceps. British Journal of Obstetrics and Gynaecology 88: 577–581
Olshan A F, Shy K K, Luthy D A, Hickok D, Weiss N S, Daling J R 1984 Cesarean birth and neonatal mortality in very low birth weight infants. Obstetrics and Gynecology 64: 267–270
O'Neil A G B, Skull E, Michael C 1981 A new method of traction for the vacuum cup. Australian and New Zealand Journal of Obstetrics and Gynaecology 21: 24–25
Paintin D B 1982 Mid-cavity forceps delivery. British Journal of Obstetrics and Gynaecology 89: 495–500
Parry-Jones E 1968 Barton's forceps: its use in transverse position of the fetal head. Journal of Obstetrics and Gynaecology of the British Commonwealth 75: 892–901
Phelan J P, Stine L E, Edwards N B, Clark S L, Horenstein J 1985 The role of external version in the intrapartum management of the transverse lie presentation. American Journal of Obstetrics and Gynecology 151: 724–726
Phillips K C, Thomas T A 1983 Second stage of labour with or without extradural analgesia. Anaesthesia 38: 972–976
Phillips R D, Freeman M 1974 The management of the persistent occiput posterior position. Obstetrics and Gynecology 43: 171–177
Philpott R H 1980 Obstructed labour. Clinics in Obstetrics and Gynaecology 7: 601–619
Pritchard C W, Sutherland H W, Carr-Hill R A 1983 Birthweight and paternal height. British Journal of Obstetrics and Gynaecology 90: 156–161

Rayburn W F, Donn S M, Kolin M G, Schork M A 1983 Obstetric care and intraventricular hemorrhage in the low birth weight infant. Obstetrics and Gynecology 62: 408–413
Reading A E, Sledmere C M, Cox D N, Campbell S 1982 How women view postepisiotomy pain. British Medical Journal 284: 243–246
Ridley W J, Jackson P, Stewart J H, Boyle P 1982 Role of antenatal radiography in the management of breech deliveries. British Journal of Obstetrics and Gynaecology 89: 342–347
Roberts A D G, McKay Hart D 1983 Polyglycolic acid and catgut sutures, with and without oral proteolytic enzymes, in the healing episiotomies. British Journal of Obstetrics and Gynaecology 90: 650–653
Russell J K 1982 Breech: vaginal delivery or caesarean section. British Medical Journal 285: 830–831
Sandberg E C 1985 The Zavanelli maneuver: a potentially revolutionary method for the resolution of shoulder dystocia. American Journal of Obstetrics and Gynecology 152: 479–484
Savona-Ventura C 1986 The role of external cephalic version in modern obstetrics. Obstetrical and Gynecological Survey 41: 393–400
Sbarra A J, Thomas G B, Cetrulo C L, Shakr C, Chaudhury A, Paul B 1987 Effect of bacterial growth on the bursting pressure of fetal membranes in vitro. Obstetrics and Gynecology 70: 107–110
Scheer K, Nubar J 1976 Variation of fetal presentation with gestational age. American Journal of Obstetrics and Gynecology 125: 269–270
Schutterman E B, Grimes D A 1983 Comparative safety of the low transverse versus the low vertical uterine incision for cesarean delivery of breech infants. Obstetrics and Gynecology 61: 593–597
Seeds J W, Cefalo R C 1982 Malpresentations. Clinical Obstetrics and Gynecology 25: 145–156
Seitchik J, Castillo M 1983 Oxytocin augmentation of dysfunctional labor. American Journal of Obstetrics and Gynecology 145: 526–529
Seitchik J, Amico J, Robinson A G, Castillo M 1984 Oxytocin augmentation of dysfunctional labor. American Journal of Obstetrics and Gynecology 150: 225–228
Singhi S, Chookang E, Hall J St E, Kalghatgi S 1985 Iatrogenic neonatal and maternal hyponatraemia following oxytocin and aqueous glucose infusion during labour. British Journal of Obstetrics and Gynaecology 92: 356–363
Smith A R B, James D K, Faragher E B, Gilfillan S 1982 Continuous lumbar epidural analgesia in labour—does delaying 'pushing' in the second stage reduce the incidence of instrumental delivery? Journal of Obstetrics and Gynaecology 2: 170–172
Steer P J, Carter M C, Beard R W 1985a The effect of oxytocin infusion on uterine activity levels in slow labour. British Journal of Obstetrics and Gynaecology 92: 1120–1126
Steer P J, Carter M C, Choong K, Hanson M, Gordon A J, Pradhan P 1985b A multicentre prospective randomised controlled trial of induction of labour with an automatic closed-loop feedback controlled oxytocin infusion system. British Journal of Obstetrics and Gynaecology 92: 1127–1133
Stewart D B 1984a The pelvis as a passageway. I. Evolution and adaptations. British Journal of Obstetrics and Gynaecology 91: 611–617
Stewart D B 1984b The pelvis as a passageway. II. The modern human pelvis. British Journal of Obstetrics and Gynaecology 91: 618–623
Stewart P, Calder A A 1984 Posture in labour: patients' choice and its effect on performance. British Journal of Obstetrics and Gynaecology 91: 1091–1095
Torgrim S, Bakke T 1986 The length of the human umbilical cord in vertex and breech presentations. American Journal of Obstetrics and Gynecology 154: 1086–1087
Traub A I, Morrow R J, Ritchie J W K, Dornan K J 1984 A continuing use for Kielland's forceps? British Journal of Obstetrics and Gynaecology 91: 894–898
Vacca A, Grant A, Wyatt G, Chalmers I 1983 Portsmouth operative delivery trial: a comparison of vacuum extraction and forceps delivery. British Journal of Obstetrics and Gynaecology 90: 1107–1112
Van Dorsten J P, Schifrin B S, Wallace R L 1981 Randomized control trial of external cephalic version with tocolysis in late pregnancy. American Journal of Obstetrics and Gynecology 141: 417–424
Wallace R L, Eglinton G S, Yonekura M L, Wallace T M 1984 Extraperitoneal cesarean section: a surgical form of infection prophylaxis? American Journal of Obstetrics and Gynecology 148: 172–177
Watson W J, Benson W L 1984 Vaginal delivery for the selected frank breech infant at term. Obstetrics and Gynecology 64: 638–640
Weaver J B 1980 Breech delivery—obstetric outcome. In: Beard R W, Paintin D B (eds) Outcomes of obstetric intervention in Britain. RCOG, London, pp 47–62
Westgren M, Paul R H 1985 Delivery of the low birthweight infant by cesarean section. Clinical Obstetrics and Gynecology 28: 752–762
Westgren M, Grundsell H, Ingemarsson I, Muhlow A, Svenningsen N W 1981 Hyperextension of the fetal head in breech presentation: a study with long-term follow-up. British Journal of Obstetrics and Gynaecology 88: 101–104
Westgren M, Ingemarsson I, Ahlstrom H, Lindroth N, Svenningsen N W 1982 Delivery and long-term outcome of very low birthweight infants. Acta Obstetricia et Gynecologica Scandinavica 61: 25–30
Westgren L M R, Songster G, Paul R H 1985a Preterm breech delivery: another retrospective study. Obstetrics and Gynecology 66: 481–484
Westgren M, Edvall H, Nordstrom L, Svalenius E, Ranstam J 1985b Spontaneous cephalic version of breech presentation in the last trimester. British Journal of Obstetrics and Gynaecology 92: 19–22
Westin B 1977 Evaluation of a feto-pelvic scoring system in the management of breech presentations. Acta Obstetricia et Gynecologica Scandinavica 56: 505–508
Wigglesworth J S, Husemeyer R P 1977 Intracranial birth trauma in vaginal breech delivery: the continued importance of injury to the occipital bone. British Journal of Obstetrics and Gynaecology 84: 684–691
Williams R M, Thom M H, Studd J W W 1980 A study of the benefits and acceptability of ambulation in spontaneous labour. British Journal of Obstetrics and Gynaecology 87: 122–126
Yu V Y H, Bajuk B, Cutting D, Orgill A A, Astbury J 1984 Effect of mode of delivery on outcome of very-low-birthweight infants. British Journal of Obstetrics and Gynaecology 91: 633–639
Yudkin P L, Redman C W G 1986 Caesarean section dissected, 1978–1983. British Journal of Obstetrics and Gynaecology 93: 135–144

54

Philip Myerscough

Cephalopelvic disproportion

Cephalopelvic dystocia has been recognized as a grave complication of human parturition since earliest times. Its more serious consequences — uterine rupture, vesicovaginal fistula, maternal and fetal death, birth injury — still exact a steady toll of suffering in the developing world. The prevalence of cephalopelvic dystocia in the human species is related to the unique size of the human brain and cranium at the time of birth in the newborn, and to the erect posture, which influences the mother's pelvic shape and size.

Most, if not all, the disasters which may result from unrecognized or unrelieved cephalopelvic dystocia can be prevented through timely and appropriate intervention. It was, therefore, an important milestone in obstetric care when the concept of cephalopelvic disproportion was first propounded in the late 19th century. The idea embodied in the concept of disproportion was that disparity in size between the head and the pelvis could be assessed and identified before labour, or early in labour before serious dystocia occurred.

In this way, the attendants are alerted to the anticipated risk of difficult labour, and delivery can be planned with appropriate skilled supervision. In historical perspective, the concept of cephalopelvic disproportion was one of the first elements in the development of preventive prenatal care.

Initially, disproportion was diagnosed through the use of relatively crude clinical assessments of the fetal head fitting in the pelvic brim. The prevalence of disproportion tended to be overestimated, and its importance was sometimes exaggerated. For many years it was a generally accepted dogma that if in a primigravida engagement of the head failed to occur by the 36th week of pregnancy, cephalopelvic disproportion should be suspected. This teaching was subsequently shown by Weekes & Flynn (1975) and by Sharma & Soni (1978) to be quite erroneous. The modal interval between engagement and the onset of labour is, in fact, less than 7 days.

Later, during the second quarter of this century, radiological methods of pelvic measurement were developed; some obstetric radiologists claimed remarkable accuracy for their predictions of the degree of mechanical difficulty which would occur in labour. Since the heyday of radiological prediction in the 1950s, the pendulum has swung back towards a more empirical outlook. This chapter will seek to present a balanced contemporary view of cephalopelvic assessment and of the management of disproportion. First it is necessary to consider the major factors influencing pelvic size and shape, so that the epidemiology of pelvic contraction can be better understood.

FACTORS INFLUENCING PELVIC MORPHOLOGY

The girdle of bone which bounds the birth canal has an important weight-bearing function throughout life. Among pronograde animals, weight-bearing is shared by all four limbs, but in the erect human posture the lower limbs, through the pelvic girdle, support the whole weight of the rest of the body.

In an infant the developing component parts of the bony pelvis are still separated by wide margins of osteogenic cartilage, and the pelvic cavity has a long oval (dolichopellic) shape. The formation and consolidation of bone depends on an adequate intake of mineral — calcium, phosphorus — and of vitamin D, which promotes mineral absorption (Table 54.1).

During normal growth, the rate of increase in the density and strength of the bones matches the progressive increase in the child's body weight at every stage. If, however, the requirement for mineral and vitamin D is not fully met during the years of growth, particularly during the growth spurts of infancy and adolescence, nutritional disease of bone is likely to develop and overall growth may be stunted. The

Table 54.1 Nutritional/metabolic bone disease. Factors influencing vitamin D metabolism

Source	Form of vitamin D	Interfering factors
Diet	Ergocalciferol Vitamin D_2	Poor nutrition Phytates
Skin	7-Dehydrocholesterol	
UV light →	↓	Lack of sunlight
	Cholecalciferol Vitamin D_3 ↓	
Liver	25-OHD_3 ↓	Liver disease Anticonvulsants
Kidney	$1,25\text{-(OH)}_2D_3$ Calcitriol	Vitamin D dependent rickets Renal osteodystrophy Renal tubular disorders

impaired strength of the affected bone will permit distortion by the stresses of weight-bearing. Obesity in childhood will increase these distorting forces so that the knock-kneed overfed child of an affluent family is only too commonly seen. Excessive load-carrying in childhood can be expected to have a similar influence.

Florid rickets and osteomalacia are now rarities in Britain but there is clear evidence from biochemical studies and measurements of bone density that nutritional bone disease occurs in less overt forms in the neonate (Lancet Editorial 1986), the infant (Amiel & Crosbie 1963), the adolescent (Ford et al 1976) and the adult (British Medical Journal Editorial 1979).

The delicacy of the balance normally maintained between weight-bearing stress and bone strength during growth is also demonstrated if the growing child suffers from disease or injury affecting one lower limb, and has an impairing gait over a period of time. Even a modest extra share of weight-bearing carried by the good leg is usually sufficient to distort the side wall of the pelvis on the healthy side, because of the extra pressure on the acetabular floor, despite normal consolidation of bone. When the condition affects the infant before he or she can stand or walk, the body weight in the sitting position is transmitted through the imperfectly ossified pelvic girdle to the ischial tuberosities, which tend to splay apart, widening the pubic arch and the transverse diameters of the lower pelvis. The upper part of the sacrum is pushed forward, but the lower sacrum rotates backwards, pivoting on the sacroiliac joints.

When, however, nutritional bone disease develops during the later growth spurt of adolescence (11–13 years old in females) the pelvis in its lower part is subjected to different compressive forces through the acetabula. The bony structure of the lower and anterior parts of the pelvis is much lighter than the dense posterior arch, and ossification is completed later; these parts are pushed medially. As a consequence, the brim of the pelvis loses its rounded contour anteriorly, the pubic arch may be narrowed, and the side walls of the mid and lower pelvis are approximated, with funnelling of the birth canal (Fig. 54.1).

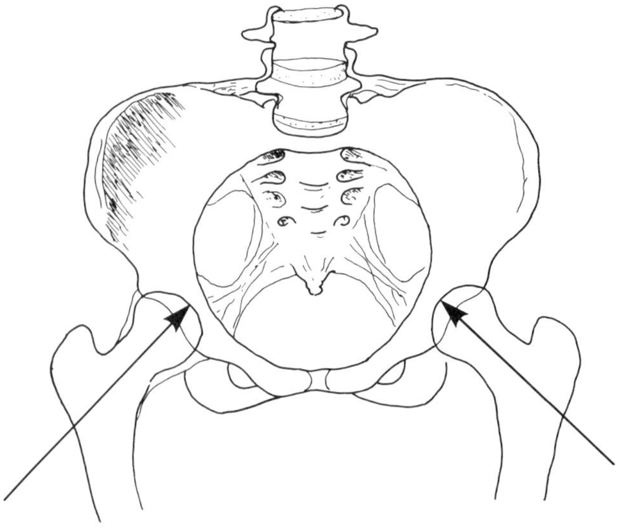

Fig. 54.1 Pelvis illustrating the almost transverse compression effect of weight-bearing. This could lead to funnelling of the lower pelvis if the compressive forces acted in the presence of nutritional bone disease.

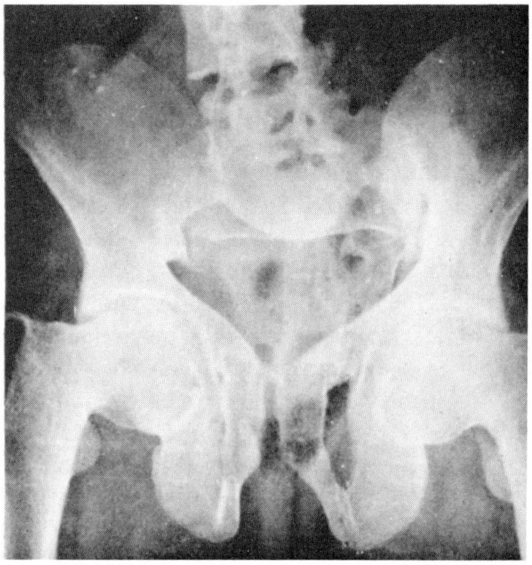

Fig. 54.2 X-ray of pelvis showing osteomalacia (from Myerscough 1982, with permission).

In rare instances of severe adult osteomalacia, the softened pelvic bones are grossly distorted into a triradiate form (Fig. 54.2), clearly illustrating the nature and direction of the main weight-bearing stresses on the pelvic girdle. However, milder forms of adult osteomalacia occur, as has been documented, for example, in Arab and Bedouin women by Fahmy (1973), Toppozada (1964) and by Chaim et al (1981). In these milder forms of nutritional bone disease in the adult, the commonest deformity is a progressive protrusion of the upper sacrum, reducing the conjugate diameter of the pelvic brim. Even a modest reduction in pelvic capacity of this nature can have disastrous obstetric consequences in a multiparous woman.

The pattern of pelvic contraction in a community, therefore, reflects the nutritional experience of the females concerned from their infant years. In Britain and similar developed countries, such bone changes in the infant have been virtually eliminated by ensuring an adequate intake of vitamin D, and are only liable to develop in the infant of very low birthweight. A surprising amount of nutritional bone disease, much of it overt, has been discovered among adolescents, mainly in immigrant Asian communities. Causal factors in these subjects include a diet rich in phytate (chapatti flour), and limited exposure of the skin to sunlight. Similarly, evidence of osteomalacia in multiparous immigrant women during pregnancy and lactation can be demonstrated. Prophylaxis with vitamin D (500 u/day) is indicated, but compliance is often poor.

In an overall view, the nutritional factors described are found to be the dominant influence on pelvic size and shape. Genetic variations certainly exist, but in practical terms are of secondary importance.

Among the tallest, best nourished women, therefore, the brim of the pelvis commonly retains a long oval (dolichopellic) shape, and all the pelvic diameters are adequate for parturition, as Greulich & Thoms first demonstrated (1939). This pelvic shape is the truly gynaecoid pelvis, if that word is to be used.

Among women of near-average stature and nutrition, the pelvic brim is rounded, and although the conjugate diameter is often less than the transverse diameter, no serious flattening has occurred during growth. Shorter women with a less favourable nutritional background include more frequent examples of brim-flattening amounting to significant deformation, which is liable to result in cephalopelvic disproportion.

Convergent funnelling of the pelvic side walls was recognized many years ago by Whitridge Williams (1941) to be a relatively common (perhaps the commonest) form of pelvic deformation then encountered in American women. This may well also be true of Britain at the present time. The configuration of this type of pelvic deformation and its associated features are consistent with the view that it results from less severe nutritional bone disease in the adolescent, often with excessive weight-bearing stress due to obesity. By the time of the adolescent growth spurt, the posterior arch of dense bone between the acetabula, formed by the thick lower part of the ilium and the ala of the sacrum, is relatively resistant to deformation, but the strut-like form of the anterior and lower pelvis renders it more malleable.

The specific deformations which may result include slight flattening of the posterior segment of the brim, beaking of the anterior segment of the brim, and convergent funnelling of the side walls in the lower parts of the pelvis. The angle of the pubic arch may thus be reduced.

Summarizing in simple outline, therefore, it is evident that more severe nutritional bone disease in infancy is liable to result in deformation maximal at the pelvic brim, with reduction in the anteroposterior diameter, while less severe forms of the condition in the older child may cause deformation mainly of the lower pelvis, reducing the transverse diameters towards the outlet. Because this latter type of deformity is the one most likely to be encountered in Britain and other developed countries, the traditional view that a lateral pelvic X-ray delineates the most important pelvic dimensions may need to be revised.

RECOGNITION OF CEPHALOPELVIC DISPROPORTION

Careful observation can alert the obstetrician to the possibility of disproportion long before progress in labour becomes arrested (obstructed labour).

General features

The relationship between stature and pelvic size has been recognized for many years. It derives from the stunting of growth which accompanies impaired nutrition in infancy and early childhood. The degree of brim-flattening is thus likely to be reflected in the degree of growth-stunting. Contraction of the outlet, however, originating at a later stage in growth, is less closely associated with restriction of stature.

Primigravidae of less than 155 cm (5′ 1″) should, therefore, be carefully assessed at or shortly before the onset of labour. Women whose height is 165 cm (5′ 5″) or greater will rarely manifest disproportion. Those women with a limp or a history of pelvic fracture will also all require careful earlier review. These guidelines are relevant to British practice. However, in the developing world, where malnutrition is rife, almost every primigravida must be regarded as having a pelvis of uncertain capacity.

Among parous patients a history of previous dystocia is always relevant, but its absence provides no firm assurance that disproportion will not develop. Birthweight tends to increase as parity advances and, besides, insidious flattening of the brim may develop in the multipara with osteomalacia.

Prelabour assessment

This is of some value as a screening procedure in primigravidae of small stature. The modal interval between engagement of the head and the onset of labour in primigravidae is less than 7 days, and in 80% of cases the interval is less than 14 days (Weekes & Flynn 1975). Non-engagement of the head is therefore unlikely to be of importance before the 39th week, but is of greater prognostic significance at the time of onset of labour.

In such cases a rough clinical assessment of possible brim-flattening can be attempted by estimating the diagonal conjugate. If the anterior surface of the first (or second) piece of the sacrum can be reached with the tip of the examining fingers, the anteroposterior dimensions of the upper pelvis are less than adequate. At the same time, the level of the head should be carefully assessed, and expressed as the amount of head (in fifths) still palpable in the abdomen (see Fig. 54.3). This simple and reproducible assessment provides a more reliable and objective guide to possible disproportion than do tests of head-brim fitting. If after the 39th week the head remains four-fifths palpable, cephalopelvic disproportion must be suspected.

A clinical assessment of the capacity of the pelvic outlet is also possible before or during labour. The angle of divergence of the pelvic rami (subpubic angle) can be felt anteriorly, and the anteroposterior diameter to the tip of the sacrum assessed with the extended fingers, in a manner similar to the diagonal conjugate estimate. However, the transverse dimensions of the lower pelvis are most significant, so that both the interischial spinous and the intertuberous diameters should be assessed. The prominence of the spine is felt vaginally; the intertuberous width can be roughly gauged with a closed fist externally. But clinical outlet assessment is of very limited accuracy as a screening test. Floberg et al (1986) screened a large group of primigravidae both clinically and radiologically. One-half of the patients with contracted outlets were not identified by clinical assessment. If the evidence from this prelabour assessment — taking into account short stature, high head, and unfavourable clinical pelvimetry — points towards possible disproportion, X-ray pelvimetry is usually of value.

Radiological pelvimetry

If as a result of clinical assessment before or during labour cephalopelvic disproportion is suspected, the wise course is to obtain accurate information about the pelvic dimensions by radiological pelvimetry. The newer imaging techniques of ultrasound and magnetic resonance imaging are also capable of depicting pelvic morphology, but have not yet replaced radiological methods.

Two films provide adequate information for a comprehensive pelvic assessment. These are a frontal view using the semi-orthodiagraphic (tube-shift) method to define the transverse diameters at both brim and outlet and a lateral view depicting the anteroposterior diameters (Borell & Radberg 1964). The techniques of X-ray pelvimetry have been refined over the years to minimize fetal exposure to radiation which, with the method described, is about 2 mGy. To reduce exposure to radiation even further, it is possible to use one film alone as the initial screening procedure. In developed countries it is logical, for the reasons outlined earlier in the chapter, to use the transverse pelvimetry film for screening. The radiation exposure involved is only a small fraction of that resulting from a lateral film. If the transverse diameters are adequate, no lateral film is required.

When both exposures are performed, the information they provide about the anteroposterior and transverse diameters at brim and outlet levels can be combined to calculate the approximate cross-sectional area of the birth canal at these levels. The area estimate ($\pi\ r_1\ r_2$), as Allan (1947) demonstrated, correlates more closely with the incidence of cephalopelvic dystocia than does any single diameter. In the lower pelvis, where the axis of the birth canal is more sharply curved and the level of the different diameters does not coincide, Borell & Fernstrom (1960) advocated the combining of three diameters — the interspinous, intertuberous and sagittal — into a single index, the sum of the outlet. This should measure more than 32 cm.

The role of pelvimetry

The value of pelvimetry lies in:

1. Identifying those patients, few in our community, whose pelvic contraction, combined with other unfavourable features, justifies elective Caesarean section. Section in labour, despite the protective use of antibiotics, still carries a maternal risk which is about three times greater than elective abdominal delivery.
2. Forewarning the obstetrician about borderline disproportion. He or she is then guided in the conduct of trial labour not only by observation of the progress of descent and dilatation, but also by knowledge of the degree of mechanical difficulty which the head would encounter at lower levels in the pelvis.
3. Influencing the mode of delivery in outlet dystocia, the most common type of disproportion in the developed world, and one which is easily overlooked. The fine judgement required in deciding between abdominal or vaginal intervention is reinforced if objective pelvic measurements are known.

It must be acknowledged that, in the past, pelvimetry has often been employed inappropriately and sometimes with indiscriminate zeal. This has led to scepticism about its value, though this is counterbalanced by medicolegal concern about the consequences of ignoring pelvimetry. A panel convened jointly by the American Colleges of Obstetrics and Gynecology and of Radiology suggested guidelines for the use of pelvimetry, which would restrict the method to about 3% of parturients in the American population (United States Department of Health Education and Welfare 1980).

Interpretation of pelvimetry findings

As with most biological measurements, it is not helpful or appropriate to attempt to define absolute limits of normality. Disproportion must take account not only of the size of the pelvis, but also of the size of the head. Formerly X-ray cephalometry was attempted, and Moir (1947) developed methods of incorporating head size in his system of pelvic assessment

Table 54.2 Borderline zone between pelvic adequacy and absolute disproportion

Variable	Measurement (cm)
Brim area	90^2–110^2
Obstetrical conjugate	9.0 –11.5
Outlet area	80^2–100^2
Sum of outlet	31.0 –33.5

as he sought to refine its predictive value. Sonar cephalometry now provides a much more accurate and safe method of measuring head size, which has yet to be applied systematically in the assessment of disproportion.

Table 54.2 sets out for various pelvic parameters the borderline zone between pelvic adequacy and absolute disproportion.

CEPHALOPELVIC DISPROPORTION IN PRIMIGRAVIDAE

First stage of labour

The alerting features in this situation include:

1. The head remains three- or four-fifths palpable abdominally.
2. The latent phase may be prolonged.
3. The active phase of dilatation is retarded. Eventually the progress of dilatation may cease, often between 7 and 9 cm.
4. The cervix may be poorly applied to the head, and in neglected cases may become oedematous.
5. As the progress of dilatation ceases, excessive head moulding is likely to become apparent and fetal heart rate decelerations during contractions tend to occur. Initially this is the result of head compression only, but ultimately it is also due to hypoxia.

Second stage of labour

When cephalopelvic dystocia only becomes evident at this late stage in labour, it is usually because the pelvis is contracted in its lower part. Although the first stage of labour may not have been unduly prolonged, often there will have been some premonitory sign of impending difficulty. Typically the partogram indicates that the rate of cervical dilatation in its later stages has slowed down, and one- or two-fifths of the head remains palpable abdominally. On vaginal examination, the arrest of descent of the head may be masked by an increasingly large caput and head moulding is pronounced. The impaction of the head prevents anterior rotation of the occiput, so a persistent occipito-posterior or occipito-transverse position may be found.

Head moulding in cephalopelvic dystocia

Philpott & Stewart (1974) described a simple system of scoring to assess the degree of head moulding quantitatively. Moulding is assessed in at least two locations, i.e. lambdoidal suture, sagittal suture and, if possible, coronal suture. It is scored in three degrees:

+ indicates closing of the suture line;
++ indicates reducible overlap;
+++ indicates irreducible overlap of the cranial bones.

When the sum of the moulding scores at two of the sites is five or six pluses, serious disproportion is present and safe vaginal delivery will rarely be possible.

FETAL DISTRESS DUE TO CEPHALOPELVIC DYSTOCIA

Two factors are responsible for the fetal distress which may arise during mechanically difficult labour:

1. Fetal head compression slows the fetal heart rate due to the rise in intracranial pressure accompanying contractions in the presence of marked head moulding. The decelerations synchronize with the contractions and are particularly likely to occur as the head, having moulded into a contracted pelvic inlet, then begins to descend more rapidly into the pelvic cavity.
2. When the progress of descent and dilatation is arrested, and labour is prolonged, fetal hypoxia is likely to develop. This causes late decelerations of the fetal heart rate typical of fetal asphyxia.

In cases of serious disproportion, both these effects may be seen together; the decelerations begin early during the contractions but reach a delayed nadir and recover slowly. This combined variable deceleration pattern is typical of the fetal distress caused by major cephalopelvic dystocia.

MANAGEMENT OF CEPHALOPELVIC DISPROPORTION IN PRIMIGRAVIDAE

It is necessary to consider primigravidae and parous women separately, because the pattern of their labours in the presence of cephalopelvic disproportion is quite different; this applies particularly to the risk of uterine rupture. The uterus of the primigravida reacts to mechanical difficulty with reduced contractility, though the myometrium may not relax normally between contractions. The undamaged primigravid uterus, therefore, can be relied on not to rupture spontaneously.

Elective Caesarean section

In the absence of other unfavourable features, elective Caesarean section is only indicated if the degree of pelvic contraction is severe, and particularly if the diameters are seriously reduced at more than one level. In other instances, complications such as malpresentation, advanced age, infertility, or diabetes will justify an elective operation, even when the pelvis is only moderately contracted. Although the maternal risk from abdominal delivery is small, it should not be forgotten that, despite antibiotic cover, section in labour carries a risk more than twice as great as an elective procedure. It also prejudices the management of future deliveries.

Trial of labour

In cases of minor or moderate cephalopelvic disproportion, which make up the great majority in this country, a trial of labour is the appropriate management. The term implies that the outcome of labour is uncertain because of mechanical difficulty, and that particularly vigilant monitoring of progress and of fetal well-being are required.

In some instances the trial will be relatively tentative, and will only be allowed to continue if there is progressive advance. But in the case of a young primigravida, where the pelvic contraction affects only one principal diameter, there should be greater persistence to achieve vaginal delivery, and augmentation of the uterine action with oxytocin infusion may be indicated if spontaneous uterine activity is not adequate.

Duration of trial of labour

It is not helpful to specify some arbitrary time limit for a trial of labour. If oxytocin augmentation of labour is utilized to maintain good uterine action, it should become clear within 12–18 hours at the most whether safe vaginal delivery will be possible. If during the active phase there is arrest of dilatation and descent over a period of 3–4 hours with good contractions, abdominal delivery is indicated. To secure adequate but not excessive uterine activity in the presence of disproportion it may be helpful to monitor intrauterine pressure with a catheter manometer, as a guide to oxytocin dosage.

Monitoring fetal well-being

Continuous electronic fetal heart rate recording should be utilized during trial of labour. External transducers can often provide an adequate signal, failing which a scalp electrode should be used. The deceleration patterns encountered during cephalopelvic dystocia have already been described. Intermittent scalp-blood sampling to check fetal pH may be necessary if the fetal heart rate tracing is of uncertain interpretation.

Monitoring the progress of labour

Regular accurate clinical observations on the partogram are essential to the proper conduct of a trial of labour. The successive observations of cervical dilatation and descent of the head should usually be made at intervals of 3–4 hours. It is important that the level of the head should be assessed both by vaginal and abdominal palpation. The abdominal findings are, in this situation, generally the more significant.

Methods of assessment of head level

The earliest clinical techniques of palpation of the head focused on head-brim fitting, and the question addressed was: 'Is the head engaged?' or 'Has the widest diameter entered the brim?' The lateral contours of the accessible portion of the head were therefore explored by deep palpation in the iliac fossae, to gain an impression whether the fingertips could feel beyond the widest part of the head.

Later, the concept of vaginal station of the head was promulgated in the USA. The level of the head was defined by a vaginal assessment, using the ischial spines as a reference level, and relating the lowest part of the head (vertex) to this level, in estimated centimetres of vertical distance. Thus a station of −2 indicated that the vertex was still 2 cm above the ischial spine level. Such an assessment of vaginal station may not correlate exactly with the findings on abdominal palpation because of the elongation of the head produced by moulding and variations in the pelvic depth.

In terms of the basic mechanics of disproportion, it is the amount of head remaining above the pelvic brim which provides the most significant indicator of difficulty yet to be overcome. This principle was recognized by the South African obstetricians Crichton (1952), Notelelowitz (1973), Lasbery (1963) and Philpott & Castle (1972) and a system of assessment was devised which defined the head level in terms of the amount — in fifths — of the head palpable abdominally (Fig. 54.3).

To define the level of the head accurately in this way, a different pattern of palpation should be adopted, aiming to define the level of the highest part of the head felt in or near the midline. The distance between this level and the top of the symphysis can be expressed as finger-breadths of an average adult hand, which in turn represents the number of fifths of the head above the brim. Figure 54.4, depicting a cross-sectional view through the mother's body at the level of the head, illustrates how close to the abdominal surface the head lies near the midline. The technique is, therefore, more definitive and less uncomfortable for the patient.

By using both vaginal examination and the method of abdominal palpation described for assessment of the descent of the head much greater accuracy will be achieved. If there appears to be a discrepancy between the two findings, it is the amount of head remaining palpable in the abdomen which has the greater significance, for the reasons already described.

Disproportion at the pelvic brim is relatively easy to diagnose, assess and manage in labour, but disproportion at lower

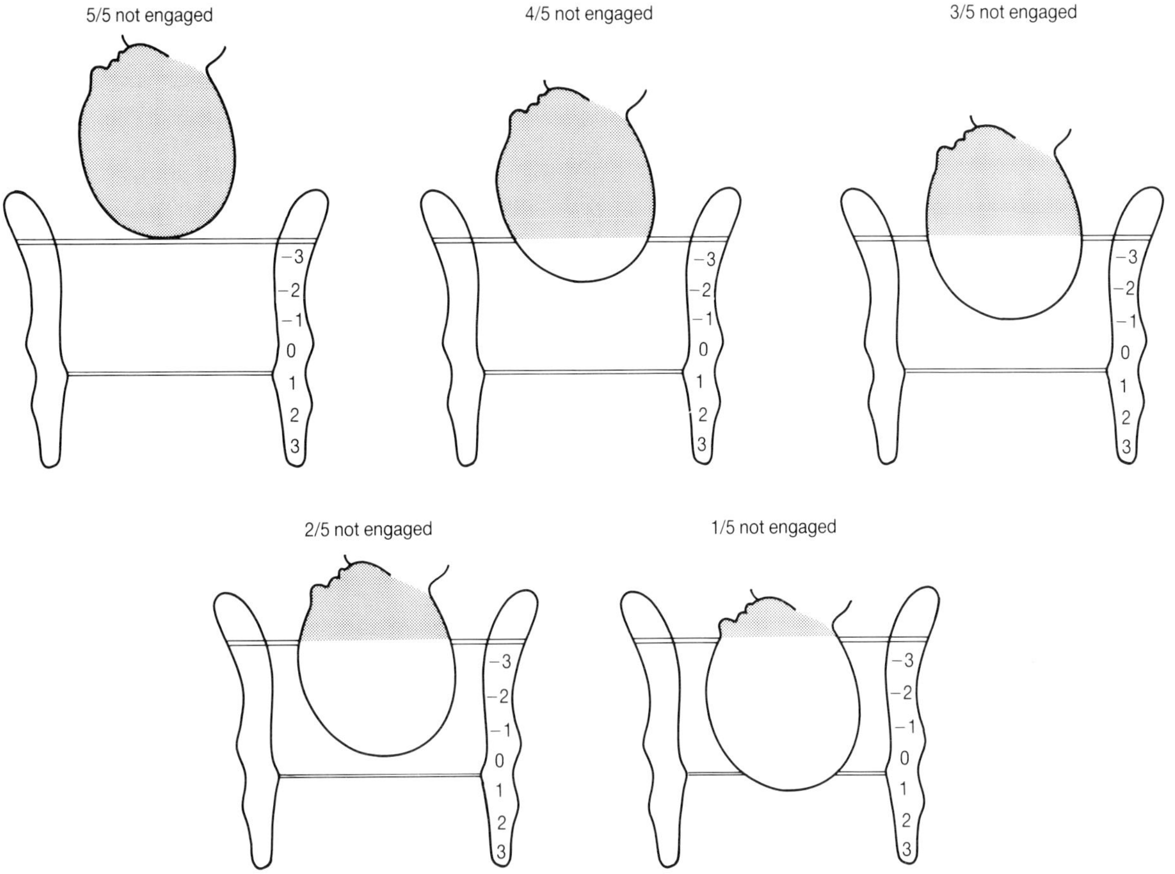

Fig. 54.3 Fifths of a head; a concept for translating clinical findings from abdominal palpation of the fetal head into degrees of descent through the mother's pelvis.

levels in the pelvis is more common in Britain, and is often unsuspected. It is therefore, in the writer's experience, the more dangerous condition, calling for skill, patience, and fine judgement in its management.

Pain relief

During a trial of labour analgesia can with advantage be secured by epidural nerve block, though other forms of pain relief are not excluded.

Outcome of a trial of labour

A trial of labour should usually be terminated if, despite active management, there is failure to progress over a period of 3–4 hours, or if a major degree of fetal distress is diagnosed. Stewart & Philpott (1980) proposed a systematic outline plan for selecting the safest mode of delivery in the presence of disproportion. Their scheme, based on a study of African women, needs to be modified for application in Britain. A simplified plan of action is shown in Table 54.3. It should be noted that:

1. in the presence of disproportion, the ventouse provides a safer method of assisted delivery than the forceps;
2. potentially difficult vaginal delivery should never be attempted in the presence of fetal distress;
3. symphysiotomy has been shown in many parts of the world to provide a safer alternative than a Caesarean section for appropriately selected cases.

CEPHALOPELVIC DISPROPORTION IN PAROUS WOMEN

For several important reasons, disproportion in parous women presents different and much more dangerous problems than in primiparae. The patient's history of uneventful delivery may falsely reassure the obstetrician, as well as the woman herself. But in a subsequent labour, the infant is likely to be bigger, or the presentation may be abnormal, or the pelvis, in some instances, smaller! Surprise dystocia may therefore occur.

The tempo of labour will be more rapid in a parous woman, and the character of uterine action in the presence of disproportion, unlike that of primigravidae, is likely to be vigorously reactive, culminating in neglected cases in tonic contraction of the uterus and uterine rupture. The pattern of progress of cervical dilatation on the partogram

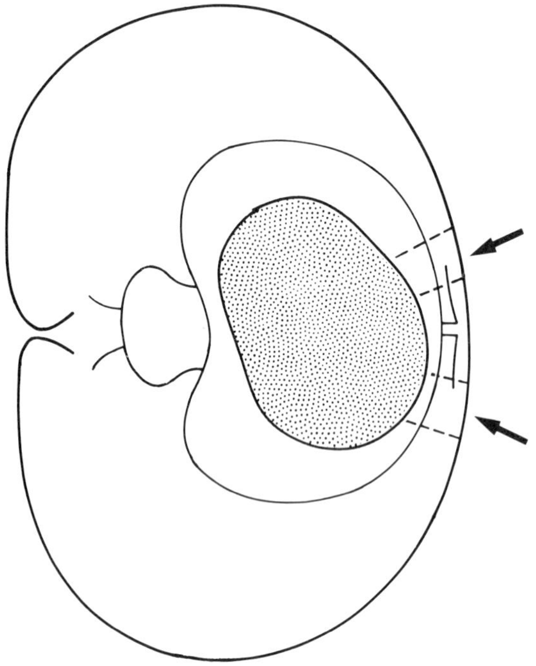

Fig. 54.4 Cross-section at level of fetal head. The head is most accessible to palpation near the midline.

Table 54.3 Scheme for selecting mode of delivery

Amount of head palpable (fifths)	Mode of delivery
0/5	Ventouse or forceps
1/5	Trial ventouse If fetal distress, Caesarean section
2/5	Caesarean section or symphysiotomy
3/5+	Caesarean section

(Soglow & Friedman 1967) is not invariably retarded, so that an important warning sign which is present in primigravidae cannot be relied on. Diagnosis of mechanical difficulty rests on other features of the labour — delay in descent of the head, exaggerated moulding, and sometimes unremitting uterine activity.

If the presence of disproportion is undetected and labour is augmented with oxytocin, the danger of uterine rupture is very real but insidious. The classical signs of impending spontaneous rupture of an unscarred uterus — frequent, violent uterine contractions and possibly an exaggerated retraction ring (Bandl's ring) — do not usually appear prior to rupture during oxytocin infusion in parous women. Often the only warning sign of impending iatrogenic rupture may be the failure of the uterus to relax between apparently normal contractions. For these reasons, labour should not be augmented in parous women where disproportion is thought to be present.

The management of disproportion in parous women therefore requires particular vigilance; careful assessment of progress, including vaginal examination, may be required at intervals of as little as 1–2 hours during the active phase of the first stage of labour. In grand multiparae, disproportion presents formidable risks, and such labours should always be supervised by an experienced obstetrician.

CONCLUSIONS

The shape and size of the bony pelvis are principally determined by nutritional factors, operating particularly during the years of growth. If progressive consolidation of the bones is not adequate to sustain the stresses of weight-bearing, distortion of the pelvis occurs.

Major degrees of pelvic contraction and serious cephalopelvic dystocia have therefore become much less common as the nutritional status of British women has improved, and their mean stature increased. In particular, marked brim-flattening is now rarely seen in the UK, but pelvic funnelling may be encountered and outlet dystocia may develop with little advance warning. The ability to anticipate difficulty and to assess accurately the degree of disproportion is all-important if correct decisions about the safe mode of delivery are to be ensured.

Cephalopelvic disproportion occurring for the first time in multigravidae can be due to either an increase in fetal size or a reduction in pelvic capacity, or both. The risk of uterine rupture in these circumstances is appreciable, and is magnified if uterine action is augmented with oxytocin.

REFERENCES

Allan E P 1947 Standardised radiological pelvimetry. British Journal of Radiology 20: 108, 164, 205, 451

Arniel G C, Crosbie J C 1963 Infantile rickets returns to Glasgow. Lancet ii: 423

Borell U, Fernstrom I 1960 Radiologic pelvimetry. Acta Radiologica suppl 191

Borell U, Radberg C 1964 Orthodiagraphic pelvimetry with special references to capacity of distal part of pelvis and pelvic outlet. Acta Radiologica (Diagnostica) 2: 273

British Medical Journal Editorial 1979 Rickets in Asian immigrants. British Medical Journal 1: 1744

Chaim W, Alroi A, Leiberman J R, Cohen A 1981 Severe contracted pelvis appearing after normal deliveries. Acta Obstetricia et Gynecologica Scandinavica 60: 131

Crichton D 1952 The accuracy of X-ray cephalometry in utero. Proceedings of the Royal Society of Medicine 45: 535

Fahmy K 1973 Disproportion in multiparae. Journal of the Kuwait Medical Association 7: 119

Floberg J, Belfrage P, Carlsson M, Ohlsen H 1986. The pelvic outlet. A comparison between clinical evaluation and radiologic pelvimetry. Acta Obstetricia et Gynecologica Scandinavica 65: 321

Ford J A, McIntosh W B, Butterfield R 1976 Clinical and subclinical vitamin D deficiency in Bradford children. Archives of Disease in Childhood 51: 939

Greulich W W, Thoms H 1939 A study of pelvis type and its relationship to body build in white women. Journal of the American Medical Association 112: 485

Lancet Editorial 1986 Metabolic bone disease of prematurity. Lancet i: 200
Lasbery A H 1963 The symptomatic sequelae of symphysiotomy. A follow-up study of 100 patients subjected to symphysiotomy. South African Medical Journal 37: 231
Moir J C 1947 The use of radiology in predicting difficult labour. Journal of Obstetrics and Gynaecology of the British Empire 54: 20
Myerscough P R 1982 Munro Kerr's operative obstetrics. Baillière Tindall, London, p 139
Notelowitz M 1973 Beware the weeping womb. South African Journal of Obstetrics and Gynaecology 47(3): 1653–1655
Philpott R, Castle W M 1972 Journal of Obstetrics and Gynaecology of the British Commonwealth 79: 592, 599
Philpott R H, Stewart K S 1974 Intensive care of the high-risk fetus in Africa. Clinics in Obstetrics and Gynaecology 1: 241
Sharma S, Soni I K 1978 The time of engagement of the fetal head. Journal of Obstetrics and Gynaecology of India 28: 410
Soglow S R, Friedman E A 1967 Feto-pelvic disproportion in multiparae. Obstetrics and Gynecology 29: 848
Stewart K S, Philpott R H 1980 Fetal response to cephalopelvic disproportion. British Journal of Obstetrics and Gynaecology 87: 641
Toppozada H K 1964 Clinical pelvimetry I. Alexandria Medical Journal 10: 287
United States Department of Health Education and Welfare Public Health Service Food and Drugs Administration 1980 The selection of patients for X-ray examination. Brown R F et al (eds)
Weekes A R L, Flynn M J 1975 Engagement of the fetal head in primigravidae and its relationship to duration of gestation and time of onset of labour. British Journal of Obstetrics and Gynaecology 82: 7
Williams W 1941 Obstetrics. Appleton-Century, New York

55

Andrew Calder

Induction and augmentation of labour

INTRODUCTION

Labour is an inevitable consequence of pregnancy. Only two events can prevent the onset of labour once pregnancy has become well established — the death of the undelivered mother or removal of the fetus by Caesarean section. The timing of the onset of labour may vary widely, but it will happen, sooner or later.

INDUCTION

Induction of labour is an obstetric procedure designed to pre-empt the natural process of labour by initiating its onset artificially before this occurs spontaneously. Many women whose labours are induced today would, left alone, labour tomorrow while for others, induction advances the process by many days or even weeks. The decision to advance the labour is taken to serve some interest — usually that of the offspring; less often it is that of the mother and rarely it is that of the obstetrician or the clinical service.

Few medical issues have generated so much controversy in the past 15 years as have the use and abuse of labour induction. In the early 1970s the media mounted a public challenge to the speciality on this issue, the impact of which can still be felt today. At the time, many obstetricians rightly felt that the presentation of the arguments by the media was dishonest and distorted. Many felt bitter that their professional judgement and competence were subjected to such public challenge, but few would now deny that the long-term effects have been beneficial. Obstetricians were made aware of the need to re-examine their motives, to be more accountable and, most of all, to explain more fully and discuss their views with the person most intimately and immediately concerned — the prospective mother.

Authoritarianism is cosy and simple, while informed discussion is time-consuming and bothersome. Nevertheless, induction of labour represents such a profound interference with natural laws that the clinician must be prepared to justify it to his or her patients, to the wider public and to him- or herself.

The obstetrician must be conscious of a feeling of power. Among a profession often accused of trying to usurp the authority of the Almighty, obstetricians may be at risk from the temptation to exercise God-like power. They have few more potent clinical weapons at their disposal and it therefore behoves them to use this power wisely and only for reasons which can be amply justified.

Putting aside the largely contentious question of intervention for the benefit of the obstetric services or of the clinical staff (which is hard to defend on purely medical grounds, but might in certain circumstances be justified on the basis of the best deployment of resources), labour induction must be seen to benefit the mother or the offspring or both. The particular challenge of obstetrics which lies in the need to care for two parties simultaneously is seen in its sharpest focus when the interests of the mother and those of the fetus may appear to be in conflict. The last few years have seen an increase in the number of mothers who yearn for what has come to be called natural childbirth and who eschew obstetric interference in any form. To such women, the induction of labour may be particularly abhorrent; often it seems that such mothers believe that if they are sufficiently determined in their mental approach they will achieve a normal and trouble-free pregnancy, labour and delivery.

There is as yet no evidence that yearning for natural childbirth is an effective protection against antepartum haemorrhage, gestational diabetes, placental insufficiency and such disorders. In consequence, it may often be necessary to insist that some mothers subordinate their aspirations for a fulfilling birth experience to the more pressing interests of their offspring. This may seem an obvious course, but few obstet-

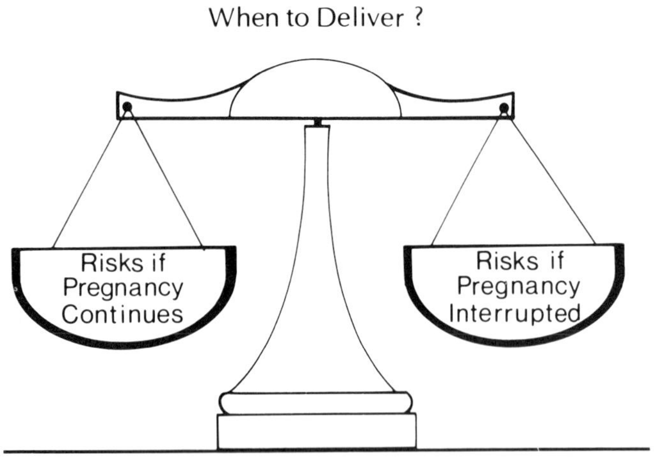

Fig. 55.1 The obstetric balance.

ricians have not had the experience of trying to convince what appears to be an infuriatingly stubborn mother that she has her priorities wrong. Happily, most mothers see the well-being of their offspring as paramount, but this emphasizes the need for the obstetrician to be on the firmest ground in giving advice and not to recommend induction lightly.

Many of the difficulties we now face date from the era when enthusiasm for our new-found ability to induce labour outstripped sound clinical judgement. It is easy to employ emotional blackmail in persuading a mother of our case for induction by suggesting that her failure to agree may put her baby at risk. We must therefore constantly strive for intellectual and clinical honesty in the advice we offer.

Indications for induction of labour

The essence of the indications for induction of labour lies in our assessment of the components which contribute to the obstetric balance (Calder 1983; Fig. 55.1). Intervention is only appropriate when its risks are judged to be fewer than those associated with non-intervention.

Fetal indications

Labour induction for fetal indications assumes that the welfare of the offspring is better served by being delivered than by remaining in utero. Certain obstetric complications are well known to carry clearcut fetal risks (e.g. rhesus disease, diabetes, severe pre-eclampsia); in others the risks are less consistent. These latter may be described as epidemiological indications in conditions such as prolonged pregnancy, mild and moderate pre-eclampsia or increased maternal age. It is this latter category which has contributed most to the widely varying rates of labour induction and to the consequent controversy. The firmer indications account for fewer than 10% of confinements in most populations (Studd & Cardozo 1985), whereas marginal indications may be identified in anything from 10 to 50% of the remainder. It is the interpretation of the significance and weight of such indications that determines the frequency with which induction is applied in any given obstetric service.

Essentially the obstetrician must assess the relative risks for the fetus of continuing in utero or being delivered. The inaccessibility of the fetus to clinical examination and assessment makes the risks in utero difficult to quantify but the risks after delivery may be no more precise. The increasing willingness of obstetricians to confer with their neonatal colleagues is greatly welcomed but ultimately the decision is a matter of judgement based on the assessment of several uncertainties. Birthweight, estimated by clinical methods or by ultrasound and gestational age are important factors in predicting neonatal problems but other factors, especially those complications which are under consideration, may have a crucial bearing on whether or not the neonate has a stormy introduction to extrauterine life.

The past two decades have witnessed increased sophistication in the methods of assessment of both types of risk. Diagnostic ultrasound has allowed more precise measurement of fetal growth and well-being. Cardiotocography may give valuable information about the fetal condition. The assessment of the fetal biophysical profile (Manning et al 1980) is gaining in popularity.

Such measures are also useful in predicting neonatal difficulties so that the value of amniocentesis to allow measurement of liquor phospholipids (Gluck & Kulovich 1973) in order that the fetal lung maturity can be determined now plays a smaller part than it once did.

A further factor concerns the skills and facilities available for the care of the newborn. Clearly the availability of the highest level of neonatal intensive care will put a very different complexion on the prospect of delivery. In the absence of such facilities there is little merit in delivering a grossly immature infant with little prospect of survival.

It is a matter of balance. In most pregnancies the balance (Fig. 55.1) remains firmly tipped against interference and remains so until the spontaneous onset of labour at term. In some instances the risks in utero may be seen to be gradually rising and delivery may be contemplated at an appropriate moment. The radical obstetrician favours early intervention in the belief that it is better to deliver the offspring before it has been seriously compromised. A conservative colleague will favour delaying intervention until evidence of fetal compromise is clearly seen, which may never happen.

Rhesus disease. Maternal rhesus isoimmunization illustrates many of the matters considered above. The risks of this complication are almost all directed towards the fetus. Haemolysis of fetal red blood cells may lead to progressive anaemia, cardiac failure and eventually to hydrops fetalis. The earlier these complications appear the greater is the likelihood that intervention will be required to prevent fetal death in utero. Such intervention may be labour induction if it is judged that the fetus is sufficiently mature; otherwise blood transfusion of the fetus in utero is required.

Hitherto the methods of assessing these factors have been fairly imprecise. The maternal antibody pattern is no more than a general pointer, while liquor bilirubin assessment is only a crude index of fetal haemoglobin levels. Methods of direct fetal blood sampling may now bring greater precision to the management of this condition and measurement of liquor phospholipids remains a useful procedure in this condition (Whitfield 1982).

The outcome of each case depends on the race between declining haemoglobin concentration and advancing fetal maturation. When it is judged that the fetus is sufficiently mature, delivery is indicated, perhaps by labour induction.

Diabetes. Maternal diabetes confers major hazards on the offspring. Poor control of the maternal blood glucose level increases the risks of fetal and maternal complications, leading to increased rates of perinatal death and morbidity. Sudden fetal demise in utero during the last weeks of gestation is less common nowadays because of improvements in diabetic control but induction of labour remains an important weapon in the battle to achieve a successful outcome to these pregnancies.

Severe pre-eclampsia. This condition may be associated with impaired placental function leading to growth retardation or even death of the fetus in utero. Timely induction of labour may be appropriate in the fetal interest.

Maternal indications

It is rare nowadays to have to consider labour induction purely in the maternal interest. Nevertheless some maternal diseases such as valvular disorders of the heart, hypertension, renal disease, liver disease and certain autoimmune disorders may, especially if deteriorating, require consideration to be given to delivery in the maternal interest. Malignant conditions present a particularly taxing challenge.

Few maternal diseases are actually improved during pregnancy; in general the extra burden of pregnancy hastens their progression. The existence of such conditions is often recognized before pregnancy but commonly may only come to light or indeed may arise de novo during the course of pregnancy.

The process of ending the pregnancy may in itself pose an added risk but as a general if not invariable rule, when a mother's life is becoming threatened by such a disease during pregnancy, it is to her benefit to have the pregnancy removed from the clinical picture. In the past, women with serious medical conditions were often strongly counselled not to embark on pregnancy at all or if they did conceive therapeutic abortion was immediately advised. This is now less common for two reasons. Firstly, the likely course of the disease states concerned and the effects of pregnancy on it are better understood. Secondly, the methods of pregnancy interruption have been steadily improved.

It remains true that the earlier a pregnancy is terminated, the safer it will be for the mother concerned but it is now more possible to intervene at any stage of gestation if the need to do so becomes apparent. Whereas formerly for the pregnancy to stand a good chance of success it had to continue for at least 36 weeks, nowadays, thanks to the advances in neonatal care, it may have a good chance of a successful outcome in many good neonatal units after only 28 weeks. In addition, in years gone by the dangers from methods of interruption rose steeply after the first trimester and did not begin to decline until the natural course of pregnancy was almost complete. Thus there was a window, or perhaps more aptly a closed door, between 12 and 36 weeks during which interruption carried greater hazards and this encouraged the view that early abortion might be best.

The advent of prostaglandins has brought the ability to induce labour throughout gestation. Thus a mother with a serious disease may now more often be allowed to embark on a pregnancy on the understanding that if her condition deteriorates dangerously as it advances the pregnancy may need to be interrupted. It may however have advanced far enough to be successful. The desire for parenthood is so strong that such women should not be forbidden the chance to reproduce on the grounds of unncertain deleterious effects. We can now more often put the question to the test without incurring unacceptable risks.

The decision to intervene

The foregoing may help to explain the reasons why induction of labour has been such a controversial procedure in recent times. Obstetricians have argued bitterly about the appropriate use of induction. The rates of induction in different hospitals and between different clinicians, differing widely, have been the subject of pride or the object of criticism. Many of these arguments have been sterile because the populations of mothers concerned have differed greatly in the risks they face.

Nevertheless, with the advance of obstetrics as a clinical science we are steadily moving away from the days of induction of labour for vague theoretical or epidemiological risks to more enlightened times where the indications are based on risks more precisely identified within the individual mother or fetus. Increased capacity for studying the condition and behaviour of the fetus in utero, although far from perfect, is assisting this process. Closer contact with the neonatologist and careful obstetric and neonatal audit allow more accurate prediction of the outlook for a particular neonate. Thus the various components in the obstetric balance can be measured with greater precision and the decision that labour induction is required reaches a sounder footing.

AUGMENTATION OF LABOUR

The need to intervene to augment labour implies two things: firstly, that labour has already begun, and secondly that its quality or progress is unsatisfactory. An additional category of indication can be included under this heading, namely, the situation in which the fetal membranes have ruptured but labour has not become established. This latter situation is conventionally described as premature rupture of the membranes, an unsatisfactory description because the term prematurity implies that the fetus is immature. Nevertheless, for want of a better description, the term premature rupture of the membranes will be used to refer to this clinical problem.

In deciding on the clinical need for augmentation of labour, two difficulties arise. First of all, the diagnosis of labour is itself far from easy. Many mothers are admitted to maternity units in what may be described as false or hesitant labour and left alone; many of these will not progress to establish in labour. It is a moot point whether in such circumstances at term it is better to apply conservative or active policies. Many obstetricians, fearing that such false or hesitant labours may be associated with unrecognized fetal compromise, may favour intervention. Others, however, are more inclined simply to observe and await the definite onset of labour.

Where the membranes have ruptured but labour has not immediately followed, there is a general belief that delivery is desirable in a relatively short period. In most such instances a conservative approach will be followed by spontaneous labour in the majority of instances within a day or two. The sword of Damocles which hangs over all such clinical situations is, however, intrauterine infection and for this reason, most obstetricians will favour stimulation of uterine contractility, if this does not itself become established within a certain number of hours.

When labour has been diagnosed, it should proceed to delivery within certain accepted time limits. In the past it was conventional to define upper time limits for the normal durations of first- and second-stage labour. Much more profitable is the application of the principle of partography, which owes its origins to the work of Friedman (1967) in the USA and Philpott (1972) in Southern Africa. Thus, the progress of labour may be plotted graphically and deviations from the normal pattern may be recognized early. Various different partograms have been described, but all share the ability to define a labour which has deviated from the normal pattern of progress and where this is slow, augmentation may be indicated (see Chapter 46).

It must, however, be remembered that there are a number of causes for unsatisfactory progress in labour and poor uterine contractility is but one of these. Fetopelvic disproportion may also be responsible for poor cervimetric progress, especially in the latter phase of cervical dilatation, and while augmentation of uterine contractility may represent a useful clinical step in reaching the diagnosis, the dangers associated with obstructed labour and augmented uterine contractility (uterine rupture and fetal demise) must never be forgotten.

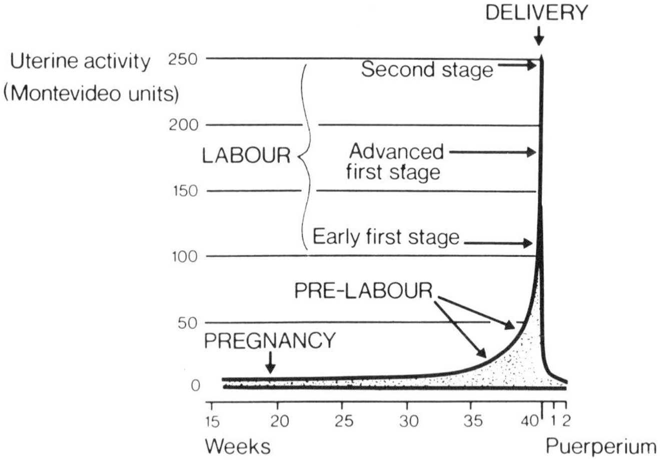

Fig. 55.2 The quantitative pattern of uterine contractility during pregnancy, prelabour and labour (from Caldeyro-Barcia 1958).

METHODS OF INDUCTION AND AUGMENTATION OF LABOUR

Although for practical reasons it will be necessary to consider induction and augmentation separately and to regard them as different types of obstetric intervention, the only important distinction between the two lies in the extent to which the process of spontaneous labour has already begun. Just as we regard the ovarian cycle as consisting of a number of phases (follicular–ovulatory–luteal–menstrual), it is important to regard each birth cycle as a continuum from pregnancy to delivery through the sequence pregnancy–prelabour–latent labour–active labour–delivery.

In physiological terms the onset of human labour is not the sudden event it often appears, but rather a culmination of a gradual process evolving over a period of several weeks. This period is well described as prelabour and it sees the critical conversion of the myometrium from a state of inhibition to one of stimulation. Less obvious than the change in the myometrium is the radical modification which takes place in the tissues of the uterine cervix to allow delivery to take place.

Uterine contractility

At no stage in its life history is the human uterus entirely at rest. In the non-pregnant state it shows episodic contractility with peaks at the time of ovulation and menstruation. In pregnancy, the pattern of contractility which was so carefully studied and beautifully described by Caldeyro-Barcia (1958) is shown in Figure 55.2. This shows the uterine contractility throughout pregnancy, parturition and the early puerperium and demonstrates that the quiescent myometrium of pregnancy begins a build-up of activity about 4–5 weeks before the onset of labour proper. This steadily evolves throughout the phase of prelabour until labour becomes fully expressed.

Cervical ripening

Just as the powerful contractions of clinical labour are preceded by a period of gradual evolution, so are the dramatic changes of effacement and dilatation which the cervix undergoes during labour. A number of careful studies (Bishop 1964, Anderson & Turnbull 1969, Hendricks et al 1970) have demonstrated that the rapid change in the shape of the cervix during labour begins imperceptibly during prelabour. Moreover, the change in the physical properties of the connective tissue which forms the main mass of the cervical stroma and which allows the shape change to take place probably begins even earlier. The non-pregnancy and early-pregnant cervix has a firm and unyielding character attributed to the collagen fibres which it possesses in abundance. These undergo radical modification to afford the massive increase in compliance in the tissue which is essential to allow the stretching and dilatation during labour necessary for delivery.

In spite of extensive studies of the nature of these modifications, the exact mechanisms are not fully elucidated. The proteoglycans of the cervical ground substance appear to undergo changes which in turn alter the physical properties of the tissue. Since these molecules are mostly responsible for the binding of the collagen fibres it seems likely that a change in such binding might contribute to the altered physical properties of the cervix. There may, however, be a more fundamental modification of the collagen consisting of a quantitative reduction or indeed a qualitative change in type.

Muscle is relatively sparse in cervical tissue and is thought to contribute little to these processes. The principal cellular element, the fibroblast, is regarded as the orchestrator of most of these tissue changes, since it seems to be the source of both collagen and proteoglycan synthesis and also of the lytic enzymes which are responsible for their removal from the tissue. The factors which control these changes and thus modify the compliance of cervical tissue have been reviewed by Liggins (1978) and Calder (1979).

The normal physiological control of the transition from pregnancy to labour thus requires the development not only of uterine contractility, but of a maturing process in the cervix which lowers its resistance to dilatation. Throughout pregnancy, the cervix functions as a closed sphincter, but as delivery approaches it must be capable of rapid opening. A normal co-ordinated and successful labour and delivery requires that the corpus and cervix of the uterus must act in synchrony, altering their roles from those required to maintain the pregnancy to those necessary to allow its culmination with delivery. This synchronous relationship between the two components of the uterus is illustrated in Figure 55.3.

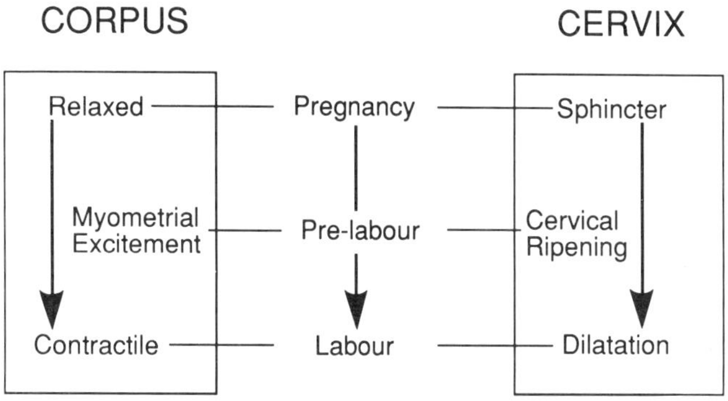

Fig. 55.3 The inter-related changes in the corpus uteri and cervix uteri during pregnancy, pre-labour and labour.

HORMONAL CONTROL OF LABOUR

The endocrine control of parturition represents a jigsaw in which many of the pieces of scientific knowledge are still missing. This has been carefully reviewed in Chapter 46. Many of the agents which have been shown to influence uterine contractility have been explored as possible agents for induction or inhibition of human labour. The list of candidates is extensive, including arginine vasopressin, corticotrophin, corticosteroids, catecholamines, oxytocin, oestrogens, progesterone, adenyl cyclase, relaxin and prostaglandins. Of these, only oxytocin and prostaglandins have been used extensively in clinical practice, although many of the others have been the subject of experimental studies.

It seems likely that the final event responsible for the onset of labour contractions in the human is an increased synthesis of prostaglandins of the E and F series within the uterine compartment, from the decidua and fetal membranes (Keirse 1979). Once this synthesis has been initiated, labour is likely to become established. Csapo & Pulkinnen (1979) described the prostaglandins as 'the ultimate uterine stimulant' and clearly their production within the uterine compartment is subject to higher endocrine control in which the placental steroids, oestrogen and progesterone, appear to play a crucial role. The role of relaxin in human parturition is as yet far from clear, but represents an exciting prospect for further study.

The uterus only becomes fully sensitive to exogenous oxytocin in late pregnancy (Fuchs 1973). The early pregnant uterus is insensitive to oxytocin, but becomes sensitive if prostaglandin E_2 or prostaglandin $F_{2\alpha}$ is administered. This favours the conclusion that the rise of prostaglandin activity in prelabour sensitizes the myometrium to the action of oxytocin.

As far as cervical ripening is concerned there is little evi-

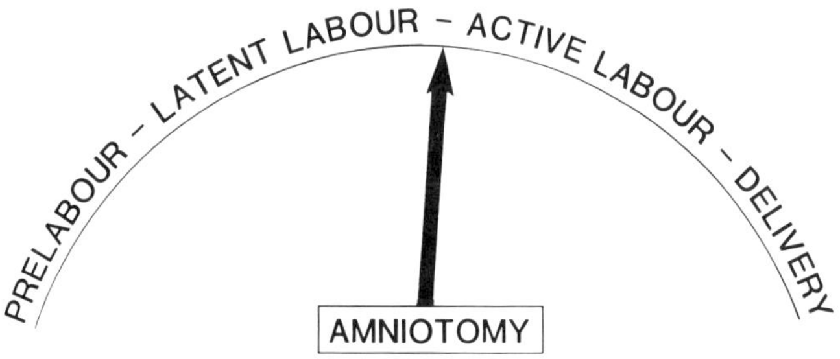

Fig. 55.4 Spectrum of phases in the transition from pregnancy to delivery. The membranes may rupture spontaneously or be ruptured artificially at any point in this spectrum.

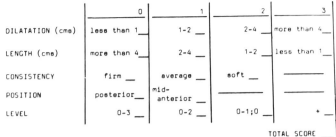

	0	1	2	3
DILATATION (cms)	less than 1	1-2	2-4	more than 4
LENGTH (cms)	more than 4	2-4	1-2	less than 1
CONSISTENCY	firm	average	soft	
POSITION	posterior	mid-anterior		
LEVEL	0-3	0-2	0-1;0	+
				TOTAL SCORE

Fig. 55.5 Modified Bishop's score (Calder et al 1974).

dence to support an important role for oxytocin. On the other hand, the prostaglandins (especially prostaglandin E_2) appear to be centrally concerned in this process and again this may be under the control of steroid hormones (Lerner 1980) and possibly relaxin (Steinetz et al 1980).

Thus, it seems likely, and perhaps not surprising, that similar endocrine control mechanisms operate for both the activation of myometrial contractility and for the induction of cervical ripening.

Practical aspects

We have considered the reasons why it may be necessary to recommend induction or augmentation of labour and the physiological background against which we must consider how to intervene. Beazley (1975) argued that all labour induction should more properly be called augmentation or acceleration of labour since, as has been stated earlier, it simply brings forward an inevitable future prospect. Clearly the physiological status of the individual mother, and in particular the position she occupies on the spectrum illustrated in Figure 55.4, will determine whether her management requires to fall into the category of induction of labour or that of augmentation. In practical terms, if she has not passed from the phase of prelabour into the phase of latent labour, we must regard intervention as induction, whereas if she has already begun latent labour, albeit unsatisfactorily, the intervention should be classified as augmentation.

It has been shown that prelabour occupies several weeks in late pregnancy and it is important to emphasize that the point occupied by the mother within that evolutionary phase has a crucial bearing on her response to labour induction. Thus, if she is still in very early prelabour she has a very different induction prospect from someone in late prelabour. In simple terms, the closer the onset of spontaneous labour, the easier and more successful will labour induction prove. The converse is even more important. Labour induction undertaken when spontaneous labour is a distant prospect is fraught with much more difficulty and many more complications.

This would be of little consequence if there was no way of judging the mother's situation within prelabour, but because cervical ripening is a central event during this phase, an assessment of the degree to which this has developed provides a helpful guide.

Assessment of cervical ripening is based on the scoring system devised by Bishop (1964); indeed, in Bishop's original study, he showed that there was a clear inverse relationship between the cervical score and the time programmed for spontaneous onset of labour. Stated simply, a high Bishop score indicates that spontaneous labour is imminent, while a low Bishop score denotes that it is a distant prospect. More importantly, a high Bishop score predicts a good response to labour induction, while a low score presages difficulties.

Clinical assessment of cervical state is an essential element in the process of considering and implementing a decision to induce labour. For this purpose we employ a slight modification of Bishop's original scoring system (Calder et al 1974) which has proved easier to apply in practice (Fig. 55.5).

Techniques of induction and augmentation

A historical review of labour induction (Donald 1972) describes a wide variety of mechanical and chemical assaults, many of them bizarre, and embraces a wide spectrum of success and failure. Such success as was achieved by mechanical interference (such as bougies or balloons passed through the cervix) was probably because they stimulated the release of endogenous prostaglandins within the uterine compartment (Keirse 1979). The only mechanical method which has stood the test of time is amniotomy.

Many chemical substances possess the ability — in varying degrees — to stimulate the myometrium, but most of these are unsatisfactory for labour induction or augmentation. Thus, ergometrine, although a potent myometrial stimulant and a valuable agent in the prevention and treatment of postpartum haemorrhage, has no place before delivery on account of its unpredictable effect and the danger of inducing myometrial spasm. Sparteine sulphate was popular for a time, but never gained an established place in clinical practice. Castor oil, an agent with a well recognized capacity to stimulate gastrointestinal smooth muscle, was widely employed until about 20 years ago, but its effects on the myometrium were uncertain and it fell from grace.

Oxytocin

The chemical substance most widely used for labour induction has been the posterior pituitary polypeptide, oxytocin. Controversy has abounded throughout the 80 years since it was discovered by Sir Henry Dale (Dale 1906) and since its first clinical application by William Blair Bell (Bell 1909). The first preparations were crude pituitary extracts of widely varying potency and unpredictable absorption from intramuscular injection sometimes led to catastrophes from violent and uncontrolled uterine stimulation. In a famous public lecture before the Second World War, the eminent American clinician Joseph Bolivar DeLee roundly condemned oxytocin and illustrated his point by holding up in one hand a ruptured uterus and in the other a dead fetus. Quoting from holy scripture (Proverbs chapter 23 verse 32) he declared: 'It biteth like a serpent and stingeth like an adder'. His dramatic declaration emphasized the dangers of inappropriate use of this powerful agent.

In spite of this, oxytocin has evolved into a safe therapeutic weapon. The three main developments which have allowed this have been firstly, the isolation of pure oxytocin, its chemical characterization (DuVigneaud et al 1953) and its subsequent commercial synthesis (Boissonas et al 1955); secondly, the acceptance that intravenous administration using controlled infusion apparatus was the safest and most reliable means of administration (supplanting intranasal, sublingual and buccal oxytocin); and thirdly, the recognition that the oxytocin sensitivity of the pregnant uterus varies widely between individuals and at differing stages of pregnancy. From this last development evolved the principle of oxytocin titration against uterine response (Turnbull & Anderson 1968).

Prostaglandins

This important group of bioactive compounds has roles in almost all body functions. Unlike oxytocin, they are not circulating hormones, but are synthesized and released at, or very close to, their target organ. Because of this and because of the rapidity with which circulating prostaglandins are inactivated, systemic administration of these agents requires large doses and is likely to provoke troublesome side-effects. Consequently, in clinical obstetric practice, local routes of administration within the genital tract have gained wider acceptance because of a greater degree of specificity, the need for a lower dosage, and consequently the virtual elimination of unwanted side-effects. Prostaglandin $F_{2\alpha}$ and prostaglandin E_2 are the two prostaglandins which have been used extensively in labour induction, and of these prostaglandin E_2 has been found to be the agent of choice.

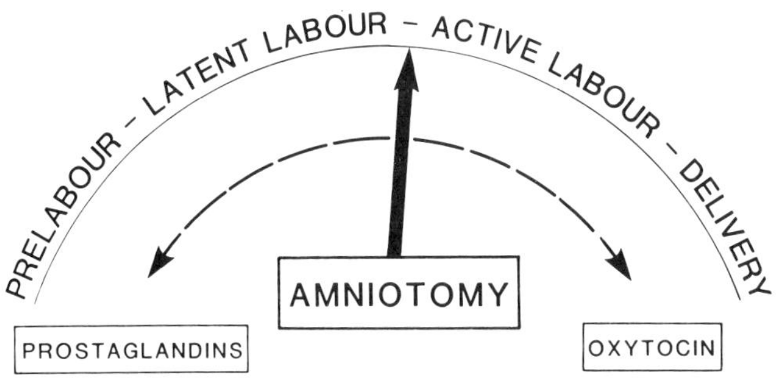

Fig. 55.6 A scheme for labour induction. Prostaglandins may be used to greatest advantage in prelabour and latent labour prior to amniotomy. Oxytocin is most effective following amniotomy. The best timing for amniotomy is after latent labour has begun.

A SCHEMATIC APPROACH TO LABOUR INDUCTION AND AUGMENTATION

In present-day obstetric practice, the clinician has at his or her disposal a triad of weapons. The three prongs of the attack are as follows:

1. Amniotomy (introduced by Thomas Denman of the Middlesex Hospital more than 200 years ago).
2. Oxytocin (introduced by Blair Bell 80 years ago).
3. Prostaglandins (introduced for labour induction within the past 20 years).

The art of labour induction and augmentation depends on a rational combination of these three weapons.

As a general rule, the prostaglandins have their greatest effect in the prelabour and latent labour phase before amniotomy. Oxytocin, in contrast, is of little value before amniotomy, but flourishes thereafter, especially in active labour. Amniotomy is the cornerstone of successful induction and its timing is paramount in relation to both the progression of the natural physiological processes and the employment or otherwise of prostaglandins and/or oxytocin (Fig. 55.6). Some clinical situations may demand the use of none of the three weapons (as in spontaneous labour, spontaneous membrane rupture and efficient progression to delivery), while others may require all three. Between these extremes lies a spectrum of situations. Some may need amniotomy alone; some prostaglandins and then amniotomy; some amniotomy and then oxytocin. The particular requirement depends on the clinical condition of the individual patient.

Assessment of the patient

The appropriate technique for labour induction or augmentation therefore depends on the point which has been reached along the physiological progression from pregnancy to delivery. In theory, it should be possible to determine whether uterine contractility is absent or present, but since the uterus is never entirely quiescent and since it is not always possible to diagnose established labour, even in the presence of apparently strong uterine contractions, this is more difficult in practice.

The most convincing evidence of progress in labour is descent of the presenting part within the birth canal. Abdominal examination allows assessment of the level of the presenting part, but in practice this is no more than a rough guide to the progress of labour.

The clinical history and abdominal examination are not in themselves sufficient. The best source of information is vaginal examination and assessment of the cervical score (Fig. 55.5). This also allows determination of whether the membranes are intact or not, if this issue is in doubt.

The place of prostaglandins

Prostaglandin E_2 is the prostaglandin which is best suited for labour induction. It is more potent and less likely to provoke side-effects than prostaglandin $F_{2\alpha}$ and achieves its best results when given locally within the genital tract. It is indicated where the cervix is unripe, with a low cervical score, especially in primigravidae (Calder 1979).

The unripe genital tract offers the choice of three routes of prostaglandin administration — extra-amniotic, endocervical or vaginal. The first two routes are effective for cervical ripening with relatively low doses, of the order of 0.5 mg prostaglandin E_2, but are more invasive than the simpler vaginal route, which requires a larger dose. Vaginal administration of prostaglandin in pessaries or gel formulations, repeated if necessary, is effective in ripening the cervix and increasing the cervical score (Calder 1986). Side-effects are rare, although care must be taken to avoid uterine hyperstimulation, and a careful watch should be kept for this complication.

Vaginal prostaglandin E_2 is also valuable for labour induction when the cervix is already ripe. A single dose of 1–2 mg prostaglandin E_2 gel is generally effective in establishing latent labour and if this is reinforced by amniotomy, the majority proceed to active labour and delivery without further stimulation (Kennedy et al 1982). Local prostaglandins may also be used for induction of labour following amniotomy or for augmentation, but in this regard their advantages over oxytocin are less clear.

Other routes of prostaglandin administration have been largely abandoned, although some clinicians continue to favour oral administration of tablets containing 0.5 mg prostaglandin E_2. These require to be given more frequently, perhaps as often as every hour, but are effective both for induction in favourable cases and for augmentation.

The main advantages of the use of prostaglandins appear to lie in their ability to reproduce many of the features of spontaneous labour. From the woman's viewpoint they are less disagreeable than the use of intravenous oxytocin, which requires complicated infusion apparatus and limits her mobility. In the case of the unfavourable induction, especially the primigravada with a low cervical score, prostaglandins result in a lower incidence of maternal and fetal complications during labour, and in particular a reduction in the Caesarean section rate compared to the rate associated with amniotomy and intravenous oxytocin. In addition, from the fetal point of view the incidence of birth asphyxia and neonatal jaundice appear to be reduced. Finally, postpartum haemorrhage is less common.

The place of amniotomy

Intact fetal membranes have been described as the biggest single hindrance to progress in labour and clearly amniotomy has a potent labour-promoting effect. Amniotomy has a central place in labour induction and augmentation, but it should not be employed until the cervix is ripe. Thereafter, it should not be delayed.

The place of oxytocin

As has already been stated, oxytocin is of little clinical value prior to amniotomy. Amniotomy stimulates the release of endogenous prostaglandins within the uterine compartment, notably from the amnion and the decidua, and this appears to sensitize the myometrium to the action of oxytocin. It is best given by intravenous infusion and should be controlled by a mechanical infusion pump, since reliance on gravity-feed can result in dangerously wild fluctuations in dose rate.

Oxytocin can be employed immediately after either spontaneous or artificial membrane rupture or its use may be delayed until the response to membrane rupture is assessed. Some clinicians prefer to wait before administering intravenous oxytocin, but most feel there is little to be gained by this and prefer to proceed without delay.

The solution of oxytocin should not be too dilute (ideally 20 iu/l) and administration should begin at the rate of 1 mu/min and increased, preferably on a logarithmic scale to a maximum of around 32 mu/min. It should rarely be necessary to go above this maximum dose. Administration of oxytocin should be controlled carefully using an infusion pump with electronic control. A paediatric infusion set ensures precise regulation. When higher doses of oxytocin are used, it is wise to record the amniotic fluid pressure by means of an intrauterine catheter connected to a pressure recorder.

Hazards of induction of labour

As was emphasized at the start of this chapter, labour induction is a potentially hazardous step. There may be hazards inherent in the fact of interruption, or in the method employed. If the fetus is immature it faces a number of dangers and may perish as a direct result of immaturity.

Amniotomy carries two particular hazards: firstly, in the absence of a well fitting presenting part, the umbilical cord may prolapse during amniotomy. Secondly, pathogenic bacteria may be introduced at the time of amniotomy, and if delivery is delayed thereafter this is likely to lead to intrauterine infection of serious clinical import for mother or offspring, or both.

There are specific hazards associated with oxytocic agents, the most obvious of which is uterine hyperstimulation and consequent fetal hypoxia.

Prostaglandins

Apart from uterine hyperstimulation, prostaglandins are relatively free of hazards, although they may be the cause of irksome side-effects. These are largely minimized by the use of local routes of administration.

Oxytocin

Oxytocin has been shown to be associated with a number of dangers, some of which may be serious. The antidiuretic action of this hormone can lead to water intoxication of the mother, and this has on occasion been fatal. There has also been an association with neonatal jaundice, although this is usually mild. There may be an increased tendency towards atonic postpartum haemorrhage, even if, as is recommended, the infusion of oxytocin is continued for 30–60 minutes after delivery.

Although these hazards are potentially very dangerous, careful adherence to appropriate guidelines in respect of induction of labour should result in their being rare.

CONCLUSIONS

Labour should not be induced or augmented unless there are clear clinical indications to do so. An understanding of the physiology of labour is crucial to good clinical practice.

The method chosen to accomplish delivery should be tailored to the obstetric features of each individual patient. If delivery is indicated when the cervix is unripe, the choice must lie between elective Caesarean section and therapeutic cervical ripening. If cervical ripening is chosen, this is best achieved by local prostaglandin E_2 therapy.

Amniotomy, the cornerstone of induction, should not be performed before the cervix is ripe. Oxytocin comes into its own following membrane rupture, whether artificial or spontaneous. The dose should be titrated against the uterine response.

REFERENCES

Anderson A B M, Turnbull A C 1969 Relationship between length of gestation and cervical dilatation, uterine contractility and other factors during pregnancy. American Journal of Obstetrics and Gynecology 105: 1207–1214

Beard R W 1968 The effect of fetal blood sampling on caesarean sections for fetal distress. British Journal of Obstetrics and Gynaecology 75: 1291–1295

Beazley J M 1975 In: Beard R, Brudenell M, Dunn P, Fairweather D (eds) The management of labour. Royal College of Obstetricians and Gynaecologists, London, pp 25–26

Bell W B 1909 The pituitary body and the therapeutic value of infundibular extract in shock, uterine atony and intestinal paresis. British Medical Journal 2: 1609–1613

Bishop E H 1964 pelvic scoring for elective induction. Obstetrics and Gynecology 24: 266–268

Boissonas R A, Guttmann S, Jaquenand P A, Waller T P 1955 A new synthesis of oxytocin. Helvetica Chimica Acta 38: 1491–1495

Calder A A 1979 Management of the unripe cervix. In: Keirse M J N C, Anderson A B M (eds) Human parturition. Leiden University Press, Leiden, pp 201–217

Calder A A 1983 Methods of induction of labour. In: Studd J (ed) Progress in obstetrics and gynaecology, vol 3. Churchill Livingstone, Edinburgh, pp 86–100

Calder A A 1986 Cervical ripening. In: Bygdeman M, Berger G S, Keith L G (eds) Prostaglandins and their inhibitors in clinical obstetrics and gynaecology. MTP Press, Lancaster, pp 145–264

Calder A A, Embrey M P, Hillier K 1974 Extra-amniotic prostaglandin E_2 for the induction of labour at term. Journal of Obstetrics and Gynaecology of the Commonwealth 81: 39–46

Caldeyro-Barcia R 1958 Uterine contractility in obstetrics. Proceedings of the Second International Congress of Gynaecology and Obstetrics, Montreal, vol 1 pp 65–78

Csapo A I, Pulkinnen 1979 The mechanisms of prostaglandin action on the pregnant human uterus. Prostaglandins 17: 283–299

Dale H H 1906 On some physiological aspects of ergot. Journal of Physiology 34: 163

Donald I 1972 A review of procedures in induction of labour. The case of prostaglandin E_2 and $F_{2\alpha}$. In obstetrics and gynaecology. Symposia Specialists, Miami, pp 5–11

DuVigneaud V, Ressler C, Trippet S 1953 The sequence of amino acid in oxytocin with a proposal for the structure of oxytocin. Journal of Biological Chemistry 205: 949–955

Friedman E A 1967 Labor. Clinical evaluation and management. Meredith, New York

Fuch F 1973 Initiation of labour. In: Klopper A, Gardner J (eds) Endocrine factors in labour. Cambridge University Press, Cambridge, pp 1–24

Gluck L, Kulovich M V 1973 Lecithin/sphingomyelin ratios in amniotic fluid in normal and abnormal pregnancies. American Journal of Obstetrics and Gynecology 115: 539–546

Hendricks C H, Brenner W E, Kvans G 1970 Normal cervical dilatation pattern in late pregnancy and labor. American Journal of Obstetrics and Gynecology 106: 1065–1082

Keirse M J N C 1979 Endogenous prostaglandins in human parturition. In: Keirse M J N C, Anderson A, Bennebroek Gravenhorst J (eds) Human parturition. Leiden University Press, Leiden, pp 101–142

Kennedy J H, Stewart P, Barlow D H, Hillan E, Calder A A 1982 Induction of labour: a comparison of a single prostaglandin E_2 vaginal tablet with amniotomy and intravenous oxytocin. British Journal of Obstetrics and Gynaecology 89: 704–707

Lerner U 1980 The uterine cervix and the initiation of labor: action of estradiol-17β. In: Naftolin F, Stubblefield P G (eds) Dilatation of the uterine cervix. Raven Press, New York, pp 301–316

Liggins G C 1978 Ripening of the cervix. Seminars in Perinatology 2: 261–271

Manning F A, Platt L D, Sipos 1980 Antepartum fetal evaluation. Development of a fetal biophysical profile score. American Journal of Obstetrics and Gynecology 136: 787–795

Philpott R H 1972 Graphic records in labour. British Medical Journal 4: 163–165

Steinetz B G, O'Byrne E M, Kroc R L 1980 The role of relaxin in cervical softening during pregnancy in mammals. In: Naftolin F, Stubblefield P G (eds) Dilatation of the uterine cervix. Raven Press, New York, pp 157–177

Studd J W W, Cardozo L 1985 Evaluation of induction of labour. In: Studd J (ed) The management of labour. Blackwell, Oxford, pp 123–132

Turnbull A C, Anderson A B M 1968 Induction of labour; results with amniotomy and oxytocin titration. Journal of Obstetrics and Gynaecology of the British Commonwealth 75: 32–41

Whitfield C R 1982 Future challenges in the management of rhesus disease. Progress in Obstetrics and Gynaecology 2: 48–61

Bryan M. Hibbard

Forceps delivery

HISTORICAL BACKGROUND

Until the 17th century all manner of instruments had been devised for bringing forth the tardy child. Midwives commonly utilized a variety of household utensils including pot hooks and ladles whilst the man-midwives used purpose-designed hooks, knives and tongs which Roesslin (1540) described in 'The Birth of Mankynde' as 'severe and harde remedies', none of which were intended to deliver a live baby. Percival Willughby (1596–1685) favoured the crotchet and recommended that midwives should be given practical instruction in its use. Others favoured the procedure of internal podalic version in cases of obstructed labour so that traction could be applied without mutilation of the fetus and with the occasional possibility of delivery of a live child.

With the advent of the obstetric forceps live births from obstructed labour became a practical possibility and it is not surprising that their inventors tried to keep the nature of the instruments a closely guarded family secret, which they succeeded in doing for three generations. The story of the Chamberlen family, Huguenot refugees, begins with William who fled to Southampton to escape the persecution of Catherine de Medici in 1569. The forceps were probably devised by his elder son, Peter, who delivered, amongst others, Queen Anne. The secret of the instruments was maintained by carrying them in a massive gilt chest, quite disproportionate to their size, and by blindfolding the patients. A nephew of Peter the Elder, Dr Peter, born in 1601, qualified in medicine and tried to organize the midwives of London into a guild. He was to receive a fee for each delivery and was to be called for all difficult cases. The intercession of the Archbishop of Canterbury put a stop to this enterprise.

Dr Peter's son Hugh tried to sell the secret to Mauriceau in Paris in 1670 but failed to accomplish the test which Mauriceau set him — the delivery of a rhachitic dwarf. Hugh was physician to King Charles the Second but fell out of favour and, in 1690, left the country in haste for Amsterdam where, in need of money, he sold the secret method for saving the lives of infants to Roger van Roonhuyze who, like Dr Peter sought to capitalize on the acquisition by selling the secret to physicians under a pledge of silence. In fact, it seems that Hugh had sold him but one of the pair of blades.

Evidently the secret leaked out or was unravelled in several places in the first half of the 18th century. In 1733 Alexander Butter presented an illustration of Dusee's forceps to the Edinburgh Medical Society. The first written description is by Giffard in his book published posthumously in 1734 but he claimed to have first used the instrument in 1726.

In 1735 Chapman published a description of the Chamberlen forceps and soon virtually all man-midwives were equipped with the new instrument or its relatives.

These mechanical aids to delivery were so successful that they gained ground in an atmosphere and philosophy which favoured humoral medicine — the use of fumigations and birth powders. Furthermore, in the middle of the 18th century there was increasing knowledge of anatomy, including the birth canal, and awareness of mechanical principles. The addition of a pelvic curve to the blades was first advocated by Smellie in 1762, a concept which was also described by Johnson (1769) in Edinburgh and Levret (1751) in France.

In order to improve the mechanical advantage of the forceps when delivering the head from high in the pelvis or above the pelvic brim various modifications of the shank and handles were made which facilitated traction in the correct axis of the birth canal. Although one of the first of these was described in 1777 by Van de Haar it was not until a century later that Tarnier described axis traction forceps as we understand them today and on which most of the subsequent instruments were based. The most successful axis traction rods were devised by Neville of Dublin in 1886 as an attachment which could be combined with various types of long forceps then in use. In particular they became wedded to the Barnes forceps and the virtually indestructible Neville-Barnes instruments are, a century later, still in use (albeit without the traction rods) in many units without thought for the original design and purpose of the instrument.

THE SELECTION OF FORCEPS

Success in forceps delivery is dependent on three factors — the accurate appraisal of the clinical situation, the manual skill of the operator and the suitability of the instrument. The training of an obstetrician is focused on the first two of these factors but critical appraisal of his or her tools is neglected; too often the obstetrician continues in his or her career tacitly accepting the instruments of his or her forefathers. It is therefore worth considering the components of the forceps, as has been done by Rhodes (1958), Forster (1971, 1975) and others (Fig. 56.1).

The blades

The instruments of the last century were designed for delivery of the long ovoid moulded head which resulted from prolonged labour and not the more spherical, less moulded head of the present day. Therefore the shape and cephalic curve of the blades is often inappropriate and results in compression of the head and a concentration rather than dispersal of the traction force (Fig. 56.1a). With the exception of Kielland's forceps there are few specified measurements for forceps blades and even within one type, wide variations may occur (Forster 1971), creating potential hazards for the fetus and the mother as well as difficulties for the obstetrician. Thus, design of the blades must take account of the average maternal pelvic size as well as the size and shape of the fetal head. Compromises may be required and there is likely to be a need for regional variations. Measurements appropriate for an average Caucasian population were suggested by Rhodes (1958, 1960) and supported by Forster (1975). These are as follows (see Fig. 56.1b):

1. Length of blade 16 cm.
2. Widest distance between blades 9 cm.
3. Distance between tips 3.5 cm.
4. Radius of cephalic curve 11.25 cm.
5. Radius of pelvic curve 17.5 cm.

The shank and lock

Long-shanked (6–9 cm) forceps of the Barnes type were generally in standard use from the mid 19th century and were necessary for delivery of the high head. They continue

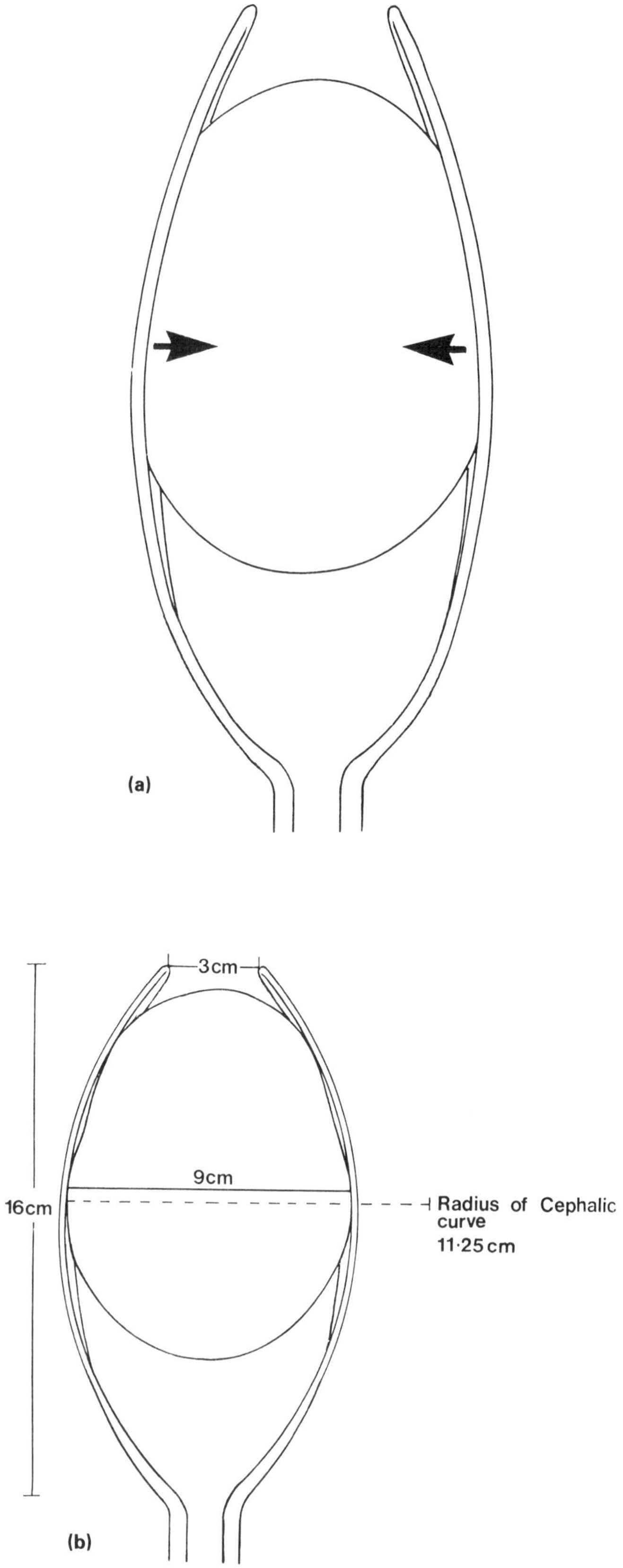

Fig. 56.1 The design of forceps blades. (**a**) Some forceps, especially those of 19th century design, have an inappropriate shape and measurements, risking fetal damage. (**b**) Measurements recommended by Rhodes (1960). From Hibbard (1988) with permission.

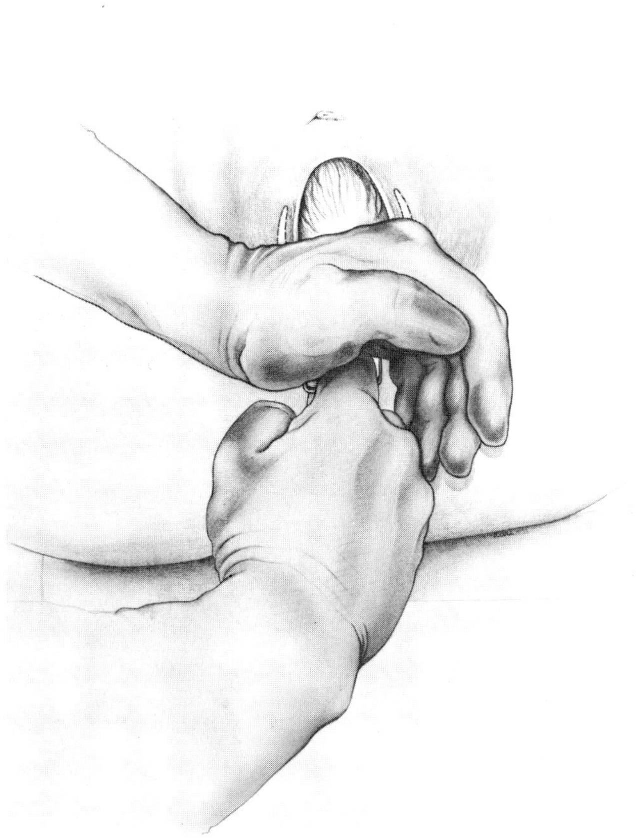

Fig. 56.2 Pajot's manoeuvre. This is rarely required. Pressure on the shank of the forceps combined with traction provides resultant force in line with the axis of the birth canal when the head is in mid-cavity. From Hibbard (1988) with permission.

to be used for delivery from the mid-cavity and also for delivery of the aftercoming head in breech presentation. The longer shank increases maternal discomfort and risk of soft-tissue trauma. At most a shank length of 6–6.25 cm is required in modern practice. Axis traction devices, now condemned, were usually attached to the shanks (e.g. Neville) but occasionally to the blades (e.g. Milne–Murray) to facilitate delivery from the pelvic brim. The same resultant traction force can be accomplished in mid-forceps delivery by the use of Pajot's manoeuvre (Fig. 56.2) but this is only occasionally required. In some cases the shanks were widened close to the lock to form a finger ring, facilitating traction at this point, rather than grasping the handles, thereby reducing the risk of unnecessary compression force on the fetal head (Fig. 56.3).

The *short shank*, typical of modern light forceps of the Wrigley type (Fig. 56.3), allows relatively painless application and a greater sensitivity in manipulation. This should be regarded as the standard instrument for the modern obstetrician.

The handle

In earlier forceps the handle was an important component to produce a compression force on the impacted head and to facilitate traction. To these ends handles tended to be large and were designed with a variety of serrated surfaces, ribs, grooves and finger lugs. These mechanical advantages are no longer necessary and constitute a temptation to use unnecessary and undesirable force. The modern Wrigley type of forceps has a very attenuated handle which is used primarily in the control of the final stage of delivery of the head, from crowning, the main traction force being exerted at the junction of the shanks.

The lock

In most forceps the two halves are linked by a lock or articulation situated between the shank and the handle. The *cross-over lock* devised by Smellie is typical of English forceps. In Europe a fixed *pivot lock* has been more widely used but allows less scope for manoeuvre when the application of the blades is less than perfect. Either of these traditional patterns is a first-class lever and close gripping of the handles is likely to have an undue compressive effect on the fetal skull. Indeed this was used deliberately and many older forceps had a handle shaped to facilitate tying the handles together with cord or kerchief. In other models the potential mechanical advantage was further enhanced by adding a compression screw lock to the handles.

An alternative design, widely used in Europe, is based on siting the lock at the end of the handles. The parent of this type of *parallel forceps* was Assalini (1811); the metal handles curve inwards at their ends to form hooks which face each other and are united by a mortice and tenon lock. Provided the traction force is applied only to the hooked end there is no direct compressive force on the head. Fitting finger-grip lugs on the outer aspects of the handles traction creates a *divergent* resultant force on the blades, with the hold on the fetal head being maintained by maternal soft-tissue pressure.

Forceps of this type have been favoured and are still used in European countries, particularly the Netherlands.

Variations

This review has been concerned with the forceps as a traction implement. Instruments used for rotation of the head from abnormal positions are discussed later.

As long ago as 1929 Das catalogued over 600 different types of obstetric forceps and many more have been described since then. His classic work and that of Laufe (1968), together with the references previously cited, provide stimulating and thought-provoking reading for the modern obstetrician.

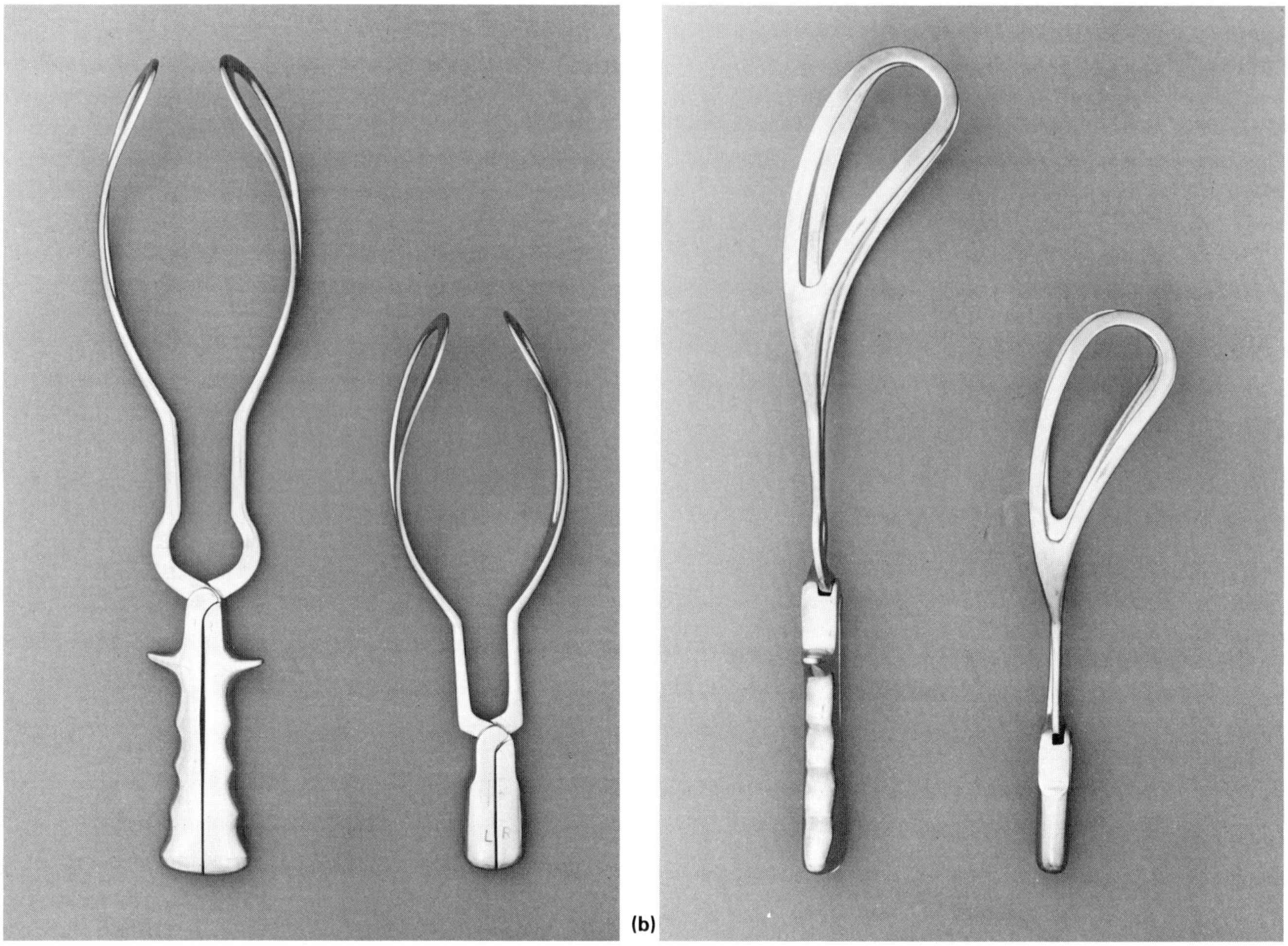

(a) (b)

Fig. 56.3 Anderson's long forceps (left) and Wrigley's forceps (right) compared. (**a**) Plan; (**b**) elevation. From Hibbard (1988) with permission.

Choice of instrument in modern practice

The historical review indicates the vast armamentarium from which the obstetrician may choose. Different instruments seem to work better in different hands. The only essential rules in the choice of forceps are that they should be appropriate to the task and that the operator should be experienced in their use. It is possible to undertake all forceps deliveries using two, or at most three, instruments. For outlet forceps delivery a short-shanked light forceps of the Wrigley type is the most suitable. For mid-cavity forceps when the sagittal suture is in the anteroposterior diameter an instrument with a longer shank is needed; it should be as light in weight as possible and should have dimensions appropriate to modern practice. For forceps rotation, if such manoeuvres are undertaken, Kielland's forceps are most widely used. For delivery of the aftercoming head in breech presentation the conventional long-shanked forceps are suitable but the Piper forceps, in which the pelvic curve is set behind the long axis, is widely used, particularly on the American continent, and its aficionados claim that application of the blades is easier.

TERMINOLOGY

Although certain terms are used to describe types of forceps deliveries the definitions of these terms vary and this makes comparison of data difficult.

A *high-forceps* delivery is one in which the fetal head is not engaged and on vaginal examination the vertex is above the level of the ischial spines. The hazards of such a procedure are so great that it should never be contemplated in modern obstetric practice.

A *mid-forceps* delivery is one in which the head is in the mid pelvic cavity with the vertex at or near the level of the ischial spines. Internal rotation of the head is often incomplete and this will need to be corrected before traction can be applied. The management of such cases is one of the most controversial current issues.

A *low-forceps* delivery usually refers to those cases in which the head is at or near the pelvic floor and is visible at the introitus, although perineal distension does not occur with contractions.

Outlet forceps refer to when the vertex has reached the

pelvic floor, the sagittal suture is in the anteroposterior diameter and only maternal soft tissues, and possibly the coccyx, are impeding the delivery of the head. It is unfortunate that the terms outlet and low are used more or less synonymously and indiscriminately by many obstetricians, because according to the definition given above, low-forceps delivery may be necessitated by some degree of cephalopelvic disproportion and the problems and hazards are more akin to those of mid-forceps delivery, although of lesser degree. Until general agreement is reached it is incumbent on units or individuals to define their use of these terms clearly.

INDICATIONS FOR FORCEPS DELIVERY

A need to expedite delivery may arise because of poor progress or because of the advent of some maternal or fetal emergency, the latter often being consequent on the former.

Delay in the second stage

It has been customary to apply arbitrary time limits for the duration of the second stage of labour, commonly 2 hours in nulliparae and 1 hour in multiparae, but these are not particularly useful, especially as it is often uncertain when the second stage actually began. Of far more importance is the progress, as judged by serial assessment of the descent of the presenting part, and the position and attitude of the head. Expulsive forces, involuntary and voluntary, may be insufficient to maintain progressive labour because they are inherently weak or because there is undue resistance to descent of the head occasioned by cephalopelvic disproportion or by soft-tissue obstruction. Disproportion is a relative concept which may be due to a relatively large head, a relatively small or misshapen pelvis, or to positional disproportion caused by malpresentation.

There are no absolute criteria as to when or how to intervene when progress is unduly slow, providing there are no other acute complicating factors. Too early interference may involve the operator in an unnecessarily difficult operative delivery, perhaps with the need for rotation of the head, whereas with a little more patience some further progress could be achieved, followed by an easier forceps delivery. On the other hand unnecessary waiting increases, to no avail, the physical and mental discomfort for the mother and the risk of asphyxia and trauma for the baby.

An outlet forceps delivery carries no significant risk for the mother or baby and is freely employed when there is delay due to relative rigidity of the maternal soft tissues or when maternal expulsive efforts are inadequate because of exhaustion, non-co-operation, or lack of the bearing-down reflex associated with epidural anaesthesia.

As long ago as 1920 De Lee proposed prophylactic forceps delivery, anticipating the inevitable, but this was generally condemned as meddlesome interference.

Even with a prolonged second stage, providing there is progress there is a reasonable chance of spontaneous delivery occurring, as has been shown in the life table analysis of Kadar & Romero (1983) which relates to primigravidae who have not had epidural analgesia. The fact that even after 2 hours in the second stage there is still a reasonable chance of spontaneous vaginal delivery does not, of course, mean that it is desirable or beneficial to wait — a test of achievement may then be replaced by a test of endurance. Again it is the degree of progress set against maternal and fetal condition which becomes the final arbiter. Friedman (1978) defined normal progress as descent of the presenting part at the rate of 1 cm/h in nulliparae and 2 cm/h in multigravidae but it is difficult in clinical practice to achieve such precision of assessment and factors such as caput formation and moulding can give a false impression of progress.

Whilst there is little or no evidence that delay uncomplicated by other factors is significantly detrimental to the fetus or neonate it is clear that a conservative policy of management must include diligent and expert monitoring to be sure that there are no adverse factors. Continuous monitoring of the fetal heart rate is required, for it is known that a progressive fetal acidaemia develops during the second stage of labour (Pearson & Davies 1974). Assessment of the presentation, position and descent of the head should be undertaken by a senior person because all too often in such cases malpresentations have been missed or an increasingly large caput has been interpreted as descent of the head.

Specific maternal and fetal indications

Although there are certain clearcut conditions which in themselves indicate the need for urgent delivery, more commonly intelligent anticipation of maternal or fetal deterioration, particularly in cases of prolonged labour, leads to obstetric intervention.

Maternal compromise

Maternal obstetric indications include eclampsia, severe pre-eclampsia and intrapartum haemorrhage. *Intercurrent illness*, such as severe cardiac or pulmonary disease, is usually regarded as an indication for early recourse to forceps delivery if progress is not rapid, in order to minimize physical strain.

Maternal distress to former generations meant a mother exhausted physically and mentally, dehydrated and ketotic, with a raised pulse rate and often mildly pyrexial. To allow such a situation to develop in modern obstetric practice is indefensible. However the term is still used and refers to circumstances where progress is slow and further beguiling and encouragement of the mother are to no avail.

Fetal compromise

There are some clearly recognized and defined complications in the second stage, such as umbilical cord prolapse and premature separation of the placenta, in which early delivery, usually by forceps, is imperative.

More commonly, there is gradually accumulating evidence of fetal distress — a clinical concept implying progressive fetal asphyxia — for which no specific cause is identified although in many cases there are defined risk factors, such as maternal age, hypertension, prolonged pregnancy and intrauterine growth retardation. Other alerting factors include the passage of meconium-stained amniotic fluid, fetal bradycardia and late deceleration patterns on a cardiotocograph. However, as in the first stage of labour, action based on fetal heart rate patterns alone will lead to many unnecessary interventions and unless the pattern is truly alarming, or delivery is likely to be achieved quickly and easily by episiotomy and outlet forceps delivery, fetal blood sampling may be performed before deciding on the need for, and mode of, delivery.

ALTERNATIVE METHODS OF MANAGEMENT

Since indications for forceps delivery are rarely, if ever, absolute, other options need to be considered.

Wait

When the head is in the mid-cavity and incompletely rotated, temporizing may result in some further progress and avoid the need for rotation as well as bringing the head lower in the pelvis. There is no case for waiting if there is arrest of progress.

Encourage stronger uterine action

This may be done by administration of oxytocin, as advocated by O'Driscoll & Meagher (1980), at least in primigravidae. The authors distinguish two phases in the second stage of labour. In phase 1 the head is high in the pelvis and the occiput is usually lateral. It is a natural extension of the first stage of labour and there is no maternal desire to push. Phase 2 begins when the head reaches the pelvic floor and the mother has a compulsive desire to push. O'Driscoll & Meagher take the extreme view that vaginal delivery with forceps should never be attempted in phase 1, when a need for urgent delivery is met by Caesarean section. If there is no urgency, adequate uterine activity can be restored by oxytocin infusion, replacing traction by propulsion. Although there may be an eventual need for forceps delivery it is likely to be easier. The other side of the coin is that oxytocin may result in further impaction and if Caesarean section is ultimately needed, displacement and delivery of the head may be more difficult. Clearly careful selection of cases for such a form of management is vital if trauma is to be avoided.

Caesarean section

Abandonment of mid-forceps operations, especially those involving rotation of the fetal head, has gained favour in recent years, not only because of the attitudes expressed by O'Driscoll & Meagher (1980) but because of increasing concern with defensive obstetrics occasioned by attitudes to litigation in the event of misfortune. The risks of Caesarean section are clear and relatively well quantified. The risks of forceps delivery from the mid-cavity are not and, in spite of an extensive literature, judgement continues to be based on common sense rather than statistical analyses of often dubious validity. From the published literature, including the review by Cohen & Friedman (1983), it is evident that judgement is confounded by many factors, including the following: there have been no prospective or controlled trials; varying definitions have been used; indications for forceps delivery vary and series may or may not include rotations performed by various means; management policies include varying degrees of conservatism; it is difficult to be certain whether many fetal complications and condition at birth are propter hoc or post hoc, cause or effect; distinction is not made between operations performed by skilled and unskilled obstetricians; the availability of senior assistance or facilities for immediate Caesarean section in case of undue difficulty is a relevant factor. Many of these problems are highlighted by the provocative papers of Cardozo et al (1982) and Chiswick & James (1979) and the extensive correspondence which followed them.

On the basis of available evidence there does not appear to be a case for absolute abandonment of mid-cavity forceps delivery, even if it involves rotation, in favour of Caesarean section but the following general guidelines should ensure that these potentially dangerous operations can be relatively safe for mother and baby and the longer-term sequelae of Caesarean section can be minimized:

1. Caesarean section should generally be carried out if there is confirmed evidence of fetal asphyxia and the head has not reached the pelvic floor, so that there is only soft-tissue resistance to be overcome. Reassessment in the operating theatre immediately prior to section is often advisable as the situation may have changed in the interim.
2. Caesarean section is indicated in mid-cavity arrest in multigravidae, with or without malpresentation as this nearly always indicates disproportion of a degree which would make vaginal delivery dangerous.
3. If mid-forceps delivery is contemplated, senior staff should always be directly involved in assessment and supervision of the delivery. If for any reason senior assistance is not immediately available or advice is available only by telephone, Caesarean section is likely to be a preferable option.
4. If the preceding labour pattern suggests the possibility of disproportion, such as a long 7–10 cm cervical dila-

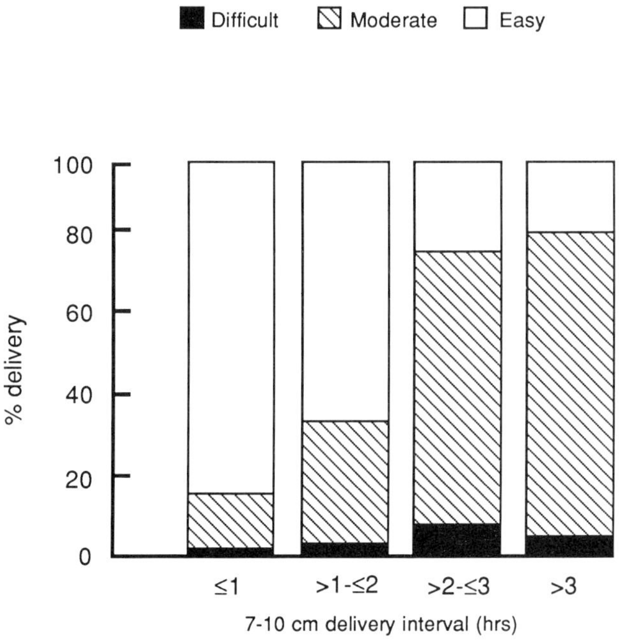

Fig. 56.4 Facility of forceps delivery related to the 7–10 cm cervical dilatation period (occipito-anterior presentations). After Davidson et al (1976).

tation interval (Davidson et al 1976; Fig. 56.4), assessment in the operating theatre with facilities immediately available for Caesarean section is required before attempting forceps application.

5. Adequate anaesthesia must be established. This usually means epidural or spinal anaesthesia — pudendal nerve block and local infiltration are inadequate.

Ventouse

The advantages and disadvantages of the ventouse are discussed in Chapter 57. Forceps and ventouse, rather than rivalling each other, should be regarded as complementary in varying circumstances and the same basic rules for their use should apply. The ventouse should not be regarded as an alternative to Caesarean section and has no useful place as an alternative to outlet forceps. In some circumstances it is a suitable option for delivery from the mid-cavity, particularly if the sagittal suture is not in the anteroposterior diameter, as traction usually results in autorotation, mimicking the normal mechanism of labour. It is certainly a safer option when no staff skilled in mid-forceps application and rotation are available.

Studies comparing the safety of the ventouse versus mid-cavity forceps are generally less helpful than those relating to Caesarean section (for review see Ryden 1986). Early papers showing markedly inferior results, particularly trauma, from ventouse delivery include cases where the instrument had been applied before full dilatation of the cervix. The Portsmouth study (Vacca et al 1983) revealed no difference in neonatal trauma although there were more cases of jaundice. In that study, ultrasound scanning for intracranial haemorrhage was not used. It was notable that the failure rate (i.e. necessitating Caesarean section) for the ventouse was 13% and for forceps 10%. It is this willing recourse to Caesarean section and the fact that most of the forceps deliveries were done by experienced obstetricians which may well account for the good neonatal results.

PREREQUISITES FOR FORCEPS DELIVERY

There are certain fundamental rules which must be fulfilled before forceps delivery is attempted, irrespective of an apparent urgency to deliver the baby. Indeed an emergency situation is just the time when discipline and adherence to well established principles are most required.

1. The cervix must be fully dilated.
2. The membranes must be ruptured.
3. The position and station of the head must be identified with certainty and the head must be in a suitable position for delivery, with prior rotation if necessary.
4. There must be no major cephalopelvic disproportion.
5. There must be adequate facilities for neonatal resuscitation and special care.

In addition it is usually recommended that the bladder should be empty. This is arguable, as the bladder is an abdominal organ at this stage and is not likely to contribute to mechanical difficulty. Neither is bladder trauma more likely if there is urine in it — indeed it might even be protective. A possible exception is when forceps rotation is being performed and it is of some importance to know that there is no pre-existing bladder injury indicated by haematuria. Certainly a catheter should be passed after delivery for the same reason.

TECHNIQUE

Occipito-anterior forceps delivery

The first essential for safe delivery of the baby is that the forceps blades should lie in correct relationship to the fetal head. To this end careful reassessment and rehearsal of the position of the blades are a desirable preliminary. The blades are designated left and right. The left blade is that which is applied on the left side of the mother's pelvis and is held in the operator's left hand. It fits comfortably into the slightly cupped right hand of the operator (Fig. 56.5).

The patient should be on an obstetric bed capable of head-down tilt or on an operating table. Most obstetricians favour the lithotomy position but necessary precautions are a wedge under one buttock to avoid aortocaval compression and minimal flexion and abduction of the thighs compatible with access.

There are three phases to the operation — application of the blades, adjustment and articulation, and traction.

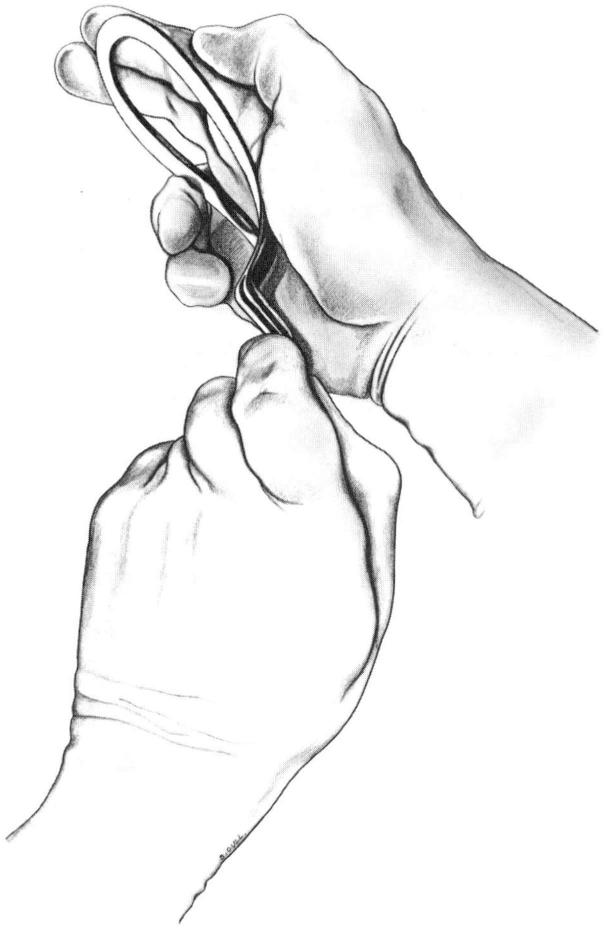

Fig. 56.5 Identification of the left blade of the forceps. The blade fits comfortably into the right hand and the fingers guard the tip. From Hibbard (1988) with permission.

Application of the blades

The left blade is selected and the handle is held between the finger and thumb of the left hand. The blade rests in the cupped right hand and the handle is approximately parallel with the right inguinal ligament (Fig. 56.6). Only two fingers of the right hand need to be inserted into the vagina to guide the tip of the blade into position alongside the fetal head as the handle is swept round in an arc. Only minimal force should be necessary and grasping the handle of the forceps like a joystick is quite unnecessary. If application and manipulation are not possible with the finger and thumb grasp something is wrong and the situation should be reassessed. The right blade is applied in like manner.

Adjustment and articulation

With proper application and positioning the forceps blades should come together and lock easily but some minor adjustments may be necessary. Optimally the blades should ultimately grasp the head along the submentovertical diameter.

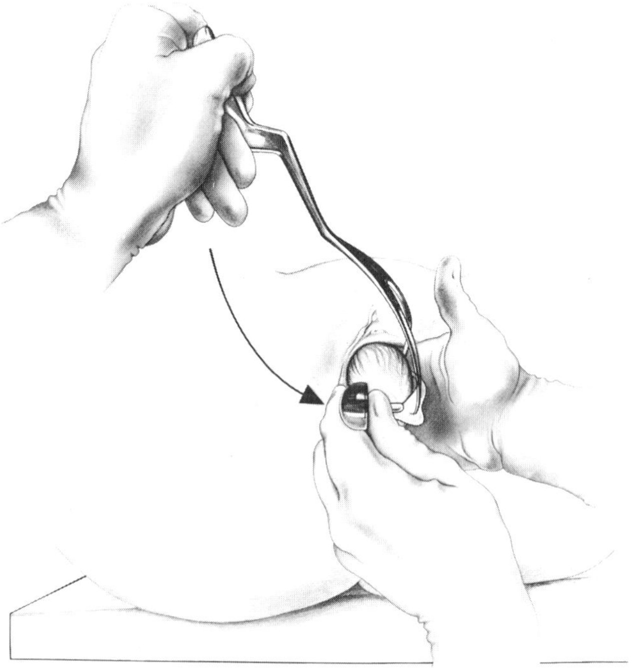

Fig. 56.6 Insertion of the left blade. The handle starts parallel with the inguinal ligament on the opposite side. From Hibbard (1988) with permission.

If the head is not quite directly in the anteroposterior diameter of the pelvis the forceps should be applied in correct relationship to the head rather than the pelvis.

The positioning is checked by feeling the lambdoid suture 2 cm from the shank of the forceps and the symmetry of the forceps in relation to the suture lines and fontanelles.

If the blades do not lock easily, undue manipulation is likely to be traumatic to mother and baby and, once more, removal and reassessment are indicated.

Traction

Traction is best applied by the fingers placed between the shanks of the forceps (Fig. 56.7). This imposes some limit to the degree of traction force which can be applied, gives a better feel of the direction of traction and avoids any risk of head compression from gripping the handles. The traction force is also limited if the forearm is kept in a flexed position.

The aim of traction is to augment the natural forces. The direction of traction should be in the axis of the birth canal, altering the angle as the head descends (Fig. 56.8). Traction is applied intermittently and synchronously with uterine contractions. There should always be some descent of the head during traction, even though it retreats in the intervening period. Lack of descent suggests a degree of dispropor-

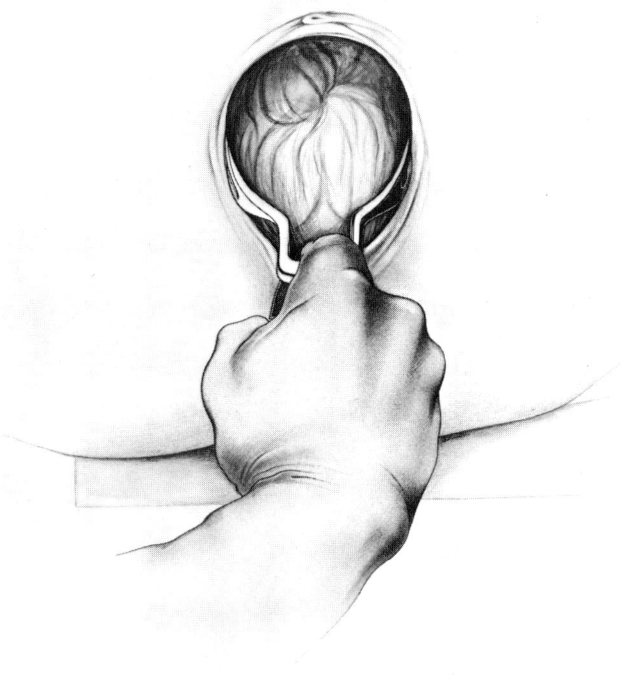

Fig. 56.7 Traction. Note the initial direction of traction which is related to the station of the head in the birth canal. The traction force is applied via the index finger between the shanks of the forceps. From Hibbard (1988) with permission.

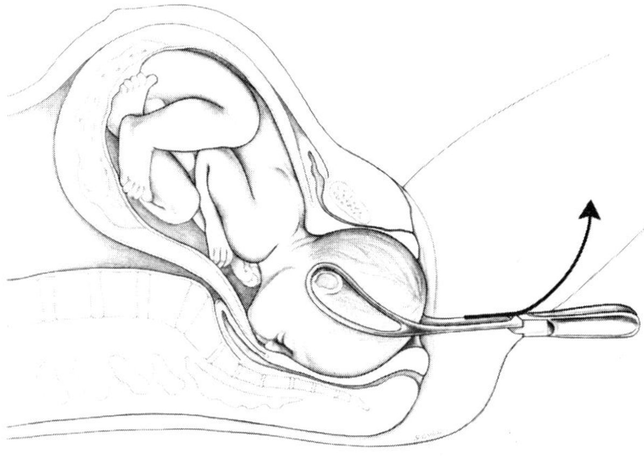

Fig. 56.8 The direction of traction follows the axis of the birth canal, reproducing the normal mechanism of labour. From Hibbard (1988) with permission.

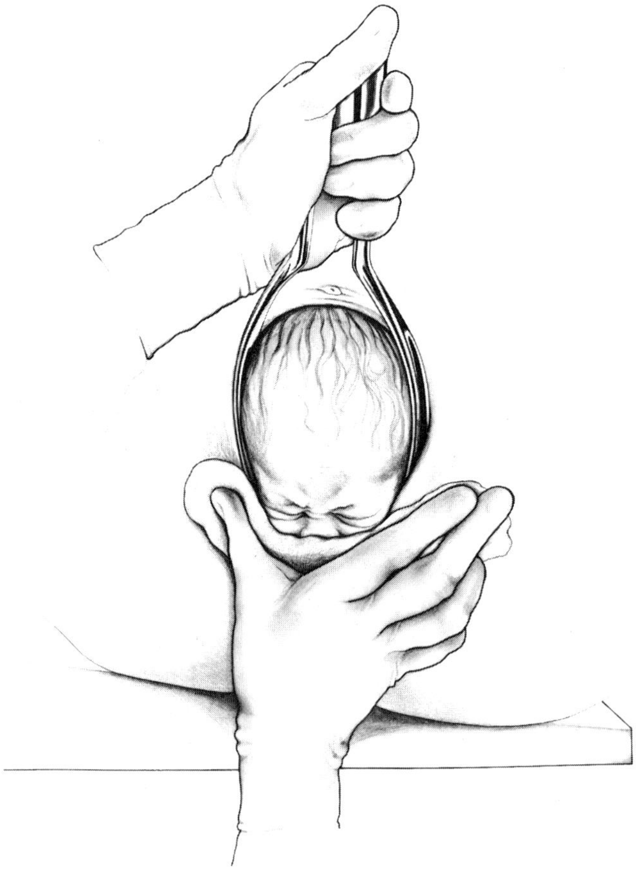

Fig. 56.9 Completion of delivery of the head by extension. The handles of the forceps are almost vertical. From Hibbard (1988) with permission.

tion incompatible with safe vaginal delivery. When the head is distending the perineum and the biparietal diameter is at the level of the ischial tuberosities an episiotomy is performed. Crowning and delivery of the head are achieved in a controlled manner by swinging the handles of the forceps upwards so that the head extends (Fig. 56.9). The blades are removed and delivery is completed in the normal manner, followed by inspection of the birth canal for lacerations and repair of the episiotomy.

FORCEPS DELIVERY FOR CEPHALIC MALPRESENTATIONS

The clinical features and general management of occipito-posterior and transverse positions are discussed elsewhere (Ch. 53). In summary, with delay associated with these malpositions the options are:

1. Caesarean section.
2. Manual rotation and forceps delivery.
3. Forceps rotation and delivery.

4. With occipito-posterior position, delivery as an occipito-posterior.
5. Ventouse delivery.

When delivering from the transverse position it is important to distinguish between true deep transverse arrest, where pelvic contraction is likely, rotation must be assisted and delivery may be difficult, and transverse position without arrest, when delivery may be required because of fetal compromise but the pelvis is of normal configuration. In the latter case the head is still in mid-cavity, but has not had time to rotate from the transverse position in which it engaged in the pelvis. In such cases traction, either by ventouse or forceps, is associated with autorotation as the head descends to the pelvic outlet. This was the desirable objective emphasized by Kielland in 1916.

The choice of operative procedure is dependent not only on the clinical conditions, but on the skills and training of the operator. All such deliveries are potentially hazardous, and increasing difficulty is related to, for example, the duration of the 7–10 cm dilatation interval (Davidson et al 1976; Fig. 56.4). Therefore such procedures must always be undertaken or supervised by the most senior person available and are often best carried out as a trial of forceps in the operating theatre with facilities immediately available for Caesarean section if conditions prove unfavourable.

Preliminaries to forceps rotation

Essential preliminaries are:

1. Assemble the full team, including anaesthetist and paediatrician.
2. Ascertain that conditions are as previously assessed and that a traumatic vaginal delivery is potentially feasible.
3. Decide on the place of delivery, i.e. delivery room or operating theatre.
4. Decide on the method of pain relief with the patient and anaesthetist.

Manual rotation

This is the least popular option and may lead to unexpected and unwanted problems.

To facilitate rotation it is usually necessary to disimpact the head by pushing it upward. This increases the risk of cord prolapse and may leave the head at a higher level after rotation, so making forceps application more difficult and more hazardous. Undue displacement may even result in the head being above the pelvic brim. Further, to have the occiput anterior when the head is high in the pelvic cavity is unanatomical and is contrary to the normal mechanism of labour. One of the basic rules of assisted delivery is to endeavour to mimic the normal mechanism of labour as closely as possible.

In general, if displacement is necessary to rotate the head, Caesarean section is a better option.

Forceps rotation and delivery

Although there is an experienced body of opinion which believes that forceps rotation of an occipito-posterior presentation should never be undertaken (O'Driscoll & Meagher 1980), the majority identify a place for forceps rotation in carefully selected cases. However, it is clear that in some units where there is ready and early recourse to forceps delivery the number of rotational forceps is unnecessarily high, and that with a little more time natural rotation often occurs and can be followed by an easier and straightforward forceps application.

Forceps of the conventional long type have been used for rotation after correct cephalic application but, because of the pelvic curve of the blades, to maintain the correct axis of the blades during rotation the handles must be swept round in a wide arc (the Scanzoni manoeuvre) which is difficult to judge accurately. It can lead to a dangerous degree of rotatory force, with risk of intracranial damage as well as trauma to the birth canal. This type of manipulation has no place in modern practice.

Kielland's forceps

Of the many types of forceps designed for rotation of the head only two have found wide favour over a long period. Kielland's forceps have been particularly popular in Europe, whilst Barton's forceps have had most support in America. The use of the former will be described in detail. Those readers who wish to make a detailed study of Barton's forceps and their modifications are referred particularly to the monograph by Parry Jones (1972).

Kielland first described his forceps in 1916 although he had publicly demonstrated them in 1910. Thus his description of their use was based on his considerable experience at the time of writing and is worthy of reconsideration. The forceps were designed primarily for extraction of the incompletely rotated head, using a correct cephalic application (oblique application had previously been a common practice). Contrary to what is often believed, Kielland condemned the use of forceps when the head was above the pelvic brim. He reiterated the observations of the previous generation who had developed axis traction forceps that: 'the extraordinary force necessary ... lay principally in the misdirected traction ... resulting from the pelvic curve'. Kielland's design might be regarded as the simplest form of axis traction because 'the bayonet-like shape permits the axis of the blade to lie parallel to the axis of the handle ... traction can therefore follow the direction of the handles' (Fig. 56.10). One potential disadvantage is that the initial direction of traction is through the perineum, so that a large and early episiotomy is required.

The other outstanding feature of the instrument is the sliding lock (Fig. 56.11) which permits satisfactory cephalic application even in cases of gross asynclitism, although in

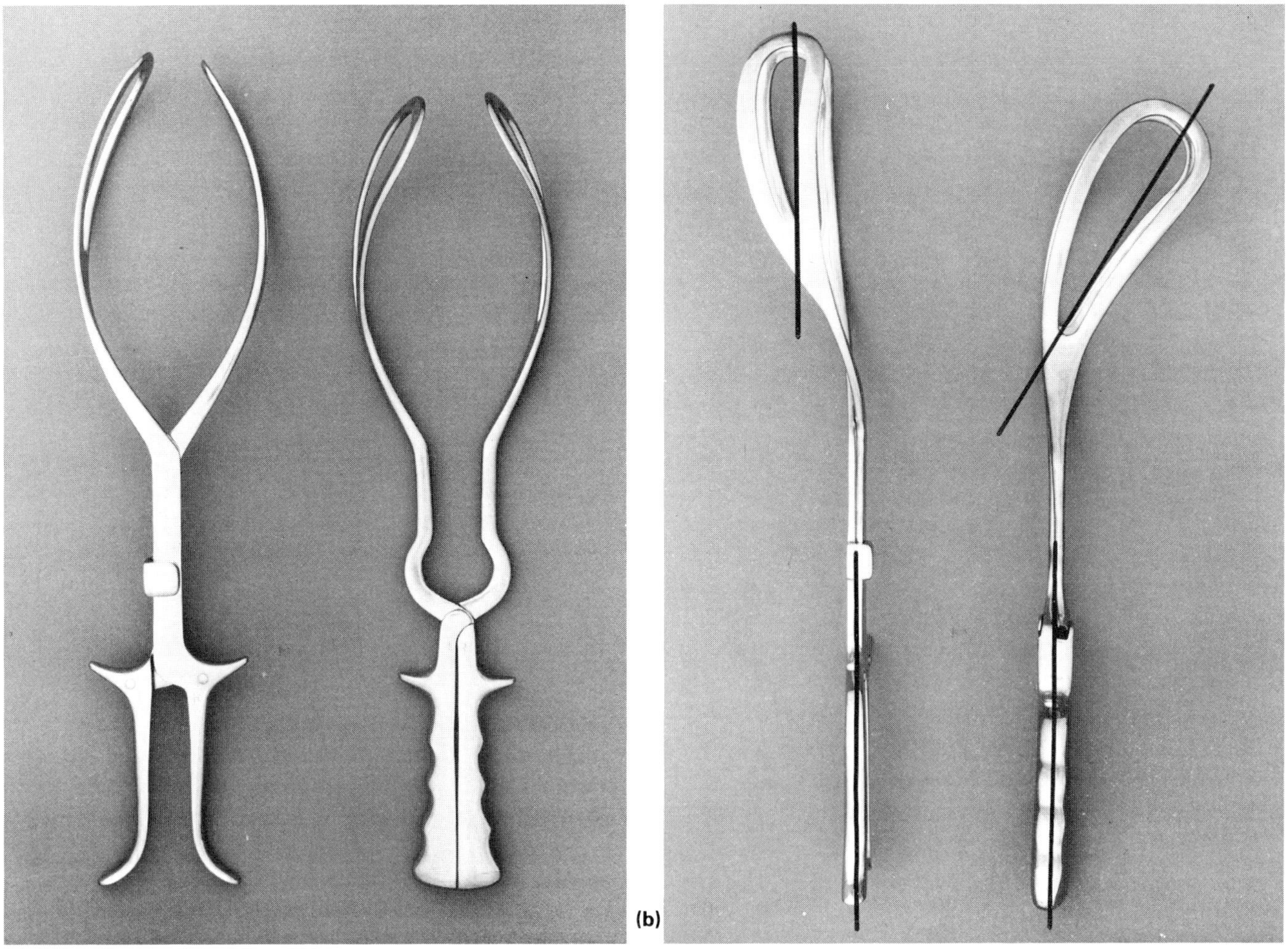

(a) (b)

Fig. 56.10 Kielland's forceps (left) and Anderson's forceps (right) compared. (**a**) Plan; (**b**) elevation. Note that in the Kielland's forceps the axes of the blades and handles are parallel. From Hibbard (1988) with permission.

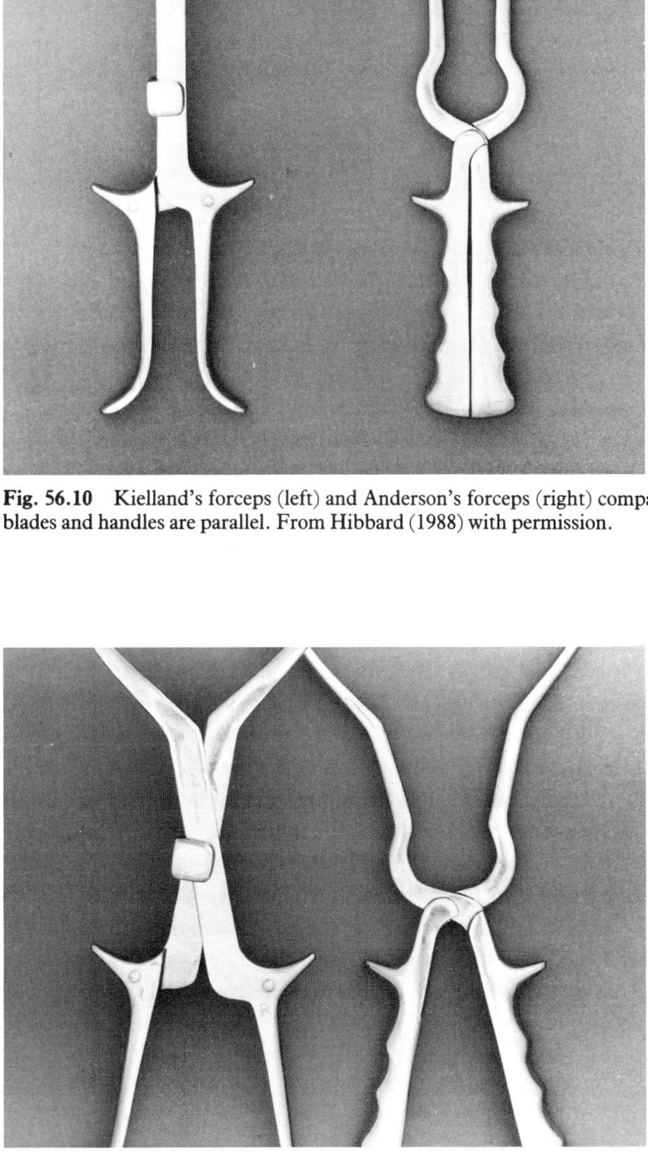

Fig. 56.11 The locks of Kielland's (left) and conventional forceps (right) compared. The sliding lock of the Kielland's forceps facilitates application when there is asymmetric moulding of the head. From Hibbard (1988) with permission.

modern practice such a condition is rarely encountered, as intervention has usually taken place at an earlier stage.

Other minor details of design are important, especially in relation to the method of application of the blades. For a detailed discussion the reader is referred to the classic monograph by Parry Jones (1952). Parry Jones defined ideal criteria for forceps which are almost fulfilled by the Kielland instrument:

1. Simple in construction.
2. Suitable for all positions of the head.
3. Require only a single application with minimal manipulation.
4. Permit true axis traction.
5. Satisfactory for rotation of the fetal head without applying excessive stressing forces.

Nevertheless, in inappropriate, unskilled hands Kielland's forceps are potentially dangerous and specialist training and continuing practice are required for their safe use. Hence there has been a growing tendency to abandon mid-cavity rotation in favour of Caesarean section. In some work-

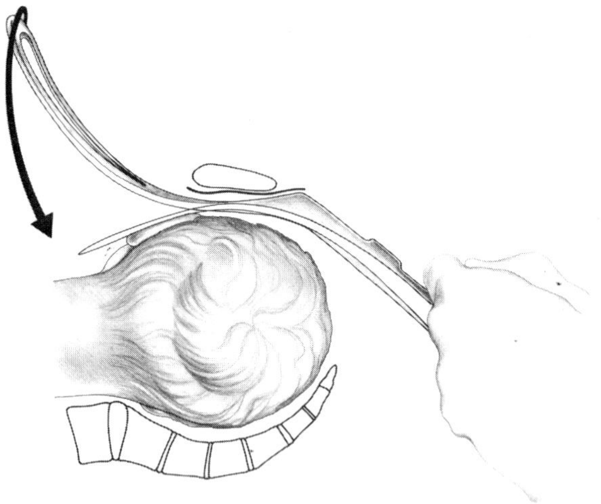

Fig. 56.12 Classic method of application of the anterior blade of Kielland's forceps. Note the position of the shank between the head and the symphysis pubis. From Hibbard (1988) with permission.

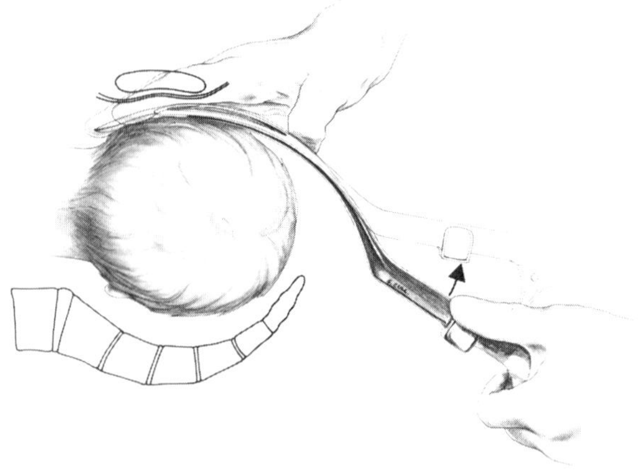

Fig. 56.13 Direct application of the anterior blade. Note the use of the operator's fingers to avoid injury to the birth canal by the tip of the forceps. From Hibbard (1988) with permission.

ing circumstances ventouse delivery may be a satisfactory or even desirable alternative, with less risk of trauma but more risk of failure. Also, the ventouse does not reduce the already limited available pelvic space.

Application of Kielland's forceps

It is helpful to rehearse the application of the blades once the station of the head and position of the occiput have been identified, remembering that the aim is to obtain a correct cephalic application with the concavity of the pelvic curve of the forceps directed towards the occiput. To aid orientation there is a raised knob on the upper surface of each finger lug and these should point in the direction of the occiput.

The anterior (superior) blade is always applied first — i.e. the left blade for a right occipito-lateral position and the right blade for a left occipito-lateral position.

Three methods of application of the anterior blade are described and the relative merits have long been debated. The most controversial is the 'classic' method recommended by Kielland himself. He was aware of criticism of what many regarded as a dangerous technique but put the counter arguments very convincingly in his original paper (1916).

Classic application. The superior blade is selected and inserted with the cephalic concavity directed anteriorly (Fig. 56.12), i.e. upside down in relation to the fetal head. The index and middle fingers of one hand are used to guide the tip of the blade and protect the fetal and maternal soft tissues. The other hand grasps the forceps 'with a full grip (like a sword, not a pen)' (Kielland 1916). The handle is initially kept nearly horizontal but when the tip of the blade encounters the fetal head the handle is depressed and the blade should then slide easily into the cavity of the uterus. Failure to recognize this can lead to damage to the lower uterine segment.

The blade is introduced until the shank impinges on the posterior vaginal wall and the narrow bevelled section between the base of the blade and the shank is between the head and the symphysis pubis. The blade is then rotated, maintaining the axis, so that it slides into correct position in relation to the head. The direction of rotation is important, as will be seen if the procedure is rehearsed. The arc which the blade describes is minimized if the concavity of the pelvic curve fits the convexity of the head, so the correct direction of rotation is always towards the concave rim of the blade. The knobs on the handles act as a guide — rotation is carried out to the side on which the knob is felt.

The available space between the head and the symphysis may not be sufficient to carry out this manoeuvre safely, particularly if the head is well down in the pelvic cavity.

Direct application. This apparently simple option is only feasible when the head is low in the pelvis because the initial position of the handle is such that it may be hampered by the perineum or the end of the operating table (Fig. 56.13).

The main force used during introduction is elevation of the handle and, as with the classic method, advancement of the blade follows naturally, with minimal effort. Again protection of the soft tissues with the operator's fingers is an essential feature.

Wandering method. This is the most popular option, perhaps because it is closer to the technique used for application of conventional forceps. The ultimate anterior blade, whether it be right or left, is inserted in the standard manner along the side wall of the pelvis and is then wandered by swinging it round to a correct cephalic relationship as insertion proceeds (Fig. 56.14). It is usually advised that it is easier to wander the blade from insertion over the forehead and this has the advantage that during the early part of inser-

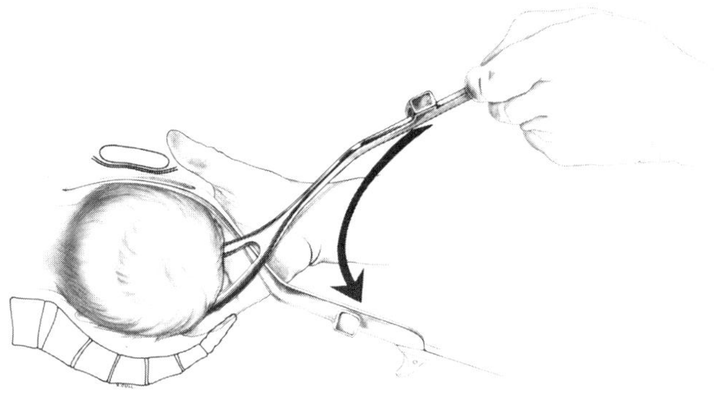

Fig. 56.14 Wandering method of application of the anterior blade. Insertion is started as with a conventional forceps application, swinging the blade round to a correct cephalic application as insertion proceeds. From Hibbard (1988) with permission.

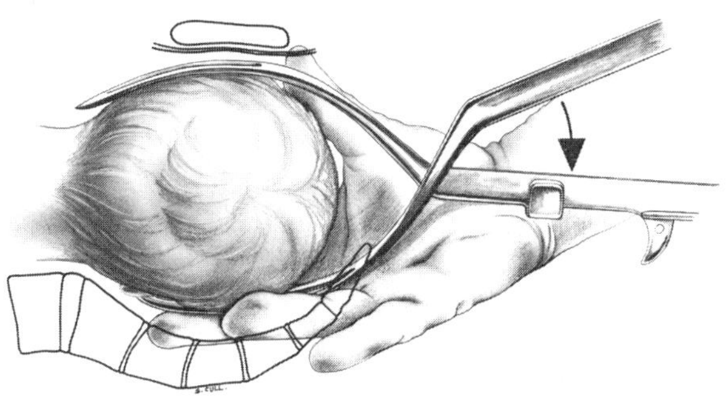

Fig. 56.15 Direct application of the posterior blade. From Hibbard (1988) with permission.

tion the pelvic curve of the blade matches the curve of the birth canal.

The posterior blade. Although it might appear from the foregoing that more difficulty is likely to be encountered with the anterior rather than the posterior blade the opposite is often the case — a point again emphasized by Kielland (1916) — because of obstruction by the sacral promontory (Fig. 56.15).

Half of the right hand is introduced into the hollow of the sacrum and is used to facilitate direct application of the blade, which often drops into position with minimal pressure. If the sacral promontory is a problem it is important for any manipulation to be carried out gently whilst the soft tissues are guarded by the operator's fingers. Sometimes in cases of difficulty a slightly oblique introduction and wandering application may be helpful.

Traction and rotation

Accepting that the desirable objective is to mimic the normal mechanism of labour as closely as possible, traction force in the exact direction of the handles should be applied first and if there is advancement of the head this can be continued without any external rotating force; the head should rotate spontaneously as it descends through the birth canal.

It must be recognized that, because of the design of the forceps, the direction of traction is more posteriorly than with conventional forceps and an early generous episiotomy is required. Also, if the patient is in the lithotomy position effective traction is difficult with the operator in a standing position or sitting on a normal operating stool. Although Kielland advocated tilting the bed to facilitate traction a better alternative is for the operator to kneel or sit on a low footstool.

Delivery is completed in the conventional manner, avoiding compression of the handles and using only the finger lugs to exert traction force (Fig. 56.16).

If the head does not descend readily during the initial traction attempt the situation should be reappraised, with the alternative options of rotation in the mid-cavity or Caesarean section.

Mid-cavity rotation must be carried out with gentleness and sensitivity. Slight upward dislodgement of the head, especially with a funnel-shaped pelvis, may facilitate rotation. Only the finger lugs should be used for applying rotational pressure, using the grip shown in Figure 56.17. Traction and rotational forces should not be applied at the same time.

FORCEPS DELIVERY AS AN OCCIPITO-POSTERIOR

The second stage of labour is likely to be prolonged with an occipito-posterior position even if spontaneous delivery eventually occurs. Generally delay which is sufficient to warrant intervention suggests the need to correct the malpresentation before applying traction, but in some cases forceps delivery as an occipito-posterior may be justified and preferable. Particular circumstances in which this option should be considered include a satisfactory bony pelvic outlet, as with an anthropoid pelvis (which favours occipito-posterior positions) and delay due to soft-tissue obstruction. The head must be below the level of the ischial spines and the position must be directly occipito-posterior (occipito-sacral).

The forceps are applied in the conventional manner, with correct pelvic application, taking care not to place the blades too far anteriorly in relation to the head as they may then

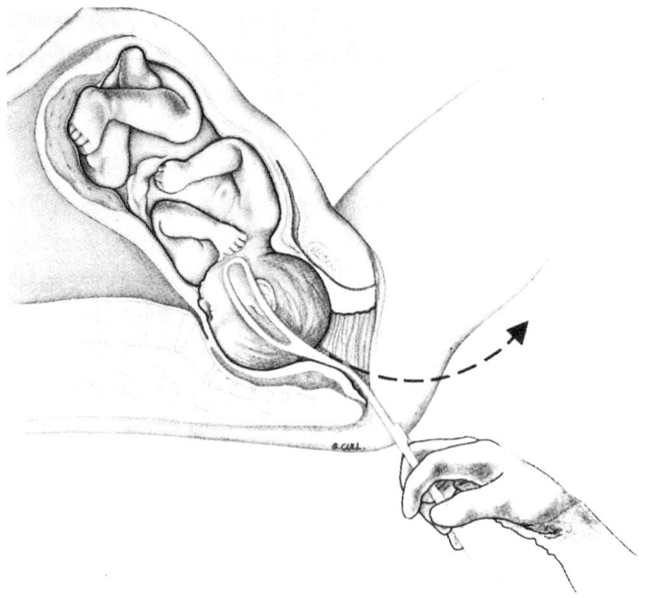

(a)

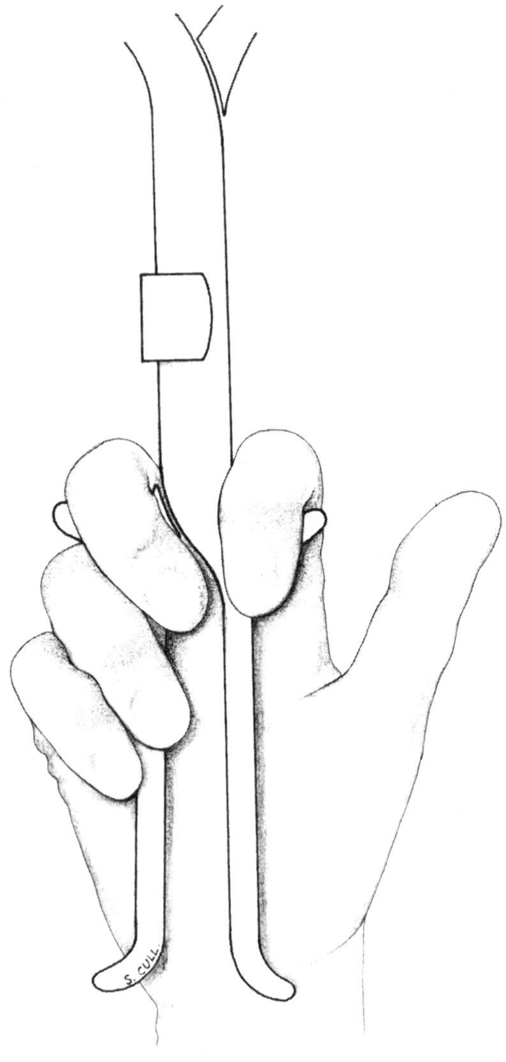

(b)

Fig. 56.16 (**a**) The direction of traction with Kielland's forceps. (**b**) The traction force is applied via the finger lugs and not by grasping the handles. From Hibbard (1988) with permission.

slip off. A generous episiotomy is usually required and traction is directed posteriorly until the glabella is under the apex of the pubic arch. The handles of the forceps are then swung upwards so that the head is delivered by flexion.

COMPLICATIONS

Most complications of forceps delivery result from errors of judgement and inexperience. The risks range from minimal for an outlet forceps delivery, to considerable for a mid-forceps delivery associated with rotation and performed by an inexperienced operator. When labour has been prolonged and difficult there is an added element of maternal tissue bruising, devitalization and risk of sepsis which is likely to increase the problems arising from any operative trauma.

The perineum and vagina

There is a risk of extension of the episiotomy and additional vaginal lacerations occurring during application of the blades and during traction, particularly if forceps of unsuitable design are used. Delivery of the occasional unrecognized occipito-posterior position increases the risk of perineal trauma and this may even extend into the anal canal. Any additional trauma makes suturing more difficult and increases the risk of painful scars and dyspareunia.

The cervix

The cervix is particularly susceptible to damage during rotational deliveries, either during the application of the blades or during the rotation. Lateral lacerations may extend upwards in the lower uterine segment, with rupture of the uterine artery or main branches. Damage anteriorly may involve the bladder, with production of a vesicocervical or vesicovaginal fistula. Traumatic haemorrhage may be severe and in any cases of doubt concerning trauma full exploration in operating theatre conditions is obligatory. Attempts at semi-blind suturing in the delivery room without adequate exposure and assistance are only likely to compound the problem.

Urinary complications

These include retention of urine and infection. In particular a careful watch should be kept to avoid retention with overflow if epidural analgesia has been used. Any difficult delivery should be followed by catheterization and if haematuria is revealed special precautions are necessary. Gross haematuria suggests the possibility of tearing and fistula formation, and detailed examination is required. Lesser degrees of haematuria are indicative of bruising and devitalization. This may be associated with tissue necrosis and the risk of late fistula formation when tissue breakdown occurs.

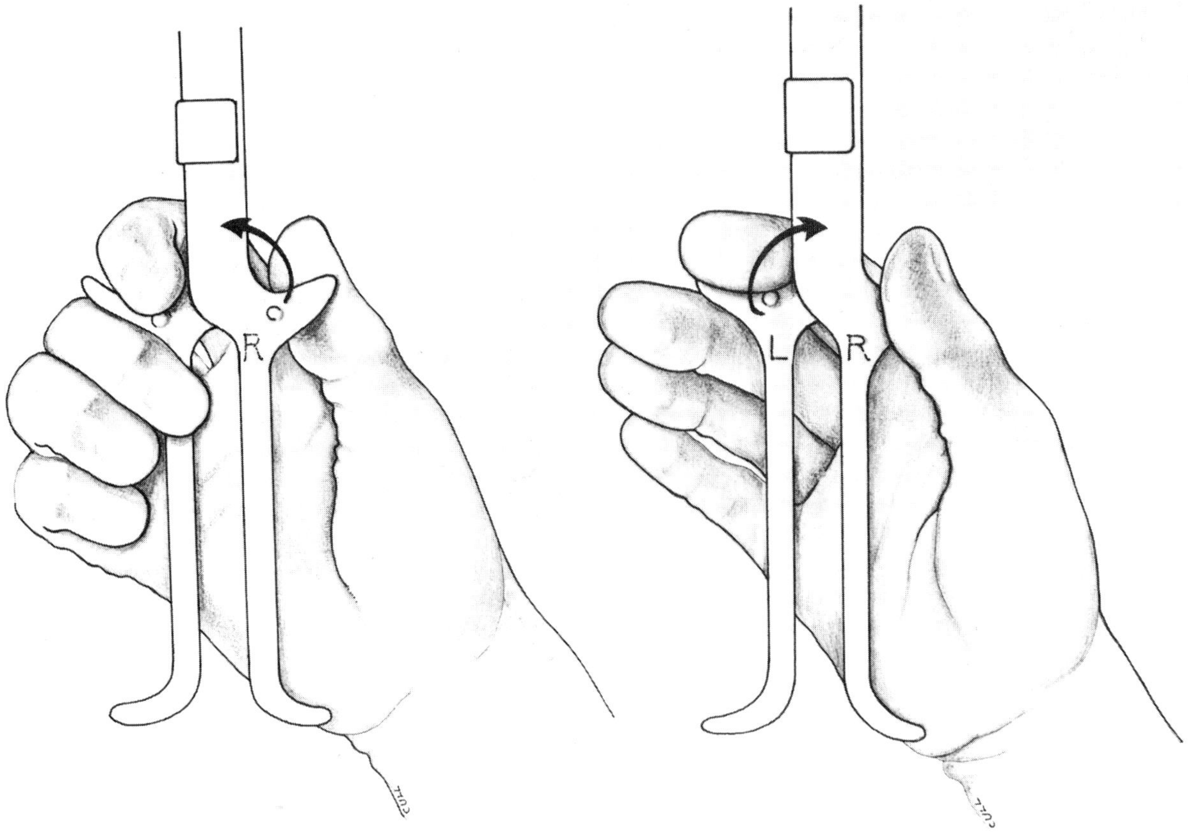

Fig. 56.17 The grip for rotation of the head with Kielland's forceps; **left:** from left occipito-lateral; **right:** from right occipito-lateral. From Hibbard (1988) with permission.

In all cases of haematuria continuous bladder drainage should be instituted and continued for some days after the urine has been macroscopically clear of blood.

Pelvic sepsis

This is usually due primarily to the conditions which led to the need for operative delivery but the risks are greatly increased by unskilled manipulations and trauma during the delivery.

The patient will be predisposed to *back strain* and nerve root or sciatic plexus damage by poor positioning during delivery, with excessive flexion and abduction of the hips, or from the use of excessive traction force.

Anaesthetic complications are discussed in Chapter 49.

Fetal injury

The infant is at particular risk of intracranial trauma and haemorrhage if forceps are abused, particularly if they are misapplied, so that there is not a true cephalic fit. Forceps of unsatisfactory design may lead to undue compression or may slip, causing facial abrasion.

Compression distortion injuries result in tears of the tentorium and rupture of the bridging veins. Rupture of the great vein of Galen leads to bleeding into the posterior fossa with compression of the brain stem, but supratentorial haemorrhages are more common.

Skull fractures are usually linear and not of lasting consequence. Depressed fractures, which may follow forceps delivery, are very uncommon but can result in subdural or subarachnoid haemorrhage.

Cephalhaematomas are seen most commonly over the parietal bone.

Facial nerve palsy is caused by pressure at the point where the nerve emerges from the stylomastoid foramen or as it passes over the mandibular ramus. The lesion is of lower motor neurone type, with paresis of the whole of the affected side of the face. Uncommonly, temporal bone fracture results in seventh nerve injury, the lesion being of upper motor neurone type and involving the lower two-thirds of the face.

FAILED FORCEPS DELIVERY

This term implies that a forceps delivery was initiated in the delivery room in the belief that it could be completed successfully but that it had to be abandoned in favour of Caesarean section. It would be more appropriate to include cases in which vaginal delivery had been achieved, but only after a second attempt by a more experienced operator, and cases in which there is undue morbidity or even mortality.

Most cases of failed forceps arise from disobeying the ground rules, inexperience and lack of discipline. The commonest contributory factors are unrecognized malpresentation, incomplete dilatation of the cervix and congenital malformations causing obstruction.

A trial of forceps which is not successful might also be regarded as failed forceps but if the trial is conducted according to defined rules — by a skilled operator, in the operating theatre, with adequate anaesthesia, and with the team and equipment ready for immediate Caesarean section — there should be no significantly increased risk of morbidity.

REFERENCES

Assalini P cited in Gervasoni G 1811 Sul' uso de' Nuovi Stromenti d'Ostetricia del Assalini. Milano
Chapman E 1735 A treatise on the improvement of midwifery, 2nd edn. Brindley, London
Cordoza L D, Gibb D, Studd J W W et al 1982 Predictive value of cervimetric labour patterns in primigravidae. British Journal of Obstetrics and Gynaecology 89: 33–38
Chiswick M L, James D K 1979 Kielland's forceps: association with neonatal morbidity and mortality. British Medical Journal 1: 7–9
Cohen W R, Friedman E A 1983 Management of labor. University Park Press, Baltimore
Das K 1929 The obstetric forceps: its history and evolution. The Art Press, Calcutta
Davidson A C, Weaver J B, Davies P, Pearson J F 1976 The relation between ease of forceps delivery and speed of cervical dilatation. British Journal of Obstetrics and Gynaecology 83: 279–283
De Lee J B 1920 The prophylactic forceps operation. American Journal of Obstetrics and Gynecology 1: 34–44
Forster F M C 1971 Robert Barnes and his obstetric forceps. Australian and New Zealand Journal of Obstetrics and Gynaecology 11: 139–147
Forster F M C 1975 On modern forceps delivery and Laufe's divergent forceps. Australian and New Zealand Journal of Obstetrics and Gynaecology 15: 209–214
Friedman E A 1978 Labor: clinical evaluation and management, 2nd edn. Appleton Century-Crofts, New York
Giffard W 1734 Cases in midwifery. E Hody, London
Hibbard B M 1988 Principles of Obstetrics. Butterworths, London
Johnson R W 1769 A new system of midwifery founded on practical observations. London
Kadar N, Romero R 1983 Prognosis for future childbearing after mid-cavity instrumental deliveries in primigravidae. Obstetrics and Gynecology 62: 166
Kielland C 1916 The application of forceps to the unrotated head. Monatsschrift für Geburtshilffe und Gynakologie 43: 48–78
Laufe L E 1968 Obstetric forceps. Harper & Row, New York
Levret A 1751 Suite des observations sur les causes et les accidens de plusieurs accouchemens laboreux. Delaguette, Paris
Neville W C 1886 Axis traction in instrumental delivery, with description of a new and simple axis traction forceps. Transactions of Academy of Medicine of Ireland 4: 192–210
O'Driscoll K, Meagher D 1980 Active management of labour. Saunders, London
Parry Jones E 1952 Kielland's forceps. Butterworths, London
Parry Jones E 1972 Barton's forceps. Sector, London
Pearson J F, Davies P 1974 The effect of continuous lumbar epidural analgesia upon fetal acid–base status during the second stage of labour. Journal of Obstetrics and Gynaecology of the British Commonwealth 81: 975–979
Rhodes P 1958 A critical appraisal of the obstetric forceps. Journal of Obstetrics and Gynaecology of the British Empire 65: 353–359
Rhodes P 1960 A standard obstetric forceps. Lancet ii: 631
Roesslin E 1540 The birth of mankynde. Translated by R Jonas. Raynalde, London
Ryden G 1986 Vacuum extraction or forceps? British Medical Journal 292: 75–76
Smellie W 1762 Treatise on the theory and practice of midwifery, 4th edn. Wilson and Durham, London
Speert H 1958 Obstetric and gynecologic milestones: essays in eponymy. Macmillan, New York
Tarnier E 1877 Description de deux nouveaux forceps. Martinet, Paris
Vacca A, Grant A, Wyatt G, Chalmers J 1983 Portsmouth operative delivery trial: a comparison of vacuum extraction and forceps delivery. British Journal of Obstetrics and Gynaecology 90: 1107–1112
Van de Laar 1777 Schets der geheele Verloskunde geschikt om derselver grondbeginzels volkomen te leeren. Gravenhaage
Willughby P 1972 Observations in midwifery. Edited from the original manuscript by Henry Blenkinsop (1863) with a new introduction by John L. Thornton. S R Publishers, Wakefield

57

Geoffrey Chamberlain

The vacuum extractor

The vacuum extractor has virtually replaced the forceps in many countries of northern Europe and in Africa. Its use however is much more limited in Britain and the Commonwealth while in the USA it is hardly used at all. Inertia is one of the hardest barriers to overcome. What one always has done is attractive and to change is difficult; probably because of this mental inertia the vacuum extractor has not been taken up more widely in the western world. It is interesting to speculate that the underemployment of this useful instrument may be associated with the skills of forceps delivery learnt traditionally over the years and which people are loath to release from their grasp.

James Simpson, Professor of Midwifery in Edinburgh, is often credited with inventing the first vacuum extractor. This is due to the Celtic influence in the teaching of obstetrics; over a century before, James Yonge, a Royal Naval surgeon, tried to draw out the fetus in 1705 using a cupping glass fitted to the scalp combined with an air pump. Possibly Simpson's description of the use of his instrument in the 1840s drew more attention because of the controversy aroused when one of his pupils claimed that he had invented the apparatus when describing the equipment in an examination paper which might have been marked by Simpson.

From then on, a steady series of improvements in the instrument took place through the latter part of the 19th century and into the mid 20th century. These are well documented in Chalmers' excellent volume on this instrument (Chalmers 1971). The definitive instrument is the one described by Malmstrom with a few modifications which have since been added. He first described his instrument in 1954 and in 1957 this was superseded by the instrument we all know now with the well known circumferential bulge, which allows a chignon of scalp to be sucked into it. The narrower ring of the edge of the extractor means a better grip is obtained on the fetal head by this cap than with any other previous instrument. It was Malmstrom's equipment and the modifications made by Bird (1969) that are now incorporated into the instruments used in the western world. Soft caps are available (O'Neil et al 1981) but these have not been shown to have any great advantage over the conventional metal ones.

INDICATIONS

The vacuum extractor has often been described as a replacement for forceps. Its use should be considered as complementary to the forceps for, although there are common indications, each instrument has its own individual criteria for use. Attempts at forceps delivery are usually contraindicated when the cervix is not yet fully dilated (see Chapter 56); one of the indications of the vacuum extractor was to bring the head down on to the cervix when there was delay in labour and so cause full dilation from 7 or 8 cm.

Because a vacuum extractor usually takes longer to assemble, apply and use properly, it is of less use when there is fetal distress in the second stage of labour; most skilled obstetricians can delivery a baby in the second stage more swiftly with forceps than they can with a vacuum extractor. However, many indications for operative vaginal delivery are not for acute fetal distress but relate to slow progress at the end of the first stage or in the second stage of labour; for these, the vacuum extractor is ideal.

First stage

Hence, in the first stage of labour the major indication for the vacuum extractor is lack of advance and delay at the end of the first stage. There should be no obvious cephalopelvic disproportion and the operator should reasonably expect to delivery the baby per vaginam. Occasionally, there may be a place for a trial of vacuum extraction, performed in an operating theatre with all facilities ready for Caesarean section.

At the latter part of the first stage, if fetal distress or a prolapsed cord occurs, delivery is usually by Caesarean section. However, if the operator is skilled in vacuum extraction and the woman is multiparous, it is likely that he could deliver the baby vaginally safely and much more swiftly than the time it takes to get an operating theatre ready and perform a Caesarean section.

Second stage

In the second stage of labour, the vacuum extractor is of major use when there has been delay. If, in the absence of overt cephalopelvic disproportion, there is no descent of the fetal head after 20 minutes of active contractions assisted by maternal effort, it is probable that the pelvic floor is holding up the fetal head. Sometimes, particularly after epidural analgesia, the head does not rotate fully and so descent is hindered; then a vacuum extractor will complete delivery very easily.

The use of the vacuum extractor for fetal distress in the second stage depends upon the degree of distress and the skill of the operator. Often a forceps delivery will be swifter but with a skilled operator and a less serious degree of fetal hypoxia, the vacuum extractor may be preferred. The skill of the operator is stressed here since an unskilled operator takes a long time to assemble the equipment of the vacuum extractor and then to raise the requisite negative pressure. All this must be done before the active process of extraction can be commenced and could take 10–15 minutes, whereas the application of the forceps blades takes a minute or so.

Another useful function of the vacuum extractor is to help the woman whom the obstetrician does not wish to have a long or fatiguing second stage, such as a mother with heart disease or raised blood pressure. Here the efforts of the second stage can be shortened very readily with a vacuum extractor. The obstetrician will be pulling with the woman's own contractions so that she can be making some small effort and does have the satisfaction of delivering her baby vaginally, although the real effort is by the obstetrician.

The vacuum extractor is used occasionally in other instances. For instance, it is a very good instrument for the delivery of a second twin when the fetal head is high and the cervix appears not to be completely dilated despite the birth of the first twin. It is an ideal instrument in these circumstances but this is rare and few operators are skilled in this procedure. It is of great use in occipito-lateral and occipito-posterior positions.

In some parts of the world a Caesarean section could lead to difficult sequelae in the woman's subsequent social and reproductive life. In parts of Central Africa, for example, a Caesarean section is considered a shameful thing and the woman's future place in the family may be jeopardized. Here the use of symphysiotomy combined with vacuum extraction has proved a boon and the literature in this specific area is well documented (Lancet Leading Article 1974).

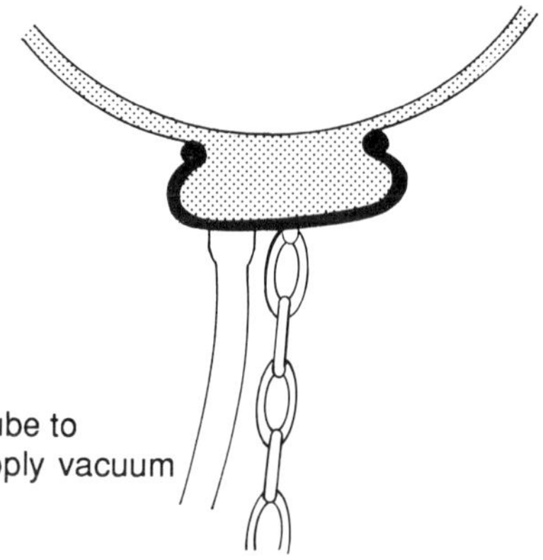

Fig. 57.1 The chignon produced on the scalp.

CONTRAINDICATIONS

The vacuum extractor is contraindicated for any presentation other than a cephalic one, preferably reasonably flexed. Hence it should not be used on a face or brow presentation, a breech or a transverse lie. If the fetus is immature (under 32 weeks' gestation), the likelihood of cephalohaematoma with the vacuum extractor rises sharply so that many would not wish to use the instrument on such small infants. Should the obstetrician think that any reasonable degree of cephalopelvic disproportion is present, the vacuum extractor must not be used to try to overcome a mechanical block.

THE APPARATUS

Most obstetricians in the western world use Malmstrom's equipment (1957) or its major modifications put forward by Bird (1969).

Caps of three diameters — 40, 50 and 60 mm — are usually provided. Although there is one of 30 mm, most hospitals do not possess this. The caps are of toughened steel, chromium-plated and shaped like a flattened hemisphere. The edge is curved in so that the rim has a smaller diameter than the cavity of the hemisphere a little higher up. Thus, if it is placed against the fetal scalp and air is evacuated from the cavity, the scalp is sucked in to fill the space of the hemisphere; the chignon, so produced, has a greater diameter above the rim than the rim itself, so that traction can be applied to the overhang (Fig. 57.1).

Air is evacuated from the cap through a thick-walled rubber tube. In the original equipment, this evacuation was from the centre of the cap and through this vacuum tube

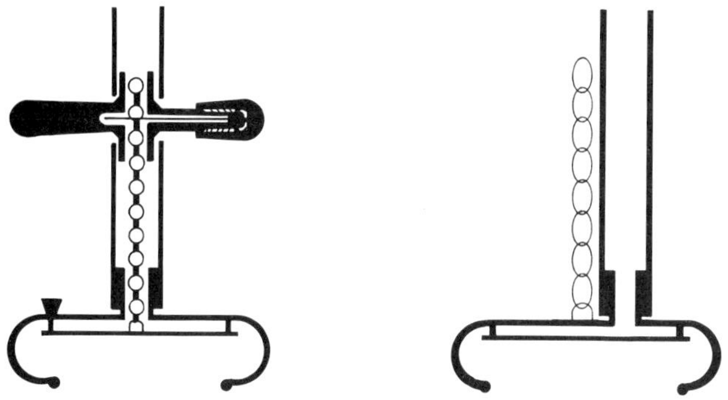

Fig. 57.2 The commonly used vacuum extraction caps. **Left**: cross-section of Malmstrom's (1957) apparatus with a central vacuum vent and the traction system through the vacuum tube. **Right**: Bird's (1969) modification showing the lateral vacuum vent and the traction chain separate.

ran the traction equipment. Bird (1969) suggested that the vacuum outlet should be to one side and independent of the traction (Fig. 57.2). This makes the cap more manoeuvrable with better application to a badly flexed head, since it can be slipped nearer to the bregma. There are also vacuum extractor caps with the tube on the side wall of the cap—an extension of the same principle. This is known as the posterior cap and was also designed by Bird (1976). Carmody et al (1986) were unable to show any great benefit for the use of this cap in a randomized controlled trial of 123 women.

If the traction chain passes down the centre of the evacuation tube, the traction handle has to be incorporated into the vacuum system. This means assembling the equipment at the time it is going to be used; this can be a fiddly business, and extremely exasperating when one wants to get on with the work in hand of delivering the baby. It is here that the experience of the operator counts since he knows that assembly has to be done in a careful and methodical way. The chain used for this type of vacuum traction usually has finer links than Bird's modification. The holding pin can be bent and links of the chain may be deformed, leading to difficulties in passing the chain down the tube. Bird's modification has a shorter, stronger chain and its shortness makes angled traction less likely.

A vacuum can be achieved by hand or mechanically; the former makes use of a small hand pump, a reverse of a bicycle pump with the valves placed the other way; hence, instead of blowing things up, each stroke removes air. The hand pump can be worked by an unskilled and unscrubbed assistant. Electrical pumps have been developed which can be controlled by a foot pedal by the operator. The more sophisticated mechanical pumps allow for small gas leakages in the equipment and automatically maintain an even negative pressure which can be preset. This is of great importance for if the operator does not notice any loss of the vacuum, he will be working with inefficient equipment; this can lead to damage of the scalp. The hand pumps are cheap and easily portable but if a vacuum extractor is to be used to any extent on a hospital unit, it is worth acquiring the larger electrical pump.

The equipment is completed by a vacuum bottle through which the air from the extractor passes before going on to the pump. This is essential for a certain amount of blood, amniotic fluid and mucus is drawn into the system and this must not be allowed to enter the pump system. The bottle must be cleaned out carefully after each delivery and sterilized with one of the liquid chemical antiseptic agents. The level of vacuum is measured from this bottle with a simple aneroid barometer, graduated from 0 to $-1.0\,\text{kg/cm}^2$. This is probably the most sensitive part of the whole apparatus and the part most likely to be damaged. It does not need sterilization because it is outside the sterile field but the rough life in the labour ward often damages it. This can lead to an under-representation of the reading which might be dangerous (Chamberlain 1965).

After use, the operators themselves should disassemble the equipment and clean it, taking it to pieces and washing all the parts exposed to blood before it is sent off for sterilization. Only then will they be sure that it is going to come back after sterilization ready for use on the next occasion. If they leave it to others, however well meaning, the equipment may be sent for sterilization in an assembled condition prepared for the last delivery; the rubber evacuation tubes are still attached to the vent lugs on the cap. When during sterilization this is heated, the metal of the lug expands and the rubber will be stretched under heat. The tube may then lose some of its elasticity and when the equipment cools, the rubber stays in an expanded position so that it is inefficient to maintain a vacuum. The equipment is robust but needs thoughtful handling and is best looked after by the operator.

USE OF THE VENTOUSE

The equipment is unpacked and assembled by the scrubbed-up operator. A cap of the most appropriate size is chosen. Generally this should be one of the larger caps (50 or 60 mm diameter) for with a larger size of chignon, less negative pressure will be applied per cm^2 over the skin, hence this will be less traumatic to the fetal scalp. If the cervix is not dilated, a 40 mm cap may be required; it is most unusual to apply a vacuum extractor these days to a woman who is less than 7 cm dilated and so the 30 mm cap is very rarely required.

No antiseptic creams should be used on the skin or at the vaginal preparation of the woman. Aqueous sterilizing solutions only should be used since cream causes too great an increased lubrication which might allow the cap to slip. This is most important.

The cap is then applied to the fetal head under sterile conditions, placing it as far back as possible. Ideally it should be over the posterior fontanelle, in the midline of the fetal

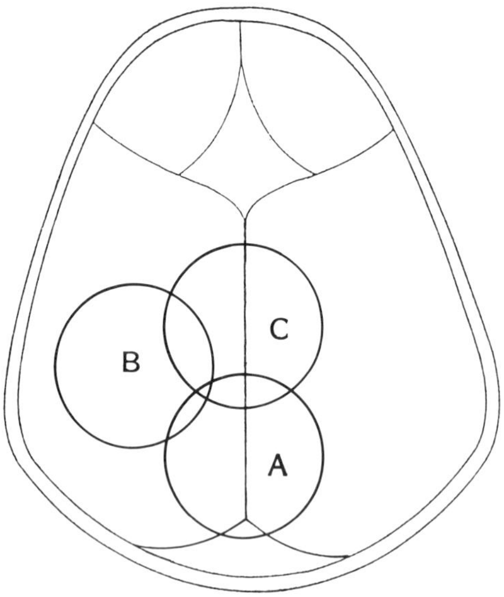

Fig. 57.3 The cap should ideally be as far back as possible over the bregma (A). If it is off the midline (B) it allows an asymmetrical pull and so larger diameters of the fetal head engage. If it is further forward than the bregma (C) the head is deflexed.

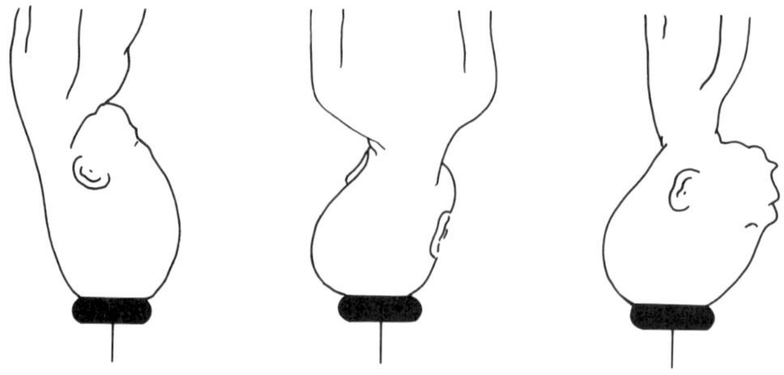

Fig. 57.4 The consequences of applications shown in Figure 57.3 are: (**a**) good application — good flexion; (**b**) off the midline — asynclitism; (**c**) too far forward — deflexion.

head (Fig. 57.3). The further forward it is from this, the more it is likely to deflect the head as tension is put on the chain. Further, if the cap is not placed in the midline, when traction occurs it causes asynclitism so that larger head diameters than necessary have to engage in the maternal pelvis (Fig. 57.4). These points are important and should be checked when the cap is first placed on the head.

Negative pressure is now applied. When done with the hand pump it is conventional to do this in stages, lowering the pressure by $-0.2\,\text{kg/cm}^2$ on each occasion. It is wise to wait 30 seconds or so between each bout of pumping. With an electrical pump, evacuation of air can be done continuously and thus the rate of induction of vacuum is quicker.

Once the cap has been attached to the scalp by the first phase of vacuum, its position must be carefully checked. It is also important that the operator runs a finger round the whole perimeter of the cap to ensure that there is no maternal tissue caught. There may be a fold of redundant vaginal wall, particularly posteriorly, which gets sucked into the cap; if a first-stage vacuum extraction is performed, part of the cervix can get caught. This step is most important and circumferential digital examination should be repeated between each bout of hand-pumping or at intervals if the continuous electrical pump is used. If this is not done, the operator will inadvertently pull down on both maternal and fetal tissues. Either the vacuum will not work since air will enter so that the cap comes off or, worse, the cap may compress the maternal tissues sufficiently to allow delivery to take place but a tear of the vagina or cervix follows as part of the delivery. Both can be avoided by checking several times that there has been no entrapment of maternal tissue.

After a vacuum of $-0.8\,\text{kg/cm}^2$ has been achieved and before traction, the operator should assess the line of pull which will be most effective. If the head is in mid-cavity or just above it, then the pull would have to be very posterior, so much so that occasionally a preliminary episiotomy must be performed to allow the line of traction to be correct. This is most important for if the operator merely pulls at right angles to the vulva, then the actual traction on the cap will be oblique and cause it to skid on the head, producing lacerations of the scalp or eventually detachment with failure of the method.

Traction is usually applied with the operator's right hand on the handle, but the function of the left hand is very important. The index finger of the left hand should be placed on the cap near the periphery if a central vent model is used, or on the opposite side from the vent if a lateral vent cap is used. This ensures that the cap does not rock or become pulled obliquely. The middle fingertip rests on the fetal head to give a guide about real descent with traction. If the uterus is contracting, then traction on the vacuum extractor is best done synchronously with these and, if the cervix is fully dilated, the mother is encouraged to bear down with each contraction in the usual way. If there are no contractions, then the operator makes his own rhythm pulling for about 30–40 seconds every 2 minutes.

Care must be taken not to dislodge the cap. If it is felt to move laterally by the index finger of the left hand, or if a sucking noise of air entering the equipment is heard, traction should stop and the position of the cap should be reassessed. It may be too lateral or more likely, too far forward on the head. There might be unsuspected cephalopelvic disproportion and the head is not going to come down; this should be considered by the operator. If these points are evaluated and it is considered that vacuum extractor delivery should continue, the negative pressure should be restored to $-0.8\,\text{kg/cm}^2$ and another attempt should be made. It is unwise to have more than one attempt at re-application of the cap and it may be that a larger size of cap should be used the second time. The method should be considered

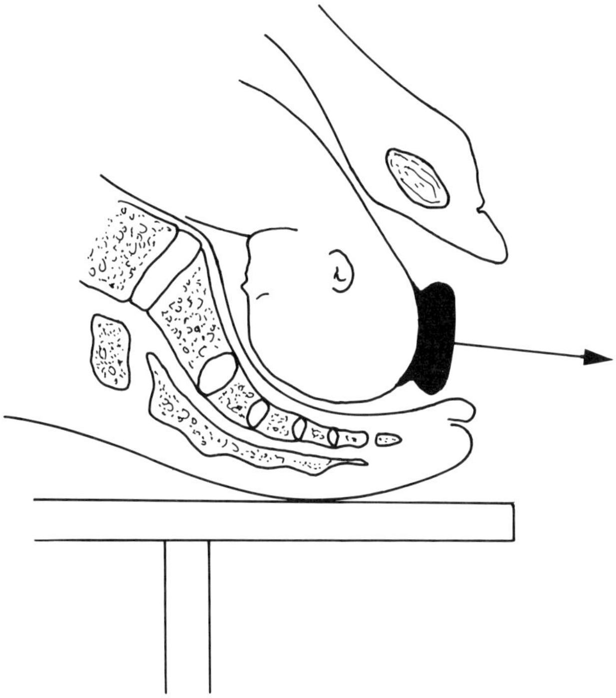

Fig. 57.5 The cap has been applied far back; the head is well flexed and progress is good. The head is now just below mid-cavity and so traction can be less posterior than when the head was higher.

to have failed if the cap comes off twice and another method of delivery should then be used.

During traction, the operator must concentrate on thinking about the level of the head in the pelvis and apply traction at right angles to that. This means that the traction will be very posterior at first, towards the mother's anus when the head is high, gradually curving round so that as the head finally enters the lower pelvis, traction is almost at right angles to the vulva (Fig. 57.5). No attempt should be made to try to rotate the fetus into an occipito-anterior position. The traction force is a linear one and the fetal head will then rotate in its own way so that its diameters engage advantageously in the various diameters of the maternal pelvis. This is the vacuum extractor's great advantage, that the head can follow its own pattern of rotation. As the head crowns, the negative pressure should be released, either by the foot pump or by the operator's assistant; the cap can then be easily detached when the negative pressure is released. There is always a chignon and there may even be a little abrasion of skin.

The operator should be on guard for shoulder dystocia which seems to be a little commoner amongst babies born by vacuum extraction. This is probably associated with the slight difficulty the woman had at delivering the head and the size of the baby in relation to the pelvis. In consequence, it is wise not to give Syntometrine until the anterior shoulder has actually appeared under the symphysis pubis.

The baby is resuscitated in the usual fashion. It is a sensible precaution before handing the baby to the parents to warn them that there will be a little bump on the head and to tell them that it will go down within 48 hours. Many operators actually swathe the baby in a sterile cloth and tactfully cover the top of the head with that cloth, claiming it is there to reduce heat loss. It is actually there to stop the parents seeing the chignon on their first view of their offspring. After the placenta is delivered and any episiotomy has been repaired, the operator will examine the baby fully with the parents; he can then show the fading chignon to them, explaining its significance and its rapid rate of disappearance.

FAILED VACUUM EXTRACTION

Failure rates are not often published, except by people who have performed large series of vacuum extractions. Hence, they are the failure rates of those who are interested and most experienced. A good example is Bird (1976) who had a failure rate of 3.2% among 1334 women when the Malmstrom classical cap was used and 0.9% among 1062 women when he used his modified cap. Bratt (1965) reported a failure rate of 2.3% among 1135 women.

Failure rates decrease with increased experience. The commonest reason for non-delivery is that the operator applies traction to the cap in an oblique fashion and not in the axis of the birth canal at the station where the fetal head is. In the first few cases, the operator may not pull hard enough and this will result in no delivery; occasionally he may pull too hard. There is a skill about vacuum extraction which tests the mind and the hands of the operator in a finer way than do forceps deliveries for this is the gentleman's way of delivering a baby. It is wise for all operators to practise vacuum extraction on easy cases first—on outlet presentations for the first few times, graduating to vacuum extraction required for mid-cavity deliveries.

In addition, the equipment can go wrong. There may be loose rubber-to-air vent connections due to ageing of the rubber following improper sterilization. The pump may be inefficient because the valve flange is not properly lubricated (a few drops of paraffin applied soon puts this right). It is essential that all equipment should be maintained properly, preferably by those who use it.

The operator may have chosen the wrong case on which to try vacuum extraction. There may actually be some cephalopelvic disproportion or a greater degree of deflection of the fetal head than the operator had first imagined, such as a brow presentation. Sometimes after a long labour when a large oedematous caput has formed, the vacuum cap does not grip so well and comes off with a more limited tractive effort.

In essence, failed vacuum extraction is due to one of two causes:

1. The cap is not gripping the scalp properly because mater-

nal tissue is trapped or there is inefficient equipment. The management is to re-apply the cap, excluding the maternal tissues, or to correct the leaks in the apparatus.
2. Although the cap will accept strong traction, the head will not descend; the commonest reason is cephalopelvic disproportion or a misapplication of the cap so that it is too far forward or off the midline.

The operator should ensure that the fetal head is descending with each tractive effort and that it is not just the scalp which comes down. Generally speaking, the operator should consider another method of delivery if, after correct application of the cap, the head is not brought into the position of crowning within three or four proper bouts of traction. If the cap comes off, it should not be re-applied more than once.

SIDE-EFFECTS

The major problem that vacuum extraction might pose for the mother is that a fold of her vagina or cervix is sucked in between the cap and the fetal head; it may then be damaged, leading to haemorrhage.

The fetus is not usually seriously affected by vacuum extraction. Any attempt to correlate fetal hypoxia with the use of the vacuum extractor is confounded by the indications for the use of the instrument. Generally, if the vacuum extraction is used for an easy, uncomplicated delivery and not more than three or four episodes of traction are required, there is no hypoxia.

Scalp injuries are moderately common. Abrasions to the scalp and skin occur; these relate to the rotation or moving of the cap on the skin which in turn is associated with a badly placed cap. If the cap is detached suddenly, this too can cause skin damage.

Cephalohaematomata can occur if a skin vein is damaged by chance; more rarely subgaleal haemorrhages have been reported (Robinson & Rossiter 1968). Again, this is probably associated with prolonged and strenuous traction which may be associated with a long and difficult labour.

Intracranial haemorrahge relates to the duration and strength of the pulling of the vacuum extractor. Plauché (1979) recorded a range of intracranial injury up to 8%. The upper end of this came from the more difficult vacuum extractions following the more difficult labours. The neurological and behavioural sequelae of such deliveries have been examined by Leijon (1980). He found that neonatal depression with later lower auditory and visual responses could occur but could often be explained by the abnormal presentations and the long labour, in addition to the long vacuum extraction. Naske et al (1976) found that there was a greater incidence of brain damage in babies born by vacuum cap delivery compared with those delivered spontaneously; there was no difference between those born with a vacuum cap as opposed to those born by forceps. Again it is hard to sort out the propter hoc from the post hoc — was the damage caused by the indication for using a vacuum extractor or its use? Generally, most workers find little adverse effect on neurological or intellectual development.

Campbell et al (1975) found an increased incidence of neonatal jaundice in mature infants born by vacuum extraction compared with those born by forceps. This is rarely a serious problem and light therapy was not often required. Jaundice follows even without apparent bruising of the infant's scalp and the workers assumed this was due to breakdown of blood in the chignon.

In the longer term, rare reports of alopecia have appeared. The author has seen two such children aged over 1 year with a distinct cleancut circle of hair loss which would have corresponded to the position and size of the vacuum cap used at their birth. However, one sees well rounded patches of alopecia occurring spontaneously.

COMPARISON OF VACUUM EXTRACTION WITH THE USE OF FORCEPS

Vacuum extraction is simple to use and, generally speaking, can be practised by less skilled people than can forceps delivery. In many parts of the underdeveloped world, midwives are perfectly competent with vacuum deliveries whereas they have not been appropriately trained to be able to use forceps. The application of forceps requires a greater knowledge of fetal and pelvic anatomy and a greater familiarity with pelvic examinations.

The vacuum extractor occupies less space at the side wall of the pelvis than do the forceps and so does not add to any potential disproportion. When traction is applied with the vacuum extractor, this is a linear pull and the head can follow its own mechanisms in the pelvis for rotation. Using a pair of forceps, the head is gripped in four places and rotation is in the control of the operator. This may be appropriate with the skilled obstetrician who has performed many forceps deliveries but with the less well trained, perhaps nature knows best and the head can be allowed to follow its own course.

The disadvantages of the vacuum extractor compared with forceps are that the equipment is marginally more likely to go wrong and that it requires maintenance whereas little can happen to two blades of a pair of forceps. The vacuum extractor is also slightly less portable than forceps.

Vacuum extraction can be performed with the help of little extra pain relief. Often it can be done without any additional analgesia since the application of the cap is not much more painful for the woman than is a vaginal examination. Putting on forceps is a more difficult art, particularly if the head is in mid-cavity. Then, a more extensive regional block is required than for a vacuum extraction. In a study of mothers randomly allocated to foreceps delivery or vacuum extraction, Garcia et al (1985) found that women required less analgesia for vacuum extraction but had more worries about their babies because of the jaundice.

Forceps delivery can be done more swiftly than vacuum extraction by most operators, provided the head is in a reasonable position in the pelvis and the cervix is fully dilated. Thus, if the baby shows signs of fetal distress in the second stage of labour — one of the major indications for operative vaginal delivery — forceps are to be preferred. However, the other major indication for accelerated delivery is delay in the second stage; for this, the vacuum extractor is an excellent instrument.

The baby nearly always has a chignon for 24–48 hours after a vacuum extraction and there is a higher prevalence of jaundice. After a forceps delivery, particularly with rotation, there are transient forceps marks on the cheeks.

It is interesting to observe how the spread of any new technique occurs in medicine. There are at first case reports from the enthusiasts; thence the technique is taken up eagerly by those who wish to try innovations. They too usually find it useful and report on it enthusiastically. After this follows a series of reports on the side-effects and complications that have occurred during the first enthusiasm of usage but have not been reported immediately; only after some years does the proper use of the technique stabilize. To some extent usage depends on the phase in the propagation of practice when an operator starts to use equipment. He may join it in the first enthusiasms or later at the complications stage. As the operator then becomes a practical teacher, he advises others what he thinks is right and teaches the wider use of what he believes in.

These mechanisms probably account for the patchy use of the vacuum extractor in the world. Earlier reports, such as by Snoeck in 1960, were that the forceps had been virtually abandoned in his hospital and vacuum extraction had taken over. Similarly, there are many Scandinavian and German hospitals where forceps are rarely used. In a large part of the Middle East where there is influence of teachers from the European area, there is also a relatively low use of forceps and a higher employment of the vacuum extractor. The incidence of operative vaginal deliveries has increased in most countries but in England and the USA these deliveries are still mostly by forceps rather than vacuum extraction.

Few comparative trials have been performed of these instruments. Greis et al (1981) compared vacuum extraction births with those by forceps delivery. Results showed that the forceps deliveries were associated with a threefold increased incidence of birth canal trauma, while anaesthesia requirements and perinatal morbidity were much less than those with vacuum extraction. Schenker & Serr (1967) compared 300 women delivered by vacuum extraction with 300 retrospectively examined forceps deliveries. Maternal complications were halved in the vacuum extraction group while the rate of fetal complications was the same in both groups; the incidence of fetal problems increased considerably when the traction time with the ventouse was longer than 15 minutes and when the cervix was not fully dilated.

A randomized controlled trial was performed in Portsmouth by Vacca et al (1983) when 304 women requiring operative delivery in the second stage of labour were randomly allocated to vacuum extraction or forceps groups. Maternal trauma, use of analgesia and blood loss at delivery were significantly less after vacuum extraction. The authors found that mild neonatal jaundice was increased in this group; more serious neonatal problems were rare in both the forceps and vacuum extraction groups. With this number of women, statistically significant conclusions could not be drawn but this is an important study and the subject deserves a wider randomized controlled trial.

CONCLUSIONS

When further research has been properly evaluated, it may well be that the vacuum extractor will be able to take its proper place. In the opinion of those who are experienced in its use, the vacuum extractor is probably most appropriate when delivering a woman, particularly multiparous, who has been shown not to have cephalopelvic disproportion but who develops delay at the end of the first stage or in the second stage of labour. The vacuum extractor should be used in parallel with forceps rather than in competition. Skills in the management of delivery with both sets of equipment should be gained in training and kept bright by constant repetition in practice.

REFERENCES

Bird G C 1969 Modifications of Malmstrom's vacuum extractor. British Medical Journal 111: 526

Bird G C 1976 The importance of flexion in vacuum extraction delivery. British Journal of Obstetrics and Gynaecology 83: 194–200

Bratt T 1965 Indications for and results of the use of the ventouse. Journal of Obstetrics and Gynaecology of the British Commonwealth 72: 883–888

Campbell N, Harvey D, Norman A P 1975 Increased frequence of neonatal jaundice. British Medical Journal 11: 548–552

Carmody F, Grant A, Somchiwang M 1986 Vacuum extraction: a randomised controlled comparison of the new generation cup with the original Bird cup. Journal of Perinatal Medicine 14: 95–100

Chalmers J A 1971 The ventouse. Year Book Medical Publishers, Chicago, p 116

Chamberlain G 1965 Vacuum extractor — a possible danger. Lancet i: 632

Garcia J, Anderson J, Vacca A, Elbourne D, Grant A, Chalmers I 1985 Views of women about instrumental delivery using vacuum extraction and forceps. Journal of Psychosomatic Obstetrics and Gynaecology 4: 1–9

Greis J B, Biermanz J, Scommegna A 1981 Comparison of maternal and fetal effects of vacuum extraction with forceps and Caesarean deliveries. Obstetrics and Gynecology 57: 571–577

Lancet Leading Article 1974 Symphysiotomy and vacuum extraction. Lancet i: 396–397

Leijon I 1980 Neurology and behaviour of the newborn infants delivered by vacuum extraction. Acta Paediatrica Scandinavica 69: 625–631

Malmstrom T 1954 Vacuum extraction. Acta Obstetricia et Gynecologica Scandinavica 33 (suppl 4): 3
Malmstrom T 1957 The vacuum extractor. An obstetrical instrument. Acta Obstetricia et Gynecologica Scandinavica 5: 153–156
Naske R V, Poustka F, Presslich J 1976 Zusammenhange zwischen operativer Geburtsbundigung und Zerebralschadigung des Kinder. Wiener Klinische Wochenschift 88: 319–324
O'Neil A G, Skull E, Michael E 1981 A new method of traction for the vacuum cup. Australian and New Zealand Journal of Obstetrics and Gynaecology 21: 24–25
Plauché W C 1979 Fetal cranial injuries related to delivery with the Malmstrom vacuum extractor. Obstetrics and Gynecology 53: 750–757
Robinson R J, Rossiter M A 1968 Massive subaponeurotic haemorrhage in babies of African origin. Archives of Disease in Childhood 43: 684–687
Schenker J C, Serr D M 1967 Comparative study of delivery by vacuum extraction and forceps. American Journal of Obstetrics and Gynecology 98: 32–35
Snoeck J 1960 The vacuum extractor (ventouse)—an alternative to the obstetric forceps. Proceedings of the Royal Society of Medicine 53: 749
Vacca A, Grant A, Wyatt G, Chalmers I 1983 A comparison of vacuum extraction and forceps delivery. British Journal of Obstetrics and Gynaecology 90: 1107–1112

58

John M. Beazley

Caesarean section

Munro Kerr, in 1921, first used a transverse incision in the anterior uterine wall, just above the level of the internal os, for Caesarean section. Both he and Eardley Holland (1921) drew attention to the risks of the classical operation, but it was St George Wilson (1931), speaking with enthusiasm about the transverse lower segment approach before the North of England Obstetrical and Gynaecological Society in 1931, who was largely responsible for popularizing the operation in Britain. Subsequently, Vernon Bailey (1934) reviewed 119 cases of the lower segment operation before the same society in 1934, and in 1939 Charles McIntosh Marshall presented an admirable historical review of the subject and wrote extensively on the operative technique for the procedure.

THE INCIDENCE OF CAESAREAN SECTION

The recent trend in the incidence of Caesarean section in the UK appears to differ significantly from that in the USA. In the USA, the incidence increased to 15.2% in 1978 and, according to Russel (1981), is continuing to increase. In 1983 the overall English Caesarean section rate was 10.1% (Office of Population Censuses and Surveys 1987) and this incidence also reflects a steady increase during the last decade.

For some years doubt has been shed upon whether the observed increase in national trends for Caesarean section can be justified in terms of perinatal statistics. For example, in 1978, Haddad & Lundy reported that in at least one important centre in the USA there had been no significant diminuition in the perinatal mortality rate since 1971 despite an increase in Caesarean section from 9 to 15%. Furthermore, the consensus view of the conference on Caesarean section at the National Institutes of Health in 1980 inferred that the increasing trend of Caesarean section might be stopped and even reversed without detriment to a continuing improvement in maternal and fetal health (British Medical Journal Leading Article 1981). As Beazley & Lobb (1983) point out, a similar view might have been expected earlier from Australia where, in 1979, attention was drawn to similar perinatal mortality rates in two widely separated centres despite very significant differences in their incidence of Caesarean section. In Western Australia the incidence of abdominal delivery was 4.2% in women aged 20 and 10.1% in women aged 40–45 years. In South Australia the comparative incidence was 22.2 and 51.3% respectively (Opit & Selwood 1979).

In specialist centres the incidence of Caesarean section may vary from 10 to 14% because of the admission of higher-risk obstetric patients. The most obvious indications for the operation include a more liberal use of Caesarean section for breech presentation, the detection of fetal distress by continuous monitoring, and the premature abdominal delivery of growth-retarded infants who are in danger of dying in utero from placental insufficiency. The increased incidence of Caesarean section in specialist centres, however, is by no means uniform. For example, in three large maternity hospitals in Dublin, the Caesarean section rate in 1983 varied between 6 and 8.9%. Interestingly, in each of these hospitals, although the Caesarean section rate has remained virtually unchanged for the last 10 years, the perinatal mortality rate has been almost halved during the same period.

The recent situation in the National Maternity Hospital, Dublin, is reflected in Figure 58.1, in which the incidence of Caesarean section and the perinatal mortality rate is compared with similar data for the USA presented by Bottoms et al (1980).

Looking at the American figures it would be tempting to conclude that there is a cause and effect relationship

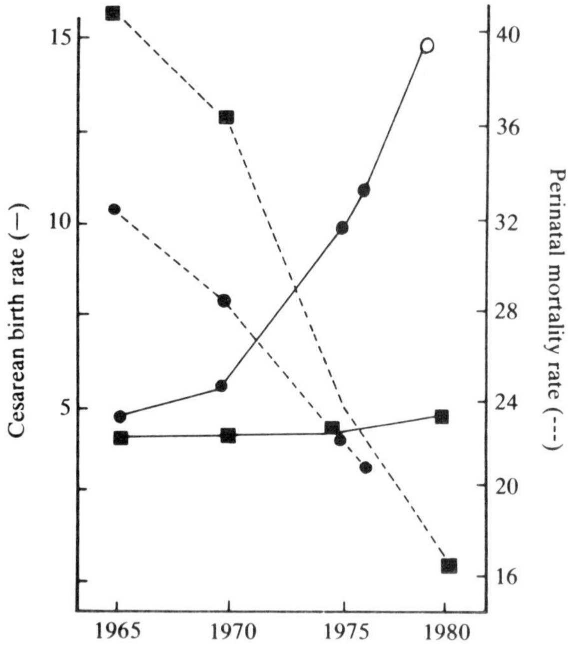

Fig. 58.1 Caesarean birth rates per 100 deliveries (solid lines) and perinatal mortality rates per 1000 deliveries (dashed lines) in the USA, according to Bottoms et al (1980) and in the National Maternity Hospital, Dublin. The US figures are represented by circles and the Dublin figures by squares. From Chamberlain et al (1985) with permission.

between the increase in the Caesarean section rate and the decrease in perinatal mortality. Looking at the Irish figures, however, it is clear that a similar decline in perinatal mortality can occur without any significant increase in Caesarean section. In the Midlands and South of England also, reports from Leicester and Oxford further indicate a 50% reduction in their perinatal mortality rate between 1979 and 1984, with no more than a 1% increase in the Caesarean section rate (Drife 1985). It seems probable that further centres will continue to review carefully their own incidence of Caesarean section with a view to keeping the increase to a minimum.

ELECTIVE CAESAREAN SECTION

In the UK cephalopelvic disproportion is not a common indication for primary elective Caesarean section. More frequently, elective abdominal delivery follows a previous trial of suspected cephalopelvic disproportion at the pelvic brim which either failed or had to be abandoned because of fetal distress. An elective operation may not be necessary if the baby in the current pregnancy is significantly smaller than the child born previously by operation.

Whenever it seems dangerous to subject the uterus to the risk of damage during labour, an elective Caesarean section is considered. Previous uterine surgery or injury normally constitutes an unacceptable hazard, but the degree of potential danger will often be determined by the site of the scar, the clinical conditions influencing previous healing (such as infection), and the present site of the placenta.

If there is a uterine abnormality or some congenital or other anomaly of the lower genital tract which precludes vaginal delivery or endangers nearby structures (e.g. ectopic anus or vesicovaginal repair or successfully treated urinary stress incontinence), elective Caesarean section may be the treatment of choice.

Placenta praevia, especially of a major degree, or fulminating pre-eclampsia provides a special indication for elective Caesarean section which is now widely recognized.

In modern obstetric practice, the indications for an elective operation are often relative rather than absolute. The indications taken into account include not only factors such as maternal age, relative infertility and past obstetric history, but also fetal age and weight. The desires expressed by the woman and her husband and their reaction to the influence of Caesarean section upon the wife's obstetric future will also be considered.

If abdominal delivery is to be performed for reasons such as cephalopelvic disproportion, breech presentation, placenta praevia, or previous Caesarean section, it is reasonable to operate any time after completion of the 37th week and usually before 40 weeks of gestation. The only safeguard required is an accurate assessment of fetal maturity, thereby avoiding the undesirable error of delivering an immature baby. When elective Caesarean section is to be utilized because fetal well-being is in jeopardy, e.g. from placental insufficiency, the timing of the operation will require particularly careful judgement. A reliable and accurate method of determining the fetal age should be used. Usually this will be evaluated by ultrasound. The head: abdomen ratio and the ultrasonic assessment of fetal weight are also helpful parameters to obtain. Antenatal cardiotocography, with the addition of an oxytocin challenge test in some centres, will help to determine the optimum time for delivery.

CAESAREAN SECTION IN LABOUR

It is sometimes necessary to abandon a proposed vaginal delivery in favour of an abdominal delivery. The indications for this change are usually fairly clear — obstructed labour occurring during labour or the appearance of fetal or maternal distress prior to full cervical dilatation. Before deciding to operate it is important for the obstetrician to confirm that fetal distress is not being caused simply by the injudicious use of oxytocics overstimulating uterine activity. Also, if maternal distress is being aggravated by pain it may be sensible to consider introducing epidural analgesia before finally deciding upon the need for Caesarean section.

Delay in the progress of labour, especially during the first stage, is probably the commonest reason for considering the need to deliver a baby abdominally. In this clinical situation it is helpful to have partographic evidence of delay, as the visual evidence of a partograph often helps the obstetrician to distinguish between any sudden onset of delay after normal progress and the slow latent or first stage of labour.

In addition to partography it is helpful to have some reliable quantitative measure of uterine activity. Simple clinical assessments of uterine activity are rather unreliable. Many potential Caesarean sections for uterine inertia can probably be avoided by recognizing quantitatively that uterine activity is suboptimal. The restoration of optimal uterine activity by oxytocic stimulation may then be attempted. If optimal activity according to quantitative criteria cannot be restored or if delay continues despite optimal uterine activity, the indications for Caesarean section become much clearer. A common example of the value of using quantitative assessments of uterine activity is the slow rotation of a fetal head from the occipito-posterior position. This will often result from uterine inertia rather than from any disadvantageous cephalopelvic relationships. If optimal uterine activity can be secured abdominal delivery may well be averted. Conversely, if delayed progress continues despite the stimulation of uterine activity which is quantitatively satisfactory, there is a clear indication to proceed to Caesarean section.

Delay in labour in a multiparous woman is to be viewed with extreme suspicion. This clinical situation always necessitates prompt and careful evaluation. Uterine inertia is a most uncommon, even a rare cause.

REPEAT CAESAREAN SECTION

Repeat Caesarean section has to be considered when a woman has once had an abdominal delivery. However, if the previous Caesarean section was performed for a non-recurrent cause, repeat Caesarean section may be unnecessary. To a large extent the decision to repeat the operation will rest upon the obstetric situation at the time of delivery. If, mechanically, the clinical situation appears satisfactory, i.e. there is a flexed cephalic presentation, a baby of reasonable size, and a maternal pelvis of adequate capacity in which the fetal head is engaged, repeat elective Caesarean section is probably unnecessary.

Following vaginal delivery it is always prudent to examine the integrity of the uterine scar digitally by the vaginal route. Any small dehiscence which, unexpectedly, may be discovered can then be repaired formally. An adverse feature which may persuade the obstetrician to repeat an abdominal delivery electively could be the insertion of part of the placenta over the site of the previous scar. The integrity of the scar and the potential risk of bleeding, should dehiscence occur, are considered by some to be sufficiently great to warrant elective surgery.

The obstetrician will bear in mind that, following a classical Caesarean section — now rare — the risks of scar rupture significantly exceed the risks following a lower segment Caesarean section. The risks of the former occurring were said to be of the order of 8.9% for those who delivered vaginally, 4.7% for those in labour, and 2.2% overall. In the case of lower segment Caesarean section, the respective risks were 1.2, 0.8 and 0.5% (Dewhurst 1957). In fact, in modern obstetric practice, the risks of rupture of a lower segment Caesarean section scar are probably nearer 0.5%, though they may occasionally rise to 2.5% (Merrill & Gibbs 1978; Demianczuk et al 1982).

The risk of maternal death arising directly from Caesarean section is less than 0.8 per 1000 cases. The operation is safer now than it has ever been. Even so, in practice, because of the risks attending abdominal delivery, Caesarean sections accounted for most maternal deaths in the triennia 1973–75, 1976–78 and 1979–1981. The immediate causes of death have varied over the years but haemorrhage, pulmonary embolism, sepsis and paralytic ileus constantly figure and emphasize the continued need for skilled surgery and the maintenance of aseptic conditions throughout labour.

About half the patients who previously had a Caesarean section may be expected to deliver safely vaginally, and patients who readily achieve 3 cm dilatation of the cervix in labour have a good prognosis. Yudkin & Redman (1986) report that in a large Oxford series repeat Caesarean sections accounted for 30% of all sections. Martin et al (1983), reporting on a prospective collaborative study of 789 women with previous Caesarean section, made clear that although vaginal delivery may be successfully completed in 62% of patients, only about 12% of American women are likely to find vaginal delivery an appealing option after abdominal delivery.

In the absence of any antenatal contraindication to vaginal delivery, a normal labour may be anticipated after Caesarean section and the process of parturition may be conducted normally. Even employing amniotomy and oxytocin infusion is reasonable, and monitoring of uterine activity in the normal way is recommended in these circumstances. Epidural analgesia should not be withheld on the grounds that significant signs of impending uterine rupture may be masked. Suprapubic tenderness as a local sign of uterine dehiscence during labour is notoriously unreliable. A much more important sign of impending or actual dehiscence is a rising maternal pulse rate, especially if this is associated with an unexpected delay in the progress of labour.

CAESAREAN SECTION FOR OBSTRUCTED LABOUR

Obstructed labour complicated by significant delay and impaction of the presenting part, together with maternal and fetal distress or even intrauterine fetal death, is now rare in obstetric practice in the UK. When the situation does occur, the patient presents a serious operative risk. Despite the need for haste in proceeding with the operation, however, adequate time must be spent in providing proper resuscitation.

Dehydration must be corrected as well as any electrolyte deficit or acidosis. If there is evidence of shock, central venous pressure monitoring will be required. In the presence of septicaemia, broad-spectrum antibiotics are necessary and probably steroid therapy. The surgeon and the anaesthetist both require to be experienced in cases of this kind.

Philpott (1982) recommends extraperitoneal Caesarean section in established or potential uterine infection in cephalic presentation. The abdominal wall is opened longitudinally but the parietal peritoneum is incised transversely, as is the visceral peritoneum. Following downward reflection of the bladder the upper edges of both the parietal and visceral peritoneum are reunited by sutures. Next, the two lower flaps are sutured together. In effect, this artificially extraperitonealizes the uterus before it is opened. Following delivery, the peritoneum is left as it is and a drain is placed over the sutured myometrium.

A low vertical (De Lee) incision in the uterus is recommended when, because of thinning and distension of the lower segment, there is a danger that any transverse incision may extend laterally and compromise major vessels or the ureters. In this regard a neglected shoulder presentation with a prolapsed arm is a particularly dangerous circumstance.

It should be remembered in cases of obstructed labour that the bladder will be bruised and friable and may extend much higher into the abdomen than is usual. If bladder damage is to be avoided the parietal peritoneum must be entered higher than usual and the bladder must be reflected downwards with extreme caution.

CAESAREAN SECTION AND CHORIOAMNIONITIS

Although obstructed labour is not common in the UK, intrauterine infection of varying degree can be encountered, especially following prolonged rupture of the membranes.

Histological evidence of fetal cord vasculitis may be discovered in about 10% of all pregnancies and leukocytic infiltration of the chorion and amnion may be found in about 10–20%. The incidence of membrane inflammation varies according to the sites examined, but the greatest incidence occurs in sections from the placental margin (Pryse-Davies et al 1973).

Clinically, the term chorioamnionitis is reserved by most obstetricians to indicate overt intrauterine infection involving the amniotic fluid and baby as well as the membranes. The clinical incidence of intra-amniotic infection has been estimated at 1–2% of pregnancies. It would seem, therefore, that only one pregnancy in 10 with histological evidence of chorioamnionitis also presents evidence of significant clinical infection (Schwarz 1982). By contrast, most — if not all — patients with severe fetal infection reveal evidence of chorioamnionitis.

Premature rupture of the membranes is the commonest antecedent of significant intra-amniotic infection. Fetal and maternal tachycardia, associated with low-grade pyrexia and, possibly, offensive liquor, may be the earliest signs of a developing infection. Caesarean section may then have to be considered if fetal maturity exceeds 26 weeks and the child is normal, but the possibility of promoting labour safely, easily and quickly is remote. (A judgement about whether to pursue vaginal delivery will be based partly upon the state of the cervix and also upon the availability of suitable obstetric and neonatal facilities to undertake controlled parturition, or to care for a compromised immature child at birth.)

Should delivery by Caesarean section be appropriate, an extraperitoneal approach might reasonably be utilized if there is anyone experienced enough to undertake it. Most frequently the approach will be via the lower uterine segment in the normal manner, special attention being paid to the placing of packs in each paracolic gutter before allowing infected liquor to escape into the peritoneum. Suction evacuation of liquor following an incision into the uterus also minimizes the risk of spreading infection by spillage. Postoperatively, peritoneal lavage is desirable, though it is debatable whether the additional application of antibiotics locally is advantageous. Moreover, Schwarz (1982) warns that inflamed surfaces might foster such rapid absorption of large quantities of antibiotics that a potential threat of toxicity may be posed. Parenteral administration therefore seems more applicable.

SURGICAL TECHNIQUES AND COMPLICATIONS

To emphasize anything more than selected points of importance in the technique of Caesarean section is beyond the scope of the present chapter. Suffice it to say initially that both the anaesthetist and the surgeon should ensure that adequate preoperative preparation has been made. In emergency cases, at the very minimum, the patient's haemoglobin should be known and blood should be cross-matched if time allows.

The use of a lateral 15° wedge at Caesarean section is now probably mandatory in order to reduce the effects of caval occlusion during surgery. The lateral tilt necessitates some reorientation for the surgeon who sees the patient's uterine and pelvic anatomy more from the side than is usual. Care has to be taken, therefore, that incisions are centred about the true midline axis of the patient and not inadvertently sited too far on one side. This can lead to difficulty, especially with transverse incisions, by approaching too near to the vasculature at the side of the uterus, an area which the surgeon normally avoids. The lateral rubber wedge can be removed as soon as the baby is born.

The Pfannenstiel incision is satisfactory for most operations; disadvantages such as increased vascularity or the operation taking longer to perform are marginal if not theoretical. Even repeat operations are not substantially more difficult by this route. The midline or paramedian approach should be reserved for potentially troublesome or hazardous operations.

Prior to entering the peritoneum special attention should be paid to the possibility of the bladder rising higher into the abdomen than expected, especially if the operation is performed during delayed labour.

Good exposure of the lower segment by blunt dissection and separation of the bladder downwards after transversely incising the visceral peritoneum is important in order not only to protect the bladder during delivery of the fetus if the lower segment tears, but also to facilitate the repair of the lower segment by clearly defining its lower edge.

Having incised the lower segment centrally with a clean scalpel, the author favours extending the incision to left and right in a slightly upwards direction with curved scissors, all the while protecting the underlying fetus by two fingers slipped through the initial wound.

To deliver the baby it is usually easy to slip a hand below the presenting part and, by allowing air to surround it, to ease and lift the head from the pelvis into the wound. There should be no undue haste. Fundal pressure can be used to assist delivery of the head. However, Wrigley's forceps are sometimes more useful if access to the head through the wound is limited. Speedy or sudden delivery of the head through a tightly fitting lower segment incision is to be avoided. This can promote intracranial haemorrhage and may well cause the wound to tear laterally at one or other of the angles. In the case of breech delivery the head can be satisfactorily controlled using the Mauriceau–Smellie–Veit procedure or delivered by forceps.

The use of an oxytocic to contract the upper segment after delivery and the removal of the placenta spontaneously or manually is now a well recognized routine.

Broad haemostatic clamps of the Green–Armytage type are applied to the angles and edges of the wounds. At this stage it is important to avoid mistaking the posterior aspect of the uterine cavity for one of the anterior edges of the uterine wound. Sometimes these three surfaces lie very close together after the uterus has been emptied.

Once sutures have been placed outside the angles of the wound, the edges are sutured, usually in two layers, and one of these is commonly inserted as a locking suture. Undue inclusion of the decidua is better omitted but does not have to be scrupulously avoided. Suture of the two layers of peritoneum and closure of the abdominal wall in layers is performed to complete the operation.

THE CLASSICAL CAESAREAN SECTION

Whenever possible the classical Caesarean section should be avoided. Nevertheless, there are occasions when its use is justifiable and even to be recommended. These circumstances include the absence of a lower segment or the impossibility of reaching the lower segment because of dense adhesions. Extreme vascularity of the lower segment may also make that approach hazardous. A classical vertical incision between the vessels may then be necessary. Rarely, the presence of a fibroid can prevent a lower segment approach. If a patient is being delivered prematurely because of the presence of carcinoma of the cervix, an upper segment incision is reasonable. Most obstetricians would also elect to perform a classical incision when the fetus lies transversely and the fetal back is immediately beneath the lower segment.

For a classical operation the abdominal approach is made via a subumbilical median or paramedian incision. Any dextrorotation of the uterus should be recognized and corrected. This should ensure that the vertical incision, to be made through the lower part of the upper segment, is performed in the midline.

Delivery of the fetus and placenta through the upper segment is usually easy but suture of the thick wall of the upper myometrium may require three layers. Thereafter there is no visceral layer of peritoneum to be repaired separately, so abdominal closure occurs in layers, beginning with the parietal peritoneum.

COMPLICATIONS OF CAESAREAN SECTION

Bleeding is a major hazard of Caesarean section. It is always difficult to estimate the loss accurately because blood is usually mixed with amniotic fluid. A blood loss of 600 ml is usual. This loss occurs chiefly from large veins in the lower segment or from large sinuses in the myometrium.

Excessive bleeding can arise from involvement of veins at the side of the uterus if a tear extends the normal wound laterally. The upward curve of the initial incision into the lower segment serves to avoid this complication. Slow delivery of the presenting part and correct central siting of the lower segment incision by prior correction of uterine dextrorotation also act as a safeguard.

A haematoma can form quickly at Caesarean section because of the vascularity and general looseness of the tissues, especially about the broad ligament. Haematoma formation must therefore be recognized early and treated while it is still relatively easy to insert a haemostatic suture.

The complications which may be associated with Caesarean section for intrapartum infection or obstructed labour have been discussed earlier. The complications associated with Caesarean section for placenta praevia are dealt with below.

Bladder damage at Caesarean section is best avoided by a careful approach to the parietal and visceral peritoneum, with gentle dissection and separation of the bladder from the lower segment. If the bladder is damaged it is important to recognize this, repair it and drain the bladder for 10 days. This usually avoids fistula formation.

Postoperatively, bowel distension is common but usually

recovers within 48 hours. Paralytic ileus is uncommon and is to be treated by gastric suction and parenteral fluids in the usual way.

Bleeding after Caesarean section

Bleeding occurring some days after a Caesarean section is most likely to be due to the lysis of a clot in a vessel by infection, occurring after absorption of the haemostatic suture. The site of bleeding is most likely to be somewhere near or in the wound itself. Retained products of conception may be associated with infection, though they usually cause bleeding to occur earlier.

The usual management of delayed postoperative bleeding is conservative. Appropriate blood replacement is recommended, as well as the administration of suitable antibiotics. Ligation of the anterior division of the internal iliac artery on one or both sides may rarely be required (Whitfield 1981).

THE INDICATIONS FOR CAESAREAN SECTION

Mention has already been made of the use of elective Caesarean section and of Caesarean section in labour. Here, attention is drawn to four additional indications for Caesarean section, about which there is often some debate — the very low birthweight (VLBW) infant, breech presentation, abruptio placentae and placenta praevia.

The VLBW infant

For the VLBW infant, especially if presenting by the breech, the best method of delivery remains controversial. Several retrospective American studies of babies weighing 1000–1499 g have suggested that Caesarean section is desirable if not mandatory (Woods 1979, Mann & Gallant 1979, De Crespigny & Pepperell 1979, Karp et al 1979, Duenhoelter et al 1979, Nissel et al 1981). The data to support the recommendation of Caesarean section in such circumstances are, however, quite scanty; the number of cases reported is often too small to allow statistical analysis (Table 58.1).

Whereas Woods (1979) reported that routine Caesarean section was not justified, Mann & Gallant (1979) revealed a slight but insignificant improvement in the Caesarean section group when compared to vaginal breech deliveries. They concluded that the VLBW baby presenting by the breech may best be managed by Caesarean section. In a series presented by De Crespigny & Pepperell (1979) the vaginal delivery of 40 VLBW babies presenting by the breech was compared with only 2 delivered by Caesarean section. Although these authors tended to favour Caesarean section, they also conceded that an alternative procedure would be a continuously monitored controlled vaginal delivery under epidural analgesia. Karp et al (1979) emphasized that Caesarean section was a safer course, particularly for the footling breech weighing less than 1500 g. Duenholter et al (1979) and Nissel et al (1981) stated that Caesarean delivery of the VLBW baby is of benefit and therefore preferable.

Table 58.1 VLBW infants in breech presentation delivered vaginally and by Caesarean section

	Vaginal delivery		Caesarean section		
Birthweight	No.	% mortality	No.	% mortality	Reference
100–1499 g	63	16	25	4	Woods (1979)
	46	15	30	10	Mann & Gallant (1979)
	55	40	0	2	De Crespigny & Pepperell (1979)
	50	12	60	5	Karp et al (1979)
	55	11	0	5	Nissell et al (1981)
	56	9	0	9	Duenholter et al (1979)
500–1500 g	37	19	0	12	Lamont et al (1983)

Table 58.2 Percentage mortality of infants of low birthweight (<2500 g) presenting by the breech according to mode of delivery

Vaginal delivery		Casarean section		
No.	% mortality	No.	% mortality	Reference
62	29	3	0	Patterson et al (1967)
38	16	9	11	Lyons & Papsin (1978)
48	15	39	5	Ingermarsson et al (1978)

It is apparent from Table 58.1 that the number of babies studied in these series is too small to permit any satisfactory statistical analysis. In the British report by Lamont et al (1983) it was confirmed that survival is dramatically better for infants weighing more than 1000 g, by whichever route they are delivered. However, a disproportionate number of infants who were delivered vaginally weighed less than 1000 g. It is therefore difficult to accept without qualification the conclusion derived from the group overall that Caesarean section improves the survival of babies weighing less than 1500 g.

Numerous other reports favouring Caesarean section collectively treat all babies weighing less than 2500 g as a homogeneous group (Table 58.2).

The view put forward by Patterson et al (1967) and to some extent endorsed by Lyons & Papsin (1978), that Caesarean section is the method of choice for breech presentation, is not now tenable. In the study by Ingermarsson et al (1978) which also favours Caesarean delivery for babies presenting by the breech and weighing less than 2500 g, it is notable that those delivered vaginally were all born between 1971 and 1974. By contrast, those delivered by Caesarean section were delivered after 1975. The obstetric care and especially the neonatal expertise given to infants in these two periods is unlikely to have been identical.

Other retrospective analyses of fetal survival in VLBW

infants according to their mode of delivery suffer from the criticism that Caesarean section is only likely to have been offered to infants deemed capable of survival. By contrast, non-viable infants stillborn prior to 28 weeks are probably recorded as vaginal breech deliveries.

As a representative review of the literature reveals no prospective randomized controlled studies, the obstetrician is left with rather a confusing hotchpotch of data upon which to base clinical judgement in a particular case. Perhaps the succinct review by Crowley & Hawkins (1980) offers the view which is most widely accepted at present. In their opinion, the present consensus is that the survival rate for infants weighing 1500–2500 g is not affected by the mode of delivery. For infants weighing 1000–1500 g, Caesarean section does appear to provide some advantage. (The assumption, of course, is that the fetal weight can be accurately estimated antenatally.)

The outcome for infants weighing less than 1000 g is largely dependent upon the facilities available in the obstetric and neonatal units concerned. In this regard, the recent prospective study performed at the Liverpool Maternity Hospital by Lobb & Morgan (personal communication) of the delivery of 104 VLBW infants presenting by the breech and matched for weight and gestational age is probably of importance. No benefit for delivery by elective Caesarean section could be demonstrated. The neonates who were delivered vaginally under epidural analgesia by a competent operator after continuous fetal heart monitoring during labour proved to be just as safe as those delivered by Caesarean section. Nor could it be shown that it was disadvantageous for the woman to labour prior to Caesarean section so long as continuous monitoring was utilized. In each group the percentage survival was of the order of 76%. Without continuous monitoring, however, the chance of survival was significantly reduced. If fetal distress is detected, therefore, prompt abdominal delivery is required.

Similar results have been reported for the management of VLBW infants presenting by the vertex as well as by the breech (Beazley & Lobb 1983). While the question: 'Do the maternal risks of Caesarean section at, say, 26 weeks' gestation outweigh the possible fetal benefit?' has not yet been finally answered, it is worth reflecting that, whereas a compromised fetus of that gestational age probably has only about a 20% chance of survival at present, a woman who suffers a perinatal loss at vaginal delivery probably has about a 90% chance of a successful pregnancy next time. Coupled with this is the practice, in some centres, of making a low vertical incision in the uterus at Caesarean section, because the lower segment has not formed properly at the time of operation. The attendant risk of such an incision awaits verification. In general, this type of incision is believed to be less hazardous than a classical Caesarean section scar, though not as safe as a lower segment Caesarean section scar. Of course at about 30 weeks' gestation, especially if severe fetal immaturity is present, any transverse incision has to be made through the lower part of the upper uterine segment and this too can be a difficult procedure. It follows, therefore, that if by continuous fetal monitoring in labour a significant number of VLBW infants can be delivered vaginally as safely as by Caesarean section, this policy has considerable maternal advantages.

Breech presentation

In the UK a persistent breech presentation is not an automatic indication for elective Caesarean section about term. Ten years ago the accepted incidence of Caesarean section for breech deliveries in Britain was 10%. Probably 40% of breech presentations are now so delivered. In the USA, the section rate for breeches is quoted as 72.5% (Russel 1982).

The reasons for the increasing trend to deliver by a Caesarean section include the relative safety of the operation, the skilled neonatal care now available for small babies, and the increasing unwillingness of obstetricians to undertake vaginal manipulative procedures because of the risk of litigation, should delivery prove difficult. According to investigations from the Netherlands, the main danger of breech presentation is in the associated complications of pregnancy. Based on a relatively long-term neurological study of 281 children delivered by the breech, Faber-Nijholt et al (1983) concluded that there is no reason to advocate a greater frequency of abdominal delivery than 20% in breech delivery.

Excluding cephalopelvic disproportion as the obvious indication for Caesarean section, most obstetricians acknowledge that a fetus aged 36–42 weeks, presenting by the breech, and weighing 2.5–4.0 kg, can be delivered vaginally with minimal danger provided certain safeguards are met (Gimovsky et al 1980). These include immediate facilities for Caesarean section and close intrapartum fetal monitoring, adequate clinical pelvimetry confirmed radiographically, no hyperextension of the fetal neck and satisfactory cervical dilatation (1 cm/h). To minimize the risk of cord prolapse during delivery perhaps the frank breech should be added to this list. If these criteria are met it is expected that 88% of vaginal breech deliveries will be successful and the remainder may be successfully delivered by Caesarean section without significant fetal problems.

The occurrence of additional maternal or fetal complications can provide sufficient cause to consider operative delivery. These may include significant maternal hypertension, diabetes mellitus, minor abruptions or marginal placental praevia. Fetal size also provides a significant factor. The small baby has been considered elsewhere, but the much larger baby estimated at 3.75 kg or more should also be considered for operative delivery unless a sufficiently large maternal pelvic capacity and a proven past obstetric performance suggest Caesarean section is unnecessary.

Obviously, the presence of any fetal abnormality will influence the decision to operate, as should potentially hazardous features of the breech presentation itself, such as a footling breech presentation or a hyperextended fetal head. This latter feature, the star-gazing fetus, provides a debatable indication for Caesarean section. It depends to some extent upon whether the head is continually hyperextended. A single X-ray film can be notoriously unreliable. Ballas & Toaf (1976) recommend that if the angle of extension exceeds 90° an elective Caesarean section should be performed.

A number of relatively minor maternal indications may provide a series of half-points which, taken together, weigh the balance in favour of Caesarean section when the fetal breech presents. Such maternal indications may include a poor obstetric history, relative infertility or a scar from a previous Caesarean section for a non-recurrent condition.

When Caesarean section is performed for breech presentation about term, the transverse lower segment incision is recommended (Schutterman & Grimes 1983). An alternative low vertical incision, is used by some, especially in preterm Caesarean section, but this is not generally advocated.

Abruptio placentae

Caesarean section has little place in the treatment of abruptio placentae. The route of choice for delivery in these circumstances is undoubtedly vaginal. There are, however, some exceptional circumstances when this policy may have to be reviewed. Green-Thompson (1982) suggests three main indications for abdominal delivery:

1. *Obstetrical indications*: apart from such absolute indications as disproportion or transverse lie, attention is drawn to the unlikely possibilities of being unable to induce labour or to secure adequate progress during parturition. Also, if the uterus contains a scar from a previous Caesarean section, thought must be directed towards the increased possibility of uterine rupture. Management will be influenced by such factors as the placental site, the extent of abruption, fetal size and the relationship of the presenting part to the maternal pelvis.
2. *Complications of abruption*: the rare complications of renal shutdown or intractable clotting defect and bleeding in a patient in whom labour cannot be initiated may, unusually, demand Caesarean section. Of course, this should not be undertaken without first securing adequate blood replacement and correcting the clotting defect.
3. *A live, viable baby*: in a useful review of this aspect, Green-Thompson emphasizes that perinatal survival rates are significantly improved by Caesarean section when the fetus is not only alive but viable. The idea is refuted that intrauterine death of the fetus is merely delayed by Caesarean section to become a neonatal death. Available evidence suggests that the babies followed up after delivery by Caesarean section for abruption are normal. Of particular importance is the advice that only beyond 35 weeks' gestation, or above a fetal weight of 1500 g, is there an improved survival with Caesarean section. At less than these parameters there is no difference in perinatal survival rate between vaginal and Caesarean delivery.

Delivery within 2–4 hours of abruption, if possible, is also reported to be associated with significantly increased fetal survival. If, therefore, the patient is seen in time, and if Caesarean section is selected in the interests of the fetus, there should be no undue delay in performing the operation. What must be avoided is compromising both the mother and the fetus by operating at the wrong time under disadvantageous, even hazardous, circumstances.

Placenta praevia

Whenever there is a major degree of placenta praevia, delivery by Caesarean section is the method of choice in the UK, even in the unusual circumstance when the baby is not alive.

Numerous problems confront the operator undertaking Caesarean section for placenta praevia. Not least of these is the foreknowledge that the operation can be a haemorrhagic procedure. It is known to be more hazardous than Caesarean section for many other indications. The experience of the operator is important in minimizing potential dangers, and surgeons in training should always have adequate assistance and appropriate supervision to support them.

The approach to the uterus is chiefly via the Pfannenstiel incision. Vertical skin incisions are rarely required, and any discussion about the significance of possible time delays in approaching the uterus, when a patient is bleeding from placenta praevia, are more theoretical than practical. Seconds are rarely vital in UK obstetric practice.

Large veins coursing over the lower segment may cause alarm. If there is no urgency, the larger veins can be ligated as necessary before being cut. In most instances, care with the incision to avoid transecting major veins will suffice and as soon as the baby is delivered the veins collapse and bleeding ceases. When the veins are too numerous to avoid, a low vertical incision between them can be used, but the need for this is rare.

If the placenta or part of it is sited anteriorly it may impede access to the baby after entering the uterus. To cut the placenta is bloody and may cause serious fetal blood loss. It is preferable, where possible, to shear the placenta off from one side and go around it. This may result in some fetal asphyxia, but the manoeuvre is preferable if expeditiously performed. In either manoeuvre early clamping and cutting of the cord is desirable so that the paediatrician can quickly assess the need for fetal transfusion.

The lower segment may bleed after placental removal, partly because the action of the living ligatures of the myometrium is minimal in the lower segment and partly because of the presence of the piecemeal decidua which remains after placental removal. An extra-careful check on postoperative vaginal bleeding must be kept to avoid missing an unexpected postpartum haemorrhage.

It is rare to have to contemplate Caesarean hysterectomy after surgery for placenta praevia, but if lower segment fails to respond to adequate suturing, pressure with warm packs or the administration of oxytocin, it may have to be done. If it is necessary, it should be tackled before the patient is in extremis.

CONCLUSIONS

There can be little doubt that the introduction and perfection of the lower segment operation has been one of the major advances in obstetric practice. The relative safety of the procedure in the hands of a skilled operator makes it an increasingly valuable method of delivery. The indications for the procedure are continually changing and in today's practice the relative indications outnumber the absolute indications. Perhaps this has led to an unacceptably high incidence of Caesarean section in recent years, but this trend is now being questioned and seems likely to be reversed. It is hoped that the correct place of abdominal delivery will shortly be established—without undue pressure from the increasing influence of litigation.

REFERENCES

Bailey K V 1934 Lower segment Caesarean section as a routine. Lancet i: 672–675
Ballas S, Toaf R 1976 Hyperextension of the fetal head in breech presentation: radiological evaluation and significance. British Journal of Obstetrics and Gynaecology 83: 201–204
Beazley J M, Lobb M O 1983 Aspects of care in labour. In: Lind T (ed) Current reviews in obstetrics and gynaecology no. 6. Churchill Livingstone, London, pp 107–110, 126–127
Bottoms S F, Rosen M G, Sokol R J 1980 The increase in the cesarean birth rate. New England Journal of Medicine 302: 559
British Medical Journal Leading Article 1981 Caesarean childbirth (summary of an NIH concensus statement) 282: 1600–1604
Crowley P, Hawkins D S 1980 Premature breech delivery—the Caesarean section debate. Journal of Obstetrics and Gynaecology 1: 2–6
De Crespigny L J C, Pepperell R J 1979 Perinatal mortality and morbidity in breech presentation. Obstetrics and Gynecology 53: 141–145
Demianczuk N N, Hunter D J S, Taylor D W 1982 Trial of labour after previous CS. American Journal of Obstetrics and Gynecology 142: 640–642
Dewhurst C J 1957 The ruptured Caesarean section scar. Journal of Obstetrics and Gynaecology of the British Empire 64: 113–118
Drife J O 1985 Operative delivery—clinical aspects. In: Chamberlain G V P, Orr J B, Sharp F (eds) Litigation and obstetrics and gynaecology. Proceedings of the 14th study group of the Royal College of Obstetricians and Gynaecologists. RCOG, London, pp 255–264
Duenhoelter J H, Wells C E, Reisch J S et al 1979 A paired controlled study of vaginal and abdominal delivery of the low birth weight breech fetus. Obstetrics and Gynecology 54: 310–313
Faber-Nijholt R, Huisjes H J, Touwen B C L, Fidler V J 1983 Neurological follow up of 281 children born in breech presentation: a controlled study. British Medical Journal 286: 9–12
Gimovsky M, Petrie R, Todd W 1980 Neonatal performance of the selected long term vaginal breech delivery. Obstetrics and Gynecology 56: 687–689
Green-Thompson R W 1982 Antepartum haemorrhage. Clinics in Obstetrics and Gynaecology 9: 493–495
Haddad H, Lundy L E 1978 Changing indications for Caesarean section: a 38 year experience at a community hospital. Obstetrics and Gynecology 51: 133–137
Holland E 1921 Methods of performing Caesarean section. Journal of Obstetrics and Gynaecology of the British Empire 28: 349–357
Ingermarsson I, Westgren M, Svenningsen N W 1978 Long term follow up of preterm infants in breech presentation delivered by Caesarean section. A prospective study. Lancet ii: 172–175
Karp L E, Doney J R, McCarthy T et al 1979 The premature breech: trial of labor or Cesarean section? Obstetrics and Gynecology 53: 88–92
Lamont R F, Dunlop P D M, Crowley P, Elder M G 1983 Spontaneous preterm labour and delivery at under 34 weeks gestation. British Medical Journal 286: 454–457
Lyons E R, Papsin F R 1978 Cesarean section in the management of breech presentation. American Journal of Obstetrics and Gynecology 130: 558–561
Mann L I, Gallant J M 1979 Modern management of the breech delivery. American Journal of Obstetrics and Gynecology 134: 611–614
Marshall C M 1939 Caesarean section. Lower segment operation. John Wright, Bristol
Martin J N, Harris B A, Huddleston J F et al 1983 Vaginal delivery following previous cesarean birth. American Journal of Obstetrics and Gynecology 146: 255–263
Merrill B S, Gibbs C E 1978 Planned vaginal delivery following CS. Obstetrics and Gynecology 52: 50–52
Munro Kerr J M 1921 The lower uterine segment incision in conservative Caesarean section. Journal of Obstetrics and Gynaecology of the British Empire 28: 475–487
Nissel H, Bistoletti P, Palme C 1981 Pre term breech delivery. Acta Obstetricia et Gynecologica Scandinavica 60: 363–366
Office of Population Censuses and Surveys 1987 HMSO, London
Opit I J, Selwood T S 1979 Caesarean section rates in Australia. Medical Journal of Australia 2: 706–709
Patterson S P, Mulliniks R C, Schreier P C 1967 Breech presentation in the primigravida. American Journal of Obstetrics and Gynecology 98: 404–410
Philpott R H 1982 Obstructed labour. Clinics in Obstetrics and Gynaecology 9: 634–635
Pryse-Davies J, Beazley J M, Leach G 1974 A study of placental size and chorio-amnionitis in a consecutive series of hospital deliveries. Journal of Obstetrics and Gynaecology of the British Commonwealth 80: 246–251
Russel J K 1981 Caesarean section. British Medical Journal 283: 1076
Russel J K 1982 Breech vaginal delivery or Caesarean section. British Medical Journal 285: 830–831
Schutterman E B, Grimes D A 1983 Comparative safety of the low transverse versus the low vertical uterine incision for Caesarean section delivery of breech infants. Obstetrics and Gynecology 61: 593–597
Schwarz R H 1982 Chorioamnionitis. In: Studd J (ed) Progress in obstetrics and gynaecology 2. Churchill Livingstone, Edinburgh, pp 18–27
Whitfield C R 1981 Complications of the third stage of labour. In: Dewhurst J (ed) Integrated obstetrics and gynaecology for postgraduates. Blackwell Scientific Publications, London, p 441
Wilson J St George 1931 Lower uterine segment Caesarean section. Journal of Obstetrics and Gynaecology of the British Empire 38: 504–515
Woods J R 1979 Effects of low birth weight breech delivery on neonatal mortality. Obstetrics and Gynecology 53: 735–740
Yudkin P L, Redman C W G 1986 Caesarean section dissected 1978–1983. British Journal of Obstetrics and Gynaecology 93: 135–144

S. S. Ratnam and Mary Rauff

Postpartum haemorrhage and abnormalities of the third stage of labour

POSTPARTUM HAEMORRHAGE

Definitions

Primary postpartum haemorrhage is defined as blood loss from the genital tract in excess of 500 ml in the first 24 hours after the delivery of the baby.

Secondary postpartum haemorrhage occurs when there is excessive bleeding from the genital tract after the first 24 hours postpartum until 6 weeks after the birth.

In some countries like Singapore and Malaysia, the definition of primary postpartum haemorrhage has for many years been taken as the loss of 300 ml or more of blood in the first 24 hours postpartum. The reasons often given for this lower figure are that Asian women are smaller built, less well nourished and generally have a lower haemoglobin level during pregnancy than their western counterparts. These attributes are believed to reduce the tolerance to the loss of a volume of blood conventionally deemed to be within physiological limits. Hence, in the Asian context, one should be alerted earlier to the dangers of postpartum haemorrhage.

Estimation of blood loss

Blood loss in the third stage of labour may be estimated by clinical or haematological means.

Haematological estimations

Recent studies have demonstrated that the average blood loss at normal delivery may be 500 ml or more. Newton (1966) assessed the blood loss in the third stage of labour and the succeeding 24 hours in 105 women by the spectrophotometric measurement of haematin in the fluid lost and the covering towels. He found that the average blood loss was at least 546 ml. The loss in the placenta was not accounted for in his study; if this had been included, the loss would have been increased by a further 100 ml. Using changes in red cell counts, De Leeuw et al (1962) demonstrated that the blood loss at normal delivery and the ensuing 24 hours was approximately 600 ml. Pritchard et al (1962) confirmed these findings with a method similar to that used by De Leeuw et al and also demonstrated that the clinically estimated blood loss was often half of the actual loss.

A case for dispensing with the standard definition of postpartum haemorrhage has been presented by Ueland (1976). This was based on his studies on the blood volume and haematocrit of patients before and during the first 5 days following delivery. Ueland felt that postpartum blood loss should be related to the fall in haematocrit 24 hours after delivery. This value would, however, be affected by the infusion of fluids during labour which would decrease the haematocrit, or the withholding of intravenous fluids with a resultant rise of the haematocrit (Taylor et al 1981).

Clinical estimation

The use of clinical parameters such as blood pressure and pulse rate changes is also not reliable. Recognition of haemorrhagic shock often comes too late since a normal healthy individual may suffer no fall in the blood pressure despite the acute loss of up to 25% of the blood volume; a loss of this amount could be fatal if unrecognized and left untreated (Hardaway 1979). Table 59.1 summarizes the clinical symptoms and signs of significant blood loss. It is evident that hypotension only occurs where there is a fall of 15% of the blood volume, i.e. considerably more than is considered dangerous in a postpartum woman with an expanded blood volume. Tachycardia only develops when blood loss reaches 10–15% of the blood volume. It is therefore not sensitive enough to alert the physician to a blood loss of 500 ml.

The average blood loss in labour is often underestimated and a loss of up to 500 ml may be considered physiological.

The commonly employed clinical methods for the estimation of blood loss are often inaccurate or unfeasible. The

Table 59.1 Clinical symptoms and signs of blood loss correlated to the amount of blood loss

Blood loss (% of blood volume)	Arterial blood pressure (systolic; mmHg)	Symptoms and signs
10–15	Normal	Postural hypotension Mild tachycardia
15–30	Slight fall	Tachycardia Thirst Weakness
30–40	60–80	Pallor Oliguria Confusion Restlessness
40+	40–60	Anuria Air hunger Coma Death

clinician usually has little choice but to accept the nurse's or midwife's estimation. If blood loss is clinically estimated to be 500 ml or more, actual loss is probably in excess of this amount; the obstetrician should be aware of this possibility.

Causes of postpartum haemorrhage

Postpartum haemorrhage is the most common cause of serious blood loss in obstetrics and an important cause of maternal mortality, accounting for 69% of deaths from haemorrhage in England and Wales (Report on Confidential Enquiries into Maternal Deaths 1976–1978).

There are three main causes of postpartum haemorrhage:

1. Uterine atony, which accounts for 90% of postpartum haemorrhages in most countries. However, Beischer & Mackay (1986) feel that in Australia uterine atony is not as important as trauma as a cause for haemorrhage.
2. Trauma to the genital tract, which accounts for about 7% of primary postpartum haemorrhage.
3. Coagulation disorders account for the remaining 3%.

Uterine atony

There are many factors in the cause of uterine atony. Some are predetermined and beyond the control of the obstetrician while others may be anticipated and therefore controllable.

Predetermined factors.

1. Uterine overdistension: overdistension of the uterus may result from polyhydramnios, multiple pregnancy or a large baby. The likelihood of a large baby causing postpartum haemorrhage was observed, according to Hellman & Pritchard (1971), as early as 1904 by Ahlfield & Aschoff; this has been confirmed by other workers (Calkins et al 1931, Reich 1939). The overdistended uterus does not contract quickly or efficiently enough after its contents have been delivered and this leads to haemorrhage. In multiple pregnancy other causes may be responsible; these include a large placental bed from which bleeding may occur or the effect of halothane anaesthesia, possibly used to relax the uterus for intervention during the delivery of the second twin.
2. Past obstetric history: a previous history of postpartum haemorrhage predisposes to an increased risk of postpartum haemorrhage in the present pregnancy (Doran et al 1955).
3. Multiparity: grand multiparae are prone to postpartum haemorrhage. One possible explanation is that with increasing multiparity there is an increasing amount of fibrous tissue in the myometrium hindering effective contraction of the uterus.
4. Antepartum haemorrhage: antepartum haemorrhage from either abruptio placentae or placenta praevia predisposes to further bleeding after delivery.

   There may be bleeding from coagulation failure following placental abruption; further, the presence of a Couvelaire uterus does not allow for efficient uterine contraction.

   The lower uterine segment has fewer muscular fibres and as a result does not contract as efficiently as the upper uterine segment. Implantation of the placenta in the lower segment therefore predisposes to postpartum haemorrhage.
5. Poor uterine contraction: uterine contraction may be inefficient in the presence of uterine fibroids or retained products of conception such as placental cotyledon, membranes, a succenturiate lobe of placenta or a morbidly adherent placenta.

Controllable factors.

1. Operative deliveries and anaesthesia: operative delivery is an important cause of controllable postpartum haemorrhage (e.g. internal podalic versions or Caesarean section). The effects are further aggravated by the use of anaesthetic agents such as chloroform or ether during the procedure. Halothane anaesthesia or the use of beta-sympathomimetics for uterine relaxation have been identified as common causes of drug-induced postpartum haemorrhage.
2. Prolonged labour: prolonged labour, associated with maternal and uterine exhaustion, is a frequent cause of postpartum haemorrhage. A big baby and uterine overdistension necessitating an operative forceps delivery, or Caesarean section can predispose to haemorrhage.
3. Mismanagement of the third stage: a common error is application of traction on an unseparated placenta to hasten the third stage. Other hazardous procedures include squeezing and kneading the uterus, which may cause incomplete placental separation.

Although Beischer & Mackay (1986) believe that

retained products of conception are the commonest cause of uterine atony, it is most likely that a combination of factors is responsible.

Trauma

This is the second most common cause of postpartum haemorrhage. It may be due to an unsutured episiotomy, multiple lacerations from precipitate labour or tears resulting from failure to perform an episiotomy when required. Uterine rupture, cervical tears from shoulder dystocia and destructive operations are less common causes of trauma.

Coagulation disorders

Patients with an inherent coagulation disorder, e.g. von Willebrand's disease or idiopathic thrombocytopenia, or those with an acquired problem such as liver disease, hepatitis or anticoagulant therapy, represent circumstances in which one can anticipate postpartum bleeding and in whom prevention is, at least to some extent, possible (Ch. 38).

However, acute coagulopathies may develop from amniotic fluid embolism, for example. These disorders require massive blood transfusions which may be difficult to manage because other complications may coexist, such as respiratory failure in amniotic fluid embolism or sepsis.

Prevention of postpartum haemorrhage

The adage that prevention is better than cure could not be more apt than when the management of postpartum haemorrhage is considered. It was the most common cause of maternal mortality in the UK (Report on Confidential Enquiries into Maternal Deaths 1976–1978), and there is an obvious need to avoid its occurrence. Furthermore, when it occurs, massive blood transfusion may be required; this can lead to further disasters like the development of coagulation failure.

Prevention of postpartum haemorrhage involves:

1. The proper management of the third stage of labour.
2. The routine use of oxytocic drugs in the management of the third stage.
3. The identification of high-risk patients and the use of more effective means to decrease bleeding in these women.

Management of the third stage

Management of the third stage of labour has been dealt with in Chapter 47. Suffice to say, mismanagement of the third stage may lead to severe postpartum haemorrhage from retained placenta and uterine inversion. The aetiology and management of these two conditions will be discussed.

Drugs

The advantages of using oxytocics to shorten the third stage of labour and reduce blood loss have been described by many authors. Daley (1951) reduced the incidence of postpartum haemorrhage with the use of ergometrine. Kimbell (1958) further confirmed this, using intramuscular ergometrine and hyaluronidase. Rowe (1962), using intravenous ergot, confirmed that postpartum haemorrhage was decreased. However, he felt that the incidence of retained placenta was higher than that reported by Kimbell although this was not statistically significant.

McGrath & Browne (1962) investigated the efficacy of intramuscular Syntometrine and found that bleeding in the third stage was reduced. Gibbons et al (1972) confirmed that intramuscular Syntometrine was as effective as intravenous oxytocics. De Villiers & du Toit (1963) reported an incidence of postpartum haemorrhage reduced from 11.98 to 2% with the use of ergometrine, Methergine or Syntometrine. Intravenous oxytocin, which is believed to be more effective than other oxytocics (Moir & Amoa 1979), has the advantages of having fewer side-effects such as nausea, retching and vomiting, which are common with ergometrine and the ergot-derived drugs. Our experience in Singapore is slightly different. We found that intravenous ergometrine was better at reducing blood loss compared with Syntometrine, prostaglandins, or no oxytocics; but the difference between the blood loss with Syntometrine and without any oxytocics was not statistically significant (Rauff, personal communication).

There are other means of decreasing the risks of postpartum haemorrhage. According to Crawford (1985), the use of epidural anaesthesia for pain relief during labour and for Caesarean section tends to decrease the amount of intraoperative bleeding. Crawford found that the incidence of postpartum haemorrhage among patients having an epidural was 12.6% compared with 15.9% in those without epidural anaesthesia. Moir & Wallace (1967) reported that the average blood loss at forceps delivery was 275 ml when the patient had an epidural anaesthesia and 400 ml when she had a pudendal block. These data were confirmed by Moodie & Moir (1976).

Read & Anderson (1977), using radioactively tagged red blood cells, found that an average of 1150 ml of blood was lost in 30 cases during a lower segment Caesarean section under general anaesthesia, using ergometrine as an oxytocic. Skovstedt et al (1973) and Crawford (1985) disagreed; they felt that a more realistic figure was 600–650 ml. Crawford used the need for blood intraoperatively as an index of the effect of the anaesthesia on postpartum haemorrhage. The need for blood transfusion fell from 8–9 to 1.7% for elective

Caesareans and 5–6 to 2.3% for emergency Caesarean section when epidural anaesthesia was used.

Takagi & co-workers (1976) found that intravenous and intramuscular prostaglandin $F_{2\alpha}$ was of little value in controlling uterine blood loss or delivery. Corson & Bolognese (1977) differed, but this was based on a single case report.

Prostaglandin analogues have been found to be useful in the control of postpartum haemorrhage. The prostaglandin commonly used is 15-S-15 methylprostaglandin, $F_{2\alpha}$-tromethamine (15-methyl $PGF_{2\alpha}$ or Prostin 15/m). It is given intramuscularly or in desperate situations directly into the uterine myometrium (Toppozada et al 1981, Bruce et al 1982, Hayashi et al 1984). One dose is adequate in most instances but repeated doses may be needed if control is not obtained. The estimated reduction in blood loss of the drug has been reported to vary between 60% (Bruce et al 1982) and 95% (Toppozada et al 1981). In Singapore the routine use of prostaglandins as an alternative to conventional oxytocics has not shown any significant reduction in blood loss, but no studies on the use of the prostaglandins in postpartum haemorrhage have been conducted (Rauff, personal communication).

Identification of high-risk patients

Just as there are patients more prone to develop postpartum haemorrhage, there are those more likely to sustain trauma to the genital tract, especially ruptured uterus.

Tears of the lower genital tract are often encountered in patients who have had a forceps delivery, though occasionally they may occur with spontaneous delivery. Forceps delivery may cause vaginal or cervical tears, possibly extending into the lateral fornices involving the uterine artery and lower uterine segment.

Uterine rupture

The incidence of ruptured uterus varies from one in 415 deliveries (Menon 1962) to one in 3869 deliveries (Chew 1984). Although uncommon, it is an important cause of maternal mortality. One of the most useful clinical classifications of uterine rupture is that given by Hellman & Pritchard (1971). It is briefly summarized as follows:

Rupture of a scarred uterus — spontaneous or traumatic
Rupture of an intact uterus — spontaneous or traumatic

The scarred uterus. With increasing resort to Caesarean section, the incidence of scar rupture is expected to rise and to become a matter of increased concern. The higher risk of rupture of the classical Caesarean section scar in subsequent pregnancy is well known. It has been quoted as approximately 2% (Delfs & Eastman 1945) as compared with 0.5% with a lower segment section scar (Hellegers & Eastman 1961). About one-third of classical Caesarean section scars rupture in the antepartum period. Repeat Caesarean section will therefore not prevent all scar ruptures.

The low incidence of scar rupture in women previously delivered by lower segment Caesarean section means that repeat section is not indicated in patients with this scar, except under the following circumstances.

1. Two previous Caesarean sections.
2. Those with previous T-shaped scars or tears extending into the bladder or other surrounding structures.
3. Where there was severe pelvic sepsis in the puerperium after Caesarean section, and uterine wound healing is suspect.
4. Where there is a maternal or fetal indication to perform a Caesarean section again.

Rupture of the uterus is also more likely in patients who have had a previous hysterotomy or perforation following a termination of pregnancy (Chew 1980, Chew & Choo 1982).

Postmyomectomy uterine rupture is not common although Pedowitz & Felmus (1952) felt that the incidence of myomectomy scar rupture is as high as after a classical Caesarean section, if the incision entered the endometrial cavity.

The intact uterus. Spontaneous rupture of the intact uterus is one of the gravest complications of obstetrics. It is seen in patients of high parity and practically never in the primigravida; it is found where cephalopelvic disproportion is undiagnosed. Rupture occurs during labour and spontaneous rupture of the intact uterus occurring before the onset of labour is extremely rare; the most common causes are previous manual removal of placenta, previous dilatation and curettage and postabortal or postpartum sepsis. Of course an occult perforation cannot be excluded in the first two causes.

Traumatic rupture is uncommon but may occur at any time during pregnancy following, say, an automobile accident. It may be the result of a direct blow or of a *contrecoup* effect. Other causes of uterine rupture are an external cephalic version performed antenatally or intrapartum, oxytocin administration in women of high parity or a difficult forceps delivery.

Management of postpartum haemorrhage

Postpartum haemorrhage can occur while the obstetrician is still conducting the delivery of the placenta or some time after he or she has left the patient's bedside. In the former situation, the uterine fundus should be palpated and the presence of uterine contraction verified. An intravenous oxytocic such as 10 units of Syntocinon should be administered if this has not been done already. Controlled cord traction with effective countertraction should be applied as soon as the uterus is well contracted; the placenta and membranes should be delivered and carefully examined for completeness.

The vulva and vagina must be examined meticulously for

any lacerations; these must be repaired as soon as possible. Arterial bleeding points should be ligated separately to prevent a vulval haematoma. Blood loss is increased when episiotomy has been performed (Brant 1966).

If an obstetrician is summoned after delivery and perineal repair has been completed, either because the patient is bleeding profusely or because the signs of impending collapse have been detected, the first observation to be made on arrival is palpation of the uterus. If the uterus is soft and atonic, rubbing up the uterus should stimulate contraction. Uterine atony, the commonest cause of postpartum haemorrhage, must be excluded by this simple test before any other procedures are contemplated. An intravenous drip should then be set up after blood has been withdrawn for blood grouping and cross-matching and an intravenous bolus injection of either Syntocinon or ergometrine given.

This approach is usually adequate to control the bleeding in most instances. Some prefer to set up an intravenous infusion of an oxytocic such as Syntocinon for a few hours to maintain uterine contraction. They take the view that during the phase of temporary atony, blood clots can accumulate in the uterine cavity, acting as retained products of conception and preventing efficient uterine contraction. If this is the case, palpating the uterus and rubbing it up should expel the clots and encourage the uterus to contract. Continuous infusion of oxytocics helps to maintain uterine contraction until clotting occurs in at the placental bed vessels.

After these procedures, the patient should be watched carefully for any signs of bleeding per vaginam or intra-abdominally. Overt intra-abdominal bleeding may be manifest by collapse of the patient with signs of haemorrhagic shock, detection of fluid in the abdominal cavity and a uterus that is poorly contracted. Other indications of intra-abdominal bleeding include peritoneal irritation, persistently low blood pressure and high pulse rate despite adequate replacement with blood and fluids. Symptoms and signs of bleeding may accompany the development of a broad ligament haematoma, pushing the uterus to the contralateral side. These events indicate obvious uterine rupture and signal the need for laparotomy after resuscitation. The signs of haemorrhage are not always so evident.

In the event that the uterus remains contracted but bleeding continues, the vagina and cervix should be examined very carefully in the operating theatre, where lighting is best, to exclude any lacerations which have hitherto been undetected at the bedside. Vaginal tears should be carefully sutured, and on completion, haemostasis ensured. Packing the vagina with gauze soaked in flavine emulsion at the end of the procedure helps maintain haemostasis. Cervical tears are more hazardous as they often extend into the uterus. On their detection, the anterior and posterior lips of the cervix should be grasped with a pair of sponge or Green Armytage forceps and the tear (usually lateral, occasionally posterior) repaired with interrupted catgut starting from the apex and working downwards. Any extension of the tear into the uterus warrants laparotomy since complete haemostasis cannot be achieved by a vaginal approach.

Bleeding may continue with the uterus contracting and relaxing intermittently. There are two possible causes: uterine atony with retained products of conception, or a ruptured uterus. Another careful inspection of the placenta, its membranes and vasculature is advisable in order to exclude the possibility of a placenta succenturiata, missing cotyledons or retained membranes. For practical purposes, this procedure may not always be adequate because the patient would still have to be taken to theatre for exploration of the uterine cavity if she continues to bleed, even if these placental findings were excluded. It is never easy to be absolutely certain of the absence of retained products and it is essential to take steps to exclude such a treatable cause.

In the operating theatre detection of products of conception warrants digital removal or curettage. Exploration of the uterine cavity is also important for the exclusion of uterine rupture. It is difficult to examine the uterine cavity digitally with the patient conscious. Examination is much easier under a general anaesthesia and tears in inaccessible positions are more easily detected; for example, in the conscious patient, a right-handed obstetrician would find it extremely difficult to detect a tear in the lower left lateral aspect of the uterus.

The management of uterine rupture hinges on two questions — the site of the rupture and the desire of the patient for future child-bearing. If the patient has had a dehiscence of a previous uterine scar, has a fundal rupture that can be repaired and desires more children, an attempt should be made to repair the rupture. The uterus can usually be conserved in these circumstances but the patient should be delivered by elective Caesarean section in any subsequent pregnancy. When the rupture occurs in, or extends into, an inaccessible position such as the broad ligament (usually as an extension of a lateral cervical tear or a lower Caesarean section scar) repair is difficult and fraught with danger as the uterine vessels and ureter are close. These tears are invariably associated with a broad ligament haematoma which further aggravates the problem of identification and repair of the rupture since the tissues are discoloured, friable and soggy and every stitch placed tears and creates more bleeding. Under such circumstances, hysterectomy with conservation of both ovaries is recommended.

In rare circumstances, the patient may continue to bleed even after the exclusion of a uterine rupture and retained products of conception. The possibility of a coagulation abnormality as the consequence of continued bleeding and transfusion with stored blood must be excluded. Blood should be sent for prothrombin, partial thromboplastin time and platelet count. If a coagulation defect is identified, the best treatment is probably replacement with fresh blood and fresh frozen plasma. Platelets should only be given if thrombocytopenia is detected (Ch. 38).

Hot douches and bimanual compression of the uterus are

other means of arresting bleeding when a coagulopathy has been excluded. The technique of bimanual compression consists of placing one hand on the patient's abdomen and introducing the other hand in the vagina. The vaginal hand is made into a fist and the whole uterus is squeezed between the fist and the external hand. This manoeuvre stimulates the uterine muscles to contract and has the additional effect of compressing the uterine veins. Success with these procedures has been reported from time to time. Packing of the uterus is generally not favoured as the uterus would merely expand to accommodate the packs. It is an unphysiological procedure which prevents effective myometrial contraction and totally contradicts the dictum that an empty uterus would contract. Furthermore, this procedure increases the risks of infection. Injection of prostaglandin directly into the uterine musculature may be attempted at this stage before a laparotomy is embarked upon.

In the rare event that the patient still continues to bleed despite the exclusion of the trauma and a coagulopathy, and there is no response to conservative measures to stop bleeding, there is little choice but to offer the patient a laparotomy with the purpose of either ligating both internal iliac arteries or performing a hysterectomy. The option depends again on the woman's desire for future child-bearing. Failure of bilateral iliac artery ligation inevitably entails hysterectomy.

ABNORMALITIES OF THE THIRD STAGE

Retained placenta

Physiologically, the uterus should contract soon after the delivery of the baby. The placenta will then separate from the uterine wall and is spontaneously expelled. Oxytocin has been used to hasten this process which may take up to half an hour or more. Despite the routine use of oxytocics the third stage may be delayed. Possible explanations for this delay are inadequate uterine contraction and retraction and, rarely, a morbidly adherent placenta.

The management of the retained placenta has varied considerably from time to time but in modern practice, manual removal of the placenta is routinely employed if there is failure to deliver the placenta half an hour after the delivery of the baby. This may be performed earlier if the patient is bleeding and the placenta has failed to separate completely. Ready resort to this procedure has been facilitated by the advent of antibiotics, the availability of blood transfusion and the safety of modern anaesthetic techniques.

Technique

The patient who has a retained placenta is often shocked, having had postpartum haemorrhage. Adequate resuscitation is mandatory before attempting manual removal. This should include giving blood if the patient is bleeding and the readministration of a second dose of the oxytocic to encourage uterine contraction and placental separation. Failure to deliver the placenta despite these measures indicates transfer of the patient to the operating theatre and the administration of a general anaesthetic.

The patient is placed in the lithotomy position. One hand is placed on the abdomen to encourage the uterus to contract and a last attempt is made with the Brandt–Andrews' method of controlled cord traction. If this fails, the abdominal hand should steady the uterus, pressing it down on to the vaginal hand. The vaginal hand should be insinuated through the cervical os and the retraction ring, if one is present, to the upper segment of the uterus, following the cord to its placental insertion. The lower edge of the placenta is then located and, with a sawing motion, the operator proceeds to detach the placenta from the uterus. When there is total separation of the placenta, it is removed and an intravenous oxytocic — preferably Syntometrine, unless contraindicated — administered to promote uterine contraction. The patient is given a course of antibiotics to prevent infection following intra-uterine manipulation.

There is an ever-present danger of uterine rupture during the procedure. This is usually because the operator fails to push the fundus down on to the vaginal hand. The inexperienced operator may mistake the lower segment for the uterine cavity, and grasp the upper segment mistaking it for the placenta! Further trauma to the lower segment may be the result of trying to force the hand through the retraction ring.

Placenta accreta

The morbid adherence of the placenta to the uterus is termed placenta accreta. The penetration of the placenta up the myometrium is termed placenta increta; when it penetrates the myometrium to the serosa, the term placenta percreta is used. The diagnosis of the latter two conditions is retrospective and is only found when laparotomy and hysterectomy are performed.

The morbidly adherent placenta is commonly associated with placenta praevia, a previous Caesarean section scar or uterine perforation.

Placenta accreta is diagnosed when difficulty is encountered during delivery of the placenta and manual removal has to be performed. When part of the placenta is morbidly adherent and not removed, there are two possible outcomes: the bleeding may be minimal or the patient may continue bleeding. When bleeding is minimal, the patient should be observed and warned of the possibility of secondary postpartum haemorrhage, which usually occurs 10–14 days after delivery. However, if bleeding continues and the patient is desirous of having more children, conservative treatment with oxytocics or prostaglandins should be tried first; internal iliac ligation or hysterectomy are the last resort. When the subject has completed her family, a hysterectomy may be considered as the method of choice.

Acute uterine inversion

This is an uncommon complication of the third stage of labour. There are three degrees of inversion.

1. The inverted fundus reaches the cervical os.
2. The whole body is inverted up to the cervical os.
3. The uterus, cervix and vagina are completely inverted.

Acute inversion may be spontaneous or the result of mismanagement of the third stage of labour. Spontaneous inversion is often associated with a fundally located adherent placenta. Other associated factors are uterine atony, an arcuate or unicornuate uterus. In patients with uterine atony, the inversion may occur following a cough, sneeze or any other act causing an increase in intra-abdominal pressure. This, unexpectedly, is seen in a number of primiparae (Das 1940).

Mismanagement of the third stage of labour may result in uterine inversion. This occurs when traction on the cord is attempted before uterine contraction and placental separation are established. However, the most common cause is resort to Credé's method of expelling the uterus when the uterus is relaxed. Rarely, it may follow a manual removal of the placenta when the abdominal hand is firmly pressed on the uterus and the vaginal hand is withdrawn too quickly. This results in the creation of a negative pressure and the uterus inverts.

The most dramatic presentation is the complaint of severe lower abdominal pain and the feeling of prolapse followed by collapse and haemorrhage. In milder degrees of prolapse the patient may complain of pain and haemorrhage. When only indentation of the fundus occurs, symptoms are minimal and it usually corrects spontaneously. The shock produced by a uterine inversion is commonly neurogenic in origin as considerable traction is placed on the infundibulopelvic and round ligaments. Haemorrhagic shock may further complicate the situation since uterine atony and partial placental separation may have occurred.

When called to see such a patient, the obstetrician should always exclude a submucous fibroid protruding from the os. The diagnosis is easy enough as the uterine body and fundus are palpable in the abdomen in this situation.

Prevention is the mainstay of management of acute uterine inversion. One should never exert traction on the cord when the uterus is still relaxed, and countertraction should be applied when the uterus finally contracts, when delivery of the placenta should be attempted. Credé's manoeuvre should not be employed.

If the inversion occurs at the time of delivery, with the obstetrician in attendance, it is probably best to replace the uterus immediately, and follow with an intravenous bolus dose of an oxytocic to initiate uterine contraction. The patient should then be sent to the operating theatre for manual removal of the placenta. If the inversion is only detected some time after the event, and the woman is in shock, it is best to resuscitate her with intravenous fluids and blood. Pain is alleviated by packing the vagina to relieve the tension on the infundibulopelvic ligaments. The patient should then be transferred to the operating theatre and a general anaesthetic administered.

Hydrostatic replacement, as described by O'Sullivan (1945), has made correction of an inversion simple. This involves infusing warm saline from a container held about 1 m above the patient via a rubber tube into the vagina. To minimize the leak of saline, an assistant will be required to use his or her hands at the vaginal orifice to block it. The hydrostatic pressure would correct the inversion quite dramatically as the uterus pops back into place. However, a considerable amount of saline may be required to replace the uterus. If the placenta is still attached to the uterus it should be removed manually and then an oxytocic should be administered to ensure uterine contraction. For obvious reasons it is most important to exclude any uterine rupture before employing O'Sullivan's technique.

Vulval haematoma

A vulval haematoma is not a common complication of the postpartum period. It is often said to be due to rupture of varicosities of the vulval region. The more likely cause is incomplete haemostasis during an episiotomy repair, especially when an artery is not ligated separately. It may occur on the lateral vaginal walls after a forceps or normal delivery and the only plausible explanation is a tear in the submucosal vessels without any break in the vaginal epithelium.

The haematoma usually occurs in the subcutaneous tissues of the labia majora but may track downwards to the perineum and the ischiorectal fossa. Occasionally the haematoma forms at a higher level, occluding the vagina, and may even extend up to the broad ligament and retroperitoneal space. The bleeding is usually quite insidious and signs and symptoms may only manifest long after the woman leaves the labour ward.

The woman may complain of severe pain at the perineal region if the haematoma is at the labia majora. More often, she complains of symptoms such as giddiness, and looks pale with all the signs of haemorrhagic shock. When a vaginal haematoma exists, the patient may complain of a feeling of defecation or 'bearing down'. The haematoma may not be obvious since it is vaginal and only an internal examination provides the answer. The haemoglobin level is often very low.

The patient must be resuscitated with fluids and adequate blood transfusion before surgery is attempted. Some of these haematomas may contain 1 litre of blood or more. When the patient is brought to the operating theatre, evacuation of the haematoma should be performed under regional or general anaesthetic. Haemostasis has to be secured with dexon or catgut sutures but the causal vessel is usually not identifiable. The space created by the evacuation of the haematoma must be packed or a corrugated drain must be left in situ. Small haematomas which do not appear to be enlarging need not be evacuated.

SECONDARY POSTPARTUM HAEMORRHAGE

Unlike primary postpartum haemorrhage, there is no quantifying factor in the amount of blood lost in secondary postpartum haemorrhage. It is merely a subjective impression of an increase in the amount of bleeding after the first 24 hours postpartum and may occur any time up to the end of puerperium. Oppenheimer et al (1986) studied the duration of lochia and concluded that mean duration was 33 days, although as many as 13% of their subjects had persistent lochia for as long as 60 days. Lochia rubra was observed to last an average of 4 days but, as a simple working principle, if bleeding continues to decrease steadily, this is deemed satisfactory.

The incidence of secondary postpartum haemorrhage has been estimated as occurring in 0.5–1.5% of all deliveries (Beischer & Mackay 1986). As in primary postpartum haemorrhage, the condition is often due to abnormal involution of the placental site and retained products of conception. Submucous fibroids may predispose the retained portion of placenta to undergo necrosis and, with the deposition of fibrin, it may become a placental polyp. This interferes with the involution of the placental site and results in secondary haemorrhage. Infection is often present. Other causes of late postpartum haemorrhage are infection and dehiscence of a Caesarean section scar, rupture of a vulval haematoma and, very rarely, the development of choriocarcinoma following a normal delivery.

Secondary postpartum haemorrhage usually occurs during the second week postdelivery. The woman may bleed quite excessively and arrive at the casualty department in a state of shock. More commonly, the patient will present herself at the postnatal clinic complaining of a return of bleeding after the development of lochia serosa. It may be a sequel of a placenta accreta that has responded to initial conservative therapy only to develop secondary infection and subinvolution of the placental site. In the former state, the patient has to be resuscitated and, if necessary, transfused with blood. Since retained placenta is almost always infected by this stage, therapy with a broad-spectrum antibiotic should be started. When the patient has been adequately resuscitated, she should be sent to the operating theatre for dilatation and curettage. Curettings should always be sent for histological analysis to exclude choriocarcinoma (Ch. 31).

Dehiscence of Caesarean section scar is usually treated by hysterectomy.

REFERENCES

Ahlfield & Aschoff 1904 Cited in Hellman L M, Pritchard J A (eds) 1971 William's textbook of obstetrics, 14th edn. Appleton Century Croft, New York, p 957

Beischer N A, Mackay E V 1986 Obstetrics and the newborn. W B Saunders, London, pp 510–518

Brant H A 1966 Blood loss at Caesarean section. Journal of Obstetrics and Gynaecology of the British Commonwealth 73: 456

Bruce B L, Richard P H, Van Dorsten J P 1982 Control of postpartum uterine atony by intramyometrial uterine prostaglandin. Obstetrics and Gynaecology 59 (suppl): 47S–50S

Calkins L A, Litzenberg J C, Plass E D 1931 Management of the third stage of labor with special reference to blood loss. American Journal of Obstetrics and Gynecology 21: 175–186

Chew S Y 1980 Uterine rupture in present day obstetrics in Singapore. Singapore Journal of Obstetrics and Gynaecology 11: 15

Chew S Y 1984 Uterine rupture in labour — a 10-year review. Singapore Medical Journal 25: 24

Chew S Y, Choo H T 1982 Spontaneous uterine rupture through perforation scar of previous currettement. Singapore Medical Journal 23: 283

Crawford J S 1985 Principles and practice of obstetric anaesthesia, Asian edn. Blackwell Scientific Publications, Singapore

Daley D 1951 The use of intramuscular ergometrine at the end of the second stage of normal labour. Journal of Obstetrics and Gynaecology of the British Empire 58: 388–391

Das K 1940 Inversion of the uterus. Journal of Obstetrics and Gynaecology of the British Empire 47: 525–548

De Leeuw N K M, Lowenstein L, Tucker E C, Dayal S 1968 Correlation of red cell loss at delivery with changes in red cell mass. American Journal of Obstetrics and Gynecology 100: 1092–1011

Delfs E, Eastman N J 1945 Rupture of the uterus (an analysis of 53 cases). Canadian Medical Association Journal 52: 376

de Villiers P D, du Toit J P 1963 The prevention of postpartum haemorrhage. South African Medical Journal 37: 237–240

Doran J R, O'Brien S A, Randall J H 1955 Repeated postpartum haemorrhage. Obstetrics and Gynecology 5: 186–192

Gibbens D, Boyd N R H, Crocker S, Baumber S, Chard T 1972 The circulating levels of oxytocin following intravenous and intramuscular administration of Syntometrine. Journal of Obstetrics and Gynaecology of the British Commonwealth 79: 644

Hardaway R M 1979 Monitoring of a patient in the state of shock. Surgery, Gynecology and Obstetrics 148: 339

Hayashi R H, Castillo M S, Noah M L 1984 Management of severe postpartum hemorrhage with a prostaglandin $F_{2\alpha}$ analogue. Obstetrics and Gynecology 63: 806–808

Hellegers A E, Eastman N J 1961 The problem of prematurity in gravidas with caesarean section scars. American Journal of Obstetrics and Gynecology 82: 679

Hellman L M, Pritchard J A 1971 William's obstetrics, 14th edn. Appleton Century Crofts, New York, p 937

Kimbell N 1958 Brandt Andrews technique of delivery of placenta. British Medical Journal 1: 203–204

McGrath J, Browne A D H 1962 Use of Syntometrine in Rotunda Hospital District Maternity Service. British Medical Journal 2: 524–525

Menon K M K 1962 Rupture of the uterus — review of 164 cases. Journal of Obstetrics and Gynaecology of the British Commonwealth 69: 18

Moir D D, Amoa A M 1979 Ergometrine or oxytocin, blood loss and side-effects at spontaneous vertex delivery. British Journal of Anaesthesia 51: 113–117

Moir D D, Wallace G 1967 Blood loss at forceps delivery. Journal of Obstetrics and Gynaecology of the British Commonwealth 74: 64

Moodie J E, Moir D D 1976 Ergometrine, oxytocin and extradural analgesia. British Journal of Anaesthesia 48: 571

Newton M 1966 Postpartum hemorrhage. American Journal of Obstetrics and Gynecology 94: 711–717

Oppenheimer L W, Sheriff E A, Goodman J D S, Shah D, James C E 1985 The duration of lochia. British Journal of Obstetrics and Gynaecology 93: 754

O'Sullivan J V 1945 A simple method of correcting puerperal uterine inversion. British Medical Journal 2: 282

Pedowitz P, Felmus L B 1952 Rupture of myomectomy scars. Obstetrical and Gynecological Survey 7: 305–313
Pritchard J A, Baldwin R M, Dickey J C, Wiggins K M 1962 Blood volume changes in pregnancy and the puerperium. American Journal of Obstetrics and Gynecology 84: 1271
Read M D, Anderson J M 1977 Radioisotope dilution technique for measurement of blood loss associated with lower segment caesarean section. British Journal of Obstetrics and Gynaecology 84: 859
Reich A M 1939 A critical analysis of blood loss following delivery. American Journal of Obstetrics and Gynecology 37: 224
Report on Confidential Enquiries into Maternal Deaths in England and Wales 1976–1978. HMSO, London, p 26
Rowe I L 1962 Postpartum haemorrhage in relation to methods of management of labour. Medical Journal of Australia 49(1): 109–116
Skovstedt P, Misfeldt B B, Mognesen J V, Brockner J 1973 Effects of anaesthesia on blood loss at caesarean section. Acta Anaesthesiologica Scandinavica 17: 153
Taylor D J, Philips P, Lind T 1981 Puerperal haematological indices. British Journal of Obstetrics and Gynaecology 88: 601
Toppozado M, El-Bossaty M, El-Rahman H A, Shams El-Din A H 1981 Control of intractable postpartum hemorrhage by 15-methyl prostaglandin. $F_{2\alpha}$. Obstetrics and Gynecology 58: 327–330
Ueland K 1976 Maternal cardiovascular dynamics VII. Intrapartum blood volume changes. American Journal of Obstetrics and Gynecology 126: 671

H. F. Seeley

Massive blood loss in obstetrics

INTRODUCTION AND HISTORY

Blood has always held a special significance for the human race. Sacrifice and the ritual shedding of blood have played an important role in many ceremonies, both sacred and secular. The life-sustaining properties of blood were certainly known to the Romans who used haemorrhage as a relatively painless means of committing suicide.

A brief, but entertaining, history of blood transfusion is given by Marshall & Bird (1983).

The first human blood transfusion may have taken place in 1492. More than 100 years before Harvey first described the circulation, Pope Innocent VII was given blood from three young men, thus ensuring the death of all four involved. Denis of Montpellier seems to have been the first to transfuse blood from an animal to man in 1667, an experiment repeated by Lower in England in the same year. Others followed their example so it was not surprising that 3 years later blood transfusions were forbidden by law in both countries (James 1982). During the 18th century the medical profession became more interested in blood-letting than blood transfusion as a therapeutic manoeuvre, and bleeding became a common treatment even for the severely injured.

During the early 19th century Blundell showed that blood of different species was incompatible. He and Cline reintroduced the practice of human blood transfusion, mainly to treat those who had suffered major haemorrhage during childbirth. Though only small volumes were transfused the procedure seems to have had some success.

Three factors were responsible for major advances in the early 20th century. First, the American surgeon Crile showed that infusions of warm saline could reduce mortality in experimental haemorrhage. Second was the discovery by Landsteiner of the ABO groups in human blood. Third was the development of an anticoagulant that could be infused safely. These advances were refined during the treatment of casualties from the First World War; armed conflict provided, as Hippocrates noted it always does, a chance to improve the treatment of the severely injured.

Once the scientific foundations of the treatment of severe haemorrhage had been established the concept of irreversible shock developed. If resuscitation was inadequate or subject to excessive delay then death ensued despite subsequent restoration of circulating volume. It seemed that prolonged hypotension could lead to a state of hypoxic tissue damage that was irretrievable. With modern techniques for the support of failing lungs, heart and kidneys the distinction between reversible and irreversible shock has become blurred. However, these techniques are expensive, time-consuming and not always successful so that early recognition and competent treatment of massive haemorrhage are essential.

Massive blood loss is usually obvious in obstetric patients. Covert haemorrhage is more insidious as almost the entire blood volume can be sequestered internally with a normal haemoglobin concentration in what little blood remains in the circulation. Though every first-aid manual lists the classic signs and symptoms of haemorrhagic shock, the diagnosis is often missed if bleeding is not obvious and the classic signs are absent or misinterpreted. A loss of 25% of blood volume may prove fatal yet in the early stages of shock the arterial pressure can remain unaltered. This illustrates how the concept of shock has changed. Shock is now defined in terms of a circulation which cannot meet the overall metabolic requirements of the cells; it should not be defined in terms of specific values of pulse or blood pressure.

MASSIVE BLOOD LOSS IN OBSTETRICS

During the period 1979–1981, 14 maternal deaths in England and Wales were directly attributed to haemorrhage (Report 1986). In 12 of these care was considered substandard. In another 12 cases haemorrhage contributed to a fatal outcome. With the inclusion of deaths from ectopic pregnancy, excessive blood loss played a part in 25% of all direct deaths during this period.

The Confidential Enquiries for this triennium (Report 1986) drew attention to three factors which were important in the deaths from haemorrhage:

1. Failure to anticipate the high risk associated with operative delivery for placenta praevia in women with previous Caesarean section.
2. Failure to deal efficiently with massive blood loss. This included underestimation of blood loss and subsequent under-transfusion of blood, and, conversely, excessive infusion of crystalloid solutions leading to pulmonary oedema.
3. Failure to anticipate, detect at an early stage, or deal efficiently with coagulation failure.

The Enquiries also reported that cumulative figures for the period 1970–1981 show that risk of death from haemorrhage increases with age. Women having their second babies are at lower risk than primigravidae, but subsequently risk increases with parity.

Though the Confidential Enquiries reports are a laudable exercise in self-audit, maternal mortality is an insensitive index of medical competence (Reynolds 1986). The victims of massive blood loss may survive more by luck than by good management. Failure to recognize and adequately to treat major blood loss remains an important cause of morbidity and mortality in obstetrics.

Massive blood loss is a phrase used in many accounts of the physiopathology and treatment of haemorrhage. However, like Lewis Carroll's Humpty Dumpty, authors understand massive to mean just what they choose it to mean—neither more nor less. One useful definition is an acute haemorrhage in which at least half the initial blood volume is lost (Horsey 1982). In obstetric practice the threat of massive blood loss should be considered once the patient has lost 1000–1500 ml.

PHYSIOPATHOLOGY OF MASSIVE BLOOD LOSS

Physiological background

Body fluid compartments

In the average adult intravascular or blood volume is about 5 litres. Blood consists of 2 litres of cellular elements suspended in plasma. Extracellular fluid consists of two components, the plasma and the interstitial space: the latter has a fluid volume of about 11 litres. The cellular elements of blood are part of the intracellular space which has a total volume of about 28 litres (Schultze 1982).

Capillary exchange takes place between plasma and the interstitial space (Ross 1982b). The barrier to exchange consists of the endothelial cells, the junctions between them and the basement membrane on which the cells lie. The exact structure of this barrier in any tissue determines the ease with which larger molecules gain access to the interstitial space. In the liver, molecules the size of albumin can cross with ease; in the central nervous system the barrier is so tight that even small molecules may have difficulty in crossing.

Lipid-soluble molecules such as oxygen and carbon dioxide will diffuse rapidly across the whole surface of the capillary wall. Water, water-soluble substances and ions pass more slowly through fenestrations and intercellular clefts. Large molecules will pass only through fenestrations, though on occasions they may be transported actively through endothelial cells. Thus the transfer of respiratory gases between plasma and the interstitial space will be very rapid; that of water, ions and small molecules rather less so, and the transfer of larger molecules such as albumin will be much slower.

Fluid is kept in the intravascular compartment by the oncotic pressure of the plasma proteins; the most important in this respect is albumin. The concentration of albumin in interstitial fluid is much lower than that in plasma, though the extravascular mass of albumin slightly exceeds that in the intravascular compartment (Marshall & Bird 1983). Though formulated some 90 years ago, Starling's hypothesis which explains capillary exchange remains fundamentally unchallenged (Guyton 1986a). At the arterial end of the capillary, hydrostatic pressure exceeds oncotic pressure and the net filtration pressure favours loss of fluid from the capillary to the interstitial space. At the venous end of the capillary the situation is reversed and the fluid moves back into the circulation. Overall, slightly more fluid leaves the circulation than enters, the surplus being returned to the intravascular compartment via the lymphatic system.

Control of arterial blood pressure

The prime function of the circulation is to provide the tissues with oxygen and nutrients and to remove metabolic waste. Thus the tissues constitute the master, with the heart and various control systems of the circulation acting as the servant (Cutfield 1983). Depending on specific activities, different tissues will have differing demands: thus blood flow to skeletal muscle will increase during exercise while that to the gut increases after a meal. All tissues have the ability to regulate blood flow in response to changing demand; this illustrates the master–servant relationship with the circulation. However, the speed with which flow and demand are matched, the process of autoregulation, varies from organ to organ.

For individual tissues blood flow is more important than blood pressure. However, circulatory control relies on maintaining a constant pressure reservoir from which organs can draw blood according to their varying needs. Blood flow is regulated by changing arteriolar tone and by opening and closing precapillary sphincters. These changes result from local build-up of metabolites; the exact metabolites which effect these changes vary from tissue to tissue.

It is a paradox that the physiological monitoring of the circulation is based largely on pressure measurement whilst the function of the system is to deliver flow (George & Winter 1985). Two suggestions have been made to explain this paradox. First, circulatory control must protect the arterial system from the destructive effects of excessive hydrostatic pressure. Second, pressure is much more easily sensed than flow.

Control of the circulation is governed by the equation:

$$\text{mean arterial pressure} = \text{cardiac output} \times \text{systemic vascular resistance.}$$

Arterial pressure is sensed by high-pressure receptors, the baroreceptors of the carotid sinuses and aortic arch. Information on arterial pressure is passed to integrating centres in the brainstem via the glossopharyngeal and vagus nerves (Ross 1982a).

Cardiac output is the product of heart rate and stroke volume. Heart rate is controlled by the opposing actions of the sympathetic and vagus nerves on the sinoatrial node. Stroke volume is controlled by changes in venous tone which determines right atrial filling pressure, and by changes in myocardial contractility; both these changes are mediated by the sympathetic nervous system.

Systemic vascular resistance is controlled by variations in arteriolar vasoconstriction; these, too, are mediated by the sympathetic nervous system. The maintenance of systemic vascular resistance may be regarded as a perpetual contest between local tissue demands which tend to reduce regional resistance, and a parsimonious central control whose tendency to vasoconstrict maintains, in conjunction with changes in cardiac output, the required value of arterial pressure.

Control of blood volume

Under normal conditions blood volume is maintained within narrow limits in spite of wide variation in fluid intake. Intravascular fluid volume is sensed by low-pressure (stretch) receptors in the atria: the response to changes in blood volume is both neural and hormonal (Ross 1982a).

Information from the atrial stretch receptors travels via the vagus nerves and is integrated within the central nervous system. Renal sympathetic tone is modified accordingly, leading to changes in urine output. An additional mechanism, which acts through nervous pathways involving the hypothalamus–pituitary axis, is the adjustment of the secretion rate of antidiuretic hormone.

Aldosterone, a hormone promoting reabsorption of water and sodium by the kidney, is also involved in the control of blood volume. One of the factors controlling the secretion of aldosterone is renin, a hormone released from the kidney in response to sympathetic stimulation and to changes in the composition of glomerular filtrate. Adrenocorticotrophic hormone and similar substances released from the pituitary may also be involved in the control of aldosterone secretion (Sawin 1982).

Other hormones participate in the control of blood volume. Atrial natriuretic peptide is released from the atria in response to stretch; this hormone promotes an increased loss of water and sodium in the urine (Kaye & Camm 1985). Further third factors which promote diuresis may also be involved (de Wardener & MacGregor 1983).

Thus blood volume is controlled by neural and hormonal mechanisms which match circulating volume to urine output. A decrease in blood volume results in a fall in urine output; an increase promotes a diuresis.

Homeostatic response to massive blood loss

The homeostatic response to massive blood loss can be discussed under three headings:

1. Physiological control systems which regulate arterial pressure and blood volume.
2. Emergency systems which come into operation when physiological controls are stretched beyond their normal operating limits.
3. Inappropriate responses which may actually jeopardize the patient's survival.

Response of physiological systems

Following massive blood loss the arterial pressure control system attempts to sustain blood pressure by intense sympathetic activity. Increases in heart rate and myocardial contractility try to maintain cardiac output; venoconstriction aims to maintain right heart filling pressure and reduce the functional volume of the circulation. Arteriolar constriction overrules local autoregulatory mechanisms which match blood flow to demand, so increasing systemic vascular resistance. However, this vasoconstriction is not uniformly distributed; it occurs mainly in the splanchnic area, kidney, skeletal muscle and skin. Flow to the brain and myocardium is preserved.

The effects of intense sympathetic nervous activity are augmented by adrenaline released from the adrenal medulla. Circulating adrenaline constricts metarterioles which, though responsive to catecholamines, are not sympathetically innervated.

As blood volume falls renal sympathetic vasoconstriction and increased levels of circulating antidiuretic hormone and aldosterone cause a marked fall in urine output. Levels of atrial natriuretic peptide and other third factors promoting diuresis are presumed to fall, although this has not yet been established.

Emergency systems

As arterial pressure and blood volume fall precipitously emergency systems come into operation. Peripheral arterial chemoreceptors are stimulated, resulting in an augmented sympathetic response and increased rate and depth of respiration. This stimulation occurs before hypoxaemia and acidaemia develop in arterial blood and results from a reduction in blood flow to the chemoreceptors. On the basis of flow per unit mass of tissue, blood supply to these organs is massive: the reduction in flow which occurs during hypovolaemia is interpreted as a fall in arterial PO_2 and pH.

During hypotension, activation of the renal baroreceptor causes release of increasing amounts of renin into the circulation. Acting through the renin cascade this hormone causes increased production of angiotensin II. Angiotensin has many actions (Miller 1981): it is an extremely powerful vasoconstrictor acting mainly on the arterioles of the skin, kidney and splanchnic area; it promotes retention of water and sodium by the kidney, both by direct action and through release of aldosterone; it facilitates sympathetic neurotransmission and promotes thirst (Guyton 1986b). The story of Sir Philip Sidney, who suffered great thirst after injury and loss of blood, is a reminder that thirst may be the overwhelming symptom of haemorrhage.

After massive blood loss antidiuretic hormone is released in large quantities from the posterior pituitary. In high dose, antidiuretic hormone increases still further the splanchnic vasoconstriction induced by sympathetic stimulation, circulating catecholamines and angiotensin. This property is used in the treatment of bleeding oesophageal varices.

Fluid moves into the circulation from the interstitial space. Intense arteriolar constriction leads to a fall in hydrostatic pressure at the arterial end of the capillary. The normal Starling equilibrium is disturbed and there is a net inward flux of fluid from the interstitial space into the capillary. In severe haemorrhage refill rates of 1000 ml/h can be achieved (Marshall & Bird 1983). Albumin also moves into the circulation from the interstitial space, although at a slower rate.

Severe haemorrhage induces a number of metabolic changes. Increased release of adrenocorticotrophic hormone causes a rise in plasma cortisol; high levels of cortisol may be necessary for the normal homeostatic response to haemorrhage. Catecholamines stimulate glucagon secretion, resulting in hyperglycaemia and increased levels of glycerol and free fatty acids in blood. In the longer term the negative nitrogen balance associated with the stress response develops.

Inappropriate responses

Fear, pain and anxiety markedly increase sympathetic activity. Thus, the response of the severely injured casualty or the obstetric patient with postpartum haemorrhage is more dramatic than that of a volunteer bled during a physiology experiment. Blood pressure and central venous pressure may be above normal in the early stages of haemorrhagic shock in spite of significant loss of circulating volume (Marshall & Bird 1983).

Bradycardia develops in some patients rendered hypotensive as a result of haemorrhage. This response, apparently inappropriate, may be due to increased vagal tone (Sander-Jensen et al 1986).

Inappropriately high blood pressures and central venous pressures, and inappropriately slow pulse rates may obscure the diagnosis, especially if haemorrhage is concealed.

The endogenous opiate, beta-endorphin, may be released with adrenocorticotrophic hormone after massive blood loss. Though endorphin may have the laudable effect of increasing pain threshold after injury, it may exacerbate arterial hypotension and even jeopardize survival (Faden & Holaday 1979).

Summary of homeostatic response to massive blood loss

The homeostatic response attempts to maintain arterial pressure and effective blood volume. Intense sympathetic activity causes venoconstriction, tachycardia and increased myocardial contractility, all of which aim to limit falls in cardiac output. Sympathetic activity also increases systemic vascular resistance; however, the arteriolar constriction is not uniformly distributed and occurs mainly in skin, skeletal muscle, the kidney and the splanchnic area. Splanchnic ischaemia is intense as sympathetic vasoconstriction is augmented by the actions of adrenaline, antidiuretic hormone and angiotensin in the circulation. The fact that blood pressure is maintained rather than overall flow means that arterial pressure is a poor guide to cardiac output (George & Winter 1985). Pulse pressure is a much better indicator since diastolic pressure depends on systemic vascular resistance and systolic pressure depends on stroke volume (George & Tinker 1983).

Blood volume is maintained by venoconstriction, which reduces the volume of the intravascular compartment, and by neural and hormonal actions on the kidney which reduce urine output. Fluid intake is promoted by thirst. Blood is diverted from regions where vasoconstriction is marked and fluid from the interstitial space is drawn into the circulation.

Certain features which may be seen during the homeostatic response appear anomalous; they may cause diagnostic confusion and even jeopardize survival.

Adverse consequences of the homeostatic response

The homeostatic response to massive blood loss involves intense splanchnic vasoconstriction. The profound ischaemia which results is exacerbated by the reduced oxygen-carrying capacity which follows loss of red cell mass.

Cells vary in their ability to withstand hypoxia; the astrocytes of the central nervous system are notoriously susceptible whilst skeletal muscle and liver cells are relatively resistant. Survival after hypoxia does not, however, imply normal cell function during the time of ischaemia. The splanchnic area can withstand a period of greatly reduced blood flow but if this is prolonged then adverse consequences are inevitable.

The pathological changes during haemorrhagic shock have been the subject of intense study. Most of the present understanding has come from animal experiments in which conditions can be carefully controlled. The brief survey which follows encompasses one written before; it is reproduced here by kind permission of the publishers (Seeley 1987). For more detailed accounts the reader should consult reviews by George & Tinker (1983), Runciman & Skowronski (1984) and Ledingham & Ramsay (1986).

The adverse consequences of massive bleeding can be considered under two headings: changes at the cellular and microcirculatory level, and effects on organ function.

Effects on cells and microcirculation

Three main disturbances of cell function can be discerned—alterations in regulation of cell volume, alterations in energy metabolism and the disruption of lysosomes (Ledingham & Ramsay 1986). Cell membrane function is disturbed with an influx of sodium, calcium and water and a loss of potassium and magnesium. The cells swell as do the mitochondria. Calcium flux within the cell is disturbed. As blood flow becomes sluggish, oxygen extraction increases so that venous oxygen content falls; ultimately metabolism becomes anaerobic with the production of large quantities of lactic acid. Lysosomal enzymes, found in particular abundance in the liver, spleen and pancreas, leak into other cell structures. These enzymes, together with peptide fragments and cellular debris, also pass into the circulation and may produce adverse effects in more distant parts of the body.

Proteolytic enzymes act on precursors present in plasma to form kinins. Kinins cause vasodilation and increase capillary permeability, so antagonizing sympathetic vasoconstriction and promoting loss of fluid from the circulation into the interstitial space. Kinins also depress myocardial contractility and initiate disseminated intravascular coagulation (DIC). Histamine released from damaged cells further increases vasodilation and capillary permeability. Serotonin (5-HT) released from platelets may contribute to the pulmonary hypertension which occurs.

The precise role of prostaglandins and leukotrienes in shock is not established. Different prostaglandins may have opposing actions, some promoting and others inhibiting platelet aggregation, some causing vasodilation and others vasoconstriction.

Hypoxic damage to endothelial cells, exposure of collagen fibres, failure of production of prostacyclin, sludging of red cells and aggregation of platelets are other factors which may initiate DIC. The obstetric patient is already at increased risk as pre-eclampsia, abruptio placentae and amniotic fluid embolism may be complicated by DIC.

Although sympathetic discharge causes intense precapillary vasoconstriction in the initial stages, build-up of local metabolites, together with kinins, histamine and other vasoactive products, ultimately overcomes the centrally mediated forces and leads to vasodilation and increased capillary permeability. The postcapillary venules appear more resistant to these local forces than the precapillary vessels so that hydrostatic pressure within the capillary rises and fluid moves into the interstitial space. Increased tissue pressure within the interstitial space compresses the capillaries, reducing still further blood flow in the microcirculation.

Effects on organ function

In the gastrointestinal tract the ischaemia is most marked in the mucosal layer. The integrity of the mucosal barrier is lost and the body is invaded by intestinal bacteria and their toxins. Although in the past there has been great emphasis on the role of absorbed endotoxin, the toxins of Gram-positive bacteria may be just as important (George & Tinker 1983). Mucosal damage is most marked in the stomach where superficial erosions and petechial bleeding may contribute to further blood loss. The large intestine appears to be much more resistant (Runciman & Skowronski 1984) although ischaemic necrosis of the right colon has been reported after haemorrhagic shock (Flynn et al 1983).

The liver suffers a reduction in blood flow from both hepatic artery and portal vein, the latter normally supplying some 60% of the liver's oxygen requirements. The hepatic reticuloendothelial system fails, allowing bacteria absorbed from the gut to gain access to the circulation. Bacterial toxins have adverse effects on cell function and vascular control, and activate the coagulation and complement cascades.

During severe haemorrhage blood flow to the pancreas may be reduced by 85%. Pancreatic lysosomes seem particularly susceptible to hypoxic disruption and at least nine myocardial depressant polypeptides of pancreatic origin have been identified during shock. Myocardial depressant factor is one such polypeptide which also impairs reticuloendothelial function.

A further myocardial depressant, passive transferable lethal factor, is released from the reticuloendothelial system during shock. Fibronectin, a serum opsonin essential for the normal functioning of the reticuloendothelial system, is depleted during haemorrhagic shock (Singer & Goldstone 1985).

During acute hypotension renal blood flow is reduced as a result of sympathetic stimulation. The kidney contributes to the homeostatic response to haemorrhage by reducing urine output. Hypotension may be followed by acute renal failure. It is likely that many factors are involved in the initiation, maintenance and recovery phases of acute renal failure: among the suggested mechanisms are afferent arteriolar vasoconstriction due to angiotensin, catecholamines and prostaglandins; alteration in the distribution of renal blood flow, and postischaemic tubular dysfunction.

As described above, intense vasoconstriction in certain regions allows cellular debris and active substances, collectively known as mediators, to enter the circulation. These products have deleterious effects on more distant organs.

The lung is involved in haemorrhagic shock. In the early stages hyperventilation occurs, probably due to the actions of catecholamines on the central nervous system, the effect of vasoactive substances on lung receptors and stimulation of the chemoreceptors. Prolonged uncorrected hypovolaemia may lead to adult respiratory distress syndrome (ARDS). A product of the complement cascade, activated complement fraction 5 (C5a), has been shown to cause leukocyte aggregation in the lung. D-antigen, a product of fibrin degradation, may play a similar role.

These leukocyte aggregates release free oxygen radicals and proteases which destroy cellular and structural elements in the lung. These changes themselves stimulate further leukocyte aggregation and activate the complement and clotting cascades. Circulating catecholamines, serotonin, histamine and prostaglandins contribute to the pulmonary hypertension observed during haemorrhagic shock. The ventilation/perfusion (V/Q) abnormalities caused by vasoactive substances lead to arterial hypoxaemia which is exacerbated by the shunting of mixed venous blood of low oxygen content.

Increases in rate and myocardial contractility are part of the normal sympathetic response of the heart to haemorrhage. However, if severe hypovolaemia persists, myocardial function is impaired by lactic acidosis and by circulating myocardial depressants such as kinins, myocardial depressant factor and passive transferable lethal factor. Myocardial oxygenation is jeopardized by tachycardia, rising ventricular end-diastolic pressure and falling arterial diastolic pressure. The subendocardial region is at particular risk.

The brain is essential for co-ordinating the autonomic response to haemorrhage. The cerebral circulation shows remarkable powers of autoregulation, matching flow to requirements within seconds over a wide range of perfusing pressures. It is surprising therefore that restlessness and clouding of consciousness may be seen at values of arterial pressure that are well tolerated in the postoperative recovery room. One explanation is that sympathetic stimulation shifts the autoregulation curve to the right; autoregulation is therefore lost at higher pressures than usual and cerebral ischaemia occurs even during mild hypotension (Lassen & Christensen 1976).

Table 60.1 Classification of haemorrhagic shock in relation to clinical criteria and percentage of total blood volume lost (from Hanson 1978 with permission)

Classification	Blood loss as a percentage of total blood volume	Blood pressure (mmHg)	Symptoms and signs
Compensated preshock	10–15	Normal	Palpitations Dizziness Tachycardia
Mild	15–30	Slight fall	Palpitations Thirst Tachycardia Weakness Sweating
Moderate	30–35	70–80	Restlessness Pallor Oliguria
Severe	35–40	50–70	Pallor Cyanosis Collapse
Profound	40–50	50	Collapse Air hunger Anuria

The physiopathology of massive blood loss: summary

The body's initial response to massive blood loss is remarkably effective. Blood flow to the heart and brain is maintained whilst that to regions more tolerant of ischaemia, such as skeletal muscle and the splanchnic area, is greatly reduced.

However, the response cannot be sustained indefinitely. Prolonged ischaemia in the splanchnic area leads to invasion of the portal system by bacteria and their toxins; these gain access to the systemic circulation because the liver fails to filter them. These invaders, together with products released from hypoxic cells, initiate the coagulation and immune cascades which proceed in an uncontrolled fashion. Mediators are formed which overcome all aspects of the homeostatic response by promoting vasodilation and loss of fluid into the interstitial space, and by depressing myocardial contractility. Many factors conspire to initiate DIC, which further impairs flow in the microcirculation whilst promoting increased bleeding from wounds. Thus a vicious circle is set up which leads to collapse of homeostatic compensation. Even if resuscitation succeeds in saving the victim's life, the running-amok of systems which have a local protective function may cause prolonged damage to kidneys and lungs.

The signs and symptoms of progressive blood loss are shown in Table 60.1.

TREATMENT OF MASSIVE BLOOD LOSS

The physiopathology of massive blood loss has been the subject of intense study. Animal experiments have identified many adverse metabolic consequences of haemorrhagic shock and as a result therapeutic regimes have been suggested which might prevent or at least modify these untoward effects. These include the administration of steroids, adrenergic agonists and antagonists, prostaglandins and prostaglandin inhibitors, clotting factors and anticoagulants, and infusions of various cocktails containing energy-rich compounds involved in cellular metabolism. Though they have shown promise in animal experiments none is yet of proven value in man.

Successful resuscitation must therefore rely on the principles succinctly stated by Ledingham & Ramsay (1986):

> The objective of treatment is to restore adequate oxygen availability for the metabolic requirements of the tissues. The immediate aims are to augment intravascular volume, optimise cardiac output and its distribution, and ensure adequate pulmonary gas exchange. These aims are achieved by minimising further fluid loss and replacing estimated loss with either colloid or crystalloid solutions and transfusion with concentrated red cells to a haematocrit of 30–35%; by the judicious use of pharmacological agents; and by the administration of oxygen together with mechanical ventilation when indicated.

Fluids available for restoring blood volume

In view of the availability of blood for transfusion in the UK it might at first seem surprising that there should be any discussion about the best fluid for the treatment of massive haemorrhage. However, blood has obvious disadvantages for immediate treatment in an emergency:

1. Bloods of donor and recipient must be tested for compatibility before transfusion. Unless blood has been previously cross-matched, delay will be inevitable.
2. Blood has a limited shelf-life (currently 35 days) and must be stored in a suitable refrigerator.
3. Functional changes occur during storage. Banked blood does not have the same properties as freshly drawn blood.

For these reasons other fluids are also used during resuscitation. The properties of all available fluids will now be discussed.

Stored blood and red cell concentrates

The changes which take place during storage of blood have been listed by Marshall & Bird (1983). A certain percentage of red cells die, initially because of the effects of transfer from the donor and subsequently through natural ageing. Levels of 2,3-diphosphoglycerate (2,3-DPG) within the red cells fall, shifting the oxygen–haemoglobin dissociation curve to the left: haemoglobin becomes more avid for oxygen and less ready to release it when required. Platelets and neutrophils lose their function and the labile clotting factors (V, VIII, IX and X) disappear. The pH falls to 6.7, the PCO_2 rises to over 14 kPa and the potassium to 20 mmol/l. The functional elements in stored blood are therefore red cells, whose haemoglobin has an increased affinity for oxygen, and albumin, much of which may already have been removed by the transfusion service. The accompanying fluid will be rich in potassium, citrate, lactic acid and ammonia.

It follows that during massive blood transfusion other elements found in fresh blood may be required. If the transfused blood has been in the form of red cell concentrate, then albumin (usually as 4.5% human albumin solution) or plasma substitutes will be needed. The logical way to assess the need for colloid is to measure plasma oncotic pressure but this technique is not widely available. The Confidential Enquiries (Report 1986) protocol for managing major haemorrhage recommends infusion of colloid if more than 3 units of red cell concentrate have been given.

Massive transfusion demands replacement of labile clotting factors in the form of fresh frozen plasma (FFP) and cryoprecipitate. Recommended doses differ; some suggest 1 unit of FFP as routine after 4 units of blood, while others recommend 1 unit after as many as 10 units of blood (Marshall & Bird 1983). More FFP and cryoprecipitate will be needed if DIC occurs. In all cases of massive transfusion the help of a haematologist is required and labile factors can be given on the basis of clotting studies.

Dilutional thrombocytopenia may be a problem during massive blood replacement but bleeding from this cause is more likely to appear 8–12 hours after transfusion (Marshall & Bird 1983). Platelet transfusion should be given on the advice of a haematologist; such expert help is of particular importance in the management of DIC.

The importance of 2,3-DPG and changes in oxygen affinity during transfusion have been reviewed by MacDonald (1977). There are theoretical reasons for believing that changes in oxygen affinity would be important in obstetric patients under two circumstances: first, if massive transfusion was required before delivery; second, during transfusion in patients with sickle cell anaemia. In such cases the use of fresh blood, or blood preserved in a medium which maintains normal levels of 2,3-DPG, might be considered if circumstances permit. However, the risks of inadequate circulating haemoglobin, whatever its oxygen affinity, far outweigh those associated with shifts in the dissociation curve.

In dire emergency, when it is considered that lack of oxygen-carrying capacity (rather than hypovolaemia) represents an immediate danger to the patient's life, group O Rh-negative blood can be given. If the patient's blood group and antibody screen are known, ABO-compatible uncross-matched blood is preferable. A patient's blood group can now be established within minutes and a satisfactory cross-match can be made in about half an hour (Singer & Goldstone 1985). It must be emphasized that these are times from arrival at the laboratory; rapid and reliable transport between labour ward or operating theatre and the laboratory is essential.

Crystalloids and colloids

These solutions have many attractions for the restoration of circulating volume. The problems of blood-grouping and incompatibility are absent, shelf-life is measured in years, and storage requirements are much less stringent than those for blood.

Crystalloids are isotonic solutions of small ions. When given intravenously equilibration between circulation and interstitial space is rapid. Hartmann's solution is probably the most popular crystalloid: its composition closely resembles that of extracellular fluid except that bicarbonate is given in the form of lactate. After infusion the liver converts the lactate ion to bicarbonate. Fears that any existing lactate acidosis might be aggravated by this solution have proved groundless (Ledingham & Ramsay 1986). Enthusiasm for the use of Hartmann's solution dates from studies of the loss of extracellular fluid during surgery by Shires and his colleagues (1961).

Colloids are solutions of large molecules whose molecular weight is sufficient to exert significant oncotic pressure. In practice this implies a molecular weight of 30 000 or above; the molecular weight of albumin is about 70 000. All colloids will increase circulating volume; those whose oncotic pressure exceeds that of plasma (for example, 25% albumin) will draw additional fluid from the interstitial space into the circulation.

Albumin, usually given in the form of 4.5% human albumin solution (HAS), is regarded as the gold standard colloid. Following infusion of albumin there is a small but significant frequency of severe reactions of about 0.003% (Twigley & Hillman 1985). The main objections to HAS are cost and limited availability. During its preparation HAS is heat-treated to inactivate hepatitis B virus (Marshall & Bird 1983); this process has been shown also to inactivate the human immunodeficiency virus responsible for acquired immune deficiency syndrome (AIDS) (Hilfenhaus et al 1986).

Several plasma substitutes are available which will maintain intravascular volume. They are readily obtainable and all are cheaper than HAS. However, severe reactions are 3 to 10 times more common, depending on the study quoted and the particular colloid. As with all rare side-effects, any quoted frequency should be interpreted with caution.

Three types of colloid are available for use as plasma substitutes: dextran 70, modified gelatins and hetastarch (hydroxyethyl starch). The properties of these colloids have been the subject of reviews (Horsey 1982, Singer & Goldstone 1985, Twigley & Hillman 1985).

Dextran 70 is a cheap and effective colloid for replacement of minor to moderate blood loss. However, adverse effects on haemostasis limit its use to a maximum of about 1 litre per day in the average adult. It is therefore not the colloid of choice after massive haemorrhage.

Modified gelatins are also cheap colloids. In hypovolaemia their half-life in the circulation is between 5 and 7 hours. Two preparations are available, a succinylated gelatin (Gelofusine) and a urea-linked gelatin (Haemaccel). The formulations of these two gelatins differ considerably; the high calcium and potassium content of Haemaccel should be noted. Gelatins do not affect haemostasis, nor do they interfere with cross-matching; however, a urea-linked gelatin has been shown to cause a fall in plasma fibronectin, although the clinical effects of this change have not been established (Brodin et al 1984).

Hetastarch (Hespan) has been available for some time in Europe and the USA but has only recently been introduced into the UK. It can claim to be a true plasma substitute as increases in oncotic pressure persist for several days after infusion (Haupt & Rackow 1982). Fears of a specific interference with blood clotting have not been substantiated (Diehl et al 1982). It is the most expensive plasma substitute, though considerably cheaper than HAS.

Fluids used for resuscitation

Restoring red cell mass

Although Olympic athletes have been known to use red cell infusions to improve their performance, most humans carry 25% more haemoglobin than they actually need (Doenicke et al 1977). Although it is tempting to try to restore haemoglobin levels to normal during resuscitation, a haematocrit of 30–35% represents the best compromise between oxygen-carrying capacity and blood viscosity (Hanson 1978, Ledingham & Ramsay 1986). Despite the recommendation that haematocrit should not be allowed to fall below 25% (Singer & Goldstone 1985), recent experience with patients who refuse blood transfusion, either for religious reasons or through fear of contracting AIDS, suggests that low levels of haemoglobin are better tolerated than was believed 10 or 15 years ago.

If more than half the circulating volume has been lost (about 2500 ml in the average adult) blood with normal haemoglobin–oxygen affinity (relatively fresh blood, or blood with special preservatives) should be given if available. If red cell concentrates are infused additional HAS or plasma substitutes will be needed to maintain oncotic pressure.

Additional fluids: colloid and crystalloid

Whilst there is general agreement on the criterion for maintaining red cell mass there is surprising dissension over the best fluids for restoring plasma volume; the arguments about the colloid/crystalloid controversy have been summarized by Ledingham & Ramsay (1986). Many clinicians use both types of fluid during resuscitation from massive haemorrhage and there is evidence from animal experiments to support this compromise (Smith & Norman 1982). The detailed arguments of the colloid/crystalloid controversy may seem somewhat arcane to the obstetrician faced with the problem of treating massive blood loss, and the following recommendations are based on those of Marshall & Bird (1983); a more detailed protocol is given by Hanson (1978).

Suggested procedure—initial resuscitation

The fluids used during initial resuscitation depend on clinical circumstances. Two groups of patients can be distinguished:

1. If resuscitation has been delayed and there has been a period of prolonged hypovolaemia (more than 30 minutes) fluid will have been lost from both circulation and interstitial space. The first fluid should be crystalloid, either Hartmann's solution or isotonic saline. The circulation should show improvement after infusion of 1–2 litres, after which 2 units of cross-matched blood are given. If blood is still not available 1 litre of colloid, either modified gelatin or hetastarch, can be given pending its arrival. Whole blood is preferable but if only red cell concentrates are available additional colloid is necessary to replace removed albumin: hetastarch is the logical plasma substitute under these circumstances.
2. If sudden severe haemorrhage occurs in hospital there is no excuse for any delay in resuscitation. The main fluid loss will be from the circulation and significant shift of fluid from the interstitial space will not yet have occurred. The first fluid should be blood or colloid. In torrential haemorrhage uncrossmatched blood may be life-saving. After 1–1.5 litres has been infused the situation can be reassessed.

Suggested procedure—subsequent fluids

Once the initial resuscitation has been completed, further blood, colloid, crystalloid and clotting factors will be needed. Subsequent fluid therapy can be based on the following measurements:

1. Central venous pressure.
2. Arterial pressure.
3. Heart rate (from electrocardiogram).
4. Haemoglobin and haematocrit.
5. Urine output.
6. Core–peripheral temperature difference.
7. Serum potassium, acid–base state, clotting studies.

Frequent measurements are needed to assess the reversal of the homeostatic response and the redistribution of fluids into various compartments and damaged tissues.

As normovolaemia (judged by central venous pressure and core–peripheral temperature difference) is approached, the haematocrit should be used to guide further red cell transfusion. Blood loss is often overestimated and patients can end up with raised haemoglobin levels (Marshall & Bird 1983). The advantages of a lowered haematocrit have already been described.

The need for colloid is more difficult to assess unless oncotic pressure can be measured. However, a ratio of infused colloid:crystalloid of 2:1 represents a useful guide.

Clotting factors and platelets should be given on the advice of a haematologist.

Oxygen administration should be routine and artificial ventilation will be needed if adequate pulmonary gas exchange cannot otherwise be maintained.

If hypotension persists despite adequate restoration of circulating volume, myocardial depression is present due to factors such as sepsis or persistence of myocardial depressant factor. Inotropic support may be required. Although rare in obstetric resuscitation, the possibility of cardiac tamponade or tension pneumothorax must always be considered.

Practical aspects

Venous access

Two intravenous lines should be set up using 14- or 16-gauge cannulae. Percutaneous cannulation can be very difficult in the hypovolaemic patient and a peripheral cut-down or insertion of internal jugular or subclavian lines may be required.

Blood-warmer

A warming device is essential whenever blood or other refrigerated fluid is infused rapidly. It is desirable even when fluid at room temperature is given in large quantity.

Infusors

Blood is a viscous fluid and pressure bag infusors are needed to maintain adequate flow. Martin's pumps and hand-pumped giving sets are clumsy and cause haemolysis; they should be considered obsolete.

Microfiltration

The need for microfiltration of stored blood during massive transfusion is being questioned (Derrington 1985). It was hoped that removal of microaggregates from stored blood would reduce the incidence of ARDS: evidence for the success of microfiltration in this respect is sparse. These filters may help to prevent post-transfusion reactions by trapping granulocytes; however, they may activate complement and promote formation of new microaggregates. Microfilters should not be used when transfusing fresh blood or platelets; they must be discarded whenever they impede flow during transfusion.

Central venous pressure and arterial line

Central venous pressure measurement is mandatory for correct management. Intra-arterial pressure monitoring is very helpful in the management of hypotensive patients; the arterial cannula also allows easy and frequent measurement of blood gases and acid–base state.

Metabolic effects

Stored blood is acid and rich in potassium and citrate. However, the classical problem of potassium intoxication is rare now that warming is routine during massive transfusion (Marshall & Bird 1983). Calcium and potassium are physiological antagonists. If there is electrocardiographic evidence of hyperkalaemia, calcium is given intravenously; otherwise it is rarely required. Citrate intoxication is unlikely unless the patient is hypothermic or has hepatic or renal disease (Doenicke et al 1977). Although a metabolic acidosis may be seen immediately after massive transfusion, the metabolism of citrate to bicarbonate results later in an alkalosis; there is therefore no case for the routine administration of bicarbonate (Horsey 1982).

Protocol for dealing with massive blood loss

The successful management of massive obstetric haemorrhage demands speed, skill and experience. The Confidential Enquiries for 1979–1981 (Report 1986) recommend that every obstetric unit should have its own agreed procedure which is well known to medical and nursing staff. Although the exact details of the procedure will vary with local circumstances, the following principles should be kept in mind during its formulation:

1. The procedure should be agreed in consultation with obstetricians, anaesthetists, haematologists, nursing staff and porters.
2. The importance of recognizing the mother at high risk cannot be overemphasized. All women attending the antenatal clinic should have their blood grouped and screened for antibodies. High-risk mothers should have blood cross-matched before delivery.
3. Once massive haemorrhage has occurred a general alert should be broadcast at the earliest opportunity. Experienced staff can be assembled and if necessary an operating theatre can be put on stand-by; elective surgery may need to be postponed.
4. The clinical management must be specified in detail, indicating the necessary equipment and the fluids to be infused. The volumes of blood samples for cross-matching and clotting studies and the type of specimen tubes required must be specified exactly. Inadequate volumes of sample delivered to the laboratory in inappropriate tubes can only introduce unacceptable delay.

The Confidential Enquiries for 1979–1981 (Report 1986) give guidelines for the management of massive haemorrhage which can form the basis of an individual contingency plan.

Acknowledgements

The author wishes to thank two colleagues at St George's Hospital for their help and advice—Dr J Parker-Williams, consultant haematologist, and Dr I Findley, consultant anaesthetist in charge of obstetric anaesthesia and analgesia.

REFERENCES

Brodin B, Hesselvik F, von Schenk H 1984 Decrease of plasma fibronectin concentration following infusion of a gelatin-based plasma substitute in man. Scandinavian Journal of Clinical and Laboratory Investigation 44: 529–533

Cutfield G R 1983 The systemic and pulmonary circulations. In: Tinker J, Rapin M (eds) Care of the critically ill patient. Springer-Verlag, Berlin, pp 19–36

Derrington M C 1985 The present status of blood filtration. Anaesthesia 40: 334–347

de Wardener H E, MacGregor G A 1983 The relation of a circulating sodium transport inhibitor (the natriuretic hormone?) to hypertension. Medicine 62: 310–326

Diehl J T, Lester III J L, Cosgrove D M 1982 Clinical comparison of hetastarch and albumin in postoperative cardiac patients. Annals of Thoracic Surgery 34: 674–679

Doenicke A, Grote B, Lorenz W 1977 Blood and blood substitutes. British Journal of Anaesthesia 49: 681–688

Faden A I, Holaday J W 1979 Opiate antagonists: a role in the treatment of hypovolaemic shock. Science 205: 317–318

Flynn T C, Rowlands B J, Gilliland M, Ward R E, Fischer R P 1983 Hypotension-induced post-traumatic necrosis of the right colon. American Journal of Surgery 146: 715–718

George R J D, Tinker J 1983 The pathophysiology of shock. In: Tinker J, Rapin M (eds) Care of the critically ill patient. Springer-Verlag, Berlin, pp 163–187

George R J D, Winter R J D 1985 The clinical value of measuring cardiac output. British Journal of Hospital Medicine 34: 89–95

Guyton A C 1986a Capillary dynamics and exchange of fluid between the blood and intestinal fluid. In: Textbook of medical physiology, 7th edn. W B Saunders, Philadelphia, pp 348–360

Guyton A C 1986b Regulation of blood volume, extracellular fluid volume, and extracellular fluid composition by the kidneys and by the thirst mechanism. In: Textbook of medical physiology, 7th edn. WB Saunders, Philadelphia, pp 425–437

Hanson G C 1978 The management of the patient suffering from severe trauma. In: Hanson G C, Wright P L (eds) Medical management of the critically ill. Academic Press, London, pp 333–354

Haupt M T, Rackow E C 1982 Colloid osmotic pressure and fluid resuscitation with hetastarch, albumin, and saline solutions. Critical Care Medicine 10: 159–162

Hilfenhaus J, Herrman A, Mauler R, Prince A M 1986 Inactivation of the AIDS-causing retrovirus and other human viruses in antihemophilic plasma protein preparations by pasteurization. Vox Sanguinis 50: 208–211

Horsey P J 1982 Blood transfusion. In: Atkinson R S, Langton-Hewer C (eds) Recent advances in anaesthesia and analgesia, vol 14. Churchill Livingstone, Edinburgh, pp 89–103

James D C O 1982 Blood transfusion and notes on related aspects of blood clotting. In: Scurr C, Feldman S A (eds) Scientific foundations of anaesthesia, 3rd edn. Heinemann Medical, London, pp 375–389

Kaye G, Camm A J 1985 The role of the atria in fluid volume control. British Journal of Hospital Medicine 34: 82–88

Lassen N A, Christensen M S 1976 Physiology of cerebral blood flow. British Journal of Anaesthesia 48: 719–734

Ledingham I McA, Ramsay G 1986 Hypovolaemic shock. British Journal of Anaesthesia 58: 169–189

MacDonald R 1977 Red cell 2,3-diphosphoglycerate and oxygen affinity. Anaesthesia 32: 544–553

Marshall M, Bird T 1983 Blood loss and replacement. Edward Arnold, London

Miller E D 1981 The role of the renin–angiotensin–aldosterone system in circulatory control and in hypertension. British Journal of Anaesthesia 53: 711–718

Report 1986 Report on confidential enquiries into maternal deaths in England and Wales 1979–1981. Report on health and social subjects 29. Department of Health and Social Security. HMSO, London

Reynolds F 1986 Obstetric anaesthetic services. British Medical Journal 293: 403–404
Ross G 1982a The arteries and arterial pressure. In: Ross G (ed) Essentials of human physiology, 2nd edn. Year Book Medical Publishers, Chicago, pp 203–218
Ross G 1982b The microcirculation and the veins. In: Ross G (ed) Essentials of human physiology, 2nd edn. Year Book Medical Publishers, Chicago, pp 219–229
Runciman W B, Skowronski G A 1984 Pathophysiology of haemorrhagic shock. Anaesthesia and Intensive Care 12: 193–205
Sander-Jensen K, Secher N H, Bie P, Warberg J, Schwartz T W 1986 Vagal slowing of the heart during haemorrhage: observations from 20 consecutive patients. British Medical Journal 292: 364–366
Sawin C T 1982 The adrenal gland. In: Ross G (ed) Essentials of human physiology, 2nd edn. Year Book Medical Publishers, Chicago, pp 626–637
Schultze R G 1982 Renal function and body fluids. In: Ross G (ed) Essentials of human physiology, 2nd edn. Year Book Medical Publishers, Chicago, pp 361–381
Seeley H F 1987 Pathophysiology of haemorrhagic shock. British Journal of Hospital Medicine 37: 14–20
Shires T, Williams J, Brown F 1961 Acute change in extracellular fluids associated with major surgical procedures. Annals of Surgery 154: 803–810
Singer C R J, Goldstone A H 1985 Recent advances in blood transfusion and blood products. In: Kaufman L (ed) Anaesthesia review, vol 3. Churchill Livingstone, Edinburgh, pp 156–182
Smith J A R, Norman J N 1982 The fluid of choice for resuscitation of severe shock. British Journal of Surgery 69: 702–705
Twigley A J, Hillman K M 1985 The end of the crystalloid era? Anaesthesia 40: 860–871

SECTION 8

Normal Puerperium

61

John Dennis

The physiology and management of the puerperium

INTRODUCTION

It takes 38 weeks for the maternal organism to respond to the structural and functional demands of pregnancy. In the newly delivered woman, all the pregnancy adaptations, except those related to lactation, suddenly become redundant. The period during which these changes return to the non-pregnant state is the puerperium. It has been traditionally taken to last 6 weeks and, in fact, most of the changes are completed within this period. These restorative processes, many of which are of considerable magnitude, take place at varying, though quite rapid, speeds, making the puerperium a period of physiological tumult.

STRUCTURAL CHANGES

Involution of the uterus

Immediately after the delivery of the placenta the uterus weighs approximately 900 g. The fundus, if the bladder is empty, is palpable 11–12 cm above the upper margin of the pubic symphysis. In an opened uterus, the rough area of the placental site, uncovered by epithelium, is clearly distinguishable. The cavity of the uterus is in direct continuity with the vagina and the cervix hangs as a circular curtain from the body of the uterus into the vagina. The vessels formerly supplying and draining the placenta are compressed by continuing uterine retraction and also contribute to haemostasis by contraction of the vessel wall. The uterine contractions of labour continue and, for some reason not as yet understood, are usually felt as afterpains mostly in women who have previously borne children.

Two systematic studies of human uterine involution (Montford & Pérez-Tamayo 1961, Sharman 1966) have both shown the rapid decrease in tissue mass, with total weight reduced by about 50% within 7 days of parturition. Total uterine weight, water, muscular protein, collagen and hexosamine were all shown to decrease in the same proportions. The exact mechanisms involved in uterine involution are the subject of debate but are probably caused by the rapid withdrawal of placental hormones. Electron microscope studies in postpartum guinea-pigs (Dessouky 1971) suggest that smooth muscle cells, macrophages and the endothelial cells of myometrial vessels may all participate in involution. There is autodigestion of cytoplasmic organelles, thus reducing the contents of the cytoplasm, and degradation of extracellular collagen and ground substance. These processes seem to be carried out by an increase in the number of lysosomes and in the activity of their hydrolytic enzymes.

By the end of 6 weeks the uterus has shrunk almost to its prepregnancy size and now weighs less than 100 g. Its content of fibrous tissue is greater than that of the prepregnant uterus and increases progressively with recurring pregnancies.

Sharman (1966) performed a meticulous study of the changes in the human endometrium and in the former placental site. Apart from studying 10 uteri obtained at postmortem, he carried out 626 endometrial biopsies from 285 women at varying times from the fifth day to 9 months after parturition.

Within 3 days of parturition, the superficial layer of the decidua becomes necrotic and is shed in the lochia. The deeper layers of the decidua, containing the base of the glands, are retained. Proliferation of epithelial cells from the glandular remnants and growth of the adjacent stroma are rapid, resulting in the reformation of an intact endometrial surface within 7–10 days of parturition, except over the former placental site. The restoration of an endometrial covering over the latter takes approximately 3 weeks. It is derived by ingrowth from the edge of the site and also from luteal islands of glandular remnants.

The full repair of the former placental site takes up to 6 weeks. The contracted blood vessels become thrombosed and later organized by fibrous tissue; in some, recanalization eventually occurs.

Serial endometrial biopsies, taken primarily to determine the onset of secretory changes, showed that the earliest these appeared was the 44th day postpartum. From this, it was deduced that ovulation can occur as early as the 40th day but is unlikely to occur any earlier in a non-lactating woman who has borne a living viable infant. In lactating women, secretory changes may not occur until 4 months or later. Small degenerate decidual remnants and focal stromal inflammatory cell infiltration may be present in the endometrium for up to 2 months postpartum. These are not signs of clinically significant infection but part of the physiological process of tissue degeneration and repair. In the myometrium the larger blood vessels are obliterated by hyaline change and replaced by new smaller vessels.

The cervix is usually torn to some extent in normal parturition, hence the difference in the shape of the external os in the parous and nulliparous cervix. The cervix is open and readily admits two fingers for a few days following parturition but in the absence of infection has narrowed by the end of the first week, making it difficult to introduce even one finger.

The lochia

This is the normal discharge from the genital tract in the puerperium. For up to 3 days it is red in colour (lochia rubra) and contains a variable amount of fresh blood as well as decidual debris. It then becomes pink in colour (lochia serosa) containing still some red cells, but predominantly leukocytes and necrotic decidua. By the end of the first week it is yellowish-white in colour (lochia alba), consisting now principally of serous fluid and leukocytes. It has a characteristic sweetish odour and gradually diminishes in amount over the following 3–6 weeks.

Other structural changes

The abdominal wall may remain soft and flabby for some weeks. The striae gravidarum gradually become paler in colour over 6–9 months. Permanent laxity of the abdominal wall, possibly with separation or divarication of the rectus abdominus muscles, tends to occur in a woman who has experienced excessive abdominal stretching during pregnancy, for example, by twins.

Baird (1935) carried out cystoscopic examinations of the bladder following parturition and found oedema and hyperaemia of the mucosa and frequently, submucous extravasation of blood. The puerperal bladder is readily distensible and relatively insensitive to volumes of urine which would ordinarily cause strong detrusor contractions. It is, therefore, vulnerable to overdistension and incomplete emptying. Residual urine — that left in the bladder following micturition — predisposes to cystitis and ascending urinary tract infection, both common complications in the puerperium. The ureters and renal pelves remain dilated and easily distensible and these changes can take as long as 8 weeks to revert to normal. Radiological investigations for structural abnormalties of the kidneys and ureters should therefore be postponed until at least 12 weeks following delivery.

In the first few days of the puerperium the vaginal walls are smooth, soft and oedematous. The distension which has resulted from labour remains for a few days but the return of normal elasticity and hence normal capacity is quick thereafter. Episiotomies and tears of the vagina and perineum usually heal well and quickly, provided adequate suturing has been undertaken. Healing may be impaired if complicated by infection or haematoma formation and the wound may break down and heal by granulation and fibrosis. Even if this happens, healing by second intention is usually satisfactory but occasionally persistent granulations may give rise to subsequent dyspareunia. If the woman is breastfeeding, the vaginal epithelium remains thinner than in the prepregnant state for several weeks or months, reflecting presumably the lower levels of circulating oestrogens.

HORMONAL CHANGES

These are also dealt with in Chapter 62.

Sex steroids

In late pregnancy, maternal serum levels and urinary output represent primarily the production of the fetoplacental unit, though the corpus luteum and the remaining ovarian tissue have been shown to produce progesterone and oestradiol respectively in late pregnancy (Weiss & Rifkin 1975, Acar et al 1981). Daily measurements in the puerperium have shown that mean serum levels of progesterone and oestradiol fall to non-pregnant levels by 72 hours and urinary excretion of oestrone and oestradiol by the fourth day (Carpenter 1967, Klopper et al 1978, West & McNeilly 1979). The urinary excretion of oestriol also falls rapidly after delivery but even by the eighth day, the levels are still measurably above non-pregnant values. This makes it likely that oestriol, since it is almost exclusively of fetoplacental origin, is bound or stored and released relatively slowly.

The return of ovarian activity has been measured in non-breastfeeding women by daily urinary assays (Gray et al 1987). Excluding one case where the authors accepted earlier ovulation but where the luteal phase lasted only 5 days, the earliest ovulation appears to have occurred 27 days postpartum. One-third of first cycles were anovulatory and among ovulatory cycles, 18 of 22 had some deficiency in the luteal phase.

Placental proteins

Because their half-life is longer than steroids, it is not surprising that plasma levels take longer to disappear. For example, human placental lactogen levels fall rapidly in the first 48 hours, then more slowly, remaining measurable in the serum at the end of the first week (Klopper et al 1978, West & McNeilly 1979).

Pituitary hormones

Follicle-stimulating hormone (FSH) and luteinizing hormone (LH) levels remain at their low late-pregnancy levels for the first 10 days of the puerperium (Marrs et al 1981). The capability of the adenohypophysis to release FSH returns faster than for LH, and FSH levels rise to normal non-pregnant levels within 3 weeks of delivery (Rolland et al 1975). If high doses of bromocriptine are administered for 4–7 days to suppress prolactin secretion and lactation, both FSH levels and the FSH response to a bolus injection of gonadotrophic hormone-releasing hormone (GnHRH) are readily measurable during the second puerperal week (Nader et al 1975, Fuchs 1983).

Of the neurohypophyseal hormones, oxytocin is considered in connection with lactation. Vasopressin, unlike oxytocin, is not secreted in rapid pulses. Basal levels of 1–5 pg/ml have been described in the non-pregnant female, at the end of labour and in the puerperium (Gupta et al 1967, Dawood 1983). The levels increase only in response to changes in circulating blood volume and plasma renin activity.

Thyroid function

Following delivery, concentrations of thyroid-binding globulin (TBG) fall slowly back to normal over 6 weeks (Man et al 1969). For this reason, the elevated total thyroid hormone level (T4) of late pregnancy also declines to normal over the same period. Total triiodothyronine (T3), being much less bound to TBG, shows an appreciable decline by the end of the first postpartum week, though not to non-pregnant levels (Rastogi et al 1974). At this time the radioactive iodine uptake is still elevated, but not at 6 weeks after delivery. By 6 weeks the renal clearance of iodine and the absolute iodine uptake have returned to normal but the thyroid clearance rate does not reach control values until the 12th week postpartum (Halnan 1958, Aboul-Khair et al 1964).

The suprarenal cortex

Immediately after parturition there is a short-lived rise in the urinary excretion of 17-ketosteroids (Appleby & Norymberski 1957) which may be due to the stress of labour. Plasma cortisol levels, raised during pregnancy and even higher during labour, fall to normal within a week of parturition (Bayliss et al 1955, Thornton et al 1976). The raised plasma levels of testosterone and androstenedione decline to normal within a few days of delivery (Mizuno et al 1968).

In late pregnancy the plasma levels of renin, angiotensin II and aldosterone are elevated and this is a reflection of both increased secretion and excretion. Frequent sampling following delivery shows a significant fall in plasma renin activity and concentration and in angiotensin II levels at 2 hours, but 2 hours later the levels increase to those characteristic of late pregnancy and subsequently fall very slowly to reach non-pregnant levels by 6 weeks (Pipkin et al 1978).

Insulin and glucose tolerance

In the early puerperium, there is a puzzling discrepancy between the response of plasma insulin and of plasma glucose to an oral glucose load. In healthy women in late pregnancy, an oral glucose challenge evokes an enhanced insulin response but in spite of this plasma glucose levels 1 and 2 hours later are higher than in the non-pregnant state. Two days postpartum, the fasting plasma insulin and insulin response curve have returned to non-pregnant values. In contrast, at this time the glucose response curve is no different from that in late pregnancy. Both insulin and glucose responses have returned to non-pregnant values by 8–10 weeks postpartum (Lind & Harris 1976).

BODY WEIGHT CHANGES AND WATER ELIMINATION

The average primigravida, eating to appetite, gains about 12.5 kg in weight during pregnancy. A number of measurements made during early labour and just after delivery have shown a weight loss due to labour (water loss) and parturition (products of conception) of on average 6 kg. This leaves a surplus of approximately 6.5 kg at the start of the puerperium.

When puerperal women are weighed daily under standard conditions, body weight usually remains steady or even rises for 3–4 days. It then begins to fall (Dennis & Bytheway 1965). In cases where oedema is present in late pregnancy (about 40% of the total; Dennis & Bytheway 1965) progressive weight loss from delivery is more common, though in these women daily weight loss is less in the first 3 than in the subsequent 7 days of the puerperium (Fig. 61.1). The early puerperal weight gain is more marked in multiparous women.

Body weight tends to stabilize about 10 weeks after delivery (Fig. 61.2, 61.3). At this time there is still a positive balance of about 2.25 kg compared with the assumed prepregnancy weight. This positive balance is on average 0.7 kg less in women whose lactation is continuing than in those who have not lactated.

It has long been assumed that a diuresis commences imme-

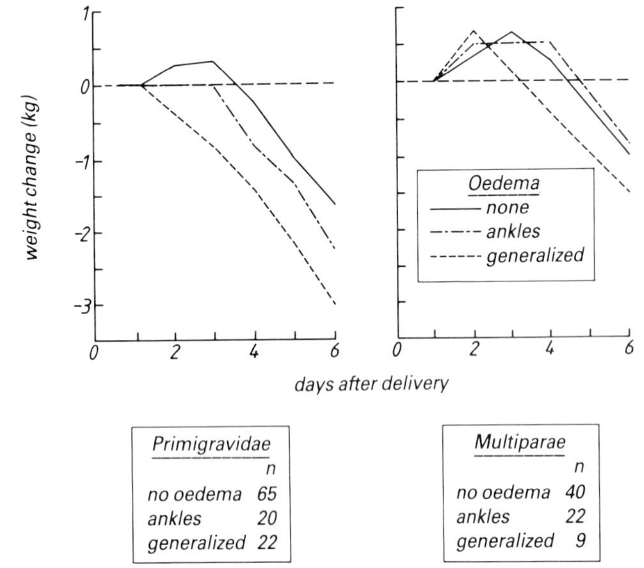

Fig. 61.1 Body weight changes in the first 6 days of the puerperium related to the presence and type of clinical oedema in late pregnancy.

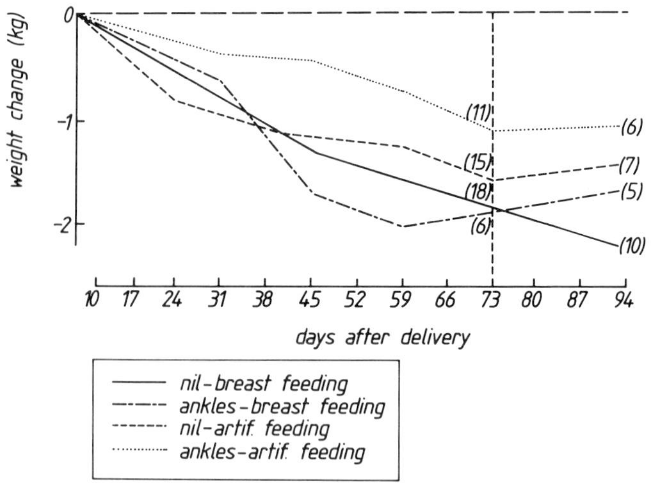

Fig. 61.3 Body weight changes between the 10th and the 94th day after delivery in a group of 50 normal primiparae related to the presence of clinical oedema in late pregnancy and to whether the subjects were breastfeeding throughout the period (number of subjects in each group in brackets).

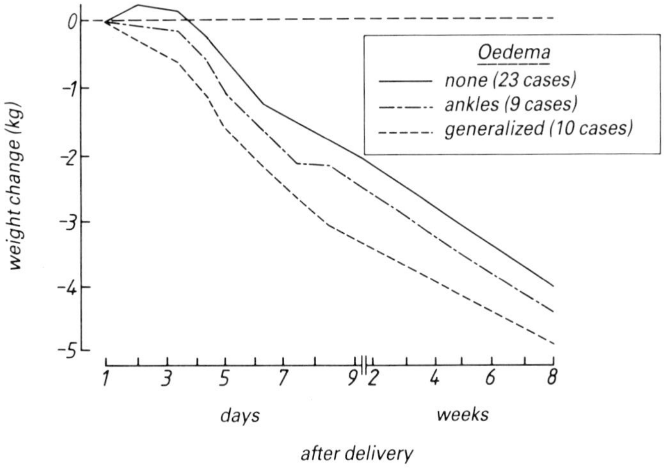

Fig. 61.2 Body weight changes from delivery until 8 weeks later in a group of 42 normal primiparae by the presence and type of clinical oedema in late pregnancy.

diately after parturition and continues for 1–2 weeks until all the additional water stored during pregnancy has been eliminated. This pattern of water shedding does indeed occur in women with clinically demonstrable oedema in late pregnancy. In the 60% who are not oedematous, however, diuresis is usually delayed until the third or fourth day of the puerperium. This means that the steady or rising body weight of the early puerperium is associated with continuing or increasing water retention at this time. The exact mechanism is not known, but it is probable that the rapid elimination of progesterone after the delivery of the placenta leaves temporarily unbalanced the activity of the aldosterone–renin–angiotensin axis which reduces more slowly than progesterone. This leads to temporary retention of sodium and water.

HAEMATOLOGICAL CHANGES

Daily estimation of the haemoglobin concentration in peripheral venous blood shows on average an initial rise on the first day of the puerperium compared with a late pregnancy measurement in the same woman. This is followed by a sharp fall to a minimum level on the fourth and fifth days. Thereafter, the haemoglobin level rises again and by the ninth day has reached about the same value as on the first day. Eight weeks postpartum there was no further change. Serial daily haematocrit measurements show parallel changes. In consequence, the mean corpuscular haemoglobin concentration remains relatively constant (Fig. 61.4). These changes occurred in women whose third-stage blood loss was within normal limits and who were given no haematinic therapy. The results suggest that the substantial fall in haemoglobin concentration and peripheral venous haematocrit in the early puerperium is due to temporary haemodilution, occurring at a time when water is being retained and when body weight is either steady or rising. In the absence of postpartum haemorrhage haemoglobin levels should therefore be measured on the first day of the puerperium rather than on the third day, if a misleading diagnosis of anaemia is to be avoided (Dennis 1976).

Serial measurements of plasma volume, using the Evans Blue dilution technique, corroborate these findings. During the first 3 days of the puerperium the plasma volume in non-oedematous women either remains static or rises

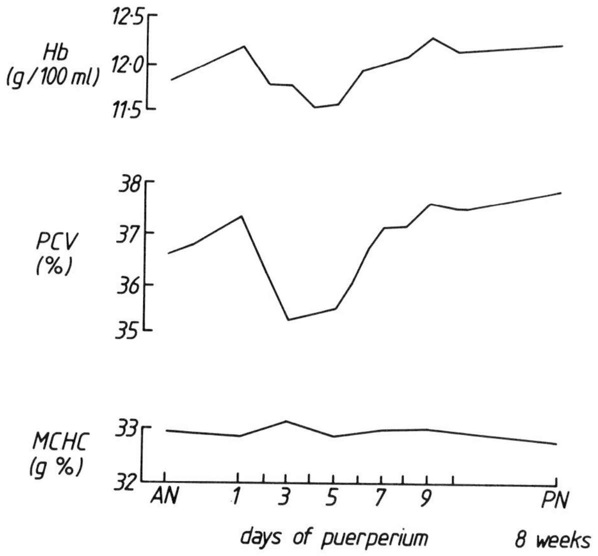

Fig. 61.4 Mean levels of haemoglobin, haematocrit and mean corpuscular haemoglobin concentration in peripheral venous blood in late pregnancy and in the puerperium in 42 normal primiparae. None of the subjects showed clinical oedema in late pregnancy.

slightly, whereas the total red cell volume falls slightly, possibly from fresh blood loss in the lochia rubra. After the third day, plasma volume falls, reaching non-pregnant values by the ninth day. Total red cell mass remains stationary.

During pregnancy there is a steadily increasing leukocytosis; the mean leukocyte count rises from 7210/μl to approximately 10 350/μl in the third trimester (Efrati et al 1964). During and immediately after labour there is a sharp further increase to between 10 000 and 40 000/μl, made up predominantly of granulocytes. The count returns to non-pregnant levels by the sixth day postpartum (Gibson 1937, Quigley et al 1960, Polishuk et al 1970).

The erythrocyte sedimentation rate (ESR) is very dependent on whole blood viscosity and upon the concentration of large molecular weight plasma proteins, of which the most important is fibrinogen. In pregnancy the plasma fibrinogen level rises substantially, though to a variable extent. The characteristic but equally variable haemodilution reduces viscosity. Consequently in the third trimester, the ESR in citrated blood ranges from 30 to 98 mm in the first hour (normal non-pregnant value < 11 mm). In the puerperium there is a further sharp rise in fibrinogen concentration and the ESR rises as high as 120 mm in the first hour in normal subjects in the first 14 days. Thereafter the rate falls and by 6 weeks has returned to normal non-pregnant values.

Plasma protein levels (other than fibrinogen and alpha$_1$-globulin) fall for the first 3 days of the puerperium but then rise steadily to return to non-pregnant values by the 10th day. Plasma osmolality, which in late pregnancy is 10 mosmol/kg below the non-pregnant value, rises after delivery and on average reaches the non-pregnant level of 290 mosmol/kg water by the fifth day.

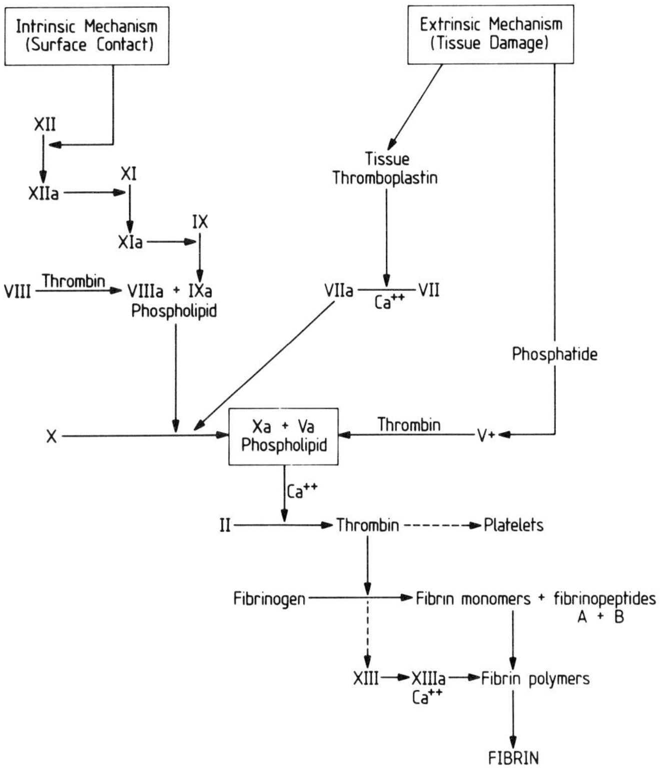

Fig. 61.5 The interaction of factors involved in blood coagulation.

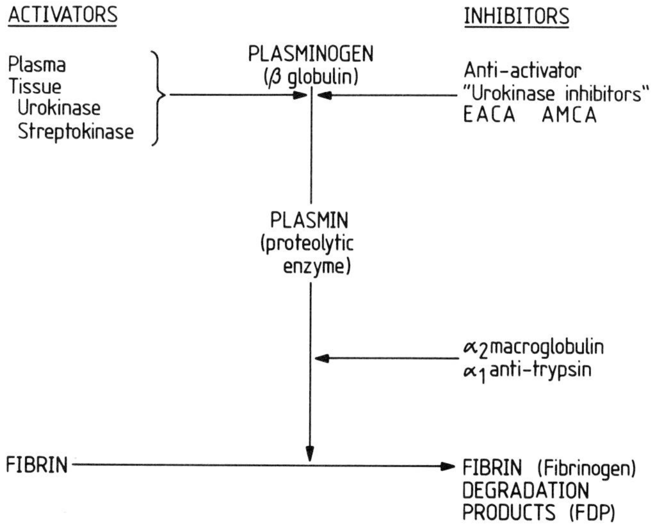

Fig. 61.6 Components of the fibrinolytic enzyme system.

HAEMOSTASIS AND FIBRINOLYSIS

The blood coagulation and fibrinolytic systems are summarized in Figures 61.5 and 61.6. To these factors must be added the initiating role of platelets, especially in injury to small vessels.

Platelet counts decrease slightly but significantly during pregnancy, but whether from haemodilution or increased platelet consumption is not known. The decrease is more marked in women developing pregnancy-induced hypertension and antedates the rise in blood pressure (Bonnar 1975, 1978). Although the average fall in normotensive women is around 20%, most women at the onset of labour have a platelet count greater than 100 000/mm^3. During the first 2 days postpartum the platelet count falls. There is then an outpouring into the circulation of fresh platelets with increased adhesiveness and a rapid rise in platelet count which remains elevated until the 50th day postpartum. The state of puerperal hypercoagulability therefore lasts about 7 weeks. This has obvious implications when planning prophylactic anticoagulant regimes for women at risk from thromboembolic disease. The duration of medication should cover the whole of this period.

HAEMODYNAMIC CHANGES

Following delivery cardiac output is increased, mainly because of the relief of inferior vena caval compression and reduced venous pooling in the uterus. The recent availability of non-invasive ultrasonic measurements and Doppler frequency shifts has allowed serial measurements of cardiac output to be made in the same subject (Robson et al 1987). These have shown that, 48 hours after delivery, resting cardiac output is still elevated to the same levels as at 38 weeks' gestation. Follow-up measurements at 14 days show a mean fall in cardiac output of 16%, suggesting that the return to non-pregnant values takes a considerable time. Since the pulse rate in the early puerperium quickly falls by about 10 beats/minute in the absence of infection and abnormally heavy blood loss, the persistent elevation in cardiac output must be due to a rise in stroke volume. Direct measurements have confirmed this. This slow return to non-pregnant cardiac output contrasts with the change in circulating blood volume which returns to non-pregnant levels by the 10th day of the puerperium.

The study of the resting blood pressure in the puerperium reflects the problems of definition. For example, many women remain normotensive during pregnancy and labour but show a rise in blood pressure in the early puerperium. Is this a manifestation of pathology and therefore outside the physiological range or is it a physiological variant? It is well known that in women developing pregnancy-induced hypertension without significant proteinuria, the blood pressure may remain elevated for 2–3 weeks postpartum and its return to normal non-pregnant levels by the 28th or 42nd day of the puerperium is used in definitions and classifications of various types of pregnancy-induced hypertensive disorders. A recent cross-sectional study (Walters et al 1986) which measured the blood pressure twice daily in normal subjects for 5 days postpartum showed that the morning levels were slightly but significantly higher than those in the afternoon (mean difference of 2.6 mmHg in diastolic pressure). There was also a slight but significant rise to the fourth day postpartum of 6 and 4 mmHg in mean systolic and diastolic pressures respectively, but there was no further rise on the fifth day. Such studies emphasize the complexity of blood pressure changes in the early puerperium and underline the need for vigilance in the care of hypertensive puerperal subjects, at least for the first 5 days of the puerperium.

Bearing in mind the magnitude of the adaptive changes which a woman has to undergo during pregnancy it is not surprising that the even more rapid de-adaptation which occurs in the puerperium may at times lead to physical illness and emotional and mental stress. A knowledge of altered physiology is essential if rational advice and appropriate care are to be provided for the newly delivered woman and her baby.

MANAGEMENT OF THE PUERPERIUM

> Although we cannot remove the patient immediately after delivery into another climate, we can qualify the air, so as to keep it in a moderate and salutary temper, by rendering it warm or cold, moist or dry, according to the circumstances of the occasion. With regard to diet women . . . even till the ninth day after delivery, ought to eat little solid food (Smellie 1752).

Smellie, the father of modern obstetrics, in his treatise merely codified the prevalent midwifery practices of his age. He accepted that the management of the puerperium has for thousands of years been the preserve of midwives in most cultures. It can justifiably be argued that, until well into the 20th century, midwives and obstetricians have done more harm than good in their advice to puerperal women. Their interference has often increased early puerperal blood loss; they have caused virulent cross-infections of the genital tract, which have at times become epidemics of mortality; and they have probably unwittingly encouraged venous thrombosis and pulmonary embolism. Possibly the first prospective randomized controlled trial in the puerperium was proposed sixty years ago by Baird (personal communication), working as an assistant obstetrician in Glasgow. His chief managed the puerperium by insisting that his patients should have their legs tied together for 14 days. Baird questioned the rationale of this regime and proposed that he might try, on alternate cases, not tying the legs and see what happens. Unfortunately, we do not know the results of Baird's proposals.

This section deals with all aspects of the management of the normal puerperium and also includes the observations needed to detect abnormalities at the earliest stage of their development. It is not concerned, however, with any aspect of the care of the breasts and the establishment of lactation (see Chapter 62).

The first few hours

Even in women who have just gone through an uncomplicated labour and delivery, an experienced obstetrician or midwife should remain in constant attendance for at least 1 hour. Occasionally uterine atony occurs and continuous bleeding may be seen from the vulva or may result in the gradual distension of the uterus with blood and clot. If this is diagnosed early, the hypovolaemia corrected and the haemorrhage controlled, all is well, but if such continuous bleeding is missed until the woman is in hypovolaemic shock, she is at risk of losing her life. The experienced attendant should therefore palpate the uterus through the abdominal wall at frequent intervals after the delivery of the placenta, checking the vulva to ensure that no more than slight bleeding is occurring. At the end of the first hour, or sooner if there is untoward bleeding, the pulse rate, blood pressure and temperature are recorded.

If the uterus becomes soft during this time a contraction should be stimulated by massaging it through the abdominal wall. If necessary an oxytocic drug, e.g. ergometrine 0.5 mg or Syntocinon 5 units or both, can be administered parenterally. If this results in the expulsion of more than 200 ml of blood and clot, an intravenous line should be established and a sample of blood taken with a request to the laboratory to cross-match 2 units of blood. In such a situation the patient will have to be observed carefully for several hours until the obstetrician is certain that no further uterine bleeding and relaxation will occur.

Bladder function

The commonest management error occurring in the first 48 hours postpartum is failure to diagnose, and therefore to treat, bladder distension. The rate of renal urinary secretion after delivery is very variable, ranging from the oliguria of the patient with severe pre-eclampsia or eclampsia to the marked diuresis of the normotensive woman who has accumulated massive generalized oedema in late pregnancy. In addition, in many women intravenous fluids are infused during labour. If the infusion contains oxytocin in moderate or high dosage the antidiuretic effect produces additional fluid retention. When after delivery the oxytocin is discontinued, the retained fluid is usually quickly eliminated, contributing to a rapid filling of the bladder. Moreover, both the sensation and the detrusor function of the bladder are reduced by the residual effect of epidural anaesthesia, by the administration of sedative and analgesic drugs, or by the presence of painful lesions in the genital tract such as episiotomy, extensive lacerations and haematoma formation. Pain from abdominal incisions or prolapsing haemorrhoids are other common causes of inability to void urine completely.

It is not surprising, therefore, that urinary distension with overflow of the bladder is a frequent complication of the early puerperium. Once overdistension has been allowed to occur, bladder sensation and detrusor muscle function are further impaired and a vicious circle is established from which the patient may take several weeks to recover. Throughout this time the stagnant pool of urine in the bladder predisposes to bacterial invasion and multiplication and to ascending infection of the urinary tract.

Prevention of overdistension demands close observation of the bladder after delivery to make sure that it does not overfill. The commonest finding on abdominal palpation is the upward displacement of the contracted body of the uterus, which is sometimes pushed to one or other side. Between the uterus and the pubic symphysis, the bladder can be felt as a boggy cystic swelling. Pressure over it may—but often does not—give rise to a desire to void urine. The main differential diagnosis, especially after abdominal delivery, is a haematoma in the broad ligament or below the uterovesical pouch. In cases of doubtful diagnosis, e.g. when palpation is difficult due to the pain of a recent abdominal incision, an ultrasound examination can readily distinguish between the distended bladder and any other cause of suprapubic swelling.

If the woman has not voided within 6 hours of delivery, it is likely that her bladder is in danger of overdistension. Conservative measures that should be tried at this stage include walking to a commode or toilet; the administration by mouth or parenterally of an analgesic to control pain; the immersion of the patient's hands into a basin of cold water, and an injection of carbachol. If these measures fail to restore adequate micturition, the bladder should be catheterized. If overdistension of the bladder has been permitted, repeat catheterization may be required. Any second or subsequent catheterization should include the measurement of the volume of residual urine. Where this exceeds 200 ml, an indwelling catheter should be left in the bladder for 48–72 hours, though this will increase the chance of urinary tract infection. This risk is reduced by inserting a fine plastic suprapubic, rather than urethral, catheter. In due course this can be clamped intermittently to retest the patient's ability to empty her own bladder per urethram and to measure the volume of residual urine. The catheter can be safely removed when the volume of residual urine is less than 60 ml.

Care of the vulva

Shortly after the completion of the third stage of labour and perineal repair, the drapings and soiled linen are removed provided there is no excessive bleeding or other reason to keep the mother in the lithotomy position on the delivery table. The external genitalia and buttocks are washed with a warm detergent antiseptic solution or soapy water in such a way that all the liquid drains from the vulva and perineum down over the anus rather than in the reverse direction. A sterile vulval pad is then applied over the genitalia and replaced by a clean pad as necessary. After each bowel movement and before any local treatment or examination, the external genitalia should be similarly cleansed.

During the early puerperium, mothers should be discouraged from using immersion baths but instead should use bidets and showers. In hospitals, toilet seats and the rims of bidets should be wiped with a swab soaked in methylated spirit or alcohol immediately prior to use (Report of the Royal College of Obstetricians and Gynaecologists 1987).

Other standard observations

Occasionally pregnancy-induced or pregnancy-associated hypertension occurs for the first time in the early puerperium. For this reason, the pulse rate and blood pressure should be checked at least four times during the first 24 hours. If these measurements show normal values, daily recordings for the first 10 days then suffice. The same frequency of measurement is adequate for body temperature in the absence of any cause which makes an elevation more likely, e.g. tender breasts, shivering, dysuria or urinary retention. A rise in body temperature above 37°C may be taken as physiological provided it occurs only in the first 24 hours and if it never exceeds 38°C. Subsequent or more serious pyrexia requires investigation.

The lochia should be observed daily for colour, volume, odour and the presence of clots. The passage of clots after the first 24 hours, the prolongation of red lochia beyond the third day or the development of an offensive odour all require further investigation, especially if associated with pyrexia, tachycardia or abdominal or vulvar tenderness.

The measurement of urinary output has already been discussed in relation to bladder function. It is important to measure total 24-hour output for at least 2 days in all cases where hypertension or ante- or postpartum haemorrhage has been a complication but this accurate measurement of urinary production is not otherwise necessary.

The daily measurement of uterine fundal height above the pubic symphysis was formerly a requirement of adequate midwifery care. It is certainly valueless unless steps are taken to ensure that the bladder is empty. Whether the measurements are recorded or not, the midwife should note her opinion of uterine involution from day to day and the presence of any uterine or vulvar pain or tenderness. The condition of any abdominal or vulvar wounds should also be assessed.

Immunizations

The rhesus-negative woman who is not isoimmunized and whose baby is rhesus-positive with a negative direct Coombs' test is given 500 iu anti-D globulin within 72 hours of delivery (Chapter 35).

Women whose early-pregnancy test showed them to be non-immune to rubella should be offered immunization in the early puerperium. This injection should however be postponed until the postnatal examination in those women who require the anti-D injection.

Diet

As mentioned above, it was formerly customary to restrict the diet of the puerperal woman who had been delivered vaginally. Such restrictions have now been removed. Following delivery, if it is unlikely that there will be any complications which may require the administration of an anaesthetic, the woman should be given something to drink if she is thirsty, or something to eat if she is hungry. A celebratory glass of champagne may, however, cause unwelcome vomiting!

The diet of the lactating mother is normally governed by local custom but should include at least a half-litre of milk per day. There is no evidence that the manipulation of food or fluid intake during the early puerperium has any effect on the quantity or quality of breast milk production or composition although, of course, the nutritional status of the mother prior to and during pregnancy can in extreme deprivation have a very significant effect. In spite of this, it is still common practice to attempt to manipulate solid and fluid intake in the first month after delivery. Such manipulations should be abandoned.

If they have not suffered a recognized postpartum haemorrhage, women who have been delivered vaginally should have their blood haemoglobin concentration or haematocrit checked within the first 36 hours of parturition, i.e. before the early haemodilution of the puerperium causes false low values. To avoid the side-effects of unnecessary iron supplementation only those with low values at this time should be treated. Following Caesarean section oral iron should be prescribed after 3 or 4 days since the blood loss is usually underestimated by the operator. When measured, it is rarely less than 400 ml and more commonly amounts to almost a litre (Pritchard et al 1962, Newton 1966).

Minor discomforts

The pain following Caesarean section, its causes, management and the management of postoperative ileus are discussed in Chapter 58. During the first few days after vaginal delivery, the mother often experiences pain or discomfort from a variety of sources. These include perineal oedema or haematoma associated with tears and episiotomy, afterpains from uterine contractions, breast engorgement, superficial thrombophlebitis, prolapsed haemorrhoids, anal fissure, constipation with gaseous distension, and, occasionally, postspinal headache. Often what is bearable discomfort by day becomes disturbing pain at night and causes sleeplessness. There should therefore be no hesitation in administering simple analgesics such as soluble aspirin 0.6 g or paracetamol 0.5–1.0 g as frequently as every 3 hours, if necessary. Although these drugs appear in breast milk, the quantity is so small that the parents can be safely reassured (Catz & Giacoia 1972, Lien et al 1974, Vorheer 1974, Briggs et al 1983).

For the relief of episiotomy pain, a heat lamp has been a standard remedy but in a hot environment it may produce more discomfort than relief. An ice bag, applied early and intermittently thereafter, tends to reduce swelling and allay discomfort and is equally useful for prolapsed, congested or thrombosed haemorrhoids. Aerosol sprays containing a local anaesthetic and a weak corticosteroid solution are helpful at times. Severe or persistent perineal pain is an indication for a careful examination of the area with a good light, since such pain is often due to a large vulvar, paravaginal or ischiorectal haematoma or abscess.

Constipation is still a common problem in spite of early ambulation. Strong purgative drugs should be avoided but the mother should be encouraged to increase the roughage content of her diet and bran may be sprinkled over her cereals or vegetables. If this is inadequate, bulk-forming drugs should be prescribed such as ispaghula husk (e.g. Fybogel, Isogel, Regulan) or methylcellulose (e.g. Celevac, Colagel). When there is associated abdominal discomfort from gaseous distension, a low-volume modern enema can give much relief.

It was formerly believed that the use of abdominal binders helped involution of the uterus and the restoration of the mother's figure. They are no longer used. If the abdomen is unusually flabby or pendulous, an ordinary girdle is more satisfactory. Exercises to help restore tone to the abdominal wall muscles may be started at any time after vaginal delivery and as soon as the abdominal soreness diminishes after Caesarean section.

Psychosocial aspects of puerperal care

More than 99% of babies are now delivered in hospital. This may be a large unit, staffed by specialist obstetricians, anaesthetists, paediatricians with full supporting services; or a small general practitioner hospital, but in both, midwives will normally be responsible for the puerperal care of the majority of mothers.

> A plan should be agreed antenatally for each mother's care to ensure that she has the support she needs both during her stay in hospital and after her return home, and that the advice she receives is consistent and that she gains confidence in her role as a parent. To ensure the plan is carried out effectively, there should be close liaison between the hospital, general practitioner, midwife and the community support services.
>
> During her postnatal stay in hospital, whether this is for a few hours or a few days, each mother should normally have her baby at her bedside and take responsibility for his or her care as soon as she is fit to do so. The baby should not be moved elsewhere unless it is at the mother's wish or unless there are over-riding medical reasons.
>
> Among the reasons for a mother remaining in hospital after the birth of her baby will be her need to rest and have time to adjust to the physiological and emotional changes and new responsibilities which follow childbirth; the aim of the staff should be to facilitate this and to help prepare her to return home as soon as she and her baby are fit and ready to do so. Until that time, staff should continue to keep mother and baby under observation to check that no unexpected complications or illnesses develop, that the baby progresses well and that his or her feeding is established.
>
> All mothers, especially those having their first baby, should be encouraged to discuss with staff anything that is worrying them and staff should find time to answer any questions. It is during the postnatal period that parental attitudes to their responsibilities for the maintenance of their health and that of their children and their expectations of professional aid may be influenced and established. Thus the relationships which are portrayed by the attitudes and actions of midwives, health visitors and doctors are of crucial importance. Openness should be encouraged to facilitate dialogue, to ensure that criticism and comment are helpful and to help parents gain confidence in caring for their family. (From Munro 1985, with permission of the Controller of Her Majesty's Stationery Office.)

Many problems in the psychosocial field can be prevented or alleviated by education and planning in the antenatal period, reinforced by support and reassurance postpartum. Pregnant women should be forewarned about the mild depression and tearfulness which afflicts 50% of mothers during the first week, and reassured that it is likely to last only a few days at most. They should also be forewarned that, on the rare occasions when it does last for more than 4 days, they should seek medical help. One study has shown that 10–13% of puerperal women suffer from a more prolonged depression (Cox 1986). This often does not start till 3 or 4 weeks postpartum and may last for several weeks. Prominent factors in the genesis of both the early transient and the later and more prolonged depressive episodes include the emotional swing away from the elation immediately following delivery; the discomforts of the early puerperium; fatigue from lack of sleep during labour and postpartum in most hospital settings; the mother's anxiety over her ability to establish breastfeeding in the early days and her capability for caring for her infant in general after leaving hospital; and fears that she has become permanently less attractive to her husband.

The modern nuclear family often means that support from relations and neighbours during the later type of depressive phase is not available. It is the midwife, health visitor or family doctor who must be vigilant and offer support and reassurance. The prescription of mild hypnotic drugs to allow adequate sleep is often necessary and sometimes the use of tricyclic antidepressants for several weeks allows the mother to recover. If taken at night, they also promote sleep.

Sexual interest and libido tend to take several weeks to return and it is important that couples should be given advice antenatally that it is quite normal for a mother, especially if she is breast-feeding, not to recover her previous sex drive for sometimes as long as 9 months (Masters & Johnson 1966, Falicov 1973, Kenny 1973, Wigfield 1981). Failure of couples to realize that it is quite normal for a new mother to be temporarily asexual often causes the husband at first to be bewildered and later disappointed; if the couple for any reason cannot discuss this problem with each other, the sexual aspect of their relationship may sustain permanent damage.

How long a mother and her baby should stay in hospital after delivery should be agreed antenatally as far as possible. The decision should take into account the parents' wishes, the adequacy of the physical home environment and the amount of help likely to be available to the mother from husband or partner, nearby relatives and friends and neighbours. Where the hospital environment is pleasant and not rushed, many mothers elect to stay for more than 2–3 days for their first baby and even for subsequent babies provided the mother is confident that the care of her other children is satisfactory.

POSTNATAL EXAMINATION

A tradition has evolved that at around 6 weeks postpartum a formal postnatal examination is undertaken. The actual physical examination is nowadays less important than the opportunity afforded to review the recent pregnancy and labour and the subsequent progress of the mother and baby. By this time the involution of the genital tract should be complete, all wounds should have healed, medical complications exacerbated by pregnancy (e.g. hypertension, diabetes) should have regressed, and menstruation may have recommenced.

The general physical condition of the mother is noted; weight and blood pressure are recorded; the urine is tested for protein and glucose, and blood is taken for haemoglobin concentration or haematocrit.

The breasts, abdomen and perineum are examined. A pelvic examination is done to check that any scars are painless, that the vagina is roomy, the cervix healthy, and the uterus involuted, non-tender and mobile. A routine cervical smear is taken unless a satisfactory normal cytological report has been issued during the preceding 3 years.

Where there have been any difficulties or complications during pregnancy, labour or the early puerperium, a full explanatory discussion is held with the mother, her questions are answered, and the likely course of the next pregnancy is explored in as much detail as seems appropriate. If there has been a perinatal death, or the birth of a low birthweight or deformed child, counselling techniques should include the reduction of parental guilt feelings as an important objective.

The method of family spacing or limitation should have been discussed antenatally and agreed in the early puerperium. This should now be reviewed and, if necessary, adjusted or revised. If the original decision was that an intrauterine device should be fitted, this is often a good opportunity for its insertion. Where desired, arrangements are made for later sterilization of husband or wife.

If it was not possible to give rubella vaccine in the early puerperium, a non-immune woman should be offered the appropriate injection.

REFERENCES

Aboul-Khair S A, Crooks J, Turnbull A C, Hytten F E 1964 The physiological changes in thyroid function during pregnancy. Clinical Science 27: 195

Acar B, Fleming R, MacNaughton M C, Coutts J R 1981 Ovarian function in women immediately post-partum. Obstetrics and Gynecology 57: 468

Appleby J I, Norymberski J K 1957 The urinary excretion of 17-hydroxy-corticosteroids in human pregnancy. Journal of Endocrinology 15: 310

Baird D 1935 The upper urinary tract in pregnancy and the puerperium. Journal of Obstetrics and Gynaecology of the British Empire 42: 733

Bayliss R I S, Browne J C McC, Round B P, Steinbeck A W 1955 Plasma-17-hydroxycorticosteroids in pregnancy. Lancet i: 62

Bonnar J 1975 The blood coagulation and fibrinolytic systems during pregnancy. Clinics in Obstetrics and Gynaecology 2: 321

Bonnar J 1978 Haemostasis in pregnancy and coagulation disorders. In: Macdonald R (ed) Scientific basis of obstetrics and gynaecology, 2nd edn. Churchill Livingstone, Edinburgh, p 250

Briggs C G, Bodendorfer T W, Freeman R K 1983 Drugs in pregnancy and lactation. A reference guide to neonatal risk. Williams & Wilkins, Baltimore

Carpenter C W 1967 Urinary estrogen excretion in the puerperium. American Journal of Obstetrics and Gynecology 99: 303

Catz C S, Giacoia G P 1972 Drugs in breast milk. Pediatric Clinics of North America 19: 151

Cox J L 1986 Postnatal depression. Churchill Livingstone, Edinburgh

Dawood M Y 1983 Neurohypophyseal hormones. In: Fuchs F, Klopper A (eds) Endocrinology of pregnancy. Harper & Row, Philadelphia, p 204

Dennis K J 1976 The puerperium. In: Walker J, MacGillivray I, MacNaughton M C (eds) Combined textbook of obstetrics and gynaecology, 9th edn. Churchill Livingstone, Edinburgh, p 397

Dennis K J, Bytheway W R 1965 Changes in body weight after delivery. Journal of Obstetrics and Gynaecology of the British Commonwealth 72: 94

Dessouky A D 1971 Myometrial changes in postpartum uterine involution. American Journal of Obstetrics and Gynecology 110: 318

Efrati P, Presentey B, MargaCith M, Rozenszajn L 1964 Leukocytes of normal pregnant women. Obstetrics and Gynecology 23: 429

Falicov C J 1973 Sexual adjustment during first pregnancy and postpartum. American Journal of Obstetrics and Gynecology 117: 991

Fuchs A R 1983 Endocrinology of lactation. In: Fuchs F, Klopper A (eds) Endocrinology of pregnancy. Harper & Row, Philadelphia, p 271

Gibson A 1937 On leucocyte changes during labour and the puerperium. Journal of Obstetrics and Gynaecology of the British Empire 44: 500

Gray R H, Campbell O M, Zacur H A, Labbok M H, Macrae S L 1987 Postpartum return of ovarian activity in non-breastfeeding women monitored by urinary assays. Journal of Clinical Endocrinology and Metabolism 64: 645

Gupta K K, Chaudhury R R, Chirtani P N 1967 Plasma anti-diuretic hormone concentration in normal subjects and in persons with edema of cardiac and renal origin and in normal pregnancy. Indian Journal of Medical Research 55: 643

Halnan K E 1958 The radioiodine uptake of the human thyroid in pregnancy. Clinical Science 17: 281

Kenny J A 1973 Sexuality of pregnant and breast-feeding women. Archives of Sexual Behaviour 2: 215

Klopper A, Buchan P, Wilson G 1978 The plasma half-life of placental hormones. British Journal of Obstetrics and Gynaecology 85: 738

Lien E J, Kuwahara J, Koda R T 1974 Diffusion of drugs into prostatic fluid and milk. Drug Intelligence and Clinical Pharmacology 8: 470

Lind T, Harris V G 1976 Changes in the oral glucose tolerance test in the puerperium. British Journal of Obstetrics and Gynaecology 83: 460

Man E B, Reid W A, Hellegers A E, Jones W S 1969 Thyroid function in human pregnancy. III Serum thyroxine binding prealbumin and thyroxine binding globulin of pregnant women aged 14 through 43 years. American Journal of Obstetrics and Gynecology 103: 338

Marrs R P, Kletzky O A, Mishell D R 1981 Functional capacity of the gonadotrophs during pregnancy and the puerperium. American Journal of Obstetrics and Gynecology 141: 658

Masters W, Johnson V 1966 Human sexual response. Little, Brown, Boston, p 141

Mizuno M, Labotsky J, Lloyd C W, Kobayashi T, Murasawa Y 1968 Plasma androstenedione and testosterone during pregnancy and in the newborn. Journal of Clinical Endocrinology and Metabolism 28: 1133

Montford I, Pérez-Tamayo R 1961 Studies on uterine collagen during pregnancy and the puerperium. Laboratory Investigation 10: 1240

Munro A 1985 Maternity care in action. Part III. Care of the mother and baby, 2.3. HMSO, London

Nader S, Kjeld J M, Blair C M, Tooley M, Gordon H, Fraser T R 1975 A study of the effect of bromocriptine on serum oestradiol, prolactin and follicle stimulating hormone levels in puerperal women. British Journal of Obstetrics and Gynaecology 82: 750

Newton M 1966 Postpartum haemorrhage. American Journal of Obstetrics and Gynecology 94: 711

Pipkin F B, Oats J J, Symonds E M 1978 Sequential changes in the human renin-angiotensin system following delivery. British Journal of Obstetrics and Gynaecology 85: 821

Polishuk W Z, Diamant Y Z, Zuckerman H, Sadovsky E 1970 Leukocyte alkaline phosphatase in pregnancy and the puerperium. American Journal of Obstetrics and Gynecology 107: 604

Pritchard J A, Baldwin R M, Dickey J C, Wiggins K M 1962 Blood volume changes in pregnancy and the puerperium. II Red blood cell loss and changes in apparent blood volume during and following vaginal delivery, caesarean section and caesarean section plus total hysterectomy. American Journal of Obstetrics and Gynecology 84: 1271

Quigley H J, Dawson E A, Hyun B H, Custer R P 1960 The activity of alkaline phosphatase in granular leukocytes during pregnancy and the puerperium — a preliminary report. American Journal of Clinical Pathology 33: 109

Rastogi G K, Sawhney R C, Sinha M K, Thomas Z, Devi P K 1974 Serum and urinary levels of thyroid hormones in normal pregnancy. Obstetrics and Gynecology 44: 176

Report of the Royal College of Obstetricians and Gynaecologists' sub-committee on problems associated with AIDS in relation to obstetrics and gynaecology 1987 Royal College of Obstetricians and Gynaecologists, London

Robson S C, Dunlop W, Hunter S 1987 Haemodynamic changes during the early puerperium. British Medical Journal 294: 1065

Rolland R, Lequin R M, Schellekens L A 1975 The role of prolactin in the restoration of ovarian function during early postpartum period in the human. Clinical Endocrinology (Oxford) 4: 15

Sharman A 1966 Reproductive physiology of the post-partum period. E & S Livingstone, Edinburgh

Smellie W 1752 A treatise on the theory and practice of midwifery. D Wilson, London

Thornton C A, Carrie L E, Sayers L, Anderson A B, Turnbull A C 1976 A comparison of the effect of extradural and parenteral anaesthesia on maternal plasma cortisol concentrations during labour and the puerperium. British Journal of Obstetrics and Gynaecology 83: 631

Vorheer H 1974 Drug excretion in breast milk. Postgraduate Medicine 56: 97

Walters B N J, Thompson M E, Lee A, de Swiet M 1986 Blood pressure in the puerperium. Clinical Science 71: 589

Weiss G, Rifkin I 1975 Progesterone and estrogen secretion by puerperal human ovaries. Obstetrics and Gynecology 46: 557

West C P, McNeilly A S 1979 Hormonal profiles in lactating and non-lactating women immediately after delivery and their relationship to breast engorgement. British Journal of Obstetrics and Gynaecology 86: 501

Wigfield R 1981 The impact of first childbirth on female sexuality. Fourth year medical student project. University of Southampton, Southampton

62

Peter Howie

Physiology of lactation

Lactation is a physiological process which is common to all mammals, strong evidence of its evolutionary importance. Despite its central place in the natural reproductive cycle, many women find breastfeeding a difficult skill to learn and the human species is the only one in which lactation has been widely replaced by artificial feeding. Indeed, this change from breast to bottle-feeding has been described as 'the largest uncontrolled in-vivo experiment in human history' (Minchen 1985). An understanding of the physiology of lactation is necessary to understand the reasons for and the consequences of this widespread change from natural to artificial infant-feeding.

ANATOMY OF THE BREAST

The breast extends from the second to the sixth rib and from the sternum to the mid axillary line with a tail extending into the axilla. It overlies the pectoralis major, serratus anterior and external oblique muscles. The main constituents of the breast are the glandular cells with their associated ducts, a very variable quantity of adipose tissue, connective tissue, blood vessels, nerves and lymphatics. The gland lies in the superficial fascia of the thorax under its overlying skin. The lactiferous ducts lead to the nipple and dilate to form sinuses immediately below the surface of the nipple. The nipple is surrounded by the areola, a pigmented area of varying size which darkens during pregnancy. The areola contains sebaceous glands which hypertrophy and become prominent during pregnancy and are called Montgomery's tubercles. The areola is richly supplied with sensory nerves which are important during suckling (for a fuller description of the functional anatomy see Gould 1983). Throughout pregnancy the areola is said to be relatively insensitive to touch but this increases greatly immediately after delivery (Robinson & Short 1977). This change ensures that the sucking of the infant sends a stream of afferent neural impulses to the hypothalamus to control not only the process of lactation itself but also other important maternal adaptations which are discussed later.

The glandular tissue of the breast is derived from the ectoderm and is arranged in 15–20 ductal–lobular–alveolar systems (Fig. 62.1). The alveolar or secreting cells are grouped in grape-like bunches around the ductules which join to form the main ducts leading to the nipple. The alveolar cells are cuboidal cells in the resting breast which develop full secretory features during lactation. The alveolar cells are surrounded by oxytocin-sensitive contractile myoepithelial cells which play an important part in milk ejection. The ducts are lined by contractile longitudinal cells which, during the milk ejection reflex, open the ducts widely to assist milk flow (McNeilly 1977).

MAMMARY GROWTH AND DEVELOPMENT

In the adult breast, four phases of mammary growth and development can be recognized. These are the resting phase, the development phase during pregnancy, the milk-secreting phase during lactation and the involutionary phase.

The human species is unusual in that a major degree of breast development occurs at puberty prior to pregnancy.

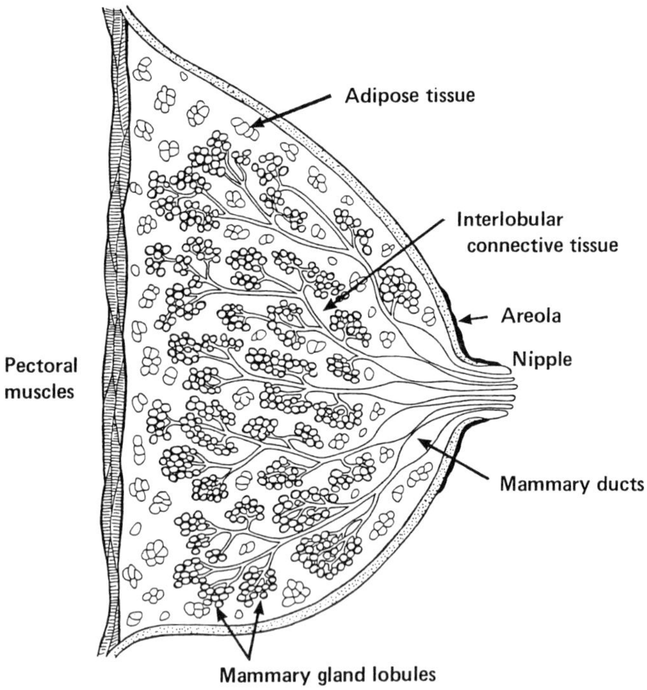

Fig. 62.1 Structure of the breast during lactation. From Gardner & Dodds (1976) with permission.

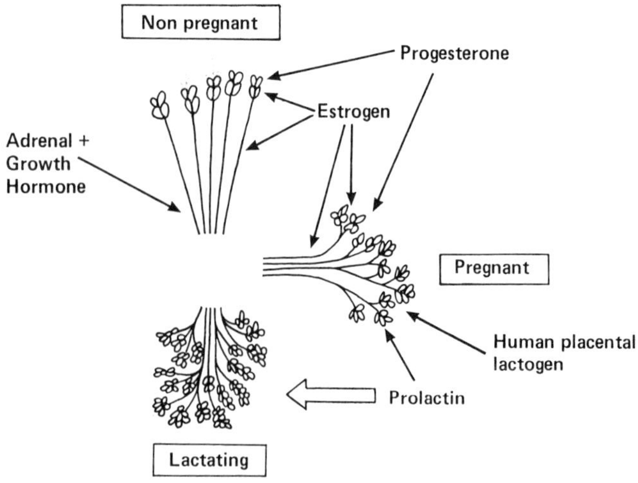

Fig. 62.2 Endocrine requirements for breast development and lactogenesis in the human. Lobulo–alveolar and ductal development appear to be steroid-dependent with an undetermined role of prolactin or placental lactogen during pregnancy. Prolactin is essential for lactogenesis. From McNeilly (1977) with permission.

It seems likely that the reason for this is that the erotic significance of the female breast plays an important part in the attraction of male to female which is essential for human reproduction. At puberty, the milk ducts leading from the nipple branch and sprout and form a modest degree of alveolar development. The control of human breast development is not fully understood and current concepts come mainly from animal experiments in which ovaries, pituitary and adrenal are removed, followed by the replacement of hormones both individually and in combination (Lyons 1958, Cowie & Tindall 1961). These experiments suggest that mammary growth and development are under the control of multiple hormones and the exact role of each has not been precisely determined. At present it seems likely that proliferation of the ducts is primarily dependent upon oestrogen in conjunction with glucocorticoids and growth hormone (Fig. 62.2). On the other hand, alveolar growth is stimulated by progesterone in the oestrogen-primed breast but may also require prolactin and prednisolone (Neville & Neifert 1983).

Once the adult breast has developed it requires only minimal stimulation by the appropriate hormones to begin milk secretion. As little as 14 days' exposure to the conjugated oestrogens followed by stimulation of prolactin secretion leads to the establishment of milk production (Tyson et al 1975). This sensitivity to endocrine stimuli has been used to encourage lactation in women who wish to suckle adopted infants (Auerbach & Avery 1981).

During early pregnancy there is a sharp increase in both ductal and alveolar elements of the mammary gland due to hyperplasia (Gould 1983) while during later pregnancy, there is alveolar cell hypertrophy and the initiation of secretory activity. These changes during pregnancy are probably dependent upon the lactogenic hormones, prolactin and human placental lactogen, with placental oestrogens and progesterone playing an important modulatory role (Gould 1983). During human pregnancy, full milk production is inhibited by the high concentrations of progesterone (and possibly oestrogen) from the placenta and the copious milk production of established lactation does not occur until after parturition (McNeilly 1977).

INITIATION OF LACTATION (LACTOGENESIS)

Following parturition, there is a progressive rise in the volume of milk secreted by the breast and this is maintained in mothers who suckle their infants. During the first 30 hours after parturition, the early milk or colostrum has high concentrations of protein relative to the concentration of lactose (Fig. 62.3). During the next 3 days, the concentrations of lactose increase sharply under the influence of prolactin stimulation and, in order to maintain ionic equilibrium, water is drawn into the breast causing an increase in milk volume (Kulski & Hartmann 1981). At the same time, the concentrations of milk proteins fall due to a dilution effect, although the absolute amounts of the individual proteins remain constant or rise slowly (Hartmann et al 1984). After this phase of transitional milk formation, a relatively stable phase of mature milk production is reached at about day 5, after which there is a slow but steady increase in milk volume to a peak around 3 weeks postpartum.

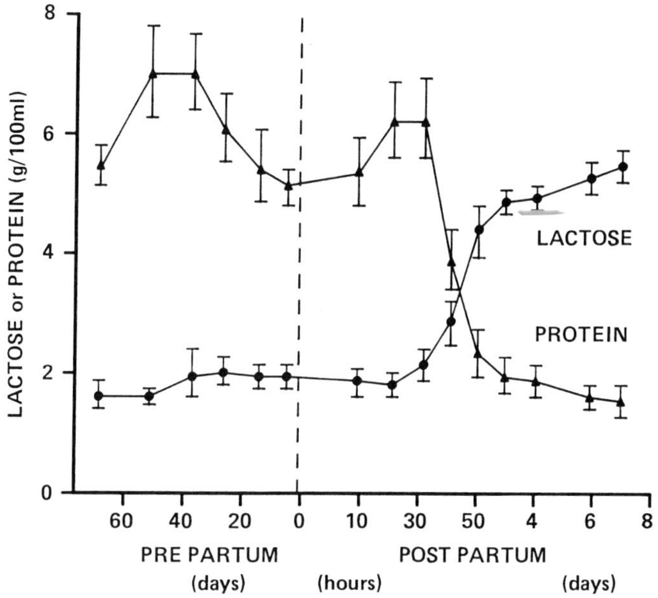

Fig. 62.3 Changes in lactose and protein concentrations in mammary secretions during the postpartum period, showing the sharp rise in lactose and the fall in protein concentration due to dilution. From Hartmann et al (1984) with permission.

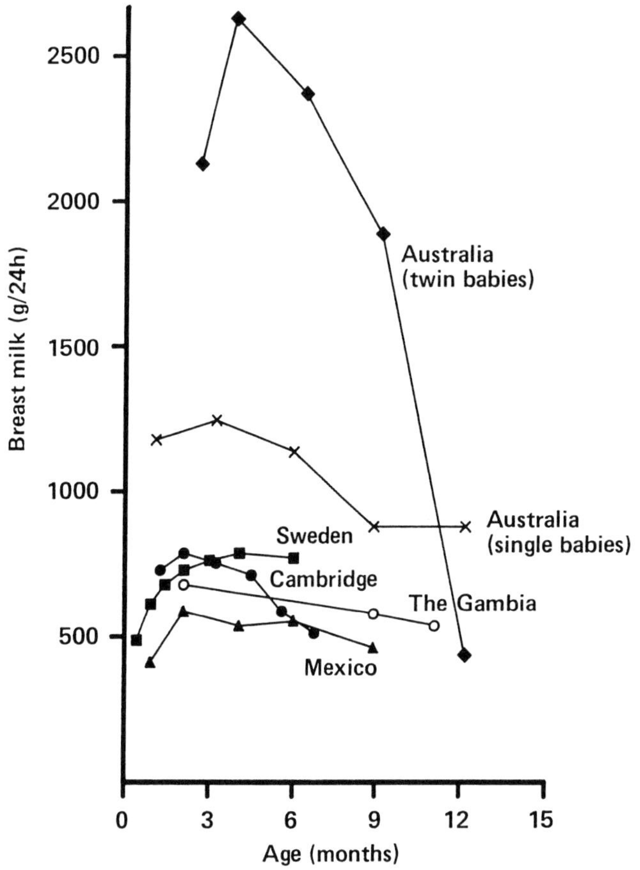

Fig. 62.4 Milk production in women from 0 to 15 months of lactation. Data from Rowland et al 1981 (Sweden, Cambridge, The Gambia and Mexico), from Rattigan et al 1981 (Australia, single babies) and from Saint & Hartmann 1982 (Australia, twins).

MAINTENANCE OF MILK SECRETION (GALACTOPOIESIS)

Mothers who do not suckle their infants secrete some milk and this may persist for 3–4 weeks postpartum (Cooke et al 1976). The suckling stimulus, which releases both prolactin and oxytocin, is essential for the maintenance of lactation and these reflexes are discussed below. Provided that the breast is emptied regularly by sucking, lactation can be maintained for long periods and in some traditional communities will continue for 2 years or more (Buchanan 1975).

Most studies have estimated that after lactation is established, the average daily volume of milk production in a healthy, well nourished mother is of the order of 750–800 ml/day (Whitehead et al 1980). More recently, studies in Australian women (Hartmann et al 1984) calculated a daily milk output of about 1200 ml/day, which was in keeping with estimates made by Nims et al in the 1930s (Nims et al 1932). A summary of the varying estimates is shown in Figure 62.4. The different methods used to measure milk volume may account for this. The most commonly used method has been the test-weighing of the baby before and after each feed; the volume of milk is calculated from the increase in infant weight, although alternatively the mother may be weighed before and after the feed (Hartmann & Saint 1984). A potential error in both methods comes from insensible fluid loss during the feed, which leads to an underestimate by infant test-weighing and an overestimate by maternal test-weighing. Furthermore, electronic integrating scales are essential to record the weights accurately and these have been used in only a few studies. Measuring expressed milk volume does not overcome the problem because it measures the capacity of the breast to secrete milk and not the amount transferred to the baby. More recent studies have measured the decay of deutrium oxide in either mother or infant (Coward et al 1979) but this method only measures average volumes over a period of several days. All methods interfere to some extent with the delicate mother–child interrelationship and this could have an important effect on physiological measurements. Differences between estimates of milk volume may also reflect the suckling practices of the populations studied, because feeding regimes involving greater mother–infant contact may increase milk production. Mothers who are feeding twins produce twice as much milk as mothers feeding singletons (Hartmann et al 1984), strongly suggesting that suckling, which is doubled in the case of twins, is the key to milk production (see Fig. 62.4).

The influence of maternal diet on milk production has not been clearly defined (Butte et al 1984) and only small differences have been observed between Swedish and Ethiopian mothers (Gebre-Medhin et al 1976) and British and Gambian mothers (Whitehead et al 1980). It may be that babies of poorly nourished mothers have to suckle more

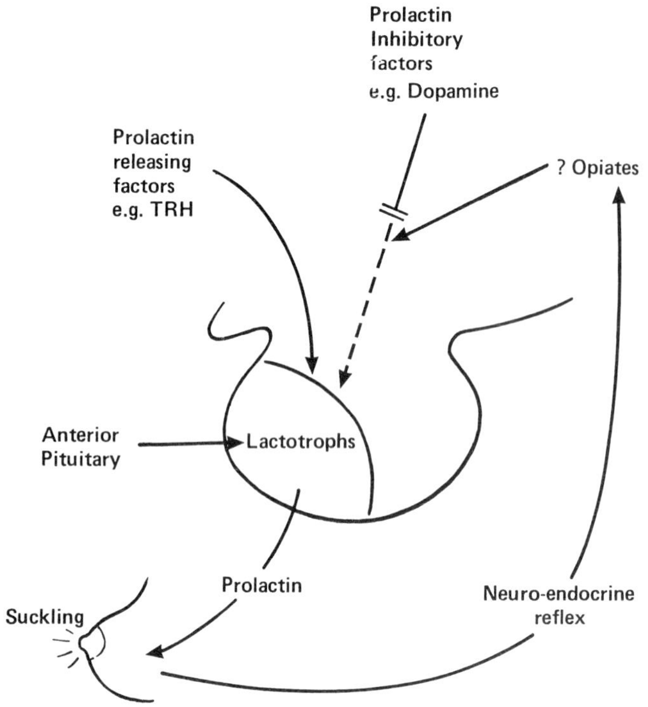

Fig. 62.5 Prolactin release is mainly under the control of prolactin inhibitory factors (dopamine) but can also be stimulated by prolactin-releasing factors (TRH = thyrotropin-releasing hormone). Sucking may release prolactin by an opiate mediate inhibitor of dopamine.

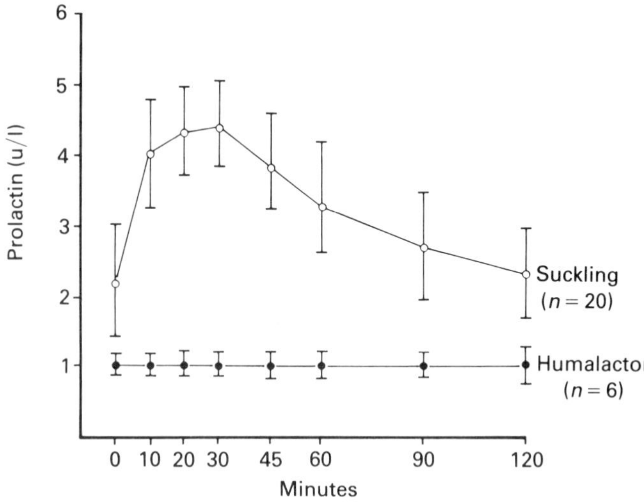

Fig. 62.6 Prolactin release in response to normal suckling and Humalactor. The Humalactor breast pump does not stimulate the nipple directly and fails to achieve effective prolactin release. Adapted from Howie et al (1980).

intensively and for longer to achieve an adequate milk supply (Lunn 1985).

PROLACTIN AND MILK PRODUCTION

Prolactin is a long-chain polypeptide hormone which is secreted from the anterior pituitary gland in response to suckling and is essential for successful lactation.

The mechanism by which prolactin secretion is controlled is a topic of much research; current knowledge is summarized in Figure 62.5. The suckling stimulus of the baby sends afferent impulses to the hypothalamus, leading to a surge of prolactin release. Prolactin release is controlled by prolactin inhibitory factors secreted into the pituitary portal blood system; dopamine is generally considered to be the most important. The suckling-induced burst of prolactin secretion from the pituitary may be induced by the inhibition of dopamine release from the hypothalamus which in turn may be controlled by opioids released locally in the hypothalamus in response to suckling. Other factors which may influence prolactin secretion include oestrogen and thyroid-stimulating hormone (TSH) (Neville & Berga 1983). Further research to clarify the control mechanisms of prolactin secretion may deepen our understanding of how breastfeeding sucking patterns can be used to maximize breast milk production.

In response to suckling, prolactin levels rise quickly to reach a peak about 30 minutes after the baby is put to the breast and then progressively decline to reach presuckling levels after about 120 minutes (Howie et al 1980). Areolar stimulation is essential for prolactin release because the Humalactor, a breast pump which empties the breast by negative pressure, does not stimulate the nipple to release prolactin (Fig. 62.6). Basal prolactin levels are high in the immediate postpartum period and progressively decline after the sixth postpartum week at a rate which is dependent upon suckling frequency and duration (Delvoye et al 1977, Howie et al 1981a). The peak levels of prolactin achieved in response to suckling also decline progressively over time (Glasier et al 1984b).

Prolactin has a diurnal variation, being higher during hours of sleep, and it has been shown that prolactin responses to suckling are higher in the evening hours compared with those achieved earlier in the same day (Glasier et al 1984b). These considerations suggest that prolactin production is increased by frequent suckling at regular intervals throughout the 24 hours, including the night time and that feeding practices which encourage such suckling patterns will produce optimal milk volumes. The relationship between prolactin and milk volume is complex.

The action of prolactin is to bind to receptors on the alveolar milk-secreting cells of the breast. Prolactin appears to act at multiple sites to stimulate the synthesis of several milk components, including casein, lactalbumin (which may regulate lactose synthesis), fatty acids and other constituents. It appears that prolactin interaction with the plasma membrane of the alveolar cells sets in motion a series of intracellular events which lead to the synthesis and secretion of all milk components (Neville & Berga 1983).

The importance of prolactin to lactogenesis can be demonstrated clinically because the administration in the early puerperium of bromocriptine, a dopamine agonist, rapidly reduces prolactin levels and abolishes milk production (Rolland & Schellekens 1973). There is conflicting evidence about the exact quantitative relationship between prolactin levels and milk production. On the one hand there is no correlation between prolactin levels and milk production in the early puerperium (Howie et al 1980) and mothers who have had pituitary surgery can breastfeed successfully despite having prolactin levels just above the non-pregnant range (Franks et al 1977). On the other hand dopamine receptor-blocking drugs, such as metoclopramide and sulpiride, raise prolactin levels and appear to improve milk production, especially in mothers with failing lactation (Aono et al 1979, Ylikorkala et al 1982). It seems that at least basal levels of prolactin are required for milk production but that above a certain threshold the absolute levels of prolactin do not by themselves dictate the volume of milk produced. Although the central role of prolactin in lactation is established, further work is required to define the exact quantitative relationships between prolactin secretion and milk volume.

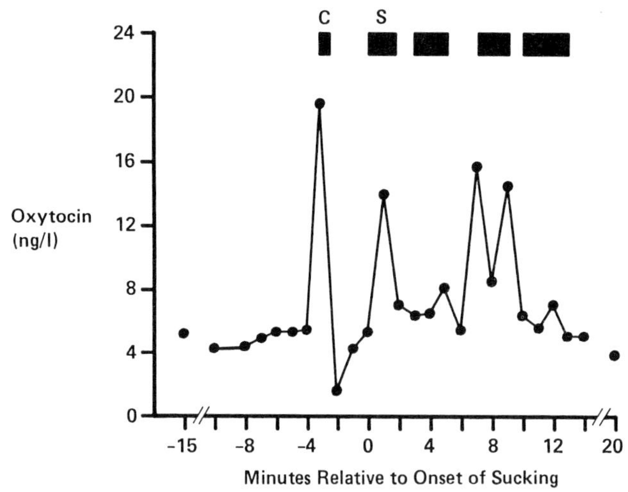

Fig. 62.7 Release of oxytocin in response to an infant's cry (C) and to suckling episodes (S), showing the importance of the presuckling stimuli in stimulating the let-down reflex. From McNeilly et al (1983) with permission.

OXYTOCIN AND THE MILK-EJECTION REFLEX

The milk-ejection reflex is responsible for transferring milk from the secreting glands of the breast to the baby. The milk-ejection reflex mimics the prolactin reflex in some respects, insofar as both are initiated by suckling and mediated by afferent neural impulses from the areola to the hypothalamus. They are, however, quite separate physiologically and have important differences.

The milk-ejection reflex is mediated by the hormone oxytocin, an octapeptide synthesized in specialized magnocellular neurones in the supraoptic and paraventricular nuclei of the hypothalamus. The neuroendocrine reflex leading to oxytocin release can be initiated not just by the suckling of the infant, but also by the mother handling the baby, hearing its cry or even just thinking of feeding. In one mother who was feeding twins, McNeilly & McNeilly (1978) noted that regular spontaneous let-down could occur even in the absence of suckling. At 2 weeks postpartum, let-down occurred at 30 minute intervals, increasing to 4-hourly intervals at 4 months postpartum. It is of interest that the frequency of these let-down reflexes has close parallels with the observed nursing frequency in traditional hunter–gathering communities such as the !Kung in the Kalahari desert (Konner & Worthman 1980). Frequent suckling may have been the true norm for the human species until relatively recent times.

In animal studies, a burst of electrical activity in oxytocic neurones can be measured 10–15 seconds prior to milk ejection, indicating that nerve depolarization is the stimulus for oxytocin release (Poulain et al 1977). In contrast to prolactin, oxytocin is released in short bursts lasting less than a minute and frequently the largest release of oxytocin occurs in response to the cry of the baby before feeding begins (McNeilly et al 1983; Fig. 62.7). This understanding of the prefeeding release of oxytocin may explain, at least in part, why rooming-in of mother and baby is associated with successful breastfeeding (Cruse et al 1978).

The action of oxytocin is to bind to specific receptors on the myoepithelial cells of the breast, thereby causing them to contract. These myoepithelial cells are placed around the milk-secreting cells of the mammary gland and longitudinally in the walls of milk ducts. When the milk-ejection reflex occurs, the contraction of the myoepithelial cells around the alveoli expels the milk into the ducts (McNeilly 1977). The flow of milk to the nipple is facilitated by the wide opening of the ducts which is induced by contraction of the longitudinal oxytocin-sensitive cells in the duct walls. When the milk-ejection reflex is well established, a mother may be aware of milk being spontaneously ejected from one breast while she suckles her baby on the other.

The milk-ejection reflex is very sensitive to emotional stress (Newton & Newton 1950) and the adverse effects of threatening or discouraging remarks to the nursing mother may act in this way. Inhibition of oxytocin release may occur but catecholamines released by stress may cause constriction of the mammary vessels and prevent oxytocin access to the myoepithelial cells.

It is clear that the milk-ejection reflex is complementary to the prolactin reflex and both pathways are required for successful lactation. Various studies have suggested that pharmacological stimulation of both the oxytocin (Huntingford 1961) and the prolactin (Aono et al 1979, Ylikorkala et al 1982) pathways can improve lactation, although more work is required to define their place in clinical practice.

INFANT SUCKING AND MILK TRANSFER

In addition to milk secretion and ejection by the mother, effective sucking by the infant is also an important part of successful breastfeeding. In contrast to bottle-feeding, where the baby obtains the milk by negative pressure, breastfeeding involves milking of the cisterns of the breast which lie deep to the nipple. To do this, the baby must take the whole nipple into its mouth and place its tongue under the adjacent areola. A baby properly fixed in this way will milk the cisterns with its tongue and, aided by the milk-ejection reflex, will establish a good milk flow. One of the most important aspects in the clinical management of breastfeeding is to ensure that the baby is properly fixed. This can be assisted by encouraging the rooting reflex of the baby with the smell and feel of the nipple round its mouth. This makes the baby open its mouth widely and fix properly on the breast.

Detailed observation of babies during breastfeeding have shown two distinct sucking patterns which have been described as nutritive and non-nutritive sucking. Nutritive sucking is characterized by a continuous stream of strong, slow sucks while non-nutritive sucking shows an alternation of rapid shallow bursts of sucking with rests (Drewett & Woolridge 1979). Nutritive sucking occurs predominantly at the beginning of the feed and is increasingly replaced by non-nutritive sucking as the feed progresses. As a result of the changing sucking pattern, the greatest proportion of milk transfer occurs in the early part of the feed (Lucas et al 1979). In one study, over 75% of milk transfer occurred in the first 10 minutes of a 20-minute feed, although considerable variation was observed among different mothers (Howie et al 1981b). The varying patterns of sucking and milk transfer indicate that it is inappropriate to manage breastfeeding on the basis of arbitrary time schedules and the duration of a feed should be determined by the infant's response.

The physiological function of non-nutritive sucking is not clearly understood. It may be that the baby derives comfort from the close mother–infant contact but the additional sucking may also be responsible for additional prolactin release and the regulation of maternal fertility and energy balance, which are discussed later.

MECHANISMS OF MILK SECRETION

A number of separate pathways are involved in the synthesis and secretion of milk products by the mammary alveolar cells. These are summarized below; a more detailed description has been given by Neville et al (1983).

Exocytosis

Many of the major components of milk, including lactose, proteins, calcium and phosphate, are packaged into secretory vesicles and secreted by exocytosis. The amino acid sequences of the milk proteins are coded in the nuclear DNA and transcribed into messenger RNA (mRNA) which moves into the cytoplasm. Under the influence of mRNA, protein synthesis occurs and the protein molecules are transferred to the Golgi system for further processing into secretory vesicles. These vesicles subsequently move to the apex of the cell and are discharged by the process of exocytosis into the alveolar lumina.

Secretion of ions and water

According to one hypothesis the major milk sugar, lactose, is synthesized when the membrane-bound enzyme, galactosyltransferase, interacts with the protein alpha-lactalbumin within the Golgi system. The Golgi system is impermeable to lactose so that an osmotic gradient is set up which attracts water into the alveolar cell. Electrolytes follow the water according to their electrochemical gradients. Chloride, however, is out of equilibrium with its concentration in the cytoplasm and it is postulated that there must be an active transport mechanism to move chloride back into the cell.

Lipid secretion

Lipid secretion is controlled by a different mechanism from the one responsible for lactose and protein synthesis. The lipids in breast milk are mainly triglycerides and are synthesized in the cytoplasm and smooth endoplasmic reticulum of the alveolar cells. The triglycerides coalesce to form fat droplets which migrate to the apex of the cell and are secreted by a mechanism which does not involve the Golgi apparatus.

Secretion of immunoglobulins

Immunoglobulin A is the principal immune protein in milk and with some other proteins can combine with specific receptors on the alveolar basement membrane before being internalized in a secretory vesicle and transported to the apex of the cell for secretion into the lumen.

Paracellular pathway

Some substances may pass between the gaps in the alveolar cells into the milk and this may be the pathway by which leukocytes and other cells enter the milk. During pregnancy and involution of the breasts, these gaps are relatively leaky but during full lactation the junctions between alveolar cells are much tighter and less permeable.

CONSTITUENTS OF BREAST MILK

The composition of milk varies greatly among different species, suggesting that evolution has developed specific milks

Table 62.1 Approximate composition of various constituents in human milk and cows' milk. From Jellife & Jelliffe (1978)

	Human milk	Cows' milk
Energy (kcal/ml)	75	66
Protein (g/100 ml)	1.1	3.5
Casein (%)	40	82
Whey protein (%)	60	18
Lactose (g/100 ml)	6.8	4.9
Fat (g/100 ml)	4.5	3.7
Sodium (mmol)	7	20
Chloride (mmol)	11	29

suited to the needs of the young of each species (Hartmann et al 1984). Studies of human milk composition also show that the concentrations of the various constituents are not constant. The constituents vary from one mother to another and in any one mother the milk content varies between one feed to another on the same day and even between the beginning and the end of the same feed. Probably the most important variable is the length of time postpartum, suggesting that the milk content adapts to meet the needs of the infant at any particular stage of development.

These considerations suggest that mothers' milk is adapted to meet the needs of the young in a sensitive way which cannot be matched by artificial feeds. It also means that any statements about milk composition merely reflect an average value, around which there is considerable individual variation.

The composition of mature human milk is used as a guide for the preparation of artificial feeds; the recommended figures for some of the major constituents are shown in Table 62.1.

Carbohydrates

Human milk contains one of the highest concentrations of carbohydrate of any mammal, mainly in the form of lactose. The dramatic rise in the synthesis of lactose in the first few days after delivery is one of the main features of the transition from colostrum to mature milk. The intestinal enzyme lactase, which is responsible for the hydrolysis and subsequent absorption of lactose, develops late in fetal life so that any intestinal inflammation which interferes with lactase function will lead to lactose intolerance and diarrhoea. When lactose is digested it yields a mixture of galactose and glucose so that lactose is not considered to be an essential sugar. The reason for the high lactose content in human milk is not clear but it may be important in controlling stool acidity and the characteristics of the intestinal flora.

Protein

Compared with cows' milk, the total protein content of human milk is much less and about 40% is in the form of casein. This means that the curds formed in human milk are much softer, more flocculent and more easily digestible for the intestinal tract. The remaining proteins are called whey proteins; they represent a mixture of soluble proteins left after the casein curd has formed. Many of these soluble proteins, such as the immunoglobulins, lactoferrin and lysozyme, are important for the anti-infective qualities of human milk and these are discussed below.

Human milk contains high concentrations of alpha-lactalbumin and, although it has been proposed as a regulator of lactose synthesis, a direct correlation between lactose and alpha-lactalbumin levels has yet to be established (Kulski & Hartmann 1981).

Fat

Lipid, which appears mainly as triglycerides, is the most variable constituent of human milk, the highest concentrations appearing in the hind-milk as milk fat globules. Fat is the major source of energy in human milk so that the estimated calorific value of 75 kcal/100 ml is at best only an approximation. The fat content of human milk is also important as the carrier of the fat-soluble vitamins A, D, E and K and of the essential fatty acids. Deficiency of vitamin D can lead to rickets, while that of vitamin K may lead to haemorrhagic disease of the newborn. The fatty acid composition of the triglycerides can vary according to the maternal diet; the influence of these dietary variations during infancy on subsequent vascular disease is a topic of interest and controversy (Hartmann et al 1984).

Minerals

Compared with cows' milk, human milk has low concentrations of sodium, chloride, iron and some other minerals. The low levels of sodium and chloride are advantageous in infants with diarrhoea because milks with a high solute load can aggravate dehydration. The concentration of iron is low (0.5 μmol/ml) in human milk and many clinicians advise iron supplements in breastfed babies. There is a much higher absorption of iron from breast milk (>75%) compared with cows' milk (30%) or iron-supplemented infant formula (10%; Saarinen & Siimes 1979) and although the reason for the greater bioavailability of iron from breast milk is not known, its binding to lactoferrin in human milk may be responsible.

NUTRITIONAL ADEQUACY OF BREAST MILK

The nutritional adequacy of breast milk is a matter of controversy. Most authorities recommend that breast milk alone is sufficient to meet infants' nutritional needs until between 4 and 6 months of age. In practice most UK mothers introduce supplementary foods before this and a World Health Organization (WHO) survey (1981) involving 27 different socioeconomic groups throughout the world showed that this was generally true. On the other hand, two studies of well nourished mothers from the USA (Ahn & McLean 1980) and Australia (Hartmann & Prosser 1984) have shown that some mothers can adequately sustain their babies on breast milk alone for longer than this. By 8 months, however, faltering in growth will occur on breast milk alone and supplements are needed. In Western Australia, 12% of nursing mothers were giving breast milk as the sole form of fluid at 1 year, indicating that breast milk can make a major contribution to infant nutrition well into infancy. The nutritional adequacy of breast milk is very variable, depending upon the success of milk production; clinical decisions must be made for individuals on the basis of the infant's progress.

MAMMARY FUNCTION DURING WEANING

During the process of weaning there is a loss of secretory activity by the mammary gland (Prosser et al 1984). When weaning is abrupt the concentrations of potassium, glucose and lactose decrease while those of sodium, chloride and protein increase. During gradual weaning the changes are similar but occur over a longer period of time. If conception occurs during lactation the rising levels of placental steroids inhibit milk secretion and this over-rides the positive stimulus of the infant's suckling.

Following the cessation of regular suckling the mammary gland quickly ceases secretory activity and enters a phase of regression. The milk in the ducts and alveoli is resorbed and although there is a decrease in parenchymal elements, the breast does not return to its prenatal state as many alveoli persist.

ANTI-INFECTIVE PROPERTIES OF BREAST MILK

Breast milk contains a number of proteins with antimicrobial activity. The anti-infective properties of breast milk are an important protection for the suckling infant, especially in areas with infected water supplies, and the antimicrobial proteins may also protect the breasts against infection and abscess formation (Hartmann et al 1984).

Lactoferrin

Lactoferrin is an iron-binding glycoprotein which inhibits bacterial growth non-specifically. *Escherichia coli* have a high requirement for free iron; lactoferrin, with its high affinity for iron, may restrict the growth of pathogenic iron-dependent bacteria. The action of lactoferrin may be low in the stomach as little iron is protein-bound in an acidic environment. In the proximal duodenum, however, bicarbonate secretion will favour the binding of iron to lactoferrin and enhance its bacteriostatic action in the intestinal tract.

Lysozyme

Lysozyme is a cationic protein which is present in concentrations of 30–40 mg/100 ml of human milk. Its bactericidal activity is mediated by its ability to cleave proteoglycans in the cell walls of a number of Gram-positive and Gram-negative bacteria. The activity is promoted by other milk components, especially IgA. Lysozyme is stable in the gut because active material is present in the faeces of breastfed babies.

Immunoglobulins

The major immunoglobulin in breast milk is IgA, with smaller amounts of IgM and IgG. The concentration of IgA is particularly high in colostrum and, although the concentration of IgA falls to about 2 mg/ml in mature milk, the daily yield remains relatively constant. The IgA in breast milk is poorly absorbed and persists in the infant's gastrointestinal tract to protect against infection. The high concentration of IgA in colostrum enables it to enter the proteoglycan lining of the gastrointestinal tract and may provide initial surface protection (Watson 1980).

Specific IgA antibodies, mostly against gastrointestinal pathogens, are also present in human milk (Bezkorovainy 1979). The mechanism of their formation is illustrated in Figure 62.8. It is suggested that if the mother meets a potential pathogen in her own gastrointestinal tract, the antigen is taken up by the gut-associated lymphoid tissue (GALT) in the Peyer's patches of her terminal ileum. Plasma cells are formed which migrate to the breast where specific IgA is secreted into the breast milk. In this way, the mother is able to give her specific protection against endemic pathogens in her environment. This remarkable interaction between mother and baby is, of course, a mechanism which cannot be replicated by artificial feeds.

Other anti-infective factors

Human milk contains a growth factor for *Lactobacillus bifidus* which facilitates colonization with this organism, which competes with intestinal pathogens. Breast milk also contains cells in the form of macrophages and leukocytes, small amounts of complement and lactoperoxidases; their importance as anti-infective agents in vivo has not been defined.

MATERNAL ADAPTATIONS DURING LACTATION

During lactation, two physiological maternal adaptations take place, both of which have important practical implications. These are, firstly, the natural inhibition of the mother's fertility and secondly, changes in maternal energy utilization which enable her to use her calories more efficiently.

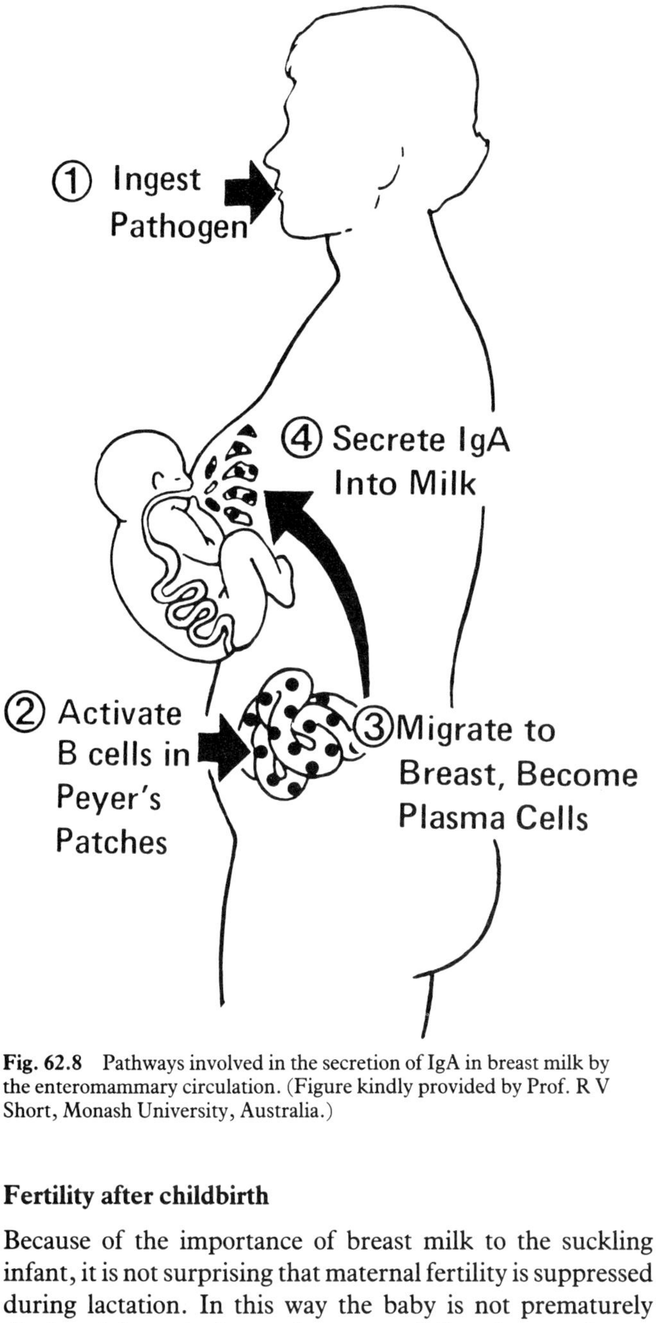

Fig. 62.8 Pathways involved in the secretion of IgA in breast milk by the enteromammary circulation. (Figure kindly provided by Prof. R V Short, Monash University, Australia.)

Fertility after childbirth

Because of the importance of breast milk to the suckling infant, it is not surprising that maternal fertility is suppressed during lactation. In this way the baby is not prematurely displaced from the breast by a new sibling, because breast milk tends to decline during pregnancy. There is also good evidence that both maternal and child health are improved by adequate interbirth intervals (Morley 1977). It is therefore important to understand and maximize the natural interbirth intervals induced by breastfeeding.

Postpartum fertility in bottle- and breastfeeding mothers

Mothers who do not breastfeed have an early resumption of menstruation, ovulation and the potential for fertility. On the basis of basal body temperature rises, the earliest that ovulation has been observed after delivery is 4 weeks (Udesky 1950), although it is unusual before 5 weeks and more commonly delayed until 8–10 weeks postpartum (Howie et al 1982). Most non-lactating mothers will have resumed ovulation and menstruation by 15 weeks postpartum. The first postpartum cycle in bottle-feeding mothers is frequently anovular (80%) or associated with an inadequate luteal phase (McNeilly et al 1982b). By the third cycle normal ovulation and luteal activity have been restored. In non-lactating women who use no contraception, 50% will have conceived by about 6–7 months postpartum (Berman et al 1972, Potter et al 1965). In contrast, breastfeeding women experience a period of lactational amenorrhoea and reduced fertility. The duration of lactational amenorrhoea varies greatly among different populations and among women within the same population. In many developing countries, lactational amenorrhoea may last for 2 years or more, whereas in developed countries menstruation and fertility may be delayed only for a few weeks (Howie & McNeilly 1982, Gross & Eastman 1985); the possible reasons for these differences are discussed below.

During the greatest part of lactational amenorrhoea, ovulation is suppressed and conception cannot occur. In the 4 weeks prior to the end of lactational amenorrhoea, ovarian activity will return and about 30–70% of these cycles will be ovulatory (Udesky 1950, Perez et al 1972). The longer the period of lactational amenorrhoea, the greater the chance of ovulation in the cycle prior to first menstruation (Howie et al 1982). The number of women conceiving during lactational amenorrhoea is reported as between 1 and 10% (Buchanan 1975). After the return of menstrual cycles during lactation, the potential for fertility increases but does not return to normal because many of the cycles are either anovular or associated with inadequate luteal function (McNeilly et al 1982b). On a global scale, lactational amenorrhoea is of great importance for fertility rates in countries where contraceptive usage is low. It has been estimated that in developing countries breastfeeding prevents more pregnancies than all other methods of family planning combined (Rosa 1975).

Endocrine changes after delivery

The normal endocrine control of ovarian function and how it may be modified by suckling are summarized in Figure 62.9. In response to the pulse generator in the hypothalamus, gonadotrophin-releasing hormone (GnRH) is released into the hypophyseal portal blood system. This provokes a pulsatile release of luteinizing hormone (LH) from the pituitary which, in combination with follicle-stimulating hormone (FSH), stimulates follicle development and oestradiol secretion in the ovary. The oestradiol promotes further follicle growth and by positive feedback stimulates the preovulatory LH surge and ovulation (McNeilly et al 1985).

During pregnancy, the high levels of placental steroids suppress the pituitary secretion of both LH and FSH to about 1% of normal (McNeilly 1979). After delivery, oestrogen and progesterone levels fall and in bottle-feeding

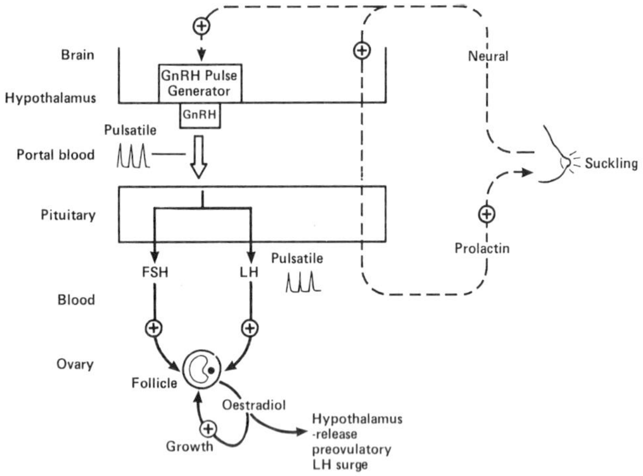

Fig. 62.9 Schematic diagram of the hypothalamic control of gonadotrophin secretion. Gonadotrophin-releasing hormone (GnRH) pulses from the hypothalamus induce luteinizing hormone (LH) pulses from the pituitary which control follicle development and ovulation. FSH = follicle-stimulating hormone. Suckling, either by a direct neural input or by increased prolactin secretion, alters LH pulse secretion through an action on the GnRH pulse generator. From McNeilly et al (1985) with permission.

mothers, plasma FSH and LH rise to early follicular phase levels by about 3 weeks postpartum to stimulate ovarian activity (Glasier et al 1983).

The mechanisms which lead to the suppression of ovarian activity during lactation are not fully understood but inhibition may occur in two ways. In the first place, suckling induces changes in the sensitivity of the hypothalamic–pituitary axis to oestrogen, making it more sensitive to the negative feedback effects of ovarian steroids and less sensitive to positive feedback (Baird et al 1979). As a result, there is inhibition of GnRH, leading to diminished or inappropriate secretion of LH (Glasier et al 1983). When there is sufficient gonadotrophin to stimulate a small follicle during lactation the oestrogen produced by the follicle will inhibit further pulsatile LH release from the pituitary because of the changed sensitivity to feedback and prevent further follicle development (Glasier et al 1984a). As the suckling stimulus declines there is progressive recovery of gonadotrophin levels and menstrual cycles may return during lactation. Many of the cycles remain abnormal, being either anovular or having inadequate luteal phases, and these may be due to suboptimal gonadotrophin stimulation (McNeilly et al 1985).

In the second place, the prolactin which is released during suckling may contribute to ovarian inhibition during lactation. Prolactin may have a direct inhibitory effect on the ovary or may, through a short-loop feedback effect, contribute to the reduced gonadotrophin secretion from the pituitary (McNeilly et al 1982a). At present there is no direct evidence that prolactin plays a part in ovarian inhibition during lactation and its exact role has yet to be defined.

In countries where contraceptive usage is low, breastfeeding makes an important contribution to birth-spacing and completed family size. For example, it has been calculated that if in Bangladesh the average duration of lactational amenorrhoea fell from 21 to 3 months, contraceptive usage would have to increase from 9 to 52% to keep fertility rates at their present level (Lesthaege et al 1981). It is clearly important not to change breastfeeding practices in countries with low contraceptive usage without fully appreciating their implications for fertility.

MATERNAL ENERGY REQUIREMENTS DURING LACTATION

For lactating mothers the daily calorie intake recommended by WHO is 2700 kcal for the first 6 months and 2950 kcal from 6 months onwards (FAO Nutritional Studies 1950). This figure is reached by the arithmetic calculation of 2200 kcal for normal non-lactating non-pregnancy requirements plus an additional 500 kcal for the overall energy cost of the milk. Assuming an average milk volume, the average calorie value of breast milk is 750 kcal/day, which is supplemented from the maternal fat stores laid down during pregnancy to the tune of 250 kcal/day. At the end of 6 months it is assumed that the available fat stores will have been used up and an additional dietary supplement of 250 kcal/day will be required.

Observational studies on healthy lactating women in developed countries have shown that their actual calorie intakes based on measured portions of food do not reach the theoretical recommendations. For example, Whitehead et al (1981) reported 2300 kcal/day and Butte et al (1984) reported 2170 kcal/day in mothers who had no limitation on food availability and successfully breastfed their babies. In developing countries the gap between theoretical and actual food intake is even greater. For example, Prentice et al (1981) found that Gambian mothers took 1773 kcal/day in the dry season and 1474 kcal/day in the less plentiful wet season and, despite the calorie shortfall, breastfed their babies successfully for prolonged periods.

One possible reason for this discrepancy between the theoretical and actual energy requirements of nursing mothers is an increase in energy efficiency during lactation. Animal studies have shown that lactation is associated with an inhibition of non-shivering thermogenesis, leading to storage of all available dietary calories to be used in milk formation. In the mouse this is achieved by physiological inhibition of brown-fat cells which, in the non-lactating state, can burn off excess calories (Trayhurn et al 1982). In this way the lactating animal becomes energy-efficient. Recent studies have shown that a similar adaptation takes place in nursing mothers (Illingworth et al 1986), although the biological mechanism in the human probably does not occur through brown fat. Compared with the bottle-feeding mother, the lactating mother shows an increased sensitivity to insulin (Illingworth et al 1986) and although the biological mechanisms have not been fully defined, it is clear that nursing itself harbours maternal energy resources for the benefit of the sucking infant.

This concept of maternal energy adaptation during lactation has two potential implications. Firstly, it means that a mother who eats according to the WHO recommendations may fail to lose weight in the postpartum period. Secondly, mothers who bottle-feed in developing countries will lose the energy-sparing effect and society will have to provide more calories to meet the needs of the mother–infant pair. Further research is required to define the biological mechanism and practical implications of this physiological adaptation in nursing mothers.

CONCLUSIONS

Lactation is an important part of natural human reproduction. Efforts by modern civilization to replace lactation by artificial substitutes do not detract from its physiological relevance or its practical importance in developing countries. The primary function of lactation is to nourish the infant and human milk is the ideal food for the human baby. Important secondary features of breastfeeding are the anti-infective, contraceptive and energy-sparing effects. Policies relating to the initiation and maintenance of breastfeeding, the appropriate use of supplements, contraceptive advice for nursing mothers and maternal diet must all be based on a sound understanding of the physiology of lactation.

REFERENCES

Ahn C H, MacLean W C 1980 Growth of the exclusively breast fed infant. American Journal of Clinical Nutrition 33: 183–192

Aono T, Shioji T, Aki T, Hirota K, Nomura K, Kurachi K 1979 Augmentation of puerperal lactation by sulpiride. Journal of Clinical Endocrinology and Metabolism 48: 478–482

Auerbach K G, Avery J L 1981 Induced lactation; a study of adoptive nursing by 240 women. American Journal of Diseases of Children 135: 340–343

Baird D T, McNeilly A S, Sawers R S, Sharpe R M 1979 Failure of estrogen-induced discharge of luteinising hormone in lactating women. Journal of Clinical Endocrinology and Metabolism 49: 500–506

Berman M L, Hanson K, Hillman I L 1972 Effect of breast feeding on post-partum menstruation, ovulation and pregnancy in Alaskan eskimos. American Journal of Obstetrics and Gynecology 114: 524–534

Bezkorovainy A 1979 Human milk and colostrum proteins: a review. Journal of Dairy Science 60: 1023–1027

Buchanan R 1975 Breast-feeding — aid to infant health and fertility control. Population Reports Series J 4: 49–66

Butte N F, Garza C, Stuff J E, Smith E O, Nichols B J 1984 Effect of maternal diet and body composition on lactational performance. American Journal of Clinical Nutrition 39: 296–306

Cooke I, Foley M, Lenton E et al 1976 The treatment of puerperal lactation with bromocriptine. Postgraduate Medical Journal 52 (suppl 1): 75–80

Coward W A, Sawyer M B, Whitehead R G, Prentice A M, Evans J 1979 New method of measuring milk intakes in breast fed babies. Lancet i: 13–14

Cowie A T, Tindall J S 1961 The maintenance of lactation in the goat after hypophysectomy. Journal of Endocrinology 23: 79–96

Cruse P, Yudkin P, Baum J D 1978 Establishing demand feeding in hospital. Archives of Disease in Childhood 53: 76–78

Delvoye P, Demaegd M, Delogne-Desnoeck J et al 1977 The influence of the frequency of nursing and of previous lactation experience on serum prolactin in lactating mothers. Journal of Biosocial Science 9: 447–451

Drewett R F, Woolridge M 1979 Sucking patterns of human babies on the breast. Early Human Development 3/4: 315–320

FAO Nutritional Studies no 5 1950 Calorie requirements. Report of the Committee on Calorie Requirements, FAO, Washington

Franks S, Kiwi R, Nabarro J D N 1977 Pregnancy and lactation after pituitary surgery. British Medical Journal 1: 882

Gardner D L, Dodds T C 1976 Human histology. Churchill Livingstone, Edinburgh

Gebre-Medhin M, Vahlquist A, Howie P W, McNeilly A S 1982 Effect of breast feeding patterns on human birth intervals. Journal of Reproduction and Fertility 65: 545–557

Glasier A, McNeilly A S, Howie P W 1983 Fertility after childbirth: changes in serum gonadotrophin levels in bottle and breast feeding women. Clinical Endocrinology 19: 493–501

Glasier A, McNeilly A S, Howie P W 1984a Pulsatile secretion of LH in relation to the resumption of ovarian activity postpartum. Clinical Endocrinology 20: 415–426

Glasier A, McNeilly A S, Howie P W 1984b The prolactin response to suckling. Clinical Endocrinology 21: 109–116

Gould S F 1983 Anatomy of the breast. In: Neville M C, Neifert M R (eds) Lactation, physiology, nutrition and breast-feeding. Plenum Press, New York, p 23

Gross B A, Eastman C J 1985 Prolactin and the return of ovulation in breast-feeding women. Journal of Biosocial Science (suppl 9): 25–42

Hartmann P E, Prosser C G 1984 Physiological basis of longitudinal changes in human milk yield and composition. Federation Proceedings 43: 2448–2453

Hartmann P E, Saint L 1984 Measurement of milk yield in women. Journal of Pediatric Gastroenterology and Nutrition 3(2): 270–274

Hartmann P E, Rattigan S, Prosser C G, Saint L, Arthur D G 1984 Human lactation: back to nature. Symposium of Zoological Society of London 51: 337–368

Howie P W, McNeilly A S 1982 Effect of breast feeding patterns on human birth intervals. Journal of Reproduction and Fertility 65: 545–557

Howie P W, McNeilly A S, McArdle T, Smart L, Houston M 1980 The relationship between suckling induced prolactin response and lactogenesis. Journal of Clinical Endocrinology and Metabolism 50: 670–673

Howie P W, McNeilly A S, Houston M J, Cook A, Boyle H 1981a Effect of supplementary food on suckling patterns and ovarian activity during lactation. British Medical Journal 283: 757–763

Howie P W, Houston M J, Cook A, Smart L, McArdle T, McNeilly A S 1981b How long should a breast feed last? Early Human Development 5: 71–77

Howie P W, McNeilly A S, Houston M J, Cook A, Boyle H 1982 Fertility after childbirth: post-partum ovulation and menstruation in bottle and breast feeding mothers. Clinical Endocrinology 17: 323–332

Huntingford P J 1961 Intranasal use of synthetic oxytocin in management of breast feeding. British Medical Journal 1: 709–711

Illingworth P J, Jung R T, Howie P W, Leslie P, Isles T E 1986 Diminution in energy expenditure during lactation. British Medical Journal 292: 437–441

Jelliffe D B, Jelliffe E F P 1978 Human milk in the modern world. Oxford University Press, Oxford

Konner M, Worthman C 1980 Nursing frequency, gonadal function and birth spacing among !Kung hunter gatherers. Science 207: 788–791

Kulski J K, Hartmann P E 1981 Changes in human milk composition during the initiation of lactation. Australian Journal of Experimental Biology and Medical Science 59: 101–114

Lesthaege R J, Shah I H, Page H J 1982 Compensating changes in intermediate fertility variables and the onset of marital fertility transition. The International Union for the Scientific Study of Population, World Conference, Manila, p 27

Lucas A, Lucas P J, Baum J D 1979 Pattern of milk flow in breast-fed infants. Lancet ii: 57–58

Lunn P G 1985 Maternal nutrition and lactational infertility: the baby in the driving seat: In: Dobbing J (ed) Maternal nutrition and lactational

infertility. Nestle nutrition workshop series, vol 9. Raven Press, New York, p 41
Lyons W R 1958 Hormonal synergism in mammary growth. Proceedings of the Royal Society of London (Series B) 149: 303–325
McNeilly A S 1977 Physiology of lactation. Journal of Biosocial Science (suppl 4): 5–21
McNeilly A S 1979 Effects of lactation on fertility. British Medical Bulletin 35: 151–154
McNeilly A S, McNeilly J R 1978 Spontaneous milk ejection during lactation and its possible relevance to success of breast-feeding. British Medical Journal 2: 466–468
McNeilly A S, Glasier A, Jonassen J, Howie P W 1982a Evidence for direct inhibition of ovarian function by prolactin. Journal of Reproduction and Fertility 65: 559–569
McNeilly A S, Howie P W, Houston M J, Cook A, Boyle H 1982b Fertility after childbirth: adequacy of post-partum luteal phases. Clinical Endocrinology 17: 609–615
McNeilly A S, Robinson I C, Houston M J, Howie P W 1983 Release of oxytocin and prolactin in response to suckling. British Medical Journal 286: 257–259
McNeilly A S, Glasier A, Howie P W 1985 Endocrine control of lactational infertility. 1. In: Dobbing J (ed) Maternal nutrition and lactational infertility. Nestle nutrition workshop series, vol 9. Raven Press, New York, p 1
Minchen M (ed) 1985 Breast feeding matters. Alma, Allen and Unwin, Sydney
Morley D 1977 Biosocial advantages of an adequate birth interval. Journal of Biosocial Science (suppl 4): 49–81
Neville M C, Berga S E 1983 Cellular and molecular aspects of the hormonal control of mammary function. In: Neville M C, Neifert M R (eds) Physiology, nutrition and breast-feeding. Plenum Press, New York, p 141
Neville M C, Neifert M R 1983 An introduction to lactation and breast-feeding. In: Neville M C, Neifert M R (eds) Physiology, nutrition and breast-feeding. Plenum Press, New York, p 3
Neville M C, Allen J C, Watters C 1983 The mechanisms of milk secretion. In: Neville M C, Neifert M R (eds) Physiology, nutrition and breast-feeding. Plenum Press, New York, p 49
Newton N, Newton M 1950 Relation of the let-down reflex to the ability to breast feed. Pediatrics 5: 726–733
Nims B, Macy I G, Hunscher H A, Brown M 1932 Human milk studies. Daily and monthly variations in milk components as observed in two successive lactation periods. American Journal of Diseases of Children 43: 1062–1077
Perez A, Vela P, Masnick G S, Potter R G 1972 First ovulation after childbirth: the effect of breast-feeding. American Journal of Obstetrics and Gynecology 114: 1041–1047
Potter R G, New M L, Wyon J B, Gordon J E 1965 Applications of field studies to research on physiology of human reproduction: lactation and its effects upon birth intervals in 11 Punjab villages, India. Journal of Chronic Diseases 18: 1125–1140
Poulain D A, Wakerley J B, Dyball R E J 1977 Electrophysiological differentiation of oxytocin and vasopressin-secreting neurons. Proceedings of the Royal Society of London (series B) 196: 367–384
Prentice A M, Whitehead R G, Roberts S B, Paul A A 1981 Long-term energy balance in child-bearing Gambian women. American Journal of Clinical Nutrition 34: 2790–2799
Prosser C G, Saint L, Hartmann P E 1984 Mammary gland function during gradual weaning and early gestation in women. Australian Journal of Experimental Biology and Medical Science 62: 215–228
Rattigan S, Ghisalberti A V, Hartmann P E 1981 Breast milk production in Australian women. British Journal of Nutrition 45: 243–249
Robinson J, Short R V 1977 Changes in human breast sensitivity at puberty, during the menstrual cycle and at parturition. British Medical Journal 2: 1188–1191
Rolland R, Schellekens L A 1973 A new approach to the inhibition of puerperal lactation. Journal of Obstetrics and Gynaecology of the British Commonwealth 80: 945–951
Rosa F W 1975 The role of breast feeding in family planning. WHO Protein Advisory Group Bulletin 5, no 3: 5–10
Rowland M G M, Paul A A, Whitehead R G 1981 Lactation and infant nutrition. British Medical Bulletin 37: 77–82
Saarinen U M, Siimes M A 1979 Iron absorption from breast milk, cow's milk and iron-supplemented formula: an opportunistic use of changes in total body iron determined by hemoglobin, ferritin and body weight in 132 infants. Pediatric Research 13: 143–147
Saint L, Hartmann P E 1982 Metabolic potential of the human mammary gland. International Congress of Biochemistry 12: 267
Trayhurn P, Douglas J B, McGuckin M M 1982 Brown adipose tissue thermogenesis is 'suppressed' during lactation in mice. Nature 298: 59–60
Tyson J E, Khojandi M, Huth J, Andreassen B 1975 The influence of prolactin secretion on human lactation. Journal of Clinical Endocrinology and Metabolism 40: 764–773
Udesky I C 1950 Ovulation in lactating women. American Journal of Obstetrics and Gynecology 59: 843–849
Watson D L 1980 Immunological functions of the mammary gland and its secretion — comparative review. Australian Journal of Biological Science 33: 403–422
Whitehead R G, Paul A A, Rowland M G M 1980 Lactation in Cambridge and the Gambia. Topics in Paediatrics 2: 22–23
Whitehead R G, Paul A A, Black A E, Wiles S J 1981 Recommended dietary amounts of energy for pregnancy and lactation in the United Kingdom. In: Torun B, Young V R, Rand W M (eds) Protein energy requirements of developing countries: evaluation of new data. United Nations University, Tokyo, pp 259–265
World Health Organization 1981 Contemporary patterns of breast-feeding. Report on the WHO collaborative study on breast feeding. World Health Organization, Geneva
Ylikorkala O, Kaupilla A, Kivinen S, Viinikka L 1982 Sulpiride improves inadequate lactation. British Medical Journal 285: 249–251

SECTION 9

Abnormal Puerperium

63

David Charles and Bryan Larsen

Puerperal sepsis

HISTORICAL BACKGROUND

Much attention today is given to the concept of nosocomial, endogenous and iatrogenic infections. Nosocomial infections are acquired in hospital and may come from the hospital environment or from the patient's own flora. In 1984 in the USA there were an estimated 2 million nosocomial infections, resulting in 300 000 deaths (Haley et al 1985a, b). Infection arising from the patient's indigenous micro-organisms is termed an endogenous infection. Exogenous infections come from external contamination. Infection resulting from medical treatment is termed iatrogenic.

Childbirth fever (puerperal infection) is one of the most striking examples of iatrogenic infection. The suggestion that this scourge of the parturient woman was iatrogenic had a stormy reception in both Europe and the USA. Epidemics of diphtheria and plague were accepted but the great epidemics of puerperal fever occurred before the principles of infectious diseases were well established. In contrast to epidemics such as diphtheria, which moved inexorably through the population, the idea that childbed fever could be carried by the obstetrician was abhorrent to those attempting to help women. It was particularly difficult for sincere physicians to accept that, despite their noble intentions, they could unwittingly harm their patients. Thomas Watson, Professor of Medicine at King's College, London, in 1842, wrote:

> The dreadful suspicion that the hand which is relied on for succour in the painful and perilous art of childbirth, and which is intended to secure the safety of both mother and child, but especially the mother, may literally become the innocent cause of her destruction; innocent no longer, however, if, after warning and knowledge of the risk, suitable means are not used to avert a catastrophe so shocking.

As the medical community began to understand that an infectious agent could be responsible for puerperal sepsis, and transmitted by physicians and nurses, fewer cases resulted from iatrogenic infection and increasingly from endogenous, pathogenic bacteria. Traditionally, women did not deliver in lying-in hospitals. Rubenstein (1983) showed that while such institutions had been established to improve obstetrical care for disadvantaged women, they actually provided a perfect setting for the spread of puerperal sepsis from patient to patient. In such institutions maternal mortality was five times the national average because of the high incidence of puerperal sepsis.

Alexander Gordon's 'Treatise on the Epidemic Puerperal Fever of Aberdeen' (1795) was the earliest report that puerperal fever was contagious. It is remarkable that, long before the recognition of the role of micro-organisms, he was able to deduce that hand-washing reduced the spread of disease. Unfortunately, childbed fever continued while Gordon's insights were largely ignored and he had to leave Aberdeen to become a naval surgeon. The cause was later taken up by Ignatz Semmelweis in Vienna and by Oliver Wendell Holmes in the USA.

Semmelweis (1861) concluded that contamination from the dissecting room was responsible for the greater prevalence of puerperal sepsis in the obstetrical division in which women were delivered by students who also attended autopsies, compared to the other division in which deliveries were performed by pupil midwives who trained on mannequins rather than cadavers. Breaking the presumed spread of cadaveric particles from the autopsy room to the obstetrical ward reduced maternal mortality from 5% of deliveries to 1.3%, a rate similar to that in the midwives' section of the hospital.

At about the same time as Semmelweis was making his contribution in Vienna, Oliver Wendell Holmes of Boston published 'The Contagiousness of Puerperal Fever' in 1843, postulating that the disease could be prevented if physicians modified their practices to avoid cross-contamination between affected and unaffected patients. He recommended that obstetrical physicians should not perform autopsies on women who died of puerperal sepsis and refrain from providing obstetrical care for a specified time after attending an autopsy for puerperal fever, or if two or more of their patients were infected.

The striking decrease in maternal mortality which accompanied the efforts of Holmes and Semmelweis indicated that the majority of cases of puerperal fever were iatrogenic. Some patients may have acquired streptococci from asymptomatic nasopharyngeal carriers or from their own genital tract microflora. Although maternal mortality in Vienna fell after Semmelweis instituted hand-washing, it remained at 1.3% of deliveries, which is high by today's standards. There is probably no way to judge today the extent to which nosocomial infection with group A streptococci accounted for puerperal infections in the 19th century (Lansing et al 1983). The success of Semmelweis implies that a major portion of the problem then was the result of iatrogenic disease.

CURRENT STATUS OF GROUP A STREPTOCOCCUS

A decade after the introduction of sulphonamides, Leonard Colebrook (1946) in an address to the Royal College of Obstetricians and Gynaecologists prophesied that haemolytic streptococcal infections were likely to remain a problem in childbirth.

Even before antibiotics, major epidemics of puerperal sepsis were largely under control, probably because of better standards of medical care or changes in the virulence of the micro-organism. Group A streptococcal sepsis is now a rare cause of puerperal infection, although sporadic outbreaks have been described. Ledger & Headington (1972) found 71 cases of postpartum endometritis among 2091 deliveries (3.4%) but only two involved the group A streptococcus. Blanco et al (1981) reported that only 4 of 123 isolates (3.3%) from blood cultures of women with puerperal endometritis were due to group A, while 24 (19.5%) were due to group B streptococci.

Although most cases of postpartum uterine infection are due to the mixed flora of the lower genital tract, do not involve septicaemia and are usually non-fatal, serious outbreaks of group A streptococcal infection have occurred during this century. In a New York epidemic the fatality rate was 36% (Watson 1928).

A subsequent outbreak in Boston was reported by Jewett et al (1968), affecting 20 mothers and 5 infants. The organism involved was virulent, as indicated by the severity of the illness in most of those affected, but there were no deaths, although extraordinary means were needed to bring the outbreak under control. Quarantine of the infected patients, cessation of elective surgery, closure of the recovery ward and penicillin prophylaxis for new patients were ultimately employed, along with thorough epidemiological investigations. Screening the hospital staff indicated that one anaesthetist might have been the source of infection.

The occasional reappearance of group A streptococci should serve as a sober reminder that the organism is still with us. The danger in complacency lies partly in failing to recognize a new uncommon disease and partly in allowing isolated cases of group A streptococcal infection to become the source of a new epidemic.

THE SIGNIFICANCE OF PUERPERAL INFECTIONS

Sweet & Ledger (1973) reported infectious morbidity in 598 (5.9%) of 10 181 puerperal patients.

In the Report on Confidential Enquiries into Maternal Deaths in England and Wales from 1973 to 1975, it was found that although mortality rate from all causes among women delivered by Caesarean section was 6.6 times greater than in those delivered vaginally, with death due to sepsis, the difference in risk with Caesarean section was 13 times as great as that with vaginal delivery.

Various reports have indicated a marked disparity between the rates of infection following vaginal delivery and Caesarean section. Sweet & Ledger (1973) found 155 cases of infectious morbidity among 5972 vaginal deliveries (0.26%), whereas among 464 Caesarean sections there were 167 cases (36%). In an Australian study, Humphrey (1972) noted 24 infections among 518 patients delivered vaginally (4.6%), but 17 in 31 Caesarean sections (55%).

Infectious morbidity is clearly increased following Caesarean section. Furthermore, puerperal infection may prevent a mother from breastfeeding her infant, because of the possible effects of therapy, resulting in loss of contact with her child.

FEBRILE MORBIDITY IN THE PUERPERIUM

Fever is frequently the main clinical signal of puerperal infection and often the basis for commencing therapy and for assessing its effectiveness. As fever and infection are not synonymous, a definition is required. Febrile morbidity is defined as a temperature of 38°C (100.4°F) or higher on any 2 of the first 10 days postpartum except in the first 24 hours.

While every febrile puerperal patient should be investigated for a source of infection, many postpartum infections do not result in this, or any other definition of morbidity, based solely on fever. Stevenson et al (1967) noted that in maternal deaths following Caesarean section, a persistent low-grade temperature which never attained 38°C could often lead to a delay in diagnosis and treatment. A small proportion of women are infected several days before their temperature rises to 38°C or more, and such infections may become severe.

Since bacteraemia is as likely to cause septic shock in the initial 24 hours postpartum as later, febrile episodes soon after delivery should not be ignored. Only 50% of puerperal women with a clinical diagnosis of endometritis actually attain the defined criteria of febrile morbidity (Sweet & Ledger 1973).

Febrile morbidity does not identify the site of infection. In obstetrics, post-Caesarean section uterine infection has emerged as the most common hospital-acquired infection nowadays. This usually results from an infection of the uterine cavity, which may have been present before labour as infection in the amniotic fluid or fetal membranes and progressed to puerperal endometritis, eventually leading to myometritis, parametritis, adnexitis, pelvic abscess and septicaemia.

Of course, not all women with postpartum fever have uterine infection. Some 5–10% of patients with postpartum fever either have no infection or infection at some site other than the genital tract. Pyrexia may be due to puerperal mastitis, urinary tract infection, episiotomy or surgical wound infection. Continuous fever in a puerperal patient who has had a genital tract infection may be the first indication of septic thrombophlebitis with its attendant risk of pulmonary embolism.

Table 63.1 summarizes the range of infectious complications encountered in the puerperal patient. Each will be discussed in greater detail in the latter part of this chapter. All potential complications must be considered in any postpartum patient with signs of infection.

Table 63.1 The range of infectious complications in the postpartum patient

Site of infection	Typical micro-organisms
Endometritis	
Postpartum	
Post-Caesarean section	Mixed flora from cervix/vagina Occasionally group B or group A streptococci
Postabortal, spontaneous	Mixed flora from cervix/vagina
Postabortal, induced	*Clostridium*
Wound infection	
Wound cellulitis	Staphylococci
Wound abscess	*Escherichia coli*
Abdominal incision, episiotomy, vaginal, cervical laceration	Mixed anaerobes Streptococci
Necrotizing fasciitis	Staphylococci and anaerobic streptococci
Septicaemia	Group B or A streptococci *Bacteroides* spp.
Septic pelvic thrombophlebitis	*Escherichia coli* *Bacteroides* spp. Anaerobic cocci *Proteus*
Urinary infection	*Escherichia coli*
Cystitis	Group B, D streptococci
Pyelonephritis	*Proteus* *Klebsiella* *Enterobacter* *Pseudomonas*
Breast infection	
Puerperal mastitis	*Staphylococcus aureus*
Breast abscess	

The organisms involved in these infections will only be identified by appropriate culture. Organisms may be found other than those listed. The predominant organism will depend on the patient population and the specific hospital.

DIFFERENTIAL DIAGNOSIS OF PUERPERAL INFECTION AND OTHER SURGICAL COMPLICATIONS

Theoretically, any surgical condition can complicate pregnancy or the puerperium, but its recognition and treatment may be elusive. Diagnosis and selective treatment of abdominal conditions form the common ground between the surgeon and the obstetrician.

Acute appendicitis and cholecystitis are the only surgical conditions which occur with any frequency during pregnancy and the puerperium. Occasionally, generalized peritonitis or intestinal obstruction are encountered and rarely, acute pancreatitis, perforation of a peptic ulcer or intraperitoneal haemorrhage from an extrauterine source.

Diagnosing these surgical conditions, especially appendicitis, is difficult and mortality associated with acute appendicitis in the gravid or postpartum patient is usually due to delayed or mistaken diagnosis. Signs and symptoms may be wrongly ascribed to the puerperal state. Free consultation between surgeon and obstetrician is important for the patient's welfare.

Repeated abdominal auscultation is important in assessing the state of the bowel and in discriminating between obstruction and peritonitis. Accentuated bowel sounds simply denote excessive intestinal activity; atony is typical of peritonitis. Intermittent bowel sounds may be heard over distended or paralysed gut. With any suspicion of intestinal obstruction, radiological examination of the abdomen is important, since distended loops of bowel and fluid levels may be readily defined. Fluid levels are not diagnostic of obstruction and radiological findings must relate to the history and clinical findings.

Occasionally, within a few hours of being delivered, a woman may complain of lower abdominal pain and pass into a state of shock inappropriate for any difficulty or bleeding encountered during parturition. If pain is the main complaint, acute appendicitis must always be considered. Unlike the intermittent pain of uterine contractions following completion of the third stage of labour (afterpains), the pain will be continuous. If shock is present, it is essential to exclude internal haemorrhage from uterine rupture and exploration of the uterus is necessary after initiating therapy. If a pelvic mass is found, differential diagnosis includes an inflammatory mass, volvulus of the caecum or ascending colon, torsion of an ovarian cyst or a broad-ligament haematoma. Volvulus of the large bowel has been reported on many occasions subsequent to parturition. There is usually rapid distension of the bowel and the mass at the site of the volvulus is not as well defined as a cyst. Symptoms of obstruction may be variable. Later in the puerperium, a lower abdominal mass with fever and signs of peritoneal irritation must be ascribed to acute appendicitis or postpartum infection.

The necessary cultures should be obtained if possible before starting treatment when genital infection is diagnosed. Prophylactic antibiotics can suppress symptoms. Antibiotics may be administered empirically while awaiting the results of the bacteriological studies and therapy subsequently corrected or modified as necessary. Anaerobic and aerobic cultures are equally important and neither should be omitted. Whenever there is a fluctuating temperature associated with rigors, blood cultures must be obtained. Even without firm bacteriological evidence, any case of postpartum pyrexia continuing for more than 10 days should be regarded as possibly the result of polymicrobial infection including anaerobic organisms.

In genital infections there may be few localizing physical signs. Any signs depend upon the nature and the extent of the inflammatory response, the health of the patient and the resistance of her tissues to infection. The possible contribution of infection in surgical agenesis such as episiotomy or laceration of the cervix must be considered. The possibility of pelvic thrombophlebitis is better detected at this stage than found at autopsy, following sudden massive pulmonary embolism.

THE HOST–PARASITE RELATIONSHIP IN THE AETIOLOGY OF POSTPARTUM INFECTIONS

Little is known about the molecular basis of host defence and the attributes of micro-organisms in relation to these defences, especially in obstetrical infections (Yonekura 1985). These are frequently caused by micro-organisms of minimal intrinsic virulence and must be due to the introduction of organisms at normally uncontaminated sites and to the inability of the host to restrict their growth in these situations. In general, of course, most tissues have mechanisms to protect themselves against microbial contamination.

Skin and mucous membranes are barriers, but if these are breached, tissue macrophages and humoral factors in the interstitial spaces limit the invasive potential of contaminating micro-organisms. Inflammation ensues and polymorphonuclear leukocytes infiltrate the injured area. If micro-organisms enter the bloodstream, macrophages of the reticuloendothelial system aid their elimination. Within a few days, specific immunological reactions trigger a variety of effects, mediated by humoral and cellular mechanisms, which further limit the infection.

Table 63.2 Host defence properties in human amniotic fluid

Property	Function
Leukocytes	Phagocytic function is limited in fluid suspension
Immunoglobulins	Opsonic and bactericidal activity; concentration about $\frac{1}{10}$ of that in serum
Lysozyme	Bacteriolytic, Gram-positive only
Transferrin	Binds iron and therefore is unavailable for bacterial growth
Phosphate-sensitive inhibitor	Zinc-associated peptide with activity against Gram-negative organisms
Beta-lysin	Primary activity against Gram-positive organisms
Sterols	Active only in high concentrations against Gram-positive bacteria

The pregnant host is a unique biological paradox. Several components of the host defence against bacterial invaders are augmented, including complement, transferrin and leukocytic activity (Larsen 1983). These alterations probably persist into the puerperium but it has not been established for how long. On the other hand, there is some depression of cell-mediated immunity — perhaps to facilitate reception of the fetal allograft? — and increased susceptibility to some viral infections. Cell-mediated immune mechanisms are of great importance in the body's defence against infection.

The relationship between nutrition and host defence in pregnancy and the puerperium remains highly unexplained. Prema et al (1982) studied anaemic Indian women during pregnancy and found that those with haemoglobin values below 8 g/dl had significantly reduced B and T lymphocytes as well as reduced levels of IgG and IgA.

The developing fetus exists in close proximity to an abundant endocervical bacterial flora, separated only by the chorioamniotic membrane and the amniotic fluid. The barrier function of the membranes is indicated by the relevant risk of intra-amniotic infection which follows rupture of the membranes. Host defence factors have been noted in amniotic fluid (Table 63.2) and their potential protective effect is apparent since membrane rupture does not always lead to intrauterine infection. If it develops, however, chorioamnionitis causes an increased risk of postpartum endometritis. The properties of the puerperal uterus which make it susceptible to infection have been discussed by Larsen (1985a) and are summarized in Table 63.3.

Table 63.3 Host defence properties of the uterus

Property	Function
Immunoglobulin A	Present in cervical secretions, destroyed by bacterial IgA proteases
Blood-borne factors	
Immunoglobulins Complement	Present as a result of bleeding but relative intrauterine effectiveness unknown
Transferrin	Present as a component of blood but becomes iron-saturated in the presence of haemoglobin
Inflammatory reaction and local leukocytosis	Presumed to occur but of unknown effectiveness

THE NATURE OF POSTOPERATIVE SOFT-TISSUE INFECTIONS

While it used to be considered that postoperative infections were due to one virulent organism, such infections are nowadays recognized to be the result of a mixture of aerobic and anaerobic organisms, individually having minimal intrinsic virulence, and therefore considered to be opportunistic organisms.

In the past 15 years anaerobic organisms have become recognized as significant components of infections arising after abdominal surgery. Recognition of the significance of these organisms, which are fragile under ordinary atmospheric conditions, has been aided by improved techniques for growing and identifying them. Swenson et al (1973) isolated anaerobes from more than two-thirds of soft-tissue infections. Anaerobes were isolated from over 25% of patients with bacteraemia associated with pelvic infection (Ledger et al 1975). Seligman & Willis (1980) also emphasized the importance of the anaerobes in female pelvic infections.

Current emphasis on anaerobes should not obscure the importance of other organisms such as *Escherichia coli* or Gram-positive cocci such as *Staphylococcus aureus*, *Staph. epidermidis*, and streptococci of groups A, B, C, F and G, as well as the enterococci (Ramsay & Gillespie 1941, Vartian et al 1985). While the relationship between different species in soft-tissue infections has not been delineated, there seems to be a co-operative, additive effect between organisms. Rarely, the relationship between organisms is synergistic and infection takes on a particularly sinister form, as with necrotizing fasciitis, an entity which is fortunately uncommon.

Experience indicates that antimicrobial therapy is most effective when it covers both aerobic and anaerobic species.

FACTORS PREDISPOSING TO PUERPERAL INFECTIONS

The development of opportunistic infections such as those which arise after parturition may help identify conditions which alter host defences and predispose to infection, and may aid in ascertaining the nature of the host defences of the puerperal uterus. A surgical procedure may serve to diminish cellular immunity, possibly by causing stress, with subsequent adrenal hormone response and resultant immunosuppression. The presence of haemoglobin at a surgical haematoma represents a source of nutrient which serves as a growth factor and enhances the virulence of a variety of micro-organisms. Suture material may form a site in which bacteria tend to multiply, and collections of serous fluid may serve as a culture medium. Necrotic decidual tissues retained in the uterus also represent a suitable culture medium for microbial replication. While viable tissues possess cellular and humoral host defence attributes, foreign bodies and devitalized tissue do not and are not perfused by blood-borne host defence factors or antibiotics.

When childbed fever was common, it was usually caused by the virulent group A beta-haemolytic streptococcus. Nowadays, most puerperal infections involve less virulent organisms, partly because modern obstetrics use procedures to prevent infections with exogenous micro-organisms and partly because the virulence of the group A streptococcus has declined (Kass 1971). Infection therefore depends on the interplay between the virulence of endogenous micro-organisms and the defences of the host. In the puerperal uterus, the normal defences are reduced and a suitable microbial culture medium is provided.

Certain clinically identifiable facts seem to be associated with the susceptibility to infection. The presence of maternal antibody against the group B streptococcus has been associated with a poor prognosis of the infant (Baker & Kasper 1976) and the probability of maternal postpartum sepsis. Platt et al (1980) found that women lacking antibody to *Mycoplasma hominis* had postpartum fever more often than did women with antibody. Lamey et al (1982) indicated that isolation of *Mycoplasma* was mainly from the blood of young nulliparous individuals who probably had little or no immunological response to the organism. Buchanan et al (1980) found that gonococcal antibody protected against the development of pelvic inflammatory disease.

Obstetric manipulation such as vaginal examination, premature rupture of the fetal membranes and internal fetal monitoring may increase susceptibility to infection following either Caesarean section or vaginal delivery.

Vaginal examinations

Apuzzio et al (1982) found postpartum endometritis in 25% of patients who had three or less vaginal examinations during labour but 34% among patients who had four or more. Although this difference was not statistically significant, the rate of endometritis was doubled in patients with ruptured membranes who had four or more vaginal examinations compared with three or less. The high overall rate of infection in these patients was attributed to their disadvantaged socio-economic status.

Internal fetal monitoring

Monitoring devices passed through the cervix should increase the risk of intrauterine infection but clinical studies do not confirm this supposition.

Rehu & Haukkamaa (1980) prospectively evaluated the role of internal monitoring as a risk factor for postpartum infection in 1778 monitored patients who delivered normally and 238 who required Caesarean section. The risk of puerperal endometritis after internal fetal monitoring was identical with the risk of infection following one vaginal examination.

Internal fetal monitoring appears to add relatively little risk of infection to Caesarean or vaginal delivery.

Premature rupture of the fetal membranes

The fetal membranes rupture before labour in about 10% of pregnancies and predispose to intra-amniotic invasion by micro-organisms from the lower genital tract. Diagnosis is usually based on a history of fluid in the vagina and confirmed by sterile speculum examination, demonstrating vaginal alkalinization using a nitrazine swab, and arborization of vaginal fluid dried on a glass slide. Ruptured membranes predispose to intrauterine infection and preterm delivery. Intrauterine infection predisposes to postpartum endometritis.

Rupture of the fetal membranes before labour removes a natural barrier to ascending bacterial contamination and chorioamnionitis. Zaaijman et al (1982) reported that bacterial colonization occurred in 41% of neonates after preterm rupture of the membranes, but in only 28% of neonates after rupture from the membranes at term and in 23% of term infants after elective amniotomy. No information on postpartum infection was provided.

Much remains to be learned about the role of intrauterine infection and chorioamnionitis as antecedents of puerperal sepsis.

Chorioamnionitis

Chorioamnionitis may cause puerperal infection. Koh et al (1979) reviewed 226 patients with a diagnosis of chorioamnionitis; of these 104 (46%) were associated with fever greater than 38°C but did not have other objective signs such as purulent or malodorous amniotic fluid. Of these, 44 (31.4%) developed problems which may have been related, including 35 with endomyometritis, 5 with Caesarean wound infections and 9 with intrapartum bacteraemia. Since there were 26 129 uninfected deliveries during this study, the overall prevalence of these complications is small but the risk of maternal infection from chorioamnionitis is significant.

THE RANGE OF POSTPARTUM INFECTIONS

Most puerperal infections involve the uterus, although other sites may of course be involved.

Caesarean section infection

The risk of infection is 10–20 times greater after Caesarean section than after normal delivery. When the uterus is incised during labour, the operative field may be contaminated with bacteria from the lower genital tract, of which the most common are group B streptococcus, *Escherichia coli* and various anaerobes.

Several aspects of abdominal delivery may predispose to infection. Blood at the operative site provides a culture medium for bacteria which may contaminate the uterus. The original choriodecidual space, or placental bed, is sometimes invaded by bacteria which provide greater than usual bacterial contamination of the surgical site.

Infection after vaginal delivery

Puerperal infection may occur after a normal vaginal delivery, although less frequently than after Caesarean section. Many of the factors which predispose to post-Caesarean section sepsis also apply to vaginal delivery. Chorioamnionitis predisposes to postpartum endometritis following any type of delivery. Lacerations of the vulva or vagina or episiotomy incisions may all become infected. Retained particles of placenta or membranes also predispose to uterine infection.

Since the same micro-organisms cause infection after vaginal delivery as after Caesarean section, the choice of chemotherapy follows the same principles.

Pelvic cellulitis

Pelvic cellulitis is one of the most important postpartum infections starting in infected lacerations of the cervix, lower uterine segment or vagina. Primary lymphangitis, frequently referred to as parametritis, occurs in the adjacent cellular tissue.

Cellulitis spreads by way of perivascular lymphatics to outside the true pelvis, possibly leading to secondary peritonitis, which might track along a ureter to the perinephric region or along large vessels to the thigh or buttock. While cellulitis can arise from an infected cervical laceration, it is the result of these infections of the body of the uterus alone, because although the parametrial tissue completely invests the supravaginal cervix, it is almost non-existent where the peritoneum covers the uterine corpus.

In the non-pregnant state, the cellular tissue between the vaginal vault and the peritoneum is approximately 1 cm thick and is significantly thicker in pregnancy. This extensive increase in cellular tissue in pregnancy means that when exudate tracks along the broad ligament, the whole uterus becomes fixed and is pushed towards the opposite side. When the cellulitis moves posteriorly, rectal examination reveals a horseshoe band of induration around the bowel and in the uterosacral ligaments.

Following completely effective treatment, recovery can be complete with no effects on future fertility. If pus forms, recovery may still be rapid if it can be drained but if it extends into other areas around the uterus, convalescence can be prolonged.

Urinary tract infection

Urinary tract infections account for approximately 40% of all hospital-acquired infections. A total of 75% of patients with urinary infection have predisposing factors such as catheterization (Feingold 1970).

The probability of bacteriuria after catheterization depends on the method of insertion, duration and type of drainage. Between 1 and 5% of patients with single, short-term catheterizations and 50% of patients with intermittent catheterizations develop bacteriuria. The idea that bacteriuria after catheterization is benign and will resolve spontaneously is erroneous.

The mucosal surface of the anterior urethra is normally colonized with bacteria present on the vaginal vestibule and perineum and these can contaminate urine samples used for the diagnosis of urinary tract infection. Significant bacteriuria is defined as greater than 10^5 colony-forming units per ml of a clean-catch midstream urine sample. This definition differentiates between contamination and true infection.

Sweet & Ledger (1973) described significant bacteriuria as one of the most common causes of puerperal fever. The prevalence of postpartum bacteriuria depends on factors such as antepartum urinary infection, catheterization during labour or type of delivery. Impaired glucose metabolism does not seem to be associated with an increased risk of bacteriuria, although diabetic patients do have an increased risk of urinary tract infections.

Catheterization is often performed in women having Caesarean section or epidural anaesthesia, and 15% of women without prior infection develop bacteriuria after catheterization. Although bladder catheterization is necessary before Caesarean section or forceps delivery, routine catheterization of all women in labour is inadvisable.

It is important to distinguish between bladder infection (cystitis) and pyelonephritis. Cystitis may or may not produce significant symptoms or present as frequency of micturition with dysuria. Most individuals respond to the commonly used antimicrobials, but tend to experience relapses during pregnancy if asymptomatic bacteriuria has not been eradicated.

Postpartum pyelonephritis is an important cause of postpartum pyrexia and is more common then than before delivery. *Escherichia coli* is the commonest organism. Unless the urine was already infected at the time of delivery, pyelonephritis characteristically does not appear before the end of the first week. Localizing symptoms are often absent and although cystitis is also present in many cases, there are often no complaints of urinary symptoms. Costovertebral tenderness is actually rather rare in such cases.

The treatment of urinary tract infection in the puerperium is the same as in pregnant or non-pregnant patients. An acute urinary tract infection can usually be eradicated if the appropriate antibiotic is administered in adequate dosage for 5 or more days. The chances of recrudescence, however, are high. While much emphasis has been placed on asymptomatic bacteriuria during pregnancy, it is also essential that postpartum bacteriuria should be adequately treated.

The fact that chronic infection has developed may only be detected later in the postnatal period. Since even 6 months of low-dose therapy with a suitable antibiotic may not provide a permanent cure, careful evaluation is needed to detect predisposing factors such as vesicoureteric reflux or renal scarring. Intravenous pyelography and micturating cystography are required for this type of investigation.

Although *E. coli* accounts for the majority of urinary tract infections, the possibility that other organisms are involved should also be borne in mind. Group B streptococcus, *Staphylococcus aureus, Klebsiella, Enterobacter, Proteus, Pseudomonas* and enterococci can all be isolated in postpartum urinary tract infections. The majority of these organisms are nosocomial pathogens, and such infections are often associated with structural abnormalities of the urinary tract.

Septic pelvic thrombophlebitis

Before antibiotics, septic thrombophlebitis and septic pulmonary emboli were frequently noted at autopsy in patients who died from fulminating puerperal sepsis. Although antibiotics have reduced the frequency of this complication, septic pelvic thrombophlebitis may still be encountered, particularly as a result of protracted and extensive cellulitis spreading to major pelvic veins.

The clinical picture may be confusing; classically, there is marked fluctuation in temperature from recurring dispersion of septic emboli throughout the body. Temperatures may reach 39.5–40.5°C with rigors, although the patient may not appear as ill as the temperature chart suggests. The pulse is consistently rapid.

When septic pelvic thrombophlebitis alone exists, abdominal findings are unimpressive and pain is mild. Pelvic examination is negative and pelvic tenderness, although common, is not marked. Since thrombosed veins are difficult to delineate, septic thrombophlebitis should be suspected in a patient with wide temperature fluctuations, elevated pulse rate and failure to respond to antimicrobial therapy. She need not appear critically ill. Abdominal and pelvic signs and symptoms mainly reflect coexistent pelvic inflammation rather than septic thrombophlebitis. Blood cultures are especially important in suspected pelvic thrombophlebitis, although they often prove negative.

In suspected cases, in addition to antibiotic therapy, a diagnostic trial of intravenous heparin should be administered. Any therapeutic response should be apparent within 48 hours. Therapy should continue for at least 1 week.

An initial loading dose of 5000 units of heparin given slowly in 10–20 ml of diluent over 10–15 minutes should be administered, followed by intravenous infusion of 400–700 units of heparin per kg body weight in 1000 ml of 5% dextrose in water over a 24-hour period.

Careful monitoring of heparin effects on coagulation is the normal way of avoiding the bleeding which is the most common complication of its administration.

Breast infection

During the past decade, breastfeeding has increased as a result of cultural factors, ethnic backgrounds and community attitudes. Prospective parents recognize lactation as the physiological completion of the experience of birth.

The majority of breast infections can be prevented by the successful establishment and maintenance of lactation. Instruction about breastfeeding is an important feature of prenatal classes and the value of human milk as the best neonatal nutrient should be stressed as well as its role in protecting against numerous neonatal infections.

The term mastitis refers to any inflammatory process in the breast, but usually implies acute breast infection during lactation. Sometimes the terms lactational mastitis or puerperal mastitis are used to refer more specifically to this distressing and painful entity. According to Marshall and his associates (1975), approximately 2.5% of nursing mothers develop mammary infections and 4.6% of these progress to a breast abscess.

Breast engorgement

Before describing true infectious mastitis, postpartum breast engorgement must be mentioned. Obstetricians are all familiar with the patient who, on the second or third postpartum day, complains of swollen, tender breasts and has a mild to moderate pyrexia. With nothing more than symptomatic therapy, the condition resolves after a day or so and lactation ensues, if the baby is being suckled. Bacteriological cultures are usually negative. Engorgement differs from true lactation, for while both entities are hormonally activated, engorgement is due to vascular and lymphatic distension and the breasts are now swollen with milk. Lactation, in contrast, depends on the suckling reflex and can occur without any engorgement.

Recently, Almeida & Kitay (1986) conducted a prospective randomized double-blind study in breastfeeding women who had puerperal fever associated with breast engorgement and were treated with bromocriptine mesylate or a placebo. In patients whose lactation was suppressed by bromocriptine within 18 hours of delivery, there was no physiological fever due to breast engorgement. This study is in accord with Roser (1966), who suggested that empiric antibiotic therapy should be withheld in unexplained puerperal pyrexia to avoid iatrogenic interference when the only complication is breast engorgement. The study demonstrates that milk fever is a true physiological entity, since suppression of lactation eliminates it. Thus puerperal fever soon after delivery in women with a normal intrapartum course may be due to physiological breast engorgement.

Infectious mastitis

Breast infection occurs in sporadic and epidemic forms. Over 30 years ago Gibberd (1953) drew attention to the fact that sporadic mastitis involving interlobular connective tissue results in cellulitis of the breast. Sporadic mastitis results from poor nursing technique, breast engorgement and milk stagnation, caused by trauma to the nipple, opening fissures into which micro-organisms migrate through the lactiferous ducts to colonize the milk and produce mammary cellulitis. This usually occurs in the second or third postpartum week, when the mother is at home and all too frequently the obstetrician is unaware of the complication. Patients with mammary cellulitis suffer from pyrexia and tachycardia. The fever may be associated with malaise, headache, anorexia and rigors. Marked systemic symptoms are rare but when a breastfeeding woman presents with an influenza-type syndrome without upper respiratory infection, the possibility of mastitis should be considered.

Epidemic mastitis is associated with mammary adenitis resulting from the introduction of micro-organisms into the mammary duct system. This form of infection usually occurs without cracked nipples and is often acquired in hospital, although it may develop after the woman has been discharged home. Frequently, pus can be expressed from the nipple and the symptomatology is similar to that of mammary cellulitis, although usually less severe. The infection is insidious in onset but has a more protracted course than true mammary cellulitis.

Both types of mastitis are often caused by *Staphylococcus aureus* which inhabits the skin and mucous membranes as a commensal organism. In cases of epidemic mastitis, localized outbreaks should be investigated by epidemiological techniques such as bacteriophage typing.

In addition to staphylococci, which account for most cases of puerperal mastitis, other bacterial species may be encountered, including beta-haemolytic streptococci of Lancefield groups B and F, and less commonly, A. *Streptococcus faecalis*, *Escherichia coli*, *Haemophilus influenzae*, *Klebsiella pneumoniae*, and *Serratia marcescens* may also be involved.

While every mother is not able to breastfeed her baby, 85% of mothers should be able to, given correct help and instruction. Many of the psychological problems about breastfeeding could be eliminated if the physiology of lactation and suckling were understood and lactation encouraged. The most consistent factor in breastfeeding difficulty is engorgement of the breasts and viscidity of the colostrum and milk in the early days after parturition. Both factors make it difficult for milk to escape and obstruction of the milk flow predisposes to breast infection. Prevention consists of teaching the patient during the last months of pregnancy manually to express fluid from her breasts and help circumvent breast infections.

The preferred therapy for breast infections due to *Staphylococcus aureus* is oral penicillin given at a dosage of 250 mg four times daily for at least 7 days, unless the patient is allergic to penicillin, when erythromycin, 250 mg four times daily, may be substituted. If the organism is not suspectible to penicillin a penicillinase-resistant penicillin such as cloxacillin at a dosage of 125 mg four times daily may be prescribed. The penicillinase-resistant penicillins are active against penicillinase- and non-penicillinase-producing strains of *Staphylococcus aureus* and *Staph. epidermidis*. The penicillinase-stable penicillins such as cloxacillin are, however, only indicated for the therapy of proven or suspected penicillin-resistant staphylococcal infections. Since more than 90% of hospital-acquired and 70% of community-acquired staphylococci are resistant to penicillin G, however, penicillinase-stable penicillins should always be considered for staphylococcal mastitis in hospital except in patients allergic to penicillin.

Breastfeeding should be discontinued from the affected breast if there is a purulent exudate or an abscess requiring drainage. If milk stasis seems to be predisposing to the infection, continued breastfeeding should be encouraged to prevent engorgement. If breastfeeding is discontinued, bromocriptine may be required to inhibit lactation although the milk flow usually settles quickly if the baby is not suckling.

If a breast abscess develops it should be drained surgically as soon as possible. Cultures should be obtained from the abscess cavity and antibiotic therapy instituted as for infectious mastitis. Antibiotic therapy without surgical drainage of a breast abscess may result in a chronic, indurated breast mass or antibioma, an indurated honeycomb of small abscess cavities. In this situation, the formation of granulation tissue and fibrosis may lead to permanent deformity of the breast.

THE MICROBIOLOGY OF PUERPERAL INFECTIONS

It is obviously essential to understand the microbiology of puerperal infection in order to prescribe rational therapy. The concept of 'one disease — one micro-organism' is so dominant that even nowadays some physicians insist on knowing which pathogen is causing the infection. While it is a valid question in some infections, it is inappropriate in obstetrical and gynaecological infections. These differ from many other infections treated by internists, in that they are usually of a polymicrobial nature. More than one bacterial species at the site of infection represents a 'mixed infection' but not necessarily synergistic infection. The micro-organisms in postpartum infections will be discussed individually, but their combined effects at the infected site should not be ignored.

Aerobic Gram-positive cocci

Group A streptococci, the organism responsible for the great epidemics of childbed fever in the last century, is no longer responsible for large outbreaks of puerperal sepsis. Yet this organism may still occasionally cause postpartum endometritis. Rarely, it may be cultured from the vagina of asymptomatic women. However, the strains most likely to cause severe infection tend to be exogenously acquired and are rarely encountered in modern obstetrical practice.

In 1935, Lancefield & Hare first isolated group B streptococci from the lower genital tract of puerperal women and in 1938, Fry found this species in vaginal cultures from both asymptomatic and symptomatic women during labour. Despite these early observations, the group B steptococcus was for years regarded as primarily responsible for bovine mastitis and named *Streptococcus agalactiae*. The report of Eickhoff et al (1964) established it as one of the important causes of neonatal meningitis in the USA.

Group B streptococcus has been isolated from the genital tract of 7–20% of gravid patients (Larsen 1985b). It probably colonizes the vagina from a rectal reservoir, although sexual transmission is also possible. Colonization of the lower genital tract is not significantly correlated with obstetric disorders (Baker & Barrett 1973) but there is a possibility of fetal infection with this organism following rupture of the fetal membranes. During the last decade, group B streptococcus has also been recognized as a cause of maternal urinary tract infections (Wood & Dillon 1981).

Colebrook & Purdie (1937) first described systemic maternal infection with the group B streptococcus. During the ensuing 20 years, only three cases of neonatal infection with this organism appeared in the literature compared with 21 cases of maternal sepsis, while in the decade from 1958 to 1968, 82 cases of neonatal sepsis were reported (Parker 1977). Since then the incidence of neonatal and postpartum infections due to this organism has increased greatly in western Europe and the USA.

Recognition of the importance of group B streptococcus as a urinary tract pathogen has occurred relatively recently. Wood & Dillon (1981) found that over 30% of significant bacteriurias in pregnancy were due to this organism and were as common as those due to *Escherichia coli*. Easmon et al (1985) also found group B streptococcus to be urinary tract pathogens in gravid patients; the authors found an association between group B streptococcus in the lower genito-urinary tract and intrapartum pyrexia. Gibbs et al (1982) found the organism to be a major cause of amnionitis and endometritis and Minkoff et al (1982) frequently detected the organism in post-Caesarean section endometritis.

Sutton et al (1985) reported the first case of extensive necrotizing fasciitis arising from an episiotomy. Group B streptococcus and *Staphylococcus aureus* were isolated from the wound. Group B streptococcus has also been found as a cause of infective endocarditis (Backes et al 1985, Gallagher & Watanakunakorn 1986). This condition is more often associated with the *viridans* group of streptococci or group D streptococcus.

Streptococci belonging to Lancefield's group D are frequent inhabitants of the vagina but their role in puerperal infections has not been established. They have been associated with endocarditis and occasionally with bacteraemia and endometritis. The role of these organisms is difficult to assess because they are frequently found in association with other organisms in surgical infections. There is a growing belief that widespread use of cephalosporins, which are generally not active against enterococci, will increase the future significance of these organisms. Jones (1985) found a marked variation in the extent of superinfection with enterococci, with different beta-lactam-type antibiotics. For example, moxalactam was associated with a 2.2–12% rate of enterococcal superinfection, while cefotaxime produced an enterococcal superinfection rate of only 0.1%.

Streptococcus pneumoniae has been reported as a rare cause of puerperal infection. McCarthy & Cho (1979) reported a case of neonatal sepsis and puerperal endometritis where a type III pneumococcus was isolated from both mother and child.

Other streptococci, both alpha-haemolytic and non-haemolytic, are frequently found in the genital tract of healthy women and as a result are commonly recovered as part of the *mélange* of organisms found in puerperal infections. These bacteria are usually considered to have minimal virulence and, as a result, their importance in infectious processes is difficult to assess. The possibility that they may contribute to the symptoms of polymicrobial infection needs to be explored, although a suitable approach to this problem has not been identified.

Of the staphylococci, *Staphylococcus epidermidis* is far more common in the lower genital flora of gravid women than is the more virulent *Staph. aureus* (Goplerud et al 1976). Endometrial infection with *Staph. aureus* is likewise uncommon, so that concern for this organism in planning antibiotic therapy is not paramount. *Staph. aureus* may produce toxic shock syndrome toxic 1 (TSST 1) and cause the toxic shock syndrome in postpartum women. *Staph. epidermidis* does not often appear as the only isolate in puerperal infections and when it occurs with other organisms its role is obscure. It is probably unwise to dismiss it as unimportant, as it can cause serious infections.

Aerobic Gram-negative bacilli

Escherichia coli is the most commonly isolated member of the Enterobacteriaciae family, present in approximately one-third of endocervical cultures from postpartum women, whereas during pregnancy it occurs in 2–11% (Goplerud et al 1976). The increase in the prevalence of *E. coli* which occurs during labour may be important in the pathogenesis of postpartum infection. *E. coli* must be considered if bacteraemia is suspected in the postpartum patient. It remains an important pathogen in postpartum infection, although it has been isolated less frequently during the past decade.

Goplerud et al (1976) reported that a variety of other organisms increase in prevalence in the early puerperium. This applies to *Klebsiella*, *Enterobacter* and *Proteus*, which are however less common in vaginal cultures than *E. coli*. Gram-negative rods other than *E. coli* are relatively uncommon causes of postpartum sepsis. *Pseudomonas* is even less common and more likely to be exogenously acquired when it occurs in an obstetrical unit.

Gardnerella vaginalis has been identified in blood cultures from postpartum women. Its more conventional setting is as a member of the vaginal flora or in association with bacterial vaginosis which is characterized by a significant overgrowth of vaginal anaerobes. The apparent symbiotic relationship of *G. vaginalis* with anaerobic bacteria and its occasional presence in blood cultures suggests that it may have a synergistic role with anaerobic bacteria in the puerperal uterus.

Anaerobic bacteria

Ledger et al (1975) reported that anaerobic bacteria can be isolated from the blood of approximately one-third of women with postpartum sepsis. Anaerobes are consistently isolated from endometrial samples in a large proportion of patients with postpartum sepsis. Peptococci and peptostreptococci are the most commonly isolated anaerobes from the uterus in endometritis cases, reflecting their high prevalence in the normal flora of the lower genital tract. These and other anaerobic species infect and grow in necrotic deciduae, producing a purulent, foul-smelling lochia.

As a class, anaerobic organisms often exist in devitalized tissue. Tissue lacking blood supply and oxygen becomes increasingly anaerobic and, as the tissue begins to die from anoxia, acidosis develops and the oxidation reduction potential decreases. This environment is excellent for the growth of anaerobic organisms; the coexistence of facultative species which utilize oxygen further enhances anaerobiosis. Thus, in mixed infections and those involving anaerobic bacteria, infection may occur without special virulence factors being required by the micro-organisms. Rather their proliferation depends on conditions which are specially conducive to their growth. Anaerobic organisms such as the clostridia possess a panoply of virulence factors; growing in suitable conditions and producing microbial toxins, they can have devastating consequences. Retained products of conception represent a very suitable medium for the growth of anaerobic organisms which normally inhabit the lower genital tract.

During the past decade increasing attention has been given to *Bacteroides* spp. which proliferate in traumatized and devitalized tissues. They produce a foul odour and predispose to protracted illness complicated by septic pelvic thrombophlebitis and, occasionally, septic pulmonary emboli. *Bacteroides bivius* is the most commonly isolated Gram-negative anaerobe cultured from women with postpartum sepsis. It is more common than either *B. disiens* or *B. fragilis*, which may also be found in serious cases of postpartum infection. Other Gram-negative anaerobic rods such as *Fusobacterium* spp. are occasionally found in cultures from women with postpartum infection.

Clostridium perfringens occurs in endocervical cultures of fewer than 5% of asymptomatic women. It is therefore occasionally responsible for puerperal endometritis but usually responds to prompt therapy. Detecting the organism in a patient who is getting better should not cause alarm. The danger of uterine gangrene must be recognized although the presence of clostridia is not synonymous with this grave complication. Failure to treat adequately non-gangrenous anaerobic infection with clostridia may lead to the serious complication of haemolytic anaemia and renal failure, as the infectious process extends beyond the endometrium and uterus. Signs of progressive infection, including uterine gas formation, haemolysis, hypotension, hyperbilirubinaemia or renal failure, should be met with prompt surgical exploration and removal of the infected uterus.

Genital mycoplasmas

Mycoplasma hominis and *Ureaplasma urealyticum* are commonly isolated from the genital tract of gravid patients. They serve as markers of sexual activity and relate to the number of sexual partners. Mycoplasmaemia is common immediaely after birth. McCormack et al (1975) isolated mycoplasmas from the blood of 15% of patients immediately after delivery, but in only 8% 10 minutes after and in only 2% 20 minutes after. Harrison et al (1983) have demonstrated an abundance of other vaginal pathogens associated with mycoplasmas, which makes it difficult to establish the significance of the mycoplasmas in comparison with other organisms.

The recovery of *M. hominis* after delivery is associated with low antibody levels. Platt et al (1980) reported that postpartum fever occurred in 40% of women with a 1:8 antibody titre to *M. hominis* but in only 14% of those with higher titres. The importance of *M. hominis* in postpartum fever was strengthened by finding significant antibody titre rises in women with otherwise unexplained febrile morbidity. Young nulligravid women are probably especially susceptible to postpartum *Mycoplasma* infection (Lamey et al 1982), possibly because they lack protective antibody. However, such patients usually only have mild symptoms and signs and are not seriously ill.

Wallace et al (1978) reported that 7 of 8 patients whose mild uterine tenderness and fever were considered to be due to infection with mycoplasmas became afebrile when antibiotics which did not inhibit *M. hominis* were administered. It is possible that postpartum infection involving *Mycoplasma* may be analogous to *M. pneumoniae* lung infections in which specific antibiotic therapy is often not necessary.

Chlamydia trachomatis

Chlamydia trachomatis may be the most common sexually transmitted infection. It is a strictly intracellular parasite which colonizes columnar mucosal epithelium. The infection it causes does not always produce symptoms. It has a long incubation period and usually causes minimal, localized clinical symptoms, contributing to diagnostic and therapeutic delays. *C. trachomatis* is now well established as an aetiological agent in endometritis and salpingitis (Mardh et al 1981) and a frequent cause of puerperal infection. Osser & Persson (1982) showed that it could cause postabortal pelvic infection. Within 1 month of induced abortion, 90 of 1101 women (8.2%) developed infection, 75 developed endometritis and 15 developed salpingitis. Of 60 women who had positive cultures for *Chlamydia*, endometritis developed in 16 and salpingitis in 10.

Paavonen et al (1985) indicated that despite the frequent presence of endometritis in postabortal and postpartum patients, pathologists may find it difficult to identify the aetiology from the curettings. There is some question as to the role of coexistent micro-organisms in the infected uterus. In the study of Paavonen et al, none in the *Chlamydia* group had mycoplasmas isolated, whereas in the non-*Chlamydia* group, *Ureaplasma urealyticum* was isolated from three women and *Mycoplasma hominis* from four. *Chlamydia* was the most prevalent isolate and may have been responsible for differences between the groups.

Harrison et al (1983) studied *Chlamydia* and *Mycoplasma* infections prospectively in pregnancy and found that 2.9% of positive women developed endometritis or postpartum fever. The prevalence among vaginal deliveries was significantly lower than among Caesarean deliveries (1.8 versus 9%). Among women who delivered vaginally, endometritis and fever correlated with black ethnicity and *Mycoplasma hominis* infection. Although risks of postpartum fever and endometritis were increased with *C. trachomatis* and *Ureaplasma urealyticum*, they were much less than with *Mycoplasma* and not statistically significant.

C. trachomatis is less commonly responsible for postpartum endometritis than the conventional bacteria which represent the indigenous biota of the lower female genital tract. Nevertheless, since antibiotics usually chosen for therapy of postpartum sepsis often lack activity against *Chlamy-*

dia, cervical cultures for *C. trachomatis* should be obtained from women with late-onset infection, especially women whose infants have had conjuctivitis or pneumonitis. Wager et al (1980) reviewed the postpartum course of women who had cervical *C. trachomatis* prior to delivery. A late, and usually mild, episode of postpartum endometritis occurred from 3 days to 6 weeks in 22% of the women with a positive culture but in only 5% of those without.

C. trachomatis is known to cause pelvic inflammatory disease by spreading from the endometrium to the Fallopian tubes. It is also responsible for perihepatitis among women with acute salpingitis (Fitz-Hugh-Curtis syndrome), a condition formerly thought to be only associated with gonococcal infection. Future studies should investigate the intrauterine environment both in the puerperium as well as in the various stages of the menstrual cycle, in order to discover the nature of the defences against chlamydial infection during the various stages of a woman's reproductive life.

DIAGNOSTIC CONSIDERATIONS

The uterus of any woman delivered by Caesarean section is tender even without infection. Malodorous lochia may be the result of infection, but this is not invariably so. Reduction of lochia 6–12 hours before the onset of fever is noted in some patients, but this is not a diagnostic feature of puerperal infection. Laboratory tests such as leukocyte counts may not be helpful because most postpartum patients have a moderate leukocytosis in any case.

The most useful diagnostic tests are adequate and timely bacteriological cultures, although they may be difficult to obtain in postpartum women. Endocervical cultures will reveal the flora which contain the organisms involved in the infectious process. They may fail to reveal which organisms are actually responsible for the uterine infection. Culture of the endometrium by means of a double-lumen catheter designed to avoid contamination by the endocervical flora has been reported (Pezzlo et al 1979) and provides more useful data for the management of the infection. However, no uterine sampling device can exclude all risks of endocervical contamination, although contamination is greatly reduced. Cervical and endometrial cultures can include organisms such as group A or B beta-haemolytic streptococci or *Neisseria gonorrhoeae*.

Attention should not be solely focused on the uterus to the neglect of other sites. Urine and blood cultures should be obtained. Blood cultures may be vital for the seriously ill patient who is not responding to the antibiotic therapy selected.

Cultures should be obtained before antimicrobial therapy is started. The possible presence of anaerobic bacteria should be considered when collecting and transporting specimens to the laboratory and in requesting anaerobic as well as aerobic cultures. Many laboratories will not process vaginal or cervical specimens because they contain normal flora and the significance of the organisms is impossible to determine. Therefore, if a culture of the endocervix is sent to the laboratory, it should be accompanied by an explanation of what is required. Direct discussion with the laboratory will often be most valuable.

Endometrial culture techniques

Cultures obtained from the cervix of women with postpartum endometritis are of limited value because such specimens will always contain many bacterial species which may not be related to the uterine infection. While Ledger et al (1976) used transfundal needle aspiration to avoid contamination by endocervical micro-organisms, negative cultures sometimes resulted from the needle missing the endometrial cavity.

Despite this, Knuppel et al (1981) showed that the endometrial cavity culture can sometimes be taken transcervically because the concentration of bacteria in an infected uterus is so high. These authors used telescoping teflon catheters housing a nylon bristle brush and retractable wire in the inner cannula. The housing was a 40 cm 10 French cannula containing a distal occluding plug made of polyethylene glycol. After passing the device into the uterus the brush was advanced to obtain the specimen, retracted and transected from the attached wire and placed into the appropriate media. In non-surgical patients, transcervical culture techniques appear to be most appropriate.

Gibbs et al (1975) passed a transcervical catheter to obtain samples by injecting the uterus with Ringer's lactate, but the results were unhelpful.

Duff et al (1983) compared four techniques for obtaining endometrial cultures from puerperal women and found careful transcervical samples could apparently reduce, but not eliminate, endometrial contamination with endocervical organisms.

Endometrial culture techniques should be accompanied by blood culture, complete blood count, urinalysis and urine culture. Positive blood cultures usually migrate in the uterus, although the organisms detected in the blood may represent only one of the species in the uterus. Chlamydial culture should be obtained from uterine specimens if culture techniques are available, as well as culture for *Mycoplasma*, although not all laboratories have the facilities to do so.

Using extremely sophisticated sampling techniques, Eschenbach et al (1986) and Rosene et al (1986) found that the cultures from afebrile controls produced only low numbers of low-virulence organisms, while in febrile patients 93% of samples grew pathogens such as *Gardnerella vaginalis*, *Peptococcus* spp. *Bacteroides* spp., *Staphylococcus epidermidis*, group B streptococcus and *Ureaplasma urealyticum*. In women with endometritis, 76% had genital mycoplasmas, but only 16% had genital mycoplasmas without other bacteria. Only 2% of cultures contained *C. trachomatis*.

WOUND INFECTIONS

Abdominal wound factors following abdominal delivery may cause considerable pain, extended hospitalization and occasionally wound dehiscence. The risk of postoperative wound sepsis is related to the extent of bacterial contamination at the time of surgery (Cruse & Foord 1973). Wound infections usually appear before the woman leaves hospital, usually within the first week. A minority are asymptomatic at this time but usually develop within 3 weeks.

Staphylococci are responsible for most superficial wound infections involving sutures. Usually exogenous, they occasionally present as multiple-resistant staphylococci. Anaerobic organisms may also be present in abdominal wound infections together with mixed Gram-negative organisms. Identification of the organisms involved is essential.

Every attempt should be made to prevent wound infection by careful aseptic technique without relying unduly on prophylactic antibiotics. Non-absorbable sutures are best for skin closure. If there is infection at the time of surgery, copious irrigation of the wound during closure is essential. If a wound does become infected, adequate drainage is the first and most important aspect of management, sometimes necessitating removal of one or two stitches. The whole superficial part of the wound may need to be opened and packed with hypochlorite(Ensol)-soaked gauze two or three times daily and irrigated as well if there is much sloughing. As soon as the dressing need only be changed once daily the patient may be allowed home to the care of the community nurse and general practitioner.

Drainage remains the keystone of management of established wound infections. Antibiotic therapy may also be essential, especially in patients who are toxic, immunosuppressed, have been on corticosteroid treatment, or have extensive cellulitis around the wound.

NECROTIZING INFECTIONS

Clostridial myositis and other gangrenous soft-tissue infections are fulminating and potentially life-threatening, being associated with profound toxicity and a high mortality. Deep infections include gas gangrene of the uterus or the abdominal wall, synergistic necrotizing fasciitis and streptococcal myositis. Prompt diagnosis, aggressive surgical debridement with an appropriate antimicrobial and general supportive treatment are essential because of the fulminating and rapidly spreading nature of these infections. More superficial infections, such as haemolytic streptococcal gangrene, are associated with a lower mortality than deep infections, but still require extensive debridement and cause considerable morbidity.

With these infections, clinical findings and bacterial cultures can be deceptive and the presence of clostridia in cultures from the postpartum uterus is not in itself ominous. The presence of clostridia coupled with clinical signs of a rapidly progressing invasive suppurative process is however extremely serious. Although the microaerophilic streptococci and staphylococci which seem to induce fulminating necrotizing fasciitis have no particular distinguishing microbiological features, they should be regarded as causal when isolated together in the symptomatic patient. These rapidly invasive factors can complicate episiotomies (Golde & Ledger 1977, Shy & Eschenbach 1979). Pudendal block anaesthesia has been complicated by necrotizing fasciitis in conjunction with a retropsoas abscess (Hibbard et al 1972).

ANTIBIOTIC THERAPY FOR PUERPERAL INFECTION

Antibiotic therapy for profound infection is similar to that prescribed for other infections of the female genital tract. Uterine infections usually involve aerobic and anaerobic organisms such as *Bacteroides bivius*. Usually cultures are not available when treatment is instituted. Effective empirical therapy is required. Combined therapy with an aminoglycoside and clindamycin is usually appropriate.

Broad-spectrum beta-lactam antibiotics, effective against enteric and most of the anaerobic species involved in female genital tract sepsis, have become popular because they lack the ototoxicity and nephrotoxicity associated with the aminoglycosides, although they have been associated with hypersensitivity reactions. Not all are active against anaerobic organisms.

Anaerobic organisms may be treated by drugs such as clindamycin, metronidazole and cefoxitin as well as some of the third-generation cephalosporins such as Moxalactam. Gram-negative enteric bacteria may be treated effectively by aminoglycosides, third-generation cephalosporins such as cefotaxime, the uriedopenicillins, or trimethoprim–sulphamethoxazole. Specific treatment for purely *Pseudomonas* infection is rarely required. The choice of treatment is influenced by the organisms detected and the severity of the infection; discussion between obstetrician and microbiologist can be of great value in difficult cases.

Antibiotic dosage is important. In about 50% of puerperal patients treated with gentamycin, therapeutic levels were not altered in serum following a standard dose based on weight (Zaske et al 1980). Altered pharmacokinetics of beta-lactam antibiotics during pregnancy persist into the puerperium (Charles & Larsen 1985, 1986). Table 63.4 shows the findings in puerperal patients. When these drugs are used to treat puerperal sepsis, therefore, more frequent administration may be necessary to attain an adequate response.

Antibiotics may be transferred to the infant in breast milk, although only with cephalosporins to a very small extent.

Table 63.4 Comparison of serum pharmacokinetic parameters in women in the puerperium and 4–6 months later

	Percentage decrease (increase) in the puerperium compared with controls			
Pharmacokinetic parameter	Piperacillin ($n = 3$)	Cefotaxime ($n = 6$)	Moxalactam ($n = 6$)	Cefoperazone ($n = 6$)
Serum level (μg/ml) 15 minutes postinfusion 1 g drug i.v.*	59.3	42.4	41.0	32.9
Volume of distribution (litres)	32.5	(98.7)	(66.2)	(48.7)
Total body clearance (litres/hour)	(1.1)	(73.7)	(73.8)	(48.7)
Half-life (hours)	33.5	(15.8)	4.6	0.7
Area under the curve time 0–infinity (μg . h/ml)	1.34	42.4	42.8	32.6

* Piperacillin levels were measured at 30 minutes instead of 15 minutes as for the other drugs.

ANTIBIOTIC PROPHYLAXIS FOR CAESAREAN SECTION

Many controlled trials have demonstrated that prophylactic antibiotic administration can reduce the incidence of surgical infections. The greatest benefit of prophylaxis is in cases where the risk of postoperative sepsis is very high or the consequences of infection are grave. Prophylaxis given after operation is ineffective. Burke (1961) demonstrated the vital importance of commencing prophylactic antibiotics before operation and continuing for only a brief perioperative period, usually no more than the day of surgery, although some continue for 48 hours.

The use of prophylactic antibiotics with Caesarean section has always been controversial because if the drug is begun before operation the fetus also receives it. An effective compromise is to administer the antibiotic only after the cord has been clamped.

Antibiotics given after cord-clamping should be administered by infusion over a 20-minute period because administration of a cephalosporin in an intravenous bolus has resulted in death from cardiovascular collapse (Spruill et al 1974). In badly infected cases an alternative to intravenous administration is peritoneal lavage; effectiveness may depend not only on the topical action but also on it being absorbed from the peritoneal cavity (Duff et al 1982). By contrast, however, Conover & Moore (1984) found antibiotic peritoneal lavage was less effective than intravenous administration.

Antibiotic prophylaxis is not indicated in elective Caesarean section unless the membranes have been ruptured for more than 12 hours, especially if pelvic examinations have been performed. Prophylactic antibiotics are never a substitute for meticulous aseptic operative technique and careful clinical observation for signs of postpartum infection.

REFERENCES

Almeida O D Jr, Kitay D Z 1986 Lactation suppression and puerperal fever. American Journal of Obstetrics and Gynecology 154: 940–941

Apuzzio J J, Reyelt C, Pelosi M, Sen P, Louria D B 1982 Prophylactic antibiotics for cesarean section: comparison of high and low risk patients for endometritis. Obstetrics and Gynecology 59: 693–698

Backes R J, Wilson W R, Geraci J E 1985 Group B streptococcal endocarditis. Archives of Internal Medicine 145: 693–696

Baker C J, Barrett F F 1973 Transmission of group B streptococci among parturient women and their neonates. Journal of Pediatrics 83: 919–925

Baker C J, Kasper D L 1976 Correlation of maternal antibody deficiency with susceptibility to neonatal group B streptococcal infection. New England Journal of Medicine 294: 753–756

Blanco J D, Gibbs R S, Castaneda Y S 1981 Bacteremia in obstetrics: clinical course. Obstetrics and Gynecology 58: 621–625

Buchanan T M, Eschenbach D A, Knall J S, Holmes K K 1980 Gonococcal salpingitis is less likely to recur with *Neisseria gonorrhoeae* of the same principal outer membrane antigenic type. American Journal of Obstetrics and Gynecology 138: 978–980

Burke J F 1961 The effective period of preventing antibiotic action in experimental incisions and dermal lesions. Surgery 50: 161–168

Charles D, Larsen B 1985 The pharmacokinetics of piperacillin in the postpartum patient. Gynecologic and Obstetric Investigation 20: 194–198

Charles D, Larsen B 1986 The pharmacokinetics of cefotaxime, Moxalactam, and cephoperazone in the early puerperium. Antimicrobial Agents and Chemotherapy 29: 873–876

Colebrook L 1946 The control of infection in obstetrics. Journal of Obstetrics and Gynaecology of the British Commonwealth 53: 114–124

Colebrook L, Purdie A W 1937 Treatment of 106 cases of puerperal fever by sulphanilamide (Streptocide). Lancet ii: 1237–1240

Conover W B, Moore T R 1984 Comparison of irrigation and intravenous antibiotic prophylaxis at cesarean section. Obstetrics and Gynecology 63: 787–791

Cruse P J E, Foord R 1973 A 5 year prospective study of 23 649 surgical wounds. Archives of Surgery 107: 206–210

Duff P, Keiser J F, Strong S L 1982 A comparative study of two antibiotic regimens for the treatment of operative site infections. American Journal of Obstetrics and Gynecology 142: 996–1003

Duff P, Gibbs R S, Blanco J D, St Clair P J 1983 Endometrial culture techniques in puerperal patients. Obstetrics and Gynecology 61: 217–222

Easmon C S F, Hastings M J G, Neill J, Bloxham B, Rivers R P A 1985 Is group B streptococcal screening during pregnancy justified? British Journal of Obstetrics and Gynaecology 92: 197–201

Eickhoff T C, Klein J O, Daly A K, Ingall D, Finland M 1964 Neonatal sepsis and other infections due to group B beta-hemolytic streptococci. New England Journal of Medicine 271: 1221–1228

Eschenbach D A, Rosene K, Tompkins L S, Watkins H, Gravett M G 1986 Endometrial cultures obtained by a triple-lumen method from afebrile and febrile postpartum women. Journal of Infectious Diseases 153: 1038–1045

Feingold D S 1970 Hospital-acquired infections. New England Journal of Medicine 283: 1384–1391

Fry R M 1938 Fatal infections by haemolytic streptococcus group B. Lancet i: 199–201

Gallagher P G, Watanakunakorn C 1986 Group B streptococcal endocarditis: report of seven cases and review of the literature, 1962–1985. Reviews of Infectious Disease 8: 175–188

Gibberd G F 1953 Sporadic and epidemic puerperal breast infections: a contrast in morbid anatomy and clinical signs. American Journal of Obstetrics and Gynecology 65: 1038–1041

Gibbs R S, O'Dell T N, MacGregor R R, Schwarz R H, Morton H 1975

Puerperal endometritis: a prospective microbiologic study. American Journal of Obstetrics and Gynecology 121: 919–925
Gibbs R S, Blanco J D, St Clair P J, Castaneda Y S 1982 Vaginal colonization with resistant aerobic bacteria after antibiotic therapy for endometritis. American Journal of Obstetrics and Gynecology 142: 130–134
Golde S, Ledger W J 1977 Necrotizing fasciitis in postpartum patients. Obstetrics and Gynecology 50: 670–673
Goplerud C P, Ohm M J, Galask R P 1976 Aerobic and anaerobic flora of the cervix during pregnancy and the puerperium. American Journal of Obstetrics and Gynecology 126: 858–868
Gordon A 1795 A treatise on the epidemic puerperal fever of Aberdeen. Robinson, London
Haley R W, Culver D H, White J W, Morgan W M, Emori T G 1985a The national nosocomial infection rate: a need for vital statistics. American Journal of Epidemiology 121: 159–167
Haley R W, Morgan W M, Culver D H et al 1985b Update from the SENIC project. Hospital infection control: recent progress and opportunities under prospective payment. American Journal of Infection Control 13: 97–108
Harrison H R, Alexander E R, Weinstein L, Lewis M, Nash M, Sim D A 1983 Cervical *Chlamydia trachomatis* and mycoplasmal infections in pregnancy. Journal of the American Medical Association 250: 1721–1727
Hibbard L T, Snyder E N, McVann R M 1972 Subgluteal and retropsoal infection in obstetrical practice. Obstetrics and Gynecology 39: 137–150
Holmes O W 1843 The contagiousness of puerperal fever. New England Quarterly Journal of Medicine and Surgery 1: 503–530
Humphrey M D 1972 Postpartum infection: a survey. Medical Journal of Australia 2: 657–659
Jewett J F, Reid D E, Safon L E, Easterday C L 1968 Childbed fever — a continuing entity. Journal of the American Medical Association 206: 344–350
Jones R N 1985 Gram positive superinfections following beta-lactam chemotherapy: the significance of the enterococcus. Infection 13 (suppl 1): s81–s88
Kass E H 1971 Infectious diseases and social change. Journal of Infectious Disease 123: 110–114
Knuppel R A, Scerbo J C, Mitchell G W, Cetrulo C L, Bartlett J 1981 Quantitative transcervical uterine cultures with a new device. Obstetrics and Gynecology 57: 243–248
Koh K S, Chan F H, Monfared A H, Ledger W J, Paul R H 1979 The changing perinatal and maternal outcome in chorioamnionitis. Obstetrics and Gynecology 53: 730–734
Lamey J R, Eschenbach D A, Mitchell S H, Blumhagen J M, Foy H M, Kenny G E 1982 Isolation of mycoplasmas and bacteria from the blood of postpartum women. American Journal of Obstetrics and Gynecology 143: 104–112
Lancefield R C, Hare R 1935 The serological differentiation of pathogenic and non-pathogenic strains of haemolytic streptococci from parturient women. Journal of Experimental Medicine 61: 335–349
Lansing D I, Penman W R, Davis D J 1983 Puerperal fever and the group B beta-hemolytic streptococcus. Bulletin of the History of Medicine 57: 70–80
Larsen B 1983 Host defense in obstetrics and gynaecology. Clinical Obstetrics and Gynecology 10: 37–64
Larsen B 1985a Host defences against intrauterine infection. In: Keith L G, Berger G S, Edelman D A (eds) Infections in reproductive health: common infections. Medical Technical Publishing, Lancaster, pp 33–48
Larsen B 1985b Normal genital microflora 1985. In: Keith L G, Berger, G S, Edelman D A (eds) Infections in reproductive health: common infections. Medical Technical Publishing, Lancaster, pp 3–32
Ledger W J, Headington J T 1972 Group A beta-hemolytic streptococcus: an important cause of serious infections in obstetrics and gynecology. Obstetrics and Gynecology 39: 474–482
Ledger W J, Norman M, Gee C, Lewis W 1975 Bacteremia on an obstetric–gynecologic service. American Journal of Obstetrics and Gynecology 121: 205–212
Ledger W J, Gee C L, Pollin P A 1976 A new approach to patients with suspected anaerobic postpartum infections. Transabdominal uterine aspiration for culture and metronidazole for treatment. American Journal of Obstetrics and Gynecology 126: 1–6
Mardh P-A, Moller B R, Ingerslev H J, Nussler E, Westrom L, Wolner-Hanssen P 1981 Endometritis caused by *Chlamydia trachomatis*. British Journal of Venereal Disease 57: 191–195
Marshall B R, Hepper J K, Zirbel C C 1975 Sporadic puerperal mastitis. An infection that need not interrupt lactation. Journal of the American Medical Association 233: 1377–1379
McCarthy V P, Cho C T 1979 Endometritis and neonatal sepsis due to *Streptococcus pneumoniae*. Obstetrics and Gynecology 53 (suppl): 475–495
McCormack W M, Rosner B, Lee Y-H, Rankin J S 1975 Isolation of genital mycoplasmas from blood obtained shortly after vaginal delivery. Lancet i: 596–599
Minkoff H L, Sierra M F, Pringle G F, Schwarz R H 1982 Vaginal colonization with group B streptococcus as a risk factor for postcesarean section febrile morbidity. American Journal of Obstetrics and Gynecology 142: 992–995
Osser S, Persson K 1982 Epidemiologic and serodiagnostic aspects of chlamydial salpingitis. Obstetrics and Gynecology 59: 206–209
Paavonen J, Kivat N, Brunham R C et al 1985 Prevalence and manifestations of endometritis among women with cervicitis. American Journal of Obstetrics and Gynecology 152: 280–286
Parker M T 1977 Neonatal streptococcal infections. Postgraduate Medical Journal 53: 598–600
Pezzlo M T, Hesser J W, Morgan T, Valter P J, Thrupp L D 1979 Improved laboratory efficiency and diagnostic accuracy with new double-lumen protected swab for endometrial specimens. Journal of Clinical Microbiology 9: 56–59
Platt R, Warren J W, Edelin K C, Lin J, Rosner B, McCormack W M 1980 Infection with *Mycoplasma hominis* in postpartum fever. Lancet ii: 1217–1221
Prema K, Ramalakshmi B A, Madhaveapeddi R, Babu S 1982 Immune status of anaemic pregnant women. British Journal of Obstetrics and Gynaecology 89: 222–225
Ramsay A M, Gillespie M 1941 Puerperal infection associated with haemolytic streptococci other than group A. Journal of Obstetrics and Gynaecology of the British Empire 48: 569–586
Rehu M, Haukkamaa M 1980 Puerperal endometritis and intrauterine fetal heart rate monitoring. Annals of Clinical Research 12: 133–135
Report on Confidential Enquiries into Maternal Deaths in England and Wales 1973–1975. Her Majesty's Stationery Office, London
Rosene K, Eschenbach D A, Tompkins L S, Kenny G E, Watkins H 1986 Polymicrobial early postpartum endometritis with facultative and anaerobic bacteria, genital mycoplasmas and *Chlamydia trachomatis:* treatment with piperacillin or cefoxitin. Journal of Infectious Disease 153: 1028–1036
Roser D M 1966 Breast engorgement and postpartum fever. Obstetrics and Gynecology 27: 73–77
Rubenstein A 1983 Subtle poison: the puerperal fever controversy in Victorian Britain. Historical Studies of Medicine 20: 420–438
Seligman S A, Willis A T 1980 Infection with non-sporing anaerobes in obstetrics and gynaecology. British Journal of Obstetrics and Gynaecology 87: 846–855
Semmelweis I P 1861 The etiology, the concept and prophylaxis. Excerpts cited in 1981 Reviews of Infectious Disease 3: 808–811
Shy K K, Eschenbach D A 1979 Fatal perineal cellulitis from an episiotomy site. Obstetrics and Gynecology 54: 292–298
Spruill F G, Minette L J, Sturner W Q 1974 Two surgical deaths associated with cephalothin. Journal of the American Medical Association 229: 440–441
Stevenson C S, Beheny C A, Miller N F 1967 Maternal death from puerperal sepsis following cesarean section. A 16 year study in Michigan. Obstetrics and Gynecology 29: 181–191
Sutton G P, Smirz L R, Clark D H, Bennett J E 1985 Group B streptococcal necrotizing fasciitis arising from an episiotomy. Obstetrics and Gynecology 66: 733–736
Sweet R L, Ledger W J 1973 Puerperal infectious morbidity — a two year review. American Journal of Obstetrics and Gynecology 117: 1093–1100
Swenson R M, Michaelson T C, Daly M J, Spaulding E H 1973 Anaerobic infections of the female genital tract. Obstetrics and Gynecology 42: 538–541
Vartian C, Lerner P I, Shales D M, Gopalakrishna K V 1985 Infections due to Lancefield group G streptococci. Medicine 64: 75–88
Wager G P, Martin D H, Koutsky L et al 1980 Puerperal infectious morbidity: relationship to route of delivery and antepartum *Chlamydia*

trachomatis infection. American Journal of Obstetrics and Gynecology 138: 1028–1033
Wallace R J Jr, Alpert S, Browne K, Lin J S-L, McCormack W M 1978 Isolation of *Mycoplasma hominis* from blood cultures in patients with postpartum fever. Obstetrics and Gynecology 51: 181–185
Watson B P 1928 An outbreak of puerperal sepsis in New York City. American Journal of Obstetrics and Gynecology 16: 157–179
Watson R 1842 Lectures on the principles and practise of physic. Delivered at King's College, London. London Medical Gazette (NS) 1: 801–808
Wood E G, Dillon H C Jr 1981 A prospective study of group B streptococcal bacteriuria in pregnancy. American Journal of Obstetrics and Gynecology 140: 515–520
Yonekura M L 1985 Risk factors for postcesarean endomyometritis. American Journal of Medicine 78 (suppl 6B): 177–187
Zaaijman J T, Wilkinson A R, Keeling J W 1982 Spontaneous premature rupture of the membranes: bacteriology, histology and neonatal outcome. Journal of Obstetrics and Gynaecology of the British Commonwealth 2: 155–160
Zaske D E, Cipolle R J, Strate R G, Malo J W, Koszalka M E Jr 1980 Rapid gentamicin elinimation in obstetric patients. Obstetrics Gynecology 56: 559–564

64

John Bonnar

Venous thrombosis and pulmonary embolism in pregnancy and the puerperium

INTRODUCTION

Thrombosis is the process by which liquid blood flowing through the vascular system turns into a solid mass of platelets, cells and fibrin within the blood vessel. The most serious vascular complication that can arise during pregnancy or the puerperium is venous thrombosis with pulmonary embolism. As maternal deaths from haemorrhage, eclampsia and sepsis have decreased over the last 30 years, pulmonary embolism has become a leading cause of maternal mortality in many obstetric services. Over the 30-year period from 1952 to 1981, the Confidential Enquiries into Maternal Deaths in England and Wales recorded nearly 1000 maternal deaths from pulmonary embolism. Since 1970, pulmonary embolism has ranked as the first or second most important cause of maternal death in England and Wales (Department of Health and Social Security 1986).

Since the majority of patients with pulmonary embolism die within 1 hour without diagnosis and treatment, the number of deaths will not be greatly reduced by improvements in treatment of the established condition. Pulmonary embolism is likely to remain a major cause of maternal death until significant advances are made both in early detection of thrombotic process and in prevention of thromboembolism. Deaths from pulmonary embolism can be kept to a minimum by more attention to predisposing factors and to selective use of effective prophylactic measures in all high-risk patients, especially in late pregnancy and the early puerperium. Thromboembolism, although the most serious complication of venous thrombosis, is only one part of the clinical problem. For many women oedema, pain, eczema and ulceration of the legs due to chronic venous insufficiency are a legacy of leg vein thrombosis associated with pregnancy.

The accurate diagnosis of venous thrombosis and pulmonary embolism is of vital importance in pregnancy. Besides the immediate threat to the mother and the possible hazards to the fetus of treatment, the diagnosis of thrombosis has long-term implications for the woman — the wisdom of having any further pregnancies and the need for prophylaxis therein, the use of the combined pill, oestrogen replacement at and after the menopause and the increased risks of future surgery.

The diagnostic problem usually lies with the less dramatic forms of the disease. It is less common to find classic presentation of iliofemoral thrombosis with a white leg (phlegmasia alba dolens) and the extreme form with intense swelling of the leg, deep cyanosis and diminished arterial pulses, with or without impending gangrene (phlegmasia caerulea dolens). The reduction of incidence of these conditions is most likely a result of the improvement in the general health of pregnant women, younger mothers and lower parity, recognition of the dangers of bedrest during pregnancy and especially after delivery, the use of prophylactic measures and the early diagnosis and treatment of the disease. Thromboembolic disease is best decribed by the term venous thrombosis, specifying the segments of the venous system involved and with pulmonary embolism as its major complication.

PATHOGENESIS OF VENOUS THROMBOSIS IN PREGNANCY

The basis for much of our understanding of the genesis of venous thrombosis was described in the mid 19th century by Virchow (1860). He postulated a triad of factors which predisposed to thrombosis:

1. Impaired blood flow resulting in venous stasis.
2. Changes in the blood coagulability.
3. Alteration or damage to the intima of the vein.

(a)

(b)

(c)

(d)

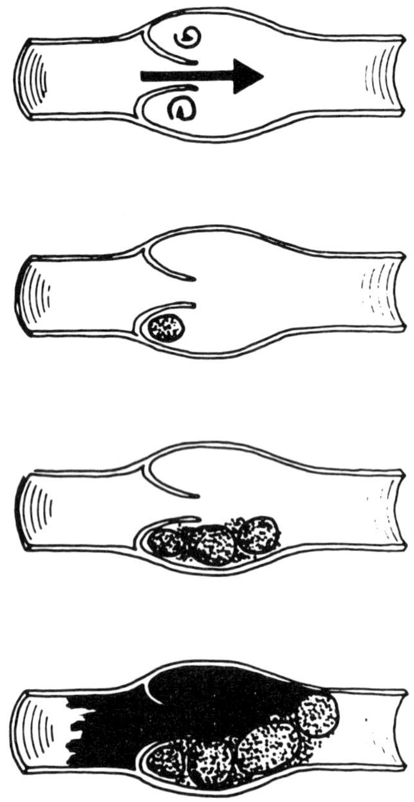

Fig. 64.1 Stages in the development of a thrombus in the valve pocket. (**a**) Vortex flow in the venous valve pocket results in an area of maximum stasis with local accumulation of activated clotting factors, platelets, leukocytes and red blood cells. (**b**) Following thrombin generation a platelet fibrin nidus forms, consisting of successive alternate layers of aggregated platelets and fibrin. (**c**) Platelet–fibrin aggregates develop on the propagating head of the thrombus and lead to thrombus growth. (**d**) Retrograde extension of the thrombus occurs when the forward propagating thrombus grows to occlude the vein. From Thomas (1987).

Changes in the vessel wall are now recognized as crucial to the understanding of arterial thrombosis but are less relevant for venous thrombogenesis. Vessel wall damage appears to be a poor stimulus to fibrin formation and has never been convincingly demonstrated as a significant aetiological factor in venous thrombosis (Thomas 1987). The only known additional factor that can rapidly transform static blood into a venous thrombosis is the generation of thrombin. If thrombin is present in areas of retarded blood flow, platelets aggregate and fibrinogen is converted to fibrin which provides the basic structure of a venous thrombus (Fig. 64.1). The degree of local fibrinolytic activity in the blood influences the extent to which fibrin will be deposited on an initial platelet nidus and whether a platelet fibrin nidus will be propagated or disappear.

Certain physiological changes of pregnancy predispose to thrombosis. The blood coagulation system undergoes physiological changes during pregnancy with marked increases in several of the plasma proteins concerned with clotting. In particular, the levels of fibrinogen, factor VII, VIII and X show a substantial rise. In late pregnancy an increased ability to neutralize heparin is also present; this disappears following delivery (Bonnar 1976). This heparin resistance is probably due to the local activation of coagulation in the uteroplacental circulation and an increased amount of platelet factor. Fibrinolytic activity in plasma decreases progressively from early pregnancy and the amount of plasminogen activator which can be released from the venous endothelium is also reduced. These changes in fibrinolysis during pregnancy can be mediated by a progressive increase of the level of fast-acting tissue-type plasminogen activator inhibitor, recently reported to increase during pregnancy (Aznar et al 1986).

In late pregnancy, the velocity of venous blood flow in the lower limbs is reduced by about 50% and this is accompanied by a rise in venous pressure by about 10 mmHg. This is due to increased venous distensibility as well as the pressure of the gravid uterus which impedes venous return. The substantial increase of venous blood flow from the gravid uterus together with internal iliac veins will also cause back pressure on the venous return in the external iliac veins draining the lower limbs.

The pathogenesis of thrombosis in pregnancy is therefore most likely to be a product of the increased tendency to venous stasis in the lower limbs, combined with a shift in the balance between coagulation and fibrinolysis towards enhanced coagulation and diminished fibrinolysis, which will encourage thrombus growth.

Incidence in pregnancy

The incidence of thromboembolic complications in pregnancy is probably greatly underestimated and in published reports varies between 2 and 5 per 1000 deliveries (Aaro & Juergens 1974, Coon 1977). In a population study in the USA, approximately one-half of all venous thromboembolic events occurring in women below the age of 40 were related to pregnancy or the puerperium (Coon et al 1973). The Confidential Enquiries into Maternal Deaths reported 28 deaths from pulmonary embolism in 1979–1981, a decrease from 45 in the previous triennia (Department of Health and Social Security 1986). Deaths in 1979–1981 included three following first-trimester abortions and two following second-trimester abortions. Eleven deaths occurred during pregnancy, one in labour and 11 after delivery. Of the latter, seven followed Caesarean section and four, vaginal delivery. Table 64.1 shows the number of deaths from pulmonary embolism from 1952 to 1981. The number of deaths following all forms of vaginal delivery has fallen steadily since 1955, but those following Caesarean section have not decreased at the same rate. Approximately one-third of the deaths have occurred during the antenatal period and these have been distributed throughout pregnancy.

Table 64.2 shows the interval between delivery and fatal pulmonary embolism following vaginal delivery and Caesarean section during the years 1970–1981. Deaths from post-

Table 64.1 Maternal death due to pulmonary embolism in England and Wales from 1952 to 1981. Rates per 10 000 deliveries or Caesarean sections are given in brackets

	After abortion or during pregnancy	After vaginal delivery	After Caesarean section	Total
1952–1954	4	104	30	138
1955–1957	24	114	26	164
1958–1960	36	80	22	138
1961–1963	47	66 (0.4)	27 (3.6)	140
1964–1966	27	43 (0.2)	25 (2.7)	95
1967–1969	28	36 (0.2)	18 (1.8)	82
1970–1972	24	23 (0.1)	15 (1.4)	62
1973–1975	17	13 (0.07)	6 (0.6)	36
1976–1978	16	20 (0.1)	9 (0.8)	45
1979–1981	17	4 (0.03)	7 (0.5)	28

From Department of Health and Social Security (1986).

Table 64.2 Interval between delivery and pulmonary embolism following vaginal delivery and Caesarean section (1970–1981)

	Vaginal delivery	Caesarean sections
Less than 24 hours	8 (13%)	7 (19%)
1–7 days	18 (30%)	8 (22%)
8–14 days	9 (15%)	9 (24%)
15–42 days	25 (42%)	13 (35%)
Total	60 (100%)	37 (100%)

From Department of Health and Social Security (1986).

partum pulmonary embolism can occur at any time, whatever the mode of delivery. The most dangerous period is the first 7 days, followed by the second week, after which the risk decreases. As shown in Table 64.2, 13% of the deaths following vaginal delivery and 19% of the deaths following Caesarean section occurred within 24 hours. This indicates that prophylactic measures against thromboembolism in high-risk patients must at least cover the period of labour and Caesarean section.

Specific aetiological factors in obstetric patients

The Confidential Enquiries indicate that where thromboembolism results in a maternal death, the following factors are important (Department of Health and Social Security 1986):

1. *Method of delivery*: the increased risk of thromboembolism after Caesarean section is clearly shown in Table 64.1. The frequency of fatal pulmonary embolism during these years was on average more than 10 times greater after Caesarean section than after vaginal delivery.
2. *Age and parity*: the risk of fatal pulmonary embolism increases more sharply with advancing age — particularly in those aged 35 years or more — than with increasing parity.
3. *Excessive obesity (exceeding 76 kg or 12 stone)*: obesity is generally accepted as an important factor in the development of thromboembolism. Approximately 1 in 5 women dying of pulmonary embolism are in this category.
4. *Hospitalization and restricted activity*: women admitted to hospital on account of obstetric complications such as diabetes, hypertension, heart disease, placenta praevia and multiple pregnancy are at increased risk, probably because of the restricted activity and prolonged bedrest associated with their management.
5. *Suppression of lactation by oestrogens*: oestrogen administration has been shown to predispose to thromboembolism in several clinical situations. The association between suppression of lactation with stilboestrol and thromboembolism was first suggested by Daniel et al (1967). These authors showed a 10-fold increase in non-fatal thromboembolism in low-parity women of 25 years and over who were not lactating compared to those who were. The evidence suggests that suppression of lactation with oestrogens can be a precipitating factor, especially in patients already at risk as a result of age and operative delivery. For this reason it seems unwise to introduce combined oestrogen–progestogen oral contraception in the immediate puerperium.
6. *History of deep vein thrombosis of pulmonary embolism in association with pregnancy, surgery or the contraceptive pill*: women with a previous proven deep vein thrombosis or pulmonary embolism must be regarded as especially at risk during pregnancy. Likewise, women undergoing a surgical operation during pregnancy are at greater risk.
7. *Lupus anticoagulant-associated thrombotic disease*: the presence of lupus anticoagulant is associated with an increased thrombotic tendency and recurrent abortions.
8. *Hereditary thrombotic disease*: women with any of the known hereditary thrombotic disorders must be considered at increased risk of thromboembolic complications during pregnancy, e.g. hereditary antithrombin III deficiency.

THE DIAGNOSIS OF DEEP VEIN THROMBOSIS AND PULMONARY EMBOLISM DURING PREGNANCY

Clinical features

Deep vein thrombosis

The normal discomforts of pregnancy can often mimic the symptoms of leg vein thrombosis. Leg cramps, swelling of the ankles, slight cyanosis of the legs and on standing an increased prominence of the superficial veins are often seen, especially in late pregnancy. Venous thrombosis when present will almost invariably cause more symptoms in one leg than the other. The diagnosis of deep vein thrombosis is almost certain when physical signs such as definite tenderness and induration of the calf muscles, unilateral oedema and increased skin temperature of the leg are present. The diagnostic problem lies in the patient in whom the clinical signs are either absent or equivocal. Examination of the lower limbs should include comparison of the minimum circumference at the calf and thighs. A difference of 2 cm or more at identical sites on the legs should be regarded as significant. In the early stages, even extensive thrombi are often asymptomatic and their presence may first be suspected with the occurrence of pulmonary embolism. Autopsy studies have shown that in almost half the patients there are no clinical signs or symptoms referable to the limbs and fatal embolism may be the first indication of thrombosis.

Unlike early or localized thrombosis, the clinical diagnosis of extensive femoral or iliofemoral thrombosis is much more accurate, as the majority of propagating venous thrombi completely occlude the lumen, causing obstruction of the venous return. The patient usually presents with pain in the calf or thigh and swelling of the leg. The onset is usually rapid but there is often a history of previous pain in the calf muscles.

Examination of the affected limb will usually show swelling and oedema with dilatation of the superficial veins. The increase in skin temperature of the affected limb is because most of the venous return is taking place through the superficial veins. The distal part of the limb may however be pale or cyanosed with absent or reduced pedal pulses. This is the result of secondary arterial spasm which often accompanies massive iliofemoral thrombosis. When thrombosis extends into the iliofemoral segment, tenderness is usually present along the course of the femoral vein.

Prospective studies using radioactive fibrinogen tests and phlebography have shown that only half the patients with early deep vein thrombosis have demonstrable clinical symptoms or signs. The reverse is also true: some 25–50% of patients with clinical signs of thrombosis have no demonstrable venous thrombi. Therefore the treatment of patients based purely on clinical signs will result in a significant proportion receiving unnecessary treatment with its attendant hazards.

Whenever possible objective diagnostic methods should be used to confirm the presence of suspected deep vein thrombosis.

Pulmonary embolism

The symptoms and signs of pulmonary embolism are predominantly associated with the cardiovascular and respiratory systems. The immediate effects vary from clinically silent to sudden death and depend on the size of the embolus and the preceding health of the patient. In the author's experience, pregnant women with iliofemoral thrombosis frequently show evidence on lung scanning of small symptomless pulmonary emboli. These small emboli are probably cleared from the pulmonary circulation within a few days by the potent fibrinolytic activity in the lung vasculature.

When pulmonary infarction occurs it is usually accompanied by the sudden onset of dyspnoea, pleural pain, haemoptysis or cough and a pleural friction rub may be detected. The classic symptoms of massive pulmonary embolism are severe chest pain, air hunger, extreme apprehension and sudden collapse. Predominant clinical signs are cyanosis, rapid breathing and jugular vein distension. Syncope is primarily a finding of massive pulmonary embolism and depends upon the degree of pulmonary vascular obstruction with the resulting decrease in cerebral blood flow.

Where pulmonary embolism occurs suddenly and unexpectedly, acute severe myocardial infarction is the principal differential diagnosis. Distended neck veins which reflect the abnormally elevated pressure of the strained right ventricle are a useful sign of massive embolism; the neck veins are usually not engorged when syncope occurs in association with severe myocardial infarction.

Where pulmonary embolism is suspected, chest X-ray, electrocardiogram (ECG) and lung scanning should be carried out. The two most common plain chest X-ray findings are the presence of a consolidation or infiltration and an elevated hemidiaphragm on the affected side. ECG changes occur in 85% of patients with pulmonary embolism. The changes include rhythm disturbances, QRS abnormalities and ST–T wave alterations. An ECG is not specific in diagnosing pulmonary embolism but is useful in excluding acute myocardial infarction, which may be confused with massive pulmonary embolism. If facilities are available, a combination of perfusion and ventilation lung scanning is a highly specific and accurate method of diagnosing or excluding pulmonary embolism in a previously healthy patient. Pulmonary angiography is also a definitive method but carries some risk.

The clinical diagnosis of both venous thrombosis and pulmonary embolism in pregnancy is so subject to error that wherever possible an objective diagnostic technique should be used. Indeed there are few situations in which diagnostic certainty is more important. An erroneous diagnosis and institution of potent but unnecessary anticoagulant therapy in pregnancy will carry significant hazards for both mother and fetus. This may not be appreciated by physicians who may be less aware of the hazard of bleeding complications in the fetus and the risk of severe haemorrhage from the placental site before, during and after delivery.

Investigations

Ascending phlebography

When carried out by a skilled radiologist, phlebography will provide the most accurate and precise diagnosis of leg vein thrombosis, giving information not only about the presence of a thrombus but also its exact position, size and whether

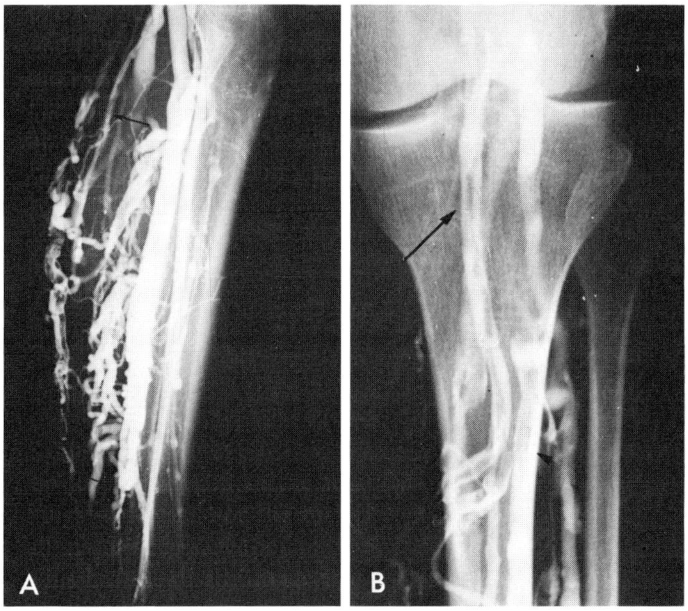

Fig. 64.2(a) Phlebogram of the veins of the calf. The small thrombi in the soleal veins are usually of no clinical significance. (**b**) Thrombi in the deep veins of the calf seen as filling defects (arrow) extending up into the popliteal vein.

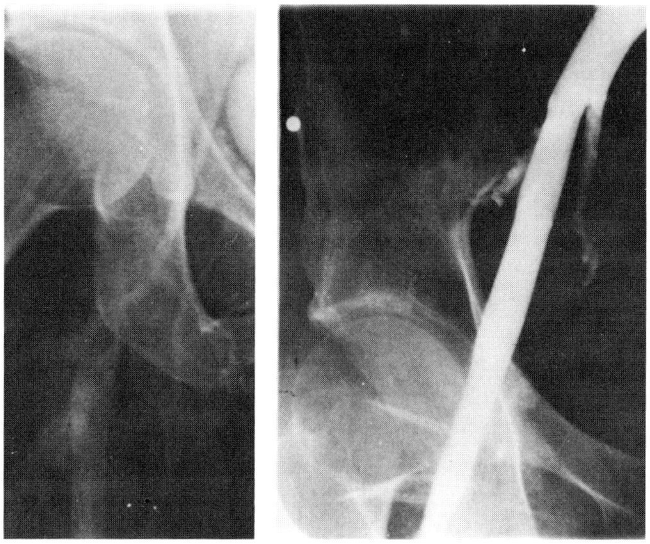

Fig. 64.3 Phlebogram showing (**left**) an occluded iliofemoral vein and (**right**) the normal appearance of the femoral, external, internal and common iliac veins.

it is loose or adherent to the vein wall. Modern X-ray diagnostic equipment, including the image intensifier and television monitor screen, has enabled venographic techniques to become a reliable method for demonstrating most venous thrombi of clinical interest. Phlebography in expert hands detects at least 95% of peripheral thrombi (Browse 1978). Satisfactory demonstration of the external and common iliac veins is achieved in approximately 90% of patients. The low-viscosity contrast medium is injected into a vein on the dorsum of the foot and the whole venous system of the leg is examined up to the external and common iliac veins (Fig. 64.2, 64.3). Lateral views of the calf are required to detect thrombi in the soleal veins. Partially occluding thrombi are seen as well defined translucent areas with a rim of contrast medium surrounding them. A sudden and sharp obstruction to the column of contrast medium and spread of the flow into a network of collateral vessels indicates obstruction of the major venous channel.

Complications of phlebography include extravasation of contrast medium at the injection site and superficial thrombophlebitis. It has also been claimed that pulmonary embolism may occur as a result of dislodgement of a thrombus during the examination. Kakkar (1987) did not observe this complication in nearly 1500 patients in whom phlebography was performed in the presence of established extensive thrombosis.

Postphlebography deep vein thrombosis has also been claimed as a complication of ascending phlebography. This complication has an incidence of less than 1% if small amounts of contrast medium are used and the deep veins are flushed out with 100 ml of isotonic saline containing 2500 units of heparin.

Contrast phlebography has often been withheld during pregnancy because of fear of the radiation hazard to the fetus. A large measure of protection to the pregnant uterus and fetus can be provided by shielding the mother's abdomen with a lead apron. Since 25–50% of patients in whom venous thrombosis is suspected from symptoms and signs do not have thrombosis, phlebography with minimum radiation will usually be indicated unless facilities are available for isotope venography. Certainly, the risk of unnecessary anticoagulant therapy to the mother and the fetus must greatly exceed any radiation risk to the fetus.

Radionuclide venography and lung scanning

Radionuclide venography was introduced by Webber et al (1969), who showed that the injection of a suitable lung scanning agent into the venous system of the foot could be used for investigating the presence not only of thrombi in the deep veins of the lower limb but also for locating pulmonary emboli. Macroaggregates of albumin (MAA) or microspheres labelled with ^{99m}Tc (technetium) have been investigated and appear to be a safe and accurate method of diagnosing thromboembolic disease during pregnancy (Johnson et al 1974, Ennis & Dowsett 1983, Lisbona et al 1987).

The technique of radionuclide venography is simple to perform but accuracy depends on meticulous attention to detail. The optimal imaging technique uses a moving scanning bed and gamma camera system to perform the venography and subsequent lung scan. A 21 gauge butterfly needle with a two-way tap is inserted into the dorsal veins of both feet. An activity of 2 mCi ^{99m}Tc–MAA is made in 5 ml of saline for each limb and injected simultaneously by hand. A tourniquet above the malleoli allows the deep veins to be filled with the radionuclide. The popliteal and femoral veins are clearly defined as wide bands of activity uniting via the iliac veins to form the vena cava. MAA have an affinity for fresh clot and adhere to its surface, resulting in a hot spot. Hot spots or increased radionuclide activity can result from causes other than thrombosis and accurate interpretation requires correlation with other scintigraphic signs. Venous obstruction with demonstration of collateral vessels is usually better demonstrated with scintigraphic techniques than with contrast venography. In late pregnancy this can occur with the vena cava because of the pressure from the uterus.

Properly carried out, radionuclide venography is reported to have a correlation with contrast phlebography of greater than 90% (Ennis & Dowsett 1983). In the iliofemoral segment, the correlation is greater than 95%.

Malone (1983) has shown that the dose to the fetus is as low as 3 mrad where there is complete tagging of the isotope and macroaggregates. Radionuclide venography is less invasive than phlebography and the radiation hazard is very much smaller. From this point of view, radionuclide venography combined with lung scanning is the investigation of choice for pregnant women with a suspected thrombosis or pulmonary embolism. Prior administration of potassium perchlorate is an obvious precaution when using ^{99m}Tc compounds in order to block the maternal and fetal thyroid.

The excretion of radiopharmaceuticals in human breast milk has been studied; discontinuation of breastfeeding following administration of a radiopharmaceutical is strongly recommended. Since about 2% of injected activity is secreted in breast milk, the technique is best avoided in lactating mothers (Malone 1983).

The main disadvantages of radionuclide venography are that the patient has to be examined by a gamma camera in an isotope department and such cameras are not readily available in isolated maternity hospitals. The chief advantage of isotope venography combined with lung scanning is that the major venous channels and the lung fields can be examined at the same time.

Ultrasonic scanning

Doppler ultrasonic examination provides a useful screening method for the diagnosis of deep vein venous thrombosis in pregnancy. The apparatus is usually readily available in obstetric units as it is widely used for listening to the fetal heart. The ultrasonic probe is placed over the femoral vein which is located immediately medial to the femoral artery. The blood flow sounds in the femoral vein may be absent if the vein is completely obstructed, and the characteristic rushing sounds due to the sudden increase in blood flow which follows gentle compression of the relaxed calf will not be heard. Because of the presence of collateral venous channels in the calf, ultrasound will not detect minor calf vein thrombosis.

Ultrasonic examination has the benefit of being non-invasive and it can now be performed readily with small portable units. These provide a most useful adjunct to clinical examination as a bedside technique for detecting thrombotic occlusion in what is potentially the most hazardous site — the iliofemoral segment. A normal or negative test represents a patent vein or at least the absence of a large thrombus in the iliofemoral venous segment. On the other hand, a positive test indicates the need for phlebography to define the exact site and extent of the thrombus. Studies comparing ultrasound with phlebography report an accuracy of 90–95% for the diagnosis of femoral or iliac vein thrombosis and a 15–20% sensitivity to calf vein thrombosis (Browse 1978).

Radioactive-labelled fibrinogen

The use of ^{125}I (iodide) fibrinogen has proved a most reliable technique for the early detection of leg vein thrombosis and provides an accurate method for assessing the efficacy of various methods of prophylaxis. The amount of radiation exposure following the injection of 100 μCi ^{125}I-labelled fibrinogen is calculated to be approximately 200 mrem delivered to blood, 20 mrem to tissues and 5 mrem to the kidneys. This is less than the acceptable annual total body absorbed radiation dose (550 mrem/year) recommended for the general population by the British National Council on Radiation Protection (Kakkar 1987). Studies carried out in antepartum and postpartum patients showed no evidence of ^{125}I-labelled fibrinogen crossing the placenta, although free ^{125}I was present in small quantities (Friend & Kakkar 1972). In the puerperium, ^{125}I-fibrinogen would also result in radioactive iodine being excreted in breast milk. For these reasons ^{125}I-fibrinogen has rarely been used in pregnancy or the puerperium. With careful precautions, the method could be used in the puerperium in non-lactating high-risk patients for the early detection of leg vein thrombosis. In postpartum women, Friend & Kakkar (1970) reported an incidence of 3% of calf vein thrombi.

The ^{125}I-labelled fibrinogen technique has been widely used as a research tool; the method has confirmed that advancing age, obesity, previous venous thromboembolism, varicose veins and malignancy increase the likelihood of developing venous thrombosis. False positive results for deep vein thrombosis will occur with conditions that lead to the accumulation of fibrinogen, fibrin or fibrin degradation products, such as bruising or haematoma formation, gross oedema and inflammatory reactions as in superficial phlebitis.

Limb impedance plethysmography

The non-invasive technique of plethysmography has been used for the diagnosis of deep vein thrombosis in the non-pregnant patient. The method involves filling the calf veins under resting conditions with a pressure cuff and measuring the rate of emptying of the calf, after releasing the cuff, to detect obstruction to the venous flow. The tests will not detect most calf vein thrombi since they do not obstruct the main outflow tract. Similarly, small non-occlusive thrombi in the popliteal and femoral veins may also be missed. We have studied the method during pregnancy and found the technique to be unreliable during the second half of pregnancy. The impedance test cannot distinguish between thrombotic and non-thrombotic venous obstruction; the pressure of the gravid uterus and the raised venous pressure of the lower limbs is a probable explanation of the false positive results.

Lung scanning

Pulmonary embolism disturbs the regional perfusion of the lungs and the use of radioactive tracer techniques allows a rapid and simple study of the perfusion pattern. Lung scanning is recommended in all patients with suspected pulmonary embolism. The exception would be the patient with massive pulmonary embolism with hypotension, when pulmonary angiography should be performed if pulmonary embolectomy is contemplated.

When a perfusion scan with multiple views is normal, the probability of pulmonary embolism is so low that clinically significant pulmonary embolism can be excluded. When the perfusion pattern or regional distribution of blood flow is abnormal, a ventilation scan should also be carried out, particularly if there is any history of other cardiopulmonary disease. Patients with pulmonary embolism show multiple lesions which have vascular configurations. An abnormal perfusion scan with a normal ventilation scan of the affected area is characteristic of pulmonary embolism. In patients with lung disease, a matched perfusion and ventilation abnormality will usually, but not always, exclude thromboembolism.

Pulmonary angiography

Selective pulmonary angiography remains the only definitive method of identifying pulmonary embolism during life. A positive diagnosis of pulmonary embolism can be made by angiography if one of two findings is present: an intravascular filling defect or a pulmonary arterial vessel cut-off (Sasahara 1987). The technique is most helpful in patients with underlying heart and lung disease who are suspected of having pulmonary embolism. These patients may present with non-specific symptoms and signs and may have an abnormal scan with doubtful lesions or matched ventilation–perfusion defects. In addition to demonstrating emboli, the pressures in the right side of the heart and pulmonary circulation can be measured. Such measurements can yield valuable information relating to severity which may influence treatment and prognosis. Many hospitals, however, do not have adequate angiographic facilities or a trained team capable of performing studies of good quality with safety.

Laboratory investigations

A number of biochemical abnormalities may occur in deep vein thrombosis and pulmonary embolism but the available laboratory tests are essentially non-specific. The levels of serum fibrin and fibrinogen degradation products, fibrin monomer and soluble complexes, plasma levels of β thromboglobulin and urinary thromboxane B_2 have been investigated but the non-specific nature of these assays renders them much less valuable in pregnancy than in the non-pregnant state. Although none of these tests can be recommended as helpful aids in diagnosis, the discovery of a readily available sensitive and specific biochemical marker would be a major advance in assisting the diagnosis of venous thromboembolism.

Where there is a family history of repeated venous thrombosis, the level of antithrombin III in plasma should be investigated. Congenital deficiencies or defects of antithrombin III occur in about 1 in 5000 of the population and are usually but not always associated with a serious thrombotic tendency. Purified preparations of antithrombin III are available and their use should be considered when a pregnant woman with congenitally deficient antithrombin III experiences a thrombotic event, or prophylactically to cover the time of maximum risk during labour and the first 2 weeks after delivery.

Diagnostic requirements for treatment

Since all hospitals do not have the same facilities and expertise, it is unrealistic to insist that all patients with venous thrombosis or suspected pulmonary embolism should be investigated in an identical manner. In dealing with a particular patient two factors should be considered: the urgency of diagnosis and the availability of the diagnostic procedures.

Ideally for the pregnant woman, a clinical picture of venous thrombosis or pulmonary embolism should be confirmed by radionuclide venography and lung scanning. Where this is not available, contrast ascending phlebography protecting the gravid uterus is recommended. If phlebography is not available the Doppler ultrasound technique should be used but the interpretation of results is highly dependent on the experience of the examiner.

Since diagnostic evaluation may be time-consuming, an intravenous bolus of 5000 units of heparin should be given if there is strong clinical suspicion of extensive thrombosis involving the iliofemoral segment or evidence of pulmonary embolism. The patient should be continued on a heparin infusion and if the diagnosis is confirmed, treatment continued. If the diagnosis is not confirmed heparin can be stopped. The only exception to administering heparin would be in patients with bleeding from placenta praevia, or in patients with suspected massive pulmonary embolism and hypotension in whom pulmonary embolectomy was contemplated.

TREATMENT OF THROMBOSIS DURING PREGNANCY

Before discussing specific antithrombotic therapy to be used in pregnancy, the general aspects of management are worth emphasizing. The pregnant woman lying on her back in late pregnancy is likely to aggravate venous stasis in the legs due to the compression of the vena cava. She should therefore be advised to rest on one side and not to lie on her back. Venous return from the lower limbs is encouraged by elevation of the foot off the bed by 15–20 cm. Exercise of the affected leg should be restricted only by pain. Mobilization and leg exercises are of vital importance in opening up collateral venous channels and are likely to be major factors in preventing long-term venous insufficiency. When effective antithrombotic treatment is instituted, active mobilization to reduce venous stasis is no longer regarded as increasing the risk of thromboembolism. The leg should be kept firmly bandaged until acute swelling has subsided and progressive ambulation should be commenced as soon as leg symptoms allow.

In several reviews of the management of thromboembolic disease during pregnancy and the puerperium, there is now general agreement on specific treatment (Bonnar 1981, Weiner 1982, 1985, Letsky & de Swiet 1984, Letsky 1985). Patients with venous thrombosis should be heparinized by continuous intravenous administration until the acute symptoms have subsided, followed by intermittent subcutaneous heparin in the long term. Warfarin should be avoided in pregnancy. Prophylactic subcutaneous heparin should be used in hereditary thrombotic disorders and in women with previous major thromboembolic complications. Fibrinolytic agents would not normally be used during pregnancy. For those at lower risk, some advocate only covering labour with dextran 70 and providing subcutaneous heparin in the puerperium; no anticoagulant is given in pregnancy (Lao et al 1985).

Anticoagulant therapy in pregnancy

The aim of specific treatment in deep vein thrombosis with or without pulmonary embolism is to prevent propagation and embolization. The choice of anticoagulant therapy lies with heparin alone or heparin in combination with oral anticoagulants.

Heparin therapy

Heparin is a sulphated polysaccharide with important anticoagulant and thrombotic properties; it is known to inhibit a number of activated clotting factors including factors XIIa, XIa, IXa, Xa and thrombin. Heparin exhibits its effect by complexing with the antithrombin III molecule, changing the latter's molecular configuration. The inhibitory activity of antithrombin III is greatly increased and its ability to neutralize activated clotting factors is enhanced. Thrombin, once formed, requires relatively large amounts of heparin to inhibit its effect; in contrast, factor Xa is inhibited by very small amounts of heparin. The inhibition of factor Xa can prevent the conversion of prothrombin to thrombin and is the basis of thrombosis prophylaxis using low-dosage heparin. Once a thrombus has developed and thrombin is present, much larger amounts of heparin are required. Other effects of heparin include potentiation of heparin co-factor II and inhibition of platelet function (Hirsh 1986).

Commercial heparin preparations for the treatment of thrombosis are prepared from bovine lungs or porcine intestines. These heterogeneous compounds have a molecular weight which varies between 3000 and 40 000 daltons. The unfractionated forms can be partially purified by depolymerization methods and show diverse functions depending upon their molecular size and binding to antithrombin III. The antithrombin activity of heparin decreases with decreasing molecular weight, whereas clotting as measured by antifactor Xa assays is unaffected by molecular weight. This has led to the suggestion that low molecular weight heparins are potential antithrombotics with low haemorrhage risks. Clinical trials with low molecular weight heparin (4000–9000 daltons) show promise in the prevention of deep vein thrombosis. Heparin analogues are also being investigated as antithrombotic agents with negligible effect on clotting tests. Neither unfractionated mucosal heparin nor the low molecular weight heparins cross the placenta to the fetus (Bonnar 1976, Forestier et al 1984, Andrew et al 1985).

Oral anticoagulants (coumarin derivatives)

Oral anticoagulants have a molecular weight of approximately 1000 and readily cross the placenta. The elevated levels of coagulation factors in the pregnant woman contrast sharply with the situation in the fetus and newborn in whom the levels of factors II, VII, IX and X are low. Although warfarin and other oral anticoagulants may be safe for the mother when she is within the therapeutic range, the fetus is likely to be considerably overdosed because of immature liver enzyme systems and the low levels of vitamin K-dependent clotting factors.

More and more women of childbearing age are receiving long-term oral anticoagulant therapy because of thrombotic complications associated with oral contraception or because of artificial heart valves. Reports in the literature indicate that in pregnant women taking oral anticoagulants, fetal mortality is around 15–30%. Tejani (1973) reported 32 pregnant women with a heart valve prosthesis who received oral anticoagulant therapy at some stage of their pregnancy. In this group 11 fetal or neonatal deaths occurred and three infants had major congenital abnormalities. In a review of world literature between 1945 and 1978, Hall et al (1980) found 418 cases which had received coumarin derivatives. Overall only two-thirds of these pregnancies had a normal fetal outcome. The abnormalities in the others were mainly due to haemorrhage, warfarin embryopathy, central nervous system effects and spontaneous abortion. The critical period of exposure for warfarin embryopathy appears to be between 6 and 9 weeks of gestation. The main features are: saddle nose, nasal and mid-face hypoplasia, frontal bossing and short stature with stippled epiphyses and short extremities, calcification of thyroid cartilage, cardiac defects, low-set ears, mental retardation and blindness (Stevenson et al 1980). The severity of the syndrome is variable and follow-up studies indicate that most survivors have a good outcome; one-half have no severe disability.

Exposure of the pregnant woman to coumarin derivatives in the second and third trimesters may be associated with an increased incidence of central nervous system abnormalities resulting in mental retardation and blindness. Intracranial bleeding in the fetus in the second and third trimester may also lead to secondary central nervous system deformities. The overall risk of central nervous system effects appears to be about 3%.

The retrospective analysis of Hall et al (1980) estimated that with the use of coumarin derivatives one-sixth of pregnancies end in abortion or stillbirth; one-sixth result in abnormal liveborn infants and about two-thirds have a relatively normal outcome. Given that the literature is biased towards reporting complicated cases, it is likely that these retrospective estimates are the worst possible and that in practice the risks are probably much less.

In an earlier review of the use of oral anticoagulants in pregnancy, Hirsh and colleagues (1970) suggested that the risk to the fetus occurred mainly at term and was related to fetal trauma arising during childbirth. In 14 patients in whom oral anticoagulants were withdrawn after the 37th week of gestation no fetal or neonatal complications were reported. Hirsh et al concluded that the main hazard of oral anticoagulant drugs resulted from their use during the first trimester or in late pregnancy prior to delivery. Although the risk to the fetus can be reduced by discontinuing oral anticoagulant therapy at the 37th week of pregnancy, premature labour and delivery are not predictable. A preterm infant delivered under the influence of oral anticoagulants is at increased risk of cerebral haemorrhage.

Oral anticoagulant therapy should therefore be avoided if at all possible during pregnancy; if a woman conceives while taking oral anticoagulants, she should be advised to discontinue them as early as 6 weeks of gestation. If anticoagulant therapy is essential during the first trimester, heparin can be used, as described later.

Neutralizing warfarin therapy

In some situations anticoagulant therapy may have to be neutralized because of bleeding. Impaired renal function and concurrent administration of drugs which inhibit platelet function increase the risk of bleeding complications with anticoagulants. If the anticoagulant effect of warfarin has to be reversed immediately, an infusion of 1–2 units of fresh plasma should be given. Aqueous vitamin K preparations reverse the effect of warfarin within 24 hours. The dosage of vitamin K given orally or intravenously depends on the clinical situation. Where there is serious haemorrhage and a firm decision is taken not to re-introduce anticoagulants, a dose of 25–50 mg should be given. This will render the patient resistant to further anticoagulant treatment for about 2 weeks. Where there is frank haemorrhage but it is intended to continue therapy, 15 mg should be given to reduce the drug effect without cancelling it. Where the routine coagulation test shows an excessive effect but the patient is not bleeding, a dose of 5 mg can be prescribed.

Fibrinolytic agents

Recent surgery or delivery is considered a contraindication to thrombolytic therapy. If streptokinase or urokinase is used when delivery is imminent or within 1 week of childbirth, severe haemorrhage from the placental site is to be expected. Likewise, extensive bleeding will occur from any genital tract lacerations or episiotomy wounds. The risk of bleeding will be greatest at the time of delivery and in the early puerperium. During pregnancy the likelihood of bleeding should be very much less and thrombolytic therapy may prove life-saving for the woman with massive thromboembolism. A small number of case reports have described the use of thrombolytic therapy in pregnancy (Hall et al 1972). The dosage schedule for thrombolytic therapy with urokinase is a loading dose of 4400 u/kg i.v. over 10 minutes followed by 4400 u/kg/h i.v. for 12–24 hours; with streptokinase the dosage is 250 000 u i.v. over 30 minutes followed by 100 000 u/h for 24–72 hours. Since these doses are standard, laboratory monitoring is recommended to ensure some degree of fibrinolysis, e.g. thrombin time, fibrinogen and plasminogen levels. Treatment with heparin should be continued following the thrombolytic therapy to prevent further thrombosis and recurrent thromboembolism.

THERAPY OF VENOUS THROMBOEMBOLISM

Pregnant women who develop venous thrombosis should be heparinized according to the protocol shown in Table

Table 64.3 Protocol for heparin therapy of thromboembolism in pregnancy (Hathaway & Bonnar 1987)

Baseline diagnostic studies
1. Venogram by ascending contrast or radionuclide venography and perfusion–ventilation lung scanning; Doppler ultrasound
2. Coagulation studies: platelet count activated partial thromboplastin time (APTT); prothrombin time; activated whole blood clotting time (ACT); hereditary disorder screening tests as indicated

Acute heparinization
Sodium heparin 50–75 u/kg i.v. bolus injection followed by 15–25 u/kg/h by continuous infusion or pump to prolong the APTT or ACT to 1.5–2 times normal; continue therapy for 5–7 days

Long-term prophylaxis
Administer 5000–10 000 units of sodium heparin subcutaneously every 12 hours. Monitor with heparin level (0.05–0.3 u/ml plasma) or APPT, ACT (1.5 times normal) at 2–4 hours postinjection and adjust dose accordingly. When a dosage of 20 000 u or greater per 24 hours is required, an 8-hourly regimen is preferable

64.3 (Hathaway & Bonnar 1987). In late pregnancy a greater amount of heparin is required for adequate anticoagulation than in the non-pregnant state (Bonnar 1976, Whitfield et al 1983). For acute heparinization 50–75 units of sodium heparin per kg should be given as an intravenous bolus injection, followed by 15–25 u/kg/h by continuous infusion to prolong the partial thromboplastin time to 1.5–2 times the baseline or mean control value. For adequate anticoagulation and avoidance of bleeding complications, strict attention to detail is essential. Intermittent bolus injections should not be used because of the increased risk of bleeding. Continuous intravenous heparin by infusion or pump should be given initially for 5–7 days. The precise duration of the initial treatment must be tailored to the individual but the objective is to maintain full anticoagulation until active thrombosis has been arrested, thrombi in the leg veins have been firmly attached to the vessel wall and the process of organization has begun. Where intravenous therapy for this period proves impossible, treatment can be given by subcutaneous injection into the flank of the anterior abdominal wall. Dosage of subcutaneous heparin of 10 000 units at 8-hourly intervals will usually provide adequate anticoagulation.

If the woman is in the puerperium, treatment with oral anticoagulants such as warfarin can be commenced and the heparin discontinued once the effect of the oral anticoagulant has been established. During pregnancy oral anticoagulants are avoided and subcutaneous heparin can be given as an alternative. Subcutaneous prophylactic heparin is an effective substitute for warfarin and can be used alone in the prevention of recurrent thrombosis both in the non-pregnant and pregnant woman (Bonnar 1976, Hellgren & Nygards 1982, Hull et al 1982). Long-term prophylaxis can be provided with sodium heparin in a dosage of 5000–10 000 units 8–12-hourly to prolong the partial thromboplastin time to 1.5 times normal at 2–4 hours following the subcutaneous injection.

Subcutaneous heparin

Particular care is required in instruction of medical and nursing staff and patients in the use of subcutaneous heparin. A concentrated aqueous solution of 25 000 iu of heparin in 1 ml is used. Ampoules containing 5000 units of heparin in 0.2 ml of solution are now available; these are safer than multidose bottles which are occasionally responsible for accidental overdosage. Preloaded syringes with 5000 and 10 000 units of heparin are also available; these are particularly useful for self-administration in pregnancy. Where these are not used a tuberculin-type syringe and a 25 or 26 gauge needle 1.5 cm in length is used.

A fold of skin is gently raised on the lateral aspect of the anterior abdominal wall in the flank. This is facilitated by the patient bending forwards. The skin is cleansed and the needle inserted to its full depth at right angles to the skin. The hub of the needle is held firmly between the thumb and index finger as the exact dose of heparin is injected. The needle is slowly removed at the same angle as it was inserted, taking care to avoid any damage to the skin and subcutaneous fat at the injection site. The injection site should not be rubbed or massaged. Subcutaneous heparin is best avoided in the arms and legs. Apart from being more painful and causing bruising in these areas, limb movements may accelerate the rate of absorption of the heparin.

For safe and effective long-term therapy with subcutaneous heparin, once- or twice-weekly measurements of the plasma heparin level or the heparin effect on plasma are advisable to ensure that adequate heparin is being given, especially during the third trimester. Increased heparin neutralization occurs in the second half of pregnancy due to the enhanced coagulation and platelet activity in the utero-placental circulation. Ideally the heparin level or partial thromboplastin time should be checked 2–4 hours after the subcutaneous injection as this is the time of the peak levels. The platelet count should also be measured, since some patients develop thrombocytopenia during heparin therapy. In view of the greater bioavailability of sodium heparin than calcium heparin, we prefer a 12-hourly regimen with sodium heparin during pregnancy (Bonnar & Ma 1979).

Wide individual variation is found in the levels of plasma heparin after subcutaneous injection; in late pregnancy some women require 10 000 units of heparin 8-hourly to produce an adequate level. When a dosage of 10 000 units subcutaneously is used, the plasma heparin levels should be monitored at weekly intervals. Our experience indicates that a plasma level of 0.1–0.3 u/ml provides effective protection against thrombosis in pregnancy without causing bleeding problems.

At the onset of labour, heparin therapy can be temporarily discontinued if the woman wishes an epidural anaesthesia. Epidural anaesthesia should preferably be avoided as it increases the operative delivery rates, and heparin should be continued during labour at a dosage of 5000 units 12-

hourly. The relative heparin resistance present in late pregnancy and labour disappears immediately after delivery. In the puerperium a dosage of 5000 units of sodium heparin 12-hourly is usually sufficient. If the risk of thrombosis in the puerperium is particularly high, 5000 iu heparin 8-hourly is advisable. Heparin therapy should be continued for 5–6 weeks after delivery. We have encountered no bleeding complications in patients during pregnancy, at vaginal delivery or at Caesarean section when the heparin level was less than 0.4 u/ml plasma.

In general, when a woman has had a previous thrombotic complication, prophylactic treatment during labour and delivery and in the puerperium is advisable. If a thromboembolic complication has occurred in the antenatal period of a previous pregnancy, prophylactic treatment from at least 4–6 weeks before the gestation time when the previous episode occurred should be considered. Lao and colleagues (1985) used no prophylactic treatment antenatally in 26 pregnant women with a previous history of thromboembolism and used treatment only at delivery with dextran 70 and for 6 weeks in the puerperium with heparin or warfarin. Of the 26, only 6 of the patients had had their original episode of thromboembolism in association with pregnancy. Using this regimen, one patient (4%) had a suspected pulmonary embolism and another patient who had had deep vein thrombosis at 38 weeks' gestation was given subcutaneous heparin from 37 weeks of pregnancy onwards.

De Sweit et al (1987) reported an extension of this study to 59 pregnancies 25 of whom had had their previous thromboembolism in pregnancy. He reported no further cases of antenatal thromboembolism and no cases postnatally using the regimen of dextran 70 infusion during labour and prophylaxis for 6 weeks postpartum with heparin or dextran. In the light of this experience de Sweit et al (1987) feel that the risk of recurrent thromboembolism in pregnancy is very low and that no prophylaxis can be justified because of the risks of subcutaneous heparin, especially bone demineralization.

The author has had experience of over 200 carefully monitored patients treated during pregnancy with subcutaneous heparin and problems with bone demineralization were not encountered. In the individual patient with a previous thromboembolism, the risk of a recurrence during pregnancy has to be weighed against the possible effects of subcutaneous heparin causing bone demineralization. Since approximately one-third of the maternal deaths due to pulmonary embolism occur during pregnancy, it would seem advisable to provide well-controlled prophylactic treatment during pregnancy with subcutaneous heparin where a patient has suffered a serious thromboembolic complication during her previous pregnancy. Possibly in the future, low molecular weight heparin may be an alternative but as yet it remains to be evaluated for use in pregnancy.

Complications of heparin therapy

Complications associated with heparin therapy include hypersensitivity reactions, osteoporosis, thrombocytopenia and bleeding. Hypersensitivity may be manifest as urticaria and in rare situations as anaphylaxis. Osteoporosis after long-term use of heparin has been reported in pregnancy (Hall et al 1980). Heparin causes demineralization of bone but this is seldom apparent unless heparin is given for more than 6 months in doses in excess of 15 000 units daily. The long-term consequences of subclinical demineralization are unknown (de Swiet et al 1983). Heparin-induced thrombocytopenia and bleeding or intravascular coagulation are rare effects of bovine lung heparin; porcine mucosal heparin, which is used mainly within the British Isles, rarely causes any significant thrombocytopenia.

Bleeding is the most important of the heparin complications and occurs in about 5–10% of patients on full-dose intravenous heparin. The risk of bleeding is particularly high in patients who have been exposed to recent surgery or trauma with bolus intravenous injections of heparin; in patients who have taken additional drug therapy such as aspirin, and in the presence of renal disease or pre-eclampsia. Partial thromboplastin times more than 2.5 times control, or plasma heparin levels over 0.5 iu/ml predispose to haemorrhage (Bonnar 1977). If bleeding occurs, stopping the heparin infusion for 8–12 hours usually allows haemostasis to recover. Where rapid reversal of the heparin effect is required, protamine sulphate can be given. For every estimated 100 units of heparin in the circulation, administer 1 mg protamine sulphate intravenously. The partial thromboplastin time or heparin assay should be repeated soon after the protamine injection; again, after 3 hours, further protamine may be required as it is eliminated faster than the heparin.

PROPHYLAXIS OF THROMBOEMBOLISM WITH DEXTRAN 70

The efficacy of dextran 70 in preventing venous thrombosis after pelvic surgery was clearly shown in double-blind controlled studies carried out in Oxford (Bonnar & Walsh 1972, Bonnar 1975). Dextran 70 (Lomodex) infusion was commenced after the induction of anaesthesia and 500 ml was given during the operation; a further 500 ml was started usually before the patient left the operating theatre and infused over the next 3–6 hours. Subsequently Kline and colleagues (1975) used the same regime in surgical patients in a randomized controlled study; these authors showed a significant reduction in fatal pulmonary embolism but not in deep vein thrombosis. Browse (1977) also found a significant reduction in pulmonary emboli as detected by ventilation–perfusion scanning in patients receiving 1 l dextran 70.

The available evidence suggests that dextran 70 has less

effect in preventing the small thrombi in the calf veins, but prevents embolism by rendering the fibrin in the thrombus much more susceptible to natural fibrinolysis and thus preventing the formation of large thrombi which produce emboli. The use of dextran 70 infusion during labour or Caesarean section would reduce puerperal pulmonary embolism. Indeed, where protection in the early puerperium is the main aim, dextran 70 infusion during labour and delivery is probably the most convenient and relatively inexpensive method of prophylaxis. Since bleeding complications are not a problem, dextran 70 can be used in patients having epidural anaesthesia. In any obstetric patient with cardiac or renal impairment or with a history of asthma or allergic reactions, dextran should be avoided; very rarely dextran can cause an anaphylactic-type reaction. In any patient receiving heparin, dextran should also be avoided as the two agents have a synergistic effect which increases the risk of bleeding.

PERIOD OF RISK IN PREGNANCY

When venous thrombosis or pulmonary embolism occurs during pregnancy, the patient must be regarded as at risk from propagation of the thrombus or recurrence of pulmonary embolism for at least 6 weeks after delivery. This emphasizes the importance of certainty in the diagnosis of thromboembolism in the pregnant woman because of the prolonged treatment required. When a pregnant woman has had a previous thromboembolic complication she must be considered as at high risk during pregnancy and the puerperium. If a thromboembolic complication has occurred in a previous pregnancy it is wise to commence prophylactic treatment at least 4–6 weeks before the gestation time when the previous episode occurred. A patient who has previously had venous thrombosis unrelated to pregnancy will be at greatest risk during the first 2 weeks of the puerperium and prophylaxis is advised during labour and for 4–6 weeks after delivery.

SPECIAL PROBLEMS DURING PREGNANCY

Massive pulmonary embolism

The use of cardiopulmonary bypass has improved the results of the surgical approach to massive thromboembolism. Surgical intervention may be indicated where the acute resuscitation measures have failed, severe hypotension persists and angiography shows that peripheral pulmonary perfusion is reduced by 75%.

The selection of patients for immediate pulmonary embolectomy remains a difficult problem. Thrombolytic therapy requires a number of hours to produce a significant resolution and time may not be on the side of the patient with severe systemic hypotension, hypoxia, elevated right heart pressures and possibly coexistent cardiorespiratory disease. A decision must be based upon the clinical and haemodynamic state of the patient as well as the ready availability of the surgical team and required facilities. If the patient survives long enough to be put on cardiopulmonary bypass, embolectomy is likely to be successful.

Vena caval occlusion

The place of surgery in interrupting the venous drainage system to prevent recurrent pulmonary emboli has not yet been clearly defined. The vena cava may be completely ligated or partially interrupted with a variety of teflon clips. Such measures are rarely indicated and should be considered only if the mother's life is threatened by recurrent thromboemboli and lower limb venography demonstrates loose thrombi. The introduction of the inferior vena cava umbrella filter, which can be positioned under fluoroscopy with local anaesthesia, has minimized the hazards of inferior vena cava interruption. This technique seems preferable in the rare situations where interruption of the vena cava is indicated.

Cerebral thrombosis

The acute onset of headaches and neurological deficits such as hemiparesis or dysphasia, focal seizures, fever and sinus tachycardia in a pregnant or postpartum patient may be the result of cerebral venous thrombosis. Computerized tomography may suggest the diagnosis but often carotid angiography is required to demonstrate the occluded vessels. Three reports emphasize the safety and efficacy of heparin treatment in this rare but serious disorder (Srinivasan 1983, Halpern et al 1984, Bousser et al 1985). Cerebral arterial thrombosis can present in pregnancy as a typical stroke (Wiebers & Whisnant 1985). The use of systemic anticoagulation is controversial in these cases but can usually be treated safely if computerized tomography shows only an ischaemic pattern without haemorrhage.

Septic pelvic vein thrombophlebitis and ovarian vein thrombosis

These thrombotic complications may present with pyrexia and non-specific signs of inflammation but accurate diagnosis is difficult. Septic pelvic vein thrombophlebitis can arise as a complication of puerperal sepsis and may lead to pulmonary embolism. Heparinization and antibiotic therapy are indicated (Weiner 1985). Acute ovarian vein thrombosis may present as severe adnexal pain and fever in the postpartum period. The condition is usually diagnosed at laparoscopy and the clot may extend into the vena cava and renal veins

(Bahnson et al 1985). Heparinization is indicated for 10–14 days.

Hereditary thrombotic disorders

The incidence of thromboembolic complications during pregnancy in women with hereditary antithrombin III deficiency has been estimated at around 70% (Hellgren et al 1982). Full therapeutic doses of heparin are recommended throughout pregnancy (Brandt & Stenbjerg 1979). Antithrombin III levels should be checked periodically. At delivery marked falls in antithrombin III and thrombocytopenia may develop even on heparin (Brandt 1981). In this situation antithrombin III concentrates of fresh frozen plasma should be given and repeated every second day during the first postpartum week.

Cardiac prosthetic valves

The optimal anticoagulation regimen for prophylaxis against thromboembolic complications in pregnant women with cardiac prosthetic valves has not yet been firmly established. In many previous reports, combinations of heparin and warfarin have been studied. The use of warfarin in the first trimester is associated with congenital anomalies and spontaneous abortion (O'Neill et al 1982). Subcutaneous low-dose heparin alone has been associated with major embolic events using a dose of 5000 units of heparin twice daily (Bennett & Oakley 1968, Wang et al 1983); this would be an inadequate dose in a pregnant woman. In 18 pregnancies treated by heparin therapy, adjusted to keep the thromboplastin time at 1.5 times control during the first and third trimester, with warfarin used between the 13th and the 36th week, no maternal thromboembolic complications or congenital malformations occurred but early abortions attributable to warfarin therapy were seen (Lee et al 1986). Our current recommendations (Hathaway & Bonnar 1987) are:

1. Pregnancy is contraindicated in women with prosthetic heart valves who have had previous thromboembolic complications and who require continuous anticoagulation with warfarin. In such patients the risk of further thrombotic episodes and fetal complications is very high.
2. In patients with cardiac valve prostheses who are at lower risk for thrombosis, warfarin should be discontinued or replaced by therapeutic heparinization prior to conception because of the high incidence of abortion in warfarin-treated patients.
3. Patients should be given subcutaneous heparin throughout pregnancy in a dosage adjusted to prolong the partial thromboplastin time to 1.5 times normal.
4. Heparin therapy should be continued for at least 1 week after delivery until the patient is re-established on warfarin. Breastfeeding is not contraindicated if the baby has received vitamin K prophylaxis.

CONCLUSIONS

In recent years the use of new diagnostic techniques has produced more information on the natural history of thrombotic disease and there is now a better understanding of methods of prevention and treatment. This chapter has attempted to evaluate the significance of these advances for those caring for pregnant women. Our first priority must be to bring proven prophylactic methods to all obstetric patients who are at high risk of thromboembolic complications. No method is likely to be 100% effective, but present evidence indicates that low-dose heparin confers a high degree of protection against venous thrombosis and if necessary can be used throughout pregnancy by the woman herself.

The time of greatest danger is the immediate puerperium, especially in patients who have been delivered by Caesarean section. The benefit of prophylaxis with either dextran 70 or low-dose heparin should be given to all mothers who are in a high-risk category for thromboembolic complications. In addition to reducing the number of maternal deaths from pulmonary embolism, the judicious use of these prophylactic methods should also decrease the incidence of the post-phlebitic syndrome.

Clinicians must accept the fallibility of the clinical diagnosis of deep vein thrombosis. Treatment based solely on the history and clinical examination will be unnecessary in as many as 50% of patients. An accurate and objective diagnostic method should therefore be used whenever possible and the most reliable methods available at present are contrast phlebography, radionuclide venography and lung scanning.

REFERENCES

Aaro L A, Juergens J L 1974 Thrombophlebitis and pulmonary embolism as complications of pregnancy. Medical Clinics of North America 58: 829–834

Andrew M, Boneu B, Cade J et al 1985 Placental transport of low molecular weight heparin in the pregnant sheep. British Journal of Haematology 59: 103–108

Aznar J, Gilabert J, Estelles A, Espana F 1986 Fibrinolytic activity and protein C in pre-eclampsia. Thrombosis and Haemostasis 55: 314–317

Bahnson R R, Wendel E F, Vogelzang R L 1985 Renal vein thrombosis following puerperal ovarian vein thrombophlebitis. American Journal of Obstetrics and Gynecology 152: 290–291

Bennett G G, Oakley C M 1968 Pregnancy in a patient with a mitral valve. Lancet i: 616–619

Bonnar J 1975 Thromboembolism in obstetric and gynaecological patients. In: Nicolaides A N (ed) Thromboembolism. MTP, Lancaster, pp 311–340

Bonnar J 1976 Long-term self-administered heparin therapy for prevention and treatment of thromboembolic complications in pregnancy. In: Kakkar V V, Thomas D P (eds) Heparin — chemistry and clinical usage. Academic Press, London, pp 247–260

Bonnar J 1977 Acute and chronic coagulation disorders in pregnancy. In: Poller L (ed) Recent advances in blood coagulation, vol 2. Churchill Livingstone, Edinburgh, pp 363–379

Bonnar J 1981 Venous thrombeombolism and pregnancy. Clinical Obstetrics and Gynecology 8: 455–473

Bonnar J, Ma P 1979 Prevention of venous thromboembolism in pregnancy with subcutaneous sodium and calcium heparin. IX World Congress of Gynecology and Obstetrics, Tokyo

Bonnar J, Walsh J J 1972 Prevention of thrombosis after pelvic surgery by British dextran 70. Lancet i: 614–616
Bousser M G, Chiras J, Bories J, Castaigne P 1985 Cerebral venous thrombosis — a review of 38 cases. Stroke 16: 199–213
Brandt P 1981 Observations during the treatment of antithrombin-III deficient women with heparin and antithrombin concentrate during pregnancy, parturition, and abortion. Thrombosis Research 22: 15–24
Brandt P, Stenbjerg S 1979 Subcutaneous heparin for thrombosis in pregnant women with hereditary antithrombin deficiency. Lancet i: 100–101
Browse N L 1977 The prevention of deep vein thrombosis and pulmonary embolism by pharmacological methods. Triangle 16: 29–32
Browse N L 1978 Diagnosis of deep vein thrombosis. British Medical Bulletin 34: 163–167
Coon W W 1977 Epidemiology of venous thromboembolism. Annals of Surgery 186: 149–164
Coon W W, Willis P W III, Keller J B 1973 Venous thromboembolism and other venous disease in the Tecumseh community health study. Circulation 48: 839–846
Daniel D G, Campbell H, Turnbull A C 1967 Puerperal thromboembolism and suppression of lactation. Lancet ii: 287–289
Department of Health and Social Security 1986 Report on confidential enquiries into maternal deaths in England and Wales, 1979–1981. Her Majesty's Stationery Office, London
de Swiet M, Ward D, Fidler S et al 1983 Prolonged heparin therapy in pregnancy causes bone demineralisation. British Journal of Obstetrics and Gynaecology 90: 1129–1134
de Swiet M, Floyd E, Letsky E 1987 Low risk of recurrent thromboembolism in pregnancy (letter). British Journal of Hospital Medicine September, p 264
Ennis J T, Dowsett D J 1983 Radionuclide venography. In: Ennis J T, Dowsett D J (eds) Vascular radionuclide imaging. A clinical atlas. Wiley, Chichester, pp 5–11
Forestier F, Daffos F, Capella-Pavlovsky M 1984 Low molecular weight heparin (PK 10169) does not cross the placenta during the second trimester of pregnancy. Study by direct fetal blood sampling under ultrasound. Thrombosis Research 34: 557–560
Friend J R, Kakkar V V 1970 The diagnosis of deep vein thrombosis in the puerperium. Journal of Obstetrics and Gynaecology of the British Commonwealth 77: 820–825
Friend J R, Kakkar V V 1972 Deep vein thrombosis in obstetric and gynaecologic patients. In: Kakkar V V, Jouhan A J (eds) Thromboembolism. Churchill Livingstone, Edinburgh, pp 131–138
Hall R J, Young C, Sutton G C, Campbell S 1972 Treatment of acute massive pulmonary embolism by streptokinase during labour and delivery. British Medical Journal 4: 647–649
Hall J G, Pauli R M, Wilson K M 1980 Maternal and fetal sequelae of anticoagulation during pregnancy. American Journal of Medicine 68: 122–140
Halpern J P, Morris J G L, Driscoll G L 1984 Anticoagulants and cerebral venous thrombosis. Australian and New Zealand Journal of Medicine 14: 643–648
Hathaway W E, Bonnar J 1987 Thrombotic disorders in pregnancy and the newborn infant. In: Haemostatic disorders of the pregnant woman and the newborn infant. Elsevier, Amsterdam, pp 151–184
Hellgren M, Nygards E B 1982 Long-term therapy with subcutaneous heparin during pregnancy. Gynecologic and Obstetric Investigations 13: 76–89
Hellgren M, Tengborn L, Abildgaard U 1982 Pregnancy in women with congenital antithrombin III deficiency: experience of treatment with heparin and antithrombin. Gynecologic and Obstetric Investigations 14: 127–141
Hirsh J 1986 Mechanism of action and monitoring of anticoagulants. Seminars in Thrombosis and Haemostasis 12: 1–11
Hirsh J, Cade J F, O'Sullivan E F 1970 Clinical experience with anticoagulant therapy during pregnancy. British Medical Journal 1: 270–273
Hull R, Delmore T, Carter C et al 1982 Adjusted subcutaneous heparin versus warfarin sodium in the long-term treatment of venous thrombosis. New England Journal of Medicine 306: 189–194
Johnson W C, Patten D H, Widrich W C, Nabseth D C 1974 Technetium 99m isotope venography. American Journal of Surgery 127: 424–428
Kakkar V V 1987 Diagnosis of deep vein thrombosis. In: Bloom A L, Thomas D P (eds) Haemostasis and thrombosis, 2nd edn. Churchill Livingstone, Edinburgh, pp 779–792
Kline A, Hughes L E, Campbell H, Williams A, Zlosnick J, Leach K G 1975 Dextran 70 in prophylaxis of thromboembolic disease after surgery: a clinically orientated randomised double blind trial. British Medical Journal 2: 109–112
Lao T T, de Swiet M, Letsky E, Walters B N J 1985 Prophylaxis of thromboembolism in pregnancy: an alternative. British Journal of Obstetrics and Gynaecology 92: 202–206
Lee P K, Wang R Y C, Chow J S F, Cheung K L, Wong V C W, Chan T K 1986 The combined use of warfarin and adjusted subcutaneous heparin during pregnancy in patients with artificial heart valves. American Journal of Cardiology 8(1): 221–224
Letsky E A 1985 Coagulation problems during pregnancy. In: Lind T (ed) Current review in obstetrics and gynaecology. Churchill Livingstone, Edinburgh, pp 29–55
Letsky E, de Swiet M 1984 Thromboembolism in pregnancy and its management. British Journal of Haematology 57: 543–552
Lisbona R, Rush C, Leparto L 1987 Technetium-99m red blood cell venography of the lower limb in symptomatic pulmonary embolization. Clinical Nuclear Medicine 12(2): 93–98
Malone L 1983 The fetus as the target organ: a special case. In: Ennis J T, Dowsett D J (eds) Vascular radionuclide imaging. A clinical atlas. Wiley, Chichester, pp 225–226
O'Neill H, Blake S, Suqure D, MacDonald D 1982 Problems in the management of patients with artificial valves during pregnancy. British Journal of Obstetrics and Gynaecology 89: 940–943
Sasahara A A 1987 Diagnosis of pulmonary embolism. In: Bloom A L, Thomas D P (eds) Haemostasis and thrombosis, 2nd edn. Churchill Livingstone, Edinburgh, pp 792–801
Srinivasan K 1983 Cerebral venous and arterial thrombosis in pregnancy and puerperium. Angiology Journal of Vascular Disease 34: 731–746
Stevenson R E, Burton O M, Ferlauto G L, Taylor H A 1980 Hazards of oral anticoagulants during pregnancy. Journal of American Medical Association 243: 1549–1551
Tejani N 1973 Anticoagulant therapy with cardiac valve prosthesis during pregnancy. Obstetrics and Gynecology 42: 785–793
Thomas D P 1987 Pathogenesis of venous thrombosis. In: Bloom A L, Thomas D P (eds) Haemostasis and thrombosis, 2nd edn. Churchill Livingstone, Edinburgh, pp 767–778
Virchow R 1860 Cited in: Cellular pathology as based upon physiological and pathological histology. Churchill Livingstone, Edinburgh, pp 197–203
Wang R Y C, Lee P K, Chow J S F, Chen W W C 1983 Efficacy of low-dose, subcutaneously administered heparin in the treatment of women with artificial heart valves. Medical Journal of Australia 2: 126–128
Webber M M, Bennet L R, Cragin M D 1969 Thrombophlebitis demonstration by scintiscanning. Radiology 92: 620–623
Weiner C P, 1982 Anticoagulants and antiplatelet agents. In: Rayburn W F, Zuspan F P (eds) Drug therapy in obstetrics and gynecology. Appleton-Century-Crofts, Norwalk, Connecticut, pp 345–358
Weiner C P 1985 Diagnosis and management of thromboembolic disease during pregnancy. Clinical Obstetrics and Gynecology 28: 107–118
Whitfield L R, Lele A S, Levy G 1983 Effect of pregnancy on the relationship between concentration and anticoagulant action of heparin. Clinical Pharmacology and Therapy 34: 23–28
Wiebers D O, Whisnant J P 1985 The incidence of stroke among pregnant women in Rochester, Minnesota, 1955 through 1979. Journal of American Medical Association 254: 3055–3057

Gillian Forrest

Parental appreciation of perinatal death

INTRODUCTION

The loss of a baby in the perinatal period is a traumatic event which has far-reaching consequences for the bereaved parents. Over the past few years, with the dramatic improvements in perinatal and infant mortality rates, parents' expectations of the safe delivery of a healthy baby have become very high. When things do go wrong therefore, they are not only confronted with the loss of their baby, but also with the loss of their faith in modern medical care. In addition, as part of industrialized western society which has lost its familiarity with death and bereavement, many parents do not even have the comfort of the mourning rituals which have traditionally helped the bereaved to cope. It is important, therefore, for professionals dealing with perinatal death to have an understanding of the bereavement process, and an awareness of the difficulties and dilemmas facing parents so that medical staff can offer the best possible care.

BEREAVEMENT

Our knowledge of bereavement is based partly on descriptive accounts of patients in psychiatric treatment, and partly on objective studies of groups of bereaved subjects. For example, Lindemann (1944) studied the acute grief reactions of the relatives of those involved in a disastrous night-club fire; Parkes (1972) has carried out a number of studies of widows and recently reviewed the literature and classification of grief reactions (Parkes 1985). Normal grief reactions vary between individuals, but there are some common features. At first, there is usually a period of shock or numbness, which may last for hours or days and is more marked after an unexpected death. This is followed by acute episodes of intense emotional distress with weeping, protestation and anger, with accompanying somatic symptoms of anxiety such as palpitations or choking sensations in the throat. These pangs of grief are precipitated by any reminders of the loss and are set against a chronic background disturbance of depressed mood, disturbances of sleep, appetite and weight and social withdrawal (Worden 1982). Vivid dreams and hallucinations of the dead person or his* voice are quite common, and often people feel compelled to carry out hopeless searches. There is an overwhelming need to rehearse the events around the death and this is one aspect of grief work, the process by which we accept the reality of the loss and withdraw psychologically from the relationship with the dead person, in order to continue our own life in a positive manner.

The chronic low mood and loss of purpose in life may continue for months or years, while the pangs of grief tend to decrease in intensity and frequency with time. There is an increase in psychosomatic and somatic illness in the year following bereavement, which may be a consequence of the disturbance of the immune system which has been reported (Bartrop et al 1977). Anniversary reactions are commonly experienced for some time.

Recovery from bereavement is marked by a return to psychological, social and physical well-being. Because of the enormous individual variations in response, it is not possible to provide a specific time scale. However, a successful outcome depends on the individual's personality and life experiences, the circumstances of the death, the relationship he had with the dead person and on the supportive network surrounding him (Raphael 1977). The style of an individual's grief reaction will be determined by his personality traits, for example, whether he grieves in private or openly expresses his emotions.

*Throughout this chapter the masculine pronoun 'he' has been used to avoid the awkward repetition of 'he or she'.

PERINATAL DEATH

Today, it is widely accepted that losing a baby late in pregnancy or soon after delivery is accompanied by the same sort of grief reaction described above. However, this was not always so and as recently as 1970, it was widely held that perinatal death was a relatively minor trauma, with recovery taking only a few weeks. Kennell et al (1970) and Giles (1970) published the first studies of grief reactions following perinatal death and dispelled this fallacious idea. Since then there has been a great deal of descriptive literature, with some objective studies on management and outcome and it is now clear that grief after perinatal death is no different, qualitatively, from that following the death of any loved person.

There are some special features. Anxiety and anger are frequently described, with blame being directed at the staff, other members of the family, or at one's self, in the form of guilt. This may be due in part to the suddenness of the death and is probably compounded when there is no scientific explanation available to help the parents understand exactly what went wrong (Newton et al 1986). Desperately seeking for a cause for the baby's death is also common. Clearly, it is easier for parents who do have an explanation such as malformations of the baby or extreme prematurity. 'Empty arms' is another common and distressing symptom after the phase of numbness has passed and mothers are frequently tormented by hearing their dead baby crying, or feeling fetal movements. Some experience negative or aggressive feelings towards other babies and are fearful of losing control, while others long to hold a baby, any baby, however painful this might be. Many mothers do not expect to lactate once the baby has died, and find the fact that they do very upsetting. Most authors emphasize the great sense of loss of self-esteem experienced by bereaved mothers; they experience failure both as women and as wives.

Most young parents will not have been bereaved before and often experience difficulties coping with the complicated registration and funeral procedures. Many mothers are unprepared for the emotional turmoil of their grief reaction and of the exacerbation of symptoms which often accompanies the expected date of delivery or the return of menstruation. They usually feel they should be over it after a few weeks. This view may be reinforced by well-meaning friends and relatives and even some medical practitioners, who may advise the couple to go ahead with another pregnancy long before they have sufficiently recovered from their loss to cope with this psychological stress. There is evidence that fathers recover from grief more quickly than mothers (Helmrath & Steinitz 1978, Clyman et al 1980, Forrest et al 1982) and this in itself may lead to relationship problems, particularly if the couple are not used to sharing their feelings, or if one is blaming the other for the baby's death. Meyer & Lewis (1979) report that sexual and marital difficulties are common sequelae, although an increase in marital breakdown rate has not been reported.

Another difficult area is the reaction of other young children in the family to the loss of the baby. They may be very confused about what has happened to the baby and even feel responsible for his disappearance (Bowlby 1979). Behavioural changes are common and may take the form of over-activity, naughtiness, regression and school problems, as well as emotional problems (Van Eerdewegh et al 1985). These reactions are usually fairly short-lived—a few weeks or months is the time noted by most authors—unless the emotional state of the parents is such that there is an absence of normal warmth in family relationships for an extended period of many months (Black & Urbanowicz 1985) or if serious relationship difficulties develop between the mother and the surviving children (Halpern 1972, Lewis 1983).

There are particular problems associated with miscarriages and stillborn babies in which iatrogenic factors undoubtedly play a part. Miscarriages are frequently regarded by professionals and others as minor setbacks in successful childbearing. For some women, however, they represent a loss as painful as that of a full-term baby (Oakley et al 1984). This is particularly so if there have been difficulties conceiving, previous miscarriages, or if the pregnancy was terminated because of fetal abnormalities (Lloyd & Laurence 1985, Iles 1986, unpublished data). Here there is the double loss of that baby and of the chance of childbearing. A previous termination of pregnancy has been reported by many clinicians as a complicating factor for normal grieving because of the associated guilt and sense of retribution that is experienced by the mothers. If the pregnancy was well advanced, beyond 20 weeks or so, some parents want to hold a funeral for their baby and this may present administrative difficulties.

Much has been written about unresolved grief after a stillborn baby, notably by Lewis (1976, 1983). He attributes this to the painful emptiness of the experience. There is no real object to mourn as the baby never lives outside the womb, and no memories to help either. It is similar to the situation in which someone is missing, believed dead. The problem is accentuated if the stillborn baby is rapidly removed from the delivery room before the parents have a chance to see or hold him, and if the hospital takes over the funeral arrangements without involving the parents as was common in the UK before about 1978. Until recently in the UK, it was not even possible to register a first name for a stillborn baby and these babies are still often buried in unmarked graves.

The attitudes of friends and relations may also contribute to the difficulties. For example, one grieving mother was told: 'You can't have postnatal depression, you haven't got a baby'! For these reasons, successful mourning after stillbirth may be harder to achieve without the guidance of well informed staff and greater understanding on the part of society in general.

Long-term effects of perinatal death

There have been few studies on the long-term effects of perinatal death. Cullberg (1971) interviewed 56 women 1–2 years after a perinatal death. Nineteen were still found to be suffering from serious maladaptive psychological symptoms. Wolff et al (1970) followed up 40 women for 3 years after a stillbirth. Although all experienced a typical grief reaction, by the end of the study 8 had resolved never to have another pregnancy and of these 4 had been sterilized.

Nicol et al (1986) followed up 110 women for 6–36 months after a perinatal death. They found 21% suffering from a pathological grief reaction, with continuing severe psychological symptoms (depression, anxiety, tiredness etc.); social adjustment problems and marital difficulties, and a resolve to have no further children. Nicol et al also found that a poor outcome was associated with a crisis in the pregnancy, an unsupportive family network and seeing but not holding the baby.

We followed up 35 women for 14 months after a perinatal death (Forrest et al 1982); these women have now been interviewed again 3–5 years later. At this more recent interview, 5 of these mothers were still showing pathological grief reactions characterized by high scores for depression and anxiety on standardized rating scales, psychosomatic symptoms and relationship problems within the family. We found that poor outcome was associated with an unsupportive marriage and social isolation. Of the remaining 30 women in the sample who were free of psychiatric symptoms and functioning well, return to good health had taken on average 24 months and was marked by a successful pregnancy. Most of these mothers reported feeling highly anxious during this pregnancy and overprotective towards the new baby in the first few months—findings which were also reported by Phipps (1985).

There have been reports of serious relationship problems with babies conceived too quickly after a loss (Cain & Cain 1964, Poznanski 1972, Lewis & Page 1978, Bourne & Lewis 1984). It seems that if the dead child has been incompletely mourned before the start of a new pregnancy, mourning may be postponed until after the delivery of the baby, when it can reappear as postnatal depression (Lewis 1979). The new baby's identity can become confused with that of the idealized dead baby, causing great emotional problems. He may never be able to live up to his parents' expectations and may also become the focus of any unresolved anger which the parents feel as a result of their loss. The survivor of twins may also be involved in very similar problems if the dead twin is not properly mourned at the time. This has been called the replacement baby syndrome.

It seems therefore that about 1 in 5 bereaved families are likely to suffer adverse long-term effects after losing a baby. Although at this stage we are not able to identify positively those most at risk, the most frequently reported factors are not seeing or holding the baby, an unsupportive partner or social network and immediately embarking on another pregnancy. Good care should therefore aim to try and prevent these long-term sequelae.

CARE

In many countries now, the recommendations for care emphasize the important role of maternity unit staff as regards families facing the loss of their baby (Giles 1970, Klaus & Kennell 1976, National Stillbirth Study Group 1979, Kowalski 1980, Fetus and Newborn Committee, Canadian Paediatric Society 1983, Rousseau & Moreau 1984, Royal College of Obstetricians and Gynaecologists 1985). In our randomized study (Forrest et al 1982) we attempted to evaluate a planned programme of care based on the National Stillbirth Study Group's recommendations. These included encouraging the parents to see, hold and name their baby and hold a funeral; arranging for them to see the senior obstetric and paediatric staff to discuss what went wrong; obtaining genetic and obstetric counselling and ensuring that parents received the autopsy results. In addition, a short series of counselling sessions with a child psychiatrist was included in the care offered to the index group. The average number of counselling contacts was three. Those mothers who had been randomly allocated to the control group received routine hospital care, which varied enormously from compassionate, individual care to rapid discharge with no further contact.

At our follow-up at 6 months, only 2 out of the 16 index mothers had high scores for measures of depression and anxiety, compared with 10 of the 19 control group of mothers ($P = 0.01$). By 14 months, this statistically significant difference between the groups had disappeared. We concluded that the provision of informed, compassionate care significantly facilitated the recovery process after perinatal death. We did not feel that bereavement counselling services were required in the majority of the group who had had a normal grief reaction.

It seems therefore that effective care for most families can and indeed should be provided by the maternity unit staff, as they are in a key position to help bereaved families by facilitating the establishment of normal grieving from the start, thus preventing abnormal reactions.

This section brings together the recommendations for care made by individual clinicians and organizations concerned with helping parents cope with perinatal death. It is generally agreed that the key task is to enable parents overcome their fear of death and dying so that they can experience the painful reality of their loss and allow mourning to begin. This involves encouraging them to have as much contact as possible with their baby, both before and after death. There is widespread agreement by authors that it is particularly important for parents of stillborn babies to see, hold and name their baby (Lewis 1976, Klaus & Kennell 1976, Morris 1976, Rousseau & Moreau 1984).

Intrauterine death and stillbirth

When an intrauterine death is suspected, the fears for the baby's condition should be shared with the parents, together if at all possible, and not denied. If the mother is at the clinic, efforts should be made to contact her partner or a friend, so that she is not left to travel home alone and unsupported. The ultrasonographers in the scanning room have an important role to play when the confirmatory scan is done. They need to be sympathetic to the situation, relaxing any rules to allow the mother to be accompanied by anyone she chooses. After intrauterine death has been confirmed, most women are very frightened at the prospect of delivering a dead baby, as well as being shocked by their loss. It helps if staff take time to explain carefully what will happen, that adequate pain relief will be available, and what the baby will look like at delivery. This is often successful in overcoming any reluctance the parents may have about seeing or holding their baby. If the baby is very malformed or macerated, it may help to show him first to the parents wrapped up. Even so, a few parents will not be able to cope with seeing and holding their baby at the time of delivery. A photograph should be taken and kept in the medical notes for possible use later and further opportunities for seeing the baby offered to parents over the next few days, as they often change their minds. Photographs and other mementos of the baby are in fact very important, as they provide tangible evidence of the reality of the baby's existence and of his loss. They should be available for parents as keepsakes, if they wish.

If a baby dies in labour, it is good practice to inform the consultant in charge immediately (or very soon if it is the middle of the night). The fact that a senior member of staff has come very promptly to try to help the parents from his own experience is nearly always deeply appreciated by parents, and can soften any resentful feelings the couple may have towards the hospital staff.

Neonatal death

When the baby lives long enough to be transferred to an intensive care unit, it is again very important for the staff to make time to keep parents as fully informed as possible about the baby's condition and encourage them to share in any possible part of the care. Photographs of the baby are very helpful, particularly for the fathers to keep at home, or if the mother is too unwell to visit the unit. In a randomized trial of the use of routine Polaroid photographs of sick babies in the first week of life (Pareira et al 1980), there was a significant increase in visiting by the parents of photographed babies compared with the non-photographed group. When the baby's condition is known to be terminal, it is important to try to involve the parents in the decision to cease life support and then to let them nurse their dying baby in their arms, free if possible from all the equipment that has been necessary until then. In describing this, authors quote parents as saying: 'It was all I could do for him, hold him in my arms as he died' (Forrest et al 1982). Guilt for removing the baby from the life support system has not been reported.

Many parents like to help with the laying-out of the baby's body and this should be encouraged. They often select special clothes or toys to be placed in the coffin with the baby.

Facilitating the parents' contact with the reality of the death of their baby in these ways facilitates their grief reactions. They also need privacy to express their grief and this should be provided, however busy the unit.

Aftercare

The choice of site of the aftercare of the mother is important as mothers differ in their requirements at this time. Some want to be on their own, far away from the sound of babies crying; others long to return to familiar faces on the ward. It is helpful if care can be as flexible as possible in this aspect; the mother will also need her partner to remain with her for the first night at least. Ideally, the hospital should provide a couch in the mother's room so that the couple can share their grief together. Help with the suppression of lactation has already been mentioned as an important issue for the mother whose baby has died. If the mother is physically fit to return home immediately and wishes to do so, it is essential to ensure that she has a good supportive network of family, friends and professionals before briskly discharging her.

The autopsy

Consent for autopsy should always be requested after a perinatal death, as it may provide invaluable information about the cause of death and help parents not only with their grief but also assist in the planning of future pregnancies. Most parents do consent although the decision is often painful. As one mother put it: 'She's been through enough; must she be cut up now as well?' There are, however, a small number of parents whose religion forbids autopsy and their dilemma needs to be acknowledged to avoid a situation in which they are subjected to intolerable pressure to obtain their consent.

Having consented, parents cherish great hopes that the findings will answer their questions about why their baby died. It is therefore very important for them to receive the results in a form which makes sense to them. The best person to do this is a senior member of staff who can interpret the pathologist's findings. This can be done as part of the follow-up interview.

Registration and funeral arrangements

Fundamental to good care is a knowledge not only of the bereavement process but also of the legal procedures required when a baby dies or is stillborn. It is also necessary to be familiar with the registration and funeral arrangements in one's own unit or locality, as these are often complicated and baffling for parents still suffering from the shock of their baby's death (Forrest et al 1981). Religious practices also vary greatly and an awareness of these and sensitivity to individual parents' wishes is crucial. A funeral may involve considerable expense and assisting parents in making difficult choices, helping those in financial straits and encouraging them to attend the funeral are therapeutic aspects of care. The unit should ensure that a suitable individual is available for this task.

Many units have prepared leaflets outlining their own procedures and providing helpful advice on various aspects of losing a baby; these can be very helpful for parents.

Communication

Good care hinges around good communication and parents often comment on communication failures in describing their experiences. Staff need to give bereaved parents opportunities for talking together about the loss of their baby and listen sympathetically to their expressions of grief. It is much harder to listen than talk oneself. In addition, staff need to try and help parents in their search for a cause of death and senior obstetric or paediatric staff need to discuss this with the parents. Seeing both parents together not only helps to strengthen their relationship as they share the experience of their baby's loss, but also helps prevent misunderstandings or inconsistencies in explanation. Arranging for the same members of staff to meet regularly with the parents also helps. Any information given in the first few days of the loss will probably have to be repeated later as the initial shock of bereavement passes. A follow-up interview a few weeks later seems to be the best way of overcoming this difficulty. Good communication between staff about the loss of the baby is also vital to prevent painful situations, such as an individual being unaware that a baby has died and breezily asking the mother when she is to be delivered. Communication between hospital and primary health care teams also needs to be good. The primary care team should be informed immediately about the baby's loss so that they can contact the family as soon as, or even before, the mother is discharged from hospital. Parents may want the support of their own religious adviser and the hospital needs to check on this and contact the person concerned.

The next pregnancy

The timing of the next pregnancy is important, as has already been discussed, to allow for the dead baby to be mourned first. From their members' experience, the Stillbirth and Neonatal Death Society (1984) recommends waiting 6–8 months. Our study (Forrest et al 1982) found that pregnancy occurring less than 6 months after the loss was strongly associated with high depression and anxiety scores at the 14-months' assessment. However, the enormous individual variation in bereavement response means that it is inappropriate to recommend a fixed time interval. The best advice appears to be to wait a while until the parents have had a chance to say goodbye to the dead baby and until the mother feels emotionally as well as physically strong enough to cope with another pregnancy. The next pregnancy will inevitably be an extremely anxious time and she will need extra support during it and in the first few months after delivery.

Follow-up

Most mothers will be discharged home within a few days of their baby's death, still too shocked to grasp properly what has happened or why. Careful follow-up is extremely important. Parents should be able to contact the staff who cared for them by telephone after they leave the hospital; and some units offer home visits by a social worker. An appointment should be made for both parents to see the consultant or a senior member of staff about 6 weeks later, as soon as the chromosomes and autopsy results are available and some form of perinatal mortality conference has taken place, to cover the following points:

1. To give the parents the opportunity of going over the events around the loss of their baby and releasing emotion.
2. To allow clarification of why the baby died, if at all possible. The autopsy results should be given to parents in an appropriate form.
3. To give obstetric counselling and in particular, advise about the timing of future pregnancies.
4. To make any necessary arrangements for genetic counselling.

Although returning to the maternity unit for these appointments is usually a harrowing prospect for parents, they almost always find it helpful. Perhaps this is because they have moved a step further in their grief work by once again facing the painful memories.

Checklists

Some units find it useful to have checklists to ensure that all practical aspects of care have been covered (White et al 1984). Although they can be helpful as *aides-mémoire*, checklists should not replace personal, compassionate contact with bereaved parents.

Care of the family at home

The general practitioner (GP), health visitor and the other primary health care workers form the professional supportive network for the family once the mother has been discharged home. These professionals can help by continuing to express concern, informing parents about the symptoms of bereavement and putting them in touch with any local support groups for parents who have lost a child (see Useful Addresses). The GP can watch for signs of a pathological grief reaction and refer for specialist help if necessary. These reactions are most likely to take the form of an inhibited reaction in which there is no sign of any sense of loss, or of a prolonged reaction, with unremitting symptoms of depression, severe anxiety or the appearance of psychosomatic illness. There may also be drug or alcohol abuse.

Unremitting anger is another feature of a pathological reaction and the GP may need to deal with anger focused on the maternity unit. To do so, he needs to have good relationships with the obstetric and paediatric staff and to be fully informed about the course of events which led to the baby's loss. The parents may also blame the GP, of course. When this happens, it is essential for him to meet the family as soon as possible so that they can ventilate their feelings, and, hopefully, re-establish their relationship. Many parents remain angry simply because they were denied any compassionate response to their situation; no one on the staff said: 'I'm so sorry your baby has died'.

The GP or health visitor will probably be the people the family turn to for help with the reactions of their other children to the baby's death. Black & Urbanowicz (1985) described the reactions of 80 bereaved children in a study of family intervention after the death of a parent and found an association between crying and talking about the dead parent with good outcome at 1 year. They concluded that the expression of mourning by children was helpful. Parents may need help in allowing their children to vent their feelings about such a painful subject and it must be remembered that young children will use play as a vehicle for expressing this emotion. Explaining death to the under-5-year-olds is also difficult, because developmentally, they are not yet able to grasp the concept (Lansdown & Benjamin 1985). Even very simple statements like: 'The baby's gone' will be interpreted literally and lead to questions about where, and when a visit can be made. The parents will need to provide more information as the child's capacity for understanding develops.

THE ROLE OF SPECIALIST COUNSELLORS

So far, this chapter has concentrated on the management of normal grief and the prevention of abnormal reactions through the care of the ordinary staff of maternity units and primary health care teams. However, about 1 in 5 families will show pathological reactions and all of these are likely to be accompanied by family relationship problems. In such cases, the help of specialist counsellors trained in grief work will be needed to advise staff on management or to take over the cases if necessary. The treatment required is often lengthy; antidepressant drugs and psychiatric surveillance may be necessary for severe depressive symptoms. Child and family psychiatrists may be particularly helpful in dealing with family relationship problems. Specialist counsellors can also help to promote normal grieving in parents who are most at risk of pathological reactions. The possible risk factors identified are a crisis in the pregnancy; an unsupportive partner or spouse, and lack of a supportive social network. Specialist counsellors can also be useful in supporting the staff of the unit through regular staff meetings, case discussions, training sessions on offering help and advice to self-help groups (Lake et al 1983, Kellner et al 1981).

SELF-HELP GROUPS

Self-help can be very effective in providing appropriate support for parents facing many different problems and perinatal bereavement is no exception. It is important that those running the group have sufficiently recovered from their own loss to be able to help others (2 years is the usual time required) and that they have access to professional help and advice as necessary. In the UK, several national organizations exist—for example, the Stillbirth and Neonatal Death Society (SANDS) and the Compassionate Friends—and there are often locally based groups as well. SANDS have played a major part in changing attitudes and practices in hospitals and in the community and have campaigned for the reform of hospital funeral arrangements and registration anomalies. Their support groups are to be found in most parts of the UK. Parents can benefit from sharing their experiences together, discovering that they are not alone in their suffering and that time helps to heal their wounds. However, not everyone can cope with group support and it is not wise to rely entirely on local self-help groups to meet all the needs of bereaved families. While it is invaluable to give parents the telephone number or address of a local contact, this should not replace follow-up by the hospital and general practitioner.

TRAINING

The training of staff in the case of families who have lost their baby or who are faced with the birth of a malformed or handicapped baby deserves as much emphasis as the development of their technical expertise. Because we have lost our familiarity with death and bereavement at a personal level, staff need to be informed about the process of mourning as well as being trained in the basic skills of interviewing and counselling. They also need to explore their own feelings about death if they are to understand and help others. A good training programme should therefore combine formal with informal teaching, such as the use of group discussions and role play. In addition, junior staff can learn a great deal from watching and listening while more experienced members of staff handle difficult and painful situations.

CONCLUSIONS

Good care does not end with a baby's death; much can be done to help the family cope with their loss and facilitate recovery from the bereavement. In this chapter, an attempt has been made to describe parental grief reactions and set out guidelines for care. But successful implementation depends on the attitudes of individual staff members and the importance attached to training in this area.

Effective care has implications for both maternity unit staff and professionals working in the community. Time needs to be spent with parents whose baby dies or is malformed, listening as well as talking. Attention also has to be paid to the details of follow-up in individual cases. The unit may have to review its procedures for postnatal care in order to be able to offer more flexibility; senior members of staff need to play a central role in caring for the parents, sharing their own experience and expertise with junior staff. Attention must be given to the practical aspects of the registration and funeral arrangements for babies and the primary health care team should monitor the bereavement process. Such changes in care improve rapport with grieving families; staff cope better with the painfulness of perinatal death because they feel able to help. Finally, families on the whole emerge from their grief able to continue functioning well, with positive attitudes towards the professionals who shared in the loss of their baby.

USEFUL ADDRESSES

Compassionate Friends, 6 Denmark Street, Bristol BS1 5D1. Tel: 0272 292778.

Stillbirth and Neonatal Death Society (SANDS), 28 Portland Place, London W1 3DE. Tel: 01 436 5881.

REFERENCES

Bartrop R W, Lazarus L, Luckhurst E, Kiloh L G, Penny R 1977 Depressed lymphocyte function after bereavement. Lancet i: 834–836

Black D, Urbanowicz A 1985 Bereaved children—family intervention. In: Stevenson J E (ed) Recent research in developmental psychopathology. Pergamon Press, Oxford

Bourne S, Lewis E 1984 Pregnancy after stillbirth or neonatal death. Lancet ii: 31–33

Bowlby J 1979 Attachment and loss, vol 3. Hogarth, London

Cain H C, Cain B S 1964 On replacing a child. Journal of the American Academy of Child Psychiatry 3: 443–455

Clyman R, Green C, Rowe J, Mikkelsen C, Ataide L 1980 Issues concerning parents after the death of their newborn. Critical Care Medicine 8: 215–218

Cullberg J 1971 Mental reactions of women to perinatal death. In: Morris N (ed) Psychosomatic medicine in obstetrics and gynaecology. Karger, Basel, pp 326–329

Fetus and Newborn Committee, Canadian Paediatric Society 1983 Support for parents experiencing perinatal loss. Canadian Medical Association Journal 129: 335–339

Forrest G C, Claridge R S, Baum J D 1981 The practical management of perinatal death. British Medical Journal 282: 31–33

Forrest G C, Standish E, Baum J D 1982 Support after perinatal death: a study of support and counselling after perinatal bereavement. British Medical Journal 285: 1475–1479

Giles P 1970 Reactions of women to perinatal death. Australian and New Zealand Journal of Obstetrics and Gynaecology 10: 207–210

Halpern W 1972 Some psychiatric sequence to crib death. American Journal of Psychiatry 129: 398–402

Helmrath T A, Steinitz E M 1978 Parental grieving and the failure of social support. Journal of Family Practice 6: 785–790

Kellner K R, Kirkley-Best E, Chessborough S, Donnelly W 1981 Perinatal mortality counseling program for families experiencing stillbirth. Death Education 5: 29–40

Kennell J H, Slyter J, Klaus M H 1970 The mourning responses of parents to the death of a newborn infant. New England Journal of Medicine 283: 344–349

Klaus M H, Kennell J H 1976 Maternal infant bonding. CV Mosby, St Louis

Kowalski K 1980 Managing perinatal loss. Clinics in Obstetrics and Gynaecology 23: 1113–1123

Lake M, Knuppel R A, Murphy J, Johnson T 1983 The role of a grief support team following stillbirth. American Journal of Obstetrics and Gynecology 146: 877–881

Lansdown R, Benjamin G 1985 The development of the concept of death in children aged 5–9 years. Child Care, Health and Development 11: 13–20

Lewis E 1976 Management of stillbirth—coping with an unreality. Lancet ii: 619–620

Lewis E 1979 Inhibition of mourning by pregnancy: psychopathology and management. British Medical Journal 11: 27–28

Lewis E 1983 Stillbirth: psychological consequences and strategies of management. In: Milunsky A (ed) Advances in perinatal medicine, vol 3. Plenum, New York

Lewis E, Page A 1978 Failure to mourn a stillbirth; an overlooked catastrophe. British Journal of Medical Psychology 51: 237–241

Lindemann E 1944 Symptomatology and management of acute grief. American Journal of Psychiatry 101: 141–148

Lloyd J, Laurence K M 1985 Sequelae and support after termination of pregnancy for fetal malformation. British Medical Journal 290: 907–909

Meyer R, Lewis E 1979 Impact of stillbirth on a marriage. Journal of Family Therapy 1: 361

Morris D 1976 Parental reactions to perinatal death. Proceedings of the Royal Society of Medicine 69: 837–838

National Stillbirth Study Group 1979 The loss of your baby. Health Education Council/Mind, London

Newton R W, Bergin R, Knowles D 1986 Parents interviewed after their child's death. Archives of Disease in Childhood 61: 711–715

Nicol M T, Tompkins J R, Campbell N A, Syme G J 1986 Maternal grieving response after perinatal death. Medical Journal of Australia 144: 287–289

Oakley A, McPherson A, Roberts H 1984 Miscarriages. Fontana, London

Pareira G R, Talbot Y R, Boatwell W R, Parina P A, Musholt K S 1980 Photographs of sick neonates prior to transport; the effect on parental visiting pattern. Pediatric Research 14: 2662–2673

Parkes C M 1972 Bereavement: studies of grief in adult life. Tavistock, London

Parkes C M 1985 Bereavement. British Journal of Psychiatry 146: 11–17

Phipps S 1985 The subsequent pregnancy after stillbirth; anticipatory parenthood in the face of uncertainty. International Journal of Psychiatry in Medicine 15: 243–263

Poznanski E O 1972 The 'replacement child'; a saga of unresolved parental grief. Behavioral Pediatrics 81: 1190–1193

Raphael B 1977 Preventive intervention with the recently bereaved. Archives of General Psychiatry 34: 1450–1454

Rousseau P, Moreau K 1984 Le deuil perinatal. Extrait de la revue L'enfant de l'ONE no 5. Jolimont, Belgium

Royal College of Obstetricians and Gynaecologists 1985 Report of the

RCOG working party on the management of perinatal deaths. RCOG, London
The Stillbirth and Neonatal Death Society 1984 Preconceptual care of preparing for your next baby. London
Van Eerdewegh M M, Clayton P, Van Eerdewegh P 1985 The bereaved child; variables influencing early psychopathology. British Journal of Psychiatry 147: 188–194
White M P, Reynolds B, Evans T J 1984 Handling of death in special care nurseries and parental grief. British Medical Journal 289: 167–169
Worden W 1982 Grief counselling and grief therapy. Tavistock, London

SECTION 10

The Normal Newborn

66

David Hull

Evaluation of the newborn

ADJUSTMENTS AT BIRTH

Lung expansion and the onset of breathing

Once the infant emerges from the birth canal and the umbilical cord is occluded, clamped and cut, the infant's immediate priority is to establish an alternative oxygen supply. For this he or she needs to fill the lungs with air and to breathe regularly at an appropriate rate and depth. The latter probably depends on the former.

At the time of birth the infant's sensory system is well in advance of the motor system, so the brain will record a kaleidoscope of new sensations as he or she is handled and squeezed and head, trunk and limbs drop into novel positions. In utero the hips are flexed — extensions of the hips may well cause a very unpleasant if not painful sensation — so it is not surprising that dangling babies by their ankles at birth provokes a gasp and crying. The sensations are such that the majority of babies gasp at birth without noxious stimulus. If the gasp occurs whilst the airway is clear, then the gas–liquid interface moves down the respiratory tree as the lung fills with air. In healthy infants no opening pressure is required, though the first inspiratory gasps can generate intrathoracic pressures of over 100 cmH_2O (Milner & Vyas 1982). The formation of the functional residual capacity depends on a number of factors, including diaphragmatic tone, but the precise mechanisms are as yet ill understood. Usually functional residual capacity is established to 70% of its final volume within a few gasps. Sometimes, despite gasps, little or no air is held. Only when the lungs are filled with air will tidal ventilation begin and only then will the infant have control of an independent oxygen supply. Most healthy infants achieve this within 1 minute (Chamberlain et al 1975; Fig. 66.1). Asphyxiated, sedated and premature infants may have problems with the initial gasps and the establishment and maintenance of a functional residual capacity.

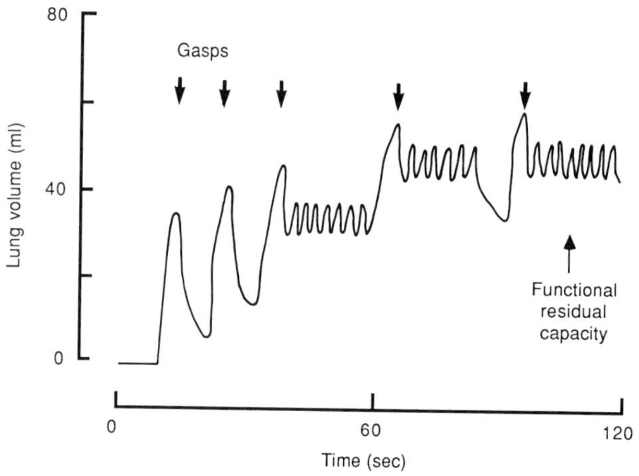

Fig. 66.1 Respiratory patterns with the onset of breathing.

The closure of the fetal channels

Consequent upon clamping the umbilical cord, the venous return from the placenta stops abruptly, the ductus venosus collapses, the pressure in the right atrium falls and the foramen ovale closes. When the lungs expand and fill with air the pulmonary vascular resistance falls, the pulmonary blood flow increases, and the increased pulmonary venous return causes a rise in the left atrium pressure which further reinforces the closure of the foramen ovale (Dawes 1968; Fig. 66.2). With the fall in pulmonary pressure, the flow through the ductus arteriosus reverses so that oxygenated blood traverses the duct; the oxygen acts on the muscle in the duct wall causing it to contract (Heymann & Rudolph 1975). The mechanism also involves reduction in fetal prostaglandin E_2, which results in ductus closure. Prostaglandin-inhibitor drugs given to mothers delivering preterm infants can cause

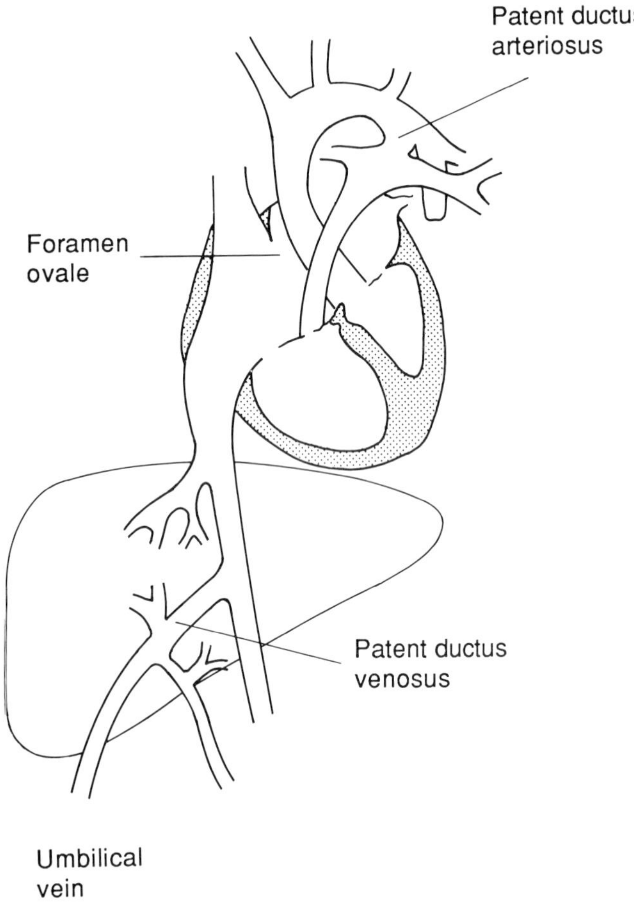

Fig. 66.2 The fetal channels.

intrauterine closure of the ductus, causing problems for the neonate, including persistent pulmonary hypotension (Friedman et al 1976). Prostaglandin E infusions can keep the ductus open in infants with congenital heart defects such as severe pulmonary stenosis and thus keep a child alive until corrective surgery can be performed (Silove 1986). With the closure of the fetal channels the chambers of the heart, previously working in series, begin to work in parallel. If one is ill formed therefore, for example hypoplasia of one ventricle, the other can no longer maintain both circulations and acute circulatory problems are precipitated.

Colour, tone and blood pressure

With birth pulmonary blood pressure falls and systemic pressure rises (Dawes 1968). Birth is a stressful experience: fetal catecholamine levels are high and peripheral vasomotor control appears to be largely untried. Thus normal, healthy infants during the first hours of life can appear to be many colours — red, white or blue and occasionally all three in patches. With oxygenation after birth, the infant's colour may change from a pasty white to a glowing pink. Some infants have blue hands and feet for some time after birth. Oxygenation also results in an increase in tone which, like the colour, improves at the top and moves downwards. Within moments of this development the infant is usually wide awake and ready to suckle.

Temperature control

Inevitably for the infant, it is a cold world. In utero the fetus is bathed in amniotic fluid at 37°C and because the fetal metabolic rate per kg is higher than the mother's, the fetal body temperature is higher by 0.3–0.6°C. At birth, as the skin dries out, the infant loses heat by evaporation; this has to be reduced to a minimum if a drop in body temperature is to be avoided. Drying down in a warm towel, followed by swaddling in a warm blanket and being cuddled by the parents is ideal. Even with precautions, an infant's rectal temperature often falls after birth and then rises slowly over the first hours of life. This subsequent rise may be in part associated with the rising minimal metabolic rate as the infant's systems begin to work to support independent existence (Smales & Kime 1978).

Even the term infant has a limited capacity to control body temperature (Hull & Chellappah 1983, Rutter 1986). Thus on exposure to cold he or she may reduce surface heat losses by vasoconstriction and double body heat production by thermogenesis in brown adipose tissue (Hull 1966) but even so, because of an infant's body weight: surface area ratio, if he or she is taken from a warm cot, undressed and prepared for a bath in a warm room at 25°C, he or she will not be able to maintain body temperature. In a hot environment a baby can sweat a little (Rutter & Hull 1979) but this capacity is limited so he or she is even more vulnerable in hot environments. Infants have always been dependent on their parents for protection and this is particularly important with respect to body warmth in the first days of life. Cuddling and swaddling are not just comforting but also important for sensing and maintaining the baby's temperature.

Swallowing, digesting and evacuation

A total of 10% of an infant's body weight at birth is formed by adipose tissue of which half is fat which can provide sufficient calories to sustain the infant for some weeks after birth (Widdowson & Spray 1981). Thus there is no great urgency for the bowel to become fully functional in the first hours of life. Indeed it has to develop and grow to accommodate its increasing workload. In utero the infant swallows amniotic fluid containing some protein (Frus-Hansen 1982). After birth, the bowel not only must accommodate a larger volume, digesting disaccharides and fats and many complex proteins, but it must also adjust to colonization with bacteria. These bacteria are usually introduced by parents or other attendants and are influenced by the intraluminal environment of the bowel, which in the main is determined by fed nutrients.

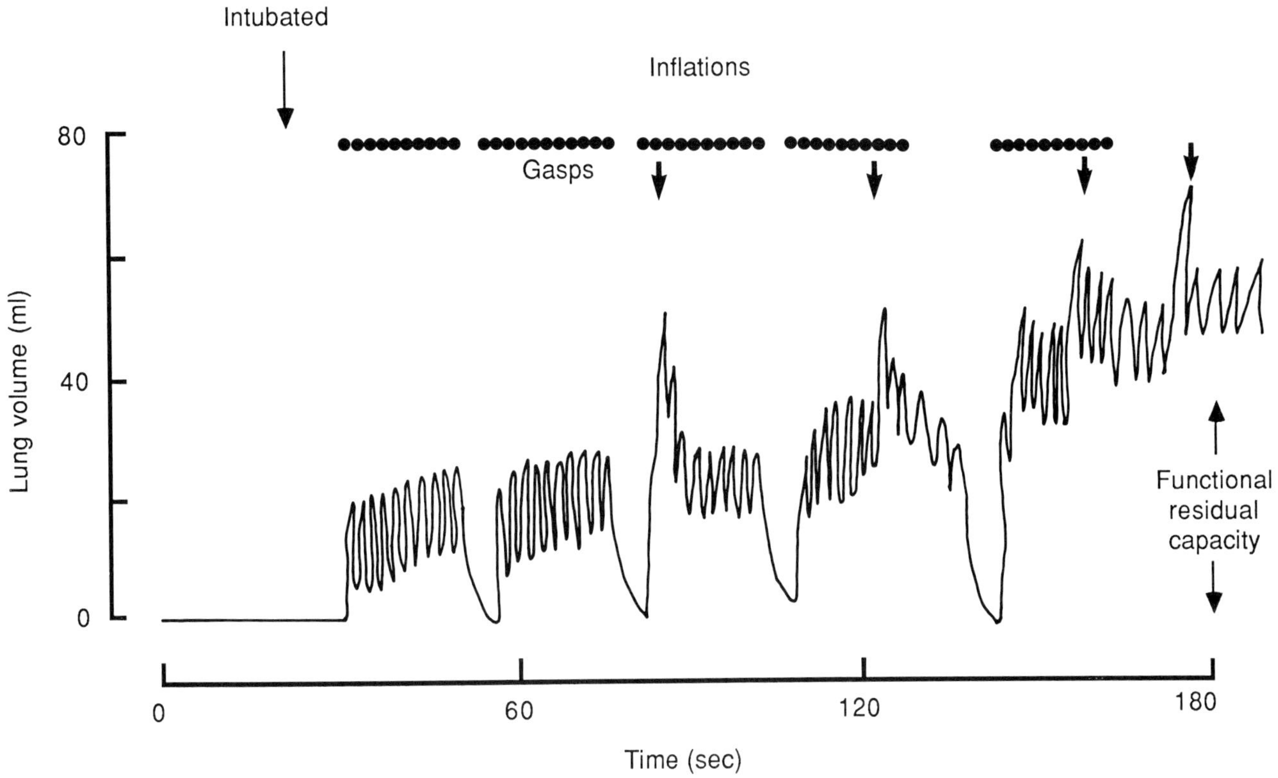

Fig. 66.3 Respiratory pattern of an asphyxiated infant.

Babies often defecate for the first time during delivery, or if not, within the first day of life. Such a remarkable event is worthy of note. By contrast, they regularly micturate in utero, making a considerable contribution to the amniotic fluid (Hytten 1985). Thus infants with obstructive problems usually declare themselves before delivery by oligohydramnios, and after birth by deformations and lung hypoplasia. However, babies who dribble urine may pass undetected, so the observation of the excretion of a good quantity of urine is also important. After birth, the kidney takes up its key role in fluid and electrolyte balance and excretion of chemical waste, a task previously performed by the placenta.

RESUSCITATION

An infant will need active resuscitation if he or she fails to gasp, expand the lungs, maintain a functional residual volume or to begin breathing rhythmically.

Failure to gasp

The risk factors include maternal sedation and anaesthesia, prolonged labour, intrauterine asphyxia, and immaturity (Chamberlain et al 1975). Perhaps the commonest factors are drugs crossing to the fetus prior to birth and suppressing brain activity, although it is amazing to see some infants bursting into life, whilst their mothers, heavily sedated or anaesthetized, are unaware of what is happening. Another cause for failure to gasp is fetal hypoxia, whatever the cause, but the fact that an infant cries immediately at birth does not mean that he or she has not been irreversibly damaged by intrauterine asphyxia. Fetal asphyxia may take any form between two extremes. At one end is the infant who suffers prolonged hypoxia which slowly drains the energy resources, particularly glycogen, causing acidosis and gradually developing widespread damage which may or may not be reversible. At the other extreme is the infant who suffers total acute asphyxia, as may occur with cord prolapse when the oxygen supply is suddenly completely cut off. Depending on the nature of the insult, infants differ both in their response to birth and in their recovery during resuscitation (Fig. 66.3). There are usually other complicating factors. Babies experiencing trauma during delivery, who may well have gasped frequently prior to delivery, may be suffering as much from shock (hypotension) and acidosis as from hypoxia.

Failure to open the lungs

An infant may gasp but fail to hold the gas in the lungs, perhaps because of the effect of drugs or hypoxia on the tone of the diaphragm and the muscles of the chest wall. The task is then to ventilate the infant, supplying oxygen

Table 66.1 Reasons why gasps may not draw air into the lungs

Problem	Cause
Airway obstruction	Aspirated vernix, meconium or blood
	Large or floppy tongue
	Laryngeal spasm or stenosis
Deformed thoracic cage	Thoracic dystrophy (many causes)
	Ill-formed or paralysed diaphragm
Thoracic cage filled with:	Pleural effusions (many causes)
	Bowel and liver (diaphragmatic hernia)
	Haematomas
Lung hypoplasia	Due to renal agenesis
	Due to chronic amniotic leak
	Associated with diaphragmatic hernia

and removing carbon dioxide until normal lung function returns.

On the other hand, it may be that with the gasp, no air enters the lungs because the airway is obstructed. With intrauterine hypoxia or because of stimulation and handling, the fetus may gasp and draw amniotic and birth canal debris, vernix and the like, into the lungs. This can occur to such an extent that aspirating the airways is both an emergency and a priority (Gregory et al 1974). Until this is performed, attempts to push oxygen into the lungs may be inappropriate. Although aspiration of lung liquid from the upper airway is to some extent unavoidable, the baby's head should be held below the level of the lungs after birth, until the airways have been cleared.

There are many other reasons why gasps may prove ineffectual, most rather rare (Table 66.1).

Failure to begin tidal breathing and persisting cyanosis

Very occasionally it is possible to ventilate a child adequately but tidal breathing still does not occur. This can be due to severe asphyxia, very heavy sedation or gross brain abnormality. It may also be a consequence of the presence of the endotracheal tube or of inadvertent hyperventilation.

Occasionally, the lungs may ventilate but the infant remains pale or cyanosed. Pallor may be due to bleeding or shock. A tentorial tear or rupture of a viscera can cause either or both. Persisting cyanosis may be due to a persistent fetal circulation or to severe congenital heart disease.

Assessment

It is common practice to have scoring systems for the assessment and resuscitation of the newborn (Curnock 1986). Whilst there are advantages in such uniformity, it is a mistake to assume that infants in need of resuscitation have similar problems and that assessment criteria have the same meaning irrespective of these problems.

An internationally respected and understood method of assessment is the Apgar score. In essence it is a numerical interpretation of the infant's heart rate, respiratory efforts,

Table 66.2 The Apgar score.

	Score		
Factors	0	1	2
Heart rate	Absent	Slow (<100 beats/min)	>100 beats/min
Respiratory effort	Absent	Slow, irregular	Good, crying
Muscle tone	Flaccid	Some limb flexion	Active motion
Reflex irritability	No response	Cry	Vigorous cry
Colour	Blue, pale	Body pink, limbs blue	Completely pink

responsiveness, colour and tone. The last three in the main reflect adequate oxygenation. It is customary to record the score at 1 and 5 minutes.

As a guide to what to do and when to do it, the infant's heart rate and respiratory efforts are the key features, however. Restoring the heart rate, expanding the chest and oxygenating the baby are the objects of the exercise. Noting the changes in response to actions such as nasal stimulation are more important than adding up the score. In fact the score at 5 minutes may well reflect more of the activities of the resuscitator than the state of the infant.

Assessment based on more pertinent criteria, such as the time to first gasp or the time to establishing regular respirations, have their own merits (Chamberlain et al 1975) but have not been generally accepted. If the Apgar score is to remain the common language, it must be interpreted correctly (Table 66.2).

Minute 0. If an infant is asphyxiated prior to birth, and is born pale or blue and floppy with a heart rate below 100 beats/min, active resuscitation must begin at birth. There is no virtue in waiting.

Minute 1. The majority of infants are not asphyxiated at birth for asphyxia is not an inevitable consequence of the birth process. However, some do not gasp and open their lungs immediately; they have primary apnoea and may need to be encouraged to gasp. Again, it is the falling heart rate and failure of the infant to make a respirating effort which signal the need for appropriate resuscitation.

Minute 5. Some babies start breathing and then give up; others do not respond to the simpler stages of resuscitation, so by 5 minutes, time becomes a premium and if the heart beat remains slow, or if blueness or pallor develop whatever the respiratory effort, informed action is required. Such a situation is a considerable challenge to the clinician.

Management

Handling

At birth, the infant, whether asphyxiated or not, should be handled gently, the cord clamped and cut, and the baby dried in warm towels as expediently as possible. If a problem is anticipated the infant should be placed on a dry, warm surface under a radiant heat source in a good light and observed closely. The clock is started at the moment of birth.

Clearing the airway

Gentle low-pressure suction is used to clear the mouth and pharynx, if necessary under direct vision using an endoscope. Injudicious prodding into the lower pharynx can cause laryngeal spasm or bradycardia from vaginal stimulation and should be avoided.

Provoking a gasp

In a cold world and in an unaccustomed position it may be assumed that the infant has been adequately stimulated. However, various powerful stimuli may provoke a response. While antirespiratory depressants like Narcan are popular, such injections should be avoided unless specifically indicated. The upper respiratory tract is the most appropriate site to stimulate. Cold oxygen blown on the nasal mucosa, for example, often works when handling has not and has the added advantage of ensuring that if the baby gasps, an oxygen-rich mixture is inhaled. The infant may also gasp during clearing of the airway. When all this has failed and artificial ventilation is required, the first inflation often provokes an inspiratory effort, a reflex response which contributes considerably to the success of the procedure (Milner et al 1984).

Oxygenation

To deliver oxygen to the infant it is necessary to fill the lungs with gas. For the majority, it is probable that air is all that is necessary though in practice, pure oxygen is used. This has the disadvantage that if it is left in the lungs after resuscitation and the infant stops breathing again, all the oxygen may be absorbed, causing secondary atelectasis which may be more difficult to reverse. It is good practice to let the infant breathe air through an endotracheal tube before removing it, so that nitrogen remains in the lung and splints the air spaces open.

Gas can be pushed into the lungs either by means of a facemask and bag or by endotracheal intubation and inflation at a controlled pressure.

Facemask and bag

This is perfectly adequate for most babies who fail to breathe. In Sweden it is the method of choice both in hospitals and in the community (Palme et al 1985). It has the advantage of being simple to apply, readily available and relatively safe. With pressure-limited systems, the stomach should not distend with gas (Vyas et al 1983). A variety of facemasks and bags are available (Palme et al 1985). If an emergency arises away from a delivery room, mouth-to-mouth resuscitation can be effective. Use only the pressure that can be generated by the cheeks.

Tracheal intubation

The most certain way for experienced staff to resuscitate the baby is to intubate the trachea with a snug-fitting tube and expand the lung with intermittent inflations at a rate of 30–40/min, holding each inflation for about 1 second and not exceeding a pressure of 30 cmH_2O. Whatever method of lung inflation is used, it is essential to watch the chest cage for expansion and to avoid over-inflation. This can occur with ball valve effects, for example from the endotracheal tube being pressed against the carina. Whilst observing the chest movement keep checking the pulse rate which is usually visible as pulsation at the root of the umbilicus.

If the infant fails to respond, ask why and respond appropriately, as follows:

1. Cardiac massage.
2. Correct acidosis.
3. Tap pneumothorax or pleural effusion.
4. Consider shock or bleeding: give plasma.

When not to resuscitate and when to stop

These are both difficult decisions, depending on clinical judgement. If an infant has a congenital abnormality incompatible with life, such as a severe meningomyelocele, renal agenesis, or gross multiple anomalies, clearly no action should be taken. With very immature infants, the decision is best left to those with experience of neonatal care. By far the majority of infants under 26 weeks' gestation die, and of those that survive under current management, many are severely handicapped. Increasingly units are drawing up guidelines for the care of infants, born technically alive by virtue of a pulsating heart, but who, as a result of prenatal pathology or immaturity, would not survive even with intensive care.

When there is doubt, or when time is required to make an informed choice, resuscitation should be performed. The additional information gained, of the infant's response to resuscitation, often helps in making decisions about whether and when to withdraw support. Such situations are often emotionally charged, due to staff concern as well as the parents' tragedy, so the timing is not solely dependent on biological factors. The following problems are not uncommon.

Severe asphyxia

An infant experiencing severe asphyxia in the last stages of delivery may be born with no sign of life, but cardiac massage and artificial ventilation may restore the heart beat. Most paediatricians can recall a miraculous recovery from such a position.

Most infants who recover probably experienced acute total asphyxia immediately prior to birth but were previously in good shape. In these cases, recovery of heart rate is usually followed quickly by gasping, and regular respirations are established within 20 minutes.

If an infant has experienced acute or chronic hypoxia then reversing a terminal situation at birth may be unrewarding for the brain may well already be irreversibly damaged. Reports based on analyses of outcomes of infants with Apgar scores of 0–1 at birth (D'Souza 1983) are difficult to interpret because the investigators are unable to adjust for the degree of prenatal asphyxia. However, in general, it has been the view that if a structurally normal mature infant is not breathing spontaneously at 30 minutes, it is unlikely that he or she will survive; if he or she does, it will be with severe brain damage. It is important in making this decision to allow the infant full opportunity to breath for him- or herself. The endotracheal tube itself may inhibit the infant's spontaneous efforts and very occasionally, an infant may begin to breathe when the tube is removed. Some units now treat cerebral oedema aggressively, guided by intracranial pressure monitoring, and it may be that some of the damage caused by asphyxia may be avoidable (Svenningsen et al 1982). If this is confirmed, the time to withdraw support may depend on the availability of such a service.

Congenital abnormality

Nothing is more challenging to the resuscitation than an apparently normally formed infant, born in good condition, who slowly dies because of failure to establish an alternative oxygen supply. While internal bleeding always has to be considered, the more likely explanation will be congenital abnormality. Always call a colleague. The possibilities include airway stenosis, bilateral lung hypoplasia, severe congenital heart abnormalities and cerebral anomalies. If the infant is pink but fails to breathe, transfer on a ventilator to the neonatal unit. If the infant remains blue or white and the heart beat slows, there is probably no point in continuing artificial ventilation after 30 minutes.

Immaturity

It is lung maturity which determines whether an infant survives the first 24 hours and lung maturity does not necessarily correspond to gestation. Lung performance can be compromised by asphyxia and aspiration. Some clinicians intubate and ventilate at birth most infants under 32 weeks' gestation to assist them to form a functional residual capacity. Only those premature infants who cry at birth, expand their chests and begin effective tidal ventilation, escape. In some premature infants born in poor condition, lung inflation is virtually impossible. Such infants should be transferred immediately to neonatal intensive care, for they will need controlled ventilating for some days if they are to survive. Their colour can be a poor guide to PaO_2, for they can look pink with a low PaO_2 or blue with a normal one. If intensive care is not available, and if they appear lifeless despite lung inflation and being kept warm, it is wise to stop after 30 minutes.

IMMEDIATE SCRUTINY

The newborn is examined under three sets of circumstances:

1. immediately at birth;
2. as a routine check within 48 hours;
3. when necessary if a problem arises.

When a baby is born everybody wants to know what he or she looks like. The parents have first claim since they need to be reassured that everything is all right. The person conducting the delivery, usually a midwife, has to answer the question whether the baby is all right — occasionally this can be very difficult. The parents do not want, nor can they reasonably expect, the whole truth.

To deal with the immediate question, it is important to check that all the external parts are present, that the head, eyes and ears appear normally formed and that the child is a boy or a girl. If there is doubt about the sex, do not guess: say that it is sometimes difficult to determine sex from the external genitalia at the time of birth and that further examination will be required. Assess the infant's adjustment to the birth and clamping the cord. Some infants cry at birth and then stop breathing. The baby can be handed on to the parents when tone and colour are good.

The next question is whether or not the infant can go with the mother to the lying-in ward or whether special care is needed. About 15% of all infants used to go to special care, but with minimal neonatal nursing skill available in the lying-in wards, this can be reduced to below 8% (Chiswick 1986). The decision will depend on local policies. It will involve some estimate of size and gestation, an evaluation of risk based on antenatal and labour records, and the state of the infant at birth.

A number of specific problems must be considered at this time.

Oesophageal atresia

In some units it is routine policy to pass a tube directly into the baby's stomach to exclude oesophageal atresia. Often the catheter which was used to aspirate the upper airways is used. The manoeuvre is certainly essential if there has been hydramnios. A firm tube which can be seen or felt in the infant's abdomen is the most certain method of excluding atresia.

Rectal agenesis

This takes many forms. In some it is obvious at a glance; in others the anal dimple is present and the problem escapes detection. It is good practice to record the infant's rectal temperature before mother and baby are transferred from the labour suite. Some babies become cool despite warm towels, while others are chilled because of complications, changed priorities and breech delivery. Asphyxiated and premature infants are at particular risk. Taking the rectal temperature is not without risk (Hull & Chellappah 1983), but properly performed it is safe and points to the need for keeping the infant warm. The need to insert the thermometer into the rectum ensures that rectal agenesis (except in the very rare high membranes) is recognized early.

Infection

It is difficult to know what to do about a baby who is born smelly or covered with turbid liquor, born after prolonged rupture of membranes. This provides grounds for careful observation rather than prophylactic antibiotics. Unfortunately these warning circumstances or signs are rarely present in infants who do contract infection from the birth canal. If a mother is known to have genital herpes, streptococcal, gonococcal or *Listeria* infections, it is essential that those responsible for the care of the newborn should be informed immediately (see Ch. 50).

Vitamin K

All infants should be given vitamin K as a prophylaxis against haemorrhagic disease of the newborn.

ROUTINE EXAMINATION

This is the service the infant receives before going out into the world. It is the first entry in a child's health records. Although it has developed casually, it is likely to become a more exacting and demanding examination. Doctors are now being sued for not doing it properly.

Ideally, it should be done at leisure, with the parents, and after appraising the essentials of the antenatal and labour records. The only way to ensure thoroughness is to complete a checklist. Inevitably, it will not be possible to follow the same routine for each infant and occasionally full examination cannot be completed at one session. If the baby is asleep, complete as much of the examination as possible without waking him or her. Leave palpitation of femoral pulses, examination for dislocation of the hip and assessment of neurological state until the end.

Minor problems

Parents often welcome reassurance about a variety of minor matters. Red marks over the eyes, bridge of nose and nape of neck (stork bites, salmon patches) usually disappear without trace within a year. White pimples in the glands on the butterfly area of the face (milia) can be prominent; these also disappear spontaneously. Cysts on the gums (ranula) pop spontaneously; primitive teeth need to be removed. Breast development with small amounts of milk secretion (witch's milk) occurs in 90% of term infants, boys and girls alike, and reflects the infant's rather than the mother's hormonal status (McKiernan & Hull 1980). In most infants, after initial swelling the breast tissue gradually disappears over a period of weeks. Girls may have a mucus plug in the vagina and a little withdrawal bleeding which has no significance. Babies develop a surprisingly wide range of rashes. Neonatal urticaria (erythema toxicum) can be very florid, with a widespread fluctuating maculopapular rash most marked on the second day. It does not appear to distress the infant and requires no treatment. A different rash, characterized by red macular patches and superficial clear vesicles (miliaria), is called a heat rash and may be precipitated by a warm humid atmosphere, but this is not always evident.

Minor abnormalities

The significance of minor congenital structural abnormalities are more difficult to assess. They may provide clues to problems elsewhere.

Fontanelles

Large fontanelles and wide sutures are not uncommon and usually have no significance if the head circumference is normal. However, a third fontanelle and prominent Vermian bones are found in some chromosome abnormalities, e.g. Down's syndrome.

Accessory auricles

These are usually isolated abnormalities but may be associated with inner ear problems and deafness, and with syndromes involving hypoplasia of mandible and/or maxilla. Abnormally formed ears are often associated with renal abnormalities and are a feature of many dysmorphic syndromes.

Palmar creases

Single creases (simian crease) occur in many normal individuals but are usually, though not invariably, a feature of Down's syndrome (trisomy 21).

Fused labia

Again these are often an isolated anomaly but may be a feature of masculinizing syndromes.

Two cord vessels

A single artery raises the question of an underlying renal abnormality. An ultrasound scan to identify the presence and size of the kidneys is indicated in infants with either abnormal ears or a single umbilical artery.

Specific conditions

Examination of the newborn is primarily a surveillance procedure aimed at identifying problems that need further attention. In some it is secondary prevention — the early identification of a disorder to minimize its expression, e.g. dislocated hips. In others, it is concerned with tertiary prevention — recognizing a handicap so that care and support can be provided, thus reducing the accumulating problems which add to the child's (and family's) disability, for example in Turner's syndrome.

Syndromes

If a child has dysmorphic features, it is important to document them precisely and if their significance is not obvious, expert advice should be sought. Occasionally the facial features of Down's syndrome are hard to recognize in the first days of life. Hypotonia and hyperextensibility are characteristic features and often help in the decision of whether to investigate further. Infants with Turner's syndrome (3/10 000) may pass undetected. Webbing of the neck, oedema of the feet or abnormal nails all indicate the need for further enquiry (Ch. 67).

Deformations

The position in utero can deform the body shape. It is often helpful to try and fold the infant into his or her fetal position. Mis-shapen heads, asymmetrical faces, torticollis, chest wall depressions, unusual dimples or distorted hands and feet may all result from restricted intrauterine movement. They usually resolve when full movement is restored after birth.

Club foot

There may be an element of deformation in all club feet. If the foot cannot be easily placed into its normal position orthopaedic opinion should be sought.

Dislocated hips

This too may be a consequence of intrauterine position. Current policy recommends that all infants should be examined. Anyone performing this examination must be well practised in the procedures: experience can be gained initially on models and then increased by examining infants under expert guidance. The more experienced the clinician, the higher the success rate; even so the diagnosis can be missed. There is still controversy as to whether late dislocation can occur in the first year of life (Dunn 1986). It seems that it does occur very rarely. Ideally the hips of those at high risk of dislocation (family history, breech delivery etc.) should be examined by ultrasound (Clarke et al 1985).

Cleft lip and palate

Cleft lip is easily identified. Cleft palate can be missed if the infant is reluctant to cry. Always ask how the infant copes with feeding. Sometimes a palatal defect can be felt when it cannot be seen easily.

Heart defects

Examination of the pulses will point to a patent ductus arteriosus (full bounding) and coarctation of the aorta (absent femoral pulses). Central cyanosis, peripheral collapse (extreme pallor) and signs of heart failure — tachycardia, tachypnoea, difficulty with feeding, excess sweating, an enlarged liver — all indicate the possibility of an underlying heart problem. The presence of a heart murmur in an otherwise healthy infant is far more difficult to interpret. Closing fetal channels lead to a variety of sounds which subsequently disappear. Conversely, in infants with severe defects no murmurs may be heard in the first days of life. If the heart is active and the murmur loud — 3/6 and above — an ECG and chest X-ray are justified. If the murmur is quiet — 2/6 or less — then clinical review is sufficient. The difficult task is to explain to the parents what you are doing without causing inappropriate anxiety.

BIOCHEMICAL SCREENING

Many inherited metabolic diseases, of which the great majority are recessive, present in the newborn period. It is pertinent to consider why this is so. For some it is because the placenta discharged the harmful metabolites; for others it is because milk feeds present a previously unfamiliar nutrient load, such as galactose in lactose and phenylalanine in milk proteins. Disorders such as galactosaemia and phenylketonuria only come to light as milk-feeding is established.

For others, it is the accelerated metabolism of independent existence which reveals the disorder. Hypothyroidism is a good example. Such disorders may be detected in three ways: firstly, by mass screening; secondly, by screening infants at risk by virtue of a family history, and thirdly, by biochemical investigation of infants with a cluster of clinical features.

Mass screening

Mass screening is appropriate if the disease is an important problem, the natural history is known and there is a latent period before irreversible damage occurs. There must be an agreed approach with recognized treatment, a suitable test and adequate resources.

Mass screening has been practised for phenylketonuria, galactosaemia, syrup urine disease, tyrosinaemia, homocystinuria, histidinaemia, arginosuccinicaciduria and for hypothyroidism, cystic fibrosis and muscular dystrophy. Only screening programmes for phenylketonuria and hypothyroidism fulfil the desirable criteria and are in common use (Danks 1981).

Phenylketonuria

This rare condition (about 1/10 000) is detected by the Guthrie procedure on heelprick blood from an infant once feeding is established, on the fourth, fifth or sixth day). It is a screening test and all positive results require further investigation, since not all will have the classical disorder which inevitably results in brain damage unless a special demanding dietary regimen is adopted.

Hypothyroidism

Hypothyroidism has an incidence of 1/4000. The same blood spot used to detect excess phenylalanine can also be used to assay thyroid-stimulating hormone, which is raised in hypothyroid states before irreversible damage has occurred. Again a raised level is an indication for further investigations to define the problem (Barnes 1985).

Familial risk

If there is a known familial risk of an inborn error of metabolism, in particular a previously affected sibling or a history of unexplained infant deaths, it is mandatory to institute appropriate investigations as soon as possible. For example, galactosaemia can be diagnosed without exposing the child to galactose, or megavitamin theory (coenzymes) can be given in an attempt to induce some enzyme systems and so avoid harm in certain inherited metabolic disorders.

Neonatal illness

Space does not allow a full description of the clinical situations in which investigations for metabolic disorders are indicated (Danks & Brown 1986). In general, they should be considered in infants who are lethargic and hypotonic; who vomit in the absence of obstruction; who convulse; who have apnoeic spells or abnormal behaviour without obvious cause; who suffer unexplained hypoglycaemia or acidaemia; who have unexplained jaundice or a haemorrhagic tendency. Suspicion will be reinforced if the infant improves when feeds are stopped or if the infant or his or her urine smells unusual. Blood glucose, calcium, acid–base status and amino acids, urinary sugars, ketones, ketoacids and amino acids would be initial estimations.

ILLNESS IN THE NEWBORN PERIOD

Parents or staff of the lying-in wards may become concerned about babies for a variety of reasons.

Grunting

It is not uncommon for infants who cry normally at birth and begin regular breathing to develop rapid or laboured respiration. The majority resolve spontaneously. The disorder has been labelled transient tachypnoea or mild respiratory distress, names which are at least descriptive and correct. If haemolytic streptococcal infection is suspected blood cultures should be taken and penicillin given immediately.

Enquiry about feeding performance is essential. If oesophageal atresia has not been excluded it should be. Babies with oesophageal atresia, unable to swallow their own saliva, are very bubbly, so the diagnosis, once considered, usually becomes clear on careful clinical assessment alone. More commonly babies have some initial difficulty with effective swallowing, whether related to asphyxia or immaturity, although often it is unrelated. Gentle skilled feeding with smaller more frequent feeds is curative and only very occasionally is tube-feeding required. There are many rare disorders resulting in oesophageal incoordination which also present at this time.

Going blue, apnoeic attacks and fits

Here again the challenge is to identify the infant with a serious problem. Cot deaths have been reported in lying-in wards, so one should not be over-confident about the survival of the apparently healthy. A clear history is very helpful. Did the episode or episodes occur with feeding or handling or whilst the baby was in the cot? Was the infant aware? Did he or she stop breathing? Did he or she cry before or after the episode? Was the baby floppy? If the body was jerking, what parts were affected?

Hypoglycaemia should be considered first and can be excluded by a quick heelprick blood test. It will have been anticipated in the dysmature type of infant described by Clifford; the child shows the features of intrauterine growth retardation with undernutrition, with low body weight for gestational age; and also in infants of diabetic mothers, although hypoglycaemia can occasionally occur in infants without any of those predisposing clinical factors (Aynsley-Green & Soltesz 1986). Perinatal asphyxia, infections and cold exposure may contribute. Once the diagnosis is made the infant needs to be transferred to the neonatal unit for management. There are a number of rare metabolic disorders which present with hypoglycaemia in the newborn (Table 66.3).

Infections, in particular meningitis, can also present with fits or blue episodes, so if there is any doubt about what happened, culture of blood and cerebrospinal fluid, and antibiotic cover until the results are to hand, is the appropriate management (see Ch. 69).

Thorough clinical examination of the infant should exclude lung disorders and heart disease. If the infant has either a serious episode or current minor episodes, obser-

Table 66.3 Rare causes of neonatal hypoglycaemia (blood level below 2.2 mmol/l)

Insulin level	Cause
Transient normal insulin levels	Small for gestational age (SGA) Asphyxia, starvation, cold, sepsis
High insulin levels	Maternal glucose infusions Infant of diabetic mother Erythroblastosis fetalis Idiopathic transient hyperinsulinism (often SGA) Beckwith–Wiedemann syndrome (macroglossia–exophthalmus)
Persistent normal or low insulin levels	Congenital hypopituitarism (small penis) Cortisol deficiency Glucagon deficiency Metabolic disorders (e.g. glycogen storage disorder)
High insulin levels	Tumours of islet cells (insulinomas) Immune-sensitive hypoglycaemia

Table 66.4 Factors which may increase neonatal jaundice

Factors	Examples
Prebirth events	Maternal drugs, e.g. oxytocin Fetal disease, e.g. rubella Blood incompatibility, e.g. rhesus
Birth events	Asphyxia Delayed clamping of cord Bruising
Postbirth events	Delayed passage of meconium Dehydration and starvation Polycythaemia Infections e.g. *Escherichia coli* and hepatitis Breast milk jaundice
Inherited disorders	In bile metabolism, e.g. Crigler–Najjar Which damage the liver e.g. galactosaemia Hypothyroidism
Obstruction to bile secretion	Extrahepatic atresia Duodenal and low bile duct obstruction

vation in the neonatal unit with an apnoea alarm is indicated until these episodes have stopped.

A clear story of convulsions demands thorough neurological assessment. If the infant shows other neurological abnormalities further investigations are indicated.

Since the majority of blue attacks or apnoeic episodes or twitchings turn out to be of no lasting importance, it becomes a nice judgement whether to reinforce parental and nursing anxiety by special observations and investigations which prove to be unnecessary, or to leave well alone and act only if new developments reinforce the initial concern. Whichever course is adopted, the parents must be kept fully informed and can make invaluable observations provided they know what is significant.

Jaundice

It is both normal and common for healthy newborn infants to become jaundiced (bilirubin above 85 μmol/l). In utero, unconjugate bilirubin is cleared by the placenta but after birth the load falls on the newborn liver so one factor is a delay in uptake by hepatocytes and the induction of glucuronyl transferase activity. Thus disorders of the liver or agents which interfere with glucuronyl transferase activity (e.g. drugs) will exaggerate the phenomenon. Another factor contributing to the raised level of unconjugated bilirubin is an increased bilirubin load due to red cell breakdown. Thus disorders which increase this burden, for example bruising or increased red cell fragility or breakdown (e.g. in rhesus incompatibility) accentuate the bilirubin levels. Bilirubin concentrations are also determined by the capacity of the serum binding proteins which may be reduced, by raised free fatty acid levels following the initial establishment of feeding and by various drugs. Bilirubin concentrations require monitoring to assess the underlying pathology and also because bilirubin is itself toxic. Further action is indicated in a healthy term infant if the unconjugated bilirubin level rises above 200 μmol/l, if clinical jaundice is present in the first 24 hours or lasts more than a week, if the conjugated level rises above 25 μmol/l or if bile is present in the urine.

The differential diagnosis of both unconjugated and conjugate bilirubin is considerable (Table 66.4) but it must again be emphasized that the majority of jaundiced infants are healthy and come to no harm and so the decision of when to investigate further is not easy.

The management of hyperbilirubinaemia has become easier with the effective use of phototherapy. Each neonatal service has its own guidelines as to when and how to use phototherapy. There is no reason why most term infants should not stay with their mothers on the lying-in wards. As a result partly of the fall in rhesus-affected infants and partly of more vigorous use of phototherapy, exchange transfusions are now rarely performed.

Temperature

The rectal temperature, measured by inserting a mercury thermometer 5 cm into the rectum and leaving it there for at least 2 minutes, is one of the parameters routinely monitored by nursing staff. The interpretation of unusual variations, whether high or low, is not straightforward. In the newborn, the body temperature is far more under the influence of environmental conditions: if the buttocks are exposed because of a nappy rash it will be lower; if the infant is near a heat source and well swaddled so that opportunities for heat loss are limited, it will rise. Clinical assessment includes both an assessment of the infant's general well-being and of the environment immediately before the temperature was taken. If the infant is otherwise normal, adjusting the environment is all that is required, with the temperature being recorded 4-hourly until it returns to the normal range.

FEEDING

Once the infant has a firm grip on independent existence, the next major step is to establish an alternative source of nutrition. While most infants root and suckle soon after birth, the volume they take is small for little is usually available and colostrum itself has relatively little energy content. Nevertheless, the experience is a first important step both in the infant's nutrition and in the induction of lactation, as well as an occasion for the emotional meeting of mother and child. In some cultures colostrum is avoided; since bottle-fed babies do not receive it and yet appear to be at no disadvantage, colostrum per se is not essential.

The breastfed baby must then await the establishment of lactation until a point is reached when infant and mother together determine the supply and demand (Ch. 62).

Breastfeeding

Breastfeeding does not appear to be instinctive; it has to be learnt. Breastfeeding is more likely to be established when the information programme before delivery has been thorough, when problems like inverted nipples have been dealt with, when mistaken notions about the effects of breastfeeding on breast shape have been discussed and when the mother knows who to turn to for advice and support.

The atmosphere in the postnatal ward and home is the key. It helps if both mother and baby are relaxed, if the baby suckles early, and if mother and infant have free and easy contact. Fixed schedules and unnecessary supplementary feeds can and often do interfere with the natural process. Babies and mothers are both individual in their feeding habits so there are many solutions, just as there are many problems. There are many excellent books and booklets on breastfeeding (Gunther 1970, Jelliffe & Jelliffe 1979).

Obstetricians, paediatricians or family doctors are not particularly expert at counselling mothers on breastfeeding, and yet their advice is often sought if problems arise. The assessment of a nursing expert on the adequacy of the mother's supply of milk, the feeding position and technique and the suckling efforts of the baby is invaluable. Clearly if the mother is uncertain, tense, depressed, frightened or in pain the problem may lie in the supply. It is most unlikely that the breast is biologically unable to perform its task. Alternatively, a lethargic or irritable baby may not be sucking effectively. Some babies have to be encouraged whilst others are so lively they would test the patience of a saint. With support and encouragement, most mothers who wish to are able to breastfeed. A feeding problem may be a symptom of the mother's mood or a sign of a disorder in the infant.

There are very few absolute contraindications to breastfeeding. Severe illness in the mother or certain infectious diseases like tuberculosis are examples. Severe mental illness or the necessity for adoption are reasons for the mother not to feed at all, either by breast or bottle. There are also rare contraindications to milk-feeding, for example galactosaemia and phenylketonuria. Only rarely do drugs given to the mother pass to the infant in significant amounts (see British National Formulary). Some exceptions are given in Table 66.5.

Table 66.5 Drugs excreted in breast milk which may harm the infant

Lithium
Cytotoxics and immunosuppressants
Phenytoin
Ergot
Radioactive pharmaceuticals

In the UK it is recommended that breastfeeding should be continued for 3–4 months before a weaning diet is introduced (Department of Health and Social Security Report 1980, 1988). In practice, most mothers begin to wean before that period. The argument is that by 4 months the infant's ability to digest, metabolize and excrete a wider range of substances has increased and he or she is beginning to be able to chew. However, milk remains a good food for a growing infant and many mothers choose to breastfeed for much longer. In third-world countries continued breastfeeding brings with it many additional benefits and is a major factor in the survival and future well-being of infants and toddlers (Jellife & Jelliffe 1979).

It is an unhappy fact however, that in the UK many mothers stop breastfeeding soon after they leave hospital. In 1980, a variety of reasons were given (Department of Health and Social Security 1980, 1988). These are probably at best only a crude index of underlying social attitudes. Insufficient milk, painful breasts, the baby not sucking or rejecting the breast — all suggest failure to establish feeding rather than secondary problems, and no doubt relate in part to the mother being unable to maintain at home what she had managed in hospital.

Breast milk

Much has been written about the unique qualities of human milk. Certainly it is more than a quantitative mixture of protein, fat, carbohydrate, minerals and vitamins. The subject is well dealt with in Chapter 62.

Bottle feeding

Nurses are the experts at artificial feeding. A deliberate ritual is followed when preparing an artificial feed: filling the bottle, selecting the teat, choosing a time and a place to suit both baby and nurse and attending to the baby before feeding begins. Some babies will only willingly take a feed from one person — usually the mother — given in a certain way; others will feed from anyone in a variety of circumstances and conditions.

If there are problems with regurgitation, vomiting or failure to thrive, it is important to watch how the infant's mother prepares a feed and how the baby takes it. Better still, ask an expert nursing sister to advise. Sometimes there are obvious problems; the infant gobbles too fast, for example, or sucks hard with little reward, or swallows air. It is a particular skill to persuade a sick infant or an infant with a congenital anomaly (e.g. cleft palate) to feed. The availability of thin plastic nasogastric tubes which can be left in situ for days on end has taken much of the anxiety out of the management of the infant who is difficult to feed, for it is now technically easy to maintain adequate nutrition.

Artificial feeds

Modern food technology is now such that virtually any recipe can be formulated. However, we are by no means certain as to what is the best recipe. Worse, we do not know what is wanted of a feed: is it rapid growth, or is it optimal growth, and is that different? Is it balanced growth, so that the increments of the body constituents are the same as those which occur with human milk feeding? Is it a feed for health which protects against infection, avoids allergies or sets the scene for longevity? No doubt there will be feeds which favour some or all of these objectives, but they will not be the same, so choices are inevitable.

In the face of this, national and international advisory bodies have recommended that infant formulas, used as the sole feed, should resemble as far as possible the constituents of average human milk (Department of Health and Social Security, 1980, 1988), and they do in quantity. It is ironic in the face of these recommendations that a soy-based feed, containing vegetable oil, vegetable protein and glucose syrup, should have been promoted so vigorously and is increasingly being offered to babies. Since there is little to choose between the other main products on the market, the price and convenience of the preparation become important factors in influencing the mother's selection.

For powdered milks the key to producing the correct mixture and the recommended calorie density is filling the scoop. It should be neither heaped nor packed but carefully levelled. It is all too easy to give extra for good measure, but this produces a feed with an electrolyte load (especially sodium) which some infants cannot handle. The resulting hypernatraemia can be potentially dangerous if the infant becomes dehydrated by gastroenteritis. Since nursing staff are as likely to make errors as mothers, prepared liquid feeds are preferred in hospital.

PROGRESS

The neurological, psychological and behavioural responses of infants around the time of birth and particularly in the following few weeks have been the subject of many detailed observations in recent years (Volpe 1981). At the same time sophisticated imaging techniques and sensitive analysis of evoked responses have become available. So far their impact on routine clinical practice has been relatively limited but is increasing.

Initial neurological assessment might involve a review of the infant's posture, feeding and sucking patterns, spontaneous activity, muscle tone and strength and his or her response to being pulled to sit or being held in ventral suspension. The infant's response to some of these manoeuvres will vary with his or her state (Prechtl 1974). Primitive reflexes might be tested; the Moro is the favourite but others include the stepping reflex, Galant's reflex, and the palmar grasp reflex. However, whilst these are of general interest, most of the essential information on tone and movement of the head, trunk and limbs can be assessed whilst handling the baby for other procedures during routine examination.

Abnormal neurological features

If the infant was damaged prior to or during the birth, or the brain is ill-formed then a variety of features may occur, which touch on most aspects of the infant's being.

Apnoea may occur at birth and hyperpnoea, hypopnoea, cyanotic episodes and irregular breathing and recurrent apnoeic attacks may follow.

Rooting and sucking may be absent, weak or ineffectual, so that tube-feeding is essential. The cry may vary in pitch and persistence but is rarely robust or easily soothed.

Extreme irritability with excessive startle response is usually accompanied by generalized hypertonia. Alternatively there may be hypotonia with little spontaneous movement. Depending on the tone, the posture varies from that of a rag doll to frightening opisthotonos.

Finally, there may be convulsions expressed as apnoeic attacks, focal fits, generalized twitching, myoclonic jerks and gross cycling movements.

The management, clinical course and prognosis will depend on the cause. If once the infant has adjusted to birth and independent existence, the features stay comparatively constant, an underlying abnormality should be considered. If they follow a sequence of hypotonia followed by hypertonia, irritability with fits followed by slow recovery, then ischaemic brain injury is more likely (Brown et al 1974). In drug withdrawal the infant is initially normal but then becomes irritable.

Everybody would wish to know whether the brain is irreversibly damaged or not. It is virtually impossible in the absence of specific syndromes with predictable clinical courses to give an informed answer at present. It may well be that with the newer imaging techniques features will become evident in term babies, as they appear to be in preterm infants, which point to a certain poor prognosis.

Specific screening

There is no doubt that newborn infants can both hear and

see. Already techniques are available and are being used in some centres to screen routinely at-risk infants for deafness. For diagnostic purposes both vision and hearing can be tested by evoked responses.

REFERENCES

Aynsley-Green A, Soltesz G 1986 Metabolic and endocrine disorders. In: Roberton N R C (ed) Textbook of neonatology. Churchill Livingstone, Edinburgh, pp 605–623

Barnes N D 1985 Screening for congenital hypothyroidism; the first decade. Archives of Disease in Childhood 60: 587–592

Brown J K, Purvis R J, Forfar J O, Cockburn F 1974 Neurological aspects of perinatal asphyxia. Developmental Medicine and Child Neurology 16: 567–580

Chamberlain R, Chamberlain G, Howlett B, Claireaux A 1975 British births 1970, vol 1. The first week of life. Heinemann Medical, London

Chiswick M L 1986 Regional organisation of perinatal care. In: Roberton N R C (ed) Textbook of neonatology. Churchill Livingstone, Edinburgh, pp 803–813

Clarke N M P, Harcke H T, Mettugh P et al 1985 Real time ultrasound in the diagnosis of congenital dislocation and dysplasia of the hip. Journal of Bone and Joint Surgery 67B: 406–412

Curnock D A 1986 Neonatal resuscitation. Hospital Update 12: 679–692

Danks D M 1981 Diagnosis of metabolic diseases after birth; neonatal screening and the investigation of symptomatic patients or babies at risk. In: Hull D (ed) Recent advances in paediatrics, vol 6. Churchill Livingstone, Edinburgh, pp 51–71

Danks D M, Brown G K 1986 Inborn errors of metabolism in the neonate. In: Roberton N R C (ed) Textbook of neonatology. Churchill Livingstone, Edinburgh, pp 644–658

Dawes G S 1968 Fetal and neonatal physiology. Year Book Medical Publishers, Chicago

Department of Health and Social Security, 1980, 1988 Present day practice in infant feeding. Report on Health and Social Subjects 20 (1980) and 32 (1988). DHSS, London

D'Souza S W 1983 Neurodevelopmental outcome after birth asphyxia. In: Chiswick M L (ed) Recent advances in perinatal medicine, vol 1. Churchill Livingstone, Edinburgh, pp 137–153

Dunn P M 1986 Screening for congenital dislocation of the hip. In: MacFarlane A (ed) Progress in child health, vol 3. Churchill Livingstone, Edinburgh, pp 1–12

Friedman W F, Hirschklau M J, Printz M P et al 1976 Pharmacologic closure of patent ductus arteriosus in the premature infant. New England Journal of Medicine 295: 526–529

Frus-Hansen B 1982 Body water metabolism in early infancy. Acta Paediatrica Scandinavica 296 (suppl): 44–48

Gregory G A, Gooding C A, Phibbs R H, Tookey W H 1974 Meconium aspiration in infants — a prospective study. Journal of Paediatrics 85: 848–852

Gunther M 1970 Infant feeding. Methuen, London

Heymann M A, Rudolph A M 1975 Control of the ductus arteriosus. Physiological Reviews 55: 62–77

Hull D 1966 The structure and function of brown adipose tissue. British Medical Bulletin 22: 92–96

Hull D, Chellappah G 1983 On keeping babies warm. Recent Advances in Perinatal Medicine 153–168

Hytten F E 1985 The physiology and pathology of amniotic fluid. In: Fox H (ed) Haines and Taylor's textbook of gynaecological and obstetrical pathology, 3rd edn. Churchill Livingstone, Edinburgh

Jelliffe D B, Jelliffe P G F 1979 Human milk in the modern world. Oxford University Press, Oxford

McKiernan J, Hull D 1981 Breast development in the newborn. Archives of Disease in Childhood 56: 525–529

Milner A D, Vyas H 1982 Lung expansion at birth. Journal of Paediatrics 101: 879–886

Milner A D, Vyas H, Hopkin I E 1984 Efficacy of face mask resuscitation at birth. British Medical Journal 289: 1563–1565

Palme C, Nystrom B, Tunnel R 1985 An evaluation of the efficiency of face mask in the resuscitation of newborn infants. Lancet i: 207–210

Precht H F R 1974 The behavioural states of the newborn infant. Brain Research 76: 185–212

Rutter N 1986 Temperature control and its disorders. In: Roberton N R C (ed) Textbook of neonatology. Churchill Livingstone, Edinburgh, pp 148–162

Rutter N, Hull D 1979 Response of term babies to a warm environment. Archives of Disease in Childhood 54: 178–183

Silove E D 1986 Pharmacological manipulation of the ductus arteriosus. Archives of Disease in Childhood 61: 827–829

Smales O R C, Kime R 1978 Thermoregulation in babies immediately after birth. Archives of Disease in Childhood 53: 58–61

Svenningsen N W, Blennow G, Lindroth M, Gaddlin P O, Alistrom H 1982 Brain-orientated intensive care treatment in severe neonatal asphyxia. Archives of Disease in Childhood 57: 176–183

Volpe J J 1981 Neurology of the newborn. W B Saunders, London

Vyas H, Hopkin I E, Milner A D 1983 Face mask resuscitation: does it lead to gastric dilatation? Archives of Disease in Childhood 58: 373–375

Widdowson E M, Spray C M 1981 Chemical composition in utero. Archives of Disease in Childhood 26: 205–214

SECTION 11

Abnormalities of the Newborn

67

Niall O'Brien

Malformations of the newborn

INTRODUCTION

Congenital malformations are structural deformations present at birth. Malformation is a faulty formation or structure of parts (Oxford Universal Dictionary 1955) and the term congenital means present at birth (Webster's 1961). The term congenital anomaly refers to abnormal behaviour, function and chemistry — when present at birth. Malformation may or may not be recognizable at birth and may emerge during the first year. The incidence of both major and minor malformations can be considerably influenced by the depth of examination of the newborn. Likewise, necropsy on an apparently normal infant may reveal structural anomalies or microscopic malformations. Defects of molecular structure give rise to inborn errors of metabolism. Investigations of malformations cover a wide range of disciplines — to include the molecular biologist, geneticist, clinician, epidemiologist and statistician. This results in many problems of differing terminology and conception (Fishbein 1970).

Incidence figures obtained in the neonatal period represent only a part of the actual incidence of congenital malformation. Frequency of major defects at birth varies from 1 to 1.7% which, if projected to 9 months and 5 years, augments the figures to 2–3% (McKeown et al 1960, Manning et al 1982). Some malformations may, however, remain silent for years.

Besides specific aetiological factors there are basic ethnic, racial and geographical problems to be considered. In general, the incidence of malformation appears to be higher in negro than in caucasian infants. The main reason for this, however, is minor abnormalities such as polydactyly and umbilical hernias (Smith 1970). But more serious malformations can also vary in ethnic groups; anencephaly occurs in 1/175 births in Ireland and only 1 in 2700 in Uganda (Coffey et al 1958, Simpkiss & Lowe 1961).

The intrauterine process of maternal selection leads to prenatal death of many deformed conceptuses, resulting in spontaneous abortion or stillbirth. More than 50% of aborted ova have been shown to be pathogenic (Stephenson 1961); 75% of spontaneously aborted conceptuses would have developed into phenotypes of little promise for adequate physical and mental development. However, many deformed fetuses grow and develop until birth, and some of these die after birth. Malformations account for 30–40% of perinatal deaths. Many abnormalities are now amenable to corrective surgery and with major advances in postoperative neonatal care, long-term results have improved dramatically.

INTRAUTERINE GROWTH RETARDATION

While factors such as maternal diabetes, drugs, radiation or intrauterine infection can raise the suspicion of possible fetal malformation in a particular pregnancy, the suspicion will have greater credibility if the fetus is not growing at the normal rate. To the paediatrician, every growth-retarded infant should raise the suspicion of associated malformations, particularly where no specific antenatal factor, such as toxaemia has been recorded and also where previous sibling birthweights were in the normal centile range. At birth, such babies should receive detailed clinical examination, including the retina. The placenta and membranes should also be checked, especially the cord vessels. Investigations should include estimation of IgM on cord blood, TORCH titres, abdominal and brain (ventricular) ultrasound. While the incidence of small-for-dates infants varies in different countries, in western Europe it is about 1–2%. The incidence of malformation among growth-retarded infants is about twice the average.

SINGLE UMBILICAL ARTERY

About 1% of all umbilical cords examined reveal this vascular anomaly (Little 1958). The congenital malformations associated with a single umbilical artery are heterogeneous in origin and morphology.

Cardiovascular, pulmonary, gastrointestinal, cerebrospinal and musculoskeletal anomalies have been observed (Seki & Strauss 1964).

INTRAUTERINE ENVIRONMENTAL SYNDROMES

Fetal alcohol syndrome

The estimated incidence is 1/600 to 1/1000 births. This condition has received considerable attention in recent years but as yet the precise amount of alcohol which can cause fetal abnormality is the subject of debate. Reported incidence varies (Clarren & Smith 1978). Virtually all these infants are growth-retarded; 80% have microcephaly and mental retardation. Other manifestations which aid diagnosis include hypotonia (50%), strabismus and myopia (25%) and occasionally neural tube defect, cleft lip and palate and Klippel–Feil anomaly (1–20%). Diagnosis, therefore, is entirely clinical and although maternal history is helpful, not all alcoholic mothers produce affected infants. Prenatal diagnosis is not possible at present.

While the expression of the disease is related to the amount of alcohol consumption during the particular pregnancy, only about 30–50% of infants of alcoholic mothers will be affected (Little & Streissguth 1981).

Fetal cytomegalovirus syndrome

This condition occurs in 0.5–2.4% of newborn infants and the infection may be subclinical or severe. Presenting signs in 70% of cases include hepatosplenomegaly, petechiae, jaundice and pneumonia. In about 25% of cases there is evidence of intrauterine growth retardation.

The most serious problem is microcephaly. This is present in approximately 50% of cases at birth, but in some of the remainder may develop during the first year. This results in mental retardation (60%), cerebral palsy (35%), epilepsy and hearing loss (33%) (Pass et al 1980). Initial investigations show elevated cord serum IgM (85%), increased cerebrospinal fluid protein (50%) and raised serum glutamic-oxalacetic transaminase (80%). Infection of the fetus occurs transplacentally around the third or fourth month and the virus may be isolated from the amniotic fluid at this time. The virus causes necrosis. There is no known effective drug therapy. Most of the infants with mild infection recover completely.

Congenital toxoplasmosis

This is due to the transplacental transmission of the protozoon *Toxoplasma gondii* to the fetus in mothers developing the infection for the first time in pregnancy. Infection occurring prior to the pregnancy does not affect the fetus. The organism causes a granulomatous inflammation and necrosis of fetal tissues, particularly in the brain. The commonest source of infection appears to be cats. The incidence of infection in the newborn varies from 1/1000 to 3/1000 births. In Europe, a high incidence is reported from France, but the incidence in Ireland is about 1/4000. Only 10–20% of infants with proven infection appear clinically sick (Dishe & Gooch 1981). The classical signs are hepatosplenomegaly, petechiae, microphthalmia, thrombocytopenia and chorioretinitis. Hydrocephalus occurs in about 30% of cases and some degree of mental retardation in a further 10%. Serologically, the diagnosis is confirmed if specific *Toxoplasma* IgM antibodies (fluorescent antibody technique) develop during pregnancy. Specific treatment is unrewarding but sulphonamides or pyrimethamine may be used.

Fetal hydantoin syndrome

This syndrome may occur in the fetus of epileptic mothers who are receiving hydantoin medication. It is not clear whether the primary cause is epilepsy or the drug, as the incidence of malformation in treated and untreated epileptic mothers is about equal. Anomalies most frequently found include cleft lip, cleft palate and congenital heart disease. A characteristic facies has been described, with depressed nasal bridge, short nose, hypertelorism, epicanthic folds and short neck (Hanson & Smith 1975). Limb anomalies may occasionally occur. The clinical picture may resemble the fetal alcohol syndrome.

Fetal rubella syndrome

This condition has now become a rare phenomenon in western communities since it was first described by Gregg in 1942. Widespread vaccination of schoolgirls has been very successful. In the rare situation where the expectant mother is not immune, the extent and seriousness of fetal involvement depends on the timing and extent of transmission across the placenta. The viraemia occurs about 1 week prior to the maternal rash. At cellular level, the virus inhibits mitosis and produces inflammation which also reduces cell growth with loss of critical cells during organogenesis. Approximately 50% of fetuses are affected if infection occurs during the first month of gestation, compared with 5–10% at 20 weeks. Cataract, retinopathy, hearing loss, congenital heart disease and microcephaly are the commonest lesions found. In some cases, the infant at birth shows stigmata of disseminated infection which include hepatosplenomegaly, purpura, bone lesions and jaundice. In many cases there is intrauterine growth retardation.

Herpes simplex virus infection

This condition is extremely rare, varying from 1 in 4000 to 1 in 30 000. There appears to be a higher incidence in social classes 1 and 2. The majority (60%) of infants are preterm and a substantial proportion (60%) of affected infants develop meningoencephalitis. The outcome is poor both for survival and for long-term development. Diagnosis may be made by culture from skin vesicles. At autopsy, the virus can usually be cultured from the brain or liver (Singer 1981).

DEVELOPMENTAL DEFECTS OF THE CENTRAL NERVOUS SYSTEM

Anencephaly

This is the most extreme example of neural tube defect. Both brain and spinal cord are completely open and the cranial vault is absent. The precise pathological picture depends on the extent of the lesion. The cerebral hemispheres and cerebellar lobes may be rudimentary or absent. Because of small orbits, the eyeballs protrude. Malformations of the limbs, thoracic cage, abdominal wall, gastrointestinal tract and genitourinary system are common associated findings. Incidence varies from 0.8 to 5.7 per 1000 births in England and Wales in 1986 (Office of Population Censuses and Surveys 1987) but the recorded incidence has been decreasing in recent years. Hydramnios is a common finding and frequently arouses suspicion; ultrasound is diagnostic from the 15th week in most cases. There is a 5% risk of recurrence but after two affected siblings the risk increases to 20–30%. Vitamin supplements prior to conception may reduce this risk.

Encephalocoele

In this condition there is herniation of brain tissue through a defect in the cranium. The lesion is called a meningocoele when no brain tissue is involved. The distribution is occipital (75%), anterior (15%), or parietal (10%). In practice, an occipital site is by far the commonest and, if a lot of brain tissue is involved, there is associated microcephaly and 100% mortality. Occasionally iniencephaly may be associated; the occiput of the excessively extended head is fused to the cervical vertebrae. Incidence varies from 1 in 2000 to 1 in 5000 livebirths and is commoner in female infants. Most encephalocoeles are sporadic. Transillumination and computerized tomography scan can outline the contents of the sac. Outcome varies, but for encephalocoele in general mortality is about 60%. Survival depends on the lesion.

Hydrocephalus

This is caused by an abnormal accumulation of fluid in the cranium. Fluid within the ventricular system signifies internal hydrocephalus while that in the subdural space around the brain signifies external hydrocephalus. If there is no obstruction within the ventricular system, the hydrocephalus is communicating, but if the flow of cerebrospinal fluid is impeded, the hydrocephalus is obstructive in type. This is the commonest form and in 75–90% of cases is of prenatal origin. In about 80% of the obstructed type there is an associated neural tube defect. The overall incidence varies from 1 per 500 to 1 per 1500 births. The enlarged cranium is detected at birth in 35% of cases and during the first 3 months in approximately 50%. Prenatal diagnosis is possible by ultrasonography. After birth, if the cerebral cortex has thinned to less than 1 cm, transillumination is positive. While computerized tomography scan is also helpful, it is often difficult to identify the exact site of obstruction.

In general, the recurrence rate is not greater than 1%, except in male infants with aqueduct stenosis who may have an X-linked recessive hydrocephaly. Approximately 50% of congenital cases are stillborn and only about 15% survive to leave hospital. However, 50% of infantile cases survive, of whom 80% have normal intelligence (Shurtleff et al 1973). Where surgery is indicated, ventriculoperitoneal shunting is the treatment of choice.

Neural tube defects

Frequency of all types is about 1/2000 but varies greatly geographically, being very high in Ireland and the rest of the British Isles. The frequency appears to have fallen in recent years (Sheridan-Pereira et al 1982). The risk of recurrence is 3–4% in a family with one affected child. Spina bifida results from abnormal closure of the neural tube at about 28 days, leaving the spinal column open. The condition varies in severity from the least severe type, spina bifida occulta with a defect in a single vertebral arch and with normal spinal cord and nerves, to a meningocoele, where there is a defect in one or two vertebrae and where the meninges extend into a sac covered by skin.

Meningomyelocoele is the most severe type and unfortunately the commonest (70% of cases; Fig. 67.1). In this condition, the defect contains both meninges and neural tissues. Often there is associated displacement of the medulla and part of the cerebellum which causes obstruction and hydrocephalus (Arnold–Chiari malformation). Spina bifida occulta requires no therapy and surgical repair of meningocoele is usually totally successful. Management of meningomyelocoele has been the subject of much debate in recent years (Stein & Ames 1975). In general terms, conservative

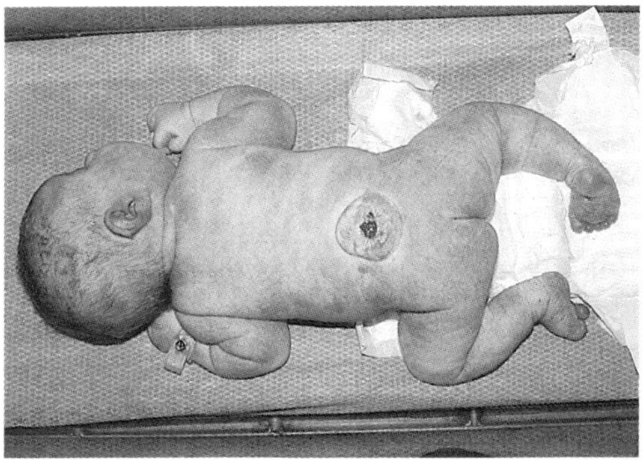

Fig. 67.1 Meningomyelocoele.

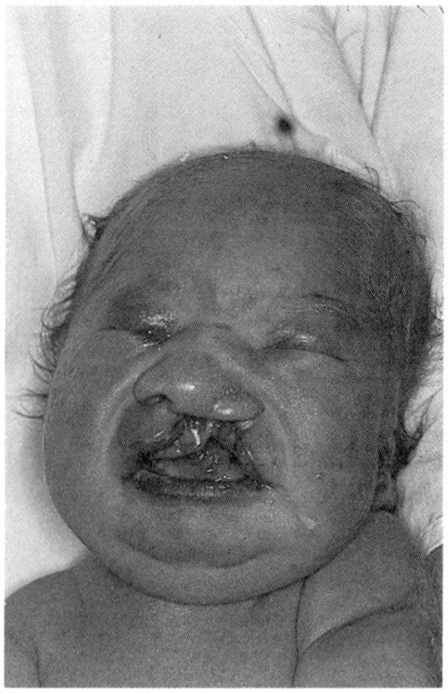

Fig. 67.2 Patau syndrome (trisomy 13–15).

management is offered where there is a gross hydrocephalus and complete paralysis of lower limbs at birth.

However, surgical centres and surgeons vary in their approach. Repair of skin defects and ventriculoperitoneal shunts are standard procedures. Long-term management is supervised by neurologists, orthopaedic surgeons, nephrologists and paediatricians.

Microcephaly

This condition is present when the head circumference is less than 3 standard deviations for age and sex. Diagnosis is therefore made by head measurement. Errors of diagnosis can easily be made in the first 48 hours, particularly when there is marked overlapping of sutures and moulding. While craniostenosis can give rise to a small head measurement, the brain in this situation is usually intrinsically normal (Qazi & Reed 1973). Failure of brain growth prenatally is either primary with probable autosomal recessive inheritance, or secondary to infections which include rubella, cytomegalovirus and toxoplasmosis. In many cases the condition is associated with other anomalies. Another notable cause is perinatal asphyxia. All genuine cases of microcephaly have mental handicap with a mean IQ of 37. Epilepsy and cerebral palsy may also be present. The overall incidence of microcephaly is about 1/10 000.

CHROMOSOMAL DISORDERS

Trisomy 21 (Down's syndrome)

By far the commonest chromosomal disorder, the overall incidence varies from 1/600 to 1/1000 and is related to maternal age (O'Brien & Crowley 1984). About 94% are due to non-dysjunction and are associated with elevated maternal age (35 years 1/350; 40 years 1/100; 45 years 1/30). About 5% are due to translocation and not related to age. While precise clinical features vary, all suffer mental retardation and generalized hypotonia. Facial characteristics include hypertelorism, epicanthic folds, palpebral fissures which slant upwards and outwards. Brushfield spots, convergent strabismus, nystagmus and brachycephaly are common. The mouth is small and the tongue readily protrudes. The hands are short and a single simian palmar crease is common, as is shortening of the fingers. Duodenal atresia is not uncommon and may even be suspected antenatally on ultrasound.

Occasionally, difficulty in diagnosis may occur at birth particularly if the infant is preterm. It is important that the most senior of the paediatric staff available should initiate discussion with parents. Congenital heart disease occurs in 40–50% of cases; the commonest are ventricular septal defect and arteriovenous conduction defect. Moderate mental handicap (30–50 IQ) is the rule, but there may be progressive deterioration to a lower level after 3 years.

Trisomy 13–15 (Patau syndrome)

This condition occurs in 1 per 12 000 births and is more commonly found where maternal age is more than 35 years. The basic defect is trisomy of 13–15 chromosome. In 75% of cases there is primary non-dysjunction and the remainder are due to translocation, involving 13, 14 or 15 chromosomes (Robertsonian) with non-dysjunction (Fig. 67.2).

Clinically, the infant often weighs less than 2500 g at birth. Microcephaly, microphthalmia coloboma, cataracts and malformed pinnae occur in approximately 80% of cases (Hodes et al 1978). Localized scalp defects in the parietal–occipital area are found in 75%. Cleft lip and palate are found in 60–70%. Congenital heart disease, genital anomalies and postaxial polydactyly are also common. More than 80% die in the neonatal period and the remainder within 6 months. Very occasionally an infant with this disorder will survive up to 2 years.

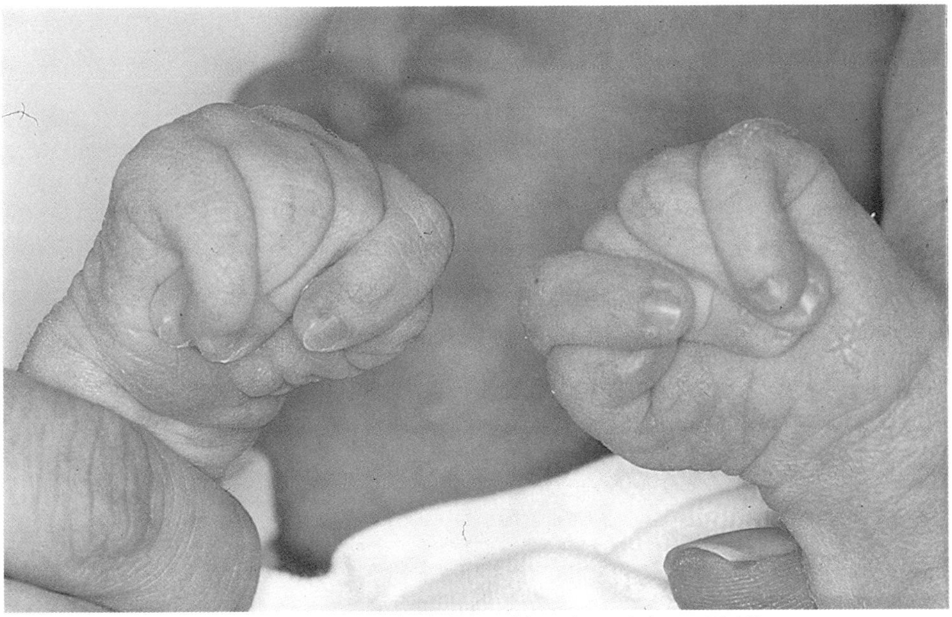

Fig. 67.3 Finger position in Edwards' syndrome (trisomy 16–18).

Trisomy 18 (Edwards' syndrome)

This condition occurs in approximately 1/4000 births and is three times more common in females. Approximately 80% of cases are caused by non-dysjunction when maternal age is more than 35 years. In about 10% translocation occurs. Fetal growth retardation is common and is associated with a small placenta and a single umbilical artery. The majority of infants weigh less than 2500 g at birth. Diagnosis is relatively easy on assessment. The clinical signs include (in the majority — 80%) narrow nasal bridge, short palpebral fissures, low-set ears, classical overlapping of flexed fingers (Fig. 67.3), hypoplastic nails, short sternum and rocker-bottom feet. Congenital heart disease occurs in about 90% of cases. More than 50% die within 4 weeks and all but 5% succumb during the first year.

Turner's syndrome

This condition occurs in 1/5000 births and is due to partial or complete monosomy X. The condition most often results from non-dysjunction in gametogenesis in either the mother or the father. In about 50% of cases there is only one X chromosome. In the 15% of cases where iso-X chromosome occurs, a large proportion are mosaics. In these cases, there is a wide clinical spectrum. Clinically, the syndrome consists of sexual infantilism, primary amenorrhoea, sterility, webbed neck and cubitus valgus (Paloner & Reichmann 1976). Low hairline occurs in 75% and the chest is shield-shaped with nipples widely spaced. Oedema of the lower limbs and dorsum of feet is common (Fig. 67.4). This is non-pitting and due to lymphoedema which may persist for some years.

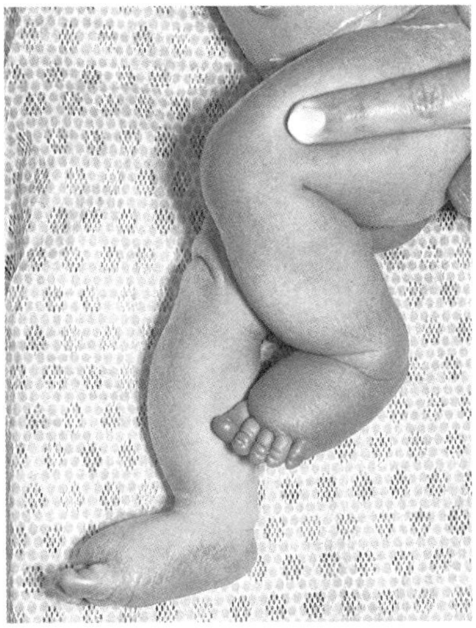

Fig. 67.4 Oedema of lower limbs in Turner's syndrome.

MALFORMATIONS OF THE FACE AND GASTROINTESTINAL TRACT

Cleft lip and palate

The incidence varies from 1 to 1.5 per 1000 births. There are racial differences and cleft lip and palate are more common in caucasians. In 50% of cases cleft lip and palate occur together, in approximately 25% cleft lip occurs alone and in the remaining 25% cleft palate occurs alone. In general, male infants are more commonly affected than females except with isolated cleft palate, which is commoner in female infants.

The left side of the palate is more commonly affected than

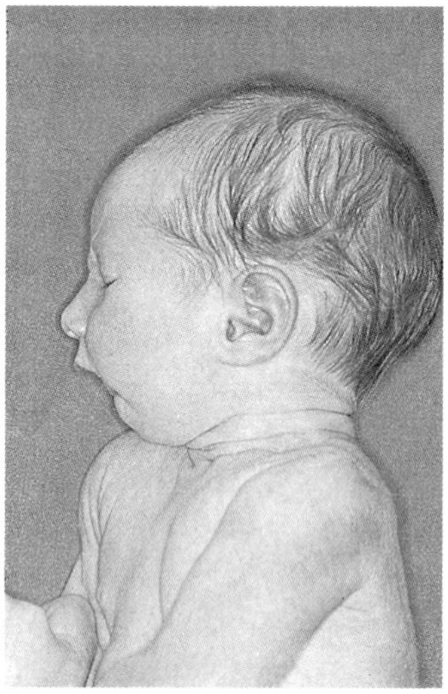

Fig. 67.5 Profile: Pierre Robin syndrome.

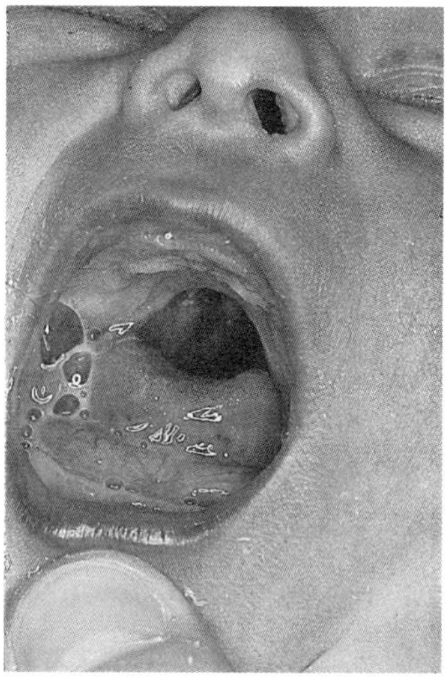

Fig. 67.6 Cleft soft palate: Pierre Robin syndrome.

the right. In approximately 20–30% of cases there is a familial factor. Parental age has also been suggested as a causative factor and the condition may also be associated with chromosomal disorders (i.e. trisomy 13–15). Drugs, including steroids and anticonvulsant agents, have also been implicated. At birth, infants with cleft lip and palate should be carefully examined for other abnormalities. Following this, early explanation and discussion with parents are extremely important to allay long-term fears. Though feeding difficulties may occur initially, the problem is readily resolved by expert nursing support.

It is imperative that the mother is involved as early as possible. Postoperative photographs may be helpful. There is still much variation in the time for surgical repair of a cleft lip. In the UK the range is from the first to the 12th week; to some extent this depends on the degree of the defect, while for the rest it depends on local surgical opinion.

Repair of cleft palate is usually commenced at 8–9 months. Following surgery, orthodontic advice and expertise are mandatory, as are speech therapy and monitoring of middle ear infections.

Pierre Robin syndrome

This anomaly consists of micrognathia, glossoptosis and cleft of the soft palate. Closure of the soft palate depends on the growth spurt of the mandible during the second month of intrauterine life; if this growth fails the tongue is not carried forward and downwards.

The condition is easily recognizable at birth (Fig. 67.5, 67.6). Associated congenital heart disease may occur in 15% of cases. Difficulties with the inspiratory phase of respiration, cyanotic episodes and feeding are common. In some cases aspiration pneumonia may occur. Failure to thrive during the first few months is common and during this time special care and nursing are necessary. The disorder should be explained in detail to the parents as they will require much patience and understanding. The majority of infants develop normally. Respiratory and feeding difficulties have usually ceased by 6 months. The condition is usually sporadic and there does not appear to be a single gene inheritance.

Oesophageal atresia with fistula

Tracheo-oesophageal fistula with oesophageal atresia occurs in about 1 in 2000 births. Infants with this condition are often growth-retarded. Though there are five different types, 90% are associated with oesophageal fistula in which the lower segment of the oesophagus communicates with the back of the trachea, the upper oesophageal segment ending in a blind pouch. Tracheo-oesophageal abnormalities are well established by the fifth week of embryonic life and probably have their beginnings as early as 21 days after fertilization. Hydramnios is present in about 90% of cases.

At birth, the infant may appear entirely normal, but excess mucus will be noted early and failure of a nasograstric tube to pass usually confirms the diagnosis. It is imperative that this procedure should be performed in every infant delivered following pregnancy complicated by hydramnios. Delayed diagnosis, permitting oral feeding, will give rise to pulmonary aspiration.

Surgical management is now so precise that results are excellent, provided multiple anomalies are not also present. In 40% of cases, associated anomalies are present.

Intestinal anomalies

Duodenal atresia occurs in about 1 in 2000 births and the highest incidence is among infants with Down's syndrome. Besides atresia, obstruction may result from malrotation of the small bowel and also from an annular pancreas. The infant may appear normal at birth (except in the case of

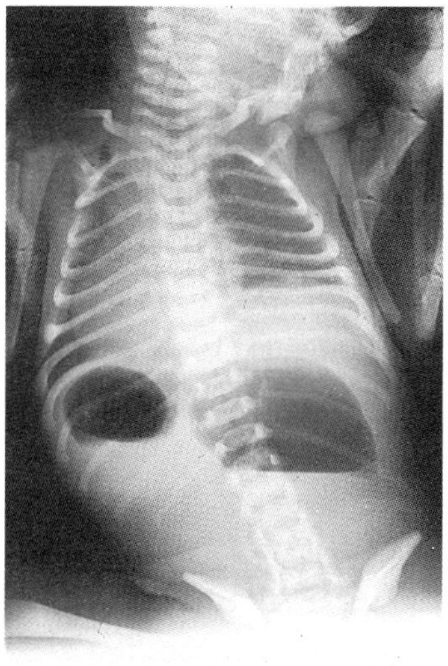

Fig. 67.7 Double bubble: duodenal atresia.

Down's syndrome), but bile-stained vomiting will inevitably commence within 24–48 hours. Mild upper abdominal distension may be present. Abdominal X-ray will reveal the classical air bubbles in both the stomach and the first part of the duodenum (Fig. 67.7). Emphasis is on keeping the infant well hydrated prior to surgery. Results of surgery are excellent and full recovery is usual. However, where Down's syndrome is present, congenital heart disease may complicate recovery.

Ileal atresia occurs in 1 in 3000 births and is usually an isolated condition. The obstruction normally occurs close to the caecum. Vomiting and generalized abdominal distension occur in the first 48 hours and the vomit is again bile-stained. Abdominal X-ray will inevitably show fluid levels. Surgery is usually successful provided the infant is in good condition and other anomalies are not present.

Congenital atresias of the colon are rare and account for about 5% of all bowel atresias.

Congenital megacolon (Hirschsprung's disease)

This condition occurs in 1 in 5000 births but may not present clinically for some months or years. Males are affected more commonly than females, in a ratio of 4:1, and although the precise genetic determination is unknown, familial cases have been reported. The basic defect is an aganglionic segment of colon and cases may be distinguished as short segment and long segment types. Approximately 2% of patients with agangliosis have Down's syndrome (Passarge 1967). Other associated malformations have been noted, in particular megaloureters and hydronephrosis (Swenson & Fisher 1955).

Symptomatically, Hirschsprung's disease usually presents shortly after birth or in early infancy. Constipation of varying degrees occurs with subsequent incomplete lower intestinal obstruction. Most cases are readily diagnosed in the neonatal period because of difficulty in passage of meconium, abdominal distension and vomiting. Occasionally the condition may go unrecognized into early childhood. Rectal biopsy usually confirms the diagnosis and resection of the aganglionic segment is the treatment of choice.

Imperforate anus

It is estimated that this condition occurs in 1 in 5000 births (Parkkulainen 1957). Though four different types are described, in 80% there is a rectal pouch reaching some distance above the anus (Orloff 1954). Approximately 70% of cases have fistulas connecting the rectum with the perineum or with the urogenital tract. Diagnosis is made at birth and treatment is surgical. Other associated anomalies include renal malformation and Down's syndrome.

Meconium ileus

This condition occurs in cystic fibrosis of the pancreas. Antenatal behaviour is usually normal and birthweight is average. Inheritance is autosomal recessive. The disorder lies somewhere between a structural congenital malformation originating during embryonic life and an inborn error of metabolism. Approximately 10–15% overall present with meconium ileus with symptoms of intestinal obstruction within 48 hours.

Plain X-ray of the abdomen frequently suggests the diagnosis. Surgery has been replaced by gastrograffin enemas in recent years. However, these infants subsequently develop recurring respiratory infections and chronic lung disease. The recent identification of the gene responsible for this condition raises hopes that carrier states may be identified in the near future.

Congenital diaphragmatic hernia

This is an anatomically simple defect (Fig. 67.8) which is easily correctable after birth by removing the herniated viscera from the chest and closing the diaphragmatic defect. However, 50–80% of all infants with this condition die as a result of pulmonary hypoplasia. This latter condition is probably due to compression by the herniated viscera since oligohydramnios is not usually present. The overall incidence is approximately 1/2200.

Clinical signs are those of severe respiratory distress, developing within 15 minutes of birth. Unfortunately, vigorous resuscitation may cause pneumothorax in the normal lung, further aggravating the situation. Prognosis depends on early surgical treatment as well as on pre- and postoperative care. Much depends on the degree of pulmonary hypo-

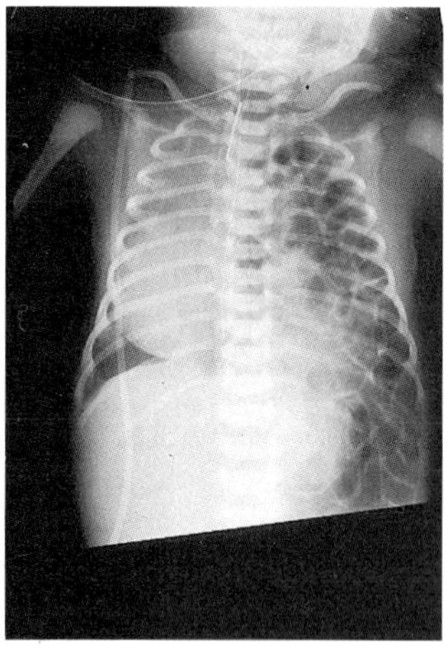

Fig. 67.8 Congenital diaphragmatic hernia.

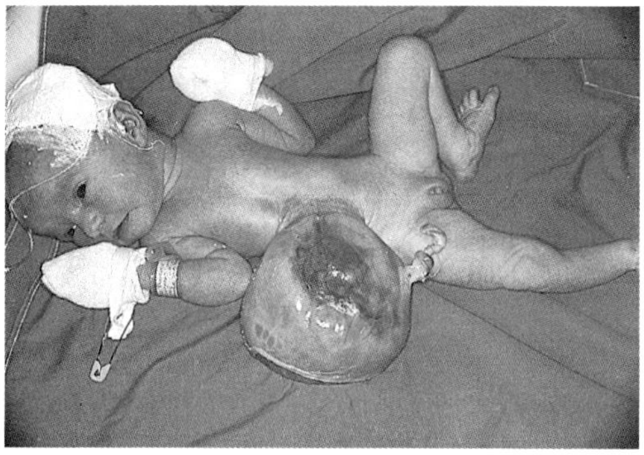

Fig. 67.9 Exomphalos.

plasia on the affected side — on the left in the majority of cases.

Exomphalos

This malformation consists of extrusion of the intestine or other abdominal contents into the extraembryonic coelomic cavity (Fig. 67.9). The incidence is 1 in 3200 (McKeown et al 1953). The size of the omphalocoele varies according to the contents; diameter may range from 2 to 15 cm. In the smaller type the hernia usually contains intestine only, but the larger types may contain other abdominal organs. In a further type called gastroschisis, there is usually a severe abdominal wall defect with extrusion of the abdominal contents without involving the umbilical cord. Prognosis in all cases depends on size and although all are amenable to surgery, postoperative complications are not uncommon and associated malformations may add further adverse influences to the outcome. Conservative medical management should be considered.

CONGENITAL HEART DISEASE

Cardiac abnormalities occur in approximately 0.08% of all newborn infants. There is a considerable variation from mild to severe types and the majority cause little disability. Aetiological factors include environmental conditions such as rubella, an intrauterine infection which has largely disappeared, hypoxia, which can give rise to a persistent ductus arteriosus, and chromosomal disorders, particularly Down's syndrome, Edwards' syndrome, Patau syndrome and Turner's syndrome (Lamy et al 1957). There may also be a family history where no other anomaly is present or it may be associated with a familial condition, for example Holt–Oram syndrome.

Despite the considerable reduction in the occurrence of congenital rubella, the overall incidence of congenital heart disease remains about 8 per 1000 births, of which approximately 90% include eight lesions — ventricular septal defect, persistent patent ductus arteriosus, atrial septal defect, pulmonary stenosis, aortic stenosis, coarctation of the aorta, tetralogy of Fallot and transposition of the great arteries.

In most cases physical examination will raise serious suspicion of a heart lesion; this impression is endorsed by the presence of a particular syndrome, or if the infant is growth-retarded. While chest X-ray, electrocardiogram and cardiac catheterization are helpful, in recent years echocardiography has revolutionized diagnosis. Recent advances in diagnostic and surgical techniques and in postoperative management have made possible repair or significant palliation of virtually all congenital heart lesions.

Ventricular septal defect

This is one of the commonest forms of heart malformation and results from failure of development of the muscular portion of the intraventricular septum, the endocardial cushions or bulbar ridges. In general the deficiency produces a left-to-right shunt and major difficulties only arise if the pulmonary vessels hypertrophy, causing an increase in pulmonary resistance. However, a high proportion of defects decrease in size or close spontaneously and require no treatment. Clinically, the most significant sign is a pansystolic murmur heard best at the fourth interspace to the left of the sternum. A palpable thrill is often associated. Chest X-ray and electrocardiogram are usually normal. If the defect is large, however, evidence of cardiac insufficiency may develop, including dyspnoea, tachycardia, gallop rhythm, hepatomegaly, and failure to thrive. This would require medical treatment initially and surgery subsequently.

Persistent patent ductus arteriosus

This condition may be associated with multiple cardiac anomalies or be present as a single disorder. The incidence has increased recently because of the aggressive management of very low birthweight infants, particularly those who require assisted ventilation for the idiopathic respiratory distress syndrome. A previously stable infant may develop hypercapnia or metabolic acidosis, a significant systolic murmur and bounding pulses. Medical therapy in the form of fluid restriction, diuretics and/or indomethacin is usually successful. In some cases, however, very early surgery may be necessary, even in the very immature baby.

Atrial septal defect

In the majority of cases this defect is in the region of the fossa ovalis and is referred to as secondum atrial septal defect. This does not usually present clinically in the newborn. In the ostium primum the defect is low in the atrial septum, just above the atrioventricular valve tissue. The aortic leaf of the mitral valve is often cleft. Because of this factor, mitral valve incompetence may result in left ventricular insufficiency early in infancy. This condition is commoner in Down's syndrome. The overall incidence of atrial septal defect is 10–15% of congenital heart disease.

Pulmonary stenosis

This results from failure of normal development of the three leaflets of the pulmonary valve, causing thickening and partial or complete fusion of the valve. This condition may occur in siblings more commonly than any other cardiac anomaly (Neel 1958). Stenosis may vary from mild to severe. In the severe form there is a loud systolic murmur at the second left interspace and an associated palpable thrill with obliteration of the pulmonary component of the second heart sound. In the mild form an ejection click with ejection systolic murmur is noted. The electrocardiogram shows varying degrees of right axis deviation and right ventricular hypertrophy. If the right ventricular pressure exceeds 70–80% of systemic pressure, pulmonary valvotomy is indicated. Pulmonary stenosis is present in about 20% of all cases of congenital heart disease.

Aortic stenosis

This is usually an isolated lesion giving rise to obstruction to left ventricular ejection. Some degree of aortic incompetence may also be present. Obstruction may also be supravalvular, in which case there may be other stigmata, including unusual facies, mental retardation and hypercalcaemia (Williams' syndrome) (Beuren 1972). Again this condition may vary from mild to severe. A systolic murmur with or without a thrill will be present at the left sternal edge with conduction to the suprasternal notch and the neck. Left ventricular hypertrophy will develop in time and cardiac failure may occur in infancy. Valvotomy is the treatment of choice.

Coarctation of the aorta

This is sometimes a difficult condition to diagnose in the newborn, particularly in the preterm infant. Classically there is reduced femoral pulse volume. A systolic murmur heard at the left sternal edge radiates to the left interscapular space.

Cardiac failure in early infancy is not uncommon, in which case early surgery may be indicated. Males are more commonly affected than females and the condition represents about 10% of all congenital heart lesions.

Tetralogy of Fallot

This malformation consists of severe pulmonary stenosis, ventricular septal defect, over-riding aorta and right ventricular hypertrophy. It is the commonest form of cyanotic heart disease in the older infant, but the newborn infant may not initially appear cyanosed. The incidence is approximately 1/2000. In general, problems do not arise in the neonatal period but progressive central cyanosis develops and corrective surgery is necessary. The outlook following surgery is good.

Transposition of the great arteries

This condition accounts for 15% of all congenital heart lesions. There is transposition of the aorta and the pulmonary artery; the aorta arises from the right ventricle and the pulmonary artery from the left. Commonly, the infant is well for 24–48 hours because there is some circulation through the ductus arteriosus and foramen ovale.

However, as blood flow diminishes through these channels, the infant becomes cyanosed and rapid deterioration occurs. A chest X-ray showing increased vascular marking should alert the clinician to the diagnosis. Urgent transfer to a paediatric cardiological unit is imperative. A Rashkind pull-through balloon procedure, widening the foramen ovale, is life-saving. Later, an arterial switch repair is carried out.

UROGENITAL SYSTEM

Bilateral renal agenesis (Potter's syndrome)

The incidence of this condition is about 1 in 3000 births (Potter 1965, Carter et al 1979). The recurrence risk is approximately 1–3%. Renal agenesis is usually associated with a characteristic facies, with ocular hypertelorism, a prominent fold of skin arising at the inner canthus and extending to the outer canthus, a squashed nose, micrognathia and flattened pinnae. Oligohydramnios or total absence of liquor is the rule. The infant is usually growth-retarded and breech presentation is common. Genital anomalies are common, as is lung hypoplasia. Gastrointestinal and skeletal anomalies may also occur. Males are three times more commonly affected than females. Overall, about 40% are stillborn and the remainder usually die within the first 24 hours. Death is due to pulmonary hypoplasia which may be associated with intrauterine compression caused by the absence of amniotic fluid. Occasionally, pulmonary function is sufficient to sustain life, but death from renal failure occurs within 48 hours.

Congenital cystic disease of the kidneys

This term relates to many forms of cystic renal disorders. Polycystic disease is the commonest type and occurs in 1 in 10 000 births. Both kidneys are involved and essentially the condition may be subdivided into infantile and adult forms. In the former, the condition presents with abdominal masses with palpable cysts. Diagnosis is confirmed by renal ultrasound and intravenous pyelography. In these cases there is hyperplasia of the interstitial portions of the collecting tubules. Such infants are either stillborn or die within 2–3 months. Cystic proliferation of hepatic bile ducts may also be found.

In the adult form there is great variability in the amount of cystic tissue. The condition may present in the neonatal period or during infancy, childhood or adult life, when hypertension and chronic renal failure may develop. This variety has an autosomal dominant mode of inheritance.

Anomalies of the urinary collecting system

Obstruction of urine flow anywhere from the urethra to the renal pelvis may give rise to hydronephrosis. This may be unilateral or bilateral, depending on the site of obstruction. Congenital urethral valves occur almost exclusively in males and are composed of mucous folds in the membranous portion of the urethra causing bladder neck obstruction. This starts in utero, so that at birth a large bladder is palpable and gross bilateral megaureter and hydronephrosis are present.

Prognosis depends on the degree of renal cortical damage. Anomalies of one or both ureters, including ureterocoele, ectopic urethral orifices, megaureter and duplication may again give rise to hydronephrosis which may be present at birth. In general, ureteric disorders are commoner than urethral ones. Fortunately, many cases present during the neonatal period with a urinary tract infection which is more common in male infants. Investigation of such cases must therefore include renal ultrasonography and a micturating cystogram. Bladder anomalies are fortunately rare and ectopic vesicae, which occurs in 1 in 30 000 births, is a very difficult condition to correct surgically.

Neurogenic bladder may occur in the newborn in association with severe neural tube defects and temporarily, secondary to ischaemic–hypoxic encephalopathy.

Wilms' tumour may occasionally present at birth (Hon & Holman 1961, Favara et al 1968). The author has observed one such case in 150 000 births. This condition may also be associated with genitourinary anomalies, hypertrophy of the liver and sporadic aniridia.

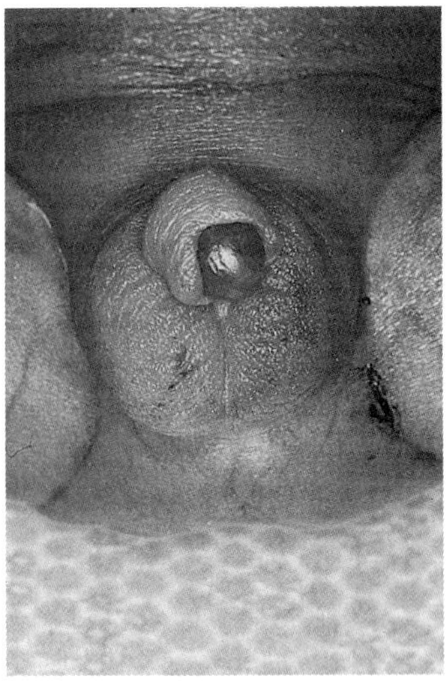

Fig. 67.10 Hypospadias.

Hypospadias

This is due to termination of the anterior urethra ventral and proximal to the normal orifice; it occurs in 1 in 500 newborn males and may be familial (Petterson 1964; Fig. 67.10). The most common site of the anomaly is at the coronal sulcus (glandular), but more serious degrees have penile, penoscrotal and perineal openings. Glandular hypospadias, the most minor degree, accounts for 80% of cases. In relation to possible surgery the presence of chordee is important. Where this is present, straightening of the curved penis, moving the meatus more distally, is the recommended treatment. If hypospadias occurs without chordee, the need for correction depends on the location of the meatus.

Epispadias

This condition is extremely rare and the author has observed only one such case in more than 100 000 live births.

Undescended testes

Though congenital absence of the testes is extremely rare, imperfect descent of the testes is common and both testes are undescended in 3% of full-term and in 30% of preterm males (Campbell 1951). In more than 50% of the former the testes reach the scrotum during the first months of life (Scorer 1956). At 1 year approximately 1% of male children have undescended testes. Unilateral maldescent is more common than bilateral. The position of a true undescended testis — as opposed to that of the retracted one — may be intra-abdominal, perineal, in the thigh or femoral area.

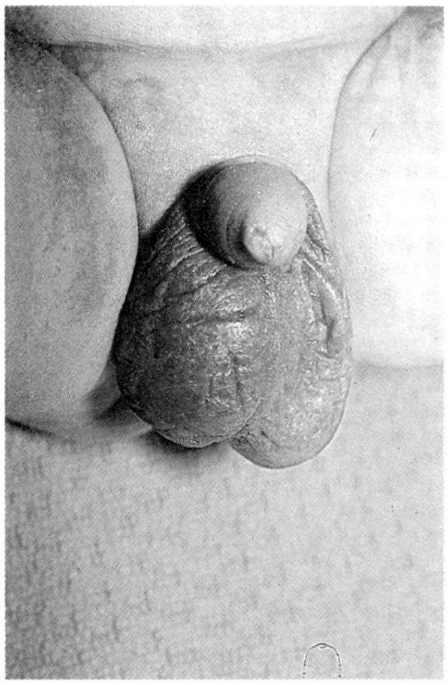

Fig. 67.11 Torsion of right testis.

Undescended testes may be smaller than normally positioned testes. Degenerative changes may also occur and because of the infrequency of spontaneous descent after 1 year, elective orchidopexy should be performed during the third year.

Torsion

This condition, although rare, may present at birth and may unfortunately be bilateral. Early surgical opinion is important. The testis affected is enlarged, discoloured, firm and tender on palpatation (Fig. 67.11).

AMBIGUOUS GENITALIA

Newborn infants with abnormal external genitalia are not uncommon. A clinical decision has to be made whether the genital malformation is an isolated defect or whether it is an indicator of an error of metabolism—an enzymatic defect.

Abnormalities of the external genitalia range from enlargement of the clitoris in a phenotypic female to hypospadias and cryptorchidism in a phenotypic male. It is essential that the infant with even a minor degree of variation from the norm should be carefully examined for other signs of disordered sex differentiation; for example, a male infant with glandular hypospadias and cryptorchidism is much more likely to have such sex differentiation defects than a similar infant in whom the testes have descended and are palpable. In cases where there is doubt, early and ongoing discussion with the parents is of the utmost importance. Detailed physical examination, buccal smear for the presence of sex chromatin (Barr body), abdominal ultrasound, karyotyping and specific hormonal determinations will facilitate a precise, early diagnosis.

Adrenogenital syndromes

In these syndromes there is a defect at one of the stages in the biosynthesis of cortisol (Simopoulos et al 1971). The 21α-hydroxylase deficiency which occurs in 90% of patients is found in 1 in 40 000 births. Because of this deficiency there is failure to convert progesterone and 17α-hydroxyprogesterone to deoxycortisocosterone and 11α-deoxycortisol. Cortisol deficiency results in an over-production of adrenocorticotrophic hormone which stimulates increased production of androgens, causing virilization. The less common types result from 11α-hydroxylase deficiency or 3β-dehydrogenase deficiency. The latter condition is associated with salt loss and this complication occurs in about 60% of cases of 21α-hydroxylase deficiency. All types are recessively inherited.

Clinically at birth the female shows varying degrees of masculinization, with clitoral enlargement and occasionally complete fusion of labioscrotal folds (Fig. 67.12). The male newborn may appear normal but penile enlargement and pigmentation of the scrotum may develop rapidly. Prior to this, however, acute dehydration and circulatory collapse may occur. In 21α-hydroxylase deficiency there is elevation of plasma and urinary 17α-oxosteroids and pregnanetriol, but the most specific test is the level of serum 17α-hydroxyprogesterone, which is markedly elevated.

Treatment consists of long-term cortisol and mineralocorticoid replacement. Long-term prognosis is good. Monitoring levels of 17α-hydroxyprogesterone and bone age reflects the adequacy of treatment.

SKELETAL ANOMALIES

Craniostenosis

Premature closure of the sutures of the skull results in deformities of the head and sometimes damage to the brain and eyes. The overall incidence is approximately 0.4–1 per 1000 births. One or more sutures may be involved and the resulting deformities of the skull vary accordingly (Fig. 67.13, 67.14). Stenosis of the sagittal suture is the commonest—60% of all cases—and may result in scaphocephaly. Apart from the altered head shape there are no other clinical stigmata and development is normal.

Stenosis of the coronal sutures occurs in 20–30% of cases and if bilateral, produces brachycephaly. In this condition there may be distortion of the face; cosmetic surgery with linear craniotomy is necessary.

In rare cases where all sutures are involved, oxycephaly may occur. In such cases, as there is rapid brain growth during the first 6 months of life, surgery should be carried out soon after birth. Diagnosis in all cases is both clinical and radiological. When making the diagnosis in the first 48 hours after birth, moulding and overlapping of cranial bones should be ruled out.

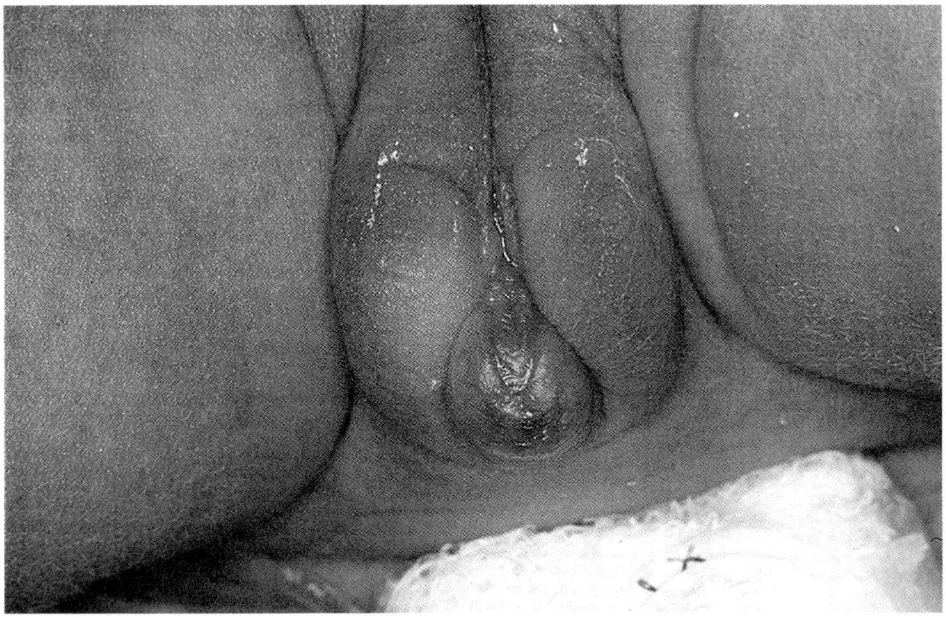

Fig. 67.12 Clitoral hypertrophy: adrenogenital syndrome.

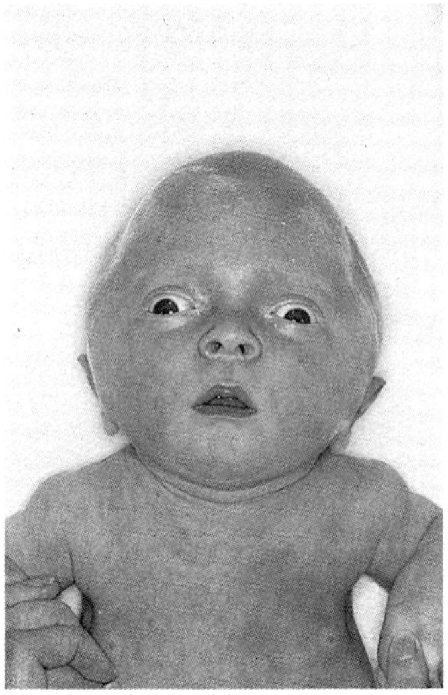

Fig. 67.13 Craniostenosis.

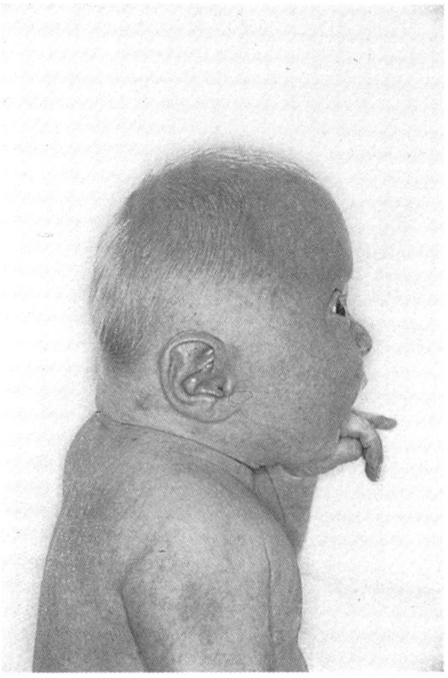

Fig. 67.14 Craniostenosis: profile.

The aetiology of craniostenosis is multifactorial (Hunter & Rudd 1977), though a single gene may be at fault. Recurrence risk is 1–2%.

Apert's syndrome is a rare condition which consists of craniostenosis with syndactyly of hands and feet. Hypertelorism is common and most patients are mentally handicapped. The skull is malformed due to early obliteration of the cranial sutures. A high arched palate is common and in 30% of cases a cleft of the soft palate is present. The hands and feet are usually symmetrically malformed. The precise cause of the defect is not known but the condition is inherited as an autosomal dominant and the overall incidence is 1 per 10 000 births.

Klippel–Feil syndrome

This anomaly is due to failure of segmentation of the cervical spine which results in a serious degree of fusion of the cervical vertebrae, causing marked limitation of neck movement and shortening (Fig. 67.15). Scoliosis occurs in about 30% of cases and deafness, due to maldevelopment of the inner ear, also occurs in 30%. Diagnosis is made by demonstrating marked limitation of neck movement clinically and radiologically. Although many newborn infants appear to have neck shortening, however, full lateral neck movement confirms normality. Virtually all cases of Klippel–Feil syndrome are sporadic and the incidence is 1 per 35 000 births (Gunderson et al 1967). There is no specific therapy.

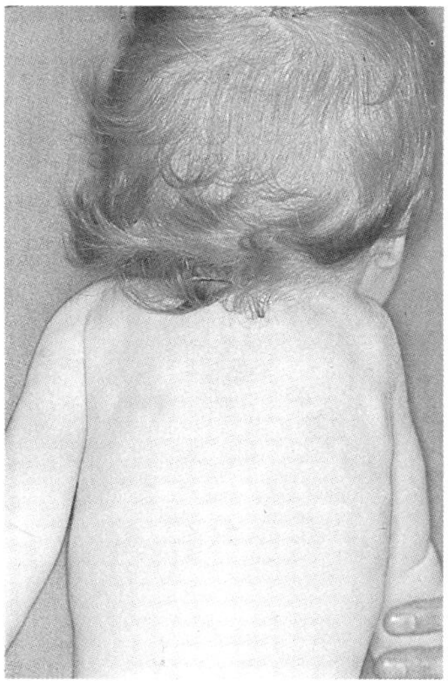

Fig. 67.15 Klippel–Feil syndrome.

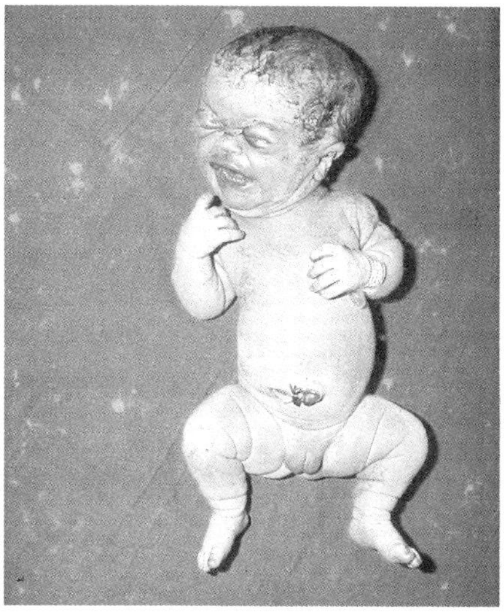

Fig. 67.16 Achondroplasia.

MALFORMATIONS OF THE MUSCULOSKELETAL SYSTEM

These anomalies can be subdivided into systemic, axial and musculoskeletal. There may be connective tissue or skeletal dysplasia. Connective tissue malformations include conditions such as Marfan's, cutis laxa, Ehlers–Danlos and osteogenesis imperfecta syndromes. Genetic disorders involving connective tissues are uncommon but some are worthy of discussion because diagnosis may be achieved in utero.

Osteogenesis imperfecta

This disorder is heterogeneous (Silence 1981) and although no specific biochemical finding has been noted, there is a decrease in collagen production. There are four distinct types and the clinical features vary in each. Type 1, which is autosomal dominant, rarely presents at birth. Fractures usually present in childhood and long-term prognosis is good, although later, otosclerosis is universal. Type II, which is autosomal recessive, is lethal. The condition may be diagnosed as early as 20 weeks and the infant has extreme bone fragility at birth. Type III, in which there are both autosomal recessive and dominant forms, may present with fractures at birth and leads to short stature and deformity. Type IV is by far the mildest form and is compatible with normal growth and stature.

Achondroplasia

Although there are many types of chondrodysplasia, achondroplasia is the commonest and occurs in about 1 in 10 000 births (Fig. 67.16). Although the precise defect is not known, there may be a decrease in endochondral ossification. The disorder is transmitted as autosomal dominant; however, 80–90% of cases result from new mutations. Increased paternal age is thought to be a contributory factor.

Clinically, the head is enlarged with frontal bossing and depression of the nasal bridge. The limb bones are shortened, particularly in the upper extremities. Lumbar lordosis is found in most cases and the hands are short and stubby. Diagnosis at birth may not be straightforward, particularly if the infant is preterm. However, the trunk-to-lower-limb length ratio is more than 2 to 1. Radiographic findings confirm the diagnosis.

After birth, although there may be transient delay in motor development, overall development is normal. Later, narrowing of the spinal canal may give rise to neurological complications (Cohen et al 1967).

MUSCULOSKELETAL CONDITIONS OF THE LIMBS

Limb deformities

Congenital amputations occur in about 1 in 6000 births and the upper limb is more commonly affected.

The condition may involve the fingers alone or the hand and/or the forearm (Fig. 67.17). In these cases no other abnormality is usually present. In contrast, where there are severe birth deformities, associated malformations are common. Amelia implies total absence of limbs, hemimelia reflects defects in the distal parts of the limbs and phocomelia signifies a reduction in size of the proximal parts of the limb. In practice, apart from the classical thalidomide phocomelias, the commonest lesion is the absence of hand and forearm and is often due simply to primary inhibition of growth. There appears to be no genetic or hereditary factor involved. In these cases, early orthopaedic and plastic surgical advice

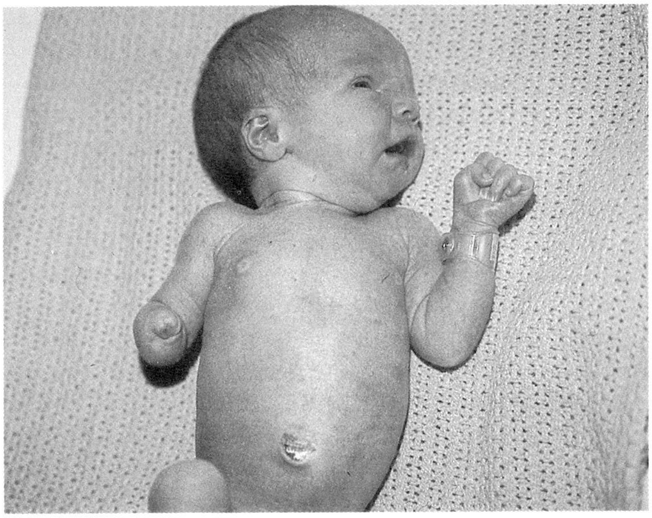

Fig. 67.17 Absent right hand and forearm.

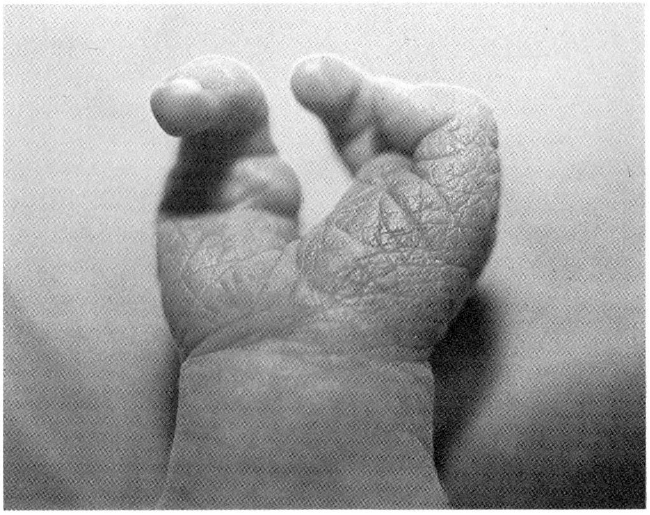

Fig. 67.18 Claw hand.

is sought and the early application of an appropriate prosthesis is advisable.

Syndactyly, split (claw) hand (Fig. 67.18) and absence of the radius and ulna are rare abnormalities which may require surgical treatment, the most important aim of which is to achieve a functional grasp. Abnormalities of the upper limb may be associated with atrial septal defect (Holt–Oram syndrome) or in association with absence of the pectoralis major muscle, as in Poland's syndrome.

A specific abnormality of both thumbs in which there is a short distal phalanx and radial deviation and limitation of opposition occurs in Rubenstein Taybi syndrome. A mild to moderate degree of mental handicap is also present.

LOWER LIMB MALFORMATIONS

Congenital dislocation of the hip

Congenital dislocation of the hip is the commonest lower limb anomaly and results from abnormal development of the acetabulum, the femoral head or the surrounding capsule and soft tissues. Though the head of the femur may be dislocated at birth, more often the capsule is lax, allowing the head of the femur to be readily dislocated and relocated. Aetiology is multifactorial; a direct family history occurs in about 20% of cases when the fetus has presented in the breech position the incidence is increased 10-fold. A total of 90% of cases occur in female infants and firstborn babies appear to be more at risk. The left hip is twice as commonly affected as the right. The incidence of dislocatable (loose) hip varies from 12 to 19 per 1000 (Manning et al 1982, Dunn et al 1985). This figure is influenced by the timing of the initial examination. It is recommended that this should be performed during the first 24 hours.

In general, Barlow's (1962) modification of Ortolani's (1948) test is an accepted method of examination. The test must be gently performed and the hips should not be forced into full abduction. Stabilization of the hip in abduction and flexion during the first 6 months is the basic principle of treatment. The Pavlik harness appears to be the most suitable stabilizing splint.

Despite normal findings on early examination, late dislocation may occur and this varies from 0.07 to 2.2 per 1000. The incidence of late dislocation may be reduced by nursing infants in the prone position during the first 6 months (Pairien 1984). While X-ray at birth is of little value, reports suggest that real-time ultrasound may be useful in locating the position of the femoral epiphysis (Hardic et al 1984). X-ray at 6 months, however, will show ossification and development of the femoral head.

Talipes equino varus (club foot)

This condition occurs in 1 per 1000 births and the male infant is twice as commonly affected as the female. One or both feet may be involved. Though often sporadic, a positive family history is common. The severity of the lesion varies and is determined clinically. The degree of mobility of the ankle joint is relevant to the timing and type of management. Where there is little or no movement, very early application of plaster boots is recommended. Despite this, orthopaedic surgery is required in about 30% of cases before the end of the first year. Club foot may be associated with other abnormalities and is also commonly found in association with meningomyelocoele.

Tarsus varus

This is by far the commonest foot abnormality. Usually a benign condition, it resolves spontaneously and only occasionally is active therapy required.

Talipes calcaneo valgus

This deformity is not uncommon and appears to be more frequent in post-term infants. Occasionally, a dislocatable hip may be associated. Spontaneous correction is the rule.

SKIN ANOMALIES

Congenital disorders of the skin range from rare hereditary disorders such as epidermolysis bullosa and ectodermal dysplasia to disorders of pigmentation and vascular anomalies. Occasionally there may be congenital defects in the skin, the most classical of which are the localized scalp defects in the parieto-occipital area found in 75% of cases of Patau syndrome (trisomy 13). Skin dimples may occur over bony prominences and are also common in the sacral area. These are benign and of no consequence. Amniotic constriction bands may occasionally produce defects in extremities and digits. Preauricular sinuses and/or skin tags are not uncommon and may be unilateral or bilateral. Minor surgery is indicated. Both cysts and sinuses in the neck may occur along the first and second branchial clefts. In some cases these anomalies are inherited as an autosomal dominant trait. Surgery is the treatment of choice. Occasionally, accessory nipples are noted. Congenital absence of an area of skin, particularly on the trunk, may rarely occur. The author has observed one such case in 150 000 live births. Happily, the large bilateral defects in the lateral abdominal walls healed spontaneously and reasonably well.

Ectodermal dysplasias

These are rare inherited conditions which include defects of the skin and teeth. The commonest type is the anhidrotic form where the sweating deficit is due to hypoplasia or absence of the eccrine glands. The skin is thin, dry and hyperpigmented. Anodontia or hypodontia is a consistent feature. Diagnosis is confirmed by skin biopsy. The condition is inherited as an X-linked recessive trait.

Epidermolysis bullosa

This consists of a heterogeneous group of hereditary skin disorders in which blistering occurs from mechanical trauma. The vesicles or bullae may occur spontaneously. Although the precise defect is not known, there appears to be an increase in collagenase in the dermis. There are three different types which include a benign form, which, though presenting in the newborn, improves with age; a more severe, dystrophic variety and a lethal form, in which secondary infection with septicaemia is a constant threat. Treatment is mainly preventive and the cardinal rule is avoidance of trauma. Phenytoin therapy has been used with some success (Bauer et al 1980).

Pigmented skin lesions

Pigmented naevi consist of melanocytes which may have originated from neural tissue (Fig. 67.19). These naevi are the most common congenital skin lesions, are benign and need to be removed only for cosmetic reasons. They are usually isolated, vary greatly in size and may be hairy. Giant hairy naevi usually occur on the back or lower trunk. Because of the possibility of the development of malignancy, early total excision and skin grafting is the treatment of choice.

Vascular lesions

The commonest of these are strawberry haemangiomas. At birth there is a demarcated area of pallor but within 1 or 2 months a telangiectasia pattern will emerge to form a red

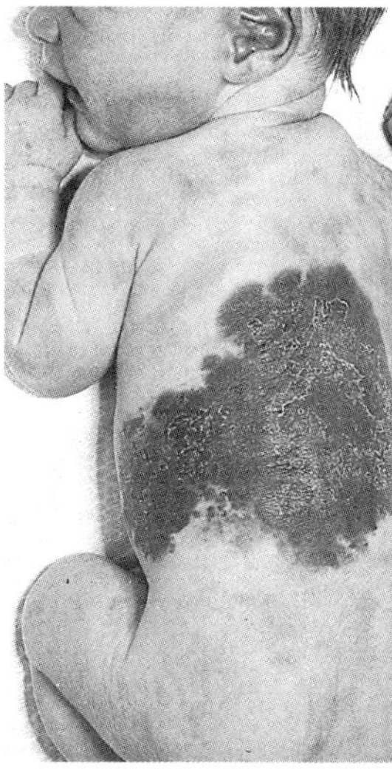

Fig. 67.19 Large pigmented naevus.

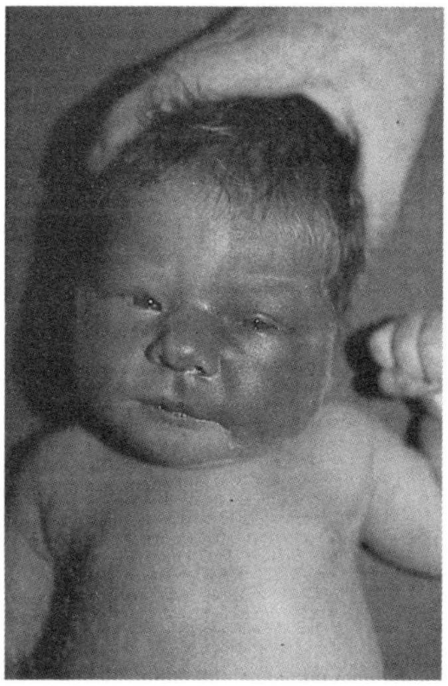

Fig. 67.20 Port-wine stain.

protuberant, soft lesion. In some cases the surface area affected may be small with a large subcutaneous element. The phase of rapid expansion is followed by a quiescent period and finally by spontaneous involution. At least 60–70% have disappeared within 5 years. The incidence is much higher in preterm infants. Occasionally large strawberry naevi may occur on the head, face or neck and may initially be very unsightly. Parents will require much support and patience.

Naevus flammeus (port-wine naevus)

These consist of mature, dilated capillaries and are permanent developmental defects (Fig. 67.20). Colour varies from pink to purple and during the first few days may be difficult to interpret because of changing skin colour. The lesion is usually unilateral and may be confined to the area of distribution of the branches of the trigeminal nerve. The possibility of an ipsilateral vascular anomaly on the surface of the brain should be considered (Sturge–Weber syndrome).

REFERENCES

Barlow T G 1962 Early diagnosis and treatment of congenital dislocation of the hip. Journal of Bone and Joint Surgery 44B: 292–301

Bauer E A, Cooper T W, Tucker D R, Esterly N B 1980 Phenytoin therapy of recessive dystrophic epidermolysis bullosa. New England Journal of Medicine 303: 776

Beuren A J 1972 Supravalvular aortic stenosis: a complex syndrome with and without mental retardation. Birth Defects 8: 45–56

Campbell M 1951 Clinical pediatric urology. W B Saunders, Philadelphia

Carter C O, Evans K, Pescia G A 1979 A family study of renal agenesis. Journal of Medical Genetics 16: 176–188

Clarren S F, Smith D W 1978 The fetal alcohol syndrome. New English Journal of Medicine 298: 1063–1067

Coffey V P, Jessop W J E 1958 A three year study of anencephaly in Dublin. Irish Journal of Medical Science 6: 39

Cohen M E, Rosenthal A D, Matson D D 1967 Neurological abnormalities in achondroplastic children. Journal of Paediatrics 71: 367–376

Dishe M R, Gooch W M III 1981 Congenital toxoplasmosis. Perspectives in Pediatric Pathology 6: 83–113

Dunn P M, Evans R E, Thearle M J et al 1985 Congenital dislocation of the hip, early and late diagnosis and management compared. Archives of Disease in Childhood 60: 407–414

Favara B E, Johnson W, Ieo J 1968 Renal tumors in the neonatal period. Cancer 22: 845

Fishbein M 1970 Third International Conference on Congenital Malformations. Excerpta Medica, Amsterdam

Gregg N 1942 Congenital cataract following German measles in mother. Transactions of the Ophthalmic Society of Australia 3: 35

Gunderson C H, Greenspan R H, Glaser G H et al 1967 The Klippel–Feil syndrome; genetic and clinical revaluation of cervical fusion. Medicine 46: 491–512

Hanson J W, Smith D W 1975 The fetal hydantoin syndrome. Journal of Pediatrics 87: 285–290

Hardic H T, Clarke M P, Myung Soo Lee et al 1984 Examination of the infant hip with real-time ultrasonography. Journal of Ultrasound Medicine 3: 131–137

Hodes M E, Cole J, Palmer C G et al 1978 Clinical experience with trisomies 18 and 13. Journal of Medical Genetics 15: 48–60

Hon L T, Holman R L 1961 Bilateral nephroblastoma in a premature infant. Journal of Pathology and Bacteriology 82: 249

Hunter A G W, Rudd N I 1976 Craniostenosis. Teratology 14: 185–193

Hunter A G W, Rudd N I 1977 Craniostenosis. Teratology 15: 301–310

Lamy M, DeGrouchy J, Schweisguth O 1957 Genetic and non-genetic factors in the etiology of congenital heart disease. A study of 1188 cases. American Journal of Human Genetics 9: 17

Little W A 1958 Aplasia of the umbilical artery. Bulletin of the Sloane Hospital for Women 4: 127

Little R E, Streissguth P 1981 Effects of alcohol on the fetus. Impact and prevention. Canadian Medical Association Journal 125: 159–164

Manning D, Hensey O, Lenehan P, O'Brien N 1982 Unstable hip in the newborn. Irish Medical Journal 75: 463–464

McKeown T, MacMahon B, Record R G 1953 An investigation of 69 cases of exomphalos. American Journal of Human Genetics 5: 169

McKeown T, Record R G 1960 Malformation in a population observed for 5 years after birth. In: Wolstenholme G E W, O'Connor C M (eds) Ciba Foundation Symposium on Congenital Malformations. J & A Churchill, London

Neel J V 1958 A study of major congenital defects in Japanese infants. American Journal of Human Genetics 10: 398

O'Brien N G, Crowley P 1984 Down's syndrome and maternal age. Irish Medical Journal 77: 10–12

Office of Population Censuses and Surveys 1987 OPCS Monitor MB3 87/1

Orloff M J 1954 Congenital anomalies of the anus and rectum. Journal of Paediatrics 45: 316

Ortolani M 1948 Lussazione congenital dell unca. Neovi criteri diagnostica — profiliatico correctio. Capelli, Bologna

Oxford universal dictionary on historical principle 1955, vol II. Clarendon Press, Oxford

Pairien K 1984 Prevention of congenital dislocation of the hip. Acta Orthopedica Scandanavica 55 (suppl): 208

Paloner C G, Reichmann A 1976 Chromosome and clinical findings in 110 females with Turner's syndrome. Human Genetics 35: 35–43

Parkkulainen K V 1957 Sacrococcygeal and urological anomalies in connection with congenital malformations of the anus and rectum. A preliminary report. Annual Pediatric Fennicae 3: 51

Pass R F, Stagno S, Myers G J et al 1980 Outcome of symptomatic CMV infection; results of long term follow-up. Pediatrics 66: 758–762

Passarge E 1967 The genetics of Hirschsprung's disease. Evidence of heterogeneous etiology and a study of 63 families. New England Journal of Medicine 276: 138

Petterson F 1964 Meclozine and congenital malformation. Lancet i: 675

Pietrzyk J J 1980 Neural tube malformations; complex segregation analysis and recurrence risk. American Journal of Medical Genetics 7: 293–300

Potter E L 1965 Bilateral absence of ureters and kidneys. A report of 50 cases. Obstetrics and Gynecology 25: 3

Qazi Q H, Reed T E 1973 A problem in diagnosis in primary versus secondary microcephaly. Clinical Genetics 4: 42–52

Scorer C G 1956 The incidence of incomplete ascent of the testes at birth. Archives of Disease in Childhood 31: 198

Seki M, Strauss L 1964 Absence of one umbilical artery. Archives of Pathology 78: 446

Sheridan-Pereira M, O'Brien N G, Hensey O 1982 Spina bifida and neural tube defects. Irish Medical Journal 75: 163–164

Shurtleff D B, Foltz E U, Loeser J D 1973 Hydrocephalus: a definition of its progression and the relationship to intellectual functions, diagnosis and complications. American Journal of Diseases of Children 125: 688–693

Silence D O 1981 Osteogenesis imperfecta; an expanding panorama of variants. Clinical Orthopedic Research 150: 11–25

Simopoulos A P, Marshall J R, Delea C S et al 1971 Studies of the deficiency of 21α-hydroxylation in patients with congenital adrenal hyperplasia. Journal of Clinical Endocrinology and Metabolism 32: 438–443

Simpkiss M, Lowe A 1961 Congenital abnormalities in the African newborn. Archives of Disease in Childhood 36: 404

Singer D B 1981 Pathology of neonatal herpes simplex virus infection. Perspectives in Paediatric Pathology 7: 243–278

Smith D W 1970 Recognisable patterns of human malformations. W B Saunders, Philadelphia

Stein S G, Ames M D 1975 Selection for early treatment of

myelomeningocoele; a retrospective analysis of selection procedures. Developmental Medicine and Child Neurology 17: 311–319
Stephenson A C 1961 Frequency of congenital and hereditary disease with special reference to mutation. British Medical Bulletin 17: 254
Swenson O, Fisher J H 1955 The relation of megacolon and megaureter. New England Journal of Medicine 253: 147
Webster's third new international dictionary of the English language 1961. G & C Merrion, Springfield, Massachusetts

Andrew R. Wilkinson

Injuries of the newborn

INTRODUCTION

An otherwise normally developed fetus may become damaged by an adverse intrauterine environment, by intrapartum factors, or by perinatal events which may compromise early neonatal adaptation (Table 68.1).

Table 68.1 Causes of injuries in the newborn

Teratogens
Irradiation
Uterine abnormalities
Oligohydramnios
Intrauterine infection
Intrapartum infection
Perinatal trauma
Perinatal hypoxic–ischaemic encephalopathy
Intracranial haemorrhage
Periventricular leukomalacia
Non-accidental injury

DRUGS AND IRRADIATION

Drugs

Drugs used in pregnancy may produce teratogenic effects during the first trimester or toxic effects in the newborn baby, particularly if taken by the mother just before delivery (Tables 68.2 and 68.3).

The adverse effects of teratogens and irradiation may be difficult to distinguish from developmental abnormalities, but in some cases are well recognized (see Ch. 67). These abnormalities are best avoided by excluding all drugs and unnecessary irradiation before conception and during pregnancy. Careful reassessment may justify the withdrawal of some chronic drug therapy or adjustment of the dose when it continues to be needed.

Table 68.2 Drugs most likely to harm the fetus (from Rylance 1986 with permission)

Period	Drug	Comment
First trimester		
Proven	Cytotoxic drugs Thalidomide	Greatest risk with alkylating agents and with folic acid antagonists
Probable	Alcohol	Chronic use
Probable	Anticonvulsants	
	Lithium	
	Warfarin	
	Live vaccines	Viraemia in fetus ?Malformation
Possible	Chloroquine	
	Oestrogens	
	Progestogens	May produce virilization of the female fetus
	Trimethoprim (+co-trimoxazole)	
Second and third trimester	Aminoglycosides	Auditory and vestibular nerve damage
	Antithyroid preparations	Goitre and hypothyroidism
	Chloroquine	Choroidoretinitis
	Diazoxide	Fetal diabetes
	Lithium	Goitre
	Tetracyclines	Discoloration of primary and secondary dentition
	Thiazides	Thrombocytopenia

Teratogenic effects

The catastrophic effects on fetal development of drugs taken during pregnancy were highlighted by the epidemic of phocomelia caused by the sedative thalidomide in the 1960s. Since then a great deal of attention has been paid to the possible effects of drugs, but restrictions in prescribing have

Table 68.3 Drugs which produce adverse effects in the newborn if administered shortly before delivery (from Rylance 1986 with permission)

Drug	Effect
Alcohol	Withdrawal syndrome
Anaesthetics	Respiratory depression
Anticoagulants (oral)	Haemorrhage (fetus or newborn)
Antimalarials	Haemolytic anaemia
Aspirin	Haemorrhage (platelet function affected and hypoprothrombinaemia)
Barbiturates	Withdrawal syndrome if given for more than a few days
Benzodiazepines	Hypotonia/hypothermia
Chloramphenicol	Grey baby syndrome
Hypnotics/sedatives	Respiratory depression
Lithium	Hypotonia/cyanosis/bradycardia
Narcotic analgesics	Respiratory depression and withdrawal syndrome
Phenothiazines	Extrapyramidal effects
Propranolol	Hyperglycaemia
Sulphonamides	Displaced unconjugated bilirubin from albumin

also reduced the potential risks. As yet there are no good tests of teratogenicity and the poor predictive value of negative experiments in animals needs to be constantly emphasized.

All drugs should be regarded as possibly harmful in pregnancy, but a sensible balance must be maintained. The omission of a drug that is clearly indicated in the management of a maternal condition could be equally harmful in other ways to both mother and fetus.

The spectrum of teratogenic effects has a wide range. Spontaneous abortion is most likely in the first 2 weeks after conception. The effect on the fetus and newborn is most likely if the drug is cleared slowly from the maternal circulation or when the drug is given repeatedly. If metabolic pathways are not fully developed, active metabolites may be produced which then exert adverse effects.

Damage as a result of teratogenesis can involve specific abnormalities of cerebral development such as the fetal hydantoin syndrome, giving rise to cleft palate, mid-face hypoplasia and mental retardation. With other drugs, specific functional defects, such as the auditory and vestibular nerve damage caused by aminoglycosides, can result. In other situations the effect of a drug may be widespread but ill-defined and give rise to non-specific microcephaly.

Drug effects may be classified into three broad categories (Hawkins 1981). The major teratogens are those with a proven serious risk of causing a congenital abnormality. Thalidomide, the cytotoxic drugs and radiochemicals are the best examples. Chronic alcohol abuse must now be considered in this category, giving rise to the syndrome of intrauterine growth retardation and particular facial features associated with a large alcohol consumption in the mother. The second group of agents is that with a therapeutic role but a known risk. Anticonvulsants are a good example, where choice of alternative drugs and careful control of dosage can minimize the risks. Finally, there is a large group of drugs which have at times been implicated on anecdotal or unconfirmed experimental evidence. It would be impossible to remove suspicion completely, but in general those drugs which have been used longest without problems should be preferred in pregnancy.

Toxic effects

Drugs such as nicotine and alcohol, if taken chronically, produce toxic effects in the newborn in terms of growth retardation and possible interference with cerebral development. When drugs of addiction such as narcotic analgesics are taken just prior to delivery, the resulting passive addiction of the newborn can give rise to a syndrome of irritability, tremulousness, diarrhoea and tachypnoea. Yawning and occasionally seizures may occur. Treatment with chlorpromazine or diazepam may be necessary (Rylance 1986).

Irradiation

Antenatal irradiation

Experiments in animals and restrospective surveys in humans suggest that irradiation can lead to death of the conceptus, malformations, mental subnormality and malignant diseases—particularly childhood leukaemia. The amount of radiation that is harmful is not known precisely, but has been estimated by Brent (1967) and Sternberg (1973) to be in the order of 50 rad (0.5 Gy) when received between the 10th and the 40th day after conception. This is 100 times the exposure received during a routine abdominal X-ray (Ministry of Health 1960). Nevertheless, as a general principle, routine radiographs of the chest can no longer be justified as tuberculosis is now less common and vital radiographic procedures should be carried out after delivery or, if this is not possible, after the first trimester.

Whether the incidence of malignancy in childhood is increased after abdominal radiographs in pregnancy is not clear. Two studies give conflicting results. Stewart & Kneale (1970) carried out a retrospective study and suggested an increase; however, the reason for the maternal X-ray and maternal age were not taken into account. Court-Brown et al (1960) found no increase in malignant disease in a study of over 40 000 women and Jablon & Kato (1970) reported that the incidence of leukaemia in children exposed antenatally in Hiroshima and Nagasaki was not increased.

Postnatal irradiation

A large number of radiographs may be taken of newborn infants, particularly those with severe respiratory disorders. However, because of the small size of the patient, the dose of radiation is small and has been calculated to be 0.07 mGy (Fletcher et al 1986). These authors estimated that the risk from neonatal radiation, excluding cardiac catheterization and computerized tomography, was that one case of childhood cancer might be caused in the whole of the UK per year. The authors of this study conclude that the risks of not using radiography in intensive care of the newborn outweigh the risks of either cancer or genetic disease.

A comprehensive review of the hazards of ionizing radiation with advice on counselling has been written by Brent (1986).

Ultrasound

No evidence has been produced to suggest that diagnostic ultrasonography is damaging to the fetus (Hellman et al 1970). However, it is still too early to be sure that absolutely no harm is ever done by this relatively new technique.

UTERINE ABNORMALITIES

Abnormalities in the shape of the uterine cavity, as, for example, when the uterus is bicornuate or when large fibroids are present, may encroach on the developing fetus. As a result, postural abnormalities may develop which postnatally appear as deformities such as marked asymmetry, particularly of the face and thoracic cage, or contractures at the hips, elbows and knees. Although sometimes quite marked, these abnormalities improve postnatally and rarely give rise to long-term problems.

OLIGOHYDRAMNIOS

A chronic deficiency of amniotic fluid may give rise to postural deformities, particularly of the limbs. If overt loss of amniotic fluid has not occurred, renal agenesis or other abnormalities of the fetal urinary tract should be suspected and investigated by careful ultrasound scanning. Talipes equino varus, scoliosis and dislocation of the hip may be present. Severe cases may be associated with hypoplasia of the lungs, giving rise to respiratory distress which may be fatal. Once any immediate neonatal problems have been dealt with, treatment of the postural abnormality with gentle physiotherapy should begin, usually within the first few days. Early consultation with an orthopaedic surgeon experienced in the care of the newborn is advisable.

The outlook for the limb abnormalities is relatively good, providing denervation and fibro-fatty changes in muscle have not occurred. This latter condition, called arthrogryposis multiplex congenita, is more resistant to treatment.

Amniotic constriction bands, thought to occur after premature rupture of the amnion, may occasionally encircle a digit or limb, resulting in soft-tissue injury with oedema or, in extreme cases, amputation. Fatal umbilical vessel occlusion by an amniotic band has also been reported (Higginbottom et al 1979).

PERINATAL TRAUMA

Some of the most noticeable advances in obstetric management have been in the reduction of physical trauma during delivery. Improved anticipation of abnormal fetal presentation and cephalopelvic disproportion has contributed greatly to the chances of a fetus being delivered without physical injury. In the past it was often difficult to distinguish between cerebral damage as a result of trauma and injury resulting from severe hypoxia. In recent years, particularly since the introduction of ultrasound scanning of the brain of babies after delivery, this distinction has become clearer. However, undoubtedly there are some babies who have suffered the effects of both trauma and hypoxia.

Soft-tissue injury

Damage to the skin is, of course, the most readily detected trauma immediately after delivery. The presenting part, whether the scalp or the buttocks, is most commonly affected. The skull may be altered in shape, usually with elongation in an occipito-frontal dimension; such moulding is often of no consequence. Oedema fluid may collect and the caput succedaneum that forms is present at birth, decreasing in size thereafter. When the periosteum is intact, oedema fluid crosses the boundaries of the cranial bones. This finding distinguishes caput from the subperiosteal haemorrhage that collects usually over one or both parietal bones. This lesion, cephalhaematoma, may develop postnatally and can take some weeks to clear. No intervention is indicated, though a progressive increase in the size of the haematoma may suggest underlying damage to the skull or a coagulation abnormality such as thrombocytopenia. Needle aspiration, with the risk of infection, is never indicated. After difficult deliveries which have given rise to these abnormalities, babies are often irritable and may improve after a small dose of chloral hydrate (50 mg/kg) though swaddling and feeding are often all that is necessary.

When the vacuum extractor is used, an iatrogenic caput is formed. Should the cup of the extractor slip, a shearing force is applied to the scalp and the periosteum. The lesion of the scalp may heal quickly but cephalhaematoma forms if the damage has been more extensive. Soft-tissue injury to the scalp may also be caused by the application of forceps or a fetal scalp electrode. Incorrect application of forceps is most likely to cause damage, particularly of the facial nerve, giving rise to facial palsy (Fig. 68.1). Bruising or minor laceration disappears quickly, but a full explanation should be given to the parents on every occasion immediately after the damage has been noticed. During breech delivery, the buttocks may become extensively bruised, particularly if labour is prolonged. The scrotum and labia may swell with oedema fluid and the testes are particularly vulnerable to damage. Preterm babies born by the breech are particularly liable to bruise easily and care must be taken to mini-

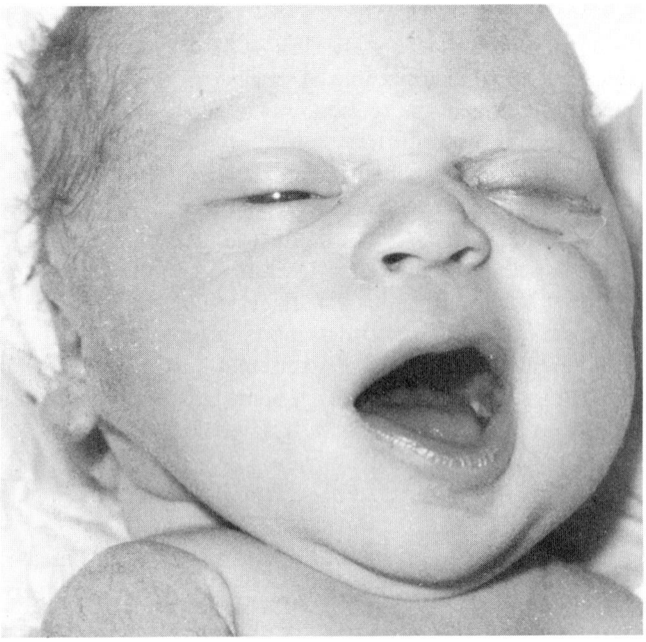

Fig. 68.1 Facial nerve palsy on the right side. The eye remains open during crying and the facial creases are absent.

mize such damage. Jaundice and hyperkalaemia may develop in the newborn and will need treatment.

Other parts of the anatomy may be exposed to soft-tissue injury during delivery. The eyelids, nose and lips, particularly after face presentation or when forceps have been incorrectly applied, may be bruised or lacerated. The sternomastoid muscle may be damaged, especially during breech delivery and haematoma may form giving rise to a palpable tumour. Providing the contraction of the sternomastoid muscle is noticed early, gentle physiotherapy can lead to a complete resolution.

Brachial plexus and spinal cord injury

Pathogenesis

Damage to the nerve roots or to the spinal cord itself is associated with difficulty during delivery leading to excessive traction. The roots of the brachial plexus, C5–C8 and T1, are vulnerable in a cephalic presentation when there is shoulder dystocia or in a breech delivery when there is cephalopelvic disproportion. In either situation undue lateral traction, particularly if the fetus is large, may lead to avulsion of the roots from the cord or to haemorrhagic oedema of the nerve sheath.

Clinical signs and diagnosis

Injury of the upper roots, C5 and C6, is more common than of the lower roots C8–T1. The former gives rise to Erb's palsy—weakness or paralysis of the proximal upper extremity, with adduction and internal rotation of the arm. The hand is pronated with fingers extended—the 'waiter's tip' posture. Sensory deficit is usually difficult to detect because of overlapping innervation. If C4 is involved, paralysis of the hemidiaphragm may be present, giving rise to respiratory distress. Isolated weakness of the distal upper extremity, Klumpke's palsy, is rare with denervation of the intrinsic muscles of the hand, wrist and finger flexors. Hyperabduction at the shoulder and arm is found. This degree of involvement is usually also associated with damage of the upper roots, giving rise to a total plexus palsy in which sensory loss is marked and Horner's syndrome may be present. Fracture of the clavicle or humerus may be associated with brachial plexus lesions.

Management

Prevention depends on good obstetric assessment and management of abnormal presentations. The newborn with a brachial plexus lesion must be nursed to prevent contractions developing by initially restraining the arm across the abdomen. After 1 week, passive movements of the shoulder, elbow and wrist are started. Splints may be required to prevent contractions of the fingers.

Prognosis

Signs of some improvement within the first month are associated with complete recovery which may be achieved by 4 months. Others—some 85–92%—with slower progress may make a complete recovery by 12 months (Eng 1971, Gordon et al 1973).

Spinal cord injury

Pathogenesis

The spinal cord of the newborn is much less able to withstand stretching than the bony spine. Difficult breech delivery is associated with injury at C6–T1 while excessive rotation during cephalic delivery may lead to injury at C1–C3.

Clinical signs and diagnosis

The damage may be so severe that the fetus is stillborn or, despite signs of life, resuscitation may be unsuccessful. Others may develop severe respiratory failure requiring artificial ventilation. Flaccidity with areflexia may be present. If the infant survives spasticity will develop with increased tendon reflexes. The history is usually suggestive but occasionally the signs may mimic a neuromuscular disorder. A sensory level may be demonstrated which excludes Werdnig–Hoffmann disease.

Management

Good obstetric care is vital, especially of breech presentation. Hyperextension of the fetal head is particularly dangerous.

Possible remediable conditions such as an extramedullary mass must be excluded but otherwise surgical decompression of the cord has not improved outcome.

Prognosis

Generally the ultimate outlook is bleak. Commonly death is due to infection of the lungs or urinary tract. Others survive with mass reflexes in the lower limbs and automatic bladder function. Some remarkable recoveries have been reported and so supportive therapy in the neonatal period is justified (Byres 1975).

Skeletal damage

Fracture of the clavicle may occur after a difficult delivery, particularly if there is shoulder dystocia in vertex presentation, or extended arms in a breech delivery. The humerus may also be the site of greenstick or full-thickness fracture. An underlying swelling may be palpated and a radiograph should be taken if there is any suspicion. Fracture of other long bones is much less common and is usually suspected by the mode of delivery and on hearing a crack. Fracture of the skull bones may occasionally underlie a cephalhaematoma and is similarly associated with a difficult delivery. Depressed fractures may be felt. Active treatment is rarely indicated. Reversing the lesion has been successfully carried out by applying the vacuum extractor to the newborn skull.

Congenital dislocation of the hip is primarily an abnormality of development of the acetabulum and is detected in most cases by routine examination of the newborn. The condition is six times more common in girls than boys and 30–50% are born by breech delivery (Salter 1968). When there is a family history, referral for ultrasonography and radiography is indicated. Routine ultrasonography of the hips of all newborns is under evaluation in some centres.

Internal injury

Compression injuries to the viscera have been described but are rare. Subcapsular haematoma of the liver may cause shock in the newborn. Indeed, the aetiology may be related to the resuscitation procedure rather than intrapartum trauma, but sometimes the precise cause is difficult to determine. Haemorrhage into the adrenal glands may also present with shock, but concurrent perinatal hypoxia is usual. Marked jaundice may develop in survivors.

PERINATAL HYPOXIC–ISCHAEMIC ENCEPHALOPATHY

The combined effects of a decreased amount of oxygen in the blood supplying the brain—hypoxaemia—and a decrease in the amount of blood supplied to the brain—ischaemia—are responsible for the clinical syndrome of encephalopathy. Intrauterine, intrapartum, and postnatal disease may all contribute and are often difficult to disentangle (Low et al 1985). Antepartum events, such as haemorrhage as a result of placental separation, often followed by maternal hypotension, are responsible for approximately one-quarter of cases. Intrapartum complications, including prolonged and difficult labours, instrumental deliveries, acute placental separation or prolapse of the umbilical cord, are present in 40%. In a further quarter, the combined effects of antepartum and intrapartum insults are seen. The remaining 10% of babies with this syndrome suffer insults that are predominantly postnatal (Brown et al 1974, Finer et al 1981).

The injury that results from the combined effects of hypoxaemia and ischaemia is an important cause of mortality and morbidity. Survivors may develop part of a spectrum of motor deficits, usually described by the term cerebral palsy. This may be predominantly spasticity, choreoathetosis or ataxia. A varying degree of mental retardation, with or without seizures, may coexist. In preterm infants, hypoxic–ischaemic encephalopathy is a common antecedent of periventricular haemorrhage and leukomalacia. The great improvements in obstetric management and the impact of modern neonatal intensive care in the last 20 years have so markedly reduced other causes of injury to the newborn that hypoxic–ischaemic encephalopathy and periventricular leukomalacia are now the most important causes of brain injury sustained in the perinatal period (Painter & Bergman 1982).

Pathogenesis

Oedema and necrosis of neurones are the hallmarks of hypoxic–ischaemic damage. However, the site of injury and the clinical syndrome depend on the gestational age of the baby (Volpe 1987).

Neuronal necrosis after hypoxic–ischaemic insult may result in the following pathology:

1. *Selective neuronal necrosis:* neurones of the cortex of the cerebrum and cerebellum may be affected. Differences in the metabolism of areas of the brain may be responsible for the patchy distribution of damage. Of particular interest clinically is the selective involvement of the motor nuclei of cranial nerves in the brain stem.
2. *Parasagittal injury:* loss of neurones of the cortex and the white matter below may result in a characteristic histological appearance with streaks of gliosis. This lesion is the hallmark of severe intrauterine asphyxia in term infants. For reasons explained below, asphyxia in the preterm infant is more likely to lead to periventricular leukomalacia.
3. *Generalized cerebral circulatory insufficiency:* a generalized disturbance of cerebral circulation may give rise to unilateral lesions in the form of porencephaly or deficient

cerebral perfusion, most commonly affecting the anterior cerebral artery, which may result in multicystic encephalomalacia.
4. *Basal ganglia and thalamic injury:* rarely the neurones near the basal ganglia and thalamus may be replaced by gliosis and hypermyelination. These areas are characterized by profuse capillary networks and a high metabolic rate. The characteristic lesion has been found at post-mortem in infants who survived for many months after a hypoxic–ischaemic event. The clinical signs of choreoathetosis and dystonia with mild or moderate mental retardation are characteristic (Malamud 1950).

Clinical signs

Studies have suggested that the initial cerebral insult leading to hypoxic–ischaemic encephalopathy was intrauterine in 9 out of 10 cases (Brown et al 1974, Volpe 1977). In cases where fetal heart rate monitoring was carried out, there was a close correlation between abnormal records and the rate of development of abnormal neurological signs. Severe asphyxia may lead to myocardial dysfunction and hypotension which, together with disturbed regulation of cerebral blood flow, may lead to additional neuronal damage.

The first signs to develop after severe hypoxic–ischaemic neuronal damage are a decreased level of consciousness with hypotonia and few, if any, spontaneous movements. Respiration may be irregular, with bursts of tachypnoea alternating with apnoea. After 6–12 hours the infant may appear unnaturally alert with permanently open eyes. Tremulousness, so-called jitteriness and clonus may be noticed. Seizure activity, which most often is initially subtle but can be myoclonic or tonic, may occur. After 24 hours, conscious level may decrease again and brain stem function may be noticeably disturbed. The papillary reactions may be absent and deviation of the eyes with absent contralateral eye movements (doll's eye response) is found.

Neurological abnormalities may persist, but in survivors the level of consciousness gradually rises. Disturbed co-ordination of sucking and swallowing leads to difficulties in establishing feeding, and intragastric tube-feeding may be required for a prolonged period. Diminished tone and proximal limb weakness, predominantly upper limb in term infants and lower limb in preterm infants, may be detected.

Investigations may lead to improvements in diagnosis and management. Ultrasound scans of the brain may show a diffuse increase in echogenicity, which represents ischaemia. Small compressed cerebral ventricles may be related to oedema and increased intracranial pressure, which can be monitored non-invasively (Rochefort et al 1987). Discrete areas of focal ischaemia related to areas of infarction have been demonstrated. This can be confirmed later when the baby is fit enough to be moved for a computerized tomography (CT) scan. The electroencephalogram (EEG) may show diminished voltage with bursts of high-voltage spike and wave activity. In the most severely affected infants, the EEG may be isoelectric. Important gestational age-related changes in the EEG must be taken into account. Seizure activity may be detected by continuous EEG monitoring and may be more prolonged than suspected from clinical observation (Eyre et al 1983).

Management

Prevention of this serious injury to the normally developed brain depends on the detection of intrauterine risk factors for abnormal labour, which should lead to appropriate monitoring and intervention (see Ch. 47). After birth, close attention must be paid to the circulating blood volume to maintain systemic blood pressure, and intra-arterial oxygenation must be kept within the normal range. This may require artificial ventilation. Hyperviscosity secondary to polycythaemia and biochemical abnormalities, such as hypoglycaemia, hypocalcaemia and hyperkalaemia, require close monitoring and therapy. Seizure activity requires therapy, though this is often difficult. Cerebral oedema may be controlled by reducing fluid intake to a minimum. Hyperosmolar infusions, barbiturates and steroids have all been used, although there are no controlled data showing any definite benefit (Eyre & Wilkinson 1986).

Prognosis

The difficulties of precisely documenting the extent of hypoxaemia inflicted on the fetus have made it difficult to compare the results of follow-up studies. Acute hypoxic episodes may do less damage than prolonged interference with oxygen supply, resulting in fetal heart rate abnormalities. Seizures, persistent irritability and the failure to establish normal feeding patterns in term babies by 10 days of age are associated with abnormal outcome (Amiel-Tison 1969, Sarnat & Sarnat 1976, Finer et al 1983, Robertson & Finer 1985). The development of extensor hypertonus after the initial period of hypertonicity is associated with a poor recovery (Brown et al 1974) and persistent neck extensor hypertonicity is also a sinister sign (Amiel-Tison et al 1977).

INTRACRANIAL HAEMORRHAGE

During the last 20 years, improvements in obstetric management have led to a large reduction in the number of term babies sustaining intracranial haemorrhage. During the same time, the improvements in survival for the preterm infant have focused attention on periventricular haemorrhage and ischaemia, which are very much more common in preterm babies and are associated with hypoxic events before, during and after birth. In some babies trauma and hypoxaemia coexist and the precise pathogenesis is complicated. This applies particularly to intracerebellar haemorrhage which has only occasionally been diagnosed before death.

Periventricular haemorrhage

Term infants

Pathogenesis. The risk of periventricular haemorrhage increases with decreasing gestational age. Although very rare in term infants, this kind of intracranial haemorrhage may accompany trauma and perinatal hypoxia. Traumatic delivery with rotation of the head by forceps and breech delivery is present in 50% of cases. The mechanisms are not yet clear, but transient changes in intracerebral blood flow and venous pressure may be important. However, in 25% of cases of term babies with intraventricular haemorrhage, no cause is found. In a few cases vitamin K_1 deficiency, particularly in breastfed babies, has been implicated.

Clinical signs. After difficult delivery, abnormal neurological signs are found in the first 24 hours. Where the perinatal history is blameless, the onset of signs is later, often in the second or third week after birth. Seizures are a common presenting sign with irritability and stupor. Apnoea may occur and some 5% progress to coma and death. Hydrocephalus requiring a shunt procedure develops in 30% and another 20% have non-progressive hydrocephalus (Cartwright et al 1979, Mitchell & O'Tuama 1980).

Diagnosis. As with preterm infants (see below) the extent of haemorrhage is shown by ultrasound scan and it is rarely necessary to resort to CT scanning.

Management. The management of term infants is similar to preterm infants (see below).

Prognosis. Term infants with intraventricular haemorrhage after trauma have a high incidence of neurological abnormality—about 40%. Those with no identifiable cause have a more benign prognosis. Overall, 55% are normal at follow-up.

Preterm infants

The survival of preterm infants in the last 20 years has increased enormously. This change in outlook has been the result of improvements in all areas of management, but particularly in the treatment of common cardiorespiratory disorders of the immature newborn. Evidence that these infants are at risk of intracranial bleeding became widespread in the early 1970s. Early studies depended first on post-mortem findings and then on series in which all babies were subjected to CT scanning. A vast increase in information has subsequently become available after the introduction of real-time ultrasound scanning at the cot-side (Volpe 1987).

Pathogenesis. The subependymal germinal layer region is the site of origin of bleeding in over 90% of cases. This cellular area, consisting of rapidly dividing neuroectodermal cells, has a rich blood supply. Between 24 and 32 weeks' gestation, the majority of the cerebral blood flow is directed to this area. From 32 weeks to term, the cells migrate to the cerebral cortex and the germinal layer gradually involutes. The capillary-like blood vessels in this area have a

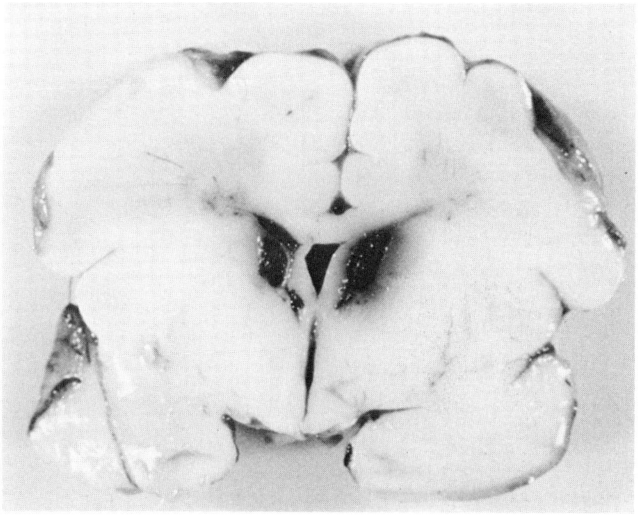

Fig. 68.2 Bilateral germinal matrix haemorrhage with intraventricular extension and periventricular leukomalacia (see Fig. 68.4).

single layer of endothelial cells and little supporting tissue. They are therefore fragile and vulnerable to damage. Cerebral blood flow is variable with poor autoregulation, particularly in preterm infants with severe respiratory disease. Sudden increases in cerebral blood flow have been shown to correlate closely with the development of periventricular haemorrhage (Perlman et al 1983). Equally sudden decreases, as cerebral blood flow fluctuates, may be responsible for ischaemic damage in this and other areas of the brain (Fig. 68.2).

Various factors are known to predispose to surges in cerebral blood flow and these may initiate bleeding within the germinal matrix. Alternating hypotension and hypertension may occur, particularly after antepartum haemorrhage and perinatal asphyxia (Weindling et al 1985a). This is exacerbated during resuscitation by rapid volume expansion with blood and plasma and hyperosmolar sodium bicarbonate. Hypercarbia, a result of poor respiratory gas exchange and the buffering effect of the bicarbonate, causes an increase in cerebral blood flow velocity.

Pneumothorax, a frequent event during mechanical ventilation, causes hypoxaemia, hypercarbia and hypotension. This may be followed by a sudden increase in blood pressure and flow when evacuation takes place (Batton et al 1984). Other suggested factors in the development of periventricular haemorrhage are abnormalities in coagulation and platelet function (Setzer et al 1982, McDonald et al 1984) and seizures. Disturbances in blood flow are also known to occur during and after nursing procedures, particularly the painful ones such as injections, but also during relatively innocuous procedures such as the installation of mydriatics and tracheal suction (Perlman & Volpe 1983, Isenberg & Everett 1984).

Haemorrhage may extend into the lateral cerebral ventricles or into the brain substance, or both (Fig. 68.3). Blood

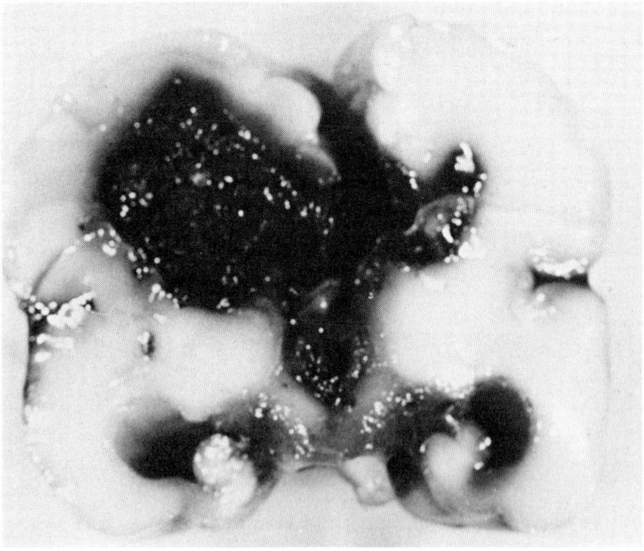

Fig. 68.3 Large intraventricular haemorrhage with dilatation of the ventricular system and extension into the left parenchyma (see Fig. 68.5, 68.6).

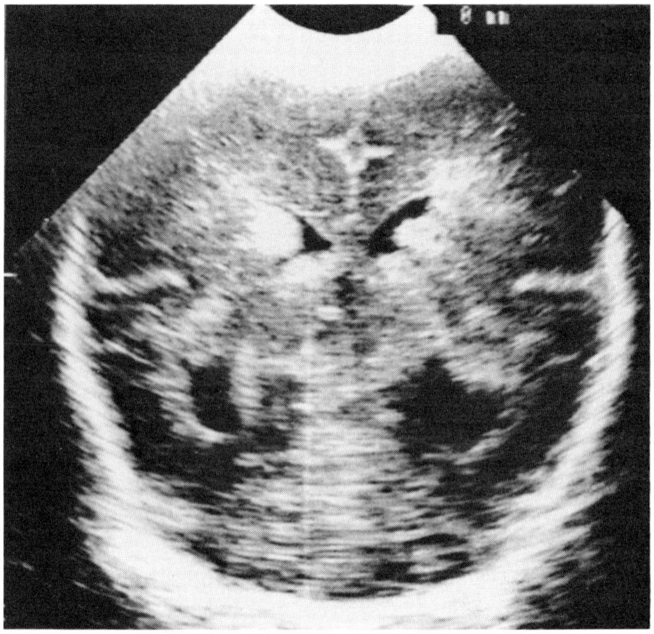

Fig. 68.4 Coronal ultrasound scan showing germinal layer and intraventricular extension.

clot in the third and fourth ventricles or arachnoiditis in the basal cisterns may block the cerebrospinal fluid pathways and may give rise to obstructive hydrocephalus.

Clinical signs. The preterm infant requiring mechanical ventilation may, when periventricular haemorrhage occurs, deteriorate rapidly, though more commonly the signs evolve over hours or days. In the former, deep coma preceded by apnoea and flaccidity alternating with tonic seizures are classical. The blood pressure falls and the anterior fontanelle becomes tense. Metabolic acidosis and temperature instability develop and a fall in haematocrit is detected. After the acute change in state, there may be a period of stabilization, particularly if resuscitation manoeuvres are initiated immediately. However, despite this, many go on to die.

More often, the signs are less obvious and nursing staff may be the first to recognize that spontaneous movements have decreased. Hypotonia and abnormal vertical drifting of the eyes are present. An abnormally tight popliteal angle which is attributed to meningeal irritation has been found to be present in 85% of babies with intraventricular haemorrhage and in only 10% of those without (Dubowitz et al 1981). These signs may fluctuate over days and, in many, clinical examination may not show any suggestive signs.

Diagnosis. Scanning at the cot-side by cranial ultrasound is the only practical routine way of detecting periventricular haemorrhage and of defining the progress (Fig. 68.4). Other methods, such as red blood-cell count and protein level in cerebrospinal fluid, or monitoring of the EEG, are too imprecise though often add extra valuable information. CT or magnetic resonance imaging are impractical as screening techniques, but may be valuable after the acute stages have past. Ultrasound scanning has the advantage of portability and because ionizing radiation is not involved, repeat studies can be made as frequently as necessary (Fig. 68.5, 68.6). The onset and progress of periventricular haemorrhage can therefore be monitored whilst intensive care continues (Levene et al 1985, Grant 1986).

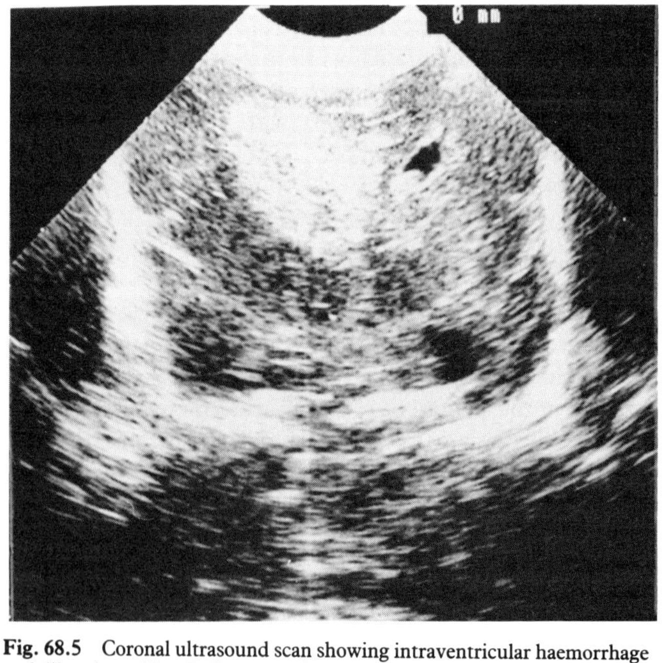

Fig. 68.5 Coronal ultrasound scan showing intraventricular haemorrhage and dilatation with echodense area in the left parenchyma.

Management. Prevention depends on antenatal and post-

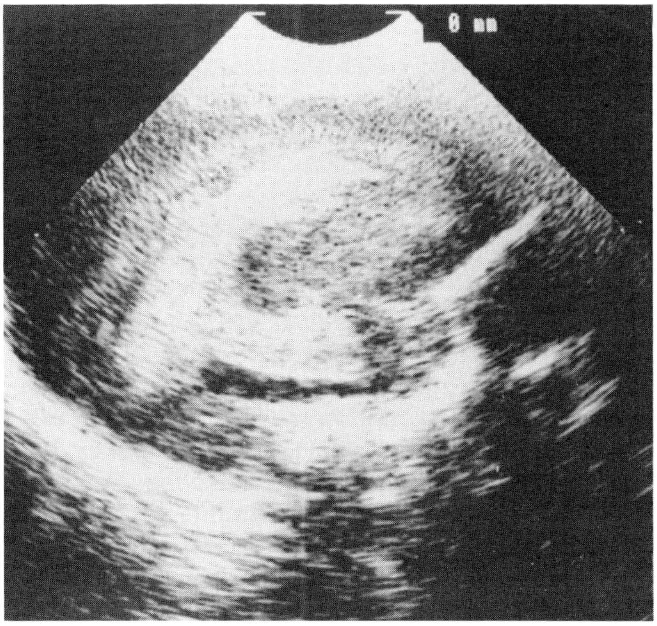

Fig. 68.6 Left parasagittal ultrasound scan showing echodense region in the parenchyma (same patient as Fig. 68.5).

natal management. Approaches to the prevention of preterm labour are dealt with in Chapter 50. Identification of high-risk pregnancies and in utero transfer to a specialized centre have improved the outcome in recent years. The factors described earlier relating to trauma and the effects of prolonged labour and breech delivery are relevant. Prompt but controlled resuscitation is vital, after which management is directed towards providing adequate oxygenation and preventing hyper- or hypocarbia. The regulation of cerebral blood flow is of vital importance, but is only partly understood at present. Volume replacement may be necessary and muscle paralysis is sometimes indicated. The merits of routine use of phenobarbitone, ethamsylate, a capillary stabilizer and vitamin E, an antioxidant, are still controversial.

No active intervention is indicated for subependymal or intraventricular haemorrhages which resolve spontaneously. Of more importance is the management of posthaemorrhagic ventricular dilatation. Two approaches are used at present. Serial lumbar punctures to control ventricular size may be initiated, but success is variable. Awaiting significant enlargement in both ventricular and head size before resorting to a shunt procedure has its advocates, but neurological signs may supervene. A multicentre randomized trial is in progress to study these approaches.

Prognosis. Severe intraventricular haemorrhage in preterm infants is often catastrophic and is associated with further cardiorespiratory deterioration. Extension of associated intracerebral haemorrhage is particularly worrying, and mortality and morbidity are correspondingly high. In uncomplicated subependymal haemorrhage or small intraventricular bleeding mortality is low and outcome is similar

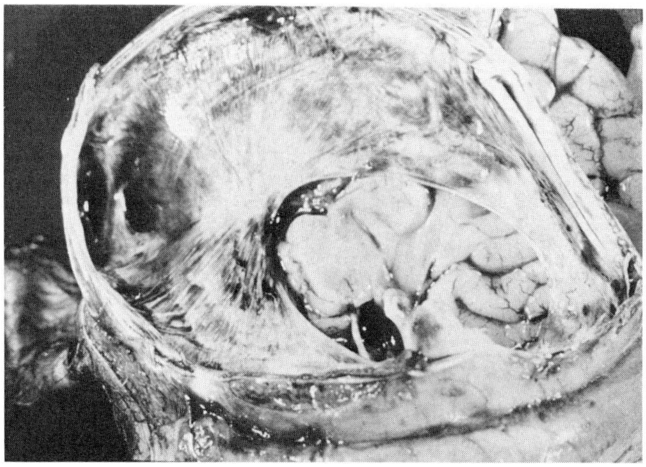

Fig. 68.7 Tear at the angle of the right tentorium cerebelli and falx. The concavity of the margin of the tentorium is lost and the surface shows irregularities. From Keeling (1987), with permission.

to that of babies without haemorrhage. Between these extremes there is considerable variation in long-term outcome, which depends as much on other complications, such as posthaemorrhagic hydrocephalus or periventricular leukomalacia, as on the haemorrhage itself (Fitzhardinge et al 1981, Stewart et al 1983, De Vries et al 1985).

Subdural haemorrhage

The great vein of Galen receives the deep venous drainage of the brain at the junction of the falx and tentorium. In the lower margin of the falx is the inferior sagittal sinus which joins the great vein to form the straight sinus. This runs posteriorly and is joined by the superior sagittal sinus in the upper margin of the falx to form the transverse or lateral sinuses. These pass in the margin of the tentorium to the jugular veins. Damage to the superficial veins or laceration of the dura leads to subdural haemorrhage (Fig. 68.7).

Pathogenesis

Subdural haemorrhage was in the past confined to the term babies who had suffered trauma during delivery, but with improvements in obstetric care the incidence has decreased. Concomitantly, the proportion recognized in preterm babies has increased. Factors predisposing to subdural haemorrhage are disproportion between fetal size and the size of the birth canal, low compliance of the birth canal in primiparous women, increased compliance of the preterm skull and either prolonged or precipitous delivery. The latter is particularly important with abnormal presentations such as foot, face, brow or breech. When delivery has to be assisted by the application of forceps with or without rotation of the head, there is an increased risk of venous contusion. Tentorial and falx laceration, particularly at their junction, may result. Superficial veins may be damaged, particularly

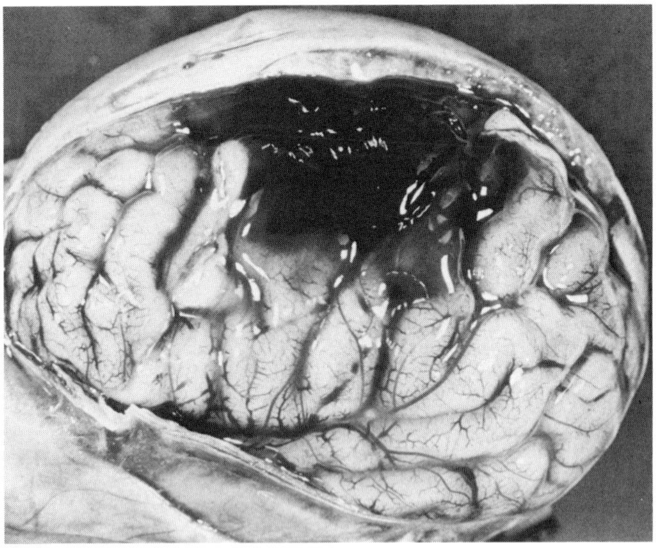

Fig. 68.8 Large left convexity subdural haemorrhage.

after marked vertical moulding and a lateral convexity subdural collection develops which is often unilateral. An important injury after breech delivery is diastasis of the occipital bone leading to damage to the occipital sinus, the dura and cerebellum. Blood collects in the posterior fossa and in most severe cases fracture of the skull may be demonstrated.

Clinical signs

When tentorial damage or occipital diastasis has occurred there are abnormal neurological signs present from birth. A depressed Apgar score of less than 5 with poor response to resuscitation is common. The baby may show signs of stupor with deviation of the eyes that does not change with the doll's eyes manoeuvre. The pupils and their response to light may be unequal. Bradycardia and tachypnoea may be noted. The collection of blood below the tentorium may enlarge rapidly and coma may develop within minutes or hours. The pupils become fixed and dilated, ocular bobbing may be seen and ultimately respiration becomes irregular, leading to arrest. Death is usual, ranging from 7 to 48 hours after birth. Infants who survive this period may later develop signs of hydrocephalus as cerebrospinal fluid is obstructed by blood clot.

When bleeding results from laceration to the falx, minor bilateral cerebral signs may be present until the clot extends below the tentorium. Few if any clinical signs are found when minor degrees of subdural blood collect over the hemispheres (Fig. 68.8). More extensive bleeding may give rise to seizures which may first be noted in the second or third day. Focal signs may develop, such as hemiparesis or ipsilateral third nerve lesion, leading to a pupil which reacts poorly or not at all to light. Finally, chronic subdural effusion detected during the first few months may be the end-result of a subdural collection of blood (Rabe et al 1968).

Diagnosis

The obstetric events are usually suggestive and once the clinical signs are recognized, a more definitive diagnosis should be sought. However, cardiorespiratory support in the form of artificial ventilation, blood and colloid replacement and suppression of seizures are priorities. Lumbar puncture should be avoided in view of the risk of precipitating herniation of the cerebellar tonsils into the foramen magnum or of the temporal lobe into the tentorial notch, when a large convexity subdural haematoma is present. Unfortunately, ultrasound scanning, which can be done in the intensive care nursery, is not at present able to detect small subdural haematomas very reliably (Levene et al 1985). Artefact signals in the near-field and from the skull at the periphery of the anterior fontanelle make the location and extent of subdural blood difficult to quantitate. CT scanning is the investigation of choice, but can usually be carried out only if the infant survives to enter a stable phase after 48–72 hours. After CT scanning, or occasionally if this is contraindicated, a subdural tap may be diagnostic. Skull X-rays may show fractures or occipital osteodiastasis in lateral views.

Management

Supportive therapy in an intensive care nursery may be lifesaving. There is little experience in the emergency neurosurgical evacuation of blood clot, but this approach is only indicated when, after early detection, deterioration has been rapid. With convexity subdural haemorrhage a tap of the collection of fluid may be of value but is indicated only if signs of increasing intracranial pressure develop and the head is enlarging.

Prognosis

Major tentorial or falx tears are almost invariably lethal either soon after birth or occasionally in the first few months, after a prolonged period of stupor. In the very few survivors, hydrocephalus is a complication. Posterior fossa collections have a better prognosis and some are amenable to surgical evacuation. Convexity subdural haemorrhage is the most benign form, needing no treatment and 60–80% of survivors are normal at follow-up. The others may have focal signs and hydrocephalus.

Subarachnoid haemorrhage

Haemorrhage from veins within and confined to the subarachnoid space is common but rarely of any importance in the newborn.

Pathogenesis

This is not clearly understood. Before CT and ultrasound scanning were developed, blood in the cerebrospinal fluid which had extended from other sites of haemorrhage was often misdiagnosed as a primary subarachnoid haemorrhage. When this has not occurred it is assumed that bleeding is from the anastomoses within the leptomeninges. Bridging veins may also be responsible. It is important to note that subarachnoid haemorrhage in the newborn is of venous origin and therefore bears no similarity to the catastrophic large arterial haemorrhage in adults. A perinatal asphyxial insult is invariably part of the history.

Clinical signs

Precise signs are difficult to enumerate as other events often occur coincidentally. Most often, particularly in preterm infants, a minimal collection of blood gives rise to no signs. More extensive bleeding in term babies results in seizures, the onset of which may be delayed until the second day. Later, hydrocephalus may develop. Finally, usually after a severe asphyxial insult and often with some degree of trauma, a massive haemorrhage may lead to a rapidly deteriorating condition which is ultimately fatal.

Diagnosis

Although suggested by a raised red blood cell count in the cerebrospinal fluid, definitive diagnosis can only be made by excluding other causes of intracerebral haemorrhage by the timely use of ultrasound and CT scanning. The former will reveal periventricular and intraparenchymal haemorrhage which may have extended. CT scanning is required, for reasons explained above, to define a collection of blood confined to the subarachnoid space.

Management

In most cases no treatment is indicated. Seizures require anticonvulsant therapy but usually this is only necessary for 5–7 days. The rare cases of severe progressive deterioration have not been amenable to intervention. Later on, hydrocephalus, which is usually of slower onset than hydrocephalus after periventricular haemorrhage, is managed by cerebrospinal fluid shunting.

Prognosis

Only the rare massive haemorrhage has a bleak outlook. The outcome from those infants without any other accompanying insult is good. Even the few who develop seizures after subarachnoid haemorrhage are usually normal at follow-up (Rose & Lombresco 1970). Those with hydrocephalus usually develop this complication insidiously. Perhaps because of this and because the aetiology is more benign, the outlook is better than in those infants who develop hydrocephalus after periventricular haemorrhage.

Intracerebellar haemorrhage

Haemorrhage into the cerebellum may be more common than was previously suspected. Massive haemorrhage has been described but the high incidence of smaller haemorrhages—15–25% reported following post-mortem examination—has not been confirmed (Martin et al 1976). These lesions may be below the resolution of the CT scanner and difficult to demonstrate by ultrasonography.

Pathogenesis

Hypoxaemia, particularly in preterm infants with severe respiratory distress, is related to intracerebellar haemorrhage in the same way as it is to periventricular haemorrhage. Perinatal trauma after breech delivery and the use of forceps are common antecedents. Of particular importance is the easily deformed skull of preterm babies. Increased longitudinal pressure displaces the squamous occipital bone under the parietal, which compresses the veins and raises venous pressure. This effect was most clearly shown in a series of babies who were ventilated with positive pressure by securing a mask to the face with a strap around the occiput. Cerebellar haemorrhage was shown post-mortem (Pape et al 1976). Mechanical forces can therefore contribute to this lesion.

Preterm infants are at risk of mechanical distortion with occipital compression when procedures such as intubation, resuscitation by bag and mask and securing of an endotracheal tube are carried out. Abnormal coagulation has been reported in some cases with vitamin K_1 deficiency (Chaou et al 1984) and thrombocytopenia (Zalneraitis et al 1979). Cerebellar haemorrhage has complicated some cases of organic acidaemia (Fischer et al 1981, Dave et al 1984). As with periventricular haemorrhage, subependymal areas of the cerebellum in the region of the fourth ventricle are particularly at risk of haemorrhage. Finally, direct extension from an intraventricular haemorrhage can occur, probably as a result of the increased pressure within the ventricular system and, in the preterm baby, as a result of the lack of fully myelinated white matter.

Clinical signs

An adverse perinatal history is usual followed by precipitous deterioration which may occur in the first few days, particularly in the preterm, but also later in the first month. Apnoea is probably related to compression of the medulla by the cerebellar mass. Signs of early hydrocephalus may develop, as may signs of brain stem involvement with skew deviation of the eyes, facial nerve palsy, intermittent tone of the limbs and flaccid quadriparesis.

Diagnosis

Intracerebellar haemorrhage is difficult to detect by ultrasound scanning because of the normal echogenicity of the cerebellum. Subdural haemorrhage may be mistaken for cerebellar haemorrhage. Parasagittal views are of most value in detecting any asymmetry. CT scanning may improve the definition of the lesion but, as noted above, it appears from post-mortem studies that present-day technology may not reveal all cases of cerebellar haemorrhage.

Management

There have been a few reports of survival after surgical evacuation in term infants, but whether surgical evacuation is necessary is unclear because equal success is reported after medical management (Fishman et al 1981). Cerebrospinal fluid shunting may be required if hydrocephalus is acute before the cerebellar clot resolves. Serious cardiorespiratory disease usually coexists in the preterm infant and often precludes anything other than supportive management.

Prognosis

In the preterm baby death is invariable. Indeed, the first series were described at post-mortem (Martin et al 1976). Conversely, in the term infant with or without surgical intervention survival is the rule. However, all develop motor abnormalities and some degree of intellectual deficit. Hydrocephalus develops in 50%. Cerebellar dysfunction in the form of intention tremor, hypotonia and truncal ataxia has been described (Volpe 1987).

Rare causes of intracranial haemorrhage

Other rare causes of intracerebral haemorrhage are vascular and coagulation defects and tumour.

PERIVENTRICULAR LEUKOMALACIA

Cystic necrosis of the white matter adjacent to the lateral ventricles is characteristically found in some preterm infants who have suffered severe respiratory illness during the first few days of life.

Pathogenesis

The lesions are found in areas of the brain where border zones between different arterial supplies exist. These areas are supplied by the penetrating branches of the middle cerebral artery and by the anterior and posterior cerebral arteries. The latter two are under-developed in the preterm baby and the anastomoses are compromised by decreased blood flow during episodes of hypotension. The most common areas are in the occipital and frontal radiations lateral and superior to the lateral ventricles (Fig. 68.9). Blood supply to the brain is regulated by variations in vascular resistance in response to changes in blood pressure and the oxygen and carbon dioxide tension in the blood, as well

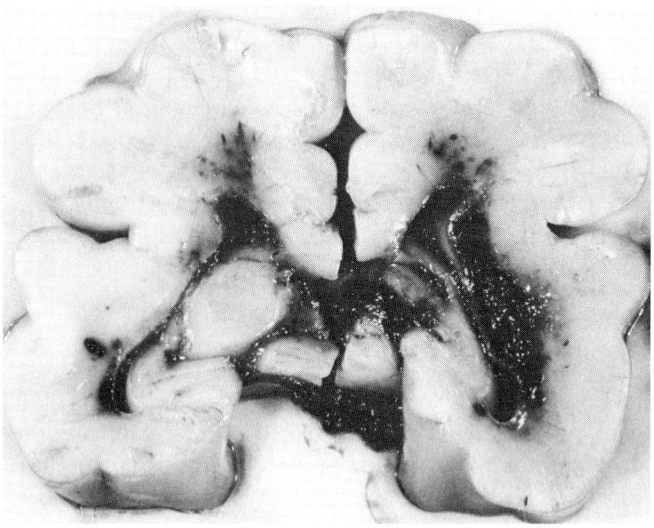

Fig. 68.9 Large intraventricular haemorrhage with extensive bilateral periventricular leukomalacia with haemorrhagic necrosis.

as other metabolic factors. When severe hypotension occurs, as for example after an antepartum haemorrhage, the cerebral blood flow is decreased, predisposing to ischaemic infarction (Weindling et al 1985a, Calvert et al 1987). The resulting lesion is a localized area of necrosis in which haemorrhage may occur. Later, cystic degeneration takes place. Multiple cysts may be present (Volpe 1987).

Clinical signs

Until recently, periventricular leukomalacia was only diagnosed at post-mortem examination. With the improved survival of preterm infants and the introduction of cerebral ultrasound scanning, the lesion is being recognized earlier. Echodense areas adjacent to the ventricles are found which correlate with post-mortem studies (Banker & Larroche 1962). Clinical findings in the neonatal period are not well documented, but are beginning to be described. Lower extremity weakness may be an early sign, but this observation requires confirmation (Volpe 1987). In survivors, spastic diplegia as a result of disruption of descending fibres from the cortex is usual. This affects the lower limbs more than the upper limbs, though more extensive lesions involve both.

Management

Prevention depends on early recognition of signs of intrauterine asphyxia and appropriate monitoring and intervention (see Ch. 47). The presence at delivery of a team of paediatric staff experienced in resuscitation is vital. Maintenance of body temperature, support of ventilation, perfusion and acid–base balance is crucial. After stabilization and transfer to the intensive care nursery, close observation and monitoring are necessary. Hypoxaemia may occur with apnoea or worsening respiratory illness and pneumothorax. Diagnostic procedures, particularly painful ones, may cause unsuspected hypoxaemia. A normal arterial carbon dioxide tension is also important in regulating cerebral blood flow and neuronal metabolism. Blood pressure may need to be supported with colloid, blood and inotropic drugs. Other factors such as seizures and cerebral oedema contribute to the postnatal injury, but to what extent is not known.

Progress

Extensive periventricular damage is commonly associated with a large intraventricular haemorrhage and the outcome is affected by both lesions. Death or severe neurological abnormality is usual. When less extensive but multiple cysts, which are often bilateral, are present in survivors, the usual outcome is moderate to severe spastic diplegia or quadriplegia. Visual abnormalities are also common. Intellectual function is affected to a varying extent (Weindling et al 1985b, Calvert et al 1986, Volpe 1987).

NON-ACCIDENTAL INJURY

Unexplained purpura, tears of the earlobe, fractures or burns from a cigarette—all common findings in non-accidental injury in older children—have been reported in the early neonatal period. Usually in these circumstances, the parent responsible is suffering from a severe psychiatric disorder.

Neglect or complete lack of mothering skills coinciding with an absence of assistance may expose some babies to neonatal cold injury (Bower et al 1960, Arneil & Kerr 1963). Clinically, babies are lethargic with a weak cry and feed poorly. Pronounced erythema of the cheeks may suggest well-being, but the skin is cold to touch and patchy sclerema may be found. If neonatal cold injury is suspected, a low-reading thermometer must be used. In most severe cases, where rectal temperature is less than 28°C, the baby may be moribund to the point of appearing dead. Recovery, however, has been known in such extreme cases.

Some reports show that child abuse is common in families where a baby has been separated from parents after admission to a neonatal intensive care unit. There is little to suggest that this is a direct relationship (Richards 1985). Rather, it is more likely that factors such as teenage pregnancy, particularly in single mothers, poor support in the community and difficulties during pregnancy and delivery may predispose to abuse (Gaines et al 1978). Much more should be done to support parents and their babies in these situations by anticipating their needs and by recognizing the social and psychological difficulties that they experience.

REFERENCES

Amiel-Tison C 1969 Cerebral damage in full-term newborn: aetiological factors, neonatal status and long-term follow up. Biologica Neonatorum 14: 234–250

Amiel-Tison C, Korobkin R, Esque-Vaucouoloux M T 1977 Neck extensor hypertonia: a clinical sign of insult to the central nervous system of the newborn. Early Human Development 1: 181–190

Arneil G C, Kerr M M 1963 Severe hypothermia in Glasgow infants in winter. Lancet ii: 756–759

Banker B Q, Larroche J-C 1962 Periventricular leukomalacia in infancy. Archives of Neurology 7: 386–410

Batton D G, Hellman J, Nardis E E 1984 Effect of pneumothorax-induced systemic blood pressure alterations on the cerebral circulation in newborn dogs. Pediatrics 74: 350–353

Bower B D, Jones L F, Weeks M N 1960 Cold injury in the newborn. British Medical Journal i: 303–309

Brent R L 1967 Medicolegal aspects of teratology. Journal of Pediatrics 71: 288–298

Brent R L 1986 The effects of embryonic and fetal exposure to X-ray, microwaves and ultrasound. Clinics in Perinatology 13: 615–648

Brown J K, Purvis R J, Forfar J O, Cockburn F 1974 Neurological aspects of perinatal asphyxia. Developmental Medicine and Child Neurology 16: 567–580

Byres R K 1975 Spinal-cord injuries during birth. Developmental Medicine and Child Neurology 17: 103–110

Calvert S A, Hoskins E M, Fong K W, Forsyth S C 1986 Periventricular leukomalacia. Acta Paediatrica Scandinavica 75: 489–496

Calvert S A, Hoskins E M, Fong K W, Forsyth S C 1987 Etiological factors associated with the development of periventricular leukomalacia. Acta Paediatrica Scandinavica 76: 254–259

Cartwright E W, Culbertson K, Schreiner R, Garg B P 1979. Changes in clinical presentation of term infants with intracranial haemorrhage. Developmental Medicine and Child Neurology 21: 730–737

Chaou W T, Chaou M L, Eitzmann D V 1984 Intracranial hemorrhage and vitamin K deficiency in early infancy. Journal of Pediatrics 105: 880–884

Court-Brown W M, Doll R, Hill A B 1960 Incidence of leukaemia after exposure to diagnostic radiation in utero. British Medical Journal ii: 1539–1545

Dave P, Curless R G, Steinmann L 1984 Cerebellar hemorrhage complicating methylmalonic and proprionic acidemia. Archives of Neurology 41: 1293–1296

De Vries L S, Dubowitz V, Lary S et al 1985 Predictive value of cranial ultrasound in the newborn baby: a reappraisal. Lancet ii: 131–134

Dubowitz L M S, Levene M I, Morante A, Palmer P, Dubowitz V 1981 Neurological signs in neonatal intraventricular haemorrhage: a correlation with real-time ultrasound. Journal of Pediatrics 99: 127–133

Eng G D 1971 Brachial plexus palsy in newborn infants. Pediatrics 48: 18–20

Eyre J A, Wilkinson A R 1986 Thiopentone induced coma after severe birth asphyxia. Archives of Disease in Childhood 61: 1084–1089

Eyre J A, Oozeer R C, Wilkinson A R 1983 Diagnosis of neonatal seizures by continuous recording and rapid analysis of the electroencephalogram. Archives of Disease in Childhood 58: 785–790

Finer N N, Robertson C M, Richards R T, Pinnell L E, Peters K L 1981 Hypoxic–ischaemic encephalopathy in term neonates: perinatal factors and outcome. Journal of Pediatrics 98: 112–117

Finer N N, Robertson C M, Peters K L, Coward J H 1983 Factors affecting outcome in hypoxic–ischaemic encephalopathy in term infants. American Journal of Disease in Children 137: 21–25

Fischer A Q, Challa V R, Burton B K, McLean W T 1981 Cerebellar hemorrhage complicating isovaleric acidemia: a case report. Neurology 31: 746–748

Fishman M A, Percy A K, Cheek W R, Speer M E 1981 Successful conservative management of cerebellar hematomas in term infants. Journal of Pediatrics 98: 466–468

Fitzhardinge P M, Flodmark O, Fitz C R, Ashby S 1981 The prognostic value of computed tomography of the brain in asphyxiated premature infants. Journal of Pediatrics 99: 476–481

Fletcher E W L, Baum D D, Draper G 1986 The risk of diagnostic radiation of the newborn. British Journal of Radiology 59: 165–170

Gaines R, Sandgrund A, Green A H, Power E 1978 Etiological factors in

child maltreatment: a multivariate study of abusing, neglecting and normal mothers. Journal of Abnormal Psychology 87: 531–540
Gordon M, Rich H, Deutschbergen J, Green M 1973 The immediate and long-term outcome of obstetric birth trauma. I. Brachial plexus paralysis. American Journal of Obstetrics and Gynecology 117: 51–56
Grant E G 1986 Neurosonography of the preterm neonate. Springer-Verlag, New York
Hawkins D F 1981 Effects of drugs in pregnancy and during lactation. In: Roberts D F, Chester R (eds) Changing patterns of conception and fertility. Academic Press, London, pp 135–163
Hellman L M, Duffins G M, Donald I, Sunden B 1970 Safety of diagnostic ultrasound in obstetrics. Lancet i: 1133–1134
Higginbottom N I C, Jones K L, Hale B D, Smith D W 1979 The amniotic band disruption complex: timing of amniotic rupture and variable spectra of consequent defects. Journal of Pediatrics 95: 544–549
Isenberg S, Everett S 1984 Cardiovascular effects of mydriatics in low birthweight infants. Journal of Pediatrics 105: 111–112
Jablon S, Kato H 1970 Childhood cancer in relation to prenatal exposure to atomic-bomb radiation. Lancet ii: 1000–1003
Keeling J W 1987 Intrapartum asphyxia and birth trauma. In: Keeling J W (ed) Fetal and neonatal pathology. Springer, London, pp 199–210
Levene M I, Williams J L, Fawer G L 1985 Ultrasound of the infant brain. Clinics in developmental medicine 92. Spastics International
Low J A, Galbraith R S, Muir D, Killen H L, Pater E A, Karchmar E J 1985 The relationship between perinatal hypoxia and newborn encephalopathy. American Journal of Obstetrics and Gynecology 152: 256–260
Malamud N 1950 Status marmoratus: form of cerebral palsy following either birth injury or inflammation of the central nervous system. Journal of Pediatrics 37: 610–619
Martin R, Roessmann U, Fanaroff A 1976 Massive intracerebellar hemorrhage in low-birthweight infants. Journal of Pediatrics 89: 290–293
McDonald M M, Johnson M L, Rumack C M et al 1984 Role of coagulopathy in newborn intracranial haemorrhage. Pediatrics 74: 26–71
Ministry of Health Department of Health for Scotland 1960 Radiological hazards in patients. Second report of the committee. Her Majesty's Stationery Office, London, p 134
Mitchell W, O'Tuama L 1980 Cerebral intraventricular hemorrhage in infants: a widening age spectrum. Pediatrics 65: 35–39
Painter M J, Bergman I 1982 Obstetrical trauma to the neonatal central nervous system and peripheral nervous system. Seminars in Perinatology 6: 89
Pape K E, Armstrong D L, Fitzhardinge P M 1976 Central nervous system pathology associated with mask ventilation in the very low birthweight infant: a new etiology for intracerebellar hemorrhages. Pediatrics 58: 473–483
Perlman J M, Volpe J J 1983 Suctioning in the preterm infant: effects on cerebral blood flow velocity, intracranial pressure, and arterial blood pressure. Pediatrics 72(3): 329–334
Perlman J M, McMenamin J B, Volpe J J 1983 Fluctuating cerebral blood-flow velocity in respiratory distress syndrome. New England Journal of Medicine 309: 204
Rabe E F, Flyn R E, Dodge P R 1968 Subdural collections of fluid in infants and children: a study of 62 patients with special reference to factors influencing prognosis and the efficacy of various forms of therapy. Neurology 18: 559–570
Richards M P M 1985 Bonding babies. Archives of Disease in Childhood 60: 293–294
Robertson C, Finer N N 1985 Term infants with hypoxic–ischaemic encephalopathy: outcome at 3.5 years. Developmental Medicine and Child Neurology 21: 473–484
Rochefort M J, Rolfe P, Wilkinson A R 1987 New fontanometer for continuous estimation of intracranial pressure in the newborn. Archives of Disease in Childhood 62: 152–155
Rose A L, Lombresco C T 1970 Neonatal seizure states: a study of clinical, pathological, and electroencephalographic features in 137 full-term babies with a long-term follow-up. Pediatrics 45: 404–425
Rylance G W 1986 Neonatal pharmacology. In: Roberton N R C (ed) Textbook of neonatology. Churchill Livingstone, Edinburgh, pp 234–235
Salter R B 1968 Etiology, pathogenesis and possible prevention of congenital dislocation of the hip. Canadian Medical Association Journal 98: 933–945
Sarnat H B, Sarnat M S 1976 Neonatal encephalopathy following fetal distress. Archives of Neurology 33: 696–705
Setzer E S, Webb I B, Wassenaat J W, Reeder J D, Mehta P S, Eitzman D V 1982 Platelet dysfunction and coagulopathy in intraventricular hemorrhage in the premature infant. Journal of Pediatrics 100: 599–605
Sternberg J 1973 Radiation risk in pregnancy. Clinical Obstetrics and Gynecology 16: 235–278
Stewart R, Kneale 1970 Radiation dose effects in relation to obstetric X-rays and childhood cancers. Lancet i: 1185–1188
Stewart A L, Thorburn R J, Hope P L, Goldsmith M, Lipscomb A P, Reynolds E O R 1983 Ultrasound appearance of the brain in very preterm infants and neurodevelopmental outcome at 18 months of age. Archives of Disease in Childhood 58: 598–604
Volpe J J 1977 Neonatal seizures. Clinics in Perinatology 4: 43–63
Volpe J J 1987 Neurology of the newborn, 2nd edn. W B Saunders, Philadelphia
Weindling A M, Wilkinson A R, Cook J, Calvert S A, Fok T-F, Rochefort M J 1985a Perinatal events which precede periventricular haemorrhage and leucomalacia in the newborn. British Journal of Obstetrics and Gynaecology 92: 1218–1223
Weindling A M, Rochefort M J, Calvert S A, Fox T-F, Wilkinson A R 1985b Development of cerebral palsy after ultrasonographic detection of perventricular cysts in the newborn. Developmental Medicine and Child Neurology 27: 800–806
Zalneraitis E L, Young R S K, Krishnamoorthy K S 1979 Intracranial haemorrhage in-utero as a complication of isoimmune thrombocytopenia. Journal of Pediatrics 95: 611–614

69

David Isaacs and E. Richard Moxon

Neonatal infections

The newborn infant, particularly if preterm, is relatively immunodeficient and the incidence of infections in the neonatal period exceeds that at all other ages. The nature of neonatal immune deficiency partly explains the increased susceptibility to some organisms. Other factors are also important. The newborn is frequently exposed to a large microbial load of bacteria or viruses colonizing or infecting the female genital tract. Babies requiring intensive care frequently undergo invasive procedures such as endotracheal intubation and the insertion of indwelling intravenous catheters. The combination of increased susceptibility and unusual exposure are important in determining the susceptibility of the newborn to severe infections, often with organisms that rarely cause major disease in older children and adults.

THE NEWBORN AS AN IMMUNODEFICIENT HOST

Humoral factors

Neonates are poor synthesizers of IgG; neonatal serum IgG derives from transplacental passage, which is dependent both on passive transfer of maternal IgG and on an active enzymatic transport (Gitlin et al 1964).

Transplacental transfer of maternal IgG varies with gestation: neonates of less than 32 weeks' gestation have less than half the maternal serum level of IgG, whereas at 40 weeks serum levels are 5–10% greater than maternal levels due to the active transport mechanism.

Activation of the alternative pathway and, to a lesser extent, the classical pathway of complement are relatively inefficient in neonates, as shown by decreased complement-mediated opsonization and generation of serum chemotactic factors against type III group B streptococci and other bacteria (Wilson 1986).

Mucosal factors

Secretory antibody production is extremely low in neonates. IgA does not cross the placenta but can be absorbed into serum from breast milk. Neonatal epithelial cells may also permit increased adherence of bacteria. For example, type III group B streptococci but not other serotypes adhere better to neonatal than to adult buccal epithelial cells (Broughton & Baker 1983). Fibronectin may also prevent bacterial adherence; newborn babies with sepsis have low serum fibronectin levels though low levels in secretions have not been demonstrated (Gerdes et al 1983). Breast milk contains secretory IgA and other antimicrobial factors, such as lactoferrin and lysozyme; breastfeeding has been shown to protect against infection with some respiratory pathogens such as respiratory syncytial virus and some gastrointestinal pathogens such as rotavirus.

Cellular factors

Defects in neonatal phagocytic function include impaired production and delivery of phagocytes to the site of infection. The neonatal polymorphonuclear pool is readily depleted in septic infants, unlike adults; neutropenia, which has a grave prognosis, may develop. Neutrophil migration is defective and this has been correlated with marked in vitro defects in neonatal neutrophil chemotaxis (Wilson 1986). Clinically this may manifest as a poor or absent inflammatory response to local sepsis.

Neonatal T-lymphocyte function is relatively normal, but decreased generation of lymphokines and interleukins which attract macrophages to the site of infection may render the neonate more susceptible to infections with viruses such as herpes simplex virus, parasites such as *Toxoplasma gondii* and intracellular bacteria such as *Listeria monocytogenes*.

OBSTETRIC FACTORS IN NEONATAL INFECTION

Chorioamnionitis

The role of chorioamnionitis in the pathogenesis of neonatal infection has been obscured by confusion over terminology. The clinical diagnosis of chorioamnionitis is based on maternal fever, foul-smelling amniotic fluid, a tender uterus and no evidence of infection outside the uterus. This situation should be distinguished from simple colonization of the vaginal tract or amniotic fluid without clinical evidence of infection. A pathological diagnosis of chorioamnionitis, such as that used by Naeye and his colleagues, as acute inflammation throughout the subchorionic plate of the placenta, occurs more frequently than demonstrable maternal infection.

Naeye & Peters (1980) found that amniotic fluid infection was two or three times more common when the membranes ruptured just prior to onset of preterm labour, compared to rupture just after onset. They interpreted this as suggesting that infection may initiate preterm labour. Regan and colleagues (1981) found a significant increase in premature rupture of membranes and delivery before 32 weeks' gestation among women colonized with group B streptococci. Behar and colleagues (1981) demonstrated phospholipase A_2 production by vaginal bacteria and have suggested that the liberation of arachidonic acid from membrane phospholipids leading to enhanced prostaglandin synthesis might cause premature labour. This work has been extended by Lamont et al (1985) who demonstrated increased prostaglandin E production by cultured amnion cells in vitro when exposed to bacterial products.

It is not generally appreciated that the vast majority of babies born to mothers with chorioamnionitis do not become infected. Siegel & McCracken (1981) have estimated that only 1–6% of infants of mothers with clinical chorioamnionitis, the highest risk group, become infected. Others have found a poor correlation between bacterial cultures from the vagina, placenta and neonate with histological chorioamnionitis (Zaaijman et al 1982).

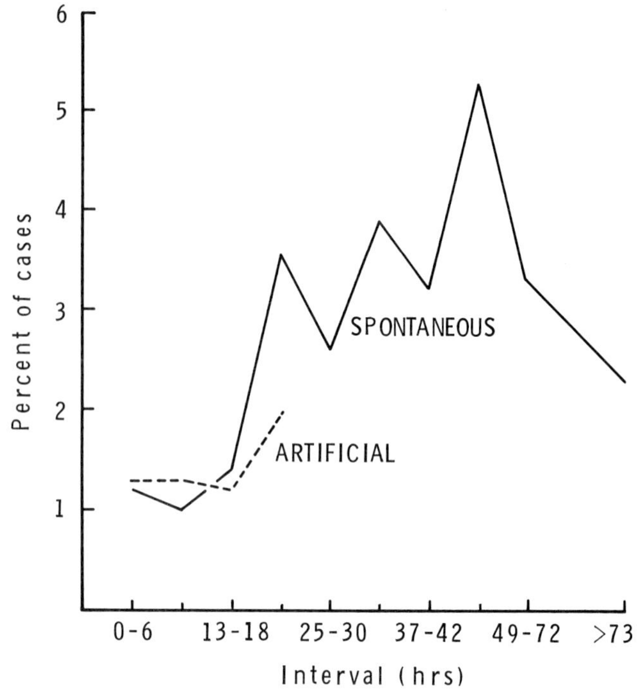

Fig. 69.1 Proportion of babies of women with clinical amnionitis developing infection in relation to interval between membrane rupture and birth. From Shubeck et al (1966), with permission from the American College of Obstetricians and Gynecologists.

Premature or prolonged rupture of the membranes

There is a complex relationship between premature rupture of the membranes and chorioamnionitis. Chorioamnionitis may predispose to premature rupture of the membranes and preterm labour (Naeye & Peters 1980). Furthermore, the risk of chorioamnionitis and perinatal infection initially increases with increasing time following premature rupture of the membranes (Shubeck et al 1966). However, the risk of infection remains low for the neonate, not exceeding 6% (Siegel & McCracken 1981), and several authors have shown that the major risks of preterm labour for the fetus are those associated with prematurity rather than with infection (Fayez et al 1978, Miller et al 1978, Kappy et al 1979, Zaaijman et al 1982).

The obstetric management is complicated by the clinical difficulty in distinguishing between premature rupture of the forewaters or hindwaters. Hindwater leak may explain the decreasing incidence of perinatal infection after greater than 72 hours of ruptured membranes (Shubeck et al 1966, Fig. 69.1). It is controversial whether premature rupture of the membranes increases fetal lung maturity. Conservative management of premature rupture of the membranes, based on the rationale that immaturity is a far greater risk than infection to the neonate, has been widely advocated (Fayez et al 1978, Kappy et al 1979, Schreiber & Benedett 1980). The reported outcome of conservative management has generally been favourable; in one study 19% of 188 pregnancies were prolonged for at least 7 days and only one non-fatal neonatal infection occurred (Kappy et al 1979), but such studies have tended to address only the situation of premature rupture of the membranes without active labour. The role of tocolytics and corticosteroids will be considered elsewhere.

There is little agreement over the place of antibiotics for women with premature or prolonged rupture of the membranes. Intravenous ampicillin given intrapartum to at-risk mothers who are colonized with group B strepotococci and have prolonged rupture of the membranes, preterm onset of labour or intrapartum fever protects neonates from systemic sepsis and decreases maternal morbidity (Boyer & Gotoff 1986). When the mother's colonization status is unknown or cultures are negative for group B streptococcus the use of intrapartum antibiotics is less clear.

Premature labour

A proportion of women in premature labour with intact membranes and no fever will have bacterial amnionitis. Some authors have advocated transabdominal amniocentesis to identify these women (Bobitt & Ledger 1978). There is some evidence that women colonized with group B streptococci are more likely to have onset of labour and rupture of membranes before 32 weeks' gestation (Regan et al 1981).

Fetal scalp monitor clips

Scalp monitor clips are a potential, albeit rare, risk for local abscesses, osteomyelitis and systemic sepsis. The older barbed monitor clip has been associated with a greater risk of infection than the newer helical electrodes (Winkel et al 1976). However, even the spiral electrode was reported to be associated with abscess in 4.5% of infants in a prospective study, though most infections were minor (Okada et al 1977). Serious infections with a variety of pathogens may rarely occur, including group A and B streptococci, gonococcus, *Escherichia coli* and anaerobes. The scalp electrode has also been described as the site of entry for herpes simplex virus (Parvey & Chi'en 1980).

Most decisions on whether or not to deliver babies early and whether or not to use antibiotics, steroids and tocolytics can be individualized to each patient. They are not usually so urgent as to preclude discussion between obstetrician and paediatrician, which is an important part of the decision-making process. It allows the best preparations for the arrival of a preterm baby and directs efforts to minimizing the risk of early-onset sepsis through rational use of cultures and antibiotics.

NEONATAL SEPSIS

Neonatal sepsis, which implies bacterial sepsis, is generally subdivided into early- and late-onset. In early-onset sepsis, which occurs within a few days of birth, the infecting organisms are likely to have been acquired by ascending infection from an infected or heavily colonized maternal genital tract, or, more rarely, transplacentally. In late-onset sepsis the infecting organisms may have been acquired by maternal organisms colonizing and later invading the neonate, or may have been acquired as a result of cross-infection from other neonates or introduced during an invasive procedure.

A large range of potential pathogens can colonize the maternal genital tract and cause neonatal sepsis. The most important organisms will depend on geographical, socio-economic and cultural factors. Host factors are important, as shown for example by the increased susceptibility of males for perinatal and neonatal sepsis (though not intrauterine infection). The virulence of the organism will also play a role in the pathogenesis and severity of infection, as shown for example by the relative importance of certain phage types of *Staphylococcus aureus* in the 1950s pandemic, and serotype III of group B streptococcus and the K1 capsular polysaccharide of *Escherichia coli* in cases of neonatal meningitis.

Early-onset sepsis

As already suggested, there will be geographical and temporal variations in the organisms causing early-onset sepsis. The rapid progression of infection precludes waiting for culture results, so that blind treatment of neonatal sepsis is the rule. The choice of antibiotic treatment should be based rationally on knowledge of the local prevalence of infection with different organisms and also on the outcome of those infections in terms of morbidity and mortality. In most industrialized societies group B streptococcus is currently the major cause of early-onset sepsis and of morbidity and mortality. In Ibadan, Nigeria, however, *Salmonella*, Enterobacteriaceae and *Streptococcus pneumoniae* were important causes of early-onset sepsis with meningitis (Barclay 1971), indicating the different spectrum of organisms causing disease in a non-industrial setting. In France, the Netherlands and West Germany, *Listeria monocytogenes* is an important cause of sepsis and, although less common in the UK, antibiotic policies need to be effective against this organism.

In western neonatal units, the high incidence and mortality of group B streptococcal sepsis means that penicillin G or ampicillin is usually given for suspected early-onset sepsis. Since Gram-negative organisms may also cause early-onset sepsis, an aminoglycoside is usually given in combination with the penicillin. The combination of a penicillin and an aminoglycoside is effective treatment for *Listeria* infections and will be effective against most of the other organisms causing early-onset sepsis. Surveillance of the organisms causing sepsis and the outcome of episodes of sepsis is important, because the prevalent organisms may change.

Late-onset sepsis

A wide variety of organisms may cause late-onset sepsis and, as for early-onset sepsis, antibiotic policies should be based not only on the organisms and their in vitro sensitivity to antibiotics but also on outcome.

In industrial countries, Gram-negative bacilli such as *Escherichia coli*, *Klebsiella*, *Pseudomonas* and *Serratia* are important causes of late-onset sepsis, sometimes causing major nursery outbreaks. *Staphylococcus epidermidis* is being increasingly recognized as a pathogen, particularly in nurseries where indwelling catheters are used for long periods. *Staph. aureus* caused major outbreaks of sepsis in the USA in the 1950s and is still an important cause of late-onset sepsis in many countries. The importance of hand-washing in preventing nursery transmission of virulent organisms cannot be over-emphasized.

The emergence of methicillin-resistant strains of *Staph.*

aureus which have caused outbreaks of neonatal sepsis in Australia and many other countries indicates the potential of bacteria to develop resistance to antibiotics and the importance of avoiding the indiscriminate use of antibiotics. Since newborn babies with sepsis can deteriorate rapidly antibiotics should be started early. On the other hand, it is also important to stop antibiotics after 48–72 hours if cultures of blood, urine and cerebrospinal fluid are sterile since the use of antibiotics for more than 72 hours increases the risk of colonization with potentially virulent Gram-negative organisms (Goldmann et al 1978).

GROUP B STREPTOCOCCAL INFECTION

Since the 1970s, streptococci of Lancefield group B have supplanted *Escherichia coli* as the organism causing most cases of neonatal septicaemia and meningitis in the USA and the UK (Baker & Edwards 1983). The incidence of proven sepsis varies from country to country and within countries, and fluctuates with time. The incidence of neonatal group B streptococcal sepsis is almost 10 times higher in the USA, where there are 2–3 cases per 1000 live births, than in the UK where the attack rate is 0.3 per 1000 (Lancet Editorial 1984).

The pattern of neonatal group B streptococcal infections is bimodal and is classically divided into early-onset and late-onset sepsis, although there is some overlap between the two categories (Anthony & Okada 1977). It has long been recognized that ascending infection is the most important route in early-onset infection (Benirschke 1960), although acquisition by passage through an infected birth canal can rarely be excluded. Maternal bacteraemia and hence haematogeneous spread are very rare. Late-onset infection, on the other hand, is usually caused by invasion of group B streptococci that have colonized the baby after passage through a colonized birth canal. Occasionally late-onset infection may result from hospital-acquired infection (Baker & Edwards 1983). Both early- and late-onset infections occur predominantly in infants with absent or low levels of specific IgG against the infecting serotype (Baker & Edwards 1983).

Serotypes

There are five recognized serotypes of group B streptococci — types Ia, Ib, Ic, II and III. Serotypes I, II and III are of approximately equal prevalence in colonizing the vagina or rectum of pregnant women and in causing early-onset neonatal sepsis without meningitis. This suggests that early-onset sepsis may result from a breach in the host defences and does not depend on the particular virulence of any serotype. In contrast, over 90% of cases of late-onset sepsis and 85% of early-onset meningitis cases are caused by serotype III, implying increased virulence of this serotype for invading the neonate's bloodstream and central nervous system. Infants with sepsis due to serotype III have low serum levels of maternally acquired opsonic antibody to the type III capsular polysaccharide (Baker et al 1981).

Early-onset group B streptococcal disease

Early-onset disease with group B streptococci is usually defined as sepsis in the first 5 days postpartum, but the mean onset of symptoms is at 20 hours (Anthony & Okada 1977) and babies are often symptomatic and septicaemic at birth. Colonization of the maternal genital tract is usually a prerequisite for early-onset sepsis and the risk of neonatal sepsis correlates with the size of the maternal genital inoculum. Maternal carriage rates for group B streptococcus of 4.6–40% have been reported, reflecting population differences but also depending on the use of selective broth media to improve sensitivity, swabbing from the anus and rectum as well as the genital tract and culturing sequentially throughout pregnancy. Higher colonization rates are found in sexually experienced women but although group B streptococci are sexually transmitted there is no correlation with promiscuity or genital symptoms in either sex.

About 1% of infants born to colonized women develop early-onset sepsis. Approximately 30–40% present with early-onset pneumonia and septicaemia; in more than half of these the radiographic features of fine granularity are indistinguishable from hyaline membrane disease. A total of 30–40% present with septicaemia alone, while 30% present with meningitis. For this reason lumbar puncture is important when investigating babies for suspected early-onset sepsis. The mortality has been over 50% and is highest in very low birthweight babies (Anthony & Okada 1977, Pyati et al 1981).

Late-onset group B streptococcal disease.

Unlike those with early-onset sepsis, babies developing group B streptococcal sepsis after 7 days and up to 12 weeks of age are mostly term babies. Some 85% present with meningitis, the remainder with bacteraemia without a recognized focus, osteomyelitis, septic arthritis and, rarely, facial cellulitis. The mortality is 15–20%; 30–50% of the survivors of meningitis have permanent neurological sequelae (Baker & Edwards 1983).

Prevention of early-onset group B streptococcal sepsis

Because of the high mortality, early-onset group B streptococcal sepsis is a major infectious cause of neonatal death and contributes significantly to perinatal mortality and morbidity. Attempts to eradicate maternal carriage by oral penicillin treatment during pregnancy have been largely unsuccessful: 20–30% of pregnant women remained infected after 2 weeks' treatment and by delivery nearly 70% were again infected (Gardner et al 1979). Furthermore, in a randomized controlled study, Pyati et al (1983) showed that treating infants of less than 2000 g birthweight with intramuscular penicillin at birth had no effect on the mortality rate from early-onset group B streptococcal infection.

If colonized women are identified at 38 weeks' gestation, vertical transmission can be greatly reduced by treating these women and their husbands with oral penicillin until delivery (Merenstein et al 1980). However, the highest incidence and mortality are in preterm babies (Pyati et al 1981). Boyer and colleagues (1983a) have shown that the incidence of early-onset sepsis is increased when there is prolonged rupture of the membranes for longer than 18 hours, maternal fever (over 37.5°C) or low birthweight (under 2500 g). The presence of one or more of these risk factors identified 74% of cases of early-onset group B streptococcal sepsis and 94% of fatal cases in Chicago. Boyer and colleagues (1983b) went on to show that vaginal or rectal cultures at delivery were positive in 67% of women with positive antenatal cultures and in 8.5% with negative cultures, indicating that antenatal cultures were barely satisfactory in indicating status at delivery. However, the authors then showed that they could usually prevent colonization of infants born to colonized women in their at-risk categories by giving intrapartum ampicillin 2 g stat then 1 g 4-hourly intravenously until delivery (Boyer et al 1983c). They subsequently showed that intrapartum ampicillin significantly reduces the occurrence of early-onset neonatal group B streptococcal bacteraemia in the babies of at-risk women (Boyer & Gotoff 1986).

The main problem with the Chicago approach is that it depends on obtaining antenatal cultures from all women, which may not be acceptable where the carriage rates are low or when there are practical and financial restraints. An alternative approach might be rapid detection of group B streptococcal antigen in vaginal swabs from mothers in high-risk groups, using a method such as latex agglutination (Lancet Editorial 1986a). The possibility of treating all women with risk factors, i.e. preterm labour, prolonged rupture of membranes or intrapartum fever, with intrapartum ampicillin without knowledge of the colonization status would need careful evaluation. In Chicago only 22.8% of women were colonized (Boyer et al 1983b) and the possible deleterious effects of antibiotics on the baby and mother might outweigh the benefits when treating large numbers of women. One disadvantage of selective chemoprophylaxis is that it does not prevent sepsis in babies born to mothers with no risk factors — 26% of all cases in Chicago and possibly more in other populations.

An immunological approach to prevention of group B streptococcal sepsis is the most promising long-term prospect. One possibility is the use of hyperimmune globulin, administered either to the neonate at birth or the mother in labour. An alternative would be active immunization of women of childbearing age with polysaccharide vaccines. Neither approach has yet been evaluated (Baker & Kasper 1985).

CONGENITAL INFECTIONS

Maternal infections during pregnancy can affect the fetus and the effects are likely to be most dramatic if infection occurs at the time of maximum organogenesis, in the first trimester. Pregnant women presenting with influenza-like or other viral illnesses during pregnancy should be investigated and counselled carefully according to current knowledge of the risk to the fetus.

Long-term effects

An association has been shown between in utero infection with the herpes viruses varicella-zoster virus and cytomegalovirus and the subsequent development of cancer. By the age of 40, 16 of 443 exposed subjects had developed cancer, compared with 7 controls (Fine et al 1985). In the same study, first-trimester exposure to mumps virus was associated with an increased risk of diabetes; 4 of 128 subjects but no controls developed diabetes by 40 years of age. There are conflicting data on a possible intrauterine link between exposure to influenza virus infection and subsequent leukaemia or lymphoid malignancy. It is not surprising that intrauterine infection might alter immunological functions, including immune surveillance. The slight increase in risk that may be associated with influenza and mumps virus infections is not sufficient to warrant termination of a pregnancy.

Rubella

Congenital rubella infection

Intrauterine infection with rubella virus can cause sensorineural deafness, blindness due to retinopathy and cataracts, cardiac defects and mental retardation; it can involve virtually every organ system (Alford & Griffiths 1983). There is no effective treatment and so the ideal is to prevent congenital infection by immunization. Failing this, it is necessary to identify non-immune mothers exposed to infection, investigate them and intervene appropriately.

Congenital infection occurs as a result of primary viraemia with placental transfer of virus which sets up a chronic infection in the fetus. Reinfections with rubella virus are rare and intrauterine transmission of virus with maternal reinfection is either exceptionally rare or does not occur. The rate of fetal infection is dependent on gestation, suggesting that the developing fetal immune response may be important in preventing infection.

Modern techniques of testing the newborn for rubella-specific IgM using immunofluorescence and radioimmunoassay have improved the sensitivity and specificity of diagnosis. The frequency of congenital infection identified using such techniques in a large prospective study of over 1000 women with proven rubella infection was 80% in the first

12 weeks of pregnancy, 54% at 13–14 weeks and 25% at the end of the second trimester (Miller et al 1982). Features of congenital rubella, primarily congenital heart disease and deafness, were found in all infants infected before 11 weeks' gestation, in 35% of those infected at 13–16 weeks who mainly developed sensorineural deafness, and none of 63 children infected after 16 weeks.

Rubella virus sets up a persistent infection in the placenta and fetus, so that even when infection occurs early in the first trimester it may be confirmed in the newborn by isolating virus from the nasopharynx, eye, urine, faeces, cerebrospinal fluid or leukocytes or by detecting specific IgM against rubella virus in the serum.

Pregnant woman exposed to rubella virus

Natural infection. If a pregnant woman is exposed to suspected or proven wild-type rubella virus infection or develops a rash up to 16 weeks' gestation, action will depend on her rubella antibody status, if known. If she is known to be immune prior to pregnancy the exceedingly low risk can be explained. Where the immune status is unknown, paired serum samples should be taken, recognizing that haemagglutination-inhibiting IgM antibodies do not appear until 14–18 days after the time of contact (Alford & Griffiths 1983). Sometimes women of unknown immune status mention a possible rubella contact which occurred several days or weeks earlier, and infection can only be confirmed or refuted by looking for specific IgM antibodies. These, as measured by haemagglutination inhibition, immunofluorescence, radioimmunoassay or enzyme-linked immunosorbent assay (ELISA) appear within 5–10 days of the rash, and persist for 50–70 days and sometimes longer (Alford & Griffiths 1983). Antenatal diagnosis by measurement of specific IgM in fetal blood samples is now possible in some centres (Daffos et al 1984).

Rubella vaccine. Each year in the UK a large number of terminations of pregnancy are performed on women accidentally immunized with live rubella vaccine. Although the vaccine is contraindicated in pregnancy and might infect the fetus, the virus is attenuated and so the risk of fetal malformations due to the vaccine is extremely low, and may even not exist. Modlin et al (1976) reported that rubella vaccine virus could be isolated from the products of conception of 9 out of 145 women who had terminations of pregnancy because of inadvertent immunization, but that none of 172 infants carried to term had clinical or serological evidence of rubella infection. Preblud et al (1981) reported no abnormalities in 94 infants of susceptible women given rubella vaccine in pregnancy. The maximum calculated risk to the fetus is approximately 3%, but may be even lower. The very low risk should be considered when counselling pregnant women who have been accidentally immunized with rubella vaccine.

Prevention

Rubella immunization is effective in preventing illness, although the tendency to waning immunity and therefore reinfections observed with natural infection is even more marked with vaccine-induced immunity. Nevertheless congenital infection rarely if ever occurs as a result of reinfections. Immunization strategies may be aimed at the total eradication of rubella by immunizing all children or the at-risk population of young girls and non-immune women postpartum. In the USA the former policy, by immunizing children at 15–18 months with a combined measles, mumps and rubella vaccine, has greatly reduced the incidence of rubella at all ages and of congenital rubella. Selective immunization of susceptible non-pregnant women of all ages in the USA has also been advocated.

In the UK and other countries, selective immunization of schoolgirls and non-immune mothers postpartum has not led to such a dramatic fall in congenital rubella. This is because epidemics of rubella continue to occur, making exposure of pregnant women more likely and necessitating a very high level of vaccination of susceptible women. In the UK even when all pregnant women are screened for rubella antibodies by haemagglutination inhibition at booking, only about 65% of non-immune women are vaccinated postpartum (Wild et al 1986). Failure to vaccinate appears to be due both to hospital and general practitioner errors and particularly to poor communication.

Cytomegalovirus infection

In developed countries congenital cytomegalovirus (CMV) infection is now the commonest intrauterine infection and a significant cause of mental retardation and sensorineural deafness. Where neonates have been screened for congenital CMV infection by attempting to isolate the virus from urine or nasopharynx and by detection of CMV-specific IgM, rates of infection of up to 5 per 1000 have been found. More than 90% of infants identified by screening are asymptomatic at birth, but follow-up studies have shown that deafness may develop postnatally as well as subtle language and learning disorders (Williamson et al 1982). Less than 5% of infected children will present at birth with some or all of the classical features of hepatosplenomegaly, purpura, jaundice, microcephaly, periventricular calcification and ocular defects such as retinopathy, cataracts or microphthalmia.

CMV, like other herpes viruses, can persist after primary infection and reactivate. Although earlier work suggested that the great majority of clinically significant congenital CMV followed primary maternal infection (Stagno et al 1982), reports from Sweden (Ahlfors et al 1982) and the UK (Preece et al 1984) have indicated that reactivation may account for a number of severe cases, particularly in low socioeconomic groups where most women of childbearing age have antibodies to CMV. These observations suggest that screening women for CMV antibody status at booking is unlikely to be effective in preventing congenital CMV infection.

Monif et al (1972) found that women who seroconverted in the first trimester gave birth to symptomatic infants whereas those who seroconverted later gave birth to infants with no apparent infection. However, Preece et al (1984) found no difference in outcome regardless of the timing of maternal infection.

CMV infection may be acquired postnatally from breast milk (Stagno et al 1980) or by intimate contact with an infected individual. Postnatal infection is generally mild, but preterm infants with chronic lung disease may acquire the disease from infected blood transfusions and can develop pneumonitis causing significant respiratory deterioration, grey pallor, hepatosplenomegaly and even death (Yeager 1974). The use of blood from donors negative for CMV antibody by haemagglutination inhibition to transfuse babies significantly reduces disease, particularly in preterm infants of seronegative mothers (Yeager et al 1981). Future hopes of preventing congenital CMV infection must rest with vaccines but only modest progress has been accomplished.

Toxoplasma gondii

Congenital infection with a protozoan parasite, *Toxoplasma gondii*, can cause clinical features which are surprisingly similar to those caused by infection with CMV and rubella virus. Classical congenital toxoplasmosis differs from congenital rubella mainly in the nature of the retinopathy, with areas of inflammation surrounded by pigment as opposed to the *pepper and salt* retinopathy of congenital rubella, and in the intracerebral calcification which consists of discrete intracerebral foci or periventricular calcification, identifiable on skull X-ray or by scan.

As with congenital rubella, the range of clinical features is from no apparent infection to the full congenital syndrome of microcephaly or, more commonly, hydrocephalus, intracerebral calcification, retinopathy, deafness, hepatosplenomegaly, pneumonitis, myocarditis, purpura, lymphadenopathy, jaundice and anaemia; rash is rare. Most children with congenital toxoplasmosis are normal at birth but may develop the features months or even years later. Ocular sequelae are the most common presentation although children may develop hydrocephalus, epilepsy or mental retardation.

Toxoplasmosis is a zoonosis, the cat being the natural host. Transmission by ingestion of undercooked meat from sheep, cows and pigs has been proven, and may explain the high incidence of congenital toxoplasmosis in France. Ingestion of cysts in cat faeces is a likely mode of infection. Other possible sources such as milk, chicken, eggs and blood transfusion have been mooted but not proven. In the UK congenital toxoplasmosis is thought to be rare, being diagnosed in about 0.2 per 1000 pregnancies, but prospective studies identifying cases by measurement of specific IgM on cord blood have shown rates from 1 to 7 per 1000 in the USA, Mexico, France, Norway, Sweden, Austria and Holland (Remington & Desmonts 1983). Even this may be an underestimate as false negatives occur when specific IgM alone is used for diagnosis.

In untreated pregnancies, serological evidence of congenital infection is more likely in the fetus the later in pregnancy that maternal infection occurs. In contrast, infection in the first trimester has the worst prognosis for the fetus while third-trimester infections are usually subclinical or mild. Thus in the first trimester, infection causes stillbirth or perinatal death in 5% and serological evidence of congenital infection in 9% with 86% of babies uninfected; in the second trimester the respective figures are 2, 27 and 71%, while in the third trimester 59% of babies have serological evidence of infection and 41% are uninfected (Remington & Desmonts 1983). In all, 76% of serologically proven infections in the first trimester result in stillbirth, perinatal death or severe congenital infection. In the second trimester, however, only 15% of infections are severe, 18% are mild and 67% are subclinical and in the third trimester 11% of infections are mild and the remaining 89% subclinical (Remington & Desmonts 1983). The increased severity with earlier gestation presumably reflects the effect of infection on the fetus at the time of maximum organogenesis. Treatment of pregnant women known to have *Toxoplasma gondii* infection with spiramycin reduces the incidence of congenital infection from 61 to 23% (Remington & Desmonts 1983).

Antenatal diagnosis of congenital toxoplasmosis with a high sensitivity and specificity is now available. This involves blood sampling to test for IgM and to look for parasitaemia by injecting blood into mice, as well as serial ultrasound examinations for hydrocephalus (Desmonts et al 1985).

Chlamydia trachomatis

Chlamydia trachomatis is probably the most common sexually transmitted pathogen in industrial societies (Schachter & Grossman 1983). Affected women may have urethritis, cervicitis, salpingitis, the urethral syndrome or may be asymptomatic.

Retrospective studies have consistently underestimated the magnitude of the problem of neonatal chlamydial infections. In prospective studies the prevalence of maternal chlamydial infection of the cervix has varied from 2 to 12.7% in industrialized countries, with 60–70% of infants born to such women acquiring infection during passage through the birth canal. Of these infants, 30–50% will develop inclusion conjunctivitis and 10–20% will develop an afebrile pneumonitis (Schachter & Grossman 1981, Preece et al 1986).

Conjunctivitis

Chlamydia trachomatis is the commonest cause of purulent conjunctivitis in the first month of life (Schachter & Grossman 1983). The incubation period is usually 5–14 days, although rarely premature rupture of the membranes will lead to conjunctivitis developing earlier. Conjunctivitis has even developed in babies born by elective Caesarean section (Barry et al 1986). A watery discharge rapidly becomes purulent with red, thickened conjunctivae and oedema of the eyelids. A pseudomembrane of inflammatory exudate may adhere to the conjunctivae and lead to scarring in sheets. As neonates do not have conjunctival lymphoid tissue, the follicular infiltration of trachoma is usually absent. Corneal involvement is rare, though micropannus may develop after 2 weeks in untreated infants. Loss of vision is rarely described but persistent conjunctivitis and occasionally florid scarring may occur.

Pneumonia

Chlamydia pneumonia was only reported in 1975 (Schachter et al 1975), although the clinical characteristics have since been beautifully described (Beem & Saxon 1977, Tipple et al 1979). Classically the infant is afebrile and at 4–8 weeks of age, though occasionally as young as 2 weeks, develops tachypnoea and a paroxysmal staccato cough. About half will have conjunctivitis or a history of it. Crepitations are commonly heard, rarely wheeze, and some infants will have apnoea. More than half will have an opaque, pearly-white tympanic membrane which may bulge forward (Tipple et al 1979). Chest X-ray shows bilateral interstitial infiltrates with hyperexpansion. The mortality is very low but the disease lasts 3–9 weeks (Beem & Saxon 1977) and co-infections with other organisms are common.

Diagnosis

The traditional diagnostic technique is tissue culture of the organism but this is time-consuming and is only performed by specialist laboratories. Culture is likely to be superseded by rapid antigen detection and serology.

When collecting swabs for culture, plain cotton-tipped swabs are preferable; calcium alignate-tipped swabs and swabs with charcoal should be avoided. The transport medium is a sucrose buffer with additives, and media used for transporting virus and gonorrhoea specimens are unsuitable. A blunt glass rod is suitable for conjunctival specimens.

For cervical cultures, the swab is inserted 1–2 cm into the cervical canal and rotated vigorously. For eyes the swab or a blunt glass rod are drawn vigorously across the conjunctiva of the lower eye. Swabbing the discharge is too insensitive a technique. Nasopharyngeal aspirates can be taken using a standard mucus aspirator; transport medium should be added if the laboratory is at a distant site.

In many laboratories antigen detection by ELISA has largely replaced tissue culture. It has been successfully evaluated for detecting *Chlamydia* in cervical and nasopharyngeal secretions but not yet for eyes. A Giemsa stain of material obtained by conjunctival scraping will often reveal the characteristic intracellular elementary body inclusions. Their presence in epithelial cells indicates the need for a scrape rather than a swab.

Specific IgM is characteristically raised in neonatal chlamydial pneumonitis (Tipple et al 1979), although about 67% of infants with uncomplicated conjunctivitis will also have IgM antibodies (Persson et al 1986), indicating the lack of specificity of the test. A microimmunofluorescence technique is usually used to measure antibodies; this technique is rarely available except in research laboratories. IgG is maternally transmitted and IgA antibodies appear in the tears late in neonatal conjunctivitis, so neither are diagnostically useful.

Treatment

When chlamydial conjunctivitis or pneumonitis is confirmed it is important to investigate and treat the infant's parents, since postpartum salpingitis and endometritis may occur and persistent infection is common, with a risk to future offspring.

Although inclusion conjunctivitis should respond to topical treatment with tetracycline, erythromycin or sulphonamide drops or ointment, failure rates of 50% or more have been reported (Schachter & Grossman 1983). For this reason, and because of the risk of pneumonitis, oral erythromycin 40 mg/kg/day for 2 weeks is recommended by Schachter & Grossman (1983). The same regime has been shown to result in clinical improvement and decreased shedding in infants with chlamydial pneumonia.

The use of screening techniques to identify chlamydial infection in pregnant women would only be justified if it could be shown that treatment eradicated carriage and prevented disease in women and their infants. This evidence is not available.

VIRAL INFECTIONS

The newborn, for reasons already discussed, is more susceptible to viral infections and, particularly in the absence of transplacentally acquired specific IgG antibody, may develop fulminating disease due to viruses which are inocuous to the mother. For this reason any perinatal virus infection occurring in the mother should be a cause for concern. The obstetrician should notify the paediatrician so that consideration can be given to isolating the mother and child, and to intervening with immune globulin or specific antiviral therapy if appropriate.

In this context, enterovirus infections occurring in women at term are an example. Poliovirus may cause paralytic poliomyelitis in the newborn. Coxsackieviruses and echoviruses can cause meningitis or disseminated infection with intravascular coagulation and massive hepatic necrosis. Not only is the child of the infected mother at risk but nursery outbreaks with multiple fatalities have occurred, particularly in South Africa (Lancet Editorial 1986b).

Herpes virus infections

Varicella-zoster virus

Varicella-zoster virus (VZV) occasionally causes a distinctive congenital infection with cicatricial scarring of the limbs, optic atrophy or microphthalmia and atrophy of the cerebellum. As chickenpox during pregnancy is rare it has been hard to gauge the size of the risk. In an 8-year prospective study of over 180 000 pregnancies, Siegel (1973) found only 4 malformations in 135 babies of mothers with chickenpox during pregnancy compared with 5 in 146 matched controls. However, of the 27 pregnancies when chickenpox occurred in the first trimester, 2 (7.4%) resulted in congenital malformations compared with 3 in 87 controls (3.4%). Paryani & Arvin (1986) reported one case of congenital varicella syndrome in 11 infants whose mothers had first-trimester varicella.

Maternal chickenpox occurring around delivery may result in fatal neonatal disease if there has been little or no transfer of maternal antibody. Reviewing all available reports, Meyers (1974) found no deaths among 23 babies whose mothers' rash developed 5 or more days before delivery, but 4 of 13 babies died when onset of maternal rash was 4 days or less before delivery (31%). Brunell (1966) has shown that when maternal varicella occurs more than a week before delivery, maternal and cord blood anti-VZV titres are the same, whereas in maternal infection 3–5 days before delivery cord blood antibodies are absent or considerably lower than maternal levels.

Zoster-immune globulin (ZIG) has been recommended for neonates whose mothers develop chickenpox within 4 days of delivery. It probably does not prevent disease but may modify infection, although the occurrence in England of three fatal cases of neonatal varicella, despite the use of ZIG, in the period from 1981 to 1986, has caused the Public Health Laboratory Service to increase the recommended dose of ZIG from 100 to 250 mg (Holland et al 1986). Acyclovir may be indicated if a neonate develops chickenpox despite ZIG, particularly for those babies at greatest risk whose mother's rash appears 4 days or less before delivery. Acyclovir does not cross the placenta so it is not indicated for treatment of the mother to prevent neonatal chickenpox.

Herpes simplex virus

Herpes simplex virus (HSV) infections may result from infection with HSV-1, which infects primarily the mouth, or HSV-2 which infects primarily the cervix. Although HSV is included in the TORCH group of agents causing congenital infection, the evidence that infection early in pregnancy causes congenital defects is very dubious. Major disease results from perinatal acquisition or from spread from contacts in the family or the nursery.

The rate of neonatal herpes infections varies geographically. In the USA the current rate is 0.1–0.3 per 1000 deliveries, which probably represents a true increase in frequency. Approximately 80% of all reported cases are due to HSV-2, and the majority of affected babies acquire their infection by passage through an infected vaginal canal. Although HSV may cause florid, painful cervical lesions and cold sores it may also be completely asymptomatic for the mother either in the cervix or the mouth.

Affected neonates occasionally have skin or eye lesions at birth, and in the USA numerically outweigh babies with overt congenital toxoplasmosis, rubella or CMV. More commonly symptoms are delayed for some days. Babies may have disease localized to one or more sites or disseminated disease involving virtually all sites. Disease usually appears in the first week, although localized central nervous system disease presents at a mean of 11 days. Skin lesions are the commonest manifestation — usually vesicles or ulcers, occasionally zosteriform eruptions, denuded skin or a generalized petechial rash. Keratoconjunctivitis, chorioretinitis or cataract are the classic eye findings which may be isolated or part of disseminated disease. Central nervous system involvement is heralded by lethargy, seizures and rapid neurological deterioration with cerebrospinal fluid pleocytosis. Hepatosplenomegaly, jaundice, oral ulceration, fever and a non-specific picture of sepsis, sometimes with disseminated intravascular coagulopathy, may occur. The natural history of neonatal HSV infections acquired as a result of primary maternal infection is that untreated localized disease progresses to involve other organs, predominantly the central nervous system, in 79% of cases (Nahmias et al 1983).

The diagnosis of HSV infection is urgent and often clinically difficult. Electron microscopy of vesicle fluid can show herpes viruses, although it will not distinguish herpes simplex from other herpes viruses such as VZV. Virus isolation usually takes 1–4 days to give the typical cytopathic effect and is still very useful where more refined techniques are not available. Papanicolaou stains on cell scrapings from the base of skin vesicles, oral ulcers or the cervix are 60–75% sensitive in diagnosing HSV infection. The use of serological assays is controversial: tests for specific IgM by immunofluorescence are not widely available and the complement fixation or passive haemagglutination tests measure IgG which may be of maternal origin. Cerebrospinal fluid antibodies to HSV result from transudation rather than local synthesis in older patients and their role in diagnosing neonatal herpes encephalitis is unknown. The most promising developments are in detecting HSV antigen using techniques such as ELISA, or detecting DNA from the virus using probes, but these are not yet widely available.

Acyclovir has been shown to be superior to adenosine arabinoside (Ara-A, vidarabine) in treating herpes simplex encephalitis at all ages (Skoldenberg et al 1984, Whitley et al 1986). Although the number of neonates treated in these studies was small, the clear superiority of acyclovir in reducing overall mortality and morbidity and the lower volume load compared to vidarabine make acyclovir the drug of choice for established neonatal HSV infection.

A classic study by Nahmias et al (1971) suggested that the risk of fetal infection when vaginal delivery was performed in the face of active primary maternal HSV infection was 54% and that this could be reduced to 7% if Caesarean section was performed within 4 hours of membrane rupture, but rose to 94% if section was performed more than 4 hours after ruptured membranes. This was a small, largely retrospective study and the authors have recently recommended that Caesarean section should be performed up to 24 hours after membrane rupture in high-risk patients, presumably those with active primary lesions (Nahmias et al 1983). Where lesions are known to be secondary, i.e. reactivation, the risk of transmission to the fetus from vaginal delivery is much lower, probably around 3–5% (Overall et al 1984) and recommendations for intervention in labour should be based accordingly. Similar considerations apply to the use of topical or systemic prophylactic antiviral agents for infants exposed to HSV at birth. Most paediatricians, given the usual delayed onset of disease, would await the results of viral cultures of the eye and nasopharynx taken at birth before making a decision on prophylaxis. When maternal disease is primary, and particularly when there are additional risk factors to the neonate, such as being preterm or lacerations resulting from scalp electrodes or forceps, some would start systemic treatment with acyclovir from birth and would also use trifluridine ophthalmic solution (Overall et al 1984).

Hepatitis B

There is a high incidence of vertical transmission of hepatitis B virus in Taiwan and Japan, but a very low incidence in western Europe and the USA. Affected infants usually become asymptomatic chronic carriers, although they occasionally develop fulminant hepatitis, often with fatal massive hepatic necrosis. Chronic carriers are at risk of chronic liver disease and hepatoma. The major risk factor for the occurrence of vertical transmission has been shown to be the presence of e-antigen in the mother, indicating a high degree of infectivity. A total of 90% of infants whose mothers are both hepatitis B surface antigen (HBsAg)- and HBeAg-positive become infected (Okada et al 1976). HBsAg carrier mothers who are HBeAg- and anti-HBe-negative are at lesser risk of vertical transmission. Mothers who are HBe antibody-positive are far less likely to have infected infants, although several instances have been described (Beasley et al 1977).

The ideal is to identify HBsAg-positive mothers antenatally and in many countries all pregnant women are screened. When screening is not routine, known risk factors such as origin from a country with a high endemic rate of hepatitis B, liver disease, multiple blood transfusions or intravenous drug abuse should suggest the need to determine maternal HBsAg status.

Passive immunization with hepatitis B immune globulin (HBIG) decreases risk of vertical transmission, but infection still occurs in 20–40% of babies of e-antigen-positive mothers in endemic areas (Beasley et al 1981). Active immunization with plasma-derived hepatitis B vaccine alone has a similar efficacy of about 70–80% in preventing perinatal transmission from e-antigen-positive mothers in endemic areas (Maupas et al 1981, Beasley et al 1983). Combined passive–active prophylaxis improves the efficacy and protects over 90% of these babies (Beasley et al 1983, Wong et al 1984). The efficacy is not 100% because some babies acquire the virus transplacentally.

There is controversy over the correct approach for babies of lower-risk mothers who are e-antibody-positive. In the UK, babies of e-antibody-positive mothers are not routinely given prophylaxis, whereas babies of HBeAg-positive mothers and HBsAg-positive mothers with no E-antigen or antibody are given combined passive–active prophylaxis. The current American recommendations are for 0.5 ml of HBIG to be given at birth and certainly before 48 hours to all infants of HBsAg-positive mothers, regardless of e-antigen status; 10 μg of hepatitis B vaccine is also given soon after birth and again at 1 and 6 months (Brunell et al 1985). The vaccine in current use is prepared from blood of HBsAg carriers treated with urea, formalin and pepsin, which inactivates viruses including retroviruses.

ACQUIRED IMMUNE DEFICIENCY SYNDROME

Approximately 1% of all cases of the acquired immune deficiency syndrome (AIDS) occur in children. The retrovirus responsible for AIDS is called human immunodeficiency virus (HIV), human T-lymphotrophic virus 3 (HTLV 3), or lymphadenopathy-associated virus (LAV). Transplacental or perinatal acquisition is one of the most important routes of infection of children.

Route of infection

Neonatal infection with HIV usually occurs transplacentally or perinatally from an infected mother. Mothers at particular risk of having been infected are intravenous drug abusers or those who are promiscuous (Oleske et al 1983, Rubinstein et al 1983). Other mothers at high risk for being infected with HIV and therefore of transmitting it to their infants are those coming from areas with a very high prevalence of AIDS such as Haiti, Central Africa and the Middle East (Scott et al 1984).

Vertical transmission is most likely to be transplacental in origin in view of the much shorter incubation period of the disease in such cases, compared with that in children infected by contaminated blood transfusion. The virus can be isolated from vaginal secretions of infected women, however, and perinatal infection from such secretions or blood is a possibility. About 75% of childhood AIDS in the USA results from vertical transmission (Centers for Disease Control 1986).

Other modes of acquisition of HIV infection by neonates and infants are much rarer. A case of AIDS has been described in an infant whose mother and haemophiliac father were both HIV antibody-positive (Ragni et al 1985). The presumed sequence of events was that the haemophiliac father was infected via contaminated factor VIII, infected his wife heterosexually, and that the infant was infected vertically or by close parental contact.

Breast milk is a possible source of infection. Ziegler et al (1985) described a woman who was infected by a postnatal blood transfusion and whose infant subsequently became infected, probably via maternal breast milk. The virus can be isolated from raw breast milk. This has important implications for breastfeeding by infected mothers and for breast-banks. Pasteurization procedures are currently being reviewed. However, standard pasteurization procedures involving heating milk at 56°C for 30 minutes completely sterilize samples of milk inoculated with live HIV (Eglin & Wilkinson 1987).

Incubation period

The mean incubation period following contaminated blood transfusion is 31 months in adults (range 4–84 months) but is only 14 months (range 4–68 months) in children. Children infected by vertical transmission, however, usually develop symptoms within the first 6 months of life (Oleske et al 1983, Rubinstein et al 1983, Scott et al 1984, Andiman et al 1985).

Risk

Studies in the USA have indicated that about two-thirds of the children of asymptomatic HIV antibody-positive mothers develop clinical symptoms before they are 2 years old.

Presentation

There are some notable differences in clinical presentation of children with HIV infection when compared to adults:

1. *Asymptomatic seroconversion*: this may occur but is less common than in adults.
2. *Non-specific*: infants and children commonly present with non-specific symptoms such as persistent oral candidiasis, chronic or recurrent diarrhoea, failure to thrive, fever, anorexia, anaemia, hepatosplenomegaly and lymphadenopathy (Scott et al 1984).
3. *Opportunistic infections*: infection with *Pneumocystis carinii* and CMV are relatively common. Infections with low-grade opportunistic organisms such as *Toxoplasma*, *Cryptosporidium* and atypical *Mycobacterium* are rare and occur late in the disease.
4. *Lymphocytic interstitial pneumonitis*: a feature common in children but rare in adults is a chronic diffuse interstitial pneumonitis with a characteristic follicular lymphocytic infiltrate. Andiman and colleagues (1985) demonstrated DNA from Epstein–Barr virus in lung biopsies from 8 of 10 affected children.
5. *Encephalopathy*: children may develop normally for 12–18 months and then regress or develop spastic quadriparesis or evidence of demyelination.
6. *Tumours*: it is rare for children to present with tumours although Kaposi's sarcoma occasionally occurs (Scott et al 1984) and central nervous system lymphoma containing Epstein–Barr virus DNA has been described (Andiman et al 1985).

Children with AIDS generally have reversed ratios of helper and suppressor T-lymphocytes with a reduced absolute number of OKT_4^+ (T-helper) lymphocytes. Marked hypergammaglobulinaemia is also common.

Prevention

Pregnancy may activate HIV, in that asymptomatic seropositive women may only become symptomatic during pregnancy. This, combined with the high risk of the fetus being infected, may lead us to counsel known seropositive women against becoming pregnant. However, it is rare to know a woman's HIV status before pregnancy. No country routinely screens expectant mothers yet. At present it would seem wise to screen at-risk groups of women for HIV antibodies at booking, although the logistics will depend on local, financial and ethical considerations. Those women most at risk are:

1. Intravenous drug abusers or consorts of intravenous drug abusers.
2. Consorts of bisexual men.
3. Prostitutes.
4. Women from endemic areas such as Haiti, Central Africa and the Middle East.
5. Wives of haemophiliacs.
6. Women who have received a blood transfusion in an endemic area.

Screening of high-risk women and a policy of counselling or termination is most likely at present to decrease the incidence of childhood AIDS; over 200 cases have already been reported in the USA (Centers for Disease Control 1986). In most countries blood donors are already being screened for HIV antibody. Although there have been rare false negatives — perhaps viraemic patients who have not yet mounted an antibody response — in practice the risk from blood transfusion is now extremely low. Donors of semen for artificial insemination should also be screened, since 4 out of 8 recipients of cryopreserved semen from an asymptomatic seropositive donor became infected (Stewart et al 1985). When intravenous drug abuse is a major cause of AIDS it has been shown that needle-sharing is a prominent factor. The provision of disposable needles to addicts may be considered politically unacceptable, but could be the single most effective preventive measure in dealing with this non-compliant population; it is being applied in certain parts of the UK.

Prospects of a vaccine seem fairly distant at present, because of the variable antigenic structure of the virus.

In view of the increasing incidence of HIV infections worldwide, and the likelihood that vertical transmission will also be increasingly recognized, it is important that obstetricians and paediatricians should be aware of the features of HIV infections.

CONCLUSIONS

It has not been possible in this chapter to cover exhaustively all the infections and infestations of the newborn infant, or even those in which vertical transmission from mother to infant is the usual route. In particular, syphilis, gonorrhoea, malaria and tuberculosis have been omitted and there is scant mention of *Listeria*, fungal infections and many virus infections. A chapter of this length can only hope to cover the basic principles of neonatal infection and we have chosen to emphasize the problems of neonatal infection in a western setting. For more extensive coverage of the omitted infections readers are referred to one of the many excellent textbooks on neonatal infections, that edited by Remington & Klein (1983).

An important message that we hope to have conveyed is the benefit of early discussion between obstetrician and paediatrician on matters relating to infection. The mother and infant are so intimately connected in infectious terms that it is vital that the physicians caring for each should try to emulate this situation.

REFERENCES

Ahlfors K, Ivarsson S A, Johnsson T, Svanberg L 1982 Primary and secondary maternal cytomegalovirus infections and their relation to congenital infection. Analysis of maternal sera. Acta Paediatrica Scandinavica 71: 109–113

Alford C A, Griffiths P D 1983 Rubella. In: Remington J S, Klein J O (eds) Infectious diseases of the fetus and newborn infant, 2nd edn. Saunders, Philadelphia, pp 69–103

Andiman W A, Eastman R, Martin K 1985 Opportunistic lymphoproliferation associated with Epstein–Barr viral DNA in infants and children with AIDS. Lancet ii: 1390–1393

Anthony B F, Okada D M 1977 The emergence of group B streptococci in infections of the newborn infants. Annual Reviews in Medicine 28: 335–369

Baker C J, Edwards M S 1983 Group B streptococcal infections. In: Remington J S, Klein J O (eds) Infectious diseases of the fetus and newborn infant, 2nd edn. Saunders, Philadelphia, pp 820–881

Baker C J, Kasper D L 1985 Group B streptococcal vaccines. Reviews in Infectious Disease 7: 458–467

Baker C J. Edwards M S, Kasper D L 1981 Role of antibody to native type III polysaccharide of group B streptococcus in infant infection. Pediatrics 68: 544–549

Barclay N 1971 High frequency of salmonella species as a cause of neonatal meningitis in Ibadan, Nigeria. A review of 38 cases. Acta Paediatrica Scandinavica 60: 540–544

Barry W C, Teare E L, Uttley A H C et al 1986 *Chlamydia trachomatis* as a cause of neonatal conjunctivitis. Archives of Disease in Childhood 61: 797–799

Beasley R P, Trepo C, Stevens C E et al 1977 The e antigen and vertical transmission of hepatitis B surface antigen. American Journal of Epidemiology 105: 94–98

Beasley R P, Hwang L-Y, Lin C-C et al 1981 Hepatitis B immune globulin (HBIG) efficacy in the interruption of perinatal transmission of hepatitis B carrier state. Lancet ii: 388–393

Beasley R P, Lee G C Y, Roan C H et al 1983 Prevention of perinatally transmitted hepatitis B virus infections with hepatitis B immune globulin and hepatitis B vaccine. Lancet ii: 1099–1102

Beem M O, Saxon E M 1977 Respiratory tract colonization and a distinctive pneumonia syndrome in infants infected with *Chlamydia trachomatis*. New England Journal of Medicine 296: 306–310

Bejar R, Curbelo V, Davis C, Gluck L 1981 Premature labour. II. Bacterial sources of phospholipase. Obstetrics and Gynecology 57: 479–482

Benirschke K 1960 Routes and types of infection in the fetus and the newborn. American Journal of Diseases in Children 99: 714–721

Bobitt J R, Ledger W J 1978 Amniotic fluid analysis. Its role in maternal and neonatal infection. Obstetrics and Gynecology 51: 56–62

Boyer K M, Gotoff S P 1986 Prevention of early-onset neonatal group B streptococcal disease with selective intrapartum chemoprophylaxis. New England Journal of Medicine 314: 1665–1669

Boyer K M, Gadzala C A, Burd L I, Fisher D E, Paton J B, Gotoff S P 1983a Selective intrapartum chemoprophylaxis of neonatal group B streptococcal early-onset disease. I. Epidemiologic rationale. Journal of Infectious Diseases 148: 795–801

Boyer K M, Gadzala C A, Kelly P D, Burd L I, Gotoff S P 1983b Selective intrapartum chemoprophylaxis of neonatal group B streptococcal early-onset disease. II. Predictive value of prenatal cultures. Journal of Infectious Diseases 148: 802–809

Boyer K M, Gadzala C A, Kelly P D, Gotoff S P 1983c Selective intrapartum chemoprophylaxis of neonatal group B streptococcal early-onset disease. III. Interruption of mother-to-infant transmission. Journal of Infectious Diseases 148: 810–816

Broughton R A, Baker C J 1983 Role of adherence in the pathogenesis of neonatal group B streptococcal infection. Infection and Immunity 39: 837–843

Brunell P A 1966 Placental transfer of varicella-zoster antibody. Pediatrics 38: 1034–1038

Brunell P A, Bass J W, Daum R S et al 1985 Prevention of hepatitis B virus infections. Pediatrics 75: 362–364

Centers for Disease Control 1986 Update: acquired immunodeficiency syndrome — United States. Morbidity and Mortality Weekly Report 35: 18–21

Daffos F, Forestier F, Grangeot-Keros L et al 1984 Prenatal diagnosis of congenital rubella. Lancet ii: 1–3

Desmonts G, Daffos F, Forestier, F, Capella-Pavlosky M, Thulliez P, Chartier M 1985 Prenatal diagnosis of congenital toxoplasmosis. Lancet i: 500–504

Eglin R P, Wilkinson A R 1987 HIV infection and pasteurisation of breast milk. Lancet i: 1093

Fayez J A, Hasan A A, Jonas H S, Miller G L 1978 Management of premature rupture of the membranes. Obstetrics and Gynecology 52: 17–21

Fine P E M, Adelstein A M, Snowman J, Clarkson J A, Evans S M 1985 Longterm effects of exposure to viral infections in utero. British Medical Journal 290: 509–511

Gardner S E, Yow M D, Leeds L J, Thompson P K, Mason E O, Clark D J 1979 Failure of penicillin to eradicate group B streptococcal colonization in the pregnant woman. American Journal of Obstetrics and Gynecology 135: 1062–1065

Gerdes J S, Yoder M C, Douglas S D, Polin R A 1983 Decreased plasma fibronectin in neonatal sepsis. Pediatrics 72: 877–881

Gitlin D, Kumate J, Urrusti J, Morales C 1964 The selectivity of the

human placenta in the transfer of plasma proteins from mother to fetus. Journal of Clinical Investigation 43: 1938–1951
Goldmann D A, Leclair J, Macon A 1978 Bacterial colonization of neonates admitted to an intensive care environment. Journal of Pediatrics 93: 288–293
Holland P, Isaacs D, Moxon E R 1986 Fatal neonatal varicella infection. Lancet ii: 1156
Kappy K A, Cetrulo C L, Knuppel R A et al 1979 Premature rupture of the membranes: a conservative approach. American Journal of Obstetrics and Gynecology 134: 655–661
Lamont R F, Rose M, Elder M G 1985 Effect of bacterial products on prostaglandin E production by amnion cells. Lancet ii: 1331–1333
Lancet Editorial 1984 Prevention of early-onset group B streptococcal infection in the newborn. Lancet i: 1056–1059
Lancet Editorial 1986a Rapid detection of beta haemolytic streptococci. Lancet i: 247–248
Lancet Editorial 1986b Avoiding the danger of enteroviruses to newborn infants. Lancet i: 194–195
Maupas P, Chiron J-P, Barim F et al 1981 Efficacy of hepatitis B vaccine in prevention of HBsAG carrier state in children. Controlled trial in an endemic area (Senegal). Lancet i: 289–292
Merenstein G B, Todd W A, Brown G, Yost C C, Luzier T 1980 Group B β-hemolytic streptococcus: randomized controlled treatment study at term. Obstetrics and Gynecology 55:315–319
Meyers J D 1974 Congenital varicella in term infants: risk reconsidered. Journal of Infectious Diseases 129: 215–217
Miller J M Jnr, Pupkin M J, Frenshaw C 1978 Premature labor and premature rupture of membranes. American Journal of Obstetrics and Gynecology 132: 1–6
Miller E, Cradock-Watson J E, Pollock T M 1982 Consequences of confirmed maternal rubella at successive stages of pregnancy. Lancet ii: 781–784
Modlin J F, Hermann K, Brandling-Bennett AD, Eddins D L, Hayden G F 1976 Risk of congenital abnormality after inadvertent rubella vaccination of pregnant women. New England Journal of Medicine 294: 972–974
Monif R G, Egan E A, Held B, Eitzman D V 1972 The correlation of maternal cytomegalovirus infection during varying stages in gestation with neonatal involvement. Journal of Pediatrics 80: 17–20
Naeye R L, Peters E C 1980 Causes and consequences of premature rupture of fetal membranes. Lancet i: 192–194
Nahmias A J, Josey W E, Naib Z M, Freeman M G, Fernandez R J, Wheeler J H 1971 Perinatal risk associated with maternal genital herpes simplex virus infection. American Journal of Obstetrics and Gynecology 110: 825–837
Nahmias A J, Keyserling H L, Kerrick G M 1983 Herpes simplex. In: Remington J S, Klein J O (eds) Infectious diseases of the fetus and newborn infant, 2nd edn. Saunders, Philadelphia, pp 636–678
Okada K, Kamiyama I, Inomata M et al 1976 E antigen and anti-e in the serum of asymptomatic carrier mothers as indicators of positive and negative transmission of hepatitis B virus to their infants. New England Journal of Medicine 294: 746–749
Okada D M, Chow A W, Bruce V T 1977 Neonatal scalp abscess and fetal monitoring: factors associated with infection. American Journal of Obstetrics and Gynecology 129: 185–189
Oleske J, Minnefor A, Cooper R et al 1983 Immune deficiency syndrome in children. Journal of American Medical Association 249: 2345–2349
Overall J C, Whitley R J, Yeager A S, McCracken G H, Nelson J D 1984 Prophylactic or anticipatory antiviral therapy for newborns exposed to herpes simplex infection. Pediatric Infectious Diseases 3: 193–195
Parvey L S, Ch'ien L T 1980 Neonatal herpes simplex virus infection introduced by fetal monitor scalp electrodes. Pediatrics 65: 1150–1153
Paryani S G, Arvin A M 1986 Intrauterine infection with varicella-zoster virus after maternal varicella. New England Journal of Medicine 314: 1542–1546
Persson K, Ronnerstam R, Svanberg L, Polberger S 1986 Neonatal chlamydial conjunctivitis. Archives of Disease in Childhood 61: 565–568
Preblud S R, Stetler H C, Frank J A, Greaves W L, Hinman A R, Herrmann K L 1981 Fetal risk associated with rubella vaccine. Journal of American Medical Association 246: 1413–1417
Preece P M, Pearl K N, Peckham C S 1984 Congenital cytomegalovirus infection. Archives of Disease in Childhood 59: 1120–1126
Preece P M, Brooks J H, Anderson J H, Thompson R 1986 The prevalence of *Chlamydia trachomatis* infection in infants following maternal infection. Archives of Disease in Childhood 61: 627–632
Pyati S P, Pildes R S, Ramamurthy R S, Jacobs N 1981 Decreasing mortality in neonates with early-onset group B streptococcal infection: reality or artifact. Journal of Pediatrics 98: 625–628
Pyati S P, Pildes R S, Jacobs N M et al 1983 Penicillin in infants weighing two kilograms or less with early-onset group B streptococcal disease. New England Journal of Medicine 308: 1383–1389
Ragni M V, Urbach A H, Kiernan S 1985 Acquired immunodeficiency syndrome in the child of a haemophiliac. Lancet i: 133–135
Regan J A, Chao L S, James L S 1981 Premature rupture of membranes, preterm delivery, and group B streptococcal colonization of mothers. American Journal of Obstetrics and Gynecology 141: 184–186
Remington J S, Desmonts G 1983 Toxoplasmosis. In: Remington J S, Klein J O (eds) Infectious diseases of the fetus and newborn infant, 2nd edn. Saunders, Philadelphia, pp 143–263
Remington J S, Klein J O (eds) 1983 Infectious diseases of the fetus and newborn, 2nd edn. Saunders, Philadelphia
Rubinstein A, Sicklick M, Gupta A et al 1983 Acquired immunodeficiency with reversed T4/T8 ratios in infants born to promiscuous and drug-addicted mothers. Journal of American Medical Association 249: 2350–2356
Schachter J, Grossman M 1981 Chlamydial infections. Annual Reviews in Medicine 32: 45–61
Schachter J, Grossman M 1983 Chlamydia. In: Remington J S, Klein J O (eds) Infectious diseases of the fetus and new born infant, 2nd edn. Saunders, Philadelphia, pp 450–461
Schachter J, Lum L, Gooding C A, Ostler B 1975 Pneumonitis following inclusion blennorhoea. Journal of Pediatrics 87: 779–780
Schreiber J, Benedett T 1980 Conservative management of preterm premature rupture of the membranes in a low socio-economic population. American Journal of Obstetrics and Gynecology 36: 92–96
Scott G B, Buck B E, Leterman J G, Bloom F L, Parks W P 1984 Acquired immunodeficiency syndrome in infants. New England Journal of Medicine 310: 76–81
Shubeck F, Benson R C, Clark W W Jr et al 1966 Fetal hazard after rupture of membranes. Obstetrics and Gynecology 28: 22–31
Siegel M 1973 Congenital malformations following chickenpox, measles, mumps and hepatitis. Results of a cohort study. Journal of American Medical Association 226: 1521–1524
Siegel J D, McCracken G H Jr 1981 Sepsis neonatorum. New England Journal of Medicine 304: 642–647
Skoldenberg B, Forsgren M, Alestig K et al 1984 Acyclovir versus vidarabine in herpes simplex encephalitis. Randomised multicentre study in consecutive Swedish patients. Lancet ii: 707–711
Stagno S, Reynolds D W, Pass R F, Alford C A 1980 Breast milk and the risk of cytomegalovirus infection. New England Journal of Medicine 302: 1073–1076
Stagno S, Pass R F, Dworsky M E et al 1982 Congenital cytomegalovirus infection. The relative importance of primary and recurrent maternal infection. New England Journal of Medicine 306: 945–949
Stewart G J, Tyler J P P, Cunningham A L et al 1985 Transmission of human T cell lymphotrophic virus type III (HTLV-III) by artificial insemination by donor. Lancet ii: 581–585
Tipple M, Beem M O, Saxon E 1979 Clinical characterisation of the afebrile pneumonia associated with *Chlamydia trachomatis* infection in infants less than 6 months of age. Pediatrics 63: 192–197
Whitley R J, Alford C A, Hirsch M S et al 1986 Vidarabine versus acyclovir therapy in herpes simplex encephalitis. New England Journal of Medicine 314: 144–149
Wild N J, Sheppard S, Smithells R W 1986 The consequences of antenatal rubella testing. Health Trends 18: 9–10
Williamson W D, Desmond M M, La Fevers N, Taber L H, Catlin F I, Weaver T B 1982 Symptomatic congenital cytomegalovirus: disorders of language, learning and hearing. American Journal of Diseases in Children 136: 902–905
Wilson C B 1986 Immunologic basis for increased susceptibility of the neonate to infection. Journal of Pediatrics 108: 1–12

Winkel C A, Snyder D L, Schlaerth J B 1976 Scalp abscess: a complication of the spiral fetal electrode. American Journal of Obstetrics and Gynecology 126: 170–172

Wong V C W, Ip H M H, Reesink H W et al 1984 Prevention of the HBsAG carrier state in newborn infants of mothers who are chronic carriers of HBsAG and HBeAG by administration of hepatitis B vaccine and hepatis B immunoglobulin. Lancet i: 939–941

Yeager A S 1974 Transfusion-acquired cytomegalovirus infections in newborn infants. American Journal of Diseases in Children 128: 478–483

Yeager A S, Hafleigh M T, Arvin A M, Bradley J S, Prober C G 1981 Prevention of transfusion-acquired cytomegalovirus infections in newborn infants. Journal of Pediatrics 98: 281–287

Zaaijman J du T, Wilkinson A R, Keeling J W, Mitchell R G, Turnbull A C 1982 Spontaneous premature rupture of the membranes: bacteriology, histology and neonatal outcome. Journal of Obstetrics and Gynecology 2: 155–169

Ziegler J B, Cooper D A, Johnson R O, Gold J 1985 Postnatal transmission of AIDS-associated retrovirus from mother to infant. Lancet i: 896–898

Anthony D. Milner and E. Wren Hoskyns

Respiratory conditions of the newborn

INTRODUCTION

A high proportion of the time of neonatal doctors and nurses is spent attempting to prevent, monitor and treat respiratory problems, particularly in those born preterm. A recent epidemiological study (Field & Milner 1986) has shown that the incidence of the idiopathic respiratory distress syndrome (IRDS), the commonest neonatal respiratory problem, has remained constant at approximately 9 per 1000 live births over the last 8–10 years. This figure hides the fact that the pattern of babies entering neonatal units has changed dramatically over this period. Babies born with a gestation of greater than 32 weeks now form only 22% of all babies presenting with IRDS, compared with 54% in 1977 (Field & Milner 1986). Mortality in this relatively mature group has been reduced by over 80% during this period. To counterbalance this, the number of babies born with a gestation of less than 32 weeks has approximately doubled over this period, so that the mean gestation of babies developing IRDS has fallen dramatically. Improvements in the more mature babies are probably due to better antenatal care and to management in the immediate neonatal period. The increased incidence of very immature babies is also probably related to improvements in obstetric care so that babies previously lost as inevitable abortions before 28 weeks are now entering the neonatal statistics and developing severe respiratory problems. Certainly over this period the need for oxygen therapy, continuous distending pressure and respiratory support has increased by over 300%.

RESPIRATORY DISTRESS SYNDROME

Definition

The definition of respiratory distress syndrome (RDS) may be clinical, pathological, radiographic or biochemical and each has its limitations.

The typical clinical features are suggestive of RDS but the diagnosis is one of exclusion, as other rare but important conditions may mimic the disease but require different management. Essential requirements for the diagnosis are tachypnoea, evidence of stiff lungs (grunting or intercostal recession) commencing within 4 hours of birth and need for supplementary oxygen for more than 24 hours.

The pathological diagnosis in the acute phase is made on the basis of patchy atelactasis and small lung volumes with hyperaemia, lymphatic dilatation and the classical hyaline membranes (Northway et al 1967). Only the most severe cases die and come to autopsy so pathological findings are based on a highly selected sample and usually reflect a combination of the disease itself and iatrogenic insults such as ventilator and oxygen damage, particularly when postnatal survival is prolonged.

Radiographic diagnosis (Donald & Steiner 1953) depends on generalized reticulogranular opacity of the lung fields, often described as a ground glass appearance; the lung fields are smaller than normal and there is an absence of other conditions with distinctive signs (Fig. 70.1).

The biochemical diagnosis is based on demonstrating surfactant deficiency in tracheal or gastric aspirate (Hallman et al 1977) soon after birth. There are several tests available but on the whole they have not become routine on neonatal units as they are expensive and, in contrast to obstetric practice, they do not alter management. The shake test (Clements et al 1972) is a cheap, simple and sensitive predictor of subsequent RDS but suffers from poor specificity. Other more elaborate tests to detect surfactant levels—lecithin, leci-

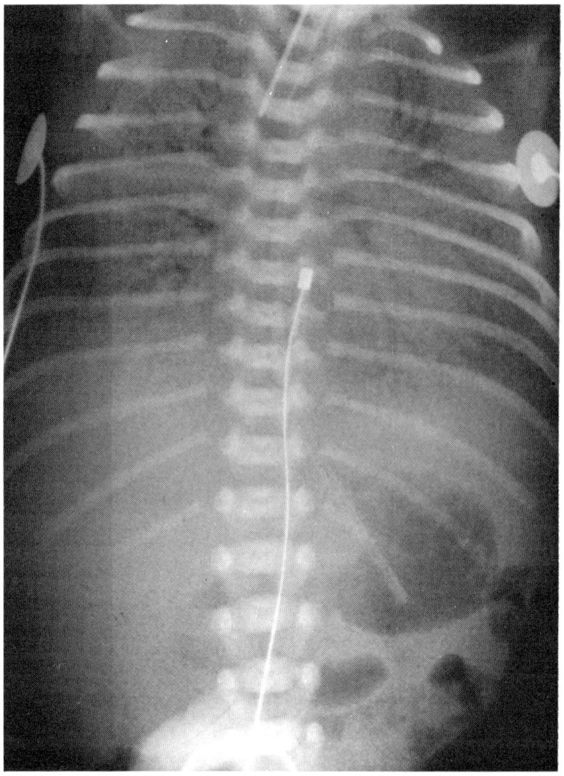

Fig. 70.1 X-ray of respiratory distress syndrome. The ground glass appearance of the lungs and air bronchogram are clearly seen and the heart borders are indistinct. The endotracheal tube is 0.5 cm above the carina and the umbilical arterial catheter is sited in the lower thoracic aorta.

thin: sphingomyelin ratio, phosphatidyl dimethyl ethanolamine and phosphatidyl glycerol — may be more specific (Gluck et al 1972, Hallman et al 1977) and are useful research tools but have little impact on clinical management.

Natural history

RDS is essentially a disease of premature infants. The overall incidence therefore depends on the incidence of premature deliveries. Two studies in geographically defined populations have assessed overall incidence at 0.33% (Hjalmarson 1981) and 0.93% (Field & Milner 1986) for a Swedish and British population respectively. Incidence with gestational age varies from 0.01% at term to 31% at 27–28 weeks' gestation. There is also doubt as to whether extremely immature infants should be considered to have RDS, as below 24 weeks' gestation the lungs have not developed any alveoli and a proportion of infants up to 28 weeks have none, so surfactant deficiency cannot be implicated in the lung disease. Many factors may affect the final common pathway which is expressed as RDS, including maternal factors (diabetes, maternal drugs), intrapartum asphyxia and postnatal management.

The typical history is of onset after the first few hours with gradual increase in severity of symptoms. The child is tachypnoeic with intercostal recession, grunting and flaring of the nostrils on inspiration. Oral feeds if attempted are not well tolerated because of the tachypnoea, and cyanosis develops as ventilation deteriorates. The severity of the disease increases over the first 24–48 hours and nearly all of the acute problems and many of the subsequent ones can be related to this critical time. Thereafter there is a gradual recovery over a period of a few days, the speed of which depends on the initial severity of the RDS and the amount of residual lung damage.

The clinical course and features can be explained on the basis of deficiency of surfactant which enhances the tendency of the alveoli to collapse and makes the lungs small and stiff. A fast breathing rate in these circumstances reduces the total work of breathing and expiration against a closed glottis, which produces grunting; it also limits the expiratory time and produces a positive pressure inside the chest which keeps alveoli open, allowing more gas exchange.

As discussed above, the diagnosis is one of exclusion and in the early stages it is important to have a full maternal, intrapartum and resuscitation history, examination and chest X-ray. The history may indicate meconium aspiration or transient tachypnoea and a term infant virtually excludes RDS as a diagnosis, although cases in term infants have been reported (Roberton et al 1967). Cardiac abnormalities may be evident on examination and a useful clinical point is that cyanosis due to cardiac anomalies rarely produces the distress seen with the equivalent amount of cyanosis in RDS, although blood gas analysis in 100% oxygen and echocardiography are usually necessary to confirm clinical suspicions.

Babies with hypoplastic lungs may be anticipated if the antenatal history and ultrasound are suggestive. Infection, particularly beta-haemolytic streptococcus group B, is an important differential diagnosis as it can be indistinguishable from RDS (French et al 1978). Some centres treat all low birthweight babies with penicillin but evidence that this affects outcome is lacking (Pyati et al 1983). The authors' practice is to give penicillin to all babies on commencing artificial ventilation for RDS. In terms of congenital malformations, diaphragmatic hernia is a relatively common condition and may occasionally be confused with RDS, although the chest X-ray is usually diagnostic.

Management

Undoubtedly the most important factor in management of babies with RDS is a high standard of general nursing care with attention to the thermoneutral environment, nutrition and minimal handling (Speidel 1978). The latter is obviously compromised by the need to perform nursing functions, medical examination and investigations. It is now possible to monitor many important parameters without disturbing the baby. Those used routinely are shown with indications

Table 70.1 Use of monitors on the neonatal unit

Type of monitor	Criteria for commencing use	Criteria for stopping use
Apnoea	All neonatal admissions	No significant apnoeas or bradycardias for 48 hours
Cardiac	All neonatal admissions	No significant apnoeas or bradycardias for 48 hours
Umbilical/arterial oxygen	All babies requiring more than 30% oxygen	After extubation or after 7 days in situ
Transcutaneous oxygen	All babies in supplementary oxygen if no arterial line is present	Discontinuation of oxygen therapy
Transuctaneous carbon dioxide	All babies on artificial ventilation in unstable clinical condition	When clinically stable with adequate blood gases
Blood pressure	All babies on artificial ventilation in unstable clinical condition	When clinically stable

for their use in Table 70.1. The place of oxygen saturation monitors is not yet established but may represent a further improvement in monitoring, as they reflect more accurately the oxygen available for tissue respiration although they are relatively insensitive to hyperoxia (Fanconi et al 1985).

In infants with anything more than mild disease, artificial ventilation is indicated. The criteria for deciding to support ventilation are not absolute and depend on the gestation of the baby and the rate of deterioration as well as the level of hypoxia, hypercapnia and blood pH. Intermittent positive pressure ventilation (IPPV) through an endotracheal tube is the method of choice. Some larger babies with good respiratory drive may be managed on continuous positive airways pressure (CPAP) via an endotracheal or nasal tube but other methods of ventilation, such as negative pressure or face-mask positive pressure, have distinct disadvantages and have been largely abandoned. The types of ventilator in common use on neonatal units are pressure-limited, continuous flow design. This means that there are five independent variables to be considered when using the ventilator — inspiratory time, expiratory time, peak pressure, and expiratory pressure and oxygen concentration. The potential number of different combinations is vast. Added to this there are changes in ventilator design and changes in the population of babies being ventilated, so the controversy over optimal ventilator settings is difficult to resolve.

Great improvements were made with the introduction of slow rates, reversed inspiratory : expiratory ratios, and positive and expiratory pressure (PEEP; Reynolds & Taghizadeh 1974), but recent trends have been towards faster rates and lower pressures in an attempt to reduce ventilator damage and pulmonary air leads (Ng & Easa 1979). It is also clear that babies who are not synchronized with the ventilator are at risk of pneumothorax (Greenough et al 1984). One way of preventing this is by increasing the ventilatory rate and decreasing the inspiratory : expiratory ratio if this is greater than one (Field et al 1985). The authors' present approach is to be flexible and attempt to synchronize the baby's breathing with the ventilator while maintaining adequate blood gas concentrations at as low a peak pressure as possible. It is still necessary on occasions to paralyse babies who fight the ventilator; these are usually more mature babies with strong respiratory drive and severe RDS.

Table 70.2 Complications of respiratory distress syndrome

Acute
Pulmonary
- Pulmonary air leaks (pneumothorax, pulmonary interstitial emphysema)
- Peristent fetal circulation
- Pulmonary haemorrhage
- Endotracheal tube blockage or misplacement

Cardiac
- Patent ductus arteriosus

Intracranial
- Intraventricular haemorrhage
- Periventricular leukomalacia

Infection

Late
Pulmonary
- Bronchopulmonary dysplasia
- Subglottic stenosis

Neurological
- Neurodevelopmental delay
- Fits
- Retinopathy of prematurity
- Sensorineural hearing loss
- Cerebral palsy

Infection

Complications

Major complications are shown in Table 70.2 and can be conveniently divided into those occurring early, during the acute illness, and those presenting during convalescence and subsequently.

Early complications

Pneumothorax. Pneumothorax is a major risk factor for mortality (Madansky et al 1979) and morbidity (Lipscomb et al 1981) in RDS. Ventilation is not the only causative factor as spontaneous pneumothorax is a relatively common event, occurring in 1–2% of term deliveries (Steele et al 1971). The extent to which ventilation causes pneumothorax or is simply a marker for lung disease is unresolved. However, it does seem that PEEP (Berg et al 1975), poor synchronization (Greenough et al 1984) and possibly slow rates contribute to an increased incidence.

Pneumothorax should be suspected in any ventilated baby with a deterioration in clinical condition or blood gases, particularly if this is sudden. It is accompanied by acidosis, hypoxia and large changes in blood pressure and cerebral

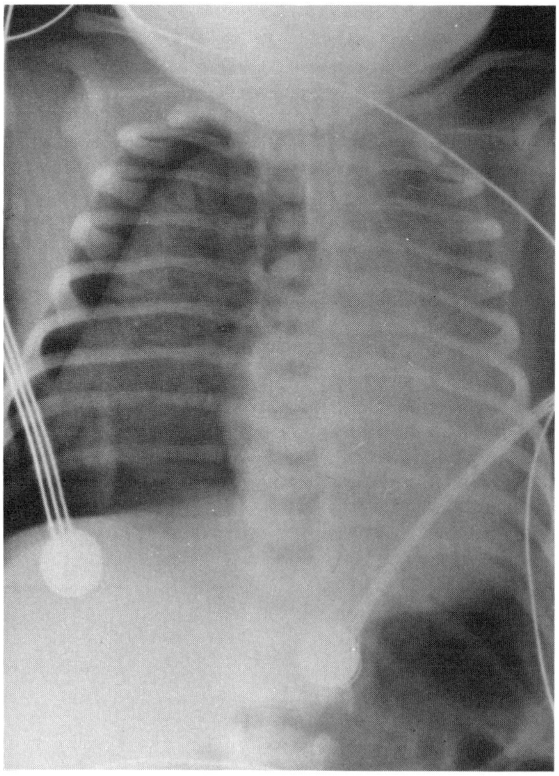

Fig. 70.2 A right-sided pneumothorax is seen on the X-ray with the lung edge clearly visible. The child has RDS, as can be seen from the left lung field.

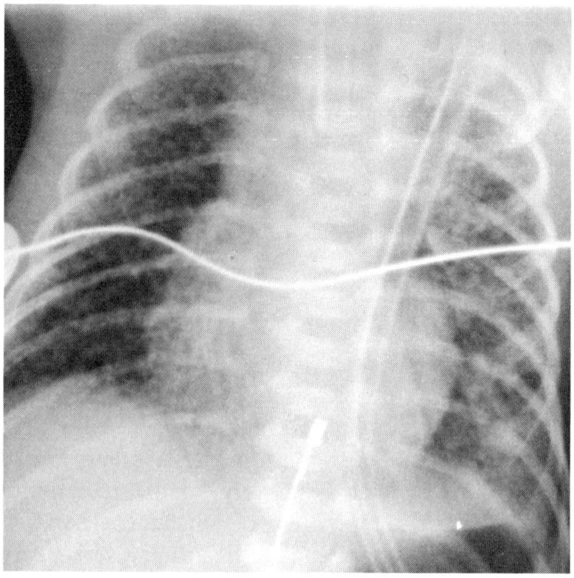

Fig. 70.3 Pulmonary interstitial emphysema shown here as multiple round or oval-shaped radiolucent areas tending to radiate out from the hilum of the lung.

blood flow. Definitive diagnosis is by chest X-ray (Fig. 70.2) but on most occasions pneumothorax occurs as an emergency and has to be treated before X-rays are available. On clinical examination, prominence of the chest wall on the affected side and decreased air entry may be present but transillumination of the chest using a cold light source is the most helpful diagnostic tool. Transillumination may give false positive results in the presence of interstitial gas and may not detect very small collections. If there is any doubt, then diagnostic aspiration using a size 21 butterfly needle attached to a three-way tap and syringe should be attempted. This will allow time for a formal chest drain insertion. Chest drains on the authors' unit are left in situ until they have stopped draining for 24 hours and are clamped intermittently before removal.

Pulmonary interstitial emphysema. This is an X-ray finding which consists of multiple oval or linear radiolucent areas radiating from the hilum of the lung (Fig. 70.3). Pathologically, this correlates with air in the lung interstitium dissecting along the tissue planes. It is much more common in extremely premature babies, with a reported incidence of 35% in babies under 1000 g (Yu et al 1986a). Pulmonary interstitial emphysema is usually bilateral and nearly always occurs in ventilated infants. The presence of interstitial air stiffens the lungs, makes ventilation more difficult and probably predisposes to chronic lung damage. Management consists of altering mechanical ventilation to decrease the peak inspiratory pressure. The ventilation rate has to be increased to maintain adequate gas exchange. This has been shown to be effective clinically and radiologically (Ng & Easa 1979).

Pulmonary haemorrhage. Pulmonary haemorrhage usually occurs in very sick infants, is often associated with bleeding at other sites and is associated with a poor prognosis. It is recognized by aspiration of blood-stained transudate from the endotracheal tube, increase in ventilatory requirements and a whiteout on chest X-ray. Management consists of replacing blood loss and clotting factors with fresh blood and fresh frozen plasma and maintaining adequate ventilation. High levels of PEEP are sometimes helpful.

Persistent fetal circulation. In utero the pressure in the pulmonary artery is high and blood entering the right side of the heart is to a large extent diverted to the systemic circulation via the foramen ovale and the ductus arteriosus. At birth, closure of the foramen ovale is effected simply by a rise in left atrial pressure. Closure of the ductus requires muscular contraction of the wall under the effect of oxygen. In preterm infants, the muscle of the ductus wall is underdeveloped and tends to remain patent. Blood flow through the lungs therefore depends on the pulmonary artery pressure which itself is determined by the pulmonary vascular resistance. The resistance in turn depends on the total cross-sectional area of the lung vasculature. Preterm infants have a smaller pulmonary bed and in RDS there is atelectasis with constriction of pulmonary vessels induced by hypoxia. All infants with RDS are thus at risk of shunting and once pulmonary vasoconstriction is established, oxygenation is difficult because blood is not reaching the alveoli.

Persistent fetal circulation is diagnosed when oxygenation cannot be maintained by increased ventilation after excluding pulmonary air leaks and congenital heart disease. The hypoxaemia is out of proportion to the hypercarbia. Management is directed towards prevention by keeping oxygenation relatively high (8–10 kPa) and by minimal handling, since in the acute phase of RDS even minor disturbance of the baby tends to precipitate shunting (Speidel 1978). Once persistent fetal circulation develops the important question is how much of it is reversible, due to constriction of smooth muscle, and how much is inevitable, due to inadequate numbers of vessels. Hyperventilation to keep arterial carbon dioxide levels below normal (2–3 kPa) reduces pulmonary vascular tone (Peckham & Fox 1978), but this is often difficult to achieve in the presence of lung disease. In this situation, after correcting pH and carbon dioxide levels, a bolus dose of tolazoline (2 mg/kg) should be given. Tolazoline has alpha-receptor blocking and histamine-blocking actions. It produces pulmonary and systemic hypotension by reducing arterial muscle tone. It will alleviate the resistance due to muscular construction, but the baby should be pretreated with plasma to counteract a potentially disastrous fall in systemic blood pressure. If effective, a continuous infusion (1 mg/kg/h) should be started with dopamine (5 mg/kg/min) to support the systemic circulation.

Intraventricular haemorrhage. Intraventricular haemorrhage in the acute phase of RDS is recognized clinically by increased ventilatory requirements, expanding head circumference, fits and fall in the haemoglobin level. It is usually associated with severe RDS in babies under 30 weeks' gestation, particularly those who have suffered a pneumothorax with accompanying acidosis and fluctuations in blood pressure and cerebral blood flow (Perlman et al 1983). Massive intraventricular haemorrhage can be treated symptomatically with transfusion and anticonvulsants. Serial lumbar punctures to reduce intracranial hypertension and remove blood-stained cerebrospinal fluid have been advocated but are of unproven efficacy (Anwar et al 1985). However, the prognosis for mortality and subsequent handicap in survivors is so poor that massive intraventricular haemorrhage is usually an indication to withdraw ventilatory support. Lesser degrees of haemorrhage can be diagnosed on ultrasound, are relatively common and have less prognostic significance but must be distinguished from periventricular leukomalacia, which is a result of pre- or postnatal ischaemia and appears to have significant neurodevelopmental consequences (Rushton et al 1985).

Late complications

Bronchopulmonary dysplasia. Bronchopulmonary dysplasia describes a group of infants who are still requiring oxygen supplementation at 30 days of age and have abnormal lungs on chest X-ray (Fig. 70.4). At autopsy, the findings are of focal emphysema and atelectasis with marked increase in

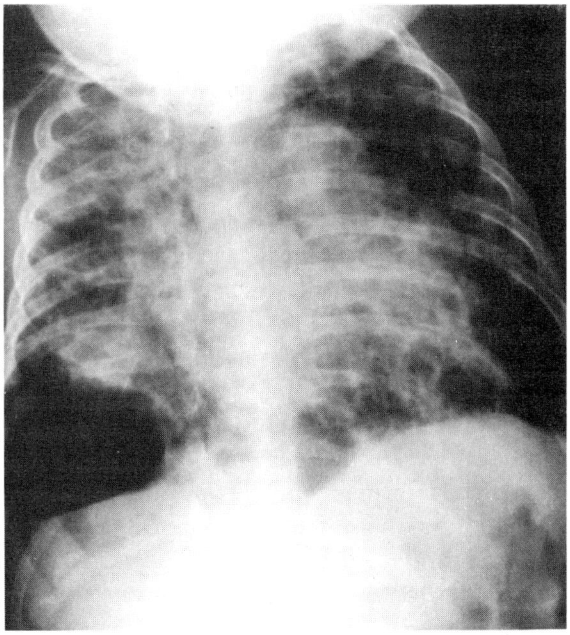

Fig. 70.4 Typical appearances of bronchopulmonary dysplasia with hyperinflation, cysts of varying sizes throughout the lung fields, with thickened walls and little normal lung tissue visible.

reticuloendothelial tissue, thickening of the alveolar basement membrane and separation of the alveolar surfaces from capillaries (Northway et al 1967). The important prerequisites for developing bronchopulmonary dysplasia are prematurity, positive pressure ventilation and oxygen supplementation. Most, but not all, babies develop bronchopulmonary dysplasia as a result of ventilation for RDS. The incidence of bronchopulmonary dysplasia in a geographically defined population has been quoted as 15% of ventilated babies who survive to 30 days of age (Field & Milner 1986). Gestational age strongly influences the risk of developing bronchopulmonary dysplasia (Greenough & Roberton 1985a) and the increased survival rate of extremely low birthweight infants (<1000 g) in the recent past has led to an increase in incidence.

Prevention has been aided by better mechanical ventilation (Reynolds & Taghizadeh 1974) and continuous monitoring of arterial or transcutaneous oxygen. Early treatment of patent ductus arteriosus may also help to reduce lung damage. Once chronic lung disease has developed a slow improvement can be expected over a period of weeks or months. In this phase it is important to achieve adequate nutrition, monitor oxygen requirements and treat the complications — chest infections and heart failure — early and aggressively. Diuretics and systemic steroids are sometimes useful but have significant complications. With infants who are hospital-bound for long periods of time, the support and involvement of the parents is of vital importance. The use of oxygen concentrators can allow some infants home on supplemental oxygen, which is of great benefit in spite of the problems and initial cost. Even when well enough to go home, infants who have had bronchopulmonary dysplasia still have very little respiratory reserve and often require readmission to hospital in the first year of life (Greenough & Roberton 1985b) following respiratory infections. Long-term consequences of the disease are not yet known.

Subglottic stenosis. This is a rare complication of prolonged intubation. The pathogenesis is an inflammatory response with concomitant fibrosis and contraction caused by repeated minor trauma to the trachea. This may occur from movement of the tip of the endotracheal tube itself with changes in head position, from high flow rates down the tube directed at the mucosa or from the trauma of repeated intubation. The condition presents with stridor, recession or even obstruction of the airway on extubation which resolves completely on re-intubation. The stenosis can often be seen at intubation with oedematous hyperaemic friable tissue at the level of the obstruction. Most infants can eventually be successfully extubated without recourse to tracheostomy. Steroid cover for the few days surrounding extubation has been advocated but is not of proven benefit; use of soft, non-shouldered endotracheal tubes may help to reduce trauma.

Retinopathy of prematurity. The epidemiology of retinopathy of prematurity is not yet clearly defined. Severe cases, formerly known as retrolental fibroplasia, result in scarring of the retina with varying degress of visual loss but milder cases with myopia or no demonstrable visual impairment are more difficult to define. In addition, many of the early changes are reversible. Ophthalmological changes can be detected at around the expected date of delivery (Fielder et al 1986), although they are related to events in the early neonatal period. There is a strong correlation between gestational age and occurrence of the disease, and oxygen is also a critical factor. However the role of oxygen therapy has probably been over-emphasized, particularly in the population of babies receiving neonatal care in the recent past (Lucey & Dangman 1984). The implication that retinopathy of prematurity is a preventable disease is an over-simplification and many other factors may influence vascular changes in the retina, the presumed pathogenesis of retinopathy of prematurity. There are no known safe levels of arterial oxygen, but even so monitoring arterial or transcutaneous oxygen of all babies receiving additional oxygen is advisable in order to reduce inspired oxygen to the minimum necessary.

Infection. This may occur at any stage of the illness and is dealt with in Chapter 69. The presence of an endotracheal tube provides a route for infection of the lower respiratory tract and prevents the normal clearance of secretions from the trachea. This, combined with the relative immunosuppression of the preterm infant, means there is often an element of infection in babies who are intubated for any length of time.

Mortality and morbidity

Because of the close relationship between gestational age and measures of outcome, mortality and handicap rates are of little value without specifying the population under study. Considerable advances have been made over the last 15 years such that it is now rare for infants over 1.5 kg to die of RDS and attention is focused on the smaller babies (<1000 g or under 30 weeks' gestation). In babies weighing under 1 kg, roughly one-third of those surviving to reach the neonatal unit will develop RDS (Yu et al 1986b). Of these, over 50% are likely to die. Overall survival of those babies under 700 g at birth is still less than 20% in the best units with significant handicap rates which are particularly related to cranial ultrasound abnormalities. Subsequent morbidity and mortality after discharge remain high with increase in number and length of hospital admissions, outpatient clinic attendances and need for surgery (Greenough & Robertson 1985a, Morgan 1985).

Future advances

Surfactant

Since surfactant deficiency was linked to RDS by Avery & Mead in 1959, there has been interest in developing a surfactant product to prevent the disease. Human, bovine and synthetic surfactant preparations have all been developed and tested in clinical trials. Human surfactant is prepared from amniotic fluid collected at Caesarean section and then purified; bovine surfactant is obtained by lavage of calf lungs. Synthetic surfactants are mixtures of the important component molecules found in human surfactant in proportions designed to reproduce the physical properties of the natural product. Results of prospective randomized controlled trials using human (Hallman et al 1985) and bovine (Enhorning et al 1985, Kwong et al 1985, Shapiro et al 1985) surfactant have shown significant improvement in gas exchange and decrease in ventilatory requirements. Trends in improved final outcome were also seen. Artificial surfactant preparations have not proved as effective (Tueusch et al 1983, Wilkinson et al 1985) although the potential advantages of lower cost, reproducible quality, sterility and lack of antigenicity make the continued search worthwhile. The reasons for this lack of effect are not known but may be related to the small lipoprotein content of the natural surfactants, although experimental evidence is lacking (Metcalfe et al 1980).

High-frequency ventilation

This term comprises three different techniques:

1. Conventional ventilation at rates of 60–150 inflations per minute where normal physiological principles of gas exchange apply.

2. Jet ventilation where a high-frequency pulse is directed down the endotracheal tube.
3. High-frequency oscillation where gas is oscillated back and forward in the circuit.

The first technique represents a modification of existing techniques which is useful in smaller babies with a faster intrinsic respiratory rate and with babies fighting the ventilator. The other two methods deliver volumes less than the dead space of the respiratory system and rely on facilitated diffusion for their action. Both methods are effective at maintaining blood gases at similar or lower mean tracheal pressures (Frantz et al 1983, Carlo et al 1984) but questions remain as to whether this will improve the eventual outcome and which group of babies are likely to benefit most.

Extracorporeal membrane oxygenation

This is theoretically an attractive solution to what is essentially transient respiratory failure. It consists of siphoning blood out of a large vein through an artificial membrane where gas exchange occurs and back into the baby through either a large vein or a carotid artery. It has been used with some success in premature infants (Bartlett et al 1985) but there are the significant technical problems of vascular access, high circuit volume to blood volume ratio, prevention of blood coagulation and platelet consumption plus the high capital and running costs.

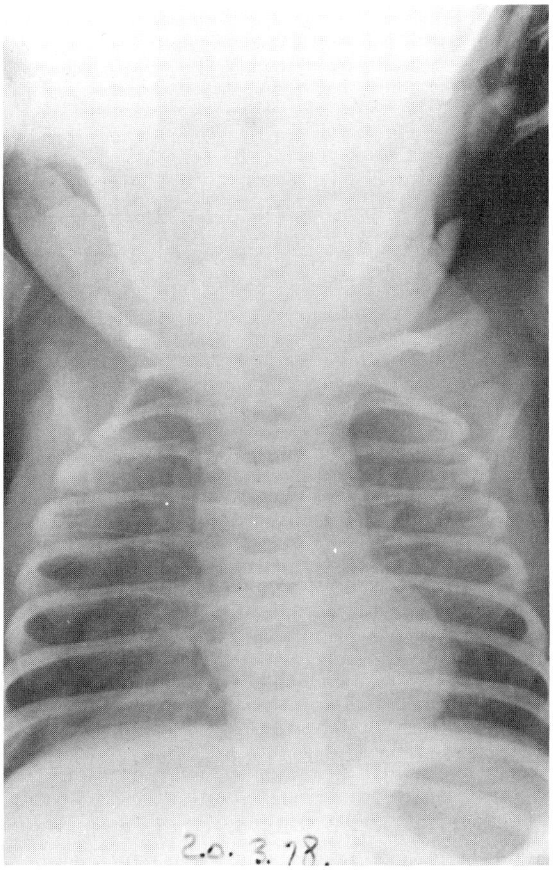

Fig. 70.5 X-ray of transient tachypnoea. The lungs are hyperinflated with streaky shadows extending from the hilum. Fluid can be seen in the horizontal fissure on the right between rib spaces 4–5.

TRANSIENT TACHYPNOEA

In utero the fetal lung is fluid-filled, probably containing about 30 ml/kg body weight. The lung secretes fluid and there is a net outflow through the trachea into the amniotic sac (Normand et al 1971). After birth, the lungs fill with air, net secretion into the alveoli ceases and any residual lung fluid needs to be resorbed. Transient tachypnoea of the newborn is a benign illness thought to be due to delayed resorbtion of lung fluid. The terms type 2 RDS, wet lung, aspiration syndrome and pulmonary maladaptation are all synonyms reflecting different approaches to aetiology and pathogenesis.

Diagnosis is based on clinical signs — tachypnoea, retraction, grunting or cyanosis — on X-ray findings of hyperinflation with evidence of lung or pleural fluid and resolution over less than 72 hours (Fig. 70.5).

The reported incidence of the condition varies widely because the diagnostic criteria, particularly in mild cases, are soft. In one population-based study with standardized diagnostic criteria (Hjalmarson 1981) the overall incidence was 0.93%.

Factors predisposing to transient tachypnoea of the newborn are prematurity, Caesarean section (especially elective operations), diabetic mothers, breech delivery and intrapartum asphyxia (Wesenberg et al 1971, Halliday et al 1981). The main differential diagnosis is between RDS, meconium aspiration, congenital heart disease, infection and extremes of normality. Differentiation of RDS from transient tachypnoea is largely based on the chest X-ray. Overinflation of the lungs is characteristic of transient tachypnoea while underinflation suggests RDS. Babies delivered near to term are more likely to have transient tachypnoea and tests of surfactant are normal.

Clinically the differentiation is unimportant as management in both cases is supportive. Meconium aspiration should be apparent at or before delivery but exclusion of congenital heart disease and streptococcal septicaemia in the early stages may be difficult and requires a high index of suspicion.

The principles of management are as for RDS. Inspired oxygen should be monitored against arterial or transcutaneous oxygen and nasogastric or intravenous fluids may be needed if tachypnoea is marked. Artificial ventilation is rarely needed and outcome is almost universally favourable.

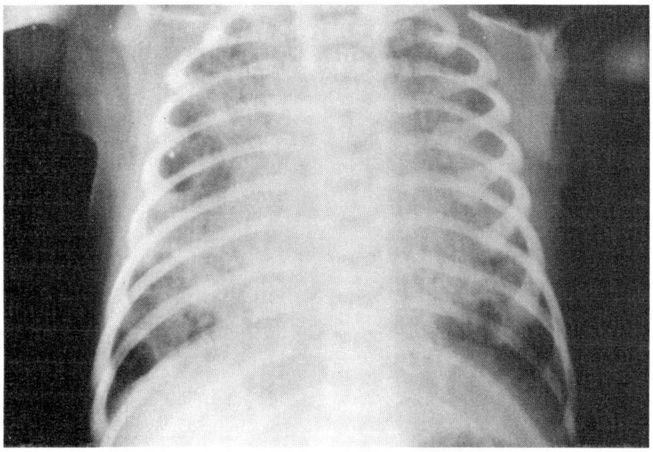

Fig. 70.6 Blotchy shadowing and hyperinflated lungs are the characteristic features of meconium aspiration, shown here.

MECONIUM ASPIRATION SYNDROME

In utero meconium is usually retained within the colon. If the fetus is exposed to a hypoxic stress, colonic peristalsis and relaxation of the anal sphincter lead to a passage of the meconium into the amniotic fluid. This occurs in 8–9% of all pregnancies (Gregory et al 1974) and in the vast number of cases represents compensated fetal distress with hypoxia but no acidosis. If the baby is exposed to a greater hypoxic stress with acidosis, inspiratory gasping will occur. Once meconium has entered the airways it tends to move peripherally, producing airways obstruction with hyperinflated barrel-shaped chest and often tension pneumothorax.

Diagnosis

Significant meconium aspiration has occurred in any baby who has had meconium-stained amniotic fluid, meconium in the trachea on direct laryngoscopy, respiratory distress and a combination of hyperinflation and dense areas of inflation on chest X-ray (Fig. 70.6; Yeh et al 1979).

Clinical features

Most babies developing meconium aspiration syndrome need resuscitation at birth. Respiratory distress with hyperinflation and tachypnoea may not be apparent for 2–4 hours after birth but tends to get progressively worse over the next 1–2 days as the meconium moves peripherally. The baby's respiratory rate often exceeds 100 breaths/min but chest wall recession is much less marked than in IRDS, due to the splinting effect of the hyperinflated lung. Cyanosis occurs relatively early, largely due to transitional circulation with right-to-left shunting at atrial and duct level. The respiratory symptoms are sometimes associated with abnormal neurological signs as a result of the hypoxic cerebral stress. These include convulsions, hypertonia and reduced level of response to stimulation; these are poor prognostic features.

Management

At delivery

Severe meconium aspiration syndrome can often be prevented by ensuring that somebody skilled at intubation is present at the delivery whenever there is meconium staining of the amniotic fluid (Gregory et al 1974). As soon as the baby's head has been delivered the nasopharynx must be sucked out. Immediately after delivery check whether there is any meconium in the trachea by direct laryngoscopy. If meconium is present, intubate the baby and apply suction to remove as much meconium as possible. One generally accepted method is to connect the endotracheal tube directly to the suction source at a negative pressure of $<50\,cmH_2O$ while withdrawing it. The endotracheal tube is then immediately replaced and the procedure repeated until meconium is no longer recovered or the baby's heart rate has fallen below 80 beats/min. Some units instil 1–2 ml of saline down the endotracheal tube between suctions. Once the baby has commenced regular respiration meconium is rapidly displaced and further suction is unlikely to be profitable.

Subsequent management

All babies who have meconium in their tracheas at birth must be admitted to the neonatal unit for observation. Respiratory and heart rate must be monitored continuously. Antibiotics are not indicated unless there is additional evidence to suggest that the baby is infected. Providing tracheal toilet has been carried out effectively, the majority of babies will show no respiratory symptoms and can be reunited with their mothers within 48–72 hours. If the baby requires additional oxygen an arterial line must be inserted so that blood gases and sugars can be analysed every 3–4 hours. These babies must be kept under careful observation as some will show progressive deterioration over the next 2–3 days, while others will develop tension pneumothorax as a result of the hyperinflation and airway plugging. Re-intubation and ventilatory support are required for those who develop carbon dioxide retention and become hypoxic despite high ambient oxygen concentrations.

These babies are particularly difficult to manage. It is preferable to commence ventilatory support with relatively low rates, 30–40 inflations per minute and inspiratory : expiratory ratios of not more than 1:2. Inflation pressures will need to be at least $20\,cmH_2O$ and the oxygen concentration between 60 and 70%. If this is insufficient, try increasing the rate up to 60–70 inflations per minute. Babies who are still fighting the ventilator and have unsatisfactory blood gases will require intravenous pancuronium to induce paralysis.

Despite this some babies will remain hypoxic due to persistent fetal circulation with a right-to-left shunting at atrial and duct level. This sometimes responds to increasing the respiratory rate up to 100 while maintaining peak pressure in an attempt to reduce the arterial carbon dioxide level to between 3 and 4 kPa, while correcting any metabolic acidosis (Peckham & Fox 1978). If this too fails, commence intravenous tolazoline (2 mg/kg stat followed by 1 mg/kg/h). It is essential to monitor arterial blood pressure at these times, as tolazoline not infrequently leads to severe systemic hypotension which can be corrected with plasma (10–20 ml/kg body weight or other vascular compartment expanders).

It is crucial to remember that the intrauterine hypoxia may have led to significant cerebral damage. This will be virtually impossible to assess during the period of paralysis. The hypoxia may also have produced temporary or even permanent renal damage and so acute renal failure is not uncommon and will obviously complicate management. Urinary output must be carefully monitored and electrolytes and urea checked at least every 24 hours.

Prognosis

Although some babies will develop pneumothorax, deaths from this condition in the UK are rare providing the baby does not have severe cerebral damage.

MILK ASPIRATION

Regurgitation of stomach contents is a common occurrence in the neonatal period, particularly in those born preterm. Often this leads purely to altered milk trickling from the baby's mouth. Sometimes however, particularly in preterm babies, the milk will enter the airways. This will lead either to the sudden onset of apnoea or aspiration of milk into the lungs.

Apnoea

There is evidence that milk other than that of human origin will stimulate laryngeal receptors, inducing apnoea. Certainly it is relatively common to find milk in the upper airways of preterm babies who are on nasogastric or oral feeds; they may develop an apnoea of sufficient severity to require an oropharyngeal suction and perhaps intubation.

Aspiration pneumonia

There is also evidence to indicate that the cough receptors of preterm babies are relatively insensitive, so that milk entering the airway is more likely to be aspirated down on to the lungs; this will lead to a pattern of respiratory distress with tachypnoea, crepitations and sometimes even cyanosis. Chest X-ray will often show patchy changes, but without the picture of hyperinflation seen with meconium aspiration syndrome.

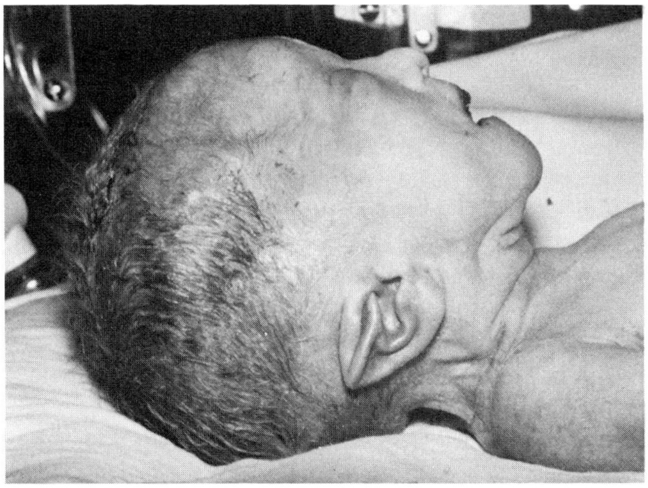

Fig. 70.7 Facial features at post-mortem of a baby with oligohydraminios and renal agenesis. Note the low-set ears and flattened nose. Marked limb deformities are often present, as well as pulmonary hypoplasia.

Management

Although most of these babies will recover satisfactorily with gentle chest physiotherapy alone, it is common practice to commence these babies on systemic antibiotics for 5–7 days on the assumption that the milk aspiration increases the risk of infection.

PULMONARY HYPOPLASIA

This term describes a generalized decrease in lung size and number of alveoli. It has been defined pathologically as a low lung to body weight ratio (Wigglesworth & Desai 1981), but there is a spectrum of severity with milder cases being fully compatible with survival. There are a number of causes which fall into three main categories:

1. Oligohydramnios either from oliguria or leak of amniotic fluid.
2. Neurological abnormalities resulting in decreased breathing movements.
3. Compression of the lungs within the chest by a diaphragmatic hernia or thoracic dystrophy.

With the possible exception of diaphragmatic herniae, the first group is by far the commonest and most important. At birth the typical appearance is of the oligohydramnios tetrad, which includes the Potter facies — low-set ears, flattened nose and micrognathia — limb deformities, growth retardation and pulmonary hypoplasia (Fig. 70.7). Respiratory difficulty is evident from birth and requires high pressures and fast rates to maintain gas exchange. In cases with oliguria or anuria the major decision is whether renal function is adequate. An antenatal diagnosis of absent or grossly dysplastic kidneys made with ultrasound is an indication to withdraw ventilatory support. Active management should be maintained if renal function is likely to be recoverable.

Prolonged rupture of the membranes with chronic amniotic fluid leak also induces pulmonary hypoplasia. As might be expected, the longer the time of ruptured membranes and the more severe the oligohydramnios, the greater the degree of pulmonary hypoplasia (Thibeault et al 1985). This has to be balanced against the advantage of continued general maturation of the fetus when contemplating delivery. Paediatric management is based on respiratory support to maintain oxygenation and prevent pulmonary hypertension and shunting. Survival depends on the underlying cause of the pulmonary hypoplasia. The survival rate for all infants with prolonged rupture of the membranes for more than 5 days was 59% in the study of Thibeault et al (1985).

Absent or dysplastic kidneys are incompatible with survival and in the other disorders survival is dependent on the degree of hypoplasia and the nature of the underlying condition. There is evidence that mild degrees of pulmonary hypoplasia are associated with amniocentesis in the second trimester. There is a 1% increase in respiratory problems at birth, an increase in limb malformations (Medical Research Council Working Party on Amniocentesis 1978) and a decrease in crying vital capacities of otherwise normal term babies (Vyas et al 1982) following amniocentesis.

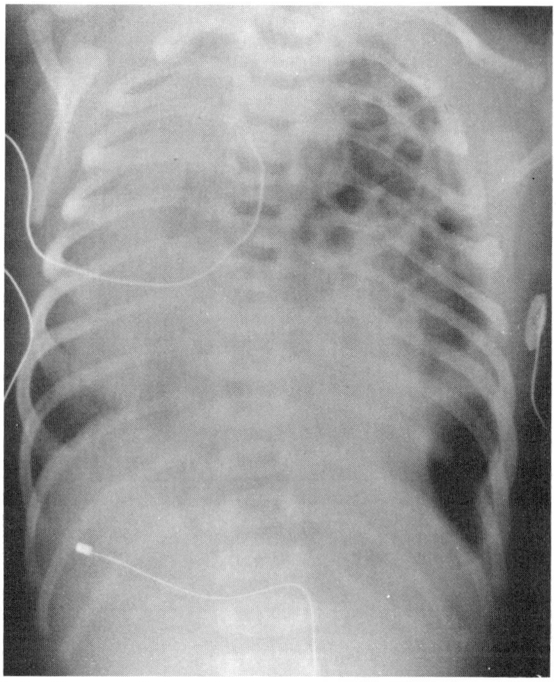

Fig. 70.8 X-ray of a baby with a diaphragmatic hernia. The left side of the chest if full of bowel shadows while the abdomen has no aerated bowel. The heart is displaced to the right but there is a relatively large amount of right lung visible, implying a good prognosis. Note that the umbilical artery catheter has been misplaced through the umbilical vein into a hepatic vein.

DIAPHRAGMATIC HERNIA

The incidence of diaphragmatic hernia is approximately 1 in 2500 births. Most result from failure of closure of the pleuroperitoneal canal (the Bochdalek-type hernia) and 85% occur on the left side (Fig. 70.8). The presence of bowel in the chest prevents the normal development of the lungs. The lung on the side of the lesion is often severely hypoplastic but more importantly, the contralateral lung is also affected. A minority of cases (10–20%) give rise to polyhydramnios associated with a kinking of the oesophago-gastric junction.

Antenatal diagnosis by ultrasound is becoming more frequent but the usual presentation is at resuscitation. The baby is usually vigorous but remains cyanosed. High pressures are needed to maintain oxygenation and the chest is hyperinflated with a scaphoid abdomen. On auscultation, air entry is absent over the affected side and the heart is displaced to the contralateral side. Presentation at a later stage implies a better prognosis.

Management consists of stabilization and control of respiration, exclusion of associated abnormalities and surgical correction. Stabilization is by mechanical ventilation combined with tolazoline, dopamine and plasma to reduce pulmonary hypertension and support the systemic circulation. It is important that the baby should be in an optimal condition before surgery, as survival can be improved (Cartlidge et al 1986). Associated congenital heart disease is common and often fatal, although some degree of left ventricular hypoplasia is to be expected. At surgery the edges of the defect can be directly apposed if the lesion is small. Larger defects can be covered with a synthetic graft. If the abdomen is too small to take all the bowel once it has been reduced from the chest, a temporary graft can be inserted into the abdominal wall.

PLEURAL EFFUSION

This is an uncommon condition which may cause respiratory difficulty at or soon after birth. The infant is tachypnoeic and often cyanosed and it may be possible to elicit dullness and reduced air entry in dependent parts of the thorax. If the effusion is unilateral there may be mediastinal shift and prominence of the affected hemithorax. Chest X-ray is diagnostic (Fig. 70.9). The main causes are hydrops fetalis, infection and chylothorax (Yancy & Spock 1967).

The treatment is to drain the effusion both to alleviate symptoms and to aid diagnosis, and then treat the underlying cause.

In hydrops fetalis the effusions are usually bilateral and are part of the generalized oedema secondary to anaemia or intrauterine heart failure.

Effusion secondary to infection is usually associated with pneumonic changes in the lungs, which will need treatment according to the clinical history and microbiology of the case.

Chylothorax is usually right-sided and thought to be due to rupture of the thoracic duct during traumatic delivery.

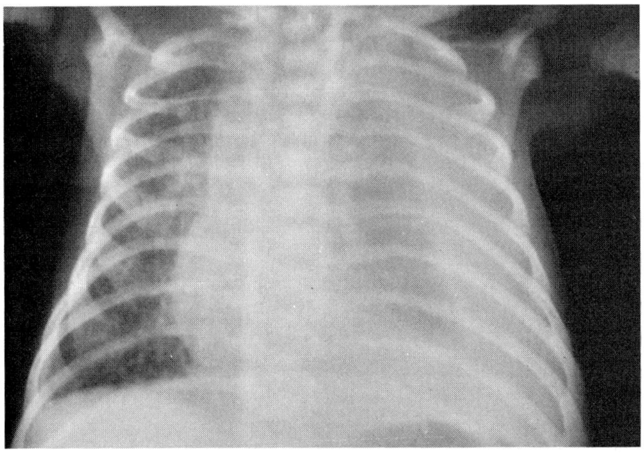

Fig. 70.9 Left pleural effusion. The outline of the left lung can be seen and, as the X-ray has been taken with the baby supine, the lung is anterior. There is no ascites to indicate generalized oedema; in fact this baby had a chylous effusion.

The effusion is initially clear with a high lymphocyte count but becomes cloudy after milk feeds are started. If the effusion reaccumulates after thoracocentesis, milk feeds containing only medium chain triglycerides are indicated. Medium chain triglycerides are absorbed from the gut directly into the blood stream rather than the lymphatics and allow the thoracic duct to heal while maintaining adequate calorie intake.

OTHER CONGENITAL ABNORMALITIES

Choanal atresia

This is an abnormality of the back of the nose in which the nasal airways do not communicate with the nasopharynx. It may be unilateral or bilateral and may be associated with other congenital anomalies. As the newborn baby breathes predominantly through the nose there is considerable respiratory difficulty if the lesion is bilateral; this difficulty disappears when the baby cries. The diagnosis is confirmed by failure to pass a nasogastric tube into the pharynx. The treatment is surgical.

Pierre Robin syndrome

Upper airway obstruction occurs in this disorder because of micrognathia which displaces the tongue backwards into the pharynx. The obstruction is less if the head is held forward and the degree of obstruction improves as the child grows. A nasopharyngeal airway is used to maintain airway patency.

Laryngeal and tracheal abnormalities

A variety of disorders give rise to narrowing of the large airways which present clinically with inspiratory stridor. Commonest of these is laryngomalacia or floppy larynx, a benign condition in which the larynx tends to collapse inwards on inspiration. The stridor is usually absent at rest, the cry is normal and chest X-ray is normal. If the clinical picture is not typical, investigation is indicated to exclude laryngeal cysts, webs and palsy or tracheal stenosis or compression.

Peripheral abnormalities

Congenital lobar emphysema is a condition which develops soon after birth and is associated with a defect in the bronchi resulting in a ball-valve effect. The affected lobe gradually hyperinflates and compresses the chest contents, causing progressive respiratory difficulty and visible chest asymmetry. The treatment is excision of the affected lobe.

Congenital cystic malformations are also localized but are a developmental anomaly which can be seen on antenatal ultrasound. The aetiology is unknown. Clinically the infant develops respiratory distress soon after birth, often with localizing chest signs. The chest X-ray shows a cystic mass in the chest but it is not always possible to distinguish this from a diaphragmatic hernia without injection of contrast. The treatment is surgical removal of the cystic portion.

APNOEA

Apnoea, the cessation of respiratory air flow, remains a major clinical problem to all those responsible for the care of preterm or sick neonates. All newborn babies, like children and adults, have episodes of apnoea lasting for up to 15 seconds, so these relatively brief periods of respiratory arrest, particularly occurring in rapid eye movement (REM) sleep, must be considered normal. However apnoea lasting for more than 20–30 seconds is frequently associated with progressive hypoxia, bradycardia and changes in blood pressure, creating conditions which may produce cerebral damage and, in the first few days of life, intraventricular haemorrhage.

Types of apnoea

Physiological studies have shown that apnoea attacks can be divided into three groups: central, obstructive and mixed (Fig. 70.10, 70.11).

Central apnoea

Central apnoea is due to a failure of the motor drive from the respiratory centre in the mid-brain. Apnoea therefore commences at the end expiratory tidal point (Milner et al 1980). Heart rate and arterial oxygen fall relatively slowly. The large majority of central apnoeas are self-terminating but if the hypoxia becomes too severe a vicious cycle may

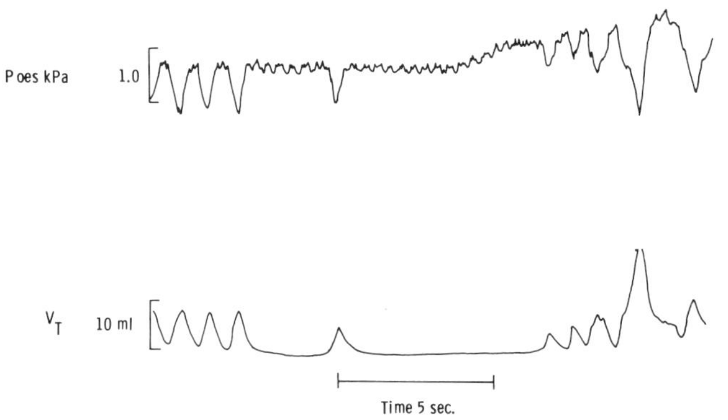

Fig. 70.10 Example of central apnoea showing a trace of intraoesophageal pressure (P oes) and simultaneous tidal volume (V_T). Oesophageal (intrathoracic) pressure changes are always associated with volume changes.

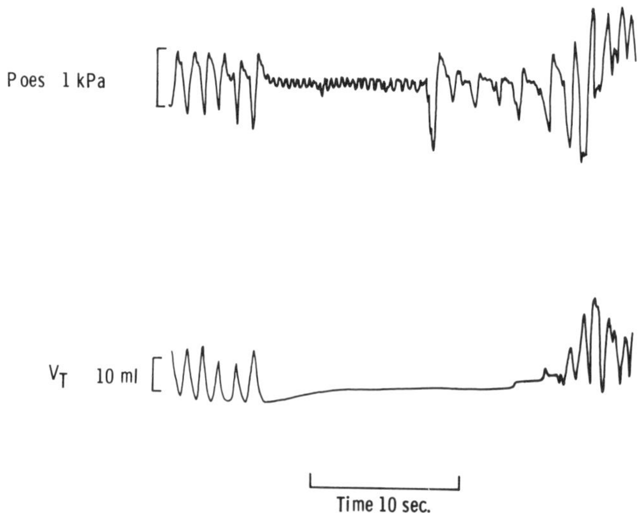

Fig. 70.11 Example of mixed apnoea. Initially the baby is making no respiratory efforts, i.e. the oesophageal pressure trace (P oes) shows only cardiac artefact. Over the later part of the apnoeic episode, the baby is making vigorous respiratory efforts with no tidal volume (V_T) change, indicating that the airway is obstructed.

result which can lead to death or severe brain damage if appropriate action is not taken. There is still considerable discussion on the mechanism of the respiratory drive failure; some evidence exists that before birth the respiratory chemoreceptors are turned off and that intrauterine respiratory movements only occur in REM sleep when breathing is predominantly a cerebral function. Certainly the balance of evidence suggests that babies having recurrent apnoea have a reduced sensitivity to inhaled carbon dioxide; there is also good evidence that even in term babies hypoxic respiratory drive is considerably reduced for the first few days of life.

A further theory is that the respiratory control mechanisms are unstable in preterm babies so that the rate and depth of respiration tend to oscillate. Certainly periodic respiration is extremely common. If the oscillations seen in periodic respiration are exaggerated the pattern of recurrent central apnoea is produced. There is also some evidence to indicate that central apnoea is more common during hypoxia and when the baby has a systemic infection.

Obstructive apnoea

Obstructive apnoea, a continuation of respiratory efforts without respiratory flow, is a relatively rare event in the neonatal unit. It occurs in babies with the Pierre Robin syndrome who have poorly developed mandibles and cleft palates so that when the baby is nursed supine the tongue tends to obstruct the airway. Obstructive apnoea also occurs in neonates who have reduced muscle tone, for example in babies with Down's syndrome. These episodes of obstructive apnoea are associated with rapid reduction in heart rate, presumably due to vagal reflexes, and are combined with rapid falls in oxygen saturation (Vyas et al 1981).

Mixed apnoea

Nearly 50% of apnoea attacks occurring in preterm babies are of mixed variety (Vyas et al 1981, Butcher-Peuch et al 1985). In these attacks part of the apnoea is due to central failure but is compounded and may sometimes be precipitated by obstruction to air flow (Milner et al 1977). The site of obstruction is under dispute but is either laryngeal or due to collapse of the pharyngeal structures (Thach & Stark 1979).

Management

Investigations

From the clinical point of view recurrent apnoea can be regarded as primary or secondary. Those who have primary apnoea will be preterm — usually less than 30 weeks' gestation. There is usually a period of up to 48 hours before the apnoea becomes apparent. Even if the attacks of apnoea are relatively severe, the baby will be pink and vigorous between episodes; the apnoea represents a physiological failure of respiratory control. For these infants the only necessary investigations are haemoglobin, since apnoea is more common in the presence of anaemia, and blood glucose level — low in apnoea.

Those with secondary apnoea are more worrying. The respiratory problem may reflect severe organic illness (Table 70.3). These babies will normally require an infection screen, consisting of a full blood picture, chest X-ray, blood, stool and urine culture and if necessary, bladder puncture and lumbar puncture. It will also be necessary to check the blood glucose and consider whether the attacks represent fits or a response to an excessively high environmental temperature. This can induce apnoea whether it is produced by pho-

Table 70.3 Cases of secondary apnoea

Systemic infections
Urinary tract infections
Pneumonia
Gastroenteritis
Meningitis
Septicaemia
Metabolic hypoglycaemia
Hyperthermia
Phototherapy
Sunlight
Hypoxia
Respiratory distress syndrome
Pneumonia
Asphyxia
Cerebral trauma
Intracranial haemorrhage
Intraventricular haemorrhage
Subdural haemorrhage

totherapy lamps or abnormally high settings on the incubator or radiant heater. Intracranial ultrasound will help identify those babies with significant intracranial haemorrhages, a not infrequent cause of severe apnoea in very preterm babies.

Therapy

Monitoring

It is obviously important to identify apnoea attacks relatively early to prevent ischaemia or haemorrhagic brain damage. For this reason babies at high risk—those born before 32 weeks' gestation, those with significant respiratory distress and babies who are acutely ill from infection, hypoxia or traumatic brain damage—will require respiratory monitoring until they are stable.

There are currently four main monitoring systems in general use in neonatal units (Special Report 1985; Fig. 70.12). The apnoea mattress has been designed so that air passes from one ripple to another as the baby breathes; this cools the temperature centre mounted at the central manifold. This device is relatively cheap but can easily be punctured. The other problems are that the degree of inflation is critical, in that it will not identify obstructive apnoea, and if set at too sensitive a level can be triggered off by the baby's heartbeat alone.

The second system is the pressure sensor. This is more expensive but less liable to be damaged; otherwise it has the same disadvantages as the apnoea mattress.

The third system is the impedance device, which requires two or three electrodes placed on the baby. It usually has an associated heart rate monitor and so will also detect periods of bradycardia. Its main disadvantage is that of expense.

The fourth device is the pressure capsule. This consists of a sensor which is attached to the abdominal wall; as the wall moves the membrane of the capsule is distorted, altering the air pressure within the device. This too can be affected by heart rate and is incapable of differentiating between obstructive or mixed apnoea and normal breathing.

Management of individual attacks

As all babies have physiological episodes of apnoea lasting for up to 15 seconds, the apnoea detector used should be set to raise the alarm after 20 or 30 seconds. Once the alarm has gone off, check to make sure the baby is indeed apnoeic as the alarm may represent a false positive response. Often simple skin stimulation will be adequate to restore regular respiration. Flicking the sole of the baby's foot or blowing cold air over the baby's face with a facemask is often enough. If these measures are ineffective suck out the oropharynx. It is important that this should be carried out gently as vigorous stimulation may actually induce apnoea. Sometimes milk will then be aspirated. Most babies who are still not breathing will respond to facemask resuscitation using a manual device. Occasionally it will be necessary to proceed to intubation and IPPV, using pressures of 15–20 cmH_2O.

Ongoing management

If infection is suspected the baby must be commenced on systemic antibiotics immediately; the antibiotic selected will depend on the sensitivity pattern of the organisms normally found in the unit and on unit policy, but will often be a combination of penicillin or cloxacillin and an aminoglycoside such as gentamicin or netilmicin. Any hypoglycaemia must be reversed with intravenous glucose 0.25–0.5 g/kg body weight as a 20% solution. If the baby is anaemic with a haemoglobin level of less than 10 g/dl, it would be well worth transfusing the baby with packed cells over 6–8 hours (20–40 ml/kg body weight).

The most effective therapy for apnoea is theophylline which increases respiratory drive and thus reduces apnoea. It is usually given in a dose of 1–2 mg/kg body weight 8-hourly. Blood levels are required as the rate of breakdown is very variable. The aim is to achieve blood levels between 5 and 15 μg/ml. Once the blood level is known, the oral dose can be altered accordingly. Alternatively, caffeine can be given (Aranda et al 1979). Those babies who are too immature to tolerate oral theophylline can be given intravenous aminophylline in similar doses.

If theophylline fails to control the apnoea the next alternative is to provide CPAP, using a facemask or a dual or even single nasal catheter. It is usually sufficient to provide distending levels of 3–4 cmH_2O. It has been shown that this eliminates mixed and obstructive central apnoea (Miller et al 1985). Those babies who fail to respond to this regime require intubation and IPPV using inspired oxygen at 25–30% and ventilation rates of 20–30 l/min, i.e. ratios of 1:2 and inflation pressure of 12–15 cmH_2O. It may be necessary to continue this for several days, usually weaning the child off by progressively reducing the respiratory rate while

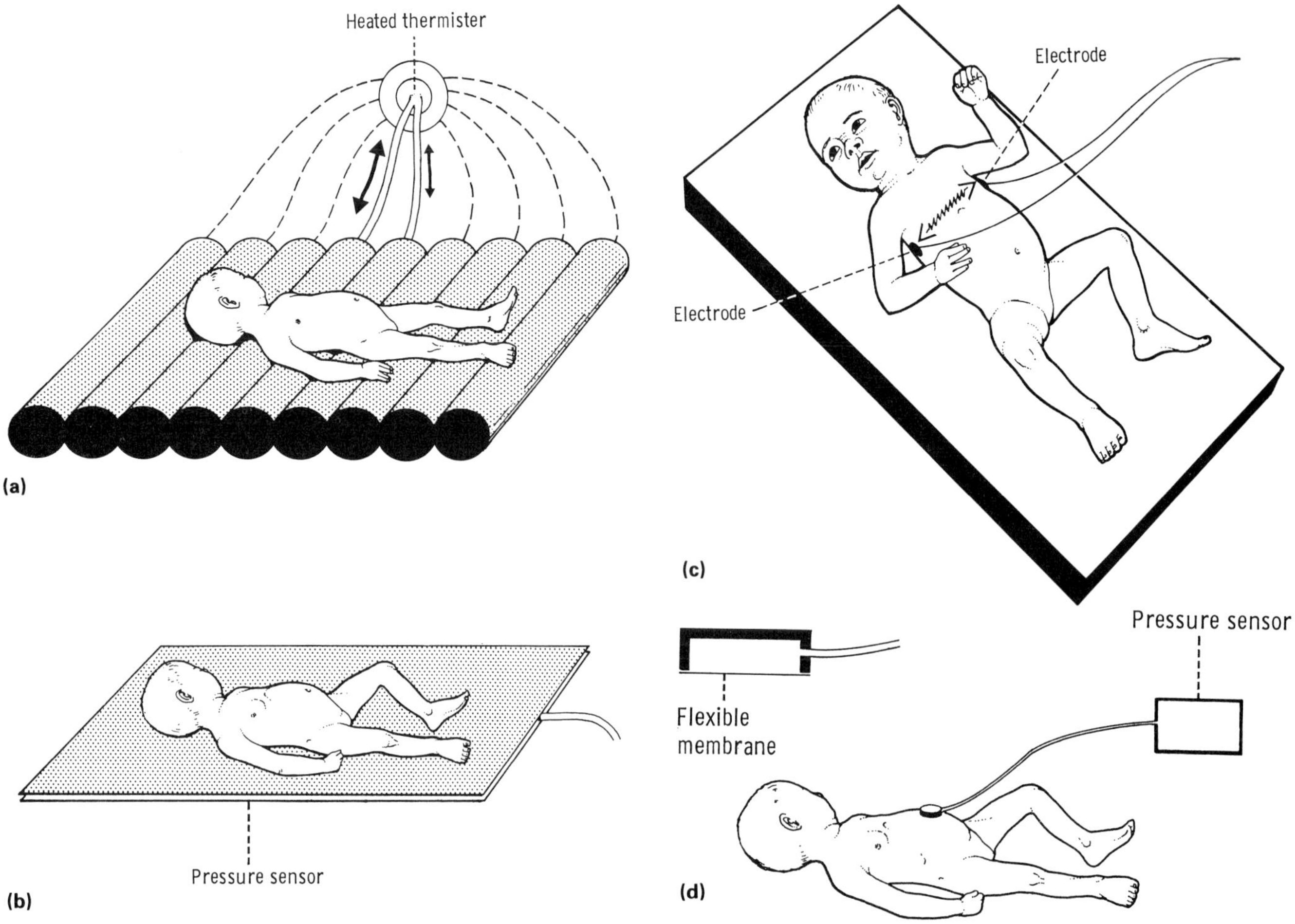

Fig. 70.12 Apnonea monitors. (**a**) Mattress; (**b**) pressure sensor; (**c**) impedance; (**d**) capsule sensor.

at the same time maintaining the blood theophylline and therapeutic levels.

Doxapram

Preliminary studies have shown that intravenous doxapram (2.5 mg/kg/h) does stimulate respiratory efforts in babies who have failed to respond to intravenous aminophylline or oral theophylline (Hayakawa et al 1986). However there are still some worries that doxapram may induce abnormal neurological states in preterm babies and until further information is available doxapram should be reserved for babies who fail to respond to conventional therapy.

REFERENCES

Anwar M, Kadam S, Hiatt I M, Hegyi T 1985 Serial lumbar punctures in prevention of post-hemorrhagic hydrocephalus in preterm infants. Journal of Pediatrics 107: 446–450

Aranda J V, Cook G E, Gorman W et al 1979 Pharmacokinetic profile of caffeine in the premature newborn infant with apnoea. Journal of Pediatrics 94: 663–668

Avery M E, Mead J 1959 Surface properties in relation to atelectasis and hyaline membrane disease. American Journal of Diseases in Children 97: 517–523

Bartlett R H, Roloff D W, Cornell R G, Andrews A F, Dillon P W, Zwischenberger J B 1985 Extracorporeal circulation in neonatal respiratory failure: a prospective randomized study. Pediatrics 76: 479–487

Berg T J, Pagtakhan R D, Reed M H, Langston C, Chernick V 1975 Bronchopulmonary dysplasia and lung rupture in hyaline membrane disease — influence of continuous distending pressure. Pediatrics 55: 51–54

Butcher-Peuch M C, Henderson-Smart D J, Holley D, Lacey J L, Edwards D 1985 Relation between apnoea duration and type and neurological status of preterm infants. Archives of Disease in Childhood 60: 953–958

Carlo W A, Chatburn R L, Martin R J et al 1984 Decrease in airway pressure during high frequency jet ventilation in infants with respiratory distress syndrome. Journal of Pediatrics 104: 101–107

Cartlidge P H T, Mann N P, Kapila L 1986 Pre-operative stabilisation in congenital diaphragmatic hernia. Archives of Disease in Childhood 61: 1226–1228

Clements J A, Platzker A C G, Tierney D F et al 1972 Assessment of the risk of the respiratory distress syndrome by a rapid test for surfactant in amniotic fluid. New England Journal of Medicine 286: 1077–1081

Donald I, Steiner R E 1953 Radiography in the diagnosis of hyaline membrane. Lancet ii: 846–849

Enhorning G, Shennan A, Possmayer F, Dunn M, Chen C P, Milligan J

1985 Prevention of neonatal respiratory distress syndrome by tracheal installation of surfactant: a randomised clinical trial. Pediatrics 76:145–153
Fanconi S, Doherty P, Edmonds J F, Barker G A, Bohn D J 1985 Pulse oximetry in pediatric intensive care: comparison with measured saturations and transcutaneous oxygen tension. Journal of Pediatrics 107: 362–366
Field D, Milner A D 1986 Respiratory disease in the neonatal period. British Medical Bulletin 42: 163–166
Field D, Milner A D, Hopkin I E 1985 Manipulation of ventilator settings to prevent active expiration against positive pressure inflation. Archives of Disease in Childhood 60: 1036–1040
Fielder A R, Ng Y K, Levene M I 1986 Retinopathy of prematurity: age of onset. Archives of Disease in Childhood 61: 774–778
Frantz III I D, Werthammer J, Stark A R 1983 High frequency ventilation in premature infants with lung disease. Adequate gas exchange at low tracheal pressure. Pediatrics 71: 483–488
French T J, Haines I L, Fleming P J, Speidel B P 1978 Early treatment of neonatal group B streptococcal infection. Lancet ii: 997–998
Gluck L, Kulovich M V, Eidelman A I, Cordero L, Khazin A F 1972 Biochemical development of surface activity in mammalian lung IV. Pulmonary lecithin synthesis in the human fetus and newborn and etiology of the respiratory distress syndrome. Pediatric Research 6: 81–99
Greenough A, Roberton N R C 1985a Morbidity and survival in neonates ventilated for the respiratory distress syndrome. British Medical Journal 290: 597–600
Greenough A, Roberton N R C 1985b Effects of a regional neonatal unit on a general paediatric ward. British Medical Journal 291: 175–176
Greenough A, Wood S, Morley C J, Davis J A 1984 Pancuronium prevents pneumothoraces in ventilated preterm infants who actively expire against positive pressure ventilation. Lancet i: 1–4
Gregory G A, Gooding C A, Phibbs R H, Tooley W H 1974 Meconium aspiration in infants — a prospective study. Journal of Pediatrics 85: 848–852
Halliday H L, McLure G, McReid M 1981 Transient tachypnoea of the newborn: two distinct clinical identities? Archives of Disease in Childhood 56: 322–325
Hallman M, Feldman B H, Kirkpatrick E, Gluck L 1977 Absence of phosplatidylglycerol (PG) in respiratory distress syndrome in the newborn. Pediatric Research 11: 714–720
Hallman M, Merritt T A, Jarvenpaa A L et al 1985 Exogenous human surfactant for treatment of severe respiratory distress syndrome: a randomised prospective clinical trial. Journal of Pediatrics 106: 963–969
Hayakawa F, Hakamada S, Kuniyushi K, Nakashima T, Miyachi Y 1986 Doxapram in the treatment of idiopathic apnoea of prematurity: desirable dosage and serum concentrations. Journal of Pediatrics 109: 138–140
Hjalmarson O 1981 Epidemiology and classification of acute neonatal respiratory disorders. Acta Paediatrica Scandinavica 70: 773–783
Kwong M S, Egan E A, Notter R M, Shapiro D L 1985 A double blind clinical trial of calf lung surfactant extract for prevention of hyaline membrane disease in extremely premature infants. Pediatrics 76:585–592
Lipscomb A P, Thorburn R J, Reynolds E O R et al 1981 Pneumothorax and cerebral haemorrhage in preterm babies. Lancet i: 416–418
Lucey J F, Dangman B 1984 A re-examination of the role of oxygen in retrolental fibroplasia. Pediatrics 73: 82–96
Madansky D L, Lawson E E, Chernick V, Taeusch H W Jr 1979 Pneumothorax and other forms of pulmonary air leak in newborns. American Review of Respiratory Disease 120: 729–737
Medical Research Council Working Party on Amniocentesis 1978 An assessment of the hazards of amniocentesis. British Journal of Obstetrics and Gynaecology 85 (suppl 2): 1–41
Metcalfe I L, Enhorning G, Possmayer F 1980 Pulmonary surfactant — associated proteins — their role in the expression of surface activity. Journal of Applied Physiology 49: 34–41
Miller M J, Carlo W A, Martin R J 1985 Continuous positive airway pressure selectively reduces obstructive apnoea in preterm infants. Journal of Pediatrics 106: 91–94
Milner A D, Saunders R A, Hopkin I E 1977 Apnoea induced by airflow obstruction. Archives of Disease in Childhood 52: 379–383
Milner A D, Boon A W, Saunders R A, Hopkin I E 1980 Upper airways obstruction and apnoea in preterm babies. Archives of Disease in Childhood 55: 22–25
Morgan M E I 1985 Late morbidity of very low birthweight infants. British Medical Journal 291: 171–173
Ng K P K, Easa D 1979 Management of interstitial emphysema by high frequency low pressure hand ventilation in neonates. Journal of Pediatrics 95: 117–118
Normand I C S, Oliver R E, Reynolds E D R, Strang L B, Welch K 1971 Permeability of lung capillaries and alveoli to non-electrolytes in the foetal lamb. Journal of Physiology 219: 303–330
Northway W H, Rosan R C, Porter D Y 1967 Pulmonary disease following respirator therapy of hyaline membrane disease. New England Journal of Medicine 276: 357–367
Peckham G J, Fox W F 1978 Physiologic factors affecting pulmonary artery pressure in infants with persistent pulmonary hypertension. Journal of Pediatrics 93: 1005–1010
Perlman J M, McMenamin J B, Volpe J J 1983 Fluctuating cerebral blood flow velocity in respiratory distress syndrome. New England Journal of Medicine 309: 204–209
Pyati S P, Pildes R S, Jacobs N M et al 1983 Penicillin in infants weighing 2 kg or less with early onset group B streptococcal disease. New England Journal of Medicine 308: 1383–1389
Reynolds E O R, Taghizadeh A 1974 Improved prognosis of infants mechanically ventilated for hyaline membrane disease. Archives of Disease in Childhood 49: 505–515
Robertson N R C, Hallidie-Smith K A, Davis J A 1967 Severe respiratory distress syndrome mimicking cyanotic heart disease in term babies. Lancet ii: 1108–1110
Rushton D I, Preston P R, Durbin G M 1985 Structure and evolution of echo dense lesions in the neonatal brain. Archives of Disease in Childhood 60: 798–800
Shapiro D L, Notter R H, Morin F C 1985 Double blind randomised trial of a calf lung surfactant extract administered at birth to very premature infants for prevention of respiratory distress syndrome. Pediatrics 76: 593–599
Special Report: Foundation for the study of infant death and the British Paediatric Respiratory Group 1985 Apnoea monitors and sudden infant death. Archives of Disease in Childhood 60: 76–80
Speidel B P 1978 Adverse effects of routine procedures on preterm infants. Lancet i: 864–866
Steele R W, Metz J R, Bass J W, Dubois J J 1971 Pneumothorax and pneumomediastinum in the newborn. Radiology 98: 624–632
Thach B, Stark A R 1979 Spontaneous neck flexion and airway obstruction during apneic spells in preterm infants. Journal of Pediatrics 94: 275–281
Thibeault D W, Beatty E C Jr, Hall R T, Bowen S K, O'Neill D H 1985 Neonatal pulmonary hypoplasia with premature rupture of fetal membranes and oligohydramnios. Journal of Pediatrics 107: 273–277
Tueusch H W, Clements J, Benson B 1983 Exogenous surfactant for human lung disease. American Review of Respiratory Disease 128: 795–799
Vyas H, Milner A D, Hopkin I E 1981 Relationship between apnoea and bradycardia in preterm infants. Acta Paediatrica Scandinavica 70: 785–790
Vyas H, Milner A D, Hopkin I E 1982 Amniocentesis and fetal lung development. Archives of Disease in Childhood 57: 627–628
Wesenberg R L, Graven S N, McCabe E B 1971 Radiological findings in wet-lung disease. Radiology 98: 69–74
Wigglesworth J S, Desai R 1981 Use of DNA estimation for growth assessment in normal and hypoplastic fetal lungs. Archives of Disease in Childhood 56: 601–605
Wilkinson A, Jenkins P A, Jeffrey J A 1985 Two controlled trials of dry artificial surfactant: early effects and late outcome in babies with surfactant deficiency. Lancet ii: 287–291
Yancy W S, Spock A 1967 Spontaneous neonatal pleural effusion. Journal of Pediatric Surgery 2: 313–319
Yeh T F, Harris V, Srinivasan Lilien L, Pyati S, Pildes R 1979 Rontgenographic finding in infants with meconium aspiration syndrome. Journal of the American Medical Association 242: 60–63
Yu V Y H, Downe L, Astbury J, Bajuk B 1986a Perinatal factors and adverse outcome in extremely low birthweight infants. Archives of Disease in Childhood 61: 554–558
Yu V Y H, Wong P Y, Bajuk B, Szymonowicz W 1986b Pulmonary air leak in extremely low birthweight infants. Archives of Disease in Childhood 61: 239–241

Low birthweight babies and their problems

Low birthweight is defined by the World Health Organization as a birthweight of less than 2500 g. Low birthweight may be due to preterm delivery (less than 37 weeks' gestation) or intrauterine growth retardation, or both. With improving neonatal care, attention is increasingly focused on infants of birthweight of 1500 g or less who have been designated as very low birthweight (VLBW) infants. Infants of birthweight 1000 g or less have even more problems and are often called extremely low birthweight (ELBW) infants. It has even been suggested that infants of birthweight of 750 g or less should be classified as incredibly low birthweight infants or ILBW! Although babies are often categorized according to birthweight, gestational age is the more important determinant of perinatal mortality and morbidity, but birthweight is still more widely used as it is more readily and accurately determined.

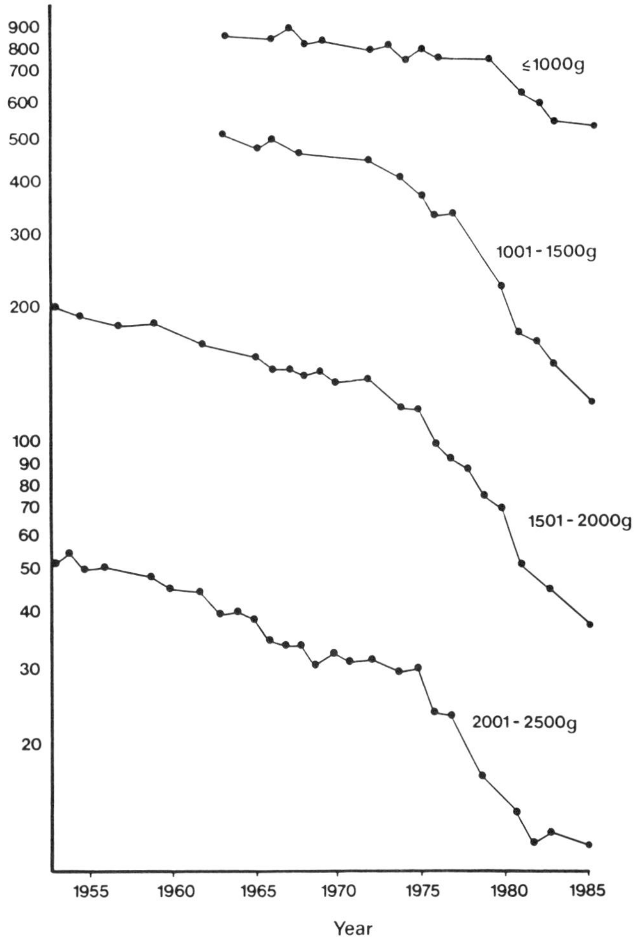

Fig. 71.1 Specific neonatal mortality rates per 1000 live births in England and Wales from 1953 to 1985, according to birthweight. From Pharoah (1986) with permission.

ORGANIZATION OF NEONATAL CARE

Although only 7% of infants in England and Wales are of low birthweight, 66% of neonatal deaths in 1988 were in this group of infants (Office of Population Censuses and Surveys 1988). There has been a steady decline in neonatal mortality for many years, but the widespread introduction of neonatal intensive care in the 1970s was accompanied by an accelerated decline in neonatal mortality in infants of birthweight 1501–2500 g and more recently in VLBW infants (Fig. 71.1). The success of neonatal intensive care in improving the survival rate for smaller and smaller babies has created the need for intensive care to be widely available. Because of the highly specialized nature of the work, requiring skilled medical and nursing staff and an extensive range of support services, intensive care has been provided in regional perinatal centres. These centres not only provide intensive care for infants, but also concentrate expertise in the prevention and management of a wide range of perinatal problems including antenatal diagnosis, the detection and management of congenital malformations and antenatal and intrapartum care of high-risk mothers. Difficult problems may require consultation with people from many different disciplines including paediatrics, obstetrics, surgery, genetics and imaging. The regional perinatal centres also need to be actively involved in the training of nurses, midwives and medical staff, both in the centre and in the district maternity and neonatal units. They should also provide facilities for research to improve perinatal care and for clinical audit.

Intensive care is now also being provided at subregional centres; this is to provide care locally, thus preventing long journeys for the parents. As relatively few mothers and infants need the services of a full perinatal centre it would be unnecessary to provide this in every district maternity unit. Infants requiring artificial ventilation, parenteral nutrition or whose condition is unstable are categorized as intensive care, whereas those needing only extra nursing care and medical supervision, such as tube-feeding or an incubator, are categorized as special care (British Paediatric Association/British Association for Perinatal Paediatrics (BPA/BAPP) 1985; Table 71.1). In the USA the terms primary, secondary and tertiary care facilities are used.

A report prepared by the Joint Standing Committee of The British Paediatric Association and Royal College of Obstetricians and Gynaecologists (BPA/RCOG 1982) suggested that five special care cots and one intensive care cot were required per 1000 births per year. They also suggested a nurse:cot ratio of 1.25:1 for special care and 4:1 for intensive care, although few units achieve these staffing ratios. The optimal ratio is higher at 1.5:1 nurses with neonatal experience for each special care cot and 5:1 nurses with neonatal intensive care experience for each intensive care cot.

With the improved results of neonatal intensive care the number of ELBW infants has increased from 2.3/1000 live births in 1976 to 3/1000 in 1986 in England and Wales (Department of Health and Social Security 1987). This is probably because some of these infants are delivered early rather than allowing the fetus to die in utero and also because many very small babies at less than 28 weeks' gestation are now resuscitated and included in the statistics whereas, in the past they were excluded as they were considered dead at birth and counted as abortions. Unfortunately in the UK there is a shortage of intensive care facilities and specially trained neonatal nurses. In addition there is a shortage of equipment, much of which is sophisticated and expensive; charitable donations have had to be relied upon to purchase it.

In contrast to the increasing requirement of neonatal intensive care the total admissions to baby units in England

Table 71.1 Categories of neonatal care

Intensive care
Babies:
1. a. Receiving assisted ventilation (including intermittent positive airway pressure, intermittent mandatory ventilation and constant positive airway pressure) and in the first 24 hours after its withdrawal
   b. Receiving total parenteral nutrition
2. With cardiorespiratory disease which is unstable, including recurrent apnoea requiring constant attention
3. Who have had major surgery, particularly in the first 24 hours after operation
4. Of less than 30 weeks' gestation during the first 48 hours after birth
5. Who are having convulsions
6. Being transported by intensive care unit staff
7. Undergoing major medical procedures

Special care
Babies:
1. Requiring continuous monitoring of respiration and heart rate, or by transcutaneous transducers
2. Receiving additional oxygen
3. Being given intravenous glucose and electrolyte solutions
4. Being tube-fed
5. Who have had minor surgery in the previous 24 hours
6. With a tracheostomy
7. Who are dying
8. Being barrier nursed
9. Undergoing phototherapy
10. Receiving special monitoring, e.g. frequent glucose or bilirubin estimations
11. Needing constant supervision, e.g. babies of mothers who are drug addicts
12. Being treated with antibiotics
13. With conditions requiring radiological examination or other methods of imaging

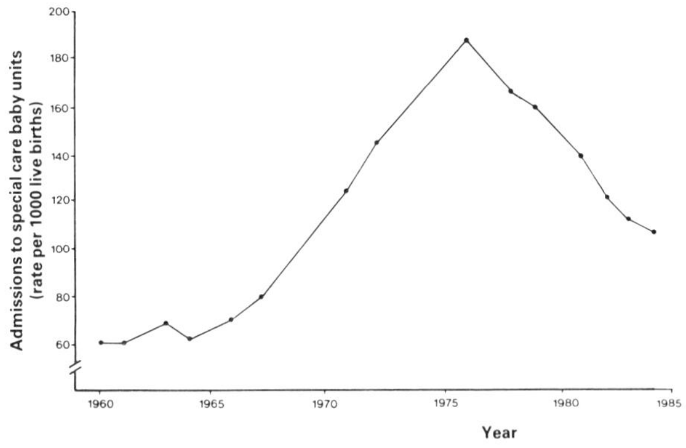

Fig. 71.2 Admission rate per 1000 live births to special care baby units (including intensive care) in England from 1960 to 1984. From Pharoah (1986) with permission.

have actually declined since 1975 (Fig. 71.2). At that time, almost one-fifth of all babies born were admitted, many for observation following an operative delivery. After concern was raised that separation of babies from their mothers could damage the relationship between them, strenuous efforts have been made to reduce the admission rate. Infants who in the past were admitted to provide additional warmth, observation for respiratory illness, monitoring of blood glucose, nasogastric feeding or treatment of jaundice, are now given this additional care on the postnatal ward beside the mother's bed.

IN UTERO OR POSTNATAL TRANSFER?

Most VLBW infants require neonatal intensive care and can only be managed properly in a perinatal centre. If these facilities are not available at the baby's place of birth the infant should be transferred postnatally. Although it is usually possible to do this successfully, there are several disadvantages. The infant needs to be kept in optimal condition before the transport team arrives; if this is not done the infant's prognosis may be jeopardized. Although even very sick infants can be transported successfully by ambulance, helicopter or plane, the journey is not without risk, is expensive and keeps trained medical and nursing staff away from the specialist unit for a considerable time. If there is a shortage of regional intensive care cots, the referring hospital may not be able to transfer the baby. It has been shown that the survival rate of babies with respiratory failure who had been refused admission to a neonatal intensive care unit was less than half that of similar babies accommodated in the intensive care unit (Sims et al 1982). In addition, the mother may be separated from her baby until she is well enough to be transferred; she will then encounter, for the first time, completely different staff.

To overcome these difficulties, high-risk mothers are now more often transferred antenatally to perinatal centres. This has potential advantages. The obstetric and midwifery staff gain experience in dealing with problems which any individual obstetrician would otherwise rarely encounter. It also provides the opportunity for more sophisticated investigation and research. The antenatal care of many of these mothers revolves around the assessment of fetal well-being to plan the optimal time of delivery, weighing the advantages of early delivery against the dangers of prematurity. On the other hand, obstetricians may also be tempted to deliver the woman too early because intensive care is available. Critical analysis and audit of perinatal practice are an essential part of the work of such a centre.

Another major advantage of in utero transfer is that the mother and her family feel reassured that everything possible is being done to help them and the infant. In addition the mother is not separated from her baby.

Whilst in utero transfer may thus appear very attractive, it does have a number of disadvantages. Although the mother may not be separated from her baby, she is often a long distance away from her home and family. In addition, it is not possible to predict accurately whether the fetus will require neonatal intensive care; between 50 and 90% of infants born to mothers transferred antenatally do not need such care. In Manchester only 20% of antenatally transferred infants needed ventilator support (Chiswick 1982). Thus, the stress from separating the mother from her family will often turn out to be unnecessary. In addition, the shortage of resources at specialist centres might mean that cots are filled by relatively well infants whilst sick infants requiring intensive care cannot be admitted.

In a number of studies it has not been possible to show an important difference in perinatal mortality rate by comparing antenatal with postnatal transfer, although the overall mortality rates in all the infants transferred to a perinatal centre were considerably lower than the national average (Crowley et al 1982, Lobb et al 1983).

In order to make an assessment of morbidity rather than mortality, comparisons have been made of the incidence of periventricular haemorrhage (PVH). In a series of infants of comparable birthweight and risk factors, inborn babies had a significantly lower rate of PVH than those transferred postnatally (Clarke et al 1981). A more recent survey from Leeds compared infants of mothers transferred antenatally, infants transferred postnatally and those born to mothers who were booked at the regional centre (Beverley et al 1986). No difference was found in the mortality or the incidence of PVH in the three study populations, after correcting for gestation, birthweight and mode of delivery. Such comparisons are limited in their value by the different selection criteria for each of the groups and the relatively small numbers.

In theory, the best pattern of care might be addressed by a randomized controlled trial, but many doubt that it would be practical to mount. This is because many obstetricians would be unhappy to have a decision about transfer to be taken out of their hands. Rather than asking whether in utero or postnatal transfer is better, we should consider the best balance of the two, since the two forms of transfer complement each other. The high-risk mother and fetus should clearly receive the benefit of referral to a specialist perinatal centre. However with improving obstetric and neonatal care in all maternity units, it should be possible for this to be highly selective. As the birth of some VLBW infants will always be unexpected, it is imperative that all maternity units should provide resuscitation and short-term intensive care. If this is provided, it should rarely be necessary to transfer mothers after 32 weeks' gestation because of preterm labour, pre-eclampsia or ruptured membranes. Better standards of neonatal care in district maternity units will also remove the temptation to transfer the mother when this would be risky. One must avoid having to manage eclampsia, severe haemorrhage or the birth of a very preterm infant during transport. In such situations, it is better for the baby to be born at the district hospital and then transferred if necessary.

RESUSCITATION

A major part of modern perinatal care is directed towards the prevention of birth asphyxia. In an unselected sample

Table 71.2 Percentage of the infants requiring intermittent positive pressure ventilation (IPPV) for resuscitation (McDonald et al 1980)

Gestation (weeks)	Number of births	% requiring IPPV
≤28	173	49
29–32	288	18
33–34	415	8
35–36	1340	2
37–38	5895	0.7
≥39	24 726	0.4

of 760 deliveries of all gestational ages at St Mary's Hospital, London, preterm infants did not have a significantly lower umbilical arterial pH or base deficit but many had a low Apgar score at 1 minute (Lissauer & Steer, unpublished data). This reflects the difficulty preterm infants have in establishing normal respiration. This is due to a combination of factors, including analgesic and anaesthetic agents given to the mother, difficulty in clearing lung liquid, a highly compliant rib cage, relatively weak respiratory muscles and stiff, surfactant-deficient lungs. All preterm deliveries should therefore be attended by a person skilled in neonatal resuscitation. When the delivery of an infant of less than 32 weeks' gestation is expected two trained staff should attend.

The labour ward must be as warm as possible, without being unpleasant for the mother and staff. A radiant heater is needed above the resuscitation table, draughts should be avoided and a warm towel should be available for the baby. As most of the immediate heat loss is by evaporation from the wet and naked infant, the assistant should dry the baby rapidly; the wet towel must then be discarded and the baby wrapped in another dry, warm towel or covered with semi-transparent bubble plastic.

Resuscitation by endotracheal ventilation is often required in preterm infants (Table 71.2). All infants under 32 weeks' gestation should be intubated unless they are pink and crying immediately after birth (Drew 1982). Active resuscitation probably prevents secondary surfactant deficiency by avoiding hypoxia and therefore reduces the incidence and severity of respiratory distress syndrome and mortality. Hypoxia and hypercarbia are implicated in PVH and cerebral ischaemia and therefore must be avoided.

In order to expand the lungs, positive pressure ventilation lasting 3–5 seconds is recommended for the first breath and 1–2 seconds for each breath thereafter. A pressure sufficient to obtain adequate chest movement is used, but should rarely be more than 30 cmH_2O.

In addition to the establishment of ventilation one must also check that the infant has an adequate cardiac output. Prompt cardiac massage is needed not only after cardiac arrest but when there is bradycardia with poor perfusion.

Drugs are very rarely needed in the labour ward. The main treatment for acidaemia is the provision of adequate ventilation and circulation to prevent hypercarbia, hypoxaemia and lactic acidaemia. As sodium bicarbonate dissociates to carbon dioxide it may make the acidaemia worse if ventilation is inadequate and the carbon dioxide is not removed. It may be thought to be useful to give sodium bicarbonate where there is a profound metabolic acidaemia in spite of adequate ventilation, such as following cardiac arrest or continuing hypoxaemia despite resuscitation. A dose of 1–2 mmol/kg can then be given as a slow injection through an umbilical venous catheter over several minutes; thereafter it is only given according to the results of blood gas analysis. Adrenaline (1 : 10 000, 0.1 ml/kg) is sometimes used for cardiac arrest which has not responded to resuscitation. It can be administered through an umbilical venous catheter or, more readily, down the endotracheal tube.

VLBW infants should be transferred to the neonatal unit in a portable incubator. If required, artificial ventilation should be maintained during the journey. If possible, the parents should be given the opportunity to see, touch and hold their baby.

Table 71.3 Stabilization of VLBW infants on arrival in the neonatal unit

1. *Warmth*
   Nurse under overhead heater or incubator
2. *Initial ventilation settings*
   Rate: 30–60 breaths/min
   Inspiratory time 0.5 seconds
   Peak pressure 18–20 cmH_2O
   End expiratory pressure 3–4 cmH_2O
   These settings are adjusted according to colour, chest wall movement, pattern of breathing and blood gas analysis
3. *Monitoring*
   Heart rate, respiratory rate and temperature are monitored continuously
   Oxygen requirements by transcutaneous PO_2 or oxygen saturation
   Transcutaneous PCO_2 is also useful
   Blood pressure
   Arterial blood gas analysis measured frequently if additional oxygen is required
   Arterial catheter inserted if oxygen concentration of more than 30% is required
4. *Circulatory support*
   Intravenous dextrose
   Colloid (10 ml/kg) as required
5. *Blood glucose*
   Monitor 4–6-hourly by glucose oxidase strips
6. *Antibiotic therapy*
   Started if respiratory distress or risk of infection, after blood culture
7. *Other initial investigations*
   Full blood count, urea and electrolytes, calcium, clotting studies if indicated, blood group; sample saved for cross-matching
8. *Radiograph*
   X-ray of chest and abdomen, including position of the endotracheal tube and arterial catheter
9. *Parents*
   The baby's condition and any change must be fully discussed with the parents

INITIAL STABILIZATION OF VLBW INFANTS (Table 71.3)

On arrival in the neonatal unit, the infant must be kept warm. The baby is weighed quickly during transfer from the transport incubator. A careful, gentle and rapid examination is very important or congenital abnormalities will be missed.

Ventilation

Many VLBW infants and the majority of infants of less than 30 weeks' gestation need initial ventilatory support whether or not they have respiratory distress syndrome (RDS). This is essential for survival as a baby who becomes hypoxic and hypercarbic develops a vicious cycle of further hypoxia, atelectasis, circulatory failure, and secondary surfactant deficiency leading to death. This can be prevented by good ventilation and adequate oxygenation.

Circulation

This should be first assessed clinically by heart rate and skin perfusion. Systolic blood pressure is best measured with a sphygmomanometer using as large a cuff as possible and Doppler ultrasound to detect the pulse. Poor peripheral perfusion may be evident from a wide central–peripheral temperature difference (greater than 2.5°C) and metabolic acidosis.

If the infant's circulation appears to be unsatisfactory in spite of adequate ventilation or if the systolic blood pressure is below 45 mmHg, the blood volume should be expanded with colloid. This may be blood if the baby is anaemic, fresh frozen plasma if there is marked bruising or clotting abnormalities, or albumin if there is none of these. If the blood pressure and perfusion do not improve, inotropic drugs, such as dopamine, may be used. An intravenous infusion of 10% dextrose is usually given to VLBW infants initially to prevent hypoglycaemia because it is not advisable to give milk and enteral feeds until these babies are stabilized.

Monitoring

Continuous monitoring of heart rate, respiratory rate and temperature is started on arrival in the unit. The infant's oxygenation should be measured to prevent hypoxia, which may result in ischaemic damage, or hyperoxaemia, which may produce retinopathy of prematurity (retrolental fibroplasia). The PaO_2 is kept between 7 and 12 kPa (50–90 mmHg).

An initial arterial sample is taken by puncture of the radial or posterior tibial arteries. Thereafter, oxygen therapy is best monitored by the insertion of an arterial catheter, either into the lower aorta through an umbilical artery, or by cannulation of a peripheral artery. The baby should be warm and stable before cannulation is performed. An umbilical arterial catheter incorporating an oxygen electrode is preferable so that a continuous record of PaO_2 is obtained. In infants less than 1 kg this may be not possible because only a smaller end-hole catheter can be inserted. When an arterial cannula has been inserted, it can also be used for continuous blood pressure measurement and to obtain blood for investigations.

Oxygen tension can also be measured transcutaneously and is now often combined with measurement of the carbon dioxide tension. The transcutaneous electrode should be placed on the right upper chest so that it measures the oxygen in blood flowing from the aorta proximal to the ductus arteriosus. This will more closely reflect the oxygenation of blood flowing to the brain if there is a right-to-left shunt through the ductus. Hypotension and poor peripheral perfusion will cause transcutaneous oxygen monitors to under-read and they should always be checked by arterial blood gas analysis at regular intervals, and after changes in the infant's condition or oxygen therapy.

Oxygen saturation monitors have recently been introduced. They have the advantage that the skin does not need to be heated but high oxygen saturation must be avoided as it may be associated with hyperoxaemia. In the immediate newborn period, a saturation of 92% is considered optimal for babies in oxygen (Southall et al 1987).

A chest X-ray will provide information not only about the infant's lungs, but will also confirm the position of the endotracheal tube and umbilical artery catheter.

Metabolic treatment

Blood glucose must be checked regularly and an intravenous infusion containing 10% dextrose given to prevent hypoglycaemia. Additional glucose is given intravenously to correct hypoglycaemia when it occurs. Hypocalcaemia is also common and calcium gluconate (1 mmol/kg/day) is often infused parenterally.

Antibiotic therapy

Preterm infants are at increased risk of infection. In addition, group B beta-haemolytic streptococcal infection can be indistinguishable from RDS. The authors therefore give appropriate intravenous antibiotics to all infants with any signs of respiratory distress or serious illness. Penicillin or ampicillin and gentamicin are widely used. A blood culture is taken and also surface swabs for culture; a swab from the auditory meatus is used as a measure of amniotic cavity colonization at birth.

Minimal handling

All procedures, expecially painful ones, have an adverse effect on oxygenation and the circulation (Speidel 1978). Handling of preterm infants should be kept to a minimum, although important investigations have to be performed and the infants' progress must be closely observed. All procedures should be done as rapidly and efficiently as possible by experienced staff; analgesia should be given before painful procedures.

Fluid balance

The fluid requirements of VLBW infants are highly variable during the first few days of life. Transepidermal water loss varies markedly with changes in the skin texture at different gestational ages and will be markedly increased if the infant is nursed under a radiant heater or has phototherapy. Usually, 40–60 ml/day of fluid is sufficient on the first day, excluding colloid support. This must be reassessed 2–3 times a day during the first few days of life. Fluid intake should be adjusted according to urine output and its specific gravity or osmolality, after assessment of the infant's peripheral circulation, oedema, acid–base balance and blood pressure. It is also important to assess the urea and electrolytes; initially this will need to be performed 1–3 times per day.

Hyponatraemia may occur in VLBW babies because of their high urinary sodium loss, as may hypernatraemia as a result of dehydration from excess water loss.

Parents

Although the initial stabilization usually keeps the medical and nursing staff fully occupied, time must be found for the parents to allow them to see their baby and for a full explanation of the various problems. When delivery has been by Caesarean section, the paediatrician must visit the mother on the labour or postnatal ward. Instant photographs of the baby and booklets about the unit and the management of preterm babies are of considerable help to parents.

SPECIFIC PROBLEMS OF LBW INFANTS

The problems of LBW infants depend on whether they are preterm or small-for-gestational-age (SGA). SGA is normally defined as an infant whose birthweight is below the tenth centile for his or her gestation; most such babies are normal. Sometimes the term is confined to infants of birthweight below the third centile as they are more likely to have problems. The infant who has been poorly nourished only in the latter part of pregnancy is likely to lack subcutaneous fat but to be of normal length and head size. Those with prolonged intrauterine growth retardation are also small in length and head size — symmetrical growth retardation.

Preterm infants have many problems due to immaturity. Problems of respiration, temperature regulation, jaundice, nutrition, neurology, patent ductus arteriosus and anaemia are described in this chapter. Some of the ethical dilemmas and problems for parents will be outlined and the results of long-term neurodevelopmental outcome reviewed. Asphyxia, birth injuries and infection are described in other chapters.

SGA infants have fewer neonatal problems, although the SGA infant is at increased risk of intrauterine hypoxia and death. Using cordocentesis, it has been shown that some very severely growth-retarded fetuses are already hypoxic and acidotic during the second trimester. The growth-retarded infant is more likely to become asphyxiated during labour and delivery. Although these babies are often thought to be at risk of meconium aspiration, this is mainly related to gestational age and it is postmaturity that places an infant at most risk, particularly when accompanied by birth asphyxia. Malformations (see Chapter 67) are commoner in SGA infants, as are chromosomal abnormalities, prenatal viral infections and dysmorphic syndromes, although they are in themselves uncommon causes of growth retardation. Hypoglycaemia is more common in SGA infants because of reduced glycogen stores to break down glucose; these babies do not have fat to produce ketones as an alternative brain metabolite. These infants should be monitored 4-hourly for 24–48 hours to detect hypoglycaemia at an early stage whilst it is still asymptomatic. Monitoring is especially important whilst breastfeeding is being established. These infants are also more prone to hypothermia and will need an appropriately warm environment. They are more likely to be polycythaemic (venous haematocrit ⩾65%), which may require treatment with an isovolaemic, dilutional exchange transfusion.

Respiratory problems

A major part of the care of LBW babies is concerned with the management of respiratory problems (see Chapter 70). Short gestation is the main factor in the incidence of RDS, although factors such as asphyxia may make it worse. The incidence of RDS at term is only 0.01%, whereas it occurs in one-third of those born at 27–28 weeks' gestation (Field & Milner 1986). Many infants under 28 weeks' gestation will require ventilation, even if the classical features of RDS are absent. This is because the alveoli are not yet sufficiently developed, respiratory muscles are feeble, atelectasis occurs and there is frequent and recurrent apnoea.

Although the overall mortality rate of infants of birthweight over 1000 g with RDS has dropped from 10% in the early 1970s (Roberton & Tizard 1975) to 5% in the 1980s (Greenough & Roberton 1985), the severity of an infant's respiratory disease remains a major determinant of his or her neonatal course and outcome. Those infants who require artificial ventilation are more likely to have pulmonary interstitial emphysema, pneumothorax and chronic lung disease (bronchopulmonary dysplasia). It also places them at increased risk of PVH and cerebral ischaemia, difficulty in establishing feeding and many of the other disorders associated with prematurity. The incidence of apnoeic attacks is also largely determined by the infant's gestation. They occur in the majority of neonates of under 30 weeks' gestation, in about 50% at 30–32 weeks but in only 7% at 34–35 weeks (Henderson-Smart 1981).

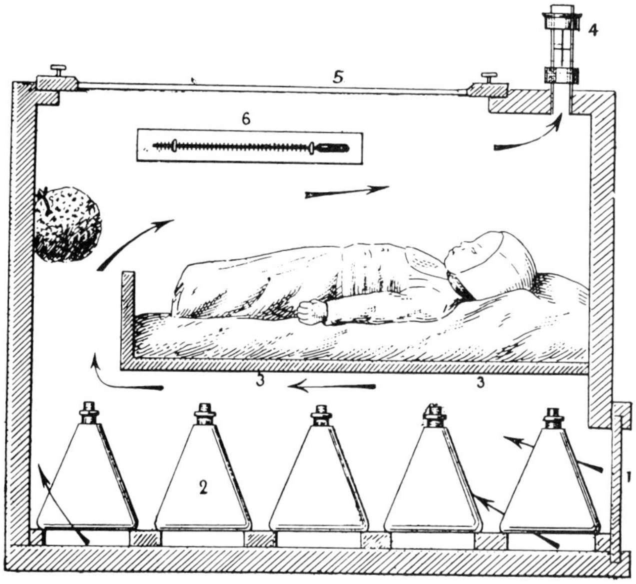

Fig. 71.3 An incubator used in Paris at the end of the 19th century.

Temperature control

Incubators and overhead radiant heaters are used to maintain the temperature of small babies but nevertheless these infants may easily develop hypothermia. Newborn infants have a larger surface area relative to their body weight than do older children. Heat production at rest per unit of surface area in a term infant is only about half of that of an adult, and it is lower still in the preterm. As the surface area determines heat loss, newborn infants require a warmer environment than older children or adults; the preterm infant needs to be kept even warmer. Such infants do not shiver, cannot curl up and are usually nursed naked to allow proper observation; this adds to their difficulties in maintaining body temperature.

The effects of hypothermia include reduced surfactant synthesis, hypoxaemia, hypoglycaemia, acidaemia, increased oxygen consumption, weight loss, deranged blood coagulation and neonatal cold injury. A cold environment increases mortality (Silverman et al 1958, Stanley & Alberman 1978) and the improved survival of preterm infants if they are kept warm has long been recognized (Fig. 71.3).

Heat production

Non-shivering thermogenesis in brown fat is the major mechanism of heat production in the first few weeks of life. Oxygen consumption is increased when the environment is too cold or hot and there is therefore a neutral temperature range when the infant's oxygen consumption is minimal; this is most suitable for nursing these babies. The neutral temperature is higher in preterm, small, young and naked babies (Fig. 71.4).

Heat loss

Heat loss is by evaporation, conduction, convection and radiation. In a term infant evaporative heat loss amounts to only a quarter of the resting heat production, mostly by transepidermal water loss (TEWL). In the preterm baby, TEWL is much higher as the skin is thin and poorly keratanized. The TEWL of an infant of 26 weeks' gestation is up to six times higher per unit surface area than in term infants (Hammarlund & Sedin 1979). Evaporative losses are further increased by exposure to a radiant warmer or phototherapy. Ambient humidity has a marked effect on TEWL; the loss of heat is lower if infants are nursed in humidified air.

Hypothermia occurs when a baby is not able to produce enough heat in a cool environment. Normal body temperature does not necessarily imply that the ambient temperature is satisfactory. However, infants are able to maintain their body temperature when subjected to cold by increasing heat production and oxygen consumption.

Incubators and radiant warmers

Healthy newborn infants weighing more than 1.5 kg at birth should preferably be clothed and nursed in a warm room. For infants of 1.5–2 kg, the room temperature will need to be about 26°C, and for those over 2 kg it should be about 24°C to achieve a neutral thermal environment. Clothing more than doubles the resistance to heat loss. In infants the head is a large part of the surface area and woollen bonnets will increase thermal insulation. An incubator or radiant warmer is needed for babies of less than 1.5 kg or sick infants who require constant observation. Infants nursed naked in an incubator lose heat by radiation and evaporation. Radiant heat loss can be reduced by keeping the neonatal unit very hot (26–28°C), by using incubators with double walls and by covering the baby with a plastic heat shield or with an insulating fabric such as bubble plastic. Evaporative heat loss can be minimized by humidification which has been recommended for infants below 30 weeks' gestation for the first week of life (Harpin & Rutter 1985). Without humidification these infants may have an evaporative heat loss which exceeds their metabolic heat production. The disadvantage of humidification is that moisture may condense on the inside of the incubator and there is a risk of colonization with *Pseudomonas* which flourishes in a damp environment.

The main disadvantage of incubators is the lack of accessibility for staff and parents. Practical procedures, especially those done in an emergency, are much more awkward to perform when babies are nursed inside incubators.

Sick or preterm infants can also be nursed naked under radiant warmers. The output of the heater is adjusted according to the infant's skin temperature. This has the considerable advantage of allowing total access to the baby; radiant heaters are more effective in keeping very immature babies warm. Their main disadvantages are that the evaporative

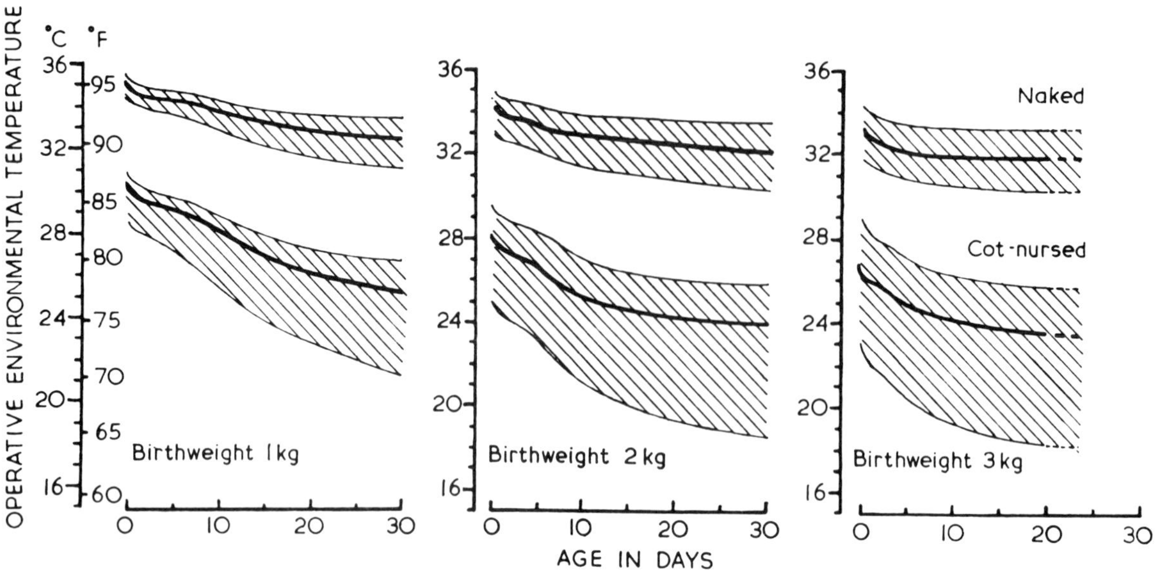

Fig. 71.4 Temperature at which to nurse newborn babies in a draught-free environment. The bold line indicates the optimal temperature; shaded areas show the range of temperature at which the baby can maintain a normal body temperature. From Hey (1971).

heat loss is considerably higher because of increased water loss from the skin, which makes the control of fluid balance more difficult. In addition heat loss by convection is increased from draught. This can be reduced by covering the infant with an insulating fabric.

Jaundice

Bilirubin is a breakdown product of haemoglobin and is produced in newborn infants at over twice the rate per kg body weight as in adults. Newborn infants are often jaundiced because of this increased bilirubin load and their metabolism of bilirubin is less well developed. The bilirubin is unconjugated and is bound to albumin in plasma. It is taken up into the liver and converted by the enzyme glucuronyl transferase to conjugated bilirubin which is excreted in bile into the gut. Within the gut some of the conjugated bilirubin is deconjugated and resorbed into the enterohepatic circulation, thus adding to the total bilirubin load. In term infants the maximum bilirubin level is reached at 60–72 hours of age and then declines. In preterm infants the maximum level is reached earlier and jaundice persists for longer.

Kernicterus is yellow staining of the basal ganglia with histological evidence of neuronal damage. It has been proposed that this is caused by unconjugated bilirubin which is not bound to albumin and circulates as free bilirubin; the free bilirubin enters brain cells and damages them. Neuronal damage may also occur when the blood–brain barrier is damaged by factors such as asphyxia. VLBW infants are at increased risk of kernicterus as jaundice is common and their plasma albumin is low. Babies with kernicterus may die in the neonatal period but if they survive they may develop cerebral palsy, usually of the choreoathetoid type, mental

Table 71.4 Bilirubin levels at which to start phototherapy or perform an exchange transfusion. The rate of rise of the bilirubin (Fig. 71.5) must also be taken into account

	Bilirubin level (μmol/l)		
		Exchange transfusion	
Gestation (weeks)	Phototherapy	Well infant	Ill infant or haemolysis
24	100	200	160
28	140	240	200
32	180	300	260
36	240	340	300
40	320	400	340

retardation and sensorineural deafness. As this high-tone deafness is seen more frequently in VLBW infants, there has been concern that it may result from a high level of prolonged hyperbilirubinaemia. However, assessing the possible damage of hyperbilirubinaemia is complicated by the other potentially ototoxic factors to which these infants are also exposed, such as aminoglycoside antibiotics, hypoxia, recurrent apnoea, sepsis, and noise from within the incubator. In term infants with haemolytic jaundice from rhesus disease kernicterus can almost always be prevented if the maximum bilirubin is kept below 340 μmol/l (20 mg/dl). Although it is not known what level of bilirubin is neurotoxic in preterm infants, the shorter the infant's gestational age, the lower the maximum level to which the bilirubin is allowed to rise. Tables and charts have been constructed as a guide in the practical management of jaundice (Table 71.4, Fig. 71.5). They will need revision as further follow-up data become available.

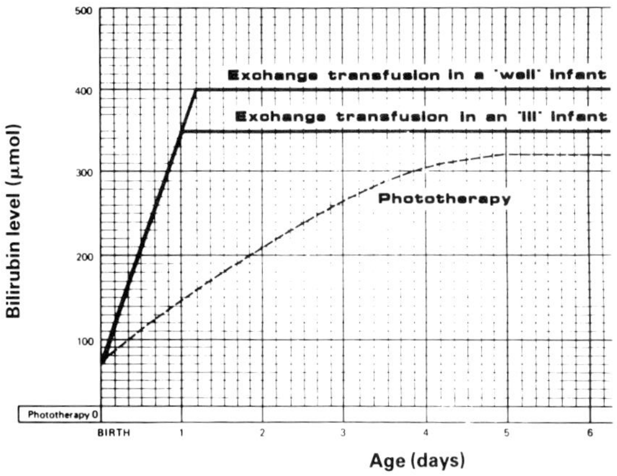

Fig. 71.5 Suggested levels of plasma bilirubin at which to treat a term infant with phototherapy or exchange transfusion. Serial bilirubin levels should be plotted to anticipate a potentially toxic level.

The treatment of jaundice is with phototherapy or exchange transfusion. Light converts bilirubin into harmless pigments; the blue wavelengths are the most effective. Although less effective, white light is often used as it does not make the baby look cyanosed or induce nausea among some of the staff. The effectiveness of phototherapy is related to the energy of the light (its irradiance); as this varies with the square root of the distance between the baby and the light source the baby needs to be nursed close to the light and the irradiance of the light source at the baby needs to be checked.

No long-term sequelae of phototherapy have been reported. However, as the baby is nursed exposed, there is a risk of hypo- or hyperthermia. An increased fluid intake is needed because of the marked fluid loss through the skin and gut. Decreased gut transit time may cause diarrhoea, probably from increased flow of bilirubin degradation products into the gut. There is often an erythematous rash. Light should not be used for infants with conjugated bilirubinaemia or the skin becomes bronzed. There are animal data suggesting that phototherapy can cause retinal damage. It is therefore standard practice to cover the eyes, despite the lack of evidence of problems in humans. Eye patches often cause considerable anxiety in mothers, particularly when they slip off; it is also distressing to see the baby naked during treatment, therefore phototherapy should not be used indiscriminately.

Phototherapy is effective in reducing the maximum serum bilirubin and the number of exchange transfusions required for physiological jaundice (Brown et al 1985). It would seem reasonable to start phototherapy early for infants of less than 30 weeks' gestation, or in any who are ill or bruised. For more mature infants the level of jaundice can be monitored and phototherapy started if the bilirubin concentration exceeds the predetermined levels. With this approach it is rarely necessary to perform an exchange transfusion unless there is a haemolytic cause of the infant's jaundice.

NUTRITION

Most preterm infants need assistance with feeding. Those of less than 34 weeks' gestation are usually unable to suck sufficiently well to feed on their own; those below 30 weeks gestation are often unable to tolerate enteral feeds initially. This is partly because of poor absorption but also as a result of respiratory or other illnesses.

Breastfeeding

It is possible to establish breastfeeding in most preterm infants even if they require intensive care. Expressed breast milk can be given straight to the infant but in most cases it will need to be stored. The establishment of full breastfeeding for VLBW infants will take several weeks, during which the mother will need to express her milk; she will have to be well motivated and be given support and encouragement by the staff. There are various methods of milk expression, using hand expression or a syringe or electrical pump. The mother's production of prolactin during expression is not as good as when infants suckle well at the breast and mothers of VLBW infants have a higher failure rate of establishing breastfeeding.

It has been reported that the milk of mothers of preterm infants has a higher protein and mineral content than that expressed by mothers of term infants (Lemons et al 1982). This was thought to correspond with the preterm infant's higher protein and sodium requirements than term infants, though some doubt has recently been cast on this. Some VLBW infants appear to tolerate breast milk somewhat better than formula, but its energy content is lower and growth is slower than on formula. Breastfed preterm infants often become hyponatraemic because of their increased urine sodium loss and sodium supplements are often required, as are additional phosphate and calcium.

Banked breast milk has the disadvantage that it contains a lower concentration of protein and minerals and fat than breast milk expressed by the infant's mother. This is particularly true of drip breast milk collected from the other breast during feeding. This milk is very dilute and is particularly low in fat. After it has been collected at home it must be frozen and samples should be tested with careful microbiological examination; milk is discarded if it is very heavily contaminated or contains dangerous organisms. All such milk should also be heat-treated, despite the disadvantage that its anti-infective properties are reduced. This heat treatment is particularly important in view of the recent concern over the possible spread of human immunodeficiency virus (HIV) by banked breast milk.

Formula feeds

Standard infant formula has been modified to make it resemble breast milk more closely, with a reduced mineral content and modified protein, amino acids and fats. To take account of the particular requirements of preterm infants special preterm infant formulae have been introduced. These contain a higher concentration of protein and minerals and additional sodium, phosphate and calcium.

Feeding preterm infants

Nasogastric feeding

In order to avoid hypoglycaemia, preterm infants should be fed with milk within 1–2 hours of birth via a nasogastric tube if necessary. Most infants of less than 30 weeks' gestation are not sufficiently well in the first 48 hours to be given enteral feeds. This is because of the risk of regurgitation and aspiration of milk, even if given into the stomach by a nasogastric tube. Respiration can be compromised by gastric distension from the feed and from nasal obstruction caused by the tube. Food absorption is also often poor under these circumstances and an intravenous infusion of glucose is usually required whilst these infants are being stabilized. Once the infant's condition has improved it may be possible to start enteral feeding. The volume of milk is steadily increased and absorption is checked by regular aspiration of the stomach to reduce the risk of complications. The milk can be infused continuously via a syringe pump or as a bolus given frequently.

Transpyloric feeding

In infants with an increased respiratory rate or apnoeic attacks it may be preferable to give the milk via a transpyloric tube to bypass the stomach. A disadvantage of this technique is that it is more difficult to position the Silastic feeding tube correctly and steatorrhoea is more likely. The maximum volume of milk infused is also usually limited to 150 ml/kg/day as larger volumes often cause abdominal distension. Enteral feeding should be discontinued if there is failure of absorption, as evidenced by increased aspiration or regurgitation, abdominal distension, significant apnoeic attacks shortly after extubation or if the baby is seriously ill.

Parenteral nutrition

Parenteral nutrition will be required to supplement or replace enteral feeding when this is inadequate or has to be discontinued. As VLBW infants may have only sufficient caloric reserves to support 4–6 days of extrauterine life, it is clearly vital to provide adequate nutrition for them when enteral feeding is not possible. This occurs most often in VLBW infants on artificial ventilation for RDS at a few days of age and in whom there is a delay in establishing full enteral feeds.

Total parenteral nutrition is also required in infants with necrotizing enterocolitis or following bowel surgery. It should not be given whilst infants are acutely ill, if they are markedly jaundiced or in renal failure. Parenteral nutrition can be given for short periods via a cannula in a peripheral vein but the infusion site needs to be observed very carefully as extravasation may result in tissue necrosis and scarring. Venous access is often very difficult as one rapidly runs out of suitable veins. Long-term parenteral nutrition is best given via a central catheter placed in the right atrium.

Parenteral nutrition in preterm infants should not be undertaken outside a fully equipped intensive care unit with experienced medical, nursing and pharmacy staff and laboratory back-up. The infants need to be meticulously monitored for complications, the commonest and most serious of which is infection, but which also include hyperglycaemia, fluid and electrolyte imbalance, metabolic acidosis and cholestatic jaundice. Parenteral feeding is also very expensive.

Rickets

Preterm infants are prone to rickets or, more correctly, osteopenia of prematurity. Their bones may become poorly mineralized and in more severe cases the metaphyses become splayed and cupped and fractures may occur. This is probably caused by a deficiency of phosphorus and calcium in milk, particularly breast milk. This is made worse by vitamin D deficiency and excessive urine loss of phosphorus and calcium. The incidence and severity can be markedly reduced by giving additional phosphate and calcium to maintain plasma levels in the normal range and by giving additional vitamin D supplements.

Growth

Most infants lose 5–10% of their body weight in the first few days of life. This may be accentuated in preterm infants with their higher body water content. Thereafter it is important to try to meet the infant's nutritional requirements, although in VLBW infants requiring prolonged artificial ventilation, growth is often static during the first few weeks. Although intrauterine growth rates are widely used as a yardstick for growth, in practice one has to accept the fastest attainable growth without causing metabolic upset. Whether these short periods of suboptimal nutrition cause long-term sequelae is unknown. Preterm infants require 215 kJ/kg/day for maintenance even when nursed in a thermoneutral environment and a further 252 kJ/kg/day to obtain the desired 10–15 g/kg/day weight gain. An intake of 180–200 ml/kg/day of infant formula should provide an infant with an energy intake of 517–574 kJ/kg/day, so any reduction in intake will result in suboptimal nutrition.

NEUROLOGY

Periventricular haemorrhage (PVH) and cerebral ischaemia are now the major causes of morbidity and mortality in low birthweight infants. PVH occurs in the rich network of fragile capillary vessels which lie alongside each lateral ventricle. The haemorrhage begins under the lining of the ventricle in the germinal matrix and then may burst into the ventricle or the parenchyma of the brain. The main complications result from this spread; intraventricular blood may lead to ventricular dilatation and hydrocephalus, while parenchymal haemorrhage destroys the brain substance. The relationship between haemorrhage and ischaemic lesions is complex and incompletely understood. Ischaemic lesions may in time become cystic and filled with cerebrospinal fluid. Cystic degeneration commonly occurs lateral to the occipital horns or the angle of the lateral ventricle and this lesion is called periventricular leukomalacia. The haemorrhage may be the primary lesion but it is now thought that it can also result from bleeding into an ischaemic area.

Pathogenesis

The more preterm the baby, the higher the incidence of PVH. About one-half of all VLBW infants have evidence of PVH on ultrasound. Most of the lesions occur within 3 days of birth. Infants most at risk are those who have experienced asphyxia or who have RDS. Episodes of hypoxia, hypotension and acidosis also increase the risk of haemorrhage. It has been proposed that these cause abrupt changes in cerebral blood flow, leading to haemorrhage from rupture of the fragile capillaries in the germinal layer, or ischaemic damage (Pape & Wigglesworth 1979). There is some evidence that changes in systemic blood flow are transmitted directly to the cerebral circulation in these small ill babies (Lou et al 1979). A pneumothorax is a common precursor of haemorrhage; it is known to cause a sudden rise in blood pressure as well as hypoxaemia, hypercarbia and increased venous pressure. Similar abrupt changes are seen following blockage or dislodgement of an endotracheal tube.

Signs and symptoms

Small haemorrhages cannot usually be recognized clinically. After a large haemorrhage, the infant may become limp, unresponsive, pale and develop convulsions—although these may be difficult to recognize without a continuous electroencephalogram record. Other signs are apnoea, hypotension, peripheral vasoconstriction and acidosis. There may be an unexplained drop in the infant's haemoglobin. After a very large haemorrhage, the fontanelle becomes tense and the head circumference increases suddenly. Such an infant may fail to respond to resuscitation.

Diagnosis

A decade ago most PVH was only diagnosed at post-mortem examination. Although computerized tomography scanning showed haemorrhage it was not until ultrasound that haemorrhage and certain ischaemic lesions could be identified regularly in all high-risk infants. The major advantage of ultrasound is that it is non-invasive and can be performed whilst the infant is undergoing intensive care. Although there are several systems of grading PVH on ultrasound they are often described as:

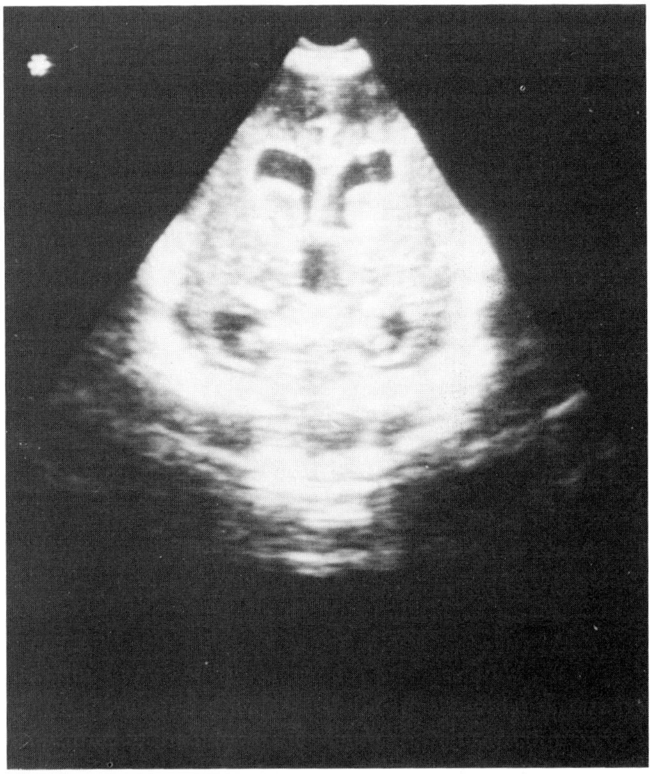

Fig. 71.6 Bilateral intraventricular haemorrhage with moderate ventricular dilatation on coronal intracranial ultrasound scans. There is echogenic clot in both lateral ventricles arising from the germinal matrix.

1. Normal.
2. Small haemorrhage where the echodense lesion is around the germinal matrix (grade I).
3. Intraventricular haemorrhage, where echoes are visible within the lateral ventricles (grades II and III; Fig. 71.6).
4. Parenchymal haemorrhage (Fig. 71.7) where the echodense area involves the parenchyma (grade IV). In surviving infants this may be replaced by a porencephalic cyst (Fig. 71.8). Ischaemic lesions may be identified by echodense areas lateral to the ventricles or as cysts (Fig. 71.9).

Ventricular dilatation

Ventricular dilatation can be readily shown and measured by ultrasound (Fig. 71.10). The dilatation may or may not progress. Aggressive ventricular dilatation usually requires treatment. If the dilatation is progressing it may be possible to keep it in check by removing cerebrospinal fluid by

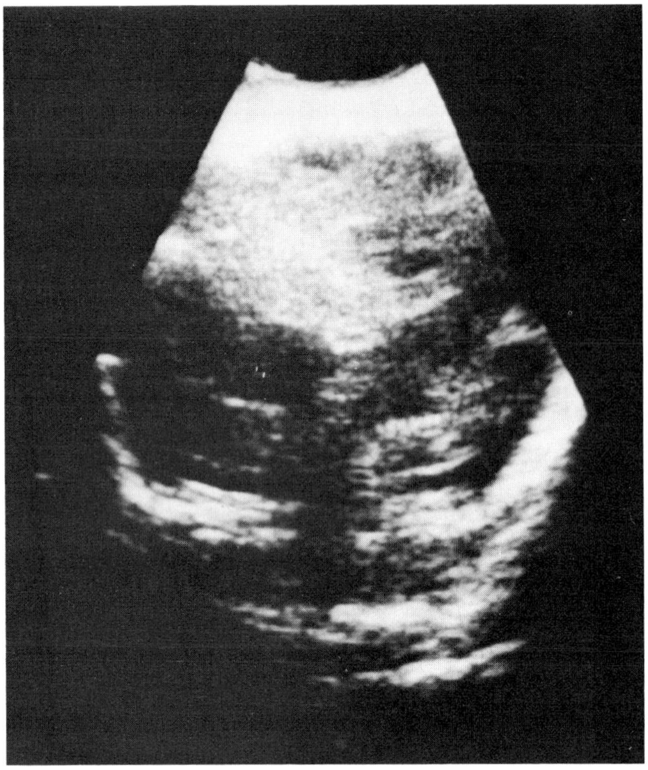

Fig. 71.7 Intracranial ultrasound showing a parenchymal haemorrhage on the right on coronal scan.

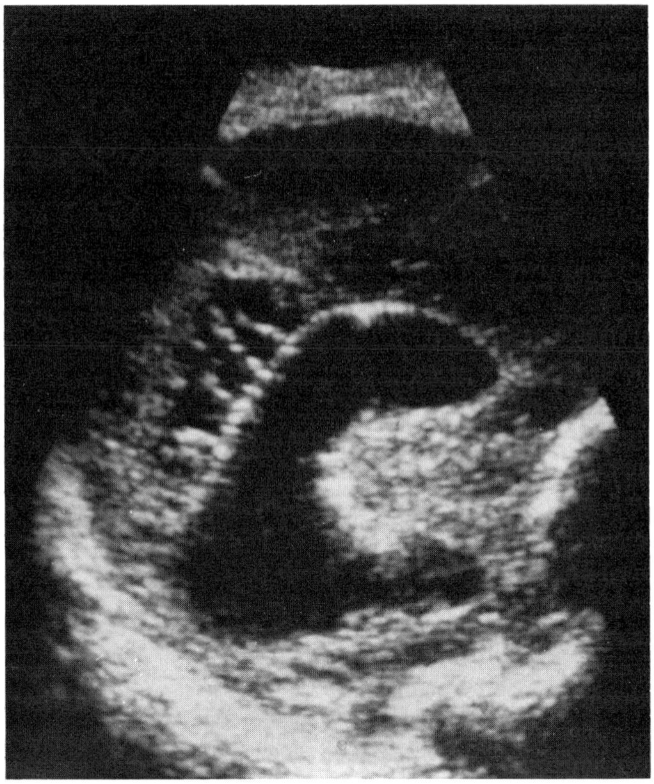

Fig. 71.8 Porencephalic cavity on coronal ultrasound scan on the right which developed following the parenchymal haemorrhage shown in Figure 71.7. The infant has a left hemiplegia.

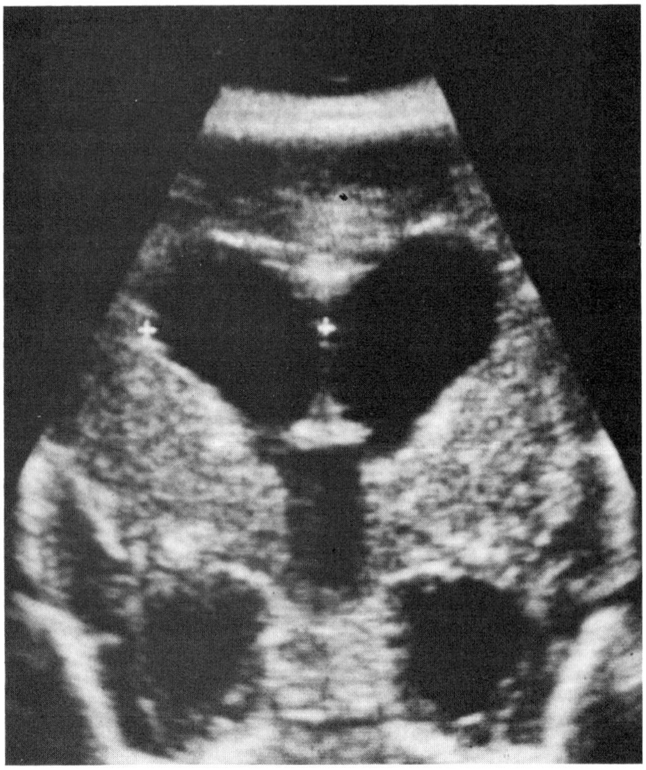

Fig. 71.9 Cystic periventricular leukomalacia on sagittal intracranial ultrasound scan. Extensive echo-free cystic areas of varying size can be seen in the periventricular white matter. The ventricle is moderately dilated.

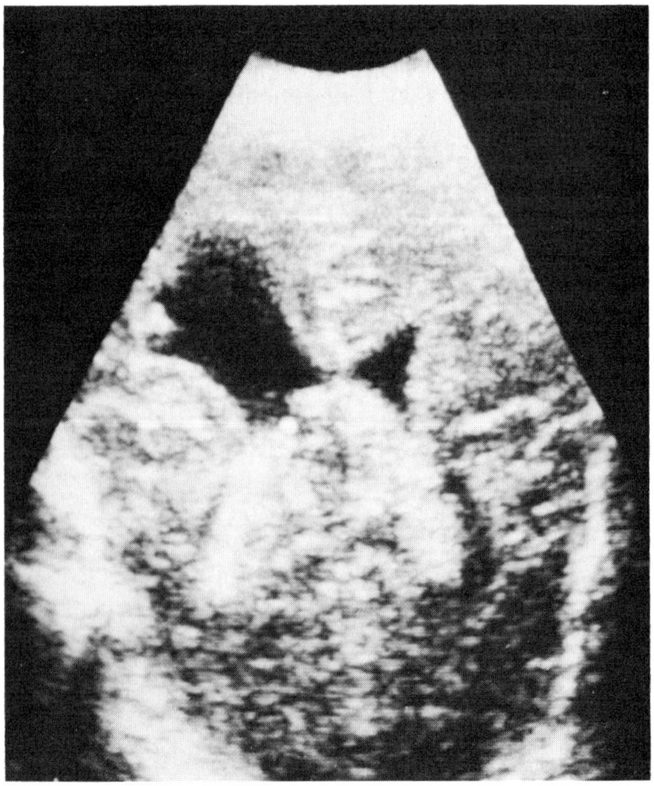

Fig. 71.10 Intracranial ultrasound showing gross dilatation of the lateral ventricles on a coronal scan.

repeated lumbar puncture. This form of therapy is currently being evaluated in a prospective randomized controlled trial. If this treatment is not successful it may be necessary to consider the removal of cerebrospinal fluid directly from the ventricle by ventricular puncture, from a drain inserted into the ventricle or with a ventriculoperitoneal shunt.

Prognosis

Intracranial ultrasound has been used as a prognostic aid. In a series of infants of less than 33 weeks' gestational age it was found at 1 year of age that infants whose ultrasound scans were normal or had germinal layer (grade 1) haemorrhage were at low risk for neurodevelopmental disorders (11% had abnormal neurodevelopment or abnormal neurological signs without disability): those with uncomplicated ventricular dilatation were in a group at intermediate risk (34%), whereas those with evidence of parenchymal haemorrhage, hydrocephalus requiring shunting or cerebral atrophy were at high risk (88%; Stewart et al 1983). However any preceding asphyxia and the presence of periventricular leukomalacia may be more important in causing disability than the haemorrhage itself. Although the ultrasound appearance allows one to place a child in a risk category it does not on its own allow one to predict accurately an individual child's neurodevelopmental outcome.

Prevention

Because rapid changes in blood pressure, PaO_2 and $PaCO_2$ result in marked fluctuations in cerebral blood flow it is postulated that PVH and cerebral ischaemia can be prevented by meticulous care with ventilation to achieve a stable circulation.

Drugs have also been tried in the prevention of PVH. Phenobarbitone has been used as it reduces cerebral metabolic rate and is a sedative but it has not proved possible consistently to show a reduction in PVH. Ethamsylate, a capillary stabilizer, has been reported in a multicentre trial to reduce the incidence and severity of PVH (Benson et al 1986). Vitamin E, a free radical scavenger, has also been reported to reduce the incidence and severity of PVH in one randomized controlled trial (Sinha et al 1987) but it was not beneficial in another (Phelps et al 1987).

PATENT DUCTUS ARTERIOSUS

The ductus arteriosus is a short, muscular vessel between the main pulmonary artery and the descending aorta, which in the fetus allows blood to bypass the lungs. Patency of the ductus during intrauterine life is thought to be maintained by the relaxant effect of low oxygen tension and locally synthesized prostaglandins. There has been some concern that drugs used in pregnancy which reduce the effect of prostaglandins, such as aspirin and indomethacin, might close the fetal ductus prematurely. In term infants, physiological closure is triggered by the rise in arterial oxygen tension which occurs when respiration is established at birth. Ductal closure may be delayed in preterm infants in whom the ductus is relatively much larger and its musculature less developed.

Incidence

In a large multicentre study, 20% of infants with a birthweight of less than 1.75 kg had a haemodynamically significant shunt (Ellison et al 1983). A significant duct was found in only 7% of infants with a birthweight of 1.5–1.75 kg, but in 42% of infants less than 1 kg, showing that the more immature the infant, the higher the incidence. It is commonest when artificial ventilation is required because of RDS in ELBW infants.

In a study of 30 infants under 30 weeks' gestation assessed by cross-sectional echocardiography, the ductus was found to have remained patent in all of them during the first 2 weeks of life; anatomical closure could only be demonstrated after the baby had reached the equivalent of 32 weeks' gestational age (Rigby et al 1984). This would suggest that there is the potential for ductal shunting in infants of less than 32 weeks' gestation. Its presence and severity will depend on the size of the ductal lumen and the difference in pulmonary and systemic vascular resistances. In the first few days of life, when the pulmonary vascular resistance is high, shunting across the patent ductus is usually from the pulmonary artery to the aorta (right-to-left). Therafter the resistance in the pulmonary circulation falls and becomes lower than in the systemic circulation and shunting is in the opposite direction, from the aorta to the pulmonary artery (left-to-right). The incidence of left-to-right shunting is increased by circulatory overload from a high fluid intake during the first few days of life.

Clinical significance

Left-to-right shunts in preterm infants may result in respiratory problems because of pulmonary oedema and venous congestion. In infants requiring artificial ventilation left-to-right shunt may cause increased ventilatory requirements and difficulty in weaning infants from the ventilator, associated with an increased incidence of chronic lung disease. Infants not on artificial ventilation may be asymptomatic or the shunting may cause respiratory distress or apnoeic attacks. It is common practice to restrict the fluid intake in infants with signs of a patent ductus and this will inevitably reduce the baby's nutrition. In addition, in infants with a left-to-right shunt there is retrograde diastolic flow of blood which mainly originates from the descending aorta. It has been suggested that this may reduce blood flow to vital organs and could result in ischaemic damage to the bowel wall, causing necrotizing enterocolitis, and to the brain, causing cerebral ischaemia.

Diagnosis

The clinical signs of ductal shunting are that the peripheral pulses become easily palpable or bounding, a systolic murmur can be heard in the pulmonary area and left sternal edge and the cardiac impulse becomes increasingly active. Additional but less specific signs are tachypnoea, tachycardia and hepatomegaly from cardiac failure. The continuous murmur characteristic of a ductus in older children is uncommon in preterm infants.

The diagnosis of a patent ductus is usually made from clinical examination. Ductal shunting occurs most often in infants with RDS, in whom the presence of a murmur or heart failure due to patent ductus arteriosus may be difficult to demonstrate.

The chest X-ray of an infant with a large ductus may show cardiomegaly and pulmonary plethora, but these may be masked by the baby's lung disease. Echocardiography has been widely used as an adjunct to clinical assessment. Left atrial enlargement from left-to-right shunting has been quantified by measuring the ratio of the left atrial diameter to aortic root diameter (Ellison et al 1983). However the sensitivity of the technique is poor as left atrial enlargement is non-specific and is affected by fluid restriction and cardiac compression from lung disease. With the high-definition cross-sectional echocardiography now available, it is often possible to identify the ductus itself to see if it is patent or not, but this does not provide information about the severity of ductal shunting.

More recently, Doppler ultrasound has been used to quantify ductal shunting from the extent of retrograde flow in the velocity waveform of peripheral arteries. More specific information can be obtained by identifying retrograde flow in the pulmonary artery using pulsed Doppler ultrasound combined with cross-sectional echocardiography, but quantifying the severity of ductal shunting remains problematic with this technique.

Management

An infant with a patent ductus may be managed by fluid restriction, diuretics, indomethacin or surgery. Some degree of fluid restriction often helps in the management of cardiac failure. This may be sufficient in an asymptomatic baby, but diuretics should be given if there are signs of cardiac failure. Oral chlorothiazide may be used and may be combined with spironolactone to reduce the frequency and severity of hypokalaemia. Preterm babies may become profoundly hyponatraemic on diuretic therapy and serum electrolytes should be monitored regularly.

Indomethacin, a prostaglandin inhibitor, has been widely used to promote ductal closure. It can be given orally or intravenously (0.2 mg/kg), in three doses at 8-hourly intervals if required. In many infants it diminishes or closes the ductus, though it is less effective in infants who are less than 28 weeks' gestation or more than 3 weeks old. Its main side-effects are oliguria and gastrointestinal haemorrhage. Indomethacin therapy is best reserved for infants with symptoms from cardiac failure despite fluid restriction and diuretic therapy.

Surgical ligation of the ductus is sometimes required in infants with resolving RDS in whom the ductus is preventing the infant from being weaned off the ventilator and in whom medical therapy has failed. It is a relatively strightforward operation, but is preferably performed without transferring the baby to another hospital.

ANAEMIA OF PREMATURITY

In the immediate newborn period blood transfusion may be required if the infant is anaemic or to replace blood taken for tests. It is preferable to maintain the haemoglobin of sick newborn infants above 12 g/dl.

As preterm infants grow, their haemoglobin levels fall to their lowest levels at 4–10 weeks of age. Their haemoglobin concentration needs to be monitored during this period and blood transfusion is usually required if the haemoglobin concentration drops below 8 g/dl or if they become symptomatic with poor feeding, poor weight gain, lethargy, tachycardia, tachypnoea or apnoea. Supplemental iron is given from 3 weeks of age, unless the infant has been recently transfused, to prevent iron deficiency anaemia from developing.

ETHICAL PROBLEMS

Ethical debate continues about the amount of medical treatment required for some of the very immature babies to ensure that they do not suffer unnecessarily from prolonged treatment and that they do not consume a disproportionate allocation of financial resources. Extreme care has to be taken to ensure that intensive therapy is not used unnecessarily to support the life of babies with such severe brain damage that it would lead to a very poor quality of life. Parents should be involved in these difficult decisions. It is also important that babies do not die or suffer damage unnecessarily because proper neonatal care is not available.

PARENTS

When a mother has a preterm baby she and her partner often feel shocked and psychologically unprepared to have a baby. Removal of the baby to the bewildering, complex world of the neonatal intensive care unit adds to their worry and stress.

It is often helpful if parents are able to meet the paediatrician and see the baby unit before delivery. They are also helped by the open visiting for parents and close family practised in neonatal units and by the efforts made by the staff to provide a friendly and caring atmosphere. Ready communication at all times with the nursing and medical staff must be encouraged. A serious problem should be discussed as it arises, otherwise trust with the parents will be undermined. Under such circumstances it is best to see both parents together and to ensure that serious and complex issues are discussed with the same members of staff so that the parents receive consistent information. Many units now have parent discussion and support groups.

Much attention has been paid during the last few years to mother–child bonding during the first few hours of birth. In common with certain animals, it was thought that there was a critical period for a bond of affection to develop between a mother and her baby during the first few hours after birth and that if a mother was separated from her baby during this critical period their relationship would be permanently damaged. It is now realized that this view is rather simplistic and, given the appropriate attitudes and understanding of the family and hospital staff, parents can overcome the psychological upset of this initial separation. However separating babies from their mothers must be avoided whenever possible.

DISCHARGE FROM HOSPITAL

LBW infants can be discharged from hospital when they are feeding well, their condition is stable and when the parents are sufficiently prepared and able to care for them. Many mothers of babies who have required prolonged hospitalization need to return to hospital for a period during which they can assume responsibility for the care of their baby prior to going home. Once home, parents initially need considerable support and advice, and this should be readily available from the hospital and community.

All LBW infants and those with neonatal problems which may have long-term sequelae are seen periodically at follow-up clinics to monitor their progress and development. Parents have to be warned that babies achieve social and motor milestones at a given time from conception, not birth, and that allowance has to be made for their prematurity. LBW infants are also given additional iron, folic acid and vitamin supplements until they are 6 months old. Immunizations should be given as for other children and started at the same age chronologically from birth, rather than from postconceptual age. The parents need to be advised whether pertussis immunization is contraindicated or not. In addition, parents are encouraged to attend their child health clinic regularly to keep a check on the infant's growth and overall development.

Infants who have had respiratory problems in the newborn period, especially those with chronic lung disease following artificial ventilation, are more prone to serious chest infections during the first year or two of life. Admission for surgical procedures, especially repair of inguinal herniae, is also markedly increased. Readmission to hospital during the first year of life is increased approximately fourfold for VLBW infants.

NEURODEVELOPMENTAL OUTCOME

Long-term follow-up is required to assess neurodevelopmental outcome. By 2 years of age, most major disabilities can be identified, but the child needs to be at least 5 years old for minor disabilities to be identified reliably.

When improved medical care of LBW and particularly VLBW infants began to be accompanied by an increasing number of survivors, it was predicted that this would be accompanied by an increased incidence in neurodevelopmental handicap (Drillien 1961). A review of the world literature of neurodevelopmental handicap rates for VLBW infants concluded that in spite of the marked improvement in survival since 1960, the prevalence of neurodevelopmental handicap amongst the liveborn VLBW population had remained static at between 6 and 8% of live births (Stewart et al 1981). Neurodevelopmental handicap denotes impairment which compromises the patient's neurological or developmental function. Since then, there has been a marked improvement in the survival rate for ELBW infants; there has also been similar concern about their long-term prognosis.

Several relatively small series have reported survival rates of 20–50% in ELBW infants, of whom 20–30% have a major neurodevelopmental disability (Britton et al 1981, Bennett et al 1983). Marlow & Chiswick (1985) studied all infants weighing 2000 g or less at birth who were admitted to the neonatal intensive care unit in Manchester from 1976 to 1980. In infants weighing 1251–2000 g a major neurodevelopmental handicap was subsequently observed in 3.6% of survivors and was not birthweight-related. Only in infants of birthweight 1250 g or less did the incidence of handicap amongst survivors rise as birthweight fell. Whereas 7% of survivors at 29–30 weeks' gestation had a major neurodevelopmental handicap, this had increased to 20% in infants of 25–26 weeks' gestation.

Survival and outcome are related to both gestational age and birthweight but gestation is more important as a determinant of mortality and adverse outcome. It is for this reason that the LBW infant who is SGA has a better chance of survival when compared to a baby of similar weight but shorter gestational age. Some studies have found that the preterm SGA baby has more problems than babies of average gestational age. Severe and prolonged growth retardation in pregnancy results in a shorter stature in childhood and a poorer intellectual development.

Range of disabilities

LBW infants are at risk of a wide range of neurodevelopmental problems. These include visual disability, hearing loss, cerebral palsy and mental handicap. Disabilities are usually classified as major when they interfere with normal daily activity or schooling, and minor when there are neurological or sensory abnormalities not affecting daily activities. A review of the major disabilities in infants weighing less or equal to 1250 g from 11 studies showed a median incidence of cerebral palsy of 7% (range 4–15%), developmental delay in 14% (range 4–30%), severe visual handicap in 5% (range 0–25%) and major auditory loss in 5% (range 0–12%, Marlow & Chiswick 1985).

Specific disabilities

Visual disability

Retinopathy of prematurity is a disorder of the retinal vasculature which commonly affects VLBW infants. Fortunately, in most cases the retinopathy is limited to early proliferation of the retinal vessels which regresses fully, but it sometimes progresses to the cicatricial stage with fibrosis, distortion and scarring of the retina which may result in retinal detachment, severe visual impairment or blindness. In VLBW infants squints and myopia are relatively common. Severe visual impairment is much less common and is mostly seen in ELBW infants requiring prolonged oxygen therapy.

In the early 1950s it was shown that the dramatic increase in blindness from retinopathy of prematurity was in preterm infants who were nursed for prolonged periods in high concentrations of oxygen. It was thought that retinopathy of prematurity could be prevented by restricting oxygen therapy to concentrations of less than 40%. Although this led to a fall in the incidence of retinopathy of prematurity it was accompanied by a rise in mortality; it was calculated that for each case prevented, there were 16 extra perinatal deaths (Cross 1973). With improved monitoring techniques which allow the oxygen concentration provided to be tailored to oxygen tension in the infant's blood, it was hoped that retinopathy of prematurity could be prevented. Unfortunately in spite of these improved methods of oxygen monitoring, the magnitude of retinopathy of prematurity in the USA is again of a similar order to that in the early 1950s (Phelps 1981).

It has been widely assumed that oxygen administration is associated with unintended hyperoxaemia and that direct oxidative damage to the developing retinal endothelium causes retinopathy of prematurity. Antioxidants, particularly vitamin E, have therefore been studied as potential preventive agents. Although there were some promising reports that vitamin E reduced the incidence and severity of retinopathy of prematurity, a recent study has failed to support its efficacy (Phelps et al 1987).

It now seems likely that oxygen toxicity is not the only factor in its aetiology (Silverman 1982, Lucey & Dangman 1984).

When VLBW infants reach the equivalent of 32–34 weeks' gestation their eyes should be checked periodically by an ophthalmologist whilst they are on the neonatal unit and also following discharge.

Hearing loss

In addition to major hearing loss, milder degrees of sensorineural hearing loss or conductive deafness are encountered relatively often in VLBW infants. Sensorineural hearing loss amongst preterm infants is often a high-frequency loss. As early detection and hearing aids are important for the severely deaf child, VLBW infants should have their hearing carefully checked. Early screening for hearing deficits can be performed using an auditory cradle, where the infant's response to sound is detected with the help of a microcomputer or by auditory-evoked potentials (Bhattacharya et al 1984). Thereafter distraction testing to sounds of various frequencies is performed.

Cerebral palsy and developmental retardation

In early follow-up studies there was a clear association between prematurity and spastic diplegia. More recent studies suggest that quadriplegia is now the commonest type of cerebral palsy, though diplegia, hemiplegia and athetosis are also seen (Marlow & Chiswick 1985). Affected infants often have developmental retardation and may have multiple disabilities.

Few of the follow-up studies of VLBW infants born since the introduction of modern methods of care have been continued long enough to provide detailed information on school performance and intellectual outcome. In a study of VLBW infants at age 8 years Stewart et al (1983) reported that 90% were attending normal schools; 76% were making satisfactory progress in regular classes and 14% required extra provision within the normal school service. Only 5% were in special schools because they were disabled, and 5% had died or could be not traced. The authors concluded that the proportion of children requiring extra provision was similar to the community as a whole, but there was a threefold increase in the proportion of seriously disabled children.

Examination of VLBW infants born in the 1960s and early 1970s suggests that they have a higher incidence of perceptual and learning disabilities and poorer fine motor co-ordination than the general population. They also appear to have more behavioural problems and are more difficult to control. In VLBW infants without a major impairment it appears that poor socioeconomic conditions operating both antenatally and postnatally are a major determinant of poor intellectual outcome. Information on the intellectual outcome of VLBW infants managed since the widespread introduction of modern intensive care is awaited.

To assess the impact of modern perinatal care on handicap in the community as a whole, Alberman et al (1982) compared infants of birthweight less than 2000 g born in the early 1950s with those born in the 1970s. They concluded that because of the overall fall in morbidity among LBW infants, the prevalence of neurodevelopmental handicap in the community as a whole had not increased as a consequence of increased survival. They also deduced that because of the relatively small numbers of LBW infants, they account for only a very small proportion of the total neurodevelopmental handicap in the population. In the UK, less than 2% of serious handicap can be accounted for by prematurity, which is less than half that attributable to birth asphyxia.

When medical staff and parents have to weigh up the risks of early delivery, particularly at 23–28 weeks' gestation, against the risks of prolonging the pregnancy in an adverse intrauterine environment, information on mortality and the incidence of neurodevelopmental handicap is required. As it is only relatively recently that infants of such very early gestation have survived, long-term follow-up data on such infants are still sparse. A study from Melbourne, Australia (Yu et al 1986) of 356 infants born at these gestational ages showed that the 1-year survival rate was only 7% at 23 weeks but was as much as 75% at 28 weeks. Boys had a significantly lower chance of normal survival than girls and multiple births had a significantly lower survival and higher incidence of impairment than singleton births. Of the 192 long-term survivors, 36 children (19%) were found to have an impairment at 1–2 years of age, of whom 11% had cerebral palsy, 7% developmental delay, 3% blindness and 3% sensorineural deafness. Table 71.5 shows the predicted outcome before birth for mortality, major disability and impairment; this is for use in counselling parents on the potential outcome of infants delivered at this gestation. Outcome data are also provided for babies who have been resuscitated successfully or have reached a week of age. Such figures need to be expanded and repeatedly revised to keep pace with the changes in neonatal care.

Table 71.5 Predicted outcome before birth of the percentage of infants born at 23–28 weeks' gestation who are likely to be normal, have a major disability or other impairments, or to die. From Yu et al (1986)

Gestation (weeks)	Predicted outcome (% of births) Normal	Major disability	Other impairment	Dead
23	5	5		90
24	31	3	3	63
25	24	8	8	60
26	44	9	5	42
27	68	4	3	25
28	64	5	2	29

REFERENCES

Alberman E, Benson J, McDonald A 1982 Cerebral palsy and severe educational subnormality in low-birthweight children: a comparison of births in 1951–53 and 1970–73. Lancet i: 606–608

Bennett F C, Robinson N M, Sells C J 1983 Growth and development of infants weighing less than 800 grams at birth. Pediatrics 71: 319–323

Benson J W T, Drayton M R, Hayward C et al 1986 Multicentre trial of ethamsylate for prevention of periventricular haemorrhage in very low birthweight infants. Lancet ii: 1297–1300

Beverley D, Foote K, Howel D, Congdon P 1986 Effect of birthplace of infants with low birth-weight. British Medical Journal 293: 981–983

Bhattacharya J, Bennett M J, Tucker S M 1984 Long term followup of infants tested with the Auditory Response Cradle. Archives of Disease in Childhood 59: 504–511

British Paediatric Association/British Association for Perinatal Paediatrics 1985 Categories of babies needing neonatal care. Archives of Disease in Childhood 60: 599–600

British Paediatric Association/Royal College of Obstetricians and Gynaecologists 1982 Midwife and nurse staffing and training for special care and intensive care of the newborn. BPA/RCOG, London

Britton S B, Fitzhardinge P M, Ashby S 1981 Is intensive care justified for infants weighing less than 801 grams at birth? Journal of Pediatrics 99: 937–943

Brown A K, Kim M H, Wo P Y K, Bryla D A 1985 Efficacy of phototherapy in prevention and management of neonatal hyperbilirubinaemia. Pediatrics 75: 393–400

Chiswick M L 1982 Perinatal referral: a time for decision. British Medical Journal 285: 83–84

Clarke C E, Glyman R I, Roth R S, Sniderman S H, Lane B, Ballard R A 1981 Risk factor analysis of intraventricular haemorrhage in low birthweight infants. Journal of Pediatrics 99: 625–628

Cross K W 1973 The cost of preventing retrolental fibroplasia? Lancet ii: 954–956

Crowley P, Lamont R, Elder M G 1982 The obstetric care of the fetus transferred in utero. Journal of Obstetrics and Gynaecology 2: 129–133

Department of Health and Social Security 1987 Birth notifications: 1976–1986. Low weight births and mortality. Summary information from LHS 27/1, 1986, England. DHSS, London

Drew J H 1982 Immediate intubation at birth of the very low birthweight infant. American Journal of Diseases in Children 136: 207–210

Drillien C M 1961 The incidence of mental and physical handicaps at school age in children of very low birthweight. Pediatrics 27: 452–464

Ellison R C, Peckham G J, Lang P et al 1983 Evaluation of the preterm infant for patent ductus arteriosus. Pediatrics 71: 364–372

Field D, Milner A D 1986 Respiratory disease in the neonatal period. British Medical Bulletin 42: 163–166

Greenough A, Roberton N R C 1985. Morbidity and survival in neonates ventilated for the respiratory distress syndrome. British Medical Journal 290: 597–600

Hammarlund K, Sedin G 1979 Transepidermal water loss in newborn infants III Relation to gestational age. Acta Paediatrica Scandinavica 68: 795–801

Harpin V A, Rutter N 1985 Humidification of incubators. Archives of Disease in Childhood 60: 219–224

Henderson-Smart D J 1981 The effect of gestational age on the incidence and duration of recurrent apnoea in newborn babies. Australian Paediatric Journal 17: 273–276

Hey E N 1971 The care of babies in incubators. In: Gardner D, Hull D (eds) Recent advances in paediatrics. J & A Churchill, London

Lemons J A, Moyle L, Hall D, Summons M 1982 Differences in composition of preterm and term human milk during early lactation. Pediatric Research 16: 113–117
Lobb M L, Morgan M E I, Bond A P, Cooke R W I 1983 Transfer before delivery in Merseyside: an analysis of the first 140 patients. British Journal of Obstetrics and Gynaecology 90: 338–341
Lou H C, Lassen N A, Friis-Hansen 1979 Impaired autoregulation of cerebral blood flow in the distressed infant. Journal of Pediatrics 94: 118–121
Lucey J F, Dangman B 1984 A re-examination of the role of oxygen in retrolental fibroplasia. Pediatrics 73: 82–96
Marlow N, Chiswick M L 1985 Neurodevelopmental outcome in extremely low birthweight survivors. In: Chiswick M L (ed) Recent advances in perinatal medicine, vol 2. Churchill Livingstone, Edinburgh, pp 181–205
McDonald H M, Mulligan J C, Allen A C, Taylor P M 1980 Neonatal asphyxia I Relationship of obstetric and neonatal complications to neonatal mortality in 38 405 consecutive deliveries. Journal of Pediatrics 96: 898–902
Office of Population Censuses and Surveys 1988 Mortality statistics 1986. DH3/20. HMSO, London
Pape K E, Wigglesworth J C 1979 Haemorrhage, ischaemia and the perinatal brain. Clinics in developmental medicine 69/70. Heinemann, London
Pharoah P O D 1986 Perspectives and patterns. British Medical Bulletin 42: 119–126
Phelps D L 1981 Retinopathy of prematurity: an estimate of vision loss in the United States — 1979. Pediatrics 67: 924–926
Phelps D L, Rosenbaum A L, Isenberg S J, Leake R D, Dorey F J 1987 Tocopherol efficacy and safety for preventing retinopathy of prematurity: a randomised, controlled, double-masked trial. Pediatrics 79: 487–500
Rigby M L, Pickering D, Wilkinson A 1984 Cross-sectional echocardiography in determining persistent patency of the ductus arteriosus in preterm infants. Archives of Disease in Childhood 59: 341–345
Roberton N R C, Tizard J P M 1975. Prognosis for infants with idiopathic respiratory distress syndrome. British Medical Journal iii: 271–274
Silverman W A 1982 Retinopathy of prematurity: oxygen dogma challenged. Archives of Disease in Childhood 57: 731–733
Silverman W A, Fertig J W, Berger A P 1958 The influence of the thermal environment upon the survival of newly born premature infants. Pediatrics 22: 876–885
Sims D J, Wynn J, Chiswick M L 1982 Outcome for newborn babies declined admission to a regional neonatal intensive care unit. Archives of Disease in Childhood 57: 334–337
Sinha S, Davies J, Toner N, Bogle S, Chiswick M 1987 Vitamin E supplementation reduces frequency of periventricular haemorrhage in very preterm infants. Lancet i: 466–470
Southall D P, Bignall S, Stebbens V A, Alexander J R, Rivers R P A, Lissauer T 1987 The clinical reliability of pulse oximeter and transcutaneous PO_2 measurements in neonatal and paediatric intensive care. Archives of Disease in Childhood 62: 882–888
Speidel B P 1978 Adverse effects of routine procedures on preterm infants. Lancet i: 864–866
Stanley F J, Alberman E D 1978 Infants of very low birthweigh I. Perinatal factors affecting survival. Developmental Medicine and Child Neurology 20: 300–312
Stewart A L, Reynolds E O R, Lipscomb A P 1981 Outcome for infants of very low birthweight: survey of the world literature. Lancet i: 1038–1041
Stewart A L, Thorburn R J, Hope P L, Goldsmith M, Lipscombe A P, Reynolds E O R 1983 Ultrasound appearance of the brain in very preterm infants and neurodevelopmental outcome at 18 months of age. Archives of Disease in Childhood 58: 598–604
Yu V Y H, Loke H L, Bajuk B, Szymonowicz W, Orgill A A, Asterbury J 1986 Prognosis for infants born at 23 to 28 weeks' gestation. British Medical Journal 293: 1200–1203

Obstetrical responsibility for abnormal fetal outcome

It seems certain that improvements in obstetrical care over the past decade or two have been substantially responsible for the well documented reduction in the perinatal mortality rate. The decrease in the fetal death component of the perinatal mortality rate is most obviously due to changes in obstetric practice, although the decrease in the neonatal death risk may also be partially due to obstetric improvements as well as to improvements in neonatal care. Much less certain is whether there has been any decrease in the risk of cerebral palsy and whether any such improvement has been mediated by obstetrical changes. The overwhelming evidence is to the contrary. A decrease in the frequency with which cerebral palsy occurs would have been expected if the 'continuum of reproductive wastage' postulated by Lilienfeld & Parkhurst (1951) actually exists. These investigators suggested that a very severe damaging fetal event would lead to fetal death (or neonatal death); a less severe event might result in severe damage (cerebral palsy) to the surviving infant, and if the event was even less severe, minimal brain damage might result. This theory has dominated medical thinking since it was first published in spite of voluminous data to refute it.

The all-or-nothing theory has been offered as an alternative, suggesting that a severe fetal event (asphyxia?) may cause death of the fetus or neonate, but if the event does not kill, the fetus/neonate will usually survive intact, i.e. without brain damage. Acceptance of the all-or-nothing theory entails an acceptance of the idea that the dominant causes of fetal/neonatal death may not be the major causes of cerebral injury. Evidence to support this view will be detailed below (Hensleigh et al 1986). If the cause of cerebral palsy is different from the dominant cause of perinatal death, i.e. asphyxia, we must search for that cause if we are to try to assess the degree of responsibility the obstetrician can be expected to have in the prevention of cerebral palsy. Thus, in this chapter we will first discuss the factors that may lead to, or at least precede, the development of cerebral palsy. As we discuss these factors, we can then postulate how obstetrical care might prevent their development or minimize their effects and thus potentially reduce the risk of the development of cerebral palsy. We will then report on certain experiments which have empirically tested the hypothesis that good obstetric care will be followed less frequently by poor short-term (e.g. newborn convulsions) or long-term (e.g. cerebral palsy) neurological outcome than will substandard obstetric care. Lastly, we will discuss the relationship between premature birth and cerebral palsy with a view to the role of obstetric care in this relationship.

ANIMAL MODELS OF BRAIN DAMAGE

Since events during labour and delivery, notably trauma and asphyxia, have long been thought to be possible causes of cerebral palsy, it is not surprising that attempts to develop brain pathology in the animal fetus similar to that seen in the human with cerebral palsy first utilized the production of elements of asphyxia — decreased blood oxygen levels and increased carbon dioxide levels leading to lactic acidosis and a lowering of blood pH. It soon became evident that anoxia of at least 10–12 minutes duration in the animal model can result in damage to the brain stem, a pathology quite unlike the pathology usually seen in the human child with cerebral palsy and therefore of little interest in this chapter (Myers 1972). Prolonged partial asphyxia of the monkey fetus, however, produced a different pathology with involvement of the cerebral hemispheres, paracentral cortical regions etc. — a pathologic picture more closely akin to that seen in the human with cerebral palsy (Myers 1972).

Thus, at least in the animal model, it appeared that severe fetal asphyxia might cause a pathological picture consistent with cerebral palsy. Of striking importance, however, was the rarity of this pathological outcome following partial asphyxia. The brain is not the only organ affected by hypoxia or asphyxia, and indeed it is probably not the first organ affected. Those animal fetuses which were severely asphyxiated usually died from the effects of the asphyxia on the heart, or they survived with an intact brain. Only a very few animals survived with the characteristic brain pathology.

At a later date and with further experiments, Myers et al (1981) concluded that the critical factors in the development of the brain damage were a very high level of lactic acid in the brain (reflected as metabolic acidosis in the blood) and poor perfusion of the brain caused by a shock-like state in the animal, probably due to the effect of asphyxia on the fetal heart. These authors also reported that a high serum glucose level seemed a critical element in the experimental production of asphyxial brain damage.

Other strategies for the induction of brain damage have also been successful in the experimental animal: these are techniques that do not depend on the presence of severe fetal asphyxia or acidosis. Clapp et al (1985) using a fetal sheep model, caused histological damage in the cortical white matter by firstly, partial intermittent cord occlusion late in pregnancy and secondly, by the induction of mild hyperglycaemia in a fetus which was growth-retarded from a technique previously shown not to induce brain damage in itself. Neither of these experimental conditions was accompanied by significant fetal hypoxia or acidosis.

Gilles et al (1976) consistently produced perinatal telencephalic leukoencephalopathy (PTL), a pathology thought to be present in many humans with cerebral palsy, in the brains of newborn kittens up to 10 days of age by exposing them to the endotoxin of *Escherichia coli*. This finding seems to have clinical relevance when one considers that human infants with terminal bacteraemia were five times more likely to have had PTL than were infants who did not have bacteraemia (Leviton & Gilles 1973). The same authors found that 85% of infants with PTL and terminal bacteraemia had Gram-negative organisms. Thus, the possibility that an endotoxin, even without clinical evidence of infection, might cause brain pathology consistent with the presence of cerebral palsy must be considered. Broman (1978) has noted an increased risk of neurological dysfunction in children of mothers who had urinary tract infections during pregnancy.

Since factors other than asphyxia in the experimental animal can produce brain damage, it is apparent that we should not theorize that asphyxia is the only mechanism, or even necessarily the primary one, for the production of brain damage in the human fetus or newborn. This is particularly true in view of the well documented fact that even very severe acidosis in the human fetus at birth is only uncommonly followed by permanent brain damage (Brown et al 1974, Scott 1976). Similarly, only a minority of children subsequently shown to have cerebral palsy were asphyxiated or acidotic at the time of birth (Nelson & Ellenberg 1981). These issues will be discussed below.

Gilles (1985) has discussed what is known and what is not known about the pathology of cerebral palsy, with special emphasis on conclusions the pathologist may draw about the cause or causes of that pathology. On the question of asphyxia Gilles wrote: 'in current textbooks of neuropathology some 28 distinct morphologic abnormalities of the neonatal brain are attributed to asphyxia, hypoxia, or anoxia.' He further points out that the 'multiple risk factors of the perinatal leucoencephalopathy characterized by focal necroses do not include markers of hypoxia, anoxia, or systemic hypotension.' Thus he concludes that the many types of pathology attributed to hypoxia or asphyxia, coupled with the lack of prominence of hypoxia or asphyxia as a possible cause of perinatal leukoencephalopathy, mean that it cannot be concluded with certainty that there is a cause and effect relationship between the presence of neonatal asphyxia and brain pathology.

In spite of this strong evidence to the contrary, fetal asphyxia, especially intrapartum fetal asphyxia, continues to be the major theoretical cause of cerebral palsy. Most of the remainder of this chapter will discuss what is known and what is not known about the asphyxia–cerebral palsy relationship.

ASPHYXIA AND CEREBRAL PALSY IN HUMANS

In studying the relationship between fetal asphyxia and cerebral palsy in humans, it is obviously impossible even to approach experimental conditions. We cannot purposely produce a certain degree of asphyxia and then wait to observe its effects. Other factors also affect any conclusions we might draw in humans regarding this relationship. We rarely know the precise degree of asphyxia or how long it has lasted; we actively interfere with any asphyxia we recognize clinically either before or after birth; we usually have no information about the intactness of the fetal brain before the time frame when the asphyxia in question is recognized. Our investigation of the matter must therefore be indirect. Nevertheless, there is a large body of data relating to the matter, and in presenting the issue several questions will be asked. The answers to these questions can be expected to clarify the relationship, if any, between asphyxia and cerebral palsy.

1. Does cerebral palsy usually follow birth asphyxia?
2. How accurate are the clinical tools we have for identifying fetal asphyxia or acidosis and do they relate to the development of cerebral palsy?
3. Does clinical evidence of asphyxia at birth usually precede the development of cerebral palsy?
4. Is the fetus who is already brain-damaged from an earlier event more likely to display evidence of intrapartum asphyxia than an intact fetus?

Table 72.1 Newborn asphyxia and cerebral palsy

Of 14 020 deliveries	
760 (5.4%)	Severely asphyxiated
83 (11%)	Abnormal newborn neurology
17	Developed cerebral palsy
17/83	= 20%
17/760	= 2.2%

From Brown et al (1974).

Table 72.2 Correlation between a low 5-minute Apgar score (0–3) and cerebral palsy in children born at term

Time period (minutes)	Percentage of survivors with cerebral palsy
1	1.5
5	4.7
10	16.7
15	36.0
20	57.1

From Nelson & Ellenberg (1981).

Does cerebral palsy usually follow birth asphyxia?

The medical literature relating to this question gives a very clear and consistent opinion. Even severe intrapartum asphyxia is rarely followed by clinical brain damage. Low et al (1978), for example, studied 42 children at 12 months of age who had suffered severe asphyxia (umbilical artery buffer base <34.0 mmol/l at birth) and compared them to a group of 69 children born without asphyxia (>36.1 mmol/l). There were no differences between the study and control babies in mental or physical development, including neurological examination.

Brown et al (1974) reported that among 14 020 women delivered in the Simpson Memorial Maternity Pavilion in Edinburgh, 760 (5.4%) liveborn babies were considered severely asphyxiated by criteria which the authors outlined — 88% required endotracheal intubation, 80% had an Apgar score of less than 5 at 5 minutes and 63% had an abnormal acid–base status (Table 72.1); 11% (83) of the 760 asphyxiated children exhibited abnormal neurological signs in the nursery and 20% (17) of these 83 asphyxiated babies who suffered an abnormal neonatal neurological course (or 2.2% (17) of the entire group of 760 asphyxiated babies) ultimately developed cerebral palsy. The study again corroborates the fact that asphyxia is common but that cerebral palsy following asphyxia is uncommon.

Scott (1976) followed 23 children born with an Apgar score of zero (seven were considered stillborn and the other 16 did not establish respiration by 20 minutes after birth). He found that 20 of the 23 had an IQ in the normal range and 17 of the 23 were without neurological deficit. D'Souza and Richards (1978) followed 53 newborns with a history of fetal distress and with severe neurological abnormality during the nursery course. Of these newborns, 58% took between 7 and 60 minutes to establish regular spontaneous breathing. At 2–5 years of age, only one child among the 53 was severely handicapped with cerebral palsy. Thomson et al (1977) followed 31 children who had scored zero on the 1-minute Apgar score or less than 4 on the 5-minute Apgar score and found that 93% (29) had no neurological handicap at between 5 and 10 years of age.

How accurate are the clinical tools we have for identifying asphyxia or acidosis and do they relate to the development of cerebral palsy?

Since asphyxia in the experimental animal can result in brain damage, and since asphyxia, either during the prenatal period or during labour, could be a cause of cerebral palsy in humans, we are faced with the necessity of appraising the tools we have for identifying fetal asphyxia before delivery. If they are accurate in this regard, the possibility exists that the labour attendant can abbreviate the fetal asphyxia thus recognized and perhaps reduce the risk of brain damage. The tools most commonly in use for recognizing fetal asphyxia at the present time are electronic fetal monitoring (EFM) and fetal scalp blood sampling (FSBS) or a combination of the two.

Since the term asphyxia has had many different meanings among the authors studying the issue of brain damage, a discussion of certain variables thought to indicate asphyxia and their relationship to outcome is necessary. *Low Apgar scores* have been used most frequently as a measure of asphyxia at and immediately after birth, and the data on these scores must be reviewed. Data *relating abnormal EFM patterns* or *fetal/neonatal acidosis* as reflected by pH levels to later outcome are sparse. One solution to this deficiency is to study the data presenting the relationship between measured acidosis or abnormal EFM patterns and near-term evidence of fetal asphyxia, notably early newborn convulsions. Such convulsions may presage the development of cerebral palsy, although the relationship between these convulsions and cerebral palsy may not be as simple as it might seem, as will be discussed shortly.

A *low Apgar score* has been the most often-used reflector of intrapartum asphyxia. The 5-minute score has enjoyed a wider use than the 1-minute score, since the effects of drugs, difficult delivery and other non-asphyxial events are thought to be reflected in the 1-minute more often than in the 5-minute measurement. The classic paper on the issue of low Apgar scores and cerebral palsy by Nelson & Ellenberg (1981) has shown a poor correlation between a low 5-minute score (0–3) and cerebral palsy in children born at term (4.7% of survivors have cerebral palsy), but there is an increasingly strong correlation with later low Apgar scores, reaching 57.1% of survivors if the 20-minute score remained at 3 or less (Table 72.2). This issue will also be discussed below.

Sykes et al (1982) reported that only 19% of babies with a 5-minute Apgar score of less than 7 had acidosis (pH <7.10 and base deficit >13 mmol/l) among 1210 consecutive deliveries who had umbilical vessel blood gas measurements at birth. Similarly, these authors reported that 86% of babies with acidosis had a 5-minute Apgar score of >7. They questioned the use of the Apgar score as an index for asphyxia.

The possibility exists that low pH values might bear a stronger relationship to poor neurological outcome than low Apgar scores. Dijxhoorn et al (1985) studied this issue among 805 appropriate-for-dates (AFD) infants delivered vaginally. While they did find a relationship between acidaemia at birth and subnormal neurological condition in the nursery, the relationship was a very weak one. They concluded: 'in AFD term infants acidemia at birth is only slightly related to neonatal neurological morbidity.' In a later study they noted no relationship between the presence of meconium-stained amniotic fluid (another frequently used index of intrapartum asphyxia) and neurological condition of the newborn and the same weak relationship between a low 3-minute Apgar score or acidaemia and neurological condition of the newborn (Dijxhoorn et al 1986). They concluded that: 'most neonatal neurological abnormalities must be due to other factors.' While Apgar scores do not correlate perfectly with fetal/neonatal asphyxia as described above, Low at al (1975) have shown that 80% of neonates with severe asphyxia have a low Apgar score. The scores enjoy the advantage that they have been widely used, thus making large banks of data available.

Banta & Thacker (1979) have extracted the available data from the literature on the ability of EFM to predict a depressed Apgar score. They reported false negative rates (1-minute Apgar score less than 7) from the literature of 7.0–13.8% and false positive rates of 18.5–79.6%. A negative EFM tracing correlated better with a high Apgar score than did a positive tracing with a low score. Similarly, Banta & Thacker tabulated the diagnostic accuracy noted by various investigators of a low pH measured by FSBS being able to predict a low 1-minute Apgar score (less than 7). False negative readings were reported in 9.0–23.6% of the cases and false positive readings occurred in 30.3–69.2%. One study utilized a 5-minute Apgar score and noted a false negative rate of 5.6% and a false positive rate of 4.6%. It appears from these studies that both EFM and FSBS are likely to be followed by the expected Apgar score if they are normal or reassuring, but that both tests carry a high false positive rate, i.e. an abnormal reading is frequently followed by the delivery of a child with normal Apgar scores.

In the largest of the randomized clinical trials (the Dublin trial, McDonald et al 1985) comparing the usefulness of continuous EFM (6474 patients) with intermittent auscultation (6490 patients), the frequency of a low Apgar score at both 1 and 5 minutes was not statistically different between the two methods of monitoring (MacDonald et al 1985). Furthermore, the mean pH of the umbilical cord blood was exactly the same in the two groupings (540 patients with EFM and 535 patients with intermittent auscultation). These observations suggest that EFM may not be superior, at least in a statistical sense, to intermittent auscultation in identifying the presence of fetal acidosis. Other possible advantages to EFM were identified, however, and will be discussed below.

Does clinical evidence of asphyxia at birth usually precede the development of cerebral palsy?

Early studies which utilized a cohort of children with cerebral palsy, usually also with a control population without cerebral palsy, were interpreted to show that asphyxiating conditions at birth were present more frequently among the babies with cerebral palsy than among the controls. Lilienfeld & Parkhurst (1951), for example, noted a higher frequency of placenta praevia, prolapse of the umbilical cord and abruptio placentae in the population of babies with cerebral palsy. Since all of these medical conditions are strongly associated with low birthweight, and since low birthweight itself shows the strongest correlation of all known factors with subsequent cerebral palsy — cerebral palsy is 22 times more likely to occur among infants weighing less than 1500 g at birth than among those infants weighing 2500 g or more (Paneth & Stark 1983) — it is entirely possible that the association noted with cerebral palsy may have been an effect of low birthweight rather than of the presumed hypoxia associated with the disease. Indeed, later investigators who controlled for low birthweight in their samples found no correlation between these potentially asphyxiating conditions and the development of cerebral palsy (Cushner 1961, Niswander et al 1975).

A more recent study which analysed one of the same data sets but with greater statistical refinements found an increased incidence of cerebral palsy after some of these obstetric complications but only in association with a very low (0–3) 5-minute Apgar score (Nelson & Ellenberg 1984). Of importance, however, was the observation that no obstetric complication among babies of mature birthweight was associated with a *high* risk of cerebral palsy; in no case was the risk of cerebral palsy following an obstetric complication greater than 2%. These authors, furthermore, cautioned that the relationship noted could not be assumed to be a causal one. 'In a fetus with abnormalities that predate labor, low Apgar scores may sometimes be the result, along with abnormalities of labor, of the underlying defect.'

Thus: 'Apgar scores seem to provide some evidence and rough quantification of abnormal status of the child soon after delivery, whether that status was the effect of an obstetric problem or its cause . . .' (Nelson & Ellenberg 1984). That most infants with cerebral palsy were probably not asphyxiated at birth is illustrated by the observation that only 13% of the cerebral palsy in the infants weighing more than 2500 g at birth occurred in infants with one or more obstetric complications and a 5-minute Apgar score of 5 or less. Or, as has been stated elsewhere by the same authors, 75% of children with cerebral palsy had 5-minute Apgar scores of 7 or greater (Nelson & Ellenberg 1981).

Table 72.3 Obstetric factors related to cerebral palsy

	Lilienfeld	Eastman	Chefetz	Durkin	Nelson
Poor reproductive history	+	++	+	++	++
Abnormality					
Prematurity	++	++		++	++
Postmaturity				++	
Placenta praevia	++				
Abruptio placentae	++	++	++	++	
Toxaemia	+	++	++		0
Placental dysfunction		0		++	+
Precipitate delivery			++	++	
Mid-cavity forceps	0	++	++		++
Anaesthesia		0	+		0
Breech or twin presentation				+	

0 = no difference noted; + = slight increase in damaged children; ++ = increase in damaged children. If left blank, not mentioned by author.
From Niswander (1983).

If asphyxia, as measured by 5-minute Apgar scores, is not a common precedent to cerebral palsy, what is? A review of the papers in the literature which have addressed this question reveals a striking lack of agreement. Table 72.3 shows that only a poor reproductive history and prematurity have been uniformly recognized by all of the authors as precedents to cerebral palsy.

In two important papers on antecedents of cerebral palsy, Nelson & Ellenberg (1985, 1986) studied in both a univariate and multivariate format the factors which preceded the appearance of cerebral palsy in the large Collaborative Perinatal Project (CPP) of the National Institute of Neurological and Communicative Disorders and Stroke. In these unusually comprehensive studies of over 400 variables, the commonly mentioned predictors for cerebral palsy were notably absent—use of oxytocin, vaginal breech delivery, precipitate or prolonged labour, etc. Relatively large increases in the cerebral palsy rate were noted with maternal mental retardation, maternal seizure disorders, maternal hyperthyroidism, or the administration of thyroid hormone and oestrogen during pregnancy, but none of these accounted for many cases of cerebral palsy because of their rarity. When the factors were subjected to a multivariate analysis, the single most important prepregnancy variable predicting cerebral palsy was maternal mental retardation. Among the prenatal predictors, the authors identified a large urinary excretion of albumin (only sometimes associated with hypertension), third-trimester bleeding and three very uncommon characteristics—unusual menstrual cycle, long menstrual cycle and mental retardation in a sibling. Once labour began, the most powerful predictor was a gestational age of 32 weeks or less. Breech presentation was also a predictor, but vaginal breech delivery was not. Severe fetal bradycardia (the study was completed before the availability of continuous EFM), chorionitis and low placental weight were also predictive. None of these factors, however, was a strong predictor, and only severe fetal bradycardia remained if only infants weighing more than 2500 g at birth were included. Among postdelivery factors, low birthweight, a delay in first cry of 5 minutes or more, neonatal seizures, and a major non-CNS malformation were predictive of cerebral palsy.

When the authors allowed the important risk factors from the prenatal period through the nursery course to compete with each other, only neonatal seizures, time to first cry of 5 minutes or more, and major non-CNS malformation were important predictors in infants weighing more than 2500 g. Even when factors from all stages were included, the ability to predict cerebral palsy was very poor. 'When information from all stages were included, children ranking in the top 5 percent according to risk contributed 37 percent of the cerebral palsy. Thus, 63 percent of the cases of cerebral palsy did not occur in the 5 percent with the highest risk' (Nelson & Ellenberg 1986). The false positive rate, furthermore, was 97% and even higher (99%) among infants weighing more than 2500 g. The authors note that the acid test of determining the cause of an outcome is the ability to predict its occurrence. Based on their data, the authors concluded: 'We probably don't know what causes most cases of cerebral palsy'. On the question of asphyxia, they noted:

> 21% of the children with cerebral palsy (40 of 189) had at least one clinical marker of asphyxia (lowest fetal heart rate <60 beats per minute, five-minute Apgar score <3, or time to first cry >5 minutes) but only 17 of that 40 did not have congenital malformations, a birth weight of 2000 gms or less, microcephaly, or an alternative explanation for the cerebral palsy . . . It is not obvious whether prevention of asphyxia could have prevented poor neurologic outcome, since there appeared to be factors present before the onset of labor that may at least have increased their vulnerability to intrapartum events . . . no foreseeable single intervention is likely to prevent a large proportion of cerebral palsy.

Is the fetus who is already brain-damaged from an earlier event more likely to display evidence of intrapartum asphyxia than an intact fetus?

Many authors who have documented a relationship between intrapartum asphyxia and subsequent neurological impairment have cautioned against assuming that this observation implies cause and effect (Nelson & Ellenberg 1986). There is substantial evidence to support an opinion that a fetus who is already brain-damaged before the onset of labour is likely to display evidence of intrapartum asphyxia leading to an unwarranted conclusion, on occasion, that the intrapartum asphyxia caused the brain damage.

Whether brain damage leading to intrapartum asphyxia is more common than intrapartum asphyxia leading to subsequent brain damage is simply unknown. It is evident, however, that there is no more justification for assuming one scenario than for assuming the other. Indirect evidence suggesting that the brain damage leading to asphyxia relationship may be more common than previously thought is, however, accumulating. An analysis of patients with congenital spastic hemiparesis by Michaelis et al (1980), for example, revealed that perinatal asphyxia related strongly to the disease. They found no correlation between the severity of handicap and perinatal complications, however, and concluded that: 'therefore one may argue that newborns with prenatal lesions are more likely to suffer perinatal asphyxia, which does not necessarily cause a further damage to the brain'.

Peters et al (1984), studying the relationship between delayed onset of regular respiration and subsequent development, noted a relationship between delayed onset of breathing and the subsequent appearance of cerebral palsy. In studying the crucial question of whether the respiratory delay may have been a factor contributing to the disease rather than just a symptom of an infant already in poor condition, they concluded that: 'it is quite possible, therefore, that the infant with a delayed onset of regular respirations is already at increased risk of . . . cerebral palsy . . . the sign of apparent asphyxia is merely a marker of other defective reactions to various insults'.

Nelson and Ellenberg (1986) noted that clinical markers of intrapartum asphyxia were present in 21% of their population of children with cerebral palsy, but less than half of these did not have an alternative explanation for the cerebral palsy. They suggest: 'a relatively small role for factors of labor and delivery in accounting for cerebral palsy' and that the cerebral palsy 'may have been related partly or wholly to defects intrinsic to the fetus'.

Gross et al (1968) attempted to correlate the brain pathology present in 891 autopsied cases with neurological disorders with the clinical diagnosis, with special emphasis on an elucidation of the aetiological factors. Perinatal brain damage represented 26% of their cases. They concluded: 'perinatal distress, therefore, may be regarded not only as the cause but also as the result of organic brain damage in a considerable proportion of cases'.

Chiswick et al (1977) studied the computerized tomography scan in seven newborn babies in an attempt to clarify the role of this laboratory tool in the diagnosis and care of newborns with neurological disease. In the three babies who suffered perinatal asphyxia and who remained neurologically abnormal on follow-up, structural lesions were found which made it unlikely that such lesions were the result of perinatal asphyxia. One possible explanation for this finding is that the structural abnormality of the brain predisposed the fetus to asphyxia, which in turn might have caused less careful investigators to conclude that the asphyxia caused the damage.

Dweck et al (1974) compared 15 children who were severely asphyxiated at birth with a group of non-asphyxiated children. At 22–40 months of age, there were no differences in IQ or motor function between the two groups except for neurological damage in three asphyxiated babies who had also displayed intrauterine growth retardation. It is possible that the newborn asphyxia noted in these three infants simply reflected the effects of intrauterine growth retardation and that these three were already brain-damaged when labour began. Certainly, the asphyxia in these children seems to have been different from the asphyxia in the remaining children. At the very least, these infants were much more sensitive to the effects of intrapartum asphyxia than the remaining children. In yet another study among 80 term infants born after intrapartum asphyxia, the five who displayed evidence of neurological damage all had prenatal suspicion of chronic intrauterine distress (Haesslein & Niswander 1980).

Goodlin (1974) reported that insisting on a fetal scalp pH before performing a Caesarean section because of an abnormal electronic fetal heart rate pattern reduced the number of rapid deliveries for fetal distress. Of 11 rapid deliveries for fetal acidosis under these circumstances, however, six of the fetuses had anomalies that were incompatible with life. The authors speculate: 'an abnormal fetus will more likely have an abnormal fetal heart rate and scalp pH during labor'.

Lastly, the finding reported by Nelson & Ellenberg (1981) that a low Apgar score at 20 minutes of age in the term infant relates strongly to the subsequent appearance of cerebral palsy — unlike a low score at 5 minutes — has been interpreted to mean that severe asphyxia (low 20-minute score) is more likely than milder asphyxia (low score at 5 minutes, better score subsequently) to cause cerebral palsy (Table 72.2). An equally plausible explanation of this finding is that the brain-damaged child cannot respond as well to the resuscitative efforts exerted immediately after birth as the child without brain damage who is merely asphyxiated. This interpretation is more in keeping with the subsequent reports (Nelson & Ellenberg 1986) on antecedents of cerebral palsy by the same authors.

RELATIONSHIP BETWEEN SUBSTANDARD OBSTETRIC CARE AND POOR NEUROLOGICAL RESULT

What has been stated regarding the causes of cerebral palsy suggests that very little is known with any degree of precision, or as Nelson & Ellenberg (1986) have written: 'a large proportion of cases of cerebral palsy remains unexplained'. Nevertheless, there is some evidence that asphyxia, either during pregnancy or during labour, may be a cause of cerebral palsy. Since an obstetrician can recognize possible asphyxia in the fetus, although only to a limited degree of accuracy, to be sure, testing the hypothesis that good obstetric care can reduce the risk of the development of cerebral palsy is warranted. This hypothesis has been tested both directly and indirectly and a synthesis of the results of these experiments will allow us to speculate further on the extent to which obstetrical care may affect the prevalence of cerebral palsy.

One approach to the problem has been to study the relationship between the quality of obstetric care and the prevalence of newborn convulsions since: 'neonatal seizures appear to be the best evidence of asphyxia and the best predictor of later damage' (Brann 1985). The possibility exists, of course, that while both parts of this statement are true, they may be unrelated. That is, neonatal seizures may reflect the presence of asphyxia in many cases, but are these the same patients who go on to develop cerebral palsy as so many do following neonatal seizures, or do the cases of cerebral palsy preceded by neonatal seizures largely reflect disease already present in the fetus even before the onset of labour? Neonatal seizures can undoubtedly reflect either recent asphyxia or neurological disease from various causes present before labour. A review of several experiments will allow us to approach an answer to these important questions.

A suggestion that the population of babies with newborn convulsions may not be homogeneous is apparent in the randomized trials on the relative efficacy of continuous EFM and intermittent auscultation of the fetal heart. The Dublin trial (McDonald et al 1985), for example, reported an incidence of very early neonatal seizures in term babies which was nearly three times as high with auscultation as with continuous EFM; this outcome was almost identical to that reported in similar earlier smaller trials (MacDonald et al 1985). Yet preliminary follow-up to 1 year of age has shown the same risk for the development of cerebral palsy in the two groups of babies. Niswander et al (1984) noted a significant relationship between obstetric failure to react to evidence of fetal asphyxia and convulsions during the first 48 hours of life in the term infant, yet there was no apparent relationship between failure to react to fetal asphyxia and cerebral palsy. These experiments suggest that early convulsions in term newborns may have two different aetiologies — one an intrapartum event which is not likely to be followed by permanent neurological damage, and the second a prenatal event which causes both the newborn convulsions and the subsequently discovered cerebral palsy. This tentative conclusion is supported by other recent experiments.

Minchom et al (1986) in the Cardiff Birth Survey studied 54 cases of neonatal seizures during the first 48 hours of life delivered between 1970 and 1979 and compared them to 41 090 controls in a geographically defined population. Follow-up information, almost always to at least 3 years of age among survivors, was available in all but three of the study cases, all of whom were known to be normal at 1 year. It was also possible to study the fetal heart rate tracings of the 33 cases delivered between 1975 and 1979 for comparison with 75 randomly selected controls delivered during the same period (Table 72.4). In 7 of 30 seizure cases for which EFM traces were available and interpretable, delivery had been preceded by prolonged abnormalities of the fetal heart rate consistent with possible severe fetal distress (bradycardia for at least 40 minutes, severe variable decelerations for at least 75 minutes or late decelerations for at least 90 minutes). No such cases were found among the 73 controls with interpretable EFM tracings. Follow-up to 3 years of age, however, revealed an equal percentage of children in the two groups who were neurologically disabled — those with presumed severe fetal asphyxia and those without evidence of severe asphyxia. Again, the explanation that newborn seizures have either an intrapartum aetiology, usually without permanent sequelae, or an earlier prenatal cause, which may also result in long-term neurological deficit, seems plausible.

Table 72.4 Prolonged abnormality of electronic fetal monitoring (EFM) and outcome from 1975 to 1979

	Prolonged abnormality of EFM	No prolonged abnormality of EFM	Total cases
Newborn			
Convulsions	7 (23.3%)	23	30 (33)
Controls	0 (0%)	73	73 (75)
At 3 years			
Neonatal death	0 (0%)	2	2
Disability	2 (28.6%)	5	7
No disability	5 (25.0%)	15	20

From Minchom et al (1986).

Lastly, Keegan et al (1985) reported a study on convulsions of the newborn. While these authors studied seizures in infants of all gestations it is possible to separate those born at term from the premature babies. They noted a strong relationship between newborn convulsions in term babies and a preceding abnormal EFM pattern. Follow-up of the children, although incomplete because of lost patients, showed a high percentage with permanent neurological damage. Assessment of the appropriateness of the reaction of the clinician to the abnormal EFM pattern showed that in all but three instances the clinical care of the patients was good. The authors thus concluded that although an abnormal EFM pattern frequently precedes newborn convulsions in the term infant, permanent neurological sequelae seem not to be prevented even when the reaction to the abnormal EFM pattern is appropriate. Again, the development of neurological sequelae following an abnormal EFM pattern (with newborn convulsions an intermediary event) even when the reaction to the abnormal pattern was deemed appropriate seems to imply that the neurological pathology was present before the occurrence of the asphyxia reflected in the EFM tape.

A study by Painter et al (1978) reported a follow-up of 12 infants with a normal EFM pattern and 22 infants who showed a severe variable or late deceleration pattern in labour. None of the 12 control infants were neurologically abnormal at 1 year while 6 of the 22 with an abnormal EFM pattern were abnormal. There was no significant difference in the time elapsed from onset of the abnormal EFM pattern and delivery between the 6 children who were abnormal at 1 year and the 16 found to be normal. At 4 years and later, none of the study children were found to be neurologically abnormal (Painter et al 1988). Thus, an abnormal EFM pattern, even when rather prolonged, does not seem to be a very good predictor of subsequent brain damage.

These observations have been confirmed by unpublished data collected by Roberto Caldeyro-Barcia, one of the earliest and most prominent advocates of EFM. Professor Caldeyro-Barcia followed children who had had grossly abnormal EFM patterns and/or low blood pH consistent with severe acidosis and found that they were likely to be severely asphyxiated at birth and that many had neurological abnormalities at a few months of age. Long-term follow-up, however, showed most of these children to be normal neurologically by clinical examination.

It has become evident to serious students of the issue that the exact cause of cerebral palsy in an individual case is usually simply not known. While there is a modest correlation between asphyxia at birth as well as early newborn convulsions in the term infant and subsequent cerebral palsy, most papers reporting these correlations warn against assuming that a cause-and-effect relationship is involved. Fiona Stanley (1984) has suggested that it is still an open question whether babies are first damaged in utero and consequently suffer perinatal asphyxia or whether brain damage is the consequence of perinatal asphyxia.

From the data outlined in this chapter, it is apparent that it is as reasonable to attribute the intrapartum asphyxia and the cerebral palsy to a common causative event as it is to implicate the asphyxia as the cause of the subsequently discovered cerebral palsy. For many reasons it may never be possible to be certain which of these scenarios is more likely. Such reasons include rarity of a bad outcome (about two cases of cerebral palsy per 1000 deliveries), varying methods of defining severity of asphyxia and the possible effect of medical intervention.

Does intrapartum asphyxia cause cerebral palsy in humans and how frequently does this happen? We need not wait for an answer to this question, however, before asking an equally important question: Does medical intervention with asphyxia lower the risk of the development of cerebral palsy? Or does substandard obstetric care increase the risk of the development of cerebral palsy?

Such an investigation was mounted under the aegis of the Oxford Cerebral Palsy Study (Niswander et al 1984). The cases from this study used in the analysis were those in which terminal apnoea was present at birth, where newborn convulsions occurred during the first 48 hours of life in term infants, and those in whom cerebral palsy was diagnosed at 18 months of age. The cases were delivered at the John Radcliffe Hospital, Oxford, between 1 January 1978 and 31 December 1980. It was possible to compare these cases with a prospectively and randomly selected control population delivered during the same period at the same hospital. The medical records of the mothers of the infants were obtained and 'blinded' by a nurse midwife to any paediatric information.

Using prearranged criteria thought to represent good contemporary obstetric care, the blinded records were reviewed by an obstetrician and categorized as receiving standard or substandard prenatal care and standard or substandard intrapartum care. The criteria emphasized the recognition and treatment of fetal asphyxia since it is this possible aetiology of cerebral palsy that has been most widely discussed in recent years. The authors also attempted to study a possible connection between difficult forceps delivery and subsequent cerebral palsy.

The issue could not be satisfactorily settled in this study, although the use of forceps did not play any apparent role in the evolution of cerebral palsy in the population analysed. This opinion is consistent with current medical thought that difficult forceps delivery is a very uncommon cause of subsequent brain damage.

The population included 92 children with terminal apnoea at birth, 34 term babies with very early neonatal seizures, and 36 children with cerebral palsy diagnosed at 18 months of age. The randomly selected controls numbered 375 for comparison with the terminally apnoeic babies and 377 for comparison with the other two study groups. The results of the analysis are given in Table 72.5. Only a few cases or controls were unclassifiable for quality of obstetric care, usually due to a very short admission-to-delivery interval or occasionally to inadequate or lost records.

In all, 4.6% of the control patients received substandard antenatal care and 14.6 received substandard care during labour. Only the mothers of the children with early convulsions were noted to have been in receipt of substandard prenatal care statistically more often than control mothers. There were no differences between the other two study groups and the controls for adequacy of prenatal care, and none of them were different from controls for quality of intrapartum care.

It was possible to identify a subgroup of mothers receiving substandard care in whom a failure to react to evidence of fetal asphyxia occurred. This was precisely defined to be present if fetal acid–base status was not made or delivery was effected in the presence of prolonged bradycardia for 40 minutes, severe unremitting variable decelerations for 75 minutes or late decelerations for 90 minutes (Table 72.6).

Table 72.5 Relationship of poor fetal outcome to substandard obstetric care

Outcome (no. of cases)	Substandard care during pregnancy			Substandard care during labour		
	n	%	Relative risk*	*n*	%	Relative risk*
Normal (random controls; 375/7)	17	4.6		53	14.6	
Fetal death (58)	8	15.1	3.7†	2	40.0	3.9
Terminal apnoea (92)	3	3.5	0.7	15	16.3	1.1
Newborn convulsions (term infants; 36)	5	13.2	3.4‡	6	16.0	1.2
Cerebral palsy (34)	1	3.1	0.7	1	2.9	0.2

* Likelihood that mother of baby with poor outcome received substandard care; † significantly different from 1 at 99% confidence level (confidence limits omitted for simplicity); ‡ significantly different from 1 at 95 *t*-confidence level.
From Niswander et al (1984).

Table 72.6 Relationship of poor fetal outcome to delayed reaction of attending personnel to intrapartum asphyxia

Outcome (no. of cases)	Cases involving delayed reaction of attending personnel		
	n	%	Relative risk*
Normal (random controls; 375/7)	5	1.4	
Fetal death (58)	1	20.0	18.0†
Terminal apnoea (92)	5	5.4	4.1†
Newborn convulsions (term infants; 36)	3	7.9	6.6‡
Cerebral palsy (34)	0	0.0	1.2

* Likelihood that mother of baby with poor outcome received substandard care; † significantly different from 1 at 95% confidence level (confidence limits omitted for simplicity); ‡ significantly different from 1 at 99% confidence level.
From Niswander et al (1984).

The authors fully realized the imprecision of these criteria in defining the failure to react to asphyxia. The relative risk of this happening with terminal apnoea compared to controls was significantly elevated, as it also was with early newborn convulsions. There was no increase in relative risk of this happening among the mothers of infants with cerebral palsy, and, indeed, a delay in reaction to fetal asphyxia was not identified in any baby who subsequently developed cerebral palsy.

This study illustrates that substandard obstetric care is at least not a common cause of cerebral palsy. It further suggests that intrapartum asphyxia is not a common cause of cerebral palsy, an observation which confirms the opinion of two National Institutes of Health publications on the matter (US Department of Health, Education and Welfare 1979, 1985). It suggests that investigators might well begin to focus on the possibility that the intrapartum or newborn asphyxia seen in a significant number of children who subsequently are found to have cerebral palsy may be a reflection of an earlier event which also caused the cerebral palsy, rather than the mechanism which causes the neurological damage. The issue continues to be an open one, but the burden of proof seems to have shifted to those who believe that the intrapartum asphyxia is the cause of the cerebral palsy and that interruption of the asphyxia will reduce the likelihood of the appearance of cerebral palsy.

PREMATURITY AND CEREBRAL PALSY

Most cerebral palsy occurs in infants born at term; as outlined above, the possible causes of cerebral palsy, especially the emphasis on intrapartum asphyxia, has primarily concerned the term infant. One of the strongest correlates, however, in all studies on the causes of cerebral palsy is the one between prematurity and cerebral palsy. While numerically the term infant accounts for most cerebral palsy simply because most pregnancies end at term, proportionately far more premature babies than term babies are eventually found to suffer from cerebral palsy. One pathological finding noted in many of the brains of these premature infants is periventricular malacia — destruction of brain tissue that lies near the third ventricle. The pathophysiology of the development of this lesion has been the subject of intense study, and several authors have attempted to see what clinical factors in these babies might predispose to the appearance of periventricular haemorrhage (PVH), probably a major precedent to the brain destruction which subsequently develops in these children.

The availability of new imaging techniques has demonstrated the frequency (about 50%) with which intraventricular haemorrhage (IVH) occurs in premature infants, especially in those of birthweight less than 1500 g. Most authors have classified these haemorrhages into three categories of severity; the most severe, grade III, is especially likely to precede the development of cerebral palsy. Grade III IVH involves extension of the haemorrhage into the periventricular tissue. What then causes IVH to occur in some premature infants while it is absent in many others? Many studies have attempted to provide an answer to this question, and we will emphasize herein the obstetrical factors studied.

Most, but not all, studies have concluded that the method of delivery shows no correlation with the development of IVH (de Crespigny & Robinson 1983, Tejani et al 1984, Low et al 1986). In most studies, Caesarean section did not prevent the occurrence of IVH and forceps usage did not increase the occurrence rate (Bada et al 1984). The presence of asphyxia and its possible relationship to IVH has been of particular interest to investigators. Almost without exception, recent reports have found no relationship between the occurrence of IVH, especially the more severe varieties, and various measurements which may denote asphyxia. Low et al (1986) found no correlation between severe metabolic acidosis at birth and risk of IVH. De Crespigny & Robinson (1983) found no correlation between low Apgar scores or the need to administer bicarbonate and the development of IVH. Beverley et al (1984) state: 'umbilical cord blood gas analysis did not support the hypothesis that hypoxia was causal [for IVH]'. Papile et al (1978) found no differences in Apgar scores or the need for respiratory assistance between the IVH group and the premature babies without IVH.

The best current theory to explain the development of IVH centres around the instability of intravascular pressure and the fragility of the vessels in the choroid plexus and the subependymal area of the brain of the premature baby. It is thought that slight changes in the blood pressure of these infants can result in rupture of the blood vessels with subsequent bleeding. One study reported a striking association in the preterm infant with the respiratory distress syndrome between a pattern of fluctuating cerebral blood flow velocity during the first day of life and IVH (Perlman et al 1983). This theory for the production of IVH was further supported by a prospective study in which newborn babies with a fluctuating pattern of cerebral blood flow velocity were randomly assigned to a control group or to a group subjected to muscle paralysis with pancuronium bromide (Perlman et al 1985). IVH developed in all 10 of the control group; 7 of the 10 had severe IVH. IVH developed in 5 of the 14 paralysed infants; in 4 of the 5 the IVH developed after cessation of the paralysis. None of the paralysed infants developed a severe form of IVH. The authors concluded: 'elimination of fluctuating cerebral blood-flow velocity in the preterm infants with respiratory distress syndrome markedly reduces the incidence and severity of intraventricular hemorrhage'.

The evidence to date thus seems to indicate that obstetrical care plays little or no role in the production of IVH. The theoretic possibility exists that either fetal asphyxia or traumatic delivery might exert an influence in this regard, however, and obstetric care of the fetus whose mother is in premature labour clearly should avoid these potentially deleterious developments, if at all possible. Similarly, the availability of various tocolytic agents has suggested the possibility that tocolysis may reduce the prevalence of premature labour and thus, potentially, the risk of IVH. One review of the subject of preterm labour, however, realistically reminds us that: 'tocolytic therapy has not ... reduced the incidence of preterm birth' (Eggleston 1986). Furthermore, the safety of the agents presently available continues to be questioned. There are far more convincing reasons — neonatal mortality, for example — for trying to prevent premature labour than the dubious decrease in the risk of IVH.

Acknowledgement

I am grateful to Dr Karin Nelson for reviewing this manuscript.

REFERENCES

Bada H, Korones S, Anderson G, Magill H, Wong S 1984 Obstetric factors and relative risk of neonatal germinal layer intraventricular hemorrhage. American Journal of Obstetrics and Gynecology 148: 798

Banta H, Thacker S 1979 Assessing the costs and benefits of electronic fetal monitoring. Obstetric and Gynecologic Survey 34: 627

Beverley D, Chance G, Coates C 1984 Intraventricular hemorrhage: timing of occurrence and relationship to perinatal events. British Journal of Obstetrics and Gynaecology 91: 1007

Brann A 1985 Factors during neonatal life that influence brain disorders. In: Freeman J (ed) Prenatal and perinatal factors associated with brain disorders. US Department of Health and Human Services NIH Publication (no. 85-1149), Bethesda, Maryland, p 53

Broman S 1978 Perinatal antecedents of severe mental retardation in school age children. Presented at the 86th Annual Convention of the American Psychological Association, Toronto

Brown J, Purvis R, Forfar J, Cockburn F 1974 Neurological aspects of perinatal asphyxia. Developmental Medicine and Child Neurology 16: 567

Chiswick M, D'Souza S, Occleshaw J 1977 Computerized transverse axial tomography in the newborn. Early Human Development 1: 171

Clapp J, Peress N, Mann L 1985 Effect of intermittent partial cord occlusion or hyperglycemia on neuropathologic outcome in the fetal lamb. Phoenix, AZ Society for Gynecologic Investigation 32nd Annual Meeting (abstract)

Cushner I 1961 Prolapse of the umbilical cord, including a late follow-up of fetal survivors. American Journal of Obstetrics and Gynecology 81: 666

de Crespigny L, Robinson H 1983 Can obstetricians prevent neonatal intraventricular hemorrhage? Australian and New Zealand Journal of Obstetrics and Gynecology 23: 146

D'Souza S, Richards B 1978 Neurological sequelae in newborn babies after asphyxia. Archives of Disease in Childhood 53: 564

Dijxhoorn M, Visser G, Huisjes H et al 1985 The relation between umbilical pH values and neonatal neurological morbidity in full term appropriate for dates infants. Early Human Development 11: 33

Dijxhoorn M, Visser G, Fidler V, Touwen B, Huisjes H 1986 Apgar score, meconium, and acidaemia at birth in relation to neonatal neurological morbidity in term infants. British Journal of Obstetrics and Gynaecology 93: 217

Dweck H, Huggins W, Dorman L, Saxon S, Benton J, Cassady G 1974 Developmental sequelae in infants having suffered severe perinatal asphyxia. American Journal of Obstetrics and Gynecology 119: 811

Eggleston M 1986 Management of preterm labor and delivery. Clinical Obstetrics and Gynecology 29: 230

Gilles F 1985 Neuropathologic indicators of abnormal development. In: Freeman J (ed) Prenatal and perinatal factors associated with brain disorders. US Department of Health and Human Services NIH Publication (no. 85-1149), Bethesda, Maryland, p 53

Gilles F, Leviton A, Kerr C 1976 Endotoxin leucoencephalopathy in the telencephalon of the newborn kitten. Journal of the Neurological Sciences 27: 183

Goodlin R 1974 Fetal monitoring. Obstetrics and Gynecology 43: 474

Gross H, Jellinger K, Kaltenback E, Rett A 1968 Infantile cerebral disorders: clinical–neuropathological correlations to elucidate the aetiological factors. Journal of the Neurological Sciences 7: 551

Haesslein H, Niswander K 1980 Fetal distress in term pregnancies. American Journal of Obstetrics and Gynecology 137: 245

Hensleigh P, Fainstat T, Spencer R 1986 Perinatal events and cerebral palsy. American Journal of Obstetrics and Gynecology 154: 978

Keegan K, Waffarn F, Quilligan E 1985 Obstetric characteristics and fetal

heart rate patterns in infants who convulse during the newborn period. American Journal of Obstetrics and Gynecology 153: 732
Leviton A, Gilles F 1973 An epidemologic study of perinatal telencephalic leucoencephalopathy in an autopsy population. Journal of Neurological Sciences 18: 53
Lilienfeld A, Parkhurst E 1951 Study of the association of factors of pregnancy and parturition with the development of cerebral palsy: a preliminary report. American Journal of Hygiene 53: 262
Low J, Pancham S, Worthington D, Boston R 1975 Clinical characteristics of pregnancies complicated by intrapartum fetal asphyxia. American Journal of Obstetrics and Gynecology 121: 452
Low J, Galbraith R, Muir D, Killen H, Karchmar J, Campbell D 1978 Intrapartum fetal asphyxia: a preliminary report in regard to long term morbidity. American Journal of Obstetrics and Gynecology 130: 525
Low J, Galbraith R, Sauerbrei E et al 1986 Maternal, fetal, and newborn complications associated with newborn intracranial hemorrhage. American Journal of Obstetrics and Gynecology 154: 345
MacDonald D, Grant A, Sheridan-Periera M, Boylan P, Chalmers I 1985 The Dublin randomized control trial of intrapartum fetal monitoring. American Journal of Obstetrics and Gynecology 152: 524
Michaelis R, Rooschuz B, Dopfer R 1980 Prenatal origins of congenital spastic hemiparesis. Early Human Development 4: 243
Minchom P, Niswander K, Chalmers I et al 1987 Antecedents and outcome of very early neonatal seizures in infants born at or after term. British Journal of Obstetrics and Gynaecology 94: 431–439
Myers R 1972 Two patterns of perinatal brain damage and their conditions of occurrence. American Journal of Obstetrics and Gynecology 112: 246
Myers R, Wagner K, de Courten G 1981 Lactic acid accumulation in tissue as cause of brain injury and death and cardiogenic shock from asphyxia. In: Lauersen N, Hochberg H (eds) Perinatal biochemical monitoring. Williams & Wilkins, Baltimore, p 11
Nelson K, Ellenberg J 1981 Apgar scores as predictors of chronic neurologic disability. Pediatrics 68: 36
Nelson K, Ellenberg J 1984 Obstetric complications as risk factors for cerebral palsy or seizure disorders. Journal of the American Medical Association 251: 1843
Nelson K, Ellenberg J 1985 Antecedents of cerebral palsy: univariate analysis of risk. American Journal of Diseases of Children 139: 1031
Nelson K, Ellenberg J 1986 Antecedents of cerebral palsy: multivariate analysis of risk. New England Journal of Medicine 315: 81
Niswander K 1983 Asphyxia in the fetus and cerebral palsy. Yearbook of Obstetrics and Gynecology. Yearbook Medical, Chicago
Niswander K, Gordon M, Drage J 1975 The effect of intrauterine hypoxia on the child surviving to 4 years. American Journal of Obstetrics and Gynecology 121: 892
Niswander K, Henson G, Elbourne D et al 1984 Adverse outcome of pregnancy and the quality of obstetric care. Lancet ii: 827
Painter M, Depp R, O'Donoghue T 1978 Fetal heart rate patterns and development in the first year of life. American Journal of Obstetrics and Gynecology 132: 271
Painter M, Scott M, Hirsch P et al 1988 Fetal heart rate patterns during labor: neurological and cognitive development at six to nine years of age. American Journal of Obstetrics and Gynecology 159: 854–858
Paneth N, Stark R 1983 Cerebral palsy and mental retardation in relation to indicators of perinatal asphyxia: an epidemiologic overview. American Journal of Obstetrics and Gynecology 147: 960
Papile L, Burstein J, Burstein R, Koffler H 1978 Incidence and evolution of subependymal and intraventricular hemorrhage: a study of infants with birth weights less than 1500 grams. Journal of Pediatrics 92: 529
Perlman J, McMenamin J, Volpe J 1983 Fluctuating cerebral blood-flow velocity in respiratory distress syndrome. New England Journal of Medicine 309: 204
Perlman J, Goodman S, Kreusser K, Volpe J 1985 Reduction in intraventricular hemorrhage by elimination of fluctuating cerebral blood-flow velocity in preterm infants with respiratory distress syndrome. New England Journal of Medicine 312: 1353
Peters T, Golding J, Lawrence C, Fryer J, Chamberlain G, Butler V 1984 Delayed onset of regular respirations and subsequent development. Early Human Development 9: 225
Scott H 1976 Outcome of very severe birth asphyxia. Archives of Diseases of Children 51: 712
Stanley F 1984 Perinatal risk factors in the cerebral palsies. Clinics of Developmental Medicine 87: 98
Sykes G, Johnson P, Ashworth F et al 1982 Do Apgar scores indicate asphyxia? Lancet i: 494
Tejani N, Rebold B, Tuck S, Ditroia D, Sutro W, Verma U 1984 Obstetric factors in the causation of early periventricular–intraventricular hemorrhage. Obstetrics and Gynecology 64: 510
Thomson A, Searle M, Russell G 1977 Quality of survival after severe birth asphyxia. Archives of Diseases of Children 52: 62
US Department of Health, Education and Welfare 1979 Predictors of intrapartum fetal distress. 79-1973
US Department of Health and Human Sciences 1985 Prenatal and perinatal factors associated with brain disorders. 85-1149

73

Tim J. Peters

Later results of obstetrical care

INTRODUCTION

It is now well over 30 years since Lilienfeld, Parkhurst and Pasamanick first introduced the concept of a continuum of reproductive casualty extending from a lethal component consisting of abortions, stillbirths and neonatal deaths to a sublethal component consisting of cerebral palsy and perhaps other developmental disorders in the children who survived (Lilienfeld & Parkhurst 1951, Lilienfeld & Pasamanick 1954). The degree of disability was postulated to be related directly to anoxia experienced as a result of complications during labour and delivery.

The implication of this concept is that factors such as pre-eclampsia and breech delivery which are associated with poor outcome of pregnancy will also be associated with later developmental problems — for example, that all the risk factors for perinatal mortality are also risk factors for cerebral palsy. Despite many reviews concluding that there is very little evidence in the literature to support this concept (Nelson 1968, Gottfried 1973, Sameroff & Chandler 1975, Sameroff 1978, Peters & Golding 1985, Ounsted 1987, Golding & Peters 1988a), it continues to influence many investigations into the long-term effects of obstetrical care (Neligan et al 1974, Steiner & Neligan 1983), including studies concerned with formal assessments of risk (Molfese & Thomson 1985). Even for cerebral palsy, the role of adverse birth events as causal factors is far from clear, with risks possibly accruing indirectly (that is, from preterm delivery and growth retardation) as well as directly from perinatal trauma (Stanley 1984b). Certainly, as regards minor developmental disorders there remains a serious question as to whether the survivors of early trauma who show no obvious brain damage fare any worse than children who have not had such an experience (Walker et al 1976, Sameroff 1978, Ounsted 1987).

The main criticism of the original work by Lilienfeld and colleagues has been that it was based entirely on retrospective analysis of children with cerebral palsy and other disorders, with no information concerning the development of the controls (Nelson 1968, Ounsted 1987). Gottfried (1973) has pointed out that prospective longitudinal studies are to be preferred when considering long-term associations, though of course quite large numbers will be required to detect subtle effects. Furthermore, any comprehensive study into brain damage at birth must consider the antecedents of problems in labour and delivery such as breech presentation and perinatal hypoxia (Illingworth 1979, 1985).

These reservations about the existence of a continuum of reproductive casualty have a number of methodological implications. Primarily, risk factors for outcome, whether perinatal or long-term, need to be investigated quantitatively in terms of specific outcomes related to specific risk factors, with adequate control for known confounding effects (Nelson 1968, Stanley 1984a). A study need not be prospective in order to achieve these objectives — indeed case control studies are more appropriate in many instances (Hagberg & Hagberg 1984), though as already noted relatively large prospective studies are preferable when investigating the relationships of pre- and perinatal factors with long-term outcomes such as physical development, the health and the educational ability of the child. It is nevertheless clear that reliable insights into the causes of impaired development are unlikely to be provided by retrospective studies with inadequate controls such as those of Lilienfeld and colleagues, and particularly by studies with no controls (Culbertson & Ferry 1982, McQueen et al 1986).

The aim of this chapter is to describe the results of investigations into child development for a nationally representative cohort of births taking place in the UK in one week of April 1970 (Chamberlain et al 1975, 1978). The members of this birth cohort were followed up at the ages of 5 and 10 years; the analyses reviewed here concern a number of aspects of their development considered in relation to obstetrical factors collected close to the time of birth. The review will cover investigations into child development following late attendance for antenatal care as well as associations with factors such as pain relief administered during labour and the residual effects of apparent neonatal asphyxia. Before discussing these results in detail, the 1970 cohort study is described and compared with various alternative designs.

THE BRITISH NATIONAL COHORT STUDIES

The 1970 study is the third in a unique series of national longitudinal studies undertaken in Britain. All three began as birth surveys of every child born in a given week, only later becoming longitudinal studies by following up the survivors at various times throughout their lives. The birth surveys were carried out in 1946, 1958 and 1970, and each consisted of a questionnaire usually completed by the midwife who attended the delivery. The midwives (or health visitors in 1946) obtained the required information both from interviews with the mother and from clinical records. The follow-up surveys involved interviews with the mother, carried out by health visitors, parental and teacher self-completion questionnaires, special tests for the children, school and health records and medical examinations by clinical medical officers (Atkins et al 1981, Fogelman & Wedge 1981, Golding 1984). The cohort studies have provided information concerning changes through time in matters such as antenatal care, obstetrical management and general characteristics of the mothers as well as birthweight, perinatal death and the development of medical conditions in childhood (Butler & Bonham 1963, Butler & Alberman 1969, Chamberlain et al 1975, 1978, Peters et al 1983, Butler & Golding 1986).

The 1970 cohort

The British Births 1970 Survey obtained information on 17 196 deliveries to 17 005 mothers (including 189 pairs of twins and one set of triplets) occurring in the UK during the week 5–11 April 1970 (Chamberlain et al 1975, 1978). It has been estimated that this represents 97.3% of all livebirths during this week and 91.4% of all stillbirths (Golding, personal communication).

Follow-up studies of this cohort began with height, weight and head circumference measurements at 22 months of age on all twins, postmature births (42 + completed weeks gestation) and small-for-dates infants together with a 10% sample of the remainder as controls. The smaller babies were observed to catch up in terms of physical growth (Chamberlain & Davey 1975). The childhood illnesses of all these selected infants have also been investigated, in a survey at 3 years of age (Chamberlain & Simpson 1979). Risk factors identified in this latter study were: family size for infectious diseases, maternal smoking for lower respiratory tract infection and maternal employment outside the home for accidents.

The first attempt to contact the entire cohort obtained information at 5 years of age on 13 135 infants, including 392 with no birth information. Generally, the children were traced to their home addresses through Family Practitioner Committees following initial identification by the registration division of the Registrar General's office of all children born during the relevant week and the acquisition of their National Health Service (NHS) numbers from the NHS Central Register (full details are given in Osborn et al 1984). Health visitors then went to the homes identified by this procedure in order to interview the mothers, at which time they measured the height and head circumference of each survey child, administered simple intellectual tests and obtained information on hospital admissions and immunizations for the child. Health visitor and child health clinic records were used to validate this information whenever possible, and in addition the mothers were given a self-completion questionnaire concerning, for example, the child's behaviour and the mother's own health and attitudes.

In all, 90% of the contacts were made within a month of the child's fifth birthday (Osborn et al 1984), and the total number represents 80% of the survivors who were resident in Britain. (Children who were resident in Northern Ireland were omitted from this and subsequent follow-up surveys because of the political situation in the province.)

The characteristics of the children lost to follow-up have been investigated in relation to information available from the birth survey and from a special survey of these children in 1977 (Osborn et al 1984, Butler & Golding 1986, Peters 1986). Although the children followed up were representative of the original cohort in many respects, the non-responders at age 5 were far less likely to be living with their natural father, whilst they were more likely to have parents from ethnic minorities, to have been taken into care and to come from geographically mobile families. It was concluded that the effects of these biases would not be expected to be large.

There have been two major volumes published on the results of the 5-year follow-up, the first concentrating on the relationship of social disadvantage, preschool education and maternal employment with the child's behaviour and performance in educational tests (Osborn et al 1984) and the second relating health and behaviour to factors such as social class, region of birth, maternal smoking, household moves, birthweight and maternal age (Butler & Golding 1986).

Many different aspects of development and environment were once again investigated when 14 906 children in the cohort were followed up at the age of 10 years (90% of the survivors). This follow-up included detailed testing of educational ability through the children's schools as well as parental self-completion questionnaires, medical examinations and information from records. Analysis of this information has to date focused upon the prevalence of disability in the cohort, presented in a number of unpublished reports by the Child Health and Education Study to the Departments of Education and Science, and Health and Social Security.

The contribution of the national cohort studies

One obvious advantage over local longitudinal studies such as the Aberdeen child development study (Illsley & Wilson 1981), the Newcastle 1000 families study (Miller et al 1974) and the Newcastle survey of child development (Neligan et al 1974) is that they are national; regional variations both in incidence/prevalence and in associations between two or more factors may then be investigated. Furthermore, despite the losses incurred, the cohorts are clearly more representative than was achieved in the collaborative perinatal project in the USA (Broman et al 1975).

On the other hand, one result of this national coverage is that only relatively infrequent follow-up studies are feasible, so that the Child Health and Education Study (1970 cohort) is essentially a series of linked cross-sectional studies carried out on the same children. In addition, the broad spectrum of issues covered by the surveys perforce limits the depth of the information obtained. As a result, specific questions concerning the effects of particular aspects of obstetrical management are more appropriately addressed by controlled trials, for which a classified bibliography is available (National Perinatal Epidemiology Unit 1985).

Nevertheless, the cohort studies are unique in their ability to provide national estimates of prevalence for many conditions. Moreover, the surveys collected information on a large number of general background factors, and simultaneously covered many different areas of either obstetrical performance or child development. Various aspects of the child's situation may therefore be taken into account in any particular investigation of the data; this is an advantage not shared by more specific studies, although again these may often examine particular hypotheses in more depth. The basic longitudinal design of cohort studies is the only reliable method of detecting subtle long-term effects on child development.

National cohort studies cannot replace smaller in-depth studies, especially for the investigation of extremely rare conditions, but may be viewed as complementing them and may be employed as hypothesis developers and eliminators to suggest where more focused studies might be worthwhile (Blaxter 1983, Golding 1984, Peters 1986). In addition, they may be used to test hypotheses suggested by each other (Peters et al 1983, Peters 1986).

OBSTETRICAL CARE AND DEVELOPMENTAL OUTCOME IN THE 1970 COHORT

Late attendance for antenatal care

In 1980 the report of the House of Commons Social Services Committee voiced a generally accepted opinion by stating: 'we unhesitatingly accept the often reiterated aim of antenatal care as a means of reducing perinatal and neonatal mortality' (Short Report 1980). As implied by this statement, however, antenatal care is promoted on the basis of benefits which are on the whole assumed rather than founded on hard scientific evidence. Whilst there are undoubtedly benefits to certain groups of high-risk pregnancies such as diabetic women and those developing eclampsia, the advantages to the majority of women not at special risk are less clear-cut; indeed both through potential side-effects of interventions and through increased anxiety many antenatal procedures may be counterproductive for large numbers of women (Enkin & Chalmers 1982).

The optimal format of antenatal care is certainly under debate (Coope & Scott 1982, Hall et al 1985) but again often in the absence of adequate evaluations of its effectiveness, and under the erroneous assumption that quantity means quality (Enkin & Chalmers 1982). Nevertheless, there is a widespread view that the first visit should take place in the first trimester.

With this background, the 1970 cohort data have been analysed first to investigate which groups of women were more likely to fail to attend for antenatal care until beyond 28 weeks' gestation (measured in completed weeks from the date of the first day of the last menstrual period), with analyses carried out for primigravidae and multigravidae separately (Thomas et al 1986). Since gestation was a crucial element of this classification, those uncertain of their dates were excluded. (These pregnancies, which together with those with unknown dates amounted to just under 20% of all singleton deliveries, are themselves to be the subject of a separate study.) The study sample thus consisted of 4492 primiparae (of whom 454 or 10.1% were late attenders) and 8635 multiparae (of whom 931 or 10.8% were late attenders). Taking account of this profile of late attenders, the authors investigated whether such delay was associated with adverse outcomes in either the mother or the child (Thomas et al 1986).

Using logistic regression methods — described briefly in the report and in more detail by Peters (1986) — applied to a large number of possible predictors, four factors were found to be independently associated with an increased proportion delaying attendance for antenatal care among both primigravidae and multigravidae: being unmarried; the father of the child being born outside England; not having used contraceptives in the 18 months prior to the conception of the survey child; residence in the West Midlands, Wales and, for first pregnancies, Scotland. For multigravidae, high parity, maternal youth and short interpregnancy interval were also associated with an increased likelihood of late attendance (Thomas et al 1986). This profile of late bookers was noted to be consistent with a number of other studies in various parts of Britain (Robertson & Carr 1970, Simpson & Walker 1980, Hall & Chng 1982, Lewis 1982), and generally to indicate a failure to plan.

Controlling for the above characteristics, the outcome of these pregnancies was not significantly different from the rest of the sample in terms of both mean birthweight and proportion of low birthweight babies, despite on average longer gestations among the late attenders. There were also no differences in perinatal mortality rate, although numbers of deaths are small, and no differences in health measures from the 5- and 10-year follow-up studies. The significant associations were predominantly measures of health behaviour (particularly significant in the larger group of multigravidae) such as failure to take the child to a dentist or have immunizations (Thomas et al 1986).

As noted by the authors, there are a number of limitations in using the cohort study to address this question; the study is observational in nature and cannot be interpreted as though it were a randomized controlled trial. No amount of 'multivariate statistical pyrotechnics' will make up for this (Enkin & Chalmers 1982, Golding & Peters 1988b). In addition, the technical advances since 1970 in the detection of fetal abnormalities and the use of ultrasound will not be covered by these data.

Nevertheless, by including only singleton pregnancies with known dates the investigation does address the question of the benefits to the low-risk majority of early monitoring of blood pressure, proteinuria and weight gain, which together with accurate history-taking remains the objective of the bulk of antenatal care. Furthermore, it is probably only feasible to address the issue of long-term advantages by considering such a study.

There is little evidence from this study of any adverse effect of late attendance on pregnancy outcome or later health and development; a more recent study of poor attenders in London has also found no differences in birthweight (Lewis 1982). Rather, late attendance appears to be an indicator of poor health behaviour which, particularly for multigravidae, continues throughout the child's early life. It remains, of course, that the group of women with uncertain or unknown dates, who were excluded from this investigation of the 1970 cohort given the difficulty in ascertaining gestation at first visit, may be more likely to benefit from early antenatal care, and it is planned to make this minority group of women the subject of further study. Nevertheless, analysis of the data from the 1970 survey and the subsequent follow-up studies led Thomas et al (1986) to question the assumption that early attendance for antenatal care optimizes pregnancy outcome, and to reiterate the call by Enkin & Chalmers (1982) for a more rigorous assessment of the components of antenatal care, taking account of their hazards as well as their benefits.

Factors relating to labour and delivery

General

In terms of relationships between the course of labour and delivery and long-term developmental outcomes identified in the 5- and 10-year follow-up studies, there have been relatively few investigations of the 1970 cohort data; most of the longitudinal analyses have concentrated on factors such as birthweight and maternal smoking at the time of the 5-year follow-up (Butler & Golding 1986). This is much the same for the follow-up reports of the previous national cohort study of a week of births in March 1958 (Davie et al 1972). On the other hand, outcome following various methods of pain relief has recently been the subject of a detailed separate study for the 1970 cohort—the results of these investigations, described in the next section, have not been published previously.

Moreover, factors such as method of delivery and length of labour have been considered in analyses of particular outcomes. For example, preliminary analyses suggested that a long second stage of labour and the administration of a narcotic analgesic during labour were both associated with an increased risk of developing eczema by the age of 5 years as assessed by the child's mother (Golding & Peters 1987). In general, however, there were few associations between labour and delivery variables and the eczema outcome, and even these two could be explained in terms of other factors (Peters & Golding 1987). Analyses of similar information from the 1958 cohort study confirmed these findings (Peters 1986).

In addition, while short second stages of labour have been found by Carpenter et al (1977) in Sheffield and Murphy et al (1982) in Cardiff to be associated with an increased risk of sudden infant death syndrome (SIDS), Golding et al (1985) concluded from an analysis of data from the Oxford record linkage study that this could be attributed to the higher average parities of the women experiencing short labours. Furthermore, the Oxford study found no associations between the risk of SIDS and a wide range of other labour and delivery variables, including pain relief during labour, method of delivery and induction or acceleration by oxytocic drugs (Golding et al 1985, Golding 1986a). As regards the 1970 cohort data, although the number of these deaths was too small to allow direct assessment of such associations, applying the risk-scoring methods derived from the Sheffield, Cardiff and Oxford investigations showed that the latter (with no labour and delivery variables) performed considerably better than the Cardiff system and marginally better than the Sheffield system at predicting the cases of SIDS in the cohort (Peters & Golding 1986).

Concerning other longitudinal studies, results from the

investigations of over 35 000 children followed up as part of the collaborative perinatal project in the USA show very little in terms of relationships between perinatal events and developmental outcomes at 4 and 7 years of age, particularly in comparison with predictors such as socioeconomic status and parental education (Broman et al 1975, Broman 1979, see also the review by Sameroff & Chandler 1975). Results of a number of smaller prospective studies in the USA have led to very similar conclusions (Sameroff 1978), even when restricted to preterm deliveries (Littman & Parmelee 1978).

In addition, while breech presentation is associated with high rates of perinatal mortality and morbidity, including cerebral palsy, many authors have concluded that this may well be a result of other complications, particularly preterm delivery and growth retardation (Faber-Nijholt et al 1983, Stanley 1984b). Indeed, it appears that the increased risks to breech deliveries are only apparent among normal-weight births; preterm and growth-retarded infants are at relatively high risk of cerebral palsy regardless of delivery method (Stanley 1984b). Certainly, studies which fail to account for these factors are unlikely to yield reliable comparisons. In any case, Stanley (1984b) concluded that only a small proportion of cases of cerebral palsy could be attributed to breech delivery, and noted that there was 'no evidence to show that any specific interventions around labour and delivery had been proven to affect the frequency of the cerebral palsies'. In terms of minor developmental problems, the relatively small effect of breech delivery on educational measures at the age of 5 years amongst boys only noted by Neligan et al (1974) was removed after controlling for social class, parity and birthweight.

The relationships of labour and delivery factors with development in childhood have also been investigated by Ounsted and colleagues in Oxford. First, neurological assessments at day 1, day 5 and 2 months were compared for 184 infants of primiparous women in four groups comprising three methods of induction and a group of spontaneous labours and deliveries (Ounsted et al 1978). Although no differences in scores at any age were found with method of delivery, and similarly in the neonatal period for method of induction, there was a significant deficit at 2 months for the group treated by amniotomy followed by intravenous oxytocin. In a separate study, methods of delivery and pain relief were found not to be associated with motor, language or comprehension scores at the age of 4 years (Ounsted et al 1980, 1981). On the other hand, elective Caesarean sections amongst a group of hypertensive pregnancies did score relatively poorly on intellectual ability scales at the age of 7 years, after controlling for confounding effects (Ounsted et al 1984).

Overall, then, there is no consistent evidence in the literature of associations between labour and delivery variables and long-term health or educational ability — those that have been found are small in relation to other effects and are often explained by factors such as birthweight. Nevertheless, the 1970 cohort study remains a unique and relatively underused source of data for these issues; the following two sections present results from recent analyses of this information.

Pain relief during childbirth and subsequent development

Although a great deal of research has been carried out on the effects of obstetrical medication on short-term behavioural outcome for the infant (Sepkoski 1985, Chantigian & Ostheimer 1986), there is relatively little in the literature concerning outcomes after the infant period (Broman 1986). Unlike the generally negative (and dose-related) immediate effects, the few investigations into long-term development have tended not to find any significant differences between the various methods of pain relief (Ounsted et al 1981, Nelson & Ellenberg 1985, Chantigian & Ostheimer 1986), although there are exceptions (Broman 1981, 1986). Once again, appropriate control for potential confounding factors is necessary in addressing this issue.

In the British Births 1970 survey, information was collected on the use of various drugs and methods of analgesia and anaesthesia, though in such a large study it was not feasible to enquire about dose of medication. With the factors considered separately in most instances, the patterns of use by variables such as maternal age, parity, social class, place of delivery and region of birth have been documented (Chamberlain et al 1978). Neonatal outcome was also considered by these authors, but with no control for confounding effects, whilst no comparisons of outcomes from the follow-up studies have been published to date.

A recent detailed investigation of the long-term effect on child development of pain relief during labour using the 1970 cohort study has therefore been conducted in two stages. First, the types of women (and labours) given the various methods were determined by considering the associations of a large number of relevant background and delivery factors with the administration of a particular medication. For example, the proportion of women receiving a narcotic analgesic was compared across various categories of women; the factors were considered simultaneously, in a series of logistic regression models, in order to ascertain the relationships with the analgesia variable that were independent of other effects. In this way, a comprehensive yet concise profile was compiled of births during which a narcotic analgesic was administered. The second stage was then to consider associations between the analgesia variable and a variety of neonatal, 5- and 10-year developmental outcomes, taking account of the potential confounding effects identified during the first stage of the analyses.

The results outlined here are for the investigations of the narcotic analgesics only.

Narcotic analgesics. Excluding the Caesarean sections and the unattended deliveries, out of a total of 15 926 women delivering singleton births in the study week, 11 756 (73.8%) were given a narcotic analgesic during labour. In the vast majority of these cases the drug was pethidine (Chamberlain et al 1978), and those not receiving such drugs included the 7% of all women in the 1970 survey for whom there was no evidence of any pain relief during labour. From amongst a large number of variables derived from the information collected in the birth survey, the following factors were found to be associated with whether or not such a drug was administered:

1. *Background variables:* region of birth; woman working or a housewife; parents' ages at completion of full-time education; marital status; parity and maternal age.
2. *Obstetrical history:* outcome of the preceding pregnancy; number of previous abortions and the number of previous Caesarean sections.
3. *Course of pregnancy:* pre-eclampsia; whether the mother was admitted as an inpatient at any time.
4. *Antenatal preparation:* persons responsible for antenatal care; attendance for mothercraft classes and labour preparation classes.
5. *Labour and delivery:* place of delivery; gestational age; method of delivery; method of induction; interval between rupture of membranes and delivery; lengths of the first and second stages of labour.

In contrast, a number of factors were found not to be significantly associated with the use of a narcotic analgesic, taking a 1% cut-off point for significance. In particular, the lower proportions for parents from the West Indies and Asia and higher for Scotland, Wales and Northern Ireland relative to England were not significant, and neither were the differences across the social class groups. Maternal height, sex of child, smoking during pregnancy, maternal diabetes, interpregnancy interval, number of previous stillbirths and of early neonatal deaths, antepartum haemorrhage, trimester of first antenatal visit and whether or not the mother was booked at the place of delivery were also not significant.

The significant factors are clearly related to each other; controlling for other variables first in the same group and then for significant factors in other groups led to a final set of characteristics independently associated with the analgesia variable. From this procedure, the following groups of women were concluded to have a relatively high chance of being given a narcotic analgesic during labour: those resident in northern England and Northern Ireland; primiparae; those delivered under consultant supervision, in a general practitioner maternity unit or private hospital; spontaneous cephalic occipito-posterior deliveries; labours induced by oxytocic drugs or artificial rupture of the membranes; deliveries taking place more than 24 hours after rupture of the membranes; long first and second stages of labour. Conversely, for example, those resident in southern regions, multiparae, home deliveries, spontaneous-onset and short labours were all relatively less likely to be given a narcotic analgesic, as were the few women who never attended for antenatal care.

Many of the associations which were initially highly significant were explained by the parity variable, in particular, maternal age, marital status, education, maternal employment and attendance at antenatal classes. The components of the obstetrical history factors not attributable to parity were explained by the labour and delivery variables, as were the two items relating to the course of pregnancy. The increased proportions of narcotic analgesics administered to post-term and very preterm deliveries were explained by the high induction rates in these two groups.

In summary, most of the statistically dominant factors predicting the proportion given a narcotic analgesic during labour relate to circumstances close to the time of delivery, that is, to the place of delivery and the course of the labour. In particular, as well as long labours, women whose labours were induced were more likely to be given such drugs, even controlling for the place of delivery. The other major factor associated with the analgesia variable was parity — almost 90% of primiparae were given a narcotic analgesic compared with 65% of multiparae. Failure to allow for this would have suggested a number of spurious associations. Even after controlling for all these variables, however, there remained a strong regional variation in the use of this form of analgesia. The significance of the relatively high rates in the northern regions of England and, in particular, in Northern Ireland was hardly altered at all by adjusting for the various other factors.

The next stage of the investigation was to compare the outcomes in the two groups of women according to whether or not they were given a narcotic analgesic, controlling for the above predisposing factors. The outcome variables were drawn from the birth, 5- and 10-year surveys, and included:

1. *Neonatal outcomes:* birthweight; perinatal and neonatal death; fetal distress (alterations in the heart rate and passage of meconium); delayed onset of regular respiration; resuscitation; cerebral irritation; child in an incubator during the first week; feeding during the first week.
2. *Outcomes at 5 years:* post-neonatal mortality; various health outcomes, including history of respiratory problems and atopic conditions; hospital admissions; cerebral palsy; sensory disorders; height and head circumference; accidents; duration of breastfeeding; assessment by the health visitor of the child's intellectual development; scores on basic educational assessments such as the English picture vocabulary test (EPVT).
3. *Outcomes at 10 years:* intellectual ability as measured by reading and mathematics tests and the British ability scales (BAS); various aspects of behaviour assessed by the mother and the child's teacher; subjective assessment by the clinical medical officer of the extent of clumsiness exhibited by the child during a series of motor co-ordination tests.

Of the neonatal outcomes listed above, alterations in the fetal heart rate (to below 120 or above 160 beats/min), delayed onset of regular respiration (more than 3 minutes), cerebral irritation (fits, convulsions or signs of cerebral irritation in the first week of life) and the need for resuscitation were the only ones which were significantly higher in the group given a narcotic analgesic, using a minimum cut-off point of 1%. All the other comparisons were not significant at this level, which was chosen as a result of the large number of significance tests performed. Controlling for the confounding variables suggested by the analyses described above led to a marked reduction in the significance levels for the resuscitation and cerebral irritation outcomes to below the 1% level. On the other hand, the associations with respiratory delay (adjusted odds ratio, that is, approximate relative risk = 2.7) and fetal heart rate alterations (adjusted odds ratio = 1.4) remained significant at beyond the 0.1% level.

Among the many 5-year outcomes, only six were even initially associated with the use of narcotic analgesics, and of these the relationships of height, EPVT, history of hayfever, frequent sore throats requiring medical attention and speech problems before the age of 5 years all became nonsignificant after controlling for the potential confounding factors. The only outcome which remained significant after this adjustment was whether or not the child had had an accident before the age of 5 years requiring medical advice or treatment. Although significant at the 1% level, the adjusted odds ratio was only 1.14; moreover, there was no trend with the number of such accidents experienced by the child.

As regards the 10-year outcomes, none of the educational measures were significantly associated with the use of narcotic analgesics after controlling for relevant confounding factors. In particular, reading and mathematics test scores, with or without adjustment for non-verbal reasoning and reading ability respectively, were not significant, even without considering confounding effects. Also not significant were measures relating to various aspects of the child's behaviour as reported by the teacher. Similar variables based on the mother's report, however, were significant at the 1% level after adjusting for confounding factors; those children whose mothers were given a narcotic analgesic during labour were, at the age of 10 years and according to their mothers, more clumsy, more antisocial, more hyperactive and more anxious than those whose mothers were not given such drugs. On the other hand, there was no significant difference between these two groups in the assessment of clumsiness made by the clinical medical officer undertaking the 10-year medical examination. (Measures of overall behaviour deviance according to the mother at the 5-year follow-up were also not significantly related to the analgesia variable.)

Overall, few outcomes were associated with the use of narcotic analgesics during labour. The relationships with fetal heart rate alterations and delayed onset of regular respiration are not surprising given previous similar investigations (Lieberman et al 1979, Belsey et al 1981) and the known effects of narcotic analgesics on respiratory function (Scialli & Fabro 1985). Maternal analgesia has also been shown to be associated with behaviour in the neonatal period (Belsey et al 1981, Rosenblatt et al 1981), in particular with responsiveness immediately after delivery. Concerning long-term behaviour, the 1970 cohort data certainly show a pattern in respect of the 10-year assessment by the mother. In the absence of associations with reports by the teacher and clinical medical officer the results suggest that this may be indicative of the mother's attitudes rather than of the child's behaviour. There is no evidence from this data set of any associations between narcotic analgesics administered during labour and the long-term health or educational ability of the child.

Delayed onset of regular respiration and subsequent development

Several methods for identifying asphyxiated neonates have been proposed in the literature but they are not equivalent. Measurement of the acid–base balance in the fetal blood, considered to be the most accurate, is not simple to determine by routine monitoring (Flynn & Kelly 1982), whilst the Apgar score and the time to onset of regular respiration are unlikely to reflect the degree of acidosis accurately (Sykes et al 1982). Nevertheless, Chamberlain et al (1975) concluded from their study of the 1970 British birth survey that a delay of over 3 minutes in the onset of regular respiration was useful as an outcome to indicate the effects of events both before and during labour. Furthermore, Chamberlain & Banks (1974) had shown that a scoring method based on measurements of the fetal heart rate and either the time to first breath or first cry was simpler but no less effective than the full Apgar score.

Many studies have observed a positive relationship between neonatal asphyxia (variously defined) and neonatal mortality, including the original study of the 1970 cohort (Chamberlain et al 1975). Moreover, MacDonald et al (1980) showed that neither gestational age nor birthweight could account for this association. Neonatal asphyxia has also been found to be associated with major abnormalities in the survivors (Mulligan et al 1980) and in particular with cerebral palsy (Nelson & Ellenberg 1981, 1984, 1985). In such instances, though, asphyxia was often regarded as a symptom and indicator of the perinatal conditions leading to such abnormalities rather than as their cause (Neligan et al 1974). Following a review of Nelson & Ellenberg's data, in particular, Stanley (1984b) concluded that asphyxia, like breech delivery, was only associated with cerebral palsy in normal-weight births.

There is much less agreement in the literature, however, regarding the possible long-term subtle effects of apparent neonatal asphyxia, though many of the studies have been small, retrospective and failed to control for confounding variables. Nevertheless, some patterns have emerged in previous reviews, namely that there is little evidence from properly conducted prospective studies to suggest that respiratory delay or low Apgar scores are associated with impaired intellectual development and motor co-ordination, particularly in follow-up studies after infancy (Gottfried 1973, Sameroff & Chandler 1975, Broman 1979).

With this background, a comprehensive study of the infants with delayed onset of regular respiration has been carried out on the 1970 cohort data (Peters et al 1984a,b, Peters 1986). In order to exclude neonates who did not or who may never have established regular respiration, only first-day survivors were considered. Multiple births and unattended deliveries were also excluded, leaving a total of 16 333 singleton deliveries with known time to onset of regular respiration, of whom 717 (4.4%) took longer than 3 minutes to breathe. Again, the first stage of the investigation was to obtain a profile of the deliveries likely to have such a delay (Peters et al 1984a), and then to consider both short- and long-term outcomes, taking this profile into account wherever possible (Peters et al 1984b).

The major characteristics of the groups identified as being independently at high risk of respiratory delay were: null and high parity; antepartum haemorrhage, particularly placenta praevia; pre-eclampsia; breech delivery; Caesarean section and low birthweight. There was no association with either smoking during pregnancy or social class (Peters et al 1984a).

In the outcome analyses, highly significant associations were found between respiratory delay and neonatal mortality, and although a detailed investigation of confounding effects was not feasible given the number of deaths, it was concluded that this relationship could not be explained by birthweight and sex. Similarly, the association with cerebral palsy was not removed by considering the low birthweights separately, though small numbers precluded further analyses. In this study, the trends in the relative risk of cerebral palsy given respiratory delay were very similar for low- and normal-weight births, though the numbers of children yielded statistical significance only in the latter group (Peters et al 1984b).

Concerning long-term development, among a large number of outcomes considered from the 5-year follow-up only a few were significantly associated with respiratory delay at birth, and most of these were explained by the confounding variables suggested by the initial birth analyses together with other relevant outcomes. In particular, the increased proportion of those with delay over 3 minutes admitted to hospital in their first 5 years (relative to those without such delay) was explained by their lower birthweights and gestations and by their higher rates of bronchitis. The increased incidence of squint was also explained by these factors, and the significant results found initially for pneumonia by the age of 5 years and for convulsions were wholly explained by the birthweight associations. The association between respiratory delay and the existence of a stammer or stutter at the time of the follow-up was removed after accounting for the relatively high proportions of males, gestations under 35 completed weeks and births to teenage mothers among both these groups.

On the other hand, the strong relationship between respiratory delay and bronchitis at some time before the age of 5 years was not accounted for by any of the potential confounding variables. Indeed, in the process of adjusting for factors such as birthweight, gestational age and parity, the odds ratio (approximate relative risk) of bronchitis for the infants with respiratory delay was only reduced from 1.53 to 1.45 (significant at the 1% level in all instances). Neither intubation nor positive pressure ventilation was responsible for this association.

The overall pattern of results from this study, like much of the literature, was consistent with little evidence of residual effects from delayed onset of regular respiration at birth, despite associations with mortality and cerebral palsy. The single exception was the raised incidence of bronchitis by the age of 5 years. Investigation of related outcomes from the 10-year follow-up would be of interest, but the general picture is unlikely to be altered by considering later outcomes.

The conclusion was that it was possible that the infant with respiratory delay was already at increased risk of neonatal death, cerebral palsy or even bronchitis: 'the sign of apparent asphyxia is merely a marker of other defective reactions to various insults' (Peters et al 1984b).

CONCLUSIONS

The general conclusion from these investigations of the 1970 national cohort data is that once the neonate has survived without obvious damage, there appear to be no residual effects of obstetrical factors on long-term development. This accords with many other studies in the literature on the associations between reproductive problems and minor developmental deficit (Sameroff & Chandler 1975). The few associations that have been found do not exclude the possibility that complications during labour and delivery act as indicators of pre-existing problems rather than being directly responsible for conditions such as cerebral palsy (Drillien 1968). In particular, delayed attendance for antenatal care appears to be an indicator of poor health behaviour generally, rather than a direct contributory factor to poor outcome, either in pregnancy or in later years.

The identification of a few associations with outcomes in studies such as these needs to be treated with some caution. Not only are they the product of analyses involving a large number of significance tests, but as discussed earlier, the data are from a purely observational study which should be followed whenever possible by further, controlled investigations. Nevertheless, the associations derived from the cohort study are informative, particularly when consistent with those from other prospective observational studies.

The results emphasize the need to control for confounding effects when considering short- or long-term outcomes in relation to obstetrical care. Moreover, when investigating cerebral palsy, Stanley (1984b) identified birthweight as an important interactive factor for this outcome; obstetrical complications were implicated more amongst normal-weight cases than amongst growth-retarded or preterm cases. Detailed consideration of both confounding and interactive effects is therefore necessary in any study of the later results of obstetrical care, to avoid spurious relationships and detect potentially illuminating interactions. Confounding factors are those which explain or inhibit the association between the outcome and the obstetrical factor of interest; an interaction is where the association of interest varies across the categories of another factor.

In summary, there is no consistent evidence of any relationship between obstetrical complications and minor developmental problems in the survivors. To determine the major influences on child development, attention should be directed towards the environment of the child, both prenatally and postnatally (Sameroff & Chandler 1975, Steiner & Neligan 1983, Golding 1986b, Ounsted 1987).

Acknowledgements

The British Births 1970 Survey was run jointly by the National Birthday Trust Fund and the Royal College of Obstetricians and Gynaecologists, and carried out under the direction of Dr Roma Chamberlain and Professor Geoffrey Chamberlain. Funding for the follow-up studies came from a variety of sources, including the Department of Health and Social Security, Department of Education and Science, Medical Research Council and National Institutes of Health. Additional support for the analyses reviewed in this chapter was received from the Health Promotion Research Trust, the Mental Health Foundation and Birthright.

The 1970 cohort study could not have been carried out without the voluntary assistance of midwives, health visitors and medical officers—I am grateful both to them and to the parents and children involved in the study.

I also thank the personnel at the Department of Child Health, University of Bristol who were responsible for the follow-up studies. In particular, I am grateful to Professor Neville Butler, Dr Sue Dowling, Dr Albert Osborn, Dr Mary Haslum, Dr Jean Golding and Brian Howlett. Jean Golding also made a number of helpful suggestions and comments regarding this chapter, and together with Peter Thomas provided useful material on the research into late attendance for antenatal care.

Computing assistance was provided by Mike Taysum and Terry Shenton, and the manuscript was typed by Shona Norrie and Julie Spiteri.

REFERENCES

Atkins E, Cherry N, Douglas J W B, Kiernan K E, Wadsworth M E J 1981 The 1946 British birth cohort: an account of the origins, progress and results of the National Survey of Health and Development. In: Mednick S A, Baert A E, Bachmann B P (eds) Prospective longitudinal research: an empirical basis for the primary prevention of psychosocial disorders. Oxford University Press for the World Health Organization Regional Office for Europe, Oxford, pp 25–30

Belsey E M, Rosenblatt D B, Lieberman B A et al 1981 The influence of maternal analgesia on neonatal behaviour: I. Pethidine. British Journal of Obstetrics and Gynaecology 88: 398–406

Blaxter M 1983 Longitudinal studies in Britain and their relevance to the study of inequalities in health. Unpublished report to the social affairs committee of the Social Science Research Council

Broman S H 1979 Perinatal anoxia and cognitive development in early childhood. In: Field T M, Miller Sostek A, Goldberg S, Shuman H H (eds) Infants born at risk: behavior and development. SP Medical and Scientific Books, Jamaica, pp 29–52

Broman S H 1981 Risk factors for deficits in early cognitive development (with discussion). In: Berg G G, Maillie H D (eds) Measurement of risks. Plenum Press, New York, pp 131–142

Broman S H 1986 Obstetric medications: a review of the literature on outcomes in infancy and childhood. In: Lewis M (ed) Learning disabilities and prenatal risk. University of Illinois Press, Urbana, pp 125–152

Broman S H, Nichols P L, Kennedy W A 1975 Preschool IQ: prenatal and early developmental correlates. Lawrence Erlbaum, New Jersey

Butler N R, Alberman E D 1969 Perinatal problems: the second report of the British Perinatal Mortality Survey. E & S Livingstone, Edinburgh

Butler N R, Bonham D G 1963 Perinatal mortality: the first report of the British Perinatal Mortality Survey. E & S Livingstone, Edinburgh

Butler N R, Golding J 1986 From birth to five: a study of the health and behaviour of Britain's five year olds. Pergamon Press, Oxford

Carpenter R G, Gardner A, McWeeny P M, Emery J L 1977 Multistage scoring system for identifying infants at risk of unexpected death. Archives of Disease in Childhood 52: 606–612

Chamberlain G, Banks J 1974 Assessment of the Apgar score. Lancet ii: 1225–1228

Chamberlain R, Davey A 1975 Physical growth in twins, postmature and small-for-dates children. Archives of Disease in Childhood 50: 437–442

Chamberlain R N, Simpson R N 1979 The prevalence of illness in childhood. Pitman Medical Publishing, Tunbridge Wells

Chamberlain R, Chamberlain G, Howlett B, Claireaux A 1975 British births 1970, vol 1: the first week of life. William Heinemann Medical Books, London

Chamberlain G, Philipp E, Howlett B, Masters K 1978 British births 1970, vol 2: obstetric care. William Heinemann Medical Books, London

Chantigian R C, Ostheimer G W 1986 Effect of maternally administered drugs on the fetus and newborn. In: Milunsky A, Friedman E A, Gluck L (eds) Advances in perinatal medicine, vol 5. Plenum Medical Books, New York, pp 181–242

Coope J K, Scott A V 1982 A programme for shared maternity and child care. British Medical Journal 284: 1936–1937

Culbertson J L, Ferry P C 1982 Neonatal asphyxia as a risk factor: early identification of developmental and medical outcome. In: Anasasiow N J, Frankenberg W K, Fanbal A W (eds) Identifying the developmentally delayed child. University Park Press, Baltimore, pp 63–72

Davie R, Butler N, Goldstein H 1972 From birth to seven. Longman, London

Drillien C M 1968 Studies in mental handicap. II: Some obstetric factors of possible aetiological significance. Archives of Disease in Childhood 43: 283–294

Enkin M, Chalmers I 1982 Effectiveness and satisfaction in antenatal care. In: Enkin M, Chalmers I (eds) Effectiveness and satisfaction in antenatal care. Clinics in developmental medicine 81/82. SIMP/William Heinemann Medical Books, London, pp 266–290

Faber-Nijholt R, Huisjes H J, Touwen B C L, Fidler V J 1983 Neurological follow-up of 281 children born in breech presentation: a controlled study. British Medical Journal 286: 9–12

Flynn A M, Kelly J 1982 Fetal monitoring in labour. In: Bonnar J (ed) Recent advances in obstetrics and gynaecology, no 14. Churchill Livingstone, Edinburgh, pp 25–45

Fogelman K, Wedge P 1981 The National Child Development Study (1958 British cohort). In: Mednick S A, Baert A E, Bachmann B P (eds) Prospective longitudinal research: an empirical basis for the primary prevention of psychosocial disorders. Oxford University Press for the World Health Organization Regional Office for Europe, Oxford, pp 30–43

Golding J 1984 Britain's national cohort studies. In: Macfarlane J A (ed) Progress in child health, vol 1. Churchill Livingstone, Edinburgh, pp 178–186

Golding J 1986a Oxytocin for induction of labor and sudden infant death syndrome (SIDS). New England Journal of Medicine 315: 192–193

Golding J 1986b Child health and the environment. British Medical Bulletin 42: 204–211

Golding J, Peters T J 1987 The epidemiology of childhood eczema: I:

A population based study of associations. Paediatric and Perinatal Epidemiology 1987 1: 67–79
Golding J, Peters T J 1988a Quantifying risk in pregnancy. In: James D K, Stirrat G M (eds) Pregnancy and risk: the basis for rational management. Wiley, Chichester, pp 7–22
Golding J, Peters T J 1988b Are hospital confinements really more dangerous for the fetus? Early Human Development 17: 29–36
Golding J, Limerick S, Macfarlane A 1985 Sudden infant death: patterns, puzzles and problems. Open Books Publishing, Shepton Mallet
Gottfried A W 1973 Intellectual consequences of perinatal anoxia. Psychological Bulletin 80: 231–242
Hagberg B, Hagberg G 1984 Prenatal and perinatal risk factors in a survey of 681 Swedish cases. In: Stanley F, Alberman E (eds) The epidemiology of the cerebral palsies. Clinics in developmental medicine 87. SIMP/Blackwell Scientific Publications, Oxford, pp 116–134
Hall M, Chng P K 1982 Antenatal care in practice. In: Enkin M, Chalmers I (eds) Effectiveness and satisfaction in antenatal care. Clinics in developmental medicine 81/82. SIMP/William Heinemann Medical Books, London, pp 60–68
Hall M, Macintyre S, Porter M 1985 Antenatal care assessed: a case study of innovation in Aberdeen. Aberdeen University Press, Aberdeen
Illingworth R S 1979 Why blame the obstetrician? A review. British Medical Journal 1: 797–801
Illingworth R S 1985 A paediatrician asks—why is it called birth injury? British Journal of Obstetrics and Gynaecology 92: 122–130
Illsley R, Wilson F 1981 Longitudinal studies in Aberdeen, Scotland. In: Mednick S A, Baert A E, Bachmann B P (eds) Prospective longitudinal research: an empirical basis for the primary prevention of psychosocial disorders. Oxford University Press for the World Health Organization Regional Office for Europe, Oxford, pp 66–68
Lewis E 1982 Attendance for antenatal care. British Medical Journal 284: 788
Lieberman B A, Rosenblatt D B, Belsey E et al 1979 The effects of maternally administered pethidine or epidural bupivacaine on the fetus and newborn. British Journal of Obstetrics and Gynaecology 86: 598–606
Lilienfeld A M, Parkhurst E 1951 A study of the association of factors of pregnancy and parturition with the development of cerebral palsy. American Journal of Hygiene 53: 262–282
Lilienfeld A M, Pasamanick B 1954 Association of maternal and fetal factors with the development of epilepsy: I. Abnormalities in the prenatal and paranatal periods. Journal of the American Medical Association 155: 719–724
Littman B, Parmelee A H 1978 Medical correlates of infant development. Pediatrics 61: 470–474
MacDonald H M, Mulligan J C, Allen A C, Taylor P M 1980 Neonatal asphyxia: I. Relationship of obstetric and neonatal complications to neonatal mortality in 38 405 consecutive deliveries. Journal of Pediatrics 96: 898–902
McQueen P C, Spence M W, Winsor E J T, Garner J B, Pereira L H 1986 Causal origins of major mental handicap in the Canadian maritime provinces. Developmental Medicine and Child Neurology 28: 697–707
Miller F J W, Court S D M, Knox E G, Brandon S 1974 The school years in Newcastle upon Tyne 1952–62. Oxford University Press, London
Molfese V J, Thomson B 1985 Optimality versus complications: assessing predictive values of perinatal scales. Child Development 56: 810–823
Mulligan J C, Painter M J, O'Donaghue P A, MacDonald H M, Allen A C, Taylor P M 1980 Neonatal asphyxia: II. Neonatal mortality and long-term sequelae. Journal of Pediatrics 96: 903–907
Murphy J F, Newcombe R G, Sibert J R 1982 The epidemiology of sudden infant death syndrome. Journal of Epidemiology and Community Health 36: 17–21
National Perinatal Epidemiology Unit 1985 A classified bibliography of controlled trials in perinatal medicine 1940–1984. Oxford University Press, Oxford
Neligan G, Prudham D, Steiner H 1974 The formative years: birth, family and development in Newcastle upon Tyne. Oxford University Press for the Nuffield Provincial Hospitals Trust, London
Nelson K B 1968 The 'continuum of reproductive casualty'. In: MacKeith R, Bax M (eds) Studies in infancy. Clinics in developmental medicine 27. SIMP/William Heinemann Medical Books, London, pp 100–109
Nelson K B, Ellenberg J H 1981 Apgar scores as predictors of chronic neurologic disability. Pediatrics 68: 36–44
Nelson K B, Ellenberg J H 1984 Obstetric complications as risk factors for cerebral palsy or seizure disorders. Journal of the American Medical Association 251: 1843–1848
Nelson K B, Ellenberg J H 1985 Antecedents of cerebral palsy I. Univariate analysis of risks. American Journal of Diseases of Children 139: 1031–1038
Osborn A F, Butler N R, Morris A C 1984 The social life of Britain's five-year-olds. Routledge & Kegan Paul, London
Ounsted M 1987 Causes, continua and other concepts: I: The 'continuum of reproductive casualty'. Paediatric and Perinatal Epidemiology 1987 1: 4–7
Ounsted M K, Boyd P A, Hendrick A M, Mutch L M M, Simons C D, Good F J 1978 Induction of labour by different methods in primiparous women II. Neuro-behavioural status of the infants. Early Human Development 2: 241–253
Ounsted M, Scott A, Moar V 1980 Delivery and development: to what extent can one associate cause and effect? Journal of the Royal Society of Medicine 73: 786–792
Ounsted M, Scott A, Moar V 1981 Pain relief during childbirth and development at 4 years. Journal of the Royal Society of Medicine 74: 629–630
Ounsted M, Moar V A, Cockburn J, Redman C W G 1984 Factors associated with the intellectual ability of children born to women with high-risk pregnancies. British Medical Journal 288: 1038–1041
Peters T J 1986 A statistical investigation of risk indicators for perinatal outcome and early child development. PhD Thesis, University of Exeter
Peters T, Golding J 1985 Assessing risk assessment. In: Milunsky A, Friedman E A, Gluck L (eds) Advances in perinatal medicine, vol 4. Plenum Medical Books, New York, pp 235–266
Peters T J, Golding J 1986 Prediction of sudden infant death syndrome: an independent evaluation of four scoring methods. Statistics in Medicine 5: 113–126
Peters T J, Golding J 1987 The epidemiology of childhood eczema: II: Statistical analyses to identify independent early predictors. Paediatric and Perinatal Epidemiology 1987 1: 80–94
Peters T J, Golding J, Butler N R, Fryer J G, Lawrence C J, Chamberlain G V P 1983 Plus ça change: predictors of birthweight in two national studies. British Journal of Obstetrics and Gynaecology 90: 1040–1045
Peters T J, Golding J, Lawrence C J, Fryer J G, Chamberlain G V P, Butler N R 1984a Factors associated with delayed onset of regular respiration. Early Human Development 9: 209–223
Peters T J, Golding J, Lawrence C J, Fryer J G, Chamberlain G V P, Butler N R 1984b Delayed onset of regular respiration and subsequent development. Early Human Development 9: 225–239
Robertson J S, Carr G 1970 Late bookers for antenatal care. In: McLachlan G, Shegog R (eds) In the beginning. Oxford University Press, London, pp 79–104
Rosenblatt D B, Belsey E M, Lieberman B A et al 1981 The influence of maternal analgesia on neonatal behaviour: II. Epidural bupivacaine. British Journal of Obstetrics and Gynaecology 88: 407–413
Sameroff A J 1978 Caretaking or reproductive casualty? Determinants in developmental deviancy. In: Horowitz F D (ed) Early developmental hazards: predictors and precautions. Westview Press, Boulder, Connecticut, pp 79–101
Sameroff A J, Chandler M J 1975 Reproductive risk and the continuum of caretaking casualty. In: Horowitz F D, Hetherington M, Scarr-Salapatek S, Siegel G (eds) Review of child development research, vol 4. University of Chicago, Chicago, pp 187–244
Scialli A R, Fabro S 1985 The toxicokinetics of anesthetics and analgesics during labor and delivery. In: Scanlon J W (ed) Contemporary issues in fetal and neonatal medicine, vol 1: Perinatal anesthesia. Blackwell Scientific Publications, Boston, pp 1–26
Sepkoski C M 1985 Maternal obstetric medication and newborn behavior. In: Scanlon J W (ed) Contemporary issues in fetal and neonatal medicine, vol 1: Perinatal anesthesia. Blackwell Scientific Publications, Boston, pp 131–173
Short Report 1980 Second report from the social services committee, vol 1. HMSO, London
Simpson H, Walker G 1980 When do pregnant women attend for antenatal care? British Medical Journal 281: 104–107

Stanley F 1984a Social and biological determinants of the cerebral palsies. In: Stanley F, Alberman E (eds) The epidemiology of the cerebral palsies. Clinics in developmental medicine 87. SIMP/Blackwell Scientific Publications, Oxford, pp 69–86
Stanley F 1984b Perinatal risk factors in the cerebral palsies. In: Stanley F, Alberman E (eds) The epidemiology of the cerebral palsies. Clinics in developmental medicine 87. SIMP/Blackwell Scientific Publications, Oxford, pp 98–115
Steiner H, Neligan G A 1983 Perinatal mortality and the quality of the survivors. In: Barron S L, Thomson A M (eds) Obstetrical epidemiology. Academic Press, London, pp 417–448
Sykes G S, Molloy P M, Johnson P et al 1982 Do Apgar scores indicate asphyxia? Lancet i: 494–496
Thomas P, Golding J, Peters T J 1986 Delayed attendance for antenatal care. Report to the Health Promotion Research Trust
Walker J, MacGillivray I, Macnaughton M C 1976 Combined textbook of obstetrics and gynaecology, 9th edn. Churchill Livingstone, Edinburgh, p 460

SECTION 12

Assisted Pregnancy

William Thompson

Artificial insemination

INTRODUCTION

Although major advances have been made in the management of female infertility particularly for ovulation induction and tubal problems, the useful treatments available for male factor infertility remain limited. In the past infertile couples faced with such a problem sought adoption to relieve their childlessness but during the 1980s as a result of improved contraception, the increased number of therapeutic abortions and single-parent families, this option is less frequently available (Traub et al 1979).

Conception by artificial insemination now provides a way of overcoming the problems of male factor infertility; increasing demand and the change in social attitudes in the western world, particularly to the use of donor semen, has undoubtedly led to an increase in these forms of treatment. The methods are confined to specialized clinics but a wider understanding of the issues involved is necessary to assist obstetricians with patient selection and counselling.

The first documented case of artificial insemination using the husband's semen (artificial insemination by husband; AIH) occurred in the late 18th century when a recently married London cloth merchant suffering from hypospadias consulted John Hunter in the hope of overcoming his disability and fathering a child (Home 1799). Hunter advised the man to insert the seminal fluid which escaped during coitus into his wife's vagina using a warm syringe. This was done and the merchant's wife bore a son. It is not recorded whether Hunter performed the AIH himself or whether he merely advised it. In 1866 J. Marion Sims reported artificial insemination performed on six women using the husband's semen; one patient conceived but later aborted. Although Sims was initially enthusiastic about the procedure he later condemned it on the grounds that it was an immoral medical practice. In the early part of the 20th century, German workers continued to attempt AIH to overcome sexual problems with reported successes (Frankel 1909). Today the indications for AIH have been extended beyond those of coital problems but its precise role and success for many remain speculative.

The first case of human donor insemination performed in 1884 in the USA was reported by Hart in 1909 in a paper entitled *Artificial impregnation*. The case caused a great deal of controversy in the medical literature; obtaining semen and then inseminating it was considered 'ridiculously criminal' and disrespectful to the laws of Nature and God (Gregoire & Mayer 1965). In spite of this, Dickenson in 1890 began using donor insemination in the utmost secrecy (Kleegman & Kaufman 1966). It was not until the 1930s when semen analysis became a routine investigation that the husband was shown to be infertile in a considerable number of childless marriages and donor insemination was seriously discussed as a treatment option.

In 1945, Barton et al first reported pregnancies using donor semen in the UK and by 1960 the Feversham Committee (Duncombe 1960) estimated that artificial insemination was being carried out by some 20 practitioners and during the previous 20 years had resulted in 1150 live births. At the same time in the USA Guttmacher (1960) reported that donor insemination was responsible for between 5000 and 7000 births annually. Since these reports the practice of artificial insemination with either husband or donor has increased dramatically and now has an established role in the management of the infertile couple. In 1983, there were at least 49 clinics offering donor insemination in the UK and in that year, 2228 patients were accepted for treatment (Thompson et al 1984).

ARTIFICIAL INSEMINATION WITH HUSBAND'S SEMEN

The literature on the subject of artificial insemination with the husband's (or consenting partner's) semen (AIH) is very extensive but despite all this documentation the precise value of AIH for the majority of claimed indications is still uncertain. The diverse methods by which AIH can be performed and the numerous regimens for semen preparation prior to insemination have made any evaluation extremely difficult. The number of variables created in any reported series is so great, in proportion to the number of patients treated, that realistic statistical analysis of the data is meaningless (Nachtigall et al 1979); virtually all reports lack control groups. It is well recognized that pregnancies occur spontaneously in cases of prolonged infertility, often of unexplained origin (Grant 1969, Bernstein et al 1979, Collins et al 1983). In these cases treatment such as AIH will often be awarded credit for achieving a pregnancy which, in effect, has occurred coincidently.

Indications for AIH

Severe vaginismus causing failure of penile penetration is almost always psychogenic in origin and AIH should only be used when exhaustive counselling fails to establish natural sexual intercourse. Although AIH may result in successful pregnancy and subsequently promote a cure of the sexual dysfunction it may also lead to a multiplicity of psychological problems (Dixon et al 1976). Some benefits may be gained if the couple perform intravaginal insemination themselves following appropriate explanation; AIH performed by the male partner at home will be more convenient for the couple and relieve some of the stress and guilt connected with the procedure.

A significant degree of hypospadias or epispadias in the male or extreme displacement of the uterine position, such as retroversion, in the female, may cause disturbed sperm deposition. If these conditions are associated with a negative postcoital test, treatment with AIH may be appropriate. A small semen volume will often exaggerate this situation and indeed may be a significant factor in its own right (Moghissi et al 1977).

Patients with impotence and premature ejaculation can also be considered for AIH. When erectile failure is due to psychological factors AIH should be instituted only after counselling and appropriate behaviour therapy have failed to solve the basic problem. In cases of organic impotence (paraplegia, diabetic neuropathy) AIH is the treatment of choice although in a high percentage of such cases it is difficult to obtain an adequate semen sample. Spontaneous nocturnal emissions are sometimes reported and a plastic sheath can be worn every night in the hope that ejaculation may occur around the time of ovulation. Unfortunately the majority of these patients have chronic infection of the lower urinary tract and this adversely affects sperm motility. Furthermore, in younger paraplegics transurethral resection is now frequently performed to assist bladder drainage and invariably this results in retrograde ejaculation. Occasionally, semen may be obtained by prostatic or vesicular massage or electrovibration, and ejaculation has also been induced by electrical stimulation with a rectal probe; such semen samples are unlikely to result in pregnancy because of poor sperm motility (Glezerman & Lunenfeld 1976).

Anejaculation may have an endocrine, psychological or anatomical basis. Even after full investigation and specific treatment, some patients still require AIH to assist conception. As with impotence, it may be difficult to obtain suitable semen samples. Retrograde ejaculation, which is often mistakenly designated as anejaculation, should be carefully sought in the infertile male as it may present a clear indication for AIH (Glezerman et al 1976). In this condition, semen passes backwards into the bladder rather than through the urethra. To confirm the diagnosis, postejaculatory urine samples will be opalescent, contain a large number of spermatozoa and show a positive fructose test. Initially, attempts should be made to achieve fertility through promotion of antegrade ejaculation by using alpha-sympathomimetic drugs (Sandler 1979) or employing the full bladder technique (Crich & Jequier 1977). If these methods fail, AIH using ejaculates recovered from the bladder can be successful. To improve sperm motility the urine should be neutralized by orally administering alkalysing agents prior to masturbation; the urine should be centrifuged and the supernatant resuspended in Tyrode's solution or the female partner's serum (Hotchkiss et al 1955, Ingerslev 1985).

The major controversy about the use of AIH concerns its effectiveness in overcoming the problem of oligospermia, a problem which is frequently also associated with lowered sperm motility and a high percentage of abnormal sperms (Pollock 1967, Hill 1970). Couples with such problems have often undergone prolonged investigations and treatment prior to referral for AIH and accept the concept of a new approach to their problem enthusiastically (Speichinger & Mattox 1976). Frequently, the expectations of the patient and indeed, the referring physician, are unrealistic as regards success. It is therefore important to define the problem accurately and present a realistic prognosis before commencing treatment.

The definition of oligospermia is not consistent in the literature. MacLeod & Gold (1951) suggested a lower limit of normal of 20 million sperms per ml and reported that only 5% of fertile men had counts below this level.

Table 74.1 shows the results of 11 studies in which AIH was performed in cases of oligospermia (sperm counts below 20 million per ml). There were 550 patients, of whom 119 (22%) became pregnant. The inseminations were performed by a variety of techniques and in view of the small numbers in the majority of reports, it is difficult to estimate the true value of a particular method of semen preparation or insemination. Intravaginal artificial insemination of whole semen containing less than 20 million sperms per ml appears to be futile.

Besides oligospermia, another major indication for AIH and specifically for intrauterine insemination is an abnormal

Table 74.1 AIH results in oligospermia (sperm count<20 million/ml)

Reference	Number of couples	Pregnancies	Success (%)
Barton et al (1945)	30	9	30
Russell (1960)	34	2	6
Barwin (1974)	20	11	55
Steinman & Taymor (1977)	22	5	23
Nunley et al (1978)	17	4	23
Barkay & Zuckerman (1978)	20	4	20
Decker (1978)	155	27	17
Whitelaw (1979)	80	10	12
Usherwood (1980)	57	19	33
Gerignon & Kunstmann (1980)	90	26	29
Corson & Batzer (1980)	25	2	8
Total	550	119	22

Table 74.2 Results of AIH in patients with a poor postcoital test

Reference	Number of couples	Pregnancies	Success (%)
Guttmacher (1943)	5	0	0
Mastroianni et al (1957)	132	7	5
Russell (1960)	10	3	30
Perez-Pelaez & Cohen (1963)	38	10	26
Barwin (1974)	18	13	72
Usherwood et al (1976)	13	4	31
White & Glass (1976)	9	5	55
Steinman & Taymor (1977)	25	8	32
Harrison (1978)	7	1	14
Ulstein (1978)	35	10	28
Kremer (1979)	22	7	32
Thompson & Boyle (1982)	34	6	18
Total	348	74	21

postcoital test. This is based on the quality and quantity of the cervical mucus obtained just prior to ovulation and/or the number of motile sperms that have successfully penetrated it. Jette & Glass (1972) showed that pregnancy rates were significantly greater when the number of motile sperms exceeded 20 per high power field (HPF); below this figure it was not possible to define specific groups and even then a substantial number of pregnancies occurred (46%). Kovacs et al (1978) studied postcoital tests in couples of proven fertility and found that four out of 50 contained no sperms, an additional six couples had less than one sperm per HPF and 20% had a sperm motility of less than 50%. This report raises serious doubts about the interpretation of postcoital tests.

Since many workers do not define what constitutes an abnormal postcoital test when it is the indication for AIH, it is difficult to evaluate the significance of the results. Table 74.2 shows the results of 12 series including 348 patients in whom the indication for AIH was an abnormal or poor postcoital test. There were 74 pregnancies (21%). If only intrauterine inseminations are considered, there were 45 pregnancies (29%) in 154 couples. Based on these figures, intrauterine insemination appears to produce improved results but it is doubtful whether the difference is significant.

The few reports on the use of AIH for poor sperm motility suggest very limited success (Usherwood et al 1976). Similarly, female patients with significant titres of antisperm antibodies associated with failure of cervical mucus penetration are unsuitable for AIH (Joyce & Vassilopoulos 1981).

Insemination techniques

Intravaginal

This is the simplest method. The whole semen sample is deposited in the upper vagina by means of a plastic syringe. It is unnecessary to expose the cervix and the procedure may be performed by the couple. Extreme care has to be taken not to inject air into the vagina or cervix as this may cause air embolism. The female partner lies on her back with the buttocks elevated by means of a pillow; sometimes advice is given that this position should be maintained for at least 10 minutes following insemination, but many consider this unnecessary. The method has no advantages over normal sexual intercourse and ejaculation and is only applicable to situations in which these are not possible, e.g. impotence, retrograde ejaculation or where semen from the partner has been stored for later use, e.g. after radiotherapy.

Intracervical and pericervical

These methods are often used together. The cervix is exposed using a Cusco's speculum with the patient in the dorsal position. The exaggerated left lateral position (Sims) can also be used and many patients find this more acceptable. A small quantity of semen (0.2–0.5 ml) is injected slowly at a depth of approximately 1 cm into the cervical canal by applying the blunt end of a plastic syringe closely applied to the external os. The remainder of the semen sample is placed in the anterior vaginal fornix and the patient remains in the dorsal or left lateral position for at least 10 minutes after the procedure.

Various cervical caps have been designed to enhance the application of semen to the cervix and reduce inactivation of sperm motility by vaginal acidity. Whitelaw (1950) used a plastic cap and reported a 40% pregnancy rate with patients who had sperm counts below 60 million per ml. The vacuum cup developed by Semm et al (1976) consists of a plastic hood, available in two sizes, connected to a flexible plastic tubing which may be closed by a roll-on clamp. Following exposure of the cervix, the cap is placed on the portio vaginalis using a grasping instrument and a vacuum is produced using a 10 ml syringe. The clamp is then closed and a syringe containing semen is attached to the plastic tubing; the clamp is opened and the sample injected. The cap remains in situ for 8–12 hours and the patient is advised to open the clamp and remove the cap by pulling on the plastic tubing. In spite of claimed advantages, the cap method, used in the presence of oligospermia, has not produced a significant improvement in pregnancy rates (Nunley et al 1978, Whitelaw 1979).

Some men have difficulty producing an ejaculate on demand; in such cases the cervical cap allows the male partner to produce a semen sample at home, fill a syringe with semen and complete the insemination procedure at a time convenient to him and his partner. Makler (1980) reported improved conception rates when cervical mucus was aspirated prior to endocervical insemination. He attributed this to improved contact between semen and mucus in the cervical crypts, increasing the rate of sperm penetration into the uterine cavity.

Intrauterine

This involves the direct insemination of semen into the uterine cavity, bypassing the cervical mucus. The theoretical advantage of intrauterine insemination over intravaginal and intracervical techniques is that a larger number of sperms is delivered to the site of fertilization in cases of oligospermia, asthenospermia, poor cervical mucus or antisperm antibodies. Fine plastic catheters, attached to a syringe containing the semen sample, have been used, including paediatric feeding catheters, Teflex intravenous catheters and a device that has been manufactured specifically for intrauterine insemination (Sefi-Medical Instruments, Haifa, Israel, Makler et al 1984). The cannulas must be able to traverse the cervical canal and reach the uterine cavity without traumatizing the cervical crypts, epithelium or endometrium. Technical difficulties are frequently encountered when the cervix is stenosed or the uterus is acutely anteverted or retroverted.

Intrauterine insemination may lead to severe cramping when untreated semen is used because of the effect of prostaglandins on the myometrium (Taylor & Kelly 1974); this complication is uncommon when the volume of fluid injected is less than 0.1 ml (White & Glass 1976). Prostaglandins, secreted by the seminal vesicles, are usually confined to the last portion of the ejaculate. Thus, by using the first portion of a split ejaculate (consisting of epididymal and prostatic secretions), uterine cramping will be reduced with the added advantage of providing a higher concentration of sperms. The risk of infection (salpingitis) with intrauterine insemination is more likely when the protective filter of the cervix is bypassed (Russell 1960). In practice, surprisingly few serious infections have been reported (Allen et al 1985) and it is therefore unnecessary to use prophylactic antibiotics, as has been advocated by some authors (Barwin 1974, Wiltbank et al 1985).

Another complication of intrauterine insemination was reported by Kremer (1979), who found a significant increase in antisperm antibody titres in sensitized women following such treatment. Women with low or negative titres did not, however, form antibodies.

Intrafallopian transfer

This technique, referred to as translaparoscopic gamete intrafallopian transfer (GIFT) was first described by Asch et al (1984). They successfully treated a couple with unexplained infertility and later reported the delivery of healthy twins (Asch et al 1985). A semen sample is prepared by centrifugation and layering to yield a concentration of 100 000 motile sperms in 25 μl and incubated in 5% carbon dioxide and air at 37°C. Following ovulation induction, using techniques similar to that employed for in vitro fertilization (IVF), oocytes are recovered by translaparoscopic follicular aspiration; the sperm preparation and oocytes are immediately transferred via a plastic catheter into the fimbriated end of the Fallopian tube to a depth of 1.5 cm.

In 1986 Asch presented his further experiences with this technique, in which four pregnancies occurred in 10 treated patients; other workers (Guastella et al 1985) have reported similar success rates.

It is obvious that GIFT is only applicable in patients with patent Fallopian tubes and it has thus been advocated for cases of idiopathic infertility, minimum endometriosis or where there are male factors.

In general, pregnancy rates with GIFT are better than with IVF; the difference may be related to the better conditions for fertilization in vivo but is more likely to be associated with patient selection.

A randomized controlled trial comparing the effectiveness of GIFT and IVF procedures showed no significant differences in pregnancy rates in the management of patients with idiopathic or male infertility (Leeton et al 1987). An obvious disadvantage of GIFT is that it failed to provide data on the fertilizing capacity of sperm, particularly in cases of oligospermia. In this series, pregnancy rates for GIFT with oligospermia (counts less than 20 million/ml and idiopathic infertility were 33 and 19% respectively.

Matson et al (1987) have reported on the use of GIFT in the treatment of oligospermic infertility. They treated 32 couples in whom the male partner had reduced sperm numbers (<12 million/ml). There were no pregnancies when the recommended 100 000 motile sperms were transferred to each Fallopian tube. When the technique was modified to increase the number of motile sperms transferred, six pregnancies were achieved from 21 attempts (29%). The lowest number of sperms associated with pregnancy in this group was 325 000 per ml.

Preparation of the semen sample

Several methods of sperm preparation prior to AIH have been used in an attempt to improve conception rates and minimize complications (Matson et al 1987). The aim is to concentrate the motile sperms, especially in cases of oligospermia, and reduce the content of seminal plasma as it contains factors that reduce sperm survival and inhibit fertilization (Lindholmer 1973). The simplest method is by centrifugation of whole semen samples and resuspension of the sperms in a smaller quantity of buffered saline solution prior to AIH (Davajan et al 1983). Unfortunately most specimens from oligospermic men react adversely to centrifugation, with a marked decrease in motility. A low sperm count is frequently associated with morphological and biochemical abnormalities and it is not surprising that poor pregnancy rates have been reported using this method (Kaskarelis & Comninos 1959).

Several workers have advocated the use of the first portion of a split ejaculate as a means of overcoming a low sperm concentration (Farris & Murphy 1960, Perez-Palaez & Cohen 1963). In at least 90% of cases the first part of the ejaculate has a higher density of sperms and a lower level of prostaglandins. Amelar & Hotchkiss (1965) reported a 56% pregnancy rate when first-part split ejaculates were used, but most of the patients had initial counts of greater than 20 million per ml. More recent studies confined to cases with oligospermia with less than 20 million/ml report pregnancy rates of below 20% and suggest no improvement over that obtained in a similar population using whole semen inseminations (Steinman & Taymor 1977, Decker 1978).

Other methods have been used in an attempt to fractionate semen and isolate a high percentage of motile sperms. Paulson & Polakoski (1978) have used glass wool columns to remove debris and agglutinated and dead sperm cells, a method which is particularly useful for the treatment of high-viscosity semen. Following filtration the percentage of abnormal sperms decreased and samples showed an increased percentage with forward progressive motility. Ericsson et al (1973) showed that when semen was layered on columns of albumin it was possible after a defined time to isolate sperm fractions which had improved motility and were free from other cellular debris in a lower part of the column. In clinical practice the use of samples so prepared for AIH has been disappointing as regards conception rates (Dmowski et al 1979). The albumin column method of sperm filtration, described by Ericsson et al, is claimed to isolate a high percentage of Y sperms and this preparation can be used for insemination in couples desiring a male infant. Quinlivan et al (1982) described a Sephadex gel filtration method used to collect fractions rich in X-bearing sperms for couples desiring a female infant. While selection of either sex can be done electively on the basis of sociological preference or to balance a perceived disproportion within a family unit, female selection has an important additional indication, namely, avoidance of a male infant to carry sex-linked diseases.

Recent reports of intrauterine AIH in association with extracorporeal sperm capacitation using preparation methods similar to those employed in IVF programmes (see Ch. 75) have shown encouraging results (Kerin et al 1984, Sher et al 1984).

In cases of reduced sperm motility, semen may be treated in vitro with stimulants prior to insemination. Kallikrein, a proteinase, releases kinins which enhance sperm metabolism and has been advocated by Schill (1975). Caffeine has been used in a similar fashion; it inhibits cyclic nucleotide phosphodinase, thus preventing degradation of cyclic nucleotides (Schoenfeld et al 1975). Although Barkay et al (1977) achieved a 40% pregnancy rate when caffeine was added to frozen semen samples prior to insemination, the drug appears to cause damage to the sperms and is no longer recommendend (Harrison et al 1981).

Different storage methods have been used in an attempt to increase the total number of sperms available for insemination at the time of ovulation. However, freezing has a deleterious effect on sperm motility, especially in patients with oligospermia (Friedman & Broder 1981) and this approach is unlikely to offer any advantage.

Infertility may be related to increased seminal viscosity, resulting in marked sperm trapping (Tjioe & Oenstoeng 1968). The semen sample can be forced through an 18 gauge needle several times or mixed with a mucolytic agent (Alevaire, Winthrop Laboratories). Both methods provide samples with highly reduced viscosity suitable for AIH (Amelar & Dubin 1977). Non-liquefaction of semen presents a similar problem and may be treated in vitro with a 4% solution of amylase (Bunge & Sherman 1954) or the proteolytic enzyme chymotrypsin (Schill 1973).

Cryopreserved semen

Cryopreservation of semen has become a widely used technique (Thachil & Jewett 1981) and in association with AIH can be used to retain fertility potential in patients about to undergo vasectomy, radiotherapy or orchidectomy. Unfortunately, many patients with testicular tumours or Hodgkin's disease have impaired sperm production (Thachil et al 1981) and it may be difficult to obtain suitable semen samples prior to treatment. However, in all cases it is worth obtaining a semen sample and examining it after storage to assess the cryosurvival rate (percentage of actively motile sperms which remain after freezing and thawing). It is then possible to give the couple a realistic prognosis. Scammell et al (1985) reported a cumulative probability of pregnancy of 45% after 6 months of AIH in patients who had received chemotherapy for malignant disease.

Timing of insemination

Performing artificial insemination as near to ovulation as possible will obviously increase the chance of conception. Basal body temperature (BBT) charts have been advocated but used alone will lead to inaccurate timing in at least one-third of cycles (Lenton et al 1977, Bauman 1981). A scoring system has been devised based on the amount and quality of cervical mucus and which provides a biological marker

Table 74.3 Spontaneous abortions in pregnancies resulting from intrauterine inseminations (AIH)

Reference	Total pregnancies	Number of abortions	%
Barwin (1974)	31	7	23
Glezerman et al (1984)	13	4	31
Sher et al (1984)	24	5	21
Ulstein (1978)	10	6	60
White & Glass (1976)	5	0	0
Total	83	22	27

of endogenous oestrogen production in the preovulatory phase of the cycle (Insler et al 1972). Abundant clear mucus exhibiting significant spinnbarkheit and ferning is indicative of impending ovulation. Ovulation occurs approximately 18 hours after the peak of luteinizing hormone (World Health Organization 1981) and the development of rapid assay methods for measurement of this hormone in serum or urine has provided an extremely accurate means of timing ovulation (Descomps et al 1980). Serial ultrasonic scanning of the ovaries can demonstrate the developing dominant follicle; a mature follicle will measure approximately 20 mm (range 17–25 mm) and ovulation is presumed to have occurred when it disappears (Heasley & Thompson 1986). This provides a simple non-invasive method method for the timing of insemination and is particularly useful in patients with some degree of cycle irregularity.

The difficulty in predicting the timing of ovulation may be overcome by more frequent inseminations each cycle, starting 2–3 days before the expected rise in the BBT chart and continuing until there is a sustained rise in temperature and a significant decrease in cervical mucus. Barwin (1974) and Glezerman et al (1984) used daily inseminations with favourable results (62 and 52% pregnancy rates respectively).

Pregnancy outcome following AIH

When AIH is used, especially in cases of oligospermia associated with poor sperm morphology, concern has been expressed about the quality of resulting pregnancies. Table 74.3 shows the rates of early spontaneous abortion with intrauterine AIH; intrauterine AIH is the most critical situation because the protective filter of the cervical mucus has been bypassed. The overall rate from the combined series is 30% (range 0–60%) in 74 patients. Nachtigall et al (1979) reviewed the literature on AIH and reported an average abortion rate of 25% (range 0–45%) compared with a rate of 15% for the normal population. They concluded that the increased surveillance of pregnancies probably accounts for the higher incidence observed.

There is no evidence that children born following AIH, regardless of the indication, have an increased risk of congenital abnormalities (Allen et al 1985).

DONOR INSEMINATION

The practice of donor insemination* has been employed with increasing frequency as a solution for couples who cannot conceive because of male factor infertility. This trend has been expedited by a decrease in the number of babies available for adoption and an increasing public acceptance of the method. However, controversy still surrounds donor insemination, particularly in relation to the selection of sperm donors, screening techniques, the use of fresh or frozen semen and ethical considerations for the rights of the child.

Professional concern about the ethics of donor insemination should have been removed by the report of the panel on human artificial insemination appointed by the British Medical Association under the Chairmanship of Sir John Peel (1973). This report recognized the role of donor semen in the treatment of clinical problems and provided guidelines under which the medical practitioner could apply the technique. The UK Government committee of enquiry into human fertilization and embryology (HMSO 1984) which examined the entire field of human-assisted reproduction broadly supported the practice of donor insemination.

Selection of recipients for donor insemination

The initial contact with the couple is made at a joint interview involving the consultant responsible for the service. The first interview must establish the indication for referral and include a wide-ranging discussion of the medical, legal and social aspects of donor insemination, confidentiality and the screening procedures for recipients and donors (Table 74.4). At this stage neither party is expected to make a commitment and it is our practice to provide the couple with relevant literature on the subject and arrange another interview after an interval of several weeks, before a decision is made regarding the initiation of treatment.

It is important to ensure that couples are at ease with their final decision and further discussion may be necessary before this can be achieved. Obviously some reject the procedure once the implications have been explained and do

Table 74.4 Investigations prior to donor insemination

Male	Female
Confirmatory semen analysis	Blood group (rhesus factor)
Blood group (rhesus factor)	Rubella antibody titre
Physical characteristics	HIV antibodies
HIV antibodies	VDRL
VDRL	Prolactin
	Progesterone (day 21)

HIV = human immunodeficiency virus; VDRL = Venereal Disease Research Laboratories test.

* It is advisable to use the term donor insemination (DI) in preference to artificial insemination by donor, which is frequently abbreviated to AID. The latter is now confused with the acquired immune deficiency syndrome (AIDS), i.e. infection with HIV (HTLV-III/LAV).

not pursue the request. In spite of careful counselling some patients change their minds after starting treatment; Friedman (1977) reported a drop-out rate of 38% within three treatment cycles.

In many instances the counselling is undertaken by the consultant gynaecologist acting on his or her own with or without reference to colleagues. Ledward et al (1976) and Stewart (1984) have recommended the involvement of a medical social worker who would interview the couple at home in order to obtain a complete picture of their environment.

Kerr & Templeton (1976) and Ledward et al (1979) have outlined their criteria for selection, suggesting that a consultation team should be available to assist with counselling. This team might include a medical social worker, psychiatrist, clergyman and lawyer. However, the more personnel involved the more worried the couple may be about confidentiality. As patients express great concern about how far the knowledge of their use of donor insemination would have to be extended beyond the doctor who referred them, they require reassurance that secrecy is respected and that the greatest care is taken over letters and transfers of records. This is especially so in small communities when the information may be unwittingly divulged to an acquaintance of the recipient.

It is a difficult and controversial task to decide whether couples are suitable to be recipients of a child by donor insemination. One view is that it is not the responsibility of anyone but the couple themselves to make the decision and therefore the treatment should be provided on demand, even to single women and lesbian couples. Those who provide a donor insemination service should take whatever steps are available to assess whether the couple's relationship is sound and whether the motives for wanting a child are genuine.

A national survey of donor insemination practice in the USA showed that the third most cited indication is to provide children to women without a male partner and 10% of practitioners would support such a request (Curie-Cohen et al 1979). The Warnock Report (HMSO 1984) concluded that as a general rule it is better for children to be born into a two-parent family with both a father and a mother. Most practitioners in the UK appear to accept these guidelines, taking due regard of the psychological sequelae and legal implications.

Table 74.5 shows the indications for referral to our own practice and these are similar in most centres. Sterility is easily defined in cases of azoospermia but is more difficult with oligospermia or disorders of sperm motility; indeed, conceptions have occurred in the latter group following the initial consultation and prior to treatment commencing.

Table 74.5 Indications for donor insemination

Azoospermia
Gross oligospermia
Disorders of sperm motility and morphology
Genetic disease
Recessive, e.g. cystic fibrosis, Huntington's chorea
X-linked, e.g. muscular dystrophy
Immunological infertility
Rhesus isoimmunization
Previous vasectomy
Sexual dysfunction
Paraplegia, impotence, ejaculatory failure

Donor selection, screening and matching

The most important requirement for a successful donor insemination programme is a plentiful supply of donor semen of good quality. In the UK donors are usually recruited from the student population or hospital staff but each clinic has to make its own ad hoc arrangements. A modest fee is often paid to reimburse donors for expenses but it is considered undesirable to increase this fee to a level where a substantial financial incentive would be created. The institution of commercial sperm banks in the USA is of concern to some who feel that it appeals to motives which may lead to suppression or falsification of information which could make the donor unacceptable.

In France central donor banks have been established and samples are distributed to centres. The advantages are that uniform standards can be applied, hazards monitored and the number of pregnancies from any one donor restricted. Central registration of donors precludes an individual giving samples to more than one centre.

The donor must be physically and mentally healthy and under 35 years of age. A full medical and personal history, including family and genetic, is obtained. The responsibilities of being a donor are carefully explained and the importance of confidentiality emphasized. A potential donor should have a sperm count of at least 20 million/ml (preferably 40 million/ml) and a progressive motility rate of at least 60%. This motility rate is essential for cryopreservation which will inevitably result in a drop of motility of at least 20%. Semen samples should be sent regularly for bacteriological culture to exclude *Neisseria gonorrhoeae* and should be rejected if they contain pus cells.

There is concern that children conceived by the same donor, and who therefore are half-brothers and sisters, might marry and have children; the progeny of genetically related individuals will show a mortality and malformation rate which is higher than normal (Nevin 1976). However, considering the population involved, the chance of such a union is extremely small (McLaren 1973). Nevertheless, it is incumbent on clinics, especially when dealing with couples in small communities, to see that a single donor does not father too many children. The Warnock report (HMSO 1984) recommended a limit of 10 children.

Blood grouping is performed along with appropriate tests to exclude syphilis and hepatitis B antigen. Some centres will obtain a karyotype in the chance of detecting a serious abnormal chromosomal constitution. However, even the most careful donor selection cannot completely eliminate the risk of a child inheriting a congenital defect (Smith 1984).

Following the report of acquired immune deficiency syndrome (AIDS) by human immunodeficiency virus (HIV) transmission through donor insemination (Stewart et al 1985) guidelines issued by the Department of Health and Social Security encourage clinic managers to ensure that all donors read an explanatory leaflet and sign a consent form indicating that they do not belong to a high-risk group, i.e. homosexuals or bisexual men, drug abusers or residents from areas where AIDS is common. All donors should be tested for HIV (HTLV/LAV) antibody on recruitment; this test is repeated at 3-monthly intervals for as long as the donor continues to attend the clinic. The small risk of AIDS transmission by semen is even further reduced if only cryopreserved quarantined semen is used for insemination; clinics are now encouraged to provide such facilities and avoid the use of fresh samples.

The degree of matching between husband and donor will depend on the number of unusual features of the husband and the size and variety of the pool of donors. Couples of ethnic groups other than Caucasian pose a particular problem; Hindu and Muslim donors are extremely difficult to recruit. The donor should be of the same race as the recipient and ideally have the same social and intellectual background. The blood group should preferably be the same as that of the husband or the wife and if the wife is rhesus-negative, a rhesus-negative donor should be used. Other characteristics should be matched with the donor, including hair colour, eye colour and body build.

Clinic management

Table 74.4 shows the screening tests which should be performed on the woman before treatment is started; if she is non-immune to rubella, vaccination is advised and treatment postponed for 3 months. The extent to which female infertility is investigated before donor insemination varies from clinic to clinic. The confirmation of ovulation by BBT or observation of preovulatory cervical mucus is essential. If the cycle is irregular it may be necessary, even when ovulation is confirmed, to use clomiphene citrate to manipulate follicular development in order to ensure that insemination is properly timed. In difficult cases ultrasonic monitoring of the follicle can be used. Many patients with regular cycles will develop irregularity after commencing treatment; this is probably associated with stress but will usually respond to therapy with clomiphene citrate.

In patients with no relevant history or evidence of pelvic disease it is probably unnecessary to perform tubal patency tests before commencing treatment (Friedman 1977). The majority of conceptions (over 80%) occur within 6 months and as delay in conception places considerable emotional pressure on the patient and is a common reason for treatment being abandoned, female fertility should be reviewed after six consecutive treatment cycles even if earlier investigations proved normal.

A donor insemination clinic should ideally have provision for treatment on a daily basis but staffing levels often preclude this and most will see patients on weekdays only. Insemination should be carried out between days 11 and 14 of a normal 28-day cycle; at least two inseminations (on separate days) in each cycle are offered to patients. The cervix is exposed and a small portion of the semen sample, loaded in a syringe, is instilled into the cervical canal while the remainder is allowed to spill over the cervix and vaginal vault; the total volume used is 0.3 ml of fresh or 0.5 ml of thawed cryopreserved semen. The patient may lie on the couch for 10 minutes after the procedure but this is probably unnecessary. Careful records of all procedures must be maintained; however, it is essential that they remain confidential to the clinic staff.

Legal and moral implications

The potential legal problems concerning donor insemination are immense and involve the mother, her husband, the biological father (the donor), the practitioner, the child and probably the relatives of both partners and the donor. The legal status of the child is the greatest concern to the parents. In the UK, such a child is at present illegitimate, although the husband, by his consent, has accepted the child as family with all the associated rights and responsibilities. The English Law Commission (HMSO 1984) recommended that the law should be reformed to remove all the legal disadvantages of illegitimacy so that there would be no legal distinction between legitimate and illegitimate children. The Commission further recommended that when a married woman has received donor insemination with her husband's consent, the husband, rather than the donor, should for all legal purposes be regarded as the father of the child so conceived. The Warnock report (HMSO 1984) supported these recommendations. Draft resolutions have also been discussed by the Council of Europe (1982) proposing that when donor artificial insemination has been administered with the consent of the husband the child should be considered as the legitimate child of the woman and her husband and nobody may contest the legitimacy on the sole ground of artificial insemination. It was further recommended that donor insemination should be administered only on the responsibility of a physician and that the physician must make appropriate enquiry and examinations in order to prevent the transmission from the donor of a hereditary condition or contagious disease or other factor which might present a danger to the health of the woman or the future child. In French law the problem has already been simplified by

French Civil Code Article 312 which states that the 'husband is considered to be the father of any child conceived during marriage' (Revillard 1973).

It is generally accepted that adopted children fare better when they are made aware as soon as possible of their adoption (Brandon 1979). It can be argued that this should also apply to children born through donor insemination (Rowland 1985). However, in practice donor insemination has tended to be surrounded by secrecy, largely due to the lack of a satisfactory legal basis. This secrecy amounts to more than a desire for confidentiality and privacy since the couple may deceive their family and friends and often the child as well. Snowden (1984) reported that 58% of couples kept donor insemination a complete secret and the main reasons given were:

1. A desire to appear as a normal family.
2. A fear of stigmatization of the husband or the child by society generally or by family members.
3. The preservation of harmonious family relationships which might be endangered if the genetic imbalance between the maternal and paternal sides of the family was made known.
4. A wish to protect the child from knowledge about his or her origins which might prove harmful.
5. A wish to protect the feelings of the older generation.

Other couples in Snowden's survey argued equally strongly for the avoidance of secrecy based on the fact that the relatives have the right to know and the couple's wish to avail themselves of family support in a stressful situation.

There seem to be good reasons for maintaining the anonymity of the donor. If the identify of the donor is known, conflicting emotional ties between the family of the recipient and the donor may arise. Without anonymity men would be less likely to become donors in view of the risk that they might subsequently be identified and forced to accept parental responsibility for the child.

The Warnock report (HMSO 1984) recommended that information about the ethnic origin and genetic health of the donors should be made available to the child at the age of 18 years and that legislation should be enacted to provide the right of access to this. A change in the law was suggested so that semen donors will have no parental rights or duties in relation to the child. Informed consent should be given by the mother and her husband and it is also advisable to request this of the donors.

In our own practice we have not been asked by any couples to enlarge on the religious view of donor insemination, although we do ask if they require advice and would recommend them to consult their own clergy for such guidance. The Roman Catholic Church has repeatedly rejected the practice of donor insemination for married as much as for unmarried couples in statements from the Holy Office in 1897 and from Pope Pius XII in 1949 and 1956 (CTS 1960); artificial insemination is condemned on the basis that the exclusive rights of procreation reside only in marriage. The Anglican Church has also expressed its disapproval; in 1948 the commission set up by the Archbishop of Canterbury declared the practice to be 'contrary to Christian principles and worthy to be considered a criminal offence'; no other Protestant faith has approved the practice. Orthodox Judaism is also opposed but several reformed Jewish groups have indicated approval (Dunstan 1976).

Table 74.6 Success rates with donor insemination

Reference	Patients	Conceptions	Pregnancy rate (%)
Chong & Taymor (1975)	142	103	72
Dixon et al (1976)	171	61	36
Jackson & Richardson (1977)	604	355	59
Friedman (1977)	227	91	40
Bromwich et al (1978)	214	82	38
Joyce (1979)	149	47	31.5
Total	1507	739	49

Pregnancy outcome with donor insemination

Table 74.6 shows the pregnancy rates in several published reports; this varies from 31.5 to 72% (overall 49%). There are several reasons for the wide variation; patients who drop out early in the treatment programme may not be included in the figures; many who are apparently lost to follow-up turn up with a request for a second child, having failed to report their first one in the interest of confidentiality, and practitioners may not attempt a positive follow-up when couples do not communicate voluntarily. Patient selection also influences results; if recipients are accepted on the basis of being under 30 years of age and having other causes of infertility excluded, results should be good. Fecundability (the chance of pregnancy per cycle of exposure) in women over 30 years is about 70% of corresponding values for those under 30 years. Whether fresh or frozen semen is used should not affect the success rate although it will take longer to achieve pregnancy using cryopreserved semen. Richter et al (1984) reported that fecundability was 18.9% with fresh semen and 5% with cryopreserved semen; fresh semen is thus more than three times as likely to induce pregnancy per cycle of treatment as is frozen semen.

There is no evidence to suggest that pregnancy loss following donor insemination is any greater than after normal conception. Table 74.7 shows the outcome of 6587 pregnancies collected by a survey of donor insemination clinics in the UK during a 7-year period (Newton 1984). The live birth rate on a yearly basis varied from 74 to 83% and the spontaneous abortion rate was between 11 and 16%. Fourteen terminations of pregnancy were carried out during this 7-year period. In the early years many of these were due to rubella contracted in early pregnancy; this emphasizes the need for relevant patient screening and immunization prior to the commencement of treatment. After 1980 the terminations

Table 74.7 Pregnancy outcome with donor insemination

	1977	1978	1979	1980	1981	1982	1983	Total
Live births*	463(83)	574(83)	653(80)	658(77)	869(78)	820(74)	1081(79)	5118
Abortions*	86(16)	98(14)	90(11)	119(14)	137(12)	134(12)	151(11)	815
Terminations	1	1	3	2	3	2	2	14
Ectopic pregnancies	5	3	4	6	6	5	10	39
Stillbirths	1	7	2	9	14	NR	9	42
Unknown outcome	2	10	63	60	76	15	192	559
Total*	556(0.4)	693(1.4)	820(8)	854(7)	1105(7)	1112(14)	1445(14)	6587

After Newton (1984).
NR = not recorded.
* Percentage in parentheses.

were mainly performed for serious fetal abnormalities diagnosed on ultrasound. The ectopic pregnancy rate was no higher than one would expect for natural conceptions. The unknown outcome was 14% in 1983 and reflects the difficulty in collecting accurate data. There is no significant evidence that donor insemination is associated with an increased rate of congenital abnormalities; theoretically the careful selection of donors should reduce numbers.

As a result of the secrecy surrounding donor insemination, long-term follow-up of children has been poor but Iizuka et al (1968) assessed the physical and mental development of 54 children and found it was superior to a control group.

DONOR OOCYTES

The use of donor oocytes raises the same ethical and legal considerations, as donor semen from the infertile patient's partner would be used for fertilization. The practice is further complicated because oocytes are not readily available and it may be necessary to recruit donors from a friend or relative.

The ovulation cycles of donor and recipient must be carefully synchronized by hormone therapy; the recent use of frozen embryos will make transfer at the correct time more easily achieved.

The indications for this practice are:

1. Adhesions and extensive pelvic disease preventing oocyte recovery.
2. Premature menopause or bilateral oophorectomy (Feichtinger & Kemeter 1985).
3. Inheritable genetic disease transmitted by the female partner, e.g. tuberosus sclerosis.

The Warnock Committee (HMSO 1984) accepted oocyte donation as a recognized technique in the treatment of infertility subject to the same regulations as donor insemination, including anonymity of the donor and limitation to 10 of the number of children born from the oocytes of one woman. However, it was suggested that an exception to the principle of anonymity would occur when the oocyte was donated by a sister or close friend; in such cases particularly careful counselling of all concerned would be necessary.

Another method of ovum donation was described by Buster et al (1985); a consenting woman was artificially inseminated with the male partner's semen and uterine lavage was then performed 5 days after the luteinizing hormone peak. Fertilized eggs were recovered and then transferred to the uterus of the infertile woman. The authors reported three intrauterine and one ectopic pregnancy from 10 treated cases. They called the procedure surrogate embryo transfer (SET). The technique carries potential risks to the donor mother in that lavage may not dislodge the pregnancy and there is a risk of pelvic sepsis.

Embryo donation involves the use of donor oocyte and sperms and constitutes a form of prenatal adoption. There is the advantage over normal adoption that the couple share the experience of pregnancy and childbirth, leading to improved bonding. The Warnock Committee (HMSO 1984) recommended that ovum or embryo donation in which the gametes were brought together in vitro was acceptable as a treatment of infertility but were opposed to the use of the lavage method pending additional information regarding its safety.

SURROGATE MOTHERHOOD

Surrogate parenting is a process by which a couple obtain a baby after the male partner's sperm is artificially inseminated into another woman who has agreed, usually for financial gain, to carry the pregnancy to term and then to relinquish any claim to the infant. The child is then adopted by the infertile couple. There are certain medical circumstances in which surrogacy would be an option for the alleviation of infertility, such as severe pelvic disease precluding access to the ovaries or if the patient had had a hysterectomy. The practice might also be used to help women who had repeated spontaneous abortions.

Utian et al (1985) reported a case of a pregnancy in which fertilization of an ovum obtained from a woman who had had a hysterectomy was followed by transfer of the embryo to a surrogate. A survey by Jones (1975) showed that at least 1000 children have been born to surrogate mothers and adopted in the USA. The practice has generated considerable public and professional debate.

The risks of surrogacy include the possibility that the commissioning father might come to believe he was not the infant's genetic father; the surrogate mother might refuse to hand over the infant; the infant might be rejected by all parties because of handicap or the mother might become ill during pregnancy or take a drug which might damage the fetus. There has been a case report of a baby born with the fetal alcohol syndrome (Friedman 1984).

The experience of conception, gestation and childbirth has a profound effect on all mothers. The surrogate mother may start out wanting to do something generous for a couple but find herself wanting to keep the baby. It is difficult to anticipate the short-term or long-term feelings that may arise. Unfortunately major discussions have tended to involve legal and logistical problems but have ignored the critical issue, namely the child so conceived (Davis & Brown 1984). The Warnock Committee (HMSO 1984) debated the question of surrogacy at length and concluded that even in compelling medical circumstances the danger of exploitation of one human being by another outweighed the potential benefits. They were strongly opposed to commercial agencies whose purposes include the recruitment of women for surrogate pregnancies. In 1985 the UK Government took steps to outlaw commercial surrogacy following further public and professional concern about such practices (Surrogacy Arrangements Act; Deitch 1985).

REFERENCES

Allen N C, Herbert C M, Maxon W S, Rogers B J, Diamond M P, Wentz A C 1985 Intrauterine insemination: a critical review. Fertility and Sterility 44: 569–580

Amelar R D, Dubin L 1977 Special problems in management. In: Amelar R D, Dubin L, Walsh P C (eds) Male infertility. Saunders, London, pp 191–214

Amelar R D, Hotchkiss R S 1965 The split ejaculate. Its use in the management of male infertility. Fertility and Sterility 16: 46–60

Asch R H, Ellsworth L R, Balmaceda J P, Wong P C 1984 Pregnancy following translaparoscopic gamete intrafallopian transfer (GIFT). Lancet ii: 1034–1035

Asch R H, Ellsworth L R, Balmaceda J P, Wong P C 1985 Birth following gamete intrafallopian transfer. Lancet i: 163

Asch R H, Balmaceda J P, Ellsworth L R, Wong P C 1986 Preliminary experiences with gamete intrafallopian transfer (GIFT). Fertility and Sterility 45: 366

Barkay J, Zuckerman H 1978 Further developed device for human sperm freezing by the 20 minute method. Fertility and Sterility 29: 304–308

Barkay J, Zuckerman H K, Sklan D, Gordon S 1977 Effect of caffeine on increasing the motility of frozen human sperm. Fertility and Sterility 28: 175–177

Barton M, Walker K, Wiesner B P 1945 Artificial insemination. British Medical Journal i: 40–43

Barwin B N 1974 Intrauterine insemination of husband's semen. Journal of Reproduction and Fertility 36: 101

Bauman J E 1981 Basal body temperature: unreliable method of ovulation detection. Fertility and Sterility 3: 729–733

Bernstein D, Levin S, Amsterdam E, Insler V 1979 Is conception in infertile couples treatment related? International Journal of Fertility 24: 65–67

Brandon J 1979 Telling the AID child. Adoption and Fostering 95: 13–14

Bromwich P, Kilpatrick M, Newton J R 1978 Artificial insemination with frozen stored donor semen. British Journal of Obstetrics and Gynaecology 85: 641–644

Bunge R G, Sherman J K 1954 Liquefaction of human semen by alpha-amylase. Fertility and Sterility 5: 353–356

Buster J E, Bustillo M, Rodi I A et al 1985 Biologic and morphologic development of donated human ova recovered by non-surgical uterine lavage. American Journal of Obstetrics and Gynecology 153: 211–217

Chong A P, Taymor M L 1975 Sixteen years of experience with therapeutic donor insemination. Fertility and Sterility 26: 791–798

Collins J A, Wrixon W, Janes L B, Wilson E H 1983 Treatment-independent pregnancy among infertile couples. New England Journal of Medicine 309: 1201–1206

Corson S L, Batzer F R 1980 Artificial insemination. Current Problems in Obstetrics and Gynaecology, vol 7

Council of Europe 1982 Artificial insemination of human beings. Medicine and Law 1: 3–10

Crich J P, Jequier A M 1977 Infertility in men with retrograde ejaculation: the action of urine on sperm motility, and a simple method for achieving antegrade ejaculation. Fertility and Sterility 30: 572–576

CTS 1960 Artificial insemination. Evidence on behalf of the Catholic Body in England and Wales (submitted to the Feversham Committee) Catholic Trust Society, London

Curie-Cohen M, Luttrell L, Shapiro S 1979 Current practice of artificial insemination by donor in the United States. New England Journal of Medicine 300(11): 585–590

Davajan V, Vargyas J M, Kletzky O A et al 1983 Intrauterine insemination with washed sperm to treat infertility. Fertility and Sterility 40: 419–422

Davis J H, Brown D W 1984 Artificial insemination by donor (AID) and the use of surrogate mothers. Western Journal of Medicine 141: 127–130

Decker W H 1978 Pooled and frozen homologous (husband) semen for artificial insemination. Infertility 1: 25–30

Deitch R 1985 The Government acts to prohibit surrogacy arrangements. Lancet i: 994–995

Descomps B, Nicholas J C, Chikhaoui Y, De Paulet A C 1980 Prediction and detection of ovulation by hormonal measurements: contribution of a new enzymatic method. Journal of Steroid Biochemistry 12: 385–393

Dixon R E, Buttrram V C, Schum C W 1976 Artificial insemination using homologous semen: a review of 158 cases. Fertility and Sterility 27: 647–654

Dmowski W P, Gaynor L, Lawrence M, Rao R, Scommegna A 1979 Artificial insemination homologous with oligospermic semen separated in albumin columns. Fertility and Sterility 31: 58–62

Duncombe C W S 1960 Report of the departmental committee on human artificial insemination. HMSO, London

Dunstan G W E 1976 Ethical issues relating to AID. In: Brundenell M, McLaren A, Short R, Symonds M (eds) Artificial insemination. Royal College of Obstetricians and Gynaecologists, London, p 182–191

Ericsson R J, Langevin C N, Nishino M 1973 Isolation of fractions rich in human Y sperm. Nature 246: 421–424

Farris E J, Murphy D P 1960 The characteristics of the two parts of the partitioned ejaculation and the advantages of its use for intrauterine insemination. A study of 100 ejaculates. Fertility and Sterility 11: 465–469

Feichtinger W, Kemeter P 1985 Clinical experience with ultrasound guided oocyte recovery. In: Thompson W, Joyce D N, Newton J R (eds) In vitro fertilisation and donor insemination. Royal College of Obstetricians and Gynaecologists, London, pp 163–168

Frankel L 1909 Uber künstliche Befruchtung beim Menschen und ihre gerichtsarztliche Beurteirlung. Arztliche Sachverst Ztg 15: 169

Friedman S 1977 Artificial donor insemination with frozen human semen. Fertility and Sterility 28: 1230–1233

Friedman S 1984 Surrogate parenting. Acta Europaea Fertilitatis 15: 441–444

Friedman S, Broder S 1981 Homologous artificial insemination after long term semen cryopreservation. Fertility and Sterility 35: 219–222

Gerignon C, Kunstmann J M 1980 AIH for semen insufficiency: 119 cases. In: David G, Price W (eds) Human artificial insemination and semen preservation. Plenum Press, New York, p 529

Glezerman M, Lunenfeld B 1976 Zur Therapie der mannlichen Anorgasmie — ein Fallbericht. Actuel Dermatologie 2: 167–169

Glezerman M, Lunenfeld B, Polashnik G, Oelsner G, Beer R 1976 Retrograde ejaculation: pathophysical aspects and report of two successfully treated cases. Fertility and Sterility 27: 796–800

Glezerman M, Bernstein D, Insler V 1984 The cervical factor of infertility

and intrauterine insemination. International Journal of Fertility 29: 16–20
Grant A 1969 The spontaneous cure rate of various infertility factors or post hoc and propter hoc. Australian and New Zealand Journal of Obstetrics and Gynaecology 9: 224–227
Gregoire A T, Mayer R C 1965 The impregnators. Fertility and Sterility 16: 130–134
Guastella G, Comparetto G, Gullo D et al 1985 Gamete intra-fallopian transfer (GIFT): a new technique for the treatment of unexplained infertility. Acta Europaea Fertilitatis 16: 311–315
Guttmacher A F 1943 The role of artificial insemination in the treatment of human sterility. Bulletin of the New York Academy of Medicine 19: 573–584
Guttmacher A F 1960 The role of artificial insemination in the treatment of sterility. Obstetrical and Gynecological Survey 15: 767–785
Harrison R F 1978 Insemination of husband's semen with and without the addition of caffeine. Fertility and Sterility 29: 532–537
Harrison R F, Sheppard B L, Kaliszer M 1980 Observations on the motility, ultrastructure and elemental composition of human spermatozoa incubated with caffeine. II A time sequence study. Andrologia 12: 434–443
Heasley R N, Thompson W 1986 The prediction and detection of ovulation in artificial insemination. In: Paulson J D, Negro-Vilar A, Lucena E, Martini L (eds) Andrology — male fertility and sterility. Academic Press, New York, pp 491–509
Hill A M 1970 Experiences with artificial insemination. Australian and New Zealand Journal of Obstetrics and Gynaecology 10: 112–116
HMSO 1984 The Warnock report. The United Kingdom Government committee of enquiry into human fertilisation and embryology. HMSO, London
Home E 1799 An account of the dissection of a hermaphrodite dog. Philosophical Transactions of the Royal Society, London 89: 157
Hotchkiss R S, Pinto A B, Kleegman S 1955 Artificial insemination with semen recovered from the bladder. Fertility and Sterility 6: 37–42
Iizuka R, Sawada Y, Nishina N, Ohi M 1968 The physical and mental development of children born following artificial insemination. International Journal of Fertility 13: 24–32
Ingerslev H J 1985 Retrograde ejaculation: successful artificial homologous insemination. Lancet i: 519
Insler V, Melmed H, Eichenbrenner I, Serr D M, Lunenfeld 1972 The cervical score: a simple semiquantitive method for monitoring of the menstrual cycle. International Journal of Gynaecology and Obstetrics 10: 223–226
Jackson M C N, Richardson D W 1977. The use of fresh and frozen semen in human artificial insemination. Journal of Biosocial Science 9: 251–256
Jette T N, Glass R H 1972 Prognostic value of the post coital test. Fertility and Sterility 23: 29–35
Jones K B 1984 Surrogate motherhood and criminal law. Pennsylvania Medicine 87: 22
Joyce D 1979 The organisation of a NHS clinic. In: Richardson D, Joyce D, Symonds M (eds) Frozen human semen: proceedings of a workshop upon the cryobiology of human semen and its role in artificial insemination by donor. Royal College of Obstetricians and Gynaecologists, London, pp 234–245
Joyce D, Vassilopoulos D 1981 Sperm–mucus interaction and artificial insemination. Clinics in Obstetrics and Gynaecology 8: 587–610
Kaskarelis E, Comninos A 1959 A critical evaluation of homologous artificial insemination. International Journal of Fertility 4: 38–42
Kerin J F P et al 1984 Improved conception rate after intrauterine insemination of washed spermatozoa from men with poor quality semen. Lancet i: 533–535
Kerr M, Templeton A 1976 Selection and counselling of recipients. In: Brundenwell M, McLaren A, Short R, Symonds S (eds) Proceedings of fourth study group of the Royal College of Obstetricians and Gynaecologists. Royal College of Obstetricians and Gynaecologists, London
Kleegman S J, Kaufman S A 1966 Infertility in women. F A Davis, Philadelphia, p 168
Kovacs G T, Newman G B, Henson G L 1978 The postcoital test: what is normal? British Medical Journal 1: 818
Kremer J 1979 A new technique for intrauterine insemination. International Journal of Fertility 24: 53
Ledward R S, Crich J, Sharp P, Cotton R E, Symonds E M 1976 The establishment of a programme of artificial insemination by donor semen within the National Health Service. British Journal of Obstetrics and Gynaecology 83: 917
Ledward R S, Crawford L, Symonds E M 1979 Social factors in patients for artificial insemination by donor AID. Journal of Biosocial Science 11: 473–479
Leeton J, Healey D, Rogers P, Yates C, Caro C 1987 A controlled study between the use of gamete intrafallopian transfer (GIFT) and in vitro fertilization and embryo transfer in the management of idiopathic and male infertility. Fertility and Sterility 48: 605–607
Lenton E A, Weston G A, Cooke I D 1977 Problems in using basal body temperature recordings in an infertility clinic. British Medical Journal 1: 803–805
Lindholmer C 1973 Survival of human spermatozoa in different fractions of split ejaculate. Fertility and Sterility 24: 521–526
MacLeod J, Gold R Z 1951 The male factor in fertility and infertility II. Spermatozoon counts in 1000 cases of known fertility and in 1000 cases of infertile marriage. Journal of Urology 66: 436–449
Makler A 1980 A simple technique to increase success rate of artificial insemination. International Journal of Obstetrics and Gynecology 18: 19–21
Makler A, De Cherney A, Naftolin F 1984 A device for injecting and retaining a small volume of concentrated spermatozoa in the uterine cavity and the cervical canal. Fertility and Sterility 42: 306–308
Mastroianni L, Laberge J L, Rock J 1957 Appraisal of the efficacy of artificial insemination with husband's semen and evaluation of insemination techniques. Fertility and Sterility 8: 260–266
Matson P L, Blackledge D G, Richardson P A, Turner S R, Yovich J M, Yovich J L 1987 The role of gamete intrafallopian transfer (GIFT) in the treatment of oligospermic infertility. Fertility and Sterility 48: 608–612
McLaren A 1973 Biological aspects of AID. Ciba Foundation Symposium. Amsterdam, Elsevier, p 3
Moghissi K S, Gruber J S, Evans S, Yanez J 1977 Homologous artificial insemination — reappraisal. American Journal of Obstetrics and Gynecology 129: 909–915
Nachtigall R D, Faure W, Glass R H 1979 Artificial insemination of husband's semen. Fertility and Sterility 32: 141–147
Nevin N C 1976 Aetiology of genetic disease. Prevention of handicap through antenatal care. In: Turnbull A C, Woodford F P (eds) Reviews of research and practice 18 of the Institute for Research into Mental and Multiple Handicap. Elsevier, Amsterdam
Newton J R 1984 Clinical results of AID. In: Thompson W, Joyce D N, Newton J R (eds) In vitro fertilisation and donor insemination. Royal College of Obstetricians and Gynaecologists, London, pp 307–315
Nunley W C, Kitchin J D, Thiagarajah S 1978 Homologous insemination. Fertility and Sterility 30: 510–517
Paulson J D, Polakoski K I 1978 The removal of extraneous material from the ejaculate. International Journal of Andrology (suppl) 1: 163
Peel J 1973 Report of Panel on Human Artificial Insemination. British Medical Journal (supplement) ii: 3
Perez-Pelaez M, Cohen M R 1963 The split ejaculate in homologous insemination. International Journal of Fertility 10: 25–30
Pollock M 1967 Sex and its problems: viii: artificial insemination. Practitioner 199: 244–252
Quinlivan W L G, Preciado K, Long T L, Sullivan H 1982 Separation of human X and Y spermatozoa by albumin gradients and Sephadex chromatography. Fertility and Sterility 37: 104–108
Revillard M 1973 Legal aspects of artificial insemination and embryo transfer. In: French domestic law and private international law, pp 77–90
Richter M A, Haning R V, Shapiro S 1984 Artificial insemination: fresh versus frozen semen: the patient as her own control. Fertility and Sterility 41: 277–280
Rowland R 1985 The social and psychological consequences of secrecy in artificial insemination by donor (AID) programmes. Social Science and Medicine 21: 391–396
Russell J K 1960 Artificial insemination (husband) in the management of childlessness. Lancet ii: 1223–1225
Sandler B 1979 Idiopathic retrograde ejaculation. Fertility and Sterility 32: 474–475
Scammell G E, White N, Stedronska J, Hendry W F, Edmonds D K, Jeffcoate S L 1985 Cryopreservation of semen in men with testicular

tumours or Hodgkin's disease: results of artificial insemination of their partners. Lancet ii: 31–32
Schill W B 1973 Probleme der homolgen und heterologen. Insemination aus adrologischer sicht. In: Braun-Falco O, Petzoldt D Fortschnitte der praktischen. Dermatologie und Venerologie. Springer, Berlin, pp 187–195
Schill W B 1975 Caffeine and kallikrein induced stimulation of human sperm motility: a comparative study. Andrologie 7: 229–236
Schoenfeld C, Amelar R D, Dubin L 1975 Stimulation of ejaculated spermatozoa by caffeine. Fertility and Sterility 26: 158–161
Semm K, Brandl E, Mettler L 1976. Vacuum insemination cap. In: Hafez E S E (ed) Human semen and fertility regulation in men. Mosby, St Louis, pp 439–441
Sher G, Knutzen V K, Stratton C J, Montakhab M M, Allenson S G 1984. In vitro sperm aspiration and transvesical intrauterine insemination for the treatment of refractory infertility phase 1. Fertility and Sterility 41: 260–263
Sims J M 1866 Clinical notes on uterine surgery, with special reference to the management of the sterile condition. Hardwicke, London
Smith P E 1984 Selection against genetic defects in semen donors. Clinical Genetics 26: 87–108
Snowden R 1984 The social implications of artificial reproduction. In: Thompson W, Joyce D N, Newton J R (eds) In vitro fertilisation and donor insemination. Royal College of Obstetricians and Gynaecologists, London, pp 319–328
Speichinger J P, Mattox J H 1976 Artificial insemination homologous and oligospermia. Fertility and Sterility 27: 135–138
Steinman R P, Taymor M L 1977 Artificial insemination homologous and its role in the management of infertility. Fertility and Sterility 28: 146–150
Stewart C R 1984 AID clinic management. In: Thompson W, Joyce D N, Newton J R (eds) In vitro fertilisation and donor insemination. Royal College of Obstetricians and Gynaecologists, London, pp 299–315
Stewart G J, Tyler J P P, Cunningham A L et al 1985 Transmission of human T-cell lymphotrophic virus type 111 (HTLV-111) by artificial insemination by donor. Lancet ii: 581–585
Taylor P L, Kelly R W 1974 19-hydroxylated E-prostaglandins as the major prostaglandins of human semen. Nature 250: 665–667
Thachil J V, Jewett M A S 1981 Preservation techniques for human semen. Fertility and Sterility 35: 546–548
Thachil J V, Jewett M A S, Rider W D 1981 The effect of cancer therapy on male infertility. Journal of Urology 126: 141–145
Thompson W, Boyle D D 1982 Counselling patients for artificial insemination and subsequent pregnancy. Clinics in Obstetrics and Gynaecology 9: 211–225
Thompson W, Joyce D, Newton J R 1984 In vitro fertilisation and donor insemination. Royal College of Obstetricians and Gynaecologists, London
Tijoe D Y, Oenstoeng S 1968 The viscosity of human semen and the percentage of motile spermatozoa. Fertility and Sterility 19: 562–565
Traub A I, Boyle D D, Thompson W 1979 The establishment of an AID clinic in Northern Ireland. Ulster Medical Journal 48: 137–141
Ulstein M 1973 Fertility of husbands at homologous insemination. Acta Obstetricia et Gynecologica Scandinavica 52: 97–101
Usherwood M McD 1980 AIH for cases of spermatozoa antibodies and oligozoospermia. In: David G, Price W (eds) Human artificial insemination and semen preservation. Plenum Press, New York, p 539
Usherwood M McD, Halim A, Evans P R 1976 Artificial insemination (AIH) for sperm antibodies and oligospermia. British Journal of Urology 48: 499–503
Utian W H, Sheean L, Goldbarb J M, Kiwi R 1985 Successful pregnancy after in vitro fertilisation and embryo transfer from an infertile woman to a surrogate. New England Journal of Medicine 313: 1351–1352
White R M, Glass R H 1976 Intrauterine insemination with husband's semen. Obstetrics and Gynecology 47: 119–121
Whitelaw W J 1950 Use of the cervical cap to increase fertility in cases of oligospermia. Fertility and Sterility 1: 33–39
Whitelaw W J 1979 The cervical cap self applied in the treatment of severe oligospermia. Fertility and Sterility 31: 86–87
Wiltbank M C, Kosasa T S, Rogers B J 1985 Treatment of infertile patients by intrauterine insemination of washed spermatozoa. Andrologia 17: 22
World Health Organization 1981 Temporal relationships between ovulation and defined changes in the concentration of plasma oestradiol-17B, luteinizing hormone, follicle stimulating hormone and progesterone II. American Journal of Obstetrics and Gynecology 139: 886–895

D. L. Healy and C. Wood

Extracorporeal fertilization (IVF)

INTRODUCTION

In vitro fertilization (IVF) and embryo transfer (ET) have resulted in more than 3000 babies being delivered throughout the world. IVF is now used for most patients with infertility in whom other treatment has failed. This includes patients with tubal disease, endometriosis, mild to moderate male infertility, unknown cause for the infertility, failed artificial insemination with donor (AID) semen and failed ovulation induction. In this chapter, we shall review the clinical aspects of extracorporeal fertilization: readers are referred to Chapter 4 for the basic science aspects of IVF and ET.

IVF may be combined with the use of donor oocytes or donor sperm. The main limitation to the use of donor oocytes at the present time is the difficulty in obtaining anonymous donors. For this reason couples are turning to donors they know who will be sympathetic, such as a friend or relative. Special counselling for such couples is provided. Known donors have the advantage that the recipient is more confident of the biological outcome of the pregnancy as the couple are aware of the genetic background of the donor. IVF has been combined with surrogacy, particularly in women who have ovaries but no uterus.

IVF is used in combination with embryo freezing, when there is an excess of embryos to be transferred or when immediate transfer of fresh embryos is impossible or contraindicated. Embryo freezing remains relatively inefficient as only about 60% of embryos withstand the process of freeze-thawing and the pregnancy rate from transfers is about 10%.

Cryobiology is a relatively new science and the current use of techniques, which are not well understood, can be expected to improve. Oocyte freezing is even more difficult and will probably remain less effective than embryo freezing because of the larger cell size of the oocyte and the unstable state of the chromosomes in the mature oocyte, which may be adversely affected either by freezing or the use of cryopreservants. Oocyte freezing will be required for specific reasons, where pelvic disease threatens the life of the ovary in a single woman and oocytes are stored to ensure future fertility, or where young single women have oocytes stored for possible use when they are older, thereby avoiding the risk of Down's syndrome. For married women, embryo freezing to ensure future fertility will be preferable.

The pregnancy rate by IVF treatment remains at 13–25% per treatment in different clinics around the world. Despite many attempts to determine the reason for differences, the variable success rates are largely unexplained. Embryotoxins may be undetectable in culture media. Improvements in culture media will occur. The success rate of experimental in vivo fertilization in animals is 2–5 times higher than the in vitro procedure. The use of amniotic fluid as a culture medium has already improved success rates from 15 to 20% in some centres. Culture of cells from the lining of animal oviducts or human tubes may also further improve the culture system, as the natural system is more closely associated.

Simplifying IVF treatment to reduce cost and stress has occurred so that couples can better cope with the repeated attempts necessary to have a reasonable chance of becoming pregnant. Outpatient treatment, reducing venepunctures, expert counselling, ready access to information and the use of vaginal ultrasound oocyte pick-ups all make treatment easier. Intrafallopian insertion of gametes by laparoscopy, the gamete intrafallopian transfer (GIFT) procedure, has improved success rates in couples with idiopathic infertility.

So far, no serious risk of malformation has arisen in IVF offspring. Perinatal mortality is about threefold higher, due to the increased number of multiple pregnancies and preterm labours, the increased age of the patients, increased incidence of pelvic disease and possibly the IVF process itself.

A limited follow-up of 52 IVF children in Melbourne between the ages of 1 and 4 years has shown no serious problems directly resulting from the IVF procedure. General levels of social, intellectual and physical development were normal. Three children had problems resulting from preterm delivery.

PREGNANCY OUTCOME

Embryology

IVF has been a watershed in providing new insights into human embryology. It is now clear in the human, as in the mouse, that all of the cells of an eight-cell embryo are totipotential and that the majority of these eight cells are normally destined to develop into the trophoblast or placenta (see Chapter 4). Embryos in vitro divide at a slower rate than in vivo and continue to grow more slowly when transferred to the recipient mother. Indeed, the birthweight of infants resulting from IVF is lower than in spontaneous pregnancies.

Results

Lancaster et al (1985) reported the outcome of 244 IVF pregnancies reported by eight units. At the present time, this represents the largest analysis of pregnancy outcome after extracorporeal fertilization. These results indicated that early pregnancy loss was common in IVF patients. In particular, 21% of all IVF pregnancies resulted in spontaneous abortion. This is approximately twice as frequent as occurs for spontaneous pregnancies in a general population (Jansen 1982). Moreover, at the end of gestation, a high proportion (43%) of IVF pregnancies were delivered by Caesarean section. Even for singleton pregnancies, Caesarean section was performed in 38% of IVF pregnancies.

Preterm delivery

Maternal age greater than 40 years is associated with a very low conception rate with IVF techniques. Few IVF programmes admit women 40 years or older for IVF therapy. Nevertheless, should pregnancy occur, there is no statistically significant greater risk of spontaneous abortion in the older woman.

The number of embryos transferred varies from one IVF programme to another. At Monash University, Melbourne, a maximum of three embryos is transferred. Multiple embryo transfer clearly increases the risk of multiple pregnancy with its attendant risks of congenital malformation, preterm labour and perinatal death (Kerin et al 1983). In the Australian IVF collaborative group study, 23% of deliveries were preterm. In single pregnancies, 20% of infants were delivered preterm; this is more than three times higher than the comparable figure (6.2%) in a general Australian population. In keeping with the high incidence of preterm births, 19% of singleton IVF babies weighed less than 2500 g.

Fetoplacental malformations

Against this background, 55% of pregnancies resulting from IVF result in a live birth; it is reassuring that the incidence of congenital malformations in one large study was 1.1%, which is of the same order as the incidence in the general Australian population of 1.5–2% (Lancaster et al 1985). Amniocentesis was strongly recommended in the first IVF pregnancies. Few couples have accepted this offer and this test is now infrequently performed for IVF patients, even those older than 37 years, when the age-related incidence of chromosomal abnormalities becomes significant. The sex ratio of IVF babies is no different from that of the general population.

Placental anomalies in IVF pregnancies were reported in a multicentre European study (Englert et al 1986). This study showed that marginal or velamentous insertions of the umbilical cord were found in 16% and 12.5% of IVF pregnancies respectively, compared with frequencies of 6 and 1% for a general obstetric population. When placentas from multiple pregnancies, known to show a high incidence of abnormal cord insertion rates, were excluded, these increased incidences of abnormal insertions of the umbilical cord remained. This report is of obstetric importance, not only because of the association with vasa praevia and the risk of fetal haemorrhage at rupture of the membranes, but also because of the potential for antenatal diagnosis by careful obstetric ultrasound evaluation.

These data also suggest that the inner cell mass of the embryo is commonly maloriented in an IVF pregnancy. The mechanism for this phenomenon is as yet unclear, but rodent studies have shown a similar phenomenon following relaxin injections and it is known that relaxin is elevated in peripheral serum during early IVF pregnancy (Bell et al 1987). Relaxin may be important in embryological orientation in the human.

ROUTINE IVF–ET

The birth of the first baby following IVF in 1978 will remain a milestone in reproductive medicine. Edwards and Steptoe (Edwards 1980) aspirated a single oocyte in a spontaneous ovarian cycle for this first IVF pregnancy. At first, it was thought critical that the natural ovarian cycle should be used for IVF treatment: no attempt was made to employ drugs or hormones in order to induce multiple follicular and oocyte development. Then Trounson and associates reported in 1981 that a high rate of singleton and multiple pregnancies could result in women following the use of clomiphene citrate and human chorionic gonadotrophin (hCG) to induce multiple follicular development in endocrine-normal patients. The impact of these two reports has stimulated a proliferation of IVF programmes worldwide. It is impossible to describe all the permutations of technique used by various groups in IVF treatments. Rather, our purpose here is to describe as an example the Monash University IVF programme technique as it has been used for the majority of patients since 1980.

Stimulation of ovulation for IVF

Following the initial report of multiple follicular development and pregnancy using clomiphene and hCG (Trounson et al 1981), a number of stimulation regimens have been described for IVF patients. These had included clomiphene alone (Wood et al 1981, Trounson & Leeton 1982, Fishel et al 1984), human menopausal gonadotrophin (hMG; Jones et al 1982, Laufer et al 1983), clomiphene plus hMG (Trounson 1983), purified follicle-stimulating hormone (FSH; Jones et al 1984, Bernadus et al 1985), pulsatile luteinizing hormone-releasing hormone (LHRH; Liu et al 1983) and LHRH agonists followed by hMG (Fleming et al 1985). At the present time, many IVF groups use a combination of clomiphene and hMG for ovarian stimulation.

To start the administration of fertility drugs, our approach has been to use the patient's previous six menstrual cycle lengths to predict the most likely day of the expected mid-cycle luteinizing hormone (LH) surge as reported by McIntosh and colleagues (1980). Their method, developed from analysing apparently endocrine-normal women receiving artificial insemination, derived linear regression equations to predict the day of the LH surge and its 95% confidence limits. At Monash University we have typically commenced IVF ovarian stimulation 10 days before this anticipated LH surge.

In our IVF programme, clomiphene 100 mg/24 hours for 5 days is usually begun 10 days before the calculated mid-point of the cycle. HMG 150 iu/24 hours is started 1 day later and continues until the plasma oestradiol (E_2) is 500–1000 pg/ml and steadily rising. The duration and daily dosage of hMG treatment is often adjusted between 0 and 150 iu/24 hours, depending on the patient's individual response as judged by E_2 and ovarian ultrasound determinations. Endocrine results are reviewed at a clinical IVF meeting each afternoon where the next day's stimulation is decided. When the E_2 exceeds 1000 pg/ml or the patient is within 2 days of the 95% confidence limits, she is admitted to hospital and blood samples are taken at 0800, 1400 and 2200 hours. Plasma E_2, LH and progesterone are determined and treatment is continued until plasma E_2 concentrations reach approximately 500 pg/ml per 18 mm follicle and provided the plasma progesterone concentration remains below 2 ng/ml. If a surge in plasma LH has not occurred within 36 hours of the predicted day of the LH surge, 5000 iu of hCG is administered and the operating theatre is booked 28–36 hours later for oocyte aspiration. This has traditionally been via laparoscopy.

In vitro fertilization

The general technical procedures for human IVF have now reached a stabilized state of development whereby the use of a careful methodology achieves very high rates of fertilization. These procedures have been described in detail (Trounson et al 1982). Various different embryo culture media have been used for human IVF. Whittingham's T6 medium and Hams F10 culture medium are amongst those most commonly used. The patient's own serum (10% v/v) is used as an additive to all media for insemination in culture, following experiments to determine whether bovine and human serum albumin inhibit embryo development. At Monash University, a very simple culture tube system is used rather than attempting fertilization and culture in droplets of medium under oil, since great care is required in the selection and treatment of oil to ensure it is appropriate for embryo development and not embryotoxic. The morphology and rate of human embryo development in vitro have been described in detail by Edwards (1980).

Fresh or frozen semen may be used for IVF with equally good results. Thawed semen containing cryoprotectant is diluted slowly with culture medium and the seminal plasma and diluent removed by a single centrifugation (200 g for 5 minutes). The sperm pellet is then incubated in culture medium at 37°C for 20 minutes and the supernatant containing mostly motile spermatozoa is used for insemination. A total of 10 000–50 000 motile fresh or frozen and then thawed spermatozoa are added to 1 ml culture medium containing the oocyte, 5–10 hours after oocyte recovery. The oocytes are examined 12 hours after insemination for the presence of pronuclei. If pronuclei are not observed and a single polar body is present, the oocytes may be reinseminated with further spermatozoa. The demonstration by Angell and colleagues (1983) of numerous chromosomal defects, including haploidy, of human embryos resulting from IVF emphasizes the importance of the pronuclear stage of the fertilized oocyte. Once cleavage is initiated, it is not possible at present to establish haploidy or polyploidy.

Pregnancies and babies have been obtained after the transfer of embryos anywhere between the 1- and 16-cell stage. Most IVF programmes transfer the majority of embryos between the 2- and 8-cell stages. In general, the Monash University programme prefers to transfer embryos at an earlier rather than later developmental stage in an attempt to preserve embryo viability.

Embryo transfer

Table 75.1 shows that the IVF pregnancy rate, when expressed as a percentage of ET procedures, is approximately 18% over 7 years. Pregnancy rates following embryo transfer are influenced by several variables, including the quality and number of embryos, their developmental age, the receptivity of the uterus and the technique of ET. The first cleavage division should occur 24–30 hours after insemination and each subsequent division should occur at 10–12 hour intervals. Pregnancy is more likely if transferred embryos are within these normal developmental time frames

Table 75.1 Details of Monash University IVF programme from 1979 to August 1986

Status	Number/percentage
Oocyte collection procedures	3194
Embryo transfer procedures	2525 (78%)
Pregnancies	440 (18% of embryo transfers)
Mean number of oocytes collected	4
Fertilization rate	64%
Pregnancy loss rate	33%

at the time of transfer. Few direct data exist on early human embryo development in vitro. In one study, 15 human embryos recovered before uterine implantation had developed to the 12- to 16-cell stage, indicating that the embryo takes approximately 72 hours to traverse the uterine tube (Croxatto et al 1979). Implantation occurs about 7 days after fertilization so that the human embryo lies unimplanted in the uterus for up to 3 days while it develops to the blastocyst stage. This information is not known for human embryos transferred in an IVF cycle setting.

At Monash University, it has been clearly demonstrated that the prospect of pregnancy is increased after the transfer of more than one embryo (Trounson 1984). Transfer of up to three embryos is routinely undertaken. This policy also indicates that the slight increase in pregnancy rate seen with multiple ET also exposes the patient to the risk of multiple pregnancy. Kerin and colleagues (1983) reported seven multiple pregnancies in a total of 20 IVF conceptions. Various case reports of IVF quadruplet pregnancies have been reported.

The only verified technique for successful human embryo transfer has been by the transcervical route. Other techniques of transfundal transfer or transfer via the medial aspect of the uterine tube have not proved reliable. At Monash University, an open-end 22 gauge catheter of 0.74 mm internal diameter and 1.33 mm external diameter made of Teflon 20 cm in length is routinely used. Embryos are aspirated into the internal catheter in 20–30 μl of culture medium. The catheter is then passed through the cervical canal into the uterine cavity within approximately 5 mm of the fundus. More accurate location of the catheter, with or without ultrasound guidance, has unfortunately not increased the pregnancy rate (Lenz, personal communication). Following expulsion of the embryos into the uterine cavity, the catheter is withdrawn and checked microscopically to ensure that embryos have not been retained. Pregnancy has been established following discharge home as early as 1 hour following ET. No controlled study of sufficient size has ever demonstrated that it is necessary to support the luteal phase following embryo transfer.

NEW CLINICAL ISSUES IN IVF

Male infertility

A clinician managing couples with male infertility bases many decisions regarding management on the results of clinical assessment, semen analysis and serum FSH levels. The importance of repeated semen analyses in the assessment of the husband of an infertile marriage cannot be overemphasized. In addition to semen analyses, the semen of each man prior to IVF is examined in the Monash University programme for the presence of sperm antibodies in semen and for the presence of pathogens on semen culture.

Once oocytes have been successfully collected as described above, the male partner is asked to report to the IVF laboratory and to produce a freshly masturbated specimen of semen. This sample is allowed to liquefy for up to 30 minutes at 37°C and, after liquefaction, an aliquot is taken for semen analysis. The volume of semen used for sperm harvesting depends upon the sperm count: whereas only 1 ml is used for normal counts, 2 ml or the complete sample divided into several tubes is used in cases of male subfertility. The volume of semen is then transferred to a plastic tube using a graduated Pasteur pipette and diluted approximately threefold with cultured medium. The diluted sample is then centrifuged at 300 **g** for 5 minutes and the supernatent is decanted. A small volume (0.1 ml) is usually left, in which the sperm pellet is gently resuspended. A small volume of culture medium (0.5 ml) is laid gently on the resuspended pellet and incubated for 45 minutes. The top half of the culture medium, containing highly motile sperm, is aspirated and an aliquot of this enriched semen sample is then taken for further semen analysis. The volume of sperm suspension to be added is calculated so that 100 000–150 000 motile sperm can be added to 1 ml of culture medium containing oocytes.

Results from the application of such procedures for couples with male subfertility were reported by de Kretser and colleagues in 1985. The fertilization rates in men with sperm in which only a single parameter (concentration, motility or morphology) was subnormal ranged from 65 to 70%, which is statistically equivalent to the fertilization rate in the complete Monash University IVF programme. In those men with two defects in their semen, the fertilization rate fell to 58% in a series of 67 oocytes inseminated. It was only when men with three defects in semen were considered that the fertilization rate fell dramatically, to 7.1% for 14 oocytes inseminated. In the group of patients with sperm antibodies, a fertilization rate of 53% was achieved despite parameters of count, motility and morphology being within the normal range. The very low fertilization rate in men with triple defects in semen was matched by the rate in patients with sperm which had bypassed the epididymis. In this special group of men, only 9% of fertilization occurred in 22 eggs inseminated. Overall, 10 patients achieved pregnancy out of the 73 couples with male subfertility in this study.

Clearly, greater experience is required in evaluation of male subfertility and IVF. A classification system of patients for uniformity between IVF groups is stressed and the classification system proposed by de Kretser and associates (1958) is recommended. The fertilization rates for couples with a single or even dual defect in semen is sufficiently well maintained to encourage further studies of the use of IVF in such couples. The possibility of pregnancy in couples where the man has azoospermia and from whom sperm is obtained by surgical aspiration from the remnant of the epididymis in cases of congenital absence of the vas deferens (Temple-Smith et al 1985) indicates the potential of IVF for various aspects of male infertility.

Oocyte recovery using ultrasound

Oocytes for in vitro fertilization are usually collected by laparoscopy under general anaesthesia. Oocytes may also be collected by means of ultrasonically guided punctures which may be performed under local anaesthesia on an outpatient basis (Lenz et al 1985). These procedures may be performed via percutaneous abdominal punctures which introduce the aspirating needles through the filled bladder or, more recently, with the use of a transvaginal approach to the ovaries through the posterior fornix (Dellenbach et al 1985).

Transvaginal ultrasound-guided oocyte recovery offers the major advantage of oocyte collection from women with extensive pelvic adhesions in whom the ovaries are inaccessible by laparoscopy. In addition, even if general anaesthesia is still employed, patient recovery appears more rapid following a transvaginal ultrasound-guided operation than does recovery following laparoscopy. A recent study in the Monash University IVF programme indicates that the number of oocytes obtained using a transvaginal ultrasound-guided technique is statistically similar to the number retrieved following laparoscopy and that both fertilization and pregnancy rates are similar in these two method groups (Lenz, personal communication). The extension of such techniques to ambulatory IVF patients on an outpatient basis could be expected to reduce the cost of IVF procedures significantly and to increase the possibility that any infertile couple is able to undergo a number of IVF procedures, thus increasing their possibility of pregnancy.

Oocyte donation

Human pregnancies and live births have been reported following the donation of oocytes, their in vitro fertilization by the sperm of the recipient's husband and the transfer of these embryos to the uterus of the infertile woman (Lutjen et al 1984). Patients who require donor oocytes fall broadly into two categories: firstly, women with non-functioning ovaries, including subjects with premature ovarian failure, congenital ovarian absence or bilateral ovariectomy and secondly, women with functioning ovaries in whom it is either impossible or unwise to attempt oocyte collection. This latter group includes patients at risk of genetic disease in their children.

For such patients, the ovarian steroids oestradiol and progesterone must be given exogenously in doses designed to mimic as closely as possible the normal steroid profile throughout the menstrual cycle. The endocrinology of such a treatment regimen has been previously described (Lutjen et al 1984, 1986, Chan et al 1986). The source of donor oocytes for such patients primarily comes from fellow IVF patients who donate oocytes anonymously for altruistic reasons. Additional sources of oocytes include the donation of oocytes from relatives or friends, the use of volunteer donors who are not otherwise involved in medical treatment and the collection of oocytes from consenting women undergoing laparoscopic sterilization (Templeton et al 1984).

In the Monash University IVF programme, oestradiol valerate (Progynova; Schering) is administered as an oral oestrogen commencing at 2 mg/24 hours and increasing up to a daily dose of 6 mg to mimic the mid-cycle oestradiol rise. Progesterone is administered via intravaginal suppositories commencing at 25 mg/24 hours from day 15 and increasing to 100 mg/24 hours in the mid luteal phase. Once ET to a recipient has been performed, the steroid replacement regimen is adjusted accordingly on the assumption that implantation has occurred and that a pregnancy has been established. The recipient remains on 2 mg/24 hours oestradiol valerate and 100 mg/24 hours intravaginal progesterone until plasma hCG concentrations are measured 10 and 12 days following transfer. Should detectable amounts of hCG be present, our policy has been to increase the dose of oestradiol valerate to 8 mg/24 hours and to administer intramuscular progesterone 50–100 mg/24 hours. Biweekly monitoring of plasma concentrations of oestradiol and progesterone are taken to maintain oestradiol and progesterone concentrations within the normal range for early pregnancy. With these procedures, seven deliveries have been undertaken in the Monash University programme, including one set of donor oocyte twins (Chan et al 1986). Delivery of these patients has been by Caesarean section for obstetric indications and it is still not clear if spontaneous labour is possible or normal in such patients. At Caesarean section, the absence of ovaries has been confirmed in all cases.

Embryo and oocyte cryopreservation

The first pregnancy resulting from the replacement in utero of frozen–thawed embryos was reported in 1983 (Trounson & Mohr 1983). Several groups have subsequently confirmed the birth of babies arising from frozen–thawed embryos (Zielmaker et al 1984, Mohr et al 1985, Cohen et al 1986). The techniques used for embryo freezing and thawing have evolved from those used for other mammalian species, in

Table 75.2 Details of Monash University IVF embryo freezing programme from 1981 to September 1986

Status	Number
Patients receiving frozen–thawed embryos	246
Patients pregnant	22
Patients delivered	14
Abortions	6

particular mouse, cattle and sheep embryos. The procedures used appear to depend upon the cell stage of embryo development with dimethyl sulphoxide (DMSO) appearing as the cryoprotectant of choice for freezing early embryos (2–8 cells) while glycerol appears more suitable for freezing of human blastocysts (Cohen et al 1986). At the present time, it appears uncertain whether the precise cell stage is an important factor in the survival and viability of cryopreserved embryos or whether the degree of regularity or fragmentation of embryos is important for cryopreservation. The time of ET relative to the age of the embryo is also still uncertain, although embryo replacement either 1 day earlier than the post-insemination age of the embryo or synchronous embryo transfer appears to be advantageous.

Details of 22 frozen–thawed IVF pregnancies obtained by the Monash University group have been reported (Trounson & Freemann 1985; Table 75.2). Pregnancies were obtained from frozen–thawed 3–12-cell embryos, including embryos with as few as 50% of the original blastomere number intact at the time of transfer. Cryostorage time varied from 2 to 21 months. There is little evidence that the length of time that embryos are stored affects their survival or viability. Children born to date following embryo cryopreservation have been normal. Clearly however, the numbers are still small and close observation of these infants is suggested.

Oocyte freezing is a technically more difficult procedure than is embryo freezing, due to the large size of the oocyte and the risks of damage to its cell membrane. Furthermore, oocyte freezing has not been possible in commercial species and therefore no animal model of oocyte freezing, unlike embryo cryopreservation, exists. Nevertheless, human birth following oocyte freeze–thawing has been reported (Chen 1986). This procedure offers the advantage that oocyte freezing is ethically more acceptable to some members of the community than is embryo freezing. It suffers from the disadvantage of increased complexity, increased cost and greater uncertainty, especially regarding the integrity of the meiotic spindle of the oocyte and its risk of structural damage with oocyte freeze–thawing.

Gamete intrafallopian transfer (GIFT)

Asch and colleagues (1986) recently reported a new technique, GIFT, as a new IVF-related procedure. In this operation, patients with idiopathic infertility undergo laparoscopic oocyte collection, then two oocytes and approximately 50 000 motile sperm are transferred into each uterine tube. In the initial report, 4 of 10 patients became pregnant with this operation. The GIFT technique is relatively simple when compared with IVF and because of the lack of contact of the unfertilized oocyte and sperm, this procedure may be more acceptable than other techniques to some cultural and religious groups in society.

Table 75.3 Comparative trial of gamete intrafallopian transfer (GIFT) with IVF

	GIFT	IVF	Male factor GIFT	Male factor IVF
Patients admitted for treatment	46	33	7	5
Patients admitted to hospital	42	26	7	5
Laparoscopies	42	26	7	5
Patients with GIFT	34	–	6	–
Number of oocytes	195	174	41	36
Number of oocytes used in GIFT	133	–	24	–
Oocytes fertilized in IVF	23/49 (47%)	105 (66%)	4/11 (36.3%)	10/22 (45%)
Number of oocytes transferred in IVF	–	62	–	9
Pregnancies	6 (17.6%)	6 (23%)	2 (33%)	2 (40%)

The Monash University IVF programme has recently undertaken a controlled randomized trial of IVF and GIFT for couples with idiopathic infertility (Table 75.3). The pregnancy rate in both groups of couples was similar in the IVF (6/26; 23%) and GIFT (6/34; 18%) groups. Much larger studies will be required to establish whether the pregnancy rate following the GIFT procedure remains equivalent to that following IVF.

IVF—THE FUTURE

At the moment the efficiency of IVF is low, as only about one in 10 embryos transferred results in the birth of a live baby. Failure of these embryos to survive may lie in defects in the embryo or in the environment in which it implants. More information is required concerning the chromosomal and genetic defects of these early embryos under a variety of circumstances. Do the stimulation regimes, the number of eggs developed, the methods of collection or the culture media affect the proportion of normal or abnormal embryos developed? Apart from chromosomal defects it is quite likely that some embryos suffer biochemical abnormality due to unfavourable conditions of culture. Microanalytical biochemical assays of embryos need to be developed to determine this.

Oocyte storage has potential for helping to solve the problem of excess oocytes at the time of collection for IVF. It will also be useful for women requiring donated eggs, synchronizing the donor and recipient's cycles, and in family planning and the treatment of early severe gynaecological diseases. Oocyte storage will be preferable for women wishing to defer childbearing to a later age and may also act as an insurance policy for women with early severe gynaecological disease in case of subsequent ovarian removal.

Knowledge of the fertilizing capacity of male sperm at the present time is limited. An intraspecies fertilization test would facilitate the development of knowledge of male sperm behaviour. The heterogeneous nature of the sperm population in terms of appearance, counts and various types of motility make conclusions between fertilizing capacity and specific sperm characteristics limited. The ability to isolate specific types of sperm with various morphological or motility characteristics and to carry out functional in vitro fertilization tests using human oocytes would rapidly advance knowledge of the physiology of spermatozoa. Even without sperm selection techniques, study of specific semen samples with characteristics demonstrating one dominant morphological abnormality may be useful. The use of human eggs and sperm and subsequent electron microscopy may answer some of the questions as to which type of abnormal sperm can fertilize oocytes.

Selection of optimum sperm populations may also reduce the risk of abortion and congenital malformation in those patients at increased risk of these complications. The microsurgical injection of sperm nuclei into eggs (Uehara & Yanagimachi 1976) may assist in the treatment of severe male infertility. Artificial fusion of egg and sperm by physical or chemical methods may also be possible.

Another area in which IVF is already contributing is in the development of new contraceptives. Compounds which affect oocyte and sperm interaction are being developed. Vaccines binding to specific zona or sperm membrane glycoproteins prevent sperm binding and penetration of the egg. Such a vaccine has been tested and found to be effective in small mammals.

Use of IVF in studying new contraceptives may be important in determining the efficacy of the contraceptive in several ways: in blocking the fertilization process, in checking the possibility of abnormal fertilization should the new contraceptive not be 100% effective, and in checking the subsequent health of gametes after the effects of the contraceptive have worn off.

The relative inefficiency of human embryogenesis in both natural conception and in IVF seems a basic question to answer. Once this is understood many applied human problems such as spontaneous abortion and congenital malformations may be more easily resolved. Early embryo experimentation and IVF have already contributed some information.

At present only about 10% of embryos used in IVF are capable of continued development after replacement in the uterus; in natural conception in the human, less than 50% of embryos are capable of normal development. About 30% of embryos are chromosomally defective at the 8-cell stage (Angell et al 1983) and about 50% of female pronuclei have chromosomal defects (Rudak et al 1984). We have no knowledge of the incidence of gene defects in embryos, although it is thought that at least one in 100 babies born carries gene defects.

It is already evident that the very high rate of chromosomal non-disjunction in our own species is responsible not only for many of the genetic defects at birth, but also for infertility in the form of early spontaneous abortion. We know nothing of its causes, but we do know that much of it arises during oocyte maturation or during the early fertilization process or cleavage division. In vitro studies of these stages of development could throw light on the aetiology of this and other chromosomal disorders.

Major malformations occur in two to three of every hundred births. It may be possible to monitor for the presence of an abnormal gene or chromosomal constitution in an early embryo. Trounson & Mohr (1983) have already shown that frozen 8-cell human conceptuses which have lost some of their cells can give rise to a normal fetus and offspring. If chromosome analysis of one cell can be done in 24 hours, the remainder of the embryo need not be frozen but may be kept in culture. A similar approach can be used to detect the presence of specific abnormal genes using gene probes. More and more DNA probes for genes responsible for severe genetic disease in man are becoming available and further advances in molecular biology will enable such genes to be detected in small cell samples. The means of preventing the transmission of certain severe inherited diseases coupled with the concomitant reduction in the requirement of abortions in the families at risk may therefore be possible.

The possibility of implanting genes missing in the human embryo is at present more distant. The manufacture of simple genes has commenced. The process of purification, insertion and carriage to specific sites and control of the expression of the implanted genes is more complex.

There may be cytotoxic and teratogenic effects of biozides on human embryogenesis. The environment has been contaminated with chemicals produced in packaging of goods, in pesticides, food preservation, and in other aspects of industry and agriculture. The effects of these chemicals (biozides) which are found in human body tissues and fluids remains uncertain. It has been reported that human follicular fluid contains considerable concentrations of biozides, including the chlorinated hydrocarbons and pesticides (Baukloh et al 1984). The human oocyte is formed in fetal development and is normally many years old when ovulated. The presence of biozides may be associated with the oocyte for a long period of time at high levels during meiotic maturation. This raises the obvious question as to whether these chemicals cause chromosomal or genetic changes in the egg, which may again lead to genetic errors. It seems important to document the various levels of biozides in human follicular fluid in different IVF groups and then correlate the levels of these chemicals to embryo viability, chromosomal abnormality rates and pregnancy rates.

The early embryo may be susceptible to damage which is only revealed later in development — the oft-quoted all-or-nothing effect of insults on the early embryo may not always apply. Genetic or chromosome damage in the early embryo or other types of injury may result in clinical abortion, preterm delivery, neonatal and perhaps even adult mortality. If this concept is partly true, it is an important reason for experiments on the early embryo, as the results may radically change attitudes to the cause of disease resulting from insults to the early embryo.

Early embryo research may lead to the reduction of spontaneous abortion, the reduction of therapeutic abortion for genetic reasons, the reduction of therapeutic abortion for social reasons with the better development of contraception, and the production of new families by the resolution of infertility.

EDITORS' NOTE

Each country has, or is moving towards, regulation of extracorporeal fertilization. In the UK the Voluntary Licensing Authority has laid down regulatory guidelines for in vitro fertilization and inspects and licenses workers and premises concerned with in vitro fertilization. The Authority was organized by the Royal College of Obstetricians and Gynaecologists and the Medical Research Council. It comprises a mixture of obstetricians, scientists and lay people, the last having the majority of members on the Authority.

In the autumn of 1987, the British Government announced that the duties of the Voluntary Licensing Authority would be taken over by the Statutory Licensing Authority, with the same composition and function; however, being statutory, it would have more power, as if its recommendations were ignored the matter would become illegal. In the spring of 1989 as the book goes to press, this has still not happened.

Other countries have different mechanisms for inspection and regulation of in vitro fertilization. In general, society has considered that it should have some input into the regulation of the scientists' work.

Alec Turnbull
Geoffrey Chamberlain

REFERENCES

Angell R R, Aitken R J, Van Look P F A, Lumsden M A, Templeton A A 1983 Chromosome abnormalities in human embryos after in vitro fertilization. Nature (London) 303: 336–338

Asch R H, Balmaceda J P, Ellsworth L R, Wong P C 1986 Preliminary experiences with gamete intrafallopian transfer (GIFT). Fertility and Sterility 45: 366–370

Baukloh V, Bohnet H G, Trapp M, Feichtinger W, Kemeter P 1984 Biozides in human follicular fluid. In Vitro Fertilization 1: 98–102

Bell R, Eddie L W, Lester A R et al 1987 Levels of relaxin in human pregnancy serum measured with a homologous radioimmunoassay for human relaxin. Obstetrics and Gynecology 69: 585–589

Bernadus R E, Jones G S, Acosta A A et al 1985 The significance of the ratio in follicle-stimulating hormone and luteinizing hormone induction of multiple follicular growth. Fertility and Sterility 43: 373

Chan C, Healy D L, Lutjen P J, Leeton J F, Trounson A O, Wood E C 1986 Oocyte donation for hypergonadotropic hypogonadism: clinical state of the art. Obstetrical and Gynecological Survey 42: 350–361

Chen C 1986 Pregnancy after human oocyte cryopreservation. Lancet i: 884–886

Cohen J, Simons R F, Edwards R G, Fehilly C B, Fishel S B 1986 Pregnancies following the frozen storage of expanding human blastocysts. Journal of In Vitro Fertilization and Embryo Transfer 2: 59–64

Croxatto H B, Otiz M E S, Diag S, Hers R 1979 Attempts to modify ovum transport in women. Journal of Reproduction and Fertility 55: 231–237

de Kretser D M, Yates C, Kovacs G T 1985 The use of IVF in the management of male infertility. Obstetrics and Gynecology 12: 767–773

Dellenbach P, Nisan I, Moreau L et al 1985 Transvaginal sonographical controlled follicle puncture for oocyte retrieval. Fertility and Sterility 44: 656–662

Edwards R G 1980 Conception in the human female. Academic Press, London

Englert Y, Iumbert M C, Van Rosendael E et al 1986 Placental anomalies in IVF pregnancy: preliminary report of a multi-centric study. Proceedings of the European Society of Human Reproduction and Embryology, June 22–25, Abstract 61

Fishel S B, Edward R G, Purdy J M 1984 Analysis of infertile patients treated consecutively by in vitro fertilization at Bourn Hall. Fertility and Sterility 42: 191

Fleming R, Haxton M J, Hamilton M P R et al 1985 Successful treatment of infertile women with oligomenorrhoea using a combination of an LHRH agonist and exogenous gonadotropins. British Journal of Obstetrics and Gynaecology 92: 369

Jansen R P A 1982 Spontaneous abortion incidence in the treatment of infertility. American Journal of Obstetrics and Gynecology 143: 451–473

Jones Jr H W, Jones G S, Andrews M C et al 1982 The program for in vitro fertilization at Norfolk. Fertility and Sterility 38: 14

Jones G S, Garcia J E, Rosenwaks Z 1984 The role of pituitary gonadotropins in follicular stimulation and oocyte maturation in the human. Journal of Clinical Endocrinology and Metabolism 59: 178

Kerin J et al 1983 Incidence of multiple pregnancy after in vitro fertilization and embryo transfer. Lancet ii: 537–540

Lancaster P A L et al 1985 High incidence of preterm births and early losses in pregnancy after in vitro fertilization. British Medical Journal 291: 1160–1163

Laufer N, DeCherney A H, Haseltine F P et al 1983 The use of high-dose human menopausal gonadotropin in an in vitro fertilization program. Fertility and Sterility 40: 734

Lenz S, Bang J, Lauritsen J G, Lindenberg S 1985 Ultrasonically guided aspiration of oocytes for in vitro fertilization using a plain needle and syringe under local anaesthesia. Infertility 7: 1–4

Liu J H, Durfee R D, Muse K, Yen S S C 1983 Induction of multiple ovulation by pulsatile administration of gonadotropin-releasing hormone. Fertility and Sterility 40: 18

Lutjen P J, Trounson A O, Leeton J, Renou P, Findlay J K, Wood E C 1984 The establishment and maintenance of pregnancy using in vitro fertilization and embryo donation in a patient with primary ovarian failure. Nature 307: 174–175

Lutjen P J, Findlay J K, Trounson A O, Chan C, Leeton J F 1986 The effect on plasma gonadotropins of cyclic steroid replacement in women with premature ovarian failure. Journal of Clinical Endocrinology and Metabolism 62: 419–424

Mohr L R, Trounson A O, Freemann L 1985 Deep freezing and transfer of human embryos. Journal of In Vitro Fertilization and Embryo Transfer 2: 1–10

Rudak E, Dor J, Mashiach S, Nebel L, Goldman B 1984 Chromosome analysis of multipronuclear human oocytes fertilized in vitro. Fertility and Sterility 41: 538–545

Temple-Smith P D, Southwick G J, Yates C, Trounson A O, de Kretser D M 1985 Human pregnancy by in vitro fertilization using sperm

aspirated from the epididymis. Journal of In Vitro Fertilization and Embryo Transfer 2: 119–122
Templeton A, Van Look P, Lumsden M A, Aitken J 1984 The recovery of pre-ovulatory oocytes using a fixed schedule of ovulation induction and follicle aspiration. British Journal of Obstetrics and Gynaecology 91: 148–154
Trounson A O 1983 In vitro fertilization at Monash University, Melbourne, Australia. In: Crosignani P G, Rubin B L (eds) In vitro fertilization and embryo transfer. Academic Press, London, p 315
Trounson A O 1984 In vitro fertilization and embryo preservation. In: Trounson A, Wood C (eds) In vitro fertilization and embryo transfer. Churchill Livingstone, Edinburgh
Trounson A O, Freemann L 1985 The use of embryo cryopreservation in human IVF programmes. Clinics in Obstetrics and Gynaecology 12: 825–833
Trounson A O, Leeton J F 1982 The endocrinology of clomiphene stimulation. In: Edwards R G, Purdy J M (eds) Human conception in vitro. Academic Press, London, p 51
Trounson A O, Mohr L R 1983 Human pregnancy following cryopreservation, thawing and transfer of an 8-cell embryo. Nature 305: 707–709
Trounson A O, Leeton J F, Wood C et al 1981 Pregnancies in humans by fertilization in vitro and embryo transfer in the controlled ovulatory cycle. Science 212: 681–684
Trounson A O, Mohr L R, Wood C, Leeton J F 1982 Effect of delayed insemination on in vitro fertilization, culture and transfer of human embryos. Journal of Reproduction and Fertility 64: 285–294
Uehara T, Yanagimachi R 1976 Microsurgical injection of spermatozoa into hamster eggs with subsequent transformation of sperm nuclei into male pronuclei. Biology of Reproduction 15: 467–470
Wood C, Trounson A, Leeton J F et al 1981 A clinical assessment of nine pregnancies obtained by in vitro fertilization and embryo transfer. Fertility and Sterility 35: 502
Zielmaker G J, Alberda A T, Van Gent I, Rykmans C M P M, Diendigh A C 1984 Two pregnancies following transfer of intact frozen-thawed embryos. Fertility and Sterility 42: 293–296

SECTION 13

Vital Statistics

76

Geoffrey Chamberlain

Birth rates

INTRODUCTION

Most countries in the developed world collect data on the numbers of births that take place; they also do regular population censuses. With these data, they can publish birth rates. In July 1837, the registration of live births started in England and Wales; from 1927 data on stillbirths were also collected. The Population (Statistics) Act 1938 was the beginning of the analysis of these data for statistical purposes and it was from this time that multiple births could first be distinguished in this country. The Population (Statistics) Act of 1960 required further questions about the father. Data from England and Wales are published regularly by the Registrar General through the Office of Population, Censuses and Surveys (OPCS), while those from Scotland and Northern Ireland came from their respective General Registry Offices.

Births have to be registered by law under the Births and Deaths Registration Act of 1836. The General Registrar Office and the Local Superintendent Registrars and Registrars were established by that Act, which requires a Registrar to inform him- or herself within 42 days of any birth occurring inside the district; it obliged the parents, or failing them the occupier of the tenement in which the birth took place, to provide such information to the local Registrar.

The amount of data collected has increased so that now details are obtained about:

1. The child
    a. date and place of birth
    b. sex
    c. legitimacy
2. The father
    a. place of birth
    b. occupation
    c. date of birth
3. The mother
    a. place of birth
    b. date of birth

For legitimate births only, further data are collected about the parents' marriage and the number of children born to the mother. These data are checked locally.

As well as the system of registration, the midwife or doctor who attended the birth must notify the District Medical Officer (England and Wales) or the Chief Administrative Medical Officer (Scotland and Northern Ireland) within 36 hours. While this and the civil registration system are quite separate, they act as a check of each other. The District Health Authority informs the local Registrar of Births of babies notified. In return, the Registrar returns the list of registered babies with their National Health Service number, a service the Registrars must initiate.

DEFINITIONS

The data about births can be expressed in various ways.

The absolute numbers of births is well known and can be expressed by various years (Fig. 76.1). This is helpful in knowing the numbers which may present in the population in coming years; these figures are refined in demograms (see below). The crude birth rate is the number of viable births (live and dead) per thousand of the total population (Fig. 76.2). This is a simple mathematical fraction that can be derived from the birth data and the Census returns.

$$\text{Birth rate} = \frac{\text{Births per year} \times 1000}{\text{Mid-year population}}$$

In the above ratio, the denominator is the total population, including men and women below and above the reproductive age group. A denominator should consist of all those, and only those, who might appear in the numerator. Hence,

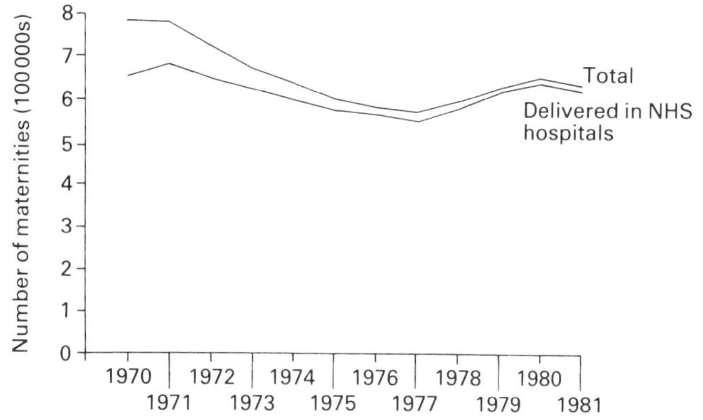

Fig. 76.1 Absolute numbers of women giving birth in England and Wales (1970–1981).

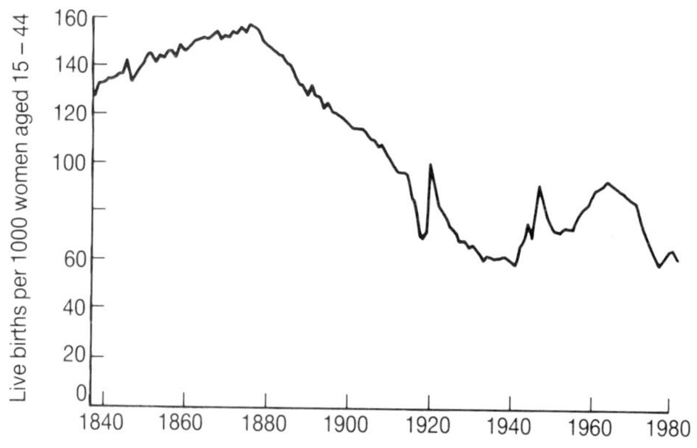

Fig. 76.3 General fertility rate for England and Wales (1838–1981).

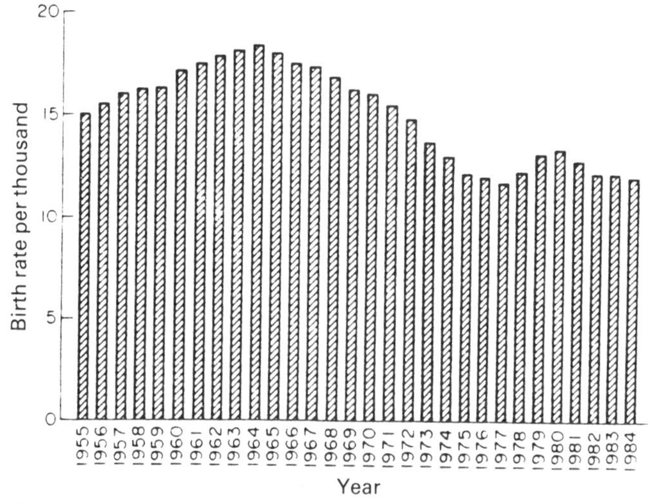

Fig. 76.2 Crude birth rates for England and Wales (1955–1984).

a more appropriate measure of birth rates can be obtained by only looking at the births in comparison to the number of women in the reproductive age group. This is taken nominally from age 15 to 44 years (Fig. 76.3). Thus the general fertility rate is derived:

$$\text{General fertility rate} = \frac{\text{Births per year} \times 1000}{\text{Women 15–44 years in mid-year population}}$$

Another measure of this is the total period fertility rate, which is the summation of the fertility rates in any given year by the years the mother has left to an age when it is considered that reproduction will probably stop (arguably taken as 50 years). This measures the average number of children that might be expected to be born to a woman if she experienced the age-specific fertility rates of the calendar year in question throughout the rest of her childbearing life.

This is a more precise measure than is that of completed family size, which can only be calculated in retrospect when a woman has completed her family. However, mean family size is an attractive index and often used in the popular press giving the coarse differences between countries. When the completed family size drops below two, replacement of the population has stopped and therefore that society is below zero population growth.

WORLD POPULATION CHANGES

Population dynamics examine how populations change in countries and between countries. The relation of this to births and deaths can be shown simply as follows:

Births ⟶ Population size ⟶ Deaths
⇅
Migration

At times of economic stability, migration is not a major feature in many countries, although it obviously has a great part to play at times of rapid economic growth, such as immigration did in the USA at the beginning of the century, or emigration in times of economic hardship, such as in Ireland at the time of the potato famines.

Leaving migration aside, one can then calculate how a country is likely to expand. A good example would be the flourishing country of Kenya which has a large agricultural and tourist industry and virtually no migration either in or out. The birth rate is 48 per thousand; the death rate is 15 per thousand. Thus there will be a natural increase of 33 per thousand in the year. From this, one can extrapolate approximately that in about 20 years' time, the population will have approximately doubled. In most countries of the western world, the birth rate and death rate are roughly equal; since migration is not a major factor, they have reached zero population growth.

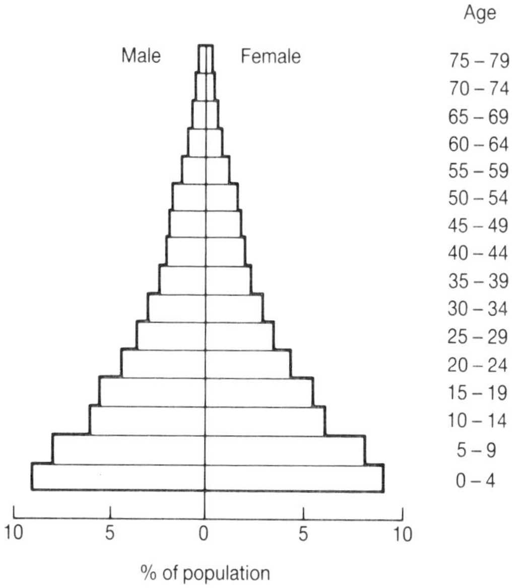

Fig. 76.4 Smoothed-off demogram for a rapidly developing country recording male and female populations in 5-year cohorts.

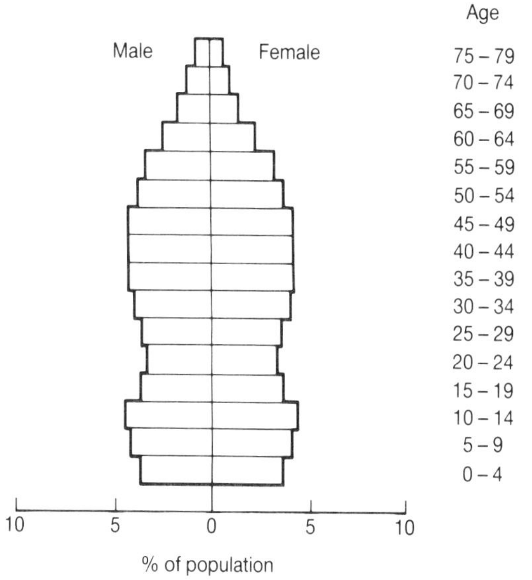

Fig. 76.5 Smoothed-off demogram for a developed country recording male and female populations in 5-year cohorts.

The classical factors which stabilized populations in the 19th century were:

1. Effects on death rate
   a. Disease
   b. Famine
   c. War
2. Effects on birth rate
   a. Celibacy of the population
   b. Restraint

While we do not live in a perfect world, the three influences which affect death rates are considerably curtailed. At the end of the 20th century, falling disease rates have been seen in the western world although many diseases, particularly the infectious ones, still need to be overcome in the developing world. The effects of famine are mostly being overcome. Agricultural policies like those in the Punjab in India are leading the world away from starvation. Despite the campaigns of Korea and Vietnam, there have been no world wars for over 40 years and so deaths from this cause are greatly reduced in both the warrior class and civilians. Hence, reduction in birth rates has now become the major instrument in altering populations. In the latter part of the 20th century, in many countries celibacy has been overtaken as an influence on birth rates by contraception and wider family spacing.

The effects of changes in the birth rate can be seen by examining the information from age-specific rates in 5-year samples of the populations. From this, population projections can be derived. Figure 76.4 depicts a typical developing country. Population data in 5-year age groups show that the numbers of the young are expanding whilst mean life expectancy is not very high. Figure 76.5 shows the same data in a more developed country where the 5-year cohorts are of approximately the same size until degenerative diseases start becoming a factor at about 55 years of age.

Figure 76.6 shows demograms from the same country (Hong Kong) over a 20-year period. Fifteen years after the war, the birth rate had been going up steadily and so in the mid 1960s, the Government began an intensive campaign to promote the use of contraception. The middle demogram shows that 10 years later this had worked, for the effect of contraception was a great reduction in the birth rate. In 1981, this reduced birth rate structure was sustained. The bulge of children born in the late 1950s had worked its way through and was represented by figures showing those aged in their 20s. The implication of this in the provision of facilities for schooling, universities and job opportunities is obvious and demograms are often used to make such social planning. If the population was to continue in this pattern, it would be expected that Hong Kong would require an enlargement in geriatric services in 30 years' time.

The demogram for the UK (Fig. 76.7) for recent years has shown a slight diminution in births from 1964 to the late 1970s. Generally, however, the demogram is straight-sided, as in other developed countries. With improvements in health and better nutrition, an ageing population will soon weigh down the upper end of this demogram. They require geriatric and social services now and over the next 30–40 years; this will be a constant strain on the social security system.

BIRTH RATES IN ENGLAND AND WALES

The birth rate in England and Wales is shown in Figure 76.3 for the last century. In the Victorian days, it was about

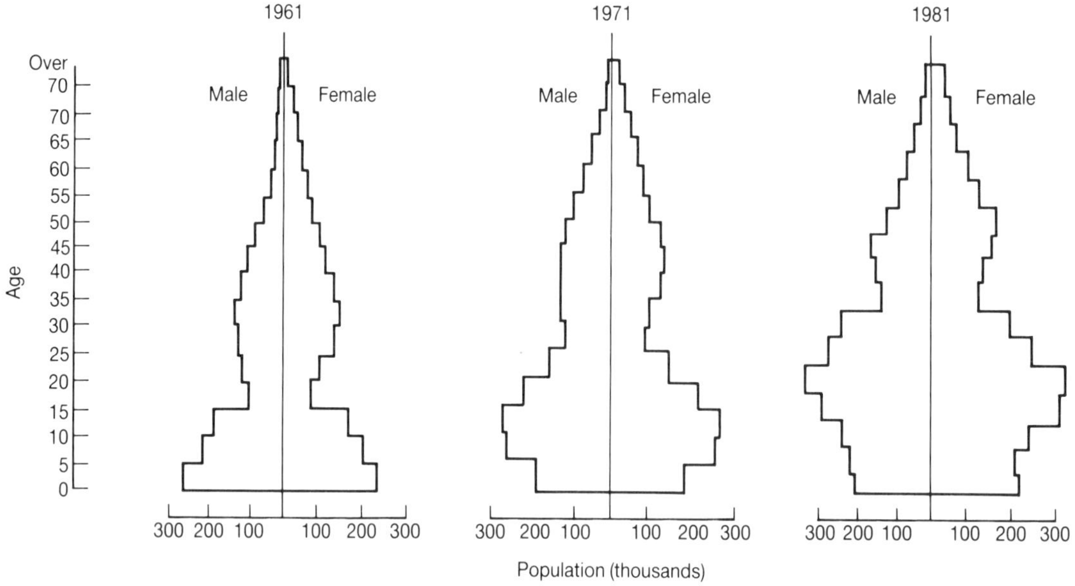

Fig. 76.6 Smoothed-off demogram of Hong Kong in 1961, 1971 and 1981 recording male and female populations in 5-year cohorts.

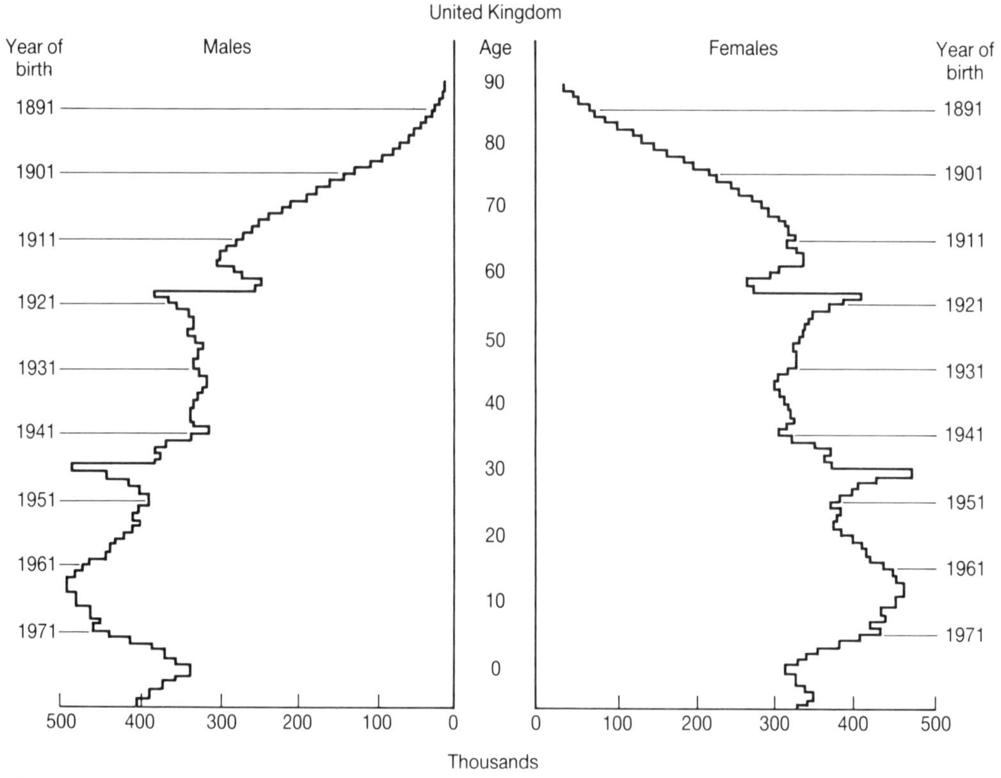

Fig. 76.7 Demogram of the UK population in 1982 in annual cohorts, i.e. data not smoothed-off. This shows changes in finer detail (redrawn from Social Trends 1983; HMSO, London).

35 per thousand. This was just after the industrial revolution when Britain was a rich nation economically. Birth rates declined from then until the 1920s, when there was the Depression. The birth rate of the 1930s was slightly boosted by the threat of war and a recovery in the activity of heavy industry. This caused a mild increase in birth rates; however, the birth rate has stayed at a generally lower level since the Second World War.

Examination of the more recent birth rate data shows that the postwar boom rose to an apex in 1964 when it was about

Table 76.1 Total fertility rates for some major regions of the world

Region	Total fertility rate
Western Europe	2.1
North America	2.2
USSR	2.4
China	3.8
India	5.2
Central America	6.4
West Africa	6.7

Total fertility rate = average number of children born per woman at current fertility rates.

17 per thousand and since then it has declined steadily (Fig. 76.2). There was a minor resurgence in 1980, when the birth rate was about 14 per thousand and the total period fertility rate 1.89—a figure still below replacement rates for a population.

In mid 1986, the estimated population of England was 47 254 000. This was an increase of 143 000 from the previous year. Whilst half of this increase was the excess of immigrants over emigrants, the other half was due to the excess of the birth rate over the death rate. Increased birth rates are also reflected in the age structure, for while the 5–15-year group has fallen by 11% since 1981, the 1–4-year group is 4% up on 1985 and 6.8% increased on 1981 data. The implications for planning educational needs in a few years' time are not lost on politicians or teachers.

FACTORS THAT MODIFY THE BIRTH RATE

Family spacing

Obviously the earlier in life couples start reproducing, the more likely they are to have a larger family. In the Pacific Islands, girls often marry at 12 or 13 years of age and so have a greater exposure to intercourse and are more likely to have more babies. The frequency of intercourse itself influences the number of children, but more important is the spacing of families. In many parts of the world, breast-feeding is the most commonly used method of contraception and so pregnancy occurs every 2 or 3 years during reproductive life. Other methods of pharmaceutical and mechanical contraception are more common in the western world and their use leads to a later start in reproduction and a wider spacing of families and so a lower birth rate.

Table 76.1 represents the average number of children born per woman at the current fertility rates in the major regions of the world. It is sharply divided into those areas where contraception is more widely used and those where it is not. Apart from conventional contraception, in many parts of Eastern Europe induced abortion is considered a method of contraception. This is frowned upon in the western world, partly because it has an unacceptable rate of medical sequelae.

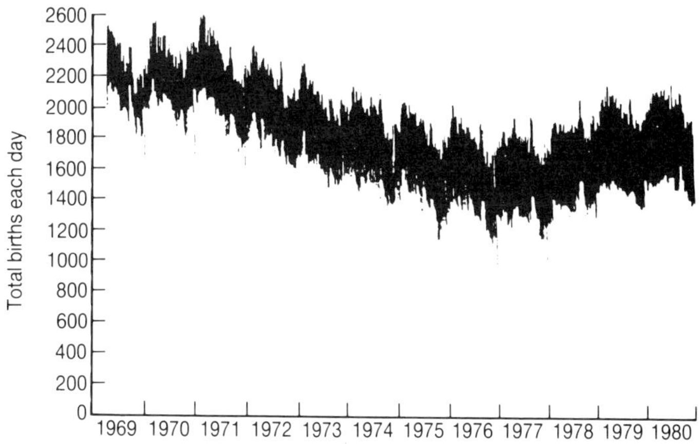

Fig. 76.8 Daily numbers of births for England and Wales (1969–1980).

Seasonal variations

There are inbuilt variations in birth rate. In the UK the seasonal pattern of birth rate changes has remained the same for over a century with only minor variations occurring during the years of World Wars I and II. The birth rate in England and Wales is highest in January to March and generally lowest from October to December. Several explanations have been put forward, including the hypothesis that intercourse may be more frequent in the spring, that the tax year finishes in early April and that trace elements are entering the diet in different rates at different times of the year. All these are hard to substantiate for there have been changes shown in other parts of the world, such as Australia, where the peak of birth rate is from the spring to the autumn. Further, limited work based on 16th century baptismal data, which bears a strong relation to birth rate data, implies that these trends were in existence long before income tax was invented—though obviously not before intercourse was invented.

Figure 76.8 shows the variation in daily births for England and Wales from 1969 to 1980. It is remarkable for its consistency. A secondary peak in birth rates can be seen in September of each year. This is commonly associated with the fact that nine months before September was Christmas and New Year with their usual festivities.

Daily variation

A short-term cycle is seen in birth rates when one examines the day of the week on which people are born. Figure 76.9 explores this in a simplified way. The birth ratio is derived by dividing by 7 the total number of births in England and Wales in 1980. Thus, if the distribution is random, the expected number of births on any day can be calculated. This is designated at 1: any figures above 1 indicate an increase in the number of births, while below 1 indicates a deficit in births on that day.

It can be seen that at the weekend there is a deficiency in the number of births; the lowest ratio is on Sunday and

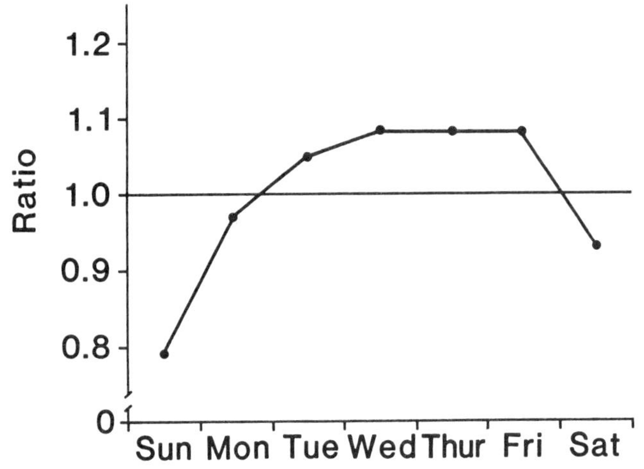

Fig. 76.9 Birth rates in 1980 by day of the week (see text).

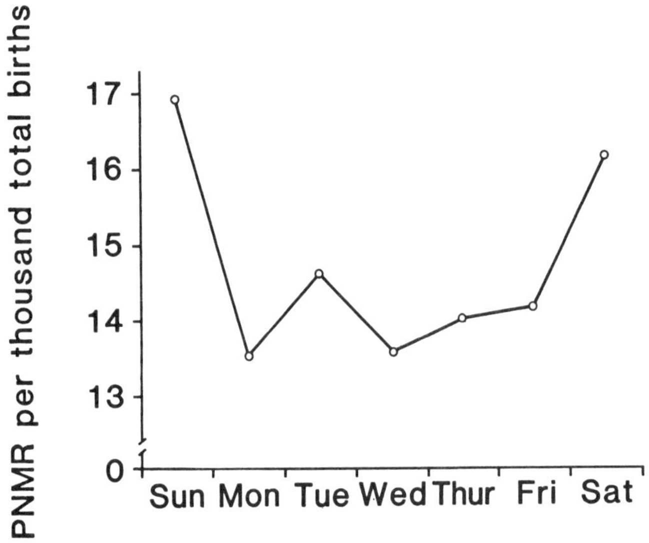

Fig. 76.10 Perinatal mortality rates (PNMR) in 1980 by day of the week (see text).

the next lowest on Saturday. It is not the purpose of this chapter to pursue the reasons for this in detail but it may be noted that the perinatal mortality rate also shows a significant increase in mortality rates at the weekend when data are broken down by day of the week (Fig. 76.10). This is difficult to explain when one considers that most obstetricians would try to induce their difficult cases (with pre-eclampsia, abruptio placentae or intrauterine growth retardation) on a weekday when maximum staff would be available.

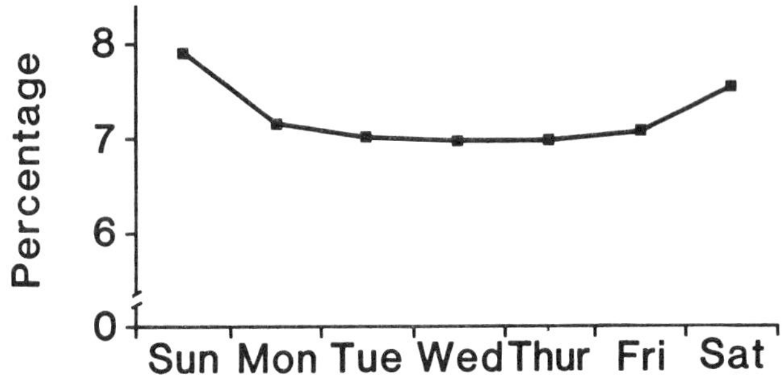

Fig. 76.11 Percentage of low birthweight babies born in 1980 by day of the week (see text).

Some clue to the high mortality rates may be seen in Figure 76.11 which shows the percentage of babies born weighing less than 2500 g. This figure is significantly raised at the weekend; again, it is unlikely that induction policies were responsible for this. It is possible that some women have a lower threshold of the uterus going into spontaneous contractions. It might be that stimulation of the cervix could cause an unusual release of prostaglandins which, whilst not enough to cause labour to start in most women, could start the process in a woman who is very close to labour with a lower-onset threshold. It is as probable that in the UK sexual intercourse is more frequent on Friday and Saturday; this might be the stimulus to the release of prostaglandins. This hypothesis is being explored at the moment.

CONCLUSIONS

Examination of birth rates is not a dull, statistical process but one that gives information in a wide range of social and medical fields. A country that keeps proper data about its births and deaths is one that usually has a good health service. If the information is not counted then the people do not count.

Acknowledgements

There are no formal references in this chapter since all the data are easily available and are constantly being updated from Government sources. The author would like to acknowledge the great help he has had from two major sources:

McFarland A, Mugford M 1984 Birth counts, the statistics of pregnancy and childbirth. Her Majesty's Stationery Office, London

Office of Population Censuses and Surveys Birth statistics 1837–1983. Series FM1 no. 13. Her Majesty's Stationery Office, London

77

Eva Alberman

Perinatal mortality

DEFINITIONS

Perinatal deaths comprise those born of at least 28 weeks' gestation but showing no signs of life and live births who die within 7 days of delivery (World Health Organization 1977). There are, however, certain anomalous features about these definitions which lead to classification problems. Firstly, such deaths include fetuses known to have died long before 28 weeks' gestation but whose delivery was after that time, for instance papyraceous twins. Secondly, in most countries there is no lower limit of gestational age for live births who, providing they are certified as having shown any sign of life, may be of much lower gestational age than 28 weeks.

It is known that policies regarding the certification as live births of very preterm deliveries vary from place to place, even within the UK, for individual judgement may be influenced by the financial implications to the mother of certifying the birth as alive in relation to burial or maternity benefits. Moreover a policy of certifying all such births as live births is likely to bring with it a higher than average mortality rate, since the risk of death in the very preterm baby is extremely high. Even greater variability of certification policies is found between countries where laws of civil registration may dictate the exclusion of live births below defined lower limits of gestational age or birthweight, or the timing of registration may determine whether a child is certified as a live or stillbirth. Efforts are now being made to try to standardize to a greater extent the definitions used, certainly within the UK (Chiswick 1986).

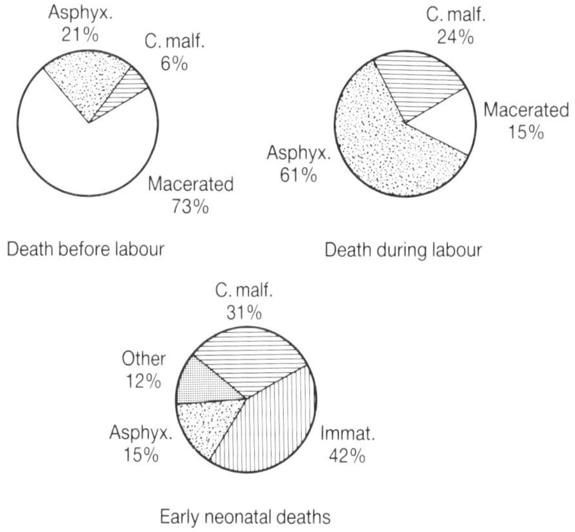

Fig. 77.1 Causes of stillbirths and early neonatal deaths. From North East Thames Regional Health Authority perinatal review group (1985).

The grouping together of stillbirths and first-week deaths has been justified on the grounds that many of the causes are the same and that it may be almost fortuitous whether a fetus dies immediately before or after delivery. There is some strength in this argument as regards fetuses who are alive at the onset of labour, particularly now when intubation and ventilation are swiftly instituted in a baby showing any delay in commencing spontaneous respiration. Nevertheless there are important differences between the causes of antepartum stillbirth and early (first-week) neonatal deaths, since a high proportion of normally formed stillbirths die before the onset of labour, often without an obvious immediate cause, while a high proportion of early neonatal deaths are due to the consequences of preterm birth (Fig. 77.1).

The perinatal death rate is the number of such deaths divided by the total births (still- plus live births) occurring

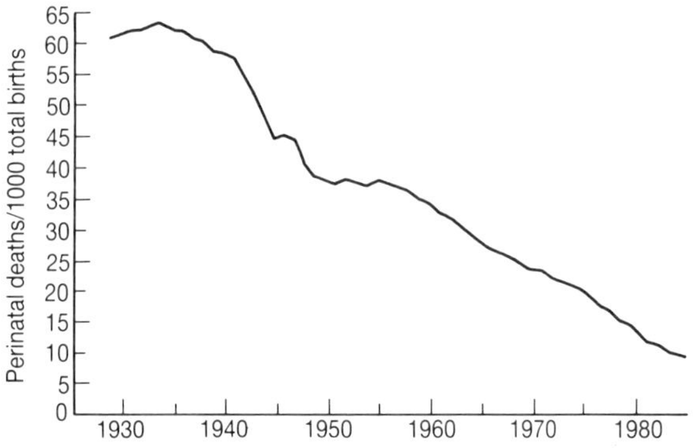

Fig. 77.2 Perinatal mortality in England and Wales from 1928 to 1985. From OPCS mortality statistics series DH3.

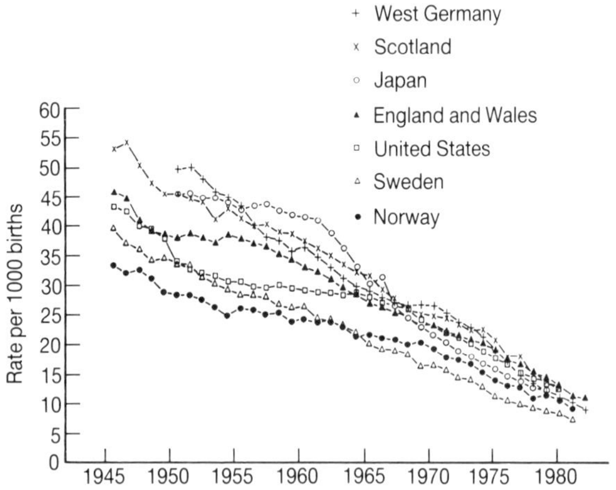

Fig. 77.3 Perinatal mortality from 1945 to 1982 in different countries (A. MacFarlane, personal communication).

over the same period. It is usually expressed as the rate per thousand total births over 1 year.

TRENDS IN PERINATAL DEATHS

Figure 77.2 shows for England and Wales the almost consistently downward trend since data have been available, a trend which has continued up to 1987, the most recent documented year when for the first time the rate was below 9 per thousand total births. Similar trends are being reported from most developed countries and although the rates between such countries have in the past been quite divergent, for reasons to be discussed later, they are now all beginning to converge at rates below 10 per thousand (Fig. 77.3). No obvious flattening out of the trend has yet occurred, although the rates of fall are beginning to slow down in some countries.

CAUSES

Immediate causes

There have been numerous attempts to classify what is known about the causes of perinatal deaths into meaningful groups, always with the aim of instituting preventive interventions. One simple classification was proposed by Wigglesworth (1980); this aims to arrange in a mutually exclusive hierarchical order all congenital malformations; remaining stillbirths which occurred before the onset of labour; neonatal deaths due to immaturity; perinatal deaths due to asphyxial conditions; other specific causes. Wigglesworth pointed out that the causes of congenital malformations and antepartum (usually macerated) stillbirths must act long before labour commences; those due to immaturity act most directly in the neonatal period and those due to asphyxial conditions during the labour and delivery. Thus, the classification directs attention to the period of most importance for preventive action for groups of immediate causes of death.

The classification of perinatal deaths in one English region (North East Thames 1985) in 1983 as suggested by Wigglesworth shows that about one-fifth were attributable to the presence of congenital malformations, about one-fifth to the effects of immaturity (none in the stillbirths, 41% in the first-week deaths) and about one-fifth to asphyxial conditions.

It is important to ask what changes in these causes have been observed over the years and whether the fall in rate can be explained by any particular intervention. Unfortunately changes in the international classification of causes of death (World Health Organization 1977) and changes in the presentation of national statistics make it difficult to analyse such trends. Nevertheless, a very simple comparison of the earliest available perinatal cause data from the 1958 British mortality survey (Butler & Bonham 1963) and the 1984 data for England and Wales (Table 77.1) shows that there have been falls in the rates of death from congenital malformations and of normally formed babies of less than 2500 g, but most of all in normally formed babies of over 2500 g, where the rates have fallen by three-quarters over the 26 years.

Figure 77.4 shows a comparison over a much shorter period, but without changes in classification, and demonstrates again that while nearly all groups of causes have shown a fall in rates, certain specific groups like deaths from haemolytic disease or difficult labour have fallen very sharply.

Predisposing causes

The explanation why these rates have fallen is not simple, and it needs to take into account changes in the prevalence of predisposing factors. Most perinatal deaths can be attributed to an interaction of several different adverse circum-

Table 77.1 Distribution and rates of perinatal deaths in 1958 and 1984

	1958		1984	
	%	Rate/1000	%	Rate/1000
All lethal malformations	18.5	6.2	18.0	1.8
Remainder				
<2500 g	43.3	16.6	54.4	5.5
⩾2500 g	38.2	12.2	27.6	2.8
Total	100	35.0	100	10.1

From Butler & Bonham (1963) and OPCS monitor DH3 86/1.
N.B. Birthweight groupings in 1958 were <2501 and ⩾2500 g.

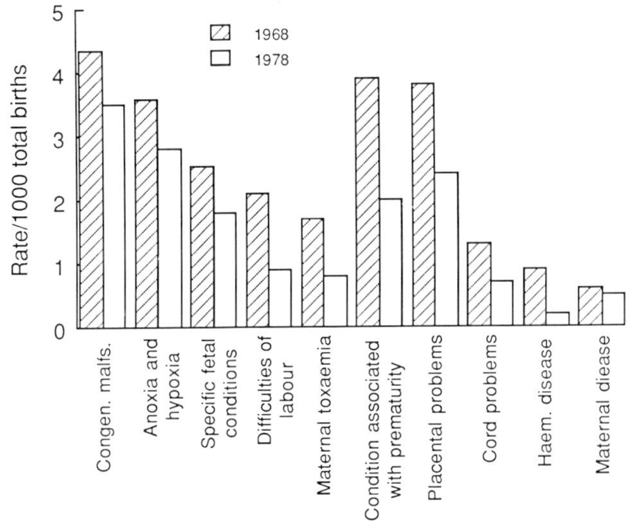

Fig. 77.4 Grouped causes of perinatal deaths derived from Annual Statistical Reviews for England and Wales, 1968 and 1978.

stances, the final insult or immediate cause frequently being the stress of labour and delivery. The predisposing causes can be of many different types—some acting before pregnancy, some early in pregnancy and some late in pregnancy.

Prepregnancy risk factors

These include parental genetic constitution which may result in the conception of a fetus with a lethal hereditary defect. They must also include those maternal infections that can be transmitted vertically from mother to child, the most obvious examples now being hepatitis B and human immunodeficiency viruses, although whether these contribute to perinatal mortality or morbidity in this country has not yet been measured.

Maternal ill health or stunted growth may conspire against a normal fetal growth rate or even, as in the case of diabetes, accelerate growth to a dangerous degree. Defects such as an abnormal uterine shape may prevent normal placentation and anomalies of the cervix predispose to incompetence of the internal os and thus to premature rupture of the membranes.

Advanced maternal age is associated with antepartum haemorrhage (Butler & Alberman 1969), possibly in part because the presence of fibroids may distort the uterus and lead to abnormalities of placentation. It is also well known that the risk of certain chromosomal anomalies, particularly trisomy 21, rises with maternal age.

Conceptional risk factors

These include errors of meiotic or early mitotic divisions which may lead to fetal chromosomal anomalies or to multiple pregnancy. These errors apparently mostly occur randomly but are also related to maternal age, particularly advanced age.

The effects on the fetus of chromosomal anomalies is largely dependent on the presence of associated anomalies which frequently include congenital heart defects or abnormalities of the brain.

Multiple births are exposed to many hazards. Multiple placentation and increased nutritional demands made by multiple fetuses may result in fetal growth retardation which is in proportion to the number of fetuses. Problems are also compounded in monozygous twinning where cords can become entangled in a single amniotic sac or competition for placental tissues may occur, so that sometimes there can be a marked difference in size between twins or indeed the death of one twin.

Environmental factors acting in pregnancy

There are many well recognized teratogens and other fetal toxins, although it is uncertain to what extent they contribute to perinatal mortality. Viral infections such as fetal rubella, cytomegalovirus or toxoplasmosis certainly contribute, both antenatally and postnatally, as do neonatal infections. However, in developed countries these probably contribute less to perinatal death than to morbidity.

The effects on the fetus of maternal smoking have been intensively studied and include deviations from normal placentation (Christianson 1979) and fetal growth retardation, possibly in part due to the direct effects of the products of cigarette smoke on the fetus (Naeye 1978). There may

Table 77.2 Birthweight distribution (%) of live births and birthweight-specific perinatal mortality risk per 1000 total births in England and Wales from 1983 to 1985

	1983		1984		1985	
Birthweight group (g)	%	PNMR/1000	%	PNMR/1000	%	PNMR/1000
<1500	0.8	384.0	0.9	365.9	0.9	350.1
1500–1999	1.3	106.9	1.3	94.7	1.3	93.7
2000–2499	4.6	29.7	4.5	30.4	4.6	28.3
2500–2999	18.6	7.5	18.4	7.3	18.4	7.2
3000–3499	38.6	2.8	38.5	2.8	38.3	2.9
3500–3999	27.3	2.2	27.6	2.1	27.5	1.8
⩾4000	8.6	2.9	8.7	2.8	8.9	3.1
Not known	0.1	228.2	0.1	242.0	0.1	195.0
Total	100	10.4	100	10.1	100	9.5

PNMR = perinatal mortality rate.
From OPCS monitors DH3 84/5; DH3 85/5; DH3 86/2 DH3 85/1; DH3 86/1; DH3 87/1.

be other effects, such as on the immune competence of the fetus of a mother who smokes. The actual contribution made by maternal smoking to the risk of perinatal death depends on the presence of other adverse factors, since the effect of smoking seems to be largely one of reducing growth rate as an added factor in adverse influences. However, its importance even in a low-risk population is illustrated by the estimate that in England and Wales in 1984, 18% of babies born weighing less than 2500 g were attributable to maternal smoking (Simpson et al 1986).

The role of maternal diet in pregnancy is still uncertain, in regard to both undernutrition and the importance of specific dietary constituents (Naismith 1981) but again this will be variable depending on the underlying health of the mother.

It seems now that alcohol, even in low quantities, can contribute to the risk of low birthweight (Mills et al 1984) and possibly to perinatal mortality.

Exposure to occupational or environmental hazards such as radiation or lead almost certainly also contributes to perinatal risk, but again the literature on this is confused. One study has shown a dose-related association between blood lead and risk of preterm delivery (McMichael et al 1986) and the role of stress per se is also still under investigation.

Complications specific to pregnancy

These include hypertensive diseases of pregnancy, still of largely unknown aetiology, and infections of the urinary tract secondary to the stasis which may occur.

Hypertension in pregnancy, whether primary or secondary to essential hypertension, is damaging to the placental vessels with a consequent reduction in blood flow and fetal growth retardation. It may also lead to a curtailment of the normal gestational age, either spontaneously or following induction of labour, and this is an additional constraint on ultimate fetal size. Urinary tract infections may also predispose to preterm labour as may infections of the amniotic sac (Peckham & Marshall 1983).

Classifications in current use

Ideally, any proposed classification should take into account the immediate cause of death, predisposing factors and pathological findings and there have been several attempts to devise classifications which incorporate these. Recent reviews of those in current use in the UK show that they fall into two main groups: one is the clinicopathological approach stemming from Aberdeen (Cole et al 1986) and the other is the pathophysiological approach expanded from the Wigglesworth classification (Hey et al 1986). Both are important, the former because it allows a classification of obstetric factors and the latter because it classifies fetal and neonatal factors. Both need to be used in conjunction with data on the maturity of the baby at birth—usually birthweight because gestational age is rarely available. The cross-tabulation of such classifications, if used in conjunction with maturity and plurality data, produces the most information about perinatal deaths and can be used to describe the situation in a defined geographical area.

FETAL GROWTH AND MATURITY

The majority of the factors which predispose to perinatal deaths do so by influencing fetal growth rate, gestational age, or both. However, over and above such pathological associations are the physiological relationships between fetal growth rate and maternal height, genetic or ethnic constitution and birth rank (Thomson 1983). All these are closely associated with socioeconomic status, as is risk of exposure to environmental hazards and personal health behaviour. Together these interactions lead to extraordinarily robust birthweight distributions which are characteristic for individual populations and their subgroups and which change only very slowly, if at all, except in the presence of major social change. It is the characteristics of these distributions which largely determine perinatal mortality risk, since birthweight is the best predictor of mortality.

Table 77.2 shows that only very slight changes have

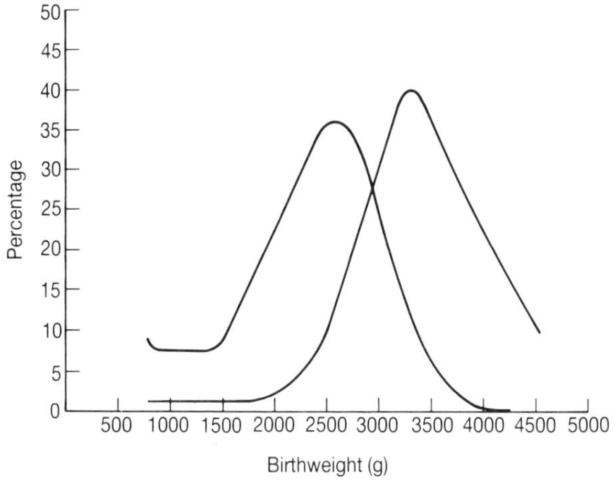

Fig. 77.5 Birthweight distribution in England and Wales of singleton and multiple births in 1984. From OPCS monitor DH 83/5.

Table 77.3 Birthweight-specific perinatal mortality rates for singleton and multiple births in England and Wales in 1985

	Rate/1000 total births	
Birthweight group (g)	Singleton	Multiple
<1500	360.0	302.3
1500–1999	107.3	43.2
2000–2499	30.8	12.2
2500–2999	7.1	10.0
3000–3499	2.9	(7.6)
3500–3999	1.8	(4.0)
>4000	3.1	—
Not known	181.7	(580.6)
Total	9.1	47.7

Rates based on less than 20 deaths or stillbirths in parentheses.
From OPCS Monitor DH3 87/1.

occurred in the birthweight distribution in England and Wales between 1983 and 1985. The fall in mortality which has occurred over these years is largely attributable to the falls in birthweight-specific mortality rates, although their sharp gradient with falling birthweight remains.

However, certain demographic changes will influence overall birthweight distribution, for instance the proportion of multiple births, since the birthweight distribution for multiple births is considerably to the left of that for singletons (Fig. 77.5) and even small reductions in multiple birth rates will reduce overall low birthweight rates. Even though birthweight-specific mortality rates for multiple births at the lower weights are lower than those for singletons (Table 77.3), this does not compensate for their disadvantageous weight distribution.

Similarly, since the distribution of birthweight is shifted to the left in primiparity and in disadvantaged socioeconomic conditions, changes in the proportions of these in the childbearing population will affect birthweight distribution and thus mortality. Hellier (1977) showed that almost a quarter of the reduction in perinatal mortality rate that occurred in England and Wales between 1953 and 1978 was explained by the demographic changes in maternal age, parity and social class that had occurred.

Certain congenital defects, notably of the neural tube, may be related to fetal growth rate and are associated with the same demographic factors, as well as having a genetic component. Some of the steep fall we are currently experiencing in the incidence of these defects—apart from the reduction of prevalence due to termination of pregnancy—may well be attributable to advantageous demographic changes, possibly secondary to improvements in diet associated with such changes (Smithells et al 1981).

CROSS-SECTIONAL AND LONGITUDINAL BIRTH DATA

Up to this point the data quoted have been derived from the compilation and analyses of cross-sectional information on the occurrence and rate of perinatal deaths in a given period, usually over a year. It has been pointed out by several authors (Roman et al 1978, Bakketeig & Hoffman 1979) that the longitudinal collection of data on births and deaths within sibships presents different demographic patterns associated with perinatal death, particularly in regard to parity. Whereas cross-sectional data suggest a U- or J-shaped pattern of risk with parity, data collected within sibships shows that within the same mothers average risk seems to fall steadily with increasing parity. The apparent artefact in cross-sectional data is probably explained by the biases caused by the over-representation of mothers in the high parity groups whose earlier pregnancies had ended in a reproductive failure. Certainly there is a need for more data to be collected longitudinally so that we may examine such patterns in different demographic subgroups. Longitudinal studies also give an opportunity to look at the effect of birth interval; what data we have on sibships suggests that close spacing of pregnancy may contribute to an increase in risk of perinatal death (Bakketeig & Hoffman 1979). Such studies also make it possible to present in a more quantifiable way, and perhaps to explain, the well known tendency for repeated perinatal death in the same mothers (Bakketeig et al 1984).

SHIFT IN AGE OF DEATH

One important question which is causing concern is whether the strong trend towards the reduction of perinatal deaths can be explained, even in part, by a shift towards a later age at death. It has been argued that if all we are doing by medical intervention is postponing death, we need to re-examine the priority given to obstetric and neonatal care. The data from the UK and elsewhere suggest that we need not be too concerned about a shift from death occurring before labour to that occurring just after delivery, since both have been showing consistent falls. More worrying is the levelling out of the post-neonatal rate, suggesting that we may indeed be postponing the death of young infants, probably particularly those of very low birthweight (Macfarlane 1982). Up to the present, the overall falls in stillbirth, first year and later childhood death rates suggest that the overall effect is still in the right direction, but it is clearly important to monitor future trends closely. There is a strong case for including late neonatal deaths in analyses of deaths occurring around the time of delivery since many deaths which previously occurred in the first week are now being shifted to later in the first month.

INTERNATIONAL, REGIONAL AND SUBREGIONAL DIFFERENCES

A source of concern as well as a powerful political weapon has been the marked difference in rates observed between and within the developed countries. In the less developed countries stillbirths are rarely registered, or incompletely so, and the neonatal mortality rates are extremely high; however, where reporting is thought to be complete the range of perinatal death rates in even neighbouring regions or countries has surprised many observers. In fact, once allowance is made for differences in demographic constitution and the consequent differences in birthweight distribution, apparently divergent crude rates become similar. In some cases there is even an apparent reversal of the gradient. Thus in the World Health Organization report (1978) of social and biological effects on perinatal mortality in seven countries, Hungary was found to have the highest crude rates, but after standardization for birthweight it fell to fifth place.

However, even though such factors explain local and international differences they do not alter the actual variations in risk of perinatal death experienced by the mothers concerned.

EFFECT OF MEDICAL CARE

One hotly debated question is to what extent improvements in the medical care of the mother and her baby can compensate for a disadvantageous birthweight distribution or other adverse features related to deprivation.

The scientific study of efficacy of obstetric and neonatal care has advanced considerably over the past 5 years or so and increasingly the tendency is to study separately the specific procedures involved in this care. These can be individually evaluated by means of randomized controlled trials looking at different outcomes, including risk of perinatal death (National Perinatal Epidemiology Unit 1986). Thus there have now been large studies evaluating the use of electronic fetal monitoring (MacDonald et al 1985, Leveno et al 1986), of different ways of managing very preterm babies and many other procedures (Chalmers & Enkin 1982, Grant & Chalmers 1985). Although this is clearly the way forward in the development and evaluation of specific measures, it is also helpful to try to weigh up the overall effect of improving the quality of staffing and facilities devoted to perinatal care.

There seems little doubt that as far as mortality is concerned excellent medical care of high-risk groups, for instance very low birthweight babies (Paneth et al 1982) or normal birthweight babies with complications (Bakketeig et al 1978) can save lives that would otherwise be lost. The benefits of this need to be balanced against possible disadvantages of the overenthusiastic introduction of medical intervention (Tew 1986).

Unfortunately it is often the case that regardless of their risk status the most socially and economically advantaged groups also procure the best medical care and vice versa. It is the latter situation that most urgently needs correcting by educational and other means; sometimes what is lacking is better organization as well as more and better equipment and medical and nursing staff.

THE COLLECTION OF DATA FOR THE DETERMINATION OF PERINATAL MORTALITY

Different countries have different methods of data collection to monitor births and perinatal deaths, but the principles and recent developments have been very similar. This section will be based largely on the situation as it is in England and Wales; for greater detail the reader is referred to volume 1 of *Birth Counts* (Macfarlane & Mugford 1984).

Civil registration of births

The first national statutory requirement to register births for civil purposes was in 1841 and since that time all births have had to be registered with the Registrar of Births and Deaths in the locality in which the birth occurred. The registration takes the form of a structured interview of the parents relating mainly to demographic factors. No medical information is collected and certain relevant demographic details, like parity, are only collected for legitimate babies, who now form a decreasing proportion of all births. Social class classification is traditionally derived from the occupation of the father, and again is available only for legitimate births.

Medical notification of births

In addition to the system for civil registration the medical attendant at the time of birth is required to notify a designated medical officer of the local health authority of any birth occurring in that authority. The opportunity has been

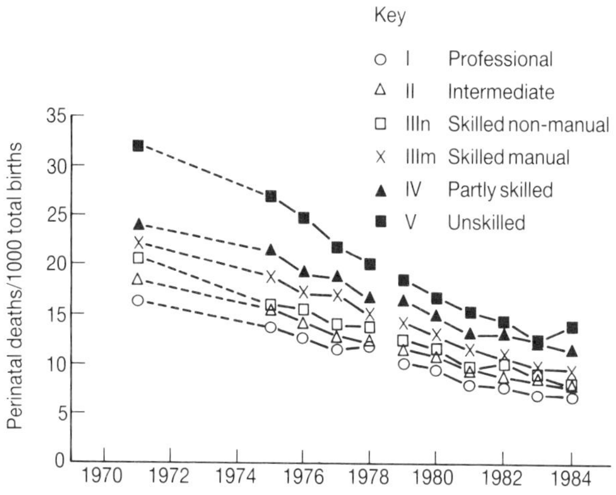

Fig. 77.6 Perinatal mortality in England and Wales by father's social class. From OPCS mortality statistics.

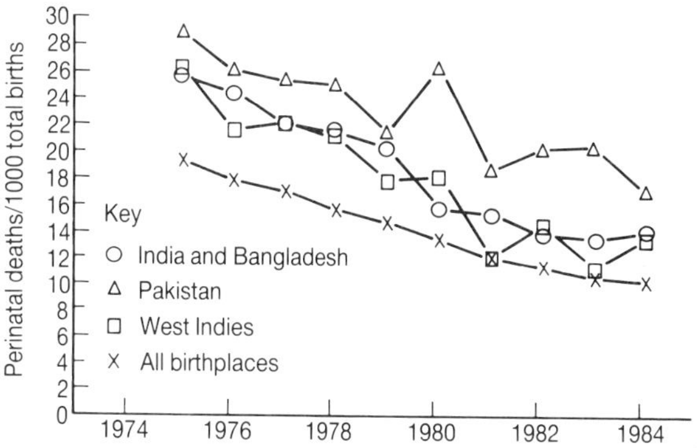

Fig. 77.7 Perinatal mortality in England and Wales by mother's country of birth. From OPCS mortality statistics.

taken of this requirement to collect on a national scale information on birthweight and the recognition of any congenital anomalies visible within 36 hours of birth. Statutory provision has been made for the exchange of information between the civil Registrars of Births and Deaths and the local authority. Since 1978 birthweight data have been transferred at local authority level from the notification forms to the birth certificates and since 1983 this has been achieved for over 98% of all births.

Death certification

Death certification of stillbirths and neonatal deaths is also a civil requirement and the certificates which are made out by the Registrars of Births and Deaths include the medical cause of death, certified by the doctor in attendance. Stillbirth certificates are in fact a combined birth and death certificate and the cause may be as certified by a midwife. Until recently neonatal deaths, no matter how early, were simply treated as deaths of any age and included no parental data. Since 1986 a new neonatal certificate has been issued which, like the stillbirth certificate, collects data on maternal causes contributing to the death. This will certainly improve the quality of information available on perinatal deaths.

Linkage of birth and death certificates

It was first demonstrated by Heady & Heasman (1959) that a linkage of the information available on the birth certificates and the death certificates of infants who subsequently died would considerably enhance the quality of information on such deaths. Such linkage allowed the calculation of death rates by those demographic factors collected for all babies at the time of birth, including place of birth of the parents as well as the place of residence and father's occupation. Among such analyses are data illustrated in Figures 77.6 and 77.7, showing the consistent gradient of risk of perinatal death with social class and mother's place of birth, gradients which are persisting even though the rates are falling within each group. This type of analysis, based on those first performed by Heady & Heasman (1959), continues to illustrate the importance of social and demographic factors. Although such data on a national scale do not allow much in the way of multivariate analyses, more intensive surveys, such as the 1958 Perinatal Mortality Survey of the National Birthday Trust Fund (Butler & Bonham 1963, Butler & Alberman 1969) showed that the important effect of social class was largely explained by its association with birthweight.

PERINATAL INQUIRIES

The persisting unacceptably large differences between developed countries and even regions of this country have acted as a spur to local inquiries or reviews into the causes of perinatal deaths (Chalmers & McIlwaine 1980). These, in part modelled on the Confidential Enquiries into Maternal Deaths (Department of Health and Social Security), have many aims, including the identification of inequalities of staffing, facilities or professional standards between different places and the sharing between professionals of new knowledge. They also serve to meet the justifiable and increasing demand from parents to understand fully the causes for their bereavement.

Inquiries into perinatal deaths have long been standard practice within many obstetric units, but they are now being undertaken within the administrative boundaries of many health authorities. The main choices of method of inquiry are between a case control study or an inquiry into cases only and a comparison with professionally agreed standards. Either method may or may not involve interviews with the bereaved parents and the primary care professionals involved with the cases, as well as reviewing the hospital history. A considerable amount of relevant data is available from statutory returns on births and deaths; this can be obtained without reference to the clinician involved (Black & Macfarlane 1982, Clarke 1982).

Both the size of the inquiry and the resources available will influence the choice of method to be adopted. Of these inquiries that have been reported from the UK, only district- or area-based inquiries have used the most costly form, a case control study including parental interviews. The Mersey inquiry (Mersey Region Working Party 1982) which covered about half a regional health authority, included parental interviews and a formal method of assessment of each case, but did not involve controls.

Different health authorities have however been experimenting with less expensive forms of inquiry, for instance, using statutory returns as control data or augmenting vital statistical data with local inquiries into staffing and facilities. The availability of resources will also govern the extension of the inquiry from perinatal to later infant deaths, or the exclusion of deaths with lethal congenital malformations, or below a lower limit of gestational maturity.

An inquiry in Exeter (Paediatric Research Unit 1973) relied more on the educational value of case conferences which included primary care workers, and nomenclature was changed so that factors contributory to the death were described as 'notable' rather than 'avoidable'. They also included in their discussions the implications of the social background of the families concerned and looked at wider aspects of management including the bereavement itself. These are all welcome advances in the development of medical audit and could do much to reduce the professional anxiety that such inquiries may engender. Well organized reviews of deaths should, where possible, involve the parents and should reduce and not increase the demand for litigation.

The actual effect of such inquiries is difficult to measure but it is the general experience of those familiar with them that they rapidly raise the quality of information available on each death. Their introduction will certainly lead to an increased awareness of the need for good perinatal pathology and its use in this form of audit.

Regions conducting such inquiries are being encouraged to use standard terminology, classifications and tabulations (Macfarlane et al 1986) so that inter-regional comparisons can be made.

PERINATALLY CAUSED MORBIDITY

The well known phrase *the continuity of reproductive casualty* was taken by many to imply that there was a continuum of disorders from those causing perinatal death through severe, moderate and mild neurological deficits including seizures, to minor learning difficulties and clumsiness. There are in fact a large number of discrete and unrelated continuities of this nature.

For instance, causes leading to malformations of the brain such as porencephalic cysts may indeed, depending on their size and site, cause a range of outcomes from perinatal death to minor neurological deficits in survivors. However, this particular continuity is probably quite rare. There are also the congenital infections such as cytomegalovirus which may cause severe illness in the perinatal period sometimes leading to death, sometimes to long-standing impairment, or may not manifest itself until much later in the child's life.

It is, however, becoming increasingly obvious that intrapartum or postpartum asphyxia, even of a very severe degree, extremely rarely leads to long-standing neurological disorder unless it is symptomatic of a prenatal pathological impairment which has caused both the asphyxia and long-term disability. This has been demonstrated anew by Nelson & Ellenberg (1986), who showed in a sample of cases of cerebral palsy that perinatal asphyxia alone probably accounted for no more than about 5%. Dennis & Chalmers (1982) also studied this question and concluded that perinatal asphyxia predictive of long-term morbidity was probably implicated only in full-term babies with early neonatal seizures, but that these occurred in only about 1 in 1000 births. Peters and colleagues (1984) followed outcome in babies in the 1970 British Births Survey who had had more than a 3-minute delay in establishing respiration and found no statistical association with long-term neurological or intellectual impairment except in the small group of children with cerebral palsy who had been of over 5 lb 8 oz (2537 g) birthweight. These accounted for 5 out of 41 children with cerebral palsy, and even in these there was no evidence that the association had been causal.

The situation in the extremely preterm but normally formed infant is different. Here we are learning that cerebral haemorrhages occurring anew in the neonatal period are far more common than was previously thought. However, it seems that many resolve, leaving only a small proportion of survivors permanently impaired. In the case of the ischaemic lesions the outlook is probably less good. In this group it is reasonable to assume that the insult which leads to these lesions may range from lethal to very mild, leaving the surviving child with only minor disabilities (see Ch. 71).

Certainly the picture is complex and we must await the results of follow-up of infants recently monitored by brain ultrasound or magnetic resonance before we know to what extent the same perinatal factors lead to mortality and morbidity (Stewart et al 1987).

Overall the messages from early studies of perinatal mortality, namely the importance of social and demographic factors, have been accepted and it is clear that major reductions in death rates will not occur without educational improvement and social change. Nevertheless, even in populations at low risk there remain possibilities for reducing the risk further, partly by modifying personal behaviour such as smoking and partly by improving the organization and quality of medical care for mothers and babies. As for the fear that by reducing the mortality of very high-risk babies we may be increasing the burden of handicap in survivors, this is clearly a complicated issue and needs to be considered separately for homogeneous aetiological subgroups. In some cases where the insult has been prenatal and severe, survivors inevitably remain impaired. In others, potentially normal at birth, as in the very preterm, excellent medical care may prevent an impairment from occurring. There remains much worthwhile work to be done in the perinatal field, since improvements in perinatal health will lead to better health in childhood and adulthood.

REFERENCES

Bakketeig L S, Hoffman H J 1979 Perinatal mortality by birth order within cohorts based on sibship size. British Medical Journal 2: 693–696

Bakketeig L S, Hoffman H J, Sternthal P M 1978 Obstetric service and perinatal mortality in Norway. Acta Obstetricia et Gynecologica Scandinavica (suppl) 77: 3–19

Bakketeig L S, Hoffman H J, Oakley A R T 1984 Perinatal mortality. In: Bracken M B (ed) Perinatal Epidemiology. Oxford University Press, New York, pp 99–151

Black N, Macfarlane A 1982 Methodological kit: monitoring mortality statistics in a health district. Community Medicine 4: 25–33

Butler N R, Alberman E D 1969 Perinatal problems. The second report of the 1958 British perinatal mortality survey. E&S Livingstone, Edinburgh

Butler N R, Bonham D G 1963 Perinatal mortality. The first report of the 1958 British perinatal mortality survey. E&S Livingstone, Edinburgh

Chalmers I, Enkin M 1982 Effectiveness and satisfaction in antenatal care. SIMP/Lavenham Press, Lavenham, Suffolk

Chalmers I, McIlwaine G (eds) Perinatal audit and surveillance. Proceedings of the 8th study group. Royal College of Obstetricians and Gynaecologists, London

Chiswick M L 1986 Commentary on current World Health Organization definitions used in perinatal statistics. British Journal of Obstetrics and Gynaecology 93: 1236–1238

Christianson R E 1979 Gross differences observed in the placentas of smokers and non-smokers. American Journal of Epidemiology 110: 178–187

Clarke M 1982 Perinatal audit: a tried and tested epidemiological method. Community Medicine 4: 104–107

Cole S K, Hey E N, Thomson A M 1986 Classifying perinatal death: an obstetric approach. British Journal of Obstetrics and Gynaecology 93: 1204–1212

Dennis J, Chalmers I 1982 Very early neonatal seizure rate: a possible epidemiological indicator of the quality of perinatal care. British Journal of Obstetrics and Gynaecology 89: 418–426

Department of Health and Social Security Triennial 1954 to 1989 Reports of confidential enquiries into maternal deaths in England and Wales. HMSO, London

Grant A, Chalmers I 1985 Some research strategies for investigating aetiology and assessing the effects of clinical practice. In: MacDonald R R (ed) Scientific basis of obstetrics and gynaecology. 3rd edn. Churchill Livingstone, London, pp 49–84

Heady J A, Heasman M A 1959 Social and biological factors in infant mortality. Studies on medical and population subjects No 15. HMSO, London

Hellier J 1977 Perinatal mortality 1950 and 1973. Population Trends 10: 13–15

Hey E N, Lloyd D J, Wigglesworth J S 1986 Classifying perinatal death: fetal and neonatal factors. British Journal of Obstetrics and Gynaecology 93: 1213–1223

Leveno K J, Cunningham G F, Nelson S et al 1986 A prospective comparison of selective and universal electronic fetal monitoring in 34 995 pregnancies. New England Journal of Medicine 315: 615–619

MacDonald D, Grant A, Sheridan-Pereira M, Boyland P, Chalmers I 1985 The Dublin randomised controlled trial of intrapartum fetal heart rate monitoring. American Journal of Obstetrics and Gynecology 152: 524–539

Macfarlane A J 1982 Infant death after 4 weeks. Lancet ii: 929–930

Macfarlane A, Mugford M 1984 Birth counts: statistics of pregnancy and childbirth. National Perinatal Epidemiology Unit, OPCS/HMSO, London

Macfarlane A, Cole S, Hey E 1986 Comparisons of data from regional perinatal mortality surveys. British Journal of Obstetrics and Gynaecology 93: 1224–1232

McMichael A J, Vimpani G V, Robertson E F, Baghurst P A, Clark P D 1986 The Port Pirie cohort study: maternal blood lead and pregnancy outcome. Journal of Epidemiology and Community Health 40: 18–25

Mersey Region Working Party on Perinatal Mortality 1982 Confidential inquiry into perinatal deaths in the Mersey region. Lancet i: 491–494

Mills J L, Graubard B I, Harley E E, Rhoads G G, Berendes H W 1984 Maternal alcohol consumption and birthweight. How much drinking during pregnancy is safe? Journal of the American Medical Association 252: 1875–1879

Naeye R 1978 Effects of maternal cigarette smoking on the fetus and placentae. British Journal of Obstetrics and Gynaecology 83: 732–737

Naismith D J 1981 Diet during pregnancy—a rationale for prescription. In: Dobbing J (ed) Maternal nutrition in pregnancy. Eating for two? Academic Press, London, pp 21–40

National Perinatal Epidemiology Unit 1986 A classified bibliography of controlled trials in perinatal medicine 1940–1984. Oxford University Press, Oxford

Nelson K B, Ellenberg J H 1986 Antecedents of cerebral palsy. Multivariate analysis of risk. New England Journal of Medicine 315: 81–86

North East Thames Regional Health Authority perinatal review group 1985 Stillbirths and neonatal deaths (1983) part I. NETRHA

Paediatric Research Unit, Royal Devon and Exeter Hospital 1973 A suggested model for inquiries into perinatal and early childhood deaths in a health care district. Children's Research Fund Report

Paneth N, Kiely J L, Wallenstein S, Marcus M, Pakter J, Susser M 1982 Newborn intensive care and neonatal mortality in low birth weight infants. New England Journal of Medicine 307: 149–155

Peckham C S, Marshall W C 1983 Infections in pregnancy. In: Barron S L, Thomson A M (eds) Obstetrical epidemiology. Academic Press, London, pp 209–262

Peters T J, Golding J, Lawrence C J, Fryer J G, Chamberlain G V P, Butler N R 1984 Delayed onset of regular respiration and subsequent development. Early Human Development 9: 225–239

Roman E, Doyle P, Beral V, Alberman E, Pharoah P 1978 Fetal loss, gravidity and pregnancy order. Early Human Development 2: 131

Simpson R J, Smith, Armand N G 1986 Maternal smoking and low birthweight: implications for antenatal care. Journal of Epidemiology and Community Health 40: 223–227

Smithells R W, Sheppard S, Schorah C J et al 1981 Apparent prevention of neural tube defects by periconceptional vitamin supplementation. Archives of Disease in Childhood 56: 911–918

Stewart A L, Reynolds E O R, Hope P L et al 1987 Probability of neurodevelopmental disorders estimated from ultrasound appearance of brains of very preterm infants. Developmental Medicine and Child Neurology 29: 3–11

Tew M 1986 Do obstetric intranatal interventions make birth safer? British Journal of Obstetrics and Gynaecology 93: 659–674

Thomson A M 1983 Fetal growth and size at birth. In: Barron S L, Thomson A M (eds) Obstetrical epidemiology. Academic Press, London, pp 89–142

Wigglesworth J S 1980 Monitoring perinatal mortality—a pathological approach. Lancet ii: 684

World Health Organization 1977 Manual of the international statistical classification of diseases, injuries and causes of death, vol 1. WHO, Geneva

World Health Organization 1978 Reports on social and biological effects on perinatal mortality, vol 1. WHO, Geneva

78

Alec Turnbull

Maternal mortality

INTRODUCTION

Today, both maternal and perinatal deaths are so rare in the developed world that standards of obstetric care cannot be assessed in terms of mortality rates. Up to the 1930s, however, the maternal mortality rate (MMR) was the dominant statistic. The downward trend in overall death rates in Britain between the second half of the 19th century and the mid 1930s is well known. Figure 78.1 shows the death rate from all causes in women aged 15–44 in England and Wales between 1838 and 1982. It illustrates the steady reduction in death rate, interrupted only by the influenza epidemic of 1920. It is now generally agreed that this decline was largely due to improvements in social and economic conditions, primarily in hygiene and nutrition, rather than in medical care (Loudon 1987).

If social and economic improvements were responsible for the fall in the general death rate, the same factors should have produced a fall in MMR. In fact, as Loudon (1987) points out, the fall in maternal deaths should have been even steeper because of advances in obstetric care; measures were introduced between the late 19th century and the 1930s which were capable of reducing MMR. These included antisepsis and asepsis in the 1870s and 1880s; Caesarean section as a safe technique for some obstetric emergencies, after 1900; the Midwives' Act of 1902; improvements in the teaching of obstetrics and the growing recognition of the import-

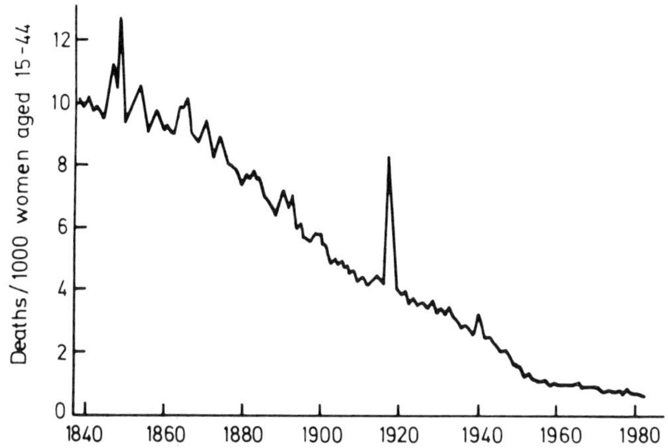

Fig. 78.1 Death rates from all causes in women aged 15–44 in England and Wales from 1838 to 1982. From Loudon (1986a) with permission.

ance of antenatal care in the 1920s and 1930s; improved organization of the specialty of obstetrics and gynaecology and higher standards of specialist care associated with the founding of the Royal College of Obstetricians and Gynaecologists in 1930.

Maternal deaths were defined as occurring in pregnancy, labour or the lying-in period. The latter was not clearly defined before the mid 19th century, and some very late deaths were included in early reports. It became the convention that the lying-in period lasted 1 month from birth: nowadays, for registration purposes, it is 6 weeks. Maternal deaths used to be classified as puerperal or associated deaths. Puerperal deaths were due either to puerperal fever (puerperal sepsis) or accidents of childbirth, the latter representing all other deaths and dominated by haemorrhage and toxaemia.

Despite the downward trend in deaths from all causes, shown in Figure 78.1, and the seeming improvements in maternity care, maternal mortality paradoxically refused to fall. Instead, it remained on a plateau from the 1850s to the mid 1930s. Table 78.1 and Figure 78.2 show the quinquennial MMR in England and Wales between 1850 and 1980.

Table 78.1 Maternal mortality rates per 1000 births in England and Wales from 1847 to 1980 (from Loudon 1986a)

5-year period	Puerperal sepsis	Accidents of childbirth	Total
(1847–1850)	1.9	3.9	5.8
1851–1855	1.5	3.4	4.9
1856–1860	1.5	3.0	4.6
1861–1865	1.6	3.2	4.8
1866–1870	1.5	3.1	4.6
1871–1875	2.4	3.0	5.4
1876–1880	1.7	2.2	3.9
1881–1885	2.8	2.1	4.9
1886–1890	2.4	2.1	4.5
1891–1895	2.5	2.9	5.4
1896–1900	2.0	2.6	4.6
1900–1905	1.9	2.3	4.2
1906–1910	1.6	2.2	3.8
1911–1915	1.5	2.3	3.8
1916–1920	1.6	2.3	3.9
1921–1925	1.5	2.2	3.7
1926–1930	1.8	2.2	4.0
1931–1935	1.6	2.7	4.3
1936–1940	0.77	2.47	3.24
1941–1945	0.36	1.90	2.26
1946–1950	0.14	0.95	1.09
1951–1955	0.098	0.60	0.702
1956–1960	0.06	0.37	0.43
1961–1965	0.04	0.28	0.32
1966–1970			0.27
1971–1975			0.13
1976–1980			0.12

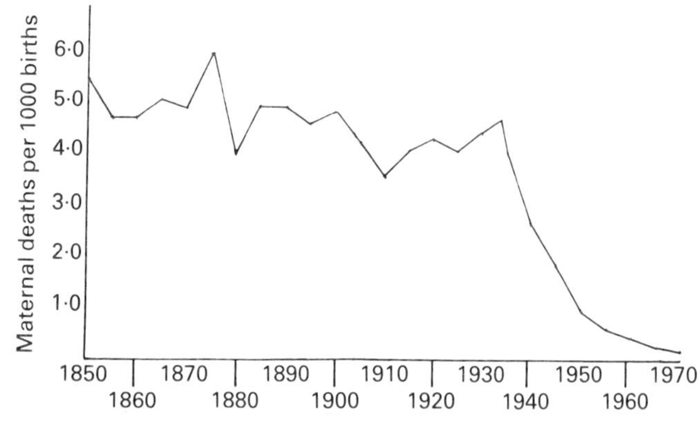

Fig. 78.2 Maternal mortality in England and Wales. Quinquennial rates per 1000 births from 1850 to 1970. From Loudon (1986a) with permission.

The persisting high MMR, which became a public and political scandal by the 1920s, was not confined to England and Wales, for the same trends were seen in Scotland, and the rates were even higher in the USA. Even in the Netherlands or Scandinavia, where maternal mortality was lower than in Britain or the USA, the rates stayed level rather than falling. The trends in maternal mortality over these years and the factors which predisposed to the lack of improvement have been reviewed in three important papers

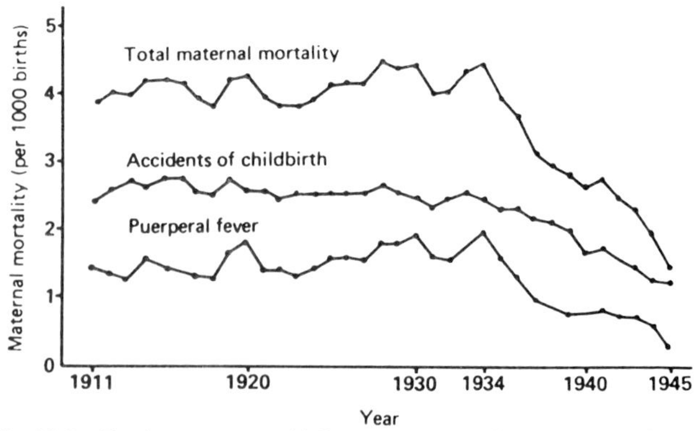

Fig. 78.3 Total maternal morbidity and mortality from puerperal fever and accidents of childbirth in England and Wales from 1911 to 1945. From Loudon (1987) with permission.

by Loudon (1986a, 1986b, 1987), and much of this introduction to the investigation of maternal mortality is taken from these publications.

In England and Wales, maternal mortality finally began to fall around 1937 and when it did, the fall was sudden, profound, and sustained, continuing up to the present time. There have been few more remarkable statistical changes during the 20th century. The same fall occurred in all the developed countries, in Europe, Scandinavia and the USA at the same time. There is little doubt that this change was first initiated by the introduction of sulphonamides, but after the first few years, they cannot have been the only explanation.

Figure 78.3 shows the importance of the reduction in deaths from puerperal fever in the overall fall in MMR after 1937. There was little reduction in deaths from accidents of childbirth between 1911 and 1934, after which a gradual fall began. By contrast, deaths from puerperal fever showed more variation, with peaks of high mortality in 1920, 1930 and 1934, and low rates in 1913 and 1918. After 1934, the reduction in deaths from puerperal fever was rapid; it accounted for 78% of the total reduction in maternal deaths in England and Wales between 1934 and 1940. Loudon (1987) argues convincingly that sulphonamides were generally available, widely used and known to be effective by late 1937. The possibility of a simultaneous decline in streptococcal virulence was suggested by several experienced observers, including Colebrooke (1936), but the most likely hypothesis is nevertheless that the improvement was due mainly to the introduction of sulphonamides. They probably brought about the sustained fall in MMR between 1937 and the early 1940s. As Loudon (1987) stresses, the first year with a notable fall in maternal mortality was 1937.

The death rates from puerperal fever were actually lower in 1913 and 1918 than they were in 1935 or 1936. Only in 1937, when deaths from puerperal fever reached a new low level, could it be said with confidence that a new factor had come into operation. After 1940, penicillin, blood transfusion and better obstetric care played increasingly import-

Table 78.2 Total maternities from 1952 to 1984 and total pregnancies in England and Wales from 1970 to 1984

Triennium	Total maternities	Total pregnancies
1952–1954	2 052 953	N/A
1955–1957	2 113 471	N/A
1958–1960	2 294 414	N/A
1961–1963	2 520 420	N/A
1964–1966	2 600 367	N/A
1967–1969	2 457 443	N/A
1970–1972	2 222 500	2 732 600
1973–1975	1 851 900	2 366 800
1976–1978	1 781 300	2 275 800
1979–1981	1 910 900	2 437 800
1982–1984	1 905 800	2 427 000

From Confidential Enquiries into Maternal Deaths (1982–1984).
N/A = not applicable.

ant roles in lowering maternal mortality and tended to eclipse the early but vital contribution of the sulphonamides.

CAUSES OF UNDIMINISHED MATERNAL MORTALITY BEFORE 1937

The high MMR in England and Wales between 1850 and 1937 was not simply the result of lack of sulphonamides or other antibiotics. In general, the persistently high maternal mortality was probably due either to poor obstetric care, resulting from poor training or poor clinical application, or to social and economic deprivation, adversely influencing the health of the mother and her ability to withstand the stresses of pregnancy and birth.

After reviewing all the evidence, Loudon (1986a) concluded that poor obstetric care was much the more important. 'Maternal mortality appears to be remarkably resistant to the ill effects of social and economic deprivation, but remarkably sensitive to the good and bad effects of medical intervention.'

Between the mid 19th century and the 1930s, maternal mortality tended to be higher in the middle and upper social classes than in the working classes (Loudon 1986b). Most births took place at home under the care of midwives or general practitioners. There was a strong association between social class and attendance by doctors. For first pregnancies, 82% of the wives of professional or salaried workers were delivered by doctors, compared with only 35% of the wives of manual workers. That study was conducted in 1946; the difference was probably even greater in the 1920s and 1930s. Because the vast majority of births were domiciliary the outcome of home delivery was largely responsible for the national level of maternal mortality.

Excessive obstetric intervention

In the second half of the 19th century there was a profound change in obstetric practice. During the preceding 80 or 90 years, practice had been extremely conservative. From the 1870s, however, obstetric practitioners, especially those in general practice, began to intervene in normal labour to an astonishing extent. They took their lead from obstetricians who advocated the active use of forceps delivery, usually under general anaesthesia. From the end of the 19th century (Loudon 1986a), forceps delivery under chloroform or anaesthesia was used in 50 or even 70% of domiciliary deliveries. This was justified on the grounds that modern women should not be expected to bear the pains of normal labour. There was also widespread disregard of antiseptic practice and little interest in antenatal care.

By contrast, extremely good results were often reported in home confinements conducted by midwives trained by charities. The poor of the great cities were delivered by midwives. The Liverpool Ladies' Charity, for example, reported an MMR of 1.3 per 1000 in over 6000 deliveries, undertaken in the poorest homes in the city (Bickerton 1936). Such good results could not have been obtained if socioeconomic deprivation was a major cause of high maternal mortality.

THE ROCHDALE EXPERIMENT

Conclusive evidence for the importance of good obstetric care came from the famous Rochdale experiment of the early 1930s. When Dr Andrew Topping was appointed Medical Officer of Health to Rochdale in 1930, the city had the highest maternal mortality in the country, just under nine per 1000 births. By vigorous reformation of the maternity services, but with no alteration to the diet or living conditions of the poor, the MMR was reduced to 1.7 per 1000 births by 1935, showing that obstetric care was the decisive factor. The measures introduced were simple. Publicity, with the help of the Press, led to a high attendance rate at specially established antenatal clinics; general practitioners were alerted to the serious hazards of interference in labour; good co-operation was established between midwives, general practitioners and a consultant, recruited from Manchester; and a puerperal fever ward was opened. When the Rochdale experiment was subsequently reviewed (Oxley et al 1935), the previously high MMR could not be attributed to economic disabilities; it had been due much more to obstetrical factors which in many instances had proved preventable.

It would be a mistake, however, to conclude that poverty and malnutrition do not influence maternal mortality. The lesson of the period between 1850 and 1930 is that the persistence of a high MMR resulted from poor obstetric care, with excessive intervention by poorly trained general practitioner obstetricians at home confinements. In this situation, the better-off who could afford a general practitioner fared worse than the poor, who were looked after by a midwife whose care was likely to be less interventionist. Obstetric care has improved a great deal over the past 50 years and analysis nowadays demonstrates the expected trend, with MMR being lower in social classes 1 and 2 and higher in 4 and 5 (Confidential Enquiries into Maternal Deaths 1979–1981).

CONFIDENTIAL AND MEDICAL ENQUIRY INTO INDIVIDUAL MATERNAL DEATHS

Although the MMR did not begin to fall significantly until 1937, an organization for recording and publicizing the causation of maternal deaths in England and Wales was originally set up in 1928 by the Minister of Health, Neville Chamberlain, when he established a Departmental Committee on Maternal Mortality and Morbidity. In that year alone there were 2920 maternal deaths in relation to 660 267 live births, an MMR of 4.42 per 1000 births. In 1930, the departmental committee introduced the concept of a primary avoidable factor in maternal deaths in its interim report and published its final report in 1932. The investigation covered 5800 cases and proved so valuable that Medical Officers of Health were asked to continue the enquiries, submitting their confidential reports to the Chief Medical Officer of the Ministry of Health. This continued up to the end of 1951; summaries of the enquiries appeared in successive annual reports on the state of the public health. A primary avoidable factor was considered to be present in 46% of the cases investigated in the first report, but the proportion with avoidable factors altered very little in subsequent years, although the number of deaths diminished markedly from 1937. The diminishing urgency of maternal mortality, combined with other problems during the war years, led to enquiries being conducted in a decreasing proportion of registered maternal deaths. By 1951, reports were received for only about 60% of known deaths. New methods were clearly needed to study preventability in the smaller number of deaths then occurring.

In 1949, maternal mortality was the subject of a discussion at the 12th British Congress on Obstetrics and Gynaecology and reference was made to a method of enquiry sometimes used in the USA—investigation by a local committee of experts, publication of case reports and comments in medical journals. The president of the congress, Sir Eardley Holland, suggested to the Minister of Health the possibility of adopting a similar method in this country. Consultations followed with the Royal College of Obstetricians and Gynaecologists and the Society of Medical Officers of Health, resulting in the adoption of a new system of enquiry involving the family doctor, the Medical Officer of Health, the midwife and the consultant obstetrician. These Confidential Enquiries into Maternal Deaths (CEMD) commenced in 1952 and the findings of the first triennial report, 1952–1954, were published in 1957 by Her Majesty's Stationery Office. Triennial reports on these confidential enquiries have been published for the 11 triennia since then. The most recent, in 1982–1984, will be the last for England and Wales, because reports from 1985–1987 are to be published on a UK basis. Previously, Scotland had produced a quinquennial report and Northern Ireland a decennial report.

CEMD in England and Wales from 1952 to 1984

These 11 confidential enquiries have provided a unique monitoring system for maternal mortality during the past 33 years in England and Wales. While studies of maternal mortality have been published in many countries, for example by Högberg (1985) on maternal mortality in Sweden, there is no national surveillance organization for the detailed investigation of every maternal death in any country outside the UK.

Constant rate of fall in maternal mortality

Figure 78.4 is similar to the graph of maternal mortality shown in Figure 78.1, but based on annual rather than quinquennial rates between 1847 and 1982. Figure 78.4 appears to indicate that the main fall in maternal mortality began in 1937 and was at first extremely rapid, particularly during the war years and immediately afterwards. When the CEMD commenced in 1952, the death rate was only a fraction of what it had been in 1937 and the fall between 1952 and 1984 looks relatively insignificant. However, such a graph is unduly influenced by the very large number of deaths in the earlier years, which must have been potentially avoidable by relatively minor improvements in care. As triennia pass and the MMR falls even lower, the number of potentially avoidable deaths inevitably becomes smaller.

To avoid the bias resulting from the larger number of deaths in earlier years, the changing MMR has to be expressed on a logarithmic scale. Figure 78.5 shows MMR between 1850 and 1970 expressed in this way and reveals that the rate of reduction in MMR has been maintained between 1937 and 1970. In other words, since the MMR first began to fall in England and Wales, the rate of improvement has been constant, approximately halving every 10 years. From over 4000 per million in 1937, the rate has fallen to 86 per million by 1982–1984, so that after almost 50 years MMR has fallen to one-fiftieth of its original level. Since the rate of reduction between 1952 and 1984 has been just as fast as it was between 1937 and 1951, the findings of the CEMD between 1952 and 1984 are clearly of the greatest relevance for achieving continued improvement in the obstetric services.

The method for conducting the CEMD

At the start, enquiry into known or suspected maternal deaths was initiated by the Medical Officer of Health of the town or district. With re-organization of the National Health Service, this post became that of Area Medical Officer and, subsequently, District Medical Officer. The enquiry form (MCW97), which has been modified, developed and

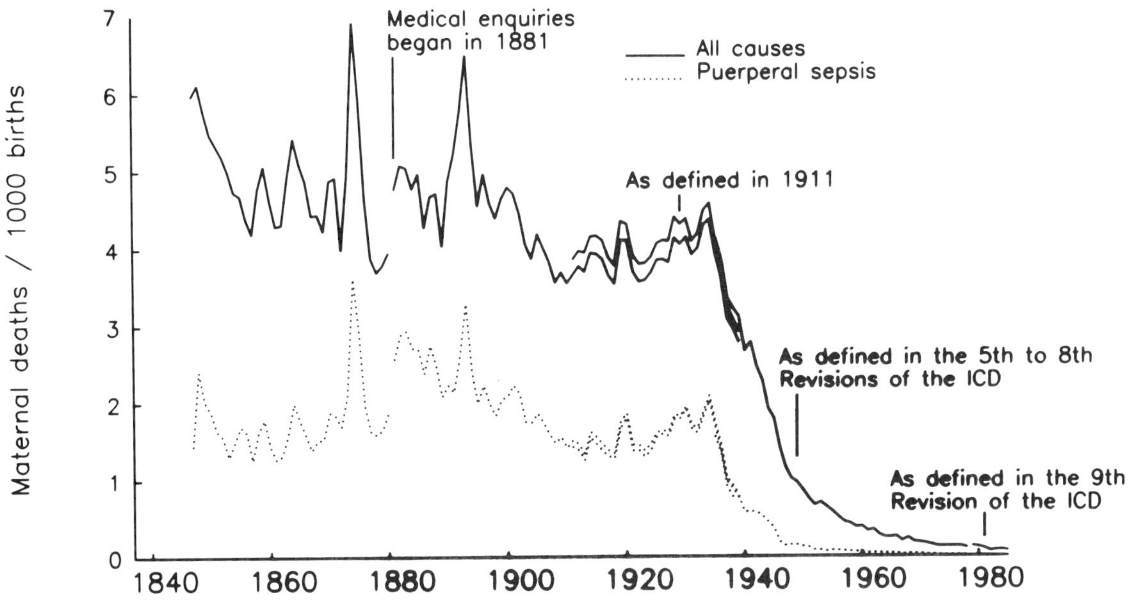

Fig. 78.4 Maternal mortality in England and Wales from 1847 to 1982. From Confidential Enquiries into Maternal Deaths in England and Wales 1982–84.

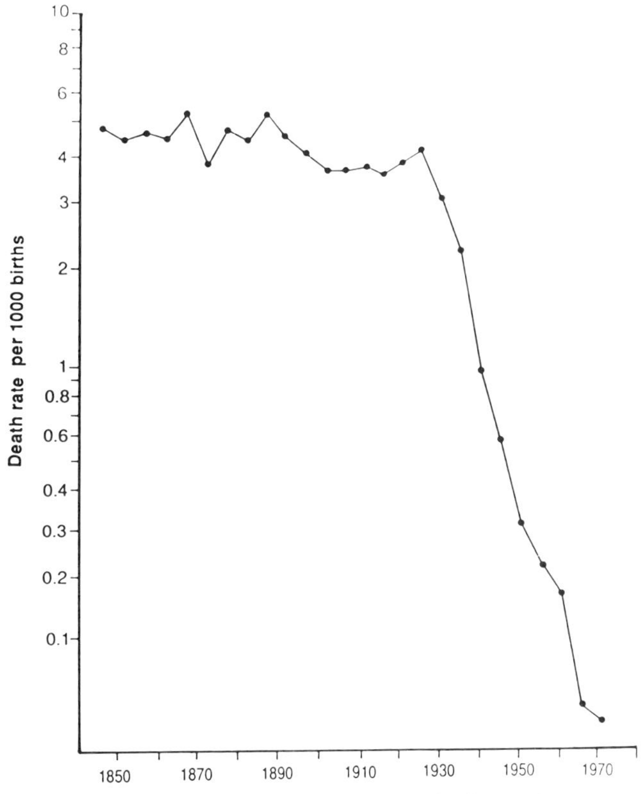

Fig. 78.5 Maternal mortality in England and Wales from 1850 to 1970. Quinquennial rates per 1000 births; semilogarithmic graph. From Loudon (1986a) with permission.

expanded over the years, is sent to all health staff concerned in the care of the woman, including the midwife, general practitioner, health visitor, community physician, consultant obstetrician and any other individual involved in the death. Every possible attempt is also made to obtain details of autopsy, including histology.

When all available local information has been collected, the District Medical Officer forwards the partially completed form to the Regional Obstetric Assessor, a senior consultant obstetrician in the region appointed by the Chief Medical Officer. The Regional Anaesthetic Assessor also reviews the enquiry forms of women who have had an anaesthetic. While there have been Regional Assessors in Obstetrics and Anaesthetics since the earliest years of the CEMD, it was only in 1981 that Regional Pathology Assessors were appointed. They also review the MCW97 forms and add their comments and opinions about the autopsy findings.

The MCW97 form is then sent to the Chief Medical Officer at the Department of Health and Social Security. The Department's Central Assessors in Obstetrics and Gynaecology, Anaesthetics and Histopathology review all facts recorded in each case and act as final arbiters in assessing the main cause of death, any contributing factors and whether or not care was of the accepted standard. Strict confidentiality is observed at all stages of the CEMD. The identity of the patient is erased from all forms so that the opinion of assessors cannot be related to a named individual. After the completion of each triennial report, all MCW97 forms are destroyed. For each death a single main cause is allotted and classified according to the WHO *International Classification of Diseases, Injuries and Causes of Death*, 9th revision (ICD 9) (1975). Although deaths are assigned to one main cause, they may be referred to in other chapters. Thus, a death assigned to hypertensive diseases of pregnancy, in which haemorrhage and anaesthesia also played a part, might be mentioned in all three chapters, but would only be counted as a death from hypertensive diseases.

CLASSIFICATION OF MATERNAL DEATHS

Until the 1973–1975 triennial report, deaths were coded under the *International Classification of Deaths*, 8th revision (WHO 1967). Up to that time, deaths classified under the heading of complications of pregnancy, childbirth and the puerperium were classified as true maternal deaths, while deaths with main causes coded elsewhere in the International Classification, in women known to have been pregnant at the time of death or to have been pregnant within 1 year of death, were classified as associated maternal deaths.

ICD 9, introduced in 1979, defined maternal deaths as:

1. *Direct*, resulting from obstetrical complications of the pregnant state (pregnancy, labour and the puerperium), from interventions, omissions, incorrect treatment or from a chain of events resulting from any of the above.
2. *Indirect*, resulting from previous existing disease, or diseases which developed during pregnancy and were not due to direct obstetric causes but aggravated by physiological effects of the pregnancy.
3. *Fortuitous*—only deaths from other causes, which fortuitously occur in pregnancy or the puerperium, are excluded from maternal mortality as internationally defined. These have been defined as fortuitous deaths in the triennial reports on CEMD from 1976 to 1978.

This new classification has helped to overcome the type of difficulty noted in previous reports, when a death could be classified as associated, even if the pregnancy had brought it to light or caused exacerbation of a pre-existing condition, making it indirect.

A further recommendation of ICD 9 is that maternal death should be defined as the death of a woman while pregnant or within 42 days of termination of pregnancy, irrespective of the duration and the site of the pregnancy, from any cause related to or aggravated by the pregnancy or its management, but not from an accidental or incidental cause. This is in line with the definition adopted by the International Federation of Gynaecology and Obstetrics (FIGO) and is included in previous reports. In the CEMD, maternal death has always been defined as one occurring during pregnancy or labour, or as a consequence of pregnancy, within 1 year of delivery or abortion. This wider definition has the advantage of including deaths in which the period of the survival is longer than 42 days but in which pregnancy played an important role. Late deaths (after 42 days) have been included in all the triennial reports but their presence has been specifically indicated since they were not included within the FIGO definition. From the 1979–1981 report onwards, late deaths have been documented separately in an additional chapter.

Denominators for calculation of incidence and rates

Historically, MMR was defined as the number of maternal deaths per 1000 total births. The CEMD has based mortality rates on the number of maternities. This is the number of mothers delivered as distinct from the number of babies born, which is larger because it includes infants from multiple births. As MMR has fallen, it has proved necessary to express the rate per 10^4, 10^5 and in the most recent reports, per 10^6 maternities. To provide realistic denominators for deaths occurring in early pregnancy, such as ectopic pregnancy or abortion, Office of Population Censuses and Surveys (OPCS) data have been used to calculate total pregnancies, a figure including legal and spontaneous abortions, ectopic pregnancies and total maternities (Table 78.2). Many rates have been calculated from this denominator since 1979–1981.

AVOIDABLE FACTORS OR SUBSTANDARD CARE

From 1930, when the Departmental Committee on Maternal Mortality identified a *primary avoidable factor* in some maternal deaths, the annual reports of the Chief Medical Officer up to 1950, and subsequently the triennial reports on the CEMD from 1952 to 1978, have included data on the incidence of avoidable factors. An avoidable factor was considered present if there was a departure from generally accepted standards of satisfactory care, or if the care provided was considered inappropriate in the circumstances. In the 1979–1981 report, the term *substandard care* was substituted for avoidable factors to take into account not only failures in clinical care but also some of the underlying factors which may have produced a low standard of care for the patient. These included shortage of resources for staffing facilities, administrative failure in the maternity services or in back-up facilities such as anaesthetic, radiological or pathology services. It was considered that the term *avoidable factors* had often been misinterpreted as meaning that avoiding these factors would have prevented the death.

In 1952–1954, the incidence of avoidable factors was approximately 45%. By 1976–1978, the incidence had increased to approximately 58%. This apparent increase resulted more from increasingly high standards of assessment than from deterioration in management.

It has proved more difficult quantitatively to assess the incidence of substandard care in 1979–1981 and 1982–1984, but apart from those due to pulmonary or amniotic fluid embolism, a high proportion of deaths due to other causes are still associated with substandard care. Considerable further improvement must therefore be possible, although maternal mortality has now fallen to such a low level.

Table 78.3 Numbers of direct deaths by cause from 1952 to 1969 in England and Wales

Causes	1952–1954	1955–1957	1958–1960	1961–1963	1964–1966	1967–1969
Hypertensive diseases of pregnancy	246	171	118	104	67	53
Pulmonary embolism	138	157	132	129	91	75
Abortion	153	141	135	139	133	117
Haemorrhage	188	138	130	92	68	41
Anaesthesia	Not classified separately				50	50
					Calculated later	Not in total
Ectopic pregnancy	No separate chapter			42	42	32
Amniotic fluid embolism	Not recognized			27	30	27
Sepsis (excluding abortion)	Included in abortion			33	57	26
Ruptured uterus	No separate chapter			38	30	18
Other direct causes	All other direct deaths					
	369	254	227	88	61	66
Total	1094	861	742	692	579	455

From Confidential Enquiries into Maternal Deaths (1982–1984).

Table 78.4 Numbers of direct deaths by cause* from 1970 to 1984 in England and Wales

Causes	1970–1972	1973–1975	1976–1978	1979–1981	1982–1984
Hypertensive diseases of pregnancy	47	39	29	36	25
Pulmonary embolism	52	33	43	23	25
Abortion	71	27	14	14	11
Haemorrhage	27	21	24	14	9
Anaesthesia	37	22	27	22	18
Ectopic pregnancy	34	19	21	20	10
Amniotic fluid embolism†	16	14	11	18	14
Sepsis (excluding abortion)	30	19	15	8	2
Ruptured uterus	13	11	14	4	3
Other direct causes	13	22	19	17	21
Total	340	227	217	176	138

* Late deaths were excluded; † confirmed histologically.
From Confidential Enquiries into Maternal Deaths (1982–1984).

Table 78.5 Rate of direct maternal deaths by cause per million maternities from 1952 to 1969 in England and Wales

Causes	1952–1954	1955–1957	1958–1960	1961–1963	1964–1966	1967–1969
Hypertensive diseases of pregnancy	119.8	80.9	50.4	41.3	25.8	21.6
Pulmonary embolism	67.2	74.3	57.5	51.2	35.0	30.5
Abortion	74.5	66.7	58.8	55.1	51.1	47.6
Haemorrhage	91.6	65.3	56.7	36.5	26.2	16.7
Anaesthesia	—	—	—	—	19.2	20.3
Ectopic pregnancy	No separate chapter			16.7	16.2	13.0
Amniotic fluid embolism	Not recognized			10.7	11.5	11.0
Sepsis (excluding abortion)	Included in abortion			13.1	21.9	10.6
Ruptured uterus	No separate chapter			15.1	11.5	7.3
Other direct causes	All other direct deaths					
	179.7	120.2	98.9	34.9	23.5	26.9
Total	532.8	407.4	323.4	274.6	222.7	185.2

From Confidential Enquiries into Maternal Deaths (1982–1984).

TRENDS IN CAUSES OF MATERNAL MORTALITY FROM 1952 TO 1984

The numbers of deaths from individual causes from 1952 to 1969 are shown in Table 78.3 and from 1970 to 1984 in Table 78.4. The direct maternal death rate by cause as a rate per million maternities from 1952 to 1969, is shown in Table 78.5 and from 1970 to 1984 in Table 78.6. The first six triennia were dominated by deaths from hypertensive diseases of pregnancy, pulmonary embolism, haemorrhage and abortion. Bearing in mind the fluctuation in the number of maternities during the triennia between 1952 and 1984 shown in Table 78.3, the rates shown in Tables 78.5 and 78.6 are more reliable indicators of trends than the numbers of deaths in Tables 78.3 and 78.4. Table 78.5 shows that there was a dramatic reduction in the MMR from hyperten-

Table 78.6 Rate of direct maternal deaths by cause per million total pregnancies* from 1970 to 1984 in England and Wales

Causes	1970–1972	1973–1975	1976–1978	1979–1981	1982–1984
Hypertensive diseases of pregnancy	16.3	15.1	12.5	41.2	10.0
Pulmonary embolism	18.0	12.8	18.5	9.0	10.0
Abortion	24.6	10.5	6.0	5.5	4.4
Haemorrhage	9.3	8.1	10.3	5.5	3.6
Anaesthesia	12.8	8.5	11.6	8.7	7.2
Ectopic pregnancy	11.8	7.4	9.0	7.9	4.0
Amniotic fluid embolism†	5.5	5.4	4.7	7.1	5.6
Sepsis (excluding abortion)	10.4	7.4	6.5	3.1	0.8
Ruptured uterus	4.5	4.3	6.0	1.6	1.2
Other direct causes	4.5	8.5	8.2	6.7	8.4
Total	117.6	88.0	93.4	69.2	55.0

* Including spontaneous and legal abortions and ectopic pregnancies; † confirmed histologically.
From Confidential Enquiries into Maternal Deaths (1982–1984).

sive diseases of pregnancy and from haemorrhage between 1952–1954 and 1958–1960, and perhaps because of this it may have been easy to improve on previously very poor standards of care. By comparison, the MMR from pulmonary embolism fell relatively little over these years. Since deaths from abortion showed no improvement, this became the main cause of death between 1958–1960 and 1970–1972. In these years, the reports comment repeatedly on the dangers of home confinement in women with a previous history of haemorrhage, of inadequate anticipation or treatment of the complications of hypertensive disease, on the need for better booking arrangements and for effective flying squad facilities.

With haemorrhage deaths, the introduction in 1962 of a combined preparation of oxytocin and ergometrine for intramuscular use must have helped to maintain the reduction in deaths from this cause over the first six triennia. Table 78.6 shows that between 1970 and 1984 deaths from haemorrhage continued to fall, perhaps because of better management, the avoidance of unwanted high-risk pregnancy in women of high parity and possibly because of better prophylaxis in second- and third-stage labour.

Perhaps the most dramatic change in the CEMD has been the effect of the Abortion Act (1967) which came into force in 1968. Abortion remained the main cause of death in 1967–1969 and although there was a marked reduction in deaths from criminal and spontaneous abortion in 1970–1972, abortion was still the main cause of death in that triennium because there was an increase in therapeutic abortion deaths associated with many relatively late abortions and the continuing use of techniques such as hysterotomy, often combined with sterilization, or hysterectomy. By 1973–1975, legal abortions were more often being performed earlier in pregnancy and more often by simple, vaginal techniques and the abortion MMR fell. By 1982–1984, the death rate from abortion was very low indeed and for the first time there were no deaths from criminal abortion.

Table 78.6 shows that in the five triennia between 1970 and 1984, there was little improvement in MMR from either hypertensive diseases of pregnancy or pulmonary embolism. As a result, these became equal main causes of death in 1982–1984. Although the MMR from hypertensive diseases of pregnancy is lower in the 1980s than in the 1950s, the slow improvement in the last 15 years has been disappointing. The recent CEMD has highlighted the serious hazards of hypertensive diseases, which can develop insidiously and progress rapidly to a dangerous stage with little warning. Death is still mainly due to cerebral haemorrhage, probably the result of failure to control severe hypertension, but can also result from disseminated intravascular coagulation, renal failure or liver necrosis. These complications can all be anticipated by appropriate investigations (repeated platelet counts, blood urea, urate, creatinine and AST). Establishment of expert teams in each region has been suggested, either to advise about management or to take over cases if requested.

Pulmonary embolism remains a major problem largely because no effective method has been developed for preventing it or for detecting deep vein thrombosis early. The triennial reports have repeatedly stressed the importance of an awareness of factors predisposing to pulmonary embolism. The 1982–1984 report draws attention to the hazard of pulmonary embolism in women delivered by elective Caesarean section for severe hypertensive diseases of pregnancy.

While the period between 1952 and 1959 was dominated by four main causes of death, the period between 1970 and 1984 has seen the emergence of new major causes of death. Thus, in 1979–1981, complications of anaesthesia were the third main cause of death, followed by ectopic pregnancy and amniotic fluid embolism. In 1982–1984, anaesthesia was again the third commonest cause of death followed by amniotic fluid embolism, abortion, ectopic pregnancy and haemorrhage.

Table 78.6 suggests that the reduction in deaths from anaesthesia has been particularly disappointing. This concern has been mirrored in a recently published report by the Association of Anaesthetists (1987). A statistical difficulty is that the MMR for anaesthesia calculated per million maternities is not a satisfactory indicator because the number of anaesthetics administered in obstetric practice has almost

Table 78.7 Estimated number of Caesarean sections performed and estimated mortality rate per 1000 Caesarean sections within 42 days in NHS hospitals in England and Wales for each triennium

	1970–1972	1973–1975	1976–1978	1979–1981	1982–1984	Total
Total maternities in NHS hospitals	2 000 612	1 799 980	1 689 670	1 876 570	1 840 970	9 270 802
Estimated number of Caesarean sections	103 310	101 410	120 570	167 020	185 820	678 130
Percentage of maternities by Caesarean sections in NHS hospitals	5.2	5.6	7.1	8.9	10.1	7.4
Deaths after Caesarean sections (direct maternal and associated deaths from enquiry series)	102	77	80	87	69	415
Estimated fatality rate per 1000 Caesarean sections	0.99	0.76	0.66	0.52	0.37	0.61

From Confidential Enquiries into Maternal Deaths (1982–1984).

certainly considerably increased in recent years. Unfortunately, there are no reliable estimates of the number of anaesthetics administered to obstetric patients, but the situation must be similar to that for Caesarean section, which is considered later. If the number of deaths from anaesthesia could be expressed as a proportion of the number of anaesthetics given, it seems likely that the MMR from obstetric anaesthesia would show a considerable fall. Although the rate of improvement in anaesthetic mortality has probably been much greater than is indicated by the rate per million maternities, the last five triennial reports have shown a high incidence of avoidable factors or substandard care; also, too often, pregnant women have not been accorded the same standard of care generally available to surgical patients, with particular respect to the facilities, equipment and seniority of anaesthetic staff, as well as the presence of trained anaesthetic assistants.

That deaths from amniotic fluid embolism are of relatively increasing importance is hardly surprising because no advance has been made in its prevention, detection or treatment. The MMR has remained practically unchanged.

Deaths from sepsis after abortion are mentioned in the CEMD chapter on genital sepsis, but are actually counted in the abortion chapter. Deaths from genital sepsis include deaths from puerperal sepsis, from sepsis after surgical procedures and from sepsis before or during labour. While the huge reduction in deaths from sepsis between 1952–1954 and 1967–1969 was impressive, the reduction in the MMR from sepsis between 1970–1972 and 1982–1984 has in fact been equally rapid.

Ectopic pregnancy has shown the most surprising and unexpected improvement in MMR in 1982–1984, having previously been static. While the incidence of ectopic pregnancy has not increased as much in England and Wales as in some European countries, the figures in the CEMD show that the incidence of ectopic pregnancy is increasing. Since many of the deaths occur very early in pregnancy, the improvement in 1982–1984 may be associated with increasingly sophisticated diagnostic tests, including rapid sensitive assays of beta-human chorionic gonadotrophin in urine or blood, improved ultrasound diagnosis including transvaginal scanning (Urquhart & Fisk 1988) and rapid recourse to laparoscopic investigation in women with pelvic pain of uncertain origin. Alternatively, it may transpire that the improvement in 1982–1984 was simply due to chance.

Ruptured uterus deaths have fallen considerably, perhaps because of increasing awareness of the dangers of excessive uterine stimulation with oxytocic drugs, especially in women previously delivered by Caesarean section, or with possible cephalopelvic disproportion in labour.

Other direct deaths, also classified as miscellaneous, show a varying incidence over the triennia, reflecting the difficulty of reliably attributing to this category direct deaths not readily attributed to other causes.

CAESAREAN SECTION

Table 78.7 is taken from the chapter on Caesarean section in the 1982–1984 CEMD report. If there was as little information about the total number of Caesarean sections as about anaesthetics, the MMR, expressed per million maternities, would show the same unsatisfactory trend. However, the increasing number of Caesarean sections in each triennium is clear; the rate has risen from 5.2% in 1970–1972 to 10.1% in 1982–1984. From these data, the fatality rate per 1000 Caesarean sections can be calculated and shows a steady rate of improvement. In 1979–1981 there was concern that despite a falling fatality rate, the number of Caesarean sections had increased so much that the number of deaths was actually increasing. However, the sharp fall in the number of Caesarean section deaths in 1982–1984 is reassuring, although the future trend must be watched. Figure 78.6 illustrates how the fatality rate has continued to fall steadily despite the rising Caesarean section rate.

Table 78.8 shows that when only direct deaths are considered, the Caesarean fatality rate over the past five triennia has fallen even more than the MMR from all causes. It is also apparent, however, that the percentage of direct deaths associated with Caesarean section has increased from 24% to 32%, probably indicating that an increasing proportion of women with severe problems in late pregnancy are delivered by Caesarean section.

Further analysis of the 1982–1984 figures shows that the incidence of direct deaths from elective Caesarean sections was only 0.09 per 1000 operations, compared with 0.37 per

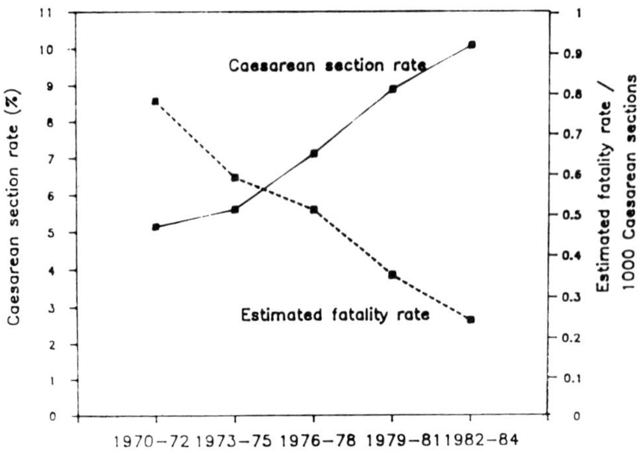

Fig. 78.6 Percentage Caesarean section rate and estimated fatality rate per 1000 Caesarean sections in England and Wales from 1970 to 1984. From Confidential Enquiries into Maternal Deaths (1982–1984) with permission.

1000 emergency operations. A similar difference was found in the previous triennium, but the 1982–1984 report stresses that the reason for the high mortality rate amongst the emergency group is not certain. Undoubtedly the conditions for which the operation is performed carry greater risks among women undergoing emergency procedures. Since it is rarely possible to predict the need for delivery by emergency Caesarean section, attempting to reduce the number by performing more elective operations would be likely merely to increase the overall Caesarean section rate. However, the comments about obstetric anaesthetic services are also relevant to the performance of Caesarean section.

Indirect, fortuitous or associated deaths and data from cardiac disease

Table 78.9 lists the numbers of direct, indirect, fortuitous, associated deaths and deaths from cardiac disease between 1952 and 1984. Up to 1973–1975, deaths not directly due to pregnancy were classified as associated and since 1976–1978 they have been classified as indirect or fortuitous. The associated group also included late deaths, occurring between 42 days and 1 year after the end of pregnancy, but since 1979–1981 the CEMD reports have provided a separate chapter for late deaths. In Table 78.9, these late deaths have been excluded from the 1967–1969 triennium onwards.

Deaths from cardiac disease are now counted as indirect or fortuitous, although cardiac deaths are described in a separate chapter. Up to 1973–1975, cardiac deaths were counted as associated deaths, although they have been described in a separate chapter since the first report in 1952–1954.

Table 78.9 shows that over the 11 triennia, direct deaths have fallen more rapidly than indirect or fortuitous deaths which have increased from around 25% of all maternal

Table 78.8 Number of direct maternal deaths within 42 days of Caesarean section

	1970–1972	1973–1975	1976–1978	1979–1981	1982–1984	Total
All direct deaths	340	227	217	175	138	1097
Direct deaths from Caesarean sections	81	60	61	59	44	305
Percentage of all direct deaths	24	26	28	34	32	28
Caesarean section rate (%)	5.16	5.63	7.14	8.90	10.09	7.36
Estimated fatality rate/1000 Caesarean sections	0.78	0.59	0.51	0.35	0.24	0.45

From Confidential Enquiries into Maternal Deaths (1982–1984).

Table 78.9 Direct, associated, indirect and fortuitous deaths and deaths from cardiac disease in England and Wales from 1952 to 1984

Triennium	Direct deaths	Associated deaths	Indirect	Fortuitous	Percentage associated	Deaths from cardiac disease: Acquired	Congenital	Total	Percentage associated due to cardiac disease
1952–1954	1094	316			22.4	121	N/A	121	38.3
1955–1957	861	339			28.3	102	N/A	102	30.1
1958–1960	742	254			25.5	66	N/A	66	26.0
1961–1963	692	244			26.1	68	13	71	29.1
1964–1966	579	176			23.3	43	7	50	28.4
1967–1969	445	218			32.9	34	15	49	22.5
Late deaths excluded									
1970–1972	340	209			33.1	33	9	42	20.1
1973–1975	227	111			32.8	14	4	18	16.2
1976–1978	217	134	78	56	38.2	14	3	17	12.7
1979–1981	176	123	92	31	41.1	12	4	16	13.0
1982–1984	138	105	71	34	43.2	11	6	17	16.2

From Confidential Enquiries into Maternal Deaths (1982–1984).

deaths in the earlier triennia to around 40% in the last three triennia.

While the main causes of associated deaths in the earlier triennia were severe generalized infections or cardiac disease, recent reports have drawn attention to deaths from disorders such as aneurysms leading to death from intracranial haemorrhage (from berry aneurysms) or intra-abdominal bleeding (from aortic, splenic or other aneurysms); severe kyphoscoliosis causing death from worsening respiratory failure; the tendency for epilepsy to worsen, causing death from uncontrolled convulsions and meriting better prophylactic control; the worsening of diabetes, with death from various metabolic complications.

Cardiac disease deaths have changed in character very markedly over the 11 triennia and Table 78.9 shows how their contribution to associated deaths has fallen. The earlier years were dominated by large numbers of deaths from acquired heart disease, almost always of rheumatic origin. Presumably because of the effective use of penicillin for the treatment of rheumatic fever, the incidence of these disorders has fallen progressively and in the last four or five triennia, the MMR for acquired heart disease has been due more often to coronary atherosclerosis with myocardial infarction, or cardiomyopathy, than to rheumatic carditis. Congenital heart disease has become increasingly important and the CEMD reports have recently drawn attention to the hazards of pregnancy in women whose congenital disease may have only been partially cured by surgery in childhood. Prepregnancy counselling is of vital importance in such women.

MATERNAL MORTALITY IN DEVELOPING COUNTRIES

While the MMR in the developed countries ranges between 6 and 150 per 100 000 live births, the MMR in developing countries still remains between 100 and 3500 deaths per 100 000 live births (Högberg 1985).

For these countries, the experience of Europe and the USA should be helpful. In general, the present problems of the developing countries have similarities to those in the developed countries before 1850. As Walker (1986) pointed out, maternal mortality must rank with some infectious diseases as among the few instances where medical care has achieved a dramatic reduction in mortality rates. In support of the proposal that effective medical care has been more important than improved socioeconomic status in reducing maternal mortality, he quoted the study of Kaunitz et al (1984) who reported that in a religious group avoiding obstetric care in the USA, MMR between 1975 and 1982 was 87 per 10 000 live births — a level over 90 times higher than in the remainder of the state of Indiana and comparable with that in many developing countries. Walker (1986) also noted that many maternal deaths in developing countries could be prevented if the number of births to older, high parity women could be reduced by appropriate family planning.

While improving living conditions is a praiseworthy aim in every country, reducing excessive MMR in developing countries is not likely to be achieved without the provision of effective obstetric care for all pregnant women.

CONCLUSIONS

This has been a brief account of the successful efforts made by the maternity services in England and Wales and in developed countries in general to overcome the once huge problem of maternal mortality. The great improvements brought about in the past 50 years have been illustrated and the factors responsible for the improvement discussed.

Inevitably, review of the 11 triennial reports of the CEMD between 1952–1954 and 1982–1984 has been extremely limited. During the period of the enquiries more than 24 million births were registered in England and Wales, and between the introduction of the 1967 Abortion Act in 1968 and the end of 1984, nearly 1.8 million legal terminations of pregnancy were performed.

Although the rate of improvement in mortality in England and Wales has been linear between 1937 and 1984, reaching its lowest level of 8.6 per 10 000 total births in 1982–1984, the high rate of substandard care shows that further improvement can and should be achieved. In Sweden, maternal mortality was only 6.6 per 100 000 total births between 1971 and 1980 (Högberg 1985).

Acknowledgements

I am grateful to the Controller of Her Majesty's Stationery Office for permission to use tables and figures from the Reports of the Confidential Enquiries into Maternal Deaths.

REFERENCES

Association of Anaesthetists 1987 Anaesthetic services for obstetrics — a plan for the future. Association of Anaesthetists of Great Britain and Ireland/Obstetric Anaesthetists' Association, London

Bickerton T H 1936 A medical history of Liverpool from the earliest days to the year 1920. John Murray, London

Colebrooke L, Kenny M (1936) Treatment with prontosil of puerperal infections due to haemolytic streptococci. Lancet ii: 1319–1322

Confidential Enquiries into Maternal Deaths in England and Wales. Eleven triennial reports from 1952–1954 to 1982–1984, inclusive. Her Majesty's Stationery Office, London

Högberg U 1985 Maternal mortality in Sweden. Umea University Medical Dissertation (new series) 156

Kaunitz A M, Spence C, Davidson T S, Rochat R W, Grieves D A 1984 Perinatal and maternal mortality in a religious group avoiding obstetric care. American Journal of Obstetrics and Gynecology 150: 826–831

Loudon I 1986a Deaths in child bed from the 18th century to 1935. Medical History 30: 1–41
Loudon I 1986b Obstetric care, social class, and maternal mortality. British Medical Journal 293: 606–608
Loudon I 1987 Puerperal fever, the streptococcus and the sulphonamides. British Journal of Medicine 295: 485–490
Oxley W H F, Philips M H, Young J 1935 Maternal mortality in Rochdale. An achievement in a black area. British Medical Journal i: 304–307
Urquhart D R, Fisk N M 1988 Transvaginal ultrasound in suspected ectopic pregnancy. British Medical Journal 296: 465–466
Walker G 1986 Family planning, maternal mortality and literacy. Lancet ii: 162
WHO (1967) Manual of the international classification of diseases, injuries and causes of death. 8th revision, vol 1. WHO, Geneva
WHO (1975) Manual of the international classification of diseases, injuries and causes of death. 9th revision, vol 1. WHO, Geneva

SECTION 14

Spacing Pregnancies

79

John Guillebaud

Contraception and sterilization

INTRODUCTION

Eighty-seven million extra humans were born in 1987 and the annual excess of births over deaths is predicted to increase by a million a year for the foreseeable future (Population Data Sheet 1987). There can be no choice about eventual stabilization of human numbers on a finite planet — the only choice is whether birth rates come down or death rates are permitted to go up. Regrettably, the issues of population and planned parenthood still feature very low on international agendas.

No textbook of obstetrics would be complete without a section on this subject. It is estimated that before the end of this century 3000 million babies will be born. No trained person will be present at 2000 million of these deliveries and between 2 and 4 million women will die as a result. 'If this carnage occurred in one place, there would be an upsurge of humanitarian concern, but because the women die one at a time, the magnitude of the problem is not recognised' (Potts & Diggory 1983). Apart from the deaths, many women suffer avoidable morbidity such as fistulae. Perinatal and infant mortality and morbidity are also high.

These problems certainly require to be tackled by better obstetric and neonatal services, but their primary prevention by the integrated provision of voluntary and culturally acceptable family planning services is also essential.

About one-third of all pregnancies in the world are unwanted (Potts & Diggory 1983). Most of these are in older women of higher parity, precisely those who, along with their infants, are at greatest risk of death and injury in childbirth (Bernard et al 1980, Fortney et al 1986). If birth intervals are shorter than 2 years the babies are twice as likely (and the older sibling is 50% more likely) to die than if there is at least a 2-year interval (Maine & McNamara 1985). Control of unwanted fertility is a basic human freedom, and saves lives.

CONTRACEPTIVE COUNSELLING

Consideration of this issue should not be an afterthought: it should be initiated antenatally. Discussion can become more specific in the closing stages of the third trimester, particularly in those cases (ideally becoming less frequent), where postpartum sterilization is planned. The final choice and initiation of the method may otherwise be delayed until the puerperium. Counselling should be non-directive, with the obstetrician acting as an adviser and facilitator but never making the decisions. It is true that most women are more motivated towards family planning just after childbirth than at any other time, and in many parts of the world postnatal follow-up is weak or non-existent. While it may therefore be correct to strike while the iron is hot, caution is necessary: for all women this is a time of emotional turmoil in varying degrees, as well as one of rapidly changing hormonal status.

SEXUAL ACTIVITY IN PREGNANCY AND THE PUERPERIUM

This subject, of great relevance to the choice and successful use of contraception, has been well reviewed by Sapire (1986). There may be anxieties about causing miscarriage or congenital abnormalities, such fears being compounded by ignorance, old wives' tales and sometimes inappropriate medical advice. These days a very relevant, unspoken fear can be fear of the husband or partner's infidelity. Sexual satisfaction correlates with both partners feeling 'happy about the pregnancy' (Reamy et al 1982). Women who are less positive about sex show a marked decline in sexual behaviour during pregnancy, a longer period of abstinence after delivery and sometimes a diminished sexual response. Other important factors include religion, taboos, cultural customs about pregnancy and previous serious obstetric problems.

Female sexual desire and coital frequency decline during the third trimester. This is not only due to fear of injury or of precipitating labour but also to increasing awkwardness in finding suitable coital positions and discomfort, once the head is engaged. In some women (Reamy et al 1982) post-orgasmic contractions are sufficiently painful to discourage coitus.

After delivery, almost 50% of women have low levels of sexual interest for 3 months postpartum (Masters & Johnson 1966). Among primiparae, Robson et al (1981) reported reduced sexual activity for up to a year after delivery.

These and related aspects need discussion during pregnancy, since forewarned is forearmed. Restrictions on sexual activity should not be imposed without a sound obstetric reason. It may be helpful to advise about various non-coital options for expressing affection when coitus is contraindicated or not desired.

After delivery

Too many obstetricians forget that the emotional and sexual interaction of many couples is sometimes seriously affected by the birth of a baby. The onset of sexual dysfunction can often be traced back to this time. Sleepless nights, exhaustion and limited time together may contribute to sexual difficulties and may affect both partners (Sapire 1986). The man may resent exclusion from the intense bond between mother and baby, compounded by his wife's fatigue and diminished libido. This may be followed by prolonged abstinence, premature ejaculation or erectile impairment, reinforced by performance anxiety. In the woman, there may be multiple anxieties about the baby, about adjustment to motherhood, resentment to being tied down. All these can be worse if there is a true postpartum depression. Physical problems include breast and nipple tenderness, or dyspareunia due to pain at the site of a perineal tear or episiotomy, monilial vaginitis or diminished vaginal lubrication.

POSTNATAL SEXUAL PROBLEMS

Episiotomy

Meticulous surgical technique with subcuticular absorbable sutures is obviously important. Coitus should not take place until healing, which is usually well before the third week. If discomfort continues beyond 3 weeks, careful examination to detect a local painful nodule or narrowing of the introitus is indicated. Surgery can be curative but is rarely necessary earlier than 6 weeks. More usually, conservative management, by massage with KY or lignocaine jelly, manual stretching of the introitus by the woman herself and pubococcygeal muscle exercises (Kegel 1952), leads in time to full recovery.

Postpartum depression or psychosis

This is treated by supportive counselling, psychotherapy and antidepressants if indicated. Depression is frequently endogenous, but may also be exogenous as a result of stillbirth, congenital abnormality, miscarriage or induced abortion (see Chapter 65). Every effort should be made to ensure that the couple are brought closer together and not driven apart by guilt and blame. Choice of contraceptive will clearly be influenced: e.g. in severe depression combined oral or injectable contraception would often be postponed, partly to avoid accusations that the contraception aggravated the condition.

Lactation

Some women experience sexual arousal even to orgasm while breastfeeding (Kolodny et al 1979) and although this may improve the sexual relationship with the partner, in others it may become a substitute or may lead to guilt feelings. It may be helpful to counsel the woman that this arousal is normal and a reflex reaction to nature, as is any associated milk ejection.

Conclusion

Coitus should not be prohibited in an uncomplicated pregnancy as there is no evidence of risk to a healthy mother or fetus. There may be religious and cultural constraints: Jews and Muslims and some African cultures prohibit coitus for varying times after delivery. If there is a reason—whether physiological or pathological—to avoid intercourse, 'displays of affection, intimacy and caressing should be encouraged, with stimulation of the male partner, throughout pregnancy as well as in the puerperium. Both partners should be made aware of the physical and emotional changes that may occur, and supportive counselling should prevent dysfunction arising before and after delivery' (Sapire 1986).

RETURN OF FERTILITY FOLLOWING PREGNANCY

The requirement for contraception depends not only on the resumption of intercourse and its frequency, but also on the timing of the return of the woman's fertility. Unfortunately, despite much research (reviewed by McCann et al 1981

Table 79.1 Published studies indicating ovulation by day 30 postpartum in women who do not breastfeed

Reference	Number of women	Method to detect ovulation	Criteria	Day of earliest ovulation	Day of next menses	Luteal phase
Cronin (1968)	93	BBT (rectal temperatures)	BBT shift	Day 27	Day 41	13 days' raised BBT
				Day 28	Day 43	14 days' raised BBT
Lamotte (1972)	50 (25 with no hormones to suppress lactation)	Secretory EB at start of menses	14 days prior to day 1 of index menses—calculated retrospectively	Day 21	Day 35	No evidence about adequacy of luteal phase (?abnormal)
Hatherley (1985)	43	Urinary pregnanediol BBT/mucus	'Standard'	Day 30	Timing not reported	
Gray et al (1987)	22	Urinary PdG and luteal phase length	See text	Day 30	Day 43	13-day luteal phase
				Day 25	Day 30	5-day luteal phase (abnormal)

BBT = basal body temperature; EB = endometrial biopsy; PdG = pregnanediol-3α-glucuronide.

and in Chapter 62), it remains impossible to predict accurately the timing of the first fertile ovulation for any individual woman. This is due not only to normal biological variation, racial or genetic factors, but also to the effects of a series of items such as the nutritional status of the woman, the stage of gestation at which the pregnancy ended, whether the woman is breastfeeding and if so the timing, frequency and duration of nipple stimulation, the amount of supplementary feeding and the time elapsed since delivery.

In any population there exists an unpredictable minority whose fertility returns early and without warning. Since accurate methods for the detection of ovulation are relatively complex and expensive, good biological studies are few and tend to be small, with the effect that the subgroup of women most at risk of early ovulation after delivery may not happen to be recruited to the studies. Hence due notice must be taken of the very earliest times of ovulation reported (Table 79.1). They could be minimal estimates.

The first fertile ovulation

The relevant question is: 'What is the earliest postpartum day that ovulation may occur?' Among 60 non-lactating women McNeilly (personal communication) failed to detect an endocrinologically normal ovulation during the first 6 weeks after delivery. But Lamotte (1972) gives the earliest published estimate (Table 79.1) and quotes studies of variable quality whose estimates range between day 25 and day 30 (Kava et al 1968). In Table 79.1 perhaps the greatest attention should be paid to the estimates by Hatherley (1985) and Gray et al (1987) who used confirmatory hormone assays.

Gray et al defined an endocrinologically normal luteal phase as one lasting more than 8 days, with values above the lower 10th percentile for urinary pregnanediol-3α-glucuronide (PdG) in their own parallel study of 16 regularly cycling women. This implied a PdG peak value of >41 μg/ml and an area under the smoothed PdG luteal phase curve of >20 μg/ml. They found that 18 out of 22 first cycles were abnormal on these criteria. However, four were normal and of these one was the day 30 ovulation shown in Table 79.1. (Their very earliest case appeared to ovulate on day 25 with PdG detectable subsequently, but the peak was only 3.33 μg/ml and the luteal phase duration only 5 days.)

Although fertilization is the only proof that an ovulation is fertile, Table 79.1 suggests that by days 27–30 fertile ovulation could occur, in rare instances, and contraception should be started before this time.

It is even more difficult when attempting to answer the same question for lactating women, because the variability in intensity and frequency of baby-induced nipple stimulation is superimposed on woman-to-woman variation (see Chapter 62). Every published study shows the first ovulation occurring later in nursing than in non-nursing mothers: among 208 of the former, Hatherley (1985) reports the earliest endocrinologically normal first cycle ovulation on day 43 despite full lactation.

Implications for contraceptive advice

For family planning programmes, a balance has to be struck. A review of 17 studies reveals that if women wait for their first warning period anything from 0 to 19% of women may conceive (McCann et al 1981). Ovulation before the first menses is even commoner: according to Perez et al (1971,

1972) this occurred eventually in as many as 78% of 170 women who breastfed with varying intensity for variable times following delivery. On the other hand, if contraception is started too soon, associated risks may be borne by a majority of women (and their infants) quite unnecessarily; moreover, side-effects may lead to women giving up the contraceptive method and this has been known to reduce birth intervals. A scheme favoured by Family Health International (FHI) is to ask the following three questions:

1. Have menses resumed?
2. Has the baby begun any supplemental feedings?
3. Does the baby sleep through the night?

If the answer is *yes* to any one of these questions, contraception should begin (Network 1986).

At some time in the future it may become possible to avoid contraceptive overkill, when an individual woman can predict ovulation reliably far enough in advance to allow for the capriciousness of sperm survival. Meanwhile, most couples prefer the risks of starting contraception too early to those of unwanted pregnancy.

The data we have reviewed suggest that a method should be used from the start of the fourth week onwards by non-lactating women and if any artificial feeds are given. This may reasonably be increased to 6 weeks during amenorrhoea with full lactation, or longer if the FHI scheme is trusted.

After an induced first-trimester abortion the earliest luteinizing hormone (LH) peak was at day 16 in the study by Lâhteenmâki & Luukkainen (1978). Contraception is therefore commenced immediately, or at the time of first coitus if the method is intercourse-related. This applies to all methods, including the oestrogen-containing pill, since the risk of thrombosis at this time is small enough to be discounted.

Which contraceptive to choose after delivery

There is a Hobson's choice to be faced by all sexually active people. The dilemma is that all the reversible methods available now or likely to become available soon are either effective and convenient (non-coitally related) but potentially dangerous because of systemic actions, or virtually risk-free but less convenient and less effective (Guillebaud 1984). The only method which achieves all these ideals is sterilization under local anaesthesia; however, this lacks easy reversibility.

Efficacy of the methods

Table 79.2 shows user failure rates for the different methods. During full lactation with frequent nipple stimulation all the methods are 100% effective, and during partial lactation the efficacy will still be greater than is shown here. However, the choice of method must take into consideration the degree of efficacy desired after as well as before weaning.

Table 79.2 User failure rates for different methods of contraception per 100 woman-years (from Guillebaud 1985)

	Range in the world literature*
Sterilization	
Male	0–0.2
Female	0–0.5
Injectable (DMPA)	0–1
Combined pills	
50 μg oestrogen	0.1–1
<50 μg oestrogen	0.2–1
Intrauterine device	0.3–4
Progestogen-only pill	0.3–4
Diaphragm	2–15
Condom	2–15
Coitus interruptus	8–17
Spermicides alone	4–25
Fertility awareness	
Pre- plus postovulation	15–30
Postovulation alone	1–6
Contraceptive sponge	9–25
During lactation, first year, no method used	c. 10–20
No method, young women	c. 80–90
No method, at age 40	c. 40–50
No method, at age 45	c. 10–20
No method, at age 50	c. 0–5

*Excludes atypical studies giving particularly poor results, and all extended-use studies.
Data are ranked in order of efficacy, but there is an overlap of ranges. Better results are obtained, for any given degree of compliance, in older women.
DMPA = depot medroxyprogesterone acetate.

Two-way interaction

Lactation is capable of altering the profile of the advantages of nearly every method of contraception. There can be a two-way interaction. Lactation can affect contraceptives, for example by greatly increasing the efficacy of barriers and spermicides, but by increasing the risk of perforation at intrauterine device (IUD) insertion. Conversely, systemic contraceptives can affect lactation by altering the quantity and constituents of breast milk.

NATURAL FAMILY PLANNING

The fundamental problem of this approach, throughout reproductive life, is how to recognize fertile ovulation far enough in advance to allow for the capriciousness of survival of the very best among the millions of sperm deposited at intercourse.

The problem is compounded after pregnancy by the very variable effects of lactation, as discussed above.

The oestrogenic changes of increased quantity, clarity, fluidity, slipperiness, elasticity and good spinnbarkheit occur well in advance of the first fertile ovulation. Hence, if cervical mucus is used there are numerous false alarms. These take the form of either symptomatic oestrogen peaks associated with follicles which grow but fail to rupture normally (Flynn et al 1983) or cycles in which ovulation occurs — according to ultrasound and biochemical criteria — but the cycle would almost certainly be infertile, with inadequate luteal phase progesterones.

Thus users of natural family planning who begin mucus observations from the cessation of lochia and who do abstain or switch to another method from the very first appearance of oestrogenic mucus onwards will most probably avoid pregnancy. But they will also be avoiding unprotected intercourse for an unnecessarily long time. Changes in the cervix — dilation, softening and elevation away from the introitus — appear to comprise the most reliable clinical indicator, at present, of the first fertile ovulation (Flynn et al 1983). It remains to be confirmed whether the woman who disregards her mucus and waits for these observer-dependent changes will obtain sufficient warning in practice. To date newer techniques using various biochemical changes are equally disappointing for ovulation prediction.

The accuracy and user-friendliness of new methods of ovulation detection (e.g. by urine dipsticks detecting the LH surge by monoclonal antibody techniques) is improving fast, however, and the postovulatory phase is truly safe, once reliably identified (Guillebaud 1985). In current practice this is deemed to commence, in the postpartum period as at other times, once the woman has identified the two signals, namely the fourth evening after peak mucus day and the third morning when the basal body temperature is higher than a coverline 0.05°C above the preceding six temperatures, whichever is the later.

If natural family planning is to be used it is essential that candidates are well selected, they and their partners are properly taught, and the teaching is supplemented by diary cards, ideally using one of the excellent practical guides which are available (e.g. Flynn & Brooks 1984). Otherwise in practice, a high failure rate is observed.

BARRIER AND CHEMICAL METHODS

Sexual activity is often resumed by 3 weeks postpartum, depending on inclination, the amount of lochia and the degree of discomfort from any healing wounds or monilial infection. These factors also influence the choice and use of the vaginal barriers, which should be refitted as appropriate at any time from 2 weeks after the end of pregnancy, in order to assess both the changes in the fitting and the user's placement technique. The latter is the sine qua non of success, far more than detailed rules about spermicide use (Guillebaud 1985).

After this, the diaphragm and other vaginal barriers, the sheath, spermicide-impregnated sponges, and spermicides alone may be supplied without any important difference in the advice given as compared with other times. Indeed, their increased efficacy in the early months of physiological infertility justifies the use of sponges and foams, in particular, despite the high failure rates which apply in cycling women (Table 79.2).

One unresolved safety issue is that of spermicide absorption. When this occurs, the quantity is minute; it appears on reviewing 17 studies up to 1985 (Bracken 1985, Mills et al 1985) to have no proven teratogenic effects on the fetus. By analogy, it might be thought that there is no harm to the newborn child caused during breastfeeding; the infant is far less vulnerable than during organogenesis. There appear however to have been no formal studies of spermicide ingestion via human breast milk (Medline search performed 1987).

Currently a more important point is the advantage that spermicides have some bactericidal and viricidal properties (Cutler et al 1977, Hicks et al 1985). The latter is particularly of interest as the human immunodeficiency virus (HIV) becomes more prevalent. The sheath, ideally used with spermicide, is more protective, however, and is being increasingly used as a supplement to whatever contraceptive is chosen (Conant et al 1986). Even with condoms, as used in practice, HIV protection is not guaranteed.

INTRAUTERINE CONTRACEPTIVE DEVICES

Once a baby has been safely delivered, an IUD is often a good choice. The method is under a woman's control, requires motivation primarily at the time of insertion, is not intercourse-related, is highly effective (Table 79.2) and is reversible. IUDs have no extrapelvic systemic side-effects and do not influence milk volume or composition (McCann et al 1981).

Progestogen-releasing IUDs may be an exception to the last statement, since Heikkila et al (1982) found that 0.1% of a daily released dose of levonorgestrel 30 μg/day would enter the breast milk during full lactation. No deleterious effects have been demonstrated from this in either mother or child.

Mode of action

This is primarily at the uterine level, by multiple effects which prevent implantation (Sapire 1986). The action begins immediately. These two points are relevant in the late postpartum period, when an IUD may usefully be inserted up to 5 days after intercourse for contraception (Sapire 1986).

Copper devices have now largely superseded the older inert IUDs. They have lower pregnancy rates, higher continuation rates, and newer versions can be used without replacement for 10 or more years. Yet in the USA they were all withdrawn in January 1986 due to the complex financial and legal situation described, together with a comprehensive review of the method, in an excellent technical report (World Health Organization 1987). Fortunately in November 1987 common sense prevailed; Gynomed Pharmaceutical launched the Copper T 380A under licence from the Population Council.

Complications

Perforation

This is the major concern in relation to postpartum IUD insertion. Its frequency was as high as 1.8% in the series reported by Ratnam & Tow (1970). Heartwell & Schlesselman (1983) found this complication to be 10 times more frequent among lactating than in non-lactating women, regardless of the type of IUD used. Any extra risk is reducible by good technique (Newton & Gee 1985). Ideally, postpartum clinics should not be used routinely for training purposes, since lack of expertise by the inserting doctor markedly increases this risk.

Infection

Infection can be caused by lack of care during insertion, or exacerbated if uterine tenderness due to postpartum endometritis is overlooked. Sexually transmitted conditions pose the main threat, however, since most devices provide no protection. Good selection of potential IUD users is essential. As a matter of sound medicine, the sexual lifestyle of the woman and her partner should always be addressed during counselling. It is hoped, though not yet proven, that the risk of pelvic infection may be reduced by use of the new progestogen-releasing devices (Nilsson et al 1983), as well as by the recommendation to use adjunctive spermicides.

Other complications

Skilful insertion reduces not only perforation rates, but also the risk of malposition of the device within the uterine cavity. The latter can cause uterine pain or lost threads, and correlates with expulsion rates (partial or complete). It is also likely that many in situ pregnancies are caused by malpositioning of the device.

A highly practical application of the last paragraph concerns failed IUD pregnancies, when no device is found at the delivery. Too often it is assumed, with potentially dangerous consequences, that the last conception must have followed unrecognized expulsion. That diagnosis can only be made if, as a minimum, puerperal abdominopelvic X-rays have excluded perforation or embedment of the IUD.

Timing of IUD insertion

Good results are reported when this is between 4 and 8 weeks after delivery (Mishell & Roy 1982), as indeed is most widely practised. In the absence of breastfeeding, 4 rather than 8 weeks is preferable in view of the increasing likelihood of fertile ovulation. After lower segment Caesarean section (LSCS) the scar will have healed by 6 weeks, and is situated at the level of the internal os. After elective LSCS the cervical canal may require gentle dilatation, often with local anaesthesia, as for nulliparae.

Early postpartum insertion

Fears that with this practice, problems would occur with the lochia or with pelvic infection, have not been confirmed, although the expulsion rate is increased. In a study from Chile the 3-month expulsion rate in 1142 women fitted with copper-bearing IUDs (TCu-200) between 8 hours and 6 days after delivery was 32% compared with 5–15% for interval insertions (Liskin & Fox 1982). Better results can be obtained by more skilful operators, particularly at the most practical time in many programmes, which is just after delivery.

Immediate postplacental insertion. Immediate IUD insertion (within minutes of delivery) has a better outcome than subsequent insertion during the first few days of the puerperium (Brenner 1983). Newton et al (1977) reported a low and acceptable expulsion rate when conventional devices were placed correctly in the fundus using special long inserters, immediately after the delivery of the placenta. FHI recommends the technique shown in Fig. 79.1 using sterile ovum or ring forceps rather than any special inserter.

To reduce further the problem of early expulsion of IUDs it was proposed that the addition of projections of biodegradable material into the cross-arms of T-shaped devices would improve their retention when inserted within 10 minutes of delivery of the placenta. It was felt that chromic catgut might be a suitable material, but this was not confirmed in a multicentre trial. Some 310 TCu220C devices and 298 identical IUDs bearing two short catgut projections on each side were inserted into 608 women chosen by random allocation (Thiery et al 1983). Though no statistically significant difference was shown between the devices, at 3 months the gross cumulative expulsion rates were very creditable: namely 6.8 per 100 women for the catgut-bearing device and 7.5 per 100 women for the controls. Wathen et al (1978) similarly reported for unmodified Multiload Cu 250 devices that expulsions occurred in only 8.3% of women, all within the first 3 weeks after insertion. In none of these studies were any cases of acute sepsis or perforation reported.

It can be concluded that immediate postplacental insertion of modern copper-bearing devices is an entirely valid option which is too rarely exercised. It is the recommended approach for high-risk mothers in populations where women are not good at returning for postnatal care. Even if expulsion does occur, the risk of pregnancy is not as great during the puerperium as with the expulsion that follows interval insertion. Follow-up arrangements should be made so that those women who do attend may have their now elongated threads shortened. A new device may be inserted if partial or complete expulsion is noted.

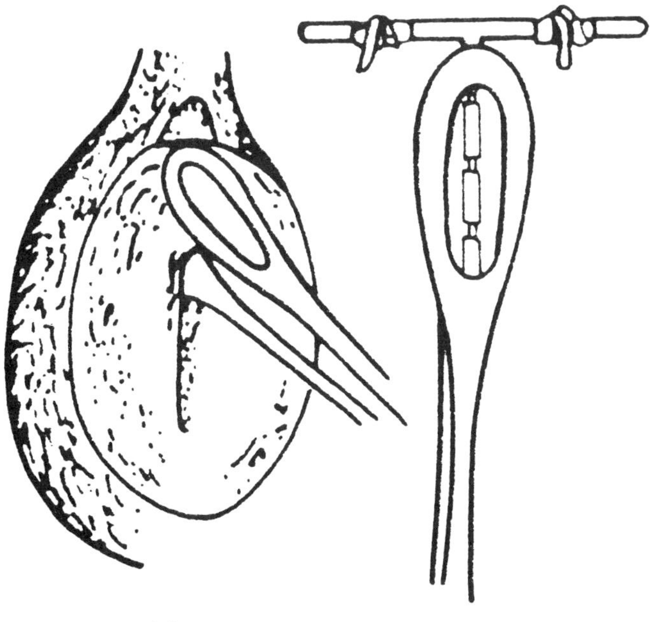

(a) (b)

Fig. 79.1 Family Health International (FHI) recommends the following technique for immediate postplacental insertion of an IUD in its clinical trials (Liskin & Fox 1982):

1. Grasp the anterior lip of the cervix at the 12 o'clock position with a sterile ring forceps (ovum or sponge-holding forceps; **a**).
2. With a second sterile ovum or ring forceps grasp the IUD (**b**) and close the lock of the forceps. Slip the distal portion of the string between the fourth and fifth fingers to keep the string straight.
3. Insert the IUD through the cervical canal. When it reaches the fundus, the operator will feel resistance. Place one hand on the abdomen and palpate the fundus to confirm that the IUD is placed as high in the uterine cavity as possible.
4. Once the IUD has reached the fundus, release the ring forceps holding the IUD, separate the blades and gently withdraw the forceps from the uterine cavity. During this procedure the strings of the IUD should not move. If more of the strings becomes visible, the IUD has dropped from its fundal placement. It must then be removed and reinserted.
5. Following removal of the ring forceps holding the IUD, release the ring forceps grasping the cervix.
6. Trim the strings 1.5 cm from the external os.

Immediate insertion after Caesarean section. Modern IUDs may similarly be inserted via the lower segment incision immediately the placenta has been delivered, with superb results reported from China (Chi et al 1986). The top of the device may be sutured at the uterine fundus with catgut, but this is not essential for good results.

Postabortion insertion. Studies have failed to confirm the increases expected in the rates of infection, perforation, expulsion, bleeding or pregnancy rates when IUDs are inserted immediately after evacuation following first-trimester abortion, whether spontaneous or induced (Liskin & Fox 1982). Expulsion rates are higher after evacuation for second-trimester abortion and the World Health Organization recommends copper-banded T-shaped devices to minimize this problem.

Despite the favourable reports, it is this author's opinion that in young women of low parity IUD insertions should be deferred to the follow-up clinic in populations which are at high risk of pelvic infection. This is because despite the greatest care at uterine evacuation, products of conception are retained in a high proportion of patients, as shown by ultrasound studies (Helm et al 1986).

Selection of method

Contraindications to some extent must be a matter of personal judgement.

Absolute contraindications

Some of these may be temporary, namely:

1. Undiagnosed irregular genital tract bleeding: uterine pathology, such as malignancy or retained products of conception, must first be excluded.
2. Pelvic infection; purulent discharge; acute vaginitis; tenderness on bimanual examination.
3. Pregnancy or suspicion of pregnancy.
4. Immunosuppression because of the infection risk and possible reduced efficacy.

Permanent contraindications

1. Past history of tubal ectopic pregnancy or current very high ectopic risk. This may be considered a relative contraindication for a woman with a family.
2. Distorted or too small uterine cavity (less than 5.5 cm on sounding).
3. True allergy to copper (Barramco 1972).

Relative contraindications

These can be found in any standard text (Guillebaud 1985) and mostly relate to the known complications threatening fertility. Heart lesions predisposing to bacterial endocarditis need special management (full antibiotic cover at insertion).

In conclusion, effective utilization of the IUD method requires:

1. Careful selection of the user, especially in regard to her own sexual lifestyle and that of her partner(s).
2. Detailed and appropriate counselling and education about the method and its possible side-effects.
3. Meticulous attention to detail at the time of insertion.
4. An open-house policy for all users who have subsequent queries or problems. Dealing promptly and effectively with unwanted effects is vital for the success of any IUD programme (Guillebaud 1980).

COMBINED ORAL CONTRACEPTIVES

Despite their efficacy, convenience and many other advantages, combined oral contraceptives (COCs) should ideally not be used during lactation (Guillebaud 1985). Most studies report some adverse impact on breastfeeding performance and milk volume composition (McCann et al 1981). A three-centre study by the World Health Organization compared the effects of a 30 μg oestrogen COC with a progestogen-only preparation and a control group. Women using the COC had a decline in milk volume of 42% after 18 weeks, whereas the progestogen-only contraceptive did not significantly affect the volume compared to controls (Tankeyoon et al 1984). Madhavepeddi & Ramachandran (1985) attributed breast enlargement in a breastfed infant to maternal ingestion of the 30 μg oestrogen COC. The latter is overtreatment anyway, since its oestrogen content is unnecessary for full contraception during lactation.

Table 79.3 Interval between delivery and pulmonary embolism following vaginal delivery from 1970 to 1981 (from DHSS 1986)

Interval	Number of cases	%
Less than 24 hours	8	13
1–7 days	18	30
7–14 days	9	15
15–42 days	25	42
Total	60	100

The weekly breakdown of the figures beyond the second week is not given but note:

1. The average would be 6 cases (10%) per week from 15–42 days.
2. The date of the causative thrombosis would be earlier than the embolism, often by many days. This implies that at least three out of four cases of thrombosis begin before day 21.

Timing of COC commencement in women who do not breastfeed

If a COC is started too late, some women will become pregnant before their first period. If it is started too early, there is the risk that the oestrogen content will increase the already increased risk of thromboembolism in the puerperium.

Despite this anxiety, one standard text recommends immediate postpartum use of oestrogen-containing pills (Hawkins & Elder 1979). Newton & Gee (1985) advised: 'non breast-feeders should start the pill between the first and second weeks', and Sapire (1986) and the British National Formulary (1987) both recommend starting after 2 weeks. Other authorities suggest 'early in the fourth week' (Guillebaud 1985) or make no definite recommendation (Family Planning Association 1981a, Potts & Diggory 1983). The pharmaceutical companies display similar uncertainty, as can be readily seen in the pages of the Data Sheet Compendium of APBI (1987). Advice ranges from that of Ortho-Cilag (1987), allowing COC initiation immediately postpartum, to that of Organon (1987) who suggest starting COCs 'on the first day of the first spontaneous menstruation or 4 to 6 weeks after delivery'. Much of this variation is related to fear of the complications of COCs.

Thromboembolism

Venous thromboembolism is a dangerous condition. In the last two Confidential Enquiries into Maternal Deaths (Department of Health and Social Security (DHSS) 1982, 1986), it was either the leading cause (1976–1978) or the second one (1979–1981). 'The most dangerous period seems to be the first seven days, then the second week, after which the risk falls' (Table 79.3). There are also reports of severe recurrent thromboembolism in higher-risk women when heparin prophylaxis in the puerperium was discontinued on the 10th day (Bonnar 1979) or at 3 weeks (de Swiet, personal communication).

The administration of oestrogens to suppress lactation has been clearly shown to increase this risk (Daniel et al 1967, Jeffcoate et al 1968). Both Howie et al (1975) and Gjonnaess et al (1975) showed that the puerperal haemostatic changes, which are interpreted as prothrombotic, were enhanced by oestrogens used in this way. Much larger doses than in current COCs were given, and they were unopposed by progestogen. Yet the COC had been prescribed to one fatal case in the 1976–1978 Confidential Enquiry (DHSS 1982) from 2 weeks after delivery. It is moreover well established epidemiologically that the oestrogen content of COCs correlates with the risk of venous thrombosis at any time (Stadel 1981).

There is a remarkable parallel between the haemostatic changes induced by pregnancy and those induced by the combined pill. If the increased coagulability of the blood of pill-takers is not associated with the usual compensatory increase in fibrinolytic activity, it is believed that clinical thrombosis is more probable (Stadel 1981).

Ideally COC-taking should not begin until the similar changes induced by pregnancy have returned to normality. This starts dramatically with delivery of the placenta, but fibrinogen concentrations actually increase at first until a decline starts around day 5 (Bonnar et al 1969, Bonnar 1979). Unfortunately there have been few serial studies beyond this first puerperal week. Near-normality by the postnatal visit at 6 weeks is well established (Howie et al 1975) and the factors studied by Gjonnaess et al (1975) were within the normal range at 4 weeks. Dahlman et al (1985) claimed that theirs was the first longitudinal study with weekly sampling during the normal puerperium. They found that both blood coagulation and fibrinolysis were significantly increased during the first 2 weeks, but by 3 weeks both were in general normal.

This literature may be interpreted as implying that oestrogen-containing pills should normally not be commenced earlier than day 21 of the puerperium, but this would be the optimum time for those perceived as being at high conception risk. In others, especially mildly overweight women, the starting day could reasonably be postponed to day 28 since, as shown earlier (Table 79.1) the risk of fertile ovulation is very low until beyond that time. If the COC is started any day before day 28, in routine cases no extra contraceptive precautions need be advised. Selective delay beyond 4 weeks using an alternative contraceptive may be safest where known risk factors apply, particularly in combination. These factors are obesity, operative delivery, especially Caesarean section, restricted activity, age above 35 and parity of four or more (DHSS 1982, 1986).

Preceding severe pre-eclampsia is a further associated factor in the database of the Confidential Enquiries (Turnbull, personal communication). Indeed, disturbances of coagulation including a rebound elevation of the platelet count have been observed 6 weeks postnatally in such cases (Redman, personal communication). Ideally therefore after severe pre-eclampsia the COC should be avoided until at least 8 weeks after delivery.

Hypertension

It has been thought that women with previous pregnancy-induced hypertension will be unusually prone to oral contraceptive-induced hypertension. In an important study by Pritchard & Pritchard (1977), blood pressure was measured before and during use of the COC in 180 young primiparous women with recent overt pre-eclampsia or eclampsia. Their subsequent mean systolic and diastolic blood pressures varied from no higher to only very slightly higher than those of 200 nulligravid women using the same formulation. The diastolic blood pressures rose to exceed 90 mmHg in nine of the women who were previously hypertensive late in their first pregnancies, compared to a similar rise in five of the nulligravid women. A total of 56 of the studied women were followed during a second pregnancy: 40 of them remained normotensive throughout, as they had been when they took the COC. Of the 16 who again developed pre-eclampsia, all but two had been normotensive while on the COC. It was concluded that the basis of hypertension that reappeared early during COC use as well as during pregnancy was underlying chronic vascular disease (essential hypertension).

Pre-eclampsia appears to have an unrelated mechanism. If it was severe at the preceding delivery, COC-taking should be delayed for at least 8 weeks; however, the past history does not otherwise contraindicate judicious use of the COC method with careful subsequent blood pressure monitoring.

Trophoblastic disease and choriocarcinoma

Stone et al (1976) found that among 611 women who had had a hydatidiform mole, the need for subsequent chemotherapy was increased two- to threefold among women who had taken oral contraceptives. COCs also delayed the fall in human chorionic gonadotrophin (hCG) excretion in women who did not need chemotherapy. This COC-related delay was not shown in a study of 194 patients from Vancouver (Yuen & Birch 1983). There are insufficient data in the latter study to rule out an effect, particularly of progestogen. Bagshawe's unit believes this may be of greater importance (Dent, personal communication). They continue to recommend that neither oestrogen nor progestogen preparations (including under this heading injectables and hormone replacement therapy) should be taken between the evacuation of a trophoblastic tumour and the return to normality of gonadotrophin values. Once hCG is undetectable, first in urine and confirmed in serum, contraceptive steroids are permitted for the remainder of the follow-up period.

This is a prudent policy, although it is not established that the modern ultralow-dose COCs would pose a significant risk. The data do not suggest that oral contraceptives increase the initial risk of trophoblastic disease itself.

Overall benefits and risks of the COC

These are discussed at length elsewhere (Potts & Diggory 1983, Guillebaud 1985, Sapire 1986). The risks of circulatory disease are well established, though reduced with modern low-dose preparations. The risk of venous disease relates to the oestrogen content, whereas that of arterial disease, including hypertension, relates to both oestrogen and progestogen.

The issue of carcinogenesis is a long way from being resolved; the literature is copious, complex and contradictory (Drife & Guillebaud 1986). The greatest difficulty relates to the phenomenon of latency (McPherson et al 1986). Best established is the protective influence of COCs on carcinoma of the endometrium and carcinoma of the ovary:

> Populations using the pill may develop different benign or malignant neoplasms from non-users, but there is no proof that the *overall* risk of either type of neoplasia is increased. (It could even be reduced, but there is no proof of that either) (Guillebaud 1985).

Absolute contraindications to COC use

The following are usually considered absolute contraindications (Guillebaud 1985):

Past or present circulatory disease

1. Past arterial or venous thrombosis of any kind.
2. Ischaemic heart disease or angina.
3. Severe or combined risk factors for arterial disease, including established hypertension.
4. Abnormal lipid profile, predisposing to atherogenesis.
5. Known thrombogenic abnormality of coagulation or fibrinolysis.
6. Other conditions predisposing to thrombosis, including 4 weeks before and a minimum of 2 weeks after elective major surgery, during immobilization of the lower limbs after trauma or any varicose vein treatment.
7. Crescendo migraine, migraine with focal abnormalities or visual field loss.

Table 79.4 Risk factors for arterial cardiovascular system disease

Nature of risk factor	Absolute contraindication	Relative contraindication	Remarks
Family history (FH) of arterial disease (heart attack or stroke) in a first-degree relative <45 years	Known atherogenic lipid profile (or strong FH and not able to be tested)	Normal blood lipid profile (or first attack was in family member over age 45 years)	If available, arrange plasma lipids if first attack in family member <45 years
Diabetes mellitus (DM)	Severe, or diabetic complications present (e.g. retinopathy, renal damage)	Not severe/labile, and no complications, young patient with short duration of DM	POP usually better choice of hormonal method
Hypertension	Diastolic blood pressure (BP) ⩾95 mmHg on repeated testing	Diastolic BP 85–95 mmHg	POP better choice
Cigarette smoking	⩾50 cigarettes/day	5–50 cigarettes/day	
Increasing age	Non-smokers ⩾45 years	Non-smokers 35–45 years	Smokers should avoid/discontinue oral contraceptives 10 years earlier
Excess weight	>50% above ideal for height	20–50% above ideal	

POP = progestogen-only pill.
Some of the numbers selected are of necessity a little arbitrary.

8. Transient cerebral ischaemic attacks causing focal abnormalities even without headaches.
9. Most types of valvular heart disease; pulmonary hypertension, with or without heart disease.

Diseases of the liver

1. Active liver disease; cholestatic jaundice of pregnancy or with previous steroid hormone treatment; congenital disorders of hepatic excretion.
2. Past liver neoplasm.
3. Gallstones — but not if past cholecystectomy.
4. The porphyrias.

History of serious condition affected by sex steroids or related to previous COC use

Possible pregnancy

Undiagnosed genital tract bleeding

Steroid-dependent neoplasms — discuss with the oncologist involved.

The woman's own continuing ambivalence about the safety of the method, even after full counselling

Note that the last four categories are not necessarily permanent.

Relative contraindications

These are listed in standard texts and follow from the known risks (Guillebaud 1985, Sapire 1986). The most important relate to risk factors for arterial disease (Table 79.4). Note that these can be absolute contraindications if severe enough or if more than one applies, for example a diabetic woman who also smokes.

Myths about method selection

Media-induced and sometimes doctor-induced myths about risks of this method abound. With modern ultralow-dose combined pills the following conditions are not contraindications despite previous medical concern:

1. Past secondary amenorrhoea, whether or not after previous COC treatment (Jacobs 1987).
2. Healthy non-smokers above 35 (Kay 1983).
3. Sickle cell trait. Even frank sickle cell disease is not now considered to contraindicate the COC in all cases (Freie 1983), although an oestrogen-free preparation is more commonly chosen.
4. Uncomplicated varicose veins. These are of relevance only if there has been past superficial venous thrombosis or phlebitis.
5. Fibroids. Ross et al (1986) showed that these are less rather than more likely to become symptomatic in users of modern pills.
6. Monilial vaginitis (Davidson & Oates 1985).
7. History of pre-eclampsia.
8. Trophoblastic disease subsequent to hCG being undetectable.

Choice of formulation and subsequent monitoring

All modern low-dose preparations contain the same oestrogen (ethinyloestradiol). In recent studies, the newer progestogens (desogestrel and gestodene), in combination with oestrogen, have been shown to be associated with fewer potentially atherogenic changes in carbohydrase and lipid metabolism than either norethisterone or levonorgestrel. Hence although the very lowest doses of the latter (as in the triphasics) are acceptable (Gaspard 1987), it is to be expected that desogestrel and gestodene-containing pills will be increasingly chosen, most particularly for women with risk factors (Table 79.4). Given the enormous individual variability in blood levels of both hormones (Back et al 1981), and the fact that low blood levels tend to manifest themselves at the uterine end-organ by breakthrough bleeding, this author has proposed (Guillebaud 1985) that each woman should be given the lowest dose formulation of a chosen progestogen that her uterus will allow. Thus at follow-up, if breakthrough bleeding occurs the next choice will be a higher-dose preparation containing the same progestogen; however, if the bleeding pattern is normal a trial will be made of a lower dose, if it is available. Each woman should finally be maintained for the long term on the preparation that is just (but only just) above her own threshold for the annoying symptom of abnormal bleeding.

If non-bleeding side-effects supervene there are two empirical rules to be followed; lowering the dose of both hormones to the greatest extent possible or switching to the use of a different progestogen. For the management of specific symptoms see Guillebaud (1985).

Follow-up

In any good programme, women should be seen initially at 3 months and subsequently at 6- to 12-monthly intervals. The frequency of visits should be increased in those with relative contraindications, or upon request for advice or reassurance. There are three main purposes of this follow-up:

1. To act on the appearance of new risk factors.
2. To monitor blood pressure. Combined pills should be discontinued if systolic blood pressure exceeds 160 mmHg or diastolic blood pressure exceeds 95 mmHg on repeated measurement. However, another method may be advised at lower levels, bearing in mind that mild hypertension may act as a higher risk marker of circulatory disease.
3. If migraine becomes severe, or is associated with symptoms of transient cerebral ischaemia, a non-oestrogen-containing type of contraceptive should be substituted (Guillebaud 1985).

PROGESTOGEN ONLY CONTRACEPTION

The progestogen only pill

The progestogen only pills (POPs) are useful but little used and even less studied. Taken on a continuous daily basis their main contraceptive actions are believed to be on cervical mucus and endometrium. They have also considerable but varying effects on the pituitary and ovary (Landgren & Diczfalusy 1980). The spectrum runs from no interference with the ovarian cycle through to abolition of all follicular activity. This explains the very varied menstrual pattern, which can be regular, chaotic or absent. Even in those with a regular bleeding pattern interference with fertile ovulation can usually be shown (Howie, personal communication).

Advantages and indications

The main advantage of the method is the very small dose of hormone being taken. Moreover, although progestogen alone is given, in most women this is not unopposed because of endogenous oestrogen from the ovaries. Aside from bleeding irregularities, side-effects are few and there is minimal alteration in metabolic variables. Efficacy is good, in the range 0.3 to 4 per 100 woman-years; the higher efficacy applies to older women (Fotherby 1982, Graham & Fraser 1982).

Effect on lactation

Unlike the combined pill, POPs have not been found to impair the quantity or (in most studies) the quality of breast milk, (McCann et al 1981). Some progestogen enters the breast milk, but the quantity is very small — 0.1% or less of the dose to the mother in 600 ml of milk (Nilsson & Nygren 1979). This equals one tablet received by the baby in 1000 days of lactation. Most women appreciate that it is unlikely, though not impossible, that this would cause any harm.

Timing of postpartum use

Since there is no anxiety about enhancing the risk of thrombosis, it has usually been suggested that the POP should be commenced in the early puerperium (British National Formulary 1987) or 7 days postpartum (Family Planning Association 1981b). However, studies have shown an increased risk of puerperal breakthrough bleeding in POP users, despite the expectation that they should have amenorrhoea during lactation (Hawkins & Elder 1979, Howie personal communication). It is therefore now suggested that breastfeeding women should begin to take the POP at about 3 weeks after delivery. Hawkins & Tothill (1979) reported that discontinuations for bleeding problems were halved by POP treatment initiated later (actually at 6 weeks) compared with the group of women who commenced it at 1 week postpartum.

Artificial feeding

Most women who do not breastfeed elect for the convenience and efficacy of the combined pill (see above). If the POP is chosen it could be commenced any time from delivery until 3 weeks and certainly no later than the fourth week, for fear of early fertile ovulation. Breakthrough bleeding problems may again be commoner if it is started earlier. Any amenorrhoeic woman in whom cyesis has definitely been excluded by a series of negative pregnancy tests may start the POP at any time, with 7 days' additional contraceptive precautions (Guillebaud 1985).

Indications

1. Lactation — at the woman's choice when a hormonal method is preferred.
2. Older women, especially smokers.
3. Diabetes mellitus — this is the hormonal method of choice in diabetics, whose compliance is particularly good since they take their POP with their evening insulin (Steel & Duncan 1981).
4. Hypertension. There is no evidence that progestogens given alone have a hypertensive effect, though a small increase in blood pressure occurs among women with previous COC-induced hypertension (Wilson et al 1984).
5. Migraine with focal symptoms due to transient cerebral ischaemia (oestrogens are contraindicated).
6. Past oestrogen-linked side-effects, including previous episodes of thrombosis. It is a myth that this past history contraindicates progestogen-only modalities of contraception.

Absolute contraindications

1. The presence of severe arterial disease or a high risk of the same (e.g. angina).
2. Serious side-effects not clearly linked to oestrogen.
3. Undiagnosed irregular bleeding.
4. Pregnancy or a suspicion of pregnancy.
5. Trophoblastic disease.
6. The woman's own continuing uncertainty about POP safety for her or for her breastfeeding child, even after full counselling.

There is also a strong relative contraindication which is specific to the POP, namely a past history of ectopic pregnancy (Tatum & Schmidt 1977). During lactation, if in conjunction with the POP ovulation is completely suppressed, ectopics are impossible. After weaning however, the woman's one precious remaining tube deserves maximum protection, e.g with the COC or an injectable.

Relative contraindications

The method should normally be avoided by patients with malabsorption syndromes or who are being treated with enzyme-inducing drugs, which predispose to pregnancy, since the dose of progestogen is already so low.

Another important relative contraindication is a history of functional ovarian cyst formation. These cysts have been shown to be commoner in POP users (Tayob et al 1986).

Choice of formulation and monitoring

As with the COC, there are no firm guidelines. Neogest is best avoided since it gives a useless dose of non-contraceptive dextronorgestrel. Otherwise, especially recalling the complex and unpredictable interaction between the POP and the woman's menstrual cycle, the initial choice of POP brand has to be arbitrary. Should bleeding or other side-effects occur, the change of brand to an alternative is also made empirically.

Maintenance of contraceptive efficacy

There are multiple contraceptive effects but one of the important ones is reduction in the sperm penetrability of cervical mucus. This effect is readily lost — hence the importance of regular POP-taking. Moreover the woman's regular time for pill-taking should preferably not be the same as her most frequent time for intercourse.

Although readily lost, the mucus effect is quickly restored. It is advised that POP users who are more than 3 hours late in taking their tablet should return to regular pill-taking but use additional contraception for the next 48 hours (Mills 1987).

Follow-up

It is usual to check blood pressure and weight and re-check at 3 and 6 months. Careful instruction is important about abdominal pain: in POP users this could herald either an ectopic pregnancy or the formation, torsion, or rupture of a functional ovarian cyst.

Injectable contraception

Two progestogens are currently given by regular deep intramuscular injection: depot medroxyprogesterone acetate (DMPA) 150 mg i.m. every 10–12 weeks, and norethisterone enanthate (NET-EN) 200 mg i.m. every 8 weeks. The latter is not licensed for long-term use in the UK but may nevertheless be used in good faith in selected cases (Sapire 1986).

Advantages

DMPA has been licensed since 1984 for use after full counselling by selected women who are unsuitable for the alternatives. The information leaflet supplied by the manufacturer should always be given, since it has been recognized by the Committee on Safety of Medicines. The advantages of injectables include: extremely high contraceptive effectiveness; most of the non-contraceptive benefits of the COC, particularly the reduction in pelvic infection (Gray 1985); a reduction in menstrual disorders in many women, with reduced risk of anaemia; and a reduction in the frequency of crises in those with sickle cell disease (de Ceulaer et al 1982).

Studies to date show no clinically important changes in carbohydrate metabolism, liver function or haemostasis. A moderate reduction in high density lipoprotein cholesterol has been reported, but the significance of this is unknown

(Kremer et al 1980). Despite the controversy about its medical safety, there are 15 million past and present users in 80 countries and no deaths have been attributed to DMPA — a statement that cannot be made about the combined pill.

Mechanisms

As with the COC there are multiple contraceptive effects. Ovulation is inhibited, but there is some endogenous oestrogen activity with oestradiol levels comparable to the early follicular phase, rising significantly towards the end of the injection period. Oestrogen deficiency is thereby avoided in most cases.

Use in lactation

Most studies of DMPA show either no change or an improvement in both quantity of milk and duration of lactation. The concentrations of lipids and proteins are the same as or higher than in non-users (McCann et al 1981, Liskin & Quillin 1983, Sapire 1986). Both DMPA and NET-EN and their metabolites cross from maternal plasma into breast milk, to a greater extent than with the POP. Dahlberg (1982) has calculated that a child would have to breastfeed for 3 years to receive as much DMPA as the mother receives in 1 day. More germanely, Sapire (1986) quotes several long-term studies of children exposed in infancy to injectables via the breast milk. To date, no morbidity and no adverse effects on growth have been found.

Timing of the first dose

Since in some countries contact with the medical personnel may be limited to delivery, the first dose of DMPA is often given within 48 hours of delivery. Injectables do not increase the risk of puerperal thrombosis and may even benefit lactation. Apart from this being much earlier than necessary for contraception, it has been noted that such early administration increases the likelihood of heavy and prolonged bleeding (Murphy 1979, Wilson 1985). Hence the first dose is now preferably delayed to 6 weeks postpartum.

Indications

1. Where a systemic method is preferred but other options are contraindicated, disliked, or unlikely to be successfully used: hence women at high risk of thrombosis, and unreliable pill-takers.
2. An excellent alternative to the IUD in women at high risk of pelvic infection.
3. In mentally handicapped women, particularly where premenstrual aggression, mood swings and increased epileptic attacks occur (Wilson 1985).
4. In sickle cell disease and to treat endometriosis.

Disadvantages and contraindications

Perhaps the greatest disadvantage is the need to reassure potential users in the face of the unjustified bad name this method has been given by adverse publicity in many countries.

For example, fears concerning breast cancer were raised when an increased incidence of benign and malignant breast nodules was noted in beagle bitches treated with DMPA. However, it is now known that beagles are particularly susceptible to progestogenic stimuli, and the resulting tumours are quite unlike human breast tumours. Most authorities have concluded that beagle dogs always were an inappropriate animal model. Moreover a World Health Organization case control study (Liskin et al 1987) of 1500 cases and 5800 controls in three countries found no link at all between DMPA use and cancer of the breast or of the endometrium, ovary or liver.

It is essential to counsel a potential user that the injection cannot be removed once given, so that it is irreversible for at least 2–3 months if early side-effects occur. Related to this is the well known delay in return of fertility. However, there is no evidence whatever of permanent impairment (Fraser 1982). In a Thai study of over 1300 women, following the first omitted dose of DMPA 95% of ex-users had conceived by 24 months — an identical rate to that of ex-users of the IUD or COC (Liskin & Quillin 1983).

Forewarned is forearmed about menstrual disturbance — the positive advantages of amenorrhoea can be stressed. Weight gain is the commonest non-menstrual side-effect but headaches, depression, loss of libido, acne and other progestogenic side-effects are reported.

Absolute contraindications

More caution is necessary than with the POP because the dose is larger and reversibility is slower. The following are absolute contraindications:

1. Past severe arterial disease or current very high risk, including current angina.
2. Serious side-effects previously occurring on the COC and not clearly due to oestrogen, e.g. liver adenoma.
3. Undiagnosed abnormal genital tract bleeding.
4. Pregnancy, whether known or suspected.
5. Recent trophoblastic disease.
6. The woman's uncertainty, which includes plans for new pregnancy within 1 year.

Relative contraindications

1. Lesser degrees of arterial disease risk (heavy smoking above the age of 40, hypertension controlled by treatment).
2. Diabetes, though the POP is preferable.
3. Steroid-dependent cancer. Take the advice of the oncologist.

4. Active liver disease: the method can be used with careful monitoring in the presence of abnormal liver function.
5. Other chronic systemic diseases. Prescribe with caution since, as with the COC, proof of absence of an adverse effect on the condition is rarely available.
6. Unacceptability of menstrual irregularities.
7. Severe obesity.
8. Severe depression.
9. In the years preceding the menopause: irregular bleeding may lead to an unnecessary curettage, among other concerns (Guillebaud 1985).

Choice of preparation

DMPA is more widely available, more effective, with longer action but slower reversibility. NET-EN is more painful as an injection but more readily reversible. It is possibly a more appropriate choice for nulliparous women, those who plan a child in the near future and those who will not tolerate amenorrhoea. With counselling, amenorrhoea is however the best state for many women and occurs with DMPA in over half the users at 1 year.

Monitoring and follow-up

A careful history and examination including cervical cytology, blood pressure and weight will exclude the contraindications. At the time of each injection the woman should be given an opportunity to discuss side-effects or problems. Weight and blood pressure should be checked annually.

Management of unacceptable bleeding

The woman must be examined to exclude retained products of conception and cervical pathology, including neoplasia. 'Bleeding from a firm, well involuted, non-tender uterus with a closed os is almost certainly not associated with significant pathology' (Wilson 1985). The next injection may be given early (though arbitrarily this is avoided within 4 weeks of the previous dose). The object of this exercise is to achieve amenorrhoea. Alternatively oestrogen can be given if not contraindicated — for example, Premarin 1.25 mg daily for 21 days.

CONTRACEPTIVE IMPLANTS AND RINGS

These new approaches share many of the advantages of injectables, including the avoidance of major impact on the liver from hormones taken via the oral route (the first-pass effect). In addition they give more stable blood levels and avoid the problem of reversibility, with regard to side-effects and return of fertility (Liskin & Quillin 1983).

Implants

Many versions, some in combination with oestrogen, are under investigation. The progestogen only one likely to achieve widespread availability in the near future is the Norplant system. Six silastic implants about the size of a matchstick are inserted with local anaesthesia under the skin of the upper arm. They slowly release levonorgestrel in a dose initially of 50 μg falling to 30 μg daily. Available data suggest efficacy greater even than that of DMPA and very high acceptability and continuation rates for 5 or more years. The method is rapidly reversible on surgical removal of the implants: 77% of women who discontinued Norplant conceived a planned pregnancy within 1 year (Liskin & Quillin 1983).

Use in lactation

Like DMPA, the progestogen enters the breast milk but does not adversely affect its quantity or quality. Pending more data, it is currently advised that Norplant is not inserted during lactation until 6 months after delivery (Network 1986).

Unwanted effects

Metabolic effects have been small, within the normal range, and mostly of no clinical importance. As with DMPA, the effects of the artificial progestogen are balanced by ovarian follicular activity. However, high density lipoprotein cholesterol is moderately depressed and functional ovarian cysts can occur (Diaz et al 1979). Infection at the site of the implants has also been reported. The main disadvantage of the method is the occurrence of menstrual disturbance.

Contraindications

These are as described for injectables with the latitude provided by immediate reversibility. An annual visit is probably sufficient for monitoring purposes, provided the user has rapid access to medical care when desired.

Contraceptive rings

These share the advantages of implants, with the addition that reversibility is under the woman's control (Liskin & Quillin 1983). The most widely tested versions are those sponsored by WHO, releasing 20 μg/day levonorgestrel for either 3 months or 1 year.

Efficacy is less than Norplant, with a failure rate of around 3 per 100 women-years. Metabolic effects are minimal; the progestogen is balanced by ovarian activity. There are the usual problems of functional ovarian cyst formation and bleeding irregularities. Other versions using newer progestogens, alone or with oestrogens, are being evaluated.

Use in lactation

This should be acceptable, but the advice for Norplant is appropriate until the safety of the method for both mothers and infants has been fully tested.

STERILIZATION

No long-term deleterious effects have been confirmed after either vasectomy (Liskin et al 1983, Petitti 1986) or female sterilization (Liskin & Rinehart 1985). The procedures themselves are minor and readily performed under local anaesthesia — but the decisions are major.

Counselling

Despite improvements in reversibility, these methods must be based on the premise of permanence and its implications, especially in the young. Counselling should begin during the preceding pregnancy, and the issue rarely, if ever, raised for the first time in the puerperium. The risk of failure of operations in either sex, however performed, must always be mentioned but put in perspective. In vasectomy, this can be even after two negative sperm counts (Philp et al 1984). The possibility of subsequent coincidental gynaecological problems, especially if the woman has used oral contraception prior to the pregnancy, must be assessed and discussed. However, Caesarean hysterectomy, which has a vogue in some countries, is not recommended solely to avoid these problems.

Who should be operated on?

Once the couple are sure after counselling that sterilization is appropriate, the main consideration is the possible impact of future loss of the partner. Though there are exceptions, most women in their late 30s have reached a decision which would remain valid even after remarriage. If the woman remarries more than 10–15 years later, the issue of reversibility becomes academic in any case. Men, on the other hand, remain fertile for many more years, and although their own views about future parenting may be definite, neither they nor the counsellor can assess the all-important views of any future female partner. Moreover, older men do in fact remarry more frequently than older women, and commonly marry women still in their childbearing years. With regards to younger women (in their late 20s and early 30s), if sterilization is performed at all in these couples, vasectomy is often the better choice — it is then more important to preserve the future childbearing options of the present wife. Thus although she often presents herself, the obstetrician should always ensure that the alternative of vasectomy has been discussed by the couple. The right operation must be performed on the right person at the right time.

Timing of the procedure

It is often convenient for all concerned if the woman is sterilized in the puerperium and if so, the earlier the better, before lactation is fully established. But the decision is more commonly regretted at this time of emotional instability for many couples (Winston 1977). So there is a welcome trend to offering the alternative of laparoscopic sterilization as an interval procedure 8–12 weeks postpartum. There then remains the risk of early death of the latest child (e.g. by the sudden infant death syndrome).

Many vasectomy services prefer to defer the procedure until the youngest child is 6–12 months of age. It is not clear why such caution is less commonly observed by obstetricians in regard to female sterilization. Female sterilization is immediately effective, whereas after vasectomy additional contraceptive precautions must be practised for 3–4 months before two sperm counts confirm success of the method.

Procedures

The procedures are well described in review articles: for vasectomy, see Blandy (1979) & Liskin et al (1983); procedures for the female are well reviewed by Liskin & Rinehart (1985) and Newton & Gee (1985). Techniques cannot be learnt from books — they must be acquired by repeated performance under supervision. Laparoscopy is unsuitable in the immediate postpartum period, although it may be performed safely after 4–6 weeks.

Of other options, minilaparotomy under local anaesthesia is the safest procedure. After involution of the uterus, a minilaparotomy requires a 3 cm incision just above the pubic hairline. The margins of the incision are separated with retractors and, with the aid of a uterine elevator, part of each Fallopian tube is delivered digitally or with a tissue-holding forceps. It may then be occluded by ligation and excision of a short segment.

Alternatively, using a vaginal speculum in the wound, the tube may be occluded in situ using either the Falope ring or a clip. The enlarged tubes found postpartum are easily torn by the application of the ring; the Filshie titanium–silastic clip can better accommodate such tubes than the Hulka-Clemens spring-loaded variety (Newton & Gee 1985). As the enclosed tubal tissue atrophies, the silicone rubber lining to the titanium clip expands, preventing the development of a fistula.

In the first days after delivery a slightly different procedure is very satisfactory. A curved incision 2–3 cm long is made in the lower margin of the umbilicus. The uterus is mobilized manually through the abdominal wall to bring each tube to the incision for its occlusion by one of the methods just described (Kleinman 1982).

Anaesthesia

Direct infiltration local anaesthesia is much safer and cheaper and allows the woman to leave the clinic or hospital 2 hours after surgery, whether by laparoscopy or minilaparotomy. Ideally general anaesthesia should be reserved for the excessively anxious, the obese, and those women likely to have pelvic adhesions.

Contraindications

There are few absolute medical contraindications to minilaparotomy postpartum, or later to interval laparoscopy, provided the woman can tolerate surgery. Active peritoneal infection should first be treated. Previous abdominal surgery or infection may cause adhesions but these are not an absolute contraindication: minilaparotomy is then safer. As with obesity, it may be necessary to enlarge the incision (Liskin & Rinehart 1985). Large fibroids, menorrhagia or marked prolapse must be detected, since these would indicate sterilization by an abdominal or vaginal hysterectomy.

The complex and contradictory literature about the post-tubal ligation syndrome of gynaecological complaints, particularly abnormal menstrual bleeding, is thoroughly reviewed by Liskin & Rinehart 1985. There were no significant differences after 6 years, in one of the largest prospective studies to date, between 2243 sterilized and 3551 unsterilized women, in rates of hospital referral for a wide range of gynaecological conditions including hysterectomy (Vessey et al 1983).

Complications

These should occur in only 1–2% of cases (Liskin & Rinehart 1985). They may include uterine perforation, mesosalpingeal tears if rings are used, haematoma, trauma to the bladder, especially at minilaparotomy, and wound infection. Major morbidity and deaths attributable to female sterilization are rare. They are mainly associated with general anaesthesia, and with gas embolism or laceration of major vessels or bowel during laparoscopy. The mortality risk associated with childbearing is far higher: it has been estimated in Bangladesh, for example, that one maternal death is prevented by every 100 sterilizations (Grimes et al 1982).

Effectiveness

The failure rate of female sterilization is higher when the procedure is performed postpartum or postabortion. Among 9399 women sterilized by diathermy or rings, the rate of pregnancies per 100 women was 0.4 after interval sterilization, 0.8 postabortion, rising to 1.4 after postpartum sterilization (Chi et al 1981). Among the resulting pregnancies, tubal ectopics are commoner: the rate is 1:8 overall (Tatum & Schmidt 1977) or 1:14 for the first year, increasing to 1:2 for failures in the third and subsequent years (Vessey et al 1983).

CONCLUSIONS

Most of the available birth control options can be offered and motivation to employ contraception may be high after recent childbirth. To ensure the best choice for each couple, the obstetrician must be fully informed about the two-way interaction of the various methods with the puerperium in general and lactation in particular. Among specific points, attention has been drawn to the advisability of delaying commencement of hormonal contraception to reduce the opposite risks of thrombosis with the oestrogen-containing combined pill and of breakthrough bleeding with progestogen-only pills or injections. Delaying the start of contraception until the first menses or the postnatal visit risks conception in a minority. Above all, a good doctor will neglect neither the particular — local physical healing after vaginal delivery — nor the general, such as the psychosexual aspects of the couple's relationship.

REFERENCES

Back D J, Breckenridge A M, Crawford F et al 1981 Interindividual variation and drug interaction with hormonal steroid contraceptives. Drugs 21: 46–61

Barramco V P 1972 Dermatitis caused by internal exposure to copper. Archives of Dermatology 106: 386–387

Bernard R P, Kendal E M, Manton K G 1980 International maternity care monitoring: a beginning. In: Aladjem A K, Brown A K, Sure A U (eds) Clinical perinatology. C V Mosby, St Louis

Blandy J P 1979 Vasectomy. British Journal of Hospital Medicine 21: 520–527

Bonnar J 1979 Gynaecology, venous thromboembolism and pregnancy. In: Stallworthy J, Bourne G (eds) Recent advances in obstetrics and gynaecology, no. 13. Churchill Livingstone, London, pp 173–192

Bonnar J, McNichol G P, Douglas A S 1969 Fibrinolytic enzyme system and pregnancy. British Medical Journal 3: 387–389

Bracken M B 1985 Spermicidal contraceptives and poor reproductive outcomes: the epidemiologic evidence against an association. American Journal of Obstetrics and Gynecology 151: 552–556

Brenner P F 1983 A clinical trial of the delta T intrauterine device: immediate post partum insertion. Contraception 28: 135–147

British National Formulary 1987 British Medical Association/Pharmaceutical Society of Great Britain, London, pp 262–266

Chi I-C, Mumford S D, Gardner S D 1981 Pregnancy risk following laparoscopic sterilisation in non-gravid and gravid women. Journal of Reproductive Medicine 26: 289–294

Chi I-C, Gao Ji, Siemens A J, Waszak C S 1986 IUD insertion at caesarean section — the Chinese experience. Advances in Contraception 2: 145–153

Conant M, Hardy D, Sernatinger J, Spicer D, Levy J A 1986 Condoms prevent transmission of AIDS-associated retrovirus. Journal of the American Medical Association 255: 1706

Cronin T J 1968 Influence of lactation upon ovulation. Lancet ii: 422–424

Cutler J C, Singh B, Carpenter U, Nickens O, Scarola A, Sussman N 1977 Vaginal contraception as prophylaxis against gonorrhoea and other sexually transmitted diseases. Advances in Planned Parenthood 12: 45

Dahlberg K 1982 Some effects of depo medroxyprogesterone acetate: observations in the nursing infant and the long-term user. International Journal of Gynecology and Obstetrics 20: 43–48

Dahlman T, Hellgren M, Blomback M 1985 Changes in blood coagulation

and fibrinolysis in the normal puerperium. Gynecologic and Obstetric Investigation 20: 37–44
Daniel D G, Campbell H, Turnbull A C 1967 Puerperal thromboembolism and suppression of lactation. Lancet ii: 287–289
Davidson F, Oates J K 1985 The pill does not cause thrush. British Journal of Obstetrics and Gynaecology 92: 1265–1266
de Ceulaer K, Gruber C, Hayes R, Serjeant G R 1982 Medroxyprogesterone acetate and homozygous sickle cell disease. Lancet ii: 229–231
Department of Health and Social Security (DHSS) 1982 The report on confidential enquiries into maternal deaths in England and Wales 1976–1978. Reports on health and social subjects. HMSO, London
Department of Health and Social Security (DHSS) 1986 The report on confidential enquiries into maternal deaths in England and Wales 1979–1981. Reports on health and social subjects. HMSO, London
Diaz S, Pavez M, Robertson D N, Croxatto H B 1979 A 3 year clinical trial with levonorgestrel silastic implants. Contraception 19: 557–573
Drife J, Guillebaud J 1986 Hormonal contraception and cancer. British Journal of Hospital Medicine 35: 25–29
Family Planning Association (FPA) 1981a Method instruction sheet: the combined pill. FPA, London
Family Planning Association (FPA) 1981b Method instruction sheet: the progestogen only pill. FPA, London
Flynn A M, Brooks M 1984 A manual of natural family planning. George Allen & Unwin, London
Flynn A M, Lynch S S, Docker M, Morris R 1983 Clinical, hormonal and ultrasonic indicators of returning fertility after childbirth. In: Harrison R F, Bonnar J, Thompson W (eds) Fertility and sterility. MTP Press, Lancaster
Fortney J, Susanti I, Gadalla S, Saleh S, Rogers F, Potts M 1986 Reproductive mortality in two developing countries. American Journal of Public Health 76: 134–138
Fotherby K 1982 The progestogen-only contraceptive pill. British Journal of Family Planning 8: 7–10
Fraser I S 1982 Long acting injectable hormonal contraceptives. Clinical Reproduction and Fertility 1: 67–88
Freie H M 1983 Sickle cell diseases and hormonal contraception. Acta Obstetricia et Gynecologica Scandinavica 62: 211–217
Gjonnaess H, Sagerhol M K, Stormorken H 1975 Studies on coagulation and fibrinolysis in blood from puerperal women with and without oestrogen treatment. British Journal of Obstetrics and Gynaecology 82: 151–157
Graham S, Fraser I S 1982 The progestogen-only mini pill. Contraception 26: 373–385
Gray R H 1985 Reduced risk of pelvic inflammatory disease with injectable contraceptives. Lancet i: 1046
Gray R H, Campbell O M, Zacur H A, Labbok M H, MacRae S L 1987 Postpartum return of ovarian activity in nonbreastfeeding women monitored by urinary assays. Journal of Clinical Endocrinology and Metabolism 64: 645–650
Grimes D A, Peterson H B, Rosenberg M J et al 1982 Sterilization attributable deaths in Bangladesh. International Journal of Gynaecology and Obstetrics 20: 149–154
Guillebaud J 1980 Intrauterine devices — present and future. International Journal of Gynecology and Obstetrics 18: 325–332
Guillebaud J 1984 Contraception: the next 20 years. Modern Medicine 29: 17–19
Guillebaud J 1985 Contraception — your questions answered. Churchill Livingstone, Edinburgh
Hatherley L I 1985 Lactation and post partum infertility: the use-effectiveness of natural family planning (NFP) after term pregnancy. Clinical Reproduction and Fertility 3: 319–334
Hawkins D F, Elder M G 1979 Human fertility control, theory and practice. Butterworth, London
Hawkins D F, Tothill A U 1979 Unpublished observations. In: Hawkins D F, Elder M G 1979 Human fertility control, theory and practice. Butterworth, London, p 391
Heartwell S S, Schlesselman S 1983 Risk of uterine perforation among users of intrauterine devices. Obstetrics and Gynecology 61: 31–36
Heikkila N, Haukkamaa M, Luukkainen T 1982 Levonorgestrel in milk plasma of breast feeding women with levonorgestrel-releasing IUDs. Contraception 25: 41–49
Helm C W, Maxwell D J, Lilford R J 1986 A prospective study of the use of ultrasound in vaginal legal abortion before 20 weeks of pregnancy. Journal of Obstetrics and Gynaecology 7: 143–145
Hicks D R, Martin L S, Getchell J P et al 1985 Inactivation of HTLV III/LAV — infected culture of normal human lymphocytes by nonoxynol-9 in vitro. Lancet ii: 1422–1423
Howie P W, Evans, K, Forbes C D, Prentice C R 1975 The effects of stilboestrol and quinestrol upon coagulation and fibrinolysis during the puerperium. British Journal of Obstetrics and Gynaecology 82: 968–975
Jacobs H S 1987 The care of patients with past and present amenorrhoea. British Journal of Family Planning 12 (suppl): 2–5
Jeffcoate T N, Miller J, Roos R F, Tindall V R 1968 Puerperal thromboembolism in relation to the inhibition of lactation by oestrogen treatment. British Medical Journal 4: 19–25
Kava H W, Klinger H P, Molnar J J, Romney S L 1968 Resumption of ovulation post partum. American Journal of Obstetrics and Gynecology 102: 122–124
Kay C R 1983 Prevention of coronary heart disease. British Medical Journal 287: 1064–1065
Kegel A 1952 Sexual functions of the pubococcygeus muscle. Western Journal of Surgery, Obstetrics and Gynecology 60: 521–524
Kleinman R 1982 Female sterilisation. International Planned Parenthood Federation (IPPF), London
Kolodny R C, Masters W H, Johnson C E 1979 Textbook of sexual medicine. Little, Brown, Boston
Kremer J, Bruijn H de, Hindriks F R 1980 Serum high density lipoprotein cholesterol levels in women using a contraceptive injection of DMPA. Contraception 22: 359–367
Lâhteenmâki P, Luukkainen T 1978 Return of ovarian function after abortion. Clinical Endocrinology 8: 123–132
Lamotte G 1972 Ovulation et post partum chez la femme non lactante. Journal of Gynecology, Obstetrics and Biological Reproduction 1: 13–20
Landgren D N, Diczfalusy E 1980 Hormonal effects of the 300 µg norethisterone (NET) minipill. Contraception 21: 87–113
Liskin L S, Fox G 1982 Intrauterine devices: an appropriate contraceptive for many women. Population Reports Series B X: 101–135
Liskin L S, Quillin W F 1983 Injectables and implants. Population Reports Series K XI: 17–55
Liskin L S, Rinehart W 1985 Minilaparotomy and laparoscopy: safe, effective and widely used. Population Reports Series C XIII: 125–167
Liskin L S, Pile J M, Quillin W F 1983 Vasectomy — safe and simple. Population Reports Series D XI: 61–100
Madhavapeddi R, Ramachandran P 1985 Side effects of oral contraceptive use in lactating women — enlargement of breast in a breast-fed child. Contraception 32: 437–443
Maine D, McNamara R 1985 Birth spacing and child survival. Center for Population and Family Health, Columbia University, New York
Masters W H, Johnson V E 1966 Human sexual response. Little, Brown, Boston
McCann M S, Liskin L S, Piotrow P T, Rinehart W, Fox G 1981 Breast-feeding, fertility and family planning. Population Reports Series J IX: 525–575
McPherson K, Coope P A, Vessey M P 1986 Early oral contraceptive use and breast cancer: theoretical effects of latency. Journal of Epidemiology and Community Health 40: 289–294
Mills A 1987 The forgotten progestogen-only pill. British Journal of Family Planning 12 (suppl): 44–46
Mills J I, Reed G F, Nugent R P, Harley E E, Berendes H W 1985 Are there adverse effects of periconceptional spermicide use? Fertility and Sterility 43: 442–446
Mishell D R, Roy S 1982 Copper IUCD event rates following insertion 4 to 8 weeks post partum. American Journal of Obstetrics and Gynecology 143: 29–35
Murphy H W 1979 Effects of depo medroxyprogesterone acetate on vaginal bleeding in the puerperium. British Medical Journal 2: 1400
Network 1986 Contraceptive needs of breast-feeding women, vol 8. Family Health International, Research Triangle Park, North Carolina, pp 1–8
Newton J, Gee H 1985 Post pregnancy and post abortion contraception. In: Studd J (eds) Progress in obstetrics and gynaecology, vol V. Churchill Livingstone, Edinburgh
Newton J, Harper N, Chan K K 1977 Immediate post placental insertion of IUCDs. Lancet ii: 272–274
Nilsson S, Nygren K 1979 Transfer of contraceptive steroids to human milk. Research in Human Reproduction II: 1–2

Nilsson C G, Allonen H, Diaz J, Luukkainen T 1983 Two years' experience with two LNG-releasing IUDs and one Cu-releasing IUD: a randomised comparative performance study. Fertility and Sterility 39: 187–192
Organon Laboratories 1987 Data sheet on Marvelon. In: ABPI data sheet compendium. Datapharm Publications, London, p 1075
Ortho-Cilag Pharmaceutical 1987 Data sheet on TriNovum. In: ABPI data sheet compendium. Datapharm Publications, London, p 1121
Perez A, Vela T, Potter R, Masnick G S 1971 Timing and sequence of resuming ovulation and menstruation after childbirth. Population Studies 25: 491–503
Perez A, Vela T, Masnick G S, Potter R 1972 First ovulation after childbirth — the effect of breastfeeding. American Journal of Obstetrics and Gynecology 114: 1041–1047
Petitti D B 1986 A review of epidemiologic studies of vasectomy. Biomedical Bulletin 5: 1–17
Philp T, Guillebaud J, Budd D 1984 Late failure of vasectomy after two documented analyses showing azoospermic semen. British Medical Journal 289: 77–79
Population Data Sheet 1987 Population Reference Bureau, New York
Potts M, Diggory T 1983 Textbook of contraceptive practice. Cambridge University Press, Cambridge, p 387
Pritchard J A, Pritchard S A 1977 Blood pressure response to estrogen–progestin oral contraceptive after pregnancy-induced hypertension. American Journal of Obstetrics and Gynecology 129: 733–739
Ratnam S S, Tow S H 1970 Translocation of the loop. In: Zatuchni G I (ed) Postpartum family planning. A report on the international program. McGraw-Hill, New York, pp 63–70
Reamy K, White S E, Daniell W C, Levine E S 1982 Sexuality and pregnancy: a prospective study. Journal of Reproductive Medicine 27: 321–327
Robson K M, Brant H A, Kumar R 1981 Maternal sexuality during the first pregnancy and after childbirth. British Journal of Obstetrics and Gynaecology 88: 882–889
Ross R K, Pike M C, Vessey M T, Bull D, Yeates D, Casagrande J 1986 Risk factors for uterine fibroids: reduced risk associated with oral contraceptives. British Medical Journal 293: 359–362
Sapire K E 1986 Contraception and sexuality in health and disease. McGraw-Hill, Isando, South Africa
Stadel B V 1981 Oral contraceptives and cardiovascular disease. New England Journal of Medicine 305: 612–618
Steel J M, Duncan L J 1981 The progestogen-only contraceptive pill in insulin dependent diabetics. British Journal of Family Planning 6: 108–110
Stone M, Dent, J, Cardana A, Bagshawe K D 1976 Relationship of oral contraception to development of trophoblastic tumour after evacuation of a hydatidiform mole. British Journal of Obstetrics and Gynaecology 83: 913–916
Tankeyoon M, Dusiesin N, Chalapati S et al 1984 WHO task force on oral contraceptives: effects of hormonal contraceptives on milk volumes and infant growth. Contraception 30: 505–521
Tatum H J, Schmidt S H 1977 Contraceptive and sterilization practices and extrauterine pregnancy — a realistic perspective. Fertility and Sterility 28: 407–421
Tayob Y, Guillebaud J, Adams J, Jacobs H S 1986 Studies on ovarian function in users of the progestogen-only contraceptive pill. Journal of Obstetrics and Gynaecology 6 (suppl 2): S91–S95
Thiery M, Laufe L, Parewijck W et al 1983 Immediate postplacental IUD insertion: a randomised trial of sutured (Lippes loop and TCu220C) and non-sutured (TCu220C) models. Contraception 28: 299–313
Vessey M, Huggins G, Lawless N, Yeats D 1983 Tubal sterilisation: findings in a large prospective study. British Journal of Obstetrics and Gynaecology 90: 203–209
Wathen N C, Sapire K E, Davey D A 1978 Post partum insertion of the combined multi-load copper intrauterine device (ML Cu 250). South African Medical Journal 54: 473–476
Wilson E S 1985 Injectable contraceptives. In: Loudon N (ed) Handbook of family planning. Churchill Livingstone, Edinburgh, pp 114–128
Wilson E S, Cruickshank J, McMaster M, Weir R J 1984 A prospective controlled study of the effect on blood pressure of contraceptive preparations containing different types and dosages of progestogen. British Journal of Obstetrics and Gynaecology 91: 1254–1260
Winston R M 1977 Why 103 women asked for a reversal of sterilisation. British Medical Journal 2: 305–307
World Health Organization 1987 Mechanism of action, safety and efficacy of intrauterine devices. Technical report series no 753, WHO, Geneva
Yuen E H, Birch H P 1983 Relationship of oral contraceptives and the intrauterine devices to the regression of concentrations of the beta subunit of human chorionic gonadotrophin and invasive complications after molar pregnancy. American Journal of Obstetrics and Gynecology 145: 214–217

SECTION 15

Medicolegal Aspects

R. N. Palmer

Medicolegal problems in obstetrics

INTRODUCTION*

Few practitioners today can be ignorant of the influence of law on medical practice. The discipline of obstetrics is, perhaps, threatened more than most medical specialties with defensive practice occasioned by fear of litigation. Whilst the scope for error is not necessarily greater than in other medical specialties, the consequences of an error may be profound in both human and financial terms.

In this chapter the author attempts to explain the course of civil litigation under English law as it affects the obstetrician. Generally, the law in Scotland is different from the law applicable to England and Wales but, at least in so far as actions for alleged obstetric negligence are concerned, the legal position in Scotland can be taken to be the same as under English law. The common law principles of English law, generally speaking, extend also to other English-speaking nations and many Commonwealth countries. There are dangers inherent in simplification which cannot be entirely avoided. The practitioner with a particular medicolegal problem is advised to seek professional legal advice at an early stage from a specialist in the field and in the country of practice concerned. The obstetrician's protection or defence organization will be able to offer such advice.

*In the interests of clarity and simplicity (and at the risk of accusations of sexism) the author has, throughout the chapter, used the masculine gender to describe obstetricians and the feminine gender to describe patients and midwives.

ENGLISH LAW

The law in England and Wales may be subdivided into criminal law and civil law, each of which may be subdivided into common law and statute law. The criminal law, whether common or statutory, represents a body of offences (crimes) against society at large, the State, for which society exacts a punitive sanction for any breach, such as a term of imprisonment or a fine. By contrast, civil law is a body of offences between individuals in which the State has no interest and for which the sanction is compensatory, not punitive. Civil law offences (torts) include defamation (libel and slander), trespass, nuisance, negligence etc.

Breaches of the criminal or civil law may be either statutory or common law in origin. Statutory offences are those created by Parliament, either as a crime proscribed by an Act of Parliament itself, or as an offence created by statutory instrument, i.e. a regulation made by a government minister under powers granted by Parliament in the parent or enabling statute. For example, the crime of theft arises from the Theft Act 1968; offences relating to drugs registers and controlled drugs are created by various regulations made under powers granted by Parliament in the Misuse of Drugs Act 1971.

English common law is that body of law which has evolved over the centuries of English legal history by case law and judicial precedent. In the criminal sphere, the law of murder is the best-known example of the evolution of the common law. In the field of civil law, the development of the law of negligence is almost entirely common law in origin, being evolved by the judges in a line of decided cases which set precedents which are binding on future cases based on similar facts.

Jury trial

Before passing to a consideration of the law of negligence it may be helpful to consider, briefly, the role of the jury. In England and Wales, jury trials are retained, for the most part, in criminal cases only. The one exception in civil cases is for cases of defamation which may be tried by jury. It is no longer possible, in England and Wales, for civil actions for alleged negligence to be tried by jury: they are tried by judge alone. (However, the exceptionally rare cases of medical manslaughter sometimes referred to as criminal negligence are, of course, tried by judge and jury.)

In Northern Ireland jury trials for civil actions were abolished in 1987. In the Republic of Ireland jury trials of civil medical negligence actions were abolished in 1988. Claims in Ireland are now tried by a single judge.

It is the role of the jury to decide issues of fact and of the judge to decide issues of law. In cases tried by judge alone, the judge decides issues of both fact and law.

The courts

Claims for compensation arising from the practise of obstetrics will be brought in the civil courts. The County Court hears cases where the value of the claims is relatively low (less than £5000, currently). Commonly, in medical cases, the County Court is used for actions to recover unpaid fees; such actions may then be met with not only a defence but also a counterclaim against the practitioner, alleging negligence or breach of contract, or both.

Claims with an estimated value in excess of £5000 will be brought in the High Court. This is part of the Supreme Court of Judicature and comprises three divisions — Chancery, Queen's Bench and Family. Negligence actions are usually brought in the Queen's Bench division but may be brought in the Chancery division. Appeals from the High Court are heard in the civil division of the Court of Appeal. From the Court of Appeal there is, with leave, a final right of appeal to (the judicial committee of) the House of Lords.

Actions in the High Court in England and Wales are heard by a single judge alone. Appeals in the Court of Appeal are heard by a bench of two or three Lords Justice of Appeal. Appeals in the House of Lords, often on matters of legal principle and issues of policy, are usually heard by five Law Lords (Lords of Appeal in Ordinary).

NEGLIGENCE

The law of negligence is that branch of English civil law which poses the most feared threat to the daily professional work of the practising obstetrician. It is important to understand what the underlying principle of the law is and to understand what it is not.

It is not a synonym for neglect, misdemeanour or reckless behaviour (all of which have overtones of criminal conduct) nor is it misconduct in the context of the term serious professional misconduct, which is the concern of the General Medical Council. Negligence is a legal concept comprising three main elements, each of which may be further subdivided.

1. A duty of care.
2. A breach of that duty of care.
3. Damage (harm) flowing from the breach.

The obstetrician undoubtedly owes a duty of care to his patients. If he falls below the standard of care demanded of him and harm (synonymous with damage) to his patient occurs, then he will be liable to pay compensation (synonym: damages) to the patient.

A large amount of judicial time has been spent on a detailed consideration of the legal test to be applied in determining the standard of care applicable to medical cases. Three cases have received consideration and analysis by our final court of appeal, the House of Lords:

1. *Whitehouse* v. *Jordan* [1981] 1 AllER 267, 1 WLR 246.
2. *Maynard* v. *West Midlands Regional Health Authority* [1985] 1 AllER 635.
3. *Sidaway* v. *Bethlem Royal Hospital and the Maudsley Hospital Health Authority and others* [1985] 2 WLR 480.

In these cases the law of medical negligence was developed in relation to advice, diagnosis and treatment.

The House of Lords has approved the principles of the law of negligence in relation to the nature of the duty owed by a doctor to a patient which were laid down in two leading cases from the 1950s — the Scottish case of *Hunter* v. *Hanley* [1955] SLT 213 and *Bolam* v. *Friern Hospital Management Committee* [1957] 2 AllER 118; [1957] 1 WLR 582. The test (widely known as the Bolam test) is 'the standard of the ordinary skilled man exercising and professing to have that special skill ... it is sufficient if (the practitioner) exercises the ordinary skill of an ordinary, competent man exercising that particular art.' If a surgeon fails to measure up to that standard in any respect ('clinical judgement' or otherwise) he has been negligent, it was said by Lord Edmund-Davies in the Whitehouse case (as above), but a practitioner is not negligent if he complies with a practice accepted as proper by a responsible body of professional opinion. So, in deciding whether on the facts of a particular case a medical practitioner has measured up to the accepted standard of skill and care, the Court will be guided and influenced by expert medical opinion.

The test, albeit judicially determined, is greatly influenced by professional medical opinion of the day. Evidence will be given as to the practice adopted by a reasonable, responsible body of professional opinion. In *Hunter* v. *Hanley* (as above, per Lord President Clyde, p 217) it was held that 'in the realm of diagnosis and treatment there is ample scope for genuine difference of opinion and one man clearly is not negligent merely because his conclusion differs from that of other professional men ... the true test for establishing negligence in diagnosis or treatment on the part of a doctor is whether he has been proved to be guilty of such failure as no doctor of ordinary skill would be guilty if acting with ordinary care.' Approving these words, Lord Scarman in

Maynard's case (as above, p 638) added: 'A case which is based on an allegation that a fully considered decision of two consultants in the field of their special skill was negligent clearly presents certain difficulties of proof. It is not enough to show that there is a body of competent professional opinion which considers that theirs was a wrong decision if there also exists a body of professional opinion, equally competent, which supports the decision as reasonable in the circumstances. It is not enough to show that subsequent events show that the operation need never have been performed if at the time the decision to operate was taken it was reasonable in the sense that a responsible body of medical opinion would have accepted it as proper.'

Later (as above, p 639) Lord Scarman added: 'I have to say that a judge's "preference" for one body of distinguished professional opinion to another also professionally distinguished is not sufficient to establish negligence in a practitioner whose actions have received the seal of approval of those whose opinions, truthfully expressed, honestly held, were not preferred... For in the realm of diagnosis and treatment negligence is not established by preferring one respectable body of professional opinion to another. Failure to exercise the ordinary skill of a doctor (in the appropriate specialty, if he be a specialist) is necessary.'

(No apology is made for quoting extensively from the actual words of the judges in the important leading cases for the meaning of words is of great importance to the lawyer and it is best that there is interposed no interpretation which might mislead.)

CAUSATION AND FORESEEABILITY

If the obstetrician falls below the standard of care of the practitioner of similar training and experience and causes avoidable harm to his patient which was reasonably foreseeable, he will be liable (personally or through his professional indemnifier) to compensate the victim of his negligent act or omission. In many negligence actions, and especially in actions alleging mismanagement of labour followed by the birth of infants with neurological damage, there may be great difficulty in establishing a causal link between the alleged negligent act or omission and the harm to the patient. The plaintiff must prove fault on the part of the defendant and that the harm flowed from the alleged fault. The nature of the harm suffered must also be a reasonably foreseeable consequence of the negligence.

If the negligent act or omission was witnessed by an onlooker and that onlooker suffers nervous shock, he or she may also be entitled to recover an award of damages.

CONSENT

Consent for diagnosis, investigation, examination and treatment is a subject of ever-increasing importance in the patient–doctor relationship. It encompasses philosophical, ethical and legal considerations but it is proposed, in this chapter, to deal only with legal aspects of consent.

Negligence and battery

Any unlawful touching of a person may give rise to a civil action for battery. It might also give rise to a criminal charge, but the criminal law of assault has almost no place in the ordinary patient–doctor relationship and is best set on one side for separate consideration in special circumstances, e.g. the rare but distressing situations in which practitioners are accused of indecent assault.

Colloquially, the term assault is in common usage but it has both civil and criminal connotations and is seldom defined with accuracy. In the context of obstetric care the term battery is more relevant and more accurate to a consideration of the evolution of the law on consent. Most professional consultations with patients involve some physical contact. If the obstetrician is to avoid legal proceedings it is essential to obtain the consent of the patient before any examination, investigation or treatment.

There are two strands in the concept of consent. Not only does the concept of consent involve the avoidance of battery (unlawful physical touching) but also it requires a sufficient explanation and discussion to take place to avoid claims alleging negligent advice. A consent obtained by getting a patient to sign a standard consent form in the absence of a proper and sufficient explanation and discussion might well afford the practitioner some protection against a claim for battery, but it will afford no protection against an action alleging negligent advice.

Informed consent

For a patient's consent to be valid in English law it must be informed. The English law concept of informed consent, as set out by the House of Lords in the case of *Sidaway* c. *Bethlem Royal Hospital and the Maudsley Hospital Health Authority and others* [1985] 2WLR 480 is very different from transatlantic doctrines of informed consent, as enunciated in cases in the USA such as the leading case of *Canterbury* v. *Spence* [1972] 464 F.2d.772.

English law, put in simple terms, basically applies the Bolam test (see above), albeit slightly modified by the House of Lords in the Sidaway case, to advice as well as to diagnosis and treatment. It is left to the medical profession to decide upon how much and what information should be given to a patient when advising on treatment and obtaining consent, i.e. a subjective test.

The American position, as enunciated in *Canterbury* v. *Spence*, is to apply an objective *prudent patient* test, to require the doctor to warn his patient of material risks inherent in the recommended treatment. A material risk is one which the court (not a responsible body of medical opinion as in the English Bolam test) is satisfied that a reasonable person in the patient's position would be likely to regard as significant. However, the American courts allow an exemption to the practitioner (called therapeutic privilege) from the duty to disclose objectively defined material risks to the patient if he takes the view that, on a reasonable assessment of the patient's condition, a warning would be detrimental to the patient's health.

However, the traditional English approach in the Bolam test is under attack, both from judges and others, not excluding the medical profession. When the issue of disclosure of risks to patients was considered by the House of Lords in the Sidaway case, a wide range of views was expressed by the five Law Lords who heard the appeal. At one end of the spectrum of views, Lord Scarman was in favour of adopting into English law the transatlantic principles of their doctrine of informed consent. At the other end of the judicial spectrum, Lord Diplock voiced a trenchant defence of the classic English law position, firmly supportive of the Bolam test, allowing the medical profession to be the judge of what, and how much, to tell the patient. Middle ground was occupied by the other three Law Lords.

It is not easy to discern a single, clear principle from the five speeches in the Sidaway case but it is respectfully submitted that the English law on informed consent can reasonably be summarized by stating that a decision about what degree of disclosure of risks is best calculated to assist a particular patient to make a rational choice as to whether or not to undergo a particular treatment must primarily be a matter of clinical judgement for the clinician. However, if there is a conflict of medical expert evidence as to whether a responsible body of medical opinion approves of non-disclosure of risks in a particular case, the trial judge would have to resolve that conflict. The doctor must decide what information and warnings as to risks should be given to the patient and the terms in which that information should be couched; his discretion is always subject to challenge by the patient and to scrutiny by the courts.

The extent of the explanation which the doctor should give when seeking consent will depend on many factors and may pose considerable problems, calling for fine clinical judgement. The factors to be taken into account will include the patient's age and maturity, physical and mental state, intellectual capacity, standard of education and the reason for the procedure, operation or treatment. For example, a routine cosmetic procedure may need to be discussed far more extensively than an emergency operation for a life-threatening condition in an ill patient. The explanation which the doctor gives will also depend upon the questions asked by the patient; some patients require to know far more than others about side-effects, complications, etc. Generally, a careful and truthful answer should be given to a particular request by a patient for information.

There is no requirement in English law that every possible complication and side-effect should be explained to the patient. Recent court cases, however, show a trend by the judges to require more detailed explanations to be given than those of a few years ago. Obviously a balance must be struck between telling patients enough to enable them to give a true consent and yet not so much as to frighten them needlessly from agreeing to treatment which is demonstrably essential to their well-being. Achieving that balance can be very difficult, even for practitioners of many years' experience.

Implied and express consent

A valid consent may be implied or express. In many consultations and procedures the patient rarely agrees explicitly but will, instead, give an implied consent, e.g. the patient will undress and lie on the examination couch when the doctor indicates a wish to examine her, or the patient may roll up a sleeve and offer an arm when the doctor indicates a wish to take the blood pressure or a blood sample.

Express consent, of course, is given when a patient states agreement in clear terms, orally or in writing, to a request.

Age of consent

In England any person of sound mind who has attained the age of 16 years may give a legally valid consent to surgical, medical or dental treatment or procedures (section 8, Family Law Reform Act 1969). What has been less clear is whether a person under the age of 16 can give consent. The Act does not say that she may not. In a case which reached the House of Lords in October 1985 (*Gillick* v. *West Norfolk and Wisbech Area Health Authority and the Department of Health and Social Security* 1985, 3AER, p 402) it was held that, save where statute otherwise provides, a minor's capacity to make his or her own decision depends upon the minor having sufficient understanding and intelligence to make the decision and is not to be determined by reference to any judicially fixed age limit. The House of Lords held that, as a matter of law, the parental right to determine whether or not a minor child below the age of 16 will have medical treatment terminates if and when the child achieves a sufficient understanding and intelligence to enable him or her to understand fully what is proposed. The House of Lords held that it will be a question of fact whether a child seeking advice has sufficient understanding of what is involved to give a consent valid in law. Until the child achieves the capacity to consent, the parental right to make the decision continues save only in exceptional circumstances.

The application of these legal principles to contraceptive advice is set out later in this chapter. The House of Lords has upheld the opinion, held by many legal authorities for many years, that a minor who is capable of appreciating fully the nature and consequences of a particular operation or of particular treatment can give an effective consent thereto and in such cases the consent of the guardian is unnecessary. However, where the infant is without that capacity any apparent consent by him or her will be a nullity, the sole right to consent being vested in the parent or guardian.

Girls under 16 years of age

In applying the legal principles to contraceptive and abortion advice and treatment it was stated by Lord Scarman in the Gillick case in the House of Lords that it has to be borne in mind that there is much that has to be understood by a girl under the age of 16 if she is to have legal capacity to consent to such treatment. It is not enough that she should understand the nature of the advice which is being given; she must also have a sufficient maturity to understand what is involved. There are moral and family questions, especially as regards her relationship with her parents; long-term problems associated with the emotional impact of pregnancy and its termination; and there are risks to health of sexual intercourse at her age, risks which contraception may diminish but cannot eliminate. It follows that a doctor will have to satisfy himself that she is able to appraise these factors before the doctor can safely proceed upon the basis that the patient has at law capacity to consent to contraceptive treatment. Ordinarily, the proper course for the doctor is first to seek to persuade the girl to bring her parents into consultation, and if she refuses, not to prescribe contraceptive treatment unless the doctor is satisfied that the patient's circumstances are such that the treatment may proceed without parental knowledge and consent.

Lord Scarman acknowledged that a criticism of this view of the law is that it will result in uncertainty and leave the law in the hands of the doctors. Lord Scarman commented that the uncertainty is the price which has to be paid to keep the law in line with social experience, which is that many girls are fully able to make a sensible decision about many matters before they reach the age of 16 years. This view of the law places great responsibilities upon the medical profession and it is pointed out that abuse of the power to prescribe contraceptive treatment for girls under the age of 16 would render a doctor liable to severe professional penalty.

Somewhat more detailed guidance was given in the House of Lords by Lord Fraser of Tullybelton who said that the doctor will be justified in proceeding without the parents' consent or even knowledge provided he is satisfied on the following matters:

1. That the girl (although under 16 years of age) will understand his advice.
2. That he cannot persuade her to inform her parents or to allow him to inform the parents that she is seeking contraceptive advice.
3. That she is very likely to begin or to continue having sexual intercourse with or without contraceptive treatment.
4. That unless she receives contraceptive advice or treatment her physical or mental health, or both, are likely to suffer.
5. That her best interests require him to give her contraceptive advice, treatment or both without parental consent. Lord Fraser commented that this result ought not to be regarded as a licence for doctors to disregard the wishes of parents on the matter whenever they find it convenient to do so.

Consent to abortion and contraception

The pregnant mother's consent alone is relevant in the case of abortion under the Abortion Act 1967. The putative father has no legal say in the matter, whether or not he is married to the mother, as was made clear in the case of *Paton* v. *Trustees* [1978] 2 AllER 987 and *C* v. *S* [1987] 1 AllER 1230. However, this is not to discourage the sound medical practice of discussing a proposed abortion with the father (provided that the mother agrees).

Similar considerations apply to contraception as to abortion. For adults there is no legal requirement to seek the consent of the spouse or consort. Many practitioners prefer to ask for the consent of both parties before fitting an intrauterine contraceptive device and, whilst there is no legal requirement to do so, it is sound medical practice.

Oral and written consent

A perfectly valid consent may be given orally and there is no absolute need for it to be in writing. However, a written consent is sometimes preferable since it provides documentary evidence of the agreement. The problem is a practical one: disputes over consent may arise months or years after the event, by which time memories of an oral consent are unreliable. A witness to an oral consent may be dead or untraceable by the time an allegation of assault or trespass is made. Thus for purely evidential reasons it is wiser to have a signed consent form, duly witnessed.

There is no magic, legal or otherwise, in a consent form. It is simply a piece of documentary evidence of the fact that a consent was sought and obtained. It would be unrealistic to insist upon a written request for all examinations and procedures and common sense is required in deciding when the consent should be evidenced in writing.

DAMAGES

The size (synonym: quantum) of the award of compensation payable to the plaintiff who can prove negligence is determined by the circumstances of the victim rather than simply by the nature of the negligent act or omission. A tiny negligent error may have the most profound consequences. For example, a negligently diagnosed or treated finger injury resulting in a stiff, functionally impaired digit will attract a modest award in a retired person but a substantial award of damages in a professional musician with an international reputation and income to match who is no longer able to enjoy a career.

Traditionally, under English law, damages were awarded on a once-and-for-all lump sum basis. This, in the words of Lord Scarman in the case of *Lim Poh Choo* v. *Camden and Islington Area Health Authority (Teaching)* [1979] 1 AllER 332, meant that in cases where the courts have to make provision for future total care in brain damage cases with an uncertain life expectancy, the courts could be sure of only one thing — that the future would prove the award to have been either too high or too low. Either too great a lump sum would be awarded so that the estate would benefit from a windfall upon the death of the victim, or else the sum would be too small, with the victim living longer than anticipated and the fund of money for her care running out prematurely.

To ameliorate this situation a statutory change in the law was enacted by an amendment to the Supreme Court Act 1981 which allows the court to make an order for provisional damages. This means that if the plaintiff proves (or the defendant admits) a chance that some time in the future, as a result of the defendant's negligence, she will develop some serious disease or suffer some serious deterioration in physical or mental condition, then the High Court can exercise its new powers, viz.:

1. To make an immediate award for pain and suffering apparent at the time of trial.
2. To give the plaintiff the right to apply for further damages at a future date if she develops the disease or suffers the deterioration in condition.

Whilst of undoubted fairness and benefit to brain-damaged and other plaintiffs, this new provision does pose problems for the insurers and indemnifiers of defendants such as health authorities and doctors, who may now have an open-ended commitment and an uncertain cut-off, leading to difficulties in making proper financial provision to fund the unknown future awards.

The assessment of damages

The amount of compensation payable depends upon the consequences for the victim, based upon the victim's personal and professional circumstances, not on the nature of the practitioner's negligent act or omission. This is the logical consequence of the object of the civil law, to compensate and not to punish.

Lawyers assess damages under several heads which are dealt with only very briefly here. (For a fuller exposition see Whitfield 1984.) The principal heads of damages are:

1. Damages for pain, suffering and loss of amenity.
2. Damages for future financial loss and expenses (together, these two heads form the bulk of 'general damages').
3. Special damages for proven financial loss already incurred such as loss of earnings, medical and nursing expenses prior to trial and cost of conversions of house or car.
4. Interest on general and special damages.

Both physical and psychiatric injuries which result from negligence are eligible for compensation. Relatives may be able to claim for nervous shock if they suffer psychiatric morbidity from having witnessed an act of negligence suffered by a patient, e.g. parents who see a negligently performed circumcision on their child. Awards of damages are based on judge-made tariffs, with straightforward injuries receiving a fairly standard award. More complex and multiple injuries may not fall within a set scale or tariff but lawyers and judges have to make an assessment based on experience and precedents, their objective being always to put the victim into the position, in so far as money can ever do this, which he or she would have been in but for the negligence and its sequelae.

Awards in England, being made by judges alone, are considered small by the standards of other countries where awards are made by juries (e.g. the USA). However, awards in England and Wales and in Scotland have risen substantially in the last decade and seem likely to continue to rise. There has been some reluctance among some senior judges in England to increase general damages too much, not least because of the effect that steep increases in compensation might have upon public health authority budgets and the fear that it might limit their ability to provide medical services to the populace and lead to the practice of defensivism in medicine. Nonetheless, the levels of awards of compensation have risen steeply in the last decade. Before 1977 no English case of medical negligence attracted an award in excess of £100 000. However, in the decade from 1977 to 1987 the level of awards rose steeply and in 1987 the courts awarded a little over £1 million to a young male adult who had suffered severe brain damage following an operation (*Abdul-Hosn* v. *Trustees of Italian Hospital*, Kemp & Kemp, vol. 2, para 1–510).

When assessing damages, the defendant must 'take his victim as he finds her' (sometimes known as the eggshell skull rule). If an injury is caused to someone of a delicate constitution or to a high-income earner rather than to a person who is of a strong constitution and temperament or to an unemployed person, that is the defendant's bad luck — or bad luck on his protection society's funds. Lost earnings and lost pension rights must be compensated. If full-time or part-time nursing care is required (e.g. for severely brain-damaged victims), that, too, must be compensated for such period of time as medical prognosticians consider to be appropriate. In trying to estimate future loss and expenses, the starting point is the victim's current net financial loss at the date of settlement or trial. The future must then be considered, taking into account any possible career progression or promotion. An attempt is made to project the estimated net loss over the period (estimated from medical prognosis) of its likely duration. So, for example, a net loss of £x per annum for an estimated 30 years is assessed as a lump sum, £$30x$. A deduction is then made to allow for the fact that the compensation is to be paid as a once-and-for-all lump sum (but see the start of this section). The discounted figure (say £$14x$) is intended to be invested to produce income and both income and capital sum are intended to be exhausted over the period prognosed.

A victim of negligence is also entitled to be compensated for her lost years, i.e. if her life expectancy is shortened, she is still entitled to recover damages for loss of net earnings for that part of a productive life denied to her, less estimated personal living expenses. The courts may also make an award for loss of earning capacity, which has to be estimated. The logical, if startling, result of the introduction of this head of damages is that an award for loss of earnings (albeit small and nominal) will be made to a brain-damaged minor (e.g. from obstetric negligence) even though it is clear that the victim's injuries are such that no gainful employment could ever be undertaken.

Notwithstanding the existence of the National Health Service (NHS), an injured patient is, by statute, entitled to claim compensation for private medical and nursing care even though he or she could enjoy comparable treatment under the NHS. If nursing care is provided by devoted relatives rather than by professional nurses, an award will be made to compensate this.

Interest on general and special damages will be awarded at statutorily fixed rates of interest and for set periods of time betweeen the dates of injury, service of writ and settlement or trial. Interest may amount to a considerable sum of money in expensive claims which have been slow to settle or come to trial.

The assessment of damages is not an exact science. Lawyers and courts attempt to apply old and new principles to the complex facts of individual cases in a logical and consistent manner, in accordance with precedents, with the purpose of doing justice to the parties in the case. Finally, the author wishes to stress that this account of damages is a very brief and simplified attempt to deal with a large and complex subject.

THE PROGRESS OF A CLAIM

The average duration of a claim for damages for personal injuries or death in England and Wales, from the date of the incident to the date of the award, is about 4 years (Report of the personal injuries litigation procedure working party 1979). Many medical negligence claims take much longer than 4 years because of a number of factors, including their complexities and the time necessary to ascertain, with reasonable accuracy, the clinical prognosis.

Not all claims for compensation will proceed to trial; quite the reverse, in fact. The report quoted above also shows that, of all personal injury actions begun by the issue of a writ, only about 1% will proceed to a hearing before a judge. Most claims are either settled between the parties out of court or are simply not pursued. Of course, it is impossible to predict for any given case whether it will be one of the 1% which will proceed to trial. Furthermore, the speed of progress of a claim is largely in the hands of the plaintiff, not the defendant. The plaintiff is able to set the pace of progress and the defendant, on the whole, can only respond to the tempo set, with little scope to force the pace.

With this statistical background, it is now proposed to outline the stages in a medical negligence action between the notification of a claim for damages and its outcome.

Disclosure of case notes or discovery of documents

The first hint or threat of a claim for compensation is very commonly a request by solicitors for access to clinical records, such as case notes, nursing records, cardiotocograph traces or scan results. Parliament has legislated to provide that when a claim for personal injuries or death is in contemplation, the prospective litigant may apply for access to the relevant case notes. Such requests are made long before the issue of a writ and the current law is set out in the Supreme Court Act 1981 at section 33. In summary, patients and their legal advisers can secure access to clinical records with comparative ease and it behoves every clinician to ensure that entries in case notes are made responsibly, objectively and in a form worthy of independent scrutiny. The days of using case notes to practise one's wit and sarcasm, or to make subjective comments of a pejorative nature, should long ago have ceased. Regrettably, bad, illegible, incomplete and defamatory notes are still too frequently seen. Such entries can prove highly embarrassing when, years later perhaps, they are scrutinized by judge and patient alike.

Writs and letters before action

The first that the individual practitioner might know about a claim is the receipt of either a solicitor's letter before action or a High Court writ. In the NHS it is usual for solicitors' letters (alleging negligence and seeking compensation) to be addressed to the hospital administrator or health authority and they will be passed to the health authority's legal adviser. Either the administrator will alert the clinicians to the problem and encourage them to seek guidance from their protection organization or alternatively the legal advisers will write to the defence or protection society and invite them to make contact with the practitioners who are thought to have had a part to play in the case.

Occasionally in NHS practice, and always in private practice, the solicitor's letter or writ will be addressed to a named practitioner and this requires prompt action. Writs may now be served by post and it is essential that service should be acknowledged within 14 days, since otherwise there is a risk of judgment being entered against the practitioner in default. The service of a writ is one of the few medicolegal emergencies, though this term is of course relative in the sense that few obstetricians would regard 14 days as being an emergency.

Time limits

The Limitation Acts enacted by Parliament provide for time limits for the issue and service of writs and generally for the initiation of litigation. Put extremely briefly, a plaintiff must bring an action in respect of personal injuries or death within 3 years—unfortunately it is not as simple as this. The time limits do not begin to run until the patient has knowledge of an entitlement to sue—classic examples being the cases of nerve deafness from noise and of pulmonary problems from asbestos.

For the obstetrician, however, there is a much greater problem and this is that, for his infant plaintiffs, time does not begin to run until the infant reaches the age of majority, currently 18 years. (The age of majority is different from the law governing the age for consent to treatment; see above.) If the infant then consults solicitors and decides to sue there is still the 3-year time limit within which the writ must be issued and a further year within which the writ must then be served and thus, in effect, the infant who is brain-damaged at birth has until her 22nd birthday to initiate litigation. If a claim is framed in contract rather than negligence then the period could be even longer. Thus it is important that good notes are not only made but retained and the Department of Health and Social Security (DHSS) circular HC(80)7 deals with retention periods for medical records. The DHSS recognizes the problems this poses in terms of storage and ultimately it must be a public policy decision as to whether health authorities would rather pay money for storing notes or money in settling claims which cannot be fought because the notes have been destroyed to ease storage problems.

Access to notes after issue of the writ

As described above, a plaintiff may gain access to medical notes before the writ is issued. In theory, once the writ is issued, she may not have access to the notes until a stage in the litigation called close of pleadings. Many a solicitor has issued a writ prematurely and then found it difficult to prepare his statement of claim; however, there is a provision by which the plaintiff's lawyers can apply to the court for early discovery (i.e. disclosure) of notes, notwithstanding the premature issue of the writ before the merits of the case have been thoroughly assessed.

Legal Aid

One of the problems of English law—and there are many—is that only the very rich and the relatively poor can afford to sue. The impoverished plaintiff may secure the assistance of Legal Aid and the problem for doctors and protection organizations is that, even if the claim is ultimately defeated, the defendant cannot recover costs against either the plaintiff or the Legal Aid Fund.

Statement of claim

After the issue of the writ the plaintiff must serve her statement of claim. In theory this should be done within a fortnight but in practice the time limits are usually waived and occasionally statements of claim do not follow the writ for two or more years. The purpose of the statement of claim is to set out in concise form the plaintiff's allegations of negligence. They are necessarily abbreviated and incomplete, but should at least give the defendants some indication of the case they have to meet. The Scottish and some foreign jurisdictions seem much more strict than the English by insisting that the plaintiff should be limited by the allegations in the document, but the fact is that in English law in recent years, High Court judges have readily given leave to amend the statement of claim during a trial, even after the close of the plaintiff's case, so as to allow new material to be used. This can make for considerable difficulties for doctors and other defendants, but if they are really taken by surprise and feel that they are unduly prejudiced by the new material it is open to them to apply for an adjournment to enable them and their advisers to consider their position.

Defence

When the statement of claim is served the allegations must be thoroughly investigated so that a written response (the defence) can be prepared, indicating which parts of the statement of claim are admitted and which are denied. This, too, must be served within weeks but usually it is possible to secure an extension of time and such extensions are essential where, for instance, several doctors had a part to play in the case and some of them have emigrated abroad or at least moved on to new posts within the UK.

In principle the object of the exercise is to interview and obtain the comments of all involved doctors, midwives and other members of staff in order that statements (or proofs of evidence as lawyers call them) can be prepared for the benefit of the defence counsel who has to prepare the defence to the claim. Strictly speaking, the service of the defence results in the closure of pleadings, but in point of fact various other stages in the paperwork of a claim may occur before the matter is set down for trial. These pieces of paperwork rejoice in various grand-sounding titles, such as requests for further and better particulars of the statement of claim, requests for further and better particulars of the defence, interrogatories, replies and the like. However, the underlying object of the exercise is to clarify the issues in a case and narrow the areas of dispute and difference between plaintiff and defendants.

The preparation of a defence to a claim requires care, thoroughness and attention to detail. The process begins by the legal equivalent of taking a good history. A defence built on poor foundations will fail at trial. It is imperative to begin by taking detailed statements from the doctors and midwives and this exercise will also involve posing a series of very probing questions on a devil's advocate basis. This exercise is generally done in private, but it is essential to the defence to know not only the strengths but also the weaknesses of the case. Where, as so often in hospital practice, numbers of doctors are involved, there has to be liaison and co-operation between their respective protection organizations. Where there is a midwife involvement there must also be co-operation between the doctor's protection organization and the health authority legal adviser, so that a full and frank exchange of factual information takes place.

Expert opinion

Once the facts are gathered (which may take many months or years, particularly when some practitioners are abroad) it is then necessary to seek expert opinion as to the defensibility of the claim. One has to bear in mind the realities of the exercise. Under English civil law the plaintiff has only to prove her case on the balance of probabilities, not beyond reasonable doubt (the criminal test) nor on the basis of statistical proof so as to satisfy the editors of learned scientific journals. The plaintiff has only to satisfy the judge that it is more likely than not that her injury was caused by the defendant's negligence for her to secure her award of damages.

Nor should there be confusion over the term negligence. As explained earlier, this is not synonymous with neglect, much less with manslaughter. Negligence is no more than a failure to come up to the standard of care which is to be expected from colleagues with similar training, skill and experience. A doctor is not negligent if he acts in accordance with a practice accepted at the time as proper by a responsible body of medical opinion, skilled in the particular form of treatment, even though there is a body of competent professional opinion which might adopt a different technique. An error of judgement may or may not be negligent: it all depends on the circumstances.

Changes in the Rules of the Supreme Court made in 1987 mean that expert evidence upon which reliance is to be placed at trial now has to be disclosed to the other parties in the action well before trial. Previously, expert evidence did not have to be disclosed until the expert took the witness stand and gave oral evidence on oath. The change in the rules, designed to prevent parties to the ligitation being taken by surprise at trial, means that cases will have to be prepared more thoroughly and at an earlier stage. Written expert opinions must be disclosed so that each party will have the advantage of knowing what the other party's experts will say. However, it is stressed that written opinions need not be disclosed unless it is intended to rely upon the evidence of that particular expert at the trial. Parties would still be able to discard unfavourable opinions and would not be under an obligation to disclose them.

The expert to whom one turns for advice should be selected with care. He should practise in the same specialty but not the same geographical area as the practitioners against whom criticism is levelled, albeit that supplementary expert opinions may need to be taken on subspecialist aspects of a case. For example, in assessing the use of drugs by gynaecologists, one's main expertise should come from a gynaecologist though it may also be necessary to have expert opinion from a pharmacologist or a medical microbiologist. It is very important that the expert should be adequately briefed, so that he understands the issues in the case and directs his mind toward the relevant points. It is also important to encourage the expert to point out the weaknesses as well as the strengths of the case. The construction of theoretical, abstruse defences may be a fascinating academic exercise worthy of a forensic clinicopathological conference, but it is of little practical assistance in civil litigation.

Occasionally an expert opinion is not necessary because the case speaks for itself—*res ipsa loquitur*. Classic examples include the retained swab or forceps, the operation on the incorrect limb or digit and the administration of the wrong drug. If the expert opinion is to the effect that the case simply is not defensible because the care provided failed to reach the required standard, it is unlikely that the matter would proceed to trial. If expert evidence cannot be found to support the doctor's actions then it is likely that authority will be given to negotiate a settlement out of court.

If it is considered by the medical experts and by legal advisers that there was no negligence (as defined above), the defence of the litigation will be continued and the protection organization's solicitors will liaise and co-operate with the health authority solicitors over the preparations for trial.

Preparations for trial

The preparations of a case for trial are long and detailed and will not be dealt with here. However, from the doctor's point of view the next event of importance will be the conference with counsel, i.e. the barrister in charge of the defence, who will be asked to advise generally and to indicate the evidence which will have to be called at trial. Every case is different but the underlying principle is always that care and thoroughness must be taken to ensure that when the matter eventually comes before the court, everything is in order and the defence is fully prepared to meet the case pleaded.

A change in the law in 1988 requires that the substance of the evidence to be given by witnesses of fact (as well as experts, see above) must now be disclosed to the other parties in the case, well in advance of trial. Therefore, written statements of doctors, midwives and others who are to be called to give evidence at the trial must be carefully and accurately prepared and disclosed by the lawyers acting for them to the lawyers acting for the other parties.

Trial

Most cases are either settled or fade away for one reason or another but about 1% of them will proceed to a hearing in court. It is important to appreciate that the English legal system provides for an adversarial contest — the 'English sporting theory of justice' — and is not an inquisition or a search for the truth. It is for the parties to the action to decide for themselves what evidence is relevant and to adduce it. The weight to be attached to that evidence is tested by cross-examination. The trial itself is usually long and slow and very expensive. From the point of view of reputations it is a truism that the worst cases never get to court because the protection organizations will settle out of court. Equally, the no-hope cases seldom get to court, though there are some counsel who will persist with legally aided lost causes all the way to trial.

It tends to be only the finely balanced cases, often where there is a genuine divergence of expert opinion, which have to be argued before the judge and it must be questionable whether this is indeed the best forum for a debate on clinical methods.

The trial process is heavily dependent upon the integrity of the expert witnesses. Fortunately, most experts are of impeccable integrity, though a few act as professional expert witnesses. However, just as when six doctors are gathered round a bed one is likely to get several opinions, so fielding a long line of experts before the court will not necessarily assist greatly in the resolution of the particular clinical problem. Ultimately of course, where there is a divergence of expert view, the judge has to balance the conflicting opinions and must make findings of fact, deciding, on the balance of probabilities, in favour of one or other party in the action.

Precedent

English law is based on a system of precedent, which means that decisions of higher courts are binding on lower courts and decisions of the courts, once made, must be followed in subsequent cases based on the same facts. However, medical negligence cases usually involve issues of fact, and not of law. Seldom does an important legal principle arise in medical cases.

If a case can be distinguished on its facts from a previous case, then the decision or precedent in the earlier case is not binding. Since two cases in medicine are seldom alike, it is not difficult to distinguish one case from a previous case and a previous precedent does not then bind the trial judge.

Thus the doctrine of precedent is not a source of great anxiety to protection societies, though it is one which seems to cause anxieties in some members of the medical profession. For example, *Whitehouse* v. *Jordan* was not a scientific debate about the comparative merits of trial of forceps or Caesarean section, though some appeared to think so. It was, as most medical negligence cases are, a trial of fact; in that case, did the obstetrician pull for too long or too hard? Very few judgments set new legal precedents which require a change of clinical practice for legal reasons.

To settle out of court does not set a precedent. In assessing whether to take a case to court, protection societies sometimes take the view that it would be better not to have a judgment which would set a precedent which might prove difficult to clinicians. Some matters, such as the post-anaesthetic hepatitis debate and the surgery-and-the-pill debate, are too subtle and contentious to be resolved sensibly by the blunt instrument of the law, with proof on the balance of probabilities and not at the level of scientific proof.

Quantum

Most cases proceeding to trial will deal not only with issues of liability but also of quantum, i.e. how much compensation is payable. Occasionally liability is admitted and a case will proceed to trial on quantum alone when there is a wide divergence of view between plaintiff and defendant as to the value of the case.

Because of the adversarial system in English law, agreement on quantum may not be reached until the door of the court, or even during trial. Defendants are sometimes blamed for this, often unfairly. The plaintiff's advisers may have adopted an unhelpful or even intransigent attitude, and may have over-inflated the value of the claim. Frequently the plaintiff does not supply until the eve of trial the documents and other information upon which an assessment of damages may be made. Sometimes a hearing before a judge is essential to achieve a fair and reasonable assessment of damages.

Results and appeals

The outcome of a trial is that one party will win and the other will lose, albeit many might question who are the true winners and losers. If a trial verdict is regarded as incorrect it is possible to lodge notice of appeal, within strict time limits, on points of law or issues of fact or mixtures of both law and fact. The defendant's legal advisers will advise on the merits and prospects for an appeal. For example, a trial result might be regarded as unfair but the judge may have made bold findings of fact in such a way as to preclude any prospect of success, on the balance of probabilities, in an appeal. Only quite exceptionally will an appeal court overrule a trial judge on issues of fact (*Whitehouse* v. *Jordan* was one such case) because only the trial judge will have had the advantage of hearing and seeing the witnesses and assessing their candour, credibility and reliability and the weight to be attached to their evidence.

With an adverse judgment it is sometimes wisest to cut one's losses and not to lodge an appeal. Although appeal hearings are usually simpler, shorter and less costly than the initial trial, it is easier to deal with trial court precedents and to distinguish them on their facts from future cases than to be bound by a precedent set by a higher, appeal court.

It is necessary also for those who represent defendant doctors and health authorities to consider trends in judicial thinking, in so far as it is possible to discern them. Many patients who suffer problems are unquestionably deserving of sympathy and support. It is often said that plaintiffs find it difficult to prove negligence against doctors and that judges are slow to censure the medical profession. However, under the common law system, for plaintiffs to recover compensation they must prove negligence—at least until such time as a system of compensation without the need to prove fault is introduced and developed, such as the systems in Sweden and New Zealand.

It is easy to be 'liberal with the lodger's loaf' and sometimes a tendency is discerned among judges to grant awards of damages from what are erroneously seen as insurance company funds on something less than the full burden and standard of proof strictly required in law. The perception of this tendency in the judiciary was reinforced, albeit in a Canadian jurisdiction, in a lecture delivered by Mr Justice Horace Krever of the Ontario Court of Appeal to students of the Faculty of Law of the University of Manitoba, Winnipeg. He is quoted as saying (Ontario Lawyers Weekly 1986, vol. 5, no. 39, p 24) that in order for totally innocent plaintiffs who suffer catastrophic injuries to be compensated by wealthy insurers of equally blameless defendants, judges will tend to find fault where none exists. Mr Justice Krever is reported as saying that judges sometimes tell themselves:

> This is a case in which everybody agrees damages should be paid to the plaintiff. I know that nothing can be paid to the plaintiff unless I can find fault, so I am going to find fault. I know perfectly well that if I find fault, even though the evidence, intellectually applied, doesn't enable me to find fault, the Court of Appeal will not interfere with my finding of fault because it is a finding of fact made by a trier of fact who saw the witnesses. So I can get away with it. I am therefore able to [make a finding of negligence].

Mr Justice Krever did not 'like to be in a position that I have to be intellectually dishonest' and found it unsatisfactory to have to continue to base compensation only on the necessity to find fault because of what he contends is a propensity toward intellectual dishonesty.

CLAIM PREVENTION AND DEALING WITH COMPLAINTS

There can surely be little argument with the proposition that claims are best prevented. A careful and caring attitude by clinicians towards high standards of professional competence, conduct and behaviour will assist in the prevention of harm to patients which might initiate litigation. Attention must be paid to specialist and consultant responsibilities, especially the training of junior medical staff in the department, and good communication, by example as well as by precept. Delegation should be allowed only after careful assessment of the abilities of those to whom tasks are delegated and the ready availability of appropriate advice and assistance is arranged. Written departmental guidance for junior staff and midwives is desirable and clear standing orders for staff are essential to the provision of a good standard of care.

Even in the best-run units, problems and complaints will arise from time to time. When complaints do arise, in a variety of ways, often through poor communication and misunderstandings, it is important that they should be taken seriously and dealt with promptly and sympathetically. It is desirable that they should be dealt with by the consultant or at least by a senior member of the team, not delegated to housemen or midwives.

A complaint which is well handled may scotch a claim. Where patients and their relatives complain about the standard of clinical care they should not be shunned and avoided. A full discussion, showing empathy and understanding, will often speedily resolve a matter which, if ignored, might develop into a claim or formal complaint.

If errors occur it is wise for the senior clinician to go and speak to the patient. It is a mistake to walk away from the problem or to send the houseman to deal with it. Patients should be given the facts of what occurred but it may be wise to avoid comment and speculation. It is certainly wrong to concede blame, or worse still, to blame others for what occurred. The factual explanation should be coupled with an assurance that everything possible will be done from a clinical point of view, and that an appropriate investigation will be made into the circumstances, with a view to the prevention of a recurrence.

Complaints may arise from ill judged comments and asides. It is better not to think aloud in the presence of patients and their relatives and preferable to voice considered comments only.

The protection and defence organizations do not seek to prohibit doctors from providing factual information to patients. Indeed, quite the reverse; the benefits of sympathetic and prompt communication are well known. Not only are they desirable qualities per se—they may also help to reduce complaints and claims. Patients who are given the facts, and an assurance that everything necessary by way of further treatment is being done, may not feel that the only means of penetrating the wall of silence is by bringing a complaint or claim.

Doctors will, of course, feel great sympathy for patients who suffer harm, and may wish to see them compensated. However, under the present tort-based system of English civil law patients must prove negligence if they are to recover damages. The protection and defence societies are trustees of their members' funds, not insurers of their members' patients' misfortunes. The doctor who, through misguided good intentions, makes an admission of legal liability where no negligence occurred may leave colleagues in difficulty, prejudicing the funds of the protection societies subscribed by the members of those societies.

TRENDS IN LITIGATION: THE FUTURE

Since the mid 1970s the UK has seen a sharp increase in the numbers of complaints against doctors and others and in the numbers of claims for compensation and the size of the compensation. There are many reasons for this trend, the more important of which are summarized below. The list is not exhaustive, but the factors listed have all contributed, to a greater or lesser degree, to the problem. It seems likely that the trend will continue for as long as the present system for compensating negligence persists and the influences on the present system continue.

Expectations

Better education, television programmes and press coverage are amongst the factors which have led the public to come to expect cures for all their ills. A fatalistic acceptance of illness, with gratitude for the doctor's efforts, has to a degree been replaced by a feeling that progress of the disease rather than cure must be the doctor's fault and a matter for monetary compensation.

Consumer groups

Help and advice are increasingly available to patients from consumer-oriented groups such as community health councils, Citizens Advice Bureaux and others.

Legal Aid

The availability of Legal Aid has made it possible for the financially disadvantaged to embark upon litigation which they could not otherwise afford.

Press and media coverage

Television programmes, magazine and newspaper articles and news coverage of medical mistakes make human-interest stories of great emotional impact and stimulate the initiation of more claims. The reporting of an award is recognized as producing a spate of 'me-too' claims.

Advances in medical science

A few years ago it was most unusual for the victims of anoxic cardiac arrest to survive for substantial periods of time. Today, the advances of medical science mean that patients may be resuscitated, only to survive for prolonged periods (perhaps 30 years or more) as 'cabbages', insentient human beings who are wholly dependent upon others for total nursing care. Such care, under our law, may be paid for on a private basis, is expensive and may be required for 20–30 years.

Monetary inflation

Monetary inflation, of course, affects the awards of compensation in many ways. The level of general damages increases and the cost of nursing care and equipment will rise. All this must be paid on behalf of the doctor who is adjudged responsible for the patient's condition. Breadwinners qualify for large awards of damages if prevented, through medical negligence, from continuing to earn their salary at pre-accident levels.

Changes in the law

In the whole of recorded English legal history no medical negligence action had attracted an award in excess of £100 000 until 1977. In November 1977 a patient who suffered anoxic brain damage during an emergency laparotomy and who survived with severe brain damage, received an award in an English court of £112 000, so breaking the £100 000 barrier. Within a month an award of a quarter of a million pounds was made to another brain-damaged survivor of a minor gynaecological procedure. In 1987 the High Court made an award slightly in excess of 1 million pounds. Having taken centuries to break the £100 000 barrier, it has taken but a decade for a further 10-fold increase in the size of the maximum award for personal injuries in England and Wales. The law has been developed and extended in the last decade to include new heads of damages, i.e. items for which patients may claim compensation, including damages for lost years, for nervous shock and for the recovery of lost estimated future income and pension rights in cases where the plaintiff is an infant who has never worked.

Solicitors' advertising

Solicitors have recently been permitted to advertise their services. Many firms have done so. Some firms have advertised specifically for medical negligence cases. The solicitors' governing body, the Law Society, is reported (The Times,

30 June 1986, p 4) to be undertaking a study of the contingency fee system as part of a review of ways to fund litigation excluded from the Legal Aid scheme. The contingency fee system, prevalent in the USA but currently unethical in England, allows a lawyer to take on a case for no charge on the understanding that if he wins the case his client then pays him a percentage of the damages recovered.

The future

A significant alteration of the trends of the last 15 years or so would probably require a radical reappraisal of the manner by which accident victims are to be compensated. It remains to be seen whether Parliament will introduce a scheme of compensation for the victims of personal injury which does not require proof of fault. If so, a further choice must be made about which system of so-called no-fault compensation is to be adopted — the Swedish insurance-based system, the New Zealand state-funded system or some other system yet to be devised. Both the Swedish and New Zealand systems have their faults and problems as well as their advantages. Many deserving cases are excluded from benefit under both schemes and arguments and problems remain over matters of definition. For example, arguments occur about causation of injuries even though there is no longer argument about fault. Problems remain over the definition of personal injury by accident.

During 1987 the British Medical Association No-Fault Working Party made recommendations to support the principle of a non-statutory scheme within defined limits which would provide compensation for medical accidents without apportionment of blame. In England, the Report of the royal commission on civil liability and compensation for personal injury (the Pearson report) recommended in 1978 that a no-fault scheme of compensation for medical accidents should not be introduced, although such a scheme was recommended for other types of accident, such as road and factory accidents. The Pearson commission recommended that the New Zealand scheme should be kept under review but it is now becoming clear that that scheme is encountering difficulties, not least of which is the adequacy of funding of the scheme. If a no-fault scheme is to be introduced in England, it would seem socially desirable for it to cover all disabilities equally, howsoever caused.

It is logically and morally indefensible that children with similar disabilities should be compensated in widely divergent ways: the child born with Down's syndrome, the child who suffers encephalopathy from pertussis vaccine and the child born with brain damage attributed to obstetric mismanagement of the mother's labour may all have similar disabilities and physical needs. Yet, under current English law, each is very differently compensated. The unfortunate victim of trisomy 21 receives no compensation; the pertussis vaccine victim stands to gain a statutorily fixed award of £20 000 under the Vaccine Damage Payments Act; the victim of a mismanaged labour stands to gain an award, by current standards, of £500 000 to £1 000 000. Such a system is neither just nor fair and deserves to be replaced by one which is.

As long as the present, fault-based tort system persists, it is as well to recognize that the standard of care demanded of obstetricians and others is ever-changing, not static. This is because the test of whether or not a doctor has been negligent is that of the reasonable practitioner of similar training, skill and experience. A judgment is made according to the state of the art at the time; since medical science and the art of medicine are ever-changing and practices change, often subtly, over time, so too does the relevant legal standard of care demanded by the profession of the doctor who considers himself as possessing the particular skills of the specialist obstetrician. When those skills come under legal challenge, the practitioner's defence may be demanding of time, expertise and resources.

REFERENCES

Report of the personal injuries litigation procedure working party 1979 Cmnd 7476. HMSO, London

Report of the royal commission on civil liability and compensation for personal injury 1978 Cmnd 7054. HMSO, London

Whitfield A 1984 In: The Medical Protection Society annual report and accounts no. 92, pp 13–15

Index